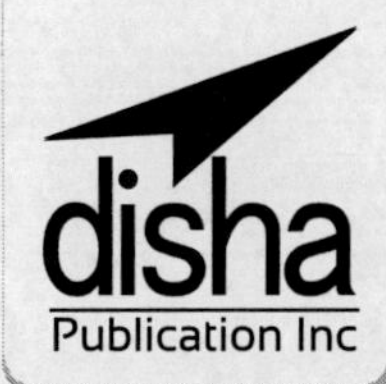

GOTO OBJECTIVE NEET Physics

Guide with DPP & CPP Sheets

Corporate Office

DISHA PUBLICATION
45, 2nd Floor, Maharishi Dayanand Marg,
Corner Market, Malviya Nagar, New Delhi - 110017
Tel : 49842349 / 49842350

Typeset by Disha DTP Team

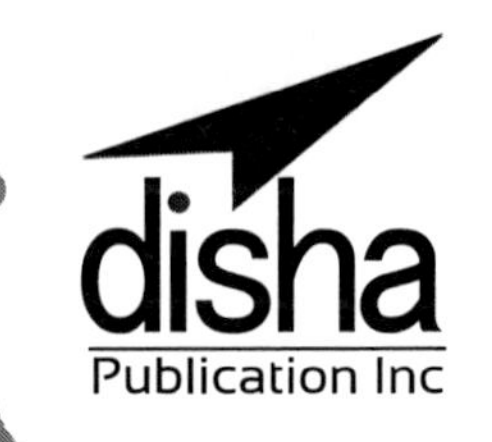

Write to us at feedback_disha@aiets.co.in

CONTENTS

NEET 2021 Solved Paper 2021-1-12

1. Physical World 1-7

Topic 1.1 : What is Science & Physics, Scope & Excitement of Physics, Physics Technology & Society, Fundamental Forces and Nature of Physical Laws
1.1 Concept Practice Problems (CPP)
Exercise 1 - Chapter Revision Problems (CRP)
Exercise 2 - Exemplar & Past Year Questions (E&PYQs)
Exercise 3 - Concept Application Problems (CAP)
Hints & Solutions

2. Units and Measurements 8-39

Topic 2.1 : Physical Quantity, Units and Dimensions
2.1 Concept Practice Problems (CPP)
Topic 2.2 : Significant Figure, Rounding off, Accuracy & Precision and Errors in Measurements
2.2 Concept Practice Problems (CPP)
Exercise 1 - Chapter Revision Problems (CRP)
Exercise 2 - Exemplar & Past Year Questions (E&PYQs)
Exercise 3 - Concept Application Problems (CAP)
Hints & Solutions

3. Motion in a Straight Line 40-74

Topic 3.1 : Distance, Displacement, Speed & Velocity
3.1 Concept Practice Problems (CPP)
Topic 3.2 : Acceleration & Equations for Uniformly Accelerated Motion
3.2 Concept Practice Problems (CPP)
Topic 3.3 : Motion under Gravity; Graphs Related to Motion & Relative Velocity
3.3 Concept Practice Problems (CPP)
Exercise 1 - Chapter Revision Problems (CRP)
Exercise 2 - Exemplar & Past Year Questions (E&PYQs)
Exercise 3 - Concept Application Problems (CAP)
Hints & Solutions

4. Motion in a Plane 75-110

Topic 4.1 : Scalars, Vectors–Addition, Subtraction, Resolution, Product of Vectors and Lami's Theorem
4.1 Concept Practice Problems (CPP)
Topic 4.2 : Motion in a Plane or Motion in Two Dimensions, Relative Velocity in two Dimensions, Projectile Motion, Projectile on an Inclined Plane
4.2 Concept Practice Problems (CPP)
Topic 4.3 : Uniform and Non-Uniform Circular Motion
4.3 Concept Practice Problems (CPP)
Exercise 1 - Chapter Revision Problems (CRP)
Exercise 2 - Exemplar & Past Year Questions (E&PYQs)
Exercise 3 - Concept Application Problems (CAP)
Hints & Solutions

5. Laws of Motion 111-155

Topic 5.1 : Newton's Laws of Motion, Equilibrium of a Particle, Constraint Motion, Free Body Diagram, Law of Conservation of Momentum and Impulse
5.1 Concept Practice Problems (CPP)
Topic 5.2 : Friction, Conservative & Non-Conservative Forces
5.2 Concept Practice Problems (CPP)
Topic 5.3 : Circular Motions & Banking of Road and Conical Pendulum
5.3 Concept Practice Problems (CPP)
Exercise 1 - Chapter Revision Problems (CRP)
Exercise 2 - Exemplar & Past Year Questions (E&PYQs)
Exercise 3 - Concept Application Problems (CAP)
Hints & Solutions

6. Work, Energy and Power 156-194

Topic 6.1 : Work
6.1 Concept Practice Problems (CPP)
Topic 6.2 : Energy, Work-Energy Theorem, Law of Conservation of Energy, Various Forms of Energy and Power
6.2 Concept Practice Problems (CPP)
Topic 6.3 : Collision
6.3 Concept Practice Problems (CPP)
Exercise 1 - Chapter Revision Problems (CRP)
Exercise 2 - Exemplar & Past Year Questions (E&PYQs)
Exercise 3 - Concept Application Problems (CAP)
Hints & Solutions

7. System of Particles and Rotational Motion 195-238

Topic 7.1 : Centre of Mass, Angular Velocity & Acceleration
7.1 Concept Practice Problems (CPP)
Topic 7.2 : Moment of Inertia, Radius of Gyration & Theorems on Moment of Inertia
7.2 Concept Practice Problems (CPP)
Topic 7.3 : Torque, Angular Momentum, Conservation of Angular Momentum, Rotational K.E. & Rolling Motion

7.3 Concept Practice Problems (CPP)
Exercise 1 - Chapter Revision Problems (CRP)
Exercise 2 - Exemplar & Past Year Questions (E&PYQs)
Exercise 3 - Concept Application Problems (CAP)
Hints & Solutions

8. Gravitation 239-271

Topic 8.1 : Newton's Universal Law of Gravitation and Acceleration due to Gravity
8.1 Concept Practice Problems (CPP)
Topic 8.2 : Gravitational-Field, Potential & Gravitational Potential Energy
8.2 Concept Practice Problems (CPP)
Topic 8.3 : Satellites-Geostationary & Polar; Orbital & Escape Speed; Keplar's Laws of Planetary Motion and Weightlessness
8.3 Concept Practice Problems (CPP)
Exercise 1 - Chapter Revision Problems (CRP)
Exercise 2 - Exemplar & Past Year Questions (E&PYQs)
Exercise 3 - Concept Application Problems (CAP)
Hints & Solutions

9. Mechanical Properties of Solids 272-293

Topic 9.1 : Interatomic & Intermolecular Force, Elasticity, Stress, Strain, Hooke's Law and Energy Stored in a Strained Body
9.1 Concept Practice Problems (CPP)
Exercise 1 - Chapter Revision Problems (CRP)
Exercise 2 - Exemplar & Past Year Questions (E&PYQs)
Exercise 3 - Concept Application Problems (CAP)
Hints & Solutions

10. Mechanical Properties of Fluids 294-320

Topic 10.1 : Fluids, Pascal's Law & Its Applications, Atmospheric, Hydrostatic, Guage Pressure, Buoyancy and Archimedes' Principle
10.1 Concept Practice Problems (CPP)
Topic 10.2 : Surface Tension, Angle of Contact, Capillarity, Shape of Liquid Meniscus
10.2 Concept Practice Problems (CPP)
Topic 10.3 : Flow of Liquids, Viscosity, Bernoulli's Theorem, Stoke's Law, Velocity of Efflux and Torricelli's Theorem
10.3 Concept Practice Problems (CPP)
Exercise 1 - Chapter Revision Problems (CRP)
Exercise 2 - Exemplar & Past Year Questions (E&PYQs)
Exercise 3 - Concept Application Problems (CAP)
Hints & Solutions

11. Thermal Properties of Matter 321-347

Topic 11.1 : Temperature, Ideal Gas Equation & Absolute Temperature and Thermal Expansion
11.1 Concept Practice Problems (CPP)
Topic 11.2 : Heat, Specific Heat Capacity, Thermal Capacity Latent Heat, Heat Transfer & Newton's Law of Cooling
11.2 Concept Practice Problems (CPP)
Exercise 1 - Chapter Revision Problems (CRP)
Exercise 2 - Exemplar & Past Year Questions (E&PYQs)
Exercise 3 - Concept Application Problems (CAP)
Hints & Solutions

12. Thermodynamics 348-372

Topic 12.1 : Thermal Equilibrium, Zeroth & First Law of Thermodynamics and Thermodynamic Processes
12.1 Concept Practice Problems (CPP)
Topic 12.2 : Reversible & Irreversible Process, Heat Engine, Refrigerator, Heat Pump, Carnot Engine and Second Law of Thermodynamics
12.2 Concept Practice Problems (CPP)
Exercise 1 - Chapter Revision Problems (CRP)
Exercise 2 - Exemplar & Past Year Questions (E&PYQs)
Exercise 3 - Concept Application Problems (CAP)
Hints & Solutions

13. Kinetic Theory 373-394

Topic 13.1 : Behaviour of Gases, Kinetic Theory of an Ideal Gas
13.1 Concept Practice Problems (CPP)
Topic 13.2 : Degree of Freedom, Mean Free Path, Law of Equipartition of Energy, Average, Root Mean Square and Most Probable Speed
13.2 Concept Practice Problems (CPP)
Exercise 1 - Chapter Revision Problems (CRP)
Exercise 2 - Exemplar & Past Year Questions (E&PYQs)
Exercise 3 - Concept Application Problems (CAP)
Hints & Solutions

14. Oscillations 395-422

Topic 14.1 : Periodic & Oscillatory Motion, Simple Harmonic Motion, Simple, Compound and Spring Pendulum
14.1 Concept Practice Problems (CPP)
Topic 14.2 : Free, Damped, Forced Oscillations and Resonance
14.2 Concept Practice Problems (CPP)
Exercise 1 - Chapter Revision Problems (CRP)
Exercise 2 - Exemplar & Past Year Questions (E&PYQs)
Exercise 3 - Concept Application Problems (CAP)
Hints & Solutions

15. Waves 423-452

Topic 15.1 : Wave Motion, Displacement Relation for Progressive Wave & Speed of Wave Motion and Interference of Waves

15.1 Concept Practice Problems (CPP)
Topic 15.2 : Beats and Doppler Effect
15.2 Concept Practice Problems (CPP)
Topic 15.3 : Stationary or Standing Waves in an Organ Pipe & on a String and Characteristics of Sound
15.3 Concept Practice Problems (CPP)
Exercise 1 - Chapter Revision Problems (CRP)
Exercise 2 - Exemplar & Past Year Questions (E&PYQs)
Exercise 3 - Concept Application Problems (CAP)
Hints & Solutions

16. Electric Charges and Fields 453-488

Topic 16.1 : Electric Charge, Conductors & Insulators, Coulomb's Law, Electric Field, Electric lines of Force, Electric Field for a Distribution of Direct & Continuous Charge and Motion of a Charged Particle in an Electric Field
16.1 Concept Practice Problems (CPP)
Topic 16.2 : Electric Dipole, Electric Flux and Gauss's Law
16.2 Concept Practice Problems (CPP)
Exercise 1 - Chapter Revision Problems (CRP)
Exercise 2 - Exemplar & Past Year Questions (E&PYQs)
Exercise 3 - Concept Application Problems (CAP)
Hints & Solutions

17. Electrostatic Potential and Capacitance 489-526

Topic 17.1 : Electrostatic Potential, Potential Energy of a System of Charges and Equipotential Surface
17.1 Concept Practice Problems (CPP)
Topic 17.2 : Electrostatics of Conductors, Capacitors & Capacitance, Energy Stored in a Capacitor, Parallel Plate Capacitor, Combination of Capacitors and Charging & Discharging a Capacitor
17.2 Concept Practice Problems (CPP)
Exercise 1 - Chapter Revision Problems (CRP)
Exercise 2 - Exemplar & Past Year Questions (E&PYQs)
Exercise 3 - Concept Application Problems (CAP)
Hints & Solutions

18. Current Electricity 527-570

Topic 18.1 : Electric Current, Current Density, Drift Velocity, Ohm's Law & Electrical Resistance, Series & Parallel Combination of Resistors and Colour Coding for Carbon Resistor
18.1 Concept Practice Problems (CPP)
Topic 18.2 : Joule's Law of Heating, Electric Power, Electromotive Force & Internal Resistance of a Cell, Combination of Cells, Kirchhoff's Law & Electrical Circuit
18.2 Concept Practice Problems (CPP)
Topic 18.3 : Wheatstone Bridge, Meter Bridges, Potentiometer, Measuring Instrument-Voltmeter and Ammeter
18.3 Concept Practice Problems (CPP)
Exercise 1 - Chapter Revision Problems (CRP)
Exercise 2 - Exemplar & Past Year Questions (E&PYQs)
Exercise 3 - Concept Application Problems (CAP)
Hints & Solutions

19. Moving Charges and Magnetism 571-602

Topic 19.1 : Oersted Experiment, Magnetic Field, Magnetic Field due to Current Carrying Conductor, Biot-Savart's Law and Ampere's circuital Law
19.1 Concept Practice Problems (CPP)
Topic 19.2 : Force on a Conductor, Torque on a Coil and Force Between two Parallel Current Carrying Conductors
19.2 Concept Practice Problems (CPP)
Topic 19.3 : Force Acting on a Charged Particle Moving in a Uniform Magnetic Field and Moving Coil Galvanometer
19.3 Concept Practice Problems (CPP)
Exercise 1 - Chapter Revision Problems (CRP)
Exercise 2 - Exemplar & Past Year Questions (E&PYQs)
Exercise 3 - Concept Application Problems (CAP)
Hints & Solutions

20. Magnetism and Matter 603-628

Topic 20.1 : Natural Magnet, Bar Magnet, Magnetic Field, Magnetic Lines of Force, Magnetic Moment, Coulomb's Law, Torque on a Magnet, Gauss's Law in Magnetism, Magnetic Field and Potential
20.1 Concept Practice Problems (CPP)
Topic 20.2 : Earth's Magnetism, Classification of Magnetic Materials and Magnetic Equipments
20.2 Concept Practice Problems (CPP)
Exercise 1 - Chapter Revision Problems (CRP)
Exercise 2 - Exemplar & Past Year Questions (E&PYQs)
Exercise 3 - Concept Application Problems (CAP)
Hints & Solutions

21. Electromagnetic Induction 629-653

Topic 21.1 : The Experiments of Faraday & Henry, Magnetic Flux, Faraday's Law, Lenz's Law, Methods of Inducing EMF and Eddy Currents
21.1 Concept Practice Problems (CPP)
Topic 21.2 : Self Inductance & Mutual Inductance, AC Generator/Dynamo/Alternator and DC Motor
21.2 Concept Practice Problems (CPP)
Exercise 1 - Chapter Revision Problems (CRP)
Exercise 2 - Exemplar & Past Year Questions (E&PYQs)
Exercise 3 - Concept Application Problems (CAP)
Hints & Solutions

22. Alternating Current 654-681

Topic 22.1 : Alternating & Direct Current, Average & RMS Value of Current, Resistance offered by various Elements to AC, Impedances and Phases of AC Circuit containing different Elements, Q-factor and Power in an AC Circuit
22.1 Concept Practice Problems (CPP)
Topic 22.2 : Varying Current, Decay of Current, LC Oscillations and Transformer
22.2 Concept Practice Problems (CPP)
Exercise 1 - Chapter Revision Problems (CRP)
Exercise 2 - Exemplar & Past Year Questions (E&PYQs)
Exercise 3 - Concept Application Problems (CAP)
Hints & Solutions

23. Electromagnetic Waves 682-697

Topic 23.1 : Displacement Current, Maxwell's Modification of Ampere's Circuital Law and Electromagnetic Waves
23.1 Concept Practice Problems (CPP)
Topic 23.2 : Electromagnetic Spectrum and Uses of Electromagnetic Waves
23.2 Concept Practice Problems (CPP)
Exercise 1 - Chapter Revision Problems (CRP)
Exercise 2 - Exemplar & Past Year Questions (E&PYQs)
Exercise 3 - Concept Application Problems (CAP)
Hints & Solutions

24. Ray Optics and Optical Instruments 698-736

Topic 24.1 : Reflection of Light, Reflection from Plane Surface and Mirror Formula
24.1 Concept Practice Problems (CPP)
Topic 24.2 : Refraction, Total Internal Reflection, Refraction at a Spherical Surface, Refraction by a Lens, Combination of Lenses and Refraction through a Prism
24.2 Concept Practice Problems (CPP)
Topic 24.3 : Optical Instruments
24.3 Concept Practice Problems (CPP)
Exercise 1 - Chapter Revision Problems (CRP)
Exercise 2 - Exemplar & Past Year Questions (E&PYQs)
Exercise 3 - Concept Application Problems (CAP)
Hints & Solutions

25. Wave Optics 737-764

Topic 25.1 : Wavefront, Huygens Wave Theory, Interference of Light and Young's Double Slit Experiment
25.1 Concept Practice Problems (CPP)
Topic 25.2 : Diffraction, Polarisation & Resolving Power of an Optical Instruments
25.2 Concept Practice Problems (CPP)
Exercise 1 - Chapter Revision Problems (CRP)
Exercise 2 - Exemplar & Past Year Questions (E&PYQs)
Exercise 3 - Concept Application Problems (CAP)
Hints & Solutions

26. Dual Nature of Radiation and Matter 765-792

Topic 26.1 : Cathode Rays, Emission of Electron and Photoelectric Effect
26.1 Concept Practice Problems (CPP)
Topic 26.2 : de-Broglie Equation, Davisson-Germer Experiment and X-rays
26.2 Concept Practice Problems (CPP)
Exercise 1 - Chapter Revision Problems (CRP)
Exercise 2 - Exemplar & Past Year Questions (E&PYQs)
Exercise 3 - Concept Application Problems (CAP)
Hints & Solutions

27. Atoms 793-815

Topic 27.1 : Thomson's Atomic Model, Alpha-Particle Scattering and Rutherford Nuclear Model of Atom
27.1 Concept Practice Problems (CPP)
Topic 27.2 : Bohr's Atomic Model, Energy Levels and the Lines Spectra of Hydrogen Atom
27.2 Concept Practice Problems (CPP)
Exercise 1 - Chapter Revision Problems (CRP)
Exercise 2 - Exemplar & Past Year Questions (E&PYQs)
Exercise 3 - Concept Application Problems (CAP)
Hints & Solutions

28. Nuclei 816-837

Topic 28.1 : Atomic Mass, Size & Composition of Nucleus, Mass Energy, Nuclear Binding Energy and Nuclear Force
28.1 Concept Practice Problems (CPP)
Topic 28.2 : Radioactivity, Radioactive Series and Nuclear Reaction
28.2 Concept Practice Problems (CPP)
Exercise 1 - Chapter Revision Problems (CRP)
Exercise 2 - Exemplar & Past Year Questions (E&PYQs)
Exercise 3 - Concept Application Problems (CAP)
Hints & Solutions

29. Semiconductor Electronics : Materials, Devices and Simple Circuits 838-876

Topic 29.1 : Energy Band Theory of Solids, Conductors, Insulators & Semiconductors, p-n. Junction Diode, Forward and Reverse Bias of p-n Junction Diode
29.1 Concept Practice Problems (CPP)
Topic 29.2 : Transistor and Logic Gates
29.2 Concept Practice Problems (CPP)
Exercise 1 - Chapter Revision Problems (CRP)
Exercise 2 - Exemplar & Past Year Questions (E&PYQs)
Exercise 3 - Concept Application Problems (CAP)
Hints & Solutions

NEET SYLLABUS

CLASS 11 PHYSICS

UNIT I Physical World and Measurement

- Physics Scope and excitement; nature of physical laws; Physics, technology and society.
- Need for measurement Units of measurement; systems of units; SI units, fundamental and derived units. Length, mass and time measurements; accuracy and precision of measuring instruments; errors in measurement; significant figures.
- Dimensions of physical quantities, dimensional analysis and its applications.

UNIT II Kinematics

- Frame of reference, Motion in a straight line; Position-time graph, speed and velocity. Uniform and non-uniform motion, average speed and instantaneous velocity. Uniformly accelerated motion, velocity-time and position-time graphs, for uniformly accelerated motion (graphical treatment).
- Elementary concepts of differentiation and integration for describing motion. Scalar and vector quantities Position and displacement vectors, general vectors, general vectors and notation, equality of vectors, multiplication of vectors by a real number; addition and subtraction of vectors. Relative velocity.
- Unit vectors. Resolution of a vector in a plane-rectangular components.
- Scalar and Vector products of Vectors. Motion in a plane. Cases of uniform velocity and uniform acceleration-projectile motion. Uniform circular motion.

UNIT III Laws of Motion

- Intuitive concept of force. Inertia, Newton's first law of motion; momentum and Newton's second law of motion; impulse; Newton's third law of motion. Law of conservation of linear momentum and its applications.
- Equilibrium of concurrent forces. Static and Kinetic friction, laws of friction, rolling friction, lubrication.
- Dynamics of uniform circular motion. Centripetal force, examples of circular motion (vehicle on level circular road, vehicle on banked road).

UNIT IV Work, Energy and Power

- Work done by a constant force and variable force; kinetic energy, work-energy theorem, power.
- Notion of potential energy, potential energy of a spring, conservative forces; conservation of mechanical energy (kinetic and potential energies); nonconservative forces; motion in a vertical circle, elastic and inelastic collisions in one and two dimensions.

UNIT V Motion of System of Particles and Rigid Body

- Centre of mass of a two-particle system, momentum conservation and centre of mass motion. Centre of mass of a rigid body; centre of mass of uniform rod.
- Moment of a force,-torque, angular momentum, conservation of angular momentum with some examples.
- Equilibrium of rigid bodies, rigid body rotation and equation of rotational motion, comparison of linear and rotational motions; moment of inertia, radius of gyration. Values of M.I. for simple geometrical objects (no derivation). Statement of parallel and perpendicular axes theorems and their applications.

UNIT VI Gravitation

- Kepler's laws of planetary motion. The universal law of gravitation. Acceleration due to gravity and its variation with altitude and depth.
- Gravitational potential energy; gravitational potential. Escape velocity, orbital velocity of a satellite. Geostationary satellites.

UNIT VII Properties of Bulk Matter

- Elastic behavior, Stress-strain relationship. Hooke's law, Young's modulus, bulk modulus, shear, modulus of rigidity, poisson's ratio; elastic energy.
- Viscosity, Stokes' law, terminal velocity, Reynold's number, streamline and turbulent flow. Critical velocity, Bernoulli's theorem and its applications.
- Surface energy and surface tension, angle of contact, excess of pressure, application of surface tension ideas to drops, bubbles and capillary rise.
- Heat, temperature, thermal expansion; thermal expansion of solids, liquids, and gases. Anomalous expansion. Specific heat capacity Cp, Cv- calorimetry; change of state – latent heat.
- Heat transfer- conduction and thermal conductivity, convection and radiation. Qualitative ideas of Black Body Radiation, Wein's displacement law, and Green House effect.
- Newton's law of cooling and Stefan's law.

UNIT VIII Thermodynamics

- Thermal equilibrium and definition of temperature (zeroth law of Thermodynamics). Heat, work and internal energy. First law of thermodynamics. Isothermal and adiabatic processes.
- Second law of the thermodynamics Reversible and irreversible processes. Heat engines and refrigerators.

UNIT IX Behaviour of Perfect Gas and Kinetic Theory

- Equation of state of a perfect gas, work done on compressing a gas.
- Kinetic theory of gases Assumptions, concept of pressure. Kinetic energy and temperature; degrees of freedom, law of equipartition of energy (statement only) and application to specific heat capacities of gases; concept of mean free path.

UNIT X Oscillations and Waves

- Periodic motion-period, frequency, displacement as a function of time. Periodic functions. Simple harmonic motion(SHM) and its equation; phase; oscillations of a spring-restoring force and force constant; energy in SHM –Kinetic and potential energies; simple pendulum-derivation of expression for its time period; free, forced and damped oscillations (qualitative ideas only), resonance.
- Wave motion. Longitudinal and transverse waves, speed of wave motion. Displacement relation for a progressive wave. Principle of superposition of waves, reflection of waves, standing waves in strings and organ pipes, fundamental mode and harmonics. Beats. Doppler effect.

CLASS 12 PHYSICS

UNIT I Electrostatics

- Electric charges and their conservation. Coulomb's law-force between two point charges, forces between multiple charges; superposition principle and continuous charge distribution.
- Electric field, electric field due to a point charge, electric field lines; electric dipole, electric field due to a dipole; torque on a dipole in a uniform electric field.
- Electric flux, statement of Gauss's theorem and its applications to find field due to infinitely long straight wire, uniformly charged infinite plane sheet and uniformly charged thin spherical shell (field inside and outside)
- Electric potential, potential difference, electric potential due to a point charge, a dipole and system of charges equipotential surfaces, electrical potential energy of a system of two point charges and of electric diploes in an electrostatic field.
- Conductors and insulators, free charges and bound charges inside a conductor. Dielectrics and electric polarization, capacitors and capacitance, combination of capacitors in series and in parallel, capacitance of a parallel plate capacitor with and without dielectric medium between the plates, energy stored in a capacitor, Van de Graaff generator.

UNIT II Current Electricity

- Electric current, flow of electric charges in a metallic conductor, drift velocity and mobility, and their relation with electric current; Ohm's law, electrical resistance, V-I characteristics (liner and non- linear), electrical energy and power, electrical resistivity and conductivity.
- Carbon resistors, color code for carbon resistors; series and parallel combinations of resistors; temperature dependence of resistance.
- Internal resistance of a cell, potential difference and emf of a cell, co mbination of cells in series and in parallel.
- Kirchhoff's laws and simple applications. Wheatstone bridge, metre bridge.
- Potentiometer-principle and applications to measure potential difference, and for comparing emf of two cells; measurement of internal resistance of a cell.

UNIT III Magnetic Effects of Current and Magnetism

- Concept of magnetic field, Oersted's experiment. Biot-Savart law and its application to current carrying circular loop.
- Ampere's law and its applications to infinitely long straight wire, straight and toroidal solenoids. Force on a moving charge in uniform magnetic and electric fields. Cyclotron.
- Force on a current-carrying conductor in a uniform magnetic field. Force between two parallel current-carrying conductors-definition of ampere. Torque experienced by a current loop in a magnetic field; moving coil galvanometer-its current sensitivity and conversion to ammeter and voltmeter.
- Current loop as a magnetic dipole and its magnetic dipole moment. Magnetic dipole moment of a revolving electron. Magnetic field intensity due to a magnetic dipole (bar magnet) along its axis and perpendicular to its axis. Torque on a magnetic dipole (bar magnet) in a uniform magnetic field; bar magnet as an equivalent solenoid, magnetic field lines; Earth's magnetic field and magnetic elements.
- Para-, dia-and ferro-magnetic substances, with examples.
- Electromagnetic and factors affecting their strengths. Permanent magnets.

UNIT IV Electromagnetic Induction and Alternating Currents

- Electromagnetic induction; Faraday's law, induced emf and current; Lenz's Law, Eddy currents. Self and mutual inductance.
- Alternating currents, peak and rms value of alternating current/ voltage; reactance and impedance; LC oscillations (qualitative treatment only), LCR series circuit, resonance; power in AC circuits, wattles current.
- AC generator and transformer.

UNIT V Electromagnetic Waves

- Need for displacement current.
- Electromagnetic waves and their characteristics (qualitative ideas only). Transverse nature of electromagnetic waves.
- Electromagnetic spectrum (radio waves, microwaves, infrared, visible, ultraviolet, x-rays, gamma rays) including elementary facts about their uses.

UNIT VI Optics

- Reflection of light, spherical mirrors, mirror formula. Refraction of light, total internal reflection and its applications optical fibres, refraction at spherical surfaces, lenses, thin lens formula, lens-maker's formula. Magnification, power of a lens, combination of thin lenses in contact combination of a lens and a mirror. Refraction and dispersion of light through a prism.
- Scattering of light- blue colour of the sky and reddish appearance of the sun at sunrise and sunset.
- Optical instruments Human eye, image formation and accommodation, correction of eye defects (myopia and hypermetropia) using lenses.
- Microscopes and astronomical telescopes (reflecting and refracting) and their magnifying powers.
- Wave optics Wavefront and Huygens' principle, reflection and refraction of plane wave at a plane surface using wavefronts.
- Proof of laws of reflection and refraction using Huygens' principle.
- Interference, Young's double hole experiment and expression for fringe width, coherent sources and sustained interference of light.
- Diffraction due to a single slit, width of central maximum.
- Resolving power of microscopes and astronomical telescopes. Polarisation, plane polarized light; Brewster's law, uses of plane polarized light and Polaroids.

UNIT VII Dual Nature of Matter and Radiation

- Photoelectric effect, Hertz and Lenard's observations; Einstein's photoelectric equation- particle nature of light.
- Matter waves- wave nature of particles, de Broglie relation. Davisson-Germer experiment (experimental details should be omitted; only conclusion should be explained).

UNIT VIII Atoms and Nuclei

- Alpha- particle scattering experiments; Rutherford's model of atom; Bohr model, energy levels, hydrogen spectrum. Composition and size of nucleus, atomic masses, isotopes, isobars; isotones.
- Radioactivity- alpha, beta and gamma particles/ rays and their properties decay law. Mass-energy relation, mass defect; binding energy per nucleon and its variation with mass number, nuclear fission and fusion.

UNIT IX Electronic Devices

- Energy bands in solids (qualitative ideas only), conductors, insulators and semiconductors; semiconductor diode- I-V characteristics in forward and reverse bias, diode as a rectifier; I-V characteristics of LED, photodiode, solar cell, and Zener diode; Zener diode as a voltage regulator. Junction transistor, transistor action, characteristics of a transistor; transistor as an amplifier (common emitter configuration) and oscillator. Logic gates (OR, AND, NOT, NAND and NOR). Transistor as a switch.

NEET 2021 Solved Paper

PHYSICS

Held on : 12th September 2021

SECTION - A

1. A body is executing simple harmonic motion with frequency 'n', the frequency of its potential energy is

[Oscillations]

(1) $4n$ (2) n (3) $2n$ (4) $3n$

2. Polar molecules are the molecules

[Electric Charges and Fields]

(1) having a permanent electric dipole moment
(2) having zero dipole moment
(3) acquire a dipole moment only in the presence of electric field due to displacement of charges
(4) acquire a dipole moment only when magnetic field is absent

3. **Column-I** gives certain physical terms associated with flow of current through a metallic conductor.
Column-II gives some mathematical relations involving electrical quantities. Match **Column-I** and **Column-II** with appropriate relations. **[Current Electricity]**

Column-I	Column-II
(A) Drift velocity	(i) $\frac{m}{ne^2\rho}$
(B) Electrical resistivity	(ii) nev_d
(C) Relaxation period	(iii) $\frac{eE}{m}\tau$
(D) Current density	(iv) $\frac{E}{J}$

(1) A - (iii), B - (ii), C - (iv), D - (i)
(2) A - (iii), B - (iv), C - (i), D - (ii)
(3) A - (iii), B - (iv), C - (ii), D - (i)
(4) A - (iii), B - (i), C - (iv), D - (ii)

4. Two charged spherical conductors of radius R_1 and R_2 are connected by a wire. Then the ratio of surface charge densities of the spheres (σ_1/σ_2) is

[Electric Charges and Fields]

(1) $\frac{R_1^2}{R_2^2}$ (2) $\frac{R_1}{R_2}$ (3) $\frac{R_2}{R_1}$ (4) $\sqrt{\left(\frac{R_1}{R_2}\right)}$

5. A parallel plate capacitor has a uniform electric field '$\vec{E}$' in the space between the plates. If the distance between the plates is 'd' and the area of each plate is 'A', the energy stored in the capacitor is (ε_0 = permittivity of free space)

[Electrostatic Potential and Capacitance]

(1) $\frac{E^2Ad}{\varepsilon_0}$ (2) $\frac{1}{2}\varepsilon_0E^2$ (3) ε_0EAd (4) $\frac{1}{2}\varepsilon_0E^2Ad$

6. An infinitely long straight conductor carries a current of 5 A as shown. An electron is moving with a speed of 10^5 m/s parallel to the conductor. The perpendicular distance between the electron and the conductor is 20 cm at an instant. Calculate the magnitude of the force experienced by the electron at that instant.

[Moving Charges and Magnetism]

Electron $v = 10^5$ m/s
20 cm
P $5A$ Q

(1) 8×10^{-20} N (2) 4×10^{-20} N
(3) $8\pi \times 10^{-20}$ N (4) $4\pi \times 10^{-20}$ N

7. If E and G respectively denote energy and gravitational constant, then $\frac{E}{G}$ has the dimensions of

[Units and Measurements]

(1) $[M^2][L^{-2}][T^{-1}]$ (2) $[M^2][L^{-1}][T^0]$
(3) $[M][L^{-1}][T^{-1}]$ (4) $[M][L^0][T^0]$

8. A lens of large focal length and large aperture is best suited as an objective of an astronomical telescope since

[Wave Optics]

(1) a large aperture contributes to the quality and visibility of the images.
(2) a large area of the objective ensures better light gathering power.
(3) a large aperture provides a better resolution.
(4) all of the above

9. Match Column - I and Column - II and choose the correct match from the given choices. **[Kinetic Theory]**

Column - I	Column - II
(A) Root mean square speed of gas molecules	(i) $\frac{1}{3}nm\bar{v}^2$
(B) Pressure exerted by ideal gas	(ii) $\sqrt{\frac{3RT}{M}}$
(C) Average kinetic energy of a molecule	(iii) $\frac{5}{2}RT$
(D) Total internal energy of 1 mole of a diatomic gas	(iv) $\frac{3}{2}k_BT$

(1) A - (iii), B - (ii), C - (i), D - (iv)
(2) A - (iii), B - (i), C - (iv), D - (ii)
(3) A - (ii), B - (iii), C - (iv), D - (i)
(4) A - (ii), B - (i), C - (iv), D - (iii)

10. Consider the following statements (1) and (2) and identify the correct answer. **[Semiconductor Electronics : Materials, Devices and Simple Circuits]**

(1) A zener diode is connected in reverse bias, when used as a voltage regulator.

(2) The potential barrier of p-n junction lies between 0.1 V to 0.3 V.

(1) (1) is incorrect but (2) is correct.
(2) (1) and (2) both are correct.
(3) (1) and (2) both are incorrect
(4) (1) is correct and (2) is incorrect.

11. A dipole is placed in an electric field as shown. In which direction will it move?

[Electrostatic Potential and Capacitance]

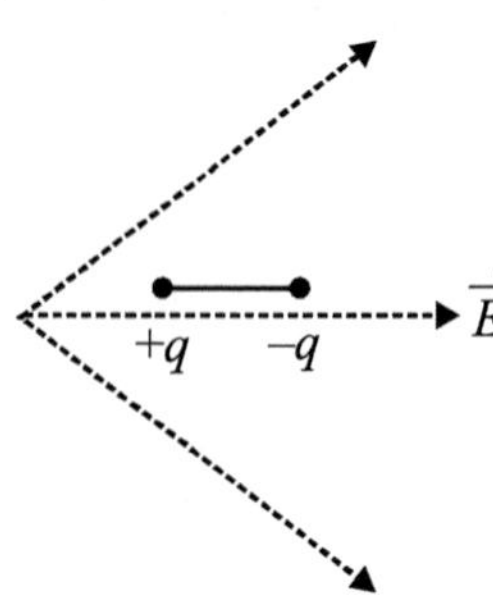

(1) Towards the right as its potential energy will increase.
(2) Towards the left as its potential energy will increase.
(3) Towards the right as its potential energy will decrease.
(4) Towards the left as its potential energy will decrease.

12. A convex lens 'A' of focal length 20 cm and a concave lens 'B' of focal length 5 cm are kept along the same axis with a distance 'd' between them. If a parallel beam of light falling on 'A' leaves 'B' as a parallel beam, then the distance 'd' in cm will be

[Ray Optics and Optical Instruments]

(1) 30 (2) 25 (3) 15 (4) 50

13. The escape velocity from the Earth's surface is v. The escape velocity from the surface of another planet having a radius, four times that of Earth and same mass density is **[Gravitation]**

(1) $4v$ (2) v (3) $2v$ (4) $3v$

14. A radioactive nucleus ${}^{A}_{Z}X$ undergoes spontaneous decay in the sequence **[Nuclei]**

${}^{A}_{Z}X \rightarrow_{Z-1} B \rightarrow_{Z-3} C \rightarrow_{Z-2} D$, where Z is the atomic number of element X. The possible decay particles in the sequence are

(1) β^-, α, β^+ (2) α, β^-, β^+
(3) α, β^+, β^- (4) β^+, α, β^-

15. A screw gauge gives the following readings when used to measure the diameter of a wire

Main scale reading : 0 mm

Circular scale reading : 52 divisions

Given that 1 mm on main scale corresponds to 100 divisions on the circular scale. The diameter of the wire from the above data is **[Units and Measurements]**

(1) 0.052 cm (2) 0.52 cm
(3) 0.026 cm (4) 0.26 cm

16. An inductor of inductance L, a capacitor of capacitance C and a resistor of resistance 'R' are connected in series to an ac source of potential difference 'V' volts as shown in figure.

Potential difference across L, C and R is 40 V, 10 V and 40 V, respectively. The amplitude of current flowing through LCR series circuit is $10\sqrt{2}\ A$. The impedance of the circuit is **[Alternating Current]**

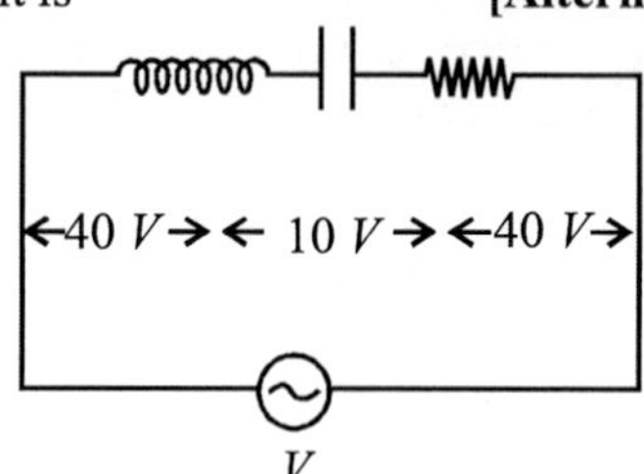

(1) $5\,\Omega$ (2) $4\sqrt{2}\,\Omega$ (3) $5\sqrt{2}\,\Omega$ (4) $4\,\Omega$

17. A particle is released from height S from the surface of the Earth. At a certain height its kinetic energy is three times its potential energy. The height from the surface of earth and the speed of the particle at that instant are respectively **[Work, Energy and Power]**

(1) $\frac{S}{4}, \sqrt{\frac{3gS}{2}}$ (2) $\frac{S}{4}, \frac{3gS}{2}$

(3) $\frac{S}{4}, \frac{\sqrt{3gS}}{2}$ (4) $\frac{S}{2}, \frac{\sqrt{3gS}}{2}$

18. A small block slides down on a smooth inclined plane, starting from rest at time $t = 0$. Let S_n be the distance travelled by the block in the interval $t = n - 1$ to $t = n$. Then, the ratio $\frac{S_n}{S_{n+1}}$ is **[Motion in a Straight Line]**

(1) $\frac{2n}{2n-1}$ (2) $\frac{2n-1}{2n}$ (3) $\frac{2n-1}{2n+1}$ (4) $\frac{2n+1}{2n-1}$

19. The half-life of a radioactive nuclide is 100 hours. The fraction of original activity that will remain after 150 hours would be **[Nuclei]**

(1) $\frac{2}{3\sqrt{2}}$ (2) $\frac{1}{2}$ (3) $\frac{1}{2\sqrt{2}}$ (4) $\frac{2}{3}$

20. The equivalent capacitance of the combination shown in the figure is **[Electrostatic Potential and Capacitance]**

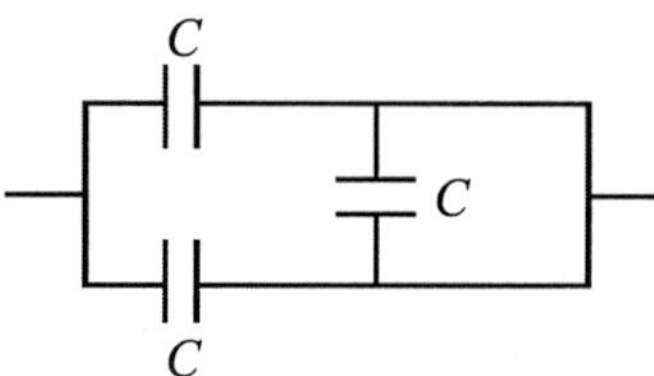

(1) $\frac{3C}{2}$ (2) $3C$ (3) $2C$ (4) $\frac{C}{2}$

21. The effective resistance of a parallel connection that consists of four wires of equal length, equal area of cross-section and same material is $0.25\ \Omega$. What will be the effective resistance if they are connected in series?

[Current Electricity]

(1) $4\,\Omega$ (2) $0.25\,\Omega$ (3) $0.5\,\Omega$ (4) $1\,\Omega$

22. A nucleus with mass number 240 breaks into two fragments each of mass number 120, the binding energy per nucleon of unfragmented nuclei is 7.6 MeV while that of fragments is 8.5 MeV. The total gain in the binding energy in the process is **[Nuclei]**

(1) 216 MeV (2) 0.9 MeV
(3) 9.4 MeV (4) 804 MeV

23. The electron concentration in an *n*-type semiconductor is the same as hole concentration in a *p*-type semiconductor. An external field (electric) is applied across each of them. Compare the currents in them. **[Semiconductor Electronics : Materials, Devices and Simple Circuits]**

(1) No current will flow in *p*-type, current will only flow in *n*-type
(2) Current in *n*-type = current in *p*-type
(3) Current in *p*-type > current in *n*-type
(4) Current in *n*-type > current in *p*-type

24. The number of photons per second on an average emitted by the source of mono-chromatic light of wavelength 600 nm, when it delivers the power of 3.3×10^{-3} watt will be ($h = 6.6 \times 10^{-34}$ J s) **[Dual Nature of Radiation]**

(1) 10^{15} (2) 10^{18} (3) 10^{17} (4) 10^{16}

25. A thick current carrying cable of radius '*R*' carries current '*I*' uniformly distributed across its cross-section. The variation of magnetic field *B*(*r*) due to the cable with the distance '*r*' from the axis of the cable is represented by **[Moving Charges and Magnetism]**

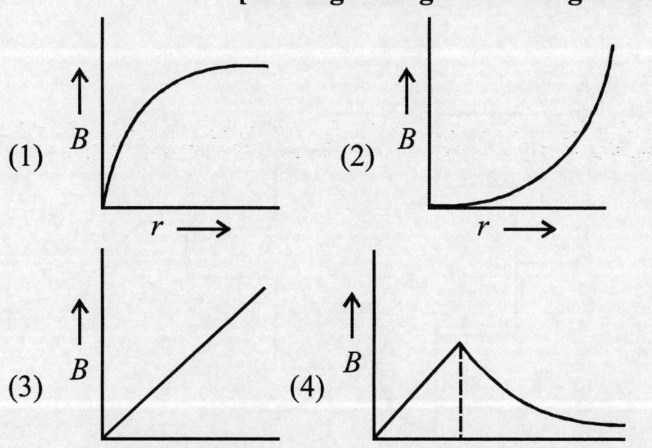

26. The velocity of a small ball of mass *M* and density *d*, when dropped in a container filled with glycerine becomes constant after some time. If the density of glycerine is $\frac{d}{2}$, then the viscous force acting on the ball will be **[Mechanical Properties of Fluids]**

(1) 2 *Mg* (2) $\frac{Mg}{2}$ (3) *Mg* (4) $\frac{3}{2}Mg$

27. Find the value of the angle of emergence from the prism. Refractive index of the glass is $\sqrt{3}$. **[Ray Optics and Optical Instruments]**

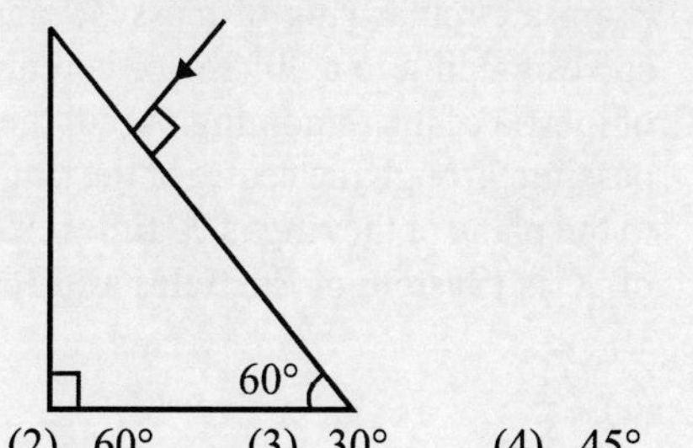

(1) 90° (2) 60° (3) 30° (4) 45°

28. A capacitor of capacitance '*C*', is connected across an ac source of voltage *V*, given by $V = V_0 \sin \omega t$
The displacement current between the plates of the capacitor, would then be given by **[Electromagnetic Waves]**

(1) $I_d = V_0 \omega C \sin \omega t$ (2) $I_d = V_0 \omega C \cos \omega t$
(3) $I_d = \frac{V_0}{\omega C} \cos \omega t$ (4) $I_d = \frac{V_0}{\omega C} \sin \omega t$

29. If force [*F*], acceleration [*A*] and time [*T*] are chosen as the fundamental physical quantities. Find the dimensions of energy. **[Units and Measurements]**

(1) $[F][A^{-1}][T]$ (2) $[F][A][T]$
(3) $[F][A][T^2]$ (4) $[F][A][T^{-1}]$

30. In a potentiometer circuit a cell of EMF 1.5 *V* gives balance point at 36 cm length of wire. If another cell of *EMF* 2.5 *V* replaces the first cell, then at what length of the wire, the balance point occurs? **[Current Electricity]**

(1) 62 cm (2) 60 cm (3) 21.6 cm (4) 64 cm

31. A spring is stretched by 5 cm by a force 10 *N*. The time period of the oscillations when a mass of 2 kg is suspended by it is **[Oscillations]**

(1) 0.628 s (2) 0.0628 s
(3) 6.28 s (4) 3.14 s

32. For a plane electromagnetic wave propagating in *x*-direction, which one of the following combination gives the correct possible directions for electric field (E) and magnetic field (2) respectively? **[Electromagnetic Waves]**

(1) $-\hat{j}+\hat{k}, -\hat{j}+\hat{k}$ (2) $\hat{j}+\hat{k}, \hat{j}+\hat{k}$
(3) $-\hat{j}+\hat{k}, -\hat{j}-\hat{k}$ (4) $\hat{j}+\hat{k}, -\hat{j}-\hat{k}$

33. A cup of coffee cools from 90°C to 80°C in *t* minutes, when the room temperature is 20°C. The time taken by a similar cup of coffee to cool from 80°C to 60°C at a room temperature same at 20°C is **[Thermal Properties of matter]**

(1) $\frac{5}{13}t$ (2) $\frac{13}{10}t$ (3) $\frac{13}{5}t$ (4) $\frac{10}{13}t$

34. An electromagnetic wave of wavelength 'λ' is incident on a photosensitive surface of negligible work function. If '*m*' mass is of photoelectron emitted from the surface has de-Broglie wavelength λ_d, then **[Dual Nature of Radiation and Matter]**

(1) $\lambda = \left(\frac{2h}{mc}\right)\lambda_d^2$ (2) $\lambda = \left(\frac{2m}{hc}\right)\lambda_d^2$
(3) $\lambda_d = \left(\frac{2mc}{h}\right)\lambda^2$ (4) $\lambda = \left(\frac{2mc}{h}\right)\lambda_d^2$

35. Water falls from a height of 60 m at the rate of 15 kg/s to operate a turbine. The losses due to frictional force are 10% of the input energy. How much power is generated by the turbine? ($g = 10$ m/s^2) **[Work, Energy and Power]**

(1) 7.0 kW (2) 10.2 kW
(3) 8.1 kW (4) 12.3 kW

SECTION - B

36. Twenty seven drops of same size are charged at 220 V each. They combine to form a bigger drop. Calculate the potential of the bigger drop.

[Electrostatic Potential and Capacitance]

(1) 1980 V (2) 660 V

(3) 1320 V (4) 1520 V

37. A point object is placed at a distance of 60 cm from a convex lens of focal length 30 cm. If a plane mirror were put perpendicular to the principal axis of the lens and at a distance of 40 cm from it, the final image would be formed at a distance of

[Ray Optics and Optical Instruments]

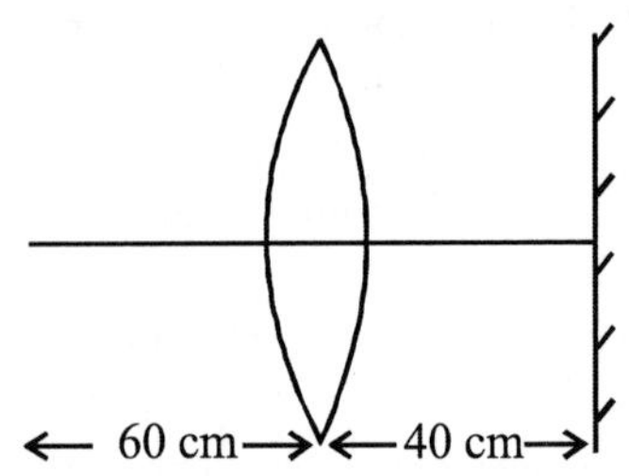

(1) 20 cm from the plane mirror, it would be a virtual image

(2) 20 cm from the lens, it would be a real image

(3) 30 cm from the lens, it would be a real image

(4) 30 cm from the plane mirror, it would be a virtual image

38. A particle of mass 'm' is projected with a velocity $v = kV_e$ $(k < 1)$ from the surface of the earth.

(V_e = escape velocity)

The maximum height above the surface reached by the particle is **[Gravitation]**

(1) $\frac{Rk^2}{1-k^2}$ (2) $R\left(\frac{k}{1-k}\right)^2$

(3) $R\left(\frac{k}{1+k}\right)^2$ (4) $\frac{R^2k}{1+k}$

39. In the product $\vec{F} = q(\vec{v} \times \vec{B})$

$= q\vec{v} \times (B\hat{i} + B\hat{j} + B_0\hat{k})$

For $q = 1$ and $\vec{v} = 2\hat{i} + 4\hat{j} + 6\hat{k}$

and $\vec{F} = 4\hat{i} - 20\hat{j} + 12\hat{k}$

What will be the complete expression for $\vec{B}$

[Moving Charges and Magnetism]

(1) $6\hat{i} + 6\hat{j} - 8\hat{k}$ (2) $-8\hat{i} - 8\hat{j} - 6\hat{k}$

(3) $-6\hat{i} - 6\hat{j} - 8\hat{k}$ (4) $8\hat{i} + 8\hat{j} - 6\hat{k}$

40. Two conducting circular loops of radii R_1 and R_2 are placed in the same plane with their centres coinciding. If $R_1 >> R_2$, the mutual inductance M between them will be directly proportional to **[Electromagnetic Induction]**

(1) $\frac{R_2^2}{R_1}$ (2) $\frac{R_1}{R_2}$ (3) $\frac{R_2}{R_1}$ (4) $\frac{R_1^2}{R_2}$

41. For the given circuit, the input digital signals are applied at the terminals A, B and C. What would be the output at the terminal y? **[Semiconductor Electronics : Materials, Devices and Simple Circuits]**

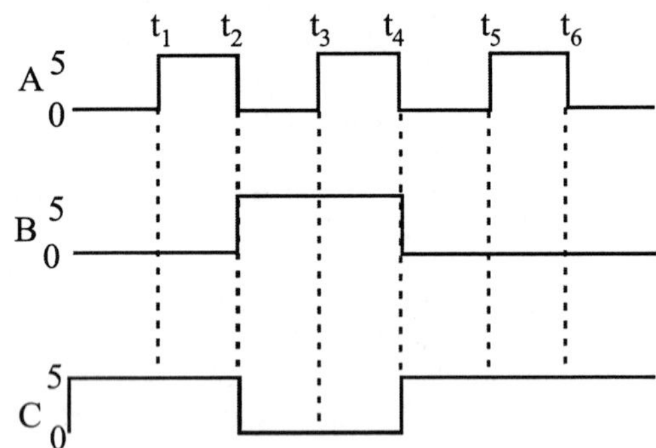

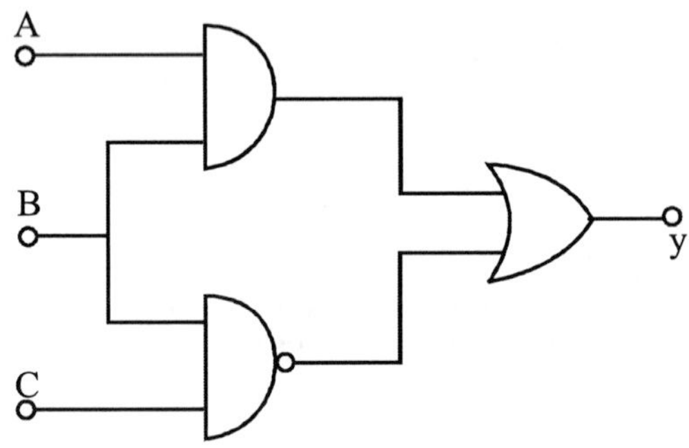

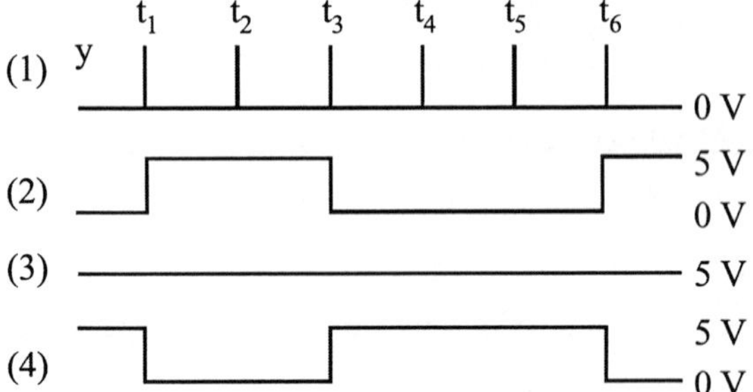

42. From a circular ring of mass 'M' and radius 'R' an arc corresponding to a 90° sector is removed. The moment of inertia of the remaining part of the ring about an axis passing through the centre of the ring and perpendicular to the plane of the ring is 'K' times 'MR^2'. Then the value of 'K' is **[System of Particles and Rotational Motion]**

(1) $\frac{1}{8}$ (2) $\frac{3}{4}$ (3) $\frac{7}{8}$ (4) $\frac{1}{4}$

43. Three resistors having resistances r_1, r_2 and r_3 are connected as shown in the given circuit. The ratio $\frac{i_3}{i_1}$ of currents in terms of resistances used in the circuit is **[Current Electricity]**

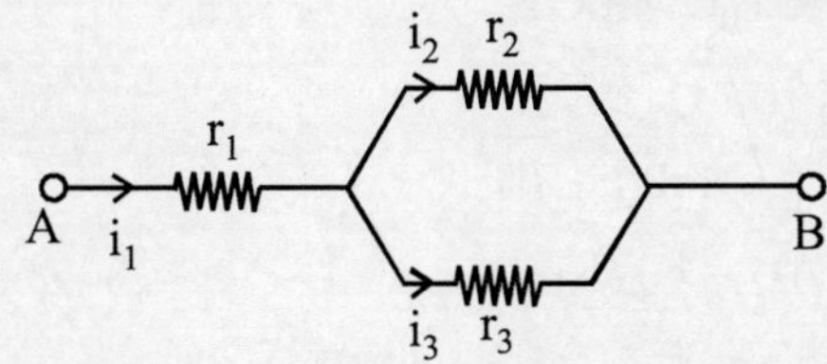

(1) $\frac{r_2}{r_1+r_3}$ (2) $\frac{r_1}{r_2+r_3}$

(3) $\frac{r_2}{r_2+r_3}$ (4) $\frac{r_1}{r_1+r_2}$

44. A car starts from rest and accelerates at 5 m/s^2. At t = 4 s, a ball is dropped out of a window by a person sitting in the car. What is the velocity and acceleration of the ball at t = 6 s? (Take g = 10 m/s^2) **[Motion in a Plane]**

(1) $20\sqrt{2}$ m/s, 10 m/s^2 (2) 20 m/s, 5 m/s^2

(3) 20 m/s, 0 (4) $20\sqrt{2}$ m/s, 0

45. A step down transformer connected to an ac mains supply of 220 V is made to operate at 11 V, 44 W lamp. Ignoring power losses in the transformer, what is the current in the primary circuit? **[Alternating Current]**

(1) 4 A (2) 0.2 A (3) 0.4 A (4) 2 A

46. A ball of mass 0.15 kg is dropped from a height 10 m, strikes the ground and rebounds to the same height. The magnitude of impulse imparted to the ball is (g = 10 m/s^2) nearly **[Laws of Motion]**

(1) 1.4 kg m/s (2) 0 kg m/s

(3) 4.2 kg m/s (4) 2.1 kg m/s

47. A series LCR circuit containing 5.0 H inductor, 80μ F capacitor and 40 Ω resistor is connected to 230V variable frequency ac source. The angular frequencies of the source at which power transferred to the circuit is half the power at the resonant angular frequency are likely to be **[Alternating Current]**

(1) 42 rad/s and 58 rad/s
(2) 25 rad/s and 75 rad/s
(3) 50 rad/s and 25 rad/s
(4) 46 rad/s and 54 rad/s

48. A uniform rod of length 200 cm and mass 500 g is balanced on a wedge placed at 40 cm mark. A mass of 2 kg is suspended from the rod at 20 cm and another unknown mass 'm' is suspended from the rod at 160 cm mark as shown in the figure. Find the value of 'm' such that the rod is in equilibrium. (g = 10 m/s^2) **[System of Particles and Rotational Motion]**

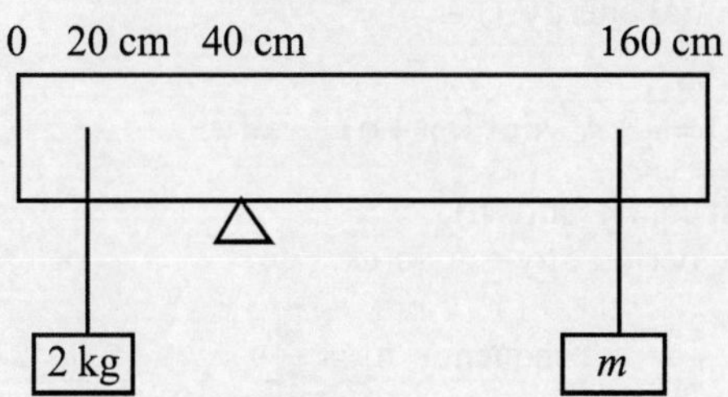

(1) $\frac{1}{12}$kg (2) $\frac{1}{2}$kg (3) $\frac{1}{3}$kg (4) $\frac{1}{6}$kg

49. A particle moving in a circle of radius R with a uniform speed takes a time T to complete one revolution. If this particle were projected with the same speed at an angle 'θ' to the horizontal, the maximum height attained by it equals 4R. The angle of projection, θ, is then given by : **[Motion in a Plane]**

(1) $\theta=\sin^{-1}\left(\frac{2gT^2}{\pi^2 R}\right)^{1/2}$

(2) $\theta=\cos^{-1}\left(\frac{gT^2}{\pi^2 R}\right)^{1/2}$

(3) $\theta=\cos^{-1}\left(\frac{\pi^2 R}{gT^2}\right)^{1/2}$

(4) $\theta=\sin^{-1}\left(\frac{\pi^2 R}{gT^2}\right)^{1/2}$

50. A uniform conducting wire of length 12a and resistance 'R' is wound up as a current carrying coil in the shape of,
(i) an equilateral triangle of side 'a'.
(ii) a square of side 'a'.
The magnetic dipole moments of the coil in each case respectively are **[Moving Charges and Magnetism]**

(1) 4 Ia^2 and 3 Ia^2 (2) $\sqrt{3}$ Ia^2 and 3 Ia^2

(3) 3 Ia^2 and Ia^2 (4) 3 Ia^2 and 4 Ia^2

ANSWER KEYS

1.	(3)	6.	(1)	11.	(3)	16.	(1)	21.	(1)	26.	(2)	31.	(1)	36.	(1)	41.	(3)	46.	(3)
2.	(1)	7.	(2)	12.	(3)	17.	(1)	22.	(1)	27.	(2)	32.	(3)	37.	(1)	42.	(2)	47.	(4)
3.	(2)	8.	(4)	13.	(1)	18.	(3)	23.	(4)	28.	(2)	33.	(3)	38.	(1)	43.	(3)	48.	(1)
4.	(3)	9.	(4)	14.	(4)	19.	(3)	24.	(4)	29.	(3)	34.	(4)	39.	(3)	44.	(1)	49.	(1)
5.	(4)	10.	(4)	15.	(1)	20.	(3)	25.	(4)	30.	(2)	35.	(3)	40.	(1)	45.	(2)	50.	(2)

HINTS & SOLUTION

1. **(3)** Displacement of particle executing SHM $y = A\sin(\omega t + \phi)$ ...(i)

Potential energy $U = \frac{1}{2}ky^2$

or, $U = \frac{1}{2}kA^2\sin^2(\omega t + \phi)$ ...(ii)

From eq. (i) and (ii),
Time period of $y = A\sin(\omega t + \phi)$

$T_1 = \frac{2\pi}{\omega}$ $\therefore$ Frequency $n_1 = \frac{\omega}{2\pi}$

and time period of $y^2 = A^2\sin^2(\omega t + \phi)$

$T_2 = \frac{\pi}{\omega}$ $\therefore$ Frequency $n_2 = \frac{\omega}{\pi}$

$\therefore n_2 = 2n_1 = 2n$

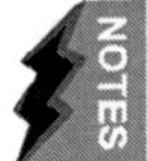

Potential energy varies periodically with double the frequency of SHM. It is maximum and equal to total energy at extreme position and minimum at mean position.

2. **(1)** In polar molecules, like $HCl \rightarrow H^{\delta+}\,Cl^{\delta-}$ the centre of positive charges does not coincide with the centre of negative charges.
Hence, permanent electric dipole exists.

3. **(2)** Drift velocity, $v_d = \frac{I}{neA} = \frac{eE\tau}{m}$

Electrical resistivity, $\rho = \frac{1}{\sigma} = \frac{E}{J}$ $\left(\because \sigma = \frac{J}{E}\right)$

Relaxation period, $\tau = \frac{m}{ne^2\rho}$

Current density, $J = \frac{I}{A} = nev_d$

(1) - (iii), (B) - (iv), (C) - (i), (D) - (ii)

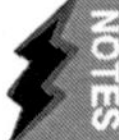

Relation between drift velocity, v_d, electrical resistivity(ρ) relaxation period (τ) and current density(J)

$$v_d = \frac{i}{neA} = \frac{J}{ne} = \frac{\sigma E}{ne} = \frac{E}{\rho ne} = \frac{V}{\rho l ne};$$

$$R = \rho\frac{1}{A} = \frac{m}{ne^2\tau}.\frac{1}{A}$$

4. **(3)** Charge density $\sigma = \frac{\text{charge}}{\text{area}}$

When two conductors are connected by a conducting wire, then they have same potential
i.e., $V_1 = V_2$

$$\therefore \frac{1}{4\pi\varepsilon_0}\frac{Q_1}{R_1} = \frac{1}{4\pi\varepsilon_0}\frac{Q_2}{R_2}$$

$$\Rightarrow \frac{1}{4\pi\varepsilon_0}\frac{Q_1}{R_1}\times\frac{R_1}{R_1} = \frac{1}{4\pi\varepsilon_0}\frac{Q_2}{R_2}\times\frac{R_2}{R_2}$$

$$\Rightarrow \frac{Q_1R_1}{4\pi R_1^2\varepsilon_0} = \frac{Q_2R_2}{4\pi R_2^2\varepsilon_0}$$

$$\therefore \frac{Q_1}{4\pi R_1^2}\Big/\frac{Q_2}{4\pi R_2^2} = \frac{R_2}{R_1}$$

or, $\sigma_1/\sigma_2 = R_2/R_1$

5. **(4)** Energy density i.e. $\frac{\text{energy}}{\text{volume}}$ with electric field

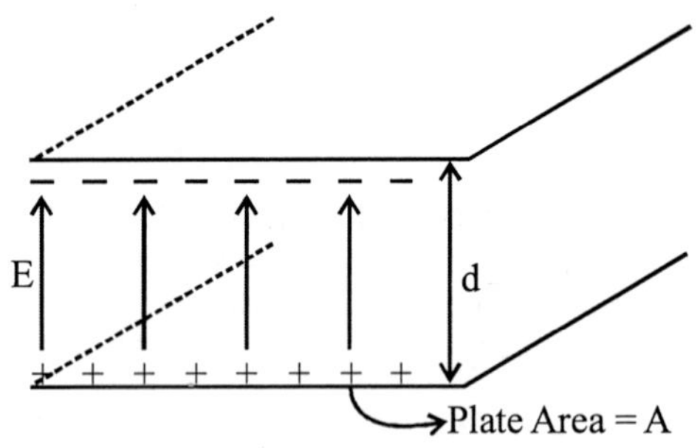

$$u = \frac{dU}{dV} = \frac{1}{2}\varepsilon_0E^2$$

$$\Rightarrow dU = \frac{1}{2}\varepsilon_0E^2dV$$

$\therefore$ Energy stored in the capacitor

$$U = \int dU = \int\frac{1}{2}\varepsilon_0E^2dV$$

$$= \frac{1}{2}\varepsilon_0E^2\int dV = \frac{1}{2}\varepsilon_0E^2V$$

$$\therefore u = \frac{1}{2}\varepsilon_0E^2Ad \qquad [\because V = Ad]$$

6. **(1)** Magnetic field due to a current carrying wire at a distance r from the wire.

$$\text{or, } B = \frac{10^{-7}\times 2\times 5}{20\times 10^{-2}} = \frac{1}{2}\times 10^{-5}$$

e
A → $v = 10^5$ m/s
r = 20cm
P 5 A Q

$$B = \frac{\mu_0}{4\pi}\frac{2I}{r} = \frac{4\pi\times 10^{-7}\times 2\times 5}{4\pi\times 20\times 10^{-2}}$$

$$\text{or, } B = \frac{10^{-7}\times 2\times 5}{20\times 10^{-2}} = \frac{1}{2}\times 10^{-5}$$

B upward to the plane of paper

Therefore, force acting on electron

$\vec{F} = q(\vec{v} \times \vec{B})$

$\Rightarrow |\vec{F}| = 1.6 \times 10^{-19} \times 10^5 \times \frac{1}{2} \times 10^{-5}$

$= 8 \times 10^{-20}$ N

7. **(2)** Dimensional formula of energy $E = \frac{1}{2}mv^2$

$[E] = [M^1 L^2 T^{-2}]$ ...(i)

Dimensional formula of gravitational constant

$G = \frac{Fr^2}{m_1 m_2}$

$[G] = [M^{-1} L^3 T^{-2}]$ ...(ii)

From eq. (i) & (ii)

$\therefore \frac{E}{G} = \frac{[M^1 L^2 T^{-2}]}{[M^{-1} L^3 T^{-2}]} = [M^2 L^{-1} T^0]$

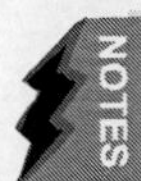

Numerical constant like, $\frac{1}{2}$, 1, 2 or 2π has no dimension.

8. **(4)** A large focal length and large aperture of an objective of an astronomical telescope, ensures better light gathering power, and resolution so contributes to the quality and visibility of the images of the far-off objects.

Resolving power of a telescope $RP = \frac{a}{1.22\lambda}$, a = aperture of the objective.

And resolving limit of telescope $d\theta = \frac{1.22\lambda}{a}$

9. **(4)** Root mean square RMS speed of gas molecule

$V_{RMS} = \sqrt{\frac{3RT}{M}}$

Pressure exerted by ideal gas $P = \frac{1}{3}nm\bar{v}^2$

Average kinetic energy of a molecule $= \frac{3}{2}k_B T$

Total internal energy of a gas is $(U) = \frac{1}{2}nfRT$

Here, for one mole n = 1 and f = 5 for diatomic

$\therefore U = \frac{5}{2}RT$

10. **(4)** • A zener diode is connected in reverse biased when used as voltage regulator as in reverse biased after breakdown, voltage becomes constant.

• Potential barrier of silicon diode is nearly 0.7V

Statement 1 is correct and statement 2 is incorrect.

11. **(3)** Potential energy of electric dipole in external electric field

$U = -\vec{P}.\vec{E} = -PE\cos\theta = -PE\cos 180°$

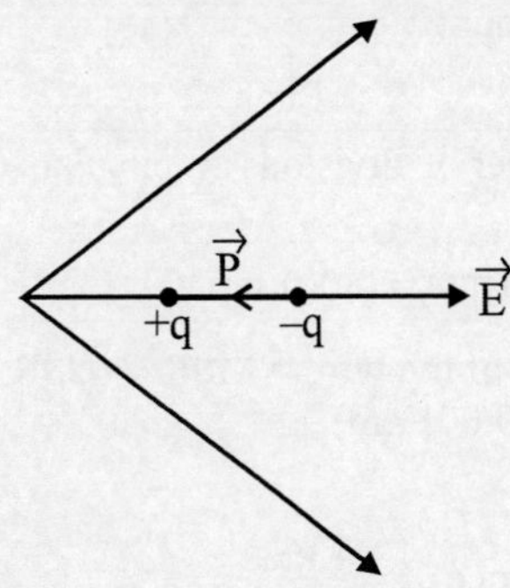

Since angle between $\vec{E}$ and $\vec{P}$ is 180°

$\therefore U = +PE$

On moving towards right electric field strength decrease

$\therefore$ U decreases.

Net force on electric dipole is towards right and net torque acting on it is zero so move towards right.

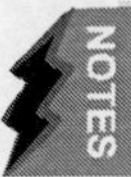

Potential energy of a dipole $U = -PE\cos\theta$, $\theta = 0° \Rightarrow$ stable equilibrium and U = –PE i.e., minimum value.
For $\theta = 90°$, U = 0 and dipole is not in equilibrium. For $\theta = 180°$, U = PE i.e., maximum value and dipole is in unstable equilibrium.

12. **(3)**

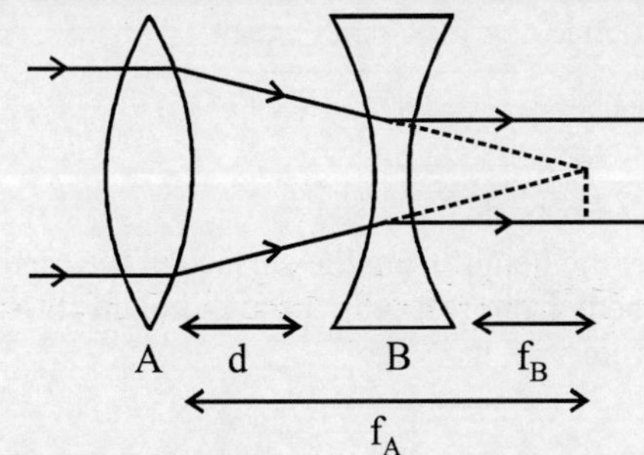

From the ray diagram light refracted from convex lens virtually meet at focus of concave lens

$\therefore d = f_A - f_B$

$= 20 - 5 = 15$ cm

13. **(1)** Escape velocity from the earth's surface

$v_e = \sqrt{\frac{2GM}{R}} = \sqrt{\frac{2G\rho\frac{4}{3}\pi R^3}{R}}$ $\left[\because \rho = \frac{M}{V}\right]$

or, $v_e = \sqrt{\frac{8G\rho\pi}{3}R^2}$ or, $v_e \propto R$ ($\because$ same density)

$\therefore \frac{v}{v_1} = \frac{R}{4R}$ or, $v_1 = 4v$

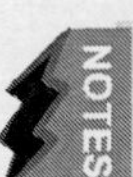

Escape velocity is double if the radius of the earth is double keeping the density unchanged. Escape velocity depends on the mass and size of the planet.

14. **(4)** Atomic number (z) decreases by 1 after one β^+ decay

Atomic number (z) increases by 1 after one β^- decay

Atomic number (z) decreases by 2 after one α decay

$^A_Z X \xrightarrow{\beta^+ \text{ decay}} {}_{z-1}B \xrightarrow{\alpha \text{ decay}} {}_{z-3}C \xrightarrow{\beta^- \text{ decay}} {}_{z-2}D$

$\therefore$ Correct order of decay is β^+, α, β^-

15. **(1)** Least count

$$LC = \frac{\text{Pitch}}{\text{Number of divisions on circular scale}}$$

$$= \frac{1}{100} = 0.01\,mm = 0.001\ cm$$

∴ Diameter of the wire = MSR + (CSR × LC)
= 0 + (52 × 0.001 cm)
= 0.052 cm

16. **(1)** Impedance $Z = \frac{V_{RMS}}{I_{RMS}}$

$$V_{RMS} = \sqrt{V_R^2 + (V_L - V_C)^2}$$

$$= \sqrt{(40)^2 + (40-10)^2} = 50\ V$$

$$I_{RMS} = \frac{I_0}{\sqrt{2}} = \frac{10\sqrt{2}}{\sqrt{2}} = 10A$$

$$\therefore Z = \frac{V_{RMS}}{I_{RMS}} = \frac{50}{10} = 5\,\Omega$$

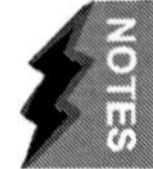

Impedance (z) is the oppsition offered by ac circuits to the flow of ac. For LCR series circuit.

Voltage $V = \sqrt{V_R^2 + (V_L - V_C)^2}$

and $Z = \sqrt{R^2 + (X_L - X_C)^2}$

17. **(1)** Let the height from the surface of the earth be x.
When body from rest falls through height (S – x)
Then from $v^2 = u^2 + 2gs$

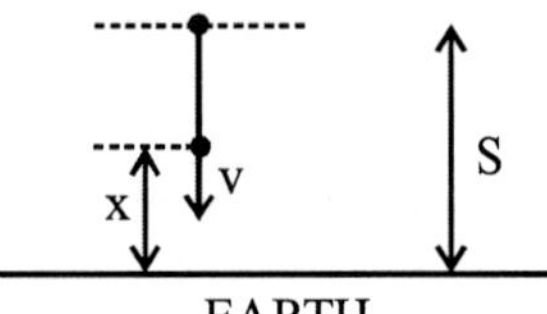

$v^2 = 0^2 + 2g(S - x)$

$\Rightarrow v = \sqrt{2g(S-x)}$ ...(i)

At this point,
U = mgx
From question, kinetic energy, K = 3U

$$\therefore \frac{1}{2}m(v)^2 = 3 \times mg(x)$$

$$\Rightarrow \frac{1}{2} \times m \times 2g(S-x) = 3 \times mgx \quad \text{(using (i))}$$

$\Rightarrow S - x = 3x$

$\therefore x = \frac{S}{4}$ ... (ii)

$$\therefore v = \sqrt{2 \times g\left(S - \frac{S}{4}\right)} = \sqrt{\frac{3gS}{2}}$$

18. **(3)** Acceleration along inclined plane,
a = gsinθ
S_n = distance travelled by object during n^{th} second.
Initial speed u = 0

$$S_n = u + \frac{a}{2}(2n-1)$$

$$\Rightarrow S_n = 0 + \frac{g\sin\theta}{2}(2n-1) = \frac{g\sin\theta}{2}(2n-1) \quad ...(i)$$

Distance travelled during $(n+1)^{th}$ second.

$$S_{n+1} = 0 + \frac{g\sin\theta}{2}\left[2(n+1) - 1\right]$$

$$= \frac{g\sin\theta}{2}(2n+1) \quad ...(ii)$$

Dividing equations (i) and (ii)

$$\frac{S_n}{S_{n+1}} = \frac{\frac{g\sin\theta}{2}(2n-1)}{\frac{g\sin\theta}{2}(2n+1)} = \frac{(2n-1)}{(2n+1)}$$

The distance covered by a body in n^{th} second i.e., $S_n \propto (2n-1)$ if body starts from rest and moves with uniform acceleration.

19. **(3)** Activity of a radioactive substance

$$A = A_0\left(\frac{1}{2}\right)^{\frac{t}{T_{1/2}}} \Rightarrow \frac{A}{A_0} = \left(\frac{1}{2}\right)^{\frac{t}{T_{1/2}}}$$

Given, $T_{1/2}$ = 100 hours & t = 150 hours

$$\Rightarrow \frac{A}{A_0} = \left(\frac{1}{2}\right)^{\frac{150}{100}} \Rightarrow \frac{A}{A_0} = \left(\frac{1}{2}\right)^{\frac{3}{2}}$$

$$\therefore \frac{A}{A_0} = \frac{1}{2\sqrt{2}}$$

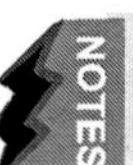

Activity of a radioactive substance is the rate of disintegration or the number of atoms of any material decaying per second.

$$\text{Activity} \propto \frac{1}{\text{half life}}$$

20. **(3)** The circuit is as shown is figure,

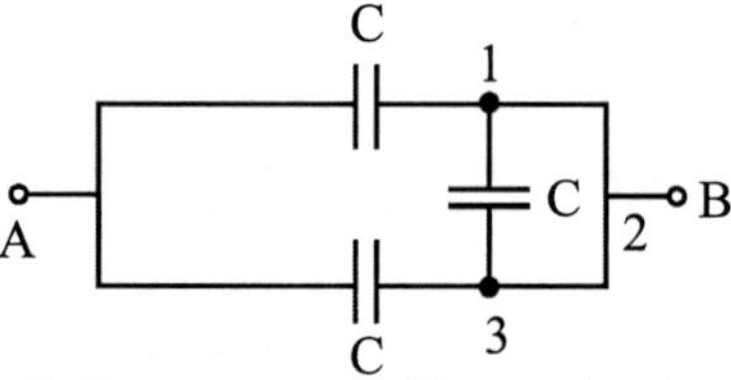

Points 1, 2, 3 are connected by conducting wire so these points are at same potential.
So the capacitor is short circuited. So it does not store any charge.
Therefore equivalent capacitance $C_{AB} = C + C = 2C$

21. **(1)** Resistance of each wire in this case will be same as l & A are same and made of same material.
$\therefore R_1 = R_2 = R_3 = R_4 = R$

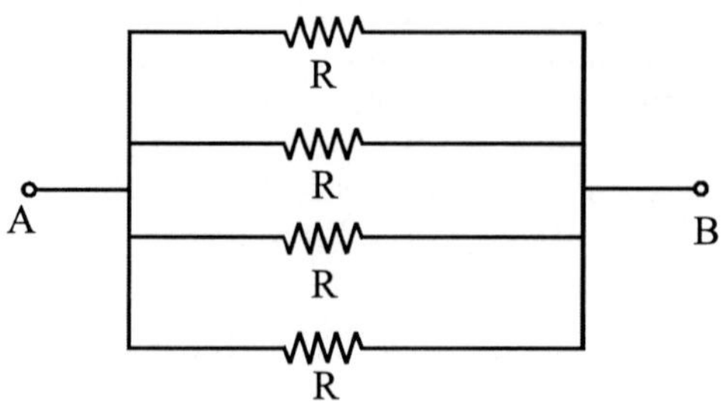

In parallel, $\frac{1}{R_p} = \frac{1}{R_1} + \frac{1}{R_2} + \frac{1}{R_3} + \frac{1}{R_4}$

$\therefore R_P = \frac{R}{4} \Rightarrow 0.25 = \frac{R}{4}$

$\therefore R = 1\ \Omega$

When arranged in series then equivalent resistance.

$R_S = R + R + R + R = 4R$

$\therefore R_S = 4 \times 1 = 4\Omega$

22. **(1)** Gain in BE = (BE) of products – (BE) of reactants.

$= [120 + 120] \times 8.5 - [240] \times 7.6$

$= (240) \times 8.5 - 240 \times 7.6$

$= (2040 - 1824)$ MeV = 216 MeV

23. **(4)** Current $\frac{I_n}{I_p} = \frac{\mu_e}{\mu_h} \because \mu_e > \mu_h$

$\therefore I_n > I_p$

Therefore current in n-type > Current in p-type

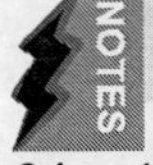

The mobility of electron is 2-3 times the mobility of holes.

24. **(4)** Power, $P = \frac{E}{t} = \frac{n}{t}\left(\frac{hc}{\lambda}\right)$

$\therefore$ No. of photons / second, $\frac{n}{t} = \frac{P}{\left(\frac{hc}{\lambda}\right)}$

$\Rightarrow \frac{n}{t} = \frac{3.3 \times 10^{-3} \times 6 \times 10^{-7}}{6.6 \times 10^{-34} \times 3 \times 10^{8}} = 10^{16}$

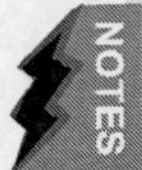

The number of photons emitted per second from a source of monochromatic radiation of wavelength λ and power P and if E = energy of each photon then,

$\frac{n}{t} = \frac{P}{E} = \frac{P}{h\nu} = \frac{P}{hc/\lambda}$

25. **(4)** From Ampere's circuital law, magnetic field

$B = \frac{\mu_0 I}{2\pi R^2}.r$ If $r < R \Rightarrow B_{inside} \propto r$

$B = \frac{\mu_0 I}{2\pi r}$ If $r \geq R \Rightarrow B_{outside} \propto \frac{1}{r}$

Hence the correct magnetic field B versus distance r graph is as shown below.

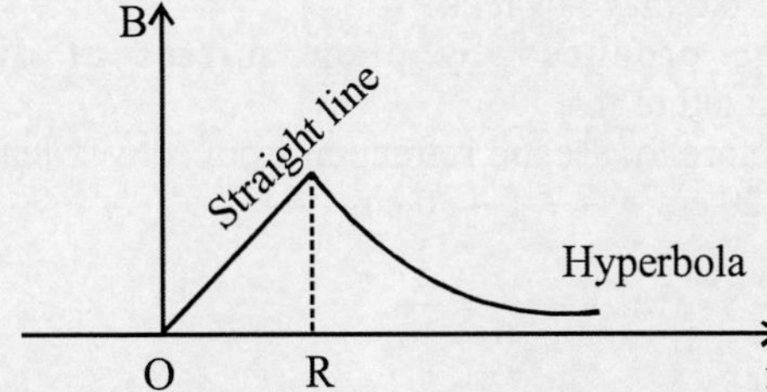

26. **(2)** Let F_v = viscous force and F_B = Bouyant force acting on the ball.

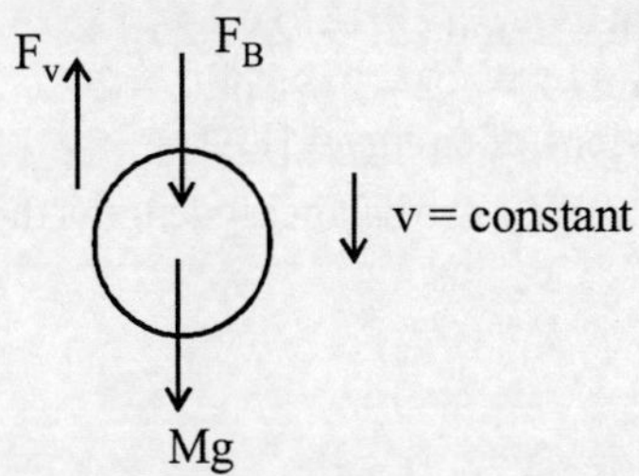

When body moves with constant velocity

$Mg = F_B + F_v$ [a = 0]

$F_v = Mg - F_B$

$= dVg - \frac{d}{2}.Vg$ (M = dVg) V = volume of ball.

or $F_v = \frac{d}{2}Vg = \frac{M}{2}g$ $[\because M = dV]$

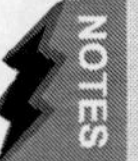

Due to motion of a body through the fluid, the fluid in contact with the body is dragged with it causes relative motion in fluid layers near the body and hence viscous force starts.

27. **(2)** From Snell's law at point P.

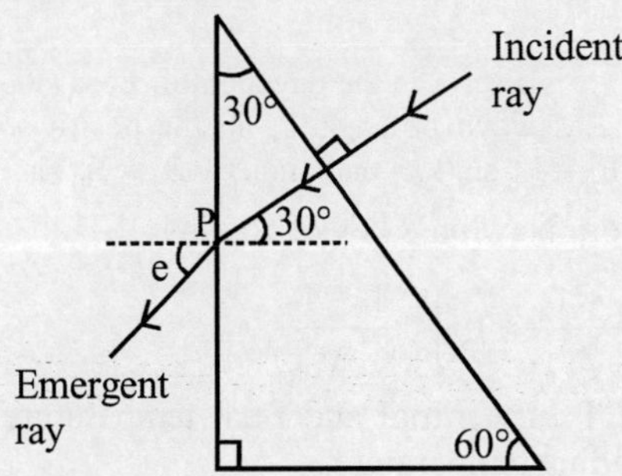

$\frac{\sin i}{\sin r} = \frac{\mu_{air}}{\mu_{Prism}}$

$\Rightarrow \frac{\sin 30°}{\sin e} = \frac{1}{\sqrt{3}}$ $(\because \angle r = \angle e$ emergent angle$)$

$\Rightarrow \sin e = \sqrt{3}.\frac{1}{2}$ $\therefore \angle e = 60°$

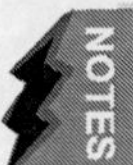

If a light ray is incident normally on first surface i.e., $\angle i = 0°$ so refraction of first surface $\angle r_1 = 0°$.

When angle of prism A > C (critical angle) then no ray emerges from second surface of the prism.

28. **(2)** Displacement current

$I_d = C\frac{dV}{dt}$

$= C\frac{d}{dt}(V_0 \sin \omega t)$ $(\because V = V_0 \sin \omega t$ given$)$

$= C(V_0\omega)\cos\omega t$

$\therefore I_d = V_0\omega C\cos\omega t$

29. **(3)** Energy, $E \propto F^a A^b T^c$

$[E] = [F^a][A^b][T^c]$

$\Rightarrow [ML^2T^{-2}] = [MLT^{-2}]^a [LT^{-2}]^b [T]^c$

$[ML^2T^{-2}] = [M^a L^{a+b} T^{-2a-2b+c}]$

Comparing dimensions on both sides.

$a = 1; a + b = 2$ and $-2 = -2a - 2b + c$
$\therefore b = 1$ and $-2 = -2 - 2 + c$ or, $c = 2$
$\therefore$ Dimensions of energy = $[FAT^2]$

30. **(2)** If ℓ_1 and ℓ_2 are balancing lengths then

$$\frac{E_1}{E_2} = \frac{\ell_1}{\ell_2}$$

$$\therefore \ell_2 = \ell_1\left(\frac{E_2}{E_1}\right) = 36\left(\frac{2.5}{1.5}\right) = 60\,\text{cm}$$

31. **(1)** Spring constant

$$k = \frac{F}{x} = \frac{10}{5\times10^{-2}} = 200\,\text{N/m}$$

And for spring-mass system undergoing SHM

$$T = 2\pi\sqrt{\frac{m}{k}} = 2\pi\sqrt{\frac{2}{200}} = \frac{2\pi}{10} = 0.628\text{s}$$

$(\because m = 2\text{kg given})$

32. **(3)** Direction of propagation along x-axis.

$$\left(-\hat{j}+\hat{k}\right)\times\left(-\hat{j}-\hat{k}\right) = 2\hat{i}$$

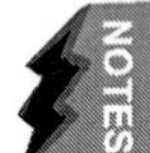

$\vec{E}\times\vec{B}$ is always in the direction of propagation of wave. The EM wave propagating in the positive x-direction $E = E_y = E_0 \sin(kx - \omega t)$ and $B = B_z = B_0 \sin(kx - \omega t)$

33. **(3)** From Newton's law of cooling

$$-K\left(\frac{T_1+T_2}{2} - T_s\right) = \frac{T_1 - T_2}{\Delta t}$$

T_1 and T_2 are initial and final temperature and T_s = surrounding temperature.

$$\Rightarrow -K\left[\frac{(90+80)}{2} - 20\right] = \frac{90-80}{t}$$

$$\Rightarrow -K(65) = \frac{10}{t} \Rightarrow K = \frac{-2}{13t}$$

When cool from 80°C to 60°C

$$-K\left(\frac{80+60}{2} - 20\right) = \frac{(80-60)}{t_1}$$

$$\Rightarrow -K(50) = \frac{20}{t_1} \Rightarrow \frac{2}{13t}(50) = \frac{20}{t_1}$$

$$\therefore t_1 = \frac{13t}{5}$$

34. **(4)** From Einstein's photoelectric equation

$$\frac{hc}{\lambda} = \phi_0 + k$$

Where ϕ_0 = work function
k = maximum kinetic energy of photoelectrons

$$\therefore \frac{hc}{\lambda} = k = \frac{P^2}{2m} \Rightarrow P = \sqrt{\frac{2mhc}{\lambda}}\ [\because \phi = \text{negligible}]$$

de-Broglie wavelength,

$$\lambda_d = \frac{h}{P} = \frac{h}{\sqrt{2mhc/\lambda}} \Rightarrow \sqrt{\lambda} = \lambda_d\sqrt{\frac{2mc}{h}}$$

$$\therefore \lambda = \left(\frac{2mc}{h}\right)\lambda_d^2$$

35. **(3)** Power on turbine $P = \frac{d(mgh)}{dt}$

$$= gh\frac{dm}{dt} = 10\times60\times15 = 9000\text{W}$$

Due to frictional force, lossses are 10%
$\therefore$ Power generated

$$= \left(1 - \frac{10}{100}\right)\times9000 = 8.1\,\text{kW}$$

36. **(1)** Let charge and radius of smaller drop is q and r respectively and R = radius of bigger drop
For smaller drop, electric potential,

$$V = \frac{kq}{r} = 220\text{ V}$$

As volume remains the same

$$\left(\frac{4}{3}\pi r^3\right)\times27 = \frac{4}{3}\pi R^3 \Rightarrow R = \sqrt[3]{27}r = 3r$$

And from conservation of charge,
$Q = 27q$
$\therefore$ Potential of bigger drop,

$$V_{\text{big drop}} = \frac{kQ}{R} = \frac{k(27q)}{3r} = 9\left(\frac{kq}{r}\right)$$

$= 9 \times 220 = 1980$ V

37. **(1)** For first refraction from convex lens
$v_1 = ?$, $u = -60$ cm, $f = 30$ cm
From lens formula,

$$\frac{1}{v_1} - \frac{1}{u} = \frac{1}{f}$$

$$\Rightarrow \frac{1}{v_1} + \frac{1}{60} = \frac{1}{30} \Rightarrow v_1 = 60\,\text{cm}$$

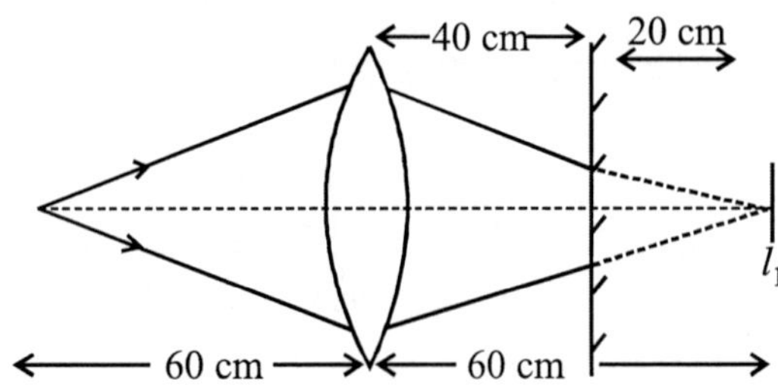

v_1 = first image by lens
Image produced by plane mirror at distance 20 cm left of it.
Therefore for second refraction from convex lens,
$u = -20$ cm, $v = ?$, $f = 30$ cm

$$\frac{1}{v} - \frac{1}{u} = \frac{1}{f} \Rightarrow \frac{1}{v} + \frac{1}{20} = \frac{1}{30}$$

$$\Rightarrow \frac{1}{v} = \frac{1}{30} - \frac{1}{20} \Rightarrow v = -60\text{cm}$$

Hence the final image which is virtual formed at a distance,
$60 - 40 = 20$ cm from plane mirror.

38. **(1)** From law of conservation of mechanical energy,

$$\frac{1}{2}mv^2 - \frac{GmM}{R} = -\frac{GmM}{(R+h)}$$

$$\Rightarrow \frac{v^2}{2} = \frac{GM}{R} - \frac{(GM)}{(R+h)} = \frac{h}{R(R+h)}GM$$

$$\Rightarrow \frac{1}{2}k^2V_e^2 = \frac{GMh}{R(R+h)}$$

We know, escape velocity $V_e = \sqrt{\frac{2GM}{R}}$

$$\Rightarrow \frac{1}{2}k^2\left(\frac{2GM}{R}\right) = \frac{(GM)}{R(R+h)} \text{ or, } k^2 = \frac{h}{(R+h)}$$

$Rk^2 + hk^2 = h \Rightarrow Rk^2 = h(1 - k^2)$

$$\therefore h = \frac{Rk^2}{(1-k^2)}$$

39. **(3)** Lorentz force, $\vec{F} = q(\vec{v} \times \vec{B})$

$= q\vec{v} \times (B\hat{i} + B\hat{j} + B_0\hat{k})$

$\therefore q = 1,\ \vec{v} = 2\hat{i} + 4\hat{j} + 6\hat{k}$ and

$\vec{F} = 4\hat{i} - 20\hat{j} + 12\hat{k}$ (given)

$\therefore (4\hat{i} - 20\hat{j} + 12\hat{k})$

$= -1 \times [(2\hat{i} + 4\hat{j} + 6\hat{k}) \times (B\hat{i} + B\hat{j} + B_0\hat{k})]$

or $(4\hat{i} - 20\hat{j} + 12\hat{k})$

$= i(4B_0 - 6B) - j(2B_0 - 6B) + \hat{k}(2B - 4B)$

Comparing L.H.S and R.H.S, we get

$4B_0 - 6B = 4 \Rightarrow 2B_0 - 3B = 2$ ...(i)

$-(2B_0 - 6B) = -20 \Rightarrow B_0 - 3B = 10$ ...(ii)

$2B - 4B = 12 \Rightarrow B = -6$ ...(iii)

From eq. (ii) and (iii)

$B = -6$ and $B_0 = -8$

$\therefore$ Complete expression for $\vec{B} = -6\hat{i} - 6\hat{j} - 8\hat{k}$

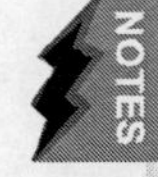

In a magnetic field a moving charged particle experiences magnetic force $\vec{F}_m = q(\vec{v} \times \vec{B})$

$\vec{F}_m = q(\vec{v} \times \vec{B})$ is called Lorentz force.

40. **(1)** Let i be the current in outer loop

Magnetic field at centre $B = \frac{\mu_0 i}{2R_1}$

Magnetic flux through inner coil $\phi_i = B \times \pi R_2^2$

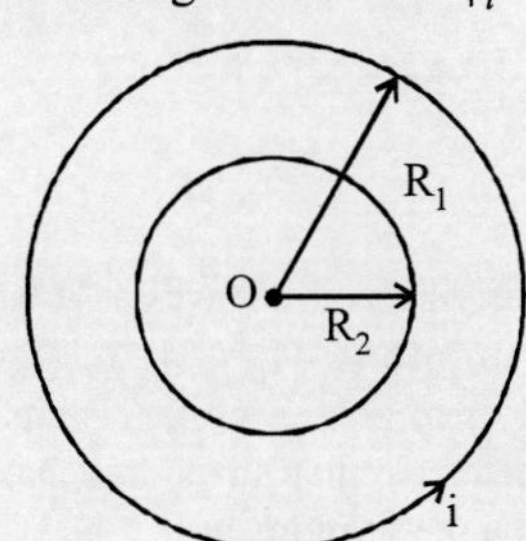

$$\phi_i = \frac{\mu_0 i}{2R_1} \times \pi R_2^2$$

$$\phi_i = \frac{\mu_0 i}{2} \times \frac{\pi R_2^2}{R_1}$$

$\because \phi = Mi$

$$\therefore M = \left(\frac{\mu_0 \pi}{2}\right)\frac{R_2^2}{R_1} \text{ or, } M \propto \frac{R_2^2}{R_1}$$

41. **(3)** Boolean expression for combination of logic gates

Output, $y = A.B + \overline{B.C}$

Time duration	Input Signals A	B	C	AB	Output Signal(y) $\overline{B.C}$	$y = A.B + \overline{B.C}$
$0 - t_1$	0	0	1	0	1	1
$t_1 - t_2$	1	0	1	0	1	1
$t_2 - t_3$	0	1	0	0	1	1
$t_3 - t_4$	1	1	0	1	1	1
$t_4 - t_5$	0	0	1	0	1	1
$t_5 - t_6$	1	0	1	0	1	1
$t_6 - t_7$	0	0	1	0	1	1

Output y is high (1) so output at the terminal y, $v_0 = 5V$

42. **(2)** As per question, 90° arc is removed from circular ring,

$\therefore$ Mass removed $= \frac{M}{4}$

$\therefore$ Mass remaining $M - \frac{M}{4} = \frac{3}{4}M$

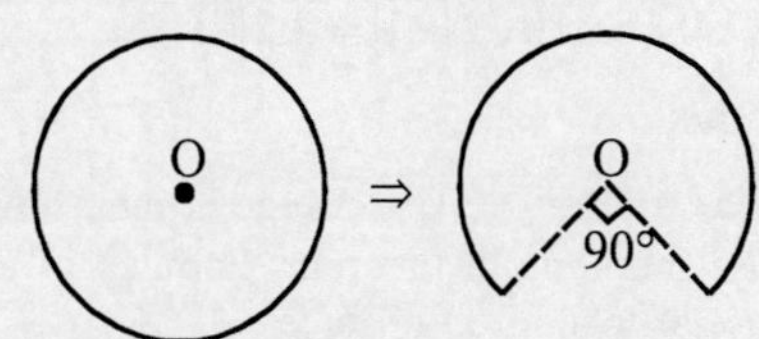

Moment of inertia of remaining $I_{remaining} = \int dmr^2$

$= R^2 \int dm \quad (\because r = R)$

$$\therefore I_{remaining} = \frac{3MR^2}{4} = KMR^2 \therefore K = \frac{3}{4}$$

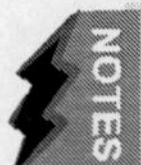

Moment of inertia of a continuous distribution of mass, treating the element of mass dm at position r as particle then $dI = dmr^2$ so $I = \int r^2 dm$

43. **(3)** Resistance r_2 and r_3 are in parallel so potential difference across $r_2 = r_3, = V$

$$\therefore i_2 r_2 = i_3 r_3 \Rightarrow i_2 = \frac{i_3 r_3}{r_2} \quad \text{... (i)}$$

Current $i_1 = i_2 + i_3 \Rightarrow i_1 = \left(\frac{r_3}{r_2} + 1\right)i_3$

$$\therefore \frac{i_3}{i_1} = \frac{r_2}{r_2 + r_3}$$

44. **(1)** Velocity of car at t = 4 s = velocity the ball dropped out of a window v = u + at

$\Rightarrow$ v = 0 + 5 × 4 = 20 ms^{-1}
$\therefore$ Velocity of ball along the horizontal and is 20ms^{-1}.
After 2 seconds of motion :
Vertical velocity of ball (v_y) = $u_y + a_y t$
$v_y = 0 + 10 \times 2 = 20$ ms^{-1} ($\because a_y = g = 10$ m/s^2)
$\therefore$ Magnitude of velocity of ball

$$(v) = \sqrt{v_x^2 + v_y^2} = 20\sqrt{2} \text{ m/s}$$

Since the ball is under free fall.
Acceleration of ball (a) at t = 6s a = g = 10 m/s^2

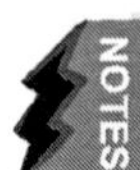
NOTES All bodies, in the absence of air resistance, irrespective of the size, weight or composition fall with same acceleration near the surface of the earth is called free fall.

45. **(2)** Power P = V × I
For an ideal transformer
Input power = Output power
$V_P I_P = V_S I_S$
or, 220 × I_P = 44 $\therefore$ I_P = 0.2 A

46. **(3)** Impulse, $\vec{I}$ = change in linear momentum
or, $I = \Delta\vec{P} = \vec{P_f} - \vec{P_i}$
or, $I = m_2v_2 - m_1v_1$
Velocity of ball at ground

$$(v) = \sqrt{2gh} \left[\because v^2 - u^2 = 2gh\right]$$

$$= \sqrt{2\times10\times10} = 10\sqrt{2} \text{ m/s}$$

$$\therefore \vec{I} = 0.15\times10\sqrt{2}\left(-\hat{j}\right) - 0.15\times10\sqrt{2}\left(\hat{j}\right)$$

$$\Rightarrow \vec{I} = 2\times0.15\times10\sqrt{2}\left(-\hat{j}\right) = 4.2\left(\hat{j}\right)$$

= 4.2 kg m/s

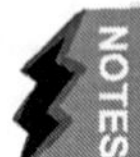
NOTES Impulse $I = \overrightarrow{\Delta P} = \vec{P}_f - \vec{P}_i$ = change in momentum is called impulse momentum theorem. Impulse of a force is a measure of total effect of force.

47. **(4)** For LCR series circuit resonance frequency

$$\omega_0 = \frac{1}{\sqrt{LC}} = \frac{1}{\sqrt{5\times80\times10^{-6}}} = 50 \text{ rad/s}$$

$\therefore$ Half power frequency, $\omega = \omega_0 \pm \frac{R}{2L}$

i.e. $\omega_L = 50 - \frac{40}{2\times5} = 46$ rad/s and

$$\omega_H = 50 + \frac{40}{2\times5} = 54 \text{ rad/s}$$

48. **(1)**

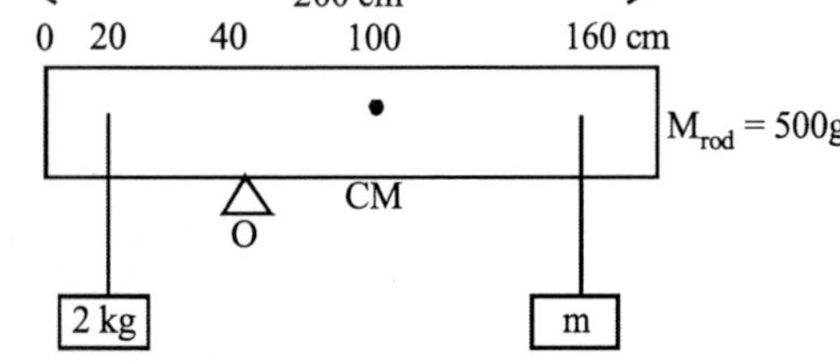

Rod will be in equilibrium, if $\vec{\tau}_{net} = 0$ about point O.
Torque at point O due to 2 kg mass

$$\vec{\tau} = \vec{r}\times\vec{F} = rF\sin\theta\left(\hat{n}\right)$$

$$\tau_1 = 20\times20\times10^{-2}\times\sin90°\left(\hat{k}\right) = 4\text{Nm}\left(\hat{k}\right)$$

Torque due to mass of rod

$$\tau_2 = 5\times60\times10^{-2}\times\sin90°\left(-\hat{k}\right) = 3\text{Nm}\left(-\hat{k}\right)$$

Torque due to mass m

$$\tau_3 = mg\times120\times10^{-2}\times\sin90°\left(-\hat{k}\right)$$

$$= 12m \text{ Nm}\left(-\hat{k}\right)$$

So $\overrightarrow{\tau_1} + \overrightarrow{\tau_2} + \overrightarrow{\tau_3} = 0 \left(\because \vec{\tau}_{net} = 0\right)$

$\Rightarrow 4 - 3 - 12m = 0 \Rightarrow 12m = 1$

$\therefore m = \frac{1}{12}$ kg

49. **(1)** Speed of particle to complete one revolution, $(U) = \frac{2\pi R}{T}$ ... (i)

Particle is projected with same speed (U) at an angle θ to the horizontal

$$\therefore \text{Maximum Height}(H) = \frac{U^2\sin^2\theta}{2g}$$

$$\text{or, } \frac{U^2\sin^2\theta}{2g} = 4R \quad [\because H = 4R \text{ given}]$$

$$\Rightarrow \sin^2\theta = \frac{8gR}{U^2}$$

$$\text{or, } \sin^2\theta = \frac{8gRT^2}{4\pi^2R^2} = \frac{2gT^2}{\pi^2R} \text{ (using equation (i))}$$

$$\therefore \theta = \sin^{-1}\left(\frac{2gT^2}{\pi^2R}\right)^{1/2}$$

50. **(2)** Current in the loop $I = \frac{V}{R}$ equal for both loops.
Magnetic moment of equilateral triangle of side a

$$M_T = \left(\frac{12a}{3a}\right).I.\frac{\sqrt{3}}{4}a^2 = \sqrt{3}Ia^2 \; [\because M = NIA]$$

Similarly magnetic moment of square of side a

$$= \left(\frac{12a}{4a}\right).I.a^2 \; [\because M = NIA]$$

$M_S = 3Ia^2$

NOTES A current carrying coil behaves as a bar magnet and its magnetic moment M = NiA, N = no, of turns, i = current through the coil, A = area of the coil. For a given perimeter circular shape has maximum area hence maximum magnetic moment.

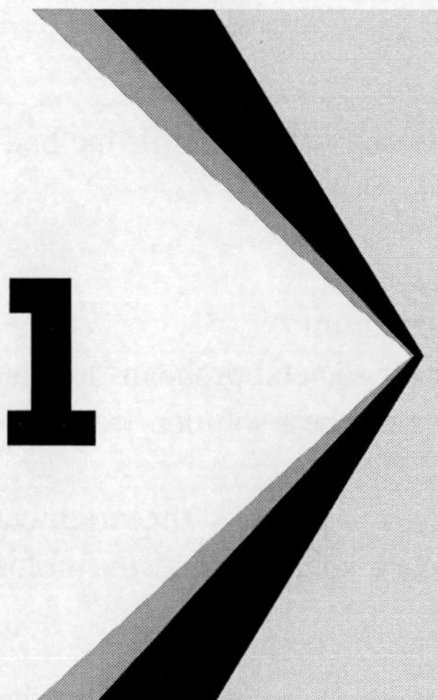

1 Physical World

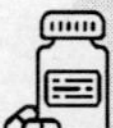

Topic 1.1 : What is Science & Physics, Scope & Excitement of Physics, Physics Technology & Society, Fundamental Forces and Nature of Physical Laws

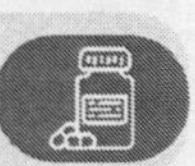

WHAT IS SCIENCE ?

Science refers to a system of acquiring knowledge. This system uses observation and experimentation to describe and explain natural phenomena. The term science also refers to the organized body of knowledge that people have gained using that system. Less formally, the word science often describes any systematic field of study or the knowledge gained from it.

The **purpose of science** is to produce useful models of reality. Most scientific investigations use some form of the scientific method.

The **scientific method** is a logical and rational order of steps by which scientists come to conclusions about the world around them. The Scientific method helps to organize thoughts and procedures so that scientists can be confident in the answers they find. Scientists use observations, hypotheses, and deductions to make these conclusions.

Science as defined above, is sometimes called pure science to differentiate it from applied science, which is the application of research to human needs. Fields of science are commonly divided into two major categories.

1. **Natural science :** The science in which we study about the natural world. Natural science includes physics, chemistry, biology, etc.
2. **Social science :** It is the systematic study of human behavior and society.

WHAT IS PHYSICS ?

The word physics originates from a Greek word which means nature. *Physics is the branch of science that deals with the study of basic laws of nature and their manifestation of various natural phenomena.*

There are two main thrusts in physics :

1. **Unification :** In physics, attempt is made to explain various physical phenomena in terms of just few concepts and laws. Attempts are being made to unify fundamental forces of nature in the persuit of unification.
2. **Reductionism.** Another attempt made in physics is to explain a macroscopic system in terms of its microsocopic constituents. This persuit is called *reductionism.*

Problem Solving Tips

1. Information received through the senses is called **observation**.
2. An idea that may explain a number of observations is called **hypothesis**.
3. A hypothesis that has been tested many times is called **scientific theory**.
4. A scientific theory that has been tested and has always proved true is called **scientific law**.

SCOPE AND EXCITEMENT OF PHYSICS

The scope of physics is very vast. It covers a tremendous range of magnitude of physical quantities like length, mass, time, energy, etc. Basically, there are two domains of interest : macroscopic and microscopic. The **macroscopic domain** includes phenomena at the laboratory, terrestrial and astronomical scales. The **microscopic domain** includes atomic, molecular and nuclear phenomena.

Classical physics deals mainly with macroscopic phenomena consisting of the study of heat, light, electricity, magnetism, optics, acoustics, and mechanics. Since the turn of the 20th century, the study of quantum mechanics and relativity has become more important. Today, physics is often divided into branches such as nuclear physics, particle physics, quantum physics, theoretical physics, and solid-state physics. The study of the planets, stars, and their interactions is known as astrophysics, the physics of the Earth is called geophysics, and the study of the physical laws relating to living organisms is called biophysics.

Physics is exciting in many ways. Application and exploitation of physical laws to make useful devices is the most interesting and exciting part and requires great ingenuity and persistence of effort.

PHYSICS, TECHNOLOGY AND SOCIETY

Physics generates new technologies and these technologies have made our lives comfortable and materially prosperous. We hear terms like science, engineering , technology all in same context though they are not exactly same.

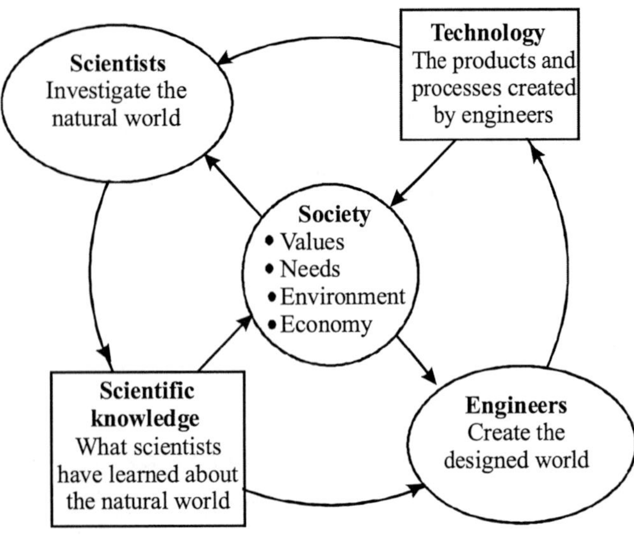

Science:

- A body of knowledge
- Seeks to describe and understand the natural world and its physical properties
- Scientific knowledge can be used to make predictions
- Science uses a process--the scientific method--to generate knowledge

Engineering:

- Design under constraint
- Seeks solutions for societal problems and needs
- Aims to produce the best solution from given resources and constraints
- Engineering uses a process–the engineering design process–to produce solutions and technologies

Technology:

- The body of knowledge, processes and artifacts that result from engineering
- Almost everything made by humans to solve a need is a technology
- Examples of technology include pencils, shoes, cell phones, and processes to treat water

In the real world, these disciplines are closely connected. Scientists often use technologies created by engineers to conduct their research. In turn, engineers often use knowledge developed by scientists to inform the design of the technologies they create.

Link between technology and physics

Technology	Scientific principle(s)
Aeroplane	Bernoulli's principle in fluid dynamics
Bose-Einstein condensate	Trapping and cooling of atoms by laser beams and magnetic fields
Computers	Digital logic
Electric generator	Faraday's laws of electromagnetic induction
Electron microscope	Wave nature of electrons
Fusion test reactor (Tokamak)	Magnetic confinement of plasma
Giant Metrewave Radio Telescope (GMRT)	Detection of cosmic radio waves
Hydroelectric power	Conversion of gravitational potential energy into electrical energy
Lasers	Light amplification by stimulated emission of radiation
Non-reflecting coatings	Thin film optical interference
Nuclear reactor	Controlled nuclear fission
Optical fibres	Total internal reflection of light
Particle accelerators	Motion of charged particles in electromagnetic fields
Photocell	Photoelectric effect
Production of ultra high magnetic fields	Superconductivity
Radio and television	Generation, propagation and detection of electromagnetic waves
Rocket propulsion	Newton's laws of motion
Sonar	Reflection of ultrasonic waves
Steam engine	Laws of thermodynamics

Some physicists from different countries of the world and their major contributions

Name of physicists	Major contribution/discovery	Country of origin
Abdus Salam	Unification of weak and electromagnetic interactions	Pakistan
Albert Einstein	Explanation of photoelectric effect; Theory of relativity	Germany
Archimedes	Principle of buoyancy; Principle of the lever	Greece
C.H. Townes	Maser; Laser	U.S.A.
Christian Huygens	Wave theory of light	Holland
C.V. Raman	Inelastic scattering of light by molecules	India
Ernest Rutherford	Nuclear model of atom	New Zealand
Galileo Galilei	Law of inertia	Italy
Heinrich Rudolf Hertz	Generation of electromagnetic waves	Germany
Homi Jehangir Bhabha	Cascade process of cosmic radiation	India
Issac Newton	Universal law of gravitation; Laws of motion; Reflecting telescope	U.K.
James Clark Maxwell	Electromagnetic theory; Light - an electromagnetic wave	U.K.
James Chadwick	Neutron	U.K.
J.C. Bose	Ultra short radio waves	India
J.J. Thomson	Electron	U.K.
John Bardeen	Transistors; Theory of super conductivity	U.S.A.
Louis Victor de Broglie	Wave nature of matter	France
Marie Sklodowska Curie	Discovery of radium and polonium; Studies on natural radioactivity	Poland
Michael Faraday	Laws of electromagnetic induction	U.K.
M.N. Saha	Thermal ionisation	India
Niels Bohr	Quantum model of hydrogen atom	Denmark
R.A. Millikan	Measurement of electronic charge	U.S.A.
S. Chandrashekhar	Chandrashekhar limit, structure and evolution of stars	India
S.N. Bose	Quantum statistics	India

Example 1. Does imagination play any role in physics?
Solution : Yes, imagination has clayed an important role in the development of physics. Huygen's principle, Bohr's theory, Maxwell equations, Heisenberg's uncertainty principle, etc. were the imaginations of the scientists which successfully explained the various natural phenomena.

Example 2. How is science different from technology?
Solution : Science is the study of natural laws while technology is the practical application of these laws to the daily life problems.

FUNDAMENTAL FORCES IN NATURE

We come across several forces in our day-to-day lives eg., frictional force, muscular force, forces exerted by springs and strings etc. These forces actually arise from four fundamental forces of nature.

Following are **the four fundamental forces in nature.**

1. *Gravitational force*
2. *Weak nuclear force*
3. *Electromagnetic force*
4. *Strong nuclear force*

Among these forces gravitational force is the weakest and strong nuclear force is the strongest force in nature.

Fundamental forces of nature

Name	Relative strength	Range	Exchange particles	Major role	Important properties
Gravitational force (Force of attraction between any two boies by virtue of their masses)	10^{-39}	Infinite	Gravitons	Large-scale structure	Universal attractive, weakest, long range, central, conservative force.
Weak nuclear force (Changes quark types as in Beta-decay of nucleus	10^{-13}	Very short, sub-nuclear size (on 10^{-16}m)	Weak bosons	Nuclear reactions	Govern process involving neutrino and antineutrino, operates only through a range of nuclear size.
Electromagnetic force (Force between particles with charge/magnetism)	10^{-2}	Infinite	Photons	Chemistry and Biology	Either attractive or repulsive, long range, central, conservative force.

Strong nuclear force (Strong attractive force which binds together the protons and neutrons in nucleus)	1	Very Short, nuclear size (on 10^{-15}m)	Gluons	Holding nuclei together	Basically an attractive becomes repulsive (when distance between nucleons < 0.5 fermi) strongest, short range, non-central, non-conservative force.

Physicists are trying to derive a unified theory that would describe all the forces in nature as a single fundamental law. So far, they have succeeded in producing a unified description of the weak and electromagnetic forces, but a deeper understanding of the strong and gravitational forces has not yet been achieved. Theories that postulate the unification of the strong, weak, and electromagnetic forces are called **Grand Unified Theories** (often known by the acronym GUTs). Theories that add gravity to the mix and try to unify all four fundamental forces into a single force are called **Superunified Theories**. The theory that describes the unified electromagnetic and weak interactions is called the **Standard Electroweak Theory**, or sometimes just the **Standard Model**.

Progress in unification of different forces/domains in nature

Name of the physicist	Year	Achievement in unification
Issac Newton	1687	Unified celestial and terrestrial mechanics; showed that the same laws of motion and the law of gravitation apply to both the domains.
Hans Christian Oersted	1820	Showed that electric and magnetic phenomena are inseparable aspects of a unified domain : electromagnetism.
Michael Faraday	1830	
James Clark Maxwell	1873	Unified electricity, magnetism and optics; showed that light is an electromagnetic wave.
Sheldon Glashow, Abdus Salam, Steven Weinberg	1979	Showed that the 'weak' nuclear force and the electromagnetic force could be viewed as different aspects of a single electro-weak force.
Carlo Rubia, Simon Vander Meer	1984	Verified experimentally the predictions of the theory of electro-weak force.

Example 3 . What is electromagnetic force?

Solution : It is the force due to interaction between two moving charges. It is caused by exchange of photons (γ) between two charged particles.

NATURE OF PHYSICAL LAWS

A physical law, scientific law, or a law of nature is a scientific generalization based on empirical observations of physical behavior. Empirical laws are typically conclusions based on repeated scientific experiments and simple observations over many years, and which have become accepted universally within the scientific community. The production of a summary description of nature in the form of such laws is a fundamental aim of science.

Physical laws are distinguished from scientific theories by their simplicity. Scientific theories are generally more complex than laws. They have many component parts, and are more likely to be changed as the body of available experimental data and analysis develops. This is because a physical law is a summary observation of strictly empirical matters, whereas a theory is a model that accounts for the observation, explains it, relates it to other observations, and makes testable predictions based upon it. Simply stated, while a law notes that something happens, a theory explains why and how something happens.

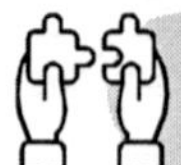

1.1 Concept Practice Problems CPP

1. A scientific way of doing things involve
   (a) identifying the problem
   (b) collecting data
   (c) hypothesising a possible theory
   (d) All of the above
2. Madam Marie Curie won Nobel Prize twice which were in the field of
   (a) Physics and chemistry (b) Chemistry only
   (c) Physics only (d) Biology only
3. Macroscopic domain includes
   (a) phenomena at the laboratory
   (b) terrestrial scales
   (c) astronomical scales
   (d) All of the above
4. Which of the following is the strongest force ?
   (a) Gravitational force
   (b) Nuclear force
   (c) Electromagnetic force
   (d) None of these
5. The scientific principle of technology, hydroelectric power is
   (a) conversion of electric energy into gravitational potential energy
   (b) conversion of kinetic energy into gravitational potential energy
   (c) conversion of gravitational potential energy into electrical energy
   (d) conversion of magnetic energy into electrical energy

ANSWER KEY

1	(d)	2	(a)	3	(d)	4	(b)	5	(c)

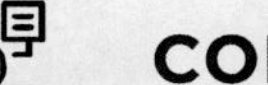

CONCEPT MAP

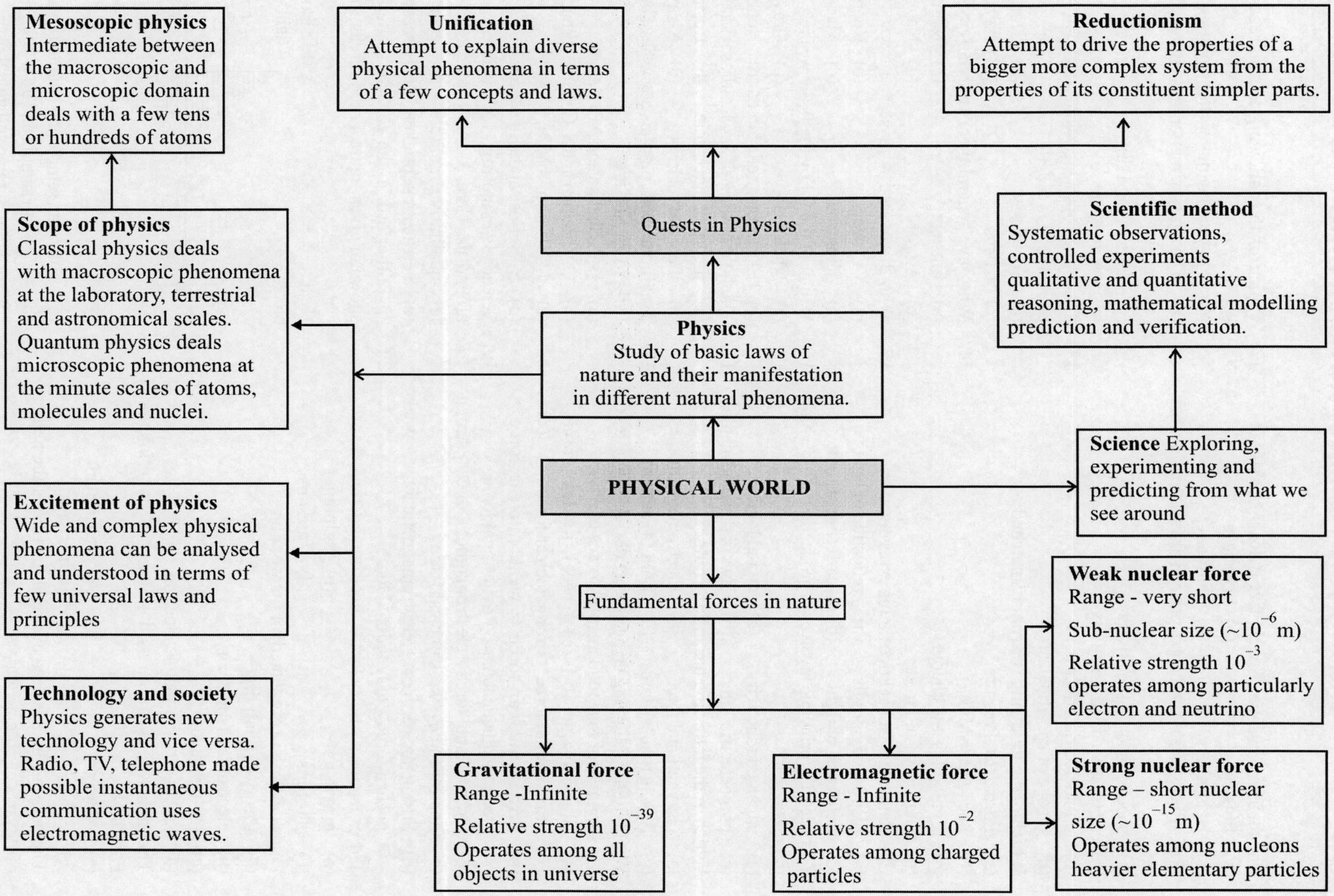

PHYSICAL WORLD

Physics
Study of basic laws of nature and their manifestation in different natural phenomena.

Quests in Physics

Unification
Attempt to explain diverse physical phenomena in terms of a few concepts and laws.

Reductionism
Attempt to drive the properties of a bigger more complex system from the properties of its constituent simpler parts.

Scope of physics
Classical physics deals with macroscopic phenomena at the laboratory, terrestrial and astronomical scales. Quantum physics deals microscopic phenomena at the minute scales of atoms, molecules and nuclei.

Mesoscopic physics
Intermediate between the macroscopic and microscopic domain deals with a few tens or hundreds of atoms

Excitement of physics
Wide and complex physical phenomena can be analysed and understood in terms of few universal laws and principles

Technology and society
Physics generates new technology and vice versa. Radio, TV, telephone made possible instantaneous communication uses electromagnetic waves.

Science Exploring, experimenting and predicting from what we see around

Scientific method
Systematic observations, controlled experiments qualitative and quantitative reasoning, mathematical modelling prediction and verification.

Fundamental forces in nature

Gravitational force
Range -Infinite
Relative strength 10^{-39}
Operates among all objects in universe

Electromagnetic force
Range - Infinite
Relative strength 10^{-2}
Operates among charged particles

Weak nuclear force
Range - very short
Sub-nuclear size ($\sim 10^{-6}$ m)
Relative strength 10^{-3}
operates among particularly electron and neutrino

Strong nuclear force
Range – short nuclear size ($\sim 10^{-15}$ m)
Operates among nucleons heavier elementary particles

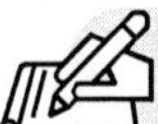

Exercise 1 - Chapter Revision Problems

CRP

1. The man who has won Nobel Prize twice in physics is
   (a) Einstein (b) Bardeen
   (c) Heisenberg (d) Faraday
2. Prof. Albert Einstein got nobel prize in physics for his work on
   (a) special theory of relativity
   (b) general theory of relativity
   (c) photoelectric effect
   (d) theory of specific heats
3. Which of the following is wrongly matched ?
   (a) Barometer-Pressure
   (b) Lactometer-Milk
   (c) Coulomb's law-charges
   (d) Humidity-Calorimeter
4. C.V. Raman got Nobel Prize for his experiment on
   (a) dispersion of light (b) reflection of light
   (c) deflection of light (d) scattering of light
5. The scientific principle involves in production of ultra high magnetic fields is
   (a) super conductivity (b) digital logic
   (c) photoelectric effect (d) laws of thermodynamics
6. Which of the following has infinite range?
   (a) Gravitational force (b) Electromagnetic force
   (c) Strong nuclear force (d) Both (a) and (b)
7. Which of the following is the correct decreasing order of the strengths of four fundamental forces of nature ?
   (a) Electromagnetic force > weak nuclear force > gravitational force > strong nuclear force
   (b) Strong nuclear force > weak nuclear force > electromagnetic force > gravitational force
   (c) Gravitational force > electromagnetic force > strong nuclear force > weak nuclear force
   (d) Strong nuclear force > electromagnetic force > weak nuclear force > gravitational force
8. The exchange particles for the electromagnetic force are
   (a) gravitons (b) gluons
   (c) photons (d) mesons
9. Louis de-Broglie is credited for his work on
   (a) theory of relativity
   (b) electromagnetic theory
   (c) matter waves
   (d) law of distribution of velocities
10. The man who is known as the Father of Experimental Physics is
   (a) Newton (b) Albert Einstein
   (c) Galileo (d) Rutherford
11. The person who has been awarded the title of the Father of Physics of 20th century is
   (a) Madame Curie (b) Sir C.V. Raman
   (c) Neils Bohar (d) Albert Einstein
12. Which of the following is true regarding the physical science?
   (a) They deal with non-living things
   (b) The study of matter are conducted at atomic or ionic levels
   (c) Both (a) and (b)
   (d) None of these
13. The branch of science which deals with nature and natural phenomena is called
   (a) Sociology (b) Biology
   (c) Civics (d) Physics
14. Who gave general theory of relativity?
   (a) Einstein (b) Marconi
   (c) Ampere (d) Newton
15. Who discovered X-rays?
   (a) Chadwick (b) Roentgen
   (c) Thomson (d) Madam Curie
16. Which of the following is the weakest force?
   (a) Nuclear force (b) Gravitational force
   (c) Electromagnetic force (d) None of these
17. The field of work of S. Chandrashekar is
   (a) theory of black hole (b) Cosmic rays
   (c) theory of relativity (d) X-rays
18. Two Indian born physicists who have been awarded Nobel Prize in Physics are
   (a) H. J. Bhabha and APJ Kalam
   (b) C.V. Raman and S. Chandrasekhar
   (c) J.C. Bose and M.N. Saha
   (d) S. N. Bose and H. J. Bhabha
19. Science is exploring, ...x... and ...y... from what we see around us. Here, x and y refer to
   (a) qualitative, modify (b) experiment, predict
   (c) verification, predict (d) reasoning, quantitative
20. In Rutherford, alpha particle scattering experiment as shown in given figure, A and B refer to

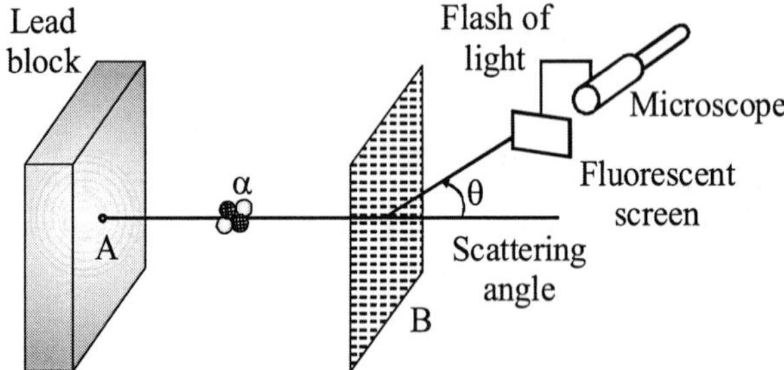

   (a) polonium sample and aluminium foil
   (b) polonium sample and gold foil
   (c) uranium sample and gold foil
   (d) uranium sample and aluminium foil

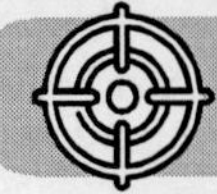

Hints & Solutions

1.1 Concept Practice Problems

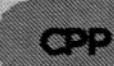

1. (d) A scientific way of doing things involve – identifying the problem, collecting data and hypothesising a possible theory.
2. (a)
3. (d) The macroscopic domain includes phenomena at the laboratory, terrestrial and astronomical scales.
4. (b)
5. (c) The principle of hydroelectric power is conversion of gravitational potential energy into electrical energy.

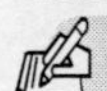

Exercise 1 - Chapter Revision Problems

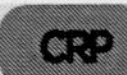

1. (b) The only person to win Nobel prize in physics twice was John Bardeen first in 1956 for the transistor and second in 1972 for his theory of superconductivity.

2. (c) 3. (d) 4. (d) 5. (a) 6. (d)

7. (d) 8. (c) 9. (c) 10. (c) 11. (d)

12. (c) 13. (d) 14. (a) 15. (b) 16. (b)

17. (a) 18. (b)

19. (b) Science is exploring, experimenting and predicting from what we see around us.
20. (b) The alpha particle scattering experiment of Rutherford gave the nuclear model of the atom as shown in figure

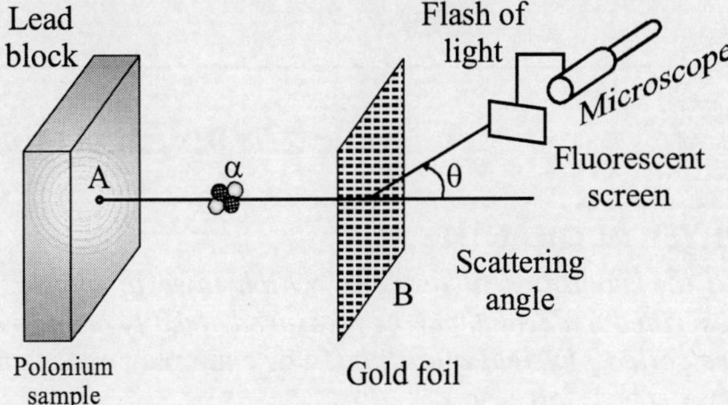

2 Units and Measurements

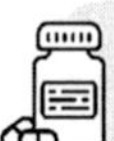

Topic 2.1 : Physical Quantity, Units and Dimensions

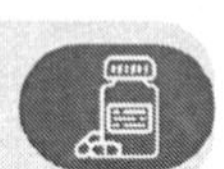

PHYSICAL QUANTITY

All the quantities in terms of which laws of physics are described and which can be measured directly or indirectly are called ***physical quantities****.* For example mass, length, time, speed, force etc.

Types of Physical Quantity

1. **Fundamental quantities :** The physical quantities which do not depend upon other physical quantities are called **fundamental** or **base physical quantities.** e.g. mass, length, time temperature electric current, luminous intensity and amount of substance.
2. **Derived quantities :**The physical quantities which depend on fundamental quantities are called **derived quantities** e.g. speed, acceleration, force, etc.

UNIT

The process of measurement is a *comparison process.*

Unit is the standard quantity used for comparision.

The chosen standard for measurement of a physical quantity, which has the same nature as that of the quantity is called the unit of that quantity.

Choice of a unit (Characteristics of a unit):

(1) It should be **suitable in size** (suitable to use)

(2) It should be **accurately defined** (so that everybody understands the unit in same way)

(3) It should be **easily reproducible**.

(4) It should **not change with time**.

(5) It should **not change with change in physical conditions** i.e., temperature, pressure, moisture etc.

(6) It should be **universally acceptable.**

Every measured quantity (its magnitude) comprises of a number and a unit. **Ex:** In the measurement of time, say

15 s ↙ ↘ Number (n) Unit (u)

If Q is the **magnitude** of the quantity (which does not depend on the selection of unit) then

$$Q = n\,u = n_1\,u_1 = n_2\,u_2 \Rightarrow n \propto \frac{1}{u}$$

Where u_1 and u_2 are the units and n_1 and n_2 are the numerical values in two different system of units.

Fundamental (or Base) and Derived Units

Fundamental units are those, which are independent of unit of other physical quantity and cannot be further resolved into any other units or the units of fundamental physical quantities are called **fundamental or base units.** e.g., kilogram, metre, second etc,

All units other than fundamental are derived units (**which are dependent on fundamental units**) e.g., unit of speed (ms^{-1}) which depends on unit of length (metre) and unit of time (second), unit of momentum ($Kgms^{-1}$) depends on unit of mass, length and time etc.

SYSTEM OF UNITS

A system of units is a complete set of fundamental and derived units for all physical quantities.

Different types of system of units

F.P.S. (Foot - Pound - Second) system. (British engineering system of units.): In this system the unit of length is foot, mass is pound and time is second.

C.G.S. (Centimetre - Gram - Second) system. (Gaussian system of units): In this system the unit of length is centimetre, mass is gram and time is second.

M.K.S (Metre - Kilogram - Second) system. This system is related to mechanics only. In this system the unit of length is metre, mass is kilogram and time is second.

S.I. (International system) units: (Introduced in 1971) Different countries use different set of units. To avoid complexity, by international agreement, seven physical quantities have been chosen as fundamental or base physical quantities and two as supplementary. These quantities are

S.No	*Base physical quantity*	*Fundamental unit*	*Symbol*
1	Mass	kilogram	kg
2	Length	metre	m
3	Time	second	s
4	Temperature	kelvin	K
5	Electric current	ampere	A
6	Luminous intensity	candela	cd
7	Amount of substance	mole	mol

S.No	Supplementary physical quantity	Supplementary unit	Symbol
1	Plane angle	radian	rad
2	Solid angle	steradian	sr

Merits of S.I. Units :

(1) SI is a **coherent system** of units: This means that all derived units are obtained by multiplication and division without introducing any numerical factor.

(2) SI is a **rational system** of units: This is because it assigns only one unit to a particular physical quantity.

(3) SI is an **absolute system** of units: There is no gravitational unit in this system.

(4) SI system is **applicable to all branches** of science.

Conventions of writing of Units and their Symbols

- Unit is **never written with capital initial letter.**
- For a **unit named after scientist the symbol is a capital letter** otherwise not.
- The unit or symbol is **never written in plural form.**
- **Punctuations marks are not written** after the symbol.

Definitions of Fundamental Units

(i) **Metre :** One metre is equal to 1650763.73 wavelength in vacuum of the radiation corresponding to transition between the levels $2p_{10}$ and $5d_5$ of the krypton – 86 atom
Or
The distance travelled by light in vacuum in $\frac{1}{299,792,458}$ second is called 1 metre.

(ii) **Kilogram :** The mass of cylinder (of height and diameter 39 cm) made of Platinum-iridium alloy kept at International Bureau of weights and measures in paris is defined as 1kg.

(iii) **Second :** It is the duration of 9,192,631,770 periods of radiation corresponding to the transition between the two hyperfine levels of the ground state of Caesium (133) atom.

(iv) **Ampere :** It is the current which when flows through two infinitely long straight conductors of negligible cross-section placed at a distance of one metre in air or vacuum produces a force of 2×10^{-7} N/m between them.

(v) **Candela :** It is the luminous intensity in a perpendicular direction, of a surface of 1/600,000 square metre of a black body at the temperature of freezing platinum under a pressure of 1.013×10^5 N/m^2.

(vi) **Kelvin :** It is the 1/273.16 part of thermodynamic temperature of triple point of water.

(vii) **Mole :** It is the amount of substance which contains as many elementary entities as there are in 0.012 kg of Carbon-12.

S.I. Prefixes :

The magnitudes of physical quantities vary over a wide range. For example, the atomic radius, is equal to 10^{-10}m, radius of earth is 6.4×10^6 m and the mass of electron is 9.1×10^{-31} kg. The internationally recommended standard prefixes for certain powers of 10 are given in the table:

Prefix	Power of 10	Symbol
exa	18	E
peta	15	P
tera	12	T
giga	9	G
mega	6	M
kilo	3	k
hecto	2	h
deca	1	da
deci	–1	d
centi	–2	c
milli	–3	m
micro	–6	μ
nano	–9	n
pico	–12	p
femto	–15	f
atto	–18	a

Some Important Practical Units :

(1) For large distance (macro-cosm)

(a) Astronomical unit: It is the average distance of the centre of the sun from the centre of the earth.
1 A.U. = 1.496×10^{11}m

(b) Light year: It is the distance travelled by the light in vacuum in one year. 1 *ly* = 9.46×10^{15}m

(c) Parsec: One parsec is the distance at which an arc 1A.U. long subtends an angle of one second.
1 parsec = 3.1×10^{16}m

(2) For small distance (micro-cosm)
1 micron = 10^{-6}m   1nanometre = 10^{-9}m
1angstorm = 10^{-10}m   1fermi = 10^{-15}m

(3) For small area   1 barn = 10^{-28}m^2

(4) For heavy mass   1 ton = 1000kg
1quintal = 100kg   1slug = 14.57kg
1 C.S.L (chandrasekhar limit) = 1.4 times the mass of the sun

(5) For small mass   1 amu = 1.67×10^{-27}kg
1 pound = 453.6g = 0.4536 kg

(6) For small time   1 shake = 10^{-8}s

(7) For large time
Lunar month: It is the time taken by the earth to complete one rotation about its axis with respect to sun.
1L.M. = 27.3 days.
Solar day: It is the time taken by the earth to complete one rotation about its axis with respect to sun.
Sedrial day: It is the time taken by earth to complete one rotation on its axis with respect to distant star.

(8) For measuring pressure
1 bar = 1atm pressure = 10^5N/m^2 = 760mmHg
1torr = 1 mmHg
1 poiseuille = 10 Poise.

DIMENSIONS

*The powers to which the fundamental units of mass, length and time must be raised to represent the physical quantity are called the **dimensions** of that physical quantity.*

For example : Force = mass × acceleration

$$= \text{mass} \times \frac{v-u}{t} = [M]\frac{[LT^{-1}]}{[T]} = [MLT^{-2}]$$

Hence the dimensions of force are 1 in mass 1 in length and (– 2) in time.

Dimensional Formula :

Unit of a physical quantity expressed in terms of M, L and T is called dimensional formula. It shows how and which of the fundamental quantities represent the dimensions.

For example, the dimensional formula of work is $[ML^2T^{-2}]$

Dimensional Equation :

When we equate the dimensional formula with the physical quantity, we get the dimensional equation.

For example Work = $[ML^2T^{-2}]$

Classification of Physical Quantities (On the basis of dimensions) :

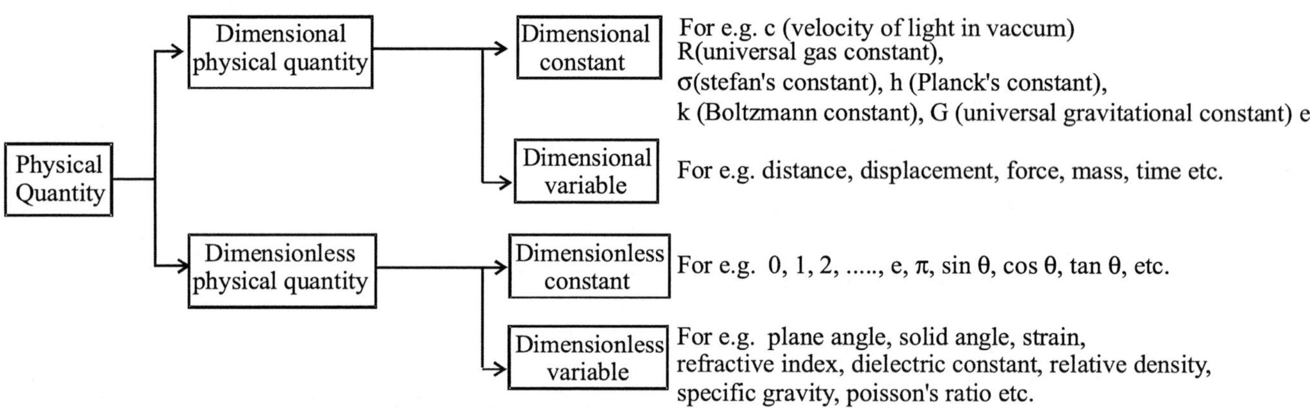

Dimensional Formula of Some Important Physical Quantities :

S.No.	*Physical quantity*	*Relation with other quantities*	*Dimensional formula*
1.	Velocity (v)	$\frac{\text{Length}}{\text{Time}}$	$[M^0LT^{-1}]$
2.	Acceleration (a)	$\frac{\text{Velocity}}{\text{Time}}$	$[M^0LT^{-2}]$
3.	Momentum (p)	Mass × velocity	$[MLT^{-1}]$
4.	Force (F)	Mass × acceleration	$[MLT^{-2}]$
5.	Work	Force × displacement	$[ML^2T^{-2}]$
6.	Power (P)	$\frac{\text{Work}}{\text{Time}}$	$[ML^2T^{-3}]$
7.	Universal gravitational constant	$G = \frac{Fr^2}{m_1 m_2}$	$[M^{-1}L^3T^{-2}]$
8.	Torque	$\vec{\tau} = \vec{r} \times \vec{F}$	$[ML^2T^{-2}]$
9.	Surface tension	$S = \frac{F}{\ell}$	$[MT^{-2}]$
10.	Gravitational potential	$V_G = \frac{W}{m}$	$[M^0L^2T^{-2}]$
11.	Coefficient of viscosity	$\eta = \frac{F}{A\frac{dv}{dx}}$	$[ML^{-1}T^{-1}]$
12.	Impulse	Force×time(F×t)	$[MLT^{-1}]$

13.	Strain	$\frac{\text{Change in length}}{\text{Original length}}\left(\frac{\Delta L}{L}\right)$	$[M^0L^0T^0]$
14.	Pressure gradient	$\frac{\text{Pressure}}{\text{Distance}}\left(\frac{P}{\ell}\right)$	$[ML^{-2}T^{-2}]$
15.	Plane angle	$\frac{\text{Arc}}{\text{Radius of circle}}\left(\frac{s}{r}\right)$	$[M^0L^0T^0]$
16.	Angular velocity	$\frac{\text{Angle}}{\text{Time}}\left(\frac{\theta}{t}\right)$	$[M^0L^0T^{-1}]$
17.	Radius of gyration	$\sqrt{\frac{\text{Moment of inertia of body}}{\text{Total mass of the body}}}\left(\sqrt{\frac{I}{\Sigma m_i}}\right)$	$[M^0L^1T^0]$
18.	Moment of force, moment of couple	Force × distance (F × s)	$[ML^2T^{-2}]$
19.	Angular frequency	2π×frequency (2πν)	$[M^0L^0T^{-1}]$
20.	Pressure	$\frac{\text{Force}}{\text{Area}}$	$[ML^{-1}T^{-2}]$
21.	Efficiency	$\frac{\text{Output work or energy}}{\text{Input work or energy}}\left(\frac{W}{Q}\right)$	$[M^0L^0T^0]$
22.	Angular impulse	forque×time (τ × t)	$[ML^2T^{-1}]$
23.	Planck's constant	$\frac{\text{Energy}}{\text{Frequency}}\left(\frac{E}{\nu}\right)$	$[ML^2T^{-1}]$
24.	Heat capacity, Entropy	$\frac{\text{Heat energy}}{\text{Temperature}}\left(\frac{Q}{T}\right)$	$[ML^2T^{-2}K^{-1}]$
25.	Specific heat capacity	$\frac{\text{Heat energy}}{\text{Mass} \times \text{temperature}}\left(\frac{Q}{m \times \Delta T}\right)$	$[M^0L^2T^{-2}K^{-1}]$
26.	Thermal conductivity, K	$\frac{\text{Heat energy} \times \text{thickness}}{\text{Area} \times \text{temperature} \times \text{time}}\left(\frac{Q}{t} = -KA\frac{\Delta T}{\Delta x}\right)$	$[MLT^{-3}K^{-1}]$
27.	Thermal Resistance, R	$\frac{\text{Length}}{\text{Thermal conductivity} \times \text{area}}$	$[M^{-1}L^{-2}T^3K]$
28.	Bulk modulus (B) or (compressibility)$^{-1}$	$\frac{\text{Volume} \times (\text{change in pressure})}{\text{Change in volume}}\left(-V\frac{\Delta P}{\Delta V}\right)$	$[ML^{-1}T^{-2}]$
29.	Stefan's constant (σ)	$\frac{(\text{Energy/area})}{\text{Time} \times (\text{temperature})^4}\left(\begin{matrix} Q = \sigma AtT^4 \\ E = Q/A.t = \sigma T^4 \end{matrix}\right)$	$[ML^0T^{-3}K^{-4}]$
30.	Universal gas constant R	$\frac{\text{Pressure} \times \text{volume}}{\text{Mole} \times \text{temperature}}\left(\frac{PV}{nT}\right)$	$[ML^2T^{-2}K^{-1}mol^{-1}]$
31.	Voltage, electric potential (V) or electromotive force (e)	$\frac{\text{Work}}{\text{Charge}}\left(\frac{W}{q}\right)$	$[ML^2T^{-3}A^{-1}]$

32.	Capacitance (C)	$\frac{\text{Charge}}{\text{Potential difference}}\left(\frac{q}{V}\right)$	$[M^{-1}L^{-2}T^4A^2]$
33.	Electric field $(\vec{E})$	$\frac{\text{Electric force}}{\text{Charge}}\left(\frac{F}{q}\right)$	$[MLT^{-3}A^{-1}]$
34.	Magnetic field($\vec{B}$), magnetic induction, magnetic flux density	$\frac{\text{Force}}{\text{Current}\times\text{length}}[F = I\ell B\sin\theta]$	$[ML^0T^{-2}A^{-1}]$
35.	Magnetic flux (ϕ_m)	$\phi = BA\cos\theta$	$[ML^2T^{-2}A^{-1}]$
36.	Inductance coefficient of self inductance (L) or coefficient of mutual inductance (M)	$\frac{\text{Magnetic flux}}{\text{Current}}\left(\frac{\phi_m}{I}\right)$	$[ML^2T^{-2}A^{-2}]$
37.	Magnetic field strength or magnetic moment density (I)	$\frac{\text{Magnetic moment}}{\text{Volume}}\left(\frac{M}{V}\right)$	$[M^0L^{-1}T^0A]$
38.	Permittivity constant in free space ε_o	$\frac{(\text{Charge})^2}{4\pi\times\text{electrostatic force(distance)}^2}\left(\frac{q^2}{4\pi\times F\times r^2}\right)$	$\left[M^{-1}L^{-3}T^4A^2\right]$
39.	Faraday constant (F), charge	Avagadro constant × elementry charge	$[M^0L^0TA\,mol^{-1}]$
40.	Mass defect, (Δm)	(Sum of masses of nucleons – mass of nucleus)$(M_P+M_N - M_{nucleus})$	$[ML^0T^0]$
41.	Resonant frequency (f_r)	$\frac{1}{T_r}$	$[M^0L^0T^{-1}]$
42.	Power of lens	$(\text{Focal length})^{-1}\left(\frac{1}{f}\right)$	$\left[M^0L^{-1}T^0\right]$
43.	Refractive index	$\frac{\text{Speed of light in vacuum}}{\text{Speed of light in medium}}$	$[M^0L^0T^0]$
44.	Wave number	$\frac{2\pi}{\text{Wavelength}}$	$\left[M^0L^{-1}T^0\right]$
45.	Binding energy of nucleus	Mass defect × (speed of light in vacuum)^2	$\left[ML^2T^{-2}\right]$
46.	Conductance (c)	$\frac{1}{\text{Resistance}}$	$\left[M^{-1}L^{-2}A^2T^3\right]$
47.	Fluid flow rate	$\left(\frac{\pi}{8}\right)\frac{(\text{Pressure})\times(\text{radius})^4}{(\text{Viscosity coefficient})\times(\text{length})}$	$\left[M^0L^3T^{-1}\right]$
48.	Inductive reactance	(Angular frequency × inductance)	$\left[ML^2T^{-3}A^{-2}\right]$
49.	Capacitive reactance	(Angular frequency × capacitance)$^{-1}$	$\left[ML^2T^{-3}A^{-2}\right]$
50.	Magnetic dipole moment	$\frac{\text{Torque}}{\text{Magnetic field}}$ or Current × area	$\left[M^0L^2T^0A\right]$

Short cuts / Time saving techniques

1. To find dimensions of a typical physical quantity which is involved in a number of formulae, try to use that formula which is easiest for you. For example if you want to find the dimensional formula of magnetic induction then you can use the following formulae

$$dB=\frac{\mu_0}{4\pi}\frac{Idl\sin\theta}{r^2},\quad B=\mu_0 nI,\ F=qvB,\ \tau=MB\sin\theta$$

Out of these the easiest is probably the third one.

2. If you have to find the dimensional formula of a combination of physical quantities, then instead of finding the dimensional formula of each, try to correlate the combination of physical quantities with a standard formula. For example, if you have to find the dimension of CV^2, then try to use formula $E=\frac{1}{2}CV^2$ where E is energy of a capacitor.

3. $\frac{1}{\sqrt{\mu_0\varepsilon_0}}=c=$ velocity of light in vacuum

- Dimensions of the following are same

$$\text{Work}=PV=nRT=qV=CV^2=\frac{q^2}{c}=\frac{V^2}{R}\times t=LI^2$$

$[ML^2T^{-2}]$

- Dimensions of the following are same
Force = Impulse / time
= q v B = q E
= Thrust
= weight = energy gradient $[MLT^{-2}]$

- The dimension of $RC=\frac{L}{R}$ is same as that of time

- Dimensions of the following are same

$$\text{velocity}=\sqrt{\frac{T}{\mu}}=\frac{1}{\sqrt{\mu_0\varepsilon_0}}=f\times\lambda \quad [M^{\circ}LT^{-1}]$$

- Dimensions of the following are same

$$\text{Frequency}=\frac{R}{L}=\sqrt{\frac{k}{m}}=\sqrt{\frac{MB}{I}}=\frac{1}{\sqrt{LC}}\ [M^{\circ}L^{\circ}T^{-1}]$$

- Dimensions of the following are same
(E) Modulus of elasticity = Y (Young's modulus)
= B (Bulk modulus)
= η (Modulus of rigidity)
= Stress

$$=\text{Pressure}=\frac{1}{\text{Compressibility}}$$

$[ML^{-1}T^{-2}]$

- Dimensions of the following are same
Acceleration, retardation, centripetal acceleration, centrifugal acceleration, gravitational intensity/strength. $[M^{\circ}LT^{-2}]$

- Dimensions of the following are same
Water equivalent, thermal capacity, entropy, Boltzmann's constant. $[ML^2T^{-2}K^{-1}]$

Problem Solving Tips

The dimensional formula of

- all trigonometric ratio is $[M^0L^0T^0]$
- x in e^x is $[M^0L^0T^0]$
- e^x is $[M^0L^0T^0]$
- x in log x is $[M^0L^0T^0]$
- log x is $[M^0L^0T^0]$

Example 1.

Find out the unit and dimensions of permittivity of free space.

Solution :

According to Coulomb's law

$$\varepsilon_0=\frac{[q^2]}{4\pi[F][r^2]}=\frac{[A^2T^2]}{[MLT^{-2}][L^2]}=[M^{-1}L^{-3}T^4A^2]$$

$$\text{Its unit}=\frac{\text{coulomb}^2}{\text{newton}\times\text{metre}^2}=\frac{(\text{coulomb})^2}{\text{joule}\times\text{metre}}=\frac{\text{coulomb}}{\text{volt}\times\text{metre}}$$

$CV^{-1}m^{-1}$

Example 2.

Find out the unit and dimensions of coefficient of self or mutual inductance of.

Solution :

$e=L\left(\frac{dI}{dt}\right)$ or $M\left(\frac{dI}{dt}\right)$, where e is induced electromotive force (e.m.f.)

$$\therefore L=e\left(\frac{dt}{dI}\right)=\frac{W}{q}\left(\frac{t}{I}\right)$$

or $$[L]=\frac{[ML^2T^{-2}][T]}{[AT][A]}=[ML^2T^{-2}A^{-2}]$$

Its unit is volt × sec/amp or ohm × sec or henry.

Example 3.

Find out the unit and dimensions of magnetic field intensity.

Solution :

As $B=\mu H$, hence $H=\frac{B}{\mu}=\frac{1}{4\pi}\frac{Id\ell\sin\theta}{r^2}$;

$$\therefore H=\frac{[A][L]}{[L^2]}=[M^{\circ}L^{-1}T^{\circ}A]$$

Its unit is ampere /metre in SI system. In c.g.s. system, the unit is oersted.

Example 4.

Find out the unit and dimensions of magnetic permeability of free space or medium.

Solution :

According to Biot-Savart's law

$$B=\frac{\mu_0}{4\pi}\frac{Idl\sin\theta}{r^2}\ \text{and}\ F=BI\,\ell\sin\theta$$

or $$\frac{F}{I\ell\sin\theta}=B=\frac{\mu_0 Id\ell\sin\theta}{4\pi r^2};$$

$\therefore \mu$ or $\mu_0 = \dfrac{Fr^2}{I^2\ell^2}$ (dimensionally)

Hence $[\mu]$ or $[\mu_0] = \dfrac{[MLT^{-2}][L^2]}{[A^2][L^2]} = [MLT^{-2}A^{-2}]$

Its units are

$$\frac{N-m^2}{amp^2-m^2} = \frac{newton}{amp^2} = \frac{joule/metre}{amp^2} = \frac{volt \times coulomb}{amp \times amp \times metre}$$

$$= \frac{ohm \times sec}{metre} = \frac{henry}{metre} = \frac{tesla \times metre}{amp.}$$

Example 5.

The dimensions of physical quantity X in the equation

Force $= \dfrac{X}{\text{Density}}$ *is given by*

(a) $[ML^4T^{-2}]$ (b) $[M^2L^{-2}T^{-1}]$
(c) $[M^2L^{-2}T^{-2}]$ (d) $[ML^{-2}T^{-1}]$

Solution :

(c) $\because$ Force $= \dfrac{X}{\text{denisty}}$

$\therefore$ X = Force × density

Hence X has dimensions

$$[MLT^{-2}]\frac{[M]}{[L^3]} = [M^2L^{-2}T^{-2}]$$

Example 6.

If force, acceleration and time are taken as fundamental quantities, then the dimensions of length will be-

(a) $[FT^2]$ (b) $[F^{-1}A^2T^{-1}]$
(c) $[FA^2T]$ (d) $[AT^2]$

Solution :

(d) $L = F^xA^yT^z$

$M^0L^1T^0 = [MLT^{-2}]^x[LT^{-2}]^yT^z$

$= M^xL^{x+y}T^{-2x-2y+z}$

$x = 0, x+y = 1, -2x-2y+z = 0$

$x = 0, y = 1, z = 2$

Hence, $L = AT^2$

DIMENSIONAL ANALYSIS AND ITS APPLICATIONS

Principle of Homogeneity :

Only those physical quantities can be added /subtracted/ equated /compared which have the same dimensions.

Uses of Dimensions :

(1) Conversion of one system of unit into another

Example : Convert a pressure of 10^6 dyne/cm² in S.I units.

Sol. We know that 1N = 10^5 dyne ⇒ 1 dyne = 10^{-5} N

Also 1m = 100 cm ⇒ 1cm = 10^{-2} m

Now, the pressure 10^6 dyne/cm² in SI unit is

$$10^6\frac{dyne}{cm \times cm} = 10^6 \times \frac{10^{-5}N}{10^{-2}m \times 10^{-2}m} = 10^5 N/m^2$$

(2) Checking the accuracy of various formulae

Example : Check the correctness of the following equation dimensionally

$F = \eta A\dfrac{dv}{dx}\sin\theta$ *where F = force, η = coefficient of viscosity, A = area, $\dfrac{dv}{dx}$ = velocity gradient w.r.t distance, θ = angle of contact*

Sol. L.H.S = force = $[MLT^{-2}]$

$$R.H.S = \eta A\frac{dv}{dx}(\sin\theta) = M^1L^{-1}T^{-1}L^2 \times \frac{LT^{-1}}{L} = \left[MLT^{-2}\right]$$

The equation is dimensionally correct.

⚠ **CAUTION :** Please note that the above equation is not correct numerically. The conclusion is that an equation, if correct dimensionally, may or may not be numerically correct. Also remember that if an equation is dimensionally incorrect, we can conclude with surety that the equation is incorrect.

(3) Derivation of formula

Example : The air bubble formed by explosion inside water performed oscillation with time period T which is directly proportional to $P^a\, d^b\, E^c$ where P is pressure, d is density and E is the energy due to explosion. Find the values of a, b and c.

Sol. Let us assume that the required expression for time period is $T = K\,P^a\,d^b\,E^c$

where K is a dimensionless constant.

Writing dimensions on both sides,

$$[M^0L^0T^1] = [ML^{-1}T^{-2}]^a[ML^{-3}]^b[ML^2T^{-2}]^c$$

$$= [M]^{a+b+c}[L]^{-a-3b+2c}[T]^{-2a-2c} = [T^1]$$

Equating the powers,

$a + b + c = 0$ ....(1)

$-a - 3b + 2c = 0$ ....(2)

$-2a - 2c = 1$ ....(3)

Solving these equations, we get,

$$a = -\frac{5}{6}, b = \frac{1}{2}, c = \frac{1}{3}.$$

Limitations of Dimensional Analysis :

(1) No information about the dimensionless constant is obtained during dimensional analysis
(2) Formula cannot be found if a physical quantity is dependent on more than three physical quantities.
(3) Formula containing trigonometrical /exponential function cannot be found.
(4) If an equation is dimensionally correct it may or may not be absolutely correct.

Example 7.

Find the dimensions of a and b in the Van der waal's equation $\left(P + \dfrac{a}{V^2}\right)(V - b) = RT$

where P is pressure and V is volume of gas.

Solution :

Dimensionally $P = \frac{a}{V^2}$ [By principle of homogeneity]

$\Rightarrow ML^{-1}T^{-2} = \frac{a}{V^2} \Rightarrow a = [ML^5T^{-2}]$

Also dimensionally V=b [By principle of homogeneity]

$\therefore \quad b = [L^3]$

Example 8.

The formula $v^2 = \frac{3mg\ell(1-\cos\theta)}{M(1+\sin^2\theta)}$ *is obtained as the solution of a problem. Use dimensions to find whether this is a reasonable solution (v is a velocity, m and M are masses,* ℓ *is a length and g is gravitational acceleration).*

Solution :

Dimensions of L.H.S. = $[LT^{-1}]^2 = [L^2T^{-2}]$

Dimensions of R.H.S. = $\frac{[M][LT^{-2}][L]}{[M]} = [L^2T^{-2}]$

Hence formula is reasonable.

Example 9.

In the formula; $N = -D\left[\frac{n_2 - n_1}{x_2 - x_1}\right]$,

D = diffusion coefficient, n_1 *and* n_2 *is number of molecules in unit volume along* x_1 *and* x_2 *which represents distances where N is number of molecules passing through per unit area per unit time calculate the dimensions of D.*

Solution :

By homogeneity theory of dimension

Dimension of (N)

$= \text{Dimension of D} \times \frac{\text{dimension of } (n_2 - n_1)}{\text{dimension of } (x_2 - x_1)}$

$\frac{1}{L^2T} = \text{Dimension of D} \times \frac{L^{-3}}{L}$

$\Rightarrow \text{Dimensions of 'D'} = \frac{L}{L^{-3} \times L^2T} = \frac{L^2}{T} = [L^2T^{-1}]$

Example 10.

Let us consider an equation $\frac{1}{2}mv^2 = mgh$ *where m is the mass of the body, v its velocity, g is the acceleration due to gravity and h is the height. Check whether this equation is dimensionally correct.*

Solution :

The dimensions of LHS are

$[M][LT^{-1}]^2 = [M][L^2T^{-2}] = [ML^2T^{-2}]$

The dimensions of RHS are

$[M][LT^{-2}][L] = [M][L^2T^{-2}] = [ML^2T^{-2}]$

The dimensions of LHS and RHS are the same and hence the equation is dimensionally correct.

Example 11.

A calorie is a unit of heat or energy and it equals about 4.2 J where $1J = 1\ kg\,m^2 s^{-2}$*. Suppose we employ a system of units in which the unit of mass equals* α *kg, the unit of length equals* β *m, the unit of time is* γ *s. Show that a calorie has a magnitude* $4.2\,\alpha^{-1}\beta^{-2}\gamma^2$ *in terms of the new units.*

Solution :

$1\ cal = 4.2\ kg\,m^2 s^{-2}$.

SI system	New system
$n_1 = 4.2$	$n_2 = ?$
$M_1 = 1$ kg	$M_2 = \alpha$ kg
$L_1 = 1$m	$L_2 = \beta$ metre
$T_1 = 1$s	$T_2 = \gamma$ second

Dimensional formula of energy is $[ML^2T^{-2}]$

Comparing with $[M^aL^bT^c]$, we find that

$a = 1, b = 2, c = -2$

Now, $n_2 = n_1\left[\frac{M_1}{M_2}\right]^a\left[\frac{L_1}{L_2}\right]^b\left[\frac{T_1}{T_2}\right]^c$

$= 4.2\left[\frac{1\ kg}{\alpha\ kg}\right]^1\left[\frac{1m}{\beta m}\right]^2\left[\frac{1s}{\gamma s}\right]^{-2}$

$= 4.2\,\alpha^{-1}\beta^{-2}\gamma^2$

2.1 Concept Practice Problems

CPP

1. Which of the following systems of units is not based on units of mass, length and time alone
   (a) SI (b) MKS
   (b) CGS (d) FPS
2. Unit of latent heat is
   (a) $J\,Kg^{-1}$ (b) $J\,mol^{-1}$
   (c) $N\,Kg^{-1}$ (d) $N\,mol^{-1}$
3. Dyne-sec is the unit of
   (a) momentum (b) force
   (c) work (d) angular momentum
4. Light year is
   (a) light emitted by the sun in one year.
   (b) time taken by light to travel from sun to earth.
   (c) the distance travelled by light in free space in one year.
   (d) time taken by earth to go once around the sun.
5. The SI unit of pressure is
   (a) atmosphere (b) bar
   (c) pascal (d) mm of Hg

6. The time of oscillation T of a small drop of liquid depends on radius r, density ρ and surface tension S. The relation between them is given by

(a) $T \propto \sqrt{\frac{S}{\rho r^3}}$ (b) $T \propto \sqrt{\frac{\rho r^3}{S}}$

(c) $T \propto \sqrt{\frac{S^2 r^3}{\rho}}$ (d) $T \propto \sqrt{\frac{\rho r^3}{S}}$

7. The potential energy of a particle varies with distance x from a fixed origin as $V = \frac{A\sqrt{x}}{x+B}$ where A and B are constants. The dimensions of AB are

(a) $[M^1 L^{5/2} T^{-2}]$ (b) $[M^1 L^2 T^{-2}]$

(c) $[M^{3/2} L^{5/2} T^{-2}]$ (d) $[M^1 L^{7/2} T^{-2}]$

8. Distance travelled by a particle at any instant 't' can be represented as $S = A(t+B) + Ct^2$. The dimensions of B are

(a) $[M^0 L^1 T^{-1}]$ (b) $[M^0 L^0 T^1]$

(c) $[M^0 L^{-1} T^{-2}]$ (d) $[M^0 L^2 T^{-2}]$

9. The deBroglie wavelength associated with a particle of mass m and energy E is $h/\sqrt{2mE}$. The dimensional formula of Planck's constant h is

(a) $[M^2 L^2 T^{-2}]$ (b) $[ML^2 T^{-1}]$

(c) $[MLT^{-2}]$ (d) $[ML^2 T^{-2}]$

10. The velocity of a body which falls under gravity varies as $g^a h^b$, where g is acc. due to gravity and h is the height. The values of a and b are

(a) a = 1, b = 1/2 (b) a = b = 1

(c) a = 1/2, b = 1 (d) a = 1/2; b = 1/2

11. The velocity v of a particle at time t is given by $v = at + \frac{b}{t+c}$

The dimensions of a, b c are respectively

(a) $[LT^{-2}]$, [L], [T] (b) $[L^2]$, [T] and $[LT^2]$

(c) $[LT^2]$, [LT] and [L] (d) [L], [LT] and $[T^2]$

12. The dimensions of $\frac{1}{\epsilon_0}\frac{e^2}{hc}$ are

(a) $M^{-1} L^{-3} T^4 A^2$ (b) $ML^3 T^{-4} A^{-2}$

(c) $M^0 L^0 T^0 A^0$ (d) $M^{-1} L^{-3} T^2 A$

13. The velocity of water waves (v) may depend on their wavelength λ, the density of water ρ and the acceleration due to gravity, g. The method of dimensions gives the relation between these quantities is

(a) v (b) $v^2 \propto g\lambda$

(c) $v^2 \propto g\lambda^2$ (d) $v^2 \propto g^{-1}\lambda^2$

14. If time T, acceleration A and force F are regarded as base units, then the dimensional formula of work is

(a) [FA] (b) [FAT]

(c) $[FAT^2]$ (d) $[FA^2T]$

15. Consider the following pairs of quantities

1. Young's modulus; pressure
2. Torque; energy
3. Linear momentum; work
4. Solar day; light year.

In which cases are the dimensions, within a pair, same?

(a) 1 and 3 (b) 1 and 4

(c) 1 and 2 (d) 2 and 4

ANSWER KEY

1	(a)	2	(a)	3	(a)	4	(c)	5	(c)	6	(b)	7	(d)	8	(b)	9	(b)	10	(d)
11	(a)	12	(c)	13	(b)	14	(c)	15	(c)										

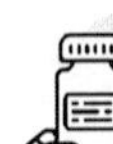

Topic 2.2 : Significant Figure, Rounding off, Accuracy & Precision and Errors in Measurements

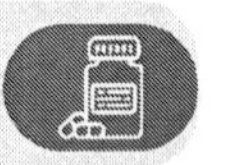

SIGNIFICANT FIGURES

The number of digits, which are known reliably in our measurement, and one digit that is uncertain are termed as significant figures.

Rules to determine the numbers of significant figures:

1. All non-zero digits are significant. 235.75 has five significant figures.
2. All zeroes between two non-zero digits are significant. 2016.008 has seven significant figures.
3. All zeroes occurring between the decimal point and the non-zero digits are not significant. provided there is only a zero to left of the decimal point. 0.00652 has three significant figures.
4. All zeroes written to the right of a non-zero digit in a number written without a decimal point are not significant. This rule does not work if zero is a result of measurement.

54000 has two significant figures whereas 54000m has five significant figures.

5. All zeroes occurring to the right of a non-zero digit in a number written with a decimal point are significant. 32.2000 has six significant figures.
6. When a number is written in the exponential form, the exponential term does not contribute towards the significant figures. 2.465×10^5 has four significant figures.

Problem Solving Tips

1. The significant figures depend upon the least count of the instrument.
2. The number of significant figure does not depend on the units chosen.

ROUNDING OFF

1. If digit to be dropped is less than 5 then preceding digit should be left unchanged.
2. If digit to be dropped is more than 5 then one should raise preceding digit by one.
3. If the digit to be dropped is 5 followed by a digit other than zero then the preceding digit is increased by one.
4. If the digit to be dropped is 5 then the preceding digit is not changed if it is even.
5. If digit to be dropped is 5 then the preceding digit is increased by one if it is odd.

Arithmetical Operations with Significant Figures and Rounding off :

(1) **For addition or subtraction**, write the numbers one below the other with all the decimal points in one line. Now locate the first column from the left that has a doubtful digit. All digits right to this column are dropped from all the numbers and rounding is done to this column. Addition subtraction is then done.

Example : Find the sum of 23.623 and 8.7 to correct significant figures.

Sol. **Step-1 :-** 23.623 + 8.7 **Step-2 :-** 23.6 + 8.7=32.3

(2) **In multiplication and division** of two or more quantities, the number of significant digits in the answer is equal to the number of significant digits in the quantity, which has minimum number of significant digits.

The insignificant digits are dropped from the result if they appear after the decimal point. They are replaced by zeroes if they appear to the left of the decimal point. The least significant digit is rounded off.

Example : 107.88 (5. S. F.)
$\times$ 0.610 (3 S. F.)
$= 65.8068 \cong 65.8$

ACCURACY, PRECISION OF INSTRUMENTS AND ERRORS IN MEASUREMENTS :

Accuracy and Precision are two terms that have very different meanings in experimental physics. We need to be able to distinguish between an accurate measurement and a precise measurement. *An **accurate** measurement is one in which the results of the experiment are in agreement with the 'accepted' value.* This only applies to experiments where this is the goal like measuring the speed of light.

*A **precise** measurement is one that we can make to a large number of decimal places.*

The following diagrams illustrate the meaning of terms accuracy and precision :

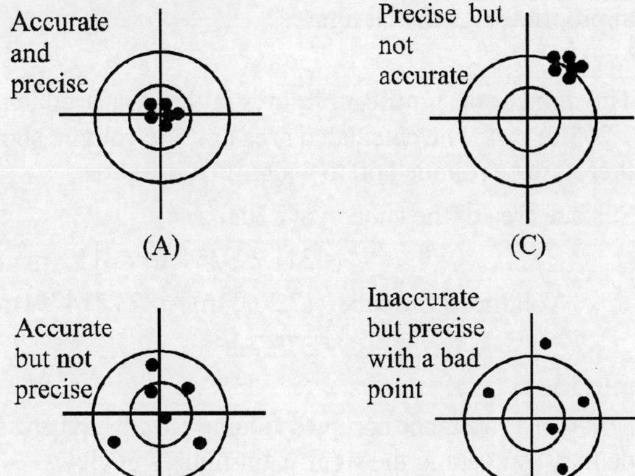

In the above figure : The centre of the target represents the accepted value. The closer to the centre, the more accurate the experiment. The extent of the scatter of the data is a measure of the precision.

A- Precise and accurate, B- Accurate but imprecise, C- Precise but not accurate, D- Not accurate nor precise

When successive measurements of the same quantity are repeated there are different values obtained. In experimental physics it is vital to be able to measure and quantify this uncertainty. (The words "error" and "uncertainty" are often used interchangeably by physicists - this is not ideal - but get used to it!)

***Error in measurements** is the difference of actual or true value and measured value.*

Error = True value – Measured value

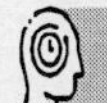

Problem Solving Tips

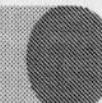

1. Accuracy depends on the least count of the instrument used for measurement.
2. In the addition and subtraction operation, the result contains the minimum number of decimal places of the figures being used
3. In the multiplication and division operation, the result contains the minimum number of significant figures.
4. Least count (L.C.) of vernier callipers = one MSD – one VSD where MSD = mains scale division
VSD = vernier scale division
5. Least count of screw gauge (or spherometer)
$$= \frac{\text{pitch}}{\text{no of divisions on circular scale}}$$
where pitch is the ratio of number of divisions moved on linear scale and number of rotations given to circular scale.
6. Pure number or unmeasured value do not have significant numbers

7. Change in the position of decimal does not change the number of significant figures.

   Similarly the change in the units of measured value does not change the significant figures.

Example 12.

Each side of a cube is measured to be 7.203 m. What are the total surface area and the volume of the cube to appropriate significant figures?

Solution :

The number of significant figures in the measured length 7.203 m is 4. The calculated area and the volume should therefore be rounded off to 4 significant figures.

Surface area of the cube $= 6(7.203)^2 \text{ m}^2$

$= 311.299254 \text{ m}^2 = 311.3 \text{ m}^2$

Volume of the cube $= (7.203)^3 \text{ m}^3 = 373.714754 \text{ m}^3$

$= 373.7 \text{ m}^3$

Example 13.

5.74 g of a substance occupies volume 1.2 cm^3. Express its density by keeping the significant figures in view.

Solution :

There are 3 significant figures in the measured mass whereas there are only 2 significant figures in the measured volume. Hence the density should be expressed to only 2 significant figures.

$$\text{Density} = \frac{\text{mass}}{\text{volume}} = \frac{5.74}{1.2} \text{gcm}^{-3} = 4.8 \text{ g cm}^{-3}.$$

Example 14.

The mass of a box measured by a grocer's balance is 2.300 kg. Two gold pieces of masses 20.15 g and 20.17 g are added to the box. What is (a) the total mass of the box, (b) the difference in the masses of the pieces to correct significant figures ?

Solution :

(a) Total mass = 2.3403 kg = 2.3 kg (upto 2 S. F.)

(b) Difference = 20.17 g – 20.15 g (upto 4 S. F.)

COMMON ERRORS IN MEASUREMENTS

It is not possible to measure the 100% correct value of any physical quantity, even after measuring it so many times. There always exists some uncertainty, which is usually referred to as experimental error.

Experimental errors :

(i) **Random error :** *It is the error that has an equal chance of being positive or negative.*

It occurs irregularly and at random in magnitude and direction. It can be caused

(a) by the lack of perfection of observer

(b) if the measuring instrument is not perfectly sensitive.

(ii) **Systematic error :** *It tends to occur in one direction either positive or negative.* It occurs due to

(a) measuring instrument having a zero error.

(b) an instrument being incorrectly calibrated (such as slow- running-stop clock)

(c) the observer persistently carrying out a mistimed action (e.g., in starting and stopping a clock)

For measuring a particular physical quantity, we take a number of readings. Let the readings be X_1, X_2............, X_n. Then the mean value is found as follows

$$X_{mean} (\text{or true value}) = \bar{X} = \frac{X_1 + X_2 + ... + X_n}{n}$$

Methods of Expressing Error:

Absolute error: *It is the difference between the mean value and the measured value of the physical quantity.*

$$|\Delta X_1| = |X_{mean} - X_1|$$

....

....

$$|\Delta X_n| = |X_{mean} - X_n|$$

Mean absolute error:

$$\Delta X_{mean} \text{ or } \overline{\Delta X} = \frac{|\Delta X_1| + |\Delta X_2| + ... + |\Delta X_n|}{n}$$

Relative error: *It is the ratio of the mean absolute error and the value of the quantity being measured.*

$$\text{Relative error } (\delta a) = \frac{\Delta X_{mean}}{X_{mean}}$$

Percentage error: *It is the relative error expressed in percent*

$$\text{Percentage error} = \frac{\overline{\Delta X}}{\bar{X}} \times 100\%$$

To find the maximum error in compound quantities we proceed as :

(i) **Sum and difference :** We have to find the sum or difference of two values given as $(a \pm \Delta a)$ and $(b \pm \Delta b)$, we do it as follows

$X \pm \Delta X = (a \pm \Delta a) + (b \pm \Delta b) = (a + b) \pm (\Delta a + \Delta b)$

$\Rightarrow X = a + b$ and $\Delta X = \Delta a + \Delta b$ in case of sum

And $X = (a - b)$ and $\Delta X = \Delta a + \Delta b$ in case of difference.

(ii) **Product and quotient :** We add the fractional or percentage errors in case of finding product or quotient.

If $P = ab$ then $\frac{\Delta P}{P} = \pm\left(\frac{\Delta a}{a} + \frac{\Delta b}{b}\right)$

If $Q = \frac{a}{b}$ then $\frac{\Delta Q}{Q} = \pm\left(\frac{\Delta a}{a} + \frac{\Delta b}{b}\right)$

(iii) **Power of a quantity :** If $x = a^n$ then $\frac{\Delta X}{X} = n\left(\frac{\Delta a}{a}\right)$

Example :

For $Q = \frac{x^2}{y}$, If $\frac{\Delta x}{x} \times 100 = 3\%$ and $\frac{\Delta y}{y} \times 100 = 4\%$

then $\frac{\Delta Q}{Q} \times 100 = (2 \times 3 + 4)\% = 10\%$

Similarly :

If $A = \frac{m^p n^q}{c^r}$ then $\frac{\Delta A}{A} = \pm\left[p\frac{\Delta m}{m} + q\frac{\Delta n}{n} + r\frac{\Delta c}{c}\right]$

Problem Solving Tips

1. More the accuracy, smaller is the error.
2. Absolute error $|\Delta X|$ is always positive.
3. $|\Delta X|$ has the same dimensions as that of X.
4. If the least count of measuring instrument is not given and the measured value is given the least error in the

measurement can be found by taking the last digit to be 1 and rest digit to be zero. For e.g. if the measured value of mass m = 2.03 kg then $\Delta m = \pm 0.01$ kg.

5. If a number of physical quantities are involved in an expression then the one with higher power contributes more in errors and therefore should be measured more accurately.
6. Relative error is a dimensionless quantity.
7. We are always interested in calculating the maximum possible error.

Example 15.

In an experiment, the refractive index of water was observed as 1.29, 1.33, 1.34, 1.35, 1.32, 1.36, 1.30 and 1.33. Calculate the mean value, mean absolute error and percentage error in the measurement.

Solution :

Mean value of refractive index,

$$\bar{\mu} = \frac{1.29 + 1.33 + 1.34 + 1.35 + 1.32 + 1.36 + 1.30 + 1.33}{8}$$

$= 1.33$

Absolute error in measurement,

$\Delta\mu_1 = 1.33 - 1.29 = +0.04$, $\Delta\mu_2 = 1.33 - 1.33 = 0.00$,

$\Delta\mu_3 = 1.33 - 1.34 = -0.01$, $\Delta\mu_4 = 1.33 - 1.35 = -0.02$,

$\Delta\mu_5 = 1.33 - 1.32 = +0.01$, $\Delta\mu_6 = 1.33 - 1.36 = -0.03$,

$\Delta\mu_7 = 1.33 - 1.30 = +0.03$, $\Delta\mu_8 = 1.33 - 1.33 = 0.00$

So, mean absolute error,

$$\overline{(\Delta\mu)} = \frac{|0.04| + |0.01| + |0.02| + |0.01| + |0.03| + |0.03| + |0|}{8}$$

$= 0.0175 \approx 0.02$

$$\text{Relative error} = \pm\frac{\overline{\Delta\mu}}{\bar{\mu}} = +\frac{0.02}{1.33} = \pm 0.015 = \pm 0.02$$

$$\text{Percentage error} = \pm\frac{0.02}{1.33} \times 100\% = \pm 1.5\%$$

Example 16.

The length and breadth of a rectangle are (5.7 ± 0.1) cm and (3.4 ± 0.2) cm. Calculate area of the rectangle with error limits.

Solution :

Here, $\ell = (5.7 \pm 0.1)$ cm, $b = (3.4 \pm 0.2)$ cm

Area $A = \ell \times b$

$= 5.7 \times 3.4 = 19.38\ \text{cm}^2$

$= 19.0\ \text{cm}^2$ (Rounding off to two significant figures)

$$\frac{DA}{A} = \pm\left(\frac{\Delta\ell}{\ell} + \frac{\Delta b}{b}\right) = \pm\left(\frac{0.1}{5.7} + \frac{0.2}{3.4}\right)$$

$$= \pm\left(\frac{0.34 + 1.14}{5.7 \times 3.4}\right)$$

$$\frac{DA}{A} = \pm\frac{1.48}{19.38} \Rightarrow \Delta A = \pm\frac{1.48}{19.38} \times A$$

$$= \pm\frac{1.48}{19.38} \times 19.38 = \pm 1.48$$

$\Delta A = \pm 1.5$ (Rounding off to two significant figures)

$\therefore$ Area = (19.0 ± 1.5) sq.cm.

Example 17.

A body travels uniformly a distance of (13.8 ± 0.2) m in a time (4.0 ± 0.3) s. Calculate its velocity with error limits. What is percentage error in velocity?

Solution :

Here, $s = (13.8 \pm 0.2)$ m, $t = (4.0 \pm 0.3)$ s

$$\text{velocity,} \quad v = \frac{s}{t} = \frac{13.8}{4.0} = 3.45\ \text{ms}^{-1} = 3.5\ \text{ms}^{-1}$$

(rounding off to two significant figures)

$$\frac{\Delta v}{v} = \pm\left(\frac{\Delta s}{s} + \frac{\Delta t}{t}\right) = \pm\left(\frac{0.2}{13.8} + \frac{0.3}{4.0}\right) = \pm\frac{(0.8 + 4.14)}{13.8 \times 4.0}$$

$$\Rightarrow \frac{\Delta v}{v} = \pm\frac{4.94}{13.8 \times 4.0} = \pm 0.0895$$

$\Delta v = \pm 0.0895 \times v = \pm 0.0895 \times 3.45 = \pm 0.3087 = \pm 0.31$

(Rounding off to two significant fig.)

Hence, $v = (3.5 \pm 0.31)\ \text{ms}^{-1}$

% age error in velocity

$$= \frac{\Delta v}{v} \times 100 = \pm 0.0895 \times 100 = \pm 8.95\% = \pm 9\%$$

Example 18.

Two resistances are expressed as $R_1 = (4 \pm 0.5)\ \Omega$ and $R_2 = (12 \pm 0.5)\ \Omega$. What is the net resistance when they are connected (i) in series and (ii) in parallel, with percentage error ?

(a) $16\Omega \pm 23\%, 3\Omega \pm 6.25\%$ (b) $3\Omega \pm 2.3\%, 3\Omega \pm 6.25\%$

(c) $3\Omega \pm 23\%, 16\Omega \pm 6.25\%$ (d) $16\Omega \pm 6.25\%, 3\Omega \pm 23\%$

Solution :

(d) $R_S = R_1 + R_2 = 16\,\Omega$;

$$R_P = \frac{R_1 R_2}{R_1 + R_2} = \frac{R_1 R_2}{R_S} = 3\,\Omega$$

$$\Delta R_S = \Delta R_1 + \Delta R_2 = 1\,\Omega$$

$$\Rightarrow \frac{\Delta R_S}{R_S} \times 100 = \frac{1}{16} \times 100\% = 6.25\%$$

$$\Rightarrow R_S = 16\Omega \pm 6.25\%$$

$$\text{Similarly,} \quad R_P = \frac{R_1 R_2}{R_S}$$

$$\frac{\Delta R_P}{R_P} = \frac{\Delta R_1}{R_1} + \frac{\Delta R_2}{R_2} + \frac{\Delta R_S}{R_S}$$

$$\Rightarrow \frac{\Delta R_P}{R_P} = \frac{0.5}{4} + \frac{0.5}{12} + \frac{1}{16} = 0.23$$

$$\Rightarrow \frac{\Delta R_P}{R_P} \times 100 = 23\% \Rightarrow R_P = 3\Omega \pm 23\%$$

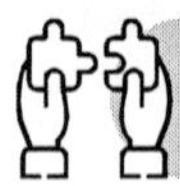

2.2 Concept Practice Problems

CPP

16. If $f = x^2$, then the relative error in f is

(a) $\frac{2\Delta x}{x}$ (b) $\frac{(\Delta x)^2}{x}$

(c) $\frac{\Delta x}{x}$ (d) $(\Delta x)^2$

17. Subtract 0.2 J from 7.26 J and express the result with correct number of significant figures.

(a) 7.1 J (b) 7.06 J

(c) 7.0 J (d) 7 J

18. Multiply 107.88 by 0.610 and express the result with correct number of significant figures.

(a) 65.8068 (b) 65.807

(c) 65.81 (d) 65.8

19. When 97.52 is divided by 2.54, the correct result is

(a) 38.3937 (b) 38.394

(c) 38.39 (d) 38.4

20. Relative density of a metal may be found with the help of spring balance. In air the spring balance reads (5.00 ± 0.05) N and in water it reads (4.00 ± 0.05) N. Relative density would be

(a) (5.00 ± 0.05)N (b) $(5.00 \pm 11\%)$

(c) (5.00 ± 0.10) (d) $(5.00 \pm 6\%)$

21. Area of a square is $(100 \pm 2)\ m^2$. Its side is

(a) (10 ± 1)m (b) (10 ± 0.1)m

(c) $(10 \pm \sqrt{2})$m (d) $10 \pm \sqrt{2}\%$

22. The least count of a stop watch is 0.2 second. The time of 20 oscillations of a pendulum is measured to be 25 second. The percentage error in the measurement of time will be

(a) 8% (b) 1.8%

(c) 0.8% (d) 0.1%

23. Which of the following is the most accurate?

(a) 200.0m (b) 20×10^1 m

(c) 2×10^2 m (d) data is inadequate

24. A quantity is represented by $X = M^a L^b T^c$. The % error in measurement of M, L and T are $\alpha\%$, $\beta\%$ and $\gamma\%$ respectively. The % error in X would be

(a) $(\alpha a + \beta b + \gamma c)\%$ (b) $(\alpha a - \beta b + \gamma c)\%$

(c) $(\alpha a - \beta b - \gamma c) \times 100\%$ (d) None of these

25. What is the fractional error in g calculated from $T = 2\pi\sqrt{\ell / g}$? Given fraction errors in T and l are $\pm$ x and $\pm$ y respectively.

(a) x + y (b) x − y

(c) 2x + y (d) 2x − y

26. The percentage errors in the measurement of mass and speed are 2% and 3% respectively. The error, in kinetic energy obtained by measuring mass and speed, will be

(a) 12% (b) 10%

(c) 8% (d) 2%

27. In a simple pendulum experiment for the determination of acceleration due to gravity, time period is measured with an accuracy of 0.2% while length was measured with an accuracy of 0.5%. The percentage accuracy in the value of g so obtained is

(a) 0.25% (b) 0.7%

(c) 0.9% (d) 1.0%

28. The dimensions of a rectangular block measured with callipers having least count of 0.01 cm are 5 mm × 10 mm × 5 mm. The maximum percentage error in the measurement of the volume of the block is

(a) 5% (b) 10%

(c) 15% (d) 20%

29. In an experiment four quantities a, b, c and d are measured with percentage error 1%, 2%, 3% and 4% respectively. Quantity P is calculated as follows

$$P = \frac{a^3 b^2}{cd}$$

% error in P is

(a) 10% (b) 7%

(c) 4% (d) 14%

30. The resistance R of a wire is given by the relation $R = \frac{\rho \ell}{\pi r^2}$. Percentage error in the measurement of ρ, ℓ and r is 1%, 2% and 3% respectively. Then the percentage error in the measurement of R is :

(a) 6 (b) 9

(c) 8 (d) 10

ANSWER KEY																			
16	(a)	17	(a)	18	(d)	19	(d)	20	(d)	21	(a)	22	(c)	23	(a)	24	(a)	25	(c)
26	(c)	27	(c)	28	(a)	29	(d)	30	(b)										

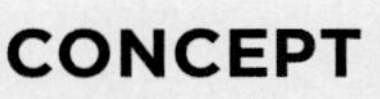

CONCEPT MAP

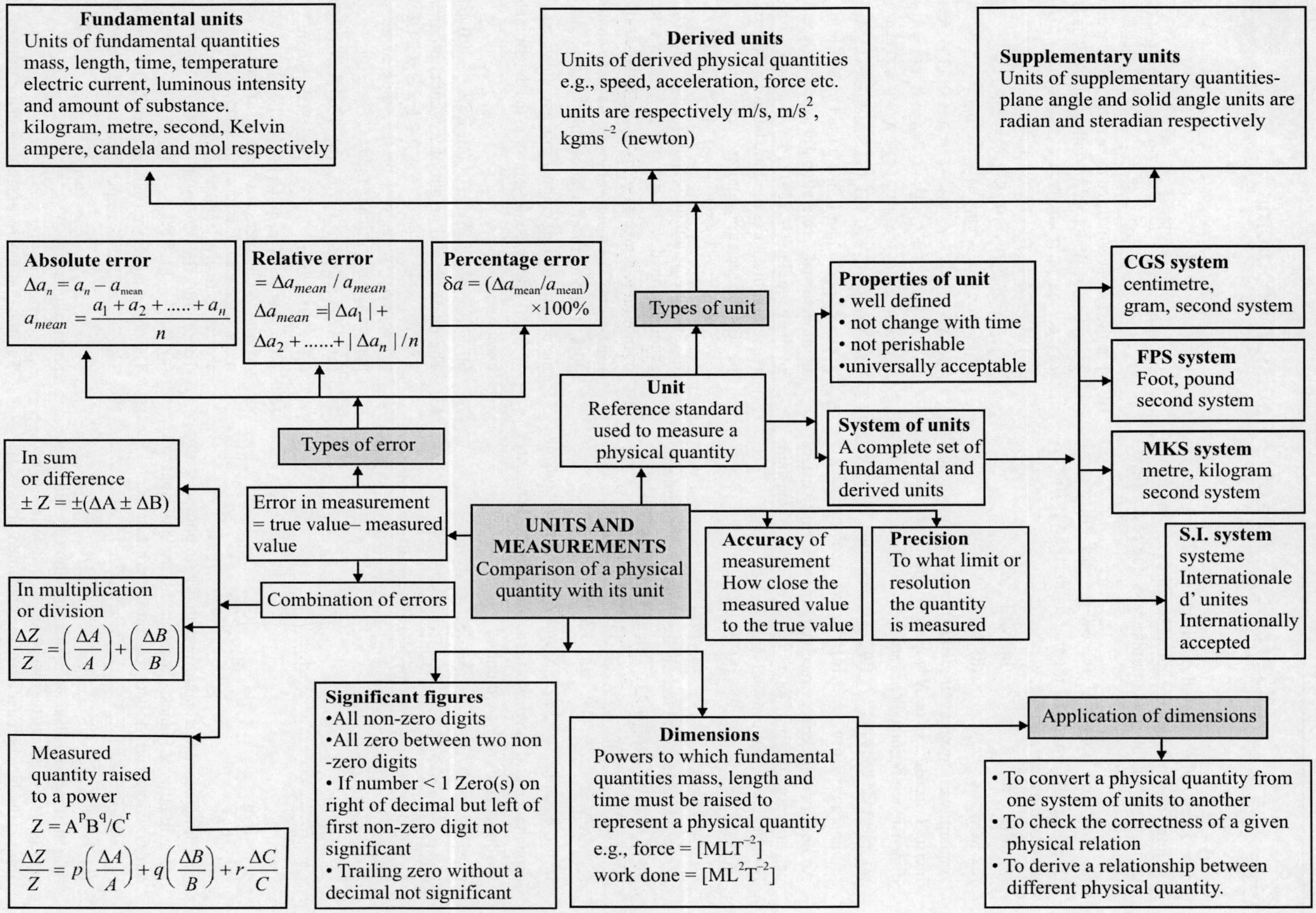

UNITS AND MEASUREMENTS
Comparison of a physical quantity with its unit

Unit
Reference standard used to measure a physical quantity

Types of unit

Fundamental units
Units of fundamental quantities mass, length, time, temperature electric current, luminous intensity and amount of substance.
kilogram, metre, second, Kelvin ampere, candela and mol respectively

Derived units
Units of derived physical quantities e.g., speed, acceleration, force etc.
units are respectively m/s, m/s^2, $kgms^{-2}$ (newton)

Supplementary units
Units of supplementary quantities-plane angle and solid angle units are radian and steradian respectively

Properties of unit
- well defined
- not change with time
- not perishable
- universally acceptable

System of units
A complete set of fundamental and derived units

CGS system
centimetre, gram, second system

FPS system
Foot, pound second system

MKS system
metre, kilogram second system

S.I. system
systeme Internationale d' unites
Internationally accepted

Accuracy of measurement
How close the measured value to the true value

Precision
To what limit or resolution the quantity is measured

Error in measurement
= true value– measured value

Types of error

Absolute error
$\Delta a_n = a_n - a_{\text{mean}}$
$a_{mean} = \dfrac{a_1 + a_2 + ... + a_n}{n}$

Relative error
$= \Delta a_{mean} / a_{mean}$
$\Delta a_{mean} = |\Delta a_1| + |\Delta a_2| + ...+ |\Delta a_n| / n$

Percentage error
$\delta a = (\Delta a_{\text{mean}}/a_{\text{mean}}) \times 100\%$

Combination of errors

In sum or difference
$\pm Z = \pm(\Delta A \pm \Delta B)$

In multiplication or division
$\dfrac{\Delta Z}{Z} = \left(\dfrac{\Delta A}{A}\right) + \left(\dfrac{\Delta B}{B}\right)$

Measured quantity raised to a power
$Z = A^p B^q / C^r$
$\dfrac{\Delta Z}{Z} = p\left(\dfrac{\Delta A}{A}\right) + q\left(\dfrac{\Delta B}{B}\right) + r\dfrac{\Delta C}{C}$

Significant figures
- All non-zero digits
- All zero between two non-zero digits
- If number < 1 Zero(s) on right of decimal but left of first non-zero digit not significant
- Trailing zero without a decimal not significant

Dimensions
Powers to which fundamental quantities mass, length and time must be raised to represent a physical quantity
e.g., force = $[MLT^{-2}]$
work done = $[ML^2T^{-2}]$

Application of dimensions
- To convert a physical quantity from one system of units to another
- To check the correctness of a given physical relation
- To derive a relationship between different physical quantity.

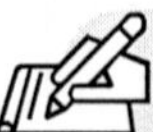

Exercise 1 - Chapter Revision Problems

CRP

1. The density of a material in SI unit is 128 kg m^{-3}. In certain units in which the unit of length is 25 cm and the unit of mass is 50 g, the numerical value of density of the material is:
   (a) 40 (b) 16 (c) 640 (d) 410
2. Dimensional formula for thermal conductivity is (here K denotes the temperature :
   (a) $MLT^{-2}K$ (b) $MLT^{-2}K^{-2}$
   (c) $MLT^{-3}K$ (d) $MLT^{-3}K^{-1}$
3. A quantity x is given by (IFv^2/WL^4) in terms of moment of inertia I, force F, velocity v, work W and Length L. The dimensional formula for x is same as that of :
   (a) planck's constant (b) force constant
   (c) energy density (d) coefficient of viscosity
4. Amount of solar energy received on the earth's surface per unit area per unit time is defined a solar constant. Dimension of solar constant is :
   (a) ML^2T^{-2} (b) ML^0T^{-3}
   (c) $M^2L^0T^{-1}$ (d) MLT^{-2}
5. If speed V, area A and force F are chosen as fundamental units, then the dimension of Young's modulus will be :
   (a) FA^2V^{-1} (b) FA^2V^{-3}
   (c) FA^2V^{-2} (d) $FA^{-1}V^0$
6. In the formula $X = 5YZ^2$, X and Z have dimensions of capacitance and magnetic field, respectively. What are the dimensions of Y in SI units ?
   (a) $[M^{-3}L^{-2}T^8A^4]$ (b) $[M^{-1}L^{-2}T^4A^2]$
   (c) $[M^{-2}L^0T^{-4}A^{-2}]$ (d) $[M^{-2}L^{-2}T^6A^3]$
7. Expression for time in terms of G (universal gravitational constant), h (Planck's constant) and c (speed of light) is proportional to:
   (a) $\sqrt{\frac{hc^5}{G}}$ (b) $\sqrt{\frac{c^3}{Gh}}$
   (c) $\sqrt{\frac{Gh}{c^5}}$ (d) $\sqrt{\frac{Gh}{c^3}}$
8. The dimensions of stopping potential V_0 in photoelectric effect in units of Planck's constant 'h', speed of light 'c' and Gravitational constant 'G' and ampere A is:
   (a) $h^{1/3}G^{2/3}c^{1/3}A^{-1}$ (b) $h^{2/3}c^{5/3}G^{1/3}A^{-1}$
   (c) $h^{-2/3}e^{-1/3}G^{4/3}A^{-1}$ (d) $h^2G^{3/2}C^{1/3}A^{-1}$
9. The characteristic distance at which quantum gravitational effects are significant, the Planck length, can be determined from a suitable combination of the fundamental physical constants G, h and c. Which of the following correctly gives the Planck length?
   (a) G^2hc (b) $\left(\frac{Gh}{c^3}\right)^{\frac{1}{2}}$ (c) $G^{\frac{1}{2}}h^2c$ (d) Gh^2c^3
10. For the four sets of three measured physical quantities as given below. Which of the following options is correct?
    (A) $A_1 = 24.36, B_1 = 0.0724, C_1 = 256.2$
    (B) $A_2 = 24.44, B_2 = 16.082, C_2 = 240.2$
    (C) $A_3 = 25.2, B_3 = 19.2812, C_3 = 236.183$
    (D) $A_4 = 25, B_4 = 236.191, C_4 = 19.5$
    (a) $A_4+B_4+C_4 < A_1+B_1+C_1 < A_3+B_3+C_3 < A_2+B_2+C_2$
    (b) $A_1+B_1+C_1 = A_2+B_2+C_2 = A_3+B_3+C_3 = A_4+B_4+C_4$
    (c) $A_4+B_4+C_4 < A_1+B_1+C_1 = A_2+B_2+C_2 = A_3+B_3+C_3$
    (d) $A_1+B_1+C_1 < A_3+B_3+C_3 < A_2+B_2+C_2 < A_4+B_4+C_4$
11. A simple pendulum is being used to determine the value of gravitational acceleration g at a certain place. The length of the pendulum is 25.0 cm and a stop watch with 1 s resolution measures the time taken for 40 oscillations to be 50 s. The accuracy in g is:
    (a) 5.40% (b) 3.40% (c) 4.40% (d) 2.40%
12. In a simple pendulum experiment for determination of acceleration due to gravity (g), time taken for 20 oscillations is measured by using a watch of 1 second least count. The mean value of time taken comes out to be 30 s. The length of pendulum is measured by using a meter scale of least count 1 mm and the value obtained is 55.0 cm. The percentage error in the determination of g is close to :
    (a) 0.7% (b) 0.2% (c) 3.5% (d) 6.8%
13. The diameter and height of a cylinder are measured by a meter scale to be 12.6 ± 0.1 cm and 34.2 ± 0.1 cm, respectively. What will be the value of its volume in appropriate significant figures?
    (a) $4264 \pm 81\ cm^3$ (b) $4264.4 \pm 81.0\ cm^3$
    (c) $4260 \pm 80\ cm^3$ (d) $4300 \pm 80\ cm^3$
14. The density of a material in the shape of a cube is determined by measuring three sides of the cube and its mass. If the relative errors in measuring the mass and length are respectively 1.5% and 1%, the maximum error in determining the density is:
    (a) 2.5% (b) 3.5% (c) 4.5% (d) 6%
15. The percentage errors in quantities P, Q, R and S are 0.5%, 1%, 3% and 1.5% respectively in the measurement of a physical quantity $A = \frac{P^3Q^2}{\sqrt{RS}}$.
    The maximum percentage error in the value of A will be
    (a) 8.5% (b) 6.0%
    (c) 7.5% (d) 6.5%

16. Temperature can be expressed as derived quantity in terms of
(a) length and mass
(b) mass and time
(c) length, mass and time
(d) None of these

17. What is the unit of "a" in Vander Waal's gas equation?
(a) Atm $litre^{-2}$ mol^2 (b) Atm $litre^2$ per mol
(c) Atm $litre^{-1}$ mol^2 (d) Atm $litre^2$ mol^{-2}

18. Random error can be eliminated by
(a) careful observation
(b) eliminating the cause
(c) measuring the quantity with more than one instrument
(d) taking large number of observations and then their mean.

19. If e is the charge, V the potential difference, T the temperature, then the units of $\frac{eV}{T}$ are the same as that of
(a) Planck's constant (b) Stefan's constant
(c) Boltzmann constant (d) gravitational constant

20. Two quantities A and B have different dimensions which mathematical operation given below is physically meaningful?
(a) A/B (b) A+B
(c) A–B (d) A=B

21. Electron volt is a unit of
(a) potential difference (b) charge
(c) energy (d) capacity

22. Dimensions of impulse are
(a) $[MLT^{-1}]$ (b) $[MLT^2]$
(c) $[MT^{-2}]$ (d) $[ML^{-1}T^{-3}]$

23. Potential is measured in
(a) joule/coulomb (b) watt/coulomb
(c) newton-second (d) None of these

24. Maxwell is the unit of
(a) magnetic susceptibility
(b) intensity of Magnetisation
(c) magnetic Flux
(d) magnetic Permeability

25. The mass of the liquid flowing per second per unit area of cross-section of the tube is proportional to (pressure difference across the ends)^n and (average velocity of the liquid)^m. Which of the following relations between m and n is correct?
(a) m = n (b) m = – n
(c) $m^2 = n$ (d) $m = -n^2$

26. Which of the following is a derived physical quantity?
(a) Mass (b) Velocity
(c) Length (d) Time

27. What are the units of magnetic permeability?
(a) $Wb\,A^{-1}\,m^{-1}$ (b) $Wb^{-1}\,Am$
(c) $Wb\,A\,m^{-1}$ (d) $Wb\,A^{-1}\,m$

28. The dimensions of pressure gradient are
(a) $[ML^{-2}T^{-2}]$ (b) $[ML^{-2}T^{-1}]$
(c) $[ML^{-1}T^{-1}]$ (d) $[ML^{-1}T^{-2}]$

29. The dimensions of Rydberg's constant are
(a) $[M^0L^{-1}T]$ (b) $[MLT^{-1}]$
(c) $[M^0L^{-1}T^0]$ (d) $[ML^0T^2]$

30. The dimensions of universal gas constant are
(a) $[L^2M^1T^{-2}K^{-1}]$ (b) $[L^1M^2T^{-2}K^{-1}]$
(c) $[L^1M^1T^{-2}K^{-1}]$ (d) $[L^2M^2T^{-2}K^{-1}]$

31. The dimensions of magnetic moment are
(a) $[L^2A^1]$ (b) $[L^2A^{-1}]$
(c) $[L^2/A^3]$ (d) $[LA^2]$

32. The dimensions of Wien's constant are
(a) $[ML^0TK]$ (b) $[M^0LT^0K]$
(c) $[M^0L^0TK]$ (d) [MLTK]

33. If L denotes the inductance of an inductor through which a current i is flowing, the dimensions of $L\,i^2$ are
(a) $[ML^2T^{-2}]$
(b) $[MLT^{-2}]$
(c) $[M^2L^2T^{-2}]$
(d) Not expressible in M, L, T

34. The dimensional formula of wave number is
(a) $[M^0L^0T^{-1}]$ (b) $[M^0L^{-1}T^0]$
(c) $[M^{-1}L^{-1}T^0]$ (d) $[M^0L^0T^0]$

35. The period of a body under S.H.M. is represented by: $T = P^a D^b S^c$ where P is pressure, D is density and S is surface tension, then values of a, b and c are
(a) $-\frac{3}{2}, \frac{1}{2}, 1$ (b) –1, – 2, 3
(c) $\frac{1}{2}, -\frac{3}{2}, -\frac{1}{2}$ (d) 1, 2 1/3

36. The dimensions of Hubble's constant are
(a) $[T^{-1}]$ (b) $[M^0L^0T^{-2}]$
(c) $[MLT^4]$ (d) $[MT^{-1}]$

37. Error in the measurement of radius of a sphere is 1%. Then error in the measurement of volume is
(a) 1% (b) 5% (c) 3% (d) 8%

38. If L and R denote inductance and resistance then dimension of L/R is
(a) $[M^0L^0T^0]$ (b) $[M^0L^0T]$
(c) $[M^2L^0T^2]$ (d) $[MLT^2]$

39. The dimensional formula for relative density is
(a) $[ML^{-3}]$ (b) $[M^0L^{-3}]$
(c) $[M^0L^0T^{-1}]$ (d) $[M^0L^0T^0]$

40. The solid angle sustended by the total surface area of a sphere, at the centre is
(a) 4π (b) 2π (c) π (d) 3π

41. The dimensions of solar constant is
(a) $[M^0L^0T^0]$ (b) $[MLT^{-2}]$
(c) $[ML^2T^{-2}]$ (d) MT^{-3}

42. The dimensional formula for entropy is
(a) $[MLT^{-2}K^1]$ (b) $[ML^2T^{-2}]$
(c) $[ML^2T^{-2}K^{-1}]$ (d) $[ML^2T^{-2}K]$

43. Dimensions of specific heat are
(a) $[ML^2T^{-2}K]$ (b) $[ML^2T^{-2}K^{-1}]$
(c) $[ML^2T^2K^{-1}]$ (d) $[L^2T^{-2}K^{-1}]$

44. L, C, R represent physical quantities inductance, capacitance and resistance respectively. The combinations which have the dimensions of frequency are

(a) 1/RC (b) R/L (c) $1/\sqrt{LC}$ (d) C/L

45. The physical quantity which has the dimensional formula $[M^1T^{-3}]$ is

(a) surface tension (b) solar constant
(c) density (d) compressibility

46. In the eqn. $\left(P+\frac{a}{V^2}\right)(V-b)=\text{constant}$, the unit of a is

(a) dyne × cm^5 (b) dyne × cm^4
(c) dyne/cm^3 (d) dyne × cm^2

47. Dimensions of 'ohm' are same as (where h is Planck's constant and e is charge)

(a) $\frac{h}{e}$ (b) $\frac{h^2}{e}$ (c) $\frac{h}{e^2}$ (d) $\frac{h^2}{e^2}$

48. The Richardson equation is given by $I = AT^2e^{-B/kT}$. The dimensional formula for AB^2 is same as that for

(a) IT^2 (b) kT (c) Ik^2 (d) Ik^2/T

49. The unit of current in C.G.S. system is

(a) 10 A (b) 1/10 A (c) 1/100 A (d) 1/1000 A

50. Which of the following do not have the same dimensional formula as the velocity?
Given that μ_0 = permeability of free space, ε_0 = permittivity of free space, ν = frequency, λ = wavelength, P = pressure, ρ = density, ω = angular frequency, k = wave number,

(a) $1/\sqrt{\mu_0\varepsilon_o}$ (b) νλ
(c) $\sqrt{P/\rho}$ (d) ωk

51. A spherical body of mass m and radius r is allowed to fall in a medium of viscosity η. The time in which the velocity of the body increases from zero to 0.63 times the terminal velocity (v) is called time constant τ. Dimensionally τ can be represented by

(a) $\frac{mr^2}{6\pi\eta}$ (b) $\sqrt{\left(\frac{6\pi m r\eta}{g^2}\right)}$

(c) $\frac{m}{6\pi\eta r v}$ (d) None of these

52. In a Vernier calliper, N divisions of vernier scale coincide with (N–1) divisions of main scale (in which one division represents 1 mm). the least count of the instrument in cm. should be

(a) N (b) N – 1

(c) $\frac{1}{10N}$ (d) $\frac{1}{N-1}$

53. Conversion of 1 MW power in a New system of units having basic units of mass, length and time as 10 kg, 1 dm and 1 minute respectively is

(a) 2.16×10^{10} unit (b) 2×10^4 unit
(c) 2.16×10^{12} unit (d) 1.26×10^{12} unit

54. Using mass (M), length(L), time (T) and electric current (A) as fundamental quantities the dimensions of permittivity will be

(a) $[MLT^{-1}A^{-1}]$ (b) $[MLT^{-2}A^{-2}]$
(c) $[M^{-1}L^{-3}T^{+4}A^2]$ (d) $[M^2L^{-2}T^{-2}A^2]$

55. The density of a cube is measured by measuring its mass and length of its sides. If the maximum error in the measurement of mass and length are 4% and 3% respectively, the maximum error in the measurement of density will be

(a) 7% (b) 9% (c) 12% (d) 13%

56. Specific gravity has .... dimensions in mass, ... dimensions in length and .... dimensions in time.

(a) 0, 0, 0 (b) 0, 1, 0 (c) 1, 0, 0 (d) 1, 1, 3

57. If I is the moment of inertia and ω the angular velocity, what is the dimensional formula of rotational kinetic energy $\frac{1}{2}I\omega^2$?

(a) $[ML^2T^{-1}]$ (b) $[M^2L^{-1}T^{-2}]$
(c) $[ML^2T^{-2}]$ (d) $[M^2L^{-1}T^{-2}]$

58. The thrust developed by a rocket-motor is given by $F = mv + A(P_1 - P_2)$ where m is the mass of the gas ejected per unit time, v is velocity of the gas, A is area of cross-section of the nozzle, P_1 and P_2 are the pressures of the exhaust gas and surrounding atmosphere. The formula is dimensionally

(a) correct
(b) wrong
(c) sometimes wrong, sometimes correct
(d) Data is not adequate

59. In a vernier callipers, ten smallest divisions of the vernier scale are equal to nine smallest division on the main scale. If the smallest division on the main scale is half millimeter, then the vernier constant is

(a) 0.5 mm (b) 0.1 mm
(c) 0.05 mm (d) 0.005 mm

60. A vernier calliper has 20 divisions on the vernier scale, which coincide with 19 on the main scale. The least count of the instrument is 0.1 mm. The main scale divisions are of

(a) 0.5 mm (b) 1 mm (c) 2 mm (d) $\frac{1}{4}$ mm

61. The pitch of the screw gauge is 0.5 mm. Its circular scale contains 50 divisions. The least count of the screw gauge is

(a) 0.001 mm (b) 0.01 mm
(c) 0.02 mm (d) 0.025 mm

62. If x = a – b, then the maximum percentage error in the measurement of x will be

(a) $\left(\frac{\Delta a}{a}+\frac{\Delta b}{b}\right)\times100\%$ (b) $\left(\frac{\Delta a}{a}-\frac{\Delta b}{b}\right)\times100\%$

(c) $\left(\frac{\Delta a}{a-b}+\frac{\Delta b}{a-b}\right)\times100\%$ (d) $\left(\frac{\Delta a}{a-b}-\frac{\Delta b}{a-b}\right)\times100\%$

63. The heat generated in a circuit is given by $Q = I^2 Rt$, where I is current, R is resistance and t is time. If the percentage errors in measuring I, R and t are 2%, 1% and 1% respectively, then the maximum error in measuring heat will be

(a) 2% (b) 3% (c) 4% (d) 6%

64. Which one of the following has the same dimension as that of time, if R is resistance, L inductance and C is capacitance?

(a) RC (b) $\sqrt{LC}$

(c) L/R (d) All of the above

65. In the equation $X = 3YZ^2$, X and Z are dimensions of capacitance and magnetic induction respectively. In MKSQ system, the dimensional formula for Y is

(a) $[M^{-3} L^{-2} T^{-2} Q^{-4}]$ (b) $[M L^{-2}]$

(c) $[M^{-3} L^{-2} Q^4 T^8]$ (d) $[M^{-3} L^{-2} Q^4 T^4]$

66. A force is given by $F = at + bt^2$, where t is time, the dimensions of a and b are

(a) $[M L T^{-4}]$ and $[M L T^{-1}]$

(b) $[M L T^{-1}]$ and $[M L T^0]$

(c) $[M L T^{-3}]$ and $[M L T^{-4}]$

(d) $[M L T^{-3}]$ and $[M L T^0]$

67. The frequency of vibration of a string is given by $f = \frac{n}{2L}\sqrt{\frac{T}{m}}$, where T is tension in the string, L is the length, n is number of harmonics. The dimensional formula for m is

(a) $[M^0 L T]$ (b) $[M^1 L^{-1} T^{-1}]$

(c) $[M^1 L^{-1} T^0]$ (d) $[M^0 L T^{-1}]$

68. Two full turns of the circular scale of a screw gauge cover a distance of 1mm on its main scale. The total number of divisions on the circular scale is 50. Further, it is found that the screw gauge has a zero error of – 0.03 mm. While measuring the diameter of a thin wire, a student notes the main scale reading of 3 mm and the number of circulr scale divisions in line with the main scale as 35. The diameter of the wire is

(a) 3.32 mm (b) 3.73 mm

(c) 3.67 mm (d) 3.38 mm

69. The time of reverberation of a room A is one second. What will be the time (in seconds) of reverberation of a room, having all the dimensions double of those of room A?

(a) 2 (b) 4 (c) $\frac{1}{2}$ (d) 1

70. Which of the following is the unit of molar gas constant?

(a) $JK^{-1} mol^{-1}$ (b) Joule

(c) JK^{-1} (d) $J mol^{-1}$

71. Density of liquid is 16.8 g cm^{-3}. Its value in the International System of Units is

(a) 16.8 kgm^{-3} (b) 168 kgm^{-3}

(c) 1680 kgm^{-3} (d) 16800 kgm^{-3}

72. The dimensional formula of couple is

(a) $[ML^2T^{-2}]$ (b) $[MLT^2]$

(c) $[ML^{-1}T^{-3}]$ (d) $[ML^{-2}T^{-2}]$

73. The refractive index of water measured by the relation $\mu = \frac{\text{real depth}}{\text{apparent depth}}$ is found to have values of 1.34, 1.38, 1.32 and 1.36; the mean value of refractive index with percentage error is

(a) $1.35 \pm 1.48\,\%$ (b) $1.35 \pm 0\,\%$

(c) $1.36 \pm 6\,\%$ (d) $1.36 \pm 0\,\%$

74. Diameter of a steel ball is measured using a Vernier callipers which has divisions of 0.1 cm on its main scale (MS) and 10 divisions of its vernier scale (VS) match 9 divisions on the main scale. Three such measurements for a ball are given below:

S.No.	MS(cm)	VS divisions
1.	0.5	8
2.	0.5	4
3.	0.5	6

If the zero error is – 0.03 cm, then mean corrected diameter is

(a) 0.52 cm (b) 0.59 cm

(c) 0.56 cm (d) 0.53 cm

75. The period of oscillation of a simple pendulum is $T = 2\pi\sqrt{\frac{L}{g}}$. Measured value of L is 20.0 cm known to 1 mm accuracy and time for 100 oscillations of the pendulum is found to be 90 s using a wrist watch of 1s resolution. The accuracy in the determination of g is

(a) 1% (b) 5% (c) 2% (d) 3%

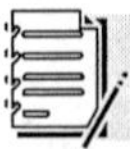

Exercise 2 - Exemplar & Past Year Questions

E&PYQs

Exemplar Questions

1. The number of significant figures in 0.06900 is
(a) 5 (b) 4 (c) 2 (d) 3

2. The sum of the numbers 436.32, 227.2 and 0.301 in appropriate significant figures is
(a) 663.821 (b) 664 (c) 663.8 (d) 663.82

3. The mass and volume of a body are 4.237 g and 2.5 cm^3, respectively. The density of the material of the body in correct significant figures is
(a) 1.6048 g cm^{-3} (b) 1.69 g cm^{-3}
(c) 1.7 g cm^{-3} (d) 1.695 g cm^{-3}

4. The numbers 2.745 and 2.735 on rounding off to 3 significant figures will give
(a) 2.75 and 2.74 (b) 2.74 and 2.73
(c) 2.75 and 2.73 (d) 2.74 and 2.74

5. The length and breadth of a rectangular sheet are 16.2 ± 0.1 cm and 10.1 ± 0.1 cm, respectively. The area of the sheet in appropriate significant figures and error is
(a) $164 \pm 3\ cm^2$ (b) $163.62 \pm 2.6\ cm^2$
(c) $163.6 \pm 2.6\ cm^2$ (d) $163.62 \pm 3\ cm^2$

6. Which of the following pairs of physical quantities does not have same dimensional forrmula?
(a) Work and torque
(b) Angular momentum and Planck's constant
(c) Tension and surface tension
(d) Impulse and linear momentum

7. Measure of two quantities along with the precision of respective measuring instrument is
$A = 2.5\ ms^{-1} \pm 0.5\ ms^{-1}$,
$B = 0.10\ s \pm 0.01\ s$. The value of AB will be
(a) (0.25 ± 0.08) m (b) (0.25 ± 0.5) m
(c) (0.25 ± 0.05) m (d) (0.25 ± 0.135) m

8. You measure two quantities as $A = 1.0\ m \pm 0.2\ m$, $B = 2.0\ m \pm 0.2\ m$. We should report correct value for $\sqrt{AB}$ as
(a) 1.4 m ± 0.4 m (b) 1.41 m ± 0.15 m
(c) 1.4 m ± 0.3 m (d) 1.4 m ± 0.2 m

9. Which of the following measurement is most precise?
(a) 5.00 mm (b) 5.00 cm (c) 5.00 m (d) 5.00 km

10. The mean length of an object is 5 cm. Which is the following measurement is most accurate?
(a) 4.9 cm (b) 4.805 cm
(c) 5.25 cm (d) 5.4 cm

11. Young's modulus of steel is 1.9×10^{11} N/m^2. When expressed in CGS units of dyne/cm^2, it will be equal to (1N = 10^5 dyne, 1 m^2 = 10^4 cm^2)
(a) 1.9×10^{10} (b) 1.9×10^{11}
(c) 1.9×10^{12} (d) 1.9×10^{13}

12. If momentum (p), area (A) and time (T) are taken to be fundamental quantities, then energy has the dimensional formula
(a) $[pA^{-1}T^{1}]$ (b) $[p^2AT]$
(c) $[pA^{-1/2}T]$ (d) $[pA^{1/2}T]$

NEET/AIPMT (2013-2020) Questions

13. In an experiment four quantities a, b, c and d are measured with percentage error 1%, 2%, 3% and 4% respectively. Quantity P is calculated as follows $P = \frac{a^3b^2}{cd}$ % error in P is:
(a) 10% (b) 7% ***[2013]***
(c) 4% (d) 14%

14. The pair of quantities having same dimensions is
(a) Young's modulus and energy ***[NEET Kar. 2013]***
(b) impulse and surface tension
(c) angular momentum and work
(d) work and torque

15. If force (F), velocity (V) and time (T) are taken as fundamental units, then the dimensions of mass are : ***[2014]***
(a) $[F V T^{-1}]$ (b) $[F V T^{-2}]$
(c) $[F V^{-1} T^{-1}]$ (d) $[F V^{-1} T]$

16. If energy (E), velocity (V) and time (T) are chosen as the fundamental quantities, the dimensional formula of surface tension will be : ***[2015]***
(a) $[EV^{-1}T^{-2}]$ (b) $[EV^{-2}T^{-2}]$
(c) $[E^{-2}V^{-1}T^{-3}]$ (d) $[EV^{-2}T^{-1}]$

17. If dimensions of critical velocity υ_c of a liquid flowing through a tube are expressed as $[\eta^x \rho^y r^x]$, where η, ρ and r are the coefficient of viscosity of liquid, density of liquid and radius of the tube respectively, then the values of x, y and z are given by : ***[2015 RS]***
(a) –1, –1, 1 (b) –1, –1, –1
(c) 1, 1, 1 (d) 1, –1, –1

18. A physical quantity of the dimensions of length that can be formed out of c, G and $\frac{e^2}{4\pi\varepsilon_0}$ is [c is velocity of light, G is universal constant of gravitation and e is charge] ***[2017]***
(a) $c^2\left[G\frac{e^2}{4\pi\varepsilon_0}\right]^{1/2}$ (b) $\frac{1}{c^2}\left[\frac{e^2}{G4\pi\varepsilon_0}\right]^{1/2}$
(c) $\frac{1}{c}G\frac{e^2}{4\pi\varepsilon_0}$ (d) $\frac{1}{c^2}\left[G\frac{e^2}{4\pi\varepsilon_0}\right]^{1/2}$

19. A student measured the diameter of a small steel ball using a screw gauge of least count 0.001 cm. The main scale reading is 5 mm and zero of circular scale division coincides with 25 divisions above the reference level. If screw gauge has a zero error of –0.004 cm, the correct diameter of the ball is ***[2018]***
(a) 0.521 cm (b) 0.525 cm
(c) 0.529 cm (d) 0.053 cm

20. The unit of thermal conductivity is : ***[2019]***
(a) $J\ m\ K^{-1}$ (b) $J\ m^{-1}\ K^{-1}$
(c) $W\ m\ K^{-1}$ (d) $W\ m^{-1}\ K^{-1}$

21. In an experiment, the percentage of error occurred in the measurement of physical quantities A, B, C an D are 1%, 2%, 3% and 4% respectively. Then the maximum percentage of error in the measurement X, where $X = \frac{A^2 B^{1/2}}{C^{1/3} D^3}$ will be: ***[2019]***

(a) $\left(\frac{3}{13}\right)\%$ (b) 16% (c) −10% (d) 10%

22. The main scale of a vernier callipers has n divisions/cm. n divisions of the vernier scale coincide with $(n-1)$ divisions of main scale. The least count of the vernier callipers is, ***[NEET Odisha, 2019]***

(a) $\frac{1}{n(n+1)}$ cm (b) $\frac{1}{(n+1)(n-1)}$ cm

(c) $\frac{1}{n}$ cm (d) $\frac{1}{n^2}$ cm

23. Dimensions of stress are : ***[2020]***

(a) $[ML^2T^{-2}]$ (b) $[ML^0T^{-2}]$
(c) $[ML^{-1}T^{-2}]$ (d) $[MLT^{-2}]$

24. Taking into account of the significant figures, what is the value of 9.99 m − 0.0099 m? ***[2020]***

(a) 9.98 m (b) 9.980 m (c) 9.9 m (d) 9.9801 m

25. A screw gauge has least count of 0.01 mm and there are 50 divisions in its circular scale. The pitch of the screw gauge is : ***[2020]***

(a) 0.25 mm (b) 0.5 mm
(c) 1.0 mm (d) 0.01 mm

Exercise 3 - Concept Application Problems

CAP

1. A metal sample carrying a current along X-axis with density J_x is subjected to a magnetic field B_z (along z-axis). The electric field E_y developed along Y-axis is directly proportional to J_x as well as B_z. The constant of proportionality has SI unit

(a) $\frac{m^2}{A}$ (b) $\frac{m^3}{As}$ (c) $\frac{m^2}{As}$ (d) $\frac{As}{m^3}$

2. The quantities $x = \frac{1}{\sqrt{\mu_0 \varepsilon_0}}$, $y = \frac{E}{B}$ and $z = \frac{1}{CR}$ are defined where C-capacitance, R-Resistance, l-length, E-Electric field, B-magnetic field and ε_0, μ_0, - free space permittivity and permeability respectively. Then :

(a) x, y and z have the same dimension.
(b) Only x and z have the same dimension.
(c) Only x and y have the same dimension.
(d) Only y and z have the same dimension.

3. If momentum (P), area (A) and time (T) are taken to be the fundamental quantities then the dimensional formula for energy is :

(a) $[P^2AT^{-2}]$ (b) $[PA^{-1}T^{-2}]$
(c) $[PA^{1/2}T^{-1}]$ (d) $[P^{1/2}AT^{-1}]$

4. Which of the following combinations has the dimension of electrical resistance ($\in_0$ is the permittivity of vacuum and μ_0 is the permeability of vacuum)?

(a) $\sqrt{\frac{\mu_0}{\varepsilon_0}}$ (b) $\frac{\mu_0}{\varepsilon_0}$ (c) $\sqrt{\frac{\varepsilon_0}{\mu_0}}$ (d) $\frac{\varepsilon_0}{\mu_0}$

5. In SI units, the dimensions of $\sqrt{\frac{\epsilon_0}{\mu_0}}$ is:

(a) $A^{-1}TML^3$ (b) $AT^2 M^{-1}L^{-1}$
(c) $AT^{-3}ML^{3/2}$ (d) $A^2T^3 M^{-1}L^{-2}$

6. Let l, r, c and v represent inductance, resistance, capacitance and voltage, respectively. The dimension of $\frac{\ell}{rcv}$ in SI units will be :

(a) $[LA^{-2}]$ (b) $[A^{-1}]$ (c) $[LTA]$ (d) $[LT^2]$

7. The force of interaction between two atoms is given by $F = \alpha\beta \exp\left(-\frac{x^2}{\alpha kT}\right)$; where x is the distance, k is the Boltzmann constant and T is temperature and α and β are two constants. The dimensions of β is:

(a) $M^0L^2T^{-4}$ (b) M^2LT^{-4}
(c) MLT^{-2} (d) $M^2L^2T^{-2}$

8. If speed (V), acceleration (A) and force (F) are considered as fundamental units, the dimension of Young's modulus will be :

(a) $V^{-2}A^2F^{-2}$ (b) $V^{-2}A^2F^2$
(c) $V^{-4}A^{-2}F$ (d) $V^{-4}A^2F$

9. A quantity f is given by $f = \sqrt{\frac{hc^5}{G}}$ where c is speed of light, G universal gravitational constant and h is the Planck's constant. Dimension of f is that of :

(a) area (b) energy
(c) momentum (d) volume

10. The dimensions of $\frac{B^2}{2\mu_0}$, where B is magnetic field and μ_0 is the magnetic permeability of vacuum, is:

(a) MLT^{-2} (b) ML^2T^{-1} (c) ML^2T^{-2} (d) $ML^{-1}T^{-2}$

11. A physical quantity z depends on four observables a, b, c and d, as $z = \frac{a^2 b^{\frac{2}{3}}}{\sqrt{c}d^3}$. The percentages of error in the measurement of a, b, c and d are 2%, 1.5%, 4% and 2.5% respectively. The percentage of error in z is :

(a) 12.25% (b) 16.5% (c) 13.5% (d) 14.5%

12. In the density measurement of a cube, the mass and edge length are measured as (10.00 ± 0.10) kg and (0.10 ± 0.01) m, respectively. The error in the measurement of density is:

(a) 0.01 kg/m³ (b) 0.10 kg/m³
(c) 0.31 kg/m³ (d) 0.07 kg/m³

13. The area of a square is 5.29 cm^2. The area of 7 such squares taking into account the significant figures is:
(a) 37cm^2 (b) 37.030 cm^2
(c) 37.03 cm^2 (d) 37.0 cm^2

14. The relative uncertainty in the period of a satellite orbiting around the earth is 10^{-2}. If the relative uncertainty in the radius of the orbit is negligible, the relative uncertainty in the mass of the earth is
(a) 3×10^{-2} (b) 10^{-2}
(c) 2×10^{-2} (d) 6×10^{-2}

15. The relative error in the determination of the surface area of a sphere is α. Then the relative error in the determination of its volume is
(a) $\frac{2}{3}\alpha$ (b) $\frac{2}{3}\alpha$ (c) $\frac{3}{2}\alpha$ (d) α

16. The following observations were taken for determining surface tensiton T of water by capillary method :
Diameter of capilary, $D = 1.25\times10^{-2}$ m
rise of water, $h = 1.45\times10^{-2}$ m
Using $g = 9.80$ m/s^2 and the simplified relation
$T = \frac{rhg}{2}\times10^3$ N/m, the possible error in surface tension is closest to :
(a) 2.4% (b) 10% (c) 0.15% (d) 1.5%

17. A physical quantity P is described by the relation
$P = a^{1/2}\, b^2\, c^3\, d^{-4}$
If the relative errors in the measurement of *a, b, c* and *d* respectively, are 2%, 1%, 3% and 5%, then the relative error in P will be :
(a) 8% (b) 12% (c) 32% (d) 25%

18. The SI unit of coefficient of mutual inductance of a coil is
(a) henry (b) volt
(c) farad (c) weber

19. The S.I. unit of pole strength is
(a) Am^2 (b) Am
(c) $A\,m^{-1}$ (d) Am^{-2}

20. Which is dimensionless?
(a) Force/acceleration (b) Velocity/acceleration
(c) Volume/area (d) Energy/work

21. Which physical quantities have same dimensions?
(a) Moment of couple and work
(b) Force and power
(c) Latent heat and specific heat
(d) Work and power

22. The expression $[ML^{-1}\,T^{-2}]$ does not represent
(a) pressure (b) power
(c) stress (d) Young's modulus

23. The unit and dimensions of impedance in terms of charge Q are
(a) mho, $[ML^2\,T^{-2}\,Q^{-2}]$ (b) ohm, $[ML^2\,T^{-1}\,Q^{-2}]$
(c) ohm, $[ML^2\,T^{-2}\,Q^{-1}]$ (d) ohm, $[MLT^{-1}\,Q^{-1}]$

24. Let Q denote the charge on the plate of a capacitor of capacitance C. The dimensional formula for $\frac{Q^2}{C}$ is
(a) $[L^2M^2T]$ (b) $[LMT^2]$
(c) $[L^2MT^{-2}]$ (d) $[L^2M^2T^2]$

25. The dimensional formula of current density is
(a) $[M^0L^{-2}T^{-1}Q]$ (b) $[M^0L^2T^1Q^{-1}]$
(c) $[MLT^{-1}Q]$ (d) $[ML^{-2}T^{-1}Q^2]$

26. If C and L denote the capacitance and inductance, the dimensions of LC are
(a) $[M^0\,L^0\,T^{-1}]$ (b) $[M^0\,L^{-1}\,T^0]$
(c) $[M^{-1}\,L^{-1}\,T^0]$ (d) $[M^0\,L^0\,T^2]$

27. The time dependence of a physical quantity p is given by $p = p_0 \exp.(-\alpha t^2)$, where α is a constant and t is the time. The constant α
(a) is dimensionless (b) has dimensions T^{-2}
(c) has dimensions T^2 (d) has dimensions of p.

28. A cube has numerically equal volume and surface area. The volume of such a cube is
(a) 1000 unit (b) 200 unit
(c) 216 unit (d) 300 unit

29. A resistor of 10 k Ω having tolerance 10% is connected in series with another resistor of 20 k Ω having tolerance 20%. The tolerance of the combination will be
(a) 10% (b) 13%
(c) 30% (d) 20%

30. The speed of sound in a gas is given by $v = \sqrt{\frac{\gamma RT}{M}}$
R = universal gas constant,
T = temperature
M = molar mass of gas
The dimensional formula of γ is
(a) $[M^0L^0T^0]$ (b) $[M^0LT^{-1}]$
(c) $[MLT^{-2}]$ (d) $[M^0L^0T^{-1}]$

31. Given that $r = m^2 \sin \pi t$, where t represents time. If the unit of m is N, then the unit of r is
(a) N (b) N^2
(c) Ns (d) N^2s

32. The dimensional formula of farad is
(a) $[M^{-1}L^{-2}TQ]$ (b) $[M^{-1}L^{-2}T^2Q^2]$
(c) $[M^{-1}L^{-2}TQ^2]$ (d) $[M^{-1}L^{-2}T^2Q]$

33. Turpentine oil is flowing through a capillary tube of length ℓ and radius r. The pressure difference between the two ends of the tube is p. The viscosity of oil is given by :
$\eta = \frac{p(r^2 - x^2)}{4v\ell}$. Here v is velocity of oil at a distance x from the axis of the tube. From this relation, the dimensional formula of η is
(a) $[ML^{-1}T^{-1}]$ (b) $[MLT^{-1}]$
(c) $[ML^2T^{-2}]$ (d) $[M^0L^0T^0]$

34. The dimensional formula of velocity gradient is

(a) $[M^0L^0T^{-1}]$ (b) $[MLT^1]$

(c) $[ML^0T^{-1}]$ (d) $[M^0LT^{-2}]$

35. If E, m, J and G represent energy, mass, angular momentum and gravitational constant respectively, then the dimensional formula of EJ^2/m^5G^2 is

(a) angle (b) length

(c) mass (d) time

36. The pressure on a square plate is measured by measuring the force on the plate and length of the sides of the plate by using the formula $P = \frac{F}{\ell^2}$. If the maximum errors in the measurement of force and length are 4% and 2% respectively, then the maximum error in the measurement of pressure is

(a) 1% (b) 2%

(c) 8% (d) 10%

37. The equation of a wave is given by

$y = a\sin\omega\left(\frac{x}{v} - k\right)$, where ω is angular velocity and v is linear velocity. The dimensions of K will be

(a) $[T^2]$ (b) $[T^{-1}]$

(c) $[T]$ (d) $[LT]$

38. The dimensions of voltage in terms of mass (M), length (L) and time (T) and ampere (A) are

(a) $[ML^2T^{-2}A^{-2}]$ (b) $[ML^2T^3A^{-1}]$

(c) $[ML^2T^{-3}A^1]$ (d) $[ML^2T^{-3}A^{-1}]$

39. Suppose the kinetic energy of a body oscillating with amplitude A and at a distance x is given by

$$K = \frac{Bx}{x^2 + A^2}$$

The dimensions of B are the same as that of

(a) work/time (b) work × distance

(c) work/distance (d) work × time

40. The dimensions of magnetic field in M, L, T and C (coulomb) are given as

(a) $[MLT^{-1}C^{-1}]$ (b) $[MT^2C^{-2}]$

(c) $[MT^{-1}C^{-1}]$ (d) $[MT^{-2}C^{-1}]$

41. If the dimensions of a physical quantity are given by $M^a L^b T^c$, then the physical quantity will be

(a) velocity if a = 1, b = 0, c = – 1

(b) acceleration if a = 1, b = 1, c = – 2

(c) force if a = 0, b = – 1, c = – 2

(d) pressure if a = 1, b = – 1, c = – 2

42. The density of a material in CGS system of units is 4g/cm^3. In a system of units in which unit of length is 10 cm and unit of mass is 100 g, the value of density of material will be

(a) 0.4 (b) 40

(c) 400 (d) 0.04

43. What is the fractional error in g calculated from $T = 2\pi\sqrt{\ell/g}$? Given fractional errors in T and *l* are ± x and ± y respectively.

(a) $x + y$ (b) $x - y$

(c) $2x + y$ (d) $2x - y$

44. What are the dimensions of permeability ?

(a) $[M^1L^1T^1A^{-2}]$ (b) $[M^1L^1T^{-2}A^{-2}]$

(c) $[M^2L^2T^1A^0]$ (d) $[M^1L^2T^2A^{-2}]$

45. The physical quantity having the dimensions $[M^{-1}L^{-3}T^3A^2]$ is

(a) resistance (b) resistivity

(c) electrical conductivity (d) electromotive force

Hints & Solutions

2.1 Concept Practice Problems

1. (a) SI is based on seven fundamental units.
2. (a) $L=\frac{Q}{m}=\frac{J}{kg}=J\,kg^{-1}$
3. (a) As force = change in momentum/time.
   $\therefore$ force × time = change in momentum
4. (c) 1 light year = speed of light in vacuum × no. of seconds in one year = $(3\times10^8)\times(365\times24\times60\times60)$ $=9.467\times10^{15}$ m.
5. (c) 1 pascal = $1\,N/m^2$.
6. (b) $\sqrt{\frac{\rho r^3}{S}}=\sqrt{\frac{ML^{-3}L^3}{MT^{-2}}}=T$
7. (d) $B=x=[L]$; $A\sqrt{x}=Vx$; $A=V\sqrt{x}$
   $=ML^2T^{-2}L^{1/2}=ML^{5/2}T^{-2}$
   $AB=(ML^{5/2}T^{-2})(L)=[M^1L^{7/2}T^{-2}]$
8. (b) In $S=A(t+B)+Ct^2$; B is added to time t. Therefore, dimensions of B are those of time.
9. (b) $h=\lambda\sqrt{2mE}=L\sqrt{M(ML^2T^{-2})}=[ML^2T^{-1}]$
10. (d) $v=g^a h^b$; $[M^0LT^{-1}]=(LT^{-2})^aL^b=L^{a+b}T^{-2a}$
    $\therefore\ a+b=1;\ -2a=-1\quad a=1/2$
    $\therefore\ b=1/2$
11. (a) As c is added to t, $\therefore\ c=[T]$
    $a=\frac{v}{t}=\frac{LT^{-1}}{T}=[LT^{-2}]$,
    $b=v(t+c)=LT^{-1}\times T=[L]$
12. (c) From $F=\frac{1}{4\pi\varepsilon_0}\frac{e^2}{r^2}$
    $\therefore\ \frac{e^2}{\varepsilon_0}=4\pi Fr^2$ (dimensionally)
    $\frac{e^2}{\varepsilon_0 hc}=\frac{4\pi Fr^2}{hc}=\frac{(MLT^{-2})L^2}{ML^2T^{-1}[LT^{-1}]}=[M^0L^0T^0A^0]$,
    $\frac{e^2}{\varepsilon_0 hc}$ is called fine structure constant & has value $\frac{1}{137}$.
13. (b) $v=k\lambda^a\rho^bg^c$
    $[M^0LT^{-1}]=L^a(ML^{-3})^b(LT^{-2})^c$
    $=M^bL^{a-3b+c}T^{-2c}$
    $\therefore\ b=0;\ a-3b+c=1$
    $-2c=-1\Rightarrow c=1/2\qquad\therefore\ a=\frac{1}{2}$
    $v\propto\lambda^{1/2}\rho^0g^{1/2}$ or $v^2\propto\lambda g$
14. (c) $[A]=[LT^{-2}]$ or $[L]=[AT^2]$
    [Work] = [Force ×Distance] = [FL] = $[FAT^2]$
15. (c)

2.2 Concept Practice Problems

16. (a) Relative error $=\frac{2\Delta x}{x}$ for $f=x^2$
17. (a) Subtraction is correct upto one place of decimal, corresponding to the least number of decimal places.
    $7.26-0.2=7.06=7.1$ J.
18. (d) Number of significant figures in multiplication is three, corresponding to the minimum number
    $107.88\times0.610=65.8068=65.8$
19. (d) $\frac{97.52}{2.54}=38.393=38.4$ (with least number of significant figures, 3).
20. (d) Relative density = $\frac{\text{Weight of body in air}}{\text{Loss of weight in water}}$
    $=\frac{5.00}{5.00-4.00}=\frac{5.00}{1.00}$
    $\frac{\Delta\rho}{\rho}\times100=\left(\frac{0.05}{5.00}+\frac{0.05}{1.00}\right)\times100$
    $=(0.01+0.05)\times100$
    $=0.06\times100=6\%$
    $\therefore$ Relative density = $5.00\pm6\%$
21. (a) Area = $(\text{Length})^2$
    or length $=(\text{Area})^{1/2}$
    $=(100\pm2)^{1/2}$
    $=(100)^{1/2}\pm\frac{1}{2}\times2$
    $=(10\pm1)$m
22. (c) $\frac{0.2}{25}\times100=0.8$
23. (a)
24. (a) $X=M^aL^bT^c$;
    $\frac{\Delta X}{X}\times100=\left(\frac{a\,\Delta M}{M}+\frac{b\,\Delta L}{L}+\frac{c\,\Delta T}{T}\right)\times100$
    $=(a\alpha+b\beta+c\gamma)\%$
25. (c) From $T=2\pi\sqrt{\frac{\ell}{g}}$; $g=4\pi^2\frac{\ell}{T^2}$
    $\frac{\Delta g}{g}=\frac{\Delta\ell}{\ell}+\frac{2\Delta T}{T}=(y+2x)$
26. (c) Percentage error in mass $\left(\frac{\Delta m}{m}\times100\right)=2\%$ and percentage error in speed $\left(\frac{\Delta v}{v}\times100\right)=3\%$.

$E=\frac{1}{2}mv^2$

$\therefore \frac{\Delta E}{E}\times 100=\frac{\Delta m}{m}\times 100+2\frac{\Delta V}{V}\times 100$

$=2\%+2\times 3\%=8\%.$

27. (c) $T=2\pi\sqrt{\frac{\ell}{g}},\ g\propto\frac{\ell}{T^2}$

$\therefore\ \frac{\Delta g}{g}\times 100=0.5\%+2\times 0.2\%=0.9\%$

28. (a) $\%\ \text{error}=\frac{0.01}{0.5}\times 100+\frac{0.01}{1.0}\times 100+\frac{0.01}{0.5}\times 100$

$=2+1+2=4+1=5$

29. (d) $P=\frac{a^3b^2}{cd},\ \frac{\Delta P}{P}\times 100\%=3\frac{\Delta a}{a}\times 100\%+2\frac{\Delta b}{b}\times$

$100\%+\frac{\Delta c}{c}\times 100\%+\frac{\Delta d}{d}\times 100\%.$

$=3\times 1\%+2\times 2\%+3\%+4\%=14\%$

30. (b) Given $=R=\frac{\rho\ell}{\pi r^2}$, then $\frac{\Delta R}{R}\times 100$

$=\frac{\Delta\rho}{\rho}\times 100+\frac{\Delta\ell}{\ell}\times 100+2\frac{\Delta r}{r}\times 100$

$=1\%+2\%+2\times 3\%=9\%$

Exercise 1 - Chapter Revision Problems CRP

1. (a) Density of material in SI unit,

$=\frac{128\text{kg}}{m^3}$

Density of material in new system

$=\frac{128(50\,g)(20)}{(25\,cm)^3(4)^3}=\frac{128}{64}(20)=40\ \text{units}$

2. (d) From formula, $\frac{dQ}{dt}=kA\frac{dT}{dx}\Rightarrow k=\frac{\left(\frac{dQ}{dt}\right)}{A\left(\frac{dT}{dx}\right)}$

$[k]=\frac{[ML^2T^{-3}]}{[L^2][KL^{-1}]}=[MLT^{-3}K^{-1}]$

3. (c) Dimension of Force $F=M^1L^1T^{-2}$

Dimension of velocity $V=L^1T^{-1}$

Dimension of work $=M^1L^2T^{-2}$

Dimension of length $=L$

Moment of inertia $=ML^2$

$\therefore x=\frac{IFv^2}{WL^4}$

$=\frac{(M^1L^2)(M^1L^1T^{-2})(L^1T^{-2})^2}{(M^1L^2T^{-2})(L^4)}$

$=\frac{M^1L^{-2}T^{-2}}{L^3}=M^1L^{-1}T^{-2}=\text{Energy density}$

4. (b) Solar constant $=\frac{\text{Energy}}{\text{Time Area}}$

Dimension of Energy, $E=ML^2T^{-2}$

Dimension of Time $=T$

Dimension of Area $=L^2$

$\therefore$ Dimension of Solar constant

$=\frac{M^1L^2T^{-2}}{TL^2}=M^1L^0T^{-3}.$

5. (d) Young's modulus, $Y=\frac{\text{stress}}{\text{strain}}$

$\Rightarrow Y=\frac{F}{A}\Big/\frac{\Delta\ell}{\ell_0}=FA^{-1}V^0$

6. (a) $X=5YZ^2$

$\Rightarrow Y\propto\frac{X}{Z^2}$ ...(i)

$X=\text{Capacitance}=\frac{Q}{V}=\frac{Q^2}{W}=\frac{[A^2T^2]}{[ML^2T^{-2}]}$

$X=[M^{-1}L^{-2}T^4A^2]$

$Z=B=\frac{F}{IL}$ $[\because F=ILB]$

$Z=[MT^{-2}A^{-1}]$

$Y=\frac{[M^{-1}L^{-2}T^4A^2]}{[MT^{-2}A^{-1}]^2}$

$Y=[M^{-3}L^{-2}T^8A^4]$ (Using (i))

7. (c) Let $t\propto G^xh^yC^z$

Dimensions of $G=[M^{-1}L^3T^{-2}]$,

$h=[ML^2T^{-1}]$ and $C=[LT^{-1}]$

$[T]=[M^{-1}L^3T^{-2}]^x[ML^2T^{-1}]^y[LT^{-1}]^z$

$[M^0L^0T^1]=[M^{-x+y}L^{3x+2y+z}T^{-2x-y-z}]$

By comparing the powers of M, L, T both the sides

$-x+y=0\Rightarrow x=y$

$3x+2y+z=0\Rightarrow 5x+z=0$ ..... (i)

$-2x-y-z=1\Rightarrow 3x+z=-1$ ..... (ii)

Solving eqns. (i) and (ii),

$x=y=\frac{1}{2},z=-\frac{5}{2}\ \therefore\ t\propto\sqrt{\frac{Gh}{C^5}}$

8. (None)

Stopping potential $(V_0)\propto h^xI^yG^ZC^r$

Here, $h=$ Planck's constant $=\left[ML^2T^{-1}\right]$

$I=$ current $=[A]$

$G=$ Gravitational constant $=[M^{-1}L^3T^{-2}]$

and $c=$ speed of light $=[LT^{-1}]$

$V_0=$ potential $=[ML^2T^{-3}A^{-1}]$

$\therefore [ML^2T^{-3}A^{-1}]=[ML^2T^{-1}]^x[A]^y[M^{-1}L^3T^{-2}]^z[LT^{-1}]^r$

$M^{x-z};\ L^{2x+3z+r};\ T^{-x-2z-r};\ A^y$

Comparing dimension of M, L, T, A, we get

$y=-1, x=0, z=-1, r=5$

$\therefore\ V_0\propto h^0I^{-1}G^{-1}C^5$

9. (b) Plank length is a unit of length, $l_p = 1.616229 \times 10^{-35}$ m

$$l_p = \sqrt{\frac{hG}{c^3}}$$

10. (None)

$D_1 = A_1 + B_1 + C_1 = 24.36 + 0.0724 + 256.2 = 280.6$

$D_2 = A_2 + B_2 + C_2 = 24.44 + 16.082 + 240.2 = 280.7$

$D_3 = A_3 + B_3 + C_3 = 25.2 + 19.2812 + 236.183 = 280.7$

$D_4 = A_4 + B_4 + C_4 = 25 + 236.191 + 19.5 = 281$

None of the option matches.

11. (c) Given, Length of simple pendulum, $l = 25.0$ cm

Time of 40 oscillation, $T = 50s$

Time period of pendulum

$$T = 2\pi\sqrt{\frac{\ell}{g}}$$

$$\Rightarrow T^2 = \frac{4\pi^2\ell}{g} \Rightarrow g = \frac{4\pi^2\ell}{T^2}$$

$$\Rightarrow \text{Fractional error in g} = \frac{\Delta g}{g} = \frac{\Delta l}{l} + \frac{2\Delta T}{T}$$

$$\Rightarrow \frac{\Delta g}{g} = \left(\frac{0.1}{25.0}\right) + 2\left(\frac{1}{50}\right) = 0.044$$

$$\therefore \text{Percentage error in } g = \frac{\Delta g}{g} \times 100 = 4.4\%$$

12. (d) We have

$$T = 2\pi\sqrt{\frac{\ell}{g}} \text{ or } g = 4\pi^2 \frac{\ell}{T^2}$$

$$\frac{\Delta g}{g} \times 100 = \frac{\Delta R}{Q} \times 100 + 2\frac{\Delta T}{T} \times 100$$

$$= \frac{0.1}{55} \times 100 + 2\left(\frac{1}{30}\right) \times 100$$

$$= 0.18 + 6.67 = 6.8\%$$

13. (c)

14. (c) = 1.5 % + 3 (1%) = 4.5%

15. (d) Maximum percentage error in A

= 3(% error in P) + 2(% error in Q)

$+\frac{1}{2}$(% error in R) + 1(% error in S)

$$= 3 \times 0.5 + 2 \times 1 + \frac{1}{2} \times 3 + 1 \times 1.5$$

$$= 1.5 + 2 + 1.5 + 1.5 = 6.5\%$$

16. (d) Temperature is one of the basic physical quantities.

17. (b) The vander Waal's gas equation is

$$(P + \frac{a}{V^2})(V - b) = RT \text{ for one mole.}$$

$$\& \left(P + \frac{\mu a}{V^2}\right)(V - \mu b) = \mu RT \text{ for } \mu \text{ mole}$$

Dimensionally in first bracket on L.H.S

$$[P] = \left[\frac{\mu a}{V^2}\right] \Rightarrow [a] = \frac{[P]V^2}{\mu}$$

$$\text{Dimension of } [a] = \left[\frac{\text{atm. litre}^2}{\text{mole}}\right]$$

18. (d)

19. (c) $\frac{eV}{T} = \frac{W}{T} = \frac{PV}{T} = R$

and $\frac{R}{N}$ = Boltzmann constant.

20. (a)

21. (c) Electron volt is a unit of energy &

1eV = 1.6×10^{-19} joule

22. (a) Impulse = force × time $= MLT^{-2} \times T = [M^1 LT^{-1}]$.

23. (a) Potential is work done per unit charge.

24. (c) Maxwell is the unit of magnetic flux in C.G.S system.

1 Wb(S.I unit) = 10^8 maxwell

25. (b) Let $M = p^n v^m$

$$ML^{-2}T^{-1} = (ML^{-1}T^{-2})^n (LT^{-1})^m$$

$$= M^n L^{-n+m} T^{-2n-m}$$

$$\therefore \ n = 1; -n + m = -2$$

$$\therefore \ m = -2 + n = -2 + 1 = -1 \qquad \therefore \ m = -n$$

26. (b)

27. (a) From Biot Savart's law

$$B = \frac{\mu_0}{4\pi}\frac{i\,dl\,\sin\theta}{r^2}$$

$$\mu_0 = \frac{4\pi\,Br^2}{i\,dl\,\sin\theta} = \frac{Wb\,m^{-2}m^2}{Am} = Wb\,A^{-1}m^{-1}$$

28. (a) Pressure gradient $= \frac{\text{Pressure difference}}{\text{distance}}$.

$$[\text{Pressure gradient}] = \frac{ML^{-1}T^{-2}}{L} = \left[ML^{-2}T^{-2}\right]$$

29. (c) From $\frac{1}{\lambda} = R\left(\frac{1}{n_1^2} - \frac{1}{n_2^2}\right)$,

dimensions of $R = \frac{1}{L} = L^{-1} = [M^0 L^{-1} T^0]$

30. (a) $R = \frac{PV}{\mu T} = \frac{W}{\mu T} = \frac{ML^2 T^{-2}}{mol\,K}$

where μ is number of mole of the gas

$= [M^1 L^2 T^{-2} K^{-1} mol^{-1}]$

31. (a) M = current × area = $AL^2 = [L^2 A^1]$

32. (b) $b = \lambda_m T = LK = [M^0 L^1 T^0 K^1]$

33. (a) Energy stored in an inductor $= \frac{1}{2} Li^2 = [ML^2 T^{-2}]$

34. (b) Wave number $\bar{\nu} = \frac{1}{\lambda} = \frac{1}{L} = [M^0 L^{-1} T^0]$.

35. (a) $T = P^a D^b S^c$

$M^0 L^0 T^1 = (ML^{-1} T^{-2})^a (ML^{-3})^b (MT^{-2})^c$

$= M^{a+b+c} L^{-a-3b} T^{-2a-2c}$

Applying principle of homogeneity

$a + b + c = 0;\ -a - 3b = 0;\ -2a - 2c = 1$

on solving, we get $a = -3/2$, $b = 1/2$, $c = 1$

36. (a) Hubble's constant, $H = \frac{\text{velocity}}{\text{distance}} = \frac{[LT^{-1}]}{[L]}$

$= [T^{-1}] = 70 \times 10^{-3}$ N/m.

37. (c) $V = \frac{4}{3}\pi r^3$;

$\frac{\Delta V}{V} \times 100 = 3\left(\frac{\Delta r}{r}\right) \times 100 = 3 \times 1\% = 3\%$

38. (b) $L/R = \frac{\text{Volt} \times \text{sec/amp.}}{\text{Volt/amp.}} = \text{sec.} = [M^0 L^0 T]$

39. (d) 40. (a)

41. (d) Solar constant = energy/sec/area

$= \frac{ML^2 T^{-2}}{TL^2} = [MT^{-3}]$

42. (c) Entropy $= \frac{Q}{T} = \frac{ML^2 T^{-2}}{K} = [ML^2 T^{-2} K^{-1}]$

43. (d) $s = \frac{Q}{m\theta} = \frac{ML^2 T^{-2}}{MK} = [L^2 T^{-2} K^{-1}]$

44. (c) $\frac{1}{\sqrt{LC}} = \frac{1}{\sqrt{(ML^2 T^{-2} A^{-2}) \times (M^{-1} L^{-2} T^4 A^2)}}$

$= \frac{1}{\sqrt{T^2}} = T^{-1}$

45. (b) Solar constant = energy/area/time

$= \frac{ML^2 T^{-2}}{L^2 T} = [M^1 T^{-3}]$.

46. (b) As $\frac{a}{V^2} = P$

$\therefore\ a = PV^2 = \frac{\text{dyne}}{\text{cm}^2}(\text{cm}^3)^2 = \text{dyne} \times \text{cm}^4$

47. (c) $\frac{h}{e^2} = \frac{ML^2 T^{-1}}{(AT)^2} = ML^2 T^{-3} A^{-2}$ = Resistance (ohm)

48. (c) $I = AT^2 e^{-B/kT}$

Dimensions of $A = I/T^2$; Dimensions of $B = kT$

($\because$ power of exponential is dimensionless)

$AB^2 = \frac{\mathbf{I}}{T^2}(kT)^2 = \mathbf{I}k^2$

49. (a) The C.G.S unit of current is called biot (Bi) i.e.,

$1A = \frac{1C}{1\,\text{sec}} = \frac{(1/10)\text{e.m.u of charge}}{\text{sec}} = \frac{1}{10}\text{Bi}$

or 1Bi = 10A

50. (d) $\omega k = \frac{1}{T} \times \frac{1}{L} = [L^{-1} T^{-1}]$

The dimensions of the quantities in a, b, c are of velocity $[LT^{-1}]$

51. (d) None of the expressions has the dimensions of time.

52. (c) N VD = (N – 1) MD

$1\ VD = \left(\frac{N-1}{N}\right) MD$

L.C. = Least count = 1MD – 1VD

$L.C. = \left(1 - \frac{N-1}{N}\right) MD$

$= \frac{1}{N} M.D. = \frac{0.1}{N} cm = \frac{1}{10N} cm$

$= \frac{\text{value of 1 part on main scale}}{\text{number of parts on vernier scale}}$

where V.D. = vernier division, M.D. Main scale division.

53. (c) We have, $n_1 u_1 = n_2 u_2$

$n_2 = n_1\left(\frac{u_1}{u_2}\right)$

$= 10^6 \times \left(\frac{M_1}{M_2}\right)\left(\frac{L_1}{L_2}\right)^2 \left(\frac{T_1}{T_2}\right)^{-3}$

$= 10^6 \times \left(\frac{1\,kg}{10\,kg}\right)\left(\frac{1\,m}{1 \times 10^{-1} m}\right)^2 \left(\frac{1\,s}{60\,s}\right)^{-3}$

$= 10^6 \times \left(\frac{1}{10}\right)(10)^2 (60)^3$

$= 10^7 \times (60)^3 = 2.16 \times 10^{12}$ units.

54. (c) Force, $F = \frac{1}{4\pi\varepsilon_0}\frac{q_1 q_2}{r^2} \Rightarrow \varepsilon_0 = \frac{q_1 . q_2}{4\pi F r^2}$

So dimension of ε_0

$$=\frac{[AT]^2}{[MLT^{-2}][L^2]}=[M^{-1}L^{-3}T^4A^2]$$

55. (d) $\text{Density}=\frac{\text{Mass}}{\text{Volume}}$

$\rho=\frac{M}{L^3}, \quad \frac{\Delta\rho}{\rho}=\frac{\Delta M}{M}+3\frac{\Delta L}{L}$

% error in density = % error in Mass + 3 (% error in length)
= 4 + 3(3) = 13%

56. (a) Specific gravity is the ratio of density of substance and density of water at 4°C. The ratio of like quantities is dimensionless.

57. (c) Dimensionally K.E = Work

58. (a) Use principle of homogeneity.

59. (c) $10\,VD = 9MD,\ 1VD=\frac{9}{10}MD$

Vernier constant = 1 MD – 1 VD

$=\left(1-\frac{9}{10}\right)MD=\frac{1}{10}MD=\frac{1}{10}\times\frac{1}{2}=0.05\,mm$

60. (c) $\frac{0.1}{10}=\left(1-\frac{19}{20}\right)MSD \Rightarrow \frac{1}{100}=\frac{1}{20}\times 1\,MSD$

$\Rightarrow 1\,MSD=\frac{1}{5}\times 10=2$

61. (b) Least count $=\frac{0.5}{50}=0.01mm$

62. (c) Maximum absolute error is $\Delta a+\Delta b$. Therefore the

$\text{percentage error}=\frac{\text{absolute error}}{\text{actual value}}\times 100$

63. (d) $\frac{\Delta Q}{Q}\times 100=\frac{2\Delta I}{I}\times 100+\frac{\Delta R}{R}\times 100+\frac{\Delta t}{t}\times 100$

$=2\times 2\%+1\%+1\%=6\%.$

64. (b) $[\sqrt{LC}]=\sqrt{ML^2T^{-2}A^{-2}.M^{-1}L^{-2}T^4A^2}=T$

65. (d) $[Y]=\frac{[X]}{[Z^2]}=\frac{M^{-1}L^{-2}T^4A^2}{M^2T^{-4}A^{-2}}=M^{-3}L^{-2}Q^4T^4$

$\left(\because A=\frac{Q}{T}\right)$

66. (c) $[at]=[F]$ amd $[bt^2]=[F]$
$\Rightarrow [a]=MLT^{-3}$ and $[b]=MLT^{-4}$

67. (c) Clearly, $m=\frac{n^2T}{4f^2L^2};\ [m]=\frac{MLT^{-2}}{T^{-2}.L^2}$

68. (d) Least count of screw gauge $=\frac{0.5}{50}mm=0.01mm$

$\therefore$ Reading = [Main scale reading + circular scale reading × L.C] – (zero error)
$=[3+35\times 0.01]-(-0.03)=3.38\,mm$

69. (a) Reverberation time,

$t=\left(\frac{d}{V}\right)_{forward}+\left(\frac{d}{V}\right)_{backward}$

when dimensions double then, $d'=2d$

$\therefore\quad t'=\frac{d'}{V}+\frac{d'}{V}=\frac{2d}{V}+\frac{2d}{V}=2\left(\frac{d}{V}+\frac{d}{V}\right)$

$\Rightarrow\quad t'=2t\ \left(\because \frac{d}{V}+\frac{d}{V}=t\right)$

70. (a) $R=\frac{PV}{nT}=\frac{J}{mol\ K}=J\ K^{-1}\ mol^{-1}$.

71. (d) $16.8\ gcm^{-3}=16800\ Kgm^{-3}$.

72. (a) Dimensionally couple = Torque = Work

73. (a) The mean value of refractive index,

$\mu=\frac{1.34+1.38+1.32+1.36}{4}=1.35$

and

$\Delta\mu=\frac{|(1.35-1.34)|+|(1.35-1.38)|+|(1.35-1.32)|+|(1.35-1.36)|}{4}$
$=0.02$

Thus $\frac{\Delta\mu}{\mu}\times 100=\frac{0.02}{1.35}\times 100=1.48$

74. (b) Least count $=\frac{0.1}{10}=0.01$ cm

$d_1=0.5+8\times 0.01+0.03=0.61$ cm
$d_2=0.5+4\times 0.01+0.03=0.57$ cm
$d_3=0.5+6\times 0.01+0.03=0.59$ cm

Mean diameter $=\frac{0.61+0.57+0.59}{3}=0.59$ cm

75. (d) As, $g=4\pi^2\frac{l}{T^2}$

So, $\frac{\Delta g}{g}\times 100=\frac{\Delta l}{l}\times 100+2\frac{\Delta T}{T}\times 100$

$=\frac{0.1}{20}\times 100+2\times\frac{1}{90}\times 100=2.72\simeq 3\%$

Exercise 2 - Exemplar & Past Year Questions E&PYQs

Exemplar Questions

1. (b) In 0.06900, the two zeroes before six are not siginificant and two zeroes on right side of 9 are significant figures. Hence, number of significant figures are four (6900).

2. (b) In addition the result will be in least number of places after decimal and minimum number of significant figure. The sum of the given numbers can be calculated as 663.821.

The number with least decimal places is 227.2 is correct to only one decimal place but in addition of numbers, the final result should be rounded off to one decimal place i.e., 664.

3. (c) As we know that in multiplication or division, the final result should retain as many significant figures as are there in the original number with the least significant figures.

The significant figure in given numbers 4.237 g and 2.5 cm^3 are four and two respectivey so, density should be reported to two significant figures.

$$\text{Density} = \frac{4.237\text{ g}}{2.5\text{ cm}^3} = 1.6948 = 1.7\text{ g.cm}^{-3}$$

∴ As rounding off the number upto 2 significant figures, we get density = 1.7.

4. (d) Rounding off 2.745 upto 3 significant figures here IVth digit is 5 and its preceding is even, so no change in 4. Thus answer would be 2.74. Rounding off 2.735 upto 3 significant figures, here IV digit is 5 and its preceding digit is 3 (odd). So 3 is increased by 1 answer become would be 2.74.

5. (a) If Δx is error in a physical quantity, then relative error is calculated as $\frac{\Delta x}{x}$.

Given that,

Length $l = (16.2 \pm 0.1)$ cm

Breadth $b = (10.1 \pm 0.1)$ cm $\because \Delta l = 0.1$ cm, $\Delta b = 0.1$ cm

Area $(A) = l \times b = 16.2 \times 10.1 = 163.62\text{ cm}^2$

In significant figure rounding off to three significant digits, area $A = 164\text{ cm}^2$

$$\frac{\Delta A}{A} = \frac{\Delta l}{l} + \frac{\Delta b}{b} = \frac{0.1}{16.2} + \frac{0.1}{10.1}$$

$$= \frac{1.01 + 1.62}{16.2 \times 10.1} = \frac{2.63}{163.62}$$

$$\text{So, } \Delta A = A \times \frac{2.63}{163.62} = 164 \times \frac{2.63}{163.62}$$

$$= 2.636\text{ cm}^2$$

Now rounding off up to one significant figure $\Delta A = 3\text{ cm}^2$.

So, Area $A = A \pm \Delta A = (164 \pm 3)\text{ cm}^2$.

6. (c) a. Work = force × distance

$= [MLT^{-2}][L] = [ML^2T^{-2}]$

Torque = F × d = $[ML^2T^{-2}]$

LHS and RHS has same dimensions.

b. Angular momentum (L)

$= mvr = [M][LT^{-1}][L]$

$= [ML^2T^{-1}]$

$$\text{Planck's constant } h = \frac{E}{\nu}$$

$$= \frac{[ML^2T^{-2}]}{[T^{-1}]} = [ML^2T^{-1}] \quad \left(\because E = h\nu \text{ and } \nu = \frac{1}{T}\right)$$

So, dimensions of h and L are equal.

c. Tension = force = $[MLT^{-2}]$

$$\text{Surface tension } = \frac{\text{force}}{\text{length}} = \frac{[MLT^{-2}]}{[L]}$$

$$= [ML^0T^{-2}]$$

d. Impulse = force × time = $[MLT^{-2}][T]$

$= [MLT^{-1}]$

Momentum = mass × velocity

$= [M][LT^{-1}] = [MLT^{-1}]$

LHS and RHS has same dimensions.

Hence only (c) options of Physical quantities does not have same dimensions.

7. (a) By applying the Rule of significant figure in multiplication and addition.

As given that,

$A = 2.5\text{ ms}^{-1} \pm 0.5\text{ ms}^{-1}, B = 0.10\text{ s} \pm 0.01\text{ s}$

$x = AB = (2.5)(0.10) = 0.25$ m (consider only significant figure value)

$$\frac{\Delta x}{x} = \frac{\Delta A}{A} + \frac{\Delta B}{B}$$

$$\frac{\Delta x}{x} = \frac{0.5}{2.5} + \frac{0.01}{0.10} = \frac{0.05 + 0.025}{0.25} = \frac{0.075}{0.25}$$

$\Delta x = 0.075 = 0.08$ m

(rounding off to two significant figures.)

$AB = (0.25 \pm 0.08)$ m

8. (d) As given that,

$A = 1.0\text{ m} \pm 0.2\text{ m}, B = 2.0\text{ m} \pm 0.2\text{ m}$

So, $X = \sqrt{AB} = \sqrt{(1.0)(2.0)} = 1.414$ m

Rounding off upto two significant digit

$X = 1.4\text{ m} = (r)$ (Let)

$$\frac{\Delta x}{x} = \frac{1}{2}\left[\frac{\Delta A}{A} + \frac{\Delta B}{B}\right] = \frac{1}{2}\left[\frac{0.2}{1.0} + \frac{0.2}{2.0}\right]$$

$$= \frac{0.6}{2 \times 2.0}$$

$$\Rightarrow \Delta x = \frac{0.6x}{2 \times 2.0} = \frac{0.6 \times 1.4}{2 \times 2.0} = 0.212$$

Rounding off upto one significant digit

$\Delta x = 0.2\text{ m} = \Delta r$ (Let)

So, correct value of

$\sqrt{AB} = r + \Delta r = (1.4 \pm 0.2)$ m

9. (a) For the most precise measurement, the unit must be least and number of digits including zeroes after decimal must be zero.

Now, take first option,

As here 5.00 mm has the smallest unit and the error in 5.00 mm is least (commonly taken as 0.01 mm if not specified), hence, 5.00 mm is most precise.

10. (a) Now, checking the errors with each options one by one,
$|\Delta l_1| = |5 - 4.9| = 0.1$ cm
$|\Delta l_2| = |5 - 4.805| = 0.195$ cm
$|\Delta l_3| = |5.25 - 5| = 0.25$ cm
$|\Delta l_4| = |5.4 - 5| = 0.4$ cm
Error Δl_1 is least or minimum.
So, 4.9 cm is most precise.

11. (c) It is given that Young's modulus (Y) is,
$Y = 1.9 \times 10^{11}$ N/m^2
1N = 10^5 dyne
So, $Y = 1.9 \times 10^{11} \times 10^5$ dyne/m^2
Convert meter to centimeter
$\because$ 1 m = 100 cm
$Y = 1.9 \times 10^{11} \times 10^5$ dyne/$(100)^2$ cm^2
$= 1.9 \times 10^{16-4}$ dyne/cm^2
$Y = 1.9 \times 10^{12}$ dyne/cm^2

12. (d) Given that fundamental quantities are momentum (p), area (A) and time (T).
Let us consider the dimensional formula for

$$E \propto [p^a A^b T^c]$$

$$E = kp^a A^b T^c]$$

where k is dimensionless constant of proportionality.
Dimensions of energy $[E] = [ML^2T^{-2}]$ and Dimension of momentum $p = mv = [MLT^{-1}]$
Dimension of Area $[A] = [L^2]$
Dimension of Time $[T] = [T]$
Dimension of energy $[E] = [K]\,[p]^a[A]^b[T]^c$
Putting all the dimensions, value
$ML^2T^{-2} = [MLT^{-1}]^a\,[L^2]^b\,[T]^c$
$= M^aL^{2b+a}T^{-a+c}$
By principle of homogeneity of dimensions,

$$a = 1,\ 2b + a = 2 \Rightarrow 2b + 1 = 2 \Rightarrow b = \frac{1}{2}$$

$$-a + c = -2$$
$$c = -2 + a = -2 + 1 = -1$$

So, Dimensional formula (of energy)
$E = [pA^{1/2}T^{-1}]$

$$E = [pA^{1/2}T^{-1}]$$

NEET/AIPMT (2013-2020) Questions

13. (d) $P = \frac{a^3b^2}{cd}$, $\frac{\Delta P}{P} \times 100\% = 3\frac{\Delta a}{a} \times 100\% + 2\frac{\Delta b}{b} \times 100\% + \frac{\Delta c}{c} \times 100\% + \frac{\Delta d}{d} \times 100\%.$
$= 3 \times 1\% + 2 \times 2\% + 3\% + 4\% = 14\%$

14. (d) Work = Force × displacement
Torque = Force × force arm
= mass × acceleration × length
$= [M] \times [LT^{-2}] \times [L] = [ML^2T^{-2}]$

15. (d) Force = mass × acceleration
$\Rightarrow$ [Mass]

$$= \left[\frac{\text{force}}{\text{acceleration}}\right]$$

$$= \left[\frac{\text{force}}{\text{velocity / time}}\right] = [FV^{-1}T]$$

16. (b) Let surface tension
$s = E^aV^bT^c$

$$\frac{MLT^{-2}}{L} = (ML^2T^{-2})^a\left(\frac{L}{T}\right)^b (T)^C$$

Equating the dimension of LHS and RHS
$ML^0T^{-2} = M^aL^{2a+b}T^{-2a-b+c}$
$\Rightarrow$ $a = 1, 2a + b = 0,\quad -2a - b + c = -2$
$\Rightarrow$ $a = 1, b = -2, c = -2$
Hence, the dimensions of surface tension are $[EV^{-2}T^{-2}]$

17. (d) Applying dimensional method :
$v_c = \eta^x\rho^y r^z$
$[M^0LT^{-1}] = [ML^{-1}T^{-1}]^x\,[ML^{-3}T^0]^y\,[M^0LT^0]^z$
Equating powers both sides
$x + y = 0; -x = -1 \therefore x = 1$
$1 + y = 0 \therefore y = -1$
$-x - 3y + z = 1$
$-1 - 3(-1) + z = 1$
$-1 + 3 + z = 1$
$\therefore z = -1$

18. (d) Let dimensions of length is related as,

$$L = [c]^x[G]^y\left[\frac{e^2}{4\pi\varepsilon_0}\right]^z$$

$$\frac{e^2}{4\pi\varepsilon_0} = ML^3T^{-2}$$

$L = [LT^{-1}]^x\,[M^{-1}L^3T^{-2}]^y[ML^3T^{-2}]^z$
$[L] = [L^{x+3y+3z}M^{-y+z}T^{-x-2y-2z}]$
Comparing both sides
$-y + z = 0 \Rightarrow y = z$ ...(i)
$x + 3y + 3z = 1$ ...(ii)
$-x - 4z = 0 \quad (\because y = z)$ ...(iii)
From (i), (ii) & (iii)

$$z = y = \frac{1}{2},\ x = -2$$

$$\text{Hence, } L = c^{-2}\left[G \cdot \frac{e^2}{4\pi\varepsilon_0}\right]^{1/2}$$

19. (c) Diameter of the ball
$= MSR + CSR \times (\ell east\ count) - zero\ error$
$= 0.5\ cm + 25 \times 0.001 - (-0.004)$
$= 0.5 + 0.025 + 0.004 = 0.529\ cm$

20. (d) In steady state, the amount of heat flowing from one face to the other face in time *dt* is given by

$$H = \frac{kA(T_1 - T_2)dt}{\ell}$$

$$\Rightarrow \frac{dH}{dt} = \frac{kA}{\ell}\Delta T\ (k = \text{coefficient of thermal conductivity})$$

$$\therefore k = \frac{\ell dH}{A\ dt\ \Delta T}$$

Unit of $k = Wm^{-1} K^{-1}$

21. (b) Given, $x = \frac{A^2 B^{1/2}}{C^{1/3} D^3}$

$$\%\ error,\ \frac{\Delta x}{x} \times 100 = 2\frac{\Delta A}{A} \times 100 + \frac{1}{2}\frac{\Delta B}{B} \times 100 + \frac{1}{3}\frac{\Delta C}{C} \times 100 + 3\frac{\Delta D}{D} \times 100$$

$$= 2 \times 1\% + \frac{1}{2} \times 2\% + \frac{1}{3} \times 3\% + 3 \times 4\%$$

$$= 2\% + 1\% + 1\% + 12\% = 16\%$$

22. (d) n VSD $= (n-1)$ MSD

$$1\ VSD = \frac{(n-1)}{n} MSD$$

$$L.C. = 1\ MSD - 1\ VSD = 1\ MSD - \frac{(n-1)}{n} MSD$$

$$= \frac{1}{n} MSD = \frac{1}{n} \times \frac{1}{n} = \frac{1}{n^2}$$

23. (c) Stress $= \frac{Force}{Area}$

Dimensions of force = $[MLT^{-2}]$
Dimensions of area = $[L^2]$

$$\therefore Stress = \frac{[MLT^{-2}]}{[L^2]} = [ML^{-1}T^{-2}]$$

24. (a) In subtraction the number of decimal places in the result should be equal to the number of decimal places of that term in the operation which contain lesser number of decimal places.

$$\begin{array}{r} 9.99 \\ -0.0099 \\ \hline 9.9801 \end{array}$$

As the least number of decimal places is 3. So, answer should be 9.98 m.

25. (b) Least count of screw gauge = 0.01 mm
Least count

$$= \frac{Pitch}{No.\ of\ divisions\ on\ circular\ scale}$$

$$\Rightarrow 0.01\ mm = \frac{Pitch}{50}$$

$\Rightarrow$ Pitch = 0.5 mm

Exercise 3 - Concept Application Problems CAP

1. (b) According to question

$E_y \propto J_x B_Z$

$\therefore$ Constant of proportionality

$$K = \frac{E_y}{B_Z J_x} = \frac{C}{J_x} = \frac{m^3}{As}$$

[As $\frac{E}{B} = C$ (speed of light) and $J = \frac{I}{Area}$]

2. (a) We know that

$$\text{Speed of light, } c = \frac{1}{\sqrt{\mu_0 \varepsilon_0}} = x$$

$$\text{Also, } c = \frac{E}{B} = y$$

Time constant, $\tau = Rc = t$

$$\therefore z = \frac{l}{Rc} = \frac{l}{t} = \text{Speed}$$

Thus, *x, y, z* will have the same dimension of speed.

3. (c) Energy, $E \propto A^a T^b P^c$

or, $E = kA^a T^b P^c$ ...(i)

where *k* is a dimensionless constant and *a, b* and *c* are the exponents.

Dimension of momentum, $P = M^1 L^1 T^{-1}$
Dimension of area, $A = L^2$
Dimension of time, $T = T^1$
Putting these value in equation (i), we get

$$M^1 L^2 T^{-2} = M^c L^{2a+c} T^{b-c}$$

by comparison
$c = 1$
$2a + c = 2$
$b - c = -2$
$c = 1, a = 1/2, b = -1$

$$\therefore E = A^{1/2} T^{-1} P^1$$

4. (a) $\sqrt{\frac{\mu_0}{\varepsilon_0}} = \sqrt{\frac{\mu_0^2}{\varepsilon_0 \mu_0}} = \mu_0 c \quad \left(\frac{1}{\sqrt{\mu_0 \varepsilon_0}} = c\right)$

$\mu_0 c \rightarrow MLT^{-2}A^{-2} \times LT^{-1}$
$ML^2T^{-3}A^{-2}$
Dimensions of resistance

5. (d) $\left[\sqrt{\frac{\varepsilon_0}{\mu_0}}\right] = \sqrt{\frac{\varepsilon_0^2}{\mu_0 \varepsilon_0}} = \left[\frac{\varepsilon_0}{\sqrt{\mu_0 \varepsilon_0}}\right] = \varepsilon_0 C[LT^{-1}] \times [\varepsilon_0]$

$$\left[\because \frac{1}{\sqrt{\mu_0 \varepsilon_0}} = C\right]$$

$\because F = \dfrac{q^2}{4\pi\varepsilon_0 r^2}$

$\Rightarrow [\varepsilon_0] = \dfrac{[AT]^2}{[MLT^{-2}]\times[L^2]} = [A^2M^{-1}L^{-3}T^4]$

$\therefore \left[\sqrt{\dfrac{\varepsilon_0}{\mu_0}}\right] = [LT^{-1}]\times[A^2M^{-1}L^{-3}T^4]$

$= [M^{-1}L^{-2}T^3A^2]$

6. (b) As we know,

$\left[\dfrac{\ell}{r}\right] = [T]$ and $[cv] = [AT]$

$\therefore \left[\dfrac{\ell}{rcv}\right] = \left[\dfrac{T}{AT}\right] = [A^{-1}]$

7. (b) Force of interaction between two atoms,

$F = \alpha\beta e^{\left(\frac{-x^2}{\alpha kT}\right)}$

Since exponential terms are dimensionless

$\therefore \left[\dfrac{x^2}{\alpha kT}\right] = M^0L^0T^0$

$\Rightarrow \dfrac{L^2}{[\alpha]ML^2T^{-2}} = M^0L^0T^0$

$\Rightarrow [\alpha] = M^{-1}T^2$

$[F] = [\alpha][\beta]$

$MLT^{-2} = M^{-1}T^2[\beta]$

$\Rightarrow [\beta] = M^2LT^{-4}$

8. (d) Let $[Y] = [V]^a[F]^b[A]^c$

$[ML^{-1}T^{-2}] = [LT^{-1}]^a[MLT^{-2}]^b[LT^{-2}]^c$

$[ML^{-1}T^{-2}] = [M^bL^{a+b+c}T^{-a-2b-2c}]$

Comparing power both side of similar terms we get,

$b = 1, a + b + c = -1, -a - 2b - 2c = -2$

solving above equations we get:

$a = -4, b = 1, c = 2$

so $[Y] = [V^{-4}FA^2] = [V^{-4}A^2F]$

9. (b) Dimension of $[h] = [ML^2T^{-1}]$

$[C] = [LT^{-1}]$

$[G] = [M^{-1}L^3T^{-2}]$

Hence dimension of

$\left[\sqrt{\dfrac{hC^5}{G}}\right] = \dfrac{[ML^2T^{-1}]\cdot[L^5T^{-5}]}{[M^{-1}L^3T^{-2}]}$

$= [ML^2T^{-2}] =$ energy

10. (d) The quantity $\dfrac{B^2}{2\mu_0}$ is the energy density of magnetic field.

$\Rightarrow \left[\dfrac{B^2}{2\mu_0}\right] = \dfrac{\text{Energy}}{\textit{Volume}} = \dfrac{\text{Force}\times\text{displacement}}{(\text{displacement})^3}$

$= \left[\dfrac{ML^2T^{-2}}{L^3}\right] = ML^{-1}T^{-2}$

11. (d) Given : $Z = \dfrac{a^2b^{2/3}}{\sqrt{cd^3}}$

Percentage error in Z,

$= \dfrac{\Delta Z}{Z} = \dfrac{2\Delta a}{a} + \dfrac{2}{3}\dfrac{\Delta b}{b} + \dfrac{1}{2}\dfrac{\Delta c}{c} + \dfrac{3\Delta d}{d}$

$= 2\times 2 + \dfrac{2}{3}\times 1.5 + \dfrac{1}{2}\times 4 + 3\times 2.5 = 14.5\%.$

12. (c) $\delta = \dfrac{M}{V} = \dfrac{M}{l^3} = Ml^{-3}$

$\dfrac{\Delta\delta}{\delta} = \dfrac{\Delta M}{M} + 3\dfrac{\Delta l}{l} = \dfrac{0.10}{10.00} + 3\left(\dfrac{0.01}{0.10}\right) = 0.31\text{ kg/m}^3$

13. (d) $A = 7\times 5.29 = 37.03\text{ cm}^2$

The result should have three significant figures, so $A = 37.0\text{ cm}^2$

14. (c) From Kepler's law, time period of a satellite,

$T = 2\pi\sqrt{\dfrac{r^3}{Gm}} \qquad T^2 = \dfrac{4\pi^2}{GM}r^3$

Relative uncertainty in the mass of the earth

$\left|\dfrac{\Delta M}{M}\right| = 2\dfrac{\Delta T}{T} = 2\times 10^{-2}$ ($\because$ 4π & G constant and relative uncertainty in radius $\dfrac{\Delta r}{r}$ negligible)

15. (c) Relative error in Surface area, $\dfrac{\Delta s}{s} = 2\times\dfrac{\Delta r}{r} = \alpha$ and relative error in volume, $\dfrac{\Delta v}{v} = 3\times\dfrac{\Delta r}{r}$

$\therefore$ Relative error in volume w.r.t. relative error in area,

$\dfrac{\Delta v}{v} = \dfrac{3}{2}\alpha$

16. (d) Surface tension, $T = \dfrac{rhg}{2}\times 10^3$

Relative error in surface tension,

$\dfrac{\Delta T}{T} = \dfrac{\Delta r}{r} + \dfrac{\Delta h}{h} + 0$ ($\because$ g, 2 & 10^3 are constant)

Percentage error

$100\times\dfrac{\Delta T}{T} = \left(\dfrac{10^{-2}\times 0.01}{1.25\times 10^{-2}} + \dfrac{10^{-2}\times 0.01}{1.45\times 10^{-2}}\right)100$

$= (0.8 + 0.689)$

$= (1.489) = 1.489\% \cong 1.5\%$

17. (c) Given, $P = a^{1/2} b^2 c^2 d^{-4}$,
Maximum relative error,

$$\frac{\Delta P}{P} = \frac{1}{2}\frac{\Delta a}{a} + 2\frac{\Delta b}{b} + 3\frac{\Delta c}{c} + 4\frac{\Delta d}{d}$$

$$= \frac{1}{2} \times 2 + 2 \times 1 + 3 \times 3 + 4 \times 5 = 32\%$$

18. (a)

19. (b) Pole strength, $m = \frac{M}{2\ell} = \frac{A\,m^2}{m} = A\,m.$

20. (d) Both energy and work have same unit.
$\therefore$ energy/work is a pure number.

21. (a) Moment of couple = force × distance = $[M^1 L^2 T^{-2}]$
work = force × distance = $[M^1 L^2 T^{-2}]$.

22. (b) Power $= \frac{\text{energy}}{\text{time}} = \frac{ML^2 T^{-2}}{T} = [ML^2 T^{-3}]$.

23. (b) Impedance $= \frac{V}{I} = \frac{W}{QI} = \frac{ML^2 T^{-2}}{Q\,QT^{-1}}$

$= [ML^2 T^{-1} Q^{-2}]$.

24. (c) We know that $\frac{Q^2}{2C}$ is energy of capacitor so it represent the dimension of energy $= [ML^2T^{-2}]$.

25. (a) Current density $= \frac{\text{Current}}{\text{area}} = \frac{Q}{\text{area} \times t}$

26. (d) From $\nu = \frac{1}{2\pi\sqrt{LC}}$

$$LC = \frac{1}{(2\pi\nu)^2} = \frac{1}{(T^{-1})^2} = T^2 = [M^0 L^0 T^2]$$

27. (b) In $p = p_0 \exp.(-\alpha t^2)$ is dimensionless

$$\therefore \alpha = \frac{1}{t^2} = \frac{1}{T^2} = [T^{-2}]$$

28. (c) Volume (L^3) = surface area $(6L^2)$
$\therefore$ L = 6, volume = $6^3 = 216$

29. (c) Effective resistance
$R_S = (10k\Omega \pm 10\%) + (20k\Omega \pm 20\%)$
$\therefore$ Tolerance of the combination = $(30k\Omega \pm 30\%)$

30. (a) Ratio of specific heat, $\gamma = \frac{C_p}{C_v}$

31. (b) Trigonometric ratio are a number and hence demensionless

32. (b) $[C] = \left[\frac{Q}{V}\right] = \left[\frac{Q^2}{W}\right] = [M^{-1}L^{-2}T^2Q^2]$

33. (a) η is the coefficient of viscosity.

34. (a) Velocity gradient is velocity per unit distance.

35. (a) $\frac{[ML^2T^{-2}][ML^2T^{-1}]^2}{[M^5][M^{-1}L^3T^{-2}]^2} = [M^0L^0T^0]$ = angle.

36. (c) $\frac{\Delta P}{P} \times 100 = \frac{\Delta F}{F} \times 100 + 2\frac{\Delta \ell}{\ell} \times 100 = 4\% + 2 \times 2\%$
$= 8\%$

37. (c) The quantity $(\frac{\omega x}{v} - \omega k)$ has dimension of angle and hence ωk is dimensionless being angle.

38. (d) $[V] = \left[\frac{W}{Q}\right] = \frac{ML^2T^{-2}}{AT} = ML^2A^{-1}T^{-3}$

39. (b) From $K = \frac{Bx}{x^2 + A^2} = \frac{Bx}{x^2} = \frac{B}{x}$

$\therefore$ B = K × x = K.E. × distance = work × distance

40. (c) We know that F = q v B

$$\therefore \ B = \frac{F}{qv} = \frac{MLT^{-2}}{C \times LT^{-1}} = MT^{-1}C^{-1}$$

41. (d) Pressure $= \frac{MLT^{-2}}{L^2} = [ML^{-1}T^{-2}]$

$\Rightarrow$ a = 1, b = − 1, c = − 2.

42. (b) In CGS system, $d = 4\frac{g}{cm^3}$
The unit of mass is 100g and unit of length is 10 cm, so

$$\text{density} = \frac{4\left(\frac{100g}{100}\right)}{\left(\frac{10}{10}cm\right)^3} = \frac{\left(\frac{4}{100}\right)}{\left(\frac{1}{10}\right)^3}\frac{(100g)}{(10cm)^3}$$

$$= \frac{4}{100} \times (10)^3 \cdot \frac{100g}{(10cm)^3} = 40 \text{ unit}$$

43. (c) From $T = 2\pi\sqrt{\frac{\ell}{g}}$; $g = 4\pi^2\frac{\ell}{T^2}$

$$\frac{\Delta g}{g} = \frac{\Delta \ell}{\ell} + \frac{2\Delta T}{T} = (y + 2x)$$

44. (b) The magnetic field at a point near a long straight conductor is given by

$$B = \frac{\mu_0}{4\pi}.\frac{2I}{r} \Rightarrow \mu_0 = \frac{4\pi r B}{2I}$$

$$\therefore \ [\mu_0] = \frac{[r][B]}{[I]} = \frac{L.MT^{-2}A^{-1}}{I} \quad \left(\because B = \frac{F}{qv}\right)$$
$$= MLT^{-2}A^{-2}$$

45. (c) Resistivity, $\rho = \frac{m}{ne^{2\tau}}$

$\rho = [ML^3T^{-3}A^{-2}]$
So, electrical conductivity

$$\sigma = \frac{1}{\rho}$$

$$\sigma = [M^{-1}L^{-3}T^3A^2]$$

3 Motion in a Straight Line

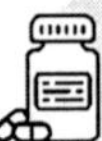

Topic 3.1 : Distance, Displacement, Speed & Velocity

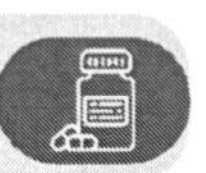

BASIC DEFINITIONS

Mechanics : Branch of physics, which deals with the study of objects in rest and in motion.

Statics : Study of objects at rest or in equilibrium.

Kinematics : Study of motion of objects without considering the cause of motion.

Dynamics : Study of motion of objects considering the cause of motion.

Rest : An object is said to be at rest if it does not change its position with time, with respect to its surrounding (a reference point which is generally taken as origin in numerical problems)

Motion : An object is said to be in motion if it changes its position with time, with respect to its surroundings.

Rest and motion are relative terms.

Point mass/Point object : An object is said to be a point mass if during its motion it covers distance much greater than its own size.

One dimensional motion : An object travels in a straight line. It is also called **rectilinear** or **linear motion**. The position change of the object with time in one dimension can be described by only one co-ordinate.

Ex. A stone falling freely under gravity.

Two dimensional motion or motion in a plane : For an object travelling in a plane two coordinates say X and Y are required to describe its motion.

Ex. An insect crawling over the floor.

Three dimensional motion : An object travels in space. To describe motion of objects in three dimension require all three coordinates x, y and z.

Ex. A kite flying in the sky.

DISTANCE AND DISPLACEMENT

Distance or Path length : *The length of the actual path travelled by an object during motion in a given interval of time is called the distance travelled by that object or path length.* It is a scalar quantity.

Displacement : *It is the shortest distance between the initial and final position of an object* and is directed from the initial position to the final position. It is a vector quantity.

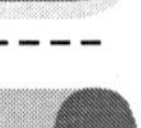

Problem Solving Tips

1. Displacement may be positive, negative or zero but distance is always positive.
2. Displacement is not affected by the shift of the coordinate axes.
3. Displacement of an object is independent of the path followed by the object but distance depends upon path.
4. Displacement and distance both have same unit as that of length i.e. metre.
5. $\frac{\text{Distance}}{|\text{Displacement}|} \geq 1$
6. For a moving body distance always increases with time
7. For a body undergoing one dimensional motion, in the same direction distance = | displacement |. For all other motion distance > | displacement |.

SPEED

It is the distance travelled per unit time by an object. It is a scalar quantity. It cannot be negative.

Uniform speed : An object is said to be moving with a uniform speed, if it covers equal distances in equal intervals of time, howsoever small the time intervals may be.

Non-uniform speed : If an object covers unequal distances in equal interval of time or equal distances in unequal interval of time.

Instantaneous speed : The speed of an object at a particular instant of time is called the instantaneous speed.

$$\textit{Instantaneous speed, } V_{inst} = \lim_{\Delta t \to 0} \frac{\Delta s}{\Delta t} = \frac{ds}{dt}.$$

Average speed : It is ratio of the total distance travelled by the object to the total time taken.

$$\textit{Average speed } V_{av} = \frac{\Delta x}{\Delta t}$$

Dimensions : $[M^0LT^{-1}]$; **Unit:** In SI systems.

VELOCITY

It is the displacement of an object per unit time. It is a vector quantity. It can be positive negative or zero.

Uniform velocity : An object is said to be moving with a uniform velocity, if it covers equal displacements in equal intervals of time, howsoever small the time intervals may be.

Non-uniform velocity : If an object covers unequal displacements in equal interval of time or equal displacements in unequal interval of time.

Instantaneous velocity : The velocity of an object at a particular instant of time is called the instantaneous velocity.

$$\textit{Instantaneous velocity, } \vec{V}_{inst} = \lim_{\Delta t \to 0} \frac{\Delta \vec{r}}{\Delta t} = \frac{d\vec{r}}{dt}.$$

Average Velocity : It is ratio of the total displacement to the total time taken.

$$\textit{Average velocity, } v_{av} = \frac{\Delta \vec{r}}{\Delta t}$$

Dimensions : $[M^0LT^{-1}]$; **Unit:** In SI system, m/s

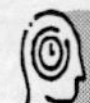

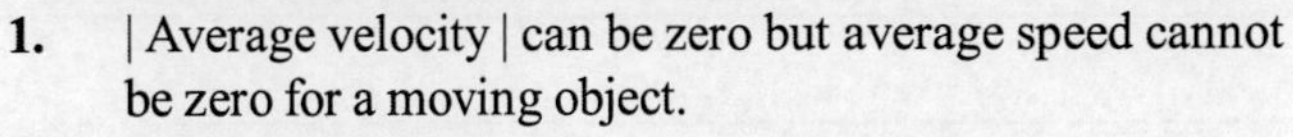

Problem Solving Tips

1. | Average velocity | can be zero but average speed cannot be zero for a moving object.
2. $\frac{|\text{Average velocity}|}{\text{Average speed}} \le 1$
3. | Instantaneous velocity | = Instantaneous speed.
4. A particle may have constant speed but variable velocity. It happens when particle travels in curvilinear path.
5. If the body covers first half distance with speed v_1 and next half with speed v_2 then

   Average speed $\bar{v} = \frac{2v_1v_2}{v_1 + v_2}$
6. If a body covers first one-third distance at a speed v_1, next one-third at speed v_2 and last one-third at speed v_3, then

   Average speed $\bar{v} = \frac{3v_1 v_2 v_3}{v_1 v_2 + v_2 v_3 + v_1 v_3}$
7. If a body travels with uniform speed v_1 for time t_1 and with uniform speed v_2 for time t_2, then

   Average speed $\bar{v} = \frac{v_1t_1 + v_2t_2}{t_1 + t_2}$

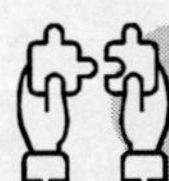

3.1 Concept Practice Problems

CPP

1. The displacement of a body is zero. The distance covered
   (a) is zero
   (b) is not zero
   (c) may or may not be zero
   (d) depends upon the acceleration
2. The slope of the velocity time graph for retarded motion is
   (a) positive (b) negative
   (c) zero (d) can be +ve, –ve or zero
3. If the displacement of a particle varies with time as $\sqrt{x} = t + 7$, the
   (a) velocity of the particle is inversely proportional to t
   (b) velocity of the particle is proportional to t
   (c) velocity of the particle is proportional to $\sqrt{t}$
   (d) the particle moves with a constant acceleration
4. The displacement-time graphs of two particles A and B are straight lines making angles of respectively 30° and 60° with the time axis. If the velocity of A is v_A and that of B is v_B, the value of v_A/v_B is
   (a) 1/2 (b) $1/\sqrt{3}$ (c) $\sqrt{3}$ (d) 1/3
5. A person travels along a straight road for the first half time with a velocity v_1 and the second half time with a velocity v_2. Then the mean velocity $\bar{v}$ is given by
   (a) $\bar{v} = \frac{v_1 + v_2}{2}$ (b) $\frac{2}{\bar{v}} = \frac{1}{v_1} + \frac{1}{v_2}$
   (c) $\bar{v} = \sqrt{v_1 v_2}$ (d) $\bar{v} = \sqrt{\frac{v_2}{v_1}}$
6. A particle covers half of the circle of radius r. Then the displacement and distance of the particle are respectively
   (a) $2\pi r, 0$ (b) $2r, \pi r$ (c) $\frac{\pi r}{2}, 2r$ (d) $\pi r, r$
7. A particle travels half the distance with a velocity of 6 ms^{-1}. The remaining half distance is covered with a velocity of 4 ms^{-1} for half the time and with a velocity of 8 ms^{-1} for the rest of the half time. What is the velocity of the particle averaged over the whole time of motion ?
   (a) 9 ms^{-1} (b) 6 ms^{-1} (c) 5.35 ms^{-1} (d) 5 ms^{-1}
8. A man leaves his house for a cycle ride. He comes back to his house after half-an-hour after covering a distance of one km. What is his average velocity for the ride ?
   (a) zero (b) 2 km h^{-1}
   (c) 10 km s^{-1} (d) $\frac{1}{2}$ km s^{-1}
9. A body moves in a straight line along Y-axis. Its distance y (in metre) from the origin is given by $y = 8t - 3t^2$. The average speed in the time interval from t = 0 second to t = 1 second is
   (a) – 4 ms^{-1} (b) zero (c) 5 ms^{-1} (d) 6 ms^{-1}
10. The displacement x of a particle varies with time t as $x = ae^{-\alpha t} + be^{\beta t}$, where a, b, α and β are positive constants. The velocity of the particle will
    (a) be independent of α and β
    (b) drop to zero when $\alpha = \beta$
    (c) go on decreasing with time
    (d) go on increasing with time

ANSWER KEY																			
1	(c)	2	(b)	3	(b)	4	(d)	5	(a)	6	(b)	7	(b)	8	(a)	9	(c)	10	(d)

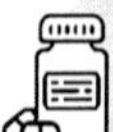

Topic 3.2 : Acceleration & Equations for Uniformly Accelerated Motion

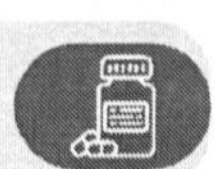

ACCELERATION

The rate of change of velocity with respect to time is called acceleration. It is a vector quantity.

Let velocity changes by $\Delta\vec{v}$ during some interval of time Δt.

Average acceleration $\vec{a}_{av}$ is given by

$$\vec{a}_{av} = \frac{\Delta\vec{v}}{\Delta t}$$

Instantaneous acceleration $\vec{a}$ is given by

$$\vec{a} = \lim_{\Delta t \to 0} \frac{\Delta\vec{v}}{\Delta t} = \frac{d\vec{v}}{dt}$$

Its **SI unit** is meter/sec^2 (ms^{-2}).

A body moving with uniform velocity has zero acceleration. It means that neither its speed nor its direction of motion is changing with time.

Uniform acceleration : If the velocity of the body changes in equal amount during same time interval, then the acceleration of the body is said to be uniform. Acceleration is uniform when neither its direction nor magnitude changes with respect to time.

Variable or non-uniform acceleration : If the velocity of body changes in different amounts during same time interval, then the acceleration of the body is known as variable acceleration. Acceleration is variable if either its direction or magnitude or both changes with respect to time. A good example of variable acceleration is the acceleration in uniform circular motion.

EQUATIONS FOR UNIFORMLY ACCELERATED MOTION

When the motion is uniformly accelerated i.e., when acceleration is constant in magnitude and direction :

(i) $v = u + at$

(ii) $s = ut + \frac{1}{2}at^2$

(iii) $v^2 - u^2 = 2as$

where u = initial velocity; v = final velocity;

a = uniform acceleration and

s = distance travelled in time t,

(iv) $s = \left(\frac{u+v}{2}\right)t$

(v) Distance travelled in nth second $s_n = u + \frac{a}{2}(2n-1)$;

s_n = distance covered in nth second

Above equations in vector form

$$\vec{v} = \vec{u} + \vec{a}t, \quad \vec{s} = \vec{u}t + \frac{1}{2}\vec{a}t^2,$$

$$\vec{v}^2 - \vec{u}^2 = 2\vec{a}.\vec{s} \quad (\text{or } \vec{v}.\vec{v} + \vec{u}.\vec{u} = 2\vec{a}.\vec{s})$$

$$\vec{s} = \frac{1}{2}(\vec{u} + \vec{v})t$$

When displacement (s) is given as a function of time t [s = f(t)] then

$s \propto t^0$	Body at rest	$v = 0$	$a = 0$
$s \propto t^1$	Uniform velocity; acceleration zero	$v \propto t^0$	$a = 0$
$s \propto t^2$	Uniform acceleration	$v \propto t^1$	$a \propto t^0$
$s \propto t^{3 \text{ or more}}$	Non uniform acceleration	$v \propto t^{2 \text{ or more}}$	$a \propto t^{1 \text{ or more}}$

We use calculus method (integration and differentiation) for displacement, velocity, acceleration as a function of time.

We know that $v = \frac{ds}{dt} \Rightarrow s = \int v\,dt$; $a = \frac{dv}{dt} \Rightarrow v = \int a\,dt$;

when a = f(s)

$$a = v\frac{dv}{ds} \Rightarrow \int a\,ds = \int v\,dv,$$

where s = displacement, v = instantaneous velocity,

a = instantaneous acceleration

Uniformly Accelerated Motion : A Discussion

While using equations of motion we can have two approaches.

Approach 1 : Take a = +ve when velocity increases and a = –ve when velocity decreases.

Take rest of physical quantities such as u, v, t and s as positive.

Approach 2 : (Vector method)

Assume one direction to be positive and other negative. Assign sign to all the vectors (u, v, a, s), +ve sign is given to a vector which is directed to the positive direction and vice-versa

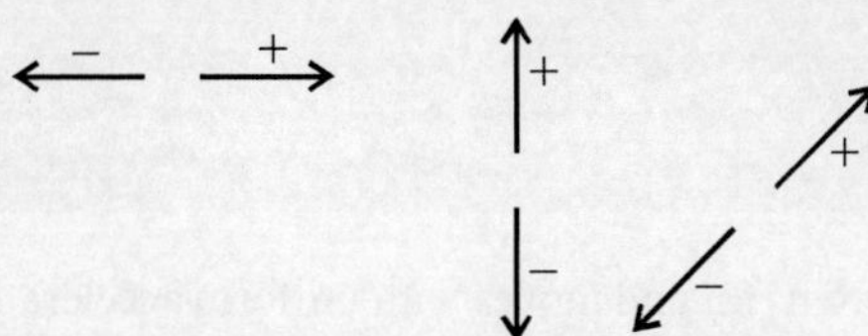

Normally the direction taken is as drawn above. But it is important to note that you can take any direction of your choice to be positive and the opposite direction to be negative.

NOTE: The second method (or approach) is useful only when there is reversal of motion during the activity concerned.

Problem Solving Tips

1. The direction of average acceleration vector is the direction of the change in velocity vector. $\vec{a} = \frac{\vec{v}_f - \vec{v}_i}{t}$

   $\vec{a}$ has a direction of $\vec{v}_f - \vec{v}_i = \vec{v}_f + (-\vec{v}_i)$

   i.e., the resultant of $\vec{v}_f$ and $-\vec{v}_i$

2. There is no definite relationship between velocity vector and acceleration vector.
3. For a body starting from rest and moving with uniform acceleration, the ratio of distances covered in t_1 sec., t_2 sec, t_3 sec, etc. are in the ratio $t_1^2 : t_2^2 : t_3^2$ etc.
4. A body moving with a velocity v is stopped by application of brakes after covering a distance *s*. If the same body moves with a velocity nv, it stops after covering a distance n^2s by the application of same retardation.

Example 1.

The displacement of particle is zero at t = 0 and displacement is 'x' at t = t. It starts moving in the positive x-direction with a velocity which varies as $v = k\sqrt{x}$ where k is constant. Show that the velocity varies with time.

Solution :

$$v = k\sqrt{x} \quad \text{or} \quad \frac{dx}{dt} = k\sqrt{x} \quad \text{or} \quad \frac{dx}{\sqrt{x}} = k\,dt$$

Given that when t = 0, x = 0 and when t = t, x = x,

$$\text{Hence} \int_0^x \frac{dx}{\sqrt{x}} = \int_0^t k\,dt\,;$$

$$\therefore \int_0^x x^{-1/2}dx = k\int_0^t dt \quad \text{or} \quad \left[\frac{x^{-\frac{1}{2}+1}}{-\frac{1}{2}+1}\right]_0^x = k[t]_0^t$$

$$\text{or } 2\sqrt{x} = kt \quad \text{or} \quad \sqrt{x} = \frac{kt}{2}$$

$$\text{Now, } v = k \times \left[\frac{kt}{2}\right] = \frac{k^2t}{2}$$

Thus the velocity varies with time.

Example 2.

A particle covers each 1/3 of the total distance with speed v_1, v_2 and v_3 respectively. Find the average speed of the particle.

Solution :

Average speed

$$\bar{v} = \frac{\text{Total distance travelled}}{\text{Total time taken}} = \frac{s}{\frac{s}{3v_1} + \frac{s}{3v_2} + \frac{s}{3v_3}}$$

$$\Rightarrow \bar{v} = \frac{3v_1v_2v_3}{v_1v_2 + v_2v_3 + v_3v_1}$$

Example 3.

A cheetah can accelerate from 0 to 96 km/h in 2 sec., whereas a cat requires 6 sec. Compute the average accelerations for the cheetah and cat.

Solution :

$$\text{For cheetah } |\vec{a}_{av}| = \frac{|\vec{v}_f - \vec{v}_i|}{\Delta t} = \frac{96\text{km/h} - 0}{2\text{sec}}$$

$$= \frac{96 \times \frac{1000\text{ m}}{3600\text{ sec}}}{2\text{ sec}} = 15 \text{ m/s}^2$$

$$\text{For cat } |\vec{a}_{av}| = \frac{96 \times \frac{10}{36}}{6} = 5 \text{ m/s}^2.$$

Example 4.

A particle is moving in east direction with speed 5 m/s. After 10 sec it starts moving in north direction with same speed. Find average acceleration.

Solution :

$|\vec{v}_f| = |\vec{v}_i| = 5$ m/s

Acceleration ≠ 0

(due to change in direction of velocity Av. acceleration,

N
W E
S

$$\Delta\vec{v} = \vec{v}_f - \vec{v}_i = \vec{v}_f + (-\vec{v}_i)$$

$$\vec{a} = \frac{\vec{v}_f - \vec{v}_i}{\Delta t} = \frac{5\hat{j} - 5\hat{i}}{10} \Rightarrow \vec{a} = -\frac{1}{2}\hat{i} + \frac{1}{2}\hat{j}$$

$$|\vec{a}| = \sqrt{\left(\frac{1}{2}\right)^2 + \left(\frac{1}{2}\right)^2} = \frac{1}{\sqrt{2}} \text{ m/s}^2.$$

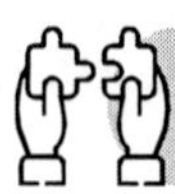

3.2 Concept Practice Problems

CPP

11. A bus starts moving with acceleration 2 m/s^2. A cyclist 96 m behind the bus starts simultaneously towards the bus at 20 m/s. After what time will he be able to overtake the bus?
(a) 4 sec (b) 8 sec
(c) 12 sec (d) 16 sec

12. When the speed of a car is v, the minimum distance over which it can be stopped is s. If the speed becomes n v, what will be the minimum distance over which it can be stopped during same retardation
(a) s/n (b) n s (c) s/n^2 (d) n^2 s

13. The two ends of a train moving with constant acceleration pass a certain point with velocities u and v. The velocity with which the middle point of the train passes the same point is
(a) $(u+v)/2$ (b) $(u^2+v^2)/2$
(c) $\sqrt{(u^2+v\upsilon^2)/2}$ (d) $\sqrt{u^2+v^2}$

14. A particle accelerates from rest at a constant rate for some time and attains a velocity of 8 m/sec. Afterwards it decelerates with the constant rate and comes to rest. If the total time taken is 4 sec, the distance travelled is
(a) 32m (b) 16m
(c) 4m (d) None of the above

15. The velocity of a particle at an instant is 10 m/s. After 5 sec, the velocity of the particle is 20 m/s. Find the velocity at 3 seconds before from the instant when velocity of a particle is 10m/s.
(a) 8 m/s (b) 4 m/s (c) 6 m/s (d) 7 m/s

16. A body covers 26, 28, 30, 32 meters in 10th, 11th, 12th and 13th seconds respectively. The body starts
(a) from rest and moves with uniform velocity
(b) from rest and moves with uniform acceleration
(c) with an initial velocity and moves with uniform acceleration
(d) with an initial velocity and moves with uniform velocity

17. The displacement x of a particle at the instant when its velocity is v is given by $v=\sqrt{3x+16}$. Its acceleration and initial velocity are
(a) 1.5 units, 4 units (b) 3 units, 4 units
(b) 16 units, 1.6 units (d) 16 units, 3 units

18. A car accelerates from rest at a constant rate α for some time after which it decelerates at a constant rate β to come to rest. If the total time elapsed is t, the maximum velocity acquired by the car is given by

(a) $\left(\dfrac{\alpha^2+\beta^2}{\alpha\beta}\right)t$ (b) $\left(\dfrac{\alpha^2-\beta^2}{\alpha\beta}\right)t$

(c) $\left(\dfrac{\alpha+\beta}{\alpha\beta}\right)t$ (d) $\left(\dfrac{\alpha\beta}{\alpha+\beta}\right)t$

19. A car moving with a speed of 40 km/hour can be stopped by applying brakes after at least 2m. If the same car is moving with a speed of 80km/hour, what is the minimum stopping distance.
(a) 8m (b) 6m (c) 4m (d) 2m

20. A body starts from rest, what is the ratio of the distance travelled by the body during the 4th and 3rd seconds ?
(a) $\frac{7}{5}$ (b) $\frac{5}{7}$ (c) $\frac{7}{3}$ (d) $\frac{3}{7}$

ANSWER KEY

11	(b)	12	(d)	13	(c)	14	(b)	15	(b)	16	(c)	17	(a)	18	(d)	19	(a)	20	(a)

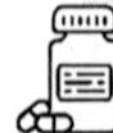

Topic 3.3 : Motion under Gravity; Graphs Related to Motion & Relative Velocity

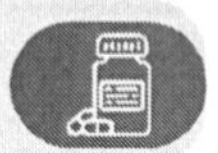

MOTION UNDER GRAVITY

(i) For a body thrown downward with initial velocity u from a height h, the equations of motion are

$$v = u + gt;\ v^2 = u^2 + 2gh$$

$$h = ut + \frac{1}{2}gt^2;\ h_{n^{th}} = u + \frac{g}{2}(2n-1)$$

(ii) If initial velocity is zero, then the equations are

$$v = gt;\ v = \sqrt{2gh}$$

$$h = \frac{1}{2}gt^2;\ h_{n^{th}} = \frac{g}{2}(2n-1)$$

(iii) When a body is thrown upwards with initial velocity u, the equations of motion are

$$v = u - gt$$

$$h = ut - \frac{1}{2}gt^2$$

$$v^2 = u^2 - 2gh.$$

To summarise :

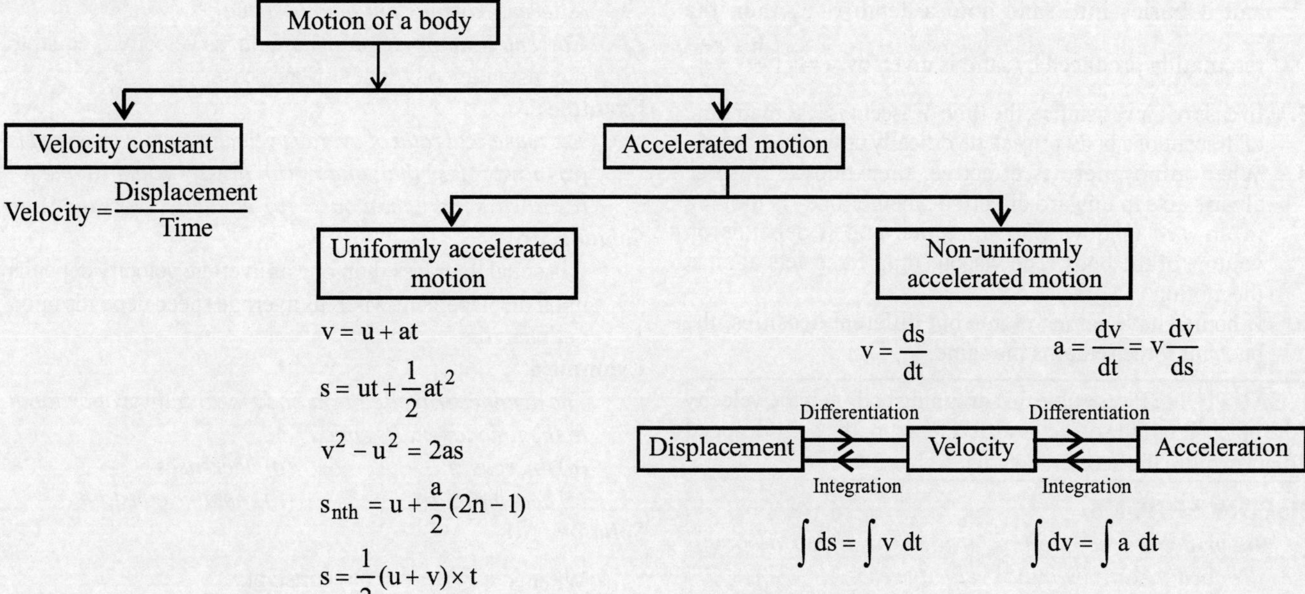

NOTE: Calculus method as shown in non-uniformly accelerated motion may also be used for uniformly accelerated motion.

Problem Solving Tips

1. An object moving under the influence of earth's gravity in which air resistance and small changes in g are neglected is called a freely falling body.
2. In the absence of air resistance, the velocity of projection is equal to the velocity with which the body strikes the ground.
3. Distance travelled by a freely falling body in 1st second is always half of the numerical value of g or 4.9 m, irrespective of height h.
4. For a freely falling body with initial velocity zero
   (i) Velocity $\propto$ time ($v = gt$)
   (ii) Velocity $\propto \sqrt{\text{Distance fallen}}$ ($v^2 = 2gs$)
   (iii) Distance fallen α (time)^2 $\left(s = \frac{1}{2}gt^2\right)$, where g is the acceleration due to gravity.
5. If maximum height attained by a body projected vertically upwards is equal to the magnitude of velocity of projection, then velocity of projection is $2g$ ms^{-1} and time of flight is 4 sec.
6. If maximum height attained by a body projected upward is equal to magnitude of acceleration due to gravity i.e., 'g', the time of ascent is $\sqrt{2}$ sec. and velocity of projection is $g\sqrt{2}$.
7. Ratio of maximum heights reached by different bodies projected with velocities u_1, u_2, u_3 etc. are in the ratio of $u_1^2 : u_2^2 : u_3^3$ etc. and ratio of times of ascent are in ratio of $u_1 : u_2 : u_3$ etc.
8. During free fall velocity increases by equal amount every decend and distance covered during 1st, 2nd, 3rd seconds of fall, are 4.9m, 14.7m, 24.5m.

   u = 0 — t = 0 — 4.9 m
   9.8 m/s — t = 1 — 14.7 m
   19.6 m/s — t = 2 — 24.5 m
   29.4 m/s — t = 3

9. If a body is projected horizontally from top of a tower, the time taken by it to reach the ground does not depend on the velocity of projection, but depends on the height of tower and is equal to $t = \sqrt{\frac{2h}{g}}$.
10. If velocity v of a body changes its direction by θ without change in magnitude then the change in velocity will be $2v\sin\frac{\theta}{2}$.
11. From the top of a tower a body is projected upward with a certain speed, 2nd body is thrown downward with same speed and 3rd is let to fall freely from same point then $t_3 = \sqrt{t_1 t_2}$
    where t_1 = time taken by the body projected upward, t_2 = time taken by the body thrown downward and t_3 = time taken by the body falling freely.

12. If a body falls freely from a height h on a sandy surface and it buries into sand upto a depth of x, then the retardation produced by sand is given by $a = g\left(\frac{h+x}{x}\right)$.
13. In case of air resistance, the time of ascent is less than time of descent of a body projected vertically upward i.e. $t_a < t_d$.
14. When atmosphere is effective, then buoyancy force always acts in upward direction whether body is moving in upward or downward direction and it depends on volume of the body. The viscous drag force acts against the motion.
15. If bodies have same volume but different densities, the buoyant force remains the same.

⚠ **CAUTION :** Please note that dropping body gets the velocity of the object but if the object is in acceleration, the body dropped will not acquire the acceleration of the object.

MISCONCEPTIONS

✘ ***Incorrect.*** *In the question, if it is given that a body is dropped, taking its initial velocity zero.*

✔ ***Correct.*** The initial velocity is zero if the object dropping the body is also at rest (zero velocity). But if the object dropping the body is having a velocity, then the body being dropped will also have initial velocity which will be same as that of the object.

For example :

(a) When an aeroplane flying horizontally drops a bomb.
(b) An ascending helicopter dropping a food packet.
(c) A stone dropped from a moving train etc.

✘ ***Incorrect.*** *Applying equations of motion in case of non-uniform acceleration of the body.*

✔ ***Correct.*** The equations of motion are for uniformly accelerated motion of the body.
Please note that when the case is of non-uniform acceleration we use calculus (differentiation and integration). $a = \frac{dv}{dt} = \frac{vdv}{ds}$; $v = \frac{ds}{dt}$.
In fact calculus method is a universal method which can be used both in case of uniform as well as non-uniform acceleration.

✘ ***Incorrect.*** *Taking average velocity same as that of instantaneous velocity.*

✔ ***Correct.*** Average velocity $= \vec{V}_{av} = \frac{\Delta\vec{r}}{\Delta t} = \frac{\vec{r}_f - \vec{r}_i}{t_f - t_i}$

(where $\vec{r}_i$ is position vector at time t_i and $\vec{r}_f$ is position vector at time t_f).
Whereas instantaneous velocity

$$\vec{V}_{inst.} = \lim_{\Delta t \to 0} \frac{\Delta\vec{r}}{\Delta t} = \frac{d\vec{r}}{dt}$$

It is important to note that average velocity is equal to instantaneous velocity only when the case is of uniform velocity.

✘ ***Incorrect.*** *Taking acceleration as negative (– a) even when acceleration is an unknown.*

✔ ***Correct.*** Take acceleration as (a) when it is unknown even if we know that the motion is a case of deceleration or retardation. On solving, we will find the value of (a) to be negative .

✘ ***Incorrect.*** *Magnitude of instantaneous velocity is different from instantaneous speed .*

✔ ***Correct.*** Magnitude of instantaneous velocity is equal to the instantaneous speed in any case.

Example 5.

The numerical ratio of average velocity to average speed is

(a) always less than one *(b) always equal to one*
(c) always more than one *(d) equal to or less than one*

Solution : **(d)**

It is equal to or less than one as average velocity depends upon displacement whereas average speed depends upon path length.

Example 6.

The distance travelled by a body is directly proportional to the time taken. Its speed

(a) increases *(b) decreases*
(c) becomes zero *(d) remains constant*

Solution : **(d)**

When $s \propto t$, so $\frac{s}{t} = v =$ constant.

Example 7.

A particle is projected vertically upwards. Prove that it will be at 3/4 of its greatest height at time which are in the ratio 1 : 3.

Solution :

If u is the initial velocity of a particle while going vertically upwards, then the maximum height attained is $h = \frac{u^2}{2g}$.

If t is the time when particle reaches at a height $\frac{3}{4}h$, then using the relation

$s = ut + \frac{1}{2}at^2$; we have $\frac{3}{4}h = ut + \frac{1}{2}(-g)t^2$

or, $\frac{3}{4}\left(\frac{u^2}{2g}\right) = ut - \frac{1}{2}gt^2$ or $t^2 - \frac{2u}{g}t + \frac{3}{4}\frac{u^2}{g^2} = 0$

Solving it for t, we have

$$t = \frac{\frac{2u}{g} \pm \sqrt{\frac{4u^2}{g^2} - 4 \times 1 \times \frac{3}{4}\frac{u^2}{g^2}}}{2} = \frac{u}{g} \pm \frac{u}{2g}$$

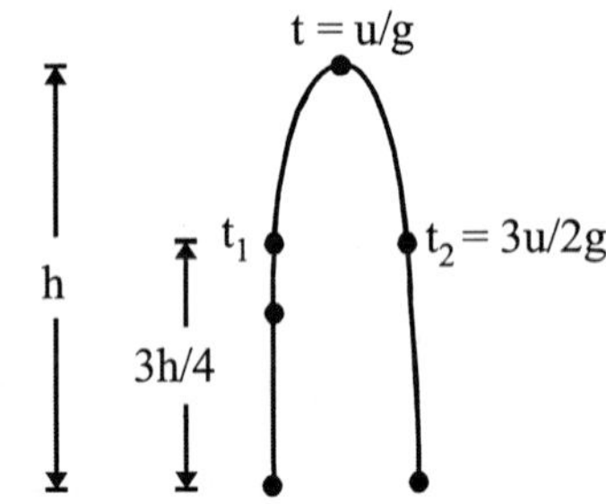

Taking negative sign, $t_1 = \frac{u}{g} - \frac{u}{2g} = \frac{u}{2g}$;

Taking positive sign, $t_2 = \frac{u}{g} + \frac{u}{2g} = 3u/2g.$

$$\frac{t_1}{t_2} = \left(\frac{u/2g}{3u/2g}\right) = \frac{1}{3}.$$

Example 8.

A police party in a jeep is chasing a dacoit on a straight road. The jeep is moving with a maximum uniform speed v. The dacoit rides on a motorcycle of his waiting friend when the jeep is at a distance d from him and the motorcycle starts with constant acceleration a. Show that the dacoit will be caught if $v \geq \sqrt{2ad}$.

Solution :

Suppose the dacoit is caught at a time t sec after the motorcycle starts. The distance travelled by the motorcycle during this interval is

$$s = \frac{1}{2}at^2 \quad ...(1)$$

During the interval, the jeep travels a distance,

$$s + d = vt \quad ...(2)$$

By (1) and (2), $\frac{1}{2}at^2 - vt + d = 0$ or $t = \frac{v \pm \sqrt{v^2 - 2ad}}{a}$

The dacoit will be caught if t is real and positive. This will be possible if $v^2 - 2ad > 0$ or $v > \sqrt{2ad}$.

Example 9.

Two trains, each of length 100 m, are running on parallel tracks. One overtakes the other in 20 second and one crosses the other in 10 second. Calculate the velocities of each train.

Solution :

Let u and v be the velocities of the trains.

The relative velocity of overtaking is u – v while the relative velocity of crossing is u + v.

Total distance = 100 + 100 = 200 m.

$$\therefore \; 20 = \frac{200}{u - v} \text{ or } u - v = 10$$

$$\text{and } 10 = \frac{200}{u + v} \text{ or } u + v = 20$$

By solving, we get, u = 15 m/sec and v = 5 m/sec.

Example 10.

A body starts from rest and moves with a uniform acceleration. The ratio of the distance covered in the nth sec to the distance covered in n sec is

(a) $\frac{2}{n} - \frac{1}{n^2}$ *(b)* $\frac{1}{n^2} - \frac{1}{n}$

(c) $\frac{2}{n^2} - \frac{1}{n^2}$ *(d)* $\frac{2}{n} + \frac{1}{n^2}$

Solution : **(a)**

The distance covered in nth second

$$s_n = u + \frac{a}{2}(2n - 1) \text{ or } s_n = 0 + \frac{a}{2}(2n - 1) \quad ...(1)$$

Further distance covered in n second

$$s = ut + \frac{1}{2}at^2 = 0 + \frac{1}{2}an^2 \quad ...(2)$$

$$\therefore \; \frac{s_n}{s} = \frac{\frac{a}{2}(2n-1)}{(an^2/2)} = \frac{2}{n} - \frac{1}{n^2}$$

Example 11.

The water drop falls at regular intervals from a tap 5 m above the ground. The third drop is leaving the tap at instant the first drop touches the ground. How far above the ground is the second drop at that instant?

(a) 1.25 m *(b) 2.50 m*

(c) 3.75 m *(d) 4.00 m*

Solution : **(c)**

See fig. Let t be the time interval between any two drops.

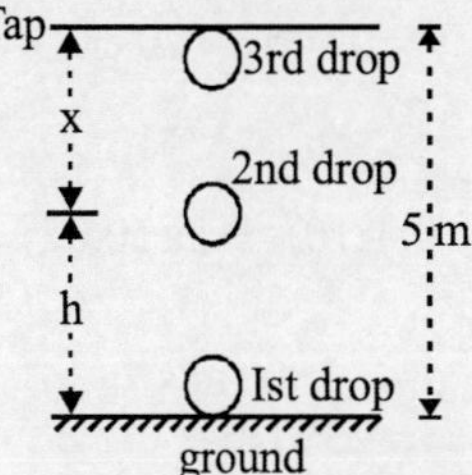

For third drop $5 = \frac{1}{2}g(2t)^2$ or $gt^2 = 5/2$

For second drop $x = \frac{1}{2}gt^2$ or $x = \frac{1}{2} \times \frac{5}{2} = \frac{5}{4} = 1.25\,m$

Therefore $h = 5 - x = 5 - 1.25 = 3.75$ m

Hence option (c)

Example 12.

The height of a tower is h metre. A body is thrown from the top of tower vertically upward with some speed, it takes t_1, second to reach the ground. Another body thrown from the top of tower with same speed downwards and takes t_2 seconds to reach the ground. If third body, released from same place takes 't' second to reach the ground, then

(a) $t = \frac{t_1 + t_2}{2}$ *(b)* $t = \frac{t_1}{t_2}$

(c) $\frac{2}{t} = \frac{1}{t_1} + \frac{1}{t_2}$ *(d)* $t = \sqrt{(t_1 t_2)}$

Solution : **(d)**

Let u be the initial velocity of the body. Then at time t_1

$$h = -ut_1 + \frac{1}{2}gt_1^2 \quad ...(1)$$

and at time t_2, $h = ut_2 + \frac{1}{2}gt_2^2$ ...(2)

From eqs. (1) and (2), we get

$$-ut_1 + \frac{1}{2}gt_1^2 = ut_2 + \frac{1}{2}gt_2^2$$

$$\text{or } \frac{1}{2}g(t_1^2 - t_2^2) = u(t_1 + t_2)$$

$$\text{or } \frac{1}{2}g(t_1 + t_2)(t_1 - t_2) = u(t_1 + t_2)$$

or $u = \frac{1}{2}g(t_1 - t_2)$ ...(3)

Substituting the value of u in eqn. (2) we get

$$h = \frac{1}{2}g(t_1 - t_2)t_2 + \frac{1}{2}gt_2^2 \quad \text{or} \quad h = \frac{1}{2}gt_1t_2 \quad ...(4)$$

For third body, $h = \frac{1}{2}gt^2$ ...(5)

From eqs. (4) and (5) we get, $t = \sqrt{t_1t_2}$

Example 13.

A bullet moving with a speed 10 m/s hits the wooden plank and is stopped when it penetrates the plank 20 cm deep. Calculate retardation of the bullet.

Solution :

$v_0 = 10$ m/s, $v = 0$ and $s = 20$ cm. $= \frac{2}{100} = 0.02$m

Using $v^2 - v_0^2 = 2ax$

$$0 - (10)^2 = 2a\,(0.02) \Rightarrow \frac{-100}{2 \times 0.02} = a$$

or $a = -2500$ m/s^2

Retardation $= 2500$ m/s^2

Example 14.

A body covers a distance of 20m in the 7th second and 24m in the 9th second. How much distance shall it cover in 15th sec?

Solution :

From formula, $S_{n^{th}} = u + \frac{1}{2}a(2n - 1)$

$S_7th = u + \frac{a}{2}(2 \times 7 - 1)$ but $S_7th = 20$m

$\therefore \quad 20 = u + \frac{a}{2} \times 13 \Rightarrow 20 = u + \frac{13a}{2}$ ... (1)

also $s_9th = 24$m $\quad \therefore \; 24 = u + \frac{17a}{2}$ ... (2)

From eq^n. (1) $u = 20 - \frac{13a}{2}$ ... (3)

Substitute this value of in eq^n. (2)

$$24 = 20 - \frac{13a}{2} + \frac{17a}{2}$$

$$24 - 20 = \frac{17a}{2} - \frac{13a}{2}$$

$$4 = \frac{4a}{2} \Rightarrow 4 = 2a \Rightarrow a = \frac{4}{2} = 2\text{ m/s}^2$$

Substituting this value of a in eqn. (3) $u = 20 - \frac{13a}{2}$

$$\Rightarrow u = 20 - \frac{13 \times 2}{2} \Rightarrow u = 20 - 13$$

$\therefore \quad u = 7$ m/s

Now, $s_{15th} = u + \frac{a}{2}(2 \times 15 - 1)$

$$= 7 + \frac{2}{2}(29) = 7 + 29 = 36\text{m}$$

Example 15.

A train starts from rest and for the first kilometer moves with constant acceleration, for the next 3 kilometers it has constant velocity and for another 2 kilometers it moves with constant retardation to come to rest after 10 min. Find the maximum velocity and the three time intervals in the three types of motion.

Solution :

Let the three time intervals be t_1 min, t_2 min, and t_3 min. respectively. Let the maximum velocity attained be v m/min.

A t_1 B v–t_2 C t_3 D
1000m 3000m 2000m

For A to B $\quad 1000 = \left(\frac{0 + v}{2}\right)t_1 \Rightarrow 2000 = vt_1$ ....(1)

For B to C $\quad 3000 = vt_2$ ....(2)

[Using in both equations disp. = mean vel. × time]

and for C to D $\quad 2000 = \left(\frac{v + 0}{2}\right)t_3 \Rightarrow 4000 = vt_3$ ...... (3)

Adding eqs. (1), (2) and (3), we get

$$9000 = v\,(t_1 + t_2 + t_3)$$

$$\therefore \; v = \frac{9000}{10} = 900\text{ m/min.} = \frac{900 \times 10^{-3}}{1/60\text{ hr.}}\text{km} = 54\text{ km/hr.}$$

Now, from eqs. (1), (2) and (3) we get

$$t_1 = \frac{2000}{900} = \frac{20}{9} = 2\frac{2}{9}\text{min.},$$

$$t_2 = \frac{3000}{900} = \frac{10}{9} = 3\frac{1}{3}\text{min.}$$

$$\text{and } t_3 = \frac{4000}{900} = \frac{40}{9} = 4\frac{4}{9}\text{min.}$$

Example 16.

A falling stone takes 0.2 seconds to fall past a window which is 1m high. From how far above the top of the window was the stone dropped ?

Solution :

$$h = \frac{1}{2}gt^2; \; h + 1 = \frac{1}{2}g(t + 0.2)^2$$

$$\frac{1}{2}gt^2 + 1 = \frac{1}{2}gt^2 + \frac{1}{2}g(0.2)^2 + \frac{1}{2}g \times 2 \times 0.2t$$

u=0
h
1m
Δt=0.2sec

$$1 = \frac{1}{5} + 0.2gt \; ; \; \frac{4}{5} = 2t \Rightarrow t = \frac{2}{5}$$

$$h = \frac{1}{2}g\frac{4}{25} = \frac{4}{5}\text{m}$$

Example 17.

From the top of a multi-storeyed building 40m tall, a boy projects a stone vertically upwards with an initial velocity of 10 ms^{-1} such that it eventually falls to the ground. (i) After how long will the stone strike the ground ? (ii) After how long will it pass through the point from where it was projected ? (iii) What will be its velocity when it strikes the ground ? Take g = 10 ms^{-2}.

Solution :

Using, $\vec{S} = \vec{u}t + \frac{1}{2}\vec{a}t^2$

(i) $-40 = 10t - \frac{1}{2}gt^2$ or $-40 = 10t - 5t^2$

[$\because$ taking $g = 10 m/s^2$]

or $5t^2 - 10t - 40 = 0$

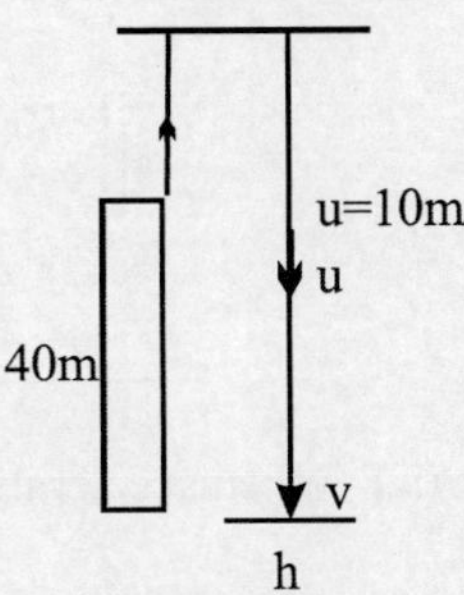

or $t = \frac{10 + \sqrt{10^2 - 4\times5(-40)}}{2\times5} = \frac{10+\sqrt{100+800}}{10}$

$= \frac{10+30}{10} = 4$ sec.

(ii) It will pass from where it was projected after

$t = \frac{2\times10}{g} = 2$ sec.

(iii) Velocity with which stone strikes the ground

$V = 10 + g\times2 = 30$ m/s

VARIOUS GRAPHS RELATED TO MOTION

(a) **Displacement-time graph -** In this graph time is plotted on x-axis and displacement on y-axis.

(i) For a stationary body (v = 0) the time-displacement graph is a straight line parallel to time axis.

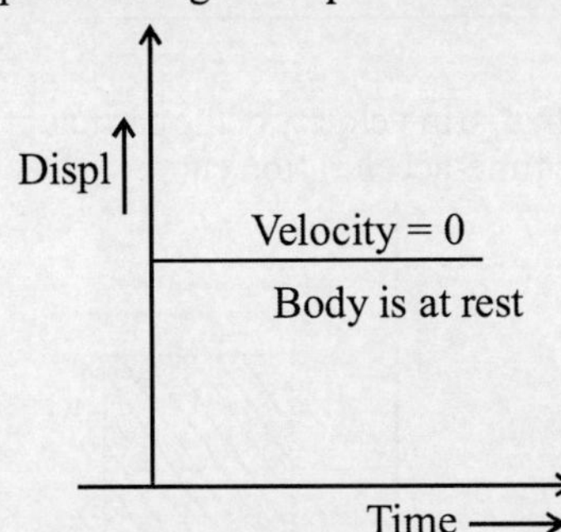

(ii) When the velocity of a body is constant then time-displacement graph will be an oblique straight line.

Greater the slope $\left(\frac{dx}{dt} = \tan\theta\right)$ of the straight line, higher will be the velocity.

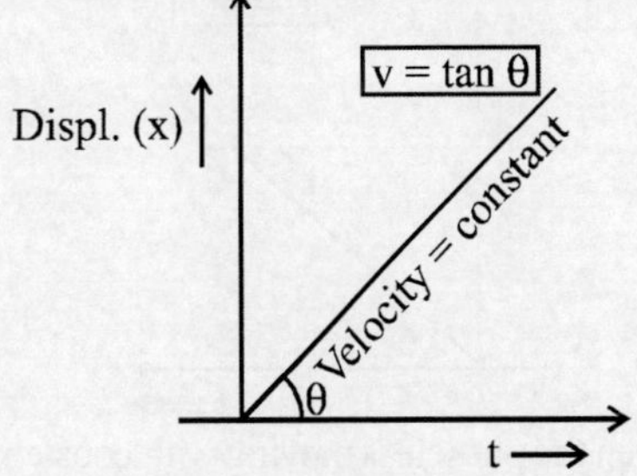

(iii) If the velocity of a body is not constant then the time-displacement curve is a zig-zag curve.

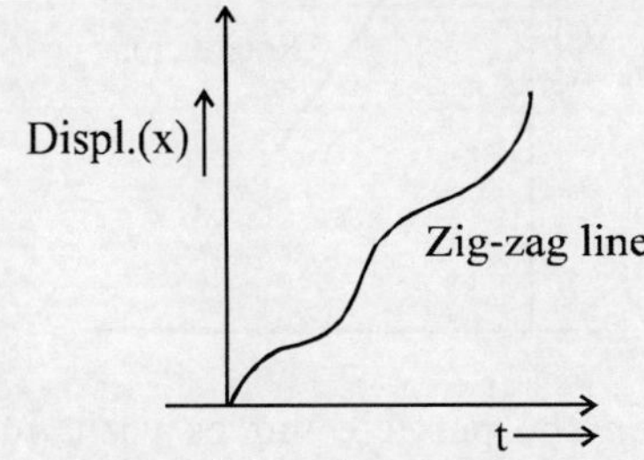

(iv) For an accelerated motion the slope of time-displacement curve increases with time while for decelerated motion it decreases with time.

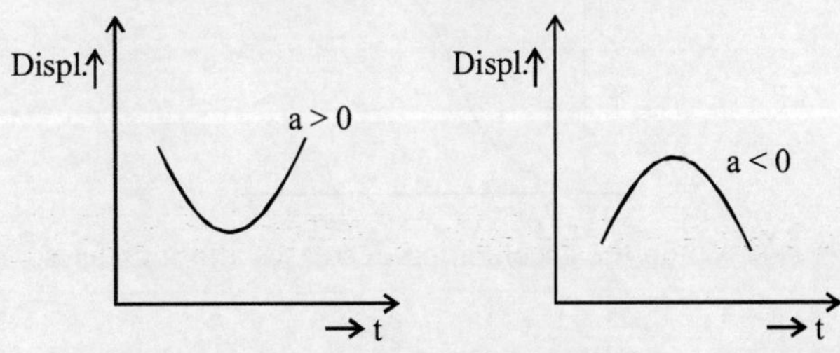

(v) When the particle returns towards the point of reference then the time-displacement line makes an angle θ > 90° with the time axis.

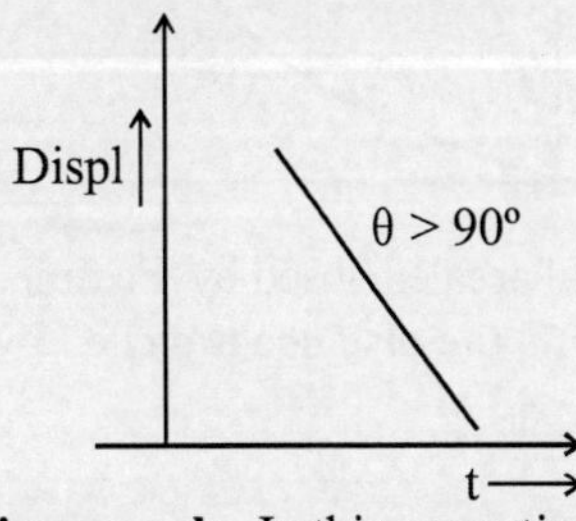

(b) **Velocity-time graph -** In this curve time is plotted along x-axis and velocity is plotted along y-axis.

(i) When the velocity of the particle is constant or acceleration is zero.

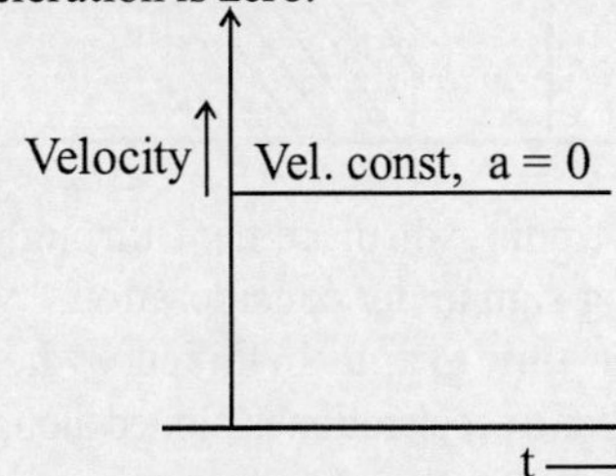

(ii) When the particle is moving with a constant acceleration and its initial velocity is zero.

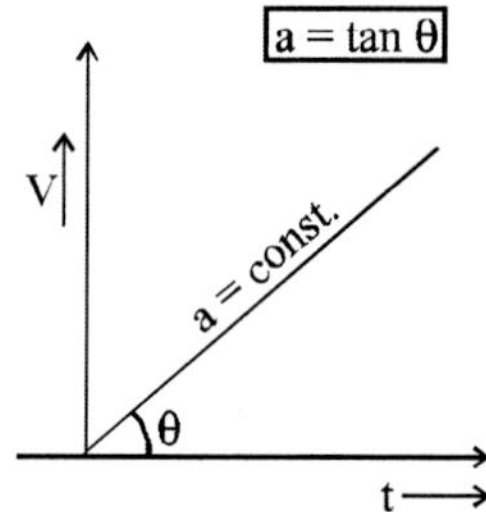

(iii) When the particle is moving with constant retardation.

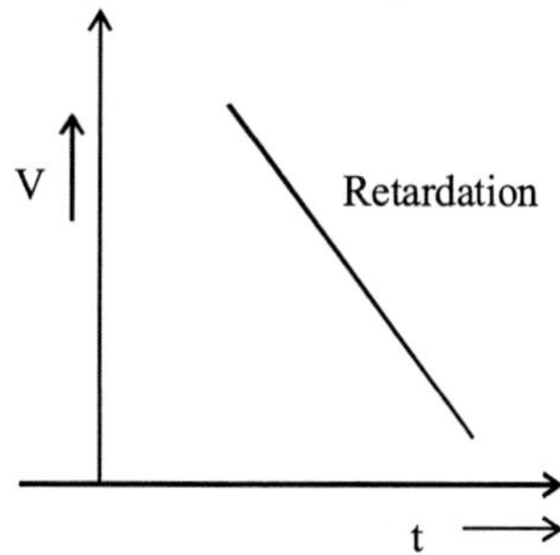

(iv) When the particle moves with non-uniform acceleration and its initial velocity is zero.

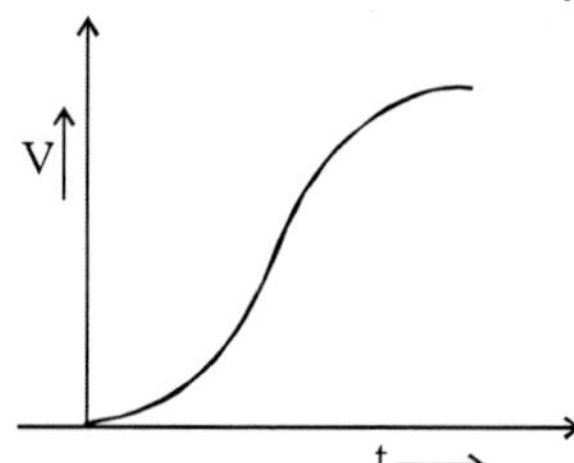

(v) When the acceleration decreases and increases.

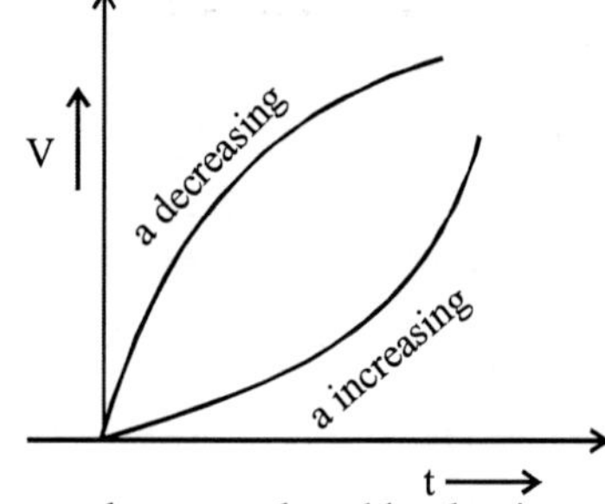

(vi) The total area enclosed by the time - velocity curve represents the distance travelled by a body.

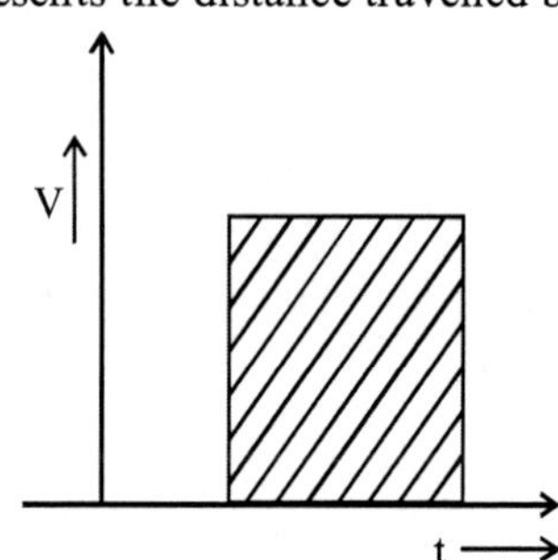

NOTE: While finding displacement through v – t graph, keeping sign under consideration.

(c) **Acceleration-time graph -** In this curve the time is plotted along X-axis and acceleration is plotted along Y-axis.

(i) When the acceleration of the particle is zero.

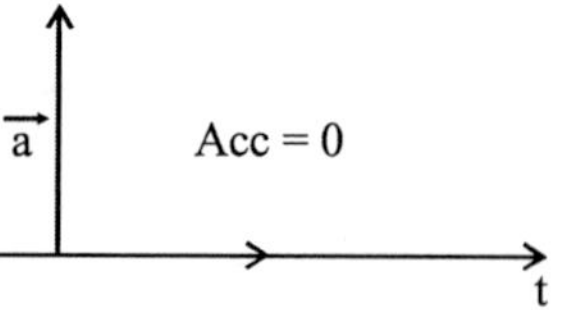

(ii) When acceleration is constant

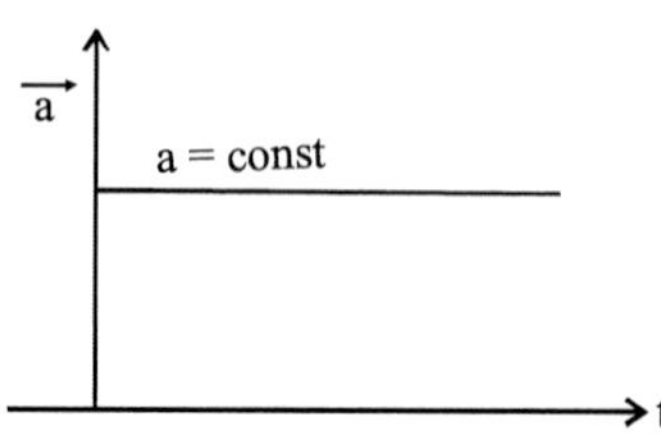

(iii) When acceleration is increasing and is positive.

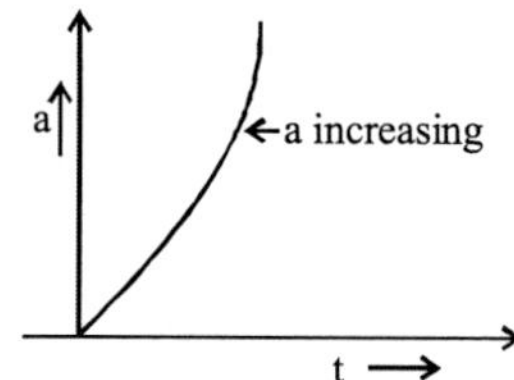

(iv) When acceleration is decreasing and is negative

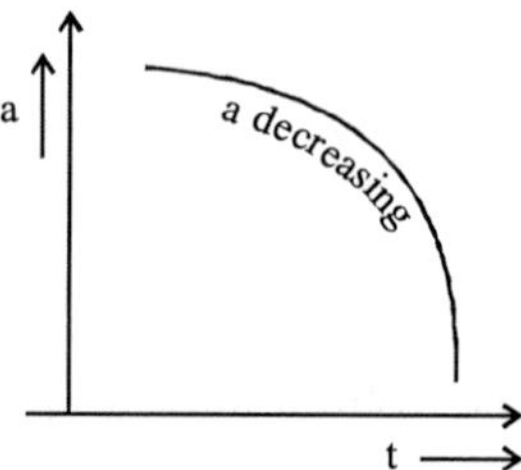

(v) When initial acceleration is zero and rate of change of acceleration is non-uniform

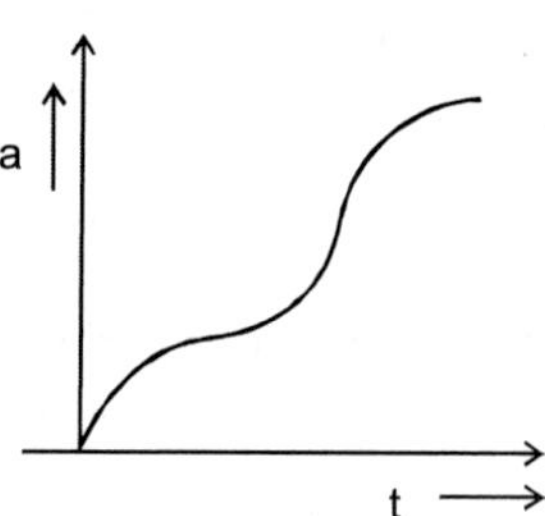

(vi) The change in velocity of the particle = area enclosed by the time-acceleration curve.

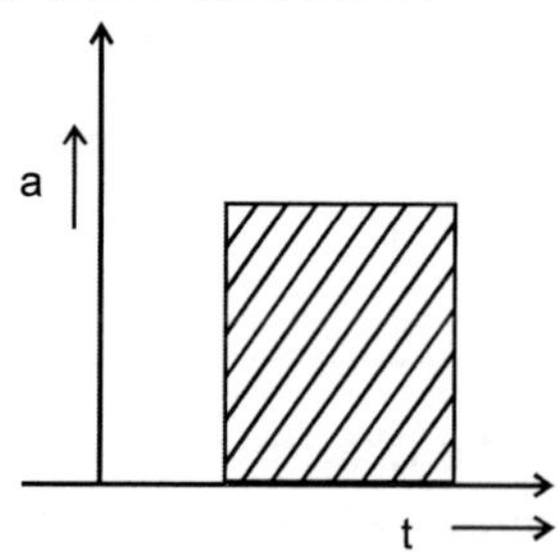

Example 18.

The velocity-time graph of a body moving in a straight line is shown in fig. Find the displacement and distance travelled by the body in 10 seconds.

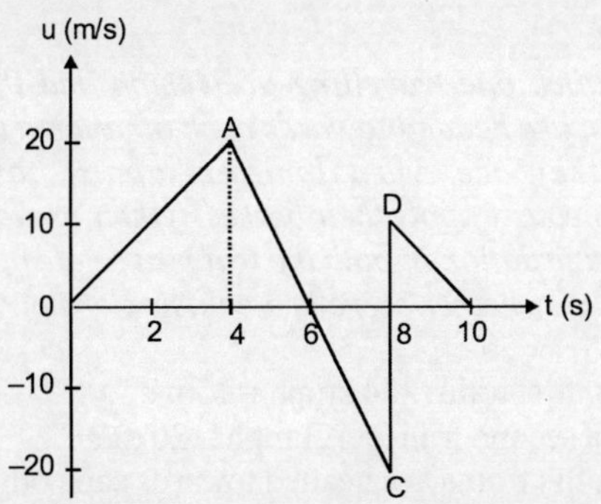

Solution :

The area enclosed by velocity-time graph with time axis measures the distance travelled in a given time. Displacement covered from 0 to 6 seconds is positive; from 6 to 8 seconds is negative and from 8 to 10 seconds is positive; whereas distance covered is always positive.

Total distance covered in 10 s

$$=\frac{1}{2}\times 6\times 20+\frac{1}{2}\times 2\times 20+\frac{1}{2}\times 2\times 10=90\,\text{m}$$

Total displacement in 10s

$$=\frac{1}{2}\times 6\times 20-\frac{1}{2}\times 2\times 20+\frac{1}{2}\times 2\times 10=50\,\text{m}$$

Example 19.

Two trains, which are moving along different tracks in opposite directions, are put on the same track due to a mistake. Their drivers, on noticing the mistake, start slowing down the trains when the trains are 300 m apart. Graphs given below show their velocities as function of time as the trains slow down, The separation, between the trains when both have stopped, is

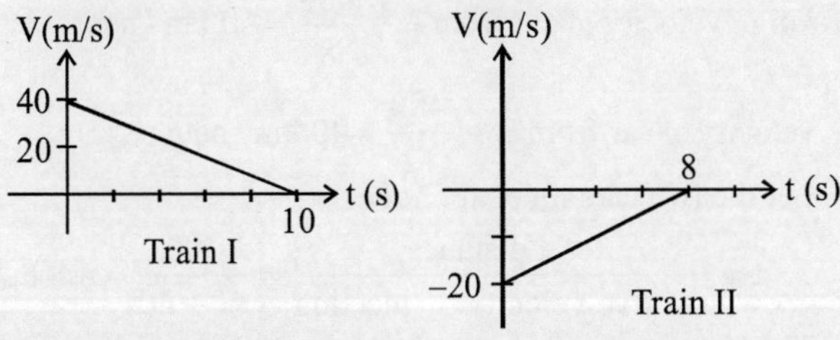

(a) 120m (b) 280m (c) 60m (d) 20m.

***Solution :* (d)**

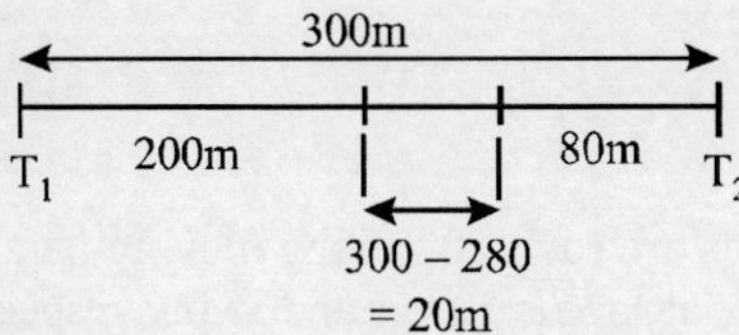

Initial distance between trains is 300m. Displacement of 1st train is calculated by area under v – t.

Curve of train I = displacement $=\frac{1}{2}\times 10\times 40=200\text{m}$

Displacement of train II $=\frac{1}{2}\times 8\times(-20)=-80\text{m}$

∴ Distance between the two trains is 20m.

Example 20.

Figure given below shows the variation of velocity of a particle with time.

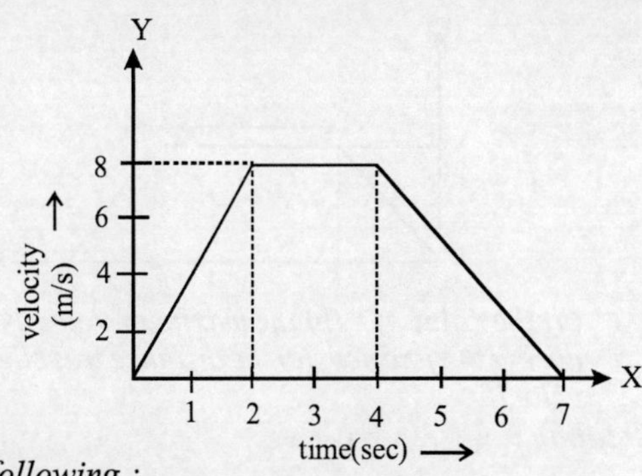

Find the following :

(i) Displacement during the time intervals
(a) 0 to 2 sec, (b) 2 to 4 sec. and (c) 4 to 7 sec.

(ii) Accelerations at –
(a) t = 1 sec, (b) t = 3 sec. and (c) t = 7 sec.

(iii) Average acceleration –
(a) between t = 0 to t = 4 sec.
(b) between t = 0 to t = 7 sec.

(iv) Average velocity during the motion.

Solution :

(i) **(a)** Displacement between t = 0 sec. to t = 2 sec.

$$\Rightarrow \frac{1}{2}\times 2\text{ sec}\times 8\text{ m/s}=8\text{m}$$

(b) Between t = 2 sec. to t = 4 sec.

$$\Rightarrow 2\text{ sec}\times 8\text{ m/s}=16\text{m}$$

(c) Between t = 4 sec. to t = 7 sec.

$$\Rightarrow \frac{1}{2}\times 3\text{ sec}\times 8\text{ m/s}=12\text{m}$$

(ii) Acceleration = slope of v – t curve

(a) At t = 1 sec,

$$\text{slope}=\frac{8\text{m/sec}}{2\text{sec}}\text{m/sec}=4\text{ m/s}^2$$

(b) At t = 3 sec, slope = 0

(c) At t = 7 sec,

$$\text{slope}=-\frac{8}{3}=-2\frac{2}{3}\text{m/s}^2$$

(iii) Average acceleration $=\dfrac{\text{Total change in velocity}}{\text{Total change in time}}$

(a) Between t = 0 to t = 4 sec.,

$$\text{Average acceleration}=\frac{8\text{m/s}}{4}=2\text{m/s}^2$$

(b) Between t = 0 to t = 7 sec.,

$$\text{Average acceleration}=\frac{0}{7}=0$$

(iv) Average velocity $=\dfrac{\text{Total displacement}}{\text{Total time}}$

$$=\frac{8+16+12}{7}=\frac{36}{7}=5\frac{1}{7}\text{m/s}$$

Example 21.

The velocity-time graph of a particle moving along a straight line is shown below.

The acceleration and deceleration are same and it is equal to 4 m/s². If the average velocity during the motion is 15 m/s and total time of motion is 20 second then find

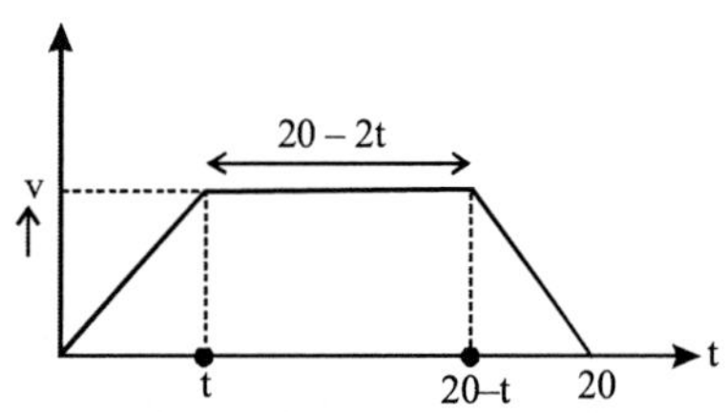

***(a)** the value of t **(b)** the maximum velocity of the particle during the journey. **(c)** the distance travelled with uniform velocity.*

Solution : $v = 0 + at$

Total displacement $= \frac{1}{2}(20 - 2t + 20) \times 4t = 2t\,(40 - 2t)$

Average velocity $= \frac{\text{Total displacement}}{\text{Total time}}$

$$15 = \frac{2t\,(40 - 2t)}{20}$$

Solving quadratic equation, $150 = 40t - 2t^2 \Rightarrow t = 5$ sec.
(another solution not acceptable think why!)
Maximum velocity $= 4t = 4 \times 5 = 20$ m/s
Distance travelled with uniform velocity
$= (20 - 2t)\,V = (20 - 2 \times 5) \times 20 = 200$ m

RELATIVE VELOCITY (In one dimension)

The velocity of A relative to B is the velocity with which A appears to be moving w.r.t.an observer who is moving with the velocity of B

Relative velocity of A w.r.t. B

$$\vec{v}_{AB} = \vec{v}_A - \vec{v}_B$$

Similarly, relative velocity of B w.r.t. A

$$\vec{v}_{BA} = \vec{v}_B - \vec{v}_A$$

Case 1: Bodies moving in same direction :

$\vec{v}_A$ → $\vec{v}_B$ →

$$\vec{v}_{AB} = \vec{v}_A - \vec{v}_B \Rightarrow v_{AB} = v_A - v_B$$

Case 2: Bodies moving in opposite direction :

$\vec{v}_A$ → ← – →+ ← $\vec{v}_B$

$$\vec{v}_{AB} = \vec{v}_A - (-\vec{v}_B) \Rightarrow v_{AB} = v_A + v_B$$

Example 22.

Two trains, one travelling at 54kmph and the other at 72kmph, are headed towards each other on a level track. When they are two kilometers apart, both drivers simultaneously apply their brakes. If their brakes produces equal retardation in both the trains at a rate of 0.15 m/s², determine whether there is a collision or not.

Solution :

Speed of first train = 54 kmph = 15m/s.
Speed of second train = 72kmph = 20 m/s
As both the trains are headed towards each other, relative velocity of one train with respect to other is given as
$v_r = 15 + 20 = 35$ m/s
Both trains are retarded by acceleration of 0.15 m/s². Relative retardation $a_r = 0.15 + 0.15 = 0.3$ m/s².
Now, we assume one train is at rest and other is coming at 35m/s retarded by 0.3 m/s² at a distance of two kilometer. The maximum distance travelled by the moving train while retarding is

$$s_{max} = \frac{v_r^2}{2a_r} = \frac{(35)^2}{2 \times 0.3} = 2041.66\text{m}$$

It is more than 2km, which shows that it will hit the second train.

Example 23.

Two cars started simultaneously towards each other from towns A and B which are 480 km apart. It took first car travelling from A to B 8 hours to cover the distance and second car travelling from B to A 12 hours. Determine when the car meet after starting and at what distance from town A. Assuming that both the cars travelled with constant speed.

Solution : Velocity of car from A $= \frac{480}{8} = 60$ km / hour

velocity of car from B $= \frac{480}{12} = 40$ km / hour

Let the two cars meet at *t* hour

$$\therefore\ t = \frac{\text{total distance}}{\text{relative velocity of meeting}} = \frac{480}{60 + 40} = 4.8 \text{ hour}$$

The distance $s = v_A \times t = 60 \times 4.8 = 288$ km.

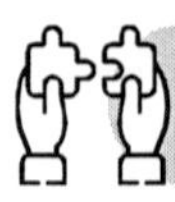

3.3 Concept Practice Problems

CPP

21. A body is thrown upwards and reaches its maximum height. At that position
(a) its acceleration is minimum
(b) its velocity is zero and its acceleration is also zero
(c) its velocity is zero but its acceleration is maximum
(d) its velocity is zero and its acceleration is the acceleration due to gravity.

22. A stone thrown upward with a speed u from the top of the tower reaches the ground with a velocity 3u. The height of the tower is
(a) $3u^2/g$ (b) $4u^2/g$ (c) $6u^2/g$ (d) $9u^2/g$

23. A ball is dropped downwards, after 1 sec another ball is dropped downwards from the same point. What is the distance between them after 3 sec?
(a) 25m (b) 20m (c) 50m (d) 9.8m

24. Two trains are each 50 m long moving parallel towards each other at speeds 10 m/s and 15 m/s respectively. After what time will they pass each other?
(a) $5\sqrt{\frac{2}{3}}$ sec (b) 4 sec (c) 2 sec (d) 6 sec

25. Similar balls are thrown vertically each with a velocity 20 ms⁻¹, one on the surface of earth and the other on the surface of moon. What will be ratio of the maximum heights attained by them? (Acceleration on moon = 1.7 ms⁻² approx)
(a) 6 (b) $\frac{1}{6}$ (c) $\frac{1}{5}$ (d) None of these

26. From a 10m high building a stone 'A' is dropped & simultaneously another stone 'B' is thrown horizontally with an initial speed of 5 m/sec^{-1}. Which one of the following statements is true?

(a) It is not possible to calculate which one of two stones will reach ground first

(b) Both stones 'A' & 'B' will reach the ground simultaneously.

(c) 'A' stones reach the ground earlier than 'B'

(d) 'B' stones reach the ground earlier than 'A'

27. From a 200 m high tower, one ball is thrown upwards with speed of 10 ms^{-1} and another is thrown vertically downwards at the same speeds simultaneously. The time difference of their reaching the ground will be nearest to

(a) 12 s (b) 6 s (c) 2 s (d) 1 s

28. A rocket is fired upward from the earth's surface such that it creates an acceleration of 19.6 $m s^{-2}$. If after 5 s, its engine is switched off, the maximum height of the rocket from earth's surface would be

(a) 980m (b) 735m (c) 490m (d) 245m

29. A food packet is released from a helicopter rising steadily at the speed of 2 m/sec. After 2 seconds the velocity of the packet is

($g = 10\ m/sec^2$)

(a) 22 m/sec (b) 20 m/sec

(c) 18 m/sec (d) none of these

30. A graph of acceleration versus time of a particle starting from rest at t = 0 is as shown in Fig. The speed of the particle at t = 14 second is

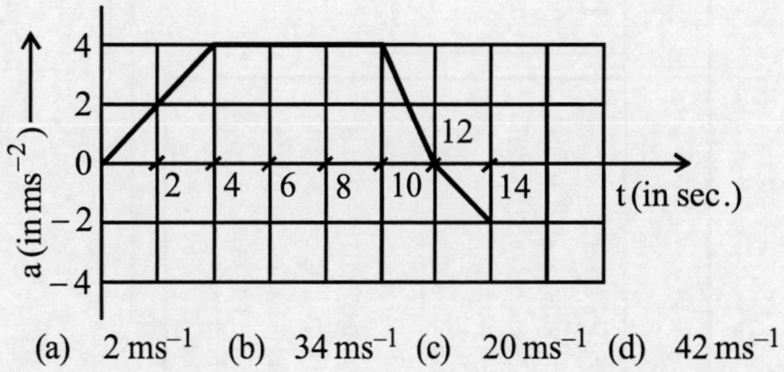

(a) 2 ms^{-1} (b) 34 ms^{-1} (c) 20 ms^{-1} (d) 42 ms^{-1}

ANSWER KEY

21	(d)	22	(b)	23	(a)	24	(b)	25	(b)	26	(b)	27	(c)	28	(b)	29	(c)	30	(b)

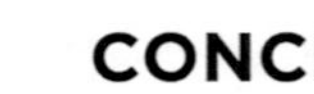

CONCEPT MAP

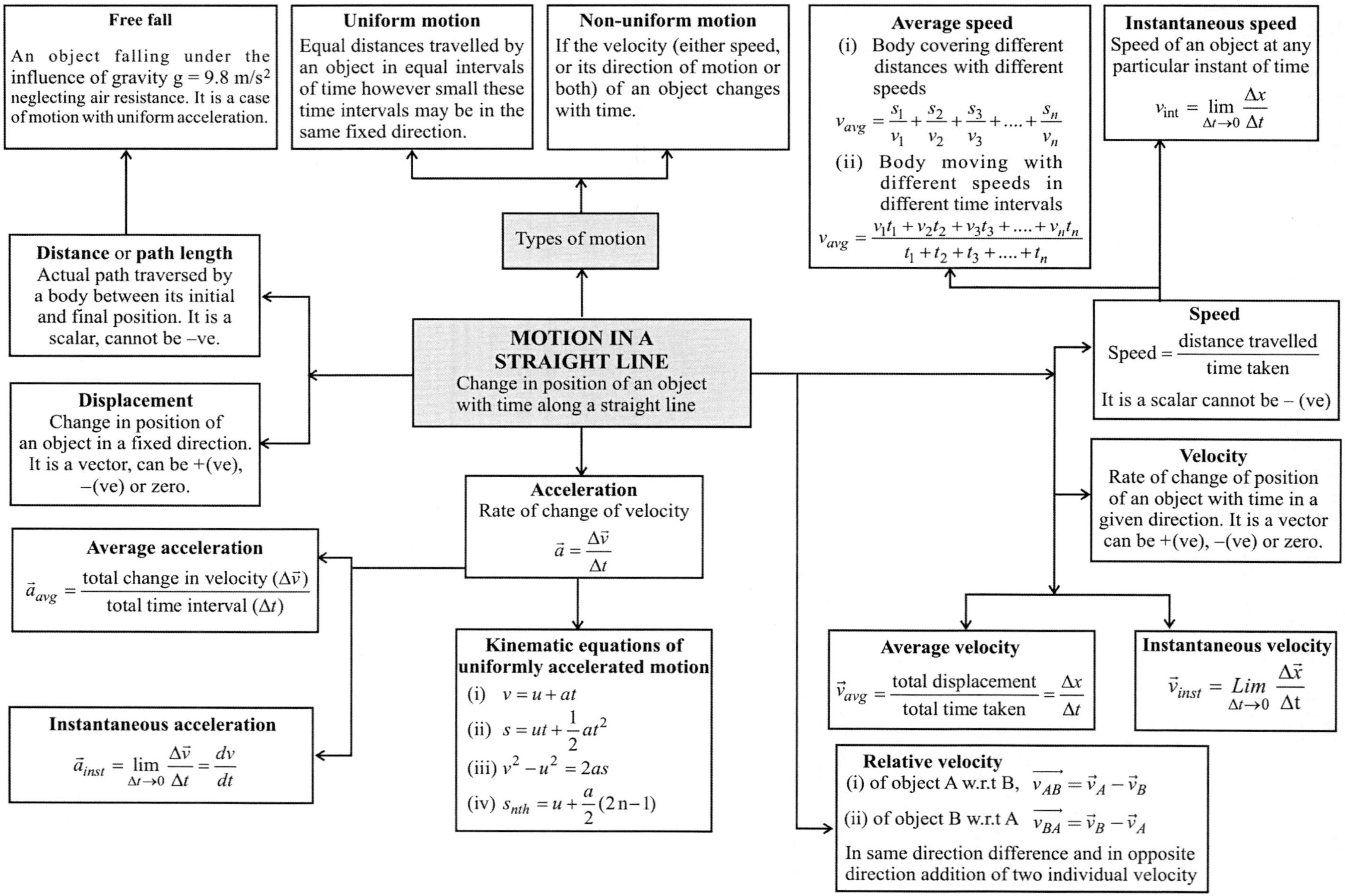

MOTION IN A STRAIGHT LINE
Change in position of an object with time along a straight line

Types of motion

Uniform motion
Equal distances travelled by an object in equal intervals of time however small these time intervals may be in the same fixed direction.

Non-uniform motion
If the velocity (either speed, or its direction of motion or both) of an object changes with time.

Distance or **path length**
Actual path traversed by a body between its initial and final position. It is a scalar, cannot be –ve.

Free fall
An object falling under the influence of gravity g = 9.8 m/s^2 neglecting air resistance. It is a case of motion with uniform acceleration.

Displacement
Change in position of an object in a fixed direction. It is a vector, can be +(ve), –(ve) or zero.

Speed

$$\text{Speed} = \frac{\text{distance travelled}}{\text{time taken}}$$

It is a scalar cannot be – (ve)

Average speed

(i) Body covering different distances with different speeds

$$v_{avg} = \frac{s_1}{v_1} + \frac{s_2}{v_2} + \frac{s_3}{v_3} + ... + \frac{s_n}{v_n}$$

(ii) Body moving with different speeds in different time intervals

$$v_{avg} = \frac{v_1 t_1 + v_2 t_2 + v_3 t_3 + ... + v_n t_n}{t_1 + t_2 + t_3 + ... + t_n}$$

Instantaneous speed
Speed of an object at any particular instant of time

$$v_{\text{int}} = \lim_{\Delta t \to 0} \frac{\Delta x}{\Delta t}$$

Velocity
Rate of change of position of an object with time in a given direction. It is a vector can be +(ve), –(ve) or zero.

Average velocity

$$\vec{v}_{avg} = \frac{\text{total displacement}}{\text{total time taken}} = \frac{\Delta x}{\Delta t}$$

Instantaneous velocity

$$\vec{v}_{inst} = \underset{\Delta t \to 0}{Lim} \frac{\Delta \vec{x}}{\Delta t}$$

Relative velocity

(i) of object A w.r.t B, $\overrightarrow{v_{AB}} = \vec{v}_A - \vec{v}_B$

(ii) of object B w.r.t A $\overrightarrow{v_{BA}} = \vec{v}_B - \vec{v}_A$

In same direction difference and in opposite direction addition of two individual velocity

Acceleration
Rate of change of velocity

$$\vec{a} = \frac{\Delta \vec{v}}{\Delta t}$$

Average acceleration

$$\vec{a}_{avg} = \frac{\text{total change in velocity } (\Delta \vec{v})}{\text{total time interval } (\Delta t)}$$

Instantaneous acceleration

$$\vec{a}_{inst} = \lim_{\Delta t \to 0} \frac{\Delta \vec{v}}{\Delta t} = \frac{dv}{dt}$$

Kinematic equations of uniformly accelerated motion

(i) $v = u + at$

(ii) $s = ut + \frac{1}{2}at^2$

(iii) $v^2 - u^2 = 2as$

(iv) $s_{nth} = u + \frac{a}{2}(2n - 1)$

Exercise 1 - Chapter Revision Problems

CRP

1. The ratio of the numerical values of the average velocity and average speed of a body is always:
(a) unity (b) unity or less
(c) unity or more (d) less than unity

2. A particle has moved from one position to another position
(a) its distance is zero
(b) its displacement is zero
(c) neither distance nor displacement is zero
(d) average velocity is zero

3. Which of the following changes when a particle is moving with uniform velocity?
(a) Speed (b) Velocity
(c) Acceleration (d) Position vector

4. The area of the acceleration-displacement curve of a body gives
(a) impulse
(b) change in momentum per unit mass
(c) change in KE per unit mass
(d) total change in energy

5. The initial velocity of a particle is u (at t = 0) and the acceleration a is given by f t.
Which of the following relation is valid?
(a) $v = u + ft^2$ (b) $v = u + ft^2/2$
(c) $v = u + ft$ (d) $v = u$

6. The distance through which a body falls in the nth second is h. The distance through which it falls in the next second is
(a) h (b) $h + \frac{g}{2}$ (c) $h - g$ (d) $h + g$

7. It is given that $t = px^2 + qx$, where x is displacement and t is time. The acceleration of particle at origin is
(a) $-\frac{2p}{q^3}$ (b) $-\frac{2q}{p^3}$ (c) $\frac{2p}{q^3}$ (d) $\frac{2q}{p^3}$

8. Figure shows the v-t graph for two particles P and Q. Which of the following statements regarding their relative motion is true ?
Their relative velocity is

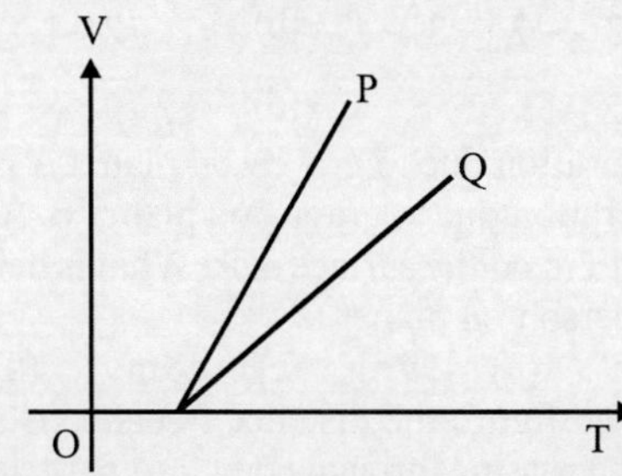

(a) is zero
(b) is non-zero but constant
(c) continuously decreases
(d) continuously increases

9. A stone is dropped into a well in which the level of water is h below the top of the well. If v is velocity of sound, the time T after which the splash is heard is given by
(a) $T = 2h/v$ (b) $T = \sqrt{\left(\frac{2h}{g}\right)} + \frac{h}{v}$
(c) $T = \sqrt{\left(\frac{2h}{v}\right)} + \frac{h}{g}$ (d) $T = \sqrt{\left(\frac{h}{2g}\right)} + \frac{2h}{v}$

10. The acceleration of a particle is increasing linearly with time t as bt. The particle starts from the origin with an initial velocity v_0. The distance travelled by the particle in time t will be
(a) $v_0 t + \frac{1}{3}bt^2$ (b) $v_0 t + \frac{1}{3}bt^3$
(c) $v_0 t + \frac{1}{6}bt^3$ (d) $v_0 t + \frac{1}{2}bt^2$

11. The displacement x of a particle varies with time according to the relation $x = \frac{a}{b}(1 - e^{-bt})$. Then select the false alternatives.
(a) At $t = \frac{1}{b}$, the displacement of the particle is nearly $\frac{2}{3}\left(\frac{a}{b}\right)$
(b) the velocity and acceleration of the particle at t = 0 are a and –ab respectively
(c) the particle cannot go beyond $x = \frac{a}{b}$
(d) the particle will not come back to its starting point at $t \to \infty$

12. The displacement of a particle is given by $\sqrt{x} = t + 1$. Which of the following statements about its velocity is true ?
(a) It is zero
(b) It is constant but not zero
(c) It increases with time
(d) It decreases with time

13. Two bodies of masses m_1 and m_2 fall from heights h_1 and h_2 respectively. The ratio of their velocities, when they hit the ground is
(a) $\frac{h_1}{h_2}$ (b) $\sqrt{\frac{h_1}{h_2}}$ (c) $\frac{m_1 h_1}{m_1 h_2}$ (d) $\frac{h_1^2}{h_2^2}$

14. The position x of a particle varies with time (t) as $x = At^2 - Bt^3$. The acceleration at time t of the particle will be equal to zero. What is the value of t?
(a) $\frac{2A}{3B}$ (b) $\frac{A}{B}$ (c) $\frac{A}{3B}$ (d) zero

15. The acceleration of a particle, starting from rest, varies with time according to the relation
$$a = -s\omega^2 \sin \omega t$$
The displacement of this particle at a time t will be
(a) $s \sin \omega t$ (b) $s\omega \cos \omega t$
(c) $s\omega \sin \omega t$ (d) $-\frac{1}{2}(s\omega^2 \sin \omega t)t^2$

16. The displacement of a particle is given by
$y = a + bt + ct^2 - dt^4$
The initial velocity and acceleration are respectively
(a) $b, -4d$ (b) $-b, 2c$ (c) $b, 2c$ (d) $2c, -4d$

17. A passenger travels along the straight road for half the distance with velocity v_1 and the remaining half distance with velocity v_2. Then average velocity is given by
(a) v_1v_2 (b) v_2^2/v_1^2
(c) $(v_1 + v_2)/2$ (d) $2v_1v_2/(v_1 + v_2)$

18. A point moves with uniform acceleration and v_1, v_2 and v_3 denote the average velocities in t_1, t_2 and t_3 sec. Which of the following relation is correct?
(a) $(v_1 - v_2):(v_2 - v_3) = (t_1 - t_2):(t_2 + t_3)$
(b) $(v_1 - v_2):(v_2 - v_3) = (t_1 + t_2):(t_2 + t_3)$
(c) $(v_1 - v_2):(v_2 - v_3) = (t_1 - t_2):(t_1 - t_3)$
(d) $(v_1 - v_2):(v_2 - v_3) = (t_1 - t_2):(t_2 - t_3)$

19. A particle experiences constant acceleration for 20 seconds after starting from rest. If it travels a distance s_1 in the first 10 seconds and distance s_2 in the next 10 seconds, then
(a) $s_2 = s_1$ (b) $s_2 = 2s_1$ (c) $s_2 = 3s_1$ (d) $s_2 = 4s_1$

20. A smooth inclined plane is inclined at an angle θ with horizontal. A body starts from rest and slides down the inclined surface.

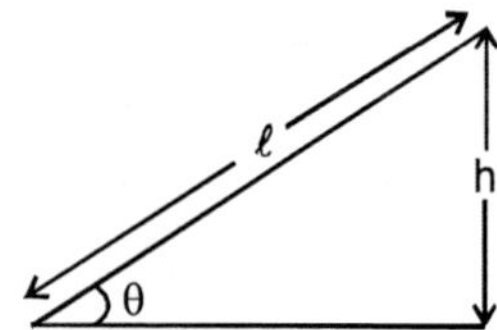

Then the time taken by it to reach the bottom is
(a) $\sqrt{\left(\frac{2h}{g}\right)}$ (b) $\sqrt{\left(\frac{2\ell}{g}\right)}$ (c) $\frac{1}{\sin\theta}\sqrt{\frac{2h}{g}}$ (d) $\sin\theta\frac{\sqrt{(2h)}}{g}$

21. A ball is projected vertically upwards with kinetic energy E. The kinetic energy of the ball at the highest point of its flight will be
(a) E (b) $E/\sqrt{2}$ (c) E/2 (d) zero

22. A particle is moving in a straight line with initial velocity and uniform acceleration a. If the sum of the distance travelled in t^{th} and $(t + 1)^{th}$ seconds is 100 cm, then its velocity after *t* seconds, in cm/s, is
(a) 80 (b) 50 (c) 20 (d) 30

23. The relative velocity V_{AB} or V_{BA} of two bodies A & B may be
(1) greater than velocity of body A
(2) greater than velocity of body B
(3) less than the velocity of body A
(4) less than the velocity of body B
(a) (1) and (2) only (b) (3) and (4) only
(c) (1), (2) and (3) only (d) (1), (2), (3) and (4)

24. A stone is thrown vertically upwards. When the particle is at a height half of its maximum height, its speed is 10m/sec, then maximum height attained by particle is ($g = 10 m/sec^2$)
(a) 8m (b) 10m (c) 15m (d) 20m

25. The motion of a particle is described by the equation $u = at$. The distance travelled by particle in first 4 sec is
(a) 4a (b) 12a (c) 6a (d) 8a

26. A body travels 2 m in the first two second and 2.20 m in the next 4 second with uniform deceleration. The velocity of the body at the end of 9 second is
(a) $-10\ ms^{-1}$ (b) $-0.20\ ms^{-1}$
(c) $-0.40\ ms^{-1}$ (d) $-0.80\ ms^{-1}$

27. A ball released from a height falls 5 m in one second. In 4 seconds it falls through
(a) 20m (b) 1.25m (c) 40m (d) 80m

28. The displacement *x* of a particle along a straight line at time t is given by : $x = a_0 + \frac{a_1t}{2} + \frac{a_2}{3}t^2$. The acceleration of the particle is
(a) $\frac{a_2}{3}$ (b) $\frac{2a_2}{3}$ (c) $\frac{a_1}{2}$ (d) $a_0 + \frac{a_2}{3}$

29. A rubber ball is dropped from a height of 5 metre on a plane where the acceleration due to gravity is same as that onto the surface of the earth. On bouncing, it rises to a height of 1.8 m. On bouncing, the ball loses its velocity by a factor of
(a) $\frac{3}{5}$ (b) $\frac{9}{25}$ (c) $\frac{2}{5}$ (d) $\frac{16}{25}$

30. A boy moving with a velocity of 20 km h^{-1} along a straight line joining two stationary objects. According to him both objects
(a) move in the same direction with the same speed of 20 km h^{-1}
(b) move in different direction with the same speed of 20 km h^{-1}
(c) move towards him
(d) remain stationary

31. Let A, B, C, D be points on a vertical line such that AB = BC = CD. If a body is released from position A, the times of descent through AB, BC and CD are in the ratio.
(a) $1:\sqrt{3}-\sqrt{2}:\sqrt{3}+\sqrt{2}$ (b) $1:\sqrt{2}-1:\sqrt{3}-\sqrt{2}$
(c) $1:\sqrt{2}-1:\sqrt{3}$ (d) $1:\sqrt{2}:\sqrt{3}-1$

32. The acceleration due to gravity on planet A is nine times the acceleration due to gravity on planet B. A man jumps to a height 2m on the surface of A. What is height of jump by same person on planet B?
(a) 2/3 m (b) 2/9 m (c) 18m (d) 6m

33. In the given figure the distance PQ is constant. SQ is a vertical line passing through point R. A particle is kept at R and the plane PR is such that angle θ can be varied such that R lies on line SQ. The time taken by particle to come down varies, as the θ increases

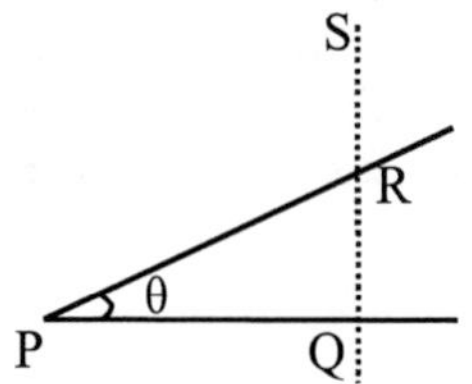

(a) decreases continuously
(b) increases
(c) increases then decreases
(d) decreases then increases

34. The dependence of velocity of a body with time is given by the equation $v = 20 + 0.1t^2$. The body is in
(a) uniform retardation
(b) uniform acceleration
(c) non-uniform acceleration
(d) zero acceleration.

35. Two stones are thrown from the top of a tower, one straight down with an initial speed u and the second straight up with the same speed u. When the two stones hit the ground, they will have speeds in the ratio
(a) 2 : 3 (b) 2 : 1 (c) 1 : 2 (d) 1 : 1

36. Figure shows the position of a particle moving along the X-axis as a function of time.

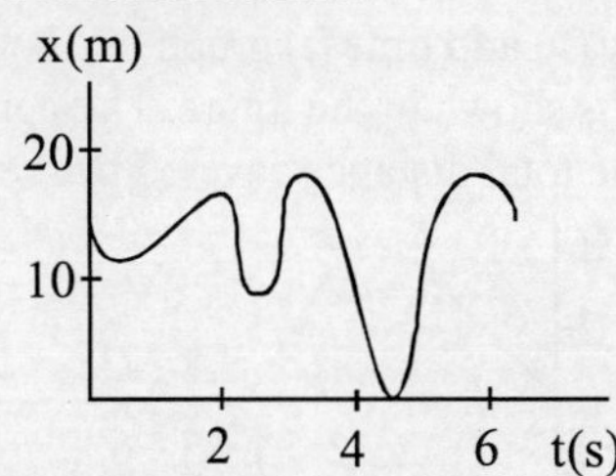

Which of the following is correct?
(a) The particle has come to the rest 6 times
(b) The maximum speed is at t = 6 s.
(c) The velocity remains positive for t = 0 to t = 6 s.
(d) The average velocity for the total period shown is negative.

37. A steel ball is bouncing up and down on a steel plate with a period of oscillation of 1 second. If $g = 10\ ms^{-2}$, then it bounces up to a height of
(a) 5m (b) 10m (c) 2.5m (d) 1.25m

38. A body starts from rest and travels a distance x with uniform acceleration, then it travels a distance 2x with uniform speed, finally it travels a distance 3x with uniform retardation and comes to rest. If the complete motion of the particle is along a straight line, then the ratio of its average velocity to maximum velocity is
(a) 2/5 (b) 3/5 (c) 4/5 (d) 6/7

39. Two bodies begin a free fall from the same height at a time interval of N s. If vertical separation between the two bodies is 1 after n second from the start of the first body, then n is equal to
(a) $\sqrt{nN}$ (b) $\frac{1}{gN}$ (c) $\frac{1}{gN}+\frac{N}{2}$ (d) $\frac{1}{gN}-\frac{N}{4}$

40. A particle starting from rest falls from a certain height. Assuming that the acceleration due to gravity remain the same throughout the motion, its displacements in three successive half second intervals are S_1, S_2 and S_3 then
(a) $S_1 : S_2 : S_3 = 1 : 5 : 9$ (b) $S_1 : S_2 : S_3 = 1 : 3 : 5$
(c) $S_1 : S_2 : S_3 = 9 : 2 : 3$ (d) $S_1 : S_2 : S_3 = 1 : 1 : 1$

41. For the velocity time graph shown in the figure below the distance covered by the body in the last two seconds of its motion is what fraction of the total distance travelled by it in all the seven seconds?

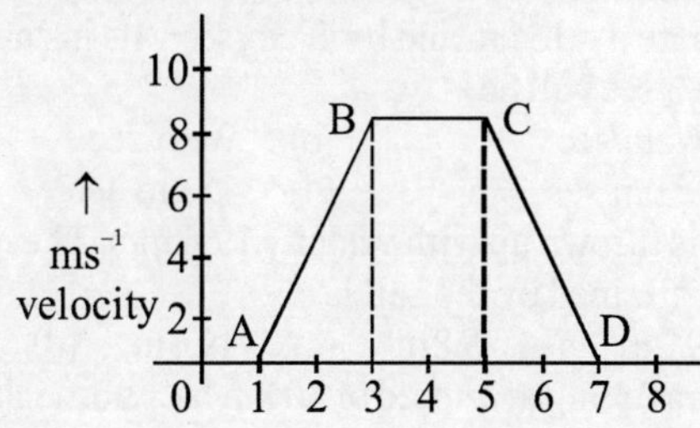

(a) $\frac{1}{2}$ (b) $\frac{1}{4}$ (c) $\frac{2}{3}$ (d) $\frac{1}{3}$

42. The distance time graph of a particle at time t makes angles 45° with the time axis. After one second, it makes angle 60° with the time axis. What is the acceleration of the particle?
(a) $\sqrt{3}-1$ (b) $\sqrt{3}+1$ (c) $\sqrt{3}$ (d) 1

43. Two particles A and B are connected by a rigid rod AB. The rod slides along perpendicular rails as shown here. The velocity of A to the left is 10 m/s. What is the velocity of B when angle $\alpha = 60°$?

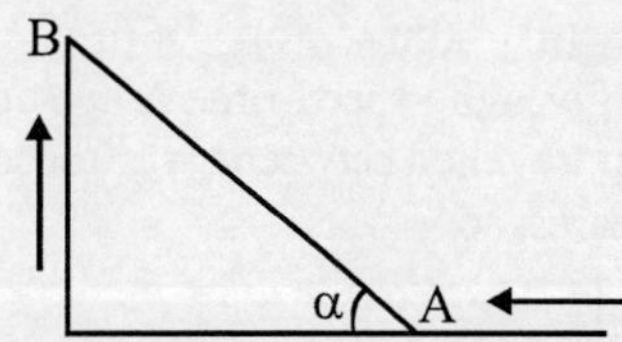

(a) 9.8 m/s (b) 10 m/s (c) 5.8 m/s (d) 17.3 m/s

44. A stone is just released from the window of a train moving along a horizontal straight track. The stone will hit the ground following a
(a) straight line path (b) circular path
(c) parabolic path (d) hyperbolic path

45. A ball is dropped from a high rise platform at t = 0 starting from rest. After 6 seconds another ball is thrown downwards from the same platform with a speed v. The two balls meet at t = 18s. What is the value of v? (take $g = 10\ m/s^2$)
(a) 75 m/s (b) 55 m/s (c) 40 m/s (d) 60 m/s

46. A particle moves a distance x in time t according to equation $x = (t + 5)^{-1}$. The acceleration of particle is proportional to
(a) $(\text{velocity})^{3/2}$ (b) $(\text{distance})^2$
(c) $(\text{distance})^{-2}$ (d) $(\text{velocity})^{2/3}$

47. A ball is released from the top of a tower of height h meters. It takes T seconds to reach the ground. What is the position of the ball at $\frac{T}{3}$ second
(a) $\frac{8h}{9}$ meters from the ground
(b) $\frac{7h}{9}$ meters from the ground
(c) $\frac{h}{9}$ meters from the ground
(d) $\frac{17h}{18}$ meters from the ground

48. The motion of particle is described by the equation x = a + bt^2, where a = 15 cm and b = 3 cm/sec^2. Its instant velocity at time 3 sec will be

(a) 36 cm/sec (b) 9 cm/sec
(c) 4.5 cm/sec (d) 18 cm/sec

49. A ball is thrown up with velocity 19.6 m/s. The maximum height attained by the ball is

(a) 29.2m (b) 9.8m (c) 19.6m (d) 15.8m

50. A car travelling at a speed of 30 km h^{-1} is brought to a halt in 8 m by applying brakes. If the same car is travelling at 60 km h^{-1}, it can be brought to a halt with the same braking power in

(a) 32m (b) 24m (c) 16m (d) 8 cm

51. A metro train starts from rest and in 5 s achieves 108 km/h. After that it moves with constant velocity and comes to rest after travelling 45 m with uniform retardation. If total distance travelled is 395 m, find total time of travelling.

(a) 12.2 s (b) 15.3 s (c) 9 s (d) 17.2 s

52. A particle moves along a straight line OX. At a time t (in second) the distance x (in metre) of the particle from O is given by x = 40 + 12t – t^3. How long would the particle travel before coming to rest?

(a) 24m (b) 40m (c) 56m (d) 16m

53. Figure here gives the speed-time graph for a body. The displacement travelled between t = 1.0 second and t = 7.0 second is nearest to

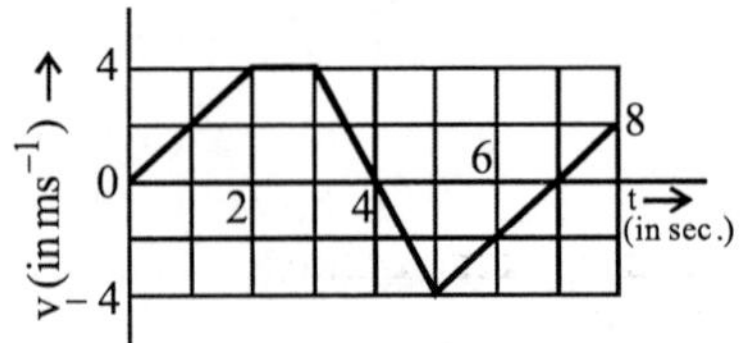

(a) 1.5m (b) 2m (c) 3m (d) 4m

54. A boat takes 2 hours to travel 8 km and back in still water lake. With water velocity of 4 km h^{-1}, the time taken for going upstream of 8 km and coming back is

(a) 160 minutes (b) 80 minutes
(c) 100 minutes (d) 120 minutes

55. A lift in which a man is standing, is moving upwards with a speed of 10 ms^{-1}. The man drops a coin from a height of 4.9 metre and if g = 9.8 ms^{-2}, then the coin reaches the floor of the lift after a time

(a) $\sqrt{2}$ s (b) 1 s (c) $\frac{1}{2}$ (d) $\frac{1}{\sqrt{2}}$

56. If a ball is thrown vertically upwards with a velocity of 40m/s, then velocity of the ball after two seconds is : (g = 10 m/sec^2)

(a) 15 m/s (b) 20 m/s (c) 25 m/s (d) 28 m/s

57. If a car at rest accelerates uniformly to a speed of 144 km/h in 20 sec., it covers a distance of

(a) 20 cm (b) 400m (c) 1440 cm (d) 2980 cm

58. The water drops fall at regular intervals from a tap 5 m above the ground. The third drop is leaving the tap at an instant when the first drop touches the ground. How far above the ground is the second drop at that instant ? (Take g = 10 m/s^2)

(a) 1.25m (b) 2.50m (c) 3.75m (d) 5.00m

59. Which of the following curve does not represent motion in one dimension?

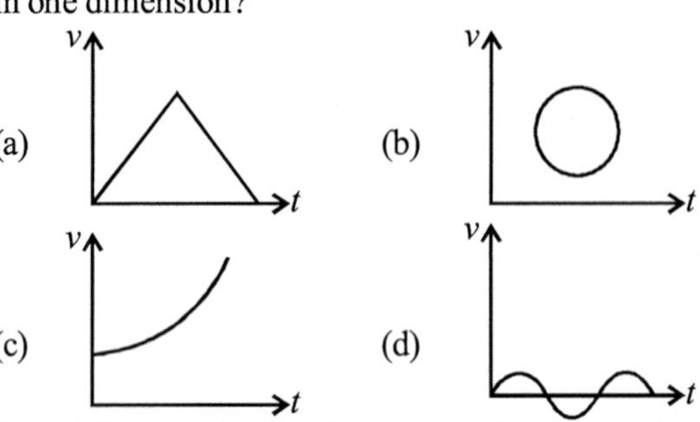

60. A particle located at $x = 0$ at time $t = 0$, starts moving along with the positive x-direction with a velocity 'v' that varies as $v = \alpha\sqrt{x}$. The displacement of the particle varies with time as

(a) t^2 (b) t (c) $t^{1/2}$ (d) t^3

61. The velocity (v) and time (t) graph of a body in a straight line motion is shown in the figure. The point S is at 4.333 seconds. The total distance covered by the body in 6 s is:

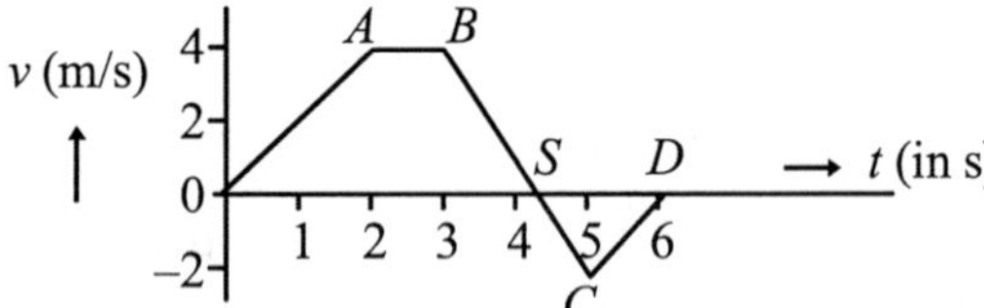

(a) $\frac{37}{3}$ m (b) 12m (c) 11m (d) $\frac{49}{4}$ m

62. A particle starts from the origin at time t = 0 and moves along the positive x-axis. The graph of velocity with respect to time is shown in figure. What is the position of the particle at time t = 5s?

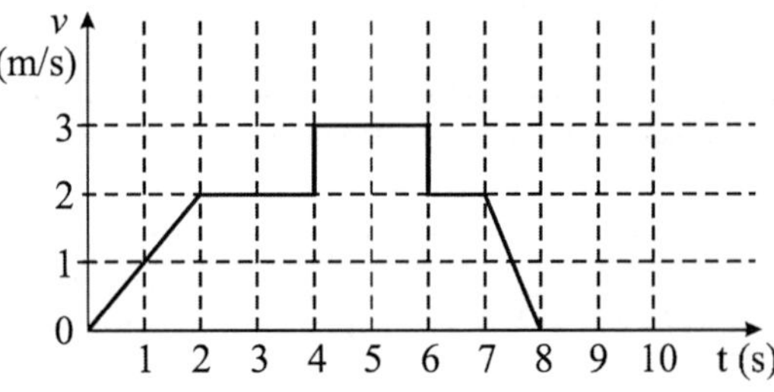

(a) 10 m (b) 6 m (c) 3 m (d) 9 m

63. The velocity-time graphs of a car and a scooter are shown in the figure. (i) the difference between the distance travelled by the car and the scooter in 15 s and (ii) the time at which the car will catch up with the scooter are, respectively

(a) 337.5m and 25s

(b) 225.5m and 10s

(c) 112.5m and 22.5s

(d) 11.2.5m and 15s

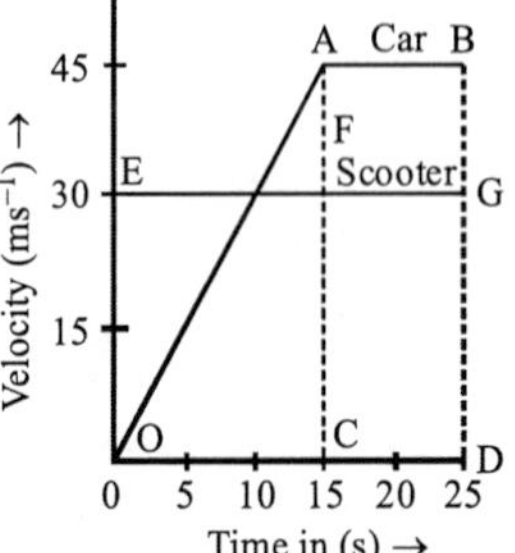

64. Which graph corresponds to an object moving with a constant negative acceleration and a positive velocity ?

(a) (b) (c) (d)

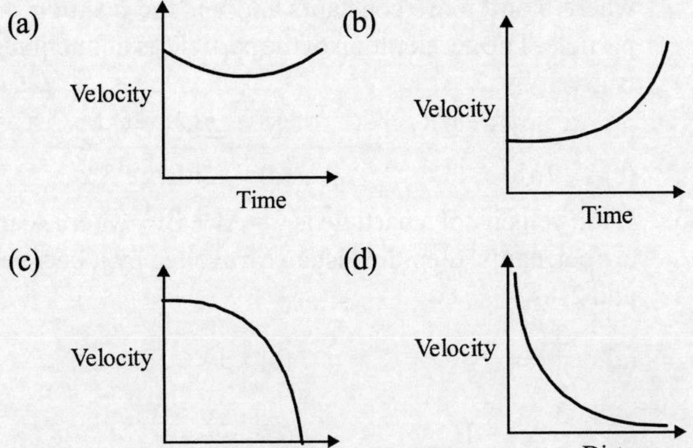

65. Train *A* and train *B* are running on parallel tracks in the opposite directions with speeds of 36 km/hour and 72 km/hour, respectively. A person is walking in train *A* in the direction opposite to its motion with a speed of 1.8 km/hour. Speed (in ms^{-1}) of this person as observed from train *B* will be close to : (take the distance between the tracks as negligible)

(a) 29.5 ms^{-1} (b) 28.5 ms^{-1}
(c) 31.5 ms^{-1q} (d) 30.5 ms^{-1}

66. A person climbs up a stalled escalator in 60 s. If standing on the same but escalator running with constant velocity he takes 40 s. How much time is taken by the person to walk up the moving escalator?

(a) 37 s (b) 27 s (c) 24 s (d) 45 s

67. A goods train accelerating uniformly on a straight railway track, approaches an electric pole standing on the side of track. Its engine passes the pole with velocity *u* and the guard's room passes with velocity *v*. The middle wagon of the train passes the pole with a velocity.

(a) $\frac{u+v}{2}$ (b) $\frac{1}{2}\sqrt{u^2+v^2}$

(c) $\sqrt{uv}$ (d) $\sqrt{\left(\frac{u^2+v^2}{2}\right)}$

68. A Tennis ball is released from a height h and after freely falling on a wooden floor it rebounds and reaches height $\frac{h}{2}$. The velocity versus height of the ball during its motion may be represented graphically by :
(graph are drawn schematically and on not to scale)

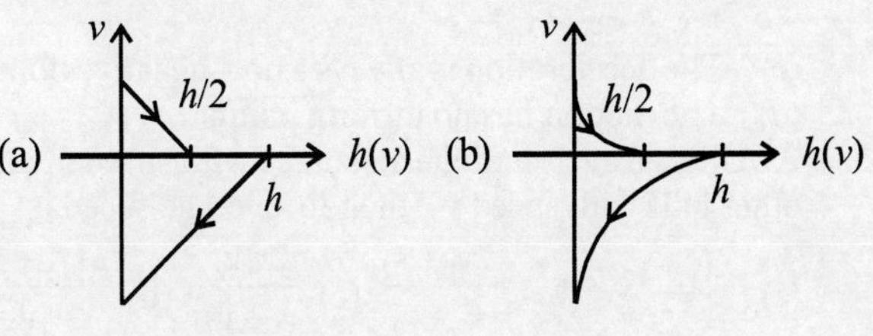

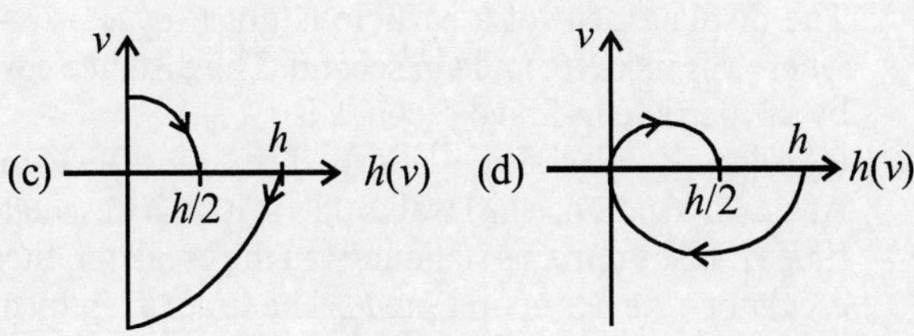

69. A body is thrown vertically upwards. Which one of the following graphs correctly represent the velocity vs time?

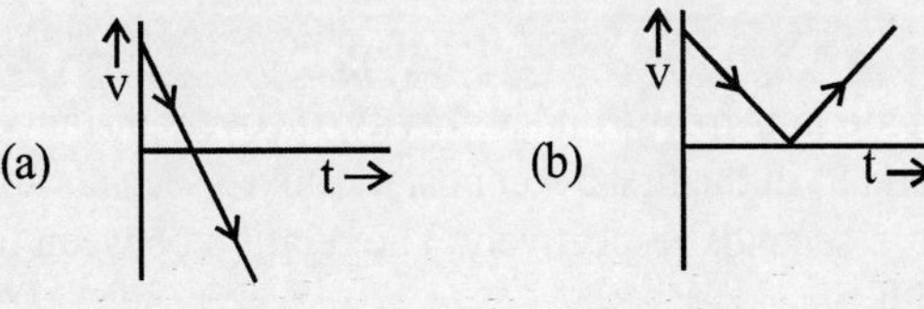

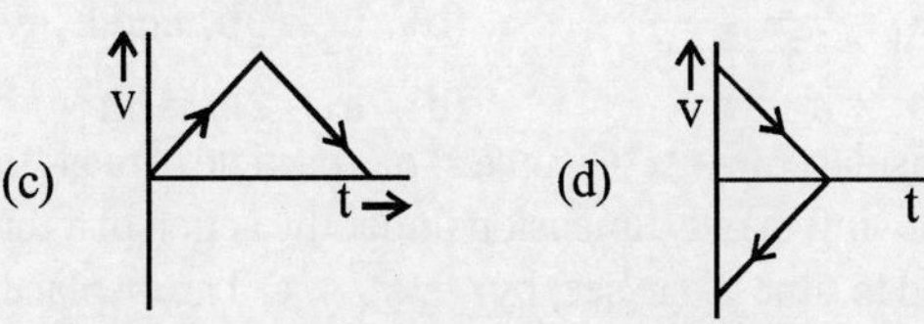

70. From a tower of height H, a particle is thrown vertically upwards with a speed u. The time taken by the particle, to hit the ground, is n times that taken by it to reach the highest point of its path. The relation between H, u and n is:

(a) $2gH = n^2u^2$ (b) $gH = (n-2)^2 u^2d$
(c) $2gH = nu^2 (n-2)$ (d) $gH = (n-2)u^2$

Exercise 2 - Exemplar & Past Year Questions

E&PYQs

Exemplar Questions

1. Among the four graph shown in the figure there is only one graph for which average velocity over the time interval (*O*, *T*) can vanish for a suitably chosen *T*. Which one is it?

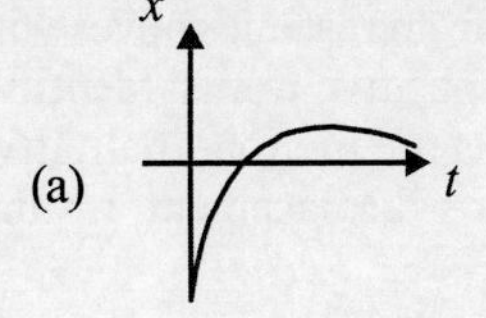

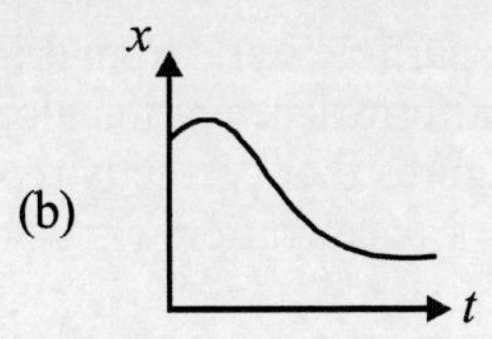

(c) (d)

2. A lift is coming from 8th floor and is just about to reach 4th floor. Taking ground floor as origin and positive direction upwards for all quantities, which one of the following is correct?

(a) $x<0, v<0, a>0$ (b) $x>0, v<0, a<0$
(c) $x>0, v<0, a>0$ (d) $x>0, v>0, a<0$

3. In one dimensional motion, instantaneous speed v satisfies $0 \le v < v_0$.
(a) The displacement in time T must always take non-negative values
(b) The displacement x in time T satisfies $-v_0T < x < v_0T$
(c) The acceleration is always a non-negative number
(d) The motion has no turning points

4. A vehicle travels half the distance l with speed v_1 and the other half with speed v_2, then its average speed is
(a) $\frac{v_1+v_2}{2}$ (b) $\frac{2v_1+v_2}{v_1+v_2}$ (c) $\frac{2v_1v_2}{v_1+v_2}$ (d) $\frac{L(v_1+v_2)}{v_1v_2}$

5. The displacement of a particle is given by $x = (t-2)^2$ where x is in metre and t in second. The distance covered by the particle in first 4 seconds is
(a) 4m (b) 8m (c) 12m (d) 16m

6. At a metro station, a girl walks up a stationary escalator in time t_1. If she remains stationary on the escalator, then the escalator take her up in time t_2. The time taken by her to walk up on the moving escalator will be
(a) $\frac{t_1+t_2}{2}$ (b) $\frac{t_1t_2}{t_2-t_1}$ (c) $\frac{t_1t_2}{t_2+t_1}$ (d) t_1-t_2

NEET/AIPMT (2013-2020) Questions

7. A stone falls freely under gravity. It covers distances h_1, h_2 and h_3 in the first 5 seconds, the next 5 seconds and the next 5 seconds respectively. The relation between h_1, h_2 and h_3 is *[2013]*
(a) $h_1 = \frac{h_2}{3} = \frac{h_3}{5}$ (b) $h_2 = 3h_1$ and $h_3 = 3h_2$
(c) $h_1 = h_2 = h_3$ (d) $h_1 = 2h_2 = 3h_3$

8. The displacement 'x' (in meter) of a particle of mass 'm' (in kg) moving in one dimension under the action of a force, is related to time 't' (in sec) by $t = \sqrt{x}+3$. The displacement of the particle when its velocity is zero, will be *[NEET Kar. 2013]*
(a) 2m (b) 4m (c) zero (d) 6m

9. A particle of unit mass undergoes one-dimensional motion such that its velocity varies according to $v(x) = bx^{-2n}$ where b and n are constants and x is the position of the particle. The acceleration of the particle as d function of x, is given by: *[2015]*
(a) $-2nb^2x^{-4n-1}$ (b) $-2b^2x^{-2n+1}$
(c) $-2nb^2e^{-4n+1}$ (d) $-2nb^2x^{-2n-1}$

10. If the velocity of a particle is $v = At + Bt^2$, where A and B are constants, then the distance travelled by it between 1s and 2s is : *[2016]*
(a) $\frac{3}{2}A+4B$ (b) $3A+7B$
(c) $\frac{3}{2}A+\frac{7}{3}B$ (d) $\frac{A}{2}+\frac{B}{3}$

11. Preeti reached the metro station and found that the escalator was not working. She walked up the stationary escalator in time t_1. On other days, if she remains stationary on the moving escalator, then the escalator takes her up in time t_2. The time taken by her to walk up on the moving escalator will be: *[2017]*
(a) $\frac{t_1t_2}{t_2-t_1}$ (b) $\frac{t_1t_2}{t_2+t_1}$ (c) t_1-t_2 (d) $\frac{t_1+t_2}{2}$

12. A person travelling in a straight line moves with a constant velocity v_1 for certain distance 'x' and with a constant velocity v_2 for next equal distance. The average velocity v is given by the relation *[NEET Odisha 2019]*
(a) $v=\sqrt{v_1v_2}$ (b) $\frac{1}{v}=\frac{1}{v_1}+\frac{1}{v_2}$
(c) $\frac{2}{v}=\frac{1}{v_1}+\frac{1}{v_2}$ (d) $\frac{v}{2}=\frac{v_1+v_2}{2}$

13. A ball is thrown vertically downward with a velocity of 20 m/s from the top of a tower. It hits the ground after some time with a velocity of 80 m/s. The height of the tower is : ($g = 10\,m/s^2$) *[2020]*
(a) 340m (b) 320m (c) 300m (d) 360m

Exercise 3 - Concept Application Problems CAP

1. A particle is moving with speed $v = b\sqrt{x}$ along positive x-axis. Calculate the speed of the particle at time $t = \tau$ (assume that the particle is at origin at t = 0).
(a) $\frac{b^2\tau}{4}$ (b) $\frac{b^2\tau}{2}$ (c) $b^2\tau$ (d) $\frac{b^2\tau}{\sqrt{2}}$

2. The velocity of a particle is $v = v_0 + gt + ft^2$. If its position is $x = 0$ at $t = 0$, then its displacement after unit time ($t = 1$) is
(a) $v_0 + g/2 + f$ (b) $v_0 + 2g + 3f$
(c) $v_0 + g/2 + f/3$ (d) $v_0 + g + f$

3. A bullet of mass 20g has an initial speed of 1 ms^{-1}, just before it starts penetrating a mud wall of thickness 20 cm. If the wall offers a mean resistance of 2.5×10^{-2} N, the speed of the bullet after emerging from the other side of the wall is close to :
(a) 0.1 ms^{-1} (b) 0.7 ms^{-1} (c) 0.3 ms^{-1} (d) 0.4 ms^{-1}

4. The position of a particle as a function of time t, is given by
$x(t) = at + bt^2 - ct^3$
where, a, b and c are constants. When the particle attains zero acceleration, then its velocity will be:
(a) $a+\frac{b^2}{4c}$ (b) $a+\frac{b^2}{3c}$ (c) $a+\frac{b^2}{c}$ (d) $a+\frac{b^2}{2c}$

5. A particle starts from origin O from rest and moves with a uniform acceleration along the positive x-axis. Identify all figures that correctly represents the motion qualitatively (a = acceleration, v = velocity, x = displacement, t = time)

(A) 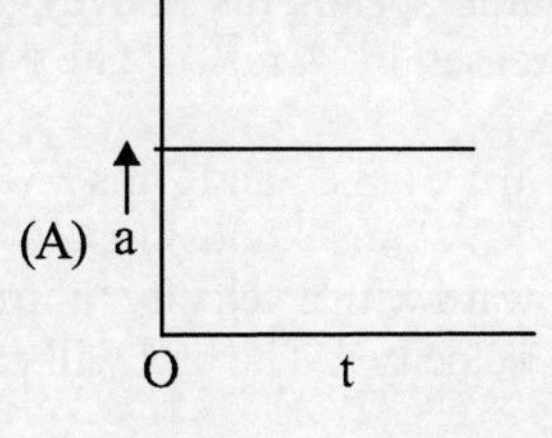

(B) 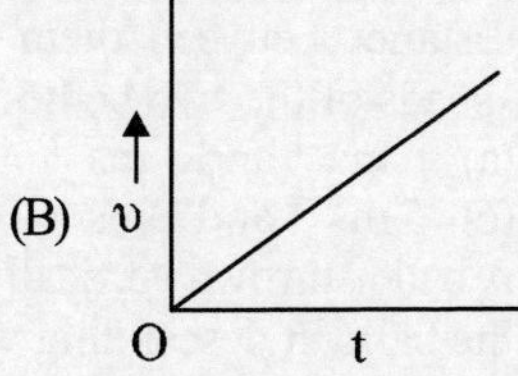

(C) 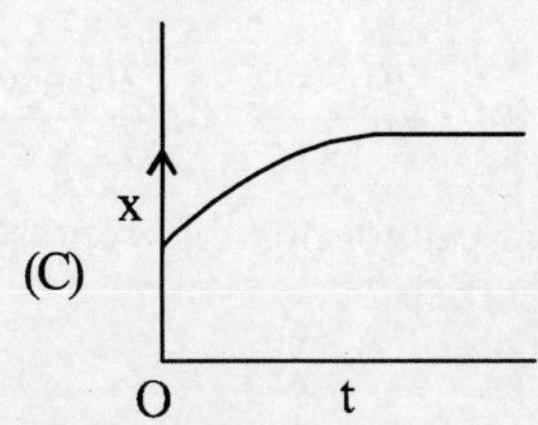

(D) 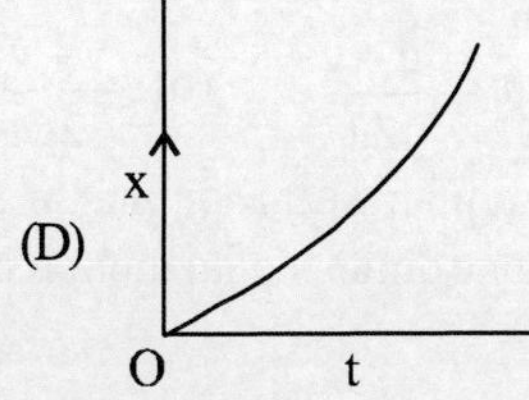

(a) (B), (C) (b) (A)

(c) (A), (B), (C) (d) (A), (B), (D)

6. In a car race on straight road, car A takes a time t less than car B at the finish and passes finishing point with a speed 'v' more than of car B. Both the cars start from rest and travel with constant acceleration a_1 and a_2 respectively. Then 'v' is equal to:

(a) $\frac{2a_1 a_2}{a_1 + a_2}t$ (b) $\sqrt{2a_1 a_2}\, t$ (c) $\sqrt{a_1 a_2}\, t$ (d) $\frac{a_1 + a_2}{2}t$

7. An automobile, travelling at 40 km/h, can be stopped at a distance of 40 m by applying brakes. If the same automobile is travelling at 80 km/h, the minimum stopping distance, in metres, is (assume no skidding)

(a) 75m (b) 160m (c) 100m (d) 150m

8. A man in a car at location Q on a straight highway is moving with speed v. He decides to reach a point P in a field at a distance d from highway (point M) as shown in the figure. Speed of the car in the field is half to that on the highway. What should be the distance RM, so that the time taken to reach P is minimum?

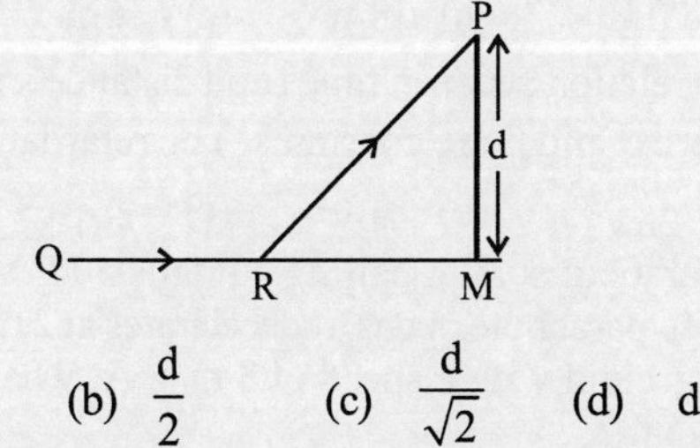

(a) $\frac{d}{\sqrt{3}}$ (b) $\frac{d}{2}$ (c) $\frac{d}{\sqrt{2}}$ (d) d

9. A passenger train of length 60 m travels at a speed of 80 km/hr. Another freight train of length 120 m travels at a speed of 30 km/h. The ratio of times taken by the passenger train to completely cross the freight train when: (i) they are moving in same direction, and (ii) in the opposite directions is:

(a) $\frac{11}{5}$ (b) $\frac{5}{2}$ (c) $\frac{3}{2}$ (d) $\frac{25}{11}$

10. A person standing on an open ground hears the sound of a jet aeroplane, coming from north at an angle 60° with ground level. But he finds the aeroplane right vertically above his position. If v is the speed of sound, speed of the plane is:

(a) $\frac{\sqrt{3}}{2}v$ (b) $\frac{2v}{\sqrt{3}}$ (c) v (d) $\frac{v}{2}$

11. A car is standing 200 m behind a bus, which is also at rest. The two start moving at the same instant but with different forward accelerations. The bus has acceleration 2 m/s^2 and the car has acceleration 4 m/s^2. The car will catch up with the bus after a time of :

(a) $\sqrt{110}$ s (b) $\sqrt{120}$ s (c) $10\sqrt{2}$ s (d) 15 s

12. A helicopter rises from rest on the ground vertically upwards with a constant acceleration g. A food packet is dropped from the helicopter when it is at a height h. The time taken by the packet to reach the ground is close to [g is the accelertion due to gravity] :

(a) $t = \frac{2}{3}\sqrt{\left(\frac{h}{g}\right)}$ (b) $t = 1.8\sqrt{\frac{h}{g}}$

(c) $t = 3.4\sqrt{\left(\frac{h}{g}\right)}$ (d) $t = \sqrt{\frac{2h}{3g}}$

13. The displacement x of a particle moving along a straight line at time t is given by

$$x = a_0 + a_1 t + a_2 t^2$$

What is the acceleration of the particle

(a) a_1 (b) a_2 (c) $2a_2$ (d) $3a_2$

14. A point traversed half of the distance with a velocity v_0. The half of remaining part of the distance was covered with velocity v_1 & second half of remaining part by v_2 velocity. The mean velocity of the point, averaged over the whole time of motion is

(a) $\frac{v_0 + v_1 + v_2}{3}$ (b) $\frac{2v_0 + v_1 + v_2}{3}$

(c) $\frac{v_0 + .2v_1 + 2v_2}{3}$ (d) $\frac{2v_0(v_1 + v_2)}{(2v_0 + v_1 + v_2)}$

15. The deceleration experienced by a moving motorboat after its engine is cut off, is given by dv/dt = – kv^3 where k is constant. If v_0 is the magnitude of the velocity at cut-off, the magnitude of the velocity at a time t after the cut-off is

(a) $\frac{v_0}{\sqrt{(2v_0{}^2 kt + 1)}}$ (b) $v_0 e^{-kt}$ (c) $v_0/2$ (d) v_0

16. Two cars A and B are travelling in the same direction with velocities v_A and v_B ($v_A > v_B$). When the car A is at a distance d behind the car B the driver of the car A applies brakes producing a uniform retardation a. There will be no collision when

(a) $d < \frac{(v_A - v_B)^2}{2a}$ (b) $d < \frac{v_A^2 - v_B^2}{2a}$

(c) $d > \frac{(v_A - v_B)^2}{2a}$ (d) $d > \frac{v_A^2 - v_B^2}{2a}$

17. A train of 150 m length is going towards north direction at a speed of 10 ms^{-1}. A parrot flies at a speed of 5 ms^{-1} towards south direction parallel to the railway track. The time taken by the parrot to cross the train is equal to

(a) 12 s (b) 8 s (c) 15 s (d) 10 s

18. A particle is moving along a straight line path according to the relation

$$s^2 = at^2 + 2bt + c$$

s represents the distance travelled in t seconds and a, b, c are constants. Then the acceleration of the particle varies as

(a) s^{-3} (b) $s^{3/2}$ (c) $s^{-2/3}$ (d) s^2

19. A stone thrown vertically upwards with a speed of 5 m/sec attains a height H_1. Another stone thrown upwards from the same point with a speed of 10 m/sec attains a height H_2. The correct relation between H_1 and H_2 is

(a) $H_2 = 4H_1$ (b) $H_2 = 3H_1$ (c) $H_1 = 2H_2$ (d) $H_1 = H_2$

20. An automobile travelling with a speed of 60 km/h, can apply brake to stop within a distance of 20m. If the car is going twice as fast i.e., 120 km/h, the stopping distance will be

(a) 60m (b) 40m (c) 20m (d) 80m

21. If you were to throw a ball vertically upward with an initial velocity of 50 m/s, approximately how long would it take for the ball to return to your hand? Assume air resistance is negligible.

(a) 2.5 s (b) 5.0 s (c) 7.5 s (d) 10 s

22. A car travels from A to B at a speed of 20 km h^{-1} and returns at a speed of 30 km h^{-1}. The average speed of the car for the whole journey is

(a) 5 km h^{-1} (b) 24 km h^{-1} (c) 25 km h^{-1} (d) 50 km h^{-1}

23. A body dropped from a height 'h' with an initial speed zero, strikes the ground with a velocity 3 km/hour. Another body of same mass dropped from the same height 'h' with an initial speed u' = 4 km/hour. Find the final velocity of second mass, with which it strikes the ground

(a) 3 km/hr (b) 4 km/hr (c) 5 km/hr (d) 6 km/hr

24. An electron starting from rest has a velocity that increases linearly with time i.e. v = kt where $k = 2\ m s^{-2}$. The distance covered in the first 3 second is

(a) 9m (b) 16m (c) 27m (d) 36m

25. A body released from the top of a tower falls through half the height of the tower in 2 s. In what time shall the body fall through the height of the tower ?

(a) 4 s (b) 3.26 s (c) 3.48 s (d) 2.828 s

26. Which one of the following equations represents the motion of a body with finite constant acceleration ? In these equations, y denotes the displacement of the body at time t and a, b and c are constants of motion.

(a) $y = at$ (b) $y = at + bt^2$

(c) $y = at + bt^2 + ct^3$ (d) $y = \frac{a}{t} + bt$

27. In the displacement d versus time t graph given below, the value of average velocity in the time interval 0 to 20 s is (in m/s)

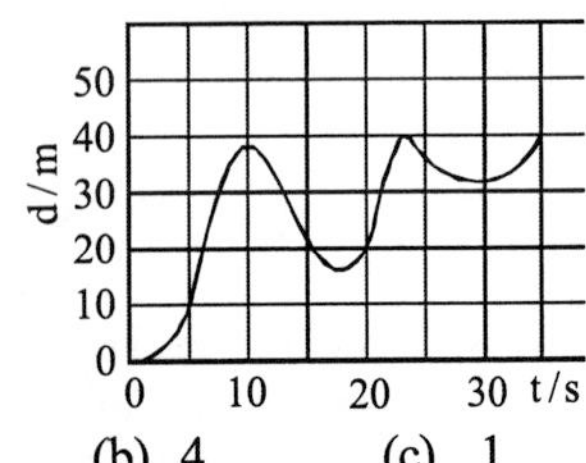

(a) 1.5 (b) 4 (c) 1 (d) 2

28. When two bodies move uniformly towards each other, the distance decreases by 6 ms^{-1}. If both bodies move in the same directions with the same speeds (as above), the distance between them increases by 4 ms^{-1}. Then the speeds of the two bodies are

(a) 3 ms^{-1} and 3 ms^{-1} (b) 4 ms^{-1} and 2 ms^{-1}

(c) 5 ms^{-1} and 1 ms^{-1} (d) 7 ms^{-1} and 3 ms^{-1}

29. A ball is thrown vertically upward with a velocity 'u' from the balloon descending with velocity v. The ball will pass by the balloon after time

(a) $\frac{u-v}{2g}$ (b) $\frac{u+v}{2g}$ (c) $\frac{2(u-v)}{g}$ (d) $\frac{2(u+v)}{g}$

30. Which of the following graph cannot possibly represent one dimensional motion of a particle?

(a) 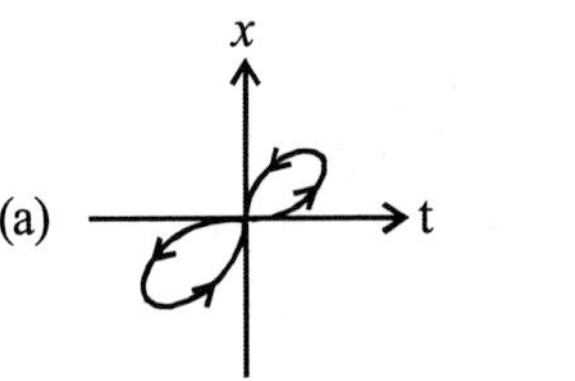

(b) x, t

(c) speed, t

(d) All of the above

31. A balloon starts rising from the ground with an acceleration of 1.25 ms^{-2}. After 8 s, a stone is released from the balloon. The stone will (Taking $g = 10\ m\,s^{-2}$)

(a) begin to move down after being released
(b) reach the ground in 4 s
(c) cover a distance of 40 m in reaching the ground
(d) will have a displacement of 50 m.

32. A point initially at rest moves along x-axis. Its acceleration varies with time as $a = (6t + 5) m/s^2$. If it starts from origin, the distance covered in 2 s is

(a) 20m (b) 18m (c) 16m (d) 25m

33. The relation between time t and distance x is $t = \alpha x^2 + \beta x$ where α and β are constants. The retardation is

(a) $2\alpha v^3$ (b) $2\beta v^3$ (c) $2\alpha\beta v^3$ (d) $2\beta^2 v^3$

34. A parachutist after bailing out falls 50 m without friction. When parachute opens, it decelerates at 2 m/s^2. He reaches the ground with a speed of 3 m/s. At what height, did he bail out ?

(a) 182m (b) 91m (c) 111m (d) 293m

35. A man throws balls with same speed vertically upwards one after the other at an interval of 2 sec. What should be the speed of throw so that more than two balls are in air at any time

(a) only with speed 19.6 m/s
(b) more than 19.6 m/s
(c) at least 9.8 m/s
(d) any speed less then 19.6 m/s.

36. A particle has initial velocity $(2\vec{i} + 3\vec{j})$ and acceleration $(0.3\vec{i} + 0.2\vec{j})$. The magnitude of velocity after 10 seconds will be

(a) $9\sqrt{2}$ units (b) $5\sqrt{2}$ units (c) 5 units (d) 9 units

37. A stone falls freely under gravity. It covers distances h_1, h_2 and h_3 in the first 5 seconds, the next 5 seconds and the next 5 seconds respectively. The relation between h_1, h_2 and h_3 is

(a) $h_1 = \frac{h_2}{3} = \frac{h_3}{5}$ (b) $h_2 = 3h_1$ and $h_3 = 3h_2$

(c) $h_1 = h_2 = h_3$ (d) $h_1 = 2h_2 = 3h_3$

38. Which one of the following equation represents the motion of a body moving with constant finite acceleration? In these equation, y denotes the displacement in time t and p, q and r are constant:

(a) $y = (p + qt)(t + pt)$ (b) $y = p + t/r$

(c) $y = (p + t)(q + t)(r + t)$ (d) $y = \frac{(p + qt)}{rt}$

39. A train *A* which is 120 m long is running with velocity 20 m/s while train *B* which is 130 m long is running in opposite direction with velocity 30 m/s. What is the time taken by train *B* to cross the train *A* ?

(a) 5 sec (b) 25 sec (c) 10 sec (d) 100 sec

40. Velocity time curve for a body projected vertically upwards is

(a) parabola (b) ellipse (c) hyperbola (d) straight line

41. A train is moving towards east and a car is along north, both with same speed. The observed direction of car to the passenger in the train is

(a) east-north direction (b) west-north direction

(c) south-east direction (d) None of the above

42. The displacement of particle is given by

$x = a_0 + \frac{a_1 t}{2} - \frac{a_2 t^2}{3}$. What is its acceleration?

(a) $\frac{2a_2}{3}$ (b) $-\frac{2a_2}{3}$ (c) a_2 (d) zero

43. The displacement time graph of a moving particle is shown below

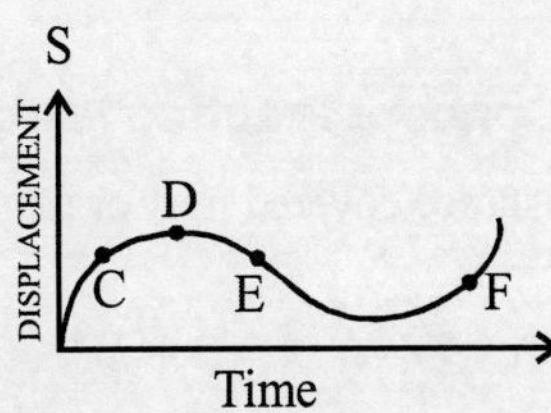

The instantaneous velocity of the particle is negative at the point

(a) D (b) F (c) C (d) E

44. A particle moves along a straight line such that its displacement at any time t is given by

$s = (t^3 - 6t^2 + 3t + 4)$ metres

The velocity when the acceleration is zero is

(a) $3\ ms^{-1}$ (b) $-12\ ms^{-1}$ (c) $42\ ms^{-2}$ (d) $-9\ ms^{-1}$

45. All the graphs below are intended to represent the same motion. One of them does it incorrectly. Pick it up.

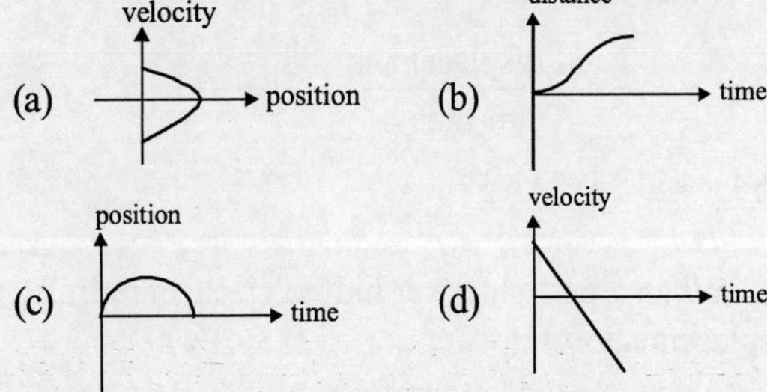

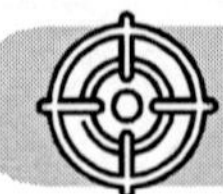

Hints & Solutions

3.1 Concept Practice Problems

1. (c) The distance covered may or may not be zero.
2. (b)
3. (b) $\sqrt{x} = (t+7)$ or $x = (t+7)^2$
$\frac{dx}{dt} = 2(t+7)$, $\therefore$ velocity $\propto$ time
4. (d) $v_A = \tan 30°$ and $v_B = \tan 60°$
$\therefore \frac{v_A}{v_B} = \frac{\tan 30°}{\tan 60°} = \frac{1/\sqrt{3}}{\sqrt{3}} = \frac{1}{3}$
5. (a) Let for the first half time t, the person travels a distance s_1. Hence $v_1 = \frac{s_1}{t}$ or $s_1 = v_1 t$
For second half time, $v_2 = \frac{s_2}{t}$ or $s_2 = v_2 t$
Now, $\bar{v} = \frac{\text{Total displacement}}{\text{Total time}} = \frac{s_1 + s_2}{2t}$
$= \frac{v_1 t + v_2 t}{2t} = \frac{v_1 + v_2}{2}$
6. (b) When a particle cover half of circle of radius r, then displacement is AB = 2r
& distance = half of circumference of circle = πr

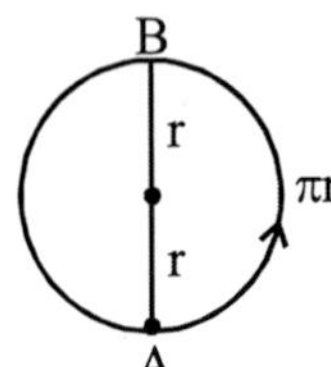

7. (b) Average velocity for the second half of the distance is $= \frac{v_1 + v_2}{2} = \frac{4+8}{2} = 6\,\text{ms}^{-1}$
Given that first half distance is covered with a velocity of $6\,\text{ms}^{-1}$. Therefore, the average velocity for the whole time of motion is $6\,\text{ms}^{-1}$
8. (a) Since displacement is zero.
9. (c) $\bar{v} = \frac{(8\times1 - 3\times1\times1) - 0}{1} = 5\,\text{ms}^{-1}$
10. (d) Given $x = ae^{-\alpha t} + be^{\beta t}$
Velocity, $v = \frac{dx}{dt} = -a\alpha e^{-\alpha t} + b\beta e^{\beta t} = -\frac{a\alpha}{e^{\alpha t}} + b\beta e^{\beta t}$
i.e., go on increasing with time.

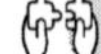

3.2 Concept Practice Problems

11. (b) Let after a time t, the cyclist overtake the bus. Then
$96 + \frac{1}{2}\times 2\times t^2 = 20\times t$ or $t^2 - 20t + 96 = 0$
$\therefore t = \frac{20 \pm \sqrt{400 - 4\times 96}}{2\times 1}$
$= \frac{20\pm 4}{2} = 8\,\text{sec. and } 12\,\text{sec.}$
12. (d) $v^2 = u^2 + 2as$ or $v^2 - u^2 = 2as$
Maximum retardation, $a = v^2/2s$
When the initial velocity is n v, then the distance over which it can be stopped is given by
$s_n = \frac{u_0^2}{2a} = \frac{(nv)^2}{2(v^2/2s)} = n^2 s$
13. (c) Let the length of train is s, then by third equation of motion, $v^2 = u^2 + 2a\times s$ ....(1)
Where v is final velocity after travelling a distance s with an acceleration a & u is initial velocity as per question
Let velocity of middle point of train at same point is v', then
$(v')^2 = u^2 + 2a\times(s/2)$ ....(2)
By equations (1) and (2), we get $v' = \sqrt{\frac{v^2 + u^2}{2}}$
14. (b) $8 = a t_1$ and $0 = 8 - a(4 - t_1)$
or $t_1 = \frac{8}{a}$ $\therefore 8 = a\left(4 - \frac{8}{a}\right)$
$8 = 4a - 8$ or $a = 4$ and $t_1 = 8/4 = 2$ sec
Now, $s_1 = 0\times 2 + \frac{1}{2}\times 4(2)^2$ or $s_1 = 8\,\text{m}$
$s_2 = 8\times 2 - \frac{1}{2}\times 4\times(2)^2$ or $s_2 = 8\,\text{m}$
$\therefore s_1 + s_2 = 16$ m
15. (b) u = 10 m/s, t = 5 sec, v = 20 m/s, a = ?
$a = \frac{20-10}{5} = 2\,\text{ms}^{-2}$
From the formula $v_1 = u_1 + at$, we have
$10 = u_1 + 2\times 3$ or $u_1 = 4$ m/sec.
16. (c) The distance covered in n^{th} second is
$S_n = u + \frac{1}{2}(2n-1)a$
where u is initial velocity & a is acceleration
then $26 = u + \frac{19a}{2}$ ....(1)
$28 = u + \frac{21a}{2}$ ....(2)
$30 = u + \frac{23a}{2}$ ....(3)
$32 = u + \frac{25a}{2}$ ....(4)
From eqs. (1) and (2) we get u = 7m/sec, a = 2m/sec^2
$\therefore$ The body starts with initial velocity u = 7m/sec and moves with uniform acceleration a = 2m/sec^2

17. (a) $v=\sqrt{3x+16} \Rightarrow v^2=3x+16$

$\Rightarrow v^2-16=3x$

Comparing with $v^2-u^2=2aS$, we get, $u=4$ units, $2a=3$ or $a=1.5$ units

18. (d) As per question,
Let max. velocity is v
then $v=\alpha t_1$ & $v-\beta t_2=0$, where $t=t_1+t_2$

Now $t_1+t_2=t$ or $\frac{v}{\alpha}+\frac{v}{\beta}=t$

$\therefore v=\frac{t}{\left(\frac{1}{\alpha}+\frac{1}{\beta}\right)}=\left(\frac{\alpha\beta}{\alpha+\beta}\right)t$ and

$s=s_1+s_2=\frac{v^2}{2\alpha}+\frac{v^2}{2\beta}=\frac{v^2}{2}\left(\frac{1}{\alpha}+\frac{1}{\beta}\right)$

19. (a) From third equation of motion : $v^2=u^2+2as$

for first case $u=\frac{40\times10}{36}$ m/sec, $v=0$, $a=?$, $s=2$ m

so, $a=\left(\frac{40\times10}{36}\right)^2\frac{1}{4}$ m/sec^2

for second case $u=\frac{80\times10}{36}$ m/sec, $v=0$,

So $s_2=\left(\frac{80\times10}{36}\right)^2/2\times\frac{1}{4}\times\left(\frac{40\times10}{36}\right)^2=8$ meter

20. (a) $\frac{D_4}{D_3}=\frac{0+\frac{a}{2}(2\times4-1)}{0+\frac{a}{2}(2\times3-1)}=\frac{7}{5}$

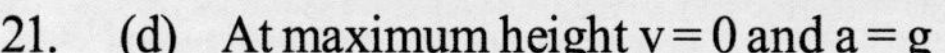

3.3 Concept Practice Problems CPP

21. (d) At maximum height $v=0$ and $a=g$

22. (b) The stone rises up till its vertical velocity is zero and again reached the top of the tower with a speed u (downward). The speed of the stone at the base is 3u.

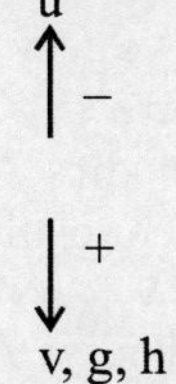

Hence $(3u)^2=(-u)^2+2gh$ or $h=\frac{4u^2}{g}$

23. (a) $S=ut+½at^2$ here $a=g$
For first body $u_1=0 \Rightarrow S_1=½g\times9$
For second body $u_2=0 \Rightarrow S_2=½g\times4$
So difference between them after 3 sec. $=S_1-S_2=½g\times5$
If $g=10$m/sec^2 then $S_1-S_2=25$ m.

24. (b) Relative speed of each train with respect to each other be, $v=10+15=25$ m/s

Here distance covered by each train = sum of their lengths $=50+50=100$ m

$\therefore$ Required time $=\frac{100}{25}=4$ sec.

25. (b) Since $v^2=u^2+2as$
For first case u_1=20m/sec, $v_1=0$, $a_1=g=10$, $s_1=?$

So $s_1=\frac{400}{2\times10}=20$m

For second case (at moon) u_2=20m/sec, v_2=0, $a_2=\frac{g}{6}=1.7$m/sec^2, $s_2=?$

$s_2=\frac{400}{2\times1.7}=\frac{400}{2\times10/6}$ so $\frac{s_1}{s_2}=\frac{1}{6}$

26. (b) Since in both case the height of building and down ward acceleration 'g' is same. So both stones reach simultaneously i.e., $S=\frac{1}{2}gt^2 \Rightarrow 10=\frac{1}{2}10\times t^2$
or $t=\sqrt{2}$ sec, for both stone.

27. (c) The ball thrown upward will lose velocity in 1s. It return back to thrown point in another 1 s with the same velocity as second. Thus the difference will be 2 s.

28. (b) Velocity when the engine is switched off
$v=19.6\times5=98\,ms^{-1}$

$h_{max}=h_1+h_2$ where $h_1=\frac{1}{2}at^2$ & $h_2=\frac{v^2}{2a}$

$h_{max}=\frac{1}{2}\times19.6\times5\times5+\frac{98\times98}{2\times9.8}$

$=245+490=735$ m

29. (c) The food packet has an initial velocity of 2 m/sec in upward direction, therefore
$v=-u+gt$ or $v=-2+10\times2=18$ m/sec.

30. (b) Area under a-t graph is change in velocity.

Area $=\frac{1}{2}(4\times4)+6\times4+\frac{1}{2}\times2\times4-\frac{1}{2}\times2\times2$

$=36-2=34\ ms^{-1}$

As initial velocity is zero therefore, the velocity at 14 second is $34\,ms^{-1}$.

Exercise 1 - Chapter Revision Problems CRP

1. (b) Velocity is a vector quantity and speed is scalar.
2. (c) 3. (d) 4. (c)
5. (b) $a=ft$, $a=\frac{dv}{dt}=ft$ at $t=0$, velocity $=u$

$\int_u^v dv=\int_0^t ft\,dt$, $v-u=f\frac{t^2}{2} \Rightarrow v=u+f\frac{t^2}{2}$

NOTE : Do not use $v=u+at$ directly because the acceleration is not constant.

6. (d) $y=\frac{1}{2}g(n+1)^2-\frac{1}{2}gn^2$

$=\frac{g}{2}[(n+1)^2-n^2]=\frac{g}{2}(2n+1)$ ......(i)

Also, $h=\frac{g}{2}(2n-1)$ ......(ii)

From (i) and (ii)

$y = h + g$

7. (a) Differentiate two times and put $x = 0$.

8. (d) The difference in velocities is increasing with time as both of them have more constant but different acceleration.

9. (b) Time taken by the stone to reach the water level

$t_1 = \sqrt{\frac{2h}{g}}$

Time taken by sound to come to the mouth of the well,

$t_2 = \frac{h}{v}$

$\therefore$ Total time $t_1 + t_2 = \sqrt{\frac{2h}{g}} + \frac{h}{v}$

10. (c) $a = bt$ or $\frac{dv}{dt} = bt$. Integrating, we get

$v = \frac{bt^2}{2} + c$, where c is a constant of integration.

At $t = 0$, $v = v_0$. Thus $v_0 = c$.

Now, $v = \frac{ds}{dt} = \frac{bt^2}{2} + v_o \therefore ds = \left(\frac{bt^2}{2} + v_o\right)dt$

Integrating we get, $s = \frac{bt^3}{6} + v_o t$

11. (d)

12. (c) $x = t^2 + 2t + 1$

Hence $v = \frac{dx}{dt} = 2t + 2$. It increases with time.

13. (b) When a body falls through a height h, it acquires a velocity $\sqrt{2gh}$.

14. (c) Given that $x = At^2 - Bt^3$

$\therefore$ velocity $= \frac{dx}{dt} = 2At - 3Bt^2$

and acceleration $= \frac{d}{dt}\left(\frac{dx}{dt}\right) = 2A - 6Bt$

For acceleration to be zero $2A - 6Bt = 0$.

$\therefore t = \frac{2A}{6B} = \frac{A}{3B}$

15. (a) $a = \frac{d^2x}{dt^2} = -s\omega^2 \sin\omega t$

On integrating, $\frac{dx}{dt} = s\omega^2 \frac{\cos\omega t}{\omega} = s\omega\cos\omega t$

Again on integrating, we get

$x = s\omega\frac{\sin\omega t}{\omega} = s\sin\omega t$

16. (c) $v = \frac{dy}{dt} = b + 2ct - 4dt^3$

$v_0 = b + 2c(0) - 4d(0)^3 = b$ ($\because$ for initial velocity, $t = 0$)

Now $a = \frac{dv}{dt} = 2c - 12dt^2$

$\therefore a_0 = 2c - 12d(0)^2 = 2c$, (at $t = 0$)

17. (d) $\dfrac{\frac{x}{2} + \frac{x}{2}}{\frac{x}{2v_1} + \frac{x}{2v_2}} = \dfrac{1}{\left(\frac{v_2 + v_1}{2v_1 v_2}\right)} = \dfrac{2v_1 v_2}{v_1 + v_2}$

18. (b)

19. (c) Let a be the constant acceleration of the particle. Then

$s = ut + \frac{1}{2}at^2$ or $\quad s_1 = 0 + \frac{1}{2} \times a \times (10)^2 = 50\,a$

and $s_2 = \left[0 + \frac{1}{2}a(20)^2\right] - 50a = 150a$

$\therefore s_2 = 3s_1$

20. (c) So by second equation of motion, we get

$S = ut + \frac{1}{2}at^2$

here $S = \ell$, $u = 0$, $a = g\sin\theta$

$t = \sqrt{\frac{2\ell}{a}} = \sqrt{\frac{2h}{g\sin^2\theta}} = \frac{1}{\sin\theta}\sqrt{\frac{2h}{g}} \left(\because \sin\theta = \frac{h}{\ell}\right)$

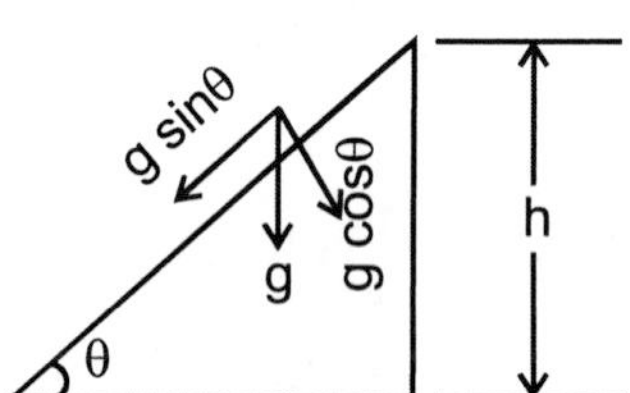

21. (d) At highest point of the trajectory velocity becomes zero and all kinetic energy changes to potential energy so at highest point, K.E. = 0

22. (b) The distance travel in n^{th} second is

$S_n = u + ½(2n-1)a$ ....(1)

so distance travel in t^{th} & $(t+1)^{th}$ second are

$S_t = u + ½(2t-1)a$ ....(2)

$S_{t+1} = u + ½(2t+1)a$ ....(3)

As per question,

$S_t + S_{t+1} = 100 = 2(u + at)$ ....(4)

Now from first equation of motion the velocity, of particle after time t, if it moves with an accleration a is

$v = u + at$ ....(5)

where u is initial velocity

So from eq(4) and (5), we get v = 50cm./sec.

23. (d) All options are correct :

(i) When two bodies A & B move in opposite directions then relative velocity between A & B either V_{AB} or V_{BA} both are greater than V_A & V_B.

(ii) When two bodies A & B move in parallel direction then $V_{AB} = V_A - V_B \Rightarrow V_{AB} < V_A$

$V_{BA} = V_B - V_A \Rightarrow V_{BA} < V_B$

24. (b) From third equation of motion

$v^2 = u^2 - 2gh$ ($\because a = -g$)

Given, v = 10 m/sec at h/2. But v = 0, when particle attained maximum height h.

Therefore $(10)^2 = u^2 - 2gh/2$

or $100 = 2gh - 2gh/2$ $\quad$ ($\because 0 = u^2 - 2gh$)

$\Rightarrow h = 10\,m$

25. (d) Equation of motion is $u = at$

we know that $u = \frac{ds}{dt} \Rightarrow \frac{ds}{dt} = at$ or $ds = atdt$

integrating it we get, $\int_0^s ds = a\int_0^4 tdt$ $\quad s = \frac{a}{2}[t^2]_0^4 = 8a$

26. (b) A B C

A to B

$2 = u \times 2 + \frac{1}{2} \times a \times 2 \times 2 \Rightarrow 1 = u + a,$

A to C

$4.20 = u \times 6 + \frac{1}{2} a \times 6 \times 6 \Rightarrow 0.7 = u + 3a$,

$2a = -0.3$ or $a = -0.15 ms^{-2}$,

$u = 1 - a = (1 + 0.15) ms^{-1} = 1.15 ms^{-1}$

Velocity at t = 9 sec.

$v = 1.15 - 0.15 \times 9 = 1.15 - 1.35 = -0.2 m s^{-1}$

27. (d) Since $S = ut + ½ gt^2$
where u is initial velocity & a is acceleration.
In this case u = 0 & a = g
so distance travelled in 4 sec is,
$S = ½ \times 10 \times 16 = 80m$

28. (b) Differentiated twice.

29. (c) Downward motion

$v^2 - 0^2 = 2 \times 9.8 \times 5$

$\Rightarrow v = \sqrt{98} = 9.9$

Also for upward motion

$0^2 - u^2 = 2 \times (-9.8) \times 1.8 \Rightarrow u = \sqrt{3528} = 5.94$

Fractional loss $= \frac{9.9 - 5.94}{9.9} = 0.4$

30. (a) Use $\vec{v}_{AB} = \vec{v}_A - \vec{v}_B$.

31. (b) $S = AB = \frac{1}{2} g t_1^2 \Rightarrow 2S = AC = \frac{1}{2} g (t_1 + t_2)^2$

and $3S = AD = \frac{1}{2} g (t_1 + t_2 + t_3)^2$

$t_1 = \sqrt{\frac{2S}{g}}$

$t_1 + t_2 = \sqrt{\frac{4S}{g}}, \ t_2 = \sqrt{\frac{4S}{g}} - \sqrt{\frac{2S}{g}}$

$t_1 + t_2 + t_3 = \sqrt{\frac{6S}{g}} \Rightarrow t_3 = \sqrt{\frac{6S}{g}} - \sqrt{\frac{4S}{g}}$

A, S, B, 2S, S, 3S, C, S, D

$t_1 : t_2 : t_3 :: 1 : (\sqrt{2} - \sqrt{1}) : (\sqrt{3} - \sqrt{2})$

32. (c) Since the initial velocity of jump is same on both planets
So $0 = u^2 - 2g_A h_A$
$0 = u^2 - 2g_B h_B$

or $\frac{g_A \times h_A}{g_B} = h_B \Rightarrow h_B = \frac{9}{1} \times 2 = 18m$

33. (d)

34. (c) On differentiating, acceleration $= 0.2t \Rightarrow a = f(t)$

35. (d) Use $v^2 - u^2 = 2aS$. In both the cases, (u positive or negative) u^2 is positive.

36. (a) At six points in the graph the tangents have zero slope i.e. velocity is zero.

37. (d) Time fall is $\frac{1}{2}$ second.

$h = \frac{1}{2} g \left(\frac{1}{2}\right)^2 = \frac{10}{8} = 1.25 m$

38. (b) $v_{av} = \frac{x + 2x + 3x}{t_1 + t_2 + t_3}$

$t_1 = \frac{2x}{v_{max}}, \ t_2 = \frac{2x}{v_{max}}, \ t_3 = \frac{6x}{v_{max}}$

$v_{av} = \frac{6x \ v_{max}}{10x}$

$\frac{v_{av}}{v_{max}} = \frac{3}{5}$

39. (c) $y_1 = \frac{1}{2} gn^2, \ y_2 = \frac{1}{2} g(n - N)^2$

$\therefore \ y_1 - y_2 = \frac{1}{2} g[n^2 - (n - N)^2]$

$\Rightarrow 1 = \frac{g}{2}(2n - N)N \qquad [\because y_1 - y_2 = 1]$

$\Rightarrow n = \frac{1}{gN} + \frac{N}{2}$

40. (b) $S_1 = \frac{1}{2} g \left(\frac{1}{2}\right)^2, \ S_1 + S_2 = \frac{1}{2} g(1)^2$

$\frac{1}{2} g \left(\frac{3}{2}\right)^2 = S_1 + S_2 + S_3$

By solving we get

$S_1 : S_2 : S_3 = 1 : 3 : 5$

41. (b) Distance in last two second

$= \frac{1}{2} \times 10 \times 2 = 10 m.$

Total distance $= \frac{1}{2} \times 10 \times (6 + 2) = 40 m.$

42. (a) Velocity at time t is tan 45° = 1. Velocity at time (t = 1) is $\tan 60° = \sqrt{3}$. Acceleration is change in velocity in one second $= \sqrt{3} - 1$.

43. (c) Here, the particle B moves upwards. Let the upward velocity of B be v then $\frac{v}{10} = \tan 60°$

44. (c) The horizontal velocity of the stone will be the same as that of the train. In this way, the horizontal motion will be uniform motion. The vertical motion will be controlled by the force of gravity, i. e., vertical motion is accelerated motion. Thus the resultant motion will be along a parabolic trajectory.

45. (a) Clearly distance moved by 1st ball in 18s = distance moved by 2nd ball in 12s.
Now, distance moved in 18 s by 1st ball

$= \frac{1}{2} \times 10 \times 18^2 = 90 \times 18 = 1620\,m$

Distance moved in 12 s by 2nd ball

$= ut + \frac{1}{2}gt^2 \quad \therefore 1620 = 12v + 5 \times 144$

$\Rightarrow v = 135 - 60 = 75\ ms^{-1}$

46. (a) $x = \frac{1}{t+5} \qquad \therefore v = \frac{dx}{dt} = \frac{-1}{(t+5)^2}$

$\therefore a = \frac{d^2x}{dt^2} = \frac{2}{(t+5)^3} = 2x^3$

Now $\frac{1}{(t+5)} \propto v^{\frac{1}{2}} \qquad \therefore \frac{1}{(t+5)^3} \propto v^{\frac{3}{2}} \propto a$

47. (a) $h = \frac{1}{2}gT^2$

now for t = T/3 second vertical distance moved is given by

$h' = \frac{1}{2}g\left(\frac{T}{3}\right)^2 \Rightarrow h' = \frac{1}{2} \times \frac{gT^2}{9} = \frac{h}{9}$

$\therefore$ position of ball from ground $= h - \frac{h}{9} = \frac{8h}{9}$

48. (d) $x = a + bt^2 = 15 + 3t^2$

$v = \frac{dx}{dt} = 3 \times 2t = 6t \Rightarrow v|_{t=3s} = 6 \times 3 = 18\text{cm/s}$

49. (c) Let the maximum height attained by the ball be h.
At maximum height, velocity of ball, $v = 0$
Given, initial velocity, $u = 19.6$ m/s
Using the equation of motion,
$v^2 = u^2 + 2gh$
We get $0 = (19.6)^2 + 2(-9.8) \times h$

$\Rightarrow h = \frac{(19.6)^2}{2 \times 9.8} = 19.6\,m$

50. (a) Retardation, $a = \frac{v^2 - u^2}{2s} = \frac{0 - (25/3)^2}{2 \times 8}$

$a = -\left(\frac{25}{3}\right)^2 \times \frac{1}{16}$

For $u = 60\ km\,h^{-1} = \frac{50}{3}\ ms^{-1}$

$s = \frac{0 - (50/3)^2}{2 \times [-(25/3)^2 \times 1/16]} = 32\,m$

51. (d)

52. (c) When particle comes to rest,

$V = 0 = \frac{dx}{dt} = \frac{d}{dt}(40 + 12t - t^3)$

$\Rightarrow 12 - 3t^2 = 0 \Rightarrow t^2 = \frac{12}{3} = 4 \therefore t = 2$ sec

Therefore distance travelled by particle before coming to rest,
$x = 40 + 12t - t^3 = 40 + 12 \times 2 - (2)^3 = 56m$

53. (b) $\frac{1}{2}(2+4) \times 2 + \frac{1}{2} \times 1 \times 4 - \frac{1}{2} \times 3 \times 4 = 2m$

54. (a) Velocity of boat $= \frac{8+8}{2} = 8\,km\,h^{-1}$

Velocity of water $= 4\,km\,h^{-1}$

$t = \frac{8}{8-4} + \frac{8}{8+4} = \frac{8}{3}h = 160$ minute

55. (b) Using relative terms

$u_{rel.} = 0\ m/s$

$a = 9.8\,ms^{-2}$, $S = 4.9\,m$, $t = ?$

$4.9 = 0 \times t + \frac{1}{2} \times 9.8 \times t^2$

$\Rightarrow 4.9t^2 = 4.9 \Rightarrow t = 1\ s$

56. (b) From first equation of motion $v = u + at$
here $u = 40$, $a = g = -10$, $t = 2$
so $v = 40 - 10 \times 2 = 20$ m/sec

57. (b) $v = [144 \times 1000/(60 \times 60)]$ m/sec.
$v = u + at$
or $(144 \times 1000)/(60 \times 60) = 0 + a \times 20$

$\therefore a = \frac{144 \times 1000}{60 \times 60 \times 20} = 2\,m/sec^2$

Now $s = ut + \frac{1}{2}at^2 = 0 + \frac{1}{2} \times 2 \times (20)^2 = 400$ m

58. (c) Height of tap = 5m and (g) = 10 m/sec^2.

For the first drop, $5 = ut + \frac{1}{2}gt^2$

$= (0 \times t) + \frac{1}{2} \times 10t^2 = 5t^2$ or $t^2 = 1$ or $t = 1$ sec.

It means that the third drop leaves after one second of the first drop. Or, each drop leaves after every 0.5 sec.
Distance covered by the second drop in 0.5 sec

$= ut + \frac{1}{2}gt^2 = (0 \times 0.5) + \frac{1}{2} \times 10 \times (0.5)^2 = 1.25\,m.$

Therefore, distance of the second drop above the ground $= 5 - 1.25 = 3.75\,m.$

59. (b) In one dimensional motion, the body can have at a time one velocity but not two values of velocities.

60. (a) $v = \alpha\sqrt{x}$,

$\Rightarrow \frac{dx}{dt} = \alpha\sqrt{x} \Rightarrow \frac{dx}{\sqrt{x}} = \alpha\,dt$

Integrating both sides,

$\int_0^x \frac{dx}{\sqrt{x}} = \alpha\int_0^t dt\ ; \left[\frac{2\sqrt{x}}{1}\right]_0^x = \alpha[t]_0^t$

$\Rightarrow 2\sqrt{x} = \alpha t \Rightarrow x = \frac{\alpha^2}{4}t^2$

61. (a)

62. (d) Position of the particle,
S = area under graph (time t = 0 to 5s)

$= \frac{1}{2} \times 2 \times 2 + 2 \times 2 + 3 \times 1 = 9m$

63. (c) Using equation, $a = \frac{v-u}{t}$ and $S = ut + \frac{1}{2}at^2$

Distance travelled by car in 15 sec $= \frac{1}{2}\frac{(45)}{15}(15)^2$

$= \frac{675}{2}$ m

Distance travelled by scooter in 15 seconds = 30 × 15 = 450

($\because$ distance = speed × time)

Difference between distance travelled by car and scooter in 15 sec, 450 – 337.5 = 112.5 m

Let car catches scooter in time t;

$\frac{675}{2} + 45(t-15) = 30t$

337.5 + 45t – 675 = 30t ⇒ 15t = 337.5

⇒ t = 22.5 sec

64. (c) According to question, object is moving with constant negative acceleration i.e., a = – constant (C)

$\frac{vdv}{dx} = -C$

vdv = – Cdx

$\frac{v^2}{2} = -Cx + k \quad x = -\frac{v^2}{2C} + \frac{k}{C}$

Hence, graph (3) represents correctly.

65. (a)

66. (c) Person's speed walking only is $\frac{1 \text{ "escalator"}}{60 \text{ second}}$

Standing the escalator without walking the speed is $\frac{1 \text{ "escalator"}}{40 \text{ second}}$

Walking with the escalator going, the speed add.

So, the person's speed is $\frac{1}{60} + \frac{1}{40} = \frac{15}{120} \frac{\text{"escalator"}}{\text{second}}$

So, the time to go up the escalator $t = \frac{120}{5} = 24$ second.

67 (d) Let '*S*' be the distance between two ends '*a*' be the constant acceleration

As we know $v^2 - u^2 = 2aS$ or, $aS = \frac{v^2 - u^2}{2}$

Let v be velocity at mid point.

Therefore, $v_c^2 - u^2 = 2a\frac{S}{2}$

$v_c^2 = u^2 + aS$

$v_c^2 = u^2 + \frac{v^2 - u^2}{2} \Rightarrow v_c = \sqrt{\frac{u^2 + v^2}{2}}$

68. (c)

69. (a) For a body thrown vertically upwards acceleration remains constant ($a = -g$) and velocity at anytime t is given by $V = u - gt$

During rise velocity decreases linearly and during fall velocity increases linearly and direction is opposite to each other.

Hence graph (a) correctly depicts velocity versus time.

70. (c) Speed on reaching ground

$v = \sqrt{u^2 + 2gh}$

Now, $v = u + at$

$\Rightarrow \sqrt{u^2 + 2gh} = -u + gt$

Time taken to reach highest point is $t = \frac{u}{g}$,

$\Rightarrow t = \frac{u + \sqrt{u^2 + 2gH}}{g} = \frac{nu}{g}$

(from question)

$\Rightarrow 2gH = n(n-2)u^2$

Exercise 2 - Exemplar & Past Year Questions E&PYQs

Exemplar Questions

1. (b) If we draw a line parallel to time axis from the point (A) on graph at $t = 0$ sec. This line can intersect graph at B.

In graph (b) for one value of displacement there are two different points of time. so, for one time, the average velocity is positive and for other time is equivalent negative.

As there are opposite velocities in the inteval 0 to T hence average velocity can vanish in (b). This can be seen in the figure given below.

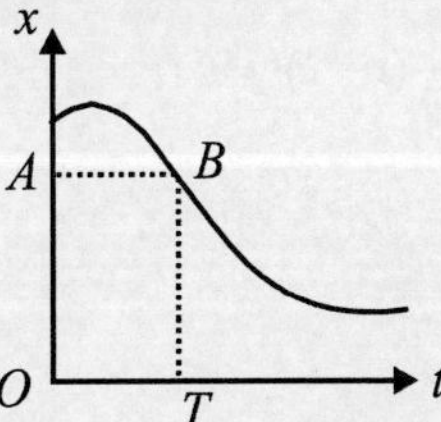

Here, $OA = BT$ (same displacement) for two different points of time.

2. (a) As the lift is moving downward directions so displacement is negative (zero). We have to see whether the motion is accelerating or retarding.

Due to downward motion displacement is negative the lift reaches 4th floor is about to stop hence, motion is retarding (–a) downward in nature hence, $x < 0$; $a > 0$.

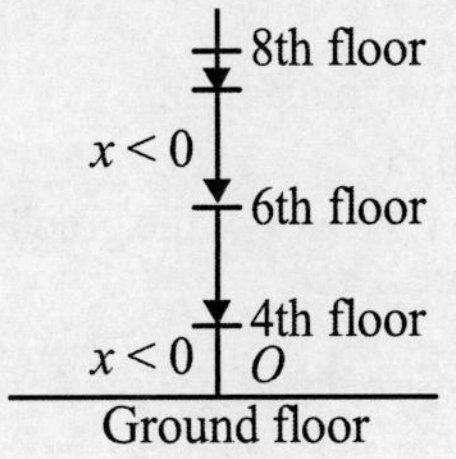

As displacement is in negative direction, $x < 0$ velocity will also be negative i.e., $v < 0$ but net acceleration is +ve $a > 0$, that can be shown in the graph.

3. (b) In one dimensional motion, for the maximum and minimum displacement we must have the magnitude and direction of maximum velocity.
As maximum velocity in positive direction is v_0, hence maximum velocity in opposite direction is also $-v_0$.
Maximum displacement in one direction $= v_0 T$
Maximum displacement in opposite directions $= -v_0 T$.
Hence, $-v_0 T < x < v_0 T$

4. (c) Time taken to travel first half distance,
$$t_1 = \frac{l/2}{v_1} = \frac{l}{2v_1} \qquad (\because L_1 = l/2)$$
Time taken to travel second half distance,
$$t_2 = \frac{l}{2v_2} \qquad (\because L_2 = l/2)$$
So, total time taken to travel full distance
$$= t_1 + t_2 = \frac{l}{2v_1} + \frac{l}{2v_2} = \frac{l}{2}\left[\frac{1}{v_1} + \frac{1}{v_2}\right]$$
$$\text{Total time} = \frac{l}{2}\left[\frac{v_2 + v_1}{v_1 v_2}\right]$$
So, average speed,
$$v_{av.} = \frac{\text{Total distance}}{\text{Total time}} \Rightarrow v_{av.} = \frac{l}{\frac{l}{2}\left[\frac{1}{v_1} + \frac{1}{v_2}\right]} = \frac{2v_1 v_2}{v_1 + v_2}$$
$$\therefore v_{av.} = \frac{2v_1 v_2}{v_1 + v_2}$$

5. (b) As given that, $x = (t-2)^2$
Now, velocity $v = \frac{dx}{dt} = \frac{d}{dt}(t-2)^2 = 2(t-2)$ m/s
Acceleration, $a = \frac{dv}{dt} = \frac{d}{dt}[2(t-2)]$
$= 2[1-0] = 2\text{ m/s}^2 = 2\text{ ms}^{-2}$
at $t = 0$; $v_0 = 2(0-2) = -4$ m/s
$t = 2$ s; $v_2 = 2(2-2) = 0$ m/s
$t = 4$ s; $v_4 = 2(4-2) = 4$ m/s

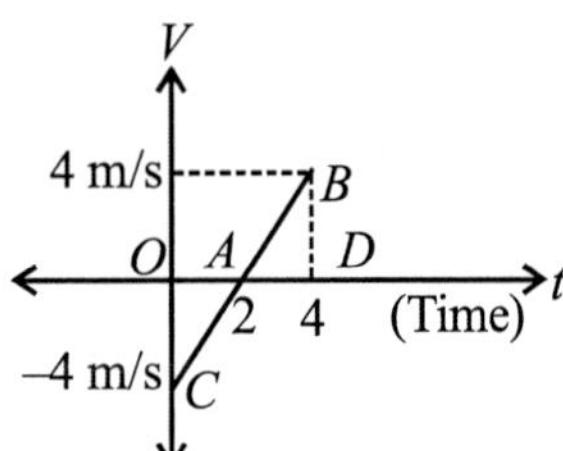

v-t graph is shown in diagram.
Distance travelled
= area between time axis of the graph
= area OAC + are ABD
$$= \frac{1}{2} OA \times OC + \frac{1}{2} AD \times BD$$
$$= \frac{4 \times 2}{2} + \frac{1}{2} \times 2 \times 4 = 8 \text{ m}$$
If displacement occurs
$$= \frac{1}{2} \times OA \times OC + \frac{1}{2} \times AD \times BD$$
$$= \frac{1}{2} \times 2(-4) + \frac{1}{2} \times 2 \times 4 = 0$$

6. (c) Let us consider, displacement is L, then velocity of girl with respect to ground,
$$v_g = \frac{L}{t_1}$$
Velocity of escalator with respect to ground,
$$v_e = \frac{L}{t_2}$$
Net velocity of the girl on moving escalator with respect to ground
$$= v_g + v_e = \frac{L}{t_1} + \frac{L}{t_2} \Rightarrow v_{ge} = L\left[\frac{t_1 + t_2}{t_1 t_2}\right]$$
Now, if t is total time taken by girl on moving escalator in covering distance L, then
$$t = \frac{\text{distance}}{\text{speed}} = \frac{L}{L\left(\frac{t_1 + t_2}{t_1 t_2}\right)} = \frac{t_1 t_2}{t_1 + t_2}$$

NEET/AIPMT (2013-2020) Questions

7. (a) $\because h = \frac{1}{2} gt^2 \qquad \therefore h_1 = \frac{1}{2} g(5)^2 = 125$
$h_1 + h_2 = \frac{1}{2} g(10)^2 = 500 \Rightarrow h_2 = 375$
$h_1 + h_2 + h_3 = \frac{1}{2} g(15)^2 = 1125$
$\Rightarrow h_3 = 625$
$h_2 = 3h_1, h_3 = 5h_1$ or $\qquad h_1 = \frac{h_2}{3} = \frac{h_3}{5}$

8. (c) $\because t = \sqrt{x} + 3$
$\Rightarrow \sqrt{x} = t - 3 \Rightarrow x = (t-3)^2$
$v = \frac{dx}{dt} = 2(t-3) = 0 \Rightarrow t = 3$
$\therefore x = (3-3)^2 \Rightarrow x = 0.$

9. (a) According to question,
$V(x) = bx^{-2n}$
So, $\frac{dv}{dx} = -2\,nb\,x^{-2n-1}$
Acceleration of the particle as function of x,
$$a = v\frac{dv}{dx} = bx^{-2n}\left\{b(-2n)x^{-2n-1}\right\}$$
$$= -2nb^2x^{-4n-1}$$

10. (c) **Given :** Velocity
$V = At + Bt^2 \Rightarrow \frac{dx}{dt} = At + Bt^2$
By integrating we get distance travelled
$$\Rightarrow \int_0^x dx = \int_1^2 (At + Bt^2)\,dt$$

Distance travelled by the particle between 1s and 2s

$$x = \frac{A}{2}(2^2 - 1^2) + \frac{B}{3}(2^3 - 1^3) = \frac{3A}{2} + \frac{7B}{3}$$

11. (b) Velocity of preeti w.r.t. elevator $v_1 = \frac{d}{t_1}$

Velocity of elevator w.r.t. ground $v_2 = \frac{d}{t_2}$ then velocity of preeti w.r.t. ground

$$v = v_1 + v_2$$

$$\frac{d}{t} = \frac{d}{t_1} + \frac{d}{t_2}$$

$$\frac{1}{t} = \frac{1}{t_1} + \frac{1}{t_2}$$

$\therefore t = \frac{t_1 t_2}{(t_1 + t_2)}$ (time taken by preeti to walk up on the moving escalator)

12. (c) As $t_1 \frac{x}{v_1} =$ and $t_2 = \frac{x}{v_2}$

$$\therefore \quad v = \frac{x + x}{t_1 + t_2} = \frac{2x}{\frac{x}{v_1} + \frac{x}{v_2}} = \frac{2v_1 v_2}{v_1 + v_2}$$

$$\therefore \quad \frac{2}{v} = \frac{1}{v_1} + \frac{1}{v_2}$$

13. (c)

$u = 20$ m/s

TOWER

g

$v = 80$ m/s

Using $v^2 = u^2 + 2gh$

$$\text{Height, } h = \frac{v^2 - u^2}{2g} = \frac{(80)^2 - (20)^2}{2 \times 10}$$

$$= \frac{6400 - 400}{20} = 300 \text{ m}$$

Exercise 3 -Concept Application Problems CAP

1. (b) Given, $v = b\sqrt{x}$

or $\frac{dx}{dt} = b\,x^{1/2}$

or $\int_0^x x^{-1/2} dx = \int_0^t b dt$

or $\frac{x^{1/2}}{1/2} = 6t$ or $x = \frac{b^2 t^2}{4}$

Differentiating w. r. t. time, we get

$$\frac{dx}{dt} = \frac{b^2 \times 2t}{4} \qquad (t = \tau)$$

or $v = \frac{b^2 \tau}{2}$

2. (c) We know that, $v = \frac{dx}{dt}$

$\Rightarrow dx = v\,dt$

Integrating, $\int_0^x dx = \int_0^t v\,dt$

or $x = \int_0^t (v_0 + gt + ft^2)\,dt = \left[v_0 t + \frac{gt^2}{2} + \frac{ft^3}{3} \right]_0^t$

or, $x = v_0 t + \frac{gt^2}{2} + \frac{ft^3}{3}$

At $t = 1$, $x = v_0 + \frac{g}{2} + \frac{f}{3}$.

3. (b) From the third equation of motion

$v^2 - u^2 = 2aS$

But, $a = \frac{F}{m}$

$$\therefore v^2 = u^2 - 2\left(\frac{F}{m}\right)S$$

$$\Rightarrow v^2 = (1)^2 - (2)\left[\frac{2.5 \times 10^{-2}}{20 \times 10^{-3}}\right]\frac{20}{100}$$

$$\Rightarrow v^2 = 1 - \frac{1}{2}$$

$$\Rightarrow v = \frac{1}{\sqrt{2}} \text{ m/s} = 0.7 \text{ m/s}$$

4. (b) $x = at + bt^2 - ct^3$

Velocity, $v = \frac{dx}{dt} = \frac{d}{dt}(at + bt^2 + ct^3)$

$= a + 2bt - 3ct^2$

Acceleration, $\frac{dv}{dt} = \frac{d}{dt}(a + 2bt - 3ct^2)$

or $0 = 2b - 3c \times 2t \quad \therefore t = \left(\frac{b}{3c}\right)$

and $v = a + 2b\left(\frac{b}{3c}\right) - 3c\left(\frac{b}{3c}\right)^2 = \left(a + \frac{b^2}{3c}\right)$

5. (d) For constant acceleration, there is straight line parallel to t-axis on $\vec{a} - t$.

Inclined straight line on $\vec{v} - t$, and parabola on $\vec{x} - t$.

6. (c) Let time taken by A to reach finishing point is t_0

$\therefore$ Time taken by B to reach finishing point $= t_0 + t$

x

$u = 0$ $\quad v_A = a_1 t_0$

$v_B = a_2(t_0 + t)$

$v_A - v_B = v$

$\Rightarrow v = a_1 t_0 - a_2(t_0 + t) = (a_1 - a_2)t_0 - a_2 t$ ...(i)

$x_B = x_A = \frac{1}{2}a_1 t_0^2 = \frac{1}{2}a_2(t_0 + t)^2$

$\Rightarrow \sqrt{a_1}t_0 = \sqrt{a_2}(t_0 + t)$

$\Rightarrow \left(\sqrt{a_1} - \sqrt{a_2}\right)t_0 = \sqrt{a_2}t$

$\Rightarrow t_0 = \frac{\sqrt{a_2}t}{\sqrt{a_1} - \sqrt{a_2}}$

Putting this value of t_0 in equation (i)

$v = (a_1 - a_2)\frac{\sqrt{a_2}t}{\sqrt{a_1} - \sqrt{a_2}} - a_2 t$

$= \left(\sqrt{a_1} + \sqrt{a_2}\right)\sqrt{a_2}t - a_2 t = \sqrt{a_1 a_2}t + a_2 t - a_2 t$

or, $v = \sqrt{a_1 a_2}\,t$

7. (b) According to question, $u_1 = 40$ km/h, $v_1 = 0$ and $s_1 = 40$ m using $v^2 - u^2 = 2as$; $0^2 - 40^2 = 2a \times 40$ ...(i)
Again, $0^2 - 80^2 = 2as$ ...(ii)
From eqn. (i) and (ii)
Stopping distance, $s = 160$ m

8. (a)

9. (a)

10. (d)

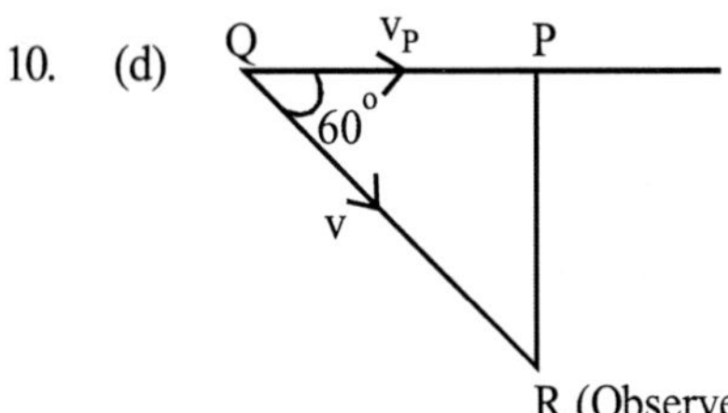

Distance, $PQ = v_p \times t$ (Distance = speed × time)
Distance, $QR = V.t$

$\cos 60° = \frac{PQ}{QR}$

$\frac{1}{2} = \frac{v_p \times t}{V.t} \Rightarrow v_p = \frac{v}{2}$

11. (c) $\longrightarrow$ 4 m/sec^2 $\quad\longrightarrow$ 2 m/sec^2

Car $\quad$ Bus

200 m

Given, $u_C = u_B = 0$, $a_C = 4$ m/s^2, $a_B = 2$ m/s^2
hence relative acceleration, $a_{CB} = 2$ m/sec^2

Now, we know, $s = ut + \frac{1}{2}at^2$

$200 = \frac{1}{2} \times 2t^2 \quad \because u = 0$

Hence, the car will catch up with the bus after time $t = 10\sqrt{2}$ second

12. (c)

13. (c) $v = \frac{dx}{dt} = a_1 + 2a_2 t \quad \therefore a = \frac{dv}{dt} = 2a_2$

14. (d) Let the total distance be d. Then for first half distance, time $= \frac{d}{2v_0}$, next distance. $= v_1 t$ and last half distance $= v_2 t$

$\therefore v_1 t + v_2 t = \frac{d}{2}$; $t = \frac{d}{2(v_1 + v_2)}$

Now average speed

$t = \frac{d}{\frac{d}{2v_0} + \frac{d}{2(v_1 + v_2)} + \frac{d}{2(v_1 + v_2)}}$

$= \frac{2v_0(v_1 + v_2)}{(v_1 + v_2) + 2v_0}$

15. (a)

16. (c) Initial relative velocity $v_A - v_B$, is reduced to 0 in distance d' (<d) with retardation a.

$\therefore 0^2 - (v_A - v_B)^2 = -2\,ad'$

$d' = \frac{(v_A - v_B)^2}{2a} \quad \therefore d > \frac{(v_A - v_B)^2}{2a}$

17. (d) So by figure the velocity of parrot w.r. t. train is = 5–(–10) = 15m/sec
so time taken to cross the train is

$= \frac{\text{length of train}}{\text{relative velocity}} = \frac{150}{15} = 10$ sec

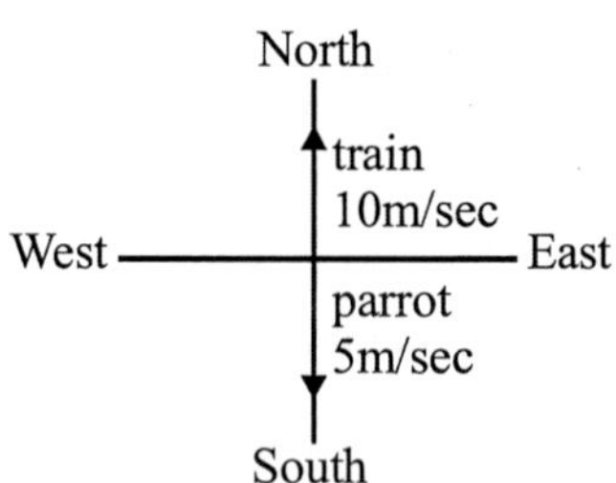

18. (a) $s^2 = at^2 + 2bt + c \quad \therefore 2s\frac{ds}{dt} = 2at + 2b$

or $\frac{ds}{dt} = \frac{at + b}{s}$, again differentiating

$\frac{d^2s}{dt^2} = \frac{a.s - (at + b)}{s^2}.\frac{ds}{dt} = \frac{as - (at + b)\left(\frac{at + b}{s}\right)}{s^2}$

$\therefore \frac{d^2s}{dt^2} = \frac{as^2 - (at + b)^2}{s^3} \quad \therefore a = \frac{d^2s}{dt^2} \propto s^{-3}$.

19. (a) From third equation of motion $v^2 = u^2 + 2ah$
In first case initial velocity $u_1 = 5$ m/sec
final velocity $v_1 = 0, a = -g$

and max. height obtained is H_1, then, $H_1 = \frac{25}{2g}$

In second case $u_2 = 10$ m/sec, $v_2 = 0, a = -g$

and max. height is H_2 then, $H_2 = \frac{100}{2g}$.

It implies that $H_2 = 4H_1$

20. (d) Speed $v_1 = 60 \times \frac{5}{18}$ m/s $= \frac{50}{3}$ m/s

$d_1 = 20$m, $v'_1 = 120 \times \frac{5}{18} = \frac{100}{3}$ m/s

Let dceleration be a

$\therefore 0 = v_1^2 - 2ad_1$ ....(1)

or $v_1^2 = 2ad_1$

$(2v_1)^2 = 2ad_2$ ...(2)

(2) divided by (1) gives,

$4 = \frac{d_2}{d_1} \Rightarrow d_2 = 4 \times 20 = 80$m

21. (d) The only force acting on the ball is the force of gravity. The ball will ascend until gravity reduces its velocity to zero and then it will descend. Find the time it takes for the ball to reach its maximum height and then double the time to cover the round trip.
Using $v_{\text{at maximum height}} = v_0 + at = v_0 - gt$, we get:
0 m/s = 50 m/s – (9.8 m/s^2) t
Therefore,
t = (50 m/s)/(9.8 m/s^2) ~ (50 m/s)/ (10 m/s^2) ~ 5s
This is the time it takes the ball to reach its maximum height. The total round trip time is 2t ~ 10s.

22. (b) Average velocity $= \frac{2 \times 20 \times 30}{20 + 30} = 24\,\text{km h}^{-1}$.

23. (c) From third equation of motion, $v^2 = u^2 + 2as$
where v & u are final & initial velocity, a is acceleration, s is distance.
For first case v_1 = 3km/hour, u_1 = 0, a_1=g & s_1=?

$s_1 = \frac{9 \times 100}{36 \times 36 \times 20}$ metre

For second case v_2=?, u_2=4km/hour,
a_2= g = 10m/sec

$\& \; s_1 = s_2 = \frac{9 \times 100}{36 \times 36 \times 20}$

so $v_2^2 = \frac{16 \times 1000 \times 1000}{3600 \times 3600} + \frac{2 \times 10 \times 9 \times 100}{20 \times 36 \times 36}$

or $v_2 = 5$ km/hour

24. (a) $\frac{ds}{dt} = kt \Rightarrow s = \frac{1}{2}kt^2 = \frac{1}{2} \times 2 \times 3 \times 3 = 9$ m.

25. (d) For constant acceleration and zero initial velocity

$h \propto t^2$

$\frac{h_1}{h_2} = \frac{t_1^2}{t_2^2} \Rightarrow t_2 = \sqrt{\frac{h_2}{h_1}} t_1 = \sqrt{2} \times t_1 = \sqrt{2} \times 2\text{s}$

26. (b) $y \propto t^2$; $v - \propto t'$; $a \propto t^{\circ}$

27. (c) At t = 20s, d = 20 m

28. (c) Let v_A and v_B are the velocities of two bodies.

In first case, $v_A + v_B = 6$m/s ....(1)

In second case, $v_A - v_B = 4$m/s ....(2)

From (1) & (2) we get, $v_A = 5$ m/s and $v_B = 1$ m/s.

29. (d) $\vec{v}_{BB}$ = Relative velocity of ball w.r.t. balloon

$= \vec{u} + \vec{v}$

$0 = -(u + v) + gt$ of $t = \frac{u + v}{g}$

Total time $= \frac{2(u + v)}{g}$

30. (d) In (a), at the same time particle has two positions which is not possible. In (b), particle has two velocities at the same time. In (c), speed is negative which is not possible.

31. (b) $v = 1.25 \times 8\,\text{ms}^{-1} = 10\,\text{ms}^{-1}$

$s = \frac{1}{2} \times 1.25 \times 8 \times 8\text{m} = 40\text{m}$

Now, $40 = -10t + \frac{1}{2} \times 10 \times t^2$

or $5t^2 - 10t - 40 = 0$

or $t^2 - 2t - 8 = 0$ or t = 4 s.

32. (b) Given acceleration $a = 6t + 5$

$\therefore a = \frac{dv}{dt} = 6t + 5$, $dv = (6t + 5)dt$

Integrating it, we have $\int_0^v dv = \int_0^t (6t + 5)dt$

$v = 3t^2 + 5t + C$, where C is constant of integration.

When t = 0, v = 0 so C = 0

$\therefore v = \frac{ds}{dt} = 3t^2 + 5t$ or $ds = (3t^2 + 5t)dt$

Integrating it within the conditions of motion, i.e., as t changes from 0 to 2 s, s changes from 0 to s, we have

$$\int_0^s ds = \int_0^2 (3t^2 + 5t)dt$$

$$\therefore s = t^3 + \frac{5}{2}t^2 \Big|_0^2 = 8 + 10 = 18\text{m}$$

33. (a) $t = \alpha x^2 + \beta x$

Differentiating w.r.t. time on both sides, we get

$$1 = 2\alpha \frac{dx}{dt}.x + \beta \frac{dx}{dt}$$

$\therefore\ v=\frac{dx}{dt}=\frac{1}{\beta+2\alpha x};\ \frac{dv}{dt}=\frac{-2\alpha v}{(\beta+2\alpha x)^2}=-2\alpha v^3$

Negative sign shows retardation.

34. (d) Initial velocity of parachute after bailing out,

$u=\sqrt{2gh}$

$u=\sqrt{2\times 9.8\times 50}=14\sqrt{5}$

50 m, v, $a=-2\,m/s^2$, 3 m/s

The velocity at ground,

$v=3m/s$

$S=\frac{v^2-u^2}{2\times 2}=\frac{3^2-980}{4}\approx 243\text{ m}$

Initially he has fallen 50 m.

$\therefore$ Total height from where he bailed out

$=243+50=293\text{ m}$

35. (b) Height attained by balls in 2 sec is

$=\frac{1}{2}\times 9.8\times 4=19.6\text{m}$

the same distance will be covered in 2 second (for descent)

Time interval of throwing balls, remaining same. So, for two balls remaining in air, the time of ascent or descent must be greater than 2 seconds. Hence speed of balls must be greater than 19.6 m/sec.

36. (b) $\vec{v}=\vec{u}+\vec{a}t$

$v=(2\hat{i}+3\hat{j})+(0.3\hat{i}+0.2\hat{j})\times 10=5\hat{i}+5\hat{j}$

$|\vec{v}|=\sqrt{5^2+5^2}\ ;\ |\vec{v}|=5\sqrt{2}$

37. (a) $\because\ h=\frac{1}{2}gt^2$

$\therefore\ h_1=\frac{1}{2}g(5)^2=125$

$h_1+h_2=\frac{1}{2}g(10)^2=500\Rightarrow h_2=375$

$h_1+h_2+h_3=\frac{1}{2}g(15)^2=1125\Rightarrow h_3=625$

$h_2=3h_1,\ h_3=5h_1$ or $h_1=\frac{h_2}{3}=\frac{h_3}{5}$

38. (a) Motion with constant acceleration is represented by a quadratic equation of t

$Y=(p+qt)(r+pt)=pr+qrt+p^2t+pqt^2$

39. (a) Here, length of train A, $L_A=120\text{ m}$

length of train B, $L_B=130\text{ m}$

velocity of train A, $v_A=20\text{ m/s}$

velocity of train B, $v_B=30\text{ m/s}$

Train B is running in opposite direction to train B,

$\therefore$ velocity of train B relative to train A,

$v_{BA}=v_B+v_A$
$=(30+20)\text{ m/s}$
$=50\text{ m/s}$

Total distance to be covered by train B

$=L_A+L_B=(120+130)\text{ m}$
$=250\text{ m}$

Hence, time required by train B to cross train A

$t=\frac{250}{50}\text{ sec}=5\text{sec}$

40. (d) Velocity time curve will be a straight line as shown:

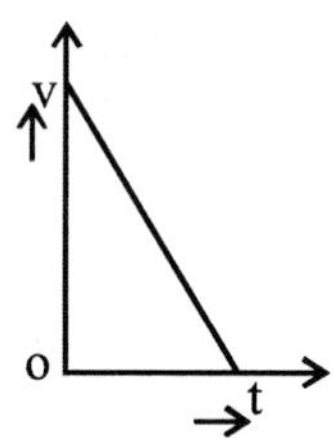

At the highest point v = 0.

41. (b) Let O be the origin, then

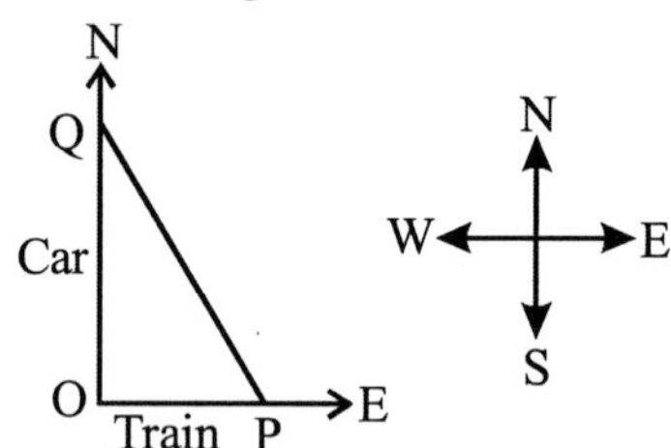

passenger in the train at P observes the car at Q along the direction PQ; i.e. west north direction.

42. (b) We get acceleration by double differentiation of displacement.

$V=\frac{dx}{dt}=\frac{d}{dt}\left(a_0+\frac{a_1t}{2}-\frac{a_2}{3}t^2\right)$

$=\frac{a_1}{2}-\frac{2}{3}a_2t$

$a=\frac{dv}{dt}=\frac{d\left(\frac{a_1}{2}-\frac{2}{3}a_2t\right)}{dt}=\frac{-2}{3}a_2$

43. (d) At E, the slope of the curve is negative.

44. (d) Velocity, $v=\frac{ds}{dt}=3t^2-12t+3$

Acceleration, $a=\frac{dv}{dt}=6t-12$; For $a=0$, we have, $0=6t-12$ or $t=2$s. Hence, at t = 2 s the velocity will be

$v=3\times 2^2-12\times 2+3=-9\text{ ms}^{-1}$

45. (b) Graphs in option (c) position-time and option (a) velocity-position are corresponding to velocity-time graph option (d) and its distance-time graph is as given below. Hence distance-time graph option (b) is incorrect.

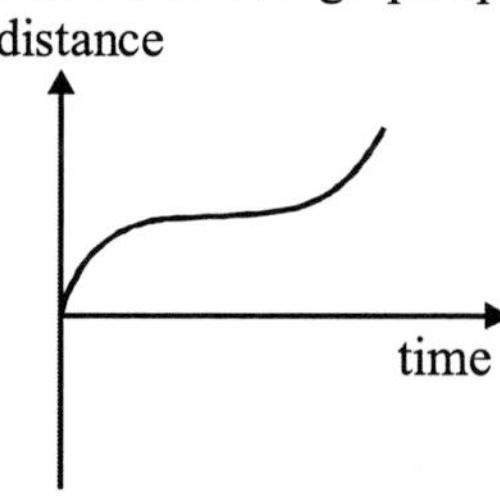

4 Motion in a Plane

Topic 4.1 : Scalars, Vectors-Addition, Subtraction, Resolution, Product of Vectors and Lami's Theorem

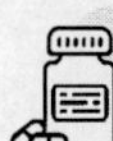

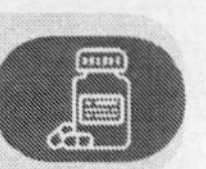

SCALARS AND VECTORS

Scalars : *The physical quantities which have only magnitude but no direction, are called scalar quantities.*

For example - distance, speed, work, temperature, mass, etc.

- Scalars are added, subtracted, multiplied and divided by ordinary laws of algebra.

Vectors: *For any quantity to be a vector,*

(i) it must have magnitude.

(ii) it must have direction.

(iii) it must satisfy parallelogram law of vector addition.

For example – displacement, velocity, force, etc.

Note : Electric current has magnitude as well as direction but still it is not treated as a vector quantity because it is added by ordinary law of algebra.

Types of Vectors

(i) Like vectors : Vectors having same direction are called like vectors. The magnitude may or may not be equal.

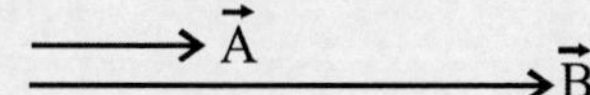

$\vec{A}$ and $\vec{B}$ are like vectors. These are also called parallel vectors or collinear vectors.

(ii) Equal vectors : Vectors having same magnitude and same direction are called equal vectors.

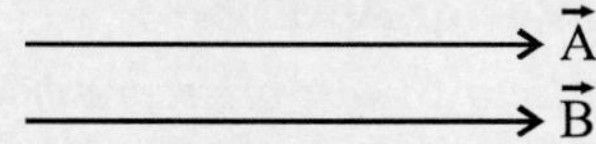

Here $\vec{A}$ and $\vec{B}$ are equal vectors $\vec{A} = \vec{B}$

Thus, equal vector is a special case of like vector.

(iii) Unlike vectors : Vectors having exactly opposite directions are called unlike vectors. The magnitude may or may not be equal.

$\vec{B}$ ⟵ ⟶ $\vec{A}$

$\vec{A}$ and $\vec{B}$ are unlike vectors.

(iv) Negative vectors : Vectors having exactly opposite direction and equal magnitudes are called negative vectors.

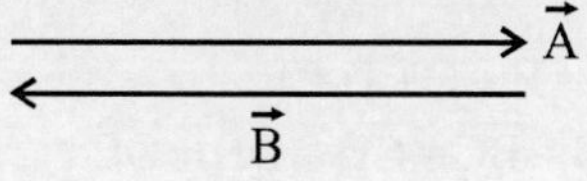

Here $\vec{A}$ and $\vec{B}$ are negative vectors, $\vec{A} = -\vec{B}$

Thus negative vectors is a special case of unlike vectors.

(v) Unit vector : Vector which has unit magnitude. It represents direction only. For example take a vector $\vec{B}$.

Unit vector in the direction of $\vec{B}$ is $\frac{\vec{B}}{|\vec{B}|}$, which is denoted as $\hat{B}$. $\hat{B}$, is read as "B cap" or "B caret".

(vi) Orthogonal unit vector : A set of unit vectors, having the directions of the positive x, y and z axes of three dimensional rectangular coordinate system are denoted by $\hat{i}, \hat{j}$ and $\hat{k}$. They are called orthogonal unit vectors because angle between any of the two unit vectors is 90°.

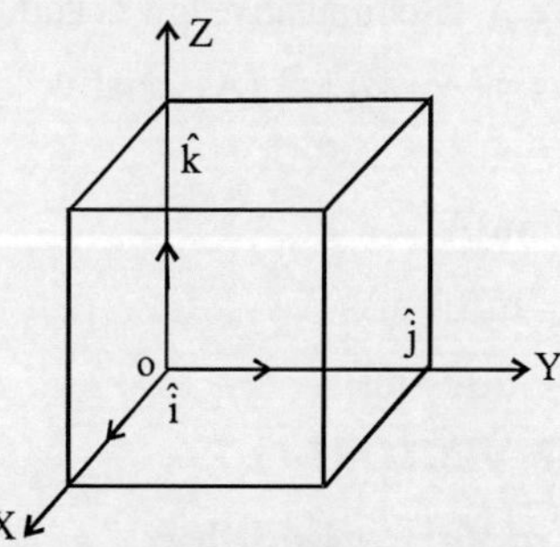

The coordinate system which has shown in fig. is called right handed coordinate system. Such a system derives its name from the fact that right threaded screw rotated through 90° from OX to OY will advance in positive Z direction as shown in the figure.

(vii) Null vector (zero vector) : A vector of zero magnitude is called a zero or null vector. Its direction is not defined. It is denoted by **0**.

Properties of Null or Zero Vector :

(a) The sum of a finite vector $\vec{A}$ and the zero vector is equal to the finite vector

i.e., $\vec{A} + \mathbf{0} = \vec{A}$

(b) The multiplication of a zero vector by a finite number n is equal to the zero vector

i.e., $\mathbf{0}\,n = 0$

(c) The multiplication of a finite $\vec{A}$ by a zero is equal to zero vector
i.e., $\vec{A}\mathbf{0} = 0$

(viii) Axial vector : Vector associated with rotation about an axis i.e., produce rotation effect is called axial vector. Examples are angular velocity, angular momentum, torque etc.

(ix) Coplanar vectors : Vectors in the same plane are called coplanar vectors.

(x) Position vectors and displacement vectors : The vector drawn from the origin of the co-ordinate axes to the position of a particle is called **position vector** of the particle. If A (x_1, y_1, z_1) and B (x_2, y_2, z_2) be the positions of the particle at two different times of its motion w.r.t. the origin O, then position vector of A and B are

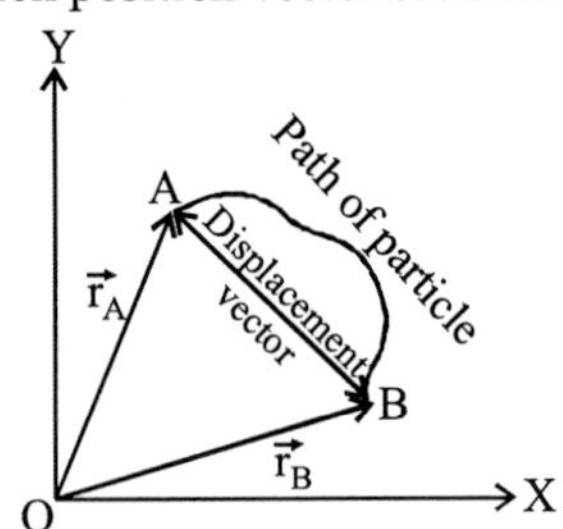

$$\vec{r_A} = \overrightarrow{OA} = x_1\hat{i} + y_1\hat{j} + z_1\hat{k}$$

$$\vec{r_B} = \overrightarrow{OB} = x_2\hat{i} + y_2\hat{j} + z_2\hat{k}.$$

The **displacement vector** is

$$\overrightarrow{AB} = \overrightarrow{OB} - \overrightarrow{OA}.$$

$$= (x_2 - x_2)\hat{i} + (y_2 - y_1)\hat{j} + (z_2 - z_1)\hat{k}$$

Laws of Vector Algebra

1. $\vec{A} + \vec{B} = \vec{B} + \vec{A}$ (Commutative law of addition)
2. $\vec{A} + (\vec{B} + \vec{C}) = (\vec{A} + \vec{B}) + \vec{C}$ (Associative law of addition)
3. $m\vec{A} = \vec{A}m$
4. $m(n\vec{A}) = (mn)\vec{A}$
5. $(m+n)\vec{A} = m\vec{A} + n\vec{A}$
6. $m(\vec{A} + \vec{B}) = m\vec{A} + m\vec{B}$

ADDITION OF VECTORS

Triangle Law of Vector Addition

It states that if two vectors acting on a particle at the same time are represented in magnitude and direction by the two sides of a triangle taken in one order, their resultant vector is represented in magnitude and direction by the third side of the triangle taken in opposite order.

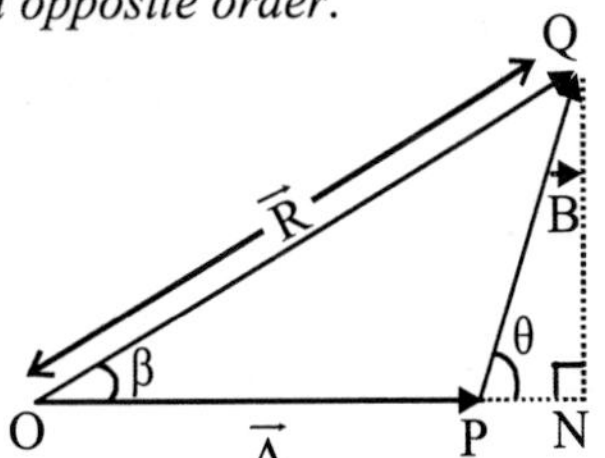

Magnitude of $\vec{R}$ is given by $R = \sqrt{A^2 + B^2 + 2AB\cos\theta}$

where θ is the angle between $\vec{A}$ and $\vec{B}$.

Direction of $\vec{R}$: Let the resultant $\vec{R}$ makes an angle β with the direction of $\vec{A}$. Then from right angle triangle QNO,

$$\tan\beta = \frac{QN}{ON} = \frac{QN}{OP + PN} = \frac{B\sin\theta}{A + B\cos\theta}$$

(i) $|\vec{R}|$ is maximum, if $\cos\theta = 1$, $\theta = 0°$ (parallel vector)

$\xrightarrow{\vec{A}} \| \xrightarrow{\vec{B}}$

$$R_{max} = \sqrt{A^2 + B^2 + 2AB} = A + B$$

(ii) $|\vec{R}|$ is minimum, if $\cos\theta = -1$, $\theta = 180°$ (opposite vector)

$\xleftarrow{\vec{B}} \xrightarrow{\vec{A}}$

$$R_{min} = \sqrt{A^2 + B^2 - 2AB} = A - B$$

(iii) If the vectors A and B are orthogonal,

i.e., $\theta = 90°, R = \sqrt{A^2 + B^2}$

Parallelogram Law of Vector Addition

It states that if two vectors are represented in magnitude and direction by the two adjacent sides of a parallelogram then their resultant is represented in magnitude and direction by the diagonal of the parallelogram.

Let the two vectors $\vec{A}$ and $\vec{B}$, inclined at angle θ are represented by sides $\overrightarrow{OP}$ and $\overrightarrow{OS}$ of parallelogram OPQS, then resultant vector $\vec{R}$ is represented by diagonal $\overrightarrow{OQ}$ of the parallelogram.

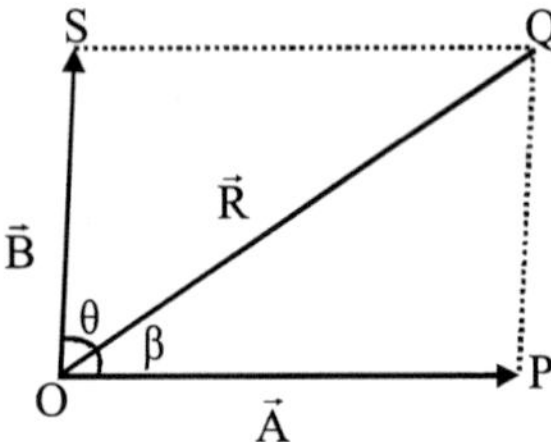

$$R = \sqrt{A^2 + B^2 + 2AB\cos\theta};\ \tan\beta = \frac{B\sin\theta}{A + B\cos\theta}$$

If $\theta < 90°$, (acute angle) $\vec{R} = \vec{A} + \vec{B}$, $\vec{R}$ is called main (major) diagonal of parallelogram

If $\theta > 90°$, (obtuse angle) $\vec{R} = \vec{A} + \vec{B}$, $\vec{R}$ is called minor diagonal.

Polygon Law of Vector Addition

If a number of non zero vectors are represented by the (n–1) sides of an n-sided polygon then the resultant is given by the closing side or the nth side of the polygon taken in opposite order.

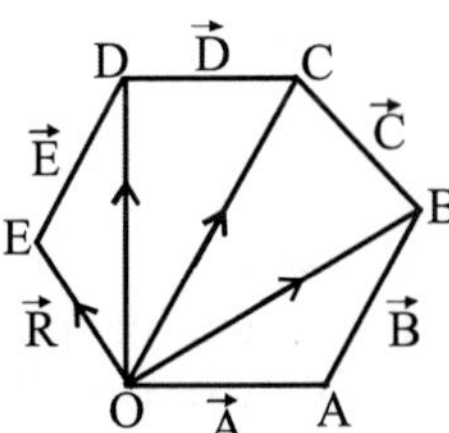

So, $\vec{R} = \vec{A} + \vec{B} + \vec{C} + \vec{D} + \vec{E}$

or, $\overrightarrow{OA} + \overrightarrow{AB} + \overrightarrow{BC} + \overrightarrow{CD} + \overrightarrow{DE} = \overrightarrow{OE}$

Note :

1. Resultant of two unequal vectors cannot be zero.
2. Resultant of three co-planar vectors may or may not be zero.
3. Minimum no. of coplanar vectors for zero resultant is 2 (for equal magnitude) and 3 (for unequal magnitude).
4. Resultant of three non coplanar vectors cannot be zero. Minimum number of non coplanar vectors whose sum can be zero is four.
5. Polygon law should be used only for diagram purpose for calculation of resultant vector (For addition of more than 2 vectors) we use components of vector.

Problem Solving Tips

1. If $\vec{A} = \vec{B}$, then $\vec{A} - \vec{B} = 0$ is a null vector.

2. Null vector or zero vector is defined as a vector whose magnitude is zero and direction indeterminate. Null vector differs from ordinary zero in the sense that ordinary zero is not associated with direction.

3. $\hat{A} = \dfrac{\vec{A}}{|\vec{A}|}$ is called a unit vector. It is unitless and dimensionless vector. Its magnitude is 1. It represents direction only.

4. If $\vec{A} = \vec{B}$, then $|\vec{A}| = |\vec{B}|$ and $\hat{A} = \hat{B}$, where $\hat{A}$ and $\hat{B}$ are unit vectors of A and B respectively.

5. A vector can be divided or multiplied by a scalar.

6. Vectors of the same kind can only be added or subtracted. It is not possible to add or subtract the vectors of different kind. This rule is also valid for scalars.

7. Vectors of same as well as different kinds can be multiplied.

8. A vector can have any number of components. But it can have only three rectangular components in space and two rectangular components in a plane. Rectangular components are mutually perpendicular.

9. The minimum number of unequal non-coplanar whose vector sum is zero is 4.

10. When $\vec{A} = A_x\hat{i} + A_y\hat{j} + A_z\hat{k}$

$|\vec{A}| = \sqrt{A_x^2 + A_y^2 + A_z^2}$, where $|\vec{A}|$ is modulus or magnitude of vector $\vec{A}$.

11. $\hat{i} + \hat{j}$ makes 45° with both X and Y-axes. It makes angle 90° with Z-axis.

12. $\hat{i} + \hat{j} + \hat{k}$ makes angle 54.74° with each of the X, Y and Z-axes.

13. $\vec{A} - \vec{B} \neq \vec{B} - \vec{A}$

14. If $|\vec{A} + \vec{B}| = |\vec{A} - \vec{B}|$ then angle between $\vec{A}$ and $\vec{B}$ is $\dfrac{\pi}{2}$.

15. Magnitude of a vector is independent of co-ordinate axes system.

16. Component of a vector perpendicular to itself is zero.

17. (a) Resultant of two vectors is maximum when angle between the vectors is zero i.e., $\theta = 0°$

$R_{max} = A + B$

(b) Resultant of two vectors is minimum when $\theta = 180°$

$R_{min} = A - B$

(c) The magnitude of resultant of $\vec{A}$ and $\vec{B}$ can vary between (A + B) and (A − B)

SUBTRACTION OF VECTORS

We convert vector subtraction into vector addition.

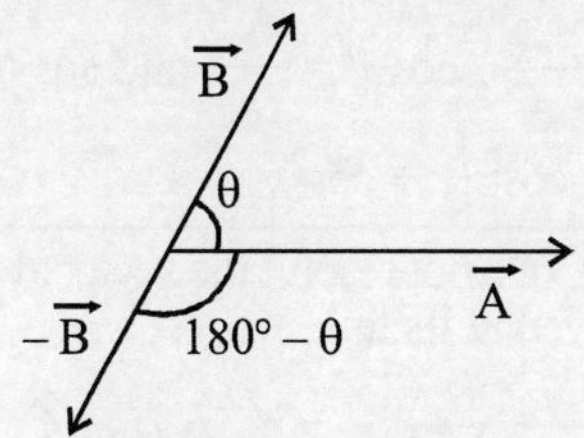

$$\vec{A} - \vec{B} = \vec{A} + (-\vec{B})$$

If the angle between $\vec{A}$ and $\vec{B}$ is θ then the angle between

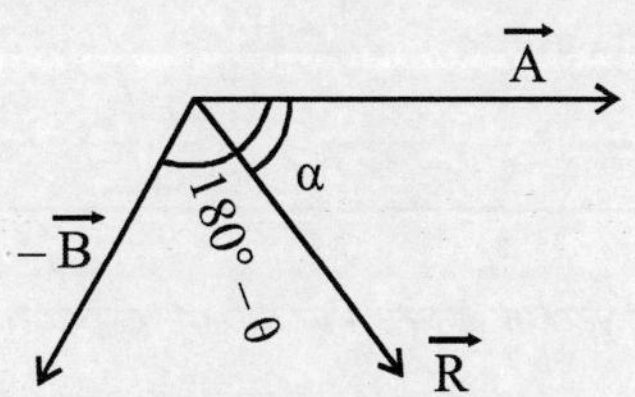

$\vec{A}$ and $-\vec{B}$ is (180° − θ).

$$|\vec{A} - \vec{B}| = \sqrt{A^2 + B^2 - 2AB\cos\theta}$$

$$\tan\alpha = \frac{B\sin(180° - \theta)}{A + B\cos(180° - \theta)} = \frac{B\sin\theta}{A - B\cos\theta}$$

RESOLUTION OF A VECTOR

Rectangular Components of a Vector in Plane

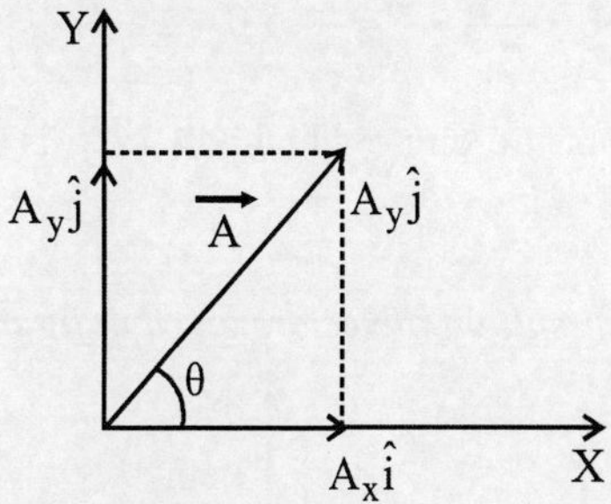

The vector $\vec{A}$ may be written as

$$\vec{A} = A_x\hat{i} + A_y\hat{j}$$

where $A_x\,\hat{i}$ is the component of vector $\vec{A}$ in X-direction and $A_y\,\hat{j}$ is the component of vector $\vec{A}$ in the Y-direction.

Also $A_x = A\cos\theta$ and $A_y = A\sin\theta$

$\therefore \vec{A} = (A\cos\theta)\,\hat{i} + (A\sin\theta)\,\hat{j}$

$\Rightarrow$ A cos θ and A sin θ are the magnitudes of the components of $\vec{A}$ in X and Y-direction respectively.

Also $|\vec{A}| = \sqrt{A_x^2 + A_y^2}$

Rectangular components of a vector in 3D : Three rectangular components along X, Y and Z direction are given by $A_x\hat{i}, A_y\hat{j}, A_z\hat{k}$. Therefore,

vector $\vec{A}$ may be written as

$$\vec{A} = A_x\hat{i} + A_y\hat{j} + A_z\hat{k} \text{ and } A = \sqrt{A_x^2 + A_y^2 + A_z^2}$$

If α, β and γ are the angles subtended by the rectangular components of vector then

$$\cos\alpha = \frac{A_x}{A},\ \cos\beta = \frac{A_y}{A} \text{ and } \cos\gamma = \frac{A_z}{A}$$

Also, $\cos^2\alpha + \cos^2\beta + \cos^2\gamma = 1$

⚠ **CAUTION :** Do not resolve the vector at its head. The vector is always resolved at its tail.

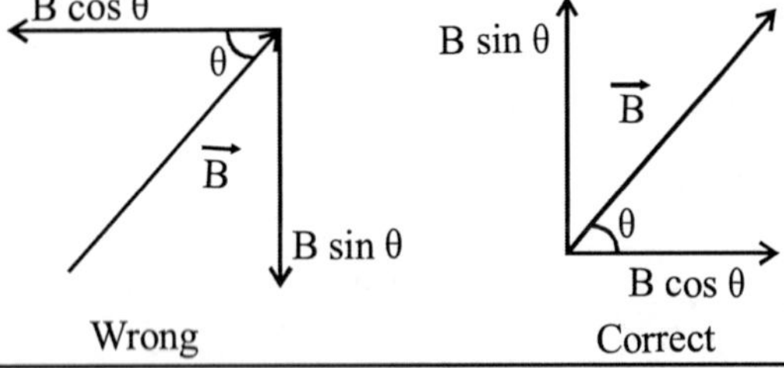

Example 1.

X and Y component of vector A are 4 and 6 m respectively. The X and Y component of $\vec{A} + \vec{B}$ are 10 m and 9 m respectively. Calculate the length of vector B and its angle with respect to X-axis

Solution :

$\vec{A} = 4\hat{i} + 6\hat{j}$ and $\vec{A} + \vec{B} = 10\hat{i} + 9\hat{j}$

$\therefore \vec{B} = (\vec{A} + \vec{B}) - \vec{A} = (10\hat{i} + 9\hat{j}) - (4\hat{i} + 6\hat{j}) = 6\hat{i} + 3\hat{j}$

$\therefore$ length of $\vec{B}$ is $|\vec{B}| = \sqrt{6^2 + 3^2} = 3\sqrt{5}$m

Also $\tan\theta = \frac{B_y}{B_x} = \frac{3}{6} = \frac{1}{2} \Rightarrow \theta = \tan^{-1}\left(\frac{1}{2}\right)$

where θ is the angle which $(\vec{A} + \vec{B})$ is making with X-axis.

Example 2.

Find the resultant of vectors given in figure

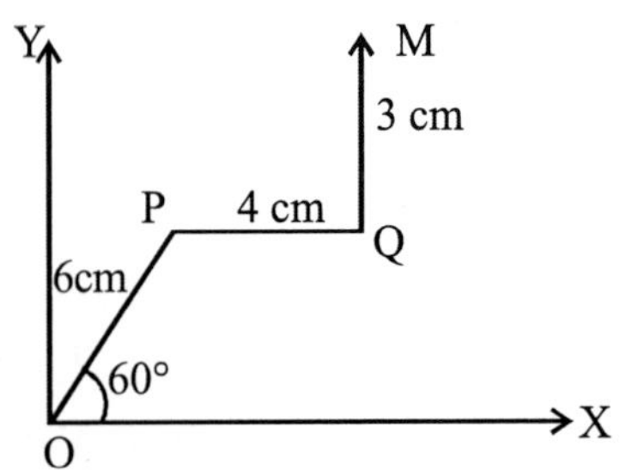

Solution :

Here $\vec{OP} = 6\cos 60°\,\hat{i} + 6\sin 60°\,\hat{j} = 3\,\hat{i} + 5.2\,\hat{j}$

$\vec{PQ} = 4\,\hat{i}$ and $QM = 3\,\hat{j}$

$\therefore \vec{OM} = \vec{OP} + \vec{PQ} + \vec{QM} = 7\,\hat{i} + 8.2\,\hat{j}$

Example 3.

The resultant of two forces F_1 and F_2 is P. If F_2 is reversed, the resultant is Q. Show that $P^2 + Q^2 = 2(F_1^2 + F_2^2)$.

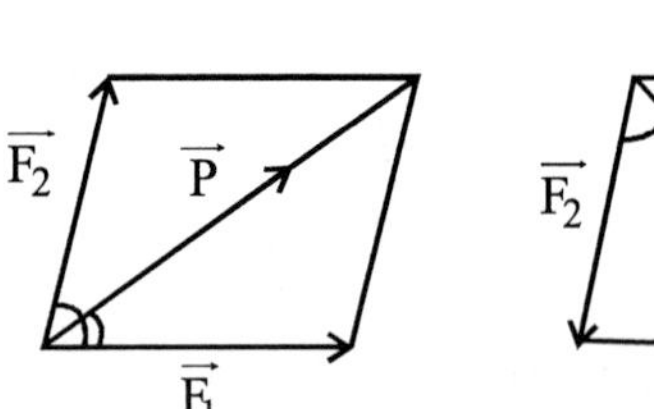

Solution :

Suppose θ be the angle between the forces $\vec{F}_1$ and $\vec{F}_2$, then $P^2 = F_1^2 + F_2^2 + 2F_1F_2\cos\theta$ ......(i)

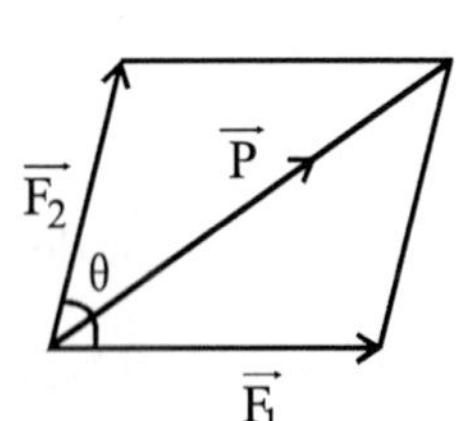

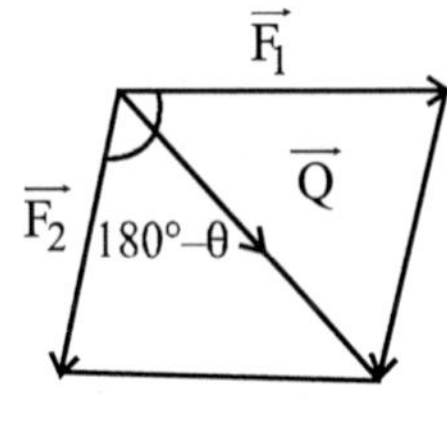

When the force F_2 is reversed, then the magnitude of their resultant is

$$Q^2 = F_1^2 + F_2^2 + 2F_1F_2\cos(180° - \theta)$$

$$= F_1^2 + F_2^2 - 2F_1F_2\cos\theta \quad \text{......(ii)}$$

Adding equations (i) and (ii),

$$P^2 + Q^2 = 2F_1^2 + 2F_2^2 = 2(F_1^2 + F_2^2)$$

Example 4.

Find the components of vector $\vec{A} = 2\hat{i} + 3\hat{j}$ along the directions of $\hat{i} + \hat{j}$ and $\hat{i} - \hat{j}$.

Solution :

Here $\vec{A} = 2\hat{i} + 3\hat{j}$

In order to find the component of $\vec{A}$ along the direction of $\hat{i} + \hat{j}$, let us find out the unit vector along $\hat{i} + \hat{j}$. If $\hat{a}$ is the unit vector along $\hat{i} + \hat{j}$, then

$$\hat{a} = \frac{\hat{i} + \hat{j}}{|\hat{i} + \hat{j}|} = \frac{\hat{i} + \hat{j}}{\sqrt{2}}$$

Hence, the magnitude of the component vector of $\vec{A}$ along $\hat{i} + \hat{j}$

$$= \vec{A}.\hat{a} = (2\hat{i} + 3\hat{j}).\frac{\hat{i} + \hat{j}}{\sqrt{2}} = \frac{1}{\sqrt{2}}(2 + 3) = \frac{5}{\sqrt{2}}$$

Therefore, component vector of A along $\hat{i}+\hat{j}$

$$= (\vec{A}.\hat{a})\hat{a} = \frac{5}{\sqrt{2}}\left(\frac{\hat{i}+\hat{j}}{\sqrt{2}}\right) = \frac{5}{2}(\hat{i}+\hat{j})$$

Similarly, if $\hat{b}$ is the unit vector along the direction of $\hat{i}-\hat{j}$, then magnitude of the component vector of $\vec{A}$ along $\hat{i}-\hat{j}$

$$= (\vec{A}.\hat{b}) = (2\hat{i}+3\hat{j}).\frac{(\hat{i}-\hat{j})}{|\hat{i}-\hat{j}|} = (2\hat{i}+3\hat{j}).\frac{(\hat{i}-\hat{j})}{\sqrt{2}} = \frac{(2-3)}{\sqrt{2}} = -\frac{1}{\sqrt{2}}$$

$\therefore$ Component vector of $\vec{A}$ along $\hat{i}-\hat{j}$

$$= (\vec{A}.\hat{b})\hat{b} = -\frac{1}{\sqrt{2}}\left(\frac{\hat{i}-\hat{j}}{\sqrt{2}}\right) = -\frac{1}{2}(\hat{i}-\hat{j})$$

Example 5.

If $0.3\hat{i}+0.4\hat{j}+c\hat{k}$ is a unit vector, then find the value of c.

Solution :

Unit vector is a vector of unit magnitude.

$$\therefore \quad \sqrt{0.3^2+0.4^2+c^2} = 1 \quad \Rightarrow 0.09+0.16+c^2 = 1$$

$$\Rightarrow c^2 = 1-0.25 = 0.75 \Rightarrow c = \sqrt{0.75}$$

Example 6.

What is the vector joining the points (3, 1, 14) and (–2, –1, –6) ?

Solution :

If P and Q be the points represented by the coordinates (3, 1, 14) and (–2, –1, –6) respectively then,

$\overrightarrow{PQ}$ = p.v. of Q – p.v. of P

$$= (-2\hat{i}-\hat{j}-6\hat{k})-(3\hat{i}+\hat{j}+14\hat{k}) = -5\hat{i}-2\hat{j}-20\hat{k}$$

and $\overrightarrow{QP} = -\overrightarrow{PQ} = 5\hat{i}+2\hat{j}+20\hat{k}$

Example 7.

Find the angle between two vectors of magnitude 12 and 18 units, if their resultant is 24 units.

Solution :

Magnitude of first vector $(\vec{A}) = 12$; Magnitude of second vector $(\vec{B}) = 18$ and resultant of the given vectors $(\vec{R}) = 24$

$$\therefore 24 = \sqrt{A^2+B^2+2AB\cos\theta}$$

$$24 = \sqrt{(12)^2+(18)^2+2\times 12\times 18\cos\theta}$$

or $(24)^2 = 144+324+432\cos\theta$ or $432\cos\theta = 108$

or $\cos\theta = \frac{108}{432} = 0.25$ or $\theta = 75°52'$

Example 8.

Two forces $\vec{F}_1 = 250$N due east and $\vec{F}_2 = 250$ N due north have their common initial point. Find the magnitude and direction of $\vec{F}_2-\vec{F}_1$

Solution :

F_2 (north), F_1 (east)

$$\vec{F}_2 = 250\hat{j},\ \vec{F}_1 = 250\hat{i}$$

$$\vec{F}_2-\vec{F}_1 = 250\hat{j}-250\hat{i},$$

$$|\vec{F}_2-\vec{F}_1| = \sqrt{250^2+250^2} = 250\sqrt{2}\text{ N}$$ (N-W direction)

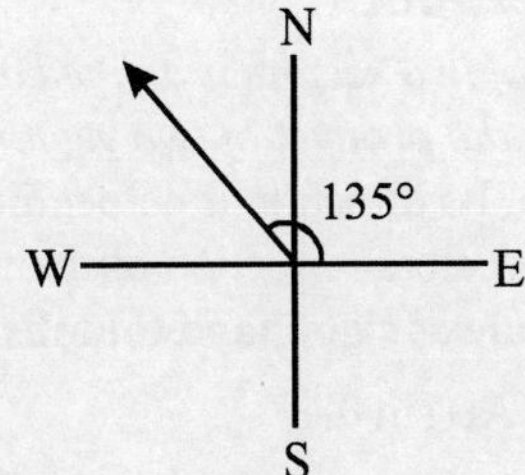

$$\tan\theta = \frac{250}{-250} = -1 \quad \Rightarrow \theta = 135°$$

Example 9.

If $\vec{a},\vec{b}$ and $\vec{c}$ are unit vectors such that $\vec{a}+\vec{b}+\vec{c} = 0$, then find the angle between $\vec{a}$ and $\vec{b}$.

Solution :

Given: $\vec{a}+\vec{b}+\vec{c} = 0 \Rightarrow \vec{c} = -(\vec{a}+\vec{b})$

Also, $|\vec{a}| = |\vec{b}| = |\vec{c}| = 1$

Let angle between $\vec{a}$ and $\vec{b} = \theta$

$$\therefore \quad 1 = \sqrt{1^2+1^2+2\times 1\times 1\times\cos\theta}$$

$$\therefore \quad \cos\theta = -1/2 \Rightarrow \theta = 120° = 2\pi/3$$

PRODUCT OF TWO VECTORS

Scalar or Dot Product

The scalar or dot product of two vectors A and B is a scalar, which is equal to the product of the magnitudes of $\vec{A}$ and $\vec{B}$ and cosine of the smaller angle between them.

i.e., $\vec{A}.\vec{B} = AB\cos\theta$

e.g. $W = \vec{F}\cdot\vec{s}; P = \vec{F}\cdot\vec{v}$

($\vec{B}$ at angle θ to $\vec{A}$ along X)

Properties of Scalar or Dot Product:

1. $\hat{i}.\hat{i} = \hat{j}.\hat{j} = \hat{k}.\hat{k} = 1$

   $\hat{i}.\hat{j} = \hat{j}.\hat{k} = \hat{k}.\hat{i} = 0$

2. $\vec{A}.\vec{B} = A(B\cos\theta) = B(A\cos\theta)$

   The dot product of two vectors can be interpreted as the product of the magnitude of one vector and the magnitude of the component of the other vector along the direction of the first vector.

3. $\vec{A}.\vec{B} = \vec{B}.\vec{A}$ Dot product of two vectors is **commutative**.

4. $\vec{A}.\vec{A} = A^2$

5. $\vec{A}.(\vec{B}+\vec{C}) = \vec{A}.\vec{B}+\vec{A}.\vec{C}$ Dot product is **distributive**.

6. $\vec{A}.\vec{B} = (A_x\hat{i}+A_y\hat{j}+A_z\hat{k}).(B_x\hat{i}+B_y\hat{j}+B_z\hat{k})$

$$= (A_x B_x + A_y B_y + A_z B_z)$$

Vector or Cross Product

The vector product of two vectors is defined as a vector having magnitude equal to the product of two vectors and sine of the angle between them. Its direction is perpendicular to the plane containing the two vectors (direction of the vector is given by **right hand screw rule** or **right hand thumb rule**.

$$\vec{C} = \vec{A}\times\vec{B} = (AB \sin\theta)\,\hat{n}$$

The direction of $(\vec{A}\times\vec{B})$ perpendicular to the plane containing vectors $\vec{A}$ and $\vec{B}$ in the sense of advance of a right handed screw rotated from $\vec{A}$ to $\vec{B}$ is through the smaller angle between them.

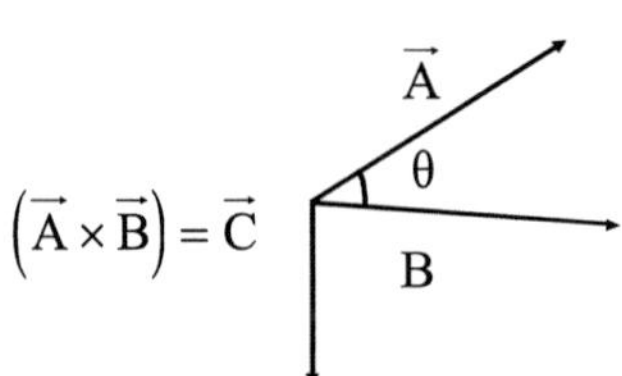

e.g., $\vec{v}=\vec{\omega}\times\vec{r};\ \vec{\tau}=\vec{r}\times\vec{F};\ \vec{L}=\vec{r}\times\vec{p}$

Properties of Vector or Cross Product

1. $\hat{i}\times\hat{i}=\hat{j}\times\hat{j}=\hat{k}\times\hat{k}=0$

2. $\hat{i}\times\hat{j}=\hat{k};\ \hat{j}\times\hat{k}=\hat{i};\ \hat{k}\times\hat{i}=\hat{j}$

3. $\vec{A}\times\vec{A}=0$

4. $\vec{A}\times\vec{B}\neq\vec{B}\times\vec{A}$ **(not commutative)** $[\because \vec{A}\times\vec{B}=-\vec{B}\times\vec{A}]$

5. $\vec{A}\times(\vec{B}+\vec{C})=(\vec{A}\times\vec{B})+(\vec{A}\times\vec{C})$ (follows **distributive** law)

6. $\vec{A}\times\vec{B}=(A_x\hat{i}+A_y\hat{j}+A_z\hat{k})\times(B_x\hat{i}+B_y\hat{j}+B_z\hat{k})$

$$= \begin{vmatrix} \hat{i} & \hat{j} & \hat{k} \\ A_x & A_y & A_z \\ B_x & B_y & B_z \end{vmatrix}$$

$$= (A_y B_z - A_z B_y)\,\hat{i} + (A_z B_x - A_x B_z)\,\hat{j} + (A_x B_y - A_y B_x)\,\hat{k}$$

7. The cross product of two vectors represents the area of the parallelogram formed by them.

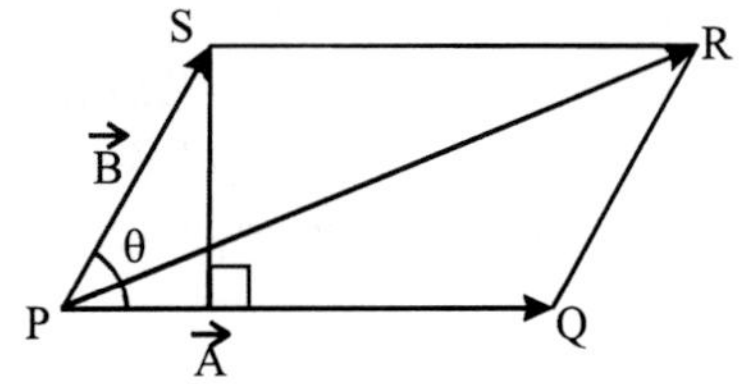

$$|\vec{A}\times\vec{B}| = A(B\sin\theta)$$

$$= \text{area of parallelogram PQRS}$$

$$= 2\,(\text{area of }\Delta PQR)$$

8. A unit vector which is perpendicular to A as well as B is

$$\frac{\vec{A}\times\vec{B}}{|\vec{A}\times\vec{B}|} = \frac{\vec{A}\times\vec{B}}{AB\sin\theta}$$

Problem Solving Tips

1. $\cos\theta = \dfrac{A_xB_x + A_yB_y + A_zB_z}{\sqrt{A_x^2+A_y^2+A_z^2}\,\sqrt{B_x^2+B_y^2+B_z^2}} = \dfrac{\vec{A}.\vec{B}}{|\vec{A}||\vec{B}|}$

2. $\tan\theta = \dfrac{|\vec{A}\times\vec{B}|}{\vec{A}\cdot\vec{B}} = \dfrac{AB\sin\theta}{AB\cos\theta}$

3. $|\vec{A}\times\vec{B}|^2 + |\vec{A}\cdot\vec{B}|^2 = A^2B^2$

4. $|\vec{A}+\vec{B}|\times|\vec{A}-\vec{B}| = 2|(\vec{B})\times(\vec{A})|$

5. If $\vec{A}+\vec{B}+\vec{C}=0$, then $\vec{A}\times\vec{B}=\vec{B}\times\vec{C}=\vec{C}\times\vec{A}$

6. $|\vec{A}\cdot\vec{B}|^2 - |\vec{A}\times\vec{B}|^2 = A^2B^2\cos 2\theta$

7. If $|\vec{A}\times\vec{B}| = \vec{A}.\vec{B}$ then angle between $\vec{A}$ and $\vec{B}$ is $\dfrac{\pi}{4}$.

8. If $\vec{A}\parallel\vec{B}$ then $\vec{A}\times\vec{B}=\vec{0}$

9. Division by a vector is not defined. Because, it is not possible to divide by a direction.

10. The sum and product of vectors is independent of co-ordinate axes system.

CONDITION OF ZERO RESULTANT VECTOR AND LAMI'S THEOREM

If the three vectors acting on a point object at the same time are represented in magnitude and direction by the three sides of a triangle taken in order, then their resultant is zero and the three vectors are said to be in equilibrium.

i.e. $\vec{F}_1+\vec{F}_2+\vec{F}_3=0$

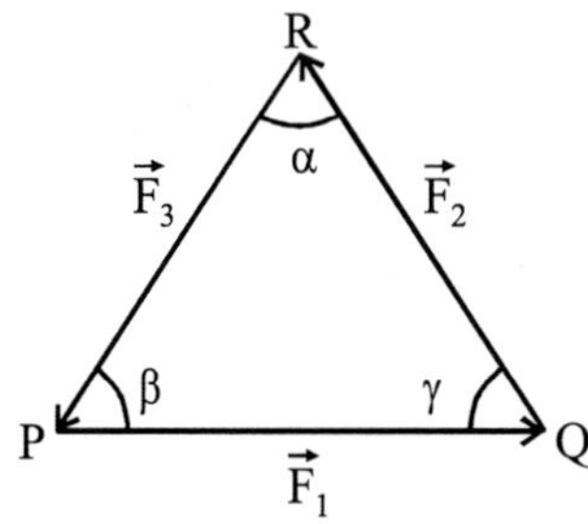

Lami's Theorem

It states that if three forces acting at a point are in equilibrium, then each force is proportional to the sine of the angle between the other two forces.

$$\frac{\vec{F_1}}{\sin\alpha} = \frac{\vec{F_2}}{\sin\beta} = \frac{\vec{F_3}}{\sin\gamma}$$

or, $$\frac{\vec{F_1}}{PQ} = \frac{\vec{F_2}}{QR} = \frac{\vec{F_3}}{PR}$$

Example 10.

Calculate the area of a parallelogram formed from the vectors $\vec{A} = \hat{i} + 2\hat{j} + 3\hat{k}$ *and* $\vec{B} = 2\hat{i} - 3j + \hat{k}$, *as adjacent sides.*

Solution :

The area of a parallelogram is given by $|\vec{A}\times\vec{B}|$

Here,

$$\vec{A}\times\vec{B} = \begin{vmatrix} \hat{i} & \hat{j} & \hat{k} \\ 1 & +2 & 3 \\ 2 & -3 & 1 \end{vmatrix}$$

$$= \hat{i}\,[(2\times 1)-(-3\times 3)] + \hat{j}\,[(3\times 2)-(1\times 1)] + \hat{k}\,[(1\times -3)-(2\times 2)]$$

$$= 11\,\hat{i} + 5\,\hat{j} - 7\,\hat{k}$$

$$\therefore\ |\vec{A}\times\vec{B}| = \sqrt{(11)^2+(5)^2+(-7)^2} \cong 14$$

Example 11.

A particle suffers three displacements 4m in the northward, 2 m in the south-east and 1 m in the south-west directions. What is the displacement of the particle and the distance covered by it?

Solution :

Taking a frame of reference with the x-axis in the eastward and the y-axis in the northward direction

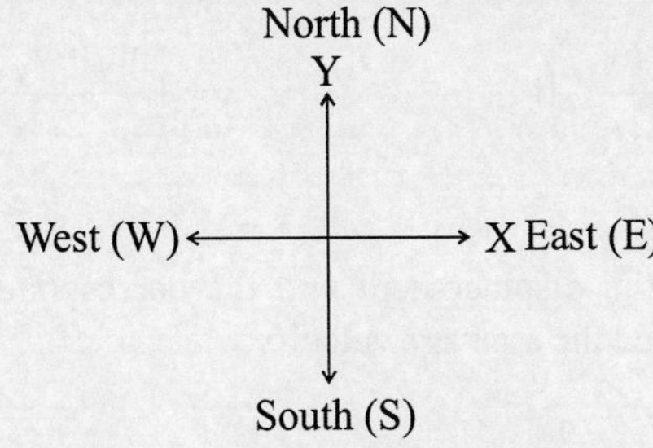

$\vec{s_1} = 4\hat{j}$, $\vec{s_2} = 2\cos 45^\circ\,\hat{i} - 2\sin 45^\circ\,\hat{j}$

$\vec{s_3} = -2\cos 45^\circ\,\hat{i} - 2\sin 45^\circ\,\hat{j}$

$\vec{s} = \vec{s_1} + \vec{s_2} + \vec{s_3} = 4\hat{j} + \sqrt{2}\,\hat{i} - \sqrt{2}\,\hat{j} - \sqrt{2}\,\hat{i} - \sqrt{2}\,\hat{j}$

$\therefore$ Displacement $\vec{s} = (4-2\sqrt{2})\hat{j} = (1.17)\hat{j} = (1.17)$ (northward)

And total distance covered $= 4 + 2 + 1 = 7$m

Example 12.

Prove that vectors $\vec{A} = \hat{i} + 2\hat{j} + 3\hat{k}$ *and* $\vec{B} = 2\hat{i} - \hat{j}$ *are perpendicular to each other.*

Solution :

Here, $\vec{A} = \hat{i} + 2\hat{j} + 3\hat{k}$ and $\vec{B} = 2\hat{i} - \hat{j}$

Two vectors are perpendicular to each other if, $\vec{A}.\vec{B} = 0$

Now $\vec{A}.\vec{B} = (\hat{i} + 2\hat{j} + 3\hat{k}).(2\hat{i} - \hat{j}) = 0$

$= 1\times 2 + 2\times(-1) + 3\times(0) = 2 - 2 + 0 = 0$

Since $\vec{A}.\vec{B} = 0$, therefore vectors $\vec{A}$ and $\vec{B}$ are perpendicular to each other.

Example 13.

Find the angle between the vectors $\vec{A} = \hat{i} + \hat{j} - 2\hat{k}$ *and* $\vec{B} = -\hat{i} + 2\hat{j} - \hat{k}$.

Solution :

Here $\vec{A} = \hat{i} + \hat{j} - 2\hat{k}$, $\vec{B} = -\hat{i} + 2\hat{j} - \hat{k}$

We know that $\vec{A}.\vec{B} = AB\cos\theta$ or $\cos\theta = \dfrac{\vec{A}.\vec{B}}{AB}$

Now $A = \sqrt{1^2 + 1^2 + (-2)^2} = \sqrt{6}$,

$B = \sqrt{(-1)^2 + 2^2 + (-1)^2} = \sqrt{6}$

$\vec{A}.\vec{B} = (\hat{i} + \hat{j} - 2\hat{k}).(-\hat{i} + 2\hat{j} - \hat{k}) = -1 + 2 + 3 = 3$

$$\cos\theta = \frac{3}{\sqrt{6}\times\sqrt{6}} = \frac{3}{6} = \frac{1}{2} \quad \text{or} \quad \theta = 60^\circ$$

Example 14.

A particle is displaced from a point (3, – 4, 5) to another point (-2, 6, – 4) under a force $2\hat{i} + 3\hat{j} - \hat{k}$. *Find the work done by the force.*

Solution :

$\vec{F} = 2\hat{i} + 3\hat{j} - \hat{k}$

The displacement of the particle is

$\vec{s}$ = position vector of point (–2, 6, – 4) – position vector of point (3, – 4, 5)

$\vec{s} = (-2\hat{i} + 6\hat{j} - 4\hat{k}) - (3\hat{i} - 4\hat{j} + 5\hat{k}) = -5\hat{i} + 10\hat{j} - 9\hat{k}$

$\therefore$ work done by the force is

$W = \vec{F}.\vec{s} = (2\hat{i} + 3\hat{j} - \hat{k}).(-5\hat{i} + 10\hat{j} - 9\hat{k})$

$W = (2)(-5) + (3)(10) + (-1)(-9) = 29$ units.

Example 15.

A force $\vec{F} = 6\hat{i} + x\hat{j}$ *acting on a particle displaces it from the point A (3, 4) to the point B (1, 1). If the work done is 3 units, then find value of x.*

Solution :

$\vec{d} = -2\hat{i} - 3\hat{j}$, $\vec{F} = 6\hat{i} + x\hat{j}$

$\therefore$ $W = \vec{F}.\vec{d}$; $3 = -12 - 3x \Rightarrow x = -5$

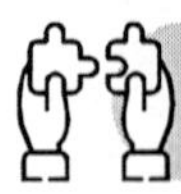

4.1 Concept Practice Problems

CPP

1. Which one of the following statements is true?
   (a) A scalar quantity is the one that is conserved in a process.
   (b) A scalar quantity is the one that can never take negative values.
   (c) A scalar quantity is the one that does not vary from one point to another in space.
   (d) A scalar quantity has the same value for observers with different orientations of the axes.
2. Which of the following is not correct ?
   (a) $\vec{A} \times \vec{B} = -\vec{B} \times A$
   (b) $\vec{A} \times \vec{B} \neq \vec{B} \times A$
   (c) $\vec{A} \times (\vec{B} + \vec{C}) = \vec{A} \times \vec{B} + \vec{A} \times \vec{C}$
   (d) $\vec{A} \times (\vec{B} + \vec{C}) = (\vec{A} \times \vec{B}) + \vec{C}$
3. If A and B are two vectors, then the correct statement is
   (a) $A + B = B + A$ (b) $A - B = B - A$
   (c) $A \times B = B \times A$ (d) None of these
4. Three vectors A, B and C satisfy the relation $A \cdot B = 0$ and $A \cdot C = 0$. The vector A is parallel to
   (a) B (b) C (c) $B \cdot C$ (d) $B \times C$
5. If $\hat{n}$ is a unit vector in the direction of the vector A, then
   (a) $\hat{n} = \frac{A}{|A|}$ (b) $\hat{n} = A|A|$
   (c) $\hat{n} = \frac{|A|}{A}$ (d) $\hat{n} = \hat{n} \times A$
6. Let $A = iA \cos\theta + jA \sin\theta$ be any vector. Another vector B, which is normal to A can be expressed as
   (a) $i\,B\cos\theta - j\,B\sin\theta$ (b) $i\,B\cos\theta + j\,B\sin\theta$
   (c) $i\,B\sin\theta - j\,B\cos\theta$ (d) $i\,B\sin\theta + j\,B\cos\theta$
7. Consider two vectors $\vec{F}_1 = 2\hat{i} + 5\hat{k}$ and $\vec{F}_2 = 3\hat{j} + 4\hat{k}$. The magnitude of the scalar product of these vectors is
   (a) 20 (b) 23 (c) $5\sqrt{33}$ (d) 26
8. Consider a vector F = 4 i – 3 j. Another vector that is perpendicular to F is
   (a) $4i + 3j$ (b) $6i$ (c) $7k$ (d) $3i - 4j$
9. If $|\vec{a} + \vec{b}| = |\vec{a} - \vec{b}|$ then angle between $\vec{a}$ & $\vec{b}$ is
   (a) 45° (b) 30° (c) 90° (d) 180°
10. If the sum of two unit vectors is a unit vector, then the magnitude of their difference is
    (a) $\sqrt{3}$ (b) $\sqrt{2}$ (c) $\sqrt{5}$ (d) $\frac{1}{\sqrt{2}}$

ANSWER KEY

1	(d)	2	(d)	3	(a)	4	(d)	5	(a)	6	(c)	7	(a)	8	(c)	9	(c)	10	(a)

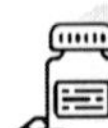

Topic 4.2 : Motion in a Plane or Motion in Two Dimensions, Relative Velocity in two Dimensions, Projectile Motion, Projectile on an Inclined Plane

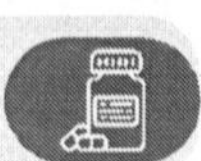

MOTION IN A PLANE OR MOTION IN TWO DIMENSIONS

The motion in which the movement of a body is restricted to a plane is called motion in a plane.

Example : A ball is thrown with some initial velocity (u) and making angle θ with harizontal.

The general approach to solve problem on this topic is to resolve the motion into two mutually perpendicular co-ordinates. One along X-axis and other along Y-axis. These two motions are independent of each other and can be treated as two separate rectilinear motions.

The velocity v and acceleration a can be resolved into its x and y components.

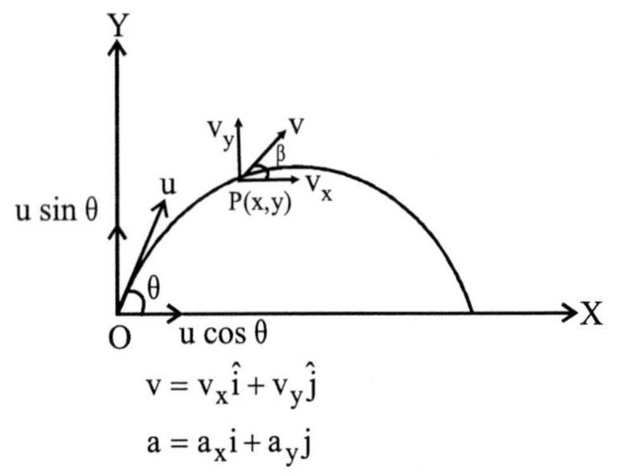

$v = v_x\hat{i} + v_y\hat{j}$

$a = a_x i + a_y j$

x-component of motion

$v_x = u_x + a_x t$

$x = u_x t + \frac{1}{2} a_x t^2$

$v_x^2 - u_x^2 = 2\,a_x x$

$x = \left(\frac{u_x + v_x}{2}\right) t$

y- component of motion

$v_y = u_y + a_y t$

$y = u_y t + \frac{1}{2} a_y t^2$

$v_y^2 - u_y^2 = 2\,a_y y$

$y = \left(\frac{u_y + v_y}{2}\right) t$

Velocity

The ratio of the displacement and the corresponding time interval is called the **average velocity**.

$\vec{v} = v_x\hat{i} + v_y\hat{j}$

Average velocity $\bar{v} = \frac{\Delta r}{\Delta t} = \hat{i}\frac{\Delta x}{\Delta t} + \hat{j}\frac{\Delta y}{\Delta t} = \bar{v}_x\hat{i} + \bar{v}_y\hat{j}$

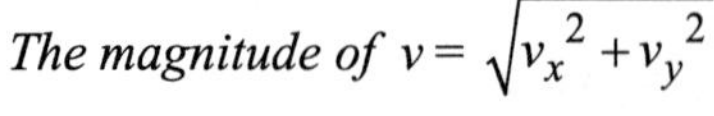

Instantaneous velocity $v_{inst} = \lim_{\Delta t \to 0} \frac{\Delta r}{\Delta t}$

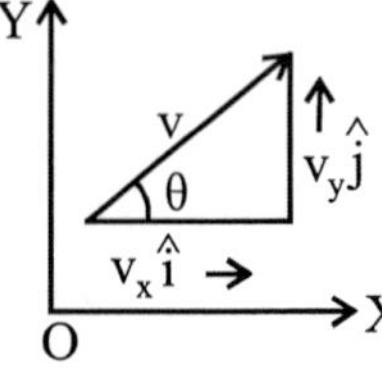

The magnitude of $v = \sqrt{v_x^2 + v_y^2}$

The direction of the velocity, $\tan\theta = \frac{v_y}{v_x}$ $\therefore$ $\theta = \tan^{-1}\frac{v_y}{v_x}$

Acceleration

The **average acceleration** in a x–y plane in time interval Δt is the change in velocity divided by the time interval.

$$\vec{a} = a_x\hat{i} + a_y\hat{j}$$

The magnitude of $a = \sqrt{a_x^2 + a_y^2}$

Average acceleration $\bar{a} = \dfrac{\Delta v}{\Delta t} = \dfrac{\Delta v_x}{\Delta t}\hat{i} + \dfrac{\Delta v_y}{\Delta t}\hat{j}$

Instantaneous acceleration

$$a_{inst} = \lim_{\Delta t \to 0} \frac{\Delta v}{\Delta t} = \lim_{\Delta t \to 0} \frac{\Delta v_x}{\Delta t}\hat{i} + \lim_{\Delta t \to 0} \frac{\Delta v_y}{\Delta t}\hat{j}$$

In two or three dimensions, the velocity and acceleration vectors may have any angle between 0°and 180° between them.

RELATIVE VELOCITY IN TWO DIMENSIONS

If two objects A and B moving with velocities V_A and V_B with respect to some common frame of reference, then :

(i) Relative velocity of A w.r.t B

$$\vec{v}_{AB} = \vec{v}_A - \vec{v}_B$$

(ii) Relative velocity of B w.r.t. A

$$\vec{v}_{BA} = \vec{v}_B - \vec{v}_A$$

Therefore, $\vec{v}_{AB} = \vec{v}_{BA}$ and $|\vec{v}_{AB}| = |\vec{v}_{BA}|$

PROJECTILE MOTION

Projectile *is the name given to a body thrown with some initial velocity in any arbitrary direction and then allowed to move under the influence of gravity alone.*

Examples : A football kicked by the player, a stone thrown from the top of building, a bomb released from a plane.

The path followed by the projectile is called a **trajectory.**

The projectile moves under the action of two velocities:

(1) A uniform velocity in the horizontal direction, which does not change (if there is no air resistance)

(2) A uniformly changing velocity in the vertical direction due to gravity.

The horizontal and vertical motions are independent of each other.

Types of Projectile:

1. **Oblique projectile :** *In this, the body is given an initial velocity making an angle θ with the horizontal and it moves under the infuence of gravity along a parabolic path.*
2. **Horizontal projectile :** *In this, the body is given an initial velocity directed along the horizontal and then it moves under the influence of gravity along a parabolic path.*

Motion along x-axis

$u_x = u,\ a_x = 0$

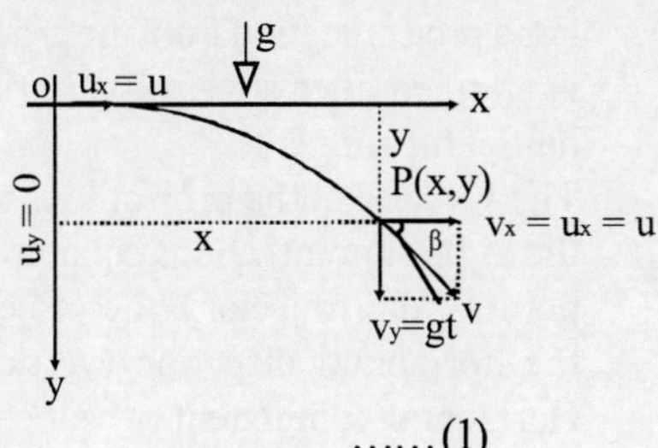

$$x = u_x t + \frac{1}{2}a_x t^2$$

$$x = ut + 0$$

$$\therefore\ t = \frac{x}{u} \qquad ......(1)$$

Motion along y-axis

$u_y = 0,\ \ a_y = g$

$$y = u_y t + \frac{1}{2}a_y t^2 \Rightarrow 0 + \frac{1}{2}gt^2$$

$$y = \frac{1}{2}gt^2 \qquad ......(2)$$

From equations (1) and (2) we get $y = \left(\dfrac{g}{2u^2}\right)x^2$

which is the equation of a **parabola.**

Velocity at any instant :

$$\vec{v} = v_x\hat{i} + v_y\hat{j}$$

$$v = \sqrt{u^2 + g^2t^2}$$

If β is the angle made by $\vec{v}$ with the horizontal, then

$$\tan\beta = \frac{v_y}{v_x} = \frac{gt}{u}$$

Time of flight and horizontal range:

If h is the distance of the ground from the point of projection, T is the time taken to strike the ground and R is the horizontal range of the projectile then

$$T = \sqrt{\frac{2h}{g}} \text{ and } R = u\sqrt{\frac{2h}{g}}$$

Case 1: If the projectile is projected from the top of the tower of height 'h', in horizontal direction, then the height of tower h, range x and time of flight t are related as :

$$h = \frac{1}{2}gt^2 \text{ and } x = vt$$

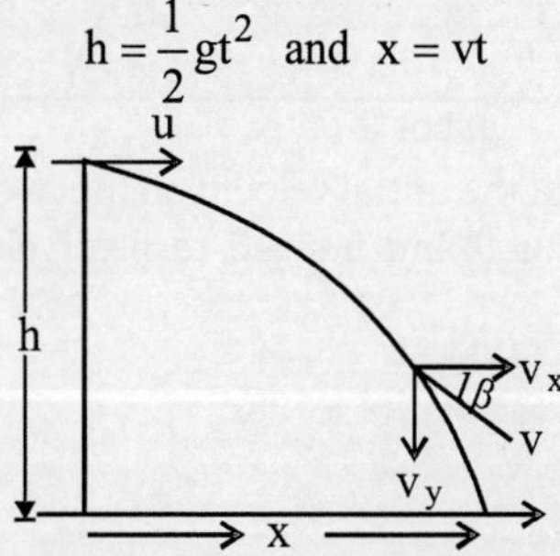

Case 2: If a particle is projected at an angle (θ) in upward direction from the top of tower of height h with velocity u, then

$u_y = u\sin\theta$

$a_y = -g$

$u_x = u\cos\theta$

$a_x = 0$

$$h = +u\sin\theta.t - \frac{1}{2}gt^2 \text{ and } x = u\cos\theta.t$$

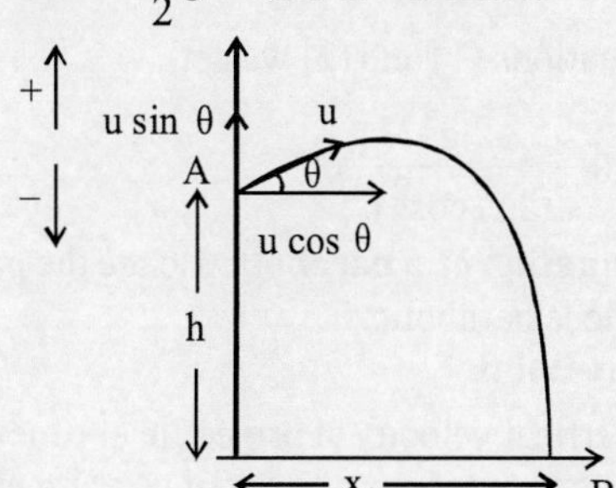

Case 3: If a body is projected at an angle (θ) from the top of tower in downward direction then

$$u_y = -u\sin\theta,\ u_x = u\cos\theta,\ a_x = 0$$

$$a_y = +g,\ -h = -u\sin\theta.t - \frac{1}{2}gt^2 \text{ and } x = u\cos q.t$$

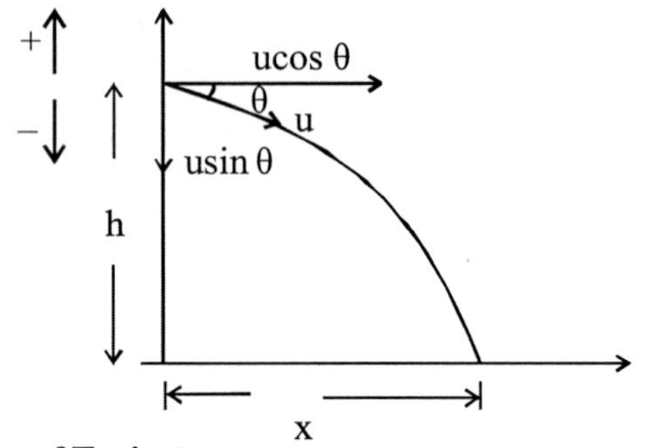

Equation of Trajectory

Let the point from which the projectile is thrown into space is taken as the origin, horizontal direction in the plane of motion is taken as the X-axis, the vertical direction is taken as the Y-axis, Let the projectile be thrown with a velocity u making an angle θ with the X-axis.

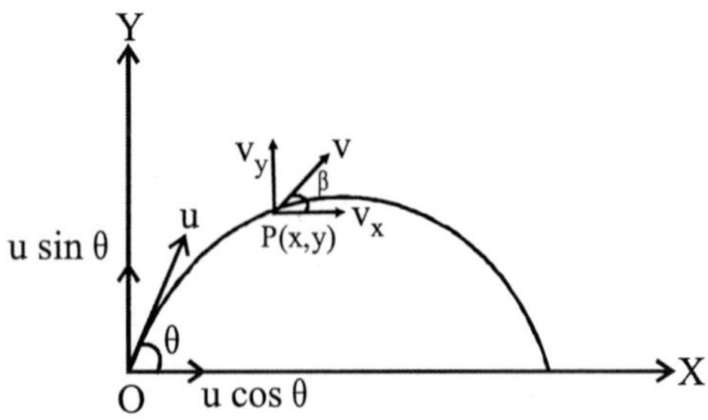

The components of the initial velocity in the X-direction and Y-direction are u cos θ and u sin θ respectively. Then at any instant of time t,

Motion along x – axis

$$u_x = u\cos\theta,\ a_x = 0$$

$$x = u_x t + \frac{1}{2}a_x t^2$$

$$x = (u\cos\theta)\,t \qquad ...(1)$$

Motion along y–axis

$$u_y = u\sin\theta,\ a_y = -g$$

$$y = u_y t + \frac{1}{2}a_y t^2$$

$$y = u\sin\theta\, t + \frac{1}{2}gt^2 \qquad ...(2)$$

From equations (1) and (2) we get

$$y = x\tan\theta - \frac{g}{2u^2\cos^2\theta}x^2$$

which is the **equation of a parabola**. Hence the path followed by the projectile is parabolic.

Velocity at any Point

Let v_y be the vertical velocity of projectile at time t. (at P)
And v_x be the horizontal component of velocity at time t.

$$\therefore\ v_y = u\sin\theta - gt \qquad ......(1)$$

$$v_x = u\cos\theta \qquad ......(2)$$

$$v = \sqrt{v_x^2 + v_y^2}$$

$$= \sqrt{u^2\cos^2\theta + u^2\sin^2\theta - 2gtu\sin\theta + g^2t^2}$$

$$\boxed{v = \sqrt{u^2 + g^2t^2 - 2gtu\sin\theta}}$$

and the instantaneous angle (β) with horizontal is given by

$$\tan\beta = \frac{v_y}{v_x} = \frac{u\sin\theta - gt}{u\cos\theta} = \tan\theta - \frac{gt}{u\cos\theta}$$

Time of Flight :

The time of flight of the projectile is given by

$$\boxed{T = 2t = \frac{2u\sin\theta}{g}},$$

where 't' is the **time of ascent** or **descent**.

Maximum Height :

Maximum height attained by the projectile is given by

$$\boxed{H = \frac{u^2}{2g}\sin^2\theta}.$$

In case of vertical motion, θ = 90° so maximum height attained

$$H = \frac{u^2}{2g}$$

Horizontal Range :

The horizontal range of the projectile is given by

$$\boxed{R = \frac{u^2\sin 2\theta}{g}} \text{ and } \boxed{R_{max} = \frac{u^2}{g}} \text{ at } \theta = 45^\circ$$

(∵ maximum value of sin2θ = 1)

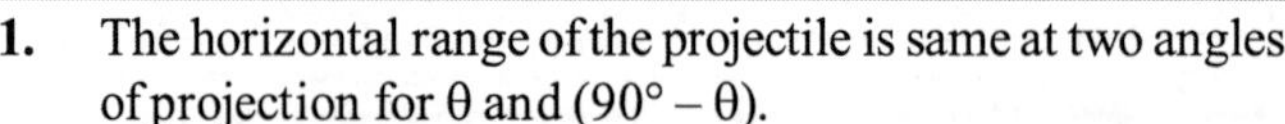

Problem Solving Tips

1. The horizontal range of the projectile is same at two angles of projection for θ and (90° – θ).
2. The height attained by the projectile above the ground is the largest when the angle of projection with the horizontal is 90° (vertically upward projection). In such a case time of flight is largest but the range is the smallest (zero).
3. If the velocity of projection is doubled. The maximum height attained and the range become 4 times, but the time of flight is doubled.
4. When the horizontal range of the projectile is maximum, (θ = 45°), then the maximum height attained is ¼th of the range.
5. For a projectile fired from the ground, the maximum height is attained after covering a horizontal distance equal to half of the range.

   The velocity of the projectile is minimum but not zero at the highest point, and is equal to *u* cosθ i.e. at the highest point of the trajectory, the projectile has net velocity in the horizontal direction (vertical component is zero). Horizontal component of velocity also remains same as the component of g in horizontal direction is zero i.e., no acceleration in horizontal direction.

Example 16.

A boat takes 2 hours to travel 8 km and back in still water lake. If the velocity of water is 4 km h^{-1}, the time taken for going upstream of 8 km and coming back is

(a) 2 hours
(b) 2 hours 40 minutes
(c) 1 hour and 20 minutes
(d) can't be estimated with given information

Solution : (b)

Total distance travelled by boat in 2 hours = 8 + 8 = 16 km.

Therefore speed of boat in still water, $v_b = 16/2 = 8 \text{ km h}^{-1}$.

Effective velocity when boat moves upstream = $v_b - v_\omega$
$= 8 - 4 = 4 \text{ km h}^{-1}$.

Therefore time taken to travel 8 km distance
$= 8/4 = 2\text{h}$.

Effective velocity when boat moves along the stream
$= v_b + v_\omega = 8 + 4 = 12 \text{ km h}^{-1}$.

The time taken to travel 8 km distance = 8/12 = 2/3h = 40 min.

Total time taken = 2h + 40 min = 2hours 40 min.

Example 17.

A boat man can row a boat with a speed of 10 km/h in still water. If the river flows at 5 km/h, the direction in which the boat man should row to reach a point on the other bank directly opposite to the point from where he started (width of the river is 2 km).

(a) is in a direction inclined at 120° to the direction of river flow
(b) is in a direction inclined at 90° to the direction of river flow.
(c) is 60° in the north-west direction
(d) is should row directly along the river flow

Solution : (a)

Refer to fig., the boat man should go along OC in order to cross the river straight (i.e. along OB).

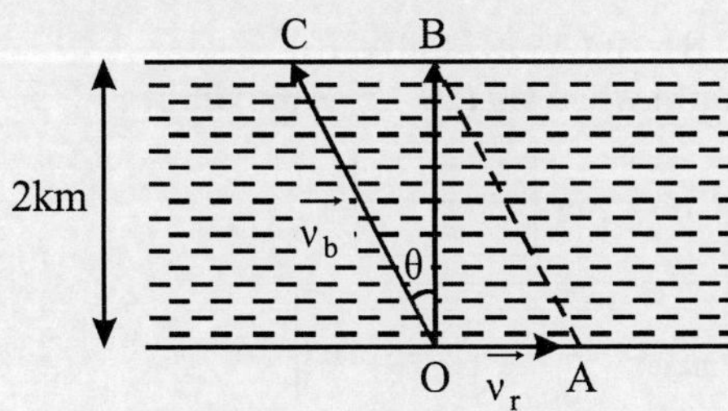

$$\sin\theta = \frac{CB}{OC} = \frac{v_r}{v_b} = \frac{5}{10} = \frac{1}{2} = \sin 30^\circ\ ;\ \theta = 30^\circ;$$

∴ Boat man should go along in a direction inclined at 90° + 30° = 120° to the direction of river flow.

Example 18.

A man swims at an angle θ = 120° to the direction of water flow with a speed v_{mw} = 5km/hr relative to water. If the speed of water v_w = 3km/hr, find the speed of the man.

Solution :

$$\vec{v}_{mw} = \vec{v}_m - \vec{v}_w$$
$$\vec{v}_m = \vec{v}_{mw} + \vec{v}_w$$

$$\Rightarrow v_m = |\vec{v}_{mw} + \vec{v}_w| = \sqrt{v_{mw}^2 + v_w^2 + 2v_{mw}.v_w\cos\theta}$$

$$\Rightarrow v_m = \sqrt{5^2 + 3^2 + 2(5)(3)\cos 120^\circ}$$

$$\Rightarrow v_m = \sqrt{25 + 9 - 15} = \sqrt{19} \text{ m/sec.}$$

Example 19.

A gun throws a shell with a muzzle speed of 98 m/sec. When the elevation is 45°, the range is found to be 900 m. How much is the range decreased by air resistance?

Solution :

Without air resistance, the expected range

$$R = \frac{u^2\sin 2\theta}{g} = \frac{(98)^2 \times \sin 90}{9.8} = \frac{(98)^2}{9.8} = 980\text{m}$$

Decrease in range = 980 m – 900 m = 80 m

Example 20.

A particle is projected with velocity u at an angle θ with the horizontal so that its horizontal range is twice the greatest height attained. The horizontal range is

(a) u^2/g *(b) $2u^2/3g$*
(c) $4u^2/5g$ *(d) None of these*

Solution : (c)

Greatest height attained

$$H = \frac{u^2\sin^2\theta}{2g} \qquad ......(1)$$

Horizontal range,

$$R = \frac{u^2\sin 2\theta}{g} = \frac{2u^2\sin\theta\cos\theta}{g} \qquad ......(2)$$

$[\because \sin 2\theta = 2\sin\theta\cos\theta]$

Given that R = 2 H

$$\therefore \frac{2u^2\sin\theta\cos\theta}{g} = \frac{2u^2\sin^2\theta}{2g}$$

Solving we get tan θ = 2 .....(3)

Hence $\sin\theta = (2/\sqrt{5})$ and $\cos\theta = (1/\sqrt{5})$

From eqn. (2) $R = \frac{2u^2}{g} \times \frac{2}{\sqrt{5}} \times \frac{1}{\sqrt{5}} = \frac{4u^2}{5g}$

Example 21.

A body is projected downwards at an angle of 30° to the horizontal with a velocity of 9.8 m/s from the top of a tower 29.4 m high. How long will it take before striking the ground?

Solution :

The situation is shown in fig.

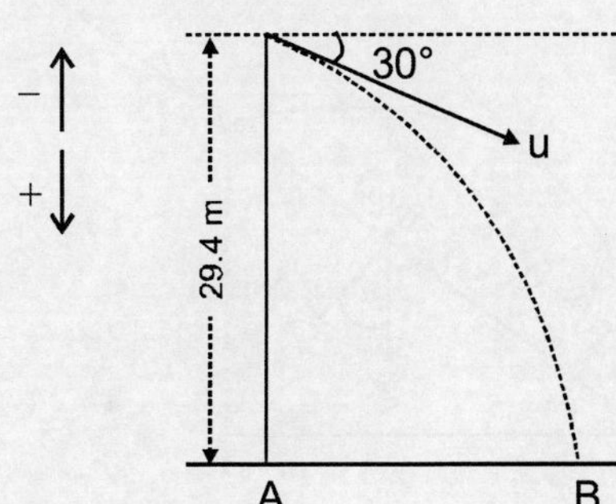

The time taken by the body is equal to the time taken by the freely falling body from the height 29.4 m with initial velocity u sin θ. This is given by

$$u\sin\theta = \frac{9.8}{2} = 4.9\ m/s$$

Applying the formula, $s = ut + \frac{1}{2}gt^2$, we have

$$29.4 = 4.9t + \frac{1}{2}(9.8)t^2 \quad \text{or} \quad 4.9t^2 + 4.9t - 29.4 = 0$$

(because s, u and g are all in downward direction)

$t^2 + t - 6 = 0$ or $t = 2$ or -3

∴ Time taken to reach ground = 2 second

Example 22.

Two boys stationed at A and B fire bullets simultaneously at a bird stationed at C. The bullets are fired from A and B at angles of 53° and 37° with the vertical. Both the bullets fire the bird simultaneously. What is the value of v_A if v_B = 60 units? (Given : tan 37° = 3/4)

Solution :

The vertical components must be equal.

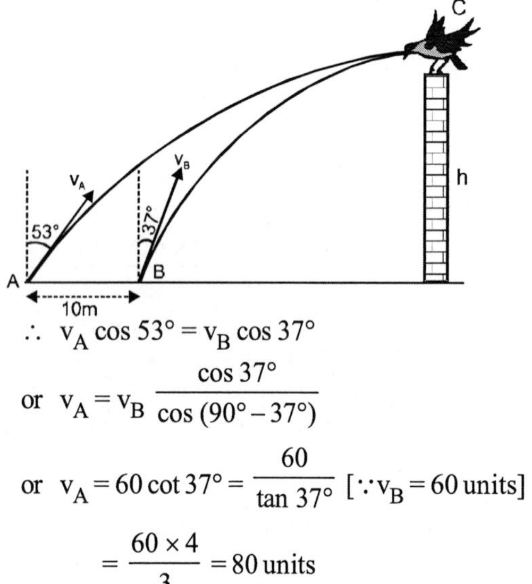

$$\therefore\ v_A \cos 53° = v_B \cos 37°$$

$$\text{or}\ v_A = v_B \frac{\cos 37°}{\cos(90° - 37°)}$$

$$\text{or}\ v_A = 60 \cot 37° = \frac{60}{\tan 37°}\ [\because v_B = 60\ \text{units}]$$

$$= \frac{60 \times 4}{3} = 80\ \text{units}$$

PROJECTILE ON AN INCLINED PLANE

Let a body is thrown from a plane OA inclined at an angle α with the horizontal, with a constant velocity u in a direction making an angle θ with the horizontal.

The body returns back on the same plane OA. Hence the net displacement of the particle in a direction normal to the plane OA is zero.

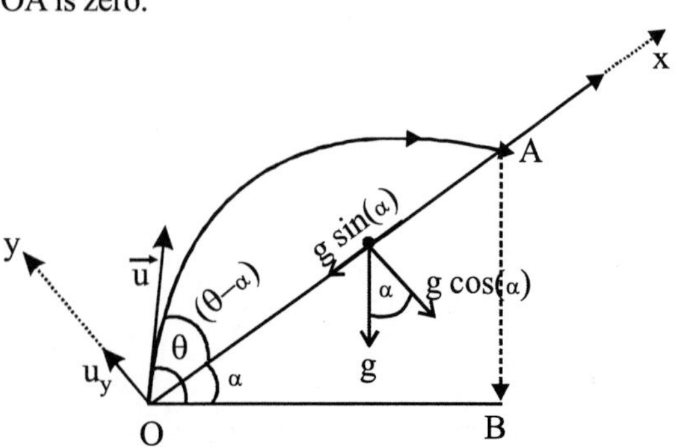

$u_x = u\cos(\theta - \alpha)$ along the incline, + x-axis)

$u_y = u\sin(\theta - \alpha)$ along the incline, + y-axis)

$a_x = g\sin\alpha$ along – x-axis, as retardation

$a_y = g\cos\alpha$ along – y-axis, as retardation

The **time of flight of the projectile** is given by

$$s = ut + \frac{1}{2}at^2$$

$$\text{or}\quad 0 = u\sin(\theta - \alpha)T - \frac{1}{2}g\cos\alpha T^2$$

$$\boxed{T = \frac{2u\sin(\theta - \alpha)}{g\cos(\alpha)}}$$

If **maximum height** above the inclined plane is H,

$$\boxed{H = \frac{u^2\sin^2(\theta - \alpha)}{2g}}$$

The **horizontal range** R of the projectile is given by

$$OB = u\cos\theta\, t = \boxed{\frac{2u^2\sin(\theta - \alpha)\cos\theta}{g\cos\alpha} = R}$$

The **range of the projectile** at the inclined plane is given by

$$OA = \boxed{\frac{OB}{\cos\alpha} = \frac{2u^2\sin(\theta - \alpha)\cos\theta}{g\cos^2\alpha} = R}$$

Condition for horizontal range R on the inclined plane to be maximum :

$$\text{Since } R = \frac{u^2}{g\cos^2\alpha}[2\sin(\theta - \alpha)\cos\theta]$$

$$= \frac{u^2}{g\cos^2\alpha}[\sin(2\theta - \alpha) - \sin\alpha]$$

{2 sin A cos B = sin(A+B)+sin(A–B)}

R is maximum when sin (2θ –α) is maximum

i.e., $\sin(2\theta - \alpha) = 1$ or $\boxed{\theta = \frac{\pi}{4} + \frac{\alpha}{2}}$

$$\Rightarrow \boxed{R_{max} = \frac{u^2}{g\cos^2\alpha}[1 - \sin\alpha]}$$

$$\text{or } R_{max}(\text{on inclined plane}) = \frac{R_{max}(\text{on horizontal plane})}{1 + \sin\alpha}$$

where R_{max} (on horizontal plane) $= \frac{u^2}{2g}$.

Condition for time of flight T to be maximum :

$T = \frac{2u\sin(\theta - \alpha)}{g\cos\alpha}$ so **T is max when sin (θ – α) is maximum**

i.e., $\sin(\theta - \alpha) = 1$ or $\boxed{\theta = \frac{\pi}{2} + \alpha \Rightarrow T = \frac{2u}{g\cos\alpha}}$

It means that if θ_1 is the angle for projectile for which T is maximum and θ_2 is the angle for which R is maximum, then $\theta_1 = 2\theta_2$.

Example 23.

The slopes of wind screen of two cars are $\beta_1 = 30°$ and $\beta_2 = 15°$ respectively. At what ratio v_1/v_2 of the velocities of the cars will their drivers see the hailstorms bounced by windscreen of their cars in the vertical direction? Assume hailstorms falling vertically.

Solution :

From the fig $\tan\alpha = \frac{v}{v_1}$ and $\alpha = 90° - 2\beta_1$

where v is velocity of hail

$$\tan(90° - 2\beta_1) = \cot 2\beta_1 = \frac{v}{v_1}$$

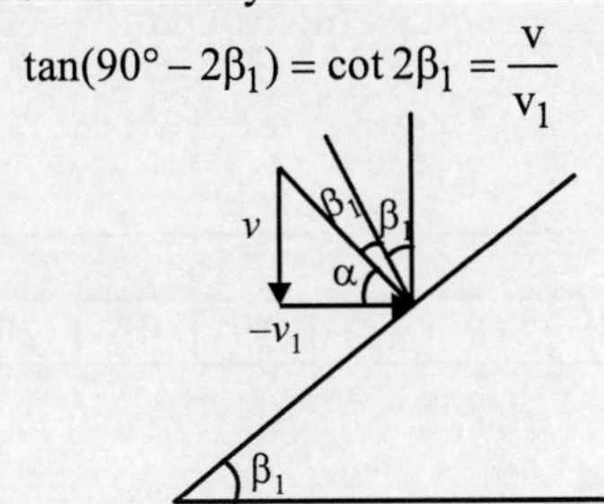

Similarly, $\cot 2\beta_2 = \frac{v}{v_2}$

$$\frac{v_1}{v_2} = \frac{\cot 2\beta_2}{\cot 2\beta_1} = \frac{\cot 30}{\cot 60} = 3.$$

Example 24.

A particle is projected up an inclined plane of inclination α to the horizontal. If the particle strikes the plane horizontally then tan α = ... Given angle of projection with the horizontal is β.

(a) 1/2 tanβ *(b) tanβ*

(c) 2 tanβ *(d) 3 tanβ*

Solution : (a)

If the projectile hits the plane horizontally then

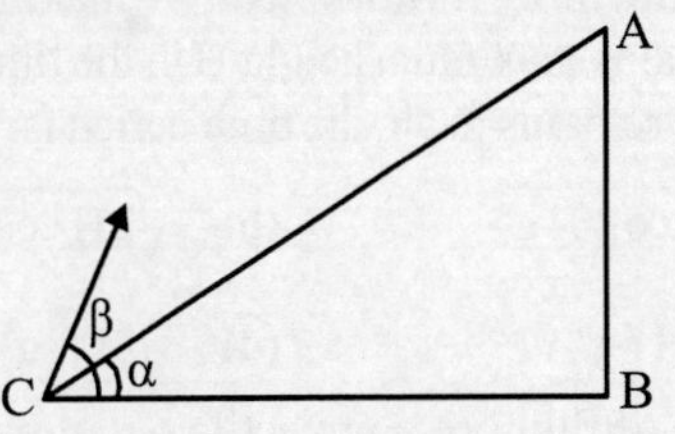

$$T_{plane} = \frac{1}{2} T_{horizontal\,plane}$$

or $$\frac{2u\sin(\beta-\alpha)}{g\cos\alpha} = \frac{u\sin\beta}{g}$$

$$2\sin\beta\cos\alpha - 2\cos\beta\sin\alpha = \cos\alpha\sin\beta$$

or $\sin\beta\cos\alpha = 2\cos\beta\sin\alpha$ or $\tan\alpha = \frac{\tan\beta}{2}$

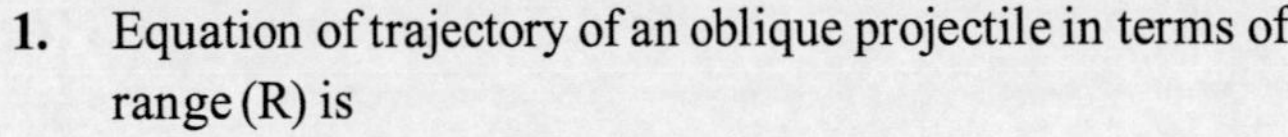

Problem Solving Tips

1. Equation of trajectory of an oblique projectile in terms of range (R) is

$$y = x\tan\theta\left(1 - \frac{x}{R}\right)$$

2. There are two unique times at which the projectile is at the same height h(< H) and the sum of these two times.

Since, $h = (u\sin\theta)t - \frac{1}{2}gt^2$ is a quadratic in time, so it has two unique roots t_1 and t_2 (say) such that sum of roots $(t_1 + t_2)$ is $\frac{2u\sin\theta}{g}$ and product $(t_1 t_2)$ is $\frac{2h}{g}$.

The time lapse $(t_1 - t_2)$ is $\sqrt{\frac{4u^2\sin^2\theta}{g^2} - \frac{8h}{g}}$.

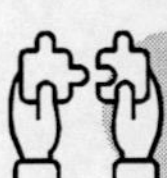

4.2 Concept Practice Problems

CPP

11. Two balls are projected at an angle θ and (90° – θ) to the horizontal with the same speed. The ratio of their maximum vertical heights is

(a) 1 : 1 (b) tanθ : 1 (c) 1 : tanθ (d) $\tan^2\theta : 1$

12. The greatest height to which a man can through a ball is *h*. What is the greatest horizontal distance to which he can throw the ball?

(a) 2h (b) $\frac{h}{4}$ (c) $\frac{h}{2}$ (d) None of these

13. A projectile thrown with a speed v at an angle θ has a range R on the surface of earth. For same v and θ, its range on the surface of moon will be $\left[g_{moon} = \frac{g_{Earth}}{6}\right]$

(a) R/6 (b) R (c) 6R (d) 36R

14. Three particles A, B and C are projected from the same point with same initial speeds making angles 30º, 45º and 60º respectively with the horizontal. Which of the following statements is correct?

(a) A, B and C have unequal ranges

(b) Ranges of A and C are equal and less than that of B

(c) Ranges of A and C are equal and greater than that of B

(d) A, B and C have equal ranges

15. A projectile can have the same range for two angles of projection. If h_1 and h_2 are maximum heights when the range in the two cases is R, then the relation between R, h_1 and h_2 is

(a) $R = 4\sqrt{h_1h_2}$ (b) $R = 2\sqrt{h_1h_2}$

(c) $R = \sqrt{h_1h_2}$ (d) None of these

16. A projectile thrown with velocity v making angle θ with vertical gains maximum height H in the time for which the projectile remains in air, the time period is

(a) $\sqrt{H\cos\theta / g}$ (b) $\sqrt{2H\cos\theta / g}$

(c) $\sqrt{4H/g}$ (d) $\sqrt{8H/g}$

17. The time of flight of a projectile on an upward inclined plane depends upon

(a) angle of inclination of the plane
(b) angle of projection
(c) the value of acceleration due to gravity
(d) all of the above.

18. At the highest point on the trajectory of a projectile, its

(a) potential energy is minimum
(b) kinetic energy is maximum
(c) total energy is maximum
(d) kinetic energy is minimum.

19. A projectile is projected with a kinetic energy E. Its range is R. It will have the minimum kinetic energy, after covering a horizontal distance equal to

(a) 0.25 R (b) 0.5 R
(c) 0.75 R (d) R

20. The range of a projectile when launched at an angle of 15° with the horizontal is 1.5 km. What is the range of the projectile when launched at an angle of 45° to the horizontal

(a) 1.5 km (b) 3.0 km
(c) 6.3 km (d) 0.75 km

ANSWER KEY

11	(d)	12	(a)	13	(c)	14	(c)	15	(a)	16	(d)	17	(d)	18	(d)	19	(b)	20	(b)

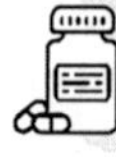

Topic 4.3 : Uniform and Non-Uniform Circular Motion

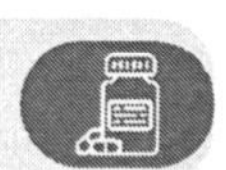

UNIFORM AND NON-UNIFORM CIRCULAR MOTION

Uniform Circular Motion

An object moving in a circle with a constant speed is said to be in uniform circular motion. **Ex.** Motion of the tip of the second hand of a clock.

Angular displacement : Change in angular position is called angular displacement (dθ).

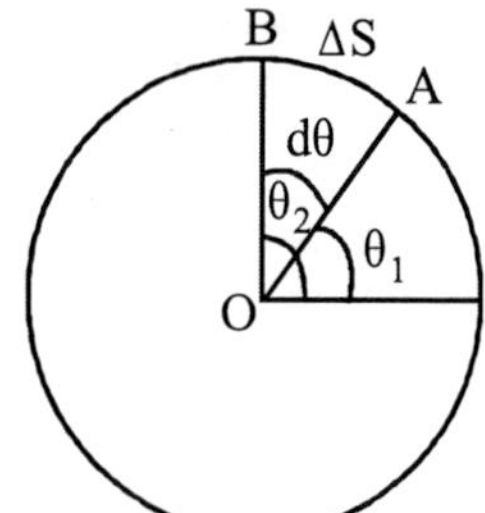

Angular velocity : Rate of change of angular displacement is called angular velocity ω

$$\text{i.e., } \omega = \frac{d\theta}{dt}$$

Relation between linear velocity (v) and angular velocity (ω).

$$\vec{v} = \vec{\omega} \times \vec{r}$$

In magnitude, $v = r\omega$

Angular acceleration : Rate of change of angular velocity is called angular accelaeration.

$$\text{i.e., } \alpha = \frac{d\omega}{dt} = \frac{d^2\theta}{dt^2}$$

Relation between linear acceleration and angular accelaration.

$$\vec{a} = \vec{\alpha} \times \vec{r}$$

In magnitude, $a = r\alpha$

Centripetal acceleration : *Acceleration acting on a body moving in uniform circular motion is called centripetal acceleration.* It arises due to the change in the direction of the velocity vector.

Magnitude of certipetal acceleration is

$$a_c = \frac{v^2}{r} = r\omega^2$$

$$\because \omega = \frac{2\pi}{T} = 2\pi\upsilon \qquad \left(\upsilon = \frac{1}{T} = \text{frequency}\right)$$

$$\therefore a_c = 4\pi^2\upsilon^2 r$$

This acceleration is always directed radially towards the centre of the circle.

Centripetal force: *The force required to keep a body moving in uniform circular motion is called centripetal force.*

$$F_c = \frac{mv^2}{r} = mr\omega^2$$

It is always directed radially inwards.

Centrifugal force : *Centrifugal force is a fictitious force which acts on a body in rotating (non-inertial frames) frame of reference.*

Magnitude of the centrifugal force $F = \frac{mv^2}{r}$.

This force is always directed radially outwards and is also called **corolious force**.

Non-uniform Circular Motion :

An object moving in a circle with variable speed is said to be in non-uniform circular motion.

If the angular velocity varies with time, the object has two accelerations possessed by it, centripetal acceleration (a_c) and Tangential accelaration (a_T) and both perpendicular to each other.

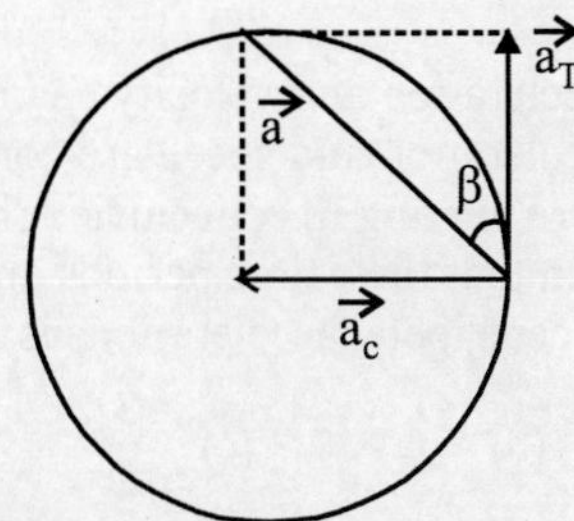

Net acceleration

$$a = \sqrt{a_c^{\ 2} + a_T^{\ 2}}$$

$$a = \sqrt{(r^2\omega^4 + r^2\alpha^2)}$$

$$a = r\sqrt{\omega^4 + \alpha^2}$$

and, $\tan\beta = \dfrac{a_c}{a_T}$

Problem Solving Tips

1. Angular displacement behaves like vector, when its magnitude is very very small. It follows laws of vector addition.
2. Angular velocity and angular acceleration are axial vectors.
3. Centripetal acceleration always directed towards the centre of the circular path and is always perpendicular to the instantaneous velocity of the particle.
4. Circular motion is uniform if $a_T = r\alpha = 0$, that is angular velocity remains constant and radial acceleration $a_c = \dfrac{v^2}{r} = r\omega^2$ is constant.
5. When a_T or α is present, angular velocity varies with time and net acceleration is
$$a = \sqrt{a_c^{\ 2} + a_T^{\ 2}}$$
6. If $a_T = 0$ or $\alpha = 0$, no work is done in circular motion.

Example 25.

A sphere of mass 0.2 kg is attached to an inextensible string of length 0.5 m whose upper end is fixed to the ceiling. The sphere is made to describe a horizontal circle of radius 0.3 m. What will be the speed of the sphere?

Solution :

Centripetal force is provided by component T sin θ, therefore

$$T\sin\theta = \frac{mv^2}{r};$$

and, $T\cos\theta = mg$;

so,

$$\tan\theta = \frac{v^2}{rg} = \frac{r}{\sqrt{\ell^2 - r^2}};$$

$$\left[\because \tan\theta = \frac{r}{\sqrt{\ell^2 - r^2}}\right]$$

$$v = \left[\frac{r^2 g}{(\ell^2 - r^2)^{1/2}}\right]^{1/2}$$

$$= \left[\frac{0.09 \times 10}{(0.25 - 0.09)^{1/2}}\right]^{1/2}$$

$= 1.5$ m/s.

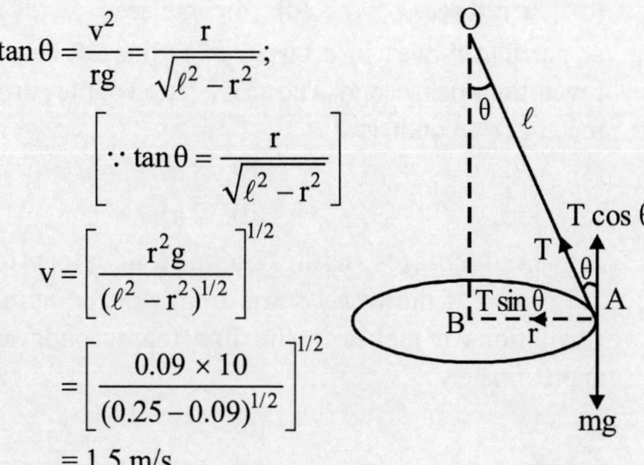

Example 26.

A cyclist is riding with a speed of 27 km/h. As he approaches a circular turn on the road of radius 80 m, he applies brakes and reduces his speed at the constant rate of 0.50 m/s every second. What is the magnitude and direction of the net acceleration of the cyclist on the circular turn ?

Solution :

Speed, $v = 27\,\text{km/h} = 27 \times \dfrac{5}{18}\,\text{ms}^{-1} = 7.5\text{ms}^{-1}$

centripetal acceleration, $a_c = \dfrac{v^2}{r}$

or $a_c = \dfrac{(7.5)^2}{80}\,\text{ms}^{-2} = 0.7\text{ms}^{-2}$

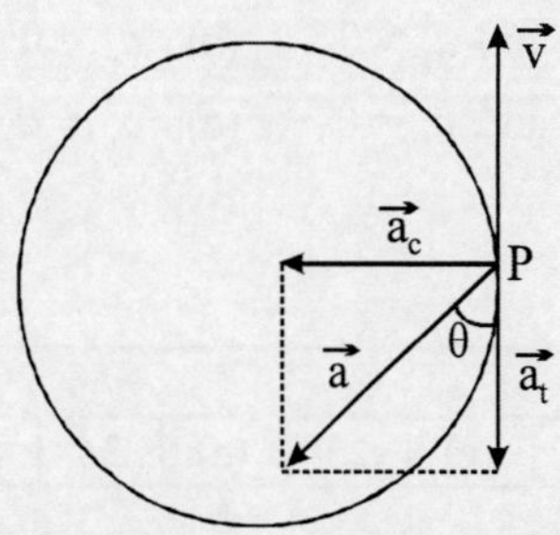

P is the point at which cyclist applies brakes. At this point, tangential acceleration a_t, being negative, will act opposite to $\vec{v}$.

Total acceleration, $a = \sqrt{a_c^2 + a_t^2}$

or, $a = \sqrt{(0.7)^2 + (0.5)^2}\,\text{ms}^{-2} = 0.86\text{ms}^{-2}$

$$\tan\theta = \frac{a_c}{a_t} = \frac{0.7}{0.5} = 1.4$$

∴ $\theta = 54°28'$

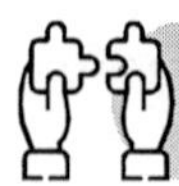

4.3 Concept Practice Problems

CPP

21. The angular speed of a fly-wheel making 120 revolutions/minute is
(a) π rad/sec (b) 4π rad/sec
(c) 2π rad/sec (d) $4\pi^2$ rad/sec

22. A particle moves in a circle of radius 25 cm at two revolutions per second. The acceleration of the particle in meter per second^2 is
(a) π^2 (b) $8\pi^2$
(c) $4\pi^2$ (d) $2\pi^2$

23. A wheel rotates with constant acceleration of 2.0 rod/s^2, if the wheel starts from rest the number of revolutions it makes in the first ten seconds will be approximately
(a) 32 (b) 24
(c) 16 (d) 8

24. A particle moves along a circle of radius $\left(\frac{20}{\pi}\right)$m with constant tangential acceleration. It the velocity of particle is 80 m/sec at end of second revolution after motion has begun, the tangential acceleration is
(a) 40π m/sec^2 (b) 40 m/sec^2
(c) 640π m/sec^2 (d) 160π m/sec^2

25. A clock has a continuously moving second's hand of 0.1 m length. The average acceleration of the tip of the hand (in units of ms^{-2}) is of the order of:
(a) 10^{-3} (b) 10^{-4}
(c) 10^{-2} (d) 10^{-1}

26. If a_r and a_t represent radial and tangential accelerations, the motion of particle will be uniformly circular, if
(a) $a_r = 0$ and $a_t = 0$ (b) $a_r = 0$ but $a_t \neq 0$
(c) $a_r \neq 0$ and $a_t = 0$ (d) $a_r \neq 0$ and $a_t \neq 0$

27. In uniform circular motion
(a) both velocity and acceleration are constant
(b) acceleration and speed are constant but velocity changes
(c) both acceleration and velocity change
(d) both acceleration and speed are constant

28. Two bodies are moving in concentric orbits of radii 2cm and 4 cm such that their time periods are the same. The ratio of their centripetal accelerations is :
(a) $\frac{1}{2}$ (b) $\frac{1}{8}$ (c) $\frac{3}{2}$ (d) $\frac{4}{9}$

29. Two particles A, B are moving on two concentric circles of radii R_1 and R_2 with equal angular speed ω. At t = 0, their positions and direction of motion are shown in the figure :

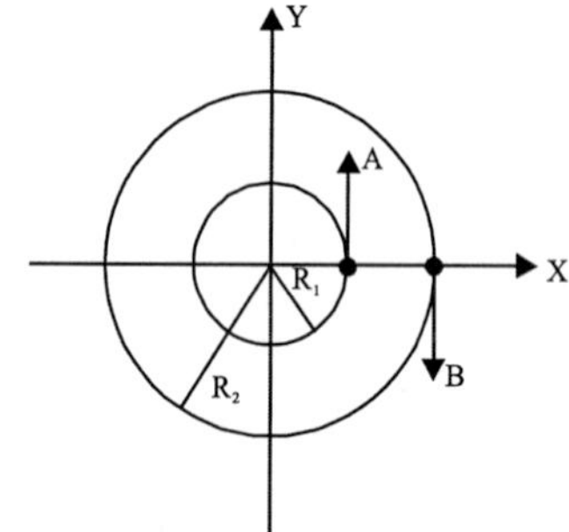

The relative velocity $\vec{v_A} - \vec{v_B}$ and $t = \frac{\pi}{2\omega}$ is given by:
(a) $\omega(R_1 + R_2)\hat{i}$ (b) $-\omega(R_1 + R_2)\hat{i}$
(c) $\omega(R_2 - R_1)\hat{i}$ (d) $\omega(R_1 - R_2)\hat{i}$

30. A particle is moving along a circular path with a constant speed of 10 ms^{-1}. What is the magnitude of the change in velocity of the particle, when it moves through an angle of 60° around the centre of the circle?
(a) $10\sqrt{3}$m/s (b) zero
(c) $10\sqrt{2}$m/s (d) 10 m/s

ANSWER KEY

21	(b)	22	(c)	23	(c)	24	(b)	25	(a)	26	(c)	27	(c)	28	(a)	29	(c)	30	(d)

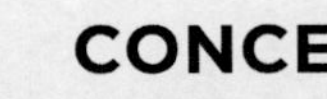

CONCEPT MAP

MOTION IN A PLANE
Vector sum of two one dimensional motions along mutually perpendicular directions

Projectile motion
Motion of an object that is in flight after being projected

Total time of flight $T_f = \frac{2u\sin\theta}{g}$

Maximum height $H_{max} = \frac{u^2\sin^2\theta}{2g}$

Horizontal range $R = \frac{u^2\sin^2\theta}{g}$

Components of initial velocity
$u_x = u\cos\theta;\ u_y = u\sin\theta$

Components of acceleration
at any instant $a_x = 0$, $a_y = -g$
Position after time t

$x = (u\cos\theta)t;\ y = (v\sin\theta)t - \frac{1}{2}gt^2$

Equation of trajectory

$y = x\tan\theta - \frac{g}{2u^2\cos^2\theta}.x^2$

Uniform circular motion
Motion along a circular path with uniform speed.
Angular velocity, $\omega = \frac{\theta}{t}$
Angular acceleration, $\alpha = \frac{\Delta\omega}{\Delta t}$

Centripetal acceleration (a_c)
A body moving along a circular path acted upon by an acceleration directed towards the centre along the radius

$a_c = \frac{v^2}{r} = r\omega^2 = 4\pi^2 rv^2$

Vectors
Quantities that have both magnitude and direction and obey triangle and parallelogram law of vector addition

Position and displacement vector in x-y plane
Position vector, $r = x\hat{i} + y\hat{j}$
Displacement vector, $\Delta r = \Delta x\hat{i} + \Delta y\hat{i}$

Velocity vector in x-y plane
$\vec{v} = v_x\hat{i} + v_y\hat{j}$ and
Magnitude $|\vec{v}| = \sqrt{v_x^2 + v_y^2}$

Acceleration vector
$\vec{a} = a_x\hat{i} + a_y\hat{j}$; $a_x = \frac{dv_x}{dt}$ and $a_y = \frac{dv_y}{dt}$
$|\vec{a}| = \sqrt{a_x^2 + a_y{}^2}$

Triangle law of vector addition
Resultant
$\vec{R} = \vec{P} + \vec{Q}$

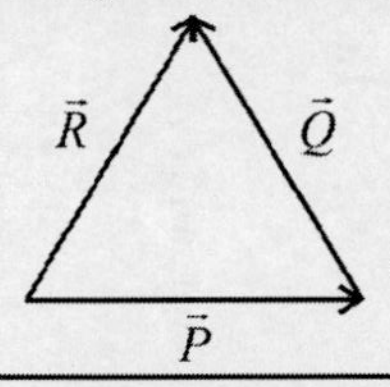

Parallelogram of law of vector addition
Resultant
$R = \sqrt{P^2 + Q^2 + 2PQ\cos\theta}$
$\tan\beta = \frac{Q\sin\theta}{P + Q\cos\theta}$

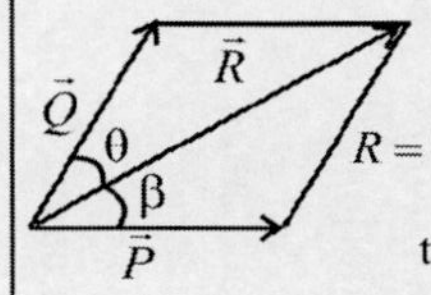

Subtraction of two vectors
$\vec{A} - \vec{B} = \vec{A} + (-\vec{B})$

Multiplication of a vector by a real number $(\lambda) = \lambda\vec{A}$

Types of vector

Zero or null vector
zero magnitude and arbitrary direction

Unit vector
A vector whose magnitude is unity $\hat{A} = \frac{\vec{A}}{|\vec{A}|}$

Equal vectors
Two vectors having same magnitude and direction

Negative vectors
$\vec{A}$ is negative of $\vec{B}$ if $\vec{A} = -\vec{B}$

Co-initial vectors
Two vectors having common starting point

Exercise 1 - Chapter Revision Problems

CRP

1. It is found that $|A+B|=|A|$. This necessarily implies,
(a) $B=0$
(b) A, B are antiparallel
(c) A, B are perpendicular
(d) $A.B \leq 0$

2. Given that A + B = R and A = B = R. What should be the angle between A and B ?
(a) 0 (b) $\pi/3$ (c) $2\pi/3$ (d) π

3. Two particles of equal masses are revolving in circular paths of radii r_1 and r_2 respectively with the same period. The ratio of their centripetal force is
(a) r_1/r_2 (b) $\sqrt{r_2/r_1}$ (c) $(r_1/r_2)^2$ (d) $(r_2/r_1)^2$

4. A bomb is released from a horizontal flying aeroplane. The trajectory of bomb is
(a) a parabola (b) a straight line
(c) a circle (d) a hyperbola

5. Two vectors A and B lie in a plane, another vector C lies outside this plane, then the resultant of these three vectors i.e., A + B + C
(a) can be zero
(b) cannot be zero
(c) lies in the plane containing A + B
(d) lies in the plane containing A – B

6. A cannon on a level plane is aimed at an angle θ above the horizontal and a shell is fired with a muzzle velocity v_0 towards a vertical cliff a distance D away. Then the height from the bottom at which the shell strikes the side walls of the cliff is
(a) $D\sin\theta - \dfrac{gD^2}{2v_0^2\sin^2\theta}$
(b) $D\cos\theta - \dfrac{gD^2}{2v_0^2\cos^2\theta}$
(c) $D\tan\theta - \dfrac{gD^2}{2v_0^2\cos^2\theta}$
(d) $D\tan\theta - \dfrac{gD^2}{2v_0^2\sin^2\theta}$

7. Three particles A, B and C are thrown from the top of a tower with the same speed. A is thrown up, B is thrown down and C is horizontally. They hit the ground with speeds v_A, v_B and v_C respectively then,
(a) $v_A = v_B = v_C$ (b) $v_A = v_B > v_C$
(c) $v_B > v_C > v_A$ (d) $v_A > v_B = v_C$

8. In uniform circular motion, the velocity vector and acceleration vector are
(a) perpendicular to each other
(b) same direction
(c) opposite direction
(d) not related to each other

9. A gun fires two bullets at 60° and 30° with horizontal. The bullets strike at some horizontal distance. The ratio of maximum height for the two bullets is in the ratio
(a) 2 : 1 (b) 3 : 1 (c) 4 : 1 (d) 1 : 1

10. If range is double the maximum height of a projectile, then θ is
(a) $\tan^{-1}4$ (b) $\tan^{-1} 1/4$ (c) $\tan^{-1} 1$ (d) $\tan^{-1} 2$

11. From a point on the ground at a distance 2 meters from the foot of a vertical wall, a ball is thrown at an angle of 45° which just clears the top of the wall and afterward strikes the ground at a distance 4 m on the other side. The height of the wall is
(a) $\frac{2}{3}$m (b) $\frac{3}{4}$m (c) $\frac{1}{3}$m (d) $\frac{4}{3}$m

12. The velocity of projection of a body is increased by 2%. Other factors remaining unchanged, what will be the percentage change in the maximum height attained?
(a) 1% (b) 2% (c) 4% (d) 8%

13. A ball is thrown from the ground with a velocity of $20\sqrt{3}$ m/s making an angle of 60° with the horizontal. The ball will be at a height of 40 m from the ground after a time t equal to ($g = 10\ ms^{-2}$)
(a) $\sqrt{2}$ sec (b) $\sqrt{3}$ sec (c) 2 sec (d) 3 sec

14. Forces of 4 N and 5 N are applied at origin along X-axis and Y-axis respectively. The resultant force will be
(a) $\sqrt{41}N, \tan^{-1}\left(\frac{5}{4}\right)$ (b) $\sqrt{41}N, \tan^{-1}\left(\frac{4}{5}\right)$
(c) $-\sqrt{41}N, \tan^{-1}\left(\frac{5}{4}\right)$ (d) $-\sqrt{41}N, \tan^{-1}\left(\frac{4}{5}\right)$

15. The vector sum of the forces of 10 N and 6 N can be
(a) 2N (b) 8 N (c) 18N (d) 20N

16. A projectile is thrown horizontally with a speed of $20\ ms^{-1}$. If g is $10\ ms^{-2}$, then the speed of the projectile after 5 second will be nearly
(a) $0.5\ ms^{-1}$ (b) $5\ ms^{-1}$ (c) $54\ ms^{-1}$ (d) $500\ ms^{-1}$

17. A ball is projected at such an angle that the horizontal range is three times the maximum height. The angle of projection of the ball is
(a) $\sin^{-1}\left(\frac{3}{4}\right)$ (b) $\sin^{-1}\left(\frac{4}{3}\right)$
(c) $\cos^{-1}\left(\frac{4}{3}\right)$ (d) $\tan^{-1}\left(\frac{4}{3}\right)$

18. A projectile of mass m is fired with velocity u making angle θ with the horizontal. Its angular momentum about the point of projection when it hits the ground is given by
(a) $\dfrac{2mu\sin^2\theta\cos\theta}{g}$ (b) $\dfrac{2mu^3\sin^2\theta\cos\theta}{g}$
(c) $\dfrac{mu\sin^2\theta\cos\theta}{2g}$ (d) $\dfrac{mu^3\sin^2\theta\cos\theta}{2g}$

19. The magnitude of the vector product of two vectors is $\sqrt{3}$ times the scalar product. The angle between vectors is

(a) $\frac{\pi}{4}$ (b) $\frac{\pi}{6}$ (c) $\frac{\pi}{3}$ (d) $\frac{\pi}{2}$

20. A rectangular sheet of material has a width of 3 m and a length of 4 m. Forces with magnitudes of 3 N and 4N. respectively, are applied parallel to two edges of the sheet, as shown in the figure below.

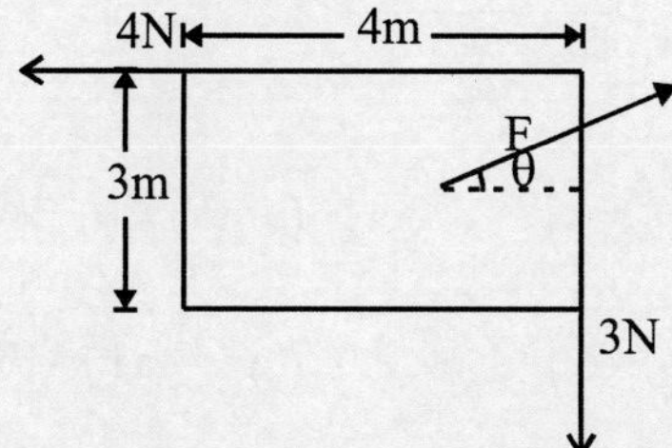

A third force F, is applied to the centre of the sheet, along a line in the plane of the sheet, at an angle $\theta = \tan 0.75$ with respect to the horizontal direction. The sheet will be in translational equilibrium when F has what value?

(a) F = 3 N (b) F = 4N (c) F = 5 N (d) F = 7N

21. The linear velocity of a rotating body is given by :

$$\vec{v} = \vec{\omega} \times \vec{r}$$

If $\vec{\omega} = \hat{i} - 2\hat{j} + 2\hat{k}$ and $\vec{r} = 4\hat{j} - 3\hat{k}$, then the magnitude of $\vec{v}$ is

(a) $\sqrt{29}$ units (b) $\sqrt{31}$ units

(c) $\sqrt{37}$ units (d) $\sqrt{41}$ units

22. Two forces are such that the sum of their magnitudes is 18 N and their resultant is 12 N which is perpendicular to the smaller force. Then the magnitudes of the forces are

(a) 12 N, 6 N (b) 13 N, 5 N (c) 10 N, 8 N (d) 16N, 2N.

23. For any two vectors $\vec{A}$ and $\vec{B}$, if $\vec{A}.\vec{B} = |\vec{A} \times \vec{B}|$, the magnitude of $\vec{C} = \vec{A} + \vec{B}$ is

(a) A + B (b) $\sqrt{A^2 + B^2 + \sqrt{2}\,AB}$

(c) $\sqrt{A^2 + B^2}$ (d) $\sqrt{A^2 + B^2 + \frac{AB}{\sqrt{2}}}$

24. The angles which the vector $\vec{A} = 3\hat{i} + 6\hat{j} + 2\hat{k}$ makes with the co-ordinate axes are :

(a) $\cos^{-1}\frac{3}{7}, \cos^{-1}\frac{4}{7}, \cos^{-1}\frac{1}{7}$

(b) $\cos^{-1}\frac{3}{7}, \cos^{-1}\frac{6}{7}, \cos^{-1}\frac{2}{7}$

(c) $\cos^{-1}\frac{4}{7}, \cos^{-1}\frac{5}{7}, \cos^{-1}\frac{3}{7}$

(d) None of these

25. The resultant of two forces 3P and 2P is R. If the first force is doubled then the resultant is also doubled. The angle between the two forces is

(a) 60º (b) 120º (c) 70º (d) 180º

26. At what angle must the two forces (x + y) and (x – y) act so that the resultant may be $\sqrt{(x^2 + y^2)}$?

(a) $\cos^{-1}[-(x^2 + y^2)/2(x^2 - y^2)]$

(b) $\cos^{-1}[-2(x^2 - y^2)/(x^2 + y^2)]$

(c) $\cos^{-1}[-(x^2 + y^2)/(x^2 - y^2)]$

(d) $\cos^{-1}[-(x^2 - y^2)/(x^2 + y^2)]$

27. A force of $-F\hat{k}$ acts on O, the origin of the coordinate system. The torque about the point (1, –1) is

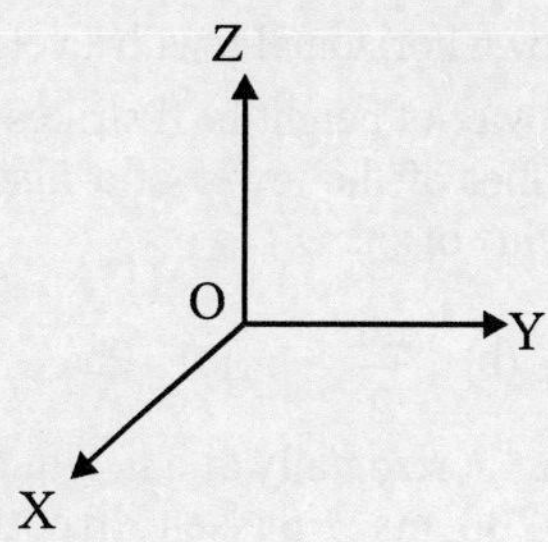

(a) $F(\hat{i} - \hat{j})$ (b) $-F(\hat{i} + \hat{j})$

(c) $F(\hat{i} + \hat{j})$ (d) $-F(\hat{i} - \hat{j})$

28. The component of vector $\vec{a} = 2\hat{i} + 3\hat{j}$ along the vector i + j is

(a) $\frac{5}{\sqrt{2}}$ (b) $10\sqrt{2}$ (c) $5\sqrt{2}$ (d) 5

29. A body is projected at an angle of 30º to the horizontal with speed 30 m/s. What is the angle with the horizontal after 1.5 seconds? Take g = 10 m/s².

(a) 0º (b) 30º (c) 60º (d) 90º

30. A large number of bullets are fired in all directions with the same speed v. What is the maximum area on the ground on which these bullets will spread?

(a) $\frac{\pi v^2}{g}$ (b) $\frac{\pi v^4}{g^2}$ (c) $\pi^2 \frac{v^2}{g^2}$ (d) $\frac{\pi^2 v^4}{g^2}$

31. A force of $(3\hat{i} + 4\hat{j})$ N acts on a body and displaces it by $(3\hat{i} + 4\hat{j})$ m. The work done by the force is

(a) 5 J (b) 30 J (c) 25 J (d) 10 J

32. If $\vec{a} = \hat{i} - \hat{j} + \hat{k}$ and $\vec{b} = 2\hat{i} + \hat{j} + 3\hat{k}$, then the unit vector along $\vec{a} + \vec{b}$ is

(a) $\frac{3i + 4k}{5}$ (b) $\frac{-3i + 4k}{5}$

(c) $\frac{-3i - 4k}{5}$ (d) None of these

33. A body is thrown with a velocity of 9.8 ms^{-1} making an angle of 30º with the horizontal. It will hit the ground after a time

(a) 3.0 s (b) 2.0 s (c) 1.5 s (d) 1 s

34. Two bullets are fired horizontally, simultaneously and with different velocities from the same place. Which bullet will hit the ground earlier ?

(a) It would depend upon the weights of the bullets.
(b) The slower one.
(c) The faster one.
(d) Both will reach simultaneously.

35. A cricket ball is hit with a velocity $25\ \text{ms}^{-1}$, 60° above the horizontal. How far above the ground, ball passes over a fielder 50 m from the bat (consider the ball is struck very close to the ground)?

Take $\sqrt{3}=1.7$ and $g=10\ \text{ms}^{-2}$

(a) 6.8m (b) 7m (c) 5m (d) 10m

36. A body is thrown horizontally with a velocity $\sqrt{2gh}$ from the top of a tower of height h. It strikes the level ground through the foot of the tower at a distance x from the tower. The value of x is

(a) gh (b) $\frac{gh}{2}$ (c) 2h (d) $\frac{2gh}{3}$

37. A plane flying horizontally at a height of 1500 m with a velocity of $200\ \text{ms}^{-1}$ passes directly overhead on antiaircraft gun. Then the angle with the horizontal at which the gun should be fired from the shell with a muzzle velocity of $400\ \text{ms}^{-1}$ to hit the plane, is

(a) 90° (b) 60° (c) 30° (d) 45°

38. The velocity of projection of oblique projectile is $(6\hat{i}+8\hat{j})\,\text{ms}^{-1}$. The horizontal range of the projectile is

(a) 4.9m (b) 9.6m (c) 19.6m (d) 14m

39. A gun is aimed at a horizontal target. It takes $\frac{1}{2}$ s for the bullet to reach the target. The bullet hits the target x metre below the aim. Then, x is equal to

(a) $\frac{9.8}{4}$m (b) $\frac{9.8}{8}$m (c) 9.8m (d) 19.6m.

40. The equation of trajectory of projectile is given by

$y=\frac{x}{\sqrt{3}}-\frac{gx^2}{20}$, where x and y are in metre.

The maximum range of the projectile is

(a) $\frac{8}{3}$m (b) $\frac{4}{3}$m (c) $\frac{3}{4}$m (d) $\frac{3}{8}$m

41. A bullet is fired with a speed of 1500 m/s in order to hit a target 100 m away. If $g=10\ \text{m/s}^2$. The gun should be aimed

(a) 15 cm above the target
(b) 10 cm above the target
(c) 2.2 cm above the target
(d) directly towards the target

42. Let $|\overrightarrow{A_1}|=3$, $|\overrightarrow{A_2}|=5$ and $|\overrightarrow{A_1}+\overrightarrow{A_2}|=5$. The value of $(2\overrightarrow{A_1}+3\overrightarrow{A_2})\bullet(3\overrightarrow{A_1}-2\overrightarrow{A_2})$ is :

(a) −106.5 (b) −99.5 (c) −112.5 (d) −118.5

43. In the cube of side 'a' shown in the figure, the vector from the central point of the face ABOD to the central point of the face BEFO will be:

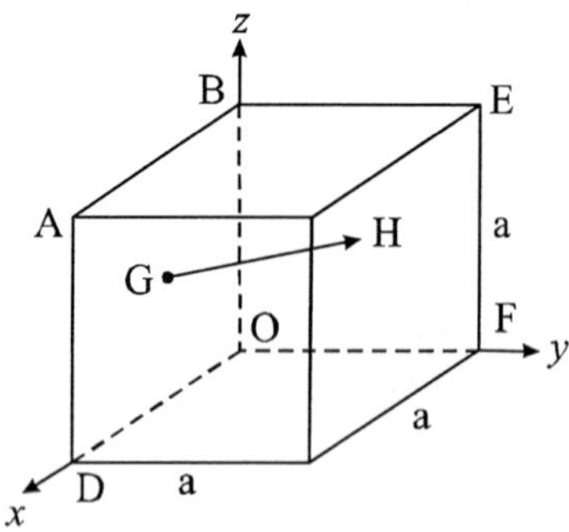

(a) $\frac{1}{2}a(\hat{k}-\hat{i})$ (b) $\frac{1}{2}a(\hat{i}-\hat{k})$

(c) $\frac{1}{2}a(\hat{j}-\hat{i})$ (d) $\frac{1}{2}a(\hat{j}-\hat{k})$

44. Two forces P and Q, of magnitude 2F and 3F, respectively, are at an angle θ with each other. If the force Q is doubled, then their resultant also gets doubled. Then, the angle θ is:

(a) 120° (b) 60° (c) 90° (d) 30°

45. A balloon is moving up in air vertically above a point A on the ground. When it is at a height h_1, a girl standing at a distance d (point B) from A (see figure) sees it at an angle 45° with respect to the vertical. When the balloon climbs up a further height h_2, it is seen at an angle 60° with respect to the vertical if the girl moves further by a distance 2.464 d (point C). Then the height h_2 is (given tan 30° = 0.5774):

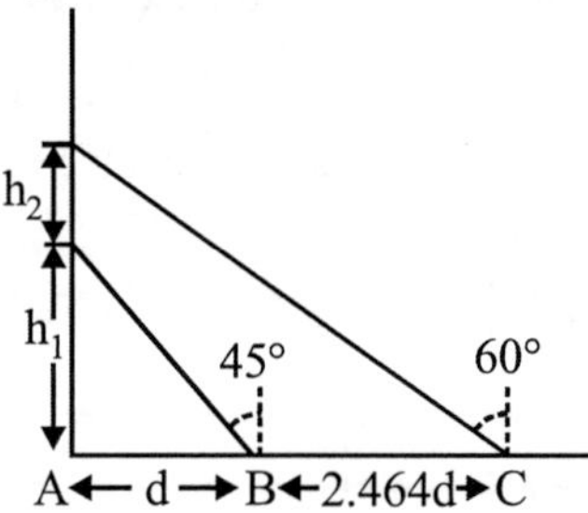

(a) 1.464d (b) 0.732d (c) 0.464d (d) d

46. Starting from the origin at time $t=0$, with initial velocity $5\hat{j}\ \text{ms}^{-1}$, a particle moves in the x–y plane with a constant acceleration of $(10\hat{i}+4\hat{j})\ \text{ms}^{-2}$. At time t, its coordiantes are (20 m, y_0 m). The values of t and y_0 are, respectively :

(a) 2 s and 18 m (b) 4 s and 52 m
(c) 2 s and 24 m (d) 5 s and 25 m

47. The position vector of a particle changes with time according to the relation $\vec{r}(t)=15t^2\hat{i}+(4-20t^2)\hat{j}$. What is the magnitude of the acceleration at $t=1$?

(a) 40 (b) 25 (c) 100 (d) 50

48. A particle is moving with a velocity $\vec{v}=K(y\hat{i}+x\hat{j})$, where K is a constant. The general equation for its path is:

(a) $y=x^2+$ constant (b) $y^2=x+$ constant
(c) $y^2=x^2+$ constant (d) $xy=$ constant

49. A particle starts from the origin at $t = 0$ with an initial velocity of $3.0\hat{i}$ m/s and moves in the x-y plane with a constant acceleration $(6.0\hat{i}+4.0\hat{j})$ m/s². The x-coordinate of the particle at the instant when its y-coordinate is 32 m is D meters. The value of D is:
(a) 32 (b) 50 (c) 60 (d) 40

50. A particle moves such that its position vector $\vec{r}(t) = \cos\omega t\,\hat{i} + \sin\omega t\,\hat{j}$ where ω is a constant and t is time. Then which of the following statements is true for the velocity $\vec{v}(t)$ and acceleration $\vec{a}(t)$ of the particle:
(a) $\vec{v}$ is perpendicular to $\vec{r}$ and $\vec{a}$ is directed away from the origin
(b) $\vec{v}$ and $\vec{a}$ both are perpendicular to $\vec{r}$
(c) $\vec{v}$ and $\vec{a}$ both are parallel to $\vec{r}$
(d) $\vec{v}$ is perpendicular to $\vec{r}$ and $\vec{a}$ is directed towards the origin

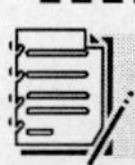

Exercise 2 - Exemplar & Past Year Questions

E&PYQs

Exemplar Questions

1. The angle between $A=\hat{i}+\hat{j}$ and $B=\hat{i}-\hat{j}$ is
(a) 45° (b) 90° (c) −45° (d) 180°

2. Which one of the following statements is true?
(a) A scalar quantity is the one that is conserved in a process
(b) A scalar quantity is the one that can never take negative values
(c) A scalar quantity is the one that does not vary from one point to another in space
(d) A scalar quantity has the same value for observers with different orientation of the axes

3. Figure shows the orientation of two vectors u and v in the xy-plane.

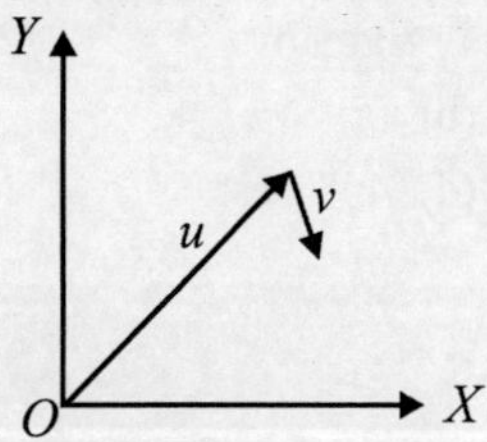

If $u = a\hat{i} + b\hat{j}$ and $v = p\hat{i} + q\hat{j}$
Which of the following is correct?
(a) a and p are positive while b and q are negative
(b) a, p and b are positive while q is negative
(c) a, q and b are positive while p is negative
(d) a, b, p and q are all positive

4. The component of a vector r along X-axis will have maximum value if
(a) r is along positive Y-axis
(b) r is along positive X-axis
(c) r makes an angle of 45° with the X-axis
(d) r is along negative Y-axis

5. The horizontal range of a projectile fired at an angle of 15° is 50 m. If it is fired with the same speed at an angle of 45°, its range will be
(a) 60 m (b) 71 m (c) 100 m (d) 141 m

6. Consider the quantities, pressure, power, energy, impulse, gravitational potential, electrical charge, temperature, area. Out of these, the only vector quantities are :
(a) impulse, pressure and area
(b) impulse and area
(c) area and gravitational potential
(d) impulse and pressure

7. In a two dimensional motion, instantaneous speed v_0 is a positive constant. Then, which of the following are necessarily true?
(a) The average velocity is not zero at any time
(b) Average acceleration must always vanish
(c) Displacements in equal time intervals are equal
(d) Equal path lengths are traversed in equal intervals

8. In a two dimensional motion, instantaneous speed v_0 is a positive constant. Then, which of the following are necessarily true?
(a) The acceleration of the particle is zero
(b) The acceleration of the particle is bounded
(c) The acceleration of the particle is necessarily in the plane of motion
(d) The particle must be undergoing a uniform circular motion

NEET/AIPMT (2013-2020) Questions

9. The velocity of a projectile at the initial point A is $(2\hat{i}+3\hat{j})$ m/s. It's velocity (in m/s) at point B is **[2013]**

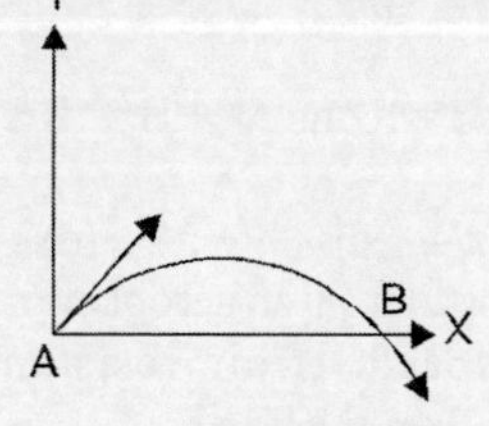

(a) $-2\hat{i}+3\hat{j}$ (b) $2\hat{i}-3\hat{j}$
(c) $2\hat{i}+3\hat{j}$ (d) $-2\hat{i}-3\hat{j}$

10. Vectors $\vec{A}, \vec{B}$ and $\vec{C}$ are such that $\vec{A}\cdot\vec{B}=0$ and $\vec{A}\cdot\vec{C}=0$. Then the vector parallel to $\vec{A}$ is **[NEET Kar. 2013]**
(a) $\vec{B}$ and $\vec{C}$ (b) $\vec{A}\times\vec{B}$ (c) $\vec{B}+\vec{C}$ (d) $\vec{B}\times\vec{C}$

11. A particle is moving such that its position coordinate (x, y) are
(2m, 3m) at time t = 0
(6m, 7m) at time t = 2 s and
(13m, 14m) at time t = 5s.
Average velocity vector $(\vec{V}_{av})$ from t = 0 to t = 5s is : **[2014]**

(a) $\frac{1}{5}(13\hat{i}+14\hat{j})$ (b) $\frac{7}{3}(\hat{i}+\hat{j})$

(c) $2(\hat{i}+\hat{j})$ (d) $\frac{11}{5}(\hat{i}+\hat{j})$

12. If vectors $\vec{A}=\cos\omega t\hat{i}+\sin\omega t\hat{j}$ and $\vec{B}=\cos\frac{\omega t}{2}\hat{i}+\sin\frac{\omega t}{2}\hat{j}$ are functions of time, then the value of t at which they are orthogonal to each other is : ***[2015 RS]***

(a) $t=\frac{\pi}{2\omega}$ (b) $t=\frac{\pi}{\omega}$ (c) $t=0$ (d) $t=\frac{\pi}{4\omega}$

13. The position vector of a particle $\vec{R}$ as a function of time is given by:

$\vec{R}=4\sin(2\pi t)\hat{i}+4\cos(2\pi t)\hat{j}$

Where R is in meter, t in seconds and $\hat{i}$ and $\hat{j}$ denote unit vectors along x-and y-directions, respectively.
Which one of the following statements is wrong for the motion of particle? ***[2015 RS]***

(a) Magnitude of acceleration vector is $\frac{v^2}{R}$, where v is the velocity of particle
(b) Magnitude of the velocity of particle is 8 meter/second
(c) path of the particle is a circle of radius 4 meter.
(d) Acceleration vector is along - $\vec{R}$

14. A ship A is moving Westwards with a speed of 10 km h^{-1} and a ship B 100 km South of A, is moving Northwards with a speed of 10 km h^{-1}. The time after which the distance between them becomes shortest, is : ***[2015]***

(a) 5 h (b) $5\sqrt{2}$ h (c) $10\sqrt{2}$ h (d) 0 h

15. A particle moves so that its position vector is given by $\vec{r}=\cos\omega t\hat{x}+\sin\omega t\hat{y}$. Where ω is a constant. Which of the following is true ? ***[2016]***
(a) Velocity and acceleration both are perpendicular to $\vec{r}$
(b) Velocity and acceleration both are parallel to $\vec{r}$
(c) Velocity is perpendicular to $\vec{r}$ and acceleration is directed towards the origin
(d) Velocity is perpendicular to $\vec{r}$ and acceleration is directed away from the origin

16. If the magnitude of sum of two vectors is equal to the magnitude of difference of the two vectors, the angle between these vectors is : ***[2016]***
(a) 0° (b) 90° (c) 45° (d) 180°

17. The x and y coordinates of the particle at any time are $x = 5t - 2t^2$ and $y = 10t$ respectively, where x and y are in meters and t in seconds. The acceleration of the particle at t = 2s is ***[2017]***
(a) 5 m/s^2 (b) –4 m/s^2
(c) –8 m/s^2 (d) 0

18. The moment of the force, $\vec{F}=4\hat{i}+5\hat{j}-6\hat{k}$ at (2, 0, –3), about the point (2, –2, –2), is given by ***[2018]***
(a) $-8\hat{i}-4\hat{j}-7\hat{k}$ (b) $-4\hat{i}-\hat{j}-8\hat{k}$
(c) $-7\hat{i}-4\hat{j}-8\hat{k}$ (d) $-7\hat{i}-8\hat{j}-4\hat{k}$

19. The speed of a swimmer in still water is 20 m/s. The speed of river water is 10 m/s and is flowing due east. If he is standing on the south bank and wishes to cross the river along the shortest path, the angle at which he should make his strokes w.r.t. north is given by : ***[2019]***
(a) 30° west (b) 0°
(c) 60° west (d) 45° west

Exercise 3 - Concept Application Problems CAP

1. Given that A + B = R and $A^2 + B^2 = R^2$. The angle between A and B is
(a) 0 (b) π/4 (c) π/2 (d) p

2. A bomb is dropped from an aeroplane moving horizontally at constant speed. If air resistance is taken into consideration, then the bomb
(a) falls on earth exactly below the aeroplane
(b) falls on the earth exactly behind the aeroplane
(c) falls on the earths ahead of the aeroplane
(d) flies with the aeroplane

3. An aeroplane flying at a constant speed releases a bomb. As the bomb moves away from the aeroplane, it will
(a) always be vertically below the aeroplane only if the aeroplane was flying horizontally
(b) always be vertically below the aeroplane only if the aeroplane was flying at an angle of 45° to the horizontal
(c) always be vertically below the aeroplane
(d) gradually fall behind the aeroplane if the aeroplane was flying horizontally.

4. A body is projected such that its KE at the top is 3/4th of its initial KE. What is the angle of projectile with the horizontal?
(a) 30° (b) 60° (c) 45° (d) 120°

5. A bomb is dropped on an enemy post by an aeroplane flying horizontally with a velocity of 60 km h^{-1} and at a height of 490 m. At the time of dropping the bomb, how far the aeroplane should be from the enemy post so that the bomb may directly hit the target ?

(a) $\frac{400}{3}$m (b) $\frac{500}{3}$m (c) $\frac{1700}{3}$m (d) 498m.

6. A body is projected horizontally from a point above the ground and motion of the body is described by the equation $x = 2t$, $y = 5t^2$ where x, and y are horizontal and vertical coordinates in metre after time t. The initial velocity of the body will be
(a) $\sqrt{29}$ m/s horizontal (b) 5 m/s horizontal
(c) 2 m/s vertical (d) 2 m/s horizontal

7. A vector $\overrightarrow{P_1}$ is along the positive x-axis. If its vector product with another vector $\overrightarrow{P_2}$ is zero then $\overrightarrow{P_2}$ could be
(a) $4\hat{j}$ (b) $-4\hat{i}$ (c) $(\hat{j}+\hat{k})$ (d) $-(\hat{i}+\hat{j})$

8. A bucket, full of water is revolved in a vertical circle of radius 2 m. What should be the maximum time-period of revolution so that the water doesn't fall out of the bucket?
(a) 1 sec (b) 2 sec (c) 3 sec (d) 4 sec

9. Out of the following sets of forces, the resultant of which cannot be zero ?
(a) 10, 10, 10 (b) 10, 10, 20
(c) 10, 20, 20 (d) 10, 20, 40

10. If A = B + C and the magnitudes of A, B and C are 5, 4 and 3 units, the angle between A and C is
(a) $\cos^{-1}(3/5)$ (b) $\cos^{-1}(4/5)$
(c) $\frac{\pi}{2}$ (d) $\sin^{-1}(3/4)$

11. Let $\vec{C} = \vec{A} + \vec{B}$
(a) $|\vec{C}|$ is always greater than $|\vec{A}|$
(b) It is possible to have $|\vec{C}| < |\vec{A}|$ and $|\vec{C}| < |\vec{B}|$
(c) $\vec{C}$ is always equal to $\vec{A} + \vec{B}$
(d) $\vec{C}$ is never equal to $\vec{A} + \vec{B}$

12. A projectile is moving at 60 m/s at its highest point, where it breaks into two equal parts due to an internal explosion. One part moves vertically up at 50 m/s with respect to the ground. The other part will move at a speed of
(a) 110 m/s (b) 120 m/s
(c) 130 m/s (d) $10\sqrt{61}$ m/s

13. A particle having a mass 0.5 kg is projected under gravity with a speed of 98 m/sec at an angle of 60°. The magnitude of the change in momentum (in N-sec) of the particle after 10 seconds is
(a) 0.5 (b) 49 (c) 98 (d) 490

14. A person aims a gun at a bird from a point at a horizontal distance of 100 m. If the gun can impact a speed of 500 ms^{-1} to the bullet. At what height above the bird must he aim his gun in order to hit it? ($g = 10\ ms^{-2}$)
(a) 10.4 cm (b) 20.35 cm
(c) 50 cm (d) 100 cms

15. The equation of a projectile is
$$y = \sqrt{3}x - \frac{gx^2}{2}$$
The angle of projection is given by
(a) $\tan\theta = \frac{1}{\sqrt{3}}$ (b) $\tan\theta = \sqrt{3}$
(c) $\frac{\pi}{2}$ (d) zero.

16. A projectile A is thrown at an angle of 30° to the horizontal from point P. At the same time, another projectile B is thrown with velocity v_2 upwards from the point Q vertically below the highest point. For B to collide with A, $\frac{v_2}{v_1}$ should be

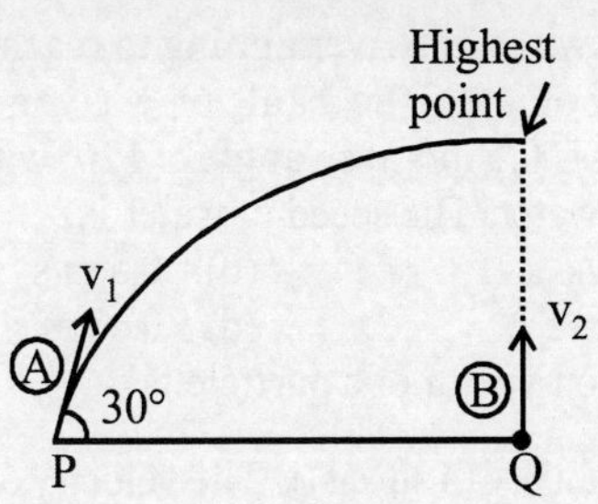

(a) 1 (b) 2 (c) $\frac{1}{2}$ (d) 4

17. A projectile of mass m is thrown with a velocity v making an angle 60° with the horizontal. Neglecting air resistance, the change in momentum from the departure A to its arrival at B, along the vertical direction is

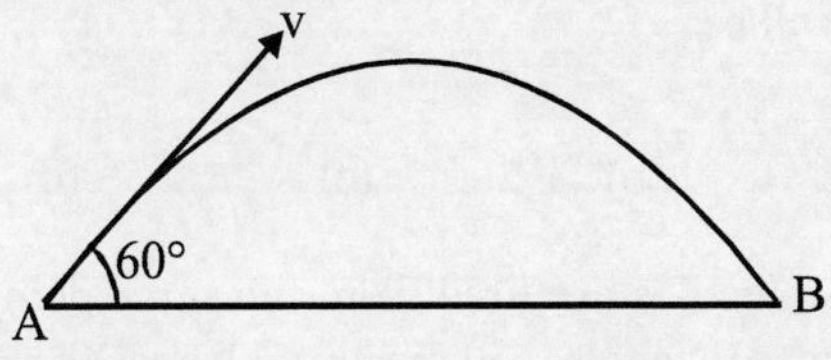

(a) 2 mv (b) $\sqrt{3}$mv (c) mv (d) $\frac{mv}{\sqrt{3}}$

18. A person sitting in the rear end of the compartment throws a ball towards the front end. The ball follows a parabolic path. The train is moving with velocity of 20 m/s. A person standing outside on the ground also observes the ball. How will the maximum heights (y_m) attained and the ranges (R) seen by the thrower and the outside observer compare with each other?
(a) Same y_m different R (b) Same y_m and R
(c) Different y_m same R (d) Different y_m and R

19. A particle moves in a circle of radius 4 cm clockwise at constant speed 2 cm/s. If $\hat{x}$ and $\hat{y}$ are unit acceleration vectors along X and Y-axis respectively (in cm/s^2), the acceleration of the particle at the instant half way between P and Q is given by

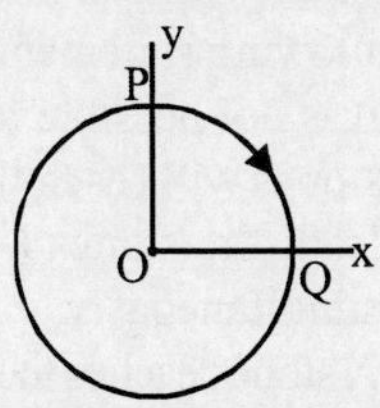

(a) $-4(\hat{x}+\hat{y})$
(b) $4(\hat{x}+\hat{y})$
(c) $-(\hat{x}+\hat{y})/\sqrt{2}$
(d) $(\hat{x}-\hat{y})/4$

20. A projectile is thrown in the upward direction making an angle of 60° with the horizontal direction with a velocity of 147 ms^{-1}. Then the time after which its inclination with the horizontal is 45°, is
(a) 15 s (b) 10.98 s (c) 5.49 s (d) 2.745 s

21. A cyclist moving at a speed of 20 m/s takes a turn, if he doubles his speed then chance of overturn
(a) is doubled (b) is halved
(c) becomes four times (d) becomes 1/4 times

22. A person swims in a river aiming to reach exactly on the opposite point on the bank of a river. His speed of swimming is 0.5 m/s at an angle of 120° with the direction of flow of water. The speed of water is
(a) 1.0 m/s (b) 0.5 m/s
(c) 0.25 m/s (d) 0.43 m/s

23. The position vector of a particle is
$\vec{r} = (a\cos\omega t)\hat{i} + (a\sin\omega t)\hat{j}$. The velocity of the particle is
(a) directed towards the origin
(b) directed away from the origin
(c) parallel to the position vector
(d) perpendicular to the position vector

24. A ball whose kinetic energy is E is thrown at an angle of 45° with horizontal. Its kinetic energy at highest point of flight will be
(a) E (b) E/2 (c) $\frac{E}{\sqrt{2}}$ (d) O

25. Two projectiles are fired from the same point with the same speed at angles of projection 60° and 30° respectively. Which one of the following is true?
(a) Their maximum height will be same
(b) Their range will be same
(c) Their landing velocity will be same
(d) Their time of flight will be same

26. A body of 3kg. moves in X-Y plane under the action of force given by $6t\hat{i} + 4t\hat{j}$. Assuming that the body is at rest at time t = 0, the velocity of body at t = 3 sec is
(a) $9\hat{i} + 6\hat{j}$ (b) $18\hat{i} + 6\hat{j}$
(c) $18\hat{i} + 12\hat{j}$ (d) $12\hat{i} + 68\hat{j}$

27. From a 10 m high building a stone A is dropped, and simultaneously another identical stone B is thrown horizontally with an initial speed of 5 ms^{-1}. Which one of the following statements is true?
(a) It is not possible to calculate which one of the two stones will reach the ground first
(b) Both the stones (A and B) will reach the ground simultaneously
(c) A stone reaches the ground earlier than B
(d) B stone reaches the ground earlier than A

28. The vector sum of two forces is perpendicular to their vector differences. In that case, the forces
(a) cannot be predicted
(b) are equal to each other
(c) are equal to each other in magnitude
(d) are not equal to each other in magnitude

29. If $|\vec{A} \times \vec{B}| = \sqrt{3}\vec{A}.\vec{B}$ then the value of $|\vec{A} + \vec{B}|$ is
(a) $(A^2 + B^2\sqrt{3}AB)^{1/2}$ (b) $(A^2 + B^2 + AB)^{1/2}$
(c) $\left(A^2 + B^2 + \frac{AB}{\sqrt{3}}\right)^{1/2}$ (d) $A + B$

30. If a vector $2\hat{i}+3\hat{j}+8\hat{k}$ is perpendicular to the vector $4\hat{j}-4\hat{i}+\alpha\hat{k}$, then the value of α is
(a) 1/2 (b) −1/2 (c) 1 (d) −1

31. Two vectors $\vec{A}$ and $\vec{B}$ have equal magnitudes. The magnitude of $(\vec{A} + \vec{B})$ is 'n' times the magnitude of $(\vec{A} - \vec{B})$. The angle between $\vec{A}$ and $\vec{B}$ is:
(a) $\cos^{-1}\left[\frac{n^2-1}{n^2+1}\right]$ (b) $\cos^{-1}\left[\frac{n-1}{n+1}\right]$
(c) $\sin^{-1}\left[\frac{n^2-1}{n^2+1}\right]$ (d) $\sin^{-1}\left[\frac{n-1}{n+1}\right]$

32. Let $\vec{A} = (\hat{i} + \hat{j})$ and $\vec{B} = (\hat{i} - \hat{j})$. The magnitude of a coplanar vector $\vec{C}$ such that $\vec{A}.\vec{C} = \vec{B}.\vec{C} = \vec{A}.\vec{B}$ is given by
(a) $\sqrt{\frac{5}{9}}$ (b) $\sqrt{\frac{10}{9}}$ (c) $\sqrt{\frac{20}{9}}$ (d) $\sqrt{\frac{9}{12}}$

33. A vector $\vec{A}$ is rotated by a small angle $\Delta\theta$ radian ($\Delta\theta << 1$) to get a new vector $\vec{B}$. In that case $|\vec{B} - \vec{A}|$ is :
(a) $|\vec{A}|\Delta\theta$ (b) $|\vec{B}|\Delta\theta - |\vec{A}|$
(c) $|\vec{A}|\left(1 - \frac{\Delta\theta^2}{2}\right)$ (d) 0

34. A particle moves from the point $(2.0\hat{i} + 4.0\hat{j})$ m, at t = 0, with an initial velocity $(5.0\hat{i} + 4.0\hat{j})$ ms^{-1}. It is acted upon by a constant force which produces a constant acceleration $(4.0\hat{i} + 4.0\hat{j})$ ms^{-2}. What is the distance of the particle from the origin at time 2s?
(a) 15m (b) $20\sqrt{2}$m (c) 5m (d) $10\sqrt{2}$m

35. The trajectory of a projectile near the surface of the earth is given as $y = 2x - 9x^2$. If it were launched at an angle θ_0 with speed v_0 then (g = 10 ms^{-2}):
(a) $\theta_0 = \sin^{-1}\frac{1}{\sqrt{5}}$ and $v_0 = \frac{5}{3}$ ms^{-1}
(b) $\theta_0 = \cos^{-1}\left(\frac{2}{\sqrt{5}}\right)$ and $v_0 = \frac{3}{5}$ ms^{-1}
(c) $\theta_0 = \cos^{-1}\left(\frac{1}{\sqrt{5}}\right)$ and $v_0 = \frac{9}{3}$ ms^{-1}
(d) $\theta_0 = \sin^{-1}\left(\frac{2}{\sqrt{5}}\right)$ and $v_0 = \frac{3}{5}$ ms^{-1}

36. Two particles are projected from the same point with the same speed u such that they have the same range R, but different maximum heights, h_1 and h_2. Which of the following is correct ?

(a) $R^2 = 4 h_1 h_2$ (b) $R^2 = 16 h_1 h_2$
(c) $R^2 = 2 h_1 h_2$ (d) $R^2 = h_1 h_2$

37. Two guns A and B can fire bullets at speeds 1 km/s and 2 km/s respectively. From a point on a horizontal ground, they are fired in all possible directions. The ratio of maximum areas covered by the bullets fired by the two guns, on the ground is:

(a) 1 : 16 (b) 1 : 2 (c) 1 : 4 (d) 1 : 8

38. A shell is fired from a fixed artillery gun with an initial speed u such that it hits the target on the ground at a distance R from it. If t_1 and t_2 are the values of the time taken by it to hit the target in two possible ways, the product $t_1 t_2$ is :

(a) R/4g (b) R/g (c) R/2g (d) 2R/g

39. A plane is inclined at an angle $\alpha = 30°$ with respect to the horizontal. A particle is projected with a speed $u = 2\ \text{ms}^{-1}$, from the base of the plane, as shown in figure. The distance from the base, at which the particle hits the plane is close to : (Take $g = 10\ \text{ms}^{-2}$)

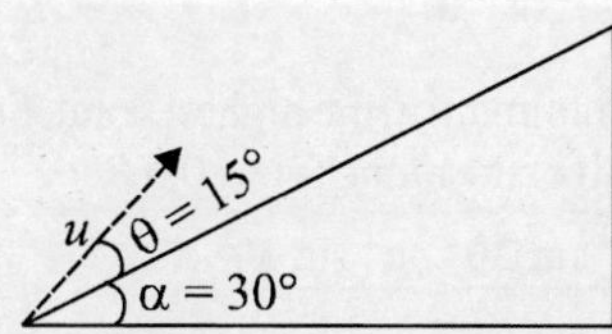

(a) 20 cm (b) 18 cm (c) 26 cm (d) 14 cm

40. A body is projected at t = 0 with a velocity 10 ms^{-1} at an angle of 60° with the horizontal. The radius of curvature of its trajectory at t = 1s is R. Neglecting air resistance and taking acceleration due to gravity g = 10 ms^{-2}, the value of R is:

(a) 10.3 m (b) 2.8 m (c) 2.5 m (d) 5.1 m

41. A particle is moving with velocity $\vec{v} = k(y\hat{i} + x\hat{j})$, where k is a constant. The general equation for its path is

(a) $y = x^2 +$ constant (b) $y^2 = x +$ constant
(c) $xy =$ constant (d) $y^2 = x^2 +$ constant

42. A particle has an initial velocity of $3\hat{i} + 4\hat{j}$ and an acceleration of $0.4\hat{i} + 0.3\hat{j}$. Its speed after 10 s is :

(a) $7\sqrt{2}$ units (b) 7 units
(c) 8.5 units (d) 10 units

43. If $\vec{A} \times \vec{B} = \vec{B} \times \vec{A}$, then the angle between A and B is

(a) $\frac{\pi}{2}$ (b) $\frac{\pi}{3}$ (c) p (d) $\frac{\pi}{4}$

44. If a body moving in circular path maintains constant speed of 10 ms^{-1}, then which of the following correctly describes relation between acceleration and radius?

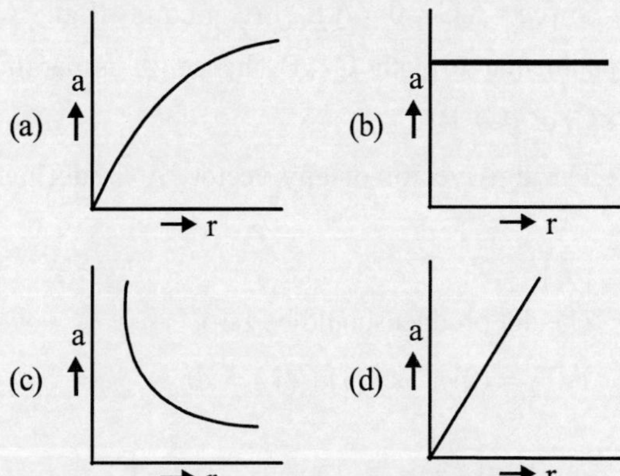

45. A particle of mass m is projected with a speed u from the ground at an angle $\theta = \frac{\pi}{3}$ w.r.t. horizontal (x-axis). When it has reached its maximum height, it collides completely inelastically with another particle of the same mass and velocity $u\hat{i}$. The horizontal distance covered by the combined mass before reaching the ground is:

(a) $\frac{3\sqrt{3}}{8}\frac{u^2}{g}$ (b) $\frac{3\sqrt{2}}{4}\frac{u^2}{g}$

(c) $\frac{5}{8}\frac{u^2}{g}$ (d) $2\sqrt{2}\frac{u^2}{g}$

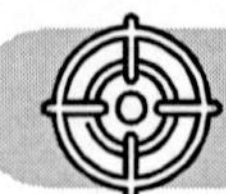

Hints & Solutions

4.1 Concept Practice Problems CPP

1. (d) A scalar quantity has the same value for observers with different orientations of the axes.
2. (d)
3. (a) In vector addition, the commutative law is obeyed

$$\text{i.e., } \vec{A}+\vec{B}=\vec{B}+\vec{A}$$

Vector subtraction does not follow commutative law.

4. (d) Since $\vec{A}.\vec{C}=0=\vec{A}.\vec{B}$, it means that $\vec{A}$ is perpendicular to both $\vec{C}\,\&\,\vec{B}$, hence $\vec{A}$ is parallel to $(\vec{B}\times\vec{C})$ or $(\vec{C}\times\vec{B})$.
5. (a) The unit vector of any vector $\vec{A}$ is defined as $\hat{A}=\dfrac{\vec{A}}{|\vec{A}|}$
6. (c) The dot product should be zero.
7. (a) $\vec{F}_1.\vec{F}_2=(2\hat{i}+5\hat{k}).(3\hat{j}+4\hat{k})=20$
8. (c)
9. (c) $|\vec{a}+\vec{b}|=|\vec{a}-\vec{b}| \Rightarrow |\vec{a}+\vec{b}|^2=|\vec{a}-\vec{b}|^2$

$\Rightarrow |a|^2+|b|^2+2\vec{a}.\vec{b}=|a|^2+|b|^2-2\vec{a}.\vec{b}$

10. (a)

4.2 Concept Practice Problems 

11. (d) $\dfrac{H_1}{H_2}=\dfrac{u^2\sin^2\theta/2g}{u^2\sin^2(90^\circ-\theta)/2g}=\tan^2\theta$
12. (a)
13. (c) On earth, $R=u^2\sin 2\theta/g$.

On moon, $g'=g/6$

$R'=u^2\sin 2\theta/g'=6u^2\sin 2\theta/g=6R$.

14. (c) $R_{30^\circ}=\dfrac{u^2\sin 60^\circ}{g}=\dfrac{\sqrt{3}}{2}(u^2/g)$

$$R_{45^\circ}=\frac{u^2\sin 90}{g}=u^2/g$$

$$R_{60^\circ}=\frac{u^2\sin 120^\circ}{g}=\frac{u^2\cos 30^\circ}{g}=\frac{u^2}{g}(\sqrt{3}/2)$$

so $R_{30^\circ}=R_{60^\circ}>R_{45^\circ}$ or $R_A=R_C>R_B$

15. (a)
16. (d) Max. height $=H=\dfrac{v^2\sin^2(90-\theta)}{2g}$ .....(i)

Time of flight, $T=\dfrac{2v\sin(90-\theta)}{g}$ ...(ii)

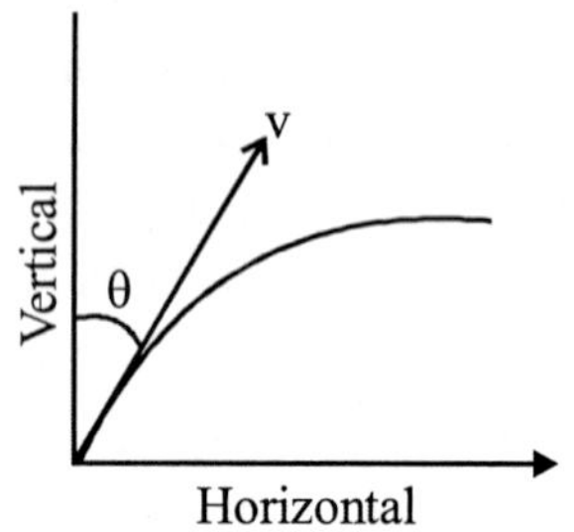

From (i), $\dfrac{v\cos\theta}{g}=\sqrt{\dfrac{2H}{g}}$,From (ii),

$$T=2\sqrt{\frac{2H}{g}}=\sqrt{\frac{8H}{g}}$$

17. (d) $T=\dfrac{2u\sin(\theta-\alpha)}{g\cos\alpha}$
18. (d) Velocity and kinetic energy is minimum at the highest point.

$$K.E=\frac{1}{2}mv^2\cos^2\theta$$

19. (b) K.E. is minimum at the highest point. So, the horizontal distance is half of the range R i.e., 0.5 R.
20. (b) $R_1=\dfrac{u^2\sin 2\theta}{g}=\dfrac{u^2\sin 30}{g}$ or $1.5=\dfrac{u^2}{2g}$ or $\dfrac{u^2}{g}=3$

$$R_2=\frac{u^2\sin 90}{g}=\frac{u^2}{g}=3\,\text{km}$$

4.3 Concept Practice Problems CPP

21. (b) $\omega=2\pi n=2\pi\times\dfrac{120}{60}=4\pi$
22. (c) Here $T=\dfrac{1}{2}$ sec the required centripetal acceleration for moving in a circle is

$$a_C=\frac{v^2}{r}=\frac{(r\omega)^2}{r}=r\omega^2=r\times(2\pi/T)^2$$

so $a_c=0.25\times(2\pi/0.5)^2=16\pi^2\times.25=4.0\pi^2$

23. (c) For circular angular motion, the formula for angular displacement θ and angular acceleration α is

$\theta=\omega t+\dfrac{1}{2}\alpha t^2$ where $\omega=$ initial velocity

or $\theta=0+\dfrac{1}{2}\alpha t^2$ or $\theta=\dfrac{1}{2}\times(2)(10)^2$

or $\theta=100$ radian

2π radian are covered in 1 revolution

$\therefore$ 1 radian is covered in $\dfrac{1}{2\pi}$ revolution or 100 radian are covered in $\frac{100}{2\pi}$ revolution

$\therefore$ Number of revolution $= \frac{50}{3.14} = 16$

24. (b) Circumference of circle is $2\pi r = 40$m
Total distance travelled in two revolution is 80m. Initial velocity u =0, final veloctiy v = 80 m/sec
so from
$v^2 = u^2 + 2as$
$\Rightarrow (80)^2 = 0^2 + 2\times 80 \times a \Rightarrow a = 40 m/sec^2$

25. (a) Here, $R = 0.1$ m

$$\omega = \frac{2\pi}{T} = \frac{2\pi}{60} = 0.105 \text{ rad/s}$$

Acceleration of the tip of the clock second's hand,

$$a = \omega^2 R = (0.105)^2 (0.1) = 0.0011 = 1.1\times 10^{-3} \text{ m/s}^2$$

Hence, average acceleration is of the order of 10^{-3}.

26. (c) When a particle moves on a circular path with a constant speed, then its motion is said to be a uniform circular motion in a plane. This motion has radial acceleration whose magnitude remains constant but whose direction changes continuously, So $a_r \neq 0$ and $a_t = 0$.
If the circular motion of the particle is not uniform but accelerated then along with the radial acceleration it will have tangential acceleration also and both these acceleration will be mutually perpendicular.

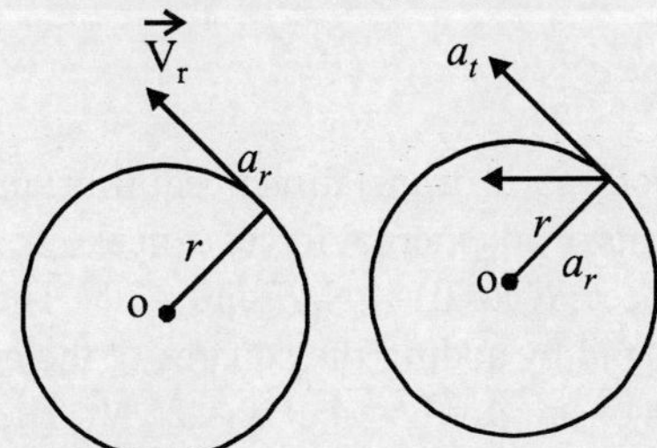

So, $a_r \neq 0$ and $a_t = 0$.
When, $a_r = 0$ and $a_t = 0$ motion is accelerated translatory.
Also, when $a_r = 0$ and then motion is uniform translatory.

27. (c) In circular motion with constant speed, acceleration is always inward, its magnitude is constant but direction changes, hence acceleration changes, so does velocity. K.E. is constant.

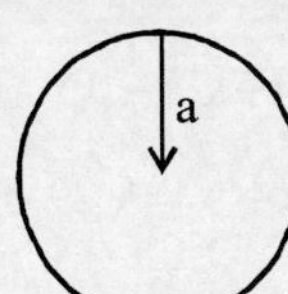

28. (a)

29. (c) From, $\theta = \omega t = \omega \frac{\pi}{2\omega} = \frac{\pi}{2}$
So, both have completed quater circle

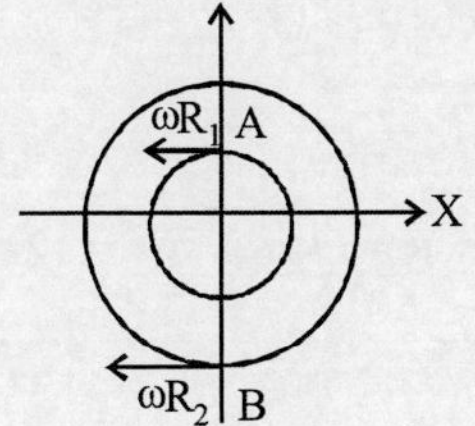

Relative velocity,

$$v_A - v_B = \omega R_1 (-\hat{i}) - \omega R_2 (-i) = \omega (R_2 - R_1) i$$

30. (d)

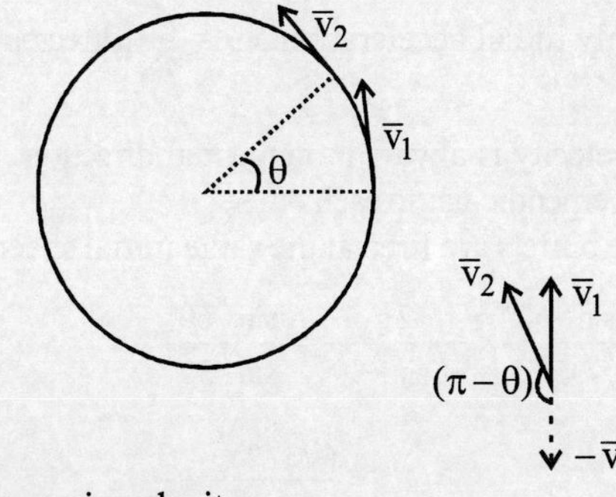

Change in velocity,

$$|\Delta \vec{v}| = \sqrt{v_1^2 + v_2^2 + 2v_1 v_2 \cos(\pi - \theta)}$$

$$= 2v\sin\frac{\theta}{2} \qquad (\because |\vec{v}_1| = |\vec{v}_2|) = v$$

$$= (2\times 10)\times \sin(30°) = 2\times 10\times \frac{1}{2}$$

$$= 10 \text{ m/s}$$

Exercise 1 - Chapter Revision Problems CRP

1. (b) If $|A+B| = A$ then A, B are anti-parallel.

2. (c) $R^2 = [A^2 + B^2 + 2AB\cos\theta]$

$$R^2 = R^2 + R^2 + 2R^2 \cos\theta$$

$$-R^2 = 2R^2\cos\theta \text{ or } \cos\theta = -1/2 \text{ or } \theta = 2\pi/3$$

3. (a) $F_1 = mr_1\omega^2$; $F_2 = mr_2\omega^2$

since period T is same, so ω is same, because $T = \frac{2\pi}{\omega}$.

Hence $\frac{F_1}{F_2} = \left(\frac{r_1}{r_2}\right)$

4. (a) A parabola
5. (b)
6. (c) From the resultant path of the particle, when it is projected at angle θ with its velocity u is

$$y = x\tan\theta - \frac{1}{2}\frac{gx^2}{u^2\cos^2\theta}$$

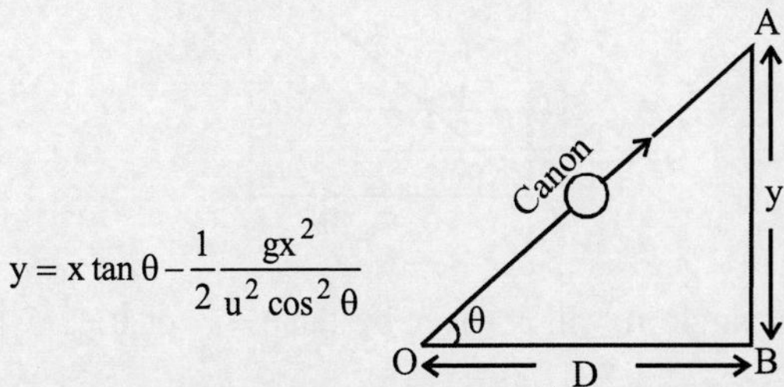

Where y denotes the instantaneous height of particle when it travels an instantaneous horizontal distance x.
here $x = D$, $u = v_0$

so $y = D\tan\theta - \frac{1}{2}\frac{gD^2}{v_0^2\cos^2\theta}$

7. (a)

8. (a) In uniform circular motion speed is constant. So, no tangential acceleration.

It has only radial acceleration $a_R = \frac{v^2}{R}$ [directed towards center]
and its velocity is always in tangential direction. So these two are perpendicular to each other.

9. (b) The bullets are fired at the same initial speed

$$\frac{H}{H'} = \frac{u^2 \sin^2 60^\circ}{2g} \times \frac{2g}{u^2 \sin^2 30^\circ} = \frac{\sin^2 60^\circ}{\sin^2 30^\circ}$$

$$= \frac{(\sqrt{3}/2)^2}{(1/2)^2} = \frac{3}{1}$$

10. (d) $\frac{u^2 2\sin\theta\cos\theta}{g} = 2 \times \frac{u^2 \sin^2\theta}{2g}$ or $\tan\theta = 2$

11. (d) $R = \frac{u^2}{g}$ or $6 = \frac{u^2}{g}$; $y = x\tan\theta - \frac{gx^2}{2u^2\cos^2\theta}$

or $h = 2\tan 45^\circ - \frac{4}{2\cos^2 45^\circ}\left(\frac{1}{6}\right) = 2 - \frac{2}{3} = \frac{4}{3}$ m

12. (c) We know that, $y_m = H = \frac{(u\sin\theta)^2}{2g} = \frac{u^2\sin^2\theta}{2g}$

$\therefore \frac{\Delta H}{H} = \frac{2\Delta u}{u}$. Given $\frac{\Delta u}{u} = 2\%$

$\therefore \frac{\Delta H}{H} = 2 \times 2 = 4\%$

13. (c) As, $s = u\sin\theta t - \frac{1}{2}gt^2$

so $40 = 20\sqrt{3} \times (\sqrt{3}/2)t - \frac{1}{2} \times 10 \times t^2$

or $5t^2 - 30t + 40 = 0$ or $t^2 - 6t + 8 = 0$

or $t = 2$ or 4.

The minimum time $t = 2$s.

14. (a) $R = \sqrt{4^2 + 5^2} = \sqrt{41}$N

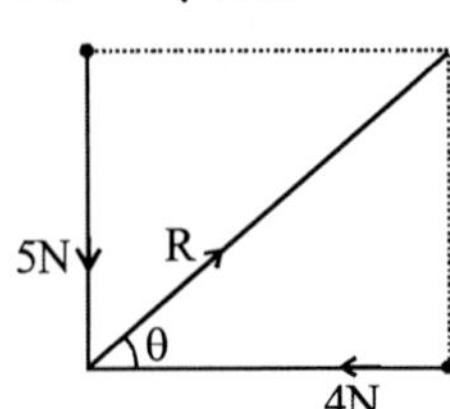

The angle θ will be given by $\tan\theta = \frac{5}{4}$ or $\theta = \tan^{-1}\left(\frac{5}{4}\right)$

15. (b) $R_{max} = (10 + 6) = 16$N, $R_{min} = (10 - 6) = 4$N

$\Rightarrow$ Values can be from 4N to 16N

16. (c) Even after 5 second, the horizontal velocity v_x will be 20 ms^{-1}. The vertical velocity v_y is given by

$v_y = 0 + 10 \times 5 = 50\,ms^{-1}$

Now, $v = \sqrt{v_x^2 + v_y^2} = \sqrt{20^2 + 50^2} \approx 54\ ms^{-1}$

17. (d) Given $\frac{u^2\sin 2\theta}{g} = 3\frac{u^2\sin^2\theta}{2g}$

$\Rightarrow \theta = \tan^{-1}\left(\frac{4}{3}\right)$

18. (b) $L = \vec{R} \times \vec{p}$

Where R = range $= \frac{u^2\sin 2\theta}{g}$

The angle between $\vec{R}$ and $\vec{p} = \theta$

Also, $p = m\,u$.

Hence, $L = \frac{u^2\sin 2\theta}{g} \times mu\sin(\theta)$

$= \frac{2mu^3\sin^2\theta\cos\theta}{g}$

19. (c) Here, $|\vec{A} \times \vec{B}| = \sqrt{3}\,|\vec{A}.\vec{B}|$

$\Rightarrow AB\sin\theta = \sqrt{3}AB\cos\theta \Rightarrow \tan\theta = \sqrt{3}$

$\Rightarrow \theta = 60^\circ = \frac{\pi}{3}$

20. (c) A body is in translational equilibrium when the components of all external forces cancel.

For the sheet : $F\cos\theta = 4$ N, $F\sin\theta = 3$ N. The magnitude of F is found by adding the squares of the components: $F^2\cos^2\theta + F^2\sin^2\theta = F^2 = 4^2 + 3^2 = 25\ N^2$. Therefore $F = 5$ N. The F vector points in the proper direction, since $\tan\theta = 0.75 = 3/4$.

21. (a) $\vec{v} = \begin{vmatrix} \hat{i} & \hat{j} & \hat{k} \\ 1 & -2 & 2 \\ 0 & 4 & -3 \end{vmatrix}$

$\vec{v} = \hat{i}[6-8] + \hat{j}[0+3] + \hat{k}[4-0]$

$\vec{v} = -2\hat{i} + 3\hat{j} + 4\hat{k} \Rightarrow |\vec{v}| = \sqrt{29}$ units.

22. (b) Use $\tan\alpha = \frac{P\sin\theta}{Q + P\cos\theta}$

$\Rightarrow \tan 90^\circ = \frac{P\sin\theta}{Q + P\cos\theta} = \infty$

$\therefore Q + P\cos\theta = 0 \Rightarrow P\cos\theta = -Q$.

$R = \sqrt{P^2 + Q^2 + 2PQ\cos\theta}$

$R = \sqrt{P^2 + Q^2 - 2Q^2}$ or $R = \sqrt{P^2 - Q^2} = 12$

$144 = (P+Q)(P-Q)$ or $P - Q = 144/18 = 8$.
$\therefore$ P = 13 N and Q = 5 N.

23. (b) $|\vec{A}.\vec{B}| = |\vec{A}\times\vec{B}| \Rightarrow AB\cos\theta = AB\sin\theta$

$$\Rightarrow \tan\theta = 1 \Rightarrow \cos\theta = \frac{1}{\sqrt{2}}$$

Now, $|\vec{A}+\vec{B}| = \sqrt{A^2+B^2+2AB\cos\theta}$

$$= \sqrt{A^2+B^2+2AB.\frac{1}{\sqrt{2}}} = \sqrt{A^2+B^2+\sqrt{2}AB}$$

24. (b) $\hat{A} = \dfrac{3\hat{i}++b\hat{j}+2\hat{k}}{\sqrt{9+36+4}} = \left(\dfrac{3}{7}\hat{i}+\dfrac{6}{7}\hat{j}+\dfrac{2}{7}\hat{k}\right)$. If α, β and γ are angles made by $\vec{A}$ with coordinate axes, then

$$\cos\alpha = \frac{3}{7}, \cos\beta = \frac{6}{7} \text{ and } \cos\gamma = \frac{2}{7}.$$

25. (b) Solve two equations : $R^2 = 9P^2 + 4P^2 + 12P^2\cos\theta$ and $4R^2 = 36P^2 + 4P^2 + 24P^2\cos\theta$.

26. (a)

$$\left(\sqrt{x^2+y^2}\right)^2 = (x+y)^2+(x-y)^2+2(x+y)(x-y)\cos\theta$$

$$\Rightarrow x^2+y^2 = x^2+y^2+2xy+x^2+y^2-2xy+2(x^2-y^2)\cos\theta$$

or $2(x^2-y^2).\cos\theta = -(x^2+y^2)$

$$\Rightarrow \theta = \cos^{-1}\left[\frac{-(x^2+y^2)}{2(x^2-y^2)}\right]$$

27. (c) Torque $\vec{\tau} = \vec{r}\times\vec{F} = (\hat{i}-\hat{j})\times(-F\hat{k})$

$$= F[-\hat{i}\times\hat{k}+\hat{j}\times\hat{k}] = F(\hat{j}+\hat{i}) = F(\hat{i}+\hat{j})$$

$$\left[\text{Since } \hat{k}\times\hat{i} = \hat{j} \text{ and } \hat{j}\times\hat{k} = \hat{i}\right]$$

28. (a) Component of $\vec{a}$ along $\vec{b} = \dfrac{\vec{a}.\vec{b}}{|\vec{b}|}$

29. (a) $u_x = 30\cos30° = 30\sqrt{3}/2,$, $u_y = 30\sin 30°$,

$v_y = 30\sin30° - gt$

$v_y = 30\sin 30° - 10\times1.5 = 0$

As vertical velocity = 0,
Angle with horizontal α = 0°
It is a state, when a particle reach to a highest point of its path.

30. (b) Maximum possible horizontal range = v^2/g
Maximum possible area of the circle

$$= \pi\left(\frac{v^2}{g}\right)^2 = \frac{\pi v^4}{g^2} \quad \left[\text{Here } r = \frac{v^2}{g}\right]$$

31. (c) Here, $\vec{F} = (3\hat{i}+4\hat{j})N$

$\vec{d} = (3\hat{i}+4\hat{j})m$ $\quad\therefore W = \vec{F}.\vec{d} = (9+16)J = 25J$

32. (a) $\vec{a}+\vec{b} = 3\hat{i}+4\hat{k}$
$\therefore$ Required unit vector

$$= \frac{\vec{a}+\vec{b}}{|\vec{a}+\vec{b}|} = \frac{3\hat{i}+4\hat{k}}{\sqrt{3^2+4^2}} = \frac{3\hat{i}+4\hat{k}}{5}.$$

33. (d) Time of flight $= \dfrac{2u\sin\theta}{g}$

$$= \frac{2\times9.8\times\sin30°}{9.8} = 2\times\frac{1}{2} = 1\,\text{sec}.$$

34. (d) The initial velocity in the vertically downward direction is zero and same height has to be covered.

35. (c) $y = x\tan\theta - \dfrac{1}{2}\dfrac{gx^2}{u^2\cos^2\theta}$

$$y = 50\tan60° - \frac{10\times50\times50}{2\times25\times25\times\cos^2 60°} = 5\,m$$

36. (c)

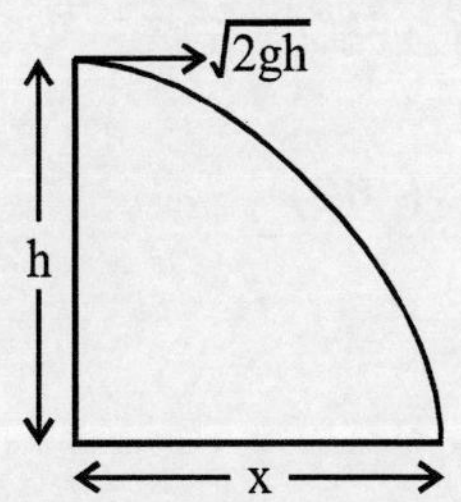

$u_y = 0$, $s_y = -h$, $a_y = -g$, $t_y = ?$

$$s = ut + \frac{1}{2}at^2$$

$$\therefore -h = -\frac{1}{2}gt^2 \Rightarrow t = \sqrt{\frac{2h}{g}}$$

$$\text{velocity} = \frac{x}{t}$$

$$\therefore x = \sqrt{2gh}\times\sqrt{\frac{2h}{g}} = 2h$$

37. (b) Horizontal distance covered should be same for the time of collision.

$$400\cos\theta = 200 \text{ or } \cos\theta = \frac{1}{2} \text{ or } \theta = 60°$$

38. (b)

39. (b) $x = \dfrac{1}{2}gt^2$

$$= \frac{1}{2}\times9.8\times\frac{1}{2}\times\frac{1}{2} = \frac{9.8}{8}\text{ m}$$

40. (b) Comparing the given equation with the equation of trajectory of a projectile,

$$y = x\tan\theta - \frac{gx^2}{2u^2\cos^2\theta}$$

we get, $\tan\theta = \dfrac{1}{\sqrt{3}} \Rightarrow \theta = 30°$

and $2u^2\cos^2\theta = 20 \Rightarrow u^2 = \dfrac{20}{2\cos^2\theta}$

$= \dfrac{10}{\cos^2 30°} = \dfrac{10}{\left(\dfrac{\sqrt{3}}{2}\right)^2} = \dfrac{40}{3}$

Now, $R_{max} = \dfrac{u^2}{g} = \dfrac{40}{3\times10} = \dfrac{4}{3}$m

41. (c)

42. (d) Using,

$R^2 = A_1^2 + A_2^2 + 2A_1A_2\cos\theta$

$5^2 = 3^2 + 5^2 + 2\times3\times5\cos\theta$

or $\cos\theta = -0.3$

$\left(2\vec{A_1} + 3\vec{A_2}\right)\cdot\left(3\vec{A_1} - 2\vec{A_2}\right) = 2A_1\times3A_1$

$+ (3A_2)(3A_1)\cos\theta - (2A_1)(2A_2)\cos\theta - 3A_2\times 2A_2$

$= 6A_1^2 + 9A_1A_2\cos\theta - 4A_1A_2\cos\theta - 6A_2^2$

$= 6A_1^2\ 6A_2^2 + 5A_1A_2\cos\theta$

$= 6\times3^2 - 6\times5^2 + 5\times3\times5(-0.3)$

$= -118.5$

43. (c) From figure,

$\vec{r}_G = \dfrac{a}{2}\hat{i} + \dfrac{a}{2}\hat{k}$

$\vec{r}_H = \dfrac{a}{2}\hat{j} + \dfrac{a}{2}\hat{k}$

$\therefore \vec{r}_H - \vec{r}_G = \left(\dfrac{a}{2}\hat{j} + \dfrac{a}{2}\hat{k}\right) - \left(\dfrac{a}{2}\hat{i} + \dfrac{a}{2}\hat{k}\right) = \dfrac{a}{2}\left(\hat{j} - \hat{i}\right)$

44. (a) Using, $R^2 = P^2 + Q^2 + 2PQ\cos\theta$

$4F^2 + 9F^2 + 12F^2\cos\theta = R^2$

When forces Q is doubled,

$4F^2 + 36F^2 + 24F^2\cos\theta = 4R^2$

$4F^2 + 36F^2 + 24F^2\cos\theta$

$= 4(13F^2 + 12F^2\cos\theta) = 52F^2 + 48F^2\cos\theta$

$\therefore \cos\theta = -\dfrac{12F^2}{24F^2} = -\dfrac{1}{2} \quad \Rightarrow \theta = 120°$

45. (d) From figure/ trigonometry,

$\dfrac{h_1}{d} = \tan 45° \qquad \therefore h_1 = d$

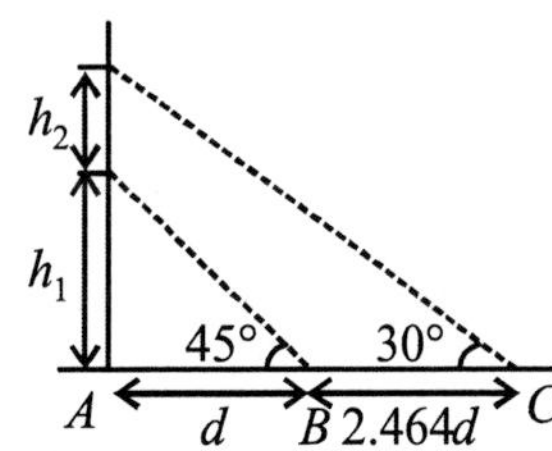

And, $\dfrac{h_1 + h_2}{d + 2.464d} = \tan 30°$

$\Rightarrow (h_1 + h_2)\times\sqrt{3} = 3.46d$

$\Rightarrow (h_1 + h_2) = \dfrac{3.46d}{\sqrt{3}} \Rightarrow d + h_2 = \dfrac{3.46d}{\sqrt{3}}$

$\therefore h_2 = d$

46. (a) Given: $\vec{u} = 5\hat{j}$ m/s

Acceleration, $\vec{a} = 10\hat{i} + 4\hat{j}$ and final coordinate $(20, y_0)$ in time t.

$S_x = u_xt + \dfrac{1}{2}a_xt^2 \qquad [\because u_x = 0]$

$\Rightarrow 20 = 0 + \dfrac{1}{2}\times10\times t^2 \Rightarrow t = 2$ s

$S_y = u_y\times t + \dfrac{1}{2}a_yt^2$

$y_0 = 5\times2 + \dfrac{1}{2}\times4\times2^2 = 18$ m

47. (d) $\vec{r} = 15t^2\hat{i} + (4 - 20t^2)\hat{j}$

$\vec{v} = \dfrac{d\vec{r}}{dt} = 30t\hat{i} - 40t\hat{j}$

Acceleration, $\vec{a} = \dfrac{d\vec{v}}{dt} = 30\hat{i} - 40\hat{j}$

$\therefore a = \sqrt{30^2 + 40^2} = 50\,\text{m/s}^2$

48. (c) From given equation,

$\vec{V} = K\left(y\hat{i} + x\hat{j}\right)$

$\dfrac{dx}{dt} = ky$ and $\dfrac{dy}{dt} = kx$

Now $\dfrac{\frac{dy}{dt}}{\frac{dx}{dt}} = \dfrac{x}{y} = \dfrac{dy}{dx}, \Rightarrow ydy = xdx$

Integrating both side

$y^2 = x^2 + c$

49. (c) Using $S = ut + \dfrac{1}{2}at^2$

$y = u_yt + \dfrac{1}{2}a_yt^2$ (along y Axis)

$\Rightarrow \quad 32 = 0\times t + \dfrac{1}{2}(4)t^2 \ \Rightarrow\ \dfrac{1}{2}\times4\times t^2 = 32$

$\Rightarrow t = 4\,s$

$S_x = u_xt + \dfrac{1}{2}a_xt^2 \qquad$ (Along x Axis)

$\Rightarrow \quad x = 3\times4 + \dfrac{1}{2}\times6\times4^2 = 60$

50. (d) Given, Position vector,

$\vec{r} = \cos\omega t\hat{i} + \sin\omega t\,\hat{j}$

Velocity, $\vec{v} = \dfrac{d\vec{r}}{dt} = \omega(-\sin\omega t\hat{i} + \cos\omega t\,\hat{j})$

Acceleration,

$$\vec{a} = \frac{d\vec{v}}{dt} = -\omega^2(\cos\omega t\hat{i} + \sin\omega t\,\hat{j})$$

$$\vec{a} = -\omega^2\vec{r}$$

$\therefore\ \vec{a}$ is antiparallel to $\vec{r}$

Also $\vec{v}.\vec{r} = 0 \quad \therefore \vec{v} \perp \vec{r}$

Thus, the particle is performing uniform circular motion.

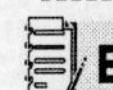

Exercise 2 - Exemplar & Past Year Questions E&PYQs

Exemplar Questions

1. (b) Given, $A = \hat{i} + \hat{j}$

$B = \hat{i} - \hat{j}$

As we know that

$$\vec{A}\cdot\vec{B} = |A||B|\cos\theta$$

$$(\hat{i}+\hat{j})\cdot(\hat{i}-\hat{j}) = (\sqrt{1^2+1^2})(\sqrt{1^2+1^2})\cos\theta$$

$$(i+j)(i-j) = \sqrt{2}\times\sqrt{2}\cos\theta$$

where θ is the angle between A and B

$$\cos\theta = \frac{1-0+0-1}{\sqrt{2}\sqrt{2}} = 0$$

$\therefore\ \theta = 90°$

2. (d) A scalar quantity does not depend on direction so it has the same value for observers with different orientations of the axes.

3. (b) From the diagram, $u = a\hat{i} + b\hat{j}$

As u is in the first quadrant, so both components a and b will be positive.

For $v = p\hat{i} + q\hat{j}$, as it is in positive x-direction and located downward so x-component p will be positive and y-component q will be negative.

Hence, a, b and p are positive but q is negative.

4. (b) Let r makes an angle θ with positive x-axis component of r along x-axis.

$$r_x = |r|\cos\theta$$

$$(r_x)_{\text{maximum}} = |r|(\cos\theta)_{\text{maximum}}$$

$$= |r|\cos 0° = |r|$$

$(\because \cos\theta$ is maximum of $\theta = 0°)$

$\theta = 0°$.

Hence the vector r has maximum value along positive x-axis.

5. (c) Consider, projectile is fired at an angle θ.

According to question,

$\theta = 15°$ and $R = 50$ m

$$\text{Range, } R = \frac{u^2\sin 2\theta}{g}$$

$$R = 50\,\text{m} = \frac{u^2\sin(2\times15°)}{g}$$

$$50\times g = u^2\sin 30° = u^2\times\frac{1}{2}$$

$$50\times g\times 2 = u^2$$

$$u^2 = 50\times9.8\times2 = 100\times9.8 = 980$$

$$u = \sqrt{980} = 31.304\text{ m/s} = 14\sqrt{5}$$

$(\because g = 9.8\text{ m/s}^2)$

Now, $\theta = 45°$;

$$R = \frac{u^2\sin 2\times45°}{g} = \frac{u^2}{g}$$

$$R = \frac{(14\sqrt{5})^2}{g} = \frac{14\times14\times5}{9.8} = 100\text{ m}$$

6. (b) As we know that,

$$\text{Impulse, } I = F\Delta t = \left(\frac{\Delta p}{\Delta t}\right)\Delta t = \Delta p$$

where F is force, Δt is time duration and Δp is change in momentum. As Δp is a vector quantity, hence impulse is also a vector quantity. Sometimes area can also be treated as vector.

7. (d) As speed is a scalar quantity, hence it will be related with path length (scalar quantity) only.

$$\text{Hence, Speed } v_0 = \frac{\text{total distance travelled}}{\text{time taken}}$$

So, total distance travelled = Path length

= (speed) × time taken

Hence, path length which is scalar and traversed in equal intervals.

8. (c) As given that in two dimensional motion the instantaneous speed v_0 is positive constant and we know that acceleration is rate of change of velocity or instantaneous speed and hence it will also be in the plane of motion.

NEET/AIPMT (2013-2020) Questions

9. (b) At point B the direction of velocity component of the projectile along Y - axis reverses.

Hence, $\vec{V}_B = 2\hat{i} - 3\hat{j}$

10. (d) Vector triple product

$$\vec{A}\times(\vec{B}\times\vec{C}) = \vec{B}(\vec{A}\cdot\vec{C}) - \vec{C}(\vec{A}\cdot\vec{B}) = 0$$

$$\Rightarrow \vec{A}\,||\,(\vec{B}\times\vec{C})$$

$[\because \vec{A}\cdot\vec{B} = 0$ and $\vec{A}\cdot\vec{C} = 0]$ 1. (a) $(\vec{A}+\vec{B})^2 = (\vec{C})^2$

$$\Rightarrow A^2 + B^2 + 2\vec{A}.\vec{B} = C^2 \Rightarrow 3^2 + 4^2 + 2\vec{A}.\vec{B} = 5^2$$

$\Rightarrow 2\vec{A}.\vec{B} = 0$

or $\Rightarrow \vec{A}.\vec{B} = 0 \;\therefore \vec{A} \perp \vec{B}$

Here $A^2 + B^2 = C^2$. Hence, $\vec{A} \perp \vec{B}$

11. (d) $\vec{v}_{av} = \dfrac{\Delta\vec{r}\text{ (displacement)}}{\Delta t\text{ (time taken)}}$

$= \dfrac{(13-2)\hat{i} + (14-3)\hat{j}}{5-0} = \dfrac{11}{5}(\hat{i}+\hat{j})$

12. (b) Two vectors are

$\vec{A} = \cos\omega t\hat{i} + \sin\omega t\hat{j}$

$\vec{B} = \cos\dfrac{\omega t}{2}\hat{i} + \sin\dfrac{\omega t}{2}\hat{j}$

For two vectors $\vec{A}$ and $\vec{B}$ to be orthogonal $\vec{A}.\vec{B} = 0$

$\vec{A}.\vec{B} = 0 = \cos\omega t.\cos\dfrac{\omega t}{2} + \sin\omega t.\sin\dfrac{\omega t}{2}$

$= \cos\left(\omega t - \dfrac{\omega t}{2}\right) = \cos\left(\dfrac{\omega t}{2}\right)$

So, $\dfrac{\omega t}{2} = \dfrac{\pi}{2}$ $\qquad \therefore\; t = \dfrac{\pi}{\omega}$

13. (b) Here, $x = 4\sin(2\pi t)$ ...(*i*)
$y = 4\cos(2\pi t)$ ...(*ii*)
Squaring and adding equation (*i*) and (*ii*)
$x^2 + y^2 = 4^2 \Rightarrow R = 4$
Motion of the particle is circular motion, acceleration vector is along $-\vec{R}$ and its magnitude $= \dfrac{V^2}{R}$
Velocity of particle, $V = \omega R = (2\pi)(4) = 8\pi$

14. (a) $\vec{V}_A = 10(-\hat{i})$

$\vec{V}_B = 10(\hat{j})$

$\vec{V}_{BA} = 10\hat{j} + 10\hat{i} = 10\sqrt{2}$ km/h

Distance OB = 100 cos 45° = $50\sqrt{2}$ km

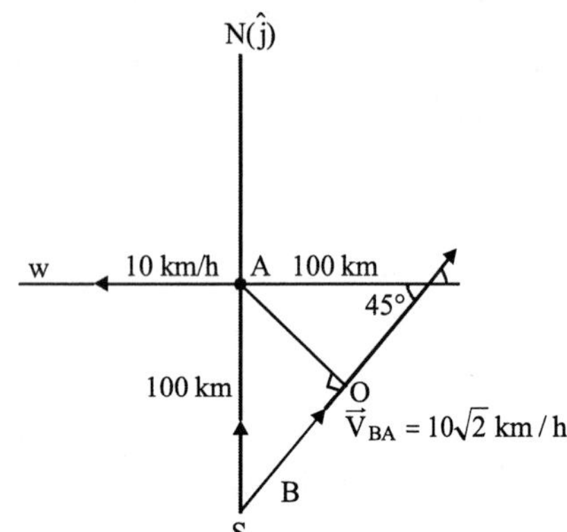

Time taken to reach the shortest distance between A and B $= \dfrac{OB}{\vec{V}_{BA}} = \dfrac{50\sqrt{2}}{10\sqrt{2}} = 5h$

15. (c) **Given:** Position vector

$\vec{r} = \cos\omega t\;\hat{x} + \sin\omega t\;\hat{y}$

$\therefore$ Velocity, $\vec{v} = -\omega\sin\omega t\;\hat{x} + \omega\cos\omega t\;\hat{y}$

and acceleration,

$\vec{a} = -\omega^2\cos\omega t\,\hat{x} - \omega^2\sin\omega t\;\hat{y} = -\omega^2\vec{r}$

$\vec{r}\cdot\vec{v} = 0$ hence $\vec{r} \perp \vec{v}$ and

$\vec{a}$ is directed towards the origin.

16. (b) $|\vec{A}+\vec{B}| = |\vec{A}-\vec{B}|$

Squaring on both sides

$|\vec{A}+\vec{B}|^2 = |\vec{A}-\vec{B}|^2$

$\Rightarrow \vec{A}\cdot\vec{A} + 2\vec{A}\cdot\vec{B} + \vec{B}\cdot\vec{B}$

$= \vec{A}\cdot\vec{A} - 2\vec{A}\cdot\vec{B} + \vec{B}\cdot\vec{B}$

$\Rightarrow 4\vec{A}\cdot\vec{B} = 0 \;\Rightarrow\; 4AB\cos\theta = 0$

$\Rightarrow \cos\theta = 0 \;\Rightarrow\; \theta = 90°$

17. (b) Given:

$x = 5t - 2t^2$ $\qquad y = 10t$

$v_x = \dfrac{dx}{dt} = 5 - 4t$ $\qquad v_y = \dfrac{dy}{dt} = 10$

$a_x = \dfrac{dv_x}{dt} = -4$ $\qquad a_y = \dfrac{dv_y}{dt} = 0$

$\vec{a} = a_x i + a_y j$ $\qquad \vec{a} = -4i\text{ m/s}^2$

Hence, acceleration of particle at (t = 2 s) = -4m/s^2

18. (c) Moment of force, $\vec{\tau} = \vec{r} \times \vec{F}$

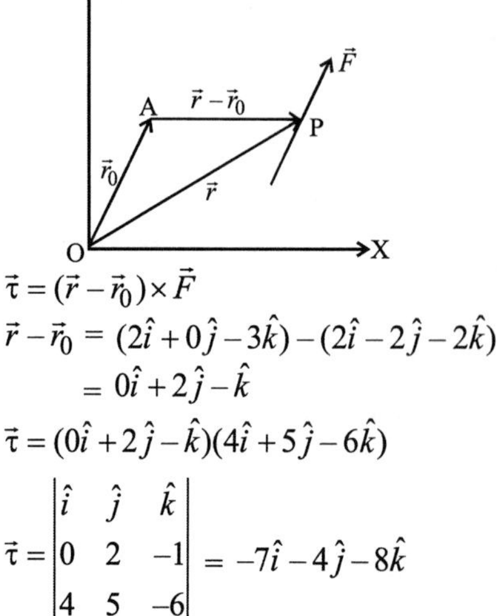

$\vec{\tau} = (\vec{r} - \vec{r}_0) \times \vec{F}$

$\vec{r} - \vec{r}_0 = (2\hat{i} + 0\hat{j} - 3\hat{k}) - (2\hat{i} - 2\hat{j} - 2\hat{k})$

$= 0\hat{i} + 2\hat{j} - \hat{k}$

$\vec{\tau} = (0\hat{i} + 2\hat{j} - \hat{k})(4\hat{i} + 5\hat{j} - 6\hat{k})$

$\vec{\tau} = \begin{vmatrix} \hat{i} & \hat{j} & \hat{k} \\ 0 & 2 & -1 \\ 4 & 5 & -6 \end{vmatrix} = -7\hat{i} - 4\hat{j} - 8\hat{k}$

19. (a) Velocity of swimmer w.r.t. river $V_{SR} = 20$ m/s
Velocity of river w.r.t. ground $V_{RG} = 10$ m/s

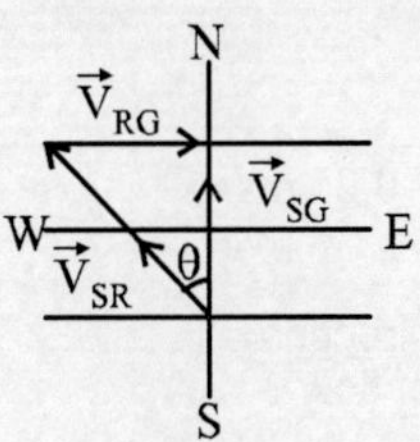

$\vec{V}_{SG} = \vec{V}_{SR} + \vec{V}_{RG}$

$\sin\theta = \left|\frac{\vec{V}_{RG}}{\vec{V}_{SR}}\right| \Rightarrow \sin\theta = \frac{10}{20}$

$\Rightarrow \sin\theta = \frac{1}{2} \quad \therefore \theta = 30°$ west

i.e.,to cross the river along the shortest path, swimmer should make his strokes 30° west.

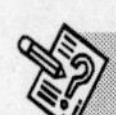

Exercise 3 - Concept Application Problems 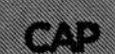

1. (c) $\cos\theta = \frac{R^2 - A^2 - B^2}{2AB} = \frac{R^2 - R^2}{2AB} = 0$

$\therefore \theta = \pi/2$

2. (b) If there is no resistance, bomb will drop at a place exactly below the flying aeroplane. But when we take into account air resistance, bomb will face deceleration in its velocity. So, it will fall on the earth exactly behind the aeroplane.
3. (c) Since horizontal component of the velocity of the bomb will be the same as the velocity of the aeroplane, therefore horizontal displacements remain the same at any instant of time.
4. (a) $\frac{1}{2}m(u\cos\theta)^2 = \frac{3}{4}\times\frac{1}{2}mu^2$

or $\cos^2\theta = \frac{3}{4}$ or $\cos\theta = \frac{\sqrt{3}}{2} = \cos 30°$.

5. (b) Time taken for vertical direction motion

$t = \sqrt{\frac{2h}{g}} = \sqrt{\frac{2\times 490}{9.8}} = \sqrt{100} = 10\,s$

The same time is for horizontal direction.

$\therefore x = vt = \left(60\times\frac{5}{18}\right)\times 10 = \frac{500}{3}$ m

6. (d) The horizontal velocity of the projectile remains constant throughout the journey.
Since the body is projected horizontally, the initial velocity will be same as the horizontal velocity at any point.

Since, $x = 2t$, $\frac{dx}{dt} = 2$

$\therefore$ Horizontal velocity = 2 m/s
$\therefore$ Initial velocity = 2 m/s

7. (b) Vector product of parallel vectors is zero.
8. (c) Let its angular velocity be ω at all points (uniform motion). At the highest point weight of the body is balanced by centrifugal force, so

$$m\omega^2 r = mg \Rightarrow \omega = \sqrt{\frac{g}{r}}$$

$$T = \frac{2\pi}{\omega} = 2\pi\sqrt{\frac{r}{g}} = 2\pi\sqrt{\frac{2}{10}} = \frac{2\pi}{\sqrt{5}}$$

$$= \frac{2\times 3.14}{2.1} = 3 \text{ sec}.$$

9. (d) $R^2 = P^2 + Q^2 - PQ\cos\theta$
$(40)^2 = (10)^2 + (20)^2 - 2\times 10\times 20\times\cos\theta$
$400\cos\theta = 500 - 1600 = -1100$

$\cos\theta = -\frac{1100}{400} = -\frac{11}{4}$ which is not possible.

In this way, the set of forces given in option (d) can not be represented both in magnitude and direction by the sides of a triangle taken in the same order. Thus their resultant can not be zero.

10. (a) See fig. Clearly **A** is the resultant of **B** and **C**. Further **B** is perpendicular to **C**

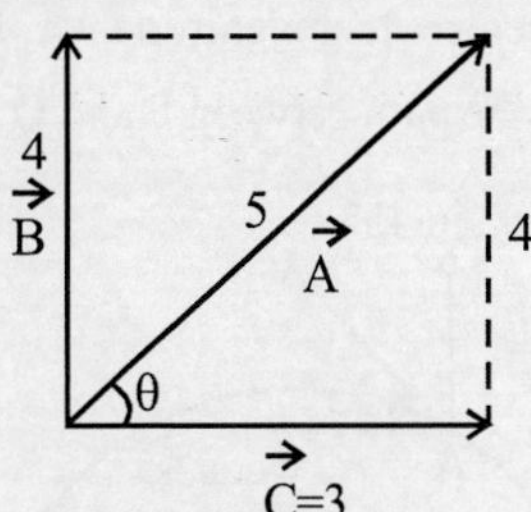

$\cos\theta = 3/5$ or $\theta = \cos^{-1}(3/5)$

11. (b)
12. (c)
13. (b) There is no change in horizontal velocity, hence no change in momentum in horizontal direction. The vertical velocity at t = 10sec is

$v = 98\times\sin 60° - (9.8)\times 10 = -13.13$ m/sec

so change in momentum in vertical direction is

$= (0.5\times 98\times\sqrt{3}/2) - [-(0.5\times 13.13)]$
$= 42.434 + 6.56 = 48.997 \approx 49$

14. (b)
15. (b) Comparing the given equation with

$y = x\tan\theta - \frac{gx^2}{2u^2\cos^2\theta}$, we get

$\tan\theta = \sqrt{3}$

16. (c) This happen when vertical velocity of both are same.

$\therefore \quad v_2 = v_1\sin 30°$ or $\frac{v_2}{v_1} = \frac{1}{2}$

17. (b)

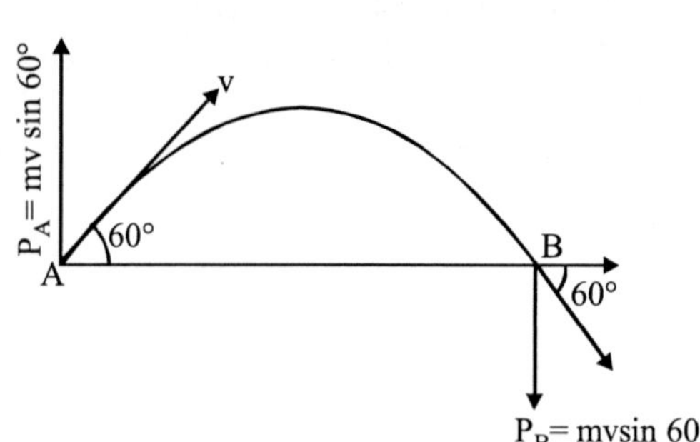

As the figure drawn above shows that at points A and B the vertical component of velocity is v sin 60° but their directions are opposite.

Hence, change in momentum is given by :

$\Delta p = mv\sin 60° - (-mv\sin 60°) = 2mv\sin 60°$

$= 2mv\dfrac{\sqrt{3}}{2} = \sqrt{3}mv$

18. (a) The motion of the train will affect only the horizontal component of the velocity of the ball. Since, vertical component is same for both observers, the y_m will be same, but R will be different.

19. (c) $a = \dfrac{v^2}{r} = 1$ cm/s. Centripetal acceleration is directed towards the centre. Its magnitude = 1. Unit vector at the mid point on the path between P and Q is $-(\hat{x}+\hat{y})/\sqrt{2}$.

20. (c)

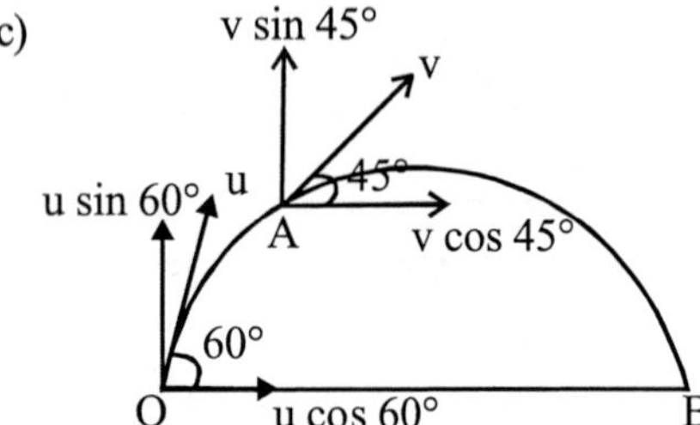

Velocity of projectile u = 147 ms^{-1}

angle of projection $\alpha = 60°$

Let, the time taken by the projectile from O to A be t where direction $\beta = 45°$. As horizontal component of velocity remains constant during the projectile motion.

$\Rightarrow v\cos 45° = u\cos 60°$

$\Rightarrow v \times \dfrac{1}{\sqrt{2}} = 147 \times \dfrac{1}{2} \Rightarrow v = \dfrac{147}{\sqrt{2}} ms^{-1}$

For Vertical motion, $v_y = u_y - gt$

$\Rightarrow v\sin 45° = 45\sin 60° - 9.8\,t$

$\Rightarrow \dfrac{147}{\sqrt{2}} \times \dfrac{1}{\sqrt{2}} = 147 \times \dfrac{\sqrt{3}}{2} - 9.8\,t$

$\Rightarrow 9.8\,t = \dfrac{147}{2}(\sqrt{3}-1) \Rightarrow t = 5.49\,s$

21. (d) When a cyclist moves on a circular path, it experiences a centrifugal force which is equal to mv^2/r. It tries to overturn the cyclist in outward direction. If speed increases twice, the value of centrifugal force too increases to 4 times its earlier value. Therefore the chance of overturning is 1/4 times.

22. (c) Here v = 0.5 m/sec. u = ?

so $\sin\theta = \dfrac{u}{v} \Rightarrow \dfrac{u}{.5} = \dfrac{1}{2}$ or $u = 0.25\ ms^{-1}$

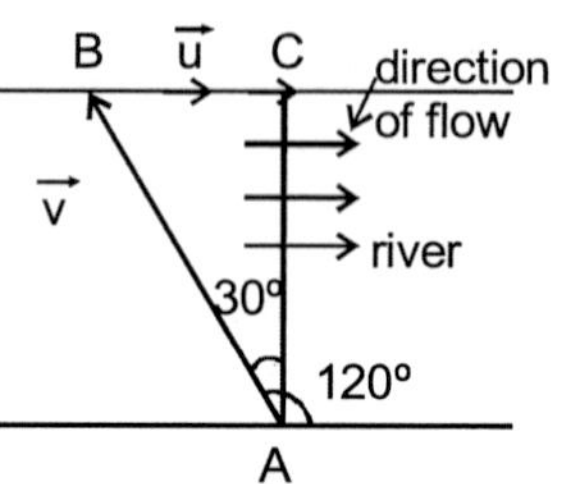

23. (d) $\vec{r} = (a\cos\omega t)\hat{i} + (a\sin\omega t)\hat{j}$

$\vec{v} = \dfrac{\vec{d}(r)}{dt} = \dfrac{d}{dt}\{(a\cos\omega t)\hat{i} + (a\sin\omega t)\hat{j}\}$

$= (-a\omega\sin\omega t)\hat{i} + (a\omega\cos\omega t)\hat{j}$

$= \omega[(-a\sin\omega t)\hat{i} + (a\cos\omega t)\hat{j}]$

$\vec{r}.\vec{v} = 0$

$\therefore$ velocity is perpendicular to the displacement.

24. (b) Since $E = \dfrac{1}{2}mv^2 \Rightarrow v = \sqrt{\dfrac{2E}{m}}$

Now at highest point of flight, the vertical component of velocity is zero & only horizontal component is non zero.

So K.E. at highest point is $E' = \dfrac{1}{2}m(v\cos 45°)^2 = E/2$

25. (b) Given, $u_1 = u_2 = u$, $\theta_1 = 60°$, $\theta_2 = 30°$

In Ist case, we know that range

$R_1 = \dfrac{u^2\sin 2(60°)}{g} = \dfrac{u^2\sin 120°}{g} = \dfrac{u^2\sin(90°+30°)}{g}$

$= \dfrac{u^2(\cos 30°)}{g} = \dfrac{\sqrt{3}u^2}{2g}$

In IInd case when $\theta_2 = 30°$, then

$R_2 = \dfrac{u^2\sin 60°}{g} = \dfrac{u^2\sqrt{3}}{2g} \Rightarrow R_1 = R_2$

(we get same value of ranges).

26. (a) $F = 6t\hat{i} + 4t\hat{j}$ or $a_x = \dfrac{6t}{3}, a_y = \dfrac{4t}{3}$

so $u_x = \int_0^t a_x dt = t^2 \Rightarrow (u_x)_{t=3} = 9$m/sec

and $u_y = \int_0^t a_y dt = \dfrac{2t^2}{3} \Rightarrow (u_y)_{t=3} = 6m/sec$

(because u_x & $u_y = 0$ at t = 0 sec)

27. (b) $s = \dfrac{1}{2}gt^2$, s and g are same for both the balls, so time of fall 't' will also be the same for both of them (s is vertical height)

28. (c) $\vec{P}$ = vector sum = $\vec{A}+\vec{B}$

$\vec{Q}$ = vector differences = $\vec{A}-\vec{B}$

Since $\vec{P}$ and $\vec{Q}$ are perpendicular

$\therefore \vec{P}.\vec{Q}=0$

$\Rightarrow (\vec{A}+\vec{B}).(\vec{A}-\vec{B})=0 \Rightarrow A^2=B^2 \Rightarrow |A|=|B|$

29. (b) $|\vec{A}\times\vec{B}|=AB\sin\theta$

$\vec{A}.\vec{B}=AB\cos\theta$

$|\vec{A}\times\vec{B}|=\sqrt{3}\ \vec{A}.\vec{B}$

$\Rightarrow AB\sin\theta=\sqrt{3}AB\cos\theta$ or $\tan\theta=\sqrt{3}$

$\therefore \theta=60^\circ$

$\therefore|\vec{A}+\vec{B}|=\sqrt{A^2+B^2+2AB\cos 60^\circ}$

$=\sqrt{A^2+B^2+AB}$

30. (b) For two vectors to be perpendicular to each other

$\vec{A}\cdot\vec{B}=0$

$(2\hat{i}+3\hat{j}+8\hat{k})\cdot(4\hat{j}-4\hat{i}+\alpha\hat{k})=0$

$-8+12+8\alpha=0$ or $\alpha=-\frac{4}{8}=-\frac{1}{2}$

31. (a)

32. (a) If $\vec{C}=a\hat{i}+b\hat{j}$ then $\vec{A}.\vec{C}=\vec{A}.\vec{B}$

$a+b=1$ ..... (i)

$\vec{B}.\vec{C}=\vec{A}.\vec{B}$

$2a-b=1$ ..... (ii)

Solving equation (i) and (ii) we get

$a=\frac{1}{3}, b=\frac{2}{3}$

$\therefore$ Magnitude of coplanar vector, $|\vec{C}|=\sqrt{\frac{1}{9}+\frac{4}{9}}=\sqrt{\frac{5}{9}}$

33. (a) Arc length = radius × angle

So, $|\vec{B}-\vec{A}|=|\vec{A}|\Delta\theta$

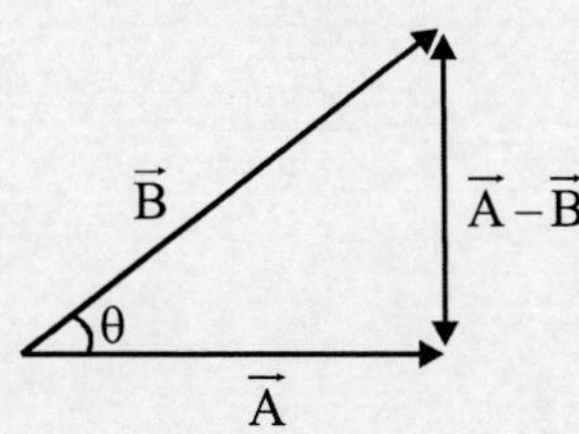

34. (b) As $\vec{S}=\vec{u}t+\frac{1}{2}\vec{a}t^2$

$\vec{S}=(5\hat{i}+4\hat{j})2+\frac{1}{2}(4\hat{i}+4\hat{j})4$

$=10\hat{i}+8\hat{j}+8\hat{i}+8\hat{j}$

$\vec{r}_f-\vec{r}_i=18\hat{i}+16\hat{j}$

[as $\vec{s}$ = change in position = $\vec{r}_f-\vec{r}_i$]

$\vec{r}_f=20\hat{i}+20\hat{j}$

$|\vec{r}_f|=20\sqrt{2}$

35. (c) Given, $y=2x-9x^2$

On comparing with,

$y=x\tan\theta-\frac{gx^2}{2u^2\cos^2\theta}$,

We have,

$\tan\theta=2$ or $\cos\theta=\frac{1}{\sqrt{5}}$

and $\frac{g}{2u^2\cos^2\theta}=9$ or $\frac{10}{2u^2(1/\sqrt{5})^2}=9$

$\therefore\quad u=5/3$ m/s

36. (b)

37. (a) As we know, range $R=\frac{u^2\sin 2\theta}{g}$

and, area $A=\pi R^2$

$\therefore A\propto R^2$ or, $A\propto u^4$

$\therefore \frac{A_1}{A_2}=\frac{u_1^4}{u_2^4}=\left[\frac{1}{2}\right]^4=\frac{1}{16}$

38. (d) R will be same for θ and $90^\circ-\theta$.

Time of flights:

$t_1=\frac{2u\sin\theta}{g}$ and

$t_2=\frac{2u\sin(90^\circ-\theta)}{g}=\frac{2u\cos\theta}{g}$

Now, $t_1t_2=\left(\frac{2u\sin\theta}{g}\right)\left(\frac{2u\cos\theta}{g}\right)$

$=\frac{2}{g}\left(\frac{u^2\sin 2\theta}{g}\right)=\frac{2R}{g}$

39. (a) On an inclined plane, time of flight (T) is given by

$T=\frac{2u\sin\theta}{g\cos\alpha}$

Substituting the values, we get

$T=\frac{(2)(2\sin 15^\circ)}{g\cos 30^\circ}=\frac{4\sin 15^\circ}{10\cos 30^\circ}$

Distance, $S=(2\cos 15^\circ)T-\frac{1}{2}g\sin 30^\circ(T)^2$

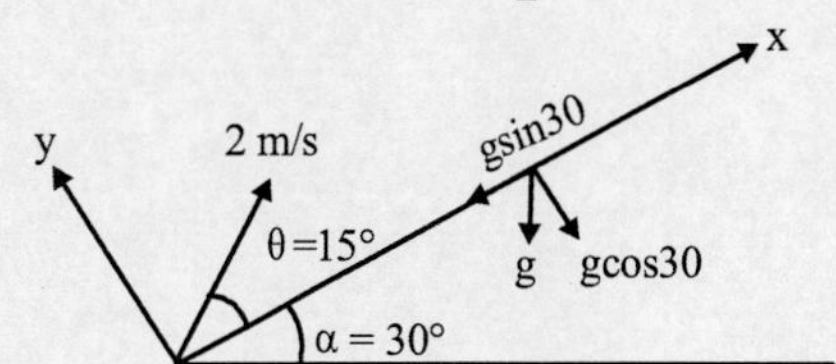

$$= (2\cos 15°)\frac{4}{10}\frac{\sin 15°}{10\cos 30°} - \left(\frac{1}{2}\times 10\sin 30°\right)\frac{16\sin^2 15°}{100\cos^2 30°}$$

$$= \frac{16\sqrt{3}-16}{60} \simeq 0.1952\text{m} \simeq 20\text{cm}$$

40. (b)

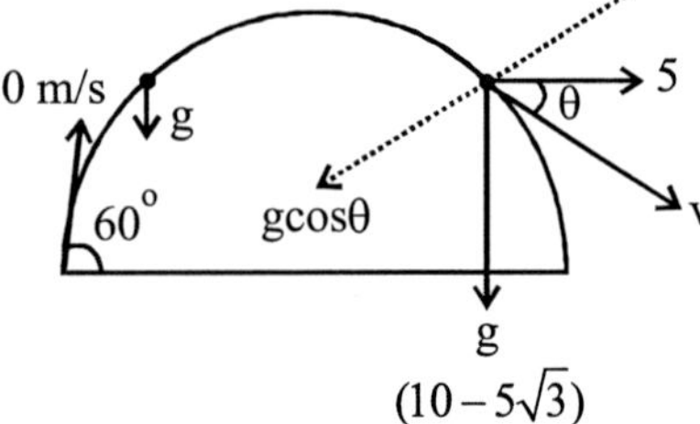

$(10-5\sqrt{3})$

Horizontal component of velocity

$v_x = 10\cos 60° = 5$ m/s

vertical component of velocity

$v_y = 10\cos 30° = 5\sqrt{3}$ m/s

After t = 1 sec.

Horizontal component of velocity $v_x = 5$ m/s

Vertical component of velocity

$v_y = |(5\sqrt{3}-10)|\ \text{m/s} = 10-5\sqrt{3}$

Centripetal, acceleration $a_n = \frac{v^2}{R}$

$$\Rightarrow R = \frac{v_x^2+v_y^2}{a_n} = \frac{25+100+75-100\sqrt{3}}{10\cos\theta} \quad ...(i)$$

From figure (using (i))

$$\tan\theta = \frac{10-5\sqrt{3}}{5} = 2-\sqrt{3} \Rightarrow \theta = 15°$$

$$R = \frac{100(2-\sqrt{3})}{10\cos 15} = 2.8\text{m}$$

41. (d) $v = k(yi+xj)$

$v = kyi + kxj$

$$\frac{dx}{dt} = ky,\ \frac{dy}{dt} = kx \text{ and } \frac{dy}{dx} = \frac{dy}{dt}\times\frac{dt}{dx}$$

$$\frac{dy}{dx} = \frac{kx}{ky}$$

$ydy = xdx$ ...(i)

Integrating equation (i)

$$\int ydy = \int x\cdot dx$$

$y^2 = x^2 + c$

42. (a) Given $\vec{u} = 3\hat{i}+4\hat{j},\ \vec{a} = 0.4\hat{i}+0.3\hat{j}, t=10$s

From 1st equatoin of motion.

$$a = \frac{v-u}{t}$$

$\therefore v = at\ tu$

$\Rightarrow v = (0.4\hat{i}+0.3\hat{j})\times 10 + (3\hat{i}+4\hat{j})$

$\Rightarrow\ 4\hat{i}+3\hat{j}+3\hat{j}+4\hat{j}$

$\Rightarrow\ v = 7\hat{i}+7\hat{j}$

$\Rightarrow\ |\vec{v}| = \sqrt{7^2+7^2} = 7\sqrt{2}$ unit.

43. (c) $\vec{A}\times\vec{B} - \vec{B}\times\vec{A} = 0 \Rightarrow \vec{A}\times\vec{B} + \vec{A}\times\vec{B} = 0$

$\therefore \vec{A}\times\vec{B} = 0$

Angle between them is 0, π, or 2 π

from the given options, $\theta = \pi$

44. (c) Speed, V = constant (from question)

Centripetal acceleration,

$$a = \frac{V^2}{r}$$

ra = constant

Hence graph (c) correctly describes relation between acceleration and radius.

45. (a) Using principal of conservation of linear momentum for horizontal motion, we have

$2mv_x = mu + mu\cos 60°$

$$v_x = \frac{3u}{4}$$

For vertical motion

$$h = 0 + \frac{1}{2}gT^2 \Rightarrow T = \sqrt{\frac{2h}{g}}$$

Let R is the horizontal distance travelled by the body.

$$R = v_x T + \frac{1}{2}(0)(T)^2 \text{ (For horizontal motion)}$$

$$R = v_x T = \frac{3u}{4}\times\sqrt{\frac{2h}{g}} \Rightarrow R = \frac{3\sqrt{3}u^2}{8g}$$

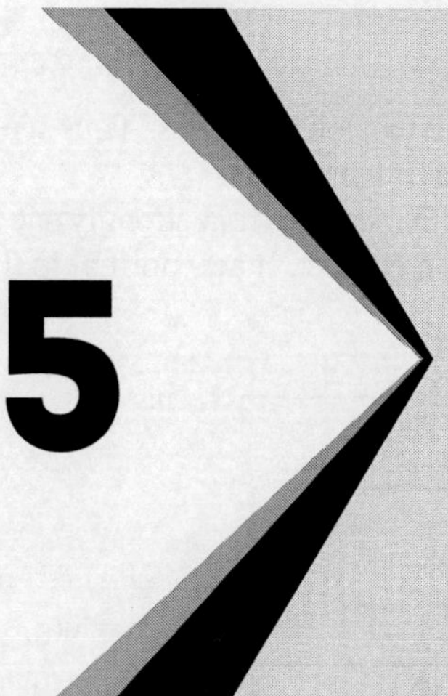

5 Laws of Motion

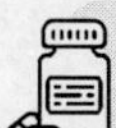

Topic 5.1 : Newton's Laws of Motion, Equilibrium of a Particle, Constraint Motion, Free Body Diagram, Law of Conservation of Momentum and Impulse

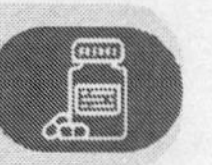

ARISTOTLE'S FALLACY

According to Aristotelian law an external force is required to keep a body in motion. However an external force is required to overcome the frictional forces in case of solids and viscous forces in fluids which are always present in nature.

LINEAR MOMENTUM (p)

Linear momentum of a body is the quantity of motion contained in the body. Momentum $\vec{p} = m\vec{v}$

It is a vector quantity having the same direction as the direction of the velocity. Its **SI unit** is kg ms^{-1}.

NEWTON'S LAWS OF MOTION

First law : *A body continues to be in a state of rest or of uniform motion, unless it is acted upon by some external force to change its state.*

Newton's first law gives the qualitative definition of force according to which *force is that external cause which tends to change or actually changes the state of rest or motion of a body*.

Newton's first law of motion is the same as **law of inertia** given by Galileo.

Inertia *is the inherent property of all bodies because of which they cannot change their state of rest or of uniform motion unless acted upon by an external force.*

Second law : *The rate of change of momentum of a body is directly proportional to the external force applied on it and the change takes place in the direction of force applied.*

$$i.e., \quad \vec{F} = \frac{d\vec{p}}{dt} = \frac{md\vec{v}}{dt} = m\vec{a}$$

This is the equation of motion of constant mass system. For variable mass system such as rocket propulsion

$$\vec{F} = \frac{d(m\vec{v})}{dt}$$

$$\text{And,} \quad \vec{F} = \frac{m(d\vec{v})}{dt} + \vec{v}\frac{dm}{dt}$$

The **SI unit** of force is newton. (One newton force is that much force which produces an acceleration of 1ms^{-2} in a body of mass 1 kg.

The **CGS unit** of force is dyne. (1N = 10^5 dyne)

The gravitational unit of force is kg-wt (kg-f) or g-wt (g-f)

$$1\ kg\text{-}wt\ (kg\text{-}f) = 9.8\ N, \qquad 1\ g\text{-}wt\ (g\text{-}f) = 980 dyne$$

Third law : *To every action there is an equal and opposite reaction.* For example – walking, swimming, a horse pulling a cart etc.

$$\vec{F}_{AB} = -\vec{F}_{BA}$$

Action and reaction act on different bodies and hence cannot balance each other. Action and reaction occur simultaneously. Forces always occur in pairs.

EQUILIBRIUM OF A PARTICLE

A body is said to be in equilibrium when no net force acts on the body.

$$i.e., \ \Sigma\vec{F} = 0$$

Then $\quad \Sigma F_x = 0, \ \Sigma F_y = 0$ and $\Sigma F_z = 0$

Stable equilibrium : If a body is slightly displaced from equilbrium position, it has the tendency to regain its original position, it is said to be in stable equilibrium.

In this case, *P.E. is minimum.* $\left(\dfrac{d^2u}{dr^2} = +ve\right)$

So, the *centre of gravity is lowest.*

Unstable equilibrium : If a body, after being displaced from the equilibrium position, moves in the direction of displacement, it is said to be in unstable equilibrium.

In this case, *P.E. is maximum.* $\left(\dfrac{d^2u}{dr^2} = -ve\right)$

So, the *centre of gravity is highest.*

Neutral equilibrium : If a body, after being slightly displaced from the equilibrium position has no tendency to come back or to move in the direction of displacement the equilibrium is known to be neutral.

In this case, *P.E. is constant* $\left(\frac{d^2u}{dr^2} = constant\right)$

The *centre of gravity remains at constant height.*

COMMON FORCES IN MECHANICS

1. **Weight :** It is the force with which the earth attracts a body and is called force of gravity, For a body of mass m, where acceleration due to gravity is g, the weight

$$W = mg$$

2. **Tension :** The force exerted by the ends of a loaded/ stretched string (or chain) is called tension. The tension has a sense of pull at its ends.

Case 1

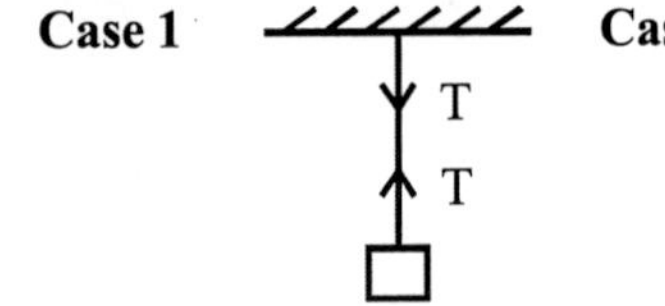

Case 2

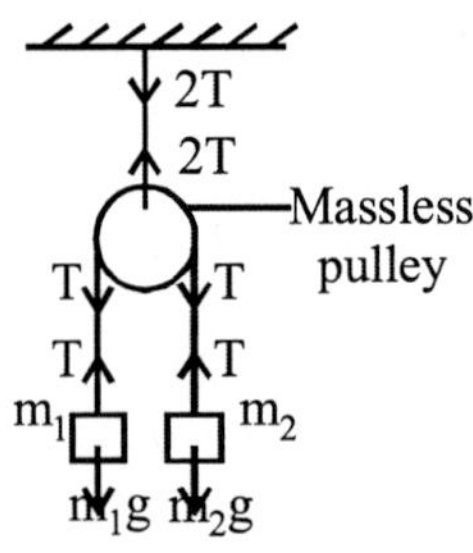

Case 3

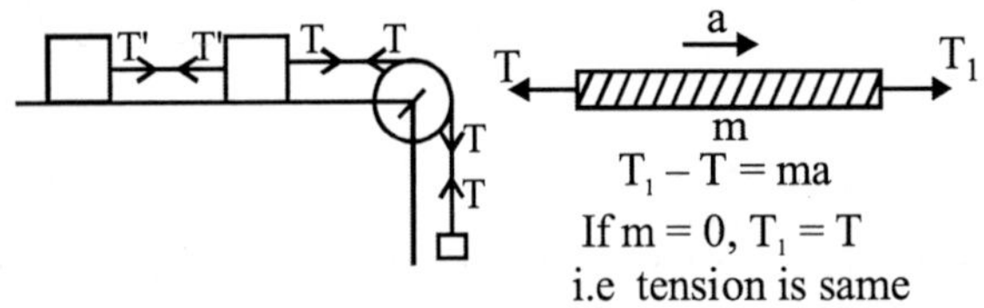

The tension in a string remains the same throughout the string if

(a) string is massless,

(b) pulley is massless or pulley is frictionless

Case 4 : String having mass

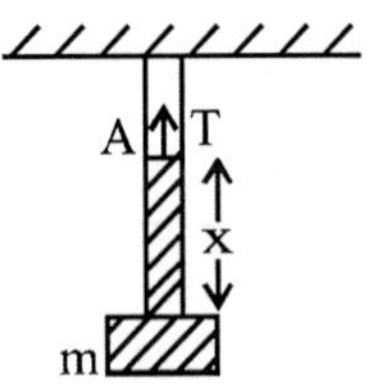

Let the total mass of the string be M and length be L. Then mass per unit length is $\frac{M}{L}$

Let x be the distance of the string from the mass m. Then the mass of the shaded portion of string is $\left(\frac{M}{L} \times x\right)$

If the string is at rest then the tension T has to balance the wt of shaded portion of string and weight of mass m.

$$\therefore T = \left(m + \frac{M}{L}x\right)g$$

$\Rightarrow$ as x increases, the tension increases. Thus tension is non-uniform in a string having mass.

3. **Normal force :** It measures how strongly one body presses the other body in contact. It acts normal to the surface of contact.

Case 1

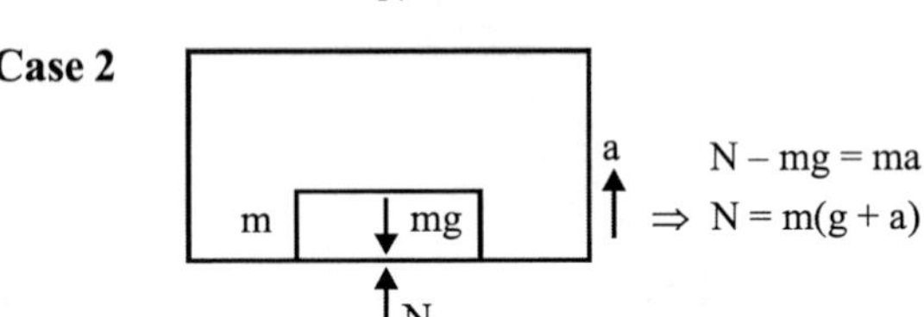

Case 2

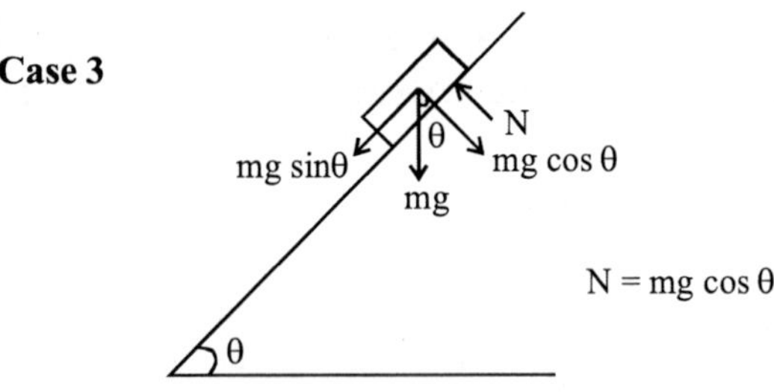

Case 3

4. **Spring force :** If an object is connected by spring and spring is stretched or compressed by a distance x, then restoring force on the object $F = -kx$

   where k is a spring contact on force constant.

5. **Frictional force :** It is a force which opposes relative motion between the surfaces in contact. $f = \mu N$

   This will be discussed in detail in later section.

6. **Pseudo force :** If a body of mass m is placed in a non-inertial frame having aceleration $\vec{a}$, then it experiences a Pseudo force acting in a direction opposite to the direction of $\vec{a}$.

$$\vec{F}_{pseudo} = -m\vec{a}$$

Negative sign shows that the pseudo force is always directed in a direction opposite to the direction of the acceleration of the frame.

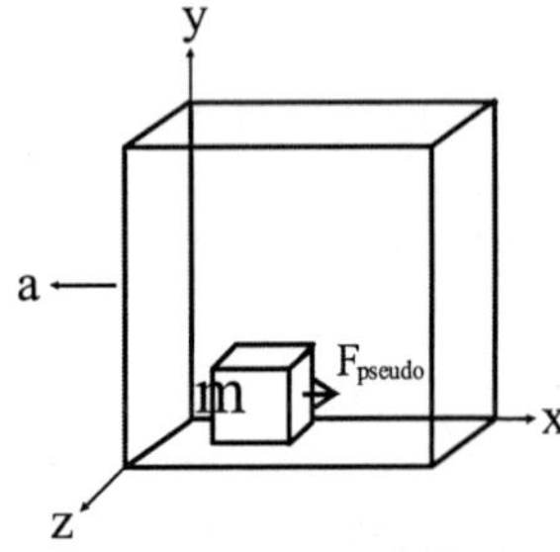

CONSTRAINT MOTION :

When the motion of one body is dependent on the other body, the relationship of displacements, velocities and accelerations of the two bodies are called constraint relationships.

Case 1 Pulley string system :

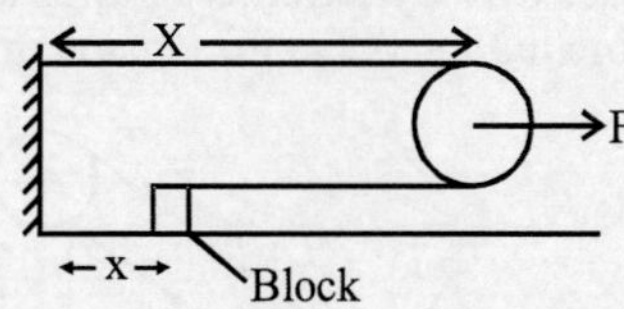

Step 1 : Find the distance of the two bodies from fixed points.

Step 2 : The length of the string remain constant. (We use of this condition)

Therefore $X + (X - x) = \text{constant} \Rightarrow 2X - x = \text{constant}$

$$\Rightarrow 2\frac{dX}{dt} - \frac{dx}{dt} = 0 \Rightarrow 2\frac{dX}{dt} = \frac{dx}{dt}$$

$$\Rightarrow 2V_p = v_B \left[\because \frac{dX}{dt} = V_p = \text{velocity of pulley}\right.$$

$$\left.\frac{dx}{dt} = v_B = \text{velocity of block}\right]$$

Again differentiating we get, $2a_p = a_B$

$$\left[a_p = \frac{dVp}{dt} \text{and } a_B = \frac{dv_B}{dt}\right]$$

a_p = acceleration of pulley, a_B = acceleration of block

Case 2 Here $\sqrt{h^2 + x^2} + y = \text{constt.}$ On differentiating w.r.t 't'

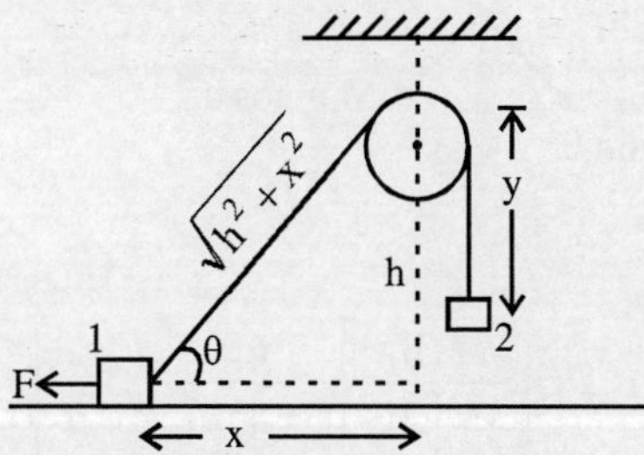

[Negative sign with dy/dt shows that with increase in time, y decreases]

$$\frac{1 \times 2x}{2\sqrt{h^2 + x^2}}\frac{dx}{dt} - \frac{dy}{dt} = 0 \Rightarrow \cos\theta\,(v_1 - v_2) = 0$$

$$\left[\because \cos\theta = \frac{x}{\sqrt{h^2 + x^2}}\right]$$

Case 3 Wedge block system : Thin lines represents the condition of wedge block at t = 0 and dotted lines at t = t

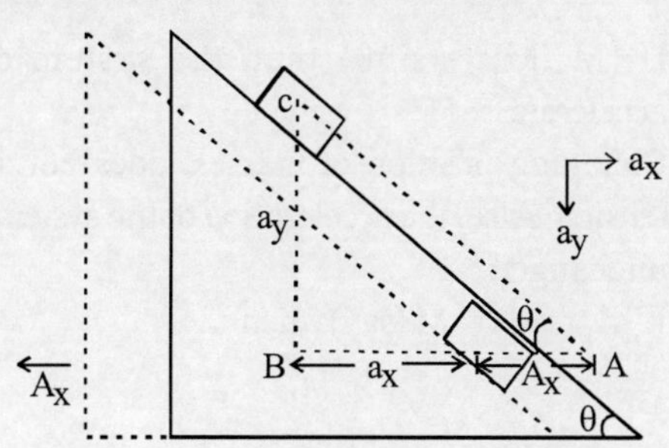

A_x = acceleration of wedge towards left

a_x, a_y = acceleration of block as shown

From ΔABC, $\tan\theta = \dfrac{a_y}{a_x + A_x}$

Frame of Reference :

Reference frames are co-ordinate systems in which an event is described.

There are two types of reference frames

(a) Inertial frame of reference: These are frames of reference in which Newton's laws hold good. These frames are at rest with each other or which are moving with uniform speed with respect to each other.
All reference frames present on surface of Earth are supposed to be inertial frame of reference.

(b) Non – inertial frame of reference: Newton's law do not hold good in non-inertial reference frame.
All accelerated and rotatory reference frames are non – inertial frame of reference. Earth is a non-intertial frame.

Note : When the observer is in non-inertial reference frame a pseudo force is applied on the body under observation.

FREE BODY DIAGRAM (FBD) :

Free body diagram of a mass is a separate diagram of that mass. All forces acting on the mass are sketched. A FBD is drawn to visualise the direct forces acting on a body.

Case 1 : Masses M_1 and M_2 are tied to a string, which goes over a frictionless pulley

(a) **If $M_2 > M_1$ and they move with acceleration a**

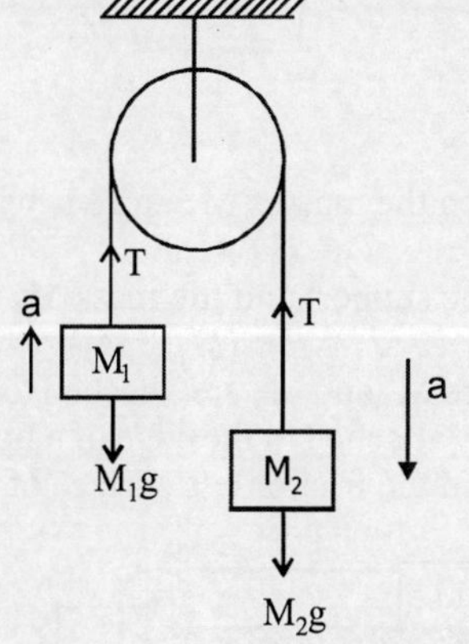

FBD of M_1, FBD of M_2

T, M_1, a, M_1g | T, M_2, a, M_2g

$T - M_1g = M_1a$ $\qquad$ $M_2g - T = M_2a$

where T is the tension in the string. It gives

$$a = \frac{M_2 - M_1}{M_1 + M_2}g \text{ and } T = \frac{2M_1M_2}{M_1 + M_2}g$$

(b) **If the pulley begins to move with acceleration f, downwards**

$$\vec{a} = \frac{M_2 - M_1}{M_1 + M_2}(\vec{g} - \vec{f}) \text{ and } \vec{T} = \frac{2M_1M_2}{M_1 + M_2}(\vec{g} - \vec{f})$$

Case 2 : Three masses M_1, M_2 and M_3 are connected with strings as shown in the figure and lie on a frictionless surface. They are pulled with a force F attached to M_1.

M_3 T_2 T_2 M_2 T_1 T_1 M_1 → F

The forces on M_2 and M_3 are as follows

$$T_1 = \frac{M_2 + M_3}{M_1 + M_2 + M_3}F \text{ and } T_2 = \frac{M_3}{M_1 + M_2 + M_3}F;$$

Acceleration of the system is $a = \dfrac{F}{M_1 + M_2 + M_3}$

Case 3 : Two blocks of masses M_1 and M_2 are suspended vertically from a rigid support with the help of strings as shown in the figure. The mass M_2 is pulled down with a force F.

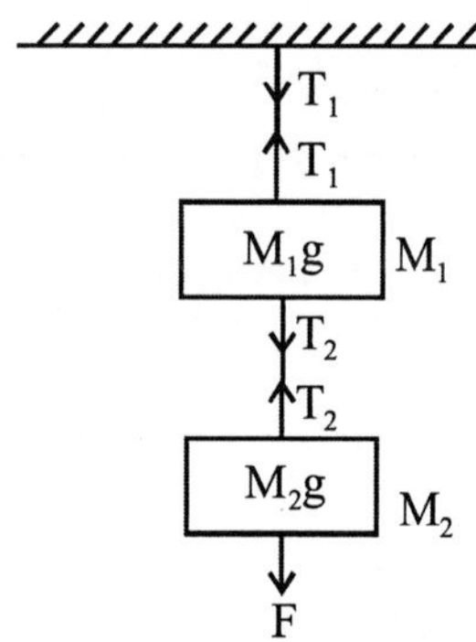

The tension between the masses M_1 and M_2 will be

$$T_2 = F + M_2g$$

Tension between the support and the mass M_1 will be

$$T_1 = F + (M_1 + M_2)g$$

Case 4 : Two masses M_1 and M_2 are attached to a string which passes over a pulley attached to the edge of a horizontal table. The mass M_1 lies on the frictionless surface of the table.

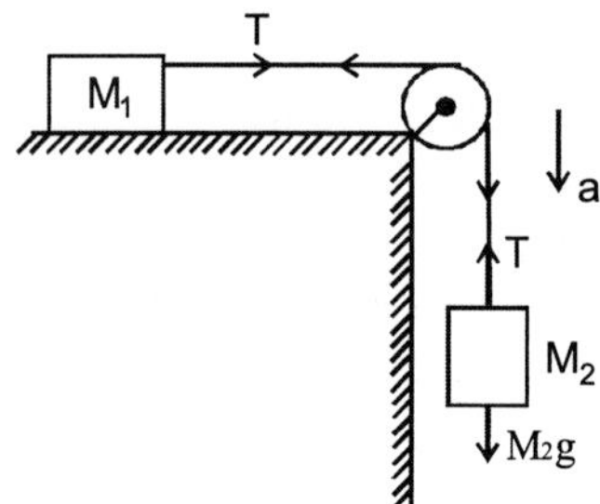

Let the tension in the string be T and the acceleration of the system be a. Then

$T = M_1a$ ...(1)

$M_2g - T = M_2a$ ...(2)

Adding eqns. (1) and (2), we get

$$a = \left[\frac{M_2}{M_1 + M_2}\right]g \text{ and } T = \left[\frac{M_1M_2}{M_1 + M_2}\right]g$$

Case 5 : Two masses M_1 and M_2 are attached to the ends of a string, which passes over a frictionless pulley at the top of the inclined plane of inclination θ. Let the tension in the string be T.

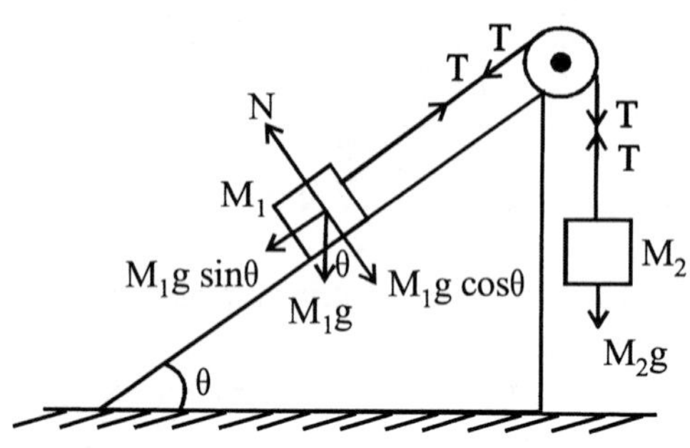

(i) **When the mass M_1 moves upwards with acceleration a.**

From the FBD of M_1 and M_2,

$T - M_1g \sin\theta = M_1a$ ...(1)

$M_2g - T = M_2a$ ...(2)

Solving eqns. (1) and (2) we get,

$$a = \left[\frac{M_2 - M_1 \sin\theta}{M_1 + M_2}\right]g$$

FBD of mass M_1

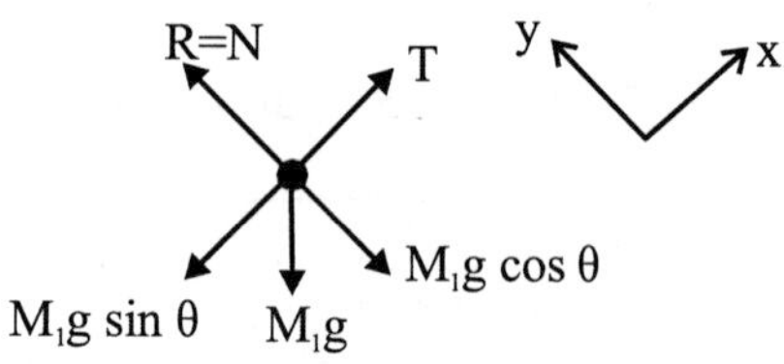

$$T = \left[\frac{M_2M_1}{M_1 + M_2}\right]\frac{g}{(1 + \sin\theta)}$$

FBD of M_2

T a M_2g

(ii) **When the mass M_1 moves downwards with acceleration a.**

Equation of motion for M_1 and M_2,

$M_1g \sin\theta - T = M_1a$ ...(1)

$T - M_2g = M_2a$ ...(2)

Solving eqns. (1) and (2) we get,

$$a = \left[\frac{M_1 \sin\theta - M_2}{M_1 + M_2}\right]g;\ T = \left[\frac{M_2M_1}{M_1 + M_2}\right]\frac{g}{(1 + \sin\theta)}$$

(a) If ($M_2/M_1 = \sin\theta$) then the system does not accelerate.

(b) Changing position of masses, does not affect the tension. Also, the acceleration of the system remains unchanged.

(c) If $M_1 = M_2 = M$ (say), then

$$a = \left(\cos\frac{\theta}{2} - \sin\frac{\theta}{2}\right)^2 \left(\frac{g}{2}\right);\ T = \left(\cos\frac{\theta}{2} + \sin\frac{\theta}{2}\right)^2 \left(\frac{Mg}{2}\right)$$

Case 6 : Two masses M_1 and M_2 are attached to the ends of a string over a pulley attached to the top of a double inclined plane of angle of inclination α and β.

Let M_2 move downwards with acceleration a and the tension in the string be T then

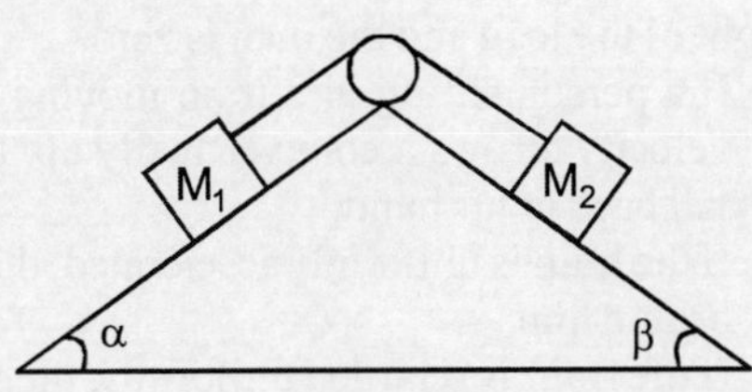

FBD of M_1

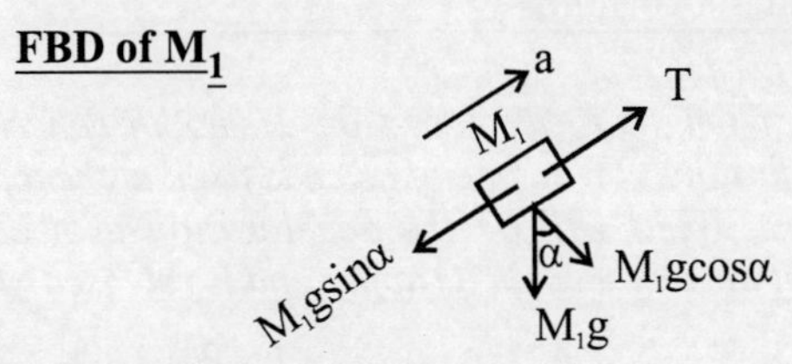

Equation of motion for M_1

$T - M_1g \sin\alpha = M_1a$

or $T = M_1g \sin\alpha + M_1a$ ...(1)

FBD of M_2

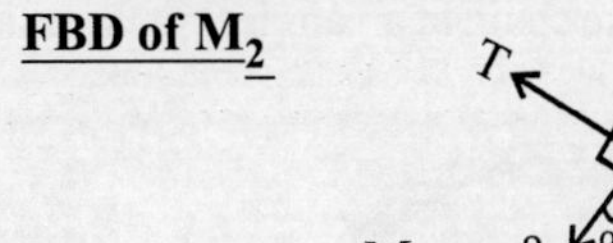

Equation of motion for M_2

$M_2g \sin\beta - T = M_2a$

or $T = M_2g \sin\beta - M_2a$ ...(2)

Using eqn. (1) and (2) we get,

$M_1g \sin\alpha + M_1a = M_2g \sin\beta - M_2a$

Solving we get,

$$a = \frac{(M_2 \sin\beta - M_1 \sin\alpha)g}{M_1 + M_2} \text{ and } T = \frac{M_1M_2g}{M_1 + M_2}[\sin\beta + \sin\alpha]$$

Case 7 : A person/monkey climbing a rope

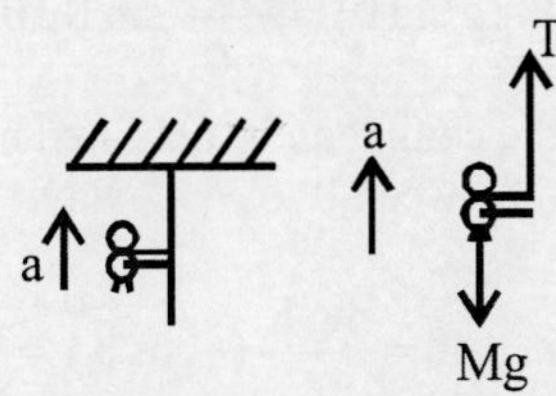

(a) A person of mass M climbs up a rope with acceleration a. The tension in the rope will be M(g+a).

$T - Mg = Ma \Rightarrow T = M(g + a)$

(b) If the person climbs down along the rope with acceleration a, the tension in the rope will be M(g–a).

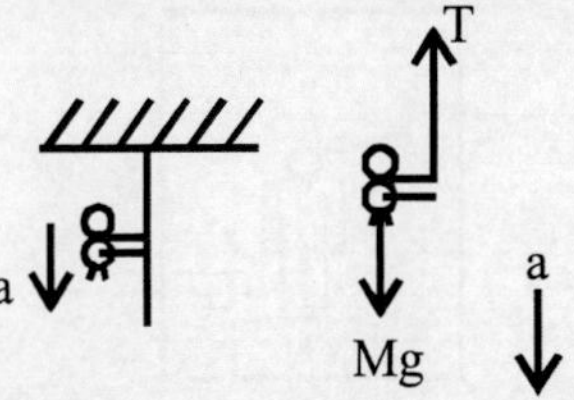

$Mg - T = Ma \Rightarrow T = M(g - a)$

(c) When the person climbs up or down with uniform speed, tension in the string will be Mg.

Case 8 : A body starting from rest moves along a smooth inclined plane of length *l*, height h and having angle of inclination θ.

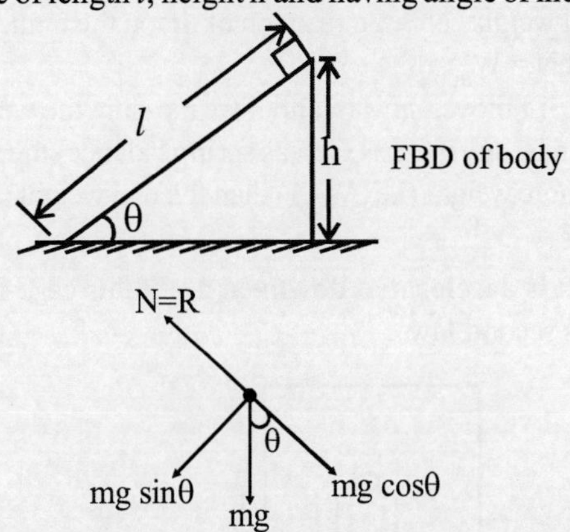

(where N=R is normal reaction applied by plane on the body of mass m)

For downward motion, along the inclined plane,

$mg \sin\theta = ma \Rightarrow a = g \sin\theta$

By work-energy theorem loss in P.E. = gain in K.E.

$$\Rightarrow mgh = \frac{1}{2}mv^2 \Rightarrow v = \sqrt{2gh}$$

Also, from the figure, $h = \ell \sin\theta$. $\therefore v = \sqrt{2gh} = \sqrt{2g\ell \sin\theta}$

(a) Acceleration down the plane is $g \sin\theta$.

(b) Its velocity at the bottom of the inclined plane will be $\sqrt{2gh} = \sqrt{2g\ell \sin\theta}$

(c) Time taken to reach the bottom will be

$$t = \left(\frac{2\ell}{g\sin\theta}\right)^{1/2} = \left(\frac{2h}{g\sin^2\theta}\right)^{1/2} = \frac{1}{\sin\theta\left(\frac{g}{2h}\right)^{1/2}} = \frac{1}{\sin\theta}\sqrt{\frac{2h}{g}}$$

(d) If angles of inclination are θ_1 and θ_2 for two inclined planes Keeping the length constant then $\frac{t_1}{t_2} = \left(\frac{\sin\theta_2}{\sin\theta_1}\right)^{1/2}$

Case 9 : Weight of a man in a lift :

(i) **When lift is accelerated upward :** In this case the man also moves in upward direction with an acceleration $\vec{a}$.

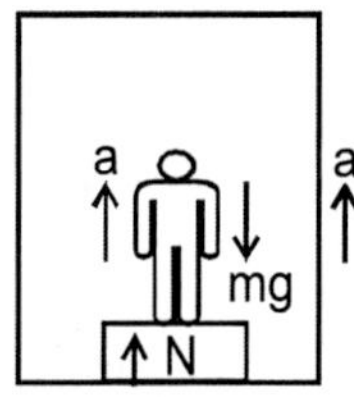

Then from Newton' second law

$N - mg = ma$ or $N = m(g + a)$

or $W_{app} = m(g + a) = W_o(1 + a/g)$ (as W = mg)

Where W_{app} is apparent weight of the man in the lift, W_o is the real weight, N is the reaction of lift on the man. It is clear that $N = W_{app}$

When the lift moves upward and if we measure the weight of the man by any means (such as spring balance) then we observe more weight (i.e., W_{app}) than the real weight (W_o)

$W_{app} > W_o$

(ii) **When lift is accelerated downward :** In this case from Newton's second law

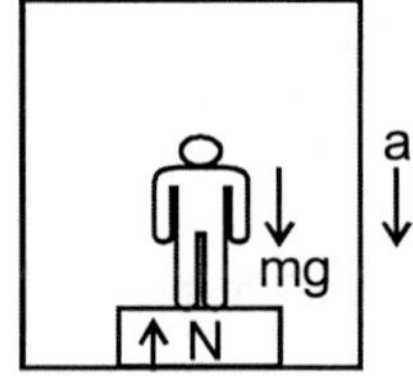

$mg - N = ma$

or $N = m(g - a) = W_0(1 - a/g)$

or $W'_{app} = W_0(1 - a/g)$ $\{\because W_o = mg\}$

If we measure the weight of man by spring balance, we observe deficiency because $W_{app} < W_0$.

(iii) **When lift is at rest or moving with constant velocity :** From Newton's second law $N - mg = 0$ or $N = mg$

In this case spring balance gives the true weight of the man.

Case 10 : Three masses M_1, M_2 and M_3 are placed on a smooth surface in contact with each other as shown in the figure. A force F pushes them as shown in the figure and the three masses move with acceleration a,

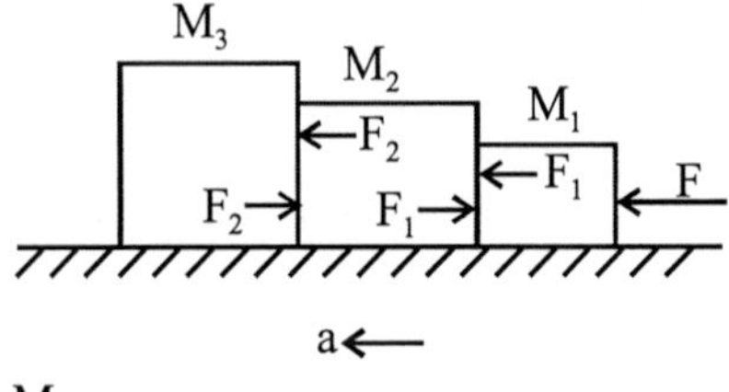

M_1: $F_1 \rightarrow \square \leftarrow F$ $\Rightarrow F - F_1 = m_1 a$ ...(i)

M_2: $F_2 \rightarrow \square \leftarrow F_1$ $\Rightarrow F_1 - F_2 = m_2 a$ ...(ii)

M_3: $\square \leftarrow F_2$ $\Rightarrow F_2 = M_3 a$ ...(iii)

Adding eqns. (i), (ii) and (iii) we get, $a = \dfrac{F}{M_1 + M_2 + M_3}$

$$\Rightarrow F_2 = \frac{M_3 F}{M_1 + M_2 + M_3} \text{ and } F_1 = \frac{(M_2 + M_3)F}{M_1 + M_2 + M_3}$$

Problem Solving Tips

1. When a man jumps with load on his head, the apparent weight of the load and the man is zero.
2. (i) If a person sitting in a train moving with uniform velocity throws a coin vertically up, then coin will fall back in his hand.
   (ii) If the train is uniformly accelerated, the coin will fall behind him.
   (iii) If the train is retarded uniformly, then the coin will fall in front of him.

Example 1.

A chain of length ℓ is placed on a smooth spherical surface of radius R with one of its ends fixed at the top of the sphere. What will be the acceleration a of each element of the chain when its upper end is released? It is assumed that the length of chain $\ell < \left(\pi \frac{R}{2}\right)$.

Solution :

Let m be the mass of the chain of length ℓ. Consider an element of length $d\ell$ of the chain at an angle θ with vertical,

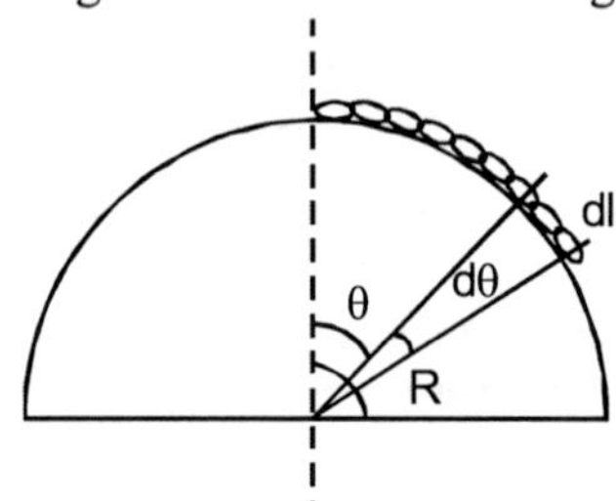

From figure, $d\ell = R\,d\theta$;

Mass of the element,

$$dm = \frac{m}{\ell} d\ell \text{ ; or } dm = \frac{m}{\ell}.R\,d\theta$$

Force responsible for acceleration, $dF = (dm)g \sin\theta$;

$$dF = \left(\frac{m}{\ell} R\,d\theta\right)(g \sin\theta) = \frac{mgR}{\ell} \sin\theta\,d\theta$$

Net force on the chain can be obtained by integrating the above relation between 0 to α, we have

$$F = \int_0^{\alpha} \frac{mg\,R}{\ell} \sin\theta\,d\theta = \frac{mg\,R}{\ell}(-\cos\theta)\Big|_0^{\alpha} = \frac{mg\,R}{\ell}[1 - \cos\alpha]$$

$$= \frac{mg\,R}{\ell}\left[1 - \cos\frac{\ell}{R}\right];$$

$$\therefore \text{ Acceleration, } a = \frac{F}{m} = \frac{gR}{\ell}\left(1 - \cos\frac{\ell}{R}\right).$$

Example 2.

A block slides down a smooth inclined plane to the ground when released at the top, in time t second. Another block is dropped vertically from the same point, in the absence of the inclined plane and reaches the ground in t/2 second. Then find the angle of inclination of the plane with the vertical.

Solution :

If θ is the angle which the inclined plane makes with the vertical direction, then the acceleration of the block sliding down the plane of length ℓ will be g cosθ.

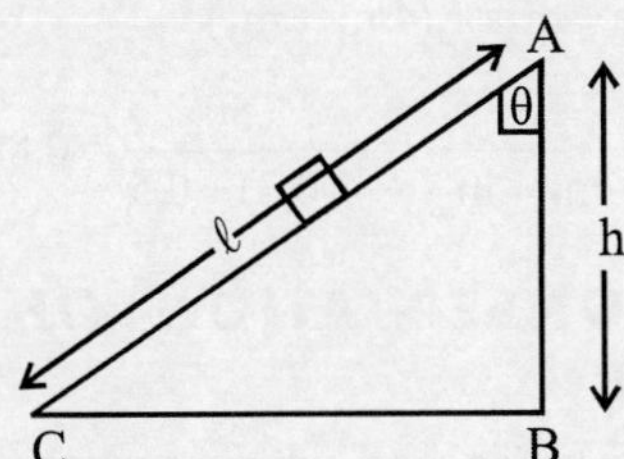

Using the formula, $s = ut + \frac{1}{2}at^2$, we have $s = \ell, u = 0, t =$ t and $a = g \cos\theta$.

so $\ell = 0 \times t + \frac{1}{2} g\cos\theta\, t^2 = \frac{1}{2}(g\cos\theta)t^2$ ...(i)

Taking vertical downward motion of the block, we get

$h = 0 + \frac{1}{2}g(t/2)^2 = \frac{1}{2}gt^2/4$ ...(ii)

Dividing eq^n. (ii) by (i), we get

$\frac{h}{\ell} = \frac{1}{4\cos\theta}$ $[\because \cos\theta = h/\ell]$

or $\cos\theta = \frac{1}{4\cos\theta}$; or $\cos^2\theta = \frac{1}{4}$; or $\cos\theta = \frac{1}{2}$

or θ = 60°

Example 3.

A large mass M and a small mass m hang at the two ends of a string that passes through a smooth tube as shown in fig. The mass m moves around a circular path in a horizontal plane. The length of the string from mass m to the top of the tube is l, and θ is the angle the string makes with the vertical. What should be the frequency (ν) of rotation of mass m so that mass M remains stationary?

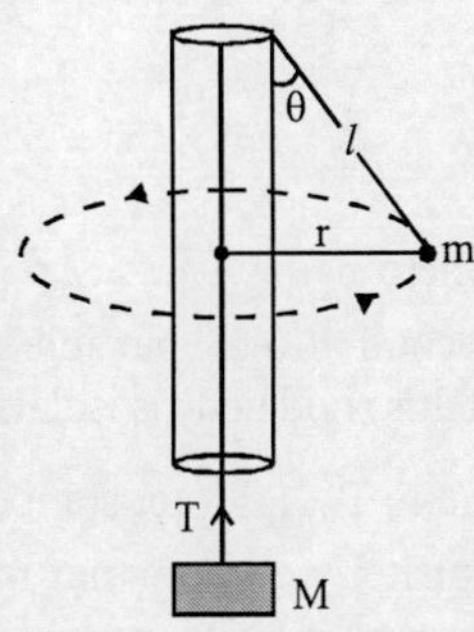

Solution :

Tension in the string T = Mg.

Centripetal force on the body = $mr\omega^2 = mr(2\pi\nu)^2$. This is provided by the component of tension acting horizontally i.e. T sinθ (= Mg sinθ).

$\therefore mr(2\pi\nu)^2 = Mg\sin\theta = Mgr/l$. or $\nu = \frac{1}{2\pi}\sqrt{\frac{Mg}{ml}}$

Example 4.

A string of negligible mass going over a clamped pulley of mass m supports a block of mass M as shown in fig. The force on the pulley by the clamp is given by

(a) $\sqrt{2}$ Mg

(b) $\sqrt{2}$ mg

(c) $[\sqrt{(M+m)^2 + m^2}]\, g$

(d) $[\sqrt{(M+m)^2 + M^2}]\, g$

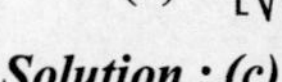

Solution : (c)

Force on the pulley by the clamp = resultant of T = (M + m)g and mg acting along horizontal and vertical respectively

$\therefore F = \sqrt{[(M+m)g]^2 + (mg)^2} = [\sqrt{(M+m)^2 + m^2}]g$

Example 5.

The masses of 10 kg and 20 kg respectively are connected by a massless spring in fig. A force of 200 newton acts on the 20 kg mass. At the instant shown, the 10 kg mass has acceleration 12 m/sec^2. What is the acceleration of 20 kg mass?

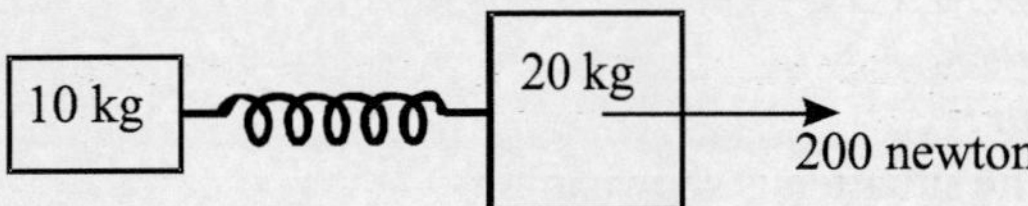

Solution :

Force on 10 kg mass = 10 × 12 = 120 N

The mass of 10 kg will pull the mass of 20 kg in the backward direction with a force of 120 N.

∴ Net force on mass 20 kg = 200 – 120 = 80 N

Its acceleration $a = \frac{\text{force}}{\text{mass}} = \frac{80\,N}{20\,kg} = 4\,m/s^2$

Example 6.

Two masses each equal to m are lying on X-axis at (–a, 0) and (+ a, 0) respectively as shown in fig. They are connected by a light string. A force F is applied at the origin and along the Y-axis. As a result, the masses move towards each other. What is the acceleration of each mass? Assume the instantaneous position of the masses as (– x, 0) and (x, 0) respectively

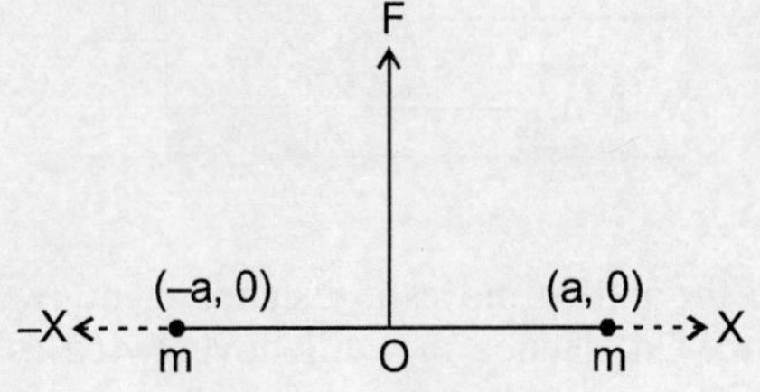

Solution :

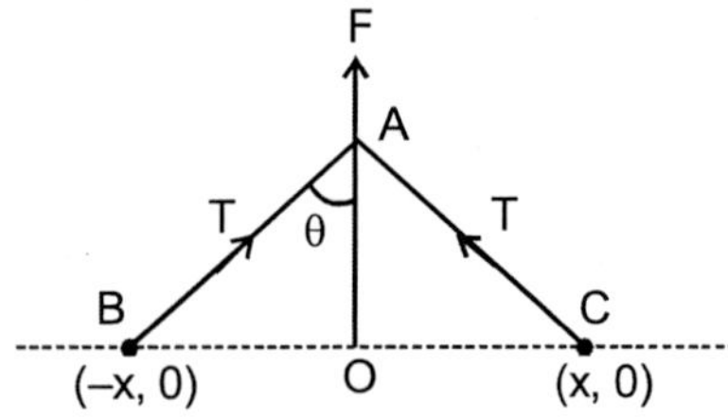

From figure $F = 2T\cos\theta$ or $T = F/(2\cos\theta)$

The force responsible for motion of masses on X-axis is T sin θ

$$\therefore ma = T\sin\theta = \frac{F}{2\cos\theta}\times\sin\theta$$

$$= \frac{F}{2}\tan\theta = \frac{F}{2}\times\frac{OB}{OA} = \frac{F}{2}\times\frac{x}{\sqrt{(a^2-x^2)}}$$

$$\text{so,} \quad a = \frac{F}{2m}\times\frac{x}{\sqrt{(a^2-x^2)}}$$

Example 7.

A block of mass M is pulled along horizontal frictionless surface by a rope of mass m. Force P is applied at one end of rope. Find the force which the rope exerts on the block.

Solution :

The situation is shown in fig

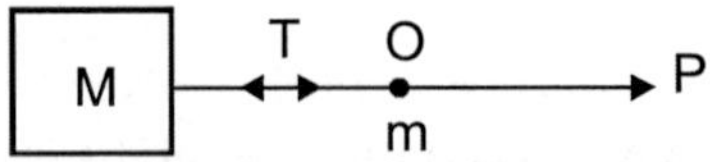

Let a be the common acceleration of the system. Here

$T = Ma$ for block

$P - T = ma$ for rope

$$\therefore P - Ma = ma \text{ or } P = a(M+m) \text{ or } a = \frac{P}{(M+m)}$$

$$\therefore T = \frac{MP}{(M+m)}$$

Example 8.

In the system shown below, friction and mass of the pulley are negligible. Find the acceleration of m_2 if $m_1 = 300$ g, $m_2 = 500$ g and $F = 1.50$ N

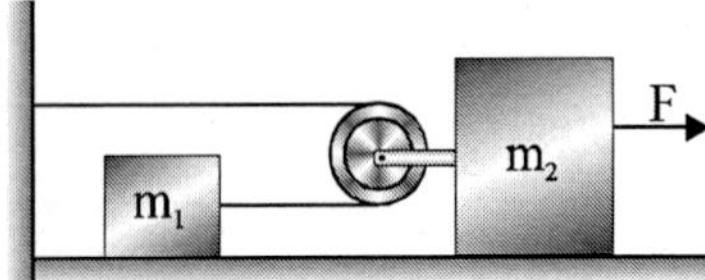

Solution :

When the pulley moves a distance d, m_1 will move a distance 2d. Hence m_1 will have twice as large an acceleration as m_2 has.

For mass m_1, $T_1 = m_1(2a)$ ...(1)

For mass m_2, $F - T_2 = m_2(a)$ ...(2)

Putting $T_1 = \frac{T_2}{2}$ in eq^n. (1) gives $T_2 = 4m_1a$

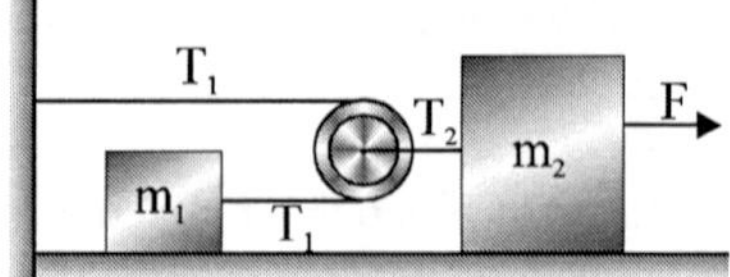

Substituting value of T_2 in equation (2),

$F = 4m_1a + m_2a = (4m_1 + m_2)a$

$$\text{Hence } a = \frac{F}{4m_1+m_2} = \frac{1.50}{4(0.3)+0.5} = 0.88 \text{ m/s}^2$$

LAW OF CONSERVATION OF LINEAR MOMENTUM

A system is said to be isolated, when no external force acts on it. For such isolated system, the linear momentum $(\vec{P} = m\vec{v})$ is constant i.e., conserved.

The linear momentum is defined as

$$\vec{P} = m\vec{v} \quad .....(1)$$

where $\vec{v}$ is the velocity of the body, whose mass is m. The direction of $\vec{P}$ is same as the direction of the velocity of the body. It is a vector quantity. From Newton's second law,

$$\vec{F}_{ext.} = \frac{d}{dt}(m\vec{v}) = \frac{d}{dt}\vec{P} \quad .....(2)$$

i.e., time rate of change in momentum of the body is equal to total external force applied on the body.

$$\text{If } \vec{F}_{ext.} = 0 \Rightarrow \frac{d}{dt}(\vec{P}) = 0 \quad \text{or } \vec{P} = \text{constant} \quad .....(3)$$

This is called **law of conservation of momentum.**

Now let us consider a rigid body consisting of a large number of particles moving with different velocities, then total linear momentum of the rigid body is equal to the summation of individual linear momentum of all particles

$$\text{i.e.,} \quad \sum_{i=1}^{n}\vec{p}_i = \vec{p}_1 + \vec{p}_2 + \vec{p}_3 + ...\vec{p}_n$$

$$\text{or} \quad \vec{P}_{total} = \sum_{i=1}^{n}\vec{p}_i = \vec{p}_1 + \vec{p}_2 + \vec{p}_3 + ... + \vec{p}_n$$

where $\vec{p}_1, \vec{p}_2 .... \vec{p}_n$ are individual linear momentum of first, second and n^{th} particle respectively.

If this rigid body is isolated i.e., no external force is applied on it, then $\vec{P}_{total}$ = constant (from Newton's second law).

Further we know that internal forces (such as intermolecular forces etc.) also act inside the body, but these can only change individual linear momentum of the particles (i.e., p_1, p_2.........), but their total momentum $\vec{P}_{total}$ remains constant.

Gun Firing a Bullet

If a gun of mass M fires a bullet of mass m with velocity v. Then from law of conservation of momentum, as initially bullet & gun are at rest position i.e., initial momentum is zero, so final momentum (gun + bullet) must also be zero.

Since on firing, the bullet moves with velocity $\vec{v}_b$ in forward direction, then from Newton's third law, the gun moves in backward direction $\vec{v}_g$. So,

Initial momentum = final momentum

$$0 = \underbrace{m\vec{v}_b}_{\text{Momentum of bullet}} + \underbrace{M\vec{V}_g}_{\text{Momentum of gun}} \quad \therefore \overrightarrow{V_g} = \frac{-m\overrightarrow{v_b}}{M}$$

(–ve sign shows that the vel. of gun will have the opposite direction to that of bullet)

IMPULSE

According to Newton's second law the rate of change of momentum of a particle is equal to the total external force applied on it (particle) i.e.,

$$\frac{d\vec{P}}{dt} = \vec{F}_{ext} \qquad ...(i)$$

$$\text{or } d\vec{P} = \vec{F}_{ext}.dt \text{ or } \Delta\vec{P} = \vec{P}_f - \vec{P}_i = \int_{t_i}^{t_f} \vec{F}_{ext}.dt \qquad ...(ii)$$

Where $\vec{P}_i$ is momentum of the particle at initial time t_i and when we apply some external force $\vec{F}_{ext}$ its final momentum is $\vec{P}_f$ at time t_f. The quantity $\vec{F}_{ext} \cdot dt$ on R.H.S in equation (ii) is called the **impulse.**

We can write equation (ii) as

$$I = \int_{t_i}^{t_f} \vec{F}_{ext} \cdot dt = \Delta\vec{P} \qquad ...(iii)$$

So, *the impulse of the force* $\vec{F}_{ext}$ *is equal to the change in momentum of the particle. It is known as* **impulse momentum theorem.**

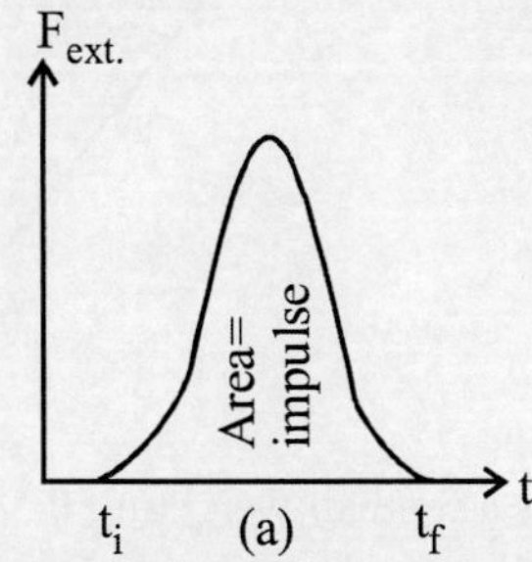

Force vary with time and impulse is area under force versus time curve

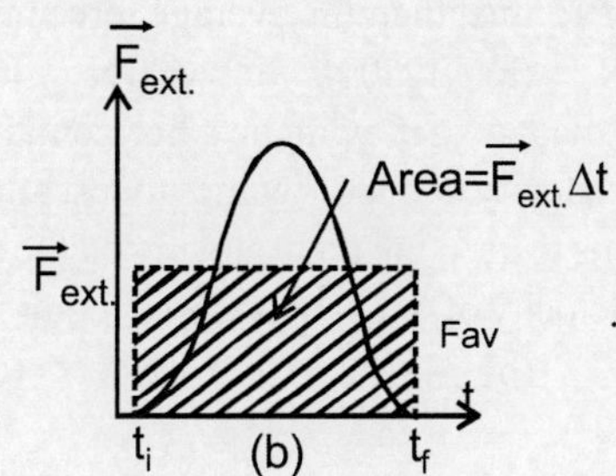

Force constant with time i.e., $\vec{F}_{ext.}$ *constant with time (shown by horizontal line) and it would give same impulse to particle* in time $\Delta t = t_f - t_i$ *as time varying force described.*

It is a vector quantity having a magnitude equal to the area under the force-time curve as shown in fig. (a). In this figure, it is assumed that force varies with time and is non-zero in time interval $\Delta t = t_f - t_i$. Fig.(b) shows the time averaged force $\vec{F}_{ext.}$ i.e., it is constant in time interval Δt, then equation (iii) can be written as

$$I = \vec{F}_{ext.}\int_{t_i}^{t_f} dt = \vec{F}_{ext.}(t_f - t_i) \qquad I = \vec{F}_{ext.}\Delta t \qquad ...(iv)$$

The direction of impulsive vector I is same as the direction of change in momentum. Impulse I has same dimensions as that of momentum i.e, $[MLT^{-1}]$

Rocket propulsion (A case of system of variable mass) : It is based on principle of conservation of linear momentum.

In rocket, the fuel burns and produces gases at high temperature. These gases are ejected out of the rocket from nozzle at the backside of rocket and the ejecting gas exerts a forward force on the rocket which accelerates it.

Let the gas ejects at a rate $r = -\frac{dM}{dt}$ and at constant velocity u w.r.t. rocket then from the conservation of linear momentum

$\frac{dv}{dt} = \frac{ru}{M} = \frac{ru}{M_0 - rt}$ where $M = M_0 - rt$ and M_0 is mass of rocket with fuel and solving this equation, we get

$v = u \log_e\left(\frac{M_0}{M_0 - rt}\right)$ where v = velocity of rocket w.r.t. ground.

Example 9.

Two skaters A and B approach each other at right angles. Skater A has a mass 30 kg and velocity 1 m/s and skater B has a mass 20 kg and velocity 2 m/s. They meet and cling together. Find the final velocity of the couple.

Solution :

Applying principle of conservation of linear momentum,

$$p = \sqrt{p_1^2 + p_2^2}; (m_1 + m_2)v = \sqrt{(m_1v_1)^2 + (m_2v_2)^2}$$

$$(30+20)v = \sqrt{(30\times1)^2 + (20\times2)^2} = 50$$

$$v = \frac{50}{50} = 1 \text{ m/s}$$

Example 10.

A hammer of mass M strikes a nail of mass m with velocity of u m/s and drives it 's' meters in to fixed block of wood. Find the average resistance of wood to the penetration of nail.

Solution :

Applying the law of conservation of momentum,

$$m\,u = (M+m)\,v_0 \Rightarrow v_0 = \left(\frac{M}{m+M}\right)u$$

There acceleration a can be obtained using the formula ($v^2 = u^2 + 2as$).

Here we have $0 - v_0^2 = 2as$ or $a = v_0^2/2s$

$$\therefore \quad a = \left(\frac{M}{m+M}\right)^2 \frac{u^2}{2s}$$

$$\text{Resistance} = (M+m)\,a = \left(\frac{M^2}{m+M}\right)\frac{u^2}{2s}$$

Example 11.

A ball of mass 0.5 kg is thrown towards a wall so that it strikes the wall normally with a speed of $10\ ms^{-1}$. If the ball bounces at right angles away from the wall with a speed of $8ms^{-1}$, what impulse does the wall exert on the ball ?

Solution :

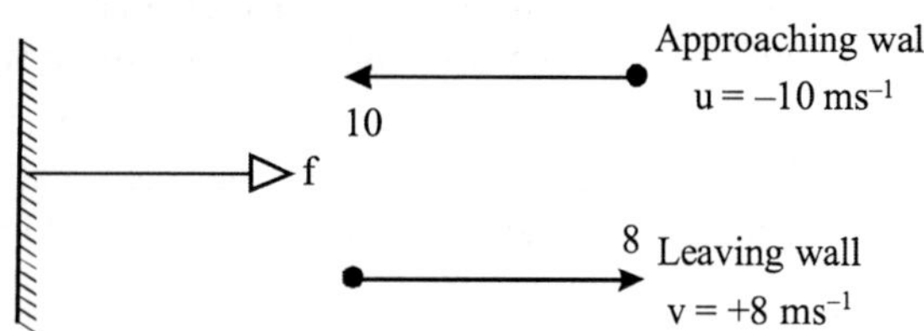

Taking the direction of the impulse J as positive and using

$$J = mv - mu$$

we have $J = \frac{1}{2} \times 8 - \frac{1}{2}(-10) = 9$ N-s

Therefore the wall exerts an impulse of 9 N-s on the ball.

Example 12.

Two particles, each of mass m, collide head on when their speeds are 2u and u. If they stick together on impact, find their combined speed in terms of u.

Solution :

Before impact m → 2u   u ← m

After impact 2m → v

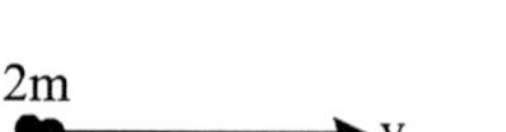

Using conservation of linear momentum (in the direction of the velocity 2u) we have

$$(m)(2u) - mu = 2m \times V \Rightarrow V = \frac{1}{2}u$$

The combined mass will travel at speed u/2.

(Note that the momentum of the second particle before impact is negative because its sense is opposite to that specified as positive.)

5.1 Concept Practice Problems

CPP

1. A particle of mass m is moving with velocity v_1, it is given an impulse such that the velocity becomes v_2. Then magnitude of impulse is equal to

   (a) $m(\vec{v}_2 - \vec{v}_1)$ (b) $m(\vec{v}_1 - \vec{v}_2)$

   (c) $m \times (\vec{v}_2 - \vec{v}_1)$ (d) $0.5m(\vec{v}_2 - \vec{v}_1)$

2. Two mass m and 2m are attached with each other by a rope passing over a frictionless and massless pulley. If the pulley is accelerated upwards with an acceleration 'a', what is the value of T?

   (a) $\frac{g+a}{3}$ (b) $\frac{g-a}{3}$

   (c) $\frac{4m(g+a)}{3}$ (d) $\frac{m(g-a)}{3}$

3. A rider on a horse back falls forward when the horse suddenly stops. This is due to

   (a) inertia of horse
   (b) inertia of rider
   (c) large weight of the horse
   (d) losing of the balance

4. A bird is in a wire cage which is hanging from a spring balance . In the first case, the bird sits in the cage and in the second case, the bird flies about inside the cage. The reading in the spring balance is

   (a) more in the first case
   (b) less in first case
   (c) unchanged
   (d) zero in second case.

5. An object of mass 10 kg moves at a constant speed of $10\ ms^{-1}$. A constant force, that acts for 4 sec on the object, gives it a speed of $2\ ms^{-1}$ in opposite direction. The force acting on the object is

   (a) –3 N (b) –30 N (c) 3 N (d) 30 N

6. A solid sphere of 2 kg is suspended from a horizontal beam by two supporting wires as shown in fig. Tension in each wire is approximately ($g = 10\ ms^{-2}$)

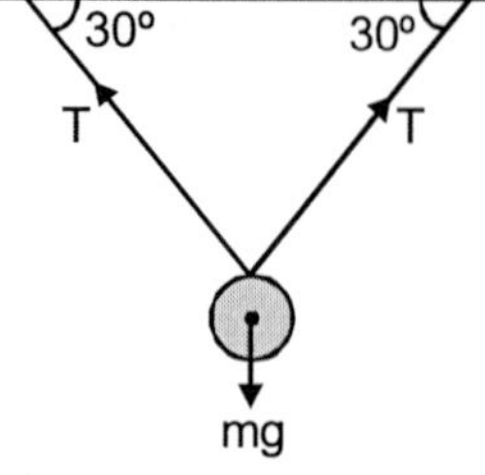

   (a) 30 N
   (b) 20 N
   (c) 10 N
   (d) 5 N

7. A player stops a football weighting 0.5 kg which comes flying towards him with a velocity of 10m/s. If the impact lasts for 1/50th sec. and the ball bounces back with a velocity of 15 m/s, then the average force involved is

   (a) 250 N (b) 1250 N (c) 500 N (d) 625 N

8. A body of mass 4 kg moving on a horizontal surface with an initial velocity of $6\ ms^{-1}$ comes to rest after 3 seconds. If one wants to keep the body moving on the same surface with the velocity of $6\ ms^{-1}$, the force required is

   (a) Zero (b) 4 N (c) 8 N (d) 16 N

9. The elevator shown in fig. is descending with an acceleration of 2 m/s^2. The mass of the block A = 0.5 kg. The force exerted by the block A on block B is

(a) 2N

(b) 4N

(c) 6N

(d) 8N

10. A rocket has a mass of 100 kg. Ninety percent of this is fuel. It ejects fuel vapors at the rate of 1 kg/sec with a velocity of 500 m/sec relative to the rocket. It is supposed that the rocket is outside the gravitational field. The initial upthrust on the rocket when it just starts moving upwards is

(a) zero (b) 500 newton

(c) 1000 newton (d) 2000 newton

ANSWER KEY																			
1	(a)	2	(c)	3	(b)	4	(a)	5	(b)	6	(b)	7	(d)	8	(c)	9	(b)	10	(b)

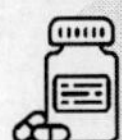

Topic 5.2 : Friction, Conservative & Non-Conservative Forces

FRICTION

When a body is in motion on a rough surface, or when an object moves through water (i.e., viscous medium), then velocity of the body decreases constantly even if no external force is applied on the body. This is due to **friction.**

So "*an opposing force which comes into existence, when two surfaces are in contact with each other and try to move relative to one another, is called friction*".

Frictional force acts along the common surface between the two bodies in such a direction so as to oppose the relative movement of the two bodies.

(a) The force of static friction f_s between book and rough surface is opposite to the applied external force $F_{ext.}$ The force of static friction $f_s = \vec{F}_{ext}$.

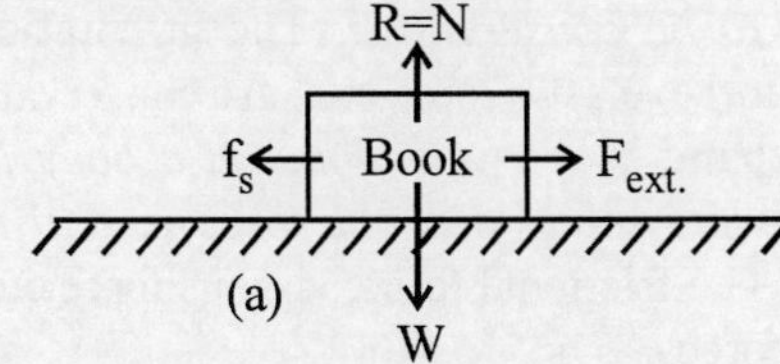

(a)

(b) When $\vec{F}_{ext}$. exceeds the certain maximum value of static friction, the book starts accelerating and during motion Kinetic frictional force is present.

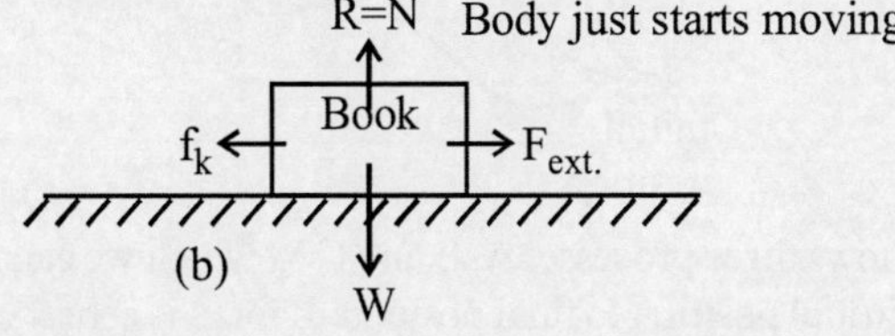

(b)

(c) *A graph $\vec{F}_{ext}$. versus | f | shown in figure. It is clear that* $f_{s,\ ,max} > f_k$

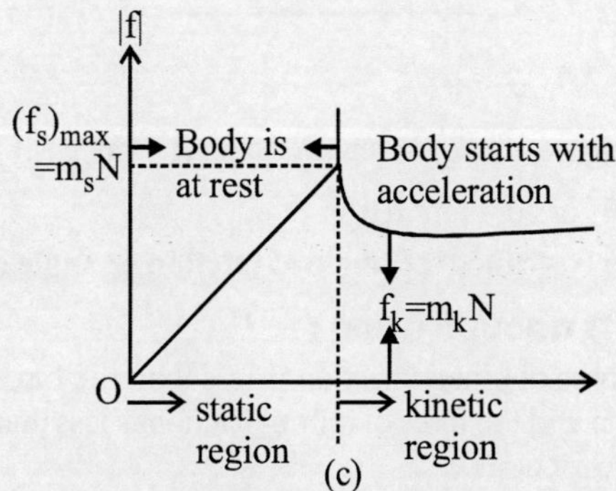

(c)

Fig.(a) shows a book on a horizontal rough surface. Now if we apply external force $\vec{F}_{ext.}$, on the book, then the book will remain stationary if $\vec{F}_{ext.}$ is not too large. If we increase $\vec{F}_{ext.}$ then frictional force f also increase up to $(f_s)_{max}$ (called maximum force of static friction or limiting friction) and $(f_s)_{max} = \mu_s N$. At any instant when $\vec{F}_{ext.}$ is slightly greater than $(f_s)_{max}$ then the book moves and accelerates to the right.

Fig.(b) when the book is in motion, the retarding frictional force become less than, $(f_s)_{max}$

Fig.(c) $(f_s)_{max}$ is equal to $\mu_k N$. When the book is in motion, we call the retarding frictional force as the force of kinetic friction f_k.

Since $f_k < (f_s)_{max}$, so it is clear that, we require more force to start motion than to maintain it against friction.

By experiment one can find that $(f_s)_{max}$ and f_k are proportional to normal force N acting on the book (by rough surface) and depends on the roughness of the two surfaces in contact.

Note :

(i) The force of static friction between any two surfaces in contact is opposite to $\vec{F}_{ext.}$ and given by $f_s \le \mu_s N$ and $(f_s)_{max} = \mu_s N$ (when the body just moves in the right direction).
where N = W = weight of book and μ_s is called coefficient of static friction, f_s is called force of static friction and $(f_s)_{max}$ is called *limiting friction or maximum value of static friction.*

(ii) The force of kinetic friction is opposite to the direction of motion and is given by $f_k = \mu_k N$
where μ_k is coefficient of kinetic friction.

(iii) The value of μ_k and μ_s depends on the nature of surfaces and μ_k is always less then μ_s.

Friction on an inclined plane : Now we consider a book on an inclined plane & it just moves or slips, then by definition

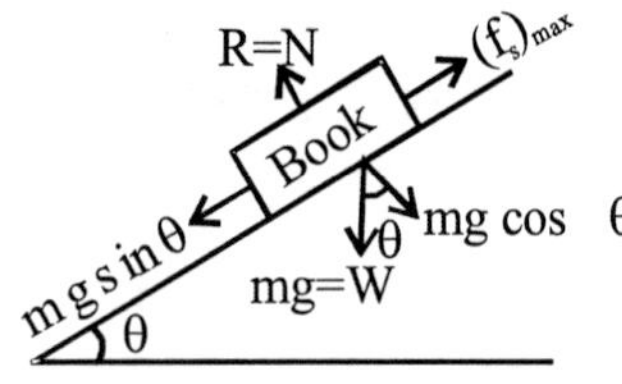

$$(f_s)_{max} = \mu_s R$$

Now from figure, $f_{s,max} = mg \sin\theta$ and $R = mg \cos\theta$

$\Rightarrow \mu_s = \tan\theta$ or $\theta = \tan^{-1}(\mu_s)$
where angle θ is called the **angle of friction** or **angle of repose**

Some facts about friction :

(1) The force of kinetic friction is less than the force of static friction and the force of rolling friction is less than force of kinetic friction i.e.,

$$f_r < f_k < f_s \quad \text{or} \quad \mu_{rolling} < \mu_{kinetic} < \mu_{static}$$

hence it is easy to roll the drum in comparison to sliding it.

(2) Frictional force does not oppose the motion in all cases, infact in some cases the body moves due to it.

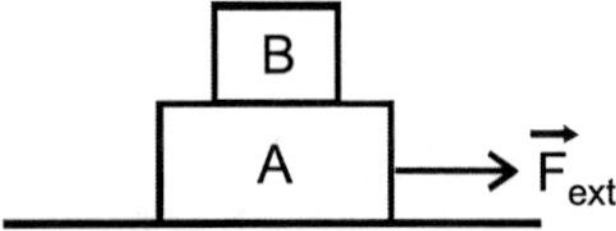

In the figure, book B moves to the right due to friction between A and B. If book A is totally smooth (i.e., frictionless) then book B does not move to the right. This is because of no force applies on the book B in the right direction.

Laws of limiting friction :

(i) The force of friction is independent of area of surfaces in contact and relative velocity between them (if it is not too high).

(ii) The force of friction depends on the nature of material of surfaces in contact (i.e., force of adhesion). μ depends upon nature of the surface. It is independent of the normal reaction.

(iii) The force of friction is directly proportional to normal reaction i.e., $F \propto N$ or $F = mn$.

While solving a problem having friction involved, follow the given methodology

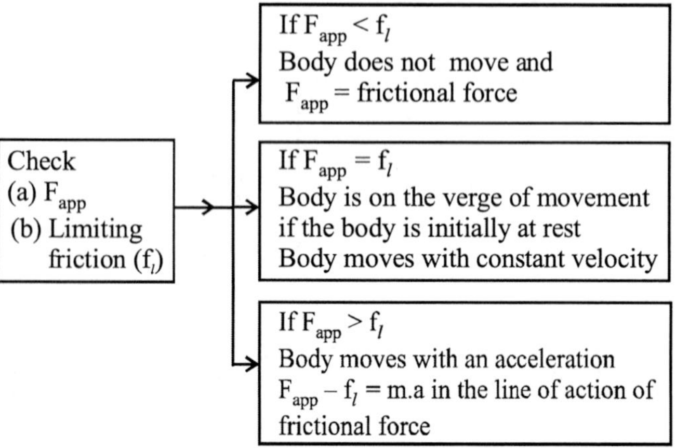

Rolling Friction :

The name rolling friction is a misnomer. Rolling friction has nothing to do with rolling. Rolling friction occurs during rolling as well as sliding operation.

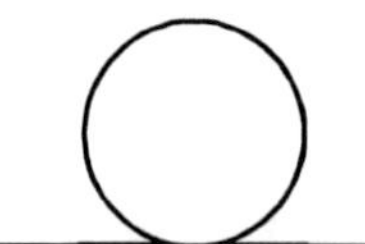

Cause of rolling friction : When a body is kept on a surface of another body it causes a depression (an exaggerated view shown in the figure). When the body moves, it has to overcome the depression. This is the cause of rolling friction.

Note : Rolling friction will be zero only when both the bodies incontact are rigid. Rolling friction is very small as compared to sliding friction. Work done by rolling friction is zero

CONSERVATIVE AND NON-CONSERVATIVE FORCES

If work done on a particle is zero in complete round trip, the force is said to be conservative. The gravitational force, electrostatics force, elastic force etc., are conservative forces. On the other hand *if the work done on a body is not zero during a complete round trip, the force is said to be non-conservative.* The frictional force, viscous force etc. are non-conservative forces.

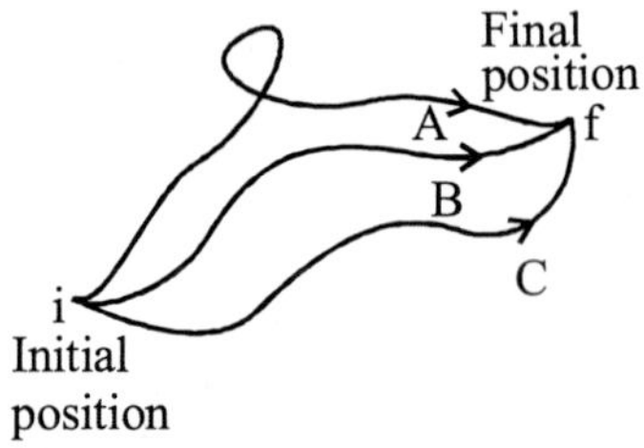

Figure shows three processes A, B and C by which we can reach from an initial position to final position. If force is conservative, then work done is same in all the three processes i.e., independent of the path followed between initial and final position.

If force is non conservative then work done from i to f is different in all three paths A,B and C.

Hence it is clear that *work done in conservative force depends only on initial & final position irrespective of the path followed between initial & final position. In case of non-conservative forces the work done depends on the path followed between initial and final position.*

We can say also that there is no change in kinetic energy of the body in complete round trip in case of conservative force. While in case of non conservative forces, when a body return to its initial position after completing the round trip, the kinetic energy of the body may be more or less than the kinetic energy with which it starts.

Example 13.

Pushing force making an angle θ to the horizontal is applied on a block of weight W placed on a horizontal table. If the angle of friction is ϕ, then determine the magnitude of force required to move the body.

Solution :

The various forces acting on the block are shown in fig.

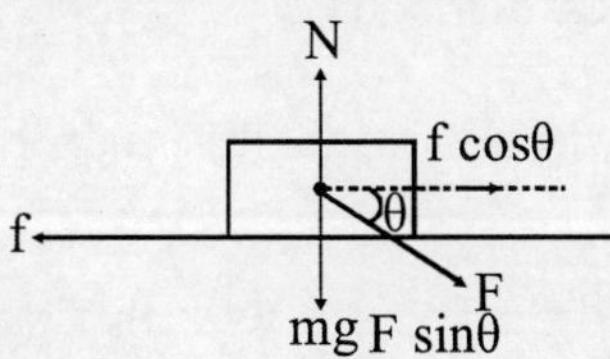

Here,

$\mu = \tan\phi = \frac{f}{N}$;   or $f = N\tan\phi$...(i)

The condition for the block just to move is

$F\cos\theta = f = N\tan\phi$ ...(ii)

and $F\sin\theta + W = N$ ...(iii)

From (ii) and (iii),

$F\cos\theta = (W + F\sin\theta)\tan\phi = W\tan\phi + F\sin\theta\tan\phi$;

or $F\cos\theta - F\sin\theta\sin\phi/\cos\phi = W\sin\phi/\cos\phi$

or $F(\cos\theta\cos\phi - \sin\theta\sin\phi) = W\sin\phi$;

or $F\cos(\theta + \phi) = W\sin\phi$ or $F = W\sin\phi/\cos(\theta + \phi)$

Example 14.

An object of weight W is resting on an inclined plane at an angle θ to the horizontal. The coefficient of static friction is μ. Find the horizontal force needed to just push the object up the plane.

Solution :

The situation is shown in fig.

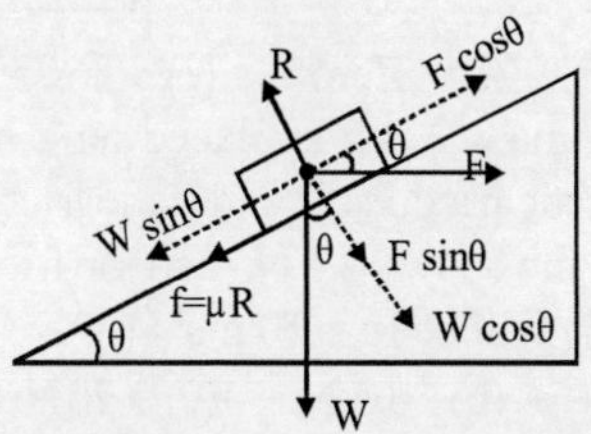

Let F be the horizontal force needed to just push the object up the plane. From figure $R = W\cos\theta + F\sin\theta$

Now $f = \mu R = \mu[W\cos\theta + F\sin\theta]$ ...(1)

Further, $F\cos\theta = W\sin\theta + f$ ...(2)

$F\cos\theta = W\sin\theta + \mu[W\cos\theta + F\sin\theta]$

$F\cos\theta - \mu F\sin\theta = W\sin\theta + \mu W\cos\theta$

$\therefore\ F = \frac{W(\sin\theta + \mu\cos\theta)}{(\cos\theta - \mu\sin\theta)}$

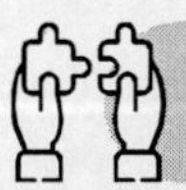

5.2 Concept Practice Problems

CPP

11. A cart of mass M has a block of mass m attached to it as shown in fig. The coefficient of friction between the block and the cart is μ. What is the minimum acceleration of the cart so that the block m does not fall?

(a) μg

(b) g/μ

(c) μ/g

(d) $M\mu g/m$

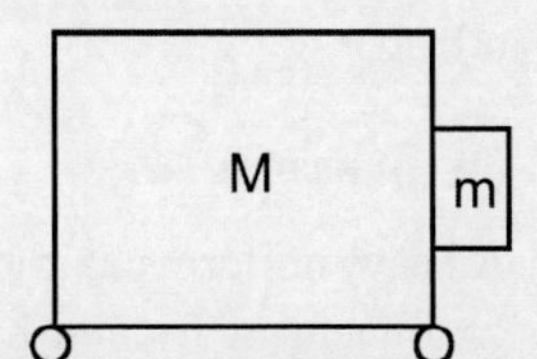

12. A weight W rests on a rough horizontal plane. If the angle of friction be θ, the least force that will move the body along the plane will be

(a) $W\cos\theta$ (b) $W\cot\theta$

(c) $W\tan\theta$ (d) $W\sin\theta$

13. A block is kept on a inclined plane of inclination θ of length ℓ. The velocity of particle at the bottom of inclined is (the coefficient of friction is μ)

(a) $[2g\ell(\mu\cos\theta - \sin\theta)]^{1/2}$ (b) $\sqrt{2g\ell(\sin\theta - \mu\cos\theta)}$

(c) $\sqrt{2g\ell(\sin\theta + \mu\cos\theta)}$ (d) $\sqrt{2g\ell(\cos\theta + \mu\sin\theta)}$

14. A block of mass m on a rough horizontal surface is acted upon by two forces as shown in figure. For equilibrium of block the coefficient of friction between block and surface is

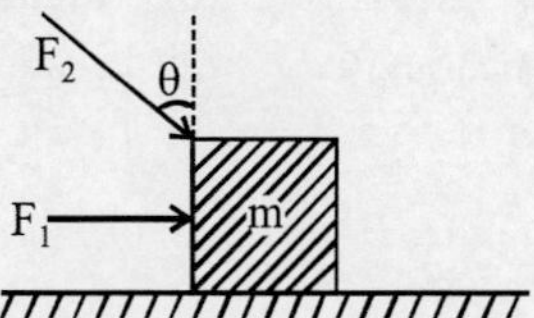

(a) $\frac{F_1 + F_2\sin\theta}{mg + F_2\cos\theta}$ (b) $\frac{F_1\cos\theta + F_2}{mg - F_2\sin\theta}$

(c) $\frac{F_1 + F_2\cos\theta}{mg + F_2\sin\theta}$ (d) $\frac{F_1\sin\theta - F_2}{mg - F_2\cos\theta}$

15. The coefficient of friction between two surfaces is 0.2. The angle of friction is

(a) $\sin^{-1}(0.2)$ (b) $\cos^{-1}(0.2)$

(c) $\tan^{-1}(0.1)$ (d) $\cot^{-1}(5)$

16. A block of mass 5 kg resting on a horizontal surface is connected by a cord, passing over a light frictionless pulley to a hanging block of mass 5 kg. The coefficient of kinetic friction between the block and the surface is 0.5. Tension in the cord is : ($g = 9.8$ m/sec^2)

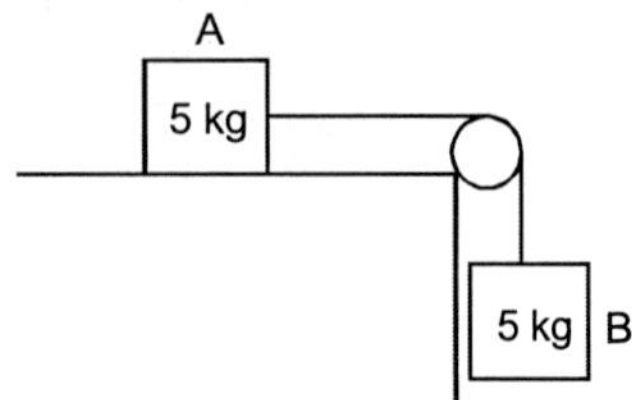

(a) 49 N (b) Zero (c) 36.75 N (d) 2.45 N

17. A body of mass 2 kg is placed on a horizontal surface having kinetic friction 0.4 and static friction 0.5. If the force applied on the body is 2.5 N, then the frictional force acting on the body will be [$g = 10$ ms^{-2}]

(a) 8 N (b) 10 N (c) 20 N (d) 2.5 N

18. For the arrangement shown in the Figure the tension in the string is [Given : $\tan^{-1}(0.8) = 39°$]

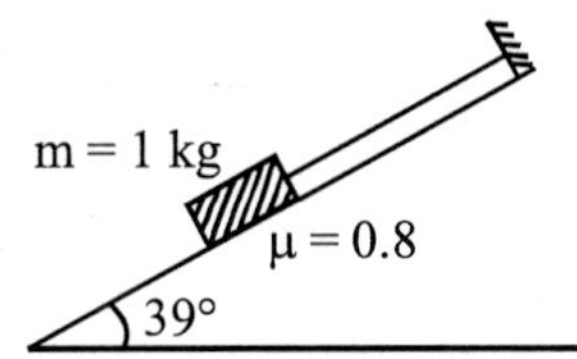

(a) 6 N (b) 6.4 N (c) 0.4 N (d) zero.

19. A horizontal force F is applied on back of mass m placed on a rough inclined plane of inclination θ. The normal reaction N is

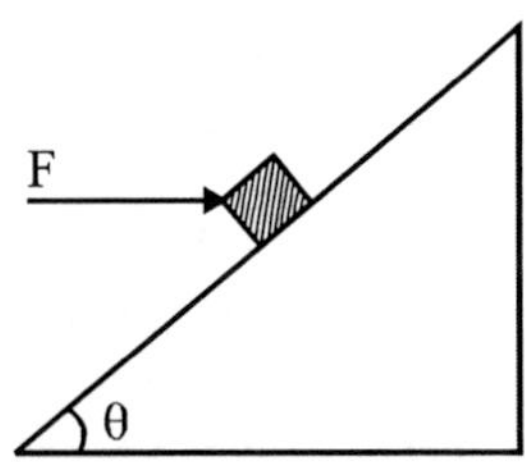

(a) $mg\cos\theta$ (b) $mg\sin\theta$

(c) $mg\cos\theta - F\cos\theta$ (d) $mg\cos\theta + F\sin\theta$

20. The coefficient of friction between the rubber tyres and the road way is 0.25. The maximum speed with which a car can be driven round a curve of radius 20 m without skidding is ($g = 9.8$ m/s^2)

(a) 5 m/s (b) 7 m/s (c) 10 m/s (d) 14 m/s

21. Block A of weight 100 kg rests on a block B and is tied with horizontal string to the wall at C. Block B is of 200 kg. The coefficient of friction between A and B is 0.25 and that between B and surface is $\frac{1}{3}$. The horizontal force F necessary to move the block B should be ($g = 10$ m/s^2)

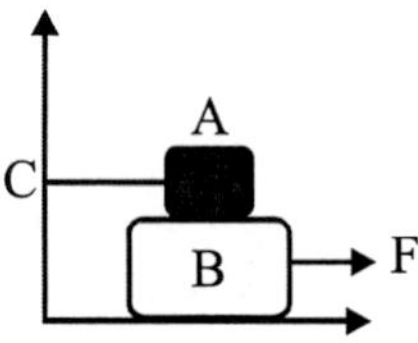

(a) 1050 N (b) 1450 N (c) 1050 N (d) 1250 N

22. A smooth block is released at rest on a 45° incline and then slides a distance 'd'. The time taken to slide is 'n' times as much to slide on rough incline than on a smooth incline. The coefficient of friction is

(a) $\mu_k = \sqrt{1-\frac{1}{n^2}}$ (b) $\mu_k = 1-\frac{1}{n^2}$

(c) $\mu_s = \sqrt{1-\frac{1}{n^2}}$ (d) $\mu_s = 1-\frac{1}{n^2}$

23. The upper half of an inclined plane with inclination ϕ is perfectly smooth while the lower half is rough. A body starting from rest at the top will again come to rest at the bottom if the coefficient of friction for the lower half is given by

(a) $2\cos\phi$ (b) $2\sin\phi$ (c) $\tan\phi$ (d) $2\tan\phi$

24. The upper half of an inclined plane of inclination θ is perfectly smooth while lower half is rough. A block starting from rest at the top of the plane will again come to rest at the bottom, if the coefficient of friction between the block and lower half of the plane is given by

(a) $\mu = \frac{2}{\tan\theta}$ (b) $\mu = 2\tan\theta$

(c) $\mu = \tan\theta$ (d) $\mu = \frac{1}{\tan\theta}$

25. A heavy uniform chain lies on horizontal table top. If the coefficient of friction between the chain and the table surface is 0.25, then the maximum fraction of the length of the chain that can hang over one edge of the table is

(a) 20% (b) 25% (c) 35% (d) 15%

ANSWER KEY

11	(b)	12	(c)	13	(b)	14	(a)	15	(d)	16	(c)	17	(d)	18	(d)	19	(d)	20	(b)
21	(d)	22	(b)	23	(d)	24	(b)	25	(a)										

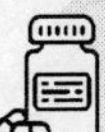

Topic 5.3 : Circular Motions & Banking of Road and Conical Pendulum

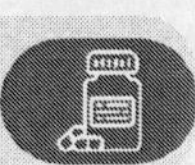

CIRCULAR MOTIONS

Motion in a Vertical Circle :

Let us consider a particle of mass m attached to a string of length R let the particle be rotated about its centre O.
At t = 0 the particle start with velocity u from the point A (lowest point of vertical circle) and at time t its position is P. Then the tension at point P is given by

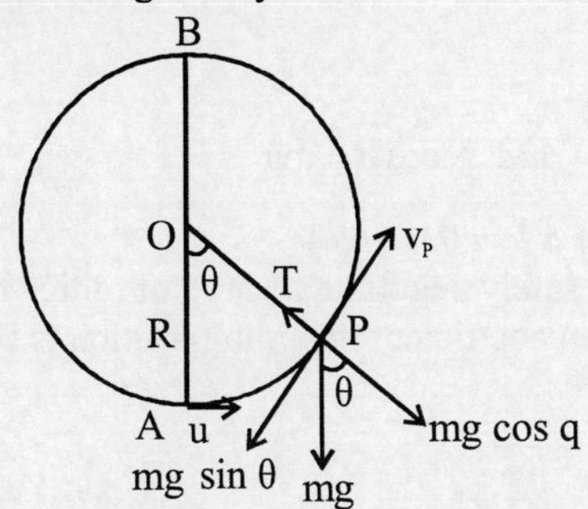

$$T_P - mg\cos\theta = \frac{mv_P^2}{R} \text{ or } T_P = mg\cos\theta + \frac{mv_P^2}{R} \quad ...(1)$$

So tension at point A (lowest point of vertical circle) is

$$T_A - mg = \frac{mv_A^2}{R} \qquad (\because \theta = 0^o) \quad ...(2)$$

and tension at point B (highest point of vertical circle) is

$$T_B + mg = \frac{mv_B^2}{R} \qquad (\because \theta = 180^o) \quad ...(3)$$

Where $\frac{mv^2}{r}$ **is centripetal force** required for the particle to move in a vertical circle.
Now from law of conservation of energy

$$\frac{1}{2}mv_A^2 - \frac{1}{2}mv_B^2 = 2mgR$$

or, $v_A^2 - v_B^2 = 4gR$ ...(4)

(change in kinetic energy of particle)
= (change in potential energy of particle)
or
(loss in kinetic energy of the particle) = (gain in potential energy)
In conservative force system (such as gravity force) the mechanical energy (i.e., kinetic energy + potential energy) must be constant.
Total energy will be constant
Now from eq^{ns}.(2) and (3), we get

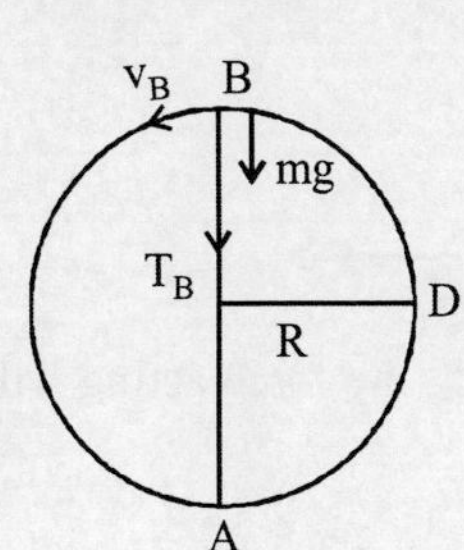

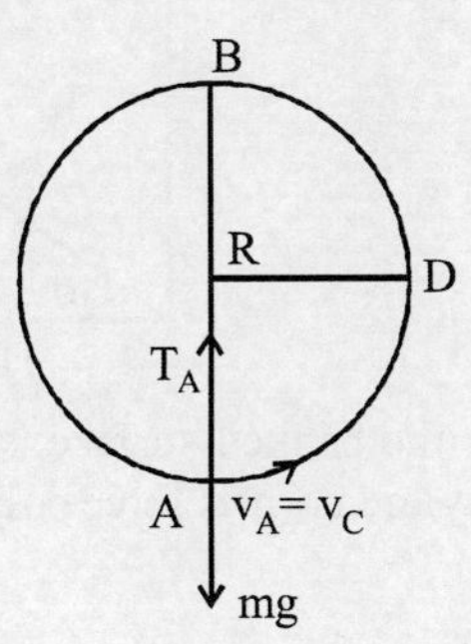

$$T_A - T_B = 2mg + \frac{m}{R}(V_A^2 - V_B^2) = 2mg + \frac{m}{R}(4gR)$$

$\Rightarrow \quad T_A - T_B = 6mg$ ...(5)

or $\quad T_A = T_B + 6mg$ ...(6)

So it is clear from eq^n. (6) that tension in string at lowest point of vertical circle is greater then the tension at highest point of vertical circle by 6mg.

Condition to complete a vertical circle :

If we reduce the velocity v_A in equation (2), then T_A will be reduce and at some critical velocity v_c, T_B will be zero, then put $T_B = 0$ and $v_B = v_C$ in equation (3) and we obtain

$$v_C = v_B = \sqrt{gR} \quad ...(7)$$

In this condition the necessary centripetal force at point B is provided by the weight of the particle [see again equation (3)] then from equation (4), we get

$$v_A^2 - gR = 4gR \Rightarrow v_A = \sqrt{5gR} \quad ...(8)$$

then the tension at the point A will be

$$T_A = mg + \frac{m(5gR)}{R} = 6mg \quad ...(9)$$

Hence if we rotate a particle in a vertical circle and tension in string at highest point is zero, then the tension at lowest point of vertical circle is 6 times of the weight of the particle.

Some Facts of Vertical Motion :

(i) The body will complete the vertical circle if its velocity at lowest point is equal to or greater then $\sqrt{5gR}$

(ii) The body will oscillate about the lowest point if its velocity at lowest point is less then $\sqrt{2gR}$. This will happen when the velocity at the halfway mark, i.e.

$$v_D = 0 \left[\because \frac{1}{2}mv_A^2 = mgR\right]$$

(iii) The string become slack and fails to describe the circle when its velocity at lowest point lies between $\sqrt{2gR}$ to $\sqrt{5gR}$

Example 15.

A mass m is revolving in a vertical circle at the end of a string of length 20 cm. By how much does the tension of the string at the lowest point exceed the tension at the topmost point?

Solution :

The tension T_1 at the topmost point is given by,

$$T_1 = \frac{m v_1^2}{20} - mg$$

Centrifugal force acting outward while weight acting downward

The tension T_2 at the lowest point, $T_2 = \frac{m v_2^2}{20} + mg$

Centrifugal force and weight (both) acting downward

$$T_2 - T_1 = \frac{m v_2^2 - m v_1^2}{20} + 2mg; \quad v_1^2 = v_2^2 - 2gh$$

or $v_2^2 - v_1^2 = 2g(40) = 80g$

$$\therefore \; T_2 - T_1 = \frac{80\,mg}{20} + 2mg = 6\,mg$$

Example 16.

A stone of mass 1 kg tied to a light inextensible string of length L = (10/3) m is whirling in a circular path of radius L in a vertical plane. If the ratio of the maximum to the minimum tension in the string is 4 and g = 10 m/s², then find the speed of the stone at the highest point of the circle.

Solution :

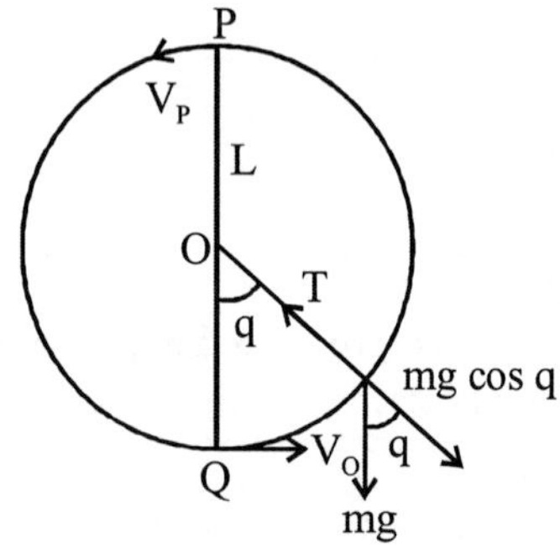

The tension T in the string is given by

$$T_{max} = m\left[g + \frac{v_Q^2}{L}\right] \text{ and } T_{min} = m\left[-g + \frac{v_P^2}{L}\right]$$

According to the given problem

$$\frac{g + (v_Q^2/L)}{-g + (v_P^2/L)} = 4 \quad \text{or} \quad g + \frac{v_Q^2}{L} = -4g + 4\frac{v_P^2}{L}$$

or $g + \frac{v_P^2 + 4gL}{L} = -4g + 4\frac{v_P^2}{L}$

$L = (10/3)$ m and $g = 10$ m/s² (given)

Solving we get $v_P = 10$ m/s.

BANKING OF ROAD

Turning of a Vehicle on Horizontal Circular Road

Negotiating a Curve :

Case of cyclist

To safely negotiate a curve of radius r, a cyclist should bend at an angle θ with the vertical.

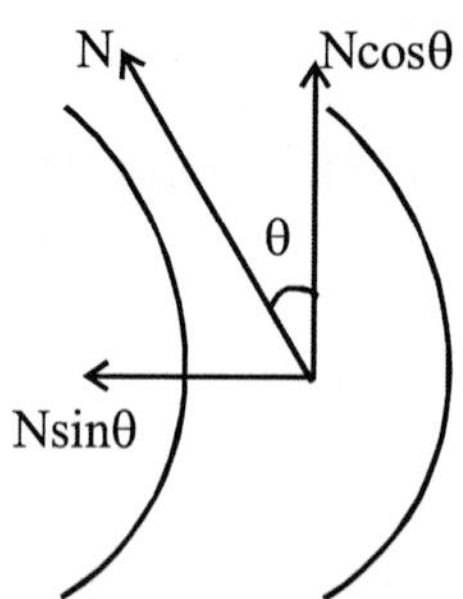

Which is given by $\tan\theta = \frac{v^2}{rg}$. Angle θ is also called as **angle of banking.**

$$N\sin\theta = \frac{mv^2}{r} \text{ and } N\cos\theta = mg$$

Case of car on a levelled road

A vehicle can safely negotiate a curve of radius r on a rough level road when coefficient of sliding friction is related to the velocity as $\mu_s \geq \frac{v^2}{rg}$.

Now consider a case when a vehicle is moving in a circle, the centrifugal force is $\frac{mv^2}{r}$ whereas m is mass of vehicle, r = radius of circle and v is its velocity.

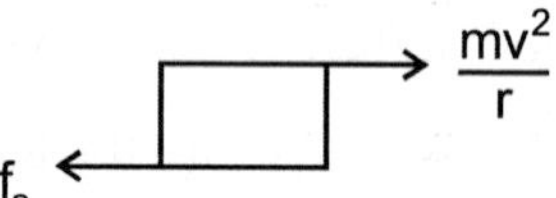

The frictional force is static since wheels are in rolling motion because point of contact with the surface is at rest

$$\therefore f_s = \frac{mv^2}{r} \qquad f_s \leq f_{max} = \mu_s mg$$

$$\frac{mv^2}{r} \leq \mu_s mg \text{ or } \mu_s \geq \frac{v^2}{rg}$$

Case of banking of road (frictionless)

A vehicle can safely negotiate a curve of radius r on a smooth (frictionless) road, when the angle θ of banking of the road is given by $\tan\theta = \frac{v^2}{rg}$.

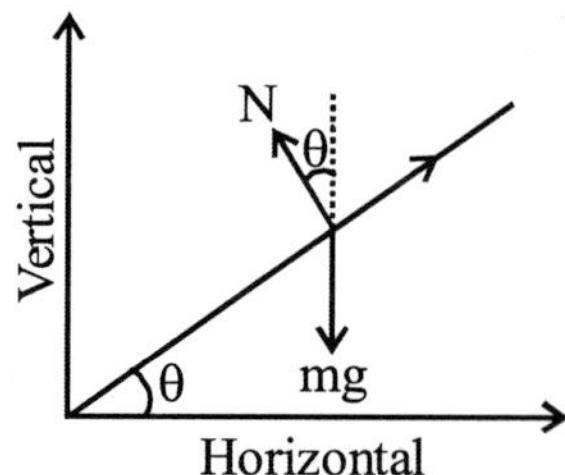

When the banked surface is smooth, the force acting will be gravity and normal force only.

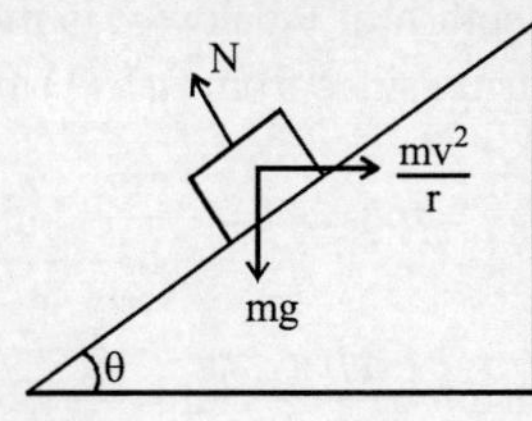

Balancing forces

$N\cos\theta = mg$ ...(1)

$N\sin\theta = \dfrac{mv^2}{r}$ ...(2)

$\dfrac{v^2}{rg} = \tan\theta$ ...(3)

Case of banking of road (with friction)

The maximum velocity with which a vehicle can safely negotiate a curve of radius r on a rough inclined road is given by

$v^2 = \dfrac{rg(\mu + \tan\theta)}{1 - \mu\tan\theta}$; where μ is the coefficient of friction of the rough surface on which the vehicle is moving, and θ is the angle of inclined road with the horizontal.

Suppose a vehicle is moving in a circle of radius r on a rough inclined road whose coefficient of friction is $\dfrac{\mu}{M}$ and angle of banking is θ.

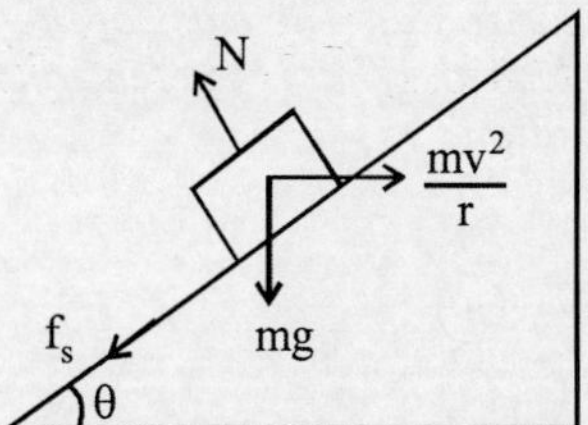

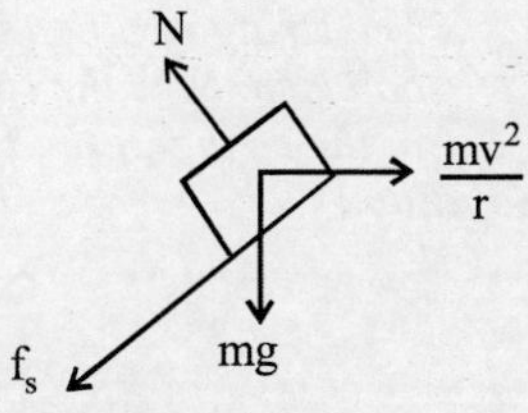

Let velocity of object (vehicle) be V.

If we apply pseudo force on body, centrifugal force is $\dfrac{mv^2}{r}$ when v is max. and friction force will be acting down the slope.

Balancing the force horizontally, $\dfrac{mv^2}{r} = f_s\cos\theta + N\sin\theta$ ...(1)

Balancing the force vertically,

$N\cos\theta = f_s\sin\theta + mg$ ...(2)

when v = maximum, $f = f_{max} = f_s = \mu N$ ...(3)

From eq^n. (2),

$N\cos\theta = \mu N\sin\theta + mg \Rightarrow N(\cos\theta - \mu\sin\theta) = mg$

or $N = \dfrac{mg}{\cos\theta - \mu\sin\theta}$

From eq^{ns}.(1) and (3), $\dfrac{mv^2}{r} = \dfrac{\mu mg\cos\theta + mg\sin\theta}{\cos\theta - \mu\sin\theta}$

$\Rightarrow \dfrac{mv^2}{r} = \dfrac{mg(\mu + \tan\theta)}{1 - \mu\tan\theta} \Rightarrow v_{max}^2 = rg\dfrac{(\mu + \tan\theta)}{1 - \mu\tan\theta}$

Now in the case of minimum velocity with which body could move in a circular motion, the direction of friction will be opposite to that one in maximum velocity case.

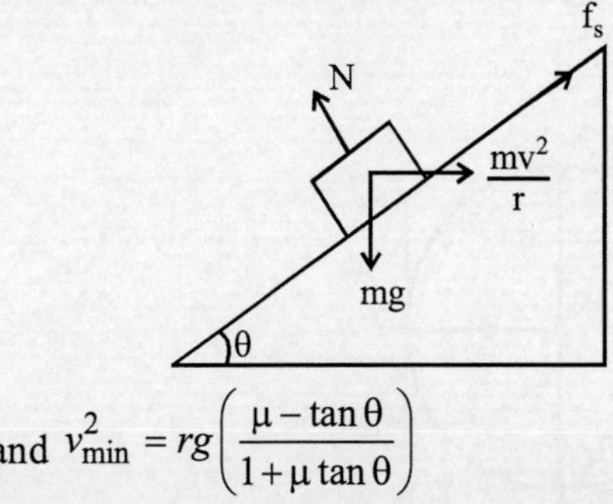

and $v_{min}^2 = rg\left(\dfrac{\mu - \tan\theta}{1 + \mu\tan\theta}\right)$

Problem Solving Tips

1. Whenever a particle is moving on the circular path then there must be some external force which will provide the necessary centripetal acceleration to the particle.

   For examples :

   (i) Motion of satellite around a planet : Here the centripetal force is provided by the gravitational force.

   i.e. $\dfrac{GMm}{r^2} = \dfrac{mv^2}{r}$

   Satellite (m), (M) Planet, V

   (ii) Motion of electron around the nucleus : Here the required centripetal force is provided by the Coulombian force

   i.e. $\dfrac{1}{4\pi\varepsilon_0}\dfrac{(ze)(e)}{r^2} = \dfrac{mv^2}{r}$

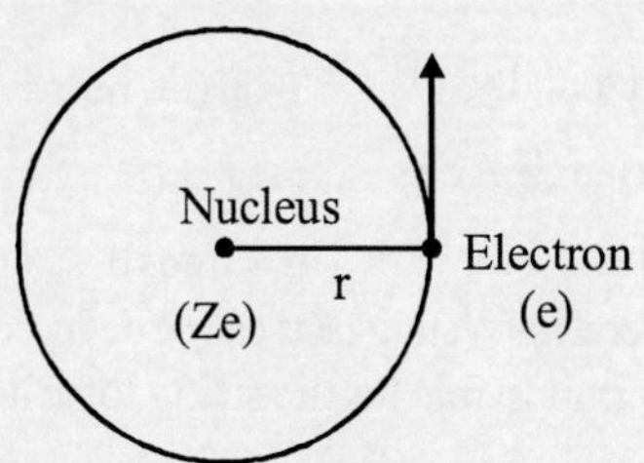

   (iii) Motion of a body in horizontal and vertical circle: Here the centripetal force is provided by the tension.

Horizontal circle

$T = \dfrac{mv^2}{r}$

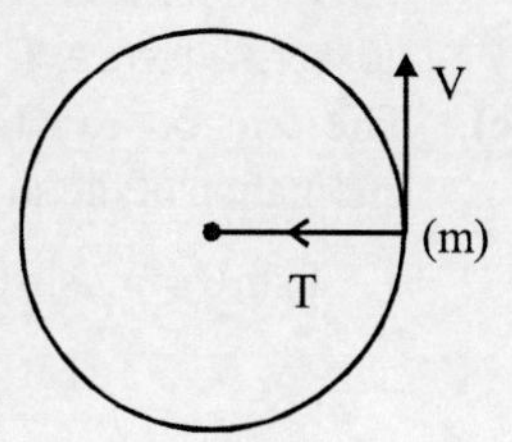

Vertical circle

At point A, $T_A = \frac{mv_A^2}{r}$; At point B, $T_B + mg = \frac{mv_B^2}{r}$

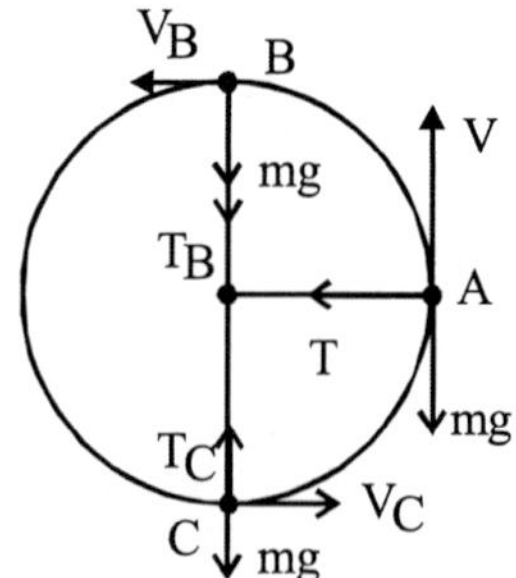

And at point C, $T_C - mg = \frac{mv_C^2}{r}$

CONICAL PENDULUM

Consider an inextensible string of length ℓ which is fixed at one end, A. At the other end is attached a particle P of mass m describing a circle with constant angular velocity ω in a horizontal plane.

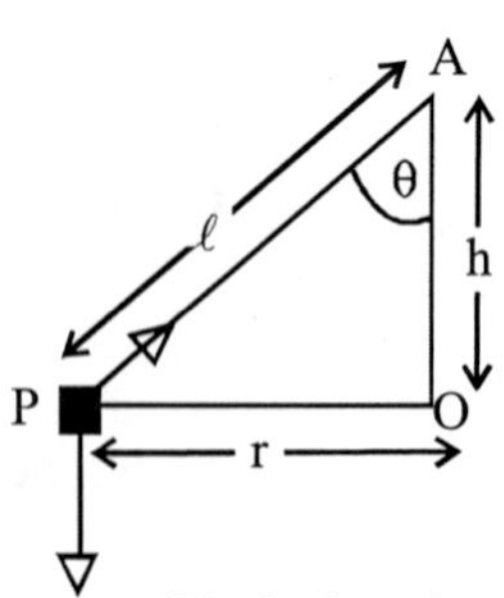

Vertical section

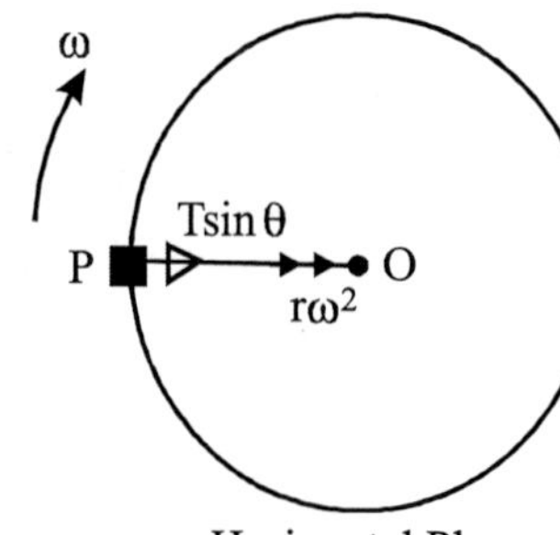

Horizontal Plane

As P rotates, the string AP traces out the surface of a cone. Consequently the system is known as a conical pendulum.

Vertically, $T\cos\theta = mg$ ...(1)

Horizontally, $T\sin\theta = mr\omega^2$ ...(2)

In triangle AOP, $r = \ell\sin\theta$ ...(3)

and $h = \ell\cos\theta$ ...(4)

Several interesting facts can be deduced from these equations:

(a) It is impossible for the string to be horizontal.

This is seen from eq^n. (1) in which $\cos\theta = \frac{mg}{T}$ cannot be zero. Hence θ cannot be 90°.

(b) The tension is always greater than mg.

This also follows from eq^n. (1) as $\cos\theta < 1$ (θ is acute but not zero). Hence, $T > mg$

(c) The tension can be calculated without knowing the inclination of the string since, from eq^n. (2) and (3)

$$T\sin\theta = m\ell\sin\theta\,\omega^2 \Rightarrow T = m\ell\omega^2$$

(d) The vertical depth h of P below A is independent of the length of the string since from eq^n. (1) and (4)

$$T\frac{h}{\ell} = mg \Rightarrow T = \frac{\ell mg}{h} \quad \text{but} \quad T = m\ell\omega^2$$

Therefore $m\ell\omega^2 = \frac{m\ell g}{h} \Rightarrow h = \frac{g}{\omega^2}$

which is independent of ℓ.

Example 17.

A particle of mass m is moving in a circular path of constant radius r such that its centripetal acceleration a_c is varying with time t as $a_c = k^2rt^2$, where k is a constant. Determine the power delivered to the particle by the forces acting on it.

Solution :

Here tangential acceleration also exists which requires power. Given that centripetal acceleration

$a_c = k^2rt^2$ also, $a_c = v^2/r$;

$\therefore v^2/r = k^2rt^2$ or $v^2 = k^2r^2t^2$ or $v = k\,r\,t$;

Tangential acceleration, $a = \frac{dv}{dt} = kr$

Now, force $F = ma = m\,k\,r$;

So, power, $P = F\,v = m\,k\,r \times k\,r\,t = m\,k^2\,r^2\,t$.

Example 18.

The string of a pendulum is horizontal. The mass of the bob is m. Now the string is released. What is the tension in the string in the lowest position?

Solution :

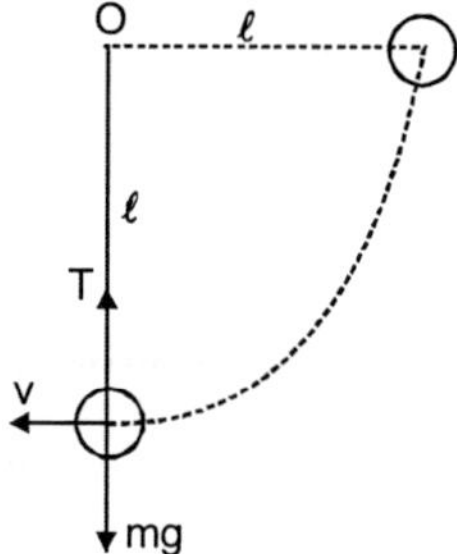

Let v be the velocity of the bob at the lowest position. In this position, The P.E. of bob is converted into K.E. Hence,

$$mg\ell = \frac{1}{2}mv^2 \quad \text{or} \quad v^2 = 2g\ell \qquad ...(1)$$

If T be the tension in the string, then

$$T - mg = \left(\frac{mv^2}{\ell}\right) \qquad ...(2)$$

From eq^{ns}. (1) and (2).

$T - mg = 2mg$ or $T = 3mg$

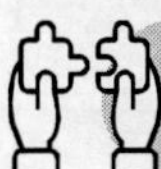

5.3 Concept Practice Problems

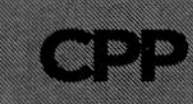

26. Centripetal force :
(a) can change speed of the body.
(b) is always perpendicular to direction of motion
(c) is constant for uniform circular motion.
(d) all of these

27. A small block is shot into each of the four tracks as shown below. Each of the tracks rises to the same height. The speed with which the block enters the track is the same in all cases. At the highest point of the track, the normal reaction is maximum in

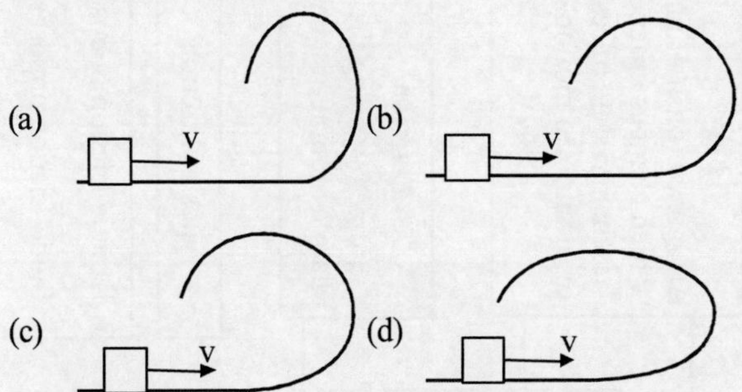

28. A bucket tied at the end of a 1.6 m long string is whirled in a vertical circle with constant speed. What should be the minimum speed so that the water from the bucket does not spill when the bucket is at the highest position?
(a) 4 m/sec (b) 6.25 m/sec
(c) 16 m/sec (d) None of the above

29. A cane filled with water is revolved in a vertical circle of radius 4 meter and the water just does not fall down. The time period of revolution will be
(a) 1 sec (b) 10 sec
(c) 8 sec (d) 4 sec

30. A circular road of radius r in which maximum velocity is v, has angle of banking
(a) $\tan^{-1}\left(\frac{v^2}{rg}\right)$ (b) $\tan^{-1}\left(\frac{rg}{v^2}\right)$
(c) $\tan^{-1}\left(\frac{v}{rg}\right)$ (d) $\tan^{-1}\left(\frac{rg}{v}\right)$

31. A small sphere is attached to a cord and rotates in a vertical circle about a point O. If the average speed of the sphere is increased, the cord is most likely to break at the orientation when the mass is at

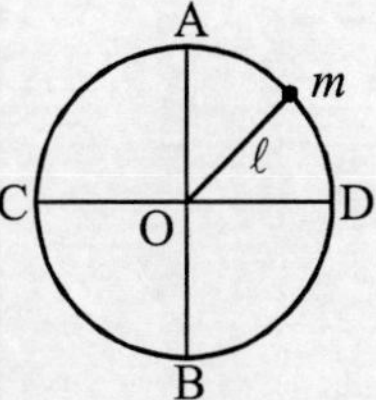

(a) bottom point B (b) the point C
(c) the point D (d) top point A

32. A person with his hand in his pocket is skating on ice at the rate of 10m/s and describes a circle of radius 50 m. What is his inclination to vertical : ($g = 10$ m/sec^2)
(a) $\tan^{-1}(½)$ (b) $\tan^{-1}(1/5)$
(c) $\tan^{-1}(3/5)$ (d) $\tan^{-1}(1/10)$

33. A particle tied to a string describes a vertical circular motion of radius r continually. If it has a velocity $\sqrt{3\,gr}$ at the highest point, then the ratio of the respective tensions in the string holding it at the highest and lowest points is
(a) 4 : 3 (b) 5 : 4 (c) 1 : 4 (d) 3 : 2

34. A motor cycle is going on an overbridge of radius *R*. The driver maintains a constant speed. As the motor cycle is ascending on the overbridge, the normal force on it
(a) increases (b) decreases
(c) remains the same (d) fluctuates erratically

35. A car of mass m moving over a concave bridge of radius 'r'. The normal reaction acting on car when it is at the lowest point of the bridge is
(a) $R = mg - \frac{mv^2}{r}$ (b) $R = mg + \frac{mv^2}{r}$
(c) $R = mg$ (d) $R = mv^2/r$

ANSWER KEY

26	(b)	27	(a)	28	(a)	29	(d)	30	(a)	31	(a)	32	(b)	33	(c)	34	(a)	35	(b)

CONCEPT MAP

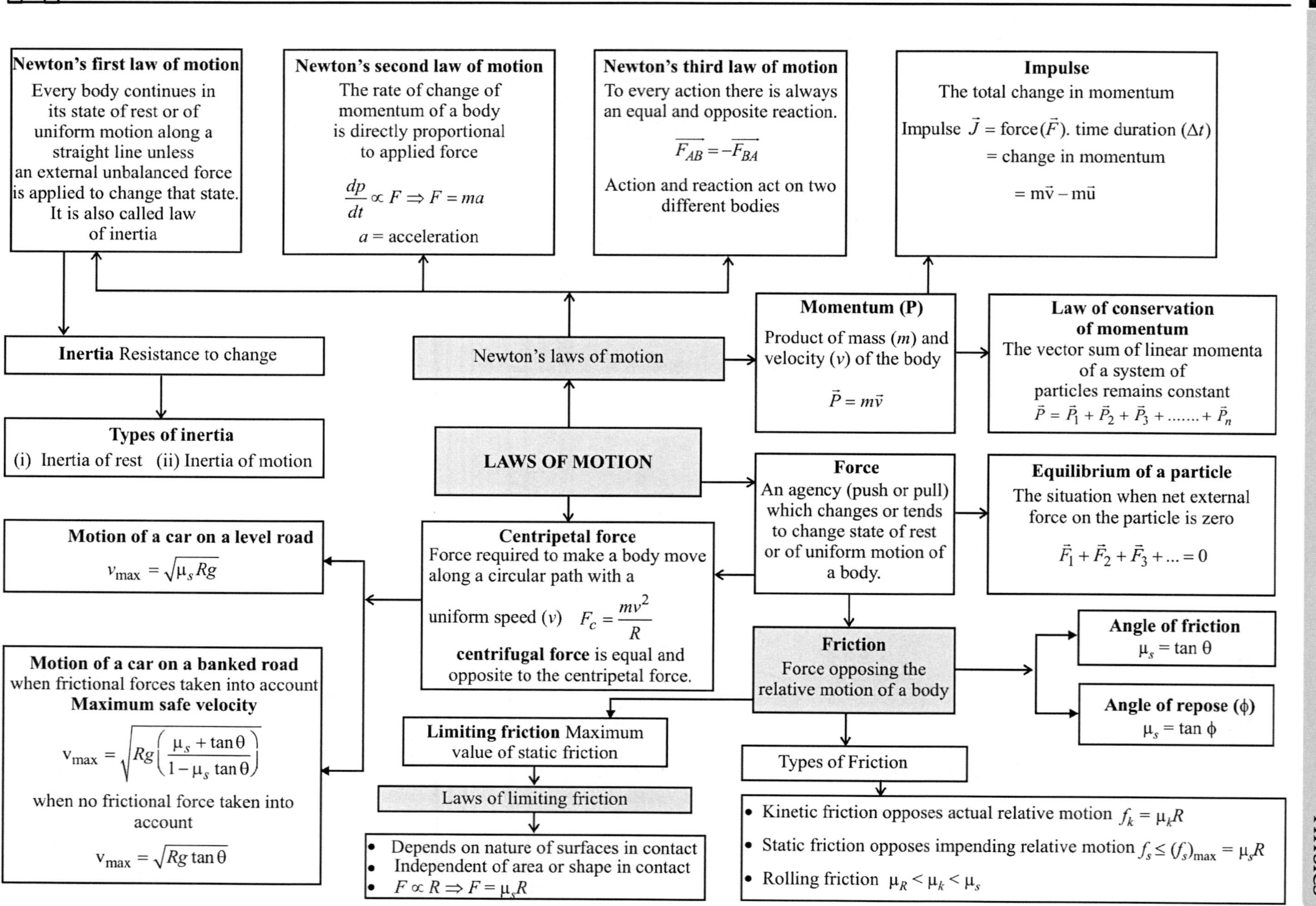
Newton's first law of motion
Every body continues in its state of rest or of uniform motion along a straight line unless an external unbalanced force is applied to change that state. It is also called law of inertia
Newton's second law of motion
The rate of change of momentum of a body is directly proportional to applied force
$\frac{dp}{dt} \propto F \Rightarrow F = ma$
a = acceleration
Newton's third law of motion
To every action there is always an equal and opposite reaction.
$\overrightarrow{F_{AB}} = -\overrightarrow{F_{BA}}$
Action and reaction act on two different bodies
Impulse
The total change in momentum
Impulse $\vec{J}$ = force($\vec{F}$). time duration (Δt)
= change in momentum
$= m\vec{v} - m\vec{u}$
Inertia Resistance to change
Types of inertia
(i) Inertia of rest (ii) Inertia of motion
Newton's laws of motion
Momentum (P)
Product of mass (m) and velocity (v) of the body
$\vec{P} = m\vec{v}$
Law of conservation of momentum
The vector sum of linear momenta of a system of particles remains constant
$\vec{P} = \vec{P}_1 + \vec{P}_2 + \vec{P}_3 + ... + \vec{P}_n$
LAWS OF MOTION
Force
An agency (push or pull) which changes or tends to change state of rest or of uniform motion of a body.
Equilibrium of a particle
The situation when net external force on the particle is zero
$\vec{F}_1 + \vec{F}_2 + \vec{F}_3 + ... = 0$
Motion of a car on a level road
$v_{max} = \sqrt{\mu_s Rg}$
Centripetal force
Force required to make a body move along a circular path with a uniform speed (v) $F_c = \frac{mv^2}{R}$
centrifugal force is equal and opposite to the centripetal force.
Friction
Force opposing the relative motion of a body
Angle of friction
$\mu_s = \tan\theta$
Angle of repose (ϕ)
$\mu_s = \tan\phi$
Motion of a car on a banked road
when frictional forces taken into account
Maximum safe velocity
$v_{max} = \sqrt{Rg\left(\frac{\mu_s + \tan\theta}{1 - \mu_s \tan\theta}\right)}$
when no frictional force taken into account
$v_{max} = \sqrt{Rg\tan\theta}$
Limiting friction Maximum value of static friction
Laws of limiting friction
Depends on nature of surfaces in contact
Independent of area or shape in contact
$F \propto R \Rightarrow F = \mu_s R$
Types of Friction
Kinetic friction opposes actual relative motion $f_k = \mu_k R$
Static friction opposes impending relative motion $f_s \leq (f_s)_{max} = \mu_s R$
Rolling friction $\mu_R < \mu_k < \mu_s$

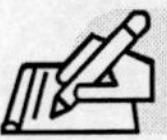

Exercise 1 - Chapter Revision Problems

CRP

1. A rectangular block is placed on a rough horizontal surface in two different ways as shown, then

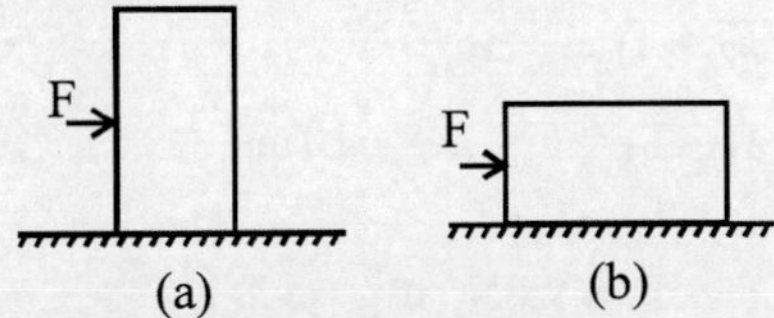

(a) friction will be more in case (a)
(b) friction will be more in case (b)
(c) friction will be equal in both the cases
(d) friction depends on the relations among its dimensions.

2. When a horse pulls a cart, the horse moves down to
(a) horse on the cart.
(b) cart on the horse.
(c) horse on the earth.
(d) earth on the horse.

3. The force of action and reaction
(a) must be of same nature
(b) must be of different nature
(c) may be of different nature
(d) may not have equal magnitude

4. A body is moving with uniform velocity, then
(a) no force must be acting on the body.
(b) exactly two forces must be acting on the body
(c) body is not acted upon by a single force.
(d) the number of forces acting on the body must be even.

5. The direction of impulse is
(a) same as that of the net force
(b) opposite to that of the net force
(c) same as that of the final velocity
(d) same as that of the initial velocity

6. A monkey is climbing up a rope, then the tension in the rope
(a) must be equal to the force applied by the monkey on the rope
(b) must be less than the force applied by the monkey on the rope.
(c) must be greater than the force applied by the monkey on the rope.
(d) may be equal to, less than or greater the force applied by the monkey on the rope.

7. A constant force $F = m_2g/2$ is applied on the block of mass m_1 as shown in fig. The string and the pulley are light and the surface of the table is smooth. The acceleration of m_1 is

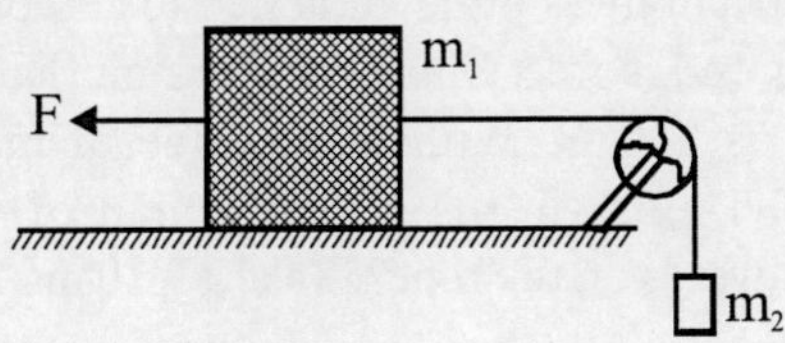

(a) $\frac{m_2g}{2(m_1+m_2)}$ towards right

(b) $\frac{m_2g}{2(m_1-m_2)}$ towards left

(c) $\frac{m_2g}{2(m_2-m_1)}$ towards right

(d) $\frac{m_2g}{2(m_2-m_1)}$ towards left

8. A ball of mass m is thrown vertically upwards. What is the rate at which the momentum of the ball changes?
(a) Zero (b) mg
(c) Infinity (d) Data is not sufficient.

9. A particle starts sliding down a frictionless inclined plane. If S_n is the distance traveled by it from time t = n – 1 sec to t = n sec, the ratio S_n/S_{n+1} is
(a) $\frac{2n-1}{2n+1}$ (b) $\frac{2n+1}{2n}$
(c) $\frac{2n}{2n+1}$ (d) $\frac{2n+1}{2n-1}$

10. In an explosion, a body breaks up into two pieces of unequal masses. In this
(a) both parts will have numerically equal momentum
(b) lighter part will have more momentum
(c) heavier part will have more momentum
(d) both parts will have equal kinetic energy

11. A plate of mass M is placed on a horizontal of frictionless surface (see figure), and a body of mass m is placed on this plate. The coefficient of dynamic friction between this body and the plate is μ . If a force 2 μ mg is applied to the body of mass m along the horizontal, the acceleration of the plate will be

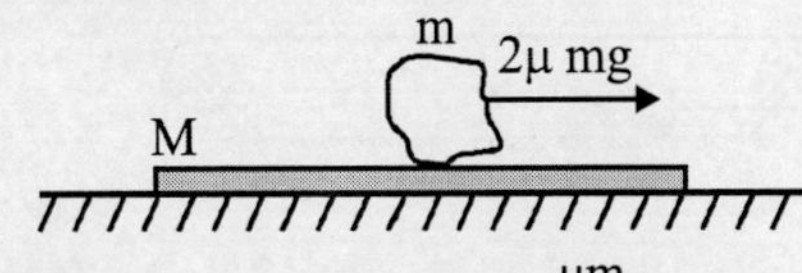

(a) $\frac{\mu m}{M}g$ (b) $\frac{\mu m}{(M+m)}g$
(c) $\frac{2\mu m}{M}g$ (d) $\frac{2\mu m}{(M+m)}g$.

12. A toy gun consists of a spring and a rubber dart of mass 16 g. When compressed by 4 cm and released, it projects the dart to a height of 2 m. If compressed by 6 cm, the height achieved is
(a) 3m (b) 4m (c) 4.5m (d) 6m

13. A car travelling at a speed of 30 km/h is brought to a halt in 4 m by applying brakes. If the same car is travelling at 60 km/h, it can be brought to halt with the same braking power in
(a) 8m (b) 16m (c) 24m (d) 32m

14. A machine gun has a mass 5 kg. It fires 50 gram bullets at the rate of 30 bullets per minute at a speed of 400 ms^{-1}. What force is required to keep the gun in position?
(a) 10N (b) 5N (c) 15N (d) 30N

15. A force time graph for the motion of a body is shown in Fig. Change in linear momentum between 0 and 8s is

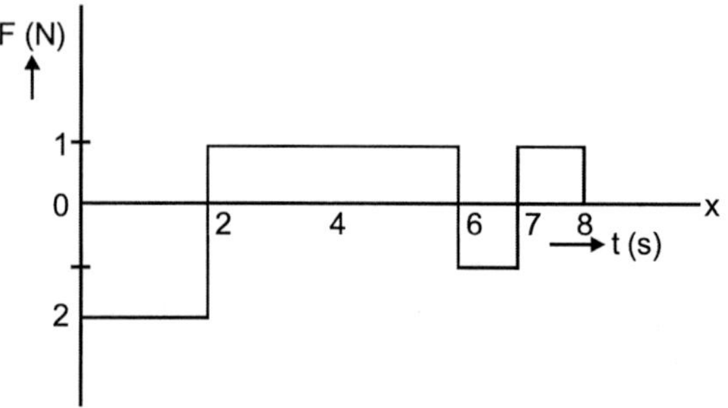

(a) zero (b) 4 N-s
(c) 8 Ns (d) None of these

16. Fig. shows a uniform rod of length 30 cm having a mass of 3.0 kg. The strings shown in the figure are pulled by constant forces of 20 N and 32 N. All the surfaces are smooth and the strings and pulleys are light. The force exerted by 20 cm part of the rod on the 10 cm part is

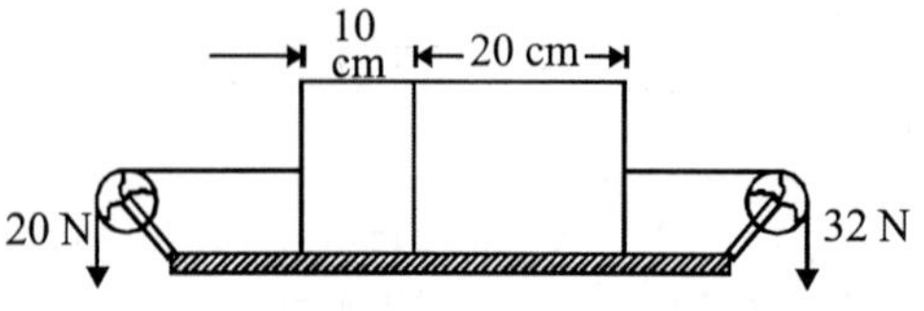

(a) 20N (b) 24N (c) 32N (d) 52N

17. A force of 10 N acts on a body of mass 20 kg for 10 seconds. Change in its momentum is
(a) 5 kg m/s (b) 100 kg m/s
(c) 200 kg m/s (d) 1000 kg m/s

18. Consider the system shown in fig. The pulley and the string are light and all the surfaces are frictionless. The tension in the string is (take g = 10 m/s^2)

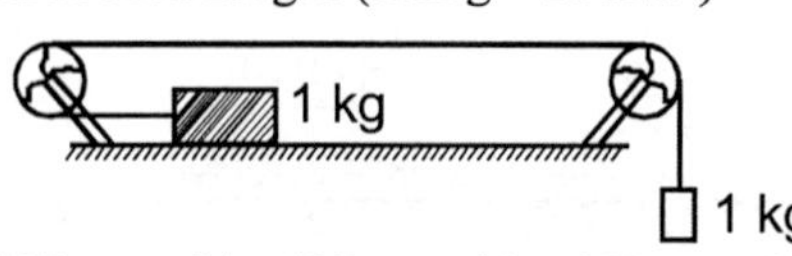

(a) 0N (b) 1N (c) 2N (d) 5N

19. Two blocks of masses 2 kg and 1 kg are placed on a smooth horizontal table in contact with each other. A horizontal force of 3 newton is applied on the first so that the block moves with a constant acceleration. The force between the blocks would be
(a) 3 newton (b) 2 newton (c) 1 newton (d) zero

20. A 4000 kg lift is accelerating upwards. The tension in the supporting cable is 48000 N. If $g = 10ms^{-2}$ then the acceleration of the lift is
(a) $1\ ms^{-2}$ (b) $2\ ms^{-2}$ (c) $4\ ms^{-2}$ (d) $6\ ms^{-2}$

21. A 0.1 kg block suspended from a massless string is moved first vertically up with an acceleration of $5ms^{-2}$ and then moved vertically down with an acceleration of $5ms^{-2}$. If T_1 and T_2 are the respective tensions in the two cases, then
(a) $T_2 > T_1$
(b) $T_1 - T_2 = 1\,N$, if $g = 10\,ms^{-2}$
(c) $T_1 - T_2 = 1kg\,f$
(d) $T_1 - T_2 = 9.8N$, if $g = 9.8\ ms^{-2}$

22. A ball of mass 0.5 kg moving with a velocity of 2 m/sec strikes a wall normally and bounces back with the same speed. If the time of contact between the ball and the wall is one millisecond, the average force exerted by the wall on the ball is :
(a) 2000 newton (b) 1000 newton
(c) 5000 newton (d) 125 newton

23. The mass of the lift is 100 kg which is hanging on the string. The tension in the string, when the lift is moving with constant velocity, is (g = 9.8 m/sec^2)
(a) 100 newton (b) 980 newton
(c) 1000 newton (d) None of these

24. In the question , the tension in the strings, when the lift is accelerating up with an acceleration 1 m/sec^2, is
(a) 100 newton (b) 980 newton
(c) 1080 newton (d) 880 newton

25. A 40 kg slab rests on frictionless floor as shown in fig. A 10 kg block rests on the top of the slab. The static coefficient of friction between the block and slab is 0.60 while the kinetic friction is 0.40. The 10 kg block is acted upon by a horizontal force of 100 N. If g = 9.8 m/s^2, the resulting acceleration of the slab will be:

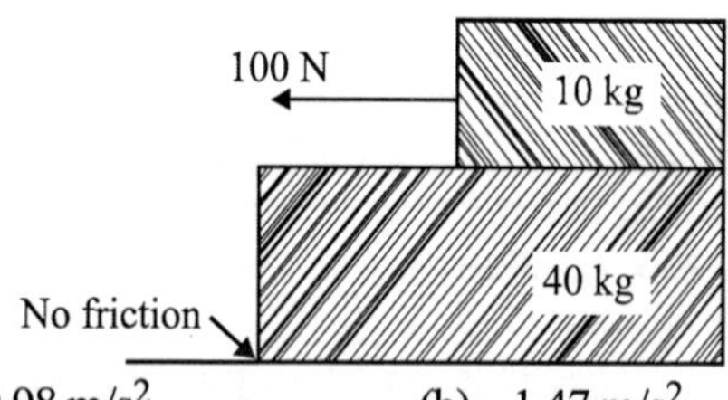

(a) 0.98 m/s^2 (b) 1.47 m/s^2
(c) 1.52 m/s^2 (d) 6.1 m/s^2

26. Two trolleys of mass m and 3m are connected by a spring. They were compressed and released at once, they move off in opposite direction and come to rest after covering a distance S_1, S_2 respectively. Assuming the coefficient of friction to be uniform, ratio of distances $S_1 : S_2$ is :
(a) 1:9 (b) 1:3 (c) 3:1 (d) 9:1

27. One end of massless rope, which passes over a massless and frictionless pulley P is tied to a hook C while the other end is free. Maximum tension that the rope can bear is 360 N. With what value of maximum safe acceleration (in ms^{-2}) can a man of 60 kg moves downwards on the rope? [Take g = 10 ms^{-2}]

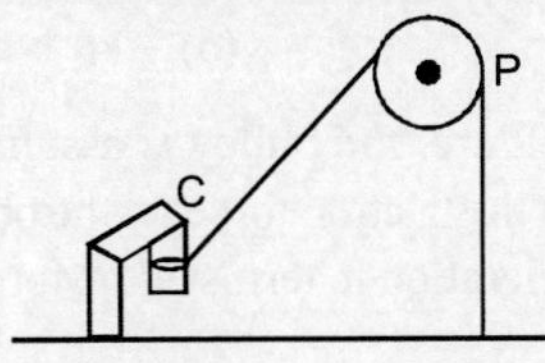

(a) 16 (b) 6 (c) 4 (d) 8

28. A force $\vec{F} = 8\hat{i} - 6\hat{j} - 10\hat{k}$ newton produces an acceleration of 1 ms^{-2} in a body. The mass of the body is

(a) 10 kg (b) $10\sqrt{2}$ kg (c) $10\sqrt{3}$ kg (d) 200 kg

29. A uniform chain of length 2 m is kept on a table such that a length of 60 cm hangs freely from the edge of the table. The total mass of the chain is 4 kg. What is the work done in pulling the entire chain on the table ?

(a) 12 J (b) 3.6 J (c) 7.2 J (d) 1200 J

30. A rocket of mass 5000 kg is to be projected vertically upward. The gases are exhausted vertically downwards with velocity 1000 ms^{-2} with respect to the rocket. What is the minimum rate of burning the fuel so as to just lift the rocket upwards against gravitational attraction ?

(a) 49 kg s^{-1} (b) 147 kg s^{-1}
(c) 98 kg s^{-1} (d) 196 kg s^{-1}

31. A 50 kg ice skater, initially at rest, throws a 0.15 kg snowball with a speed of 35 m/s. What is the approximate recoil speed of the skater?

(a) 0.10 m/s (b) 0.20 m/s (c) 0.70 m/s (d) 1.4 m/s

32. A force F is used to raise a 4-kg mass M from the ground to a height of 5 m.

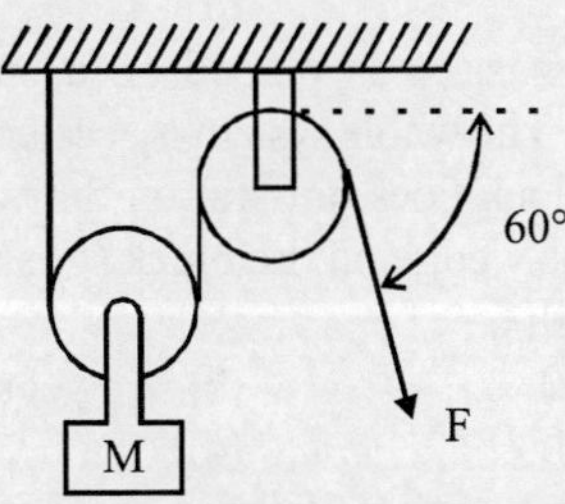

What is the work done by the force F? (Note : sin 60° = 0.87; cos 60° = 0.50. Ignore friction and the weights of the pulleys)

(a) 50 J (b) 100 J (c) 174 J (d) 200 J

33. A bullet is fired from a gun. The force on the bullet is given by $F = 600 - 2 \times 10^5 t$

Where, F is in newtons and t in seconds. The force on the bullet becomes zero as soon as it leaves the barrel. What is the average impulse imparted to the bullet?

(a) 1.8 N-s (b) Zero (c) 9 N-s (d) 0.9 N-s

34. The minimum velocity (in ms^{-1}) with which a car driver must traverse a flat curve of radius 150 m and coefficient of friction 0.6 to avoid skidding is

(a) 60 (b) 30 (c) 15 (d) 25

35. A bag of sand of mass m is suspended by a rope. A bullet of mass $\frac{m}{20}$ is fired at it with a velocity v and gets embedded into it. The velocity of the bag finally is

(a) $\frac{v}{20} \times 21$ (b) $\frac{20v}{21}$ (c) $\frac{v}{20}$ (d) $\frac{v}{21}$

36. A 1 kg block and a 0.5 kg block move together on a horizontal frictionless surface . Each block exerts a force of 6 N on the other. The block move with a uniform acceleration of

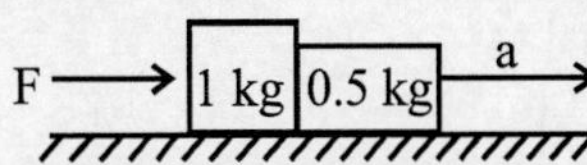

(a) 3 ms^{-2} (b) 6 ms^{-2} (c) 9 ms^{-2} (d) 12 ms^{-2}

37. A body of mass 32 kg is suspended by a spring balance from the roof of a vertically operating lift and going downward from rest. At the instant the lift has covered 20 m and 50 m, the spring balance showed 30 kg and 36 kg respectively. Then the velocity of the lift is

(a) decreasing at 20 m, and increasing at 50 m
(b) increasing at 20m and decreasing at 50 m
(c) continuously decreasing at a steady rate throughout the journey
(d) constantly increasing at constant rate throughout the journey.

38. An object at rest in space suddenly explodes into three parts of same mass. The momentum of the two parts are $2p\hat{i}$ and $p\hat{j}$. The momentum of the third part

(a) will have a magnitude $p\sqrt{3}$
(b) will have a magnitude $p\sqrt{5}$
(c) will have a magnitude p
(d) will have a magnitude 2p.

39. A body of mass 1.0 kg is falling with an acceleration of 10 m/sec^2. Its apparent weight will be (g = 10 m/sec^2)

(a) 1.0 kg wt (b) 2.0 kg wt
(c) 0.5 kg wt (d) zero

40. In the figure a smooth pulley of negligible weight is suspended by a spring balance. Weight of 1 kg f and 5 kg f are attached to the opposite ends of a string passing over the pulley and move with acceleration because of gravity, During their motion, the spring balance reads a weight of

(a) 6 kg f
(b) less then 6 kg f
(c) more than 6 kg f
(d) may be more or less then 6 kg f

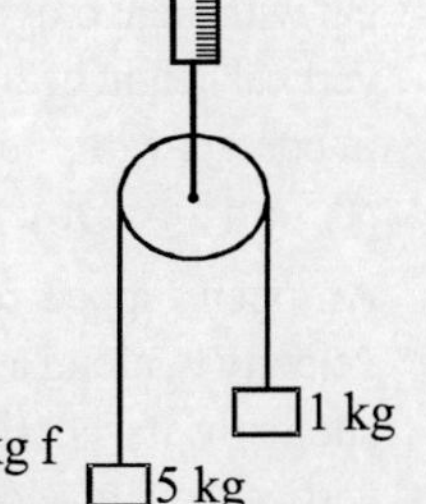

41. A particle moves so that its acceleration is always twice its velocity. If its initial velocity is 0.1 ms^{-1}, its velocity after it has gone 0.1 m is

(a) 0.3 ms^{-1} (b) 0.7 ms^{-1} (c) 1.2 ms^{-1} (d) 3.6 ms^{-1}

42. A ball of mass 0.4 kg thrown up in air with velocity 30 ms^{-1} reaches the highest point in 2.5 second. The air resistance encountered by the ball during upward motion is
(a) 0.88N (b) 8800N (c) 300 dyne (d) 300 N.

43. A player caught a cricket ball of mass 150 g moving at a rate of 20 m/s. If the catching process is completed in 0.1s, the force of the blow exerted by the ball on the hand of the player is equal to
(a) 150 N (b) 3 N (c) 30 N (d) 300 N

44. When the road is dry and the coefficient of the friction is μ, the maximum speed of a car in a circular path is 10 ms^{-1}.

If the road becomes wet and $\mu' = \frac{\mu}{2}$, what is the maximum speed permitted?
(a) 5 ms^{-1} (b) 10 ms^{-1} (c) $10\sqrt{2}$ ms^{-1} (d) $5\sqrt{2}$ ms^{-1}

45. Two pulley arrangements of figure given are identical. The mass of the rope is negligible. In fig (a), the mass m is lifted by attaching a mass 2m to the other end of the rope. In fig (b), m is lifted up by pulling the other end of the rope with a constant downward force F = 2mg. The acceleration of m in the two cases are respectively

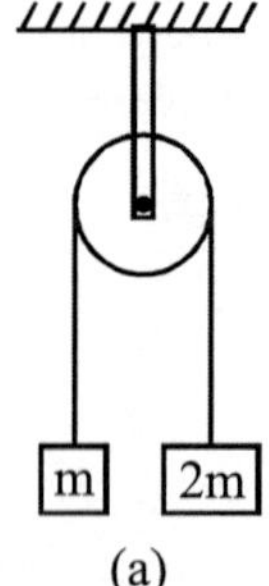

(a)

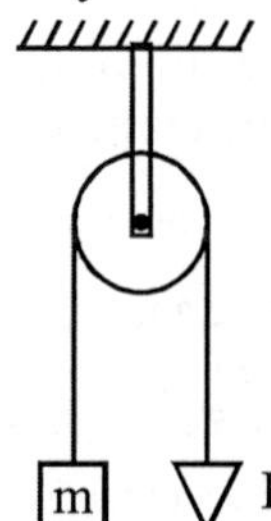

(b)

(a) 3g, g (b) g/3, g (c) g/3, 2g (d) g, g/3

46. The linear momentum p of a body moving in one dimension varies with time according to the equating P = a + bt^2 where a and b are positive constants. The net force acting on the body is
(a) proportional to t^2
(b) a constant
(c) proportional to t
(d) inversely proportional to t

47. A ball of mass 400 gm is dropped from a height of 5 m. A boy on the ground hits the ball vertically upwards with a bat with an average force of 100 newton so that it attains a vertical height of 20 m. The time for which the ball remains in contact with the bat is (g = 10 m/s^2)
(a) 0.12 s (b) 0.08 s (c) 0.04 s (d) 12 s

48. An open topped rail road car of mass M has an initial velocity v_0 along a straight horizontal frictionless track. It suddenly starts raising at time t = 0. The rain drops fall vertically with velocity u and add a mass m kg/sec of water. The velocity of car after t second will be (assuming that it is not completely filled with water)

(a) $v_0 + m\frac{u}{M}$ (b) $\frac{mv_0}{M+mt}$

(c) $\frac{Mv_0+ut}{M+ut}$ (d) $v_0 + \frac{mut}{M+ut}$

49. In the given figure, the pulley is assumed massless and frictionless. If the friction force on the object of mass m is f, then its acceleration in terms of the force F will be equal to

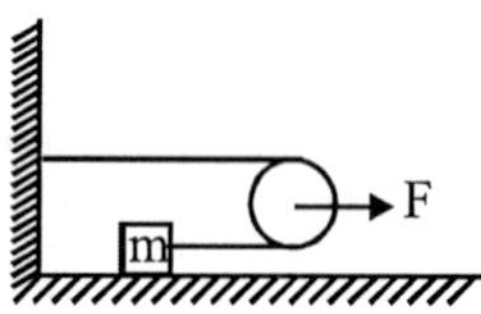

(a) (F – f)/m (b) $\left(\frac{F}{2}-f\right)/m$
(c) F/m (d) None of these

50. A particle of mass 0.3 kg subject to a force F = – kx with k = 15 N/m. What will be its initial acceleration if it is released from a point 20 cm away from the origin ?
(a) 15 m/s^2 (b) 3 m/s^2 (c) 10 m/s^2 (d) 5 m/s^2

51. A block is kept on a frictionless inclined surface with angle of inclination 'α'. The incline is given an acceleration 'a' to keep the block stationary. Then a is equal to

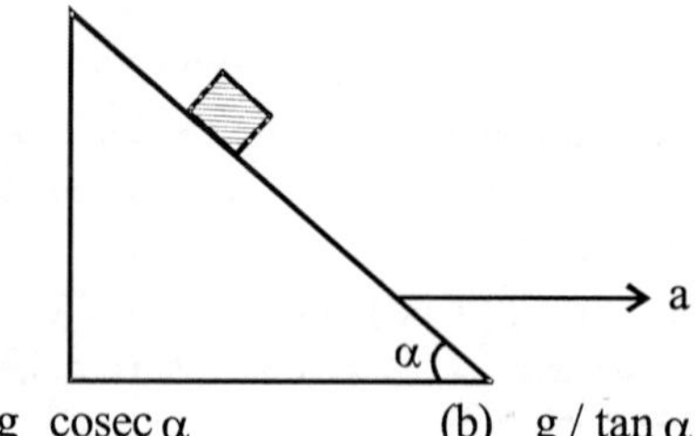

(a) g cosec α (b) g / tan α
(c) g tan α (d) g

52. A block of mass *m* is placed on a smooth wedge of inclination θ. The whole system is accelerated horizontally so that the block does not slip on the wedge. The force exerted by the wedge on the block (g is acceleration due to gravity) will be
(a) mg/cos θ (b) mg cos θ
(c) mg sin θ (d) mg

53. The coefficient of static friction, μ_s, between block A of mass 2 kg and the table as shown in the figure is 0.2. What would be the maximum mass value of block B so that the two blocks do not move? The string and the pulley are assumed to be smooth and massless. (g = 10 m/s^2)

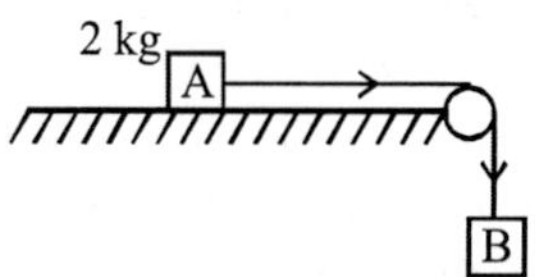

(a) 0.4 kg (b) 2.0 kg (c) 4.0 kg (d) 0.2 kg

54. A body under the action of a force

$\vec{F} = 6\hat{i} - 8\hat{j} + 10\hat{k}$, acquires an acceleration of 1 m/s^2. The mass of this body must be
(a) 10 kg (b) 20 kg
(c) $10\sqrt{2}$ kg (d) $2\sqrt{10}$ kg

55. An explosion breaks a rock into three parts in a horizontal plane. Two of them go off at right angles to each other. The first part of mass 1 kg moves with a speed of 12 ms^{-1} and the second part of mass 2 kg moves with speed 8 ms^{-1}. If the third part flies off with speed 4 ms^{-1} then its mass is
(a) 5 kg (b) 7 kg (c) 17 kg (d) 3 kg

56. A spring of force constant k is cut into two pieces whose lengths are in the ratio 1 : 2. What is the force constant of the longer piece ?
(a) $\frac{k}{2}$ (b) $\frac{3k}{2}$ (c) $2k$ (d) $3k$

57. A body of mass M hits normally a rigid wall with velocity V and bounces back with the same velocity. The impulse experienced by the body is
(a) MV (b) 1.5MV (c) 2MV (d) zero

58. A body of mass 5 kg explodes at rest into three fragments with masses in the ratio 1 : 1 : 3. The fragments with equal masses fly in mutually perpendicular directions with speeds of 21 m/s. The velocity of heaviest fragment in m/s will be
(a) $7\sqrt{2}$ (b) $5\sqrt{2}$ (c) $3\sqrt{2}$ (d) $\sqrt{2}$

59. Two bodies of masses m and 4m are moving with equal kinetic energies. The ratio of their linear momenta will be
(a) 1 : 4 (b) 4 : 1 (c) 1 : 2 (d) 2 : 1

60. A particle moving in the xy plane experiences a velocity dependent force $\vec{F} = k(v_y\hat{i} + v_x\hat{j})$, where v_x and v_y are x and y components of its velocity $\vec{v}$. if $\vec{a}$ is the acceleration of the particle, then which of the following statements is true for the particle?
(a) quantity $\vec{v} \times \vec{a}$ is constant in time
(b) $\vec{F}$ arises due to a magnetic field
(c) kinetic energy of particle is constant in time
(d) quantity $\vec{v} \cdot \vec{a}$ is constant in time

61. A ball is thrown upward with an initial velocity V_0 from the surface of the earth. The motion of the ball is affected by a drag force equal to $m\gamma v^2$ (where m is mass of the ball, v is its instantaneous velocity and γ is a constant). Time taken by the ball to rise to its zenith is :
(a) $\frac{1}{\sqrt{\gamma g}}\tan^{-1}\left(\sqrt{\frac{\gamma}{g}}V_0\right)$ (b) $\frac{1}{\sqrt{\gamma g}}\sin^{-1}\left(\sqrt{\frac{\gamma}{g}}V_0\right)$
(c) $\frac{1}{\sqrt{\gamma g}}ln\left(1+\sqrt{\frac{\gamma}{g}}V_0\right)$ (d) $\frac{1}{\sqrt{2\gamma g}}\tan^{-1}\left(\sqrt{\frac{2\gamma}{g}}V_0\right)$

62. A ball is thrown vertically up (taken as + z-axis) from the ground. The correct momentum-height (p-h) diagram is:

(a) 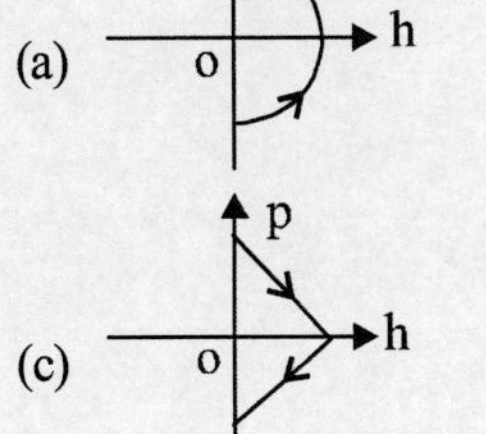

(b)

(c)

(d) 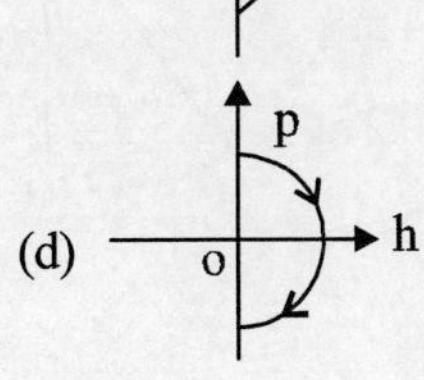

63. A particle of mass m is at rest at the origin at time $t = 0$. It is subjected to a force $F(t) = F_0e^{-bt}$ in the x direction. Its speed $v(t)$ is depicted by which of the following curves?

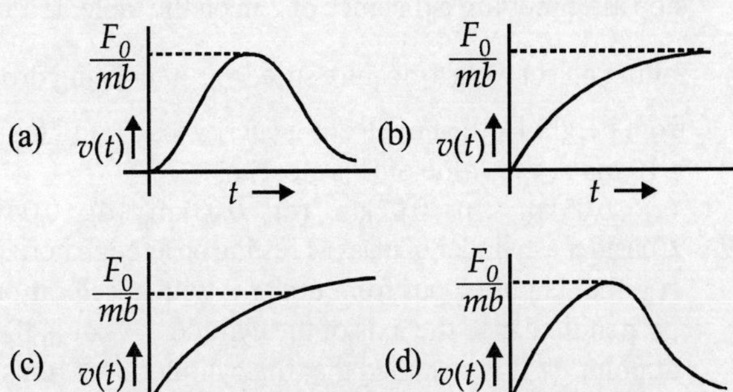

64. A mass of 10 kg is suspended by a rope of length 4 m, from the ceiling. A force F is applied horizontally at the mid-point of the rope such that the top half of the rope makes an angle of 45° with the vertical. Then F equals: (Take $g = 10$ ms^{-2} and the rope to be massless)
(a) 100 N (b) 90 N (c) 70 N (d) 75 N

65. A block of mass 5 kg is (i) pushed in case (A) and (ii) pulled in case (B), by a force F=20 N, making an angle of 30° with the horizontal, as shown in the figures. The coefficient of friction between the block and floor is μ = 0.2. The difference between the accelerations of the block, in case (B) and case (A) will be : (g =10 ms^{-2})

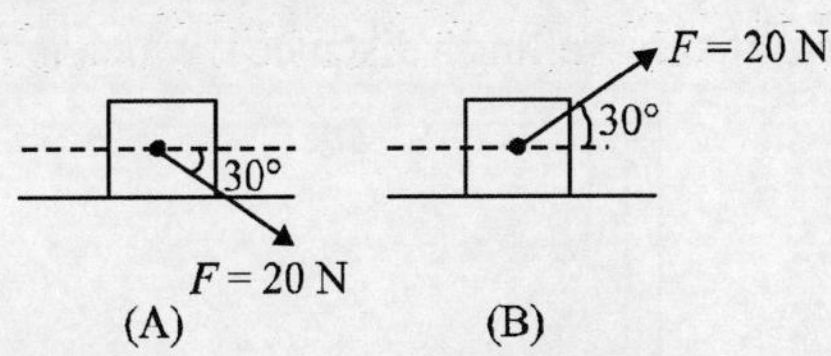

(a) 0.4 ms^{-2} (b) 3.2 ms^{-2}
(c) 0.8 ms^{-2} (d) 0 ms^{-2}

66. A block of mass 10 kg is kept on a rough inclined plane as shown in the figure. A force of 3 N is applied on the block. The coefficient of static friction between the plane and the block is 0.6. What should be the minimum value of force P, such that the block doesnot move downward? (take g = 10 ms^{-2})

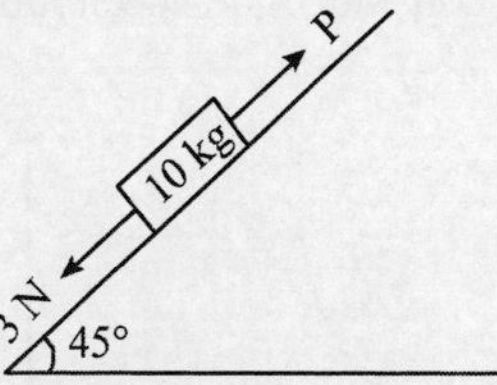

(a) 32 N (b) 18 N (c) 23 N (d) 25 N

67. A body of mass 2kg slides down with an acceleration of 3m/s^2 on a rough inclined plane having a slope of 30°. The external force required to take the same body up the plane with the same acceleration will be: (g = 10m/s^2)
(a) 4N (b) 14N (c) 6N (d) 20N

68. A block of mass m = 10 kg rests on a horizontal table. The coefficient of friction between the block and the table is 0.05. When hit by a bullet of mass 50 g moving with speed v, that gets embedded in it, the block moves and comes to stop after moving a distance of 2 m on the table. If a freely falling object were to acquire speed $\frac{v}{10}$ after being dropped from height H, then neglecting energy losses and taking g = 10 ms^{-2}, the value of H is close to:

(a) 0.05 km (b) 0.02 km (c) 0.03 km (d) 0.04 km

69. Consider a cylinder of mass M resting on a rough horizontal rug that is pulled out from under it with acceleration 'a' perpendicular to the axis of the cylinder. What is $F_{friction}$ at point P? It is assumed that the cylinder does not slip.

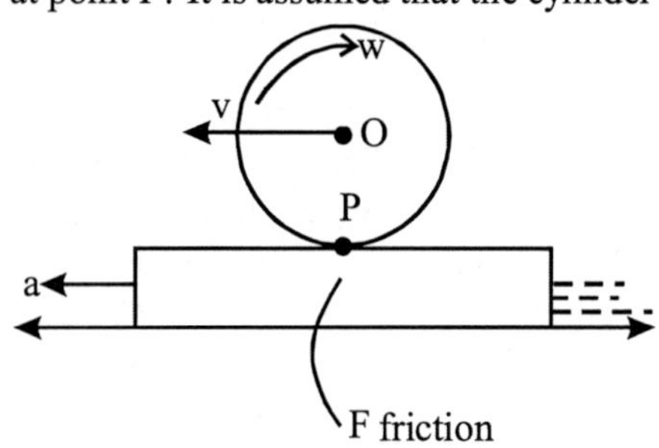

(a) Mg (b) Ma (c) $\frac{Ma}{2}$ (d) $\frac{Ma}{3}$

70. A small ball of mass m starts at a point A with speed v_o and moves along a frictionless track AB as shown. The track BC has coefficient of friction μ. The ball comes to stop at C after travelling a distance L which is:

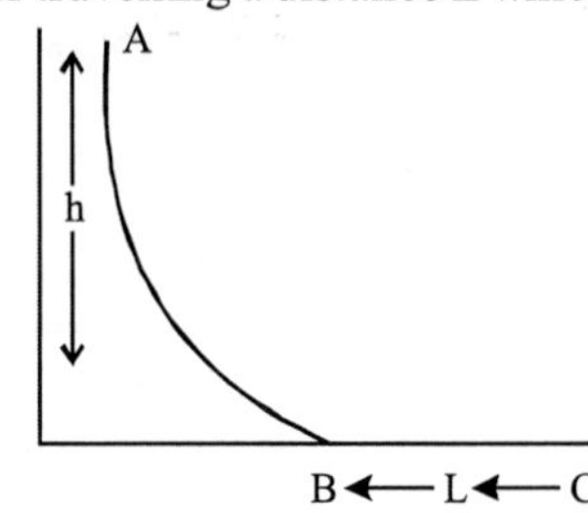

(a) $\frac{2h}{\mu}+\frac{v_o^2}{2\mu g}$ (b) $\frac{h}{\mu}+\frac{v_o^2}{2\mu g}$ (c) $\frac{h}{2\mu}+\frac{v_o^2}{\mu g}$ (d) $\frac{h}{2\mu}+\frac{v_o^2}{2\mu g}$

71. A block is placed on a rough horizontal plane. A time dependent horizontal force F = kt acts on the block, where k is a positive constant. The acceleration - time graph of the block is :

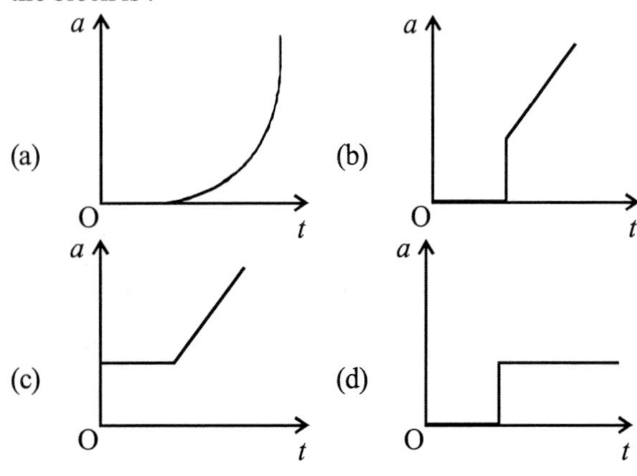

72. A block of weight W rests on a horizontal floor with coefficient of static friction μ. It is desired to make the block move by applying minimum amount of force. The angle θ from the horizontal at which the force should be applied and magnitude of the force F are respectively.

(a) $\theta=\tan^{-1}(\mu), F=\frac{\mu W}{\sqrt{1+\mu^2}}$

(b) $\theta=\tan^{-1}\left(\frac{1}{\mu}\right), F=\frac{\mu W}{\sqrt{1+\mu^2}}$

(c) $\theta=0, F=\mu W$

(d) $\theta=\tan^{-1}\left(\frac{\mu}{1+\mu}\right), F=\frac{\mu W}{1+\mu}$

73. An insect crawls up a hemispherical surface very slowly. The coefficient of friction between the insect and the surface is 1/3. If the line joining the centre of the hemispherical surface to the insect makes an angle α with the vertical, the maximum possible value of α so that the insect does not slip is given by

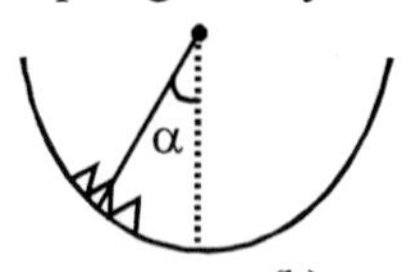

(a) cot α = 3 (b) sec α = 3
(c) cosec α = 3 (d) cos α = 3

74. A particle is released on a vertical smooth semicircular track from point X so that OX makes angle θ from the vertical (see figure). The normal reaction of the track on the particle vanishes at point Y where OY makes angle ϕ with the horizontal. Then:

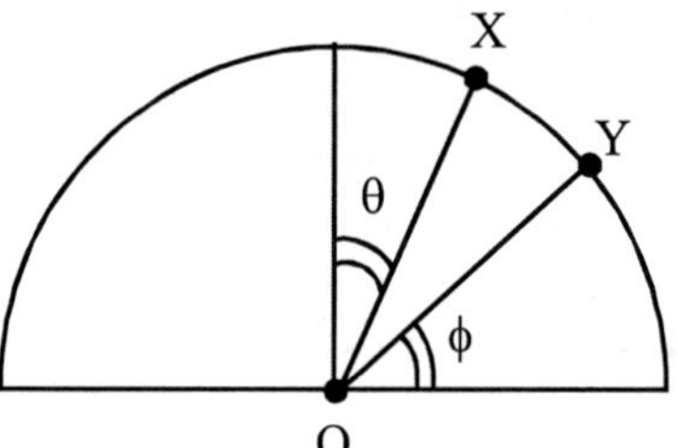

(a) sin ϕ = cos ϕ (b) $\sin\phi=\frac{1}{2}\cos\theta$

(c) $\sin\phi=\frac{2}{3}\cos\theta$ (d) $\sin\phi=\frac{3}{4}\cos\theta$

75. A conical pendulum of length 1 m makes an angle θ = 45° w.r.t. Z-axis and moves in a circle in the XY plane. The radius of the circle is 0.4 m and its centre is vertically below O. The speed of the pendulum, in its circular path, will be : (Take g = 10 ms^{-2})

(a) 0.4 m/s
(b) 4 m/s
(c) 0.2 m/s
(d) 2 m/s

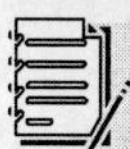

Exercise 2 - Exemplar & Past Year Questions

E&PYQs

Exemplar Questions

1. A ball is travelling with uniform translatory motion. This means that

(a) it is at rest

(b) the path can be a straight line or circular and the ball travels with uniform speed

(c) all parts of the ball have the same velocity (magnitude and direction) and the velocity is constant

(d) the centre of the ball moves with constant velocity and the ball spins about its centre uniformly

2. A metre scale is moving with uniform velocity. This implies

(a) the force acting on the scale is zero, but a torque about the centre of mass can act on the scale

(b) the force acting on the scale is zero and the torque acting about centre of mass of the scale is also zero

(c) the total force acting on it need not be zero but the torque on it is zero

(d) neither the force nor the torque need to be zero

3. A cricket ball of mass 150 g has an initial velocity $\vec{u} = (3\hat{i} + 4\hat{j})\text{ms}^{-1}$ and a final velocity $\vec{v} = -(3\hat{i} + 4\hat{j})\text{ms}^{-1}$, after being hit. The change in momentum (final momentum-initial momentum) is (in kgms^{-1})

(a) zero (b) $-(0.45\hat{i} + 0.6\hat{j})$

(c) $-(0.9\hat{j} + 1.2\hat{j})$ (d) $-5(\hat{i} + \hat{j})\hat{i}$

4. In the previous problem (3), the magnitude of the momentum transferred during the hit is

(a) zero (b) 0.75 kg-m s^{-1}

(c) 1.5 kg-m s^{-1} (d) 1.4 kg-m s^{-1}

5. Conservation of momentum in a collision between particles can be understood from

(a) Conservation of energy

(b) Newton's first law only

(c) Newton's second law only

(d) both Newton's second and third law

6. A hockey player is moving northward and suddenly turns westward with the same speed to avoid an opponent. The force that acts on the player is

(a) frictional force along westward

(b) muscle force along southward

(c) frictional force along sotuh-west

(d) muscle force along south-west

7. A body of mass 2 kg travels according to the law $x(t) = pt + qt^2 + rt^3$ where, $q = 4\text{ ms}^{-2}$, $p = 3\text{ ms}^{-1}$ and $r = 5\text{ ms}^{-3}$. The force acting on the body at $t = 2$s is

(a) 136 N (b) 134 N

(c) 158 N (d) 68 N

8. A body with mass 5 kg is acted upon by a force $\vec{F} = (-3\hat{i} + 4\hat{j})$ N. If its initial velocity at $t = 0$ is $v = (6\hat{i} - 12\hat{j})\text{ ms}^{-1}$, the time at which it will just have a velocity along the y-axis is

(a) never (b) 10 s

(c) 2 s (d) 15 s

9. A car of mass m starts from rest and acquires a velocity along east, $\vec{v} = v\hat{i}$ $(v > 0)$ in two seconds. Assuming the car moves with uniform acceleration, the force exerted on the car is

(a) $\frac{mv}{2}$ eastward and is exerted by the car engine

(b) $\frac{mv}{2}$ eastward and is due to the friction on the tyres exerted by the road

(c) more than $\frac{mv}{2}$ eastward exerted due to the engine and overcomes the friction of the road

(d) $\frac{mv}{2}$ exerted by the engine

NEET/AIPMT (2013-2020) Questions

10. Three blocks with masses m, 2 m and 3 m are connected by strings as shown in the figure. After an upward force F is applied on block m, the masses move upward at constant speed v. What is the net force on the block of mass 2m? (g is the acceleration due to gravity) ***[2013]***

(a) 2 mg

(b) 3 mg

(c) 6 mg

(d) zero

11. A car is moving in a circular horizontal track of radius 10 m with a constant speed of 10 m/s. A bob is suspended from the roof of the car by a light wire of length 1.0 m. The angle made by the wire with the vertical is ***[NEET Kar. 2013]***

(a) 0° (b) $\frac{\pi}{3}$ (c) $\frac{\pi}{6}$ (d) $\frac{\pi}{4}$

12. A balloon with mass 'm' is descending down with an acceleration 'a' (where a < g). How much mass should be removed from it so that it starts moving up with an acceleration 'a'? ***[2014]***

(a) $\frac{2ma}{g+a}$ (b) $\frac{2ma}{g-a}$ (c) $\frac{ma}{g+a}$ (d) $\frac{ma}{g-a}$

13. The force 'F' acting on a particle of mass 'm' is indicated by the force-time graph shown below. The change in momentum of the particle over the time interval from zero to 8 s is : *[2014]*

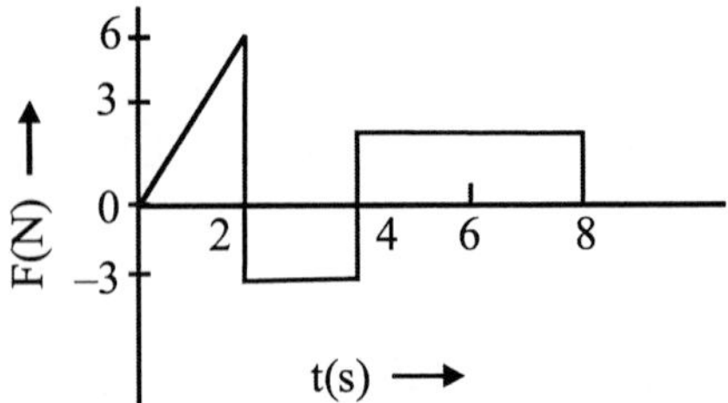

(a) 24 Ns (b) 20 Ns
(c) 12 Ns (d) 6 Ns

14. A system consists of three masses m_1, m_2 and m_3 connected by a string passing over a pulley P. The mass m_1 hangs freely and m_2 and m_3 are on a rough horizontal table (the coefficient of friction = μ). The pulley is frictionless and of negligible mass. The downward acceleration of mass m_1 is : (Assume $m_1 = m_2 = m_3 = m$) *[2014]*

P m_2 m_3 m_1

(a) $\frac{g(1-g\mu)}{g}$

(b) $\frac{2g\mu}{3}$

(c) $\frac{g(1-2\mu)}{3}$

(d) $\frac{g(1-2\mu)}{2}$

15. Two stones of masses m and 2 m are whirled in horizontal circles, the heavier one in radius $\frac{r}{2}$ and the lighter one in radius r. The tangential speed of lighter stone is n times that of the value of heavier stone when they experience same centripetal forces. The value of n is : *[2015 RS]*

(a) 3 (b) 4
(c) 1 (d) 2

16. A plank with a box on it at one end is gradually raised about the other end. As the angle of inclination with the horizontal reaches 30° the box starts to slip and slides 4.0 m down the plank in 4.0s. The coefficients of static and kinetic friction between the box and the plank will be, respectively : *[2015 RS]*

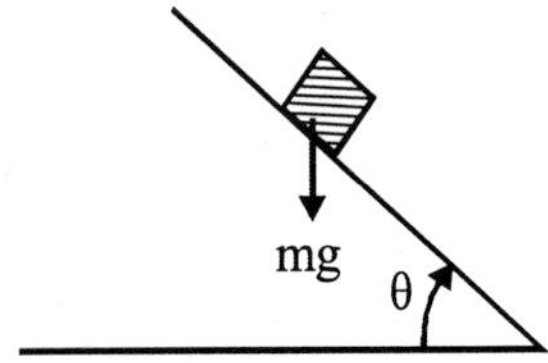

(a) 0.6 and 0.5 (b) 0.5 and 0.6
(c) 0.4 and 0.3 (d) 0.6 and 0.6

17. Three blocks A, B and C of masses 4 kg, 2 kg and 1 kg respectively, are in contact on a frictionless surface, as shown. If a force of 14 N is applied on the 4 kg block then the contact force between A and B is *[2015]*

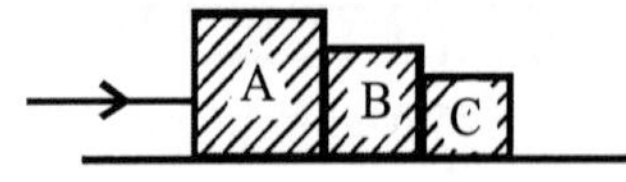

(a) 6N (b) 8N
(c) 18N (d) 2N

18. A block A of mass m_1 rests on a horizontal table. A light string connected to it passes over a frictionless pulley at the edge of table and from its other end another block B of mass m_2 is suspended. The coefficient of kinetic friction between the block and the table is μ_k. When the block A is sliding on the table, the tension in the string is *[2015]*

(a) $\frac{(m_2 - \mu k\, m_1)g}{(m_1 + m_2)}$ (b) $\frac{m_1 m_2 (1 + \mu_k)g}{(m_1 + m_2)}$

(c) $\frac{m_1 m_2 (1 - \mu_k)g}{(m_1 + m_2)}$ (d) $\frac{(m_2 + \mu_k\, m_1)g}{(m_1 + m_2)}$

19. What is the minimum velocity with which a body of mass m must enter a vertical loop of radius R so that it can complete the loop ? *[2016]*

(a) $\sqrt{gR}$ (b) $\sqrt{2gR}$
(c) $\sqrt{3gR}$ (d) $\sqrt{5gR}$

20. One end of string of length l is connected to a particle of mass 'm' and the other end is connected to a small peg on a smooth horizontal table. If the particle moves in circle with speed 'v' the net force on the particle (directed towards centre) will be (T represents the tension in the string): *[2017]*

(a) $T + \frac{mv^2}{l}$ (b) $T - \frac{mv^2}{l}$
(c) Zero (d) T

21. Two blocks A and B of masses 3 m and m respectively are connected by a massless and inextensible string. The whole system is suspended by a massless spring as shown in figure. The magnitudes of acceleration of A and B immediately after the string is cut, are respectively : *[2017]*

(a) $\frac{g}{3}, g$

(b) g, g

(c) $\frac{g}{3}, \frac{g}{3}$

(d) $g, \frac{g}{3}$

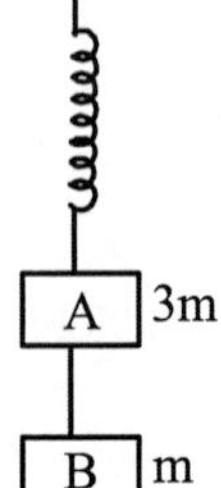

22. Which one of the following statements is incorrect? *[2018]*
(a) Rolling friction is smaller than sliding friction.
(b) Limiting value of static friction is directly proportional to normal reaction.
(c) Coefficient of sliding friction has dimensions of length.
(d) Frictional force opposes the relative motion.

23. A block of mass m is placed on a smooth inclined wedge ABC of inclination θ as shown in the figure. The wedge is given an acceleration 'a' towards the right. The relation between a and θ for the block to remain stationary on the wedge is *[2018]*

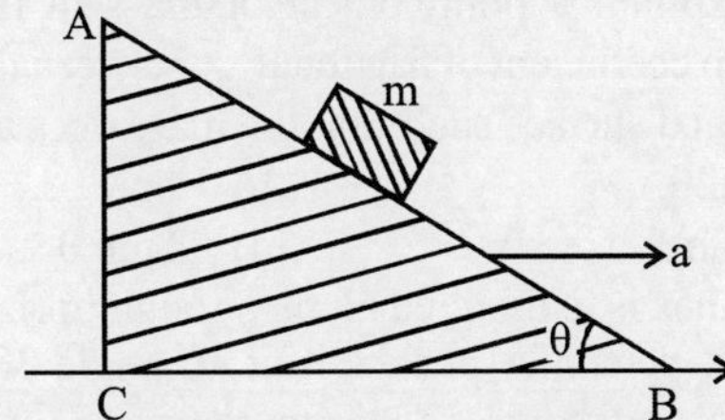

(a) $a = \frac{g}{\text{cosec}\,\theta}$ (b) $a = \frac{g}{\sin\theta}$
(c) $a = g\tan\theta$ (d) $a = g\cos\theta$

24. A block of mass 10 kg is in contact against the inner wall of a hollow cylindrical drum of radius 1 m. The coefficient of friction between the block and the inner wall of the cylinder is 0.1. The minimum angular velocity needed for the cylinder to keep the block stationary when the cylinder is vertical and rotating about its axis, will be : ($g = 10\ m/s^2$) *[2019]*
(a) $\sqrt{10}$ rad/s (b) $\frac{10}{2\pi}$ rad/s
(c) 10 rad/s (d) 10π rad/s

25. A particle moving with velocity is acted by three forces shown by the vector triangle PQR. The velocity of the particle will : *[2019]*
(a) increase
(b) decrease
(c) remain constant
(d) change according to the smallest force

26. A body of mass m is kept on a rough horizontal surface (coefficient of friction = ∝). A horizontal force is applied on the body, but it does not move. The resultant of normal reaction and the frictional force acting on the object is given by *F*, where *F* is, *[NEET Odisha 2019]*
(a) $|\vec{F}| = mg$ (b) $|\vec{F}| = mg + \propto mg$
(c) $|\vec{F}| = \propto mg$ (d) $|\vec{F}| \le mg\sqrt{1+\mu^2}$

27. Two bodies of mass 4 kg and 6 kg are tied to the ends of a massless string. The string passes over a pulley which is frictionless (see figure). The acceleration of the system in terms of acceleration due to gravity (g) is: *[2020]*

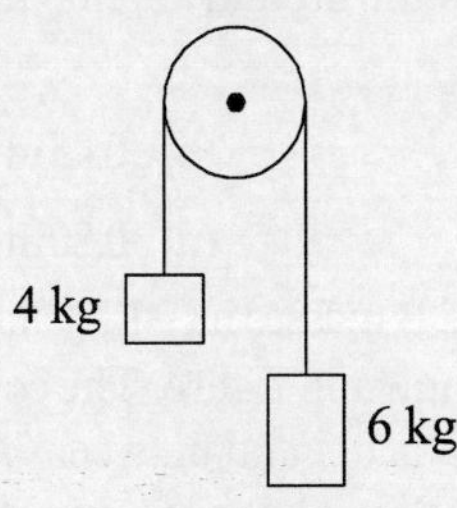

(a) g/2 (b) g/5
(c) g/10 (d) g

Exercise 3 - Concept Application Problems CAP

1. A spaceship in space sweeps stationary interplanetary dust. As a result, its mass increases at a rate $\frac{dM(t)}{dt} = bv^2(t)$, where $v(t)$ is its instantaneous velocity. The instantaneous acceleration of the satellite is :
(a) $-bv^3(t)$ (b) $-\frac{bv^3}{M(t)}$
(c) $-\frac{2bv^3}{M(t)}$ (d) $-\frac{bv^3}{2M(t)}$

2. A small ball of mass *m* is thrown upward with velocity *u* from the ground. The ball experiences a resistive force mkv^2 where *v* is its speed. The maximum height attained by the ball is :
(a) $\frac{1}{2k}\tan^{-1}\frac{ku^2}{g}$ (b) $\frac{1}{k}\ln\left(1+\frac{ku^2}{2g}\right)$
(c) $\frac{1}{k}\tan^{-1}\frac{ku^2}{2g}$ (d) $\frac{1}{2k}\ln\left(1+\frac{ku^2}{g}\right)$

3. A particle of mass m is moving in a straight line with momentum p. Starting at time t = 0, a force F = *k*t acts in the same direction on the moving particle during time interval T so that its momentum changes from p to 3p. Here *k* is a constant. The value of T is :
(a) $2\sqrt{\frac{k}{p}}$ (b) $2\sqrt{\frac{p}{k}}$ (c) $\sqrt{\frac{2k}{p}}$ (d) $\sqrt{\frac{2p}{k}}$

4. A particle of mass m is acted upon by a force F given by the empirical law $F = \frac{R}{t^2}v(t)$. If this law is to be tested experimentally by observing the motion starting from rest, the best way is to plot :
(a) log v(t) against $\frac{1}{t}$ (b) v(t) against t^2
(c) log v(t) against $\frac{1}{t^2}$ (d) log v(t) against t

5. An elevator in a building can carry a maximum of 10 persons, with the average mass of each person being 68 kg. The mass of the elevator itself is 920 kg and it moves with a constant speed of 3 m/s. The frictional force opposing the motion is 6000 N. If the elevator is moving up with its full capacity, the power delivered by the motor to the elevator ($g = 10$ m/s^2) must be at least:
(a) 56300 W (b) 62360 W
(c) 48000 W (d) 66000 W

6. A mass of 10 kg is suspended vertically by a rope from the roof. When a horizontal force is applied on the rope at some point, the rope deviated at an angle of 45° at the roof point. If the suspended mass is at equilibrium, the magnitude of the force applied is (g = 10 ms^{-2})
(a) 200 N (b) 140 N
(c) 70 N (d) 100 N

7. An insect is at the bottom of a hemispherical ditch of radius 1 m. It crawls up the ditch but starts slipping after it is at height h from the bottom. If the coefficient of friction between the ground and the insect is 0.75, then h is : (g = 10 ms^{-2})
(a) 0.20m (b) 0.45m
(c) 0.60m (d) 0.80m

8. Two blocks A and B masses $m_A = 1$ kg and $m_B = 3$ kg are kept on the table as shown in figure. The coefficient of friction between A and B is 0.2 and between B and the surface of the table is also 0.2. The maximum force F that can be applied on B horizontally, so that the block A does not slide over the block B is : [Take g = 10 m/s^2]

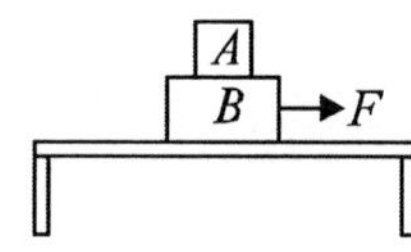

(a) 8 N (b) 16 N (c) 40 N (d) 12 N

9. A block kept on a rough inclined plane, as shown in the figure, remains at rest upto a maximum force 2 N down the inclined plane. The maximum external force up the inclined plane that does not move the block is 10 N. The coefficient of static friction between the block and the plane is : [Take g = 10 m/s^2]

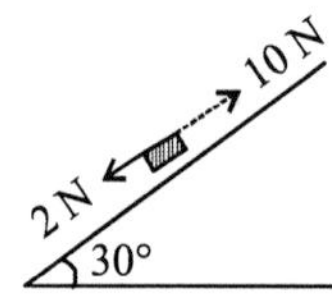

(a) $\frac{\sqrt{3}}{2}$ (b) $\frac{\sqrt{3}}{4}$
(c) $\frac{1}{2}$ (d) $\frac{2}{3}$

10. Two masses $m_1 = 5$ kg and $m_2 = 10$ kg, connected by an inextensible string over a frictionless pulley, are moving as shown in the figure. The coefficient of friction of horizontal surface is 0.15. The minimum weight m that should be put on top of m_2 to stop the motion is:
(a) 18.3 kg
(b) 27.3 kg
(c) 43.3 kg
(d) 10.3 kg

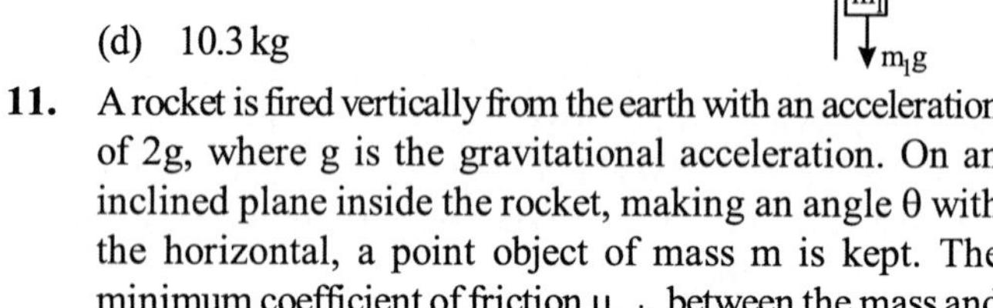

11. A rocket is fired vertically from the earth with an acceleration of 2g, where g is the gravitational acceleration. On an inclined plane inside the rocket, making an angle θ with the horizontal, a point object of mass m is kept. The minimum coefficient of friction μ_{min} between the mass and the inclined surface such that the mass does not move is:
(a) tan2θ (b) tanθ
(c) 3 tanθ (d) 2 tan θ

12. A heavy box is to dragged along a rough horizontal floor. To do so, person A pushes it at an angle 30° from the horizontal and requires a minimum force F_A, while person B pulls the box at an angle 60° from the horizontal and needs minimum force F_B. If the coefficient of friction between the box and the floor is $\frac{\sqrt{3}}{5}$, the ratio $\frac{F_A}{F_B}$ is
(a) $\sqrt{3}$ (b) $\frac{5}{\sqrt{3}}$ (c) $\sqrt{\frac{3}{2}}$ (d) $\frac{2}{\sqrt{3}}$

13. A block A of mass 4 kg is placed on another block B of mass 5 kg, and the block B rests on a smooth horizontal table. If the minimum force that can be applied on A so that both the blocks move together is 12 N, the maximum force that can be applied to B for the blocks to move together will be:
(a) 30 N (b) 25 N (c) 27 N (d) 48 N

14. A body starts from rest on a long inclined plane of slope 45°. The coefficient of friction between the body and the plane varies as $\mu = 0.3\,x$, where x is distance travelled down the plane. The body will have maximum speed (for g = 10 m/s^2) when x =
(a) 9.8 m (b) 27 m (c) 12 m (d) 3.33 m

15. A horizontal force of 10 N is necessary to just hold a block stationary against a wall. The coefficient of friction between the block and the wall is 0.2. The weight of the block is

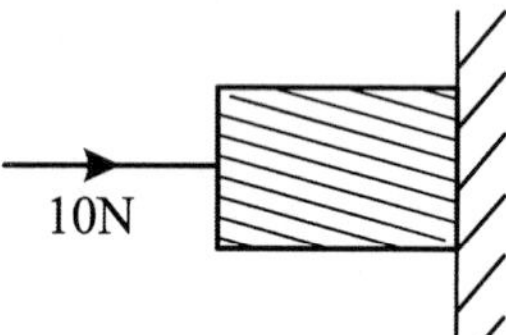

(a) 20 N (b) 50 N (c) 100 N (d) 2 N

16. A disc rotates about its axis of symmetry in a hoizontal plane at a steady rate of 3.5 revolutions per second. A coin placed at a distance of 1.25cm from the axis of rotation remains at rest on the disc. The coefficient of friction between the coin and the disc is (g = 10m/s^2)
(a) 0.5 (b) 0.7 (c) 0.3 (d) 0.6

17. An annular ring with inner and outer radii R_1 and R_2 is rolling without slipping with a uniform angular speed. The ratio of the forces experienced by the two particles situated on the inner and outer parts of the ring, $\frac{F_1}{F_2}$ is

(a) $\left(\frac{R_1}{R_2}\right)^2$ (b) $\frac{R_2}{R_1}$ (c) $\frac{R_1}{R_2}$ (d) 1

18. A uniform rope of length L resting on a frictionless horizontal surface is pulled at one end by a force F. What is the tension in the rope at a distance ℓ from the end where the force is applied.

(a) F (b) $F(1+\ell/L)$
(c) F/2 (d) $F(1-\ell/L)$

19. A mass is hanging on a spring balance which is kept in a lift. The lift ascends. The spring balance will show in its readings

(a) an increase
(b) a decrease
(c) no change
(d) a change depending on its velocity

20. A particle of mass m moving eastward with a speed v collides with another particle of the same mass moving northward with the same speed v. The two particles coalesce on collision. The new particle of mass 2m will move in the north-external direction with a velocity :

(a) v/2 (b) 2v
(c) $v/\sqrt{2}$ (d) None of these

21. A spring is compressed between two toy carts of mass m_1 and m_2. When the toy carts are released, the springs exert equal and opposite average forces for the same time on each toy cart. If v_1 and v_2 are the velocities of the toy carts and there is no friction between the toy carts and the ground, then :

(a) $v_1/v_2 = m_1/m_2$ (b) $v_1/v_2 = m_2/m_1$
(c) $v_1/v_2 = -m_2/m_1$ (d) $v_1/v_2 = -m_1/m_2$

22. A man weighing 80 kg is standing on a trolley weighing 320 kg. The trolley is resting on frictionless horizontal rails. If the man starts walking on the trolley along the rails at a speed of one metre per second, then after 4 seconds, his displacement relative to the ground will be :

(a) 5 metres (b) 4.8 metres
(c) 3.2 metres (d) 3.0 metres

23. Starting from rest, a body slides down a 45º inclined plane in twice the time it takes to slide down the same distance in the absence of friction. The coefficient of friction between the body and the inclined plane is:

(a) 0.33 (b) 0.25 (c) 0.75 (d) 0.80

24. Two blocks are connected over a massless pulley as shown in fig. The mass of block A is 10 kg and the coefficient of kinetic friction is 0.2. Block A slides down the incline at constant speed. The mass of block B in kg is:

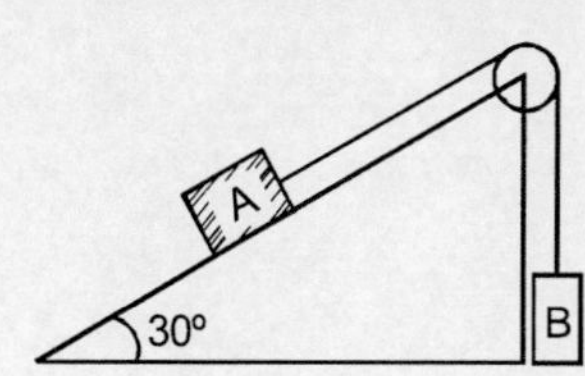

(a) 3.5 (b) 3.3 (c) 3.0 (d) 2.5

25. A particle of mass 10 kg is moving in a straight line. If its displacement, x with time t is given by $x = (t^3 - 2t - 10)$ m, then the force acting on it at the end of 4 seconds is

(a) 24 N (b) 240 N (c) 300 N (d) 1200 N

26. When forces F_1, F_2, F_3 are acting on a particle of mass m such that F_2 and F_3 are mutually perpendicular, then the particle remains stationary. If the force F_1 is now removed then the acceleration of the particle is

(a) F_1/m (b) F_2F_3/mF_1
(c) $(F_2 - F_3)/m$ (d) F_2/m

27. A body of mass 1 kg moving with a uniform velocity of $1\,ms^{-1}$. If the value of g is $5\,ms^{-2}$, then the force acting on the frictionless horizontal surface on which the body is moving is

(a) 5 N (b) 1 N (c) 0 N (d) 10N

28. A trailer of mass 1000 kg is towed by means of a rope attached to a car moving at a steady speed along a level road. The tension in the rope is 400 N. The car starts to accelerate steadily. If the tension in the rope is now 1650 N, with what acceleration is the trailer moving ?

(a) $1.75\,ms^{-2}$ (b) $0.75\,ms^{-2}$
(c) $2.5\,ms^{-2}$ (d) $1.25\,ms^{-2}$

29. Blocks A and B of masses 15 kg and 10 kg, respectively, are connected by a light cable passing over a frictionless pulley as shown below. Approximately what is the acceleration experienced by the system?

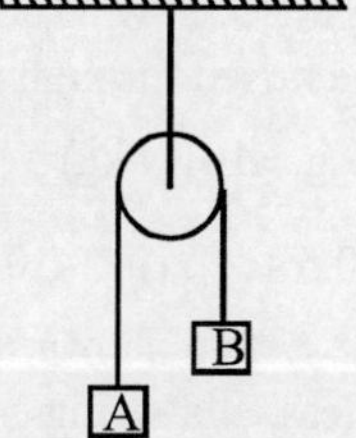

(a) $2.0\,m/s^2$

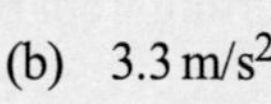
(b) $3.3\,m/s^2$

(c) $4.9\,m/s^2$

(d) $9.8\,m/s^2$

30. Block A is moving with acceleration A along a frictionless horizontal surface. When a second block, B is placed on top of Block A the acceleration of the combined blocks drops to 1/5 the original value. What is the ratio of the mass of A to the mass of B?

(a) 5 : 1 (b) 1 : 4 (c) 3 : 1 (d) 2 : 1

31. A 5000 kg rocket is set for vertical firing. The exhaust speed is 800 m/s. To give an initial upward acceleration of 20 m/s^2, the amount of gas ejected per second to supply the needed thrust will be (Take g = 10 m/s^2)

(a) 127.5 kg/s (b) 137.5 kg/s
(c) 155.5 kg/s (d) 187.5 kg/s

32. A rifle man, who together with his rifle has a mass of 100 kg, stands on a smooth surface and fires 10 shots horizontally. Each bullet has a mass 10 g and a muzzle velocity of $800\,ms^{-1}$. The velocity which the rifle man attains after firing 10 shots is

(a) $8\,ms^{-1}$ (b) $0.8\,ms^{-1}$ (c) $0.08\,ms^{-1}$ (d) $-0.8\,ms^{-1}$

33. A block of mass 4 kg rests on an inclined plane. The inclination to the plane is gradually increased. It is found that when the inclination is 3 in 5, the block just begins to slidedown the plane. The coefficient of friction between the block and the plane is

(a) 0.4 (b) 0.6 (c) 0.8 (d) 0.75.

34. A triangular block of mass M with angles 30°, 60°, and 90° rests with its 30°–90° side on a horizontal table. A cubical block of mass m rests on the 60°–30° side. The acceleration which M must have relative to the table to keep m stationary relative to the triangular block assuming frictionless contact is

(a) g (b) $\frac{g}{\sqrt{2}}$ (c) $\frac{g}{\sqrt{3}}$ (d) $\frac{g}{\sqrt{5}}$

35. An object is resting at the bottom of two strings which are inclined at an angle of 120° with each other. Each string can withstand a tension of 20N. The maximum weight of the object that can be supported without breaking the string is

(a) 5 N (b) 10 N (c) 20 N (d) 40 N

36. On a smooth plane surface (figure) two block A and B are accelerated up by applying a force 15 N on A. If mass of B is twice that of A, the force on B is

(a) 30 N (b) 15 N (c) 10 N (d) 5 N

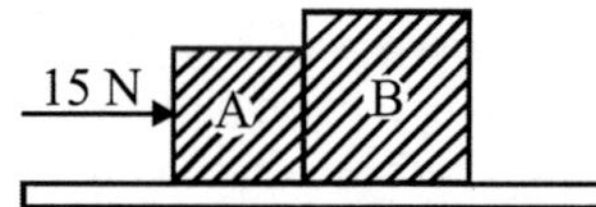

37. A 10 kg stone is suspended with a rope of breaking strength 30 kg-wt. The minimum time in which the stone can be raised through a height 10 m starting from rest is (Take $g = 10 N/kg$)

(a) 0.5 s (b) 1.0 s (c) $\sqrt{2/3}$ s (d) 2 s

38. In the system shown in figure, the pulley is smooth and massless, the string has a total mass 5g, and the two suspended blocks have masses 25 g and 15 g. The system is released from state $\ell = 0$ and is studied upto stage $\ell' = 0$ During the process, the acceleration of block A will be

(a) constant at $\frac{g}{9}$

(b) constant at $\frac{g}{4}$

(c) increasing by factor of 3

(d) increasing by factor of 2

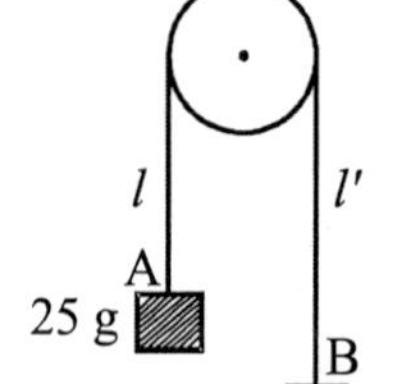

39. Three blocks of masses m_1, m_2 and m_3 are connected by massless strings, as shown, on a frictionless table. They are pulled with a force $T_3 = 40$ N. If $m_1 = 10$ kg, $m_2 = 6$ kg and $m_3 = 4$kg, the tension T_2 will be

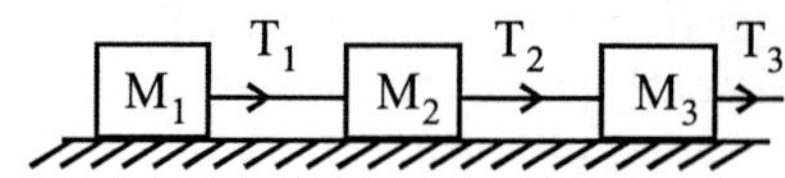

(a) 20 N (b) 40 N

(c) 10 N (d) 32 N

40. A ball mass m falls vertically to the ground from a height h_1 and rebounds to a height h_2. The change in momentum of the ball of striking the ground is

(a) $m\sqrt{2g(h_1 + h_2)}$ (b) $n\sqrt{2g(m_1 + m_2)}$

(c) $mg(h_1 - h_2)$ (d) $m(\sqrt{2gh_1} - \sqrt{2gh_2})$

41. Consider a car moving on a straight road with a speed of 100 m/s . The distance at which car can be stopped is $[\mu_k = 0.5]$

(a) 1000 m (b) 800 m (c) 400 m (d) 100 m

42. A conveyor belt is moving at a constant speed of 2m/s. A box is gently dropped on it. The coefficient of friction between them is $\mu = 0.5$. The distance that the box will move relative to belt before coming to rest on it taking $g = 10\ ms^{-2}$, is

(a) 1.2m (b) 0.6m (c) zero (d) 0.4m

43. A person of mass 60 kg is inside a lift of mass 940 kg and presses the button on control panel. The lift starts moving upwards with an acceleration $1.0\ m/s^2$. If $g = 10\ ms^{-2}$, the tension in the supporting cable is

(a) 8600N (b) 9680N (c) 11000N (d) 1200N

44. Two particles of masses m and M $(M > m)$ are connected by a cord that passes over a massless, frictionless pulley. The tension T in the string and the acceleration a of the particles is

(a) $T = \frac{2mM}{(M-m)}g; a = \frac{Mm}{(M+m)}g$

(b) $T = \frac{2mM}{(M+m)}g; a = \left(\frac{M-m}{(M+m)}\right)g$

(c) $T = \left(\frac{m-M}{(M+m)}\right)g; a = \left(\frac{Mm}{(M+m)}\right)g$

(d) $T = \left(\frac{mM}{(M+m)}\right)g; a = \left(\frac{2Mm}{(M+m)}\right)g$

45. A bullet of mass m is fired from a gun of mass M. The recoiling gun compresses a spring of force constant k by a distance d. Then the velocity of the bullet is

(a) $kd\sqrt{M/m}$ (b) $\frac{d}{M}\sqrt{km}$

(c) $\frac{d}{m}\sqrt{kM}$ (d) $\frac{kM}{m}\sqrt{d}$

Hints & Solutions

5.1 Concept Practice Problems

1. (a) Impulse = change in momentum = $m\vec{v}_2 - m\vec{v}_1$
2. (c) The equations of motion are
$2\,mg - T = 2ma$
$T - mg = ma \Rightarrow T = 4ma$ & $a = g/3$ so $T = 4mg/3$
If pulley is accelerated upwards with an accleration a, then tension in string is
$$T = \frac{4m}{3}(g+a)$$
3. (b) Inertia is resistance to change.
4. (a) Based on Newton's third law of motion.
5. (b) Here $u = 10\ ms^{-1}$, $v = -2\ ms^{-1}$, $t = 4$ s, $a = ?$
Using $a = \frac{v-u}{t} = \frac{-2-10}{4} = -3\ m/s^2$
$\therefore$ Force, $F = ma = 10\times(-3) = -30$ N
6. (b) $2\,T\cos 60^\circ = mg$
or $T = mg = 2\times10 = 20$ N.
7. (d) Here $m = 0.5$ kg ; $u = -10$ m/s ;
$t = 1/50$ s ; $v = +15\ ms^{-1}$
Force $= m(v-u)/t = 0.5\,(10+15)\times 50 = 625$ N
8. (c) Acceleration, $a = \frac{v-u}{t} = \frac{0-6}{3} = -2\ ms^{-2}$
Force $= m\times a = 4\times2 = 8$ N
9. (b) $R = mg - ma = 0.5\times10 - 0.5\times2 = 5-1 = 4$ N
10. (b) Initial thrust on the rocket $= \frac{\Delta m}{\Delta t}v_{rel} = 500\times1 = 500$ N
where $\frac{\Delta m}{\Delta t}$ = rate of ejection of fuel.

5.2 Concept Practice Problems

11. (b) See fig.

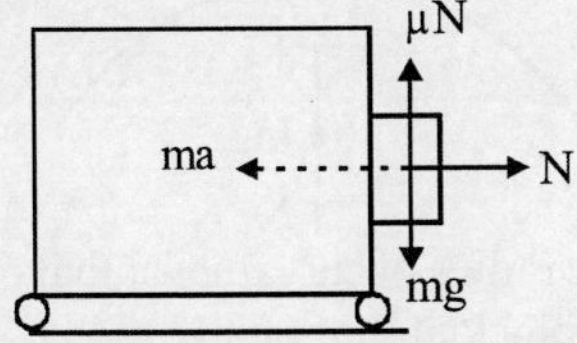

If a = acceleration of the cart, then N = ma
$\therefore \mu N = mg$ or $\mu\,ma = mg$ or $a = g/\mu$
12. (c) $f = \mu W$
$f = W\tan\theta\ [\therefore \mu = \tan\theta]$
13. (b) From the F.B.D.
$N = mg\cos\theta$
$F = ma = mg\sin\theta - \mu N$
$\Rightarrow\ a = g(\sin\theta - \mu\cos\theta)$
Now using, $v^2 - u^2 = 2as$

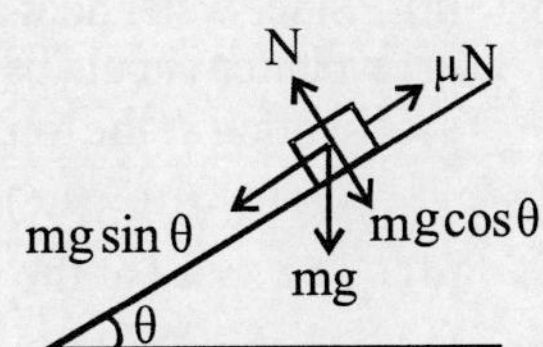

or, $v^2 = 2\times g(\sin\theta - \mu\cos\theta)\ell$
(ℓ = length of incline)
or, $v = \sqrt{2g\ell(\sin\theta - \mu\cos\theta)}$
14. (a) Here, on resolving force F_2 and applying the concept of equilibrium

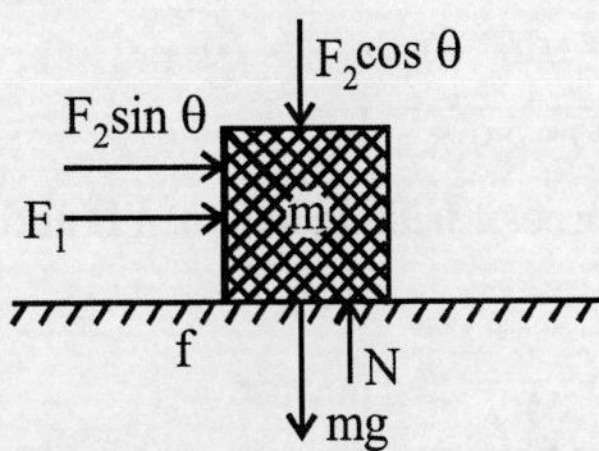

$N = mg + F_2\cos\theta$, and $f = \mu N$
$\therefore\ f = \mu[mg + F_2\cos\theta]$ ...(i)
Also $f = F_1 + F_2\sin\theta$ ...(ii)
From (i) and (ii)
$\mu[mg + F_2\cos\theta] = F_1 + F_2\sin\theta$
$$\Rightarrow \mu = \frac{F_1 + F_2\sin\theta}{mg + F_2\cos\theta}$$
15. (d) Angle of friction = $\tan^{-1}\mu$
16. (c) For block A, $T - \mu N = 5a$ and $N = 5g$

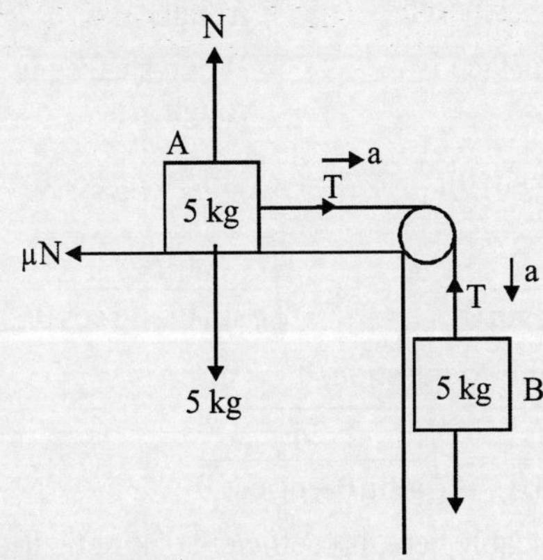

for block B, $5g - T = 5a$
$\Rightarrow T = 36.75$N, $a = 2.45$ m/sec²
17. (d) Limiting friction $= 0.5\times2\times10 = 10$N
The applied force is less than force of friction, therefore the force of friction is equal to the applied force.
18. (d) Here $\tan\theta = 0.8$
where θ is angle of repose
$\theta = \tan^{-1}(0.8) = 39^\circ$
The given angle of inclination is equal to the angle of repose. So the 1 kg block has no tendency to move.
$\therefore\ mg\sin\theta$ = force of friction
$\Rightarrow T = 0$

19. (d)

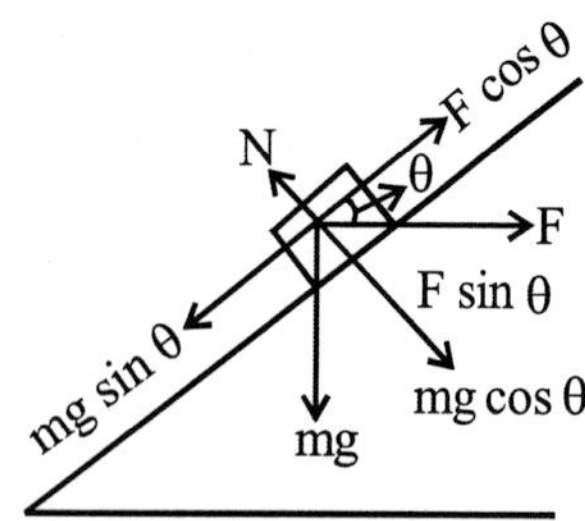

From figure $N = mg\cos\theta + F\sin\theta$

20. (b) $\mu mg = mv^2/r$ or $v = \sqrt{\mu g r}$

or $v = \sqrt{(0.25 \times 9.8 \times 20)} = 7\ m/s$

21. (d) F_1 = Force of friction between B and A

$= \mu_1 m_1 g$

$= 0.25 \times 100 \times g = 25\ g$ newton

F_2 = Force of friction between (A + B) and surface

$= \mu_2 m_2 g = \mu_2$ (mass of A and B) g

$= \frac{1}{3}(100+200)g = \frac{300}{3}g = 100g$ newton $\therefore\ F = F_1 + F_2$

$= 25\ g + 100\ g = 25g = 125 \times 10\ N \qquad \therefore F = 1250\ N$

22. (b)

d, $g\sin\theta$, d, 45°, smooth

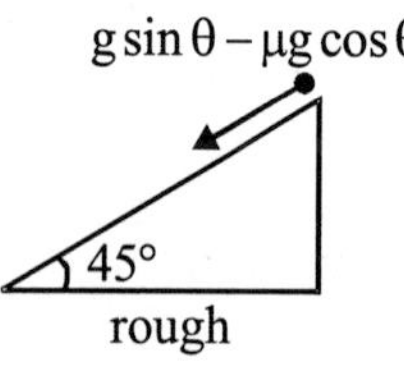

When surface is smooth

When surface is rough

$d = \frac{1}{2}(g\sin\theta)t_1^2, \quad d = \frac{1}{2}(g\sin\theta - \mu g\cos\theta)t_2^2$

$t_1 = \sqrt{\frac{2d}{g\sin\theta}}, \qquad t_2 = \sqrt{\frac{2d}{g\sin\theta - \mu g\cos\theta}}$

According to question, $t_2 = nt_1$

$n\sqrt{\frac{2d}{g\sin\theta}} = \sqrt{\frac{2d}{g\sin\theta - \mu g\cos\theta}}$

μ, applicable here, is coefficient of kinetic friction as the block moves over the inclined plane.

$n = \frac{1}{\sqrt{1-\mu_k}} \qquad \left(\because \cos 45° = \sin 45° = \frac{1}{\sqrt{2}}\right)$

$n^2 = \frac{1}{1-\mu_k} \qquad$ or $1 - \mu_k = \frac{1}{n^2}$

or $\mu_k = 1 - \frac{1}{n^2}$

23. (d) Acceleration of block while sliding down upper half $= g\sin\phi$;

retardation of block while sliding down lower half = – $(g\sin\phi - \mu g\cos\phi)$

For the block to come to rest at the bottom, acceleration in I half = retardation in II half.

$g\sin\phi = -(g\sin\phi - \mu g\cos\phi)$

$\Rightarrow \mu = 2\tan\phi$

24. (b)

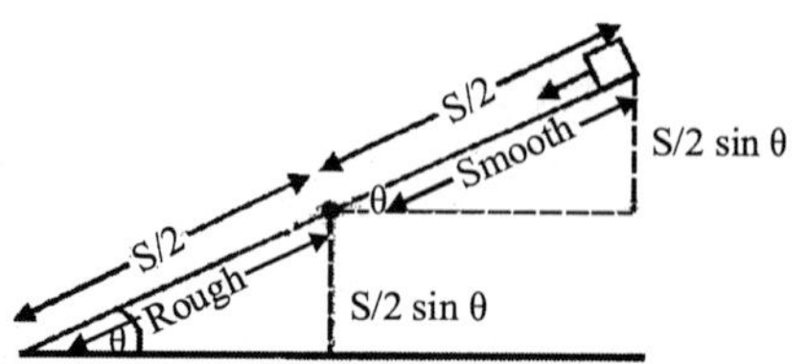

For upper half of inclined plane

$v^2 = u^2 + 2a\ S/2 = 2\ (g\sin\theta)\ S/2 = gS\sin\theta$

For lower half of inclined plane

$0 = u^2 + 2\ g\ (\sin\theta - \mu\cos\theta)\ S/2$

$\Rightarrow -gS\sin\theta = gS\ (\sin\theta - \mu\cos\theta) \Rightarrow 2\sin\theta = \mu\cos\theta$

$\Rightarrow \mu = \frac{2\sin\theta}{\cos\theta} = 2\tan\theta$

25. (a) The force of friction on the chain lying on the table should be equal to the weight of the hanging chain. Let

ρ = mass per unit length of the chain

μ = coefficient of friction

l = length of the total chain

x = length of hanging chain

Now, $\mu(l-x)\rho g = x\rho g$ or $\mu(l-x) = x$

or $\mu l = (\mu+1)x$ or $x = \mu l/(\mu+1)$

$\therefore\ x = \frac{0.25l}{(0.25+1)} = \frac{0.25l}{1.25} = 0.2l$

$\frac{x}{l} = 0.2 = 20\%$

5.3 Concept Practice Problems CPP

26. (b) Centripetal force is always perpendicular to direction of motion.

27. (a) At the highest point of the track, $N + mg = \frac{mv'^2}{r}$

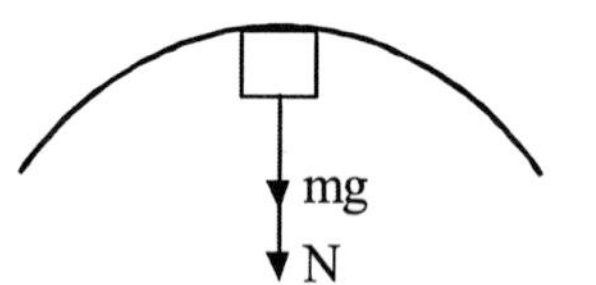

where r is the radius of curvature at that point and v′ is the speed of the block at that point.

Now $N = \frac{mv'^2}{r} - mg$

N will be maximum when r is minimum (v′ is the same for all cases). Of the given tracks, (a) has the smallest radius of curvature at the highest point.

28. (a) Since water does not fall down, therefore the velocity of revolution should be just sufficient to provide centripetal acceleration at the top of vertical circle. So,

$v = \sqrt{(gr)} = \sqrt{\{10 \times (1.6)\}} = \sqrt{(16)} = 4$ m/sec.

29. (d) The speed at the highest point must be $v \geq \sqrt{rg}$

Now $v = r\omega = r(2\pi/T)$

$\therefore\ r(2\pi/T) > \sqrt{rg}$ or $T < \frac{2\pi r}{\sqrt{rg}} < 2\pi\sqrt{\left(\frac{r}{g}\right)}$

$\therefore\ T = 2\pi\sqrt{\left(\frac{4}{9.8}\right)} = 4\,\text{sec}$

30. (a) From figure,

$N\sin\theta = \frac{mv^2}{r}$ .... (i)

$N\cos\theta = mg$ ...... (ii)

Dividing, we get

$\tan\theta = \frac{v^2}{rg}$ or $\theta = \tan^{-1}\frac{v^2}{rg}$

31. (a) In the case of a body describing a vertical circle,

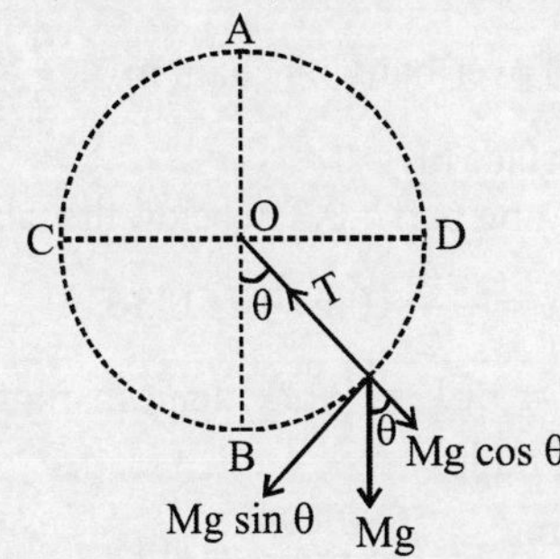

$T - mg\cos\theta = \frac{mv^2}{l}$ $\quad T = mg\cos\theta + \frac{mv^2}{l}$

Tension is maximum when $\cos\theta = +1$ and velocity is maximum

Both conditions are satisfied at $\theta = 0°$ (i.e. at lowest point B)

32. (b) Since surface (ice) is frictionless, so the centripetal force required for skating will be provided by inclination of boy with the vertical and that angle is given as

$\tan\theta = \frac{v^2}{rg}$ where v is speed of skating & r is radius of circle in which he moves.

33. (c)

34. (a) $R = mg\cos\theta - \frac{mV^2}{r}$

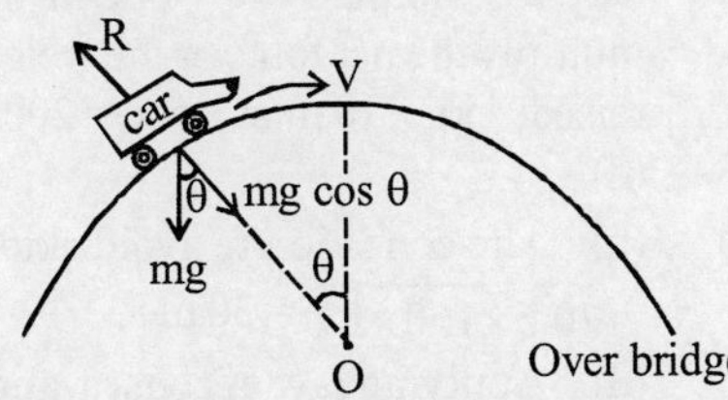

When θ decreases, cosθ increases i.e. R increases

35. (b) When car is at the lowest point of the concave bridge, then $R = mg + \frac{mv^2}{r}$.

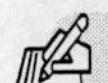 Exercise 1 - Chapter Revision Problems CRP

1. (c) Friction does not depend on the area of surfaces in contact.
2. (d) 3. (a) 4. (c) 5. (a) 6. (a)
7. (a) Let a be the acceleration of mass m_2 in the downward direction. Then

$T - m_2(g/2) = m_1 a$ ....(i)

and $m_2 g - T = m_2 a$ ....(ii)

Adding eqs. (1) and (2), we get

$(m_1 + m_2)a = m_2 g - m_2(g/2) = m_2 g/2$

$\therefore\ a = \frac{m_2 g}{2(m_1 + m_2)}$

8. (b) The time rate of change of momentum is force.

9. (a) $S_n = \frac{a}{2}(2n-1)$

$S_{n+1} = \frac{a}{2}(2n+1)$

$\frac{S_n}{S_{n+1}} = \frac{2n-1}{2n+1}$

10. (a) If m_1, m_2 are masses and u_1, u_2 are velocity then by conservation of momentum $m_1u_1 + m_2u_2 = 0$ or $|m_1u_1| = |m_2u_2|$

11. (a) The frictional force acting on M is μmg

$\therefore$ Acceleration $= \frac{\mu mg}{M}$

12. (c) If k is the spring factor, then P.E. of the spring compressed by distance x $\left(= \frac{1}{2}kx^2\right)$ will equal to gain in P.E. of the dart (= mgh) i.e. $\frac{1}{2}kx^2 = mgh$

$\therefore\ \frac{1}{2}k(4)^2 = 16\times g\times 200$ ....(i)

and $\frac{1}{2}k(6)^2 = 16\times g\times h$ ...(ii)

On solving, (i) and (ii), we get h = 450 cm = 4.5 m.

13. (b) As, $(1/2)mv^2 = Fs$

So $\frac{1}{2}m(30)^2 = F\times 4$ and $\frac{1}{2}m(60)^2 = F\times s$

$\therefore\ s/4 = (60)^2/(30)^2 = 4$ or $s = 4\times 4 = 16$ m.

14. (a) Force required $= \frac{\text{change in momentum}}{\text{time taken}}$

$= \frac{(50\times 10^{-3}\times 30)\times 400 - (5\times 0)}{60} = 10$ N

15. (a) Change in momentum = Force × time = Area which the force-time curve encloses with time axis.

16. (b)

10cm 20cm

20N(F_1) ← F ← | → F → 32N(F_2)

l_1 l_2

→ L ←

It is clear $F_2 > F_1$, so rod moves in right direction with an acceleration a, whereas a is given by

$(F_2 - F_1) = mL\times a$...............(i)

where m is mass of rod per unit length.

Now consider the motion of length l_1 from first end, then

$F - F_1 = ml_1 a$.................(ii)

Dividing eq (ii) by (i), we get

$\frac{F - F_1}{F_2 - F_1} = \frac{l_1}{L}$ or $F = (F_2 - F_1)\times\frac{l_1}{L} + F_1$

here $l_1 = 10$ cm., $L = 30$ cm., $F_1 = 20$ N, $F_2 = 32$N
so $F = 24$ N

17. (b) Change in momentum $= F \times t$
$= 10 \times 10 = 100$ Ns or 100 kg. m/s

18. (d) See fig.

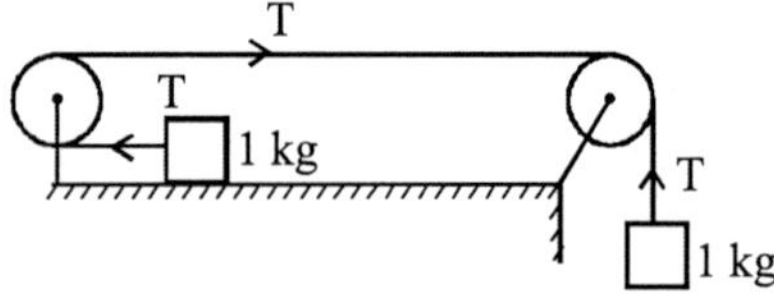

From figure, $1\,g - T = 1\,a$ ...(i)
and $T = 1\,a$ ....(ii)
From eqs. (i) and (ii), we get
$1g - 1a = 1a$ or $2a = g$
$\therefore a = (g/2) = (10/2) = 5\ m/s^2$
So, $T = ma = 1 \times 5 = 5$ N

19. (c) See fig. Let F be the force between the blocks and a their common acceleration. Then for 2 kg block,

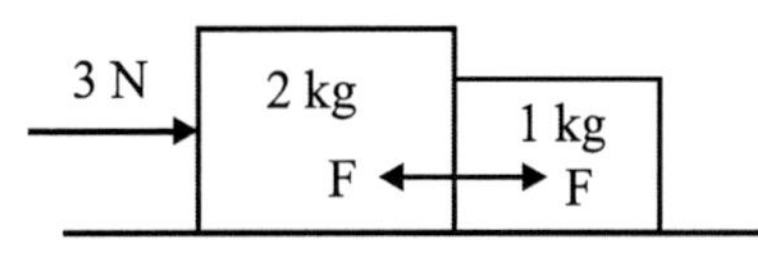

$3 - F = 2\,a$ ...(1)
for 1 kg block, $F = 1 \times a = a$ ....(2)
$\therefore 3 - F = 2\,F$ or $3\,F = 3$ or $F = 1$ newton

20. (b) $T = m(g + a)$

$48000 = 4000(10 + a) \Rightarrow a = 2\ ms^{-2}$

21. (b) $T_1 = m(g + a) = 0.1(10 + 5) = 1.5N$
$T_2 = m(g - a) = 0.1(10 - 5) = 0.5N$
$\Rightarrow T_1 - T_2 = (1.5 - 0.5)N = 1N$

22. (a) $F = \dfrac{mv - (-mv)}{t} = \dfrac{2mv}{t} = \dfrac{2 \times 0.5 \times 2}{10^{-3}} = 2 \times 10^3 N$

23. (b) $T = m\,(g + a) = 100\,(9.8 + 0) = 980$ N

24. (c) $T = m(g+a) = 100(9.8+1) = 1080N$

25. (a) Force on the slab ($m = 40$ kg) = reaction of frictional force on the upper block

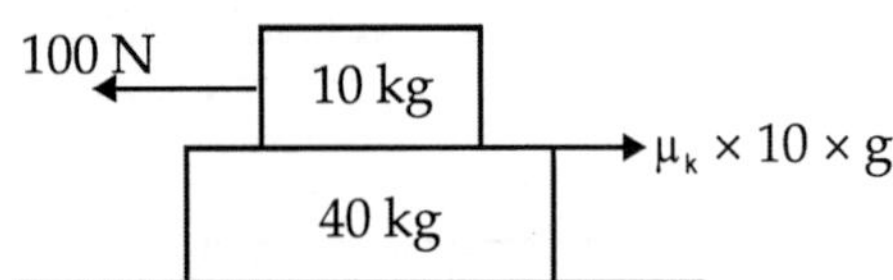

$\therefore 40a = \mu_k \times 10 \times g$ or $a = 0.98\ m/sec^2$

26. (d) $mv_1 + 3mv_2 = 0$ or $\dfrac{v_1}{v_2} = -3$

Now $\dfrac{1}{2}mv_1^2 = F.S_1 = \mu.mg.S_1$

$\dfrac{1}{2}(3m)\,v_2^2 = F.S_2 = \mu.3mg.S_2$

or $\dfrac{S_1}{S_2} = \dfrac{v_1^2}{v_2^2} = \dfrac{9}{1}$

27. (c)

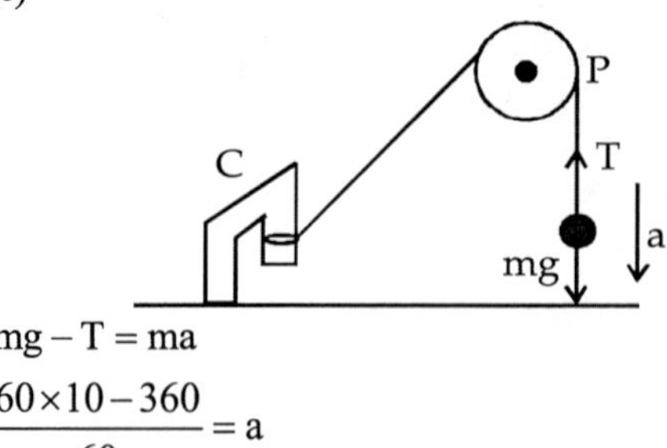

$mg - T = ma$

$\dfrac{60 \times 10 - 360}{60} = a$

$a = 4\ ms^{-2}$

28. (b) $m = \dfrac{\sqrt{8^2 + (-6)^2 + (-10)^2}}{1} = 10\sqrt{2}$kg

29. (b) Mass of over hanging chain $m' = \dfrac{4}{2} \times (0.6)$kg

Let at the surface PE = 0
C.M. of hanging part = 0.3 m below the table

$U_i = -m'gx = -\dfrac{4}{2} \times 0.6 \times 10 \times 0.30$

$\Delta U = m'gx = 3.6J$ = Work done in putting the entire chain on the table

30. (a) $\dfrac{dm}{dt} = \dfrac{mg}{v_r} = \dfrac{5000 \times 9.8}{1000} = 49\text{kg}\,s^{-1}$

31. (a) Momentum is always conserved. Since the skater and snowball are initially at rest, the initial momentum is zero. Therefore, the final momentum after the toss must also be zero.

$P_{skater} + P_{snowball} = 0$

or $m_{skater}v_{skater} + m_{snowball}v_{snowball} = 0$

$v_{skater} = -m_{snowball}v_{snowball} / m_{skater}$

$= \dfrac{-(0.15kg)(35m/s) =}{(50kg)} - 0.10m/s$

The negative sign indicates that the momenta of the skater and the snowball are in opposite directions.

32. (d) Work is the product of force and distance. The easiest way to calculate the work in this pulley problem is to multiply the net force or the weight *mg* by the distance it is raised: 4 kg x 10 m/s^2 x 5 m = 200 J.

33. (d)

34. (b) The condition to avoid skidding, $v = \sqrt{\mu rg}$
$= \sqrt{0.6 \times 150 \times 10} = 30$ m/s.

35. (d) Applying law of conservation of momentum
Momentum of bullet = Momentum of sand-bullet system

$\dfrac{m}{20}v = \left(m + \dfrac{m}{20}\right)V = \dfrac{21}{20}mV$

36. (d) For 0.5 kg block, $6 = 0.5\,a$

37. (b) While moving down, when the lift is accelerating the weight will be less and when the lift is decelerating the weight will be more.

38. (b) Total momentum $= 2p\hat{i} + p\hat{j}$
Magnitude of total momentum

$= \sqrt{(2p)^2 + p^2} = \sqrt{5p^2} = \sqrt{5}p$

This must be equal to the momentum of the third part.

39. (d) Apparent weight when mass is falling down is given by $W' = m(g-a)$

$\therefore \quad W' = 1 \times (10-10) = 0$

40. (b) Reading of spring balance

$2T = \frac{4m_1m_2}{m_1+m_2} = \frac{4\times5\times1}{6} = \frac{10}{3}$ kgf

41. (a) $a = 2v$ (given)

$\Rightarrow \quad v\frac{dv}{ds} = 2v$ or $dv = 2ds$

$\int_{0.1}^{v} dv = 2[s]_0^{0.1} = 0.2$

$v - 0.1 = 0.2 \Rightarrow v = 0.3\text{ms}^{-1}$

42. (a) Let the air resistance be F. Then

$mg + F = ma \Rightarrow F = m[a-g]$

Here $a = \frac{30}{2.5} = 12\text{ms}^{-2}$

43. (c) $F = \frac{m(v-u)}{t} = \frac{0.15(0-20)}{0.1} = 30\text{ N}$

44. (d) $v_{max} = \sqrt{\mu gr}$

45. (b)

46. (c) Linear momentum, $P = a + bt^2$

$\frac{dP}{dt} = 2bt$ (on differentiation)

$\therefore$ Rate of change of momentum, $\frac{dP}{dt} \propto t$

By 2nd law of motion, $\frac{dP}{dt} \propto F \qquad \therefore \; F \propto t$

47. (a) Velocity of ball after dropping it from a height of 5 m

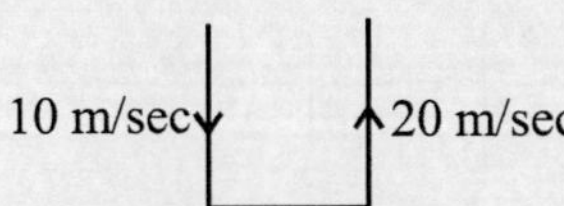

(using $v^2 = u^2 + 2gh$)

$v^2 = 0 + 2 \times 10 \times 5 \Rightarrow v = 10$ m/s

Velocity gained by ball by force exerted by bat

$0 = u^2 - 2gh$

$u^2 = 2 \times 10 \times 20$ or $u = 20$ m/s

Change in momentum $= m(u+v) = 0.4(20+10) = 12$ kg m/s

$F = \frac{\Delta P}{\Delta t}$ or $\Delta t = \frac{\Delta P}{F}$

$\Delta t = \frac{12}{100} = 0.12\text{ sec}$

48. (b) The rain drops falling vertically with velocity u do not affect the momentum along the horizontal track. A vector has no component in a perpendicular direction

Rain drops add to the mass of the car

Mass added in t sec = (mt) kg

Momentum is conserved along horizontal track.

Initial mass of car = M

Initial velocity of car $= v_0$

Final velocity of (car + water) = v

Mass of (car + water) after time t = (M + mt)

$\therefore$ final momentum = initial momentum

$(M+mt)v = Mv_0 \qquad \therefore \; v = \frac{Mv_0}{(M+mt)}$

49. (b) T = tension is the string

$\therefore$ Applied force F = 2T

$T = F/2 \qquad \ldots$(i)

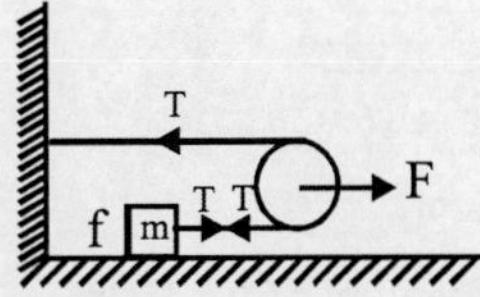

For block of mass m, force of friction due to surface f.

For sliding the block

T – f = force on the block = mass × acceleration

or acceleration of block $= \frac{T-f}{m}$. Put T from (i)

$\therefore \quad$ Acceleration $= \frac{\frac{F}{2} - f}{m}$

50. (c) Mass (m) = 0.3 kg $\Rightarrow F = m.a = -15x$

$a = -\frac{15}{0.3}x = \frac{-150}{3}x = -50x$

$a = -50 \times 0.2 = 10\text{ m/s}^2$

51. (c) From free body diagram,

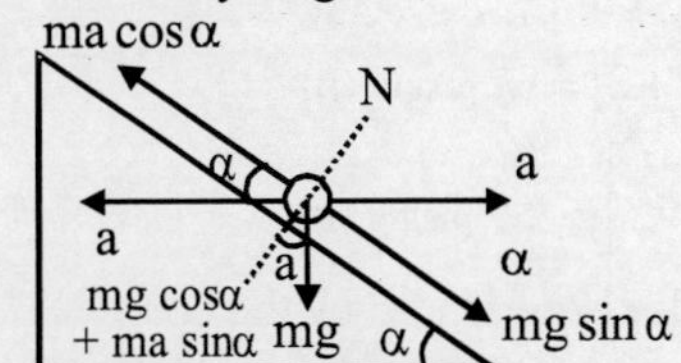

For block to remain stationary,

$mg\sin\alpha = ma\cos\alpha \Rightarrow a = g\tan\alpha$

52. (a) $N = ma\sin\theta + mg\cos\theta$ ......(1)

also $mg\sin\theta = ma\cos\theta$ ......(2)

from (2) $a = g\tan\theta$

$\therefore N = mg\frac{\sin^2\theta}{\cos\theta} + mg\cos\theta$,

or $N = \frac{mg}{\cos\theta}$

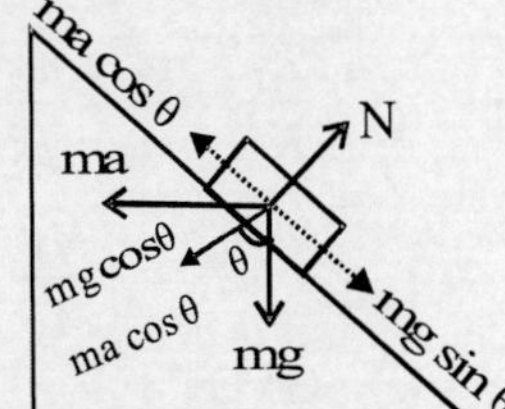

53. (a) $m_Bg = \mu_s m_Ag \quad \{\because m_Ag = \mu_s m_Ag\}$

$\Rightarrow m_B = \mu_s m_A$

or $m_B = 0.2 \times 2 = 0.4$ kg

54. (c) $\vec{F} = 6\hat{i} - 8\hat{j} + 10\hat{k}$,

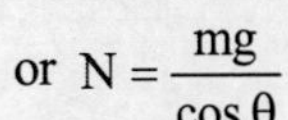

$|F| = \sqrt{36+64+100} = 10\sqrt{2}$ N $\quad \left(\because F = \sqrt{F_x^2 + F_y^2 + F_z^2}\right)$

$a = 1\text{ ms}^{-2} \qquad \because F = ma$

$\therefore \quad m = \frac{10\sqrt{2}}{1} = 10\sqrt{2}$ kg

55. (a)

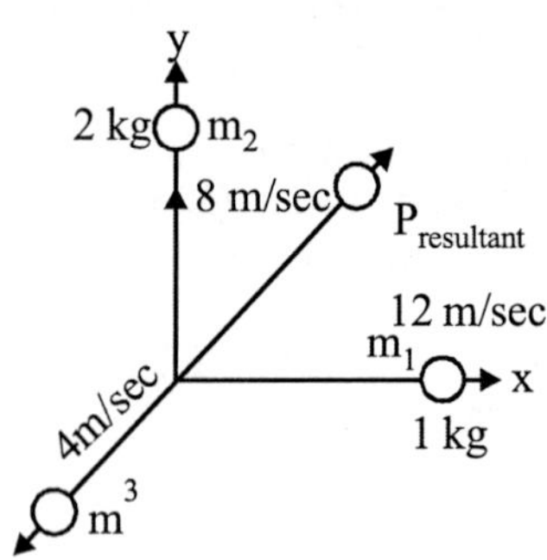

$P_{resultant} = \sqrt{12^2 + 16^2}$

$= \sqrt{144+256} = 20$

$m_3 v_3 = 20$ (momentum of third part)

or, $m_3 = \frac{20}{4} = 5$ kg

56. (b) Here, $l_2 = 2l_1$

As for a spring, force constant $k \propto \frac{1}{l}$

$\therefore k_1 \propto \frac{1}{l_1}, k_2 \propto \frac{1}{l_2}, k \propto \frac{1}{l_1 + l_2}$

$\frac{k_1}{k} = \frac{l_1 + l_2}{l_1}$ and $\frac{k_2}{k} = \frac{l_1 + l_2}{l_2}$

or $k_1 = k\left[1 + \frac{l_2}{l_1}\right]$ and $k_2 = k\left[1 + \frac{l_1}{l_2}\right]$

$\therefore k_1 = k[1+2] = 3k$ [using (i)]

$k_2 = k\left[1 + \frac{1}{2}\right] = \frac{3}{2}k$ [using (i)]

57. (c) Impulse experienced by the body
= change in momentum = MV – (–MV) = 2MV.

58. (a) Masses of the pieces are 1, 1, 3 kg. Hence

$(1 \times 21)^2 + (1 \times 21)^2 = (3 \times V)^2$

That is, $V = 7\sqrt{2}$ m/s

59. (c) $\frac{K_1}{K_2} = \frac{p_1^2}{m_1} \times \frac{m_2}{p_2^2}$ $[\because p = mv \Rightarrow K = \frac{p^2}{2m}]$

Hence, $\frac{p_1}{p_2} = \sqrt{\frac{M_1}{M_2}} = \sqrt{\frac{1}{4}} = \frac{1}{2}$

60. (a) GIVEN

$\vec{F} = k(v_y \hat{i} + v_x \hat{j})$

$\therefore F_x = k v_y \hat{i},\ F_y = k v_x \hat{j}$

$\frac{m dv_x}{dt} = k v_y \Rightarrow \frac{dv_x}{dt} = \frac{k}{m} v_y$

Similarly, $\frac{dv_y}{dt} = \frac{k}{m} v_x$

$\frac{dv_y}{dv_x} = \frac{v_x}{v_y} \Rightarrow \int v_y dv_y = \int v_x dv_x$

$v_y^2 = v_x^2 + C$

$v_y^2 - v_x^2 = \text{constant}$

$\vec{v} \times \vec{a} = (v_x \hat{i} + v_y \hat{j}) \times \frac{k}{m}(v_y \hat{i} + v_x \hat{j})$

$= (v_x^2 \hat{k} - v_y^2 \hat{k})\frac{k}{m} = (v_x^2 - v_y^2)\frac{k}{m}\hat{k} = \text{constant}$

61. (a) Net acceleration

$\frac{dv}{dt} = a = -(g + \gamma v^2)$

Let time t required to rise to its zenith (v = 0) so,

$\int_{v_0}^{0} \frac{-dv}{g + \gamma v^2} = \int_0^t dt$ [for H_{max}, v = 0]

$\therefore t = \frac{1}{\sqrt{\gamma g}} \tan^{-1}\left(\frac{\sqrt{\gamma} v_0}{\sqrt{g}}\right)$

62. (d) $v^2 = u^2 - 2gh$

or $v = \sqrt{u^2 - 2gh}$

Momentum, $P = mv = m\sqrt{u^2 - 2gh}$

At h = 0, P = mu and at $h = \frac{u^2}{f}, P = 0$

upward direction is positive and downward direction is negative.

63. (c) Given that $F(t) = F_0 e^{-bt}$

$\Rightarrow m\frac{dv}{dt} = F_0 e^{-bt}$

$\frac{dv}{dt} = \frac{F_0}{m} e^{-bt}$

$\int_0^v dv = \frac{F_0}{m} \int_0^t e^{-bt} dt$

$v = \frac{F_0}{m}\left[\frac{e^{-bt}}{-b}\right]_0^t = \frac{F_0}{mb}\left[-\left(e^{-bt} - e^{-0}\right)\right]$

$\Rightarrow v = \frac{F_0}{mb}\left[1 - e^{-bt}\right]$

64. (a) From the free body diagram

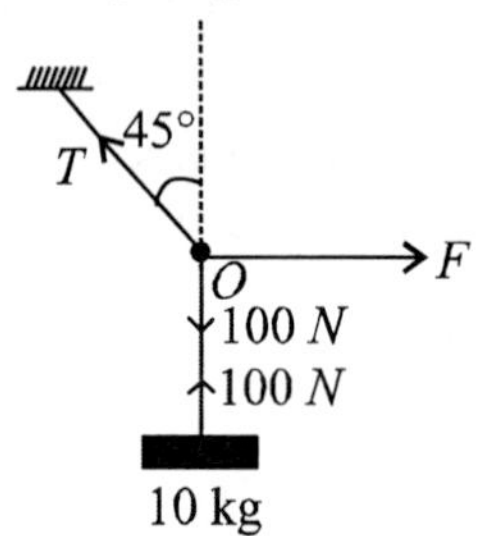

$T\cos 45° = 100\,N$ ...(i)

$T\sin 45° = F$ ...(ii)

On dividing (i) by (ii) we get

$\frac{T\cos 45°}{T\sin 45°} = \frac{100}{F} \Rightarrow F = 100\,\text{N}$

65. (c)

66. (a)

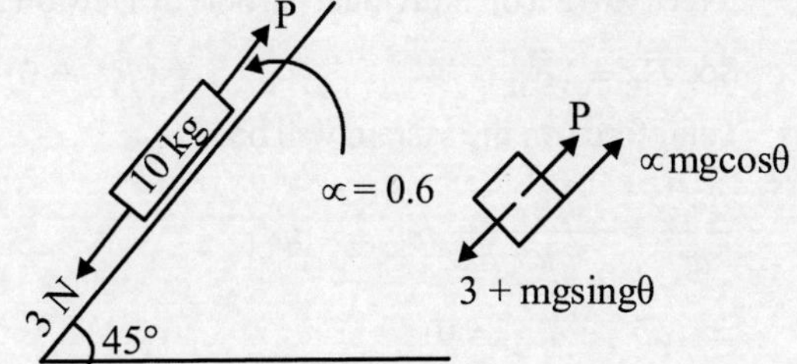

$mg \sin 45^\circ = \dfrac{100}{\sqrt{2}} = 50\sqrt{2}$ [$\because m = 10 kg, g = 9.8 ms^{-2}$]

$\mu mg \cos\theta = 0.6 \times mg \times \dfrac{1}{\sqrt{2}} = 0.6 \times 50\sqrt{2}$

$3 + mg \sin\theta = P + \mu mg \cos\theta$

$3 + 50\sqrt{2} = P + 30\sqrt{2}$

$\therefore P = 31.28 = 32 N$

67. (d) Equation of motion when the mass slides down

$Mg \sin\theta - f = Ma$

$\Rightarrow 10 - f = 6$ ($M = 2$ kg, $a = 3$ m/s^2, $\theta = 30°$ given)

$\therefore f = 4N$

Equation of motion when the block is pushed up

Let the external force required to take the block up the plane with same acceleration be F

$F - Mg \sin\theta - f = Ma$

$\Rightarrow F - 10 - 4 = 6$

$F = 20 N$

68. (d) $f = \mu(M + m) g$

$$a = \frac{f}{M+m} = \frac{\mu(M+m)g}{(M+m)} = \mu g = 0.05 \times 10 = 0.5 \text{ ms}^{-2}$$

$$V_0 = \frac{\text{Initial momentum}}{(M+m)} = \frac{0.05V}{10.05}$$

$v^2 - u^2 = 2as \Rightarrow 0 - u^2 = 2as \Rightarrow u^2 = 2as$

$$\left(\frac{0.05v}{10.05}\right)^2 = 2 \times 0.5 \times 2$$

Solving we get $v = 201\sqrt{2}$

Object falling from height H.

$$\frac{V}{10} = \sqrt{2gH} \Rightarrow \frac{201\sqrt{2}}{10} = \sqrt{2 \times 10 \times H}$$

$H = 40$ m $= 0.04$ km

69. (d) Force of friction at point P,

$$F_{friction} = \frac{1}{3} Ma \sin\theta$$

$$= \frac{1}{3} Ma \sin 90° \quad [\text{here } \theta = 90°] = \frac{Ma}{3}$$

70. (b) Initial speed at point A, $u = v_0$

Speed at point B, $v = ?$

$v^2 - u^2 = 2gh$

$v^2 = v_0^2 + 2gh$

Let ball travels distance 'S' before coming to rest

$$S = \frac{v^2}{2\mu g} = \frac{v_0^2 + 2gh}{2\mu g}$$

$$= \frac{v_0^2}{2\mu g} + \frac{2gh}{2\mu g} = \frac{h}{\mu} + \frac{v_0^2}{2\mu g}$$

71. (b) Graph (b) correctly dipicts the acceleration-time graph of the block.

72. (a)

73. (a)

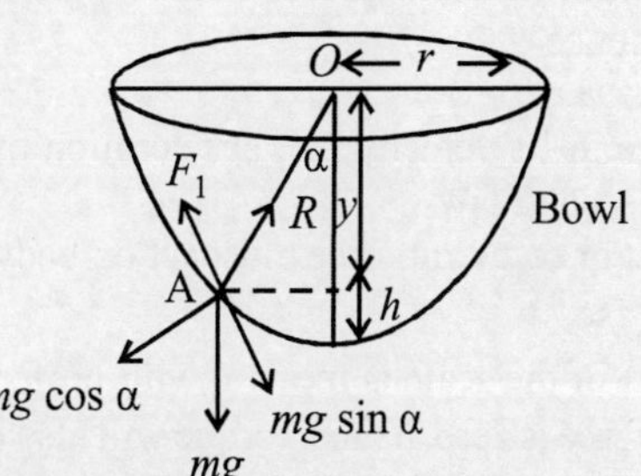

The insect crawls up the bowl upto a certain height h only till the component of its weight along the bowl is balanced by limiting frictional force.

For limiting condition at point A

$R = mg \cos\alpha$ ...(i)

$F_1 = mg \sin\alpha$ ...(ii)

Dividing eq. (ii) by (i)

$$\tan\alpha = \frac{1}{\cot\alpha} = \frac{F_1}{R} = \mu \left[As\ F_1 = \mu R\right]$$

$$\Rightarrow \tan\alpha = \mu = \frac{1}{3}\left[\because \mu = \frac{1}{3}(\text{Given})\right]$$

$\therefore \cot\alpha = 3$

74. (c)

75. (d) Given, $\theta = 45°$, $r = 0.4$ m, $g = 10$ m/s^2

$$T \sin\theta = \frac{mv^2}{r} \quad \text{...... (i)}$$

$$T \cos\theta = mg \quad \text{...... (ii)}$$

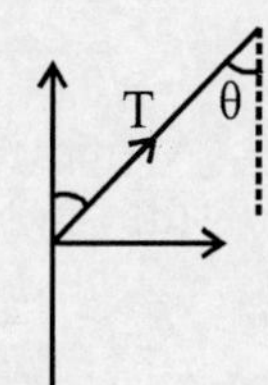

From equation (i) & (ii) we have,

$$\tan\theta = \frac{v^2}{rg}$$

$v^2 = rg \quad \because \theta = 45°$

Hence, speed of the pendulum in its circular path,

$v = \sqrt{rg} = \sqrt{0.4 \times 10} = 2$ m/s

Exercise 2 - Exemplar & Past Year Questions

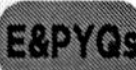

Exemplar Questions

1. (c) In a uniform translatory motion if all the parts of the body moves with (same velocity in same straight line, so the velocity is constant.

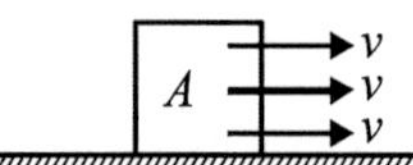

The situation is shown in (figure) where a body *A* is in unfirom translatory motion.

2. (b) According to question we have to apply Newton's second law of motion, in terms of force and change in momentum.

We know that $F = \dfrac{dp}{dt}$

As given that the meter scale is moving with uniform velocity, hence

Force $(F) = m \times 0 = 0$

No change in its velocity i.e., acceleration of it zero by Newton's second law.

Hence, net or resultant force must act on body is zero.

$\vec{\tau} = \vec{r} \times \vec{F}$, so,

As all part of the scale is moving with uniform velocity and total force is zero, hence, torque will also be zero.

3. (c) As given that,

Mass of the ball = 150 g = 0.15 kg

$\vec{u} = (3\hat{i} + 4\hat{j})$ m/s

$\vec{v} = -(3\hat{i} + 4\hat{j})$ m/s

(Δp) Change in momentum

= Final momentum – Initial momentum

$= m\vec{v} - m\vec{u} = m(\vec{v} - \vec{u}) = (0.15)[-(3\hat{i} + 4\hat{j}) - (3\hat{i} + 4\hat{j})]$

$= (0.15)[-6\hat{i} - 8\hat{j}] = -[0.15 \times 6\hat{i} + 0.15 \times 8\hat{j}]$

$= -[0.9\hat{i} + 1.20\hat{j}]$

$\Delta p = -[0.9\hat{i} + 1.2\hat{j}]$

Hence verifies option (c).

4. (c) From previous solution

$\Delta p = -(0.9\hat{i} + 1.2\hat{j}) = -0.9\hat{i} - 1.2\hat{j}$

Magnitude of $|\Delta p| = \sqrt{(-0.9)^2 + (-1.2)^2}$

$= \sqrt{0.81 + 1.44} = \sqrt{2.25} = 1.5$ kg-m s^{-1}

Verifies the option (c).

5. (d) By Newton's second law :

$\vec{F}_{ext} = \dfrac{dp}{dt}$

As $\vec{F}_{ext}$ in law of conservation of momentum is zero.

If $F_{ext} = 0$, $dp = 0 \Rightarrow p =$ constant

Hence, momentum of a system will remain conserve if external force on the system is zero.

In case of collision between particle equal and opposite forces will act on individual particle by Newton's third law.

So, $\vec{F}_{12} = -\vec{F}_{21}$ $\qquad (\because \vec{F}_{ext} = 0)$

Total force on the system will be zero.

$\dfrac{d\vec{p}_{12}}{dt} = -\dfrac{d\vec{p}_{21}}{dt}$ or $d\vec{p}_{12} = -d\vec{p}_{21}$

$\Rightarrow (d\vec{p}_{12} + d\vec{p}_{21} = 0)$

So prove the law of conservation of momentum and verifies the option (d).

6. (c) Consider the adjacent diagram.

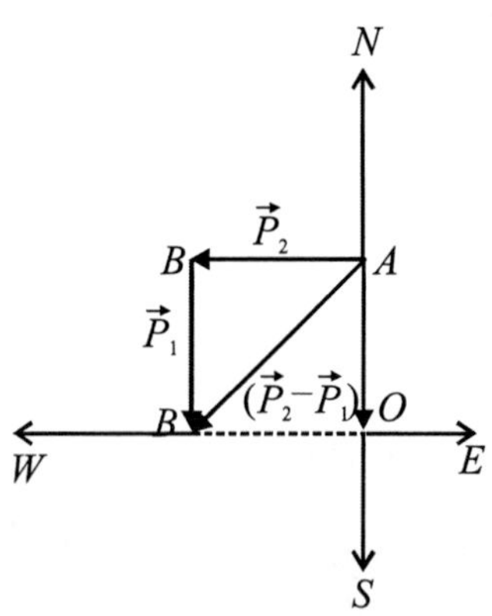

The force on player is due to rate of change of momentum. The direction of force acting on player will be the same as the direction of change in momentum.

Let $OA = P_1$ i.e., Initial momentum of player northward

$AB = P_2$ i.e., Final momentum of player towards west.

Clearly, $OB = OA + OB$

Change in momentum

$= P_2 - P_1 = AB - OA = AB + (-OA)$

= Clearly resultant *AR* will be along south-west.

So, it will be also the direction of force on player.

7. (a) As given that, mass = 2 kg

$p = 3$ m/s, $q = 4$ m/s^2, $r = 5$ m/s^3

As given equation is

$x(t) = pt + qt^2 + rt^3$

$v = \dfrac{ds(t)}{dt} = p + 2qt + 3rt^2$

$a = \dfrac{dv}{dt} = \dfrac{d^2x(t)}{dt^2} = 0 + 2q + 6rt$

$\left[\dfrac{d^2x(t)}{dt^2}\right]_{(t=2)} = 2q + 12r$

$= 2q + 12r = 2 \times 4 + 12 \times 5 = 8 + 60 = 68$ m/s^2

Force acting on body $(\vec{F}) = ma = 2 \times 68 = 136$ N.

8. (b) As given that mass = m = 5 kg

Acting force = $\vec{F} = (-3\hat{i} + 4\hat{j})$ N

Initial velocity at $t = 0$, $\vec{u} = (6\hat{i} - 12\hat{j})$ m/s

Retardation, $\hat{a} = \dfrac{\vec{F}}{m} = \left(-\dfrac{3\hat{i}}{5} + \dfrac{4\hat{j}}{5}\right)$ m/s^2

As the final velocity along Y-component only. So its x-component must be zero.

From $v_x = u_x + a_x t$, for X-component only,

$0 = 6\hat{i} + \frac{-3\hat{i}}{5}t \Rightarrow \frac{3\hat{i}}{5}(t) = 6\hat{i}$

$t = \frac{5 \times 6}{3} = 10$ s

$t = 10$ sec. Hence verifies the option (b).

9. (b) As given that mass of the car $= m$

As car starts from rest, $u = 0$

Velocity acquired along east $(\vec{v}) = v\hat{i}$

Time $(t) = 2$ s.

We know that, $v = u + at$

$\Rightarrow v\hat{i} = 0 + a \times 2 \Rightarrow \vec{a} = \frac{v}{2}\hat{i}$

(Force, by engine is internal force)

$\vec{F} = m\vec{a} = \frac{mv}{2}\hat{i}$

Hence, force acting on the car is $\frac{mv}{2}$ towards east due to force of friction is $\frac{mv}{2}\hat{i}$ which moves the car in eastward direction. Hence, force by engine is internal force.

NEET/AIPMT (2013-2020) Questions

10. (d)

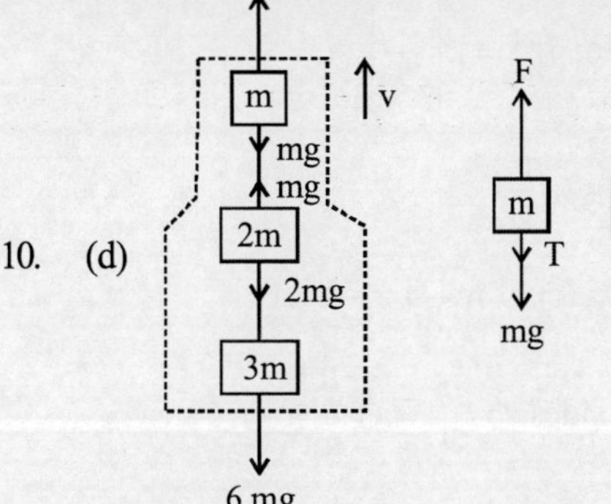

From figure

$F = 6$mg,

As speed is constant, acceleration a = 0

$\therefore$ 6 mg = 6ma = 0, F = 6 mg $\therefore$ T = 5 mg, T′ = 3 mg

$T'' = 0$

F_{net} on block of mass 2 m

$= T - T' - 2$ mg $= 0$

ALTERNATE :

$\because$ v = constant

so, a = 0, Hence, $F_{net} = ma = 0$

11. (d) Given; speed = 10 m/s; radius $r = 10$ m

Angle made by the wire with the vertical

$\tan\theta = \frac{v^2}{rg} = \frac{10^2}{10 \times 10} = 1 \Rightarrow \theta = 45° = \frac{\pi}{4}$

12. (a) Let upthrust of air be F_a then

For downward motion of balloon

$F_a = mg - ma$

$mg - F_a = ma$

For upward motion

$F_a - (m - \Delta m)g = (m - \Delta m)a$

Therefore $\Delta m = \frac{2ma}{g + a}$

13. (c) Change in momentum,

$\Delta p = \int F dt$

= Area of F-t graph = ar of Δ – ar of ▭ + ar of ▭

$= \frac{1}{2} \times 2 \times 6 - 3 \times 2 + 4 \times 3 = 12$ N-s

14. (c) Acceleration

$= \frac{\text{Net force in the direction of motion}}{\text{Total mass of system}}$

$= \frac{m_1 g - \mu(m_2 + m_3)g}{m_1 + m_2 + m_3} = \frac{g}{3}(1 - 2\mu)$

$(\because m_1 = m_2 = m_3 = m \text{ given})$

15. (d) According to question, two stones experience same centripetal force

i.e. $F_{C_1} = F_{C_2}$

or, $\frac{mv_1^2}{r} = \frac{2mv_2^2}{(r/2)}$ or, $V_1^2 = 4V_2^2$

So, $V_1 = 2V_2$ i.e., n = 2

16. (a) Coefficient of static friction,

$\mu_s = \tan 30° = \frac{1}{\sqrt{3}} = 0.577 \cong 0.6$

$S = ut + \frac{1}{2}at^2$

$4 = \frac{1}{2}a(4)^2 \Rightarrow a = \frac{1}{2} = 0.5$ [$\because$ s = 4m and t = 4s given]

$a = g\sin\theta - \mu_k(g)\cos\theta$

$\Rightarrow \mu_k = \frac{0.9}{\sqrt{3}} = 0.5$

17. (a) Acceleration of system $a = \frac{F_{net}}{M_{total}}$

$= \frac{14}{4 + 2 + 1} = \frac{14}{7} = 2 \text{ m/s}^2$

14N A 4kg B 2kg C 1kg

The contact force between A and B

$= (m_B + m_C) \times a = (2 + 1) \times 2 = 6$N

18. (b) For the motion of both the blocks

$m_1 a = T - \mu_k m_1 g$

$m_2 g - T = m_2 a$

a, T, $\mu_k m_1 g$, m_1, μ_k, m_2, a, $m_2 g$

$a = \frac{m_2 g - \mu_k m_1 g}{m_1 + m_2}$

$$m_2g - T = (m_2)\left(\frac{m_2g - \mu_k m_1g}{m_1 + m_2}\right)$$

solving we get tension in the string

$$T = \frac{m_1m_2g(1+\mu_k)g}{m_1 + m_2}$$

19. (d) To complete the loop a body must enter a vertical loop of radius R with the minimum velocity $v = \sqrt{5gR}$.

20. (d) Net force on particle in uniform circular motion is centripetal force $\left(\frac{mv^2}{l}\right)$ which is provided by tension in string so the net force will be equal to tension i.e., T.

21. (a)

22. (c) Coefficient of friction or sliding friction has no dimension.

$f = \mu_s N \Rightarrow \mu_s = \frac{f}{N} = [M^0L^0T^0]$

23. (c) Let the mass of block is m. It will remains stationary if forces acting on it are in equilibrium. *i.e.*, ma cos θ = mg sin θ ⇒ a = g tan θ

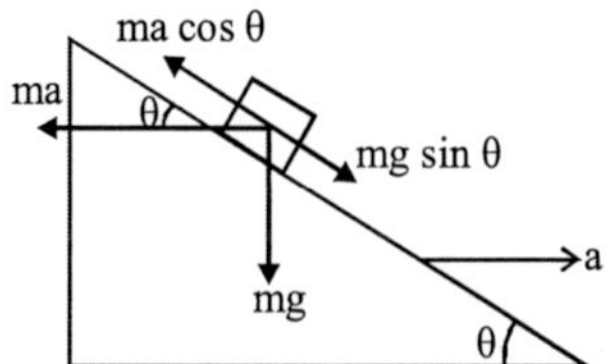

Here ma = Pseudo force on block, mg = weight.

24. (c) Given mass of block, m = 10 kg; radius of cylindrical drum, r = 1m; coefficient of friction between the block and the inner wall of the cylinder μ = 0.1;

Minimum angular velocity ω_{min}

For equilibrium of the block limiting friction

$f_L \geq mg \Rightarrow \mu N \geq mg \Rightarrow \mu r\omega^2 \geq mg$

Hrere, $N = mr\omega^2$

or, $m \geq \sqrt{\frac{g}{r\mu}}$ or, $\omega_{min} = \sqrt{\frac{g}{r\mu}}$

$\therefore \omega_{min} = \sqrt{\frac{10}{0.1 \times 1}} = 10$ rad/s

25. (c) As three forces are forming closed loop in same order, so net force is zero.

i.e., $\vec{F}_{net} = 0$

or $m\frac{d\vec{v}}{dt} = 0$

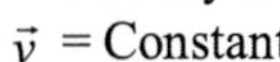

∴ Velocity of the particle

$\vec{v}$ = Constant

P R Q

26. (b) Given : Mass $M_1 = 4$ kg and $M_2 = 6$ kg.

Acceleration of the system,

$a = \frac{(m_1 - m_2)g}{(m_1 + m_2)}$ where $m_1 > m_2$

$\therefore a = \frac{(6-4)g}{6+4} = \frac{g}{5}$

27. (d) Since body does not move hence it is in equilibrium. f_r = frictional force which is less than or equal to limiting friction.

Now $N = mg$

Hence $\vec{F} = \vec{N} + \vec{f_r}$

$|\vec{F}| \leq \sqrt{(mg)^2 + (\mu mg)^2} \Rightarrow |\vec{F}| \leq mg\sqrt{1+\mu^2}$

Exercise 3 - Concept Application Problems CAP

1. (b) From the Newton's second law,

$$F = \frac{dp}{dt} = \frac{d(mv)}{dt} = v\left(\frac{dm}{dt}\right) \quad ...(i)$$

We have given, $\frac{dM(t)}{dt} = bv^2(t)$ ...(ii)

Thrust on the satellite,

$$F = -v\left(\frac{dm}{dt}\right) = -v(bv^2) = -bv^3 \text{ [Using (i) and (ii)]}$$

$$\Rightarrow F = M(t)a = -bv^3 \Rightarrow a = \frac{-bv^3}{M(t)}$$

2. (d)

3. (b) From Newton's second law

$\frac{dp}{dt} = F = kt$

Integrating both sides we get,

$$\int_p^{3p} dp = \int_0^T kt\,dt \Rightarrow [p]_p^{3p} = k\left[\frac{t^2}{2}\right]_0^T$$

$$\Rightarrow 2p = \frac{kT^2}{2} \Rightarrow T = 2\sqrt{\frac{p}{k}}$$

4. (a) From $F = \frac{R}{t^2}v(t) \Rightarrow m\frac{dv}{dt} = \frac{R}{t^2}v(t)$

Integrating both sides $\int \frac{dv}{dt} = \int \frac{Rdt}{mt^2}$

In $v = -\frac{R}{mt}$ $\therefore \ln v \propto \frac{1}{t}$

5. (d) Net force on the elevator = force on elevator + frictional force

⇒ $F = (10m + M)g + f$

where, m = mass of person, M = mass of elevator, f = frictional force

⇒ $F = (10 \times 68 + 920) \times 9.8 + 600 \Rightarrow F = 22000\,N$

⇒ $P = FV = 22000 \times 3 = 66000\,W$

6. (d)

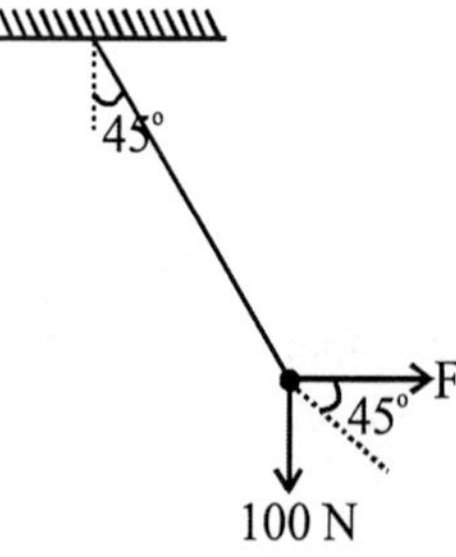

At equilibrium,

$\tan 45° = \frac{mg}{F} = \frac{100}{F}$ $\quad \therefore F = 100\,N$

7. (a)
8. (b) Taking (A + B) as system

$F - \mu(M+m)g$

$= (M+m)a \Rightarrow a = \frac{F-\mu(M+m)g}{(M+m)}$

$a = \frac{F-(0.2)4\times 10}{4} = \left(\frac{F-8}{4}\right)$ ...(i)

But, $a_{max} = \mu g = 0.2 \times 10 = 2$

$\therefore \frac{F-8}{4} = 2 \Rightarrow F = 16\,N$

9. (a) From figure, $2 + mg \sin 30° = \mu mg \cos 30°$ and

$10 = mg \sin 30° + \mu\, mg \cos 30°$
$= 2\mu mg \cos 30° - 2 \Rightarrow 6 = \mu mg \cos 30°$ and
$4 = mg \cos 30°$

By dividing above two $\Rightarrow \frac{3}{2} = \mu \times \sqrt{3}$

$\therefore$ Coefficient of friction, $\mu = \frac{\sqrt{3}}{2}$

10. (b) Given : $m_1 = 5kg$; $m_2 = 10kg$; $\mu = 0.15$
FBD for m_1, $m_1g - T = m_1a$
$\Rightarrow 50 - T = 5 \times a$
and, $T - 0.15\,(m+10)g = (10+m)a$
For rest $a = 0$
or, $50 = 0.15\,(m+10)\,10$

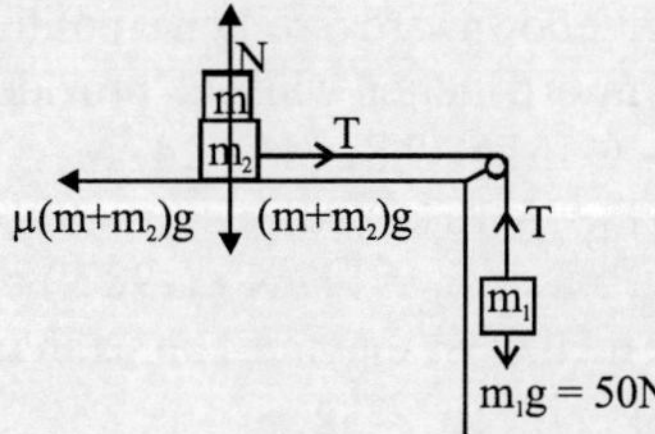

$\Rightarrow 5 = \frac{3}{20}(m+10)$

$\frac{100}{3} = m + 10 \;\therefore\; m = 23.3kg$; close to option (b)

11. (b) Let μ be the minimum coefficient of friction

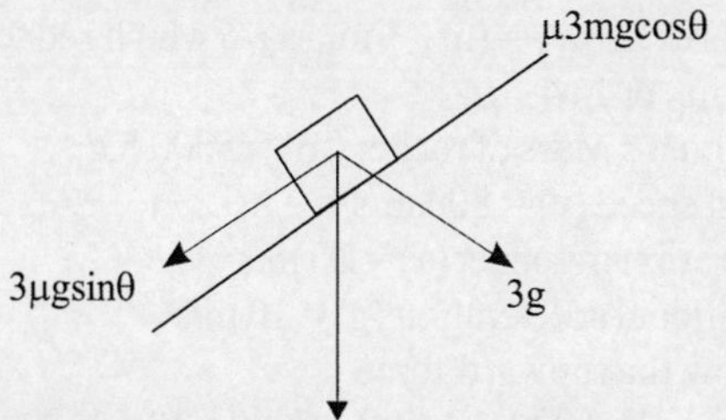

At equilibrium, mass does not move so,
$3mg \sin\theta = \mu 3mg \cos\theta$

\ $\mu_{min} = \tan\theta$

12. (d)
13. (c) Minimum force on A
= frictional force between the surfaces = 12 N

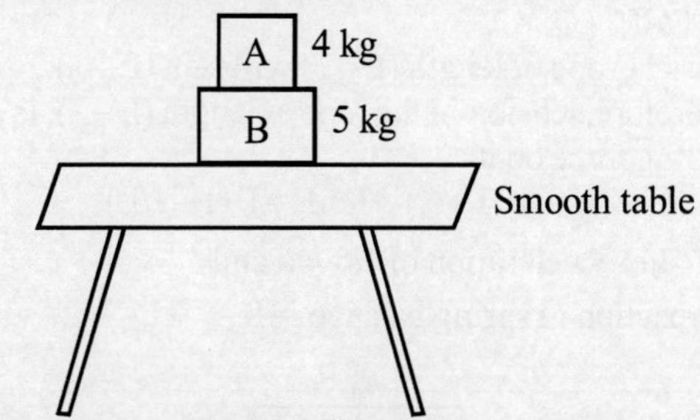

Therefore maximum acceleration

$a_{max} = \frac{12N}{4kg} = 3m/s^2$

Hence maximum force,

F_{max} = total mass × a_{max}
$= 9 \times 3 = 27\,N$

14. (d) When the body has maximum speed then
$\mu = 0.3x = \tan 45°$ $\quad \therefore x = 3.33\,m$
15. (d) Horizontal force, $N = 10\,N$.
Coefficient of friction $\mu = 0.2$.

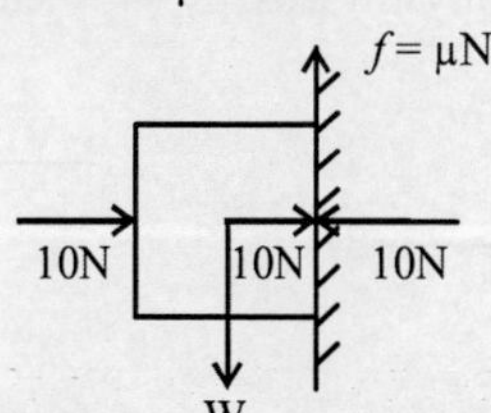

The block will be stationary so long as
Force of friction = weight of block
$\therefore \quad \mu N = W$
$\Rightarrow 0.2 \times 10 = W \Rightarrow W = 2N$

16. (d)
17. (c)

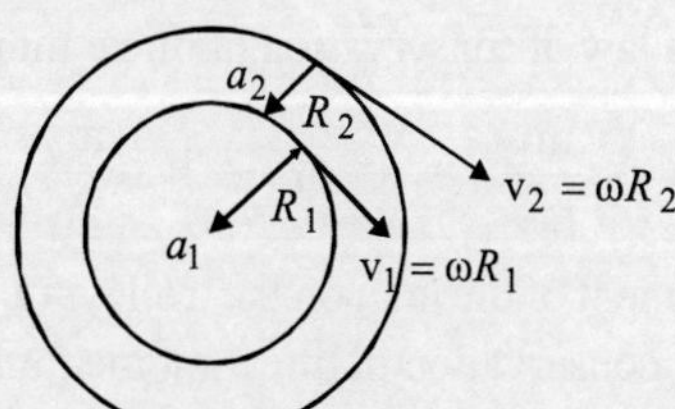

Let m is the mass of each particle and ω is the angular speed of the annular ring.

$a_1 = \frac{v_1^2}{R_1} = \frac{\omega^2 R_1^2}{R_1} = \omega^2 R_1 \Rightarrow a_2 = \frac{v_2^2}{R_2} = \omega^2 R_2$

Taking particle masses equal

$\frac{F_1}{F_2} = \frac{ma_1}{ma_2} = \frac{mR_1\omega^2}{mR_2\omega^2} = \frac{R_1}{R_2}$

NOTE :

The force experienced by any particle is only along radial direction.

Force experienced by the particle, $F = m\omega^2 R$

$\therefore \frac{F_1}{F_2} = \frac{R_1}{R_2}$

18. (d) Let n be the mass per unit length of rope. Therefore, mass of rope = nL.
Acceleration in the rope due to force F will be a = F/nL.
Mass of rope of length $(L-\ell)$ will be $n(L-\ell)$.
Therefore, tension in the rope of length $(L-\ell)$, is equal to pulling force on it
$= n(L-\ell)a = n(L-\ell)\times F/nL = F(1-\ell/L)$

19. (a) Let acceleration of lift = a and
let reaction at spring balance = R

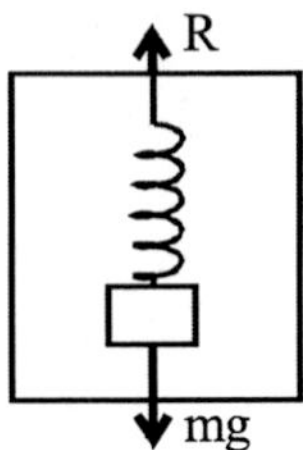

Applying Newton's law
$R - mg = ma \Rightarrow R = m(g+a)$
thus net weight increases,
So reading of spring balance increases.

20. (c) $p_1 = mv$ northwards, $p_2 = mv$ eastwards

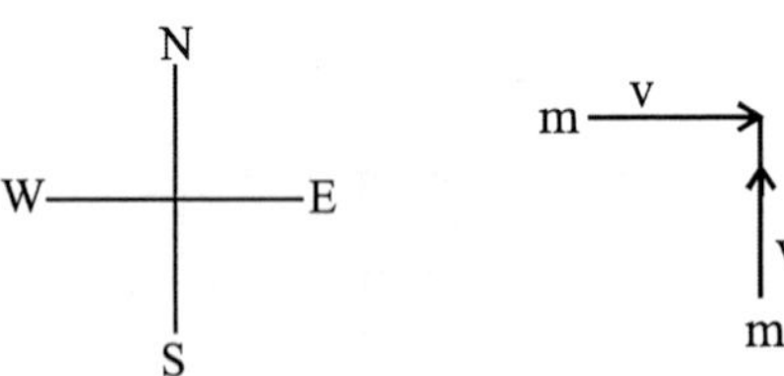

Let p = momentum after collision. Then,

$\vec{p} = \vec{p}_1 + \vec{p}_2$ or $|\vec{p}| = \sqrt{(mv)^2 + (mv)^2}$

$2mv' = mv\sqrt{2}$ or $v' = \frac{v}{\sqrt{2}}$ m/sec

21. (c) Applying law of conservation of linear momentum

$m_1v_1 + m_2v_2 = 0,\ \frac{m_1}{m_2} = -\frac{v_2}{v_1}$ or $\frac{v_1}{v_2} = -\frac{m_2}{m_1}$

22. (c) Displacement of the man on the trolley = 1 × 4 = 4m
Now applying conservation of linear momentum

$80\times 1 + 400\,v = 0$ or $v = -\frac{1}{5}$ m/sec.

The distance travelled by the trolley
$= -0.2\times 4 = -0.8$ m.
(In opposite direction to the man.)
Thus, the relative displacement of the man with the ground $= (4-0.8) = 3.2$ m.

23. (c) In presence of friction $a = (g\sin\theta - \mu g\cos\theta)$
∴ Time taken to slide down the plane

$$t_1 = \sqrt{\frac{2s}{a}} = \sqrt{\frac{2s}{g(\sin\theta - \mu\cos\theta)}}$$

In absence of friction $t_2 = \sqrt{\frac{2s}{g\sin\theta}}$

Given : $t_1 = 2t_2$

$\therefore\ t_1^2 = 4t_2^2$ or $\frac{2s}{g(\sin\theta-\mu\cos\theta)} = \frac{2s\times 4}{g\sin\theta}$

$\sin\theta = 4\sin\theta - 4\mu\cos\theta$

$\mu = \frac{3}{4}\tan\theta = \frac{3}{4} = 0.75$ (since $\theta = 45°$)

24. (b)

25. (b) $m = 10$ kg, $x = (t^3 - 2t - 10)$ m

$\frac{dx}{dt} = v = 3t^2 - 2 \qquad \frac{d^2x}{dt^2} = a = 6t$

At the end of 4 seconds, $a = 6\times 4 = 24$ m/s^2
$F = ma = 10\times 24 = 240$ N

26. (a)

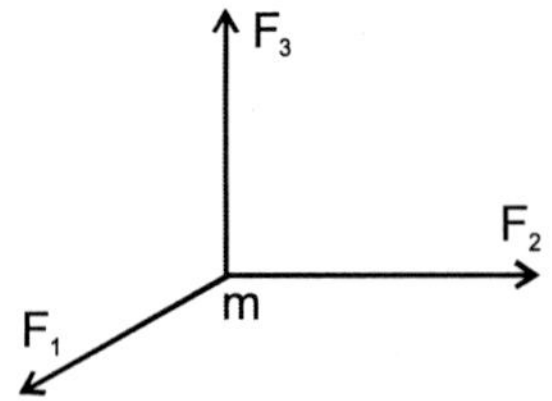

The formula for force is given by $F_1 = ma$

Acceleration of the particle $a = \frac{F_1}{m}$,

because F_1 is equal to the vector sum of F_2 & F_3.

27. (a) Weight of body = m g = 5 N

28. (d) Here, the force of friction is 400N.

$F_{net} = (1650 - 400) = 1250$N

$\therefore\ a = \frac{1250}{1000} = 1.25\,ms^{-2}$

29. (a) Two external forces, F_A and F_B, act on the system and move in opposite direction. Let's arbitrarily assume that the downward direction is positive and that F_A provides downward motion while F_B provides upward motion.
$F_A = (+15\text{ kg})(9.8\text{ m/s}^2) = 147$ N
and $F_B = (-10\text{ kg})(9.8\text{ m/s}^2) = -98$ N
$F_{total} = F_A + F_B = 147\text{ N} + (-98\text{ N}) = 49$ N
The total mass that must be set in motion is
15 kg + 10 kg = 25kg

Since $F_{total} = m_{total}a,\ a = F_{total}/m_{total}$
$= 49\text{ N}/25\text{ kg} \cong 2$ m/s^2

30. (b) Apply Newton's second law
$F_A = F_{AB}$, therefore :
$m_A a_A = (m_A + m_B)a_{AB}$ and $a_{AB} = a_A/5$
Therefore : $m_A a_A = (m_A + m_B)a_A/5$ which reduces to
$4m_A = m_B$ or 1 : 4

31. (d) **Given :** Mass of rocket (m) = 5000 Kg
Exhaust speed (v) = 800 m/s
Acceleration of rocket (a) = 20 m/s^2
Gravitational acceleration (g) = 10 m/s^2
We know that upward force
$F = m(g+a) = 5000(10+20) = 5000\times 30 = 150000$ N.
We also know that amount of gas ejected

$$\left(\frac{dm}{dt}\right) = \frac{F}{v} = \frac{150000}{800} = 187.5\text{ kg/s}$$

32. (b) According to law of conservation of momentum,

$$100v = -\frac{10}{1000} \times 10 \times 800$$

ie, $v = 0.8\ ms^{-1}$.

33. (d) $\sin\theta = \frac{3}{5}$

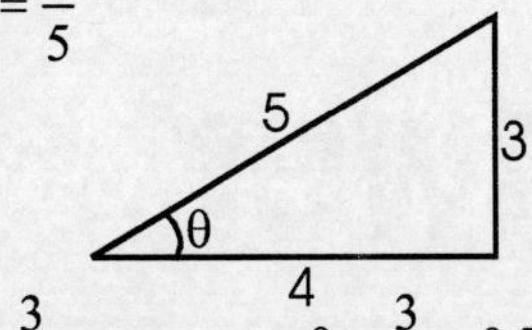

$\therefore\ \tan\theta = \frac{3}{4} \Rightarrow \mu = \tan\theta = \frac{3}{4} = 0.75$

34. (c)

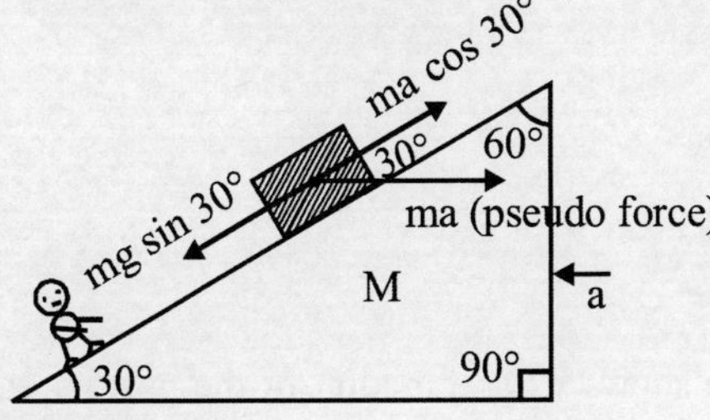

$ma\cos 30° = mg\sin 30°$

$\therefore\ a = \frac{g}{\sqrt{3}}$

35. (c) If W is the maximum weight, then
$W = 2T\cos 60°$
or $W = T = 20N$

36. (c) The acceleration of both the blocks $= \frac{15}{3x} = \frac{5}{x}$

$\therefore$ Force on $B = \frac{5}{x} \times 2x = 10\ N$

37. (b) The maximum acceleration that can be given is a

$\therefore 30g = 10g + 10a$

$\Rightarrow\ a = 2g = 20ms^{-2}$

We know that $s = ut + \frac{1}{2}at^2$

$\therefore\ t = \sqrt{\frac{2s}{a}} = \sqrt{\frac{2 \times 10}{20}} = 1\ s$

38. (c) Considering the two masses and the rope a system, then

Initial net force $= [25 - (15+5)]g = 5g$

Final net force $= [(25+5) - 15]g = 15\ g$

$\Rightarrow$ (acceleration)$_{final}$ = 3 (acceleration)$_{initial}$

39. (d)

40. (d) Let v_1 = velocity when height of free fall is h_1
v_2 = velocity when height of free rise is h_2

$\therefore\ v_1^2 = u^2 + 2gh_1$ for free fall

or For free rise after impact on ground

$0 = v_2^2 - 2gh_2$ or $v_2^2 = 2gh_2$

Initial momentum $= mv_1$

Final momentum $= mv_2$

$\therefore$ Change in momentum $= m(v_1 - v_2)$

$= m(\sqrt{2gh_2} - \sqrt{gh_2})$

41. (a) $v^2 - u^2 = 2as$ or $0^2 - u^2 = 2(-\mu_k g)s$

$$-100^2 = 2 \times -\frac{1}{2} \times 10 \times s$$

$s = 1000\ m$

42. (d) Frictional force on the box $f = \mu mg$

$\therefore$ Acceleration in the box

$a = \mu g = 5\ ms^{-2}$

$v^2 = u^2 + 2as$

$\Rightarrow\ 0 = 2^2 + 2 \times (5)\,s \Rightarrow\ s = -\frac{2}{5}$ w.r.t. belt

$\Rightarrow$ distance = 0.4 m

43. (c)

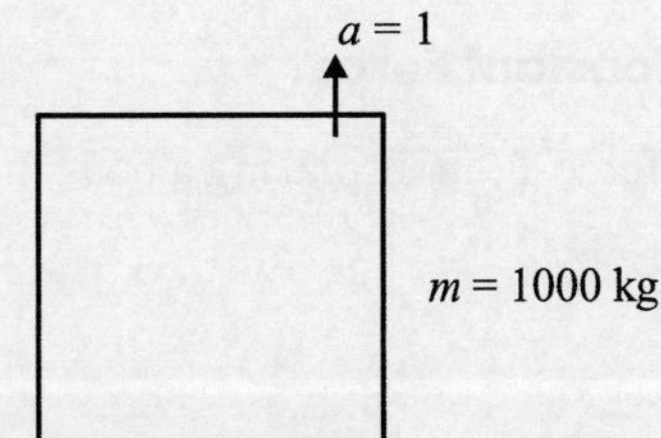

Total mass = (60 + 940) kg = 1000 kg

Let T be the tension in the supporting cable, then

$T - 1000g = 1000 \times 1$

$\Rightarrow T = 1000 \times 11 = 11000\ N$

44. (b) $Mg - T = Ma$

$T - mg = ma$

On solving, we get

$$a = \frac{(M-m)g}{M+m}$$

and $T = \frac{2Mmg}{M+m}$

45. (c) Let velocity of bullet be v. If velocity of gun is V, then

$mv + MV = 0$

$\Rightarrow\ V = -\frac{mv}{M}$

As spring compresses by d, so

$$\frac{1}{2}kd^2 = \frac{1}{2}MV^2$$

or $\frac{1}{2}kd^2 = \frac{1}{2}M\left(\frac{mv}{M}\right)^2$

$\Rightarrow\ v = \frac{d}{m}\sqrt{kM}$

6 Work, Energy and Power

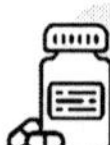

Topic 6.1 : Work

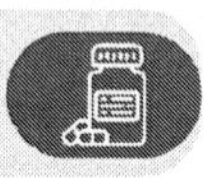

WORK

Work Done by a Constant Force

Work done (W) by a force $\vec{F}$ in displacing a body through a displacement x is given by

$W = \vec{F}.\vec{x} = Fx \cos\theta$

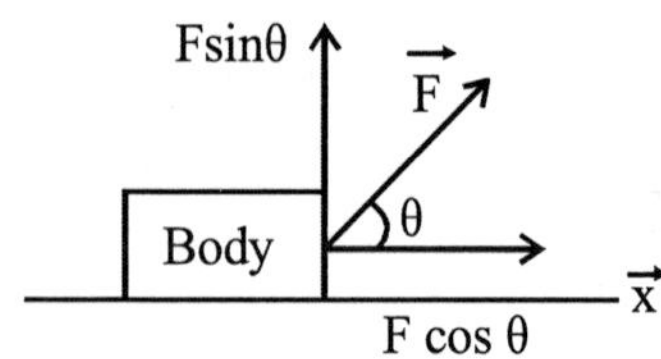

Where θ is the angle between the applied force $\vec{F}$ and displacement $\vec{x}$.

The **S.I. unit** of work is joule, **CGS unit** is erg and its **dimensions** are $[ML^2T^{-2}]$.

1 joule $= 10^7$ erg

(a) When $\theta = 0°$ then $W = Fx$

(b) When θ is between 0 and π/2 then
$W = Fx \cos\theta =$ **positive**

(c) When $\theta = \pi/2$ then $W = Fx \cos 90° = 0$ **(zero)**
Work done by centripetal force is zero as in this case angle $\theta = 90°$

(d) ∴ When θ is between $\pi/2$ and π then
$W = Fx \cos\theta =$ **negative**

Work Done by a Variable Force

When the force is an arbitrary function of position, we need the techniques of calculus to evaluate the work done by it. The figure shows F_x as function of the position x. We begin by replacing the actual variation of the force by a series of small steps.

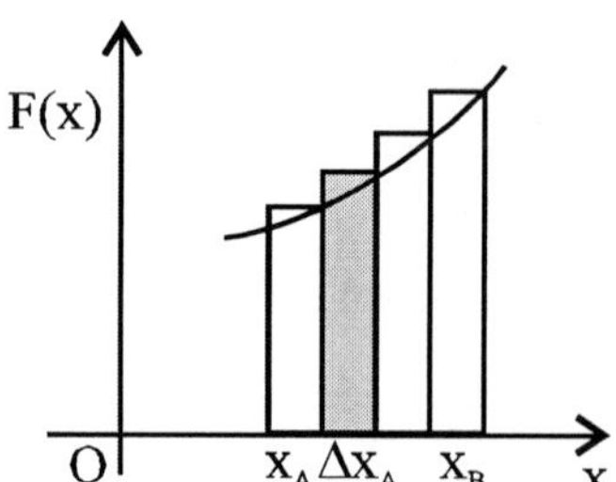

The area under each segment of the curve is approximately equal to the area of a rectangle. The height of the rectangle is a constant value of force, and its width is a small displacement Δx. Thus, the step involves an amount of work $\Delta W_n = F_n \Delta x_n$. The total work done is approximately given by the sum of the areas of the rectangles.

i.e., $W \approx \sum F_n \Delta x_n$.

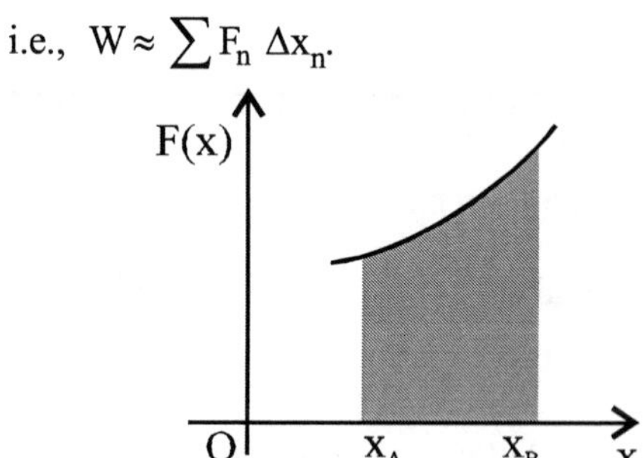

As the size of the steps is reduced, the tops of the rectangle more closely trace the actual curve shown in figure. If the limit $\Delta x \to 0$, which is equivalent to letting the number of steps tend to infinity, the discrete sum is replaced by a continuous integral.

$$W = \lim_{\Delta x_n \to 0} \sum F_n \Delta x_n = \int F_x dx$$

Thus, the work done by a force F_x from an initial point A to final point B is $W_{A \to B} = \int_{x_A}^{x_n} F_x dx$

The work done by a variable force in displacing a particle from x_1 to x_2

$W = \int_{x_1}^{x_2} F dx$ = area under force displacement graph

⚠ **CAUTION :** When we find work, we should be cautious about the question, work done by which force? Let us take an example to understand this point. Suppose you are moving a body up without acceleration.

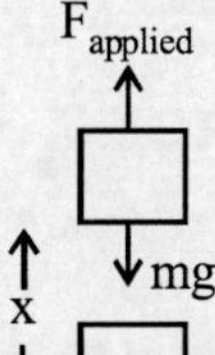

Work done by applied force

$W_{app} = \vec{F}_{app} \cdot \vec{x} = F_{app}x$

Work done by gravitational force

$\vec{W}_{grav} = \vec{F_g}\,\vec{x} = -mgx$

6.1 Concept Practice Problems

CPP

1. The magnitude of work done by a force :
   (a) depends on frame of reference
   (b) does not depend on frame of reference
   (c) cannot be calculated in non-inertial frames.
   (d) both (a) and (b)
2. When the force retards the motion of body, the work done is
   (a) zero
   (b) negative
   (c) positive
   (d) Positive or negative depending upon the magnitude of force and displacement
3. The vessels A and B of equal volume and weight are immersed in water to depth h. The vessel A has an opening at the bottom through which water can enter. If the work done in immersing A and B are W_A and W_B respectively, then
   (a) $W_A = W_B$ (b) $W_A < W_B$
   (c) $W_A > W_B$ (d) $W_A \gtrless W_B$
4. A block is acted upon by a force, which is inversely proportional to the distance covered (x). The work done will be proportional to
   (a) x (b) $x^{1/2}$
   (c) x^2 (d) None of these
5. A particle describe a horizontal circle of radius 0.5 m with uniform speed. The centripetal force acting is 10 N. The work done in describing a semicircle is
   (a) zero (b) 5 J
   (c) 5π J (d) 10π J
6. A cord is used to lower vertically a block of mass M, a distance d at a constant downward acceleration of g/4. The work done by the cord on the block is
   (a) $Mg\frac{d}{4}$ (b) $3Mg\frac{d}{4}$
   (c) $-3Mg\frac{d}{4}$ (d) Mg d
7. A boy pushes a toy box 2.0 m along the floor by means of a force of 10 N directed downward at an angle of 60º to the horizontal. The work done by the boy is
   (a) 6 J (b) 8 J
   (c) 10 J (d) 12 J
8. A particle moving in the xy plane undergoes a displacement of $\vec{s} = (2\hat{i} + 3\hat{j})$ while a constant force $\vec{F} = (5\hat{i} + 2\hat{j})$ N acts on the particle. The work done by the force F is
   (a) 17 joule (b) 18 joule
   (c) 16 joule (d) 15 joule
9. A particle moves under the effect of a force F = cx from x = 0 to x = x_1, the work done in the process is
   (a) cx_1^2 (b) $\frac{1}{2}cx_1^2$
   (c) $2cx_1^2$ (d) zero
10. A force $\vec{F} = (5\vec{i} + 3\vec{j} + 2\vec{k})$N is applied over a particle which displaces it from its origin to the point $\vec{r} = (2\vec{i} - \vec{j})$m. The work done on the particle in joule is
   (a) +10 (b) +7
   (c) −7 (d) +13

ANSWER KEY

1	(a)	2	(b)	3	(b)	4	(d)	5	(a)	6	(c)	7	(c)	8	(c)	9	(b)	10	(b)

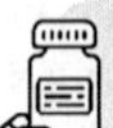

Topic 6.2 : Energy, Work-Energy Theorem, Law of Conservation of Energy Various Forms of Energy and Power

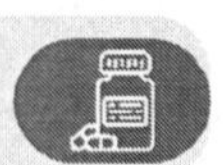

ENERGY

It is the capacity of doing work. Its units and dimensions are same as that of work.

Potential Energy

The energy possessed by a body by virtue of its position or configuration is called potential energy. Potential energy is defined only for conservative forces. It does not exist for non conservative forces.

(a) **Elastic potential energy (Potential energy of a spring)** : Let us consider a spring, its one end is attached to a rigid wall and other is fixed to a mass m. We apply an external force $\vec{F}_{ext.}$ on mass m in the left direction, so that the spring is compressed by a distance x.

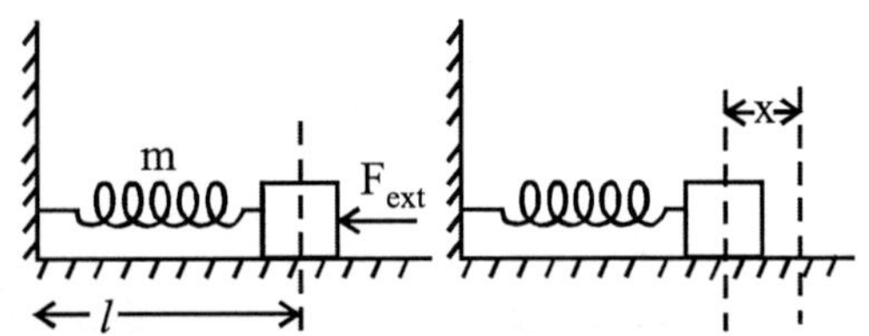

If spring constant is k, then energy stored in spring is given by

P.E. of compressed spring $= \frac{1}{2}kx^2$

Now if the external force is removed, the mass m is free to move then due to the stored energy in the spring, it starts oscillating

(b) **Gravitational potential energy :** When a body is raised to some height, above the ground, it acquires some potential energy, due to its position. The potential energy due to height is called gravitational potential energy. Let us consider a ball B, which is raised by a height h from the ground.

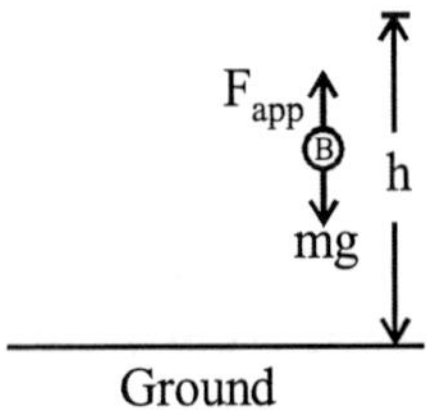

In doing so, we do work against gravity and this work is stored in the ball B in the form of gravitational potential energy and is given by

$W = F_{app}.\ h = mgh$ = *gravitational potential energy* ...(i)

Further if ball B has gravitational P.E. (potential energy) U_o at ground and at height h, U_h, then

$$U_h - U_o = mgh \qquad ...(ii)$$

If we choose $U_o = 0$ at ground (called reference point) then absolute gravitational P.E of ball at height h is

$$U_h = mgh \qquad ...(iii)$$

In general, if two bodies of masses m_1 and m_2 are separated by a distance r, then the gravitational potential energy is

$$U = -G\frac{m_1 m_2}{r}$$

Kinetic Energy

The energy possessed by a body by virtue of its motion is called kinetic energy.

The kinetic energy E_k is given by

$$E_k = \frac{1}{2}mv^2 \qquad ...(i)$$

Where m is mass of body, which is moving with velocity v. We know that linear momentum (p) of a body which is moving with a velocity v is given by

$$p = mv \qquad ...(ii)$$

So from eqs. (i) and (ii), we have

$$E_k = \frac{p^2}{2m} \qquad ...(iii)$$

This is the **relation between momentum and kinetic energy.**

The graph between $\sqrt{E_k}$ and p is **a straight line**

$\because p = \sqrt{2m\,E_k}$

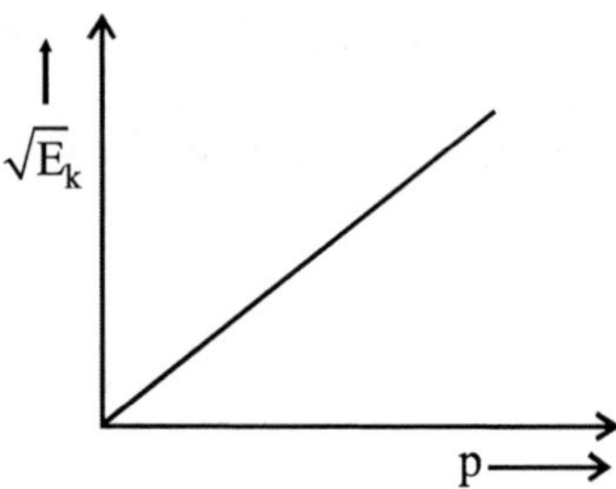

The graph between $\sqrt{E_k}$ and $\frac{1}{p}$ is a **rectangular hyperbola**

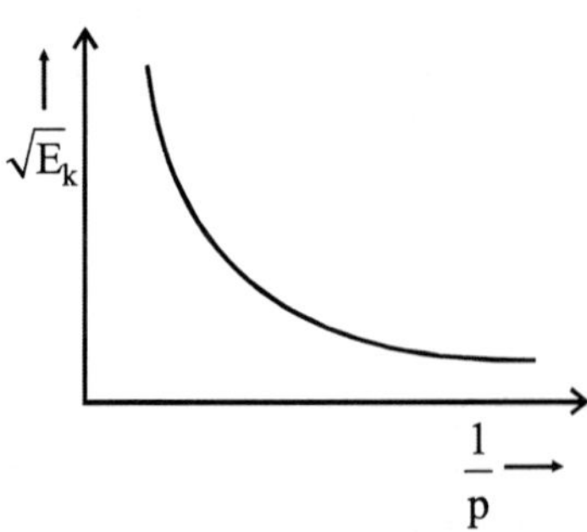

The graph between E_k and $\frac{1}{m}$ is a **rectangular hyperbola**

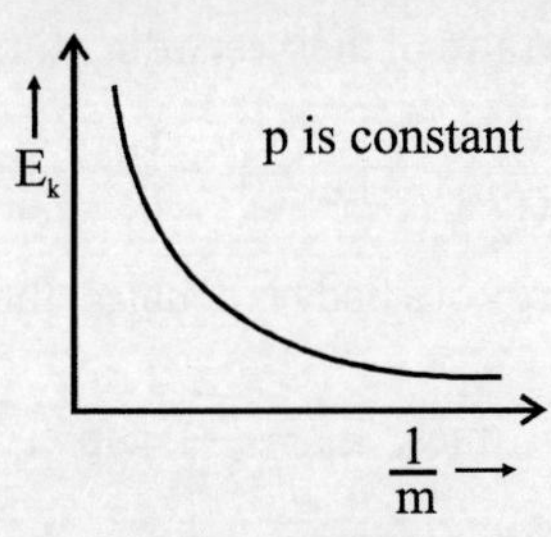

Problem Solving Tips

1. Work done by the conservative force in moving a body in a closed loop is zero.
   Work done by the non-conservative force in moving a body in a closed loop is non-zero.
2. If the momenta of two bodies are equal then the kinetic energy of lighter body will be more.

$$\because \quad p_1 = p_2 \text{ or } \sqrt{2m_1E_1} = \sqrt{2m_2E_2}$$

$$\therefore \quad \frac{E_1}{E_2} = \frac{m_2}{m_1}$$

3. If the kinetic energies of two bodies are same then the momentum of heavier body will be more.

$$\because E_1 = E_2 \qquad \therefore \frac{p_1}{p_2} = \sqrt{\frac{m_1}{m_2}}$$

WORK-ENERGY THEOREM

Let a number of forces acting on a body of mass m have a resultant force $\vec{F}_{ext.}$ And by acting over a displacement x (in the direction of $\vec{F}_{ext.}$), $\vec{F}_{ext.}$ does work on the body, and there by changing its velocity from u (initial velocity) to v (final velocity). Kinetic energy of the body changes.

So, work done by force on the body is equal to the change in kinetic energy of the body.

$$\boxed{W = \tfrac{1}{2} mv^2 - \tfrac{1}{2} mu^2}$$

This expression is called **Work energy (W.E.) theorem.**

LAW OF CONSERVATION OF MECHANICAL ENERGY

The sum of the potential energy and the kinetic energy is called the total mechanical energy.

The total mechanical energy of a system remains constant if only conservative forces are acting on a system of particles and the work done by all other forces is zero.

i.e., $\Delta K + \Delta U = 0$

or $K_f - K_i + U_f - U_i = 0$

or $K_f + U_f = K_i + U_i = \text{constant}$

VARIOUS FORMS OF ENERGY : THE LAW OF CONSERVATION OF ENERGY

Energy is of many types – mechanical energy, sound energy, heat energy, light energy, chemical energy, atomic energy, nuclear energy etc.

In many processes that occur in nature energy may be transformed from one form to other. Mass can also be transformed into energy and vice-versa. This is according to Einstein's **mass-energy equivalence relation,** $E = mc^2$.

In dynamics, we are mainly concerned with purely mechanical energy.

Law of Conservation of Energy :

The study of the various forms of energy and of transformation of one kind of energy into another has led to the statement of a very important principle, known as the law of conservation of energy.

"Energy cannot be created or destroyed, it may only be transformed from one form into another. As such the total amount of energy never changes".

Problem Solving Tips

1. Work done against friction on horizontal surface $= \mu$ mgx and work done against force of friction on inclined plane = $(\mu mg \cos\theta)$ x where μ = coefficient of friction.
2. If a body moving with velocity v comes to rest after covering a distance 'x' on a rough surface having coefficient of friction μ, then (from work energy theorem), $2\mu gx = v^2$. Here retardation is $\vec{a} = -\mu \vec{g}$
3. Work done by a centripetal force is always zero.
4. Potential energy of a system decreases when a conservative force does work on it.
5. If the speed of a vehicle is increased by n times, then its stopping distance becomes n^2 times and if momentum is increased by n times then its kinetic energy increases by n^2 times.
6. Stopping distance of the vehicle $= \frac{\text{Kinetic energy}}{\text{Stopping force}}$
7. Two vehicles of masses M_1 and M_2 are moving with velocities u_1 and u_2 respectively. When they are stopped by the same force, their stopping distance are in the ratio as follows :
   Since the retarding force F is same in stopping both the vehicles. Let x_1 and x_2 are the stopping distances of vehicles of masses M_1 & M_2 respectively, then

$$\frac{F.x_1 (\text{work done in stopping the mass } M_1)}{F.x_2 (\text{work done in stopping the mass } M_2)}$$

$$= \frac{\frac{1}{2}M_1u_1^2}{\frac{1}{2}M_2u_2^2} = \frac{E_{k_1}}{E_{k_2}} \quad ....(i)$$

where u_1 and u_2 are initial velocity of mass M_1 & M_2 respectively & final velocity of both mass is zero.

$$\Rightarrow \frac{x_1}{x_2} = \frac{E_{k_1}}{E_{k_2}} \quad ....(ii)$$

Let us apply a retarding force F on M_1 & M_2, a_1 & a_2 are the decelerations of M_1 & M_2 respectively. Then from third equation of motion $\left(v^2 = u^2 + 2ax\right)$:

$$0 = u_1^2 - 2a_1x_1 \Rightarrow a_1 = \frac{u_1^2}{2x_1} \quad ....(iii\ a)$$

$$\text{and } 0 = u_2^2 - 2a_2x_2 \Rightarrow a_2 = \frac{u_2^2}{2x_2} \quad ....(iii\ b)$$

If t_1 & t_2 are the stopping time of vehicles of masses M_1 & M_2 respectively, then from first equation of motion

$$(v = u + at)\ 0 = u_1 - a_1t_1 \Rightarrow t_1 = \frac{u_1}{a_1} \quad ....(iv\ a)$$

$$\text{and } 0 = u_2 - a_2t_2 \Rightarrow t_2 = \frac{u_2}{a_2} \quad ....(iv\ b)$$

Then by rearranging equation (i), (iii) & (iv), we get

$$\frac{t_1}{t_2} = \frac{u_1/a_1}{u_2/a_2} = \left(\frac{x_1}{x_2}\right) \times \left(\frac{u_2}{u_1}\right)$$

$$\Rightarrow \frac{t_1}{t_2} = \frac{(\frac{1}{2}M_1u_1^2)}{(\frac{1}{2}M_2u_2^2)} \times \frac{u_2}{u_1} = \left(\frac{M_1u_1}{M_2u_2}\right)$$

(a) If $u_1 = u_2 \Rightarrow \frac{t_1}{t_2} = \frac{M_1}{M_2}$

(b) If $M_1 = M_2 \Rightarrow \frac{t_1}{t_2} = \frac{u_1}{u_2}$

(c) If $M_1u_1 = M_2u_2 \Rightarrow t_1 = t_2$

and $\frac{x_1}{x_2} = \frac{(M_1u_1)^2}{(M_2u_2)^2} \times \frac{M_2}{M_1} \Rightarrow \frac{x_1}{x_2} = \frac{M_2}{M_1}$

(d) Consider two vehicles of masses M_1 & M_2 respectively.
If they are moving with same velocities, then the ratio of their stopping distances by the application of same retarding force is given by

$\frac{x_1}{x_2} = \frac{M_1}{M_2}$ and let $M_2 > M_1$ then $x_1 < x_2$

$\Rightarrow$ lighter mass will cover less distance then the heavier mass

And the ratio of their retarding times are as follows

$: \frac{t_1}{t_2} = \frac{M_1}{M_2}$ i.e $\frac{x_1}{x_2} = \frac{t_1}{t_2}$

8. If kinetic energy of a body is doubled, then its momentum becomes $\sqrt{2}$ times, $E_k = \frac{p^2}{2m} \Rightarrow p \propto \sqrt{E_k}$

9. If two bodies of masses m_1 and m_2 have equal kinetic energies, then their velocities are inversely proportional to the square root of the respective masses. i.e.

$$\frac{1}{2}m_1{v_1}^2 = \frac{1}{2}m_2{v_2}^2 \text{ then } \frac{v_1}{v_2} = \sqrt{\frac{m_2}{m_1}}$$

10. (a) The spring constant of a spring is inversely proportional to the no. of turns i.e. $K \propto \frac{1}{n}$ or kn = const.
(b) Greater the no. of turns in a spring, greater will be the work done i.e. $W \propto n$
(c) The greater is the elasticity of the spring, the greater is the spring constant.

11. **Spring constant :** The spring constant of a spring is inversely proportional to length i.e., $K \propto \frac{1}{l}$ or Kl = constant.
(a) If a spring is divided into *n* equal parts, the spring constant of each part = *nK*.
(b) If spring of spring constant K_1, K_2, K_3 .... are connected in series, then effective force constant

$$\frac{1}{K_{eff}} = \frac{1}{K_1} + \frac{1}{K_2} + \frac{1}{K_3} + ...$$

(c) If spring of spring constant K_1, K_2, K_3........... are connected in parallel, then effective spring constant $K_{eff} = K_1 + K_2 + K_3 + ...$

POWER

Power of the body is defined as the time rate of doing work by the body.

The average power P_{av} over the time interval Δt is defined by

$$P_{av} = \frac{\Delta W}{\Delta t} \quad ...(i)$$

And the instantaneous power P is defined by

$$P = \lim_{\delta t \to 0} \frac{\Delta W}{\Delta t} = \frac{dW}{dt} \quad ...(ii)$$

Power is a scalar quantity

The **S.I. unit** of power is joule per second

1 joule/sec = 1 watt

The **dimensions** of power are $[ML^2T^{-3}]$

$$P = \frac{dW}{dt} = \frac{d}{dt}(\vec{F}.\vec{S}) = \vec{F}.\frac{d\vec{S}}{dt} = \vec{F}.\vec{v}$$

(force is constant over a small time interval)

So instantaneous power (or instantaneous rate of working) of a man depends not only on the force applied to body, but also on the instantaneous velocity of the body.

Example 1.

A metre stick of mass 600 mg, is pivoted at one end and displaced through an angle of 60°. The increase in its potential energy is (g = 10 ms^{-2})

(a) 1.5 J *(b) 15 J*

(c) 150 J *(d) 0.15 J*

Solution : (a)

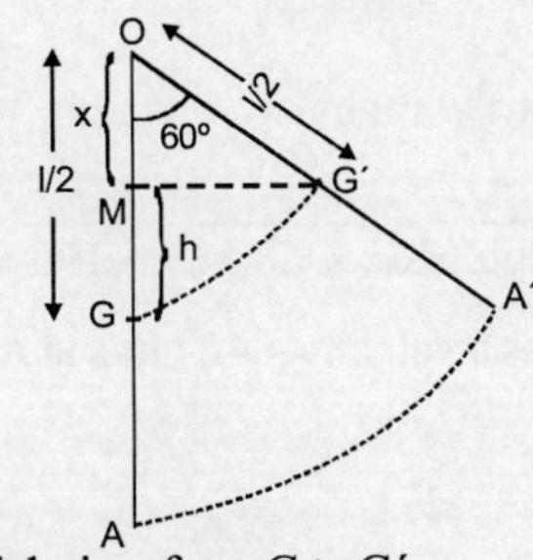

The C.G of stick rises from G to G′.

$\therefore$ Increase in P.E. = mgh

$$= mg\,(\ell/2 - x) = \frac{mg\ell}{2}(1 - \cos 60°)$$

$$= \frac{0.6 \times 10 \times 1}{2}\left[1 - \frac{1}{2}\right] = 1.5\,J$$

Example 2.

A block of mass M slides along the sides of a flat bottomed bowl. The sides of the bowl are frictionless and the base has a coefficient of friction 0.2. If the block is released from the top of the side which is 1.5 m high, where will the block come to rest if, the length of the base is 15 m ?

(a) 1 m from P (b) Mid point of flat part PQ

(c) 2 m from P (d) At Q

Solution : (b)

P.E. of the block at top of side = 1.5 mg.

This is wasted away in doing work on the rough flat part,

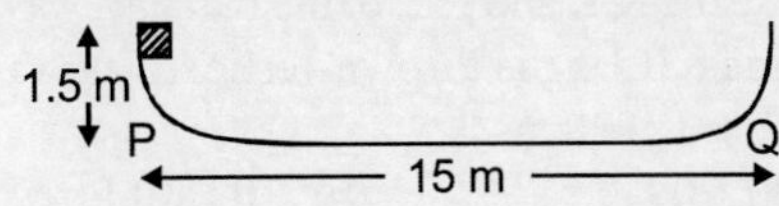

$\therefore$ 1.5 mg = μ mg.x or $x = \frac{1.5}{\mu} = 7.5\,m.$

i.e, the block comes to rest at mid-point of PQ.

Example 3.

Fig. given below shows a smooth curved track terminating in a smooth horizontal part. A spring of spring constant 400 N/m is attached at one end to the wedge fixed rigidly with the horizontal part. A 40 g mass is released from rest at a height of 4.9 m on the curved track. Find the maximum compression of the spring.

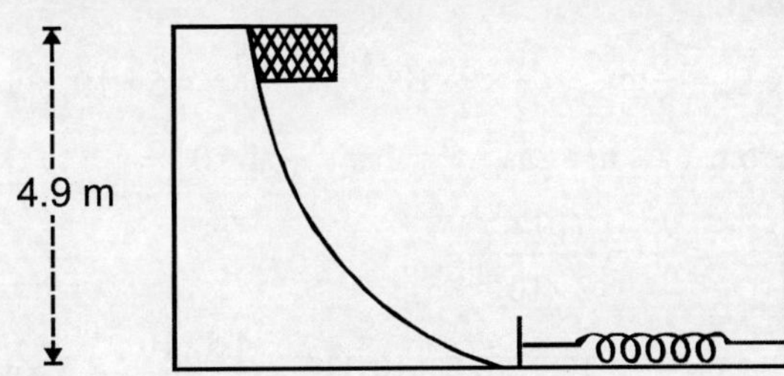

Solution :

According to the law of conservation of energy,

$$mgh = \frac{1}{2}kx^2$$

where x is maximum compression.

$$\therefore\ x = \sqrt{\left(\frac{2mgh}{k}\right)}$$

$$\text{or}\ \ x = \sqrt{\left\{\frac{2 \times (0.4\,kg) \times (9.8\,m/s^2)0 \times (4.9\,m)}{(400\,N/m)}\right\}} = 9.8\,cm.$$

Example 4.

The K.E. of a body decreases by 19%. What is the percentage decrease in momentum?

Solution :

As $p = \sqrt{2m\,K.E}$

$$\frac{p_f - p_i}{p_i} \times 100 = \frac{\sqrt{K.E_f} - \sqrt{K.E_i}}{\sqrt{K.E_i}} \times 100$$

$$= \left(\frac{\sqrt{81} - \sqrt{100}}{\sqrt{100}}\right) \times 100$$

$$= -10\%$$

Example 5.

A particle of mass m is moving along a circular path of constant radius R. The centripetal acceleration varies as a = $K^2 Rt^2$, where K is a constant and t is the time elapsed. What is the power delivered to the particle by the force acting on it?

Sol. For circular motion, $a_c = v^2/R$ here $K^2 Rt^2 = \frac{v^2}{R}$ or $v^2 = K^2 R^2 t^2$

Now, $KE = \frac{1}{2}mv^2 = \frac{1}{2}m.K^2R^2t^2$

Work done in time t = W = ΔK

(from work energy theorem)

$$\therefore \Delta K = \frac{m}{2}(K^2R^2t^2) - 0 = \frac{m}{2}K^2R^2t^2$$

$$\text{Power} = \frac{dW}{dt} = \frac{m}{2}K^2.R^2.2t = mK^2R^2t$$

Example 6.

An electron of mass 9.0 × 10^{-28} g is moving at a speed of 1000 m/sec. Calculate its kinetic energy if the electron takes up this speed after moving a distance of 10 cm from rest. Also calculate the force in kg weight acting on it.

Solution :

$$K.E. = \frac{1}{2}mv^2 = \frac{1}{2}\times 9\times 10^{-31}\ (10^3)^2 = 4.5\times 10^{-25}\ J;$$

From $v^2 - u^2 = 2as,\ v^2 = 2as \quad \because u = 0$

$$\therefore\ a = \frac{v^2}{2s} = \frac{(10^3)^2}{2\times 10^{-1}}$$

$$F = ma = 9\times 10^{-31}\ (0.5\times 10^7)\ N = \frac{4.5\times 10^{-24}}{9.8}\ kg\ wt.$$

$$= 0.46\times 10^{-24}\ kg\ wt.$$

Example 7.

The bob of a simple pendulum of length 1 m is drawn aside until the string becomes horizontal. Find the velocity of the bob, after it is released, at the equilibrium position.

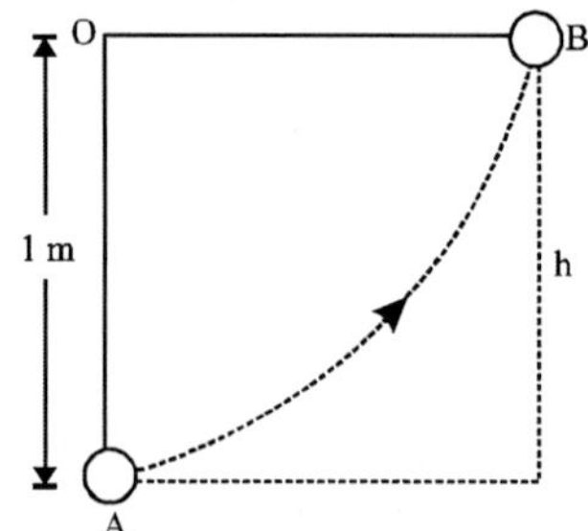

Solution :

When the bob is raised from A to B the height through which it is raised is the length of the pendulum. h = 1m

Taking A as the standard level.

P.E. at B = mgh = m × 9.8 × 1 = (9.8) m joule, where m is the mass of the bob.

Since it is at rest at B it has no K.E.

When the bob reaches A after it is released from B, its energy at A is kinetic one. P.E. at A is zero.

If v be the velocity at A, from the law of conservation of energy

K.E. at A = P.E. at B

$$\frac{1}{2}mv^2 = mgh \quad \text{or} \quad v^2 = 2gh$$

$$\Rightarrow v = \sqrt{2gh} = \sqrt{2\times 9.8\times 1} = \sqrt{196} = 4.427\ m/s$$

The bob has a velocity 4.427 m/s at A.

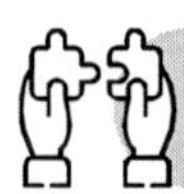

6.2 Concept Practice Problems

CPP

11. A ball of mass m and a ball B of mass $2m$ are projected with equal kinetic energies. Then at the highest point of their respective trajectories.
(a) P.E. of A will be more than that of B
(b) P.E of B will be more than that of B
(c) P.E of A will be equal to that of B
(d) can't be predicted.

12. The engine of a vehicle delivers constant power. If the vehicle is moving up the inclined plane then, its velocity,
(a) must remain constant
(b) must increase
(c) must decrease
(d) may increase, decrease or remain same.

13. A metallic wire of length L metre extends by ℓ metre when stretched by suspending a weight Mg from it. The mechanical energy stored in the wire is
(a) $2\,Mg\,\ell$ (b) $Mg\,\ell$ (c) $\frac{Mg\ell}{2}$ (b) $\frac{Mg\ell}{4}$

14. A vehicle is moving with a uniform velocity on a smooth horizontal road, then power delivered by its engine must be
(a) uniform (b) increasing
(c) decreasing (d) zero

15. A small body is projected in a direction inclined at 45° to the horizontal with kinetic energy K. At the top of its flight, its kinetic energy will be
(a) Zero (b) K/2 (c) K/4 (d) $K/\sqrt{2}$

16. If the force acting on a body is inversely proportional to its velocity, then the kinetic energy acquired by the body in time t is proportional to
(a) t^0 (b) t^1 (c) t^2 (d) t^4

17. A simple pendulum 1 metre long has a bob of 10 kg. If the pendulum swings from a horizontal position, the K.E. of the bob, at the instant it passes through the lowest position of its path is
(a) 89 joule (b) 95 joule
(c) 98 joule (d) 85 joule

18. Calculate the K.E and P.E. of the ball half way up, when a ball of mass 0.1 kg is thrown vertically upwards with an initial speed of 20 ms^{-1}.
(a) 10 J, 20 J (b) 10 J, 10 J
(c) 15 J, 8 J (d) 8 J, 16 J

19. If the linear momentum is increased by 5%, the kinetic energy will increase by
(a) 50% (b) 100% (c) 125% (d) 10%

20. A long string is stretched by 2 cm and the potential energy is V. If the spring is stretched by 10 cm, its potential energy will be
(a) V/25 (b) V/5 (c) 5V (d) 25V

ANSWER KEY

11	(c)	12	(a)	13	(c)	14	(d)	15	(b)	16	(b)	17	(c)	18	(b)	19	(d)	20	(d)

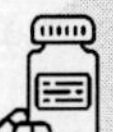

Topic 6.3 : Collision

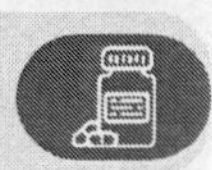

COLLISION

Collision between two bodies is said to take place if either of two bodies come in physical contact with each other or even when path of one body is affected by the force exerted due to the other.

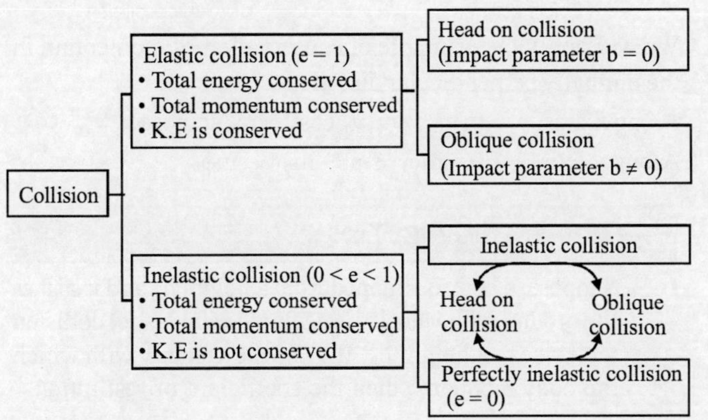

(1) Elastic collision : *The collision in which both the momentum and kinetic energy of the system remains conserved is called elastic collision.*

Forces involved in the interaction of elastic collision are conservative in nature.

(2) Inelastic collision : *The collision in which only the momentum of the system is conserved but kinetic energy is not conserved is called inelastic collision.*

Perfectly inelastic collision is one in which the two bodies stick together after the collision.

Forces involved in the interaction of inelastic collision are non-conservative in nature.

Coefficient of Restitution (or coefficient of resilience) :

It is the ratio of velocity of separation after collision to the velocity of approach before collision.

i.e., $e = |v_1 - v_2| / |u_1 - u_2|$

Here u_1 and u_2 are the velocities of two bodies before collision and v_1 and v_2 are the velocities of two bodies after collision.

1. $0 < e < 1$ (Inelastic collision)

   Collision between two ivory balls, steel balls or quartz ball is nearly elastic collision.
2. For perfectly elastic collision, $e = 1$
3. For a perfectly inelastic collision, $e = 0$

Oblique Elastic Collision :

When a body of mass m collides obliquely against a stationary body of same mass then after the collision the angle between these two bodies is always 90°.

Elastic Collision in One Dimension (Head on)

Let two bodies of masses M_1 and M_2 moving with velocities u_1 and u_2 along the same straight line, collide with each other. Let $u_1 > u_2$. Suppose v_1 and v_2 respectively are the velocities after the elastic collision, then:

According to law of conservation of momentum

$$M_1u_1 + M_2u_2 = M_1v_1 + M_2v_2 \quad ...(1)$$

M_1 u_1 M_2 u_2 Before collision M_1 v_1 M_2 v_2 After collision

From law of conservation of energy

$$\frac{1}{2}M_1u_1^2 + \frac{1}{2}M_2u_2^2 = \frac{1}{2}M_1v_1^2 + \frac{1}{2}M_2v_2^2 \quad ...(2)$$

$$u_1 - u_2 = -(v_1 - v_2) \quad ...(3)$$

Relative velocity of a body before collision   Relative velocity of a body after collision

Solving eqs. (1) and (2) we get,

$$v_1 = \frac{(M_1 - M_2)u_1}{(M_1 + M_2)} + \frac{2M_2u_2}{(M_1 + M_2)} \quad ...(4)$$

$$v_2 = \frac{(M_2 - M_1)u_2}{(M_1 + M_2)} + \frac{2M_1u_1}{(M_1 + M_2)} \quad ...(5)$$

From eqns. (4) and (5), it is clear that :

(i) If $M_1 = M_2$ and $u_2 = 0$ then $v_1 = 0$ and $v_2 = u_1$. Under this condition the first particle comes to rest and the second particle moves with the velocity of first particle after collision. In this state there occurs maximum transfer of energy.

(ii) If $M_1 >> M_2$ and ($u_2 = 0$) then, $v_1 = u_1$, $v_2 = 2u_1$ under this condition the velocity of first particle remains unchanged and velocity of second particle becomes double that of first.

(iii) If $M_1 << M_2$ and ($u_2 = 0$) then $v_1 = -u_1$ and $v_2 = \frac{2M_1}{M_2}u_1 \approx 0$ under this condition the second particle remains at rest while the first particle moves with the same velocity in the opposite direction.

(iv) If $M_1 = M_2 = M$ but $u_2 \neq 0$ then $v_1 = u_2$ i.e., the particles mutually exchange their velocities.

(v) If second body is at rest i.e., $u_2 = 0$, then fractional decrease in kinetic energy of mass M_1, is given by

$$\frac{E_{k_1}-E'_{k_1}}{E_{k_1}}=1-\frac{v_1^2}{u_1^2}=\frac{4M_1M_2}{(M_1+M_2)^2}$$

Inelastic Collision :

Let two bodies A and B collide inelastically. Then from law of conservation of linear momentum

$$M_1u_1 + M_2u_2 = M_1v_1+M_2v_2 \quad ...(i)$$

$$\text{Coefficient of restitution} = -\left(\frac{\text{velocity of separation}}{\text{velocity of approach}}\right)$$

$$e = -\frac{(v_1-v_2)}{(u_1-u_2)} \quad ...(ii)$$

From eqns.(i) and (ii), we have,

$$v_1=\left(\frac{M_1-eM_2}{M_1+M_2}\right)u_1+\left(\frac{M_2(1+e)}{M_1+M_2}\right)u_2 \quad ...(iii)$$

$$v_2=\left(\frac{(1+e)M_1}{M_1+M_2}\right)u_1+\left(\frac{M_2-eM_1}{M_1+M_2}\right)u_2 \quad ...(iv)$$

Loss in kinetic energy $(-\Delta E_k)$ = initial K.E. – final K.E

$$\Rightarrow -\Delta E_k=\left[\frac{1}{2}M_1u_1^2+\frac{1}{2}M_2u_2^2\right]-\left[\frac{1}{2}M_1v_1^2+\frac{1}{2}M_2v_2^2\right]$$

$$\Rightarrow -\Delta E_k=\frac{1}{2}\left(\frac{M_1M_2}{M_1+M_2}\right)(e^2-1)(u_1-u_2)^2 \quad ...(v)$$

Negative sign indicates that the final kinetic energy is less than initial kinetic energy.

Perfectly Inelastic Collision

In this collision, the individual bodies A and B move with velocities u_1 and u_2 but after collision move as a one single body with velocity v.

So from law of conservation of linear momentum, we have

$$M_1u_1+M_2u_2=(M_1+M_2)V \quad ...(i)$$

$$\text{or } V=\left(\frac{M_1u_1+M_2u_2}{M_1+M_2}\right) \quad ...(ii)$$

M_1 u_1 (A) M_2 u_2 (B) M_1+M_2 $\rightarrow V$ (A)(B)

Before collision $(u_1 > u_2)$ After collision

And loss in kinetic energy, $-\Delta E_k$ = total initial K.E – total final K.E

$$=\frac{1}{2}M_1u_1^2+\frac{1}{2}M_2u_2^2-\frac{1}{2}(M_1+M_2)\left(\frac{M_1u_1+M_2u_2}{M_1+M_2}\right)^2$$

$$\text{or, } -\Delta E_k=\frac{1}{2}\frac{M_1M_2}{(M_1+M_2)}(u_1-u_2)^2 \quad ...(iii)$$

Oblique Collision :

This is the case of collision in two dimensions. After the collision, the particles move at different angle.

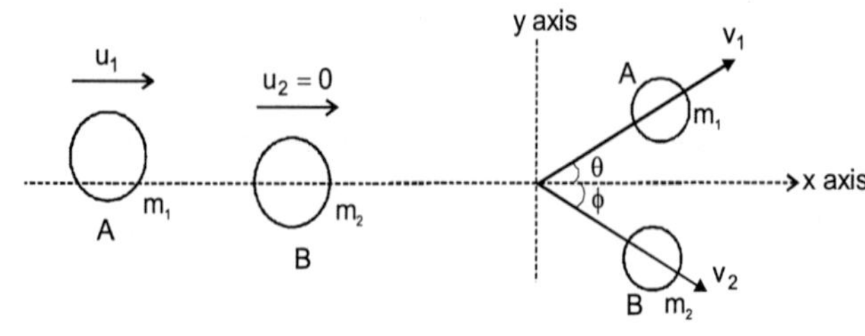

Before collision After collision

We will apply the principle of conservation of momentum in the mutually perpendicular direction.

Along x-axis, $m_1u_1 = m_1v_1\cos\theta + m_2v_2\cos\phi$

Along y-axis, $0 = m_1v_1\sin\theta - m_2v_2\sin\phi$

Problem Solving Tips

1. Suppose, a body is dropped from a height h_0 and it strikes the ground with velocity v_0. After the (inelastic) collision let it rise to a height h_1. If v_1 be the velocity with which the body rebounds, then the coefficient of restitution.

$$e=\frac{v_1}{v_0}=\left(\frac{2gh_1}{2gh_0}\right)^{\frac{1}{2}}=\left(\frac{h}{h_0}\right)^{\frac{1}{2}}$$

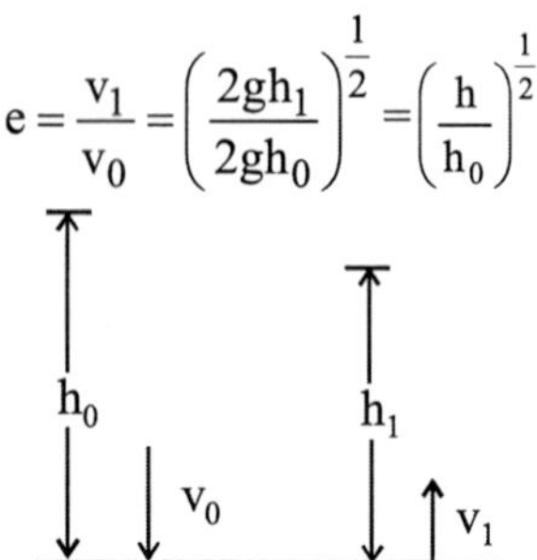

2. If after n collisions with the ground, the velocity is v_n and the height to which it rises be h_n, then

$$e^n=\frac{v_n}{v_o}=\left(\frac{h_n}{h_o}\right)^{\frac{1}{2}}$$

3. When a ball is dropped from a height *h* on the ground, then after striking the ground *n* times, it rises to a height $h_n = e^{2n}h_0$ where *e* = coefficient of restitution.
4. If a body of mass m moving with velocity v, collides elastically with a rigid ball, then the change in the momentum of the body is *2 m v*.
   (i) If the collision is elastic then we can conserve the energy as

   $$\frac{1}{2}m_1u_1^2=\frac{1}{2}m_1v_1^2+\frac{1}{2}m_2v_2^2$$

   (ii) If two particles having same mass and moving at right angles to each other collide elastically then after the collision they also move at right angles to each other.
   (iii) If a body A collides elastically with another body of same mass at rest obliquely, then after the collision the two bodies move at right angles to each other, i.e. $(\theta+\phi)=\frac{\pi}{2}$

5. In an elastic collision of two equal masses, their kinetic energies are exchanged.
6. When two bodies collide obliquely, their relative velocity resolved along their common normal after impact is in constant ratio to their relative velocity before impact (resolved along common normal), and is in the opposite direction.

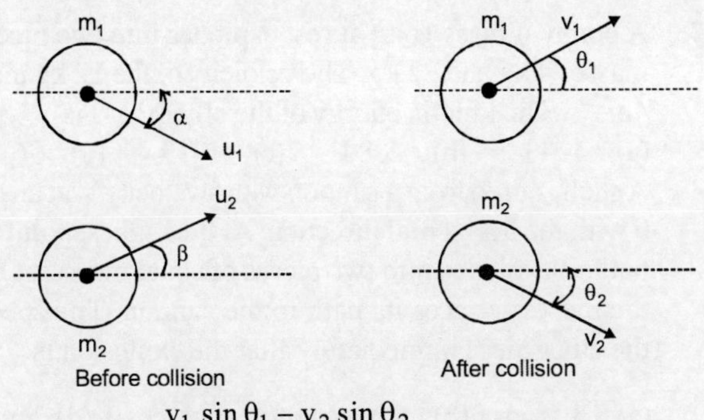

$$\frac{v_1 \sin\theta_1 - v_2 \sin\theta_2}{u_1 \sin\alpha - u_2 \sin\beta} = -e$$

Example 8.

A body of mass m moving with velocity v collides head on with another body of mass 2m which is initially at rest. What will be the ratio of K.E. of colliding body before and after collision?

Solution :

$mv + 2m \times 0 = mv_1 + 2mv_2$;

$v = v_1 + 2v_2$ or $v_2 = \frac{v - v_1}{2}$;

$$\frac{1}{2}mv^2 = \frac{1}{2}mv_1^2 + \frac{1}{2}2mv_2^2$$

$$v^2 = v_1^2 + 2v_2^2 = v_1^2 + 2\left(\frac{v - v_1}{2}\right)^2$$

$$v^2 = v_1^2 + \frac{v_1^2 + v^2 - 2vv_1}{2} \text{ or } 2v^2 = 2v_1^2 + v_1^2 + v^2 - 2vv_1$$

or $3v_1^2 - 2vv_1 - v^2 = 0$; $v_1 = -\frac{v}{3}$

$$\frac{\text{K.E. of colliding body before collision}}{\text{K.E. of colliding body after collision}} = \frac{\frac{1}{2}mv^2}{\frac{1}{2}m\left(\frac{v}{3}\right)^2} = 9:1$$

Example 9.

A bullet of mass m moving horizontally with velocity v hits a block of wood of mass M, resting on a smooth horizontal plane. Find the fraction of energy of the bullet dissipated in the collision itself (assume collision to be inelastic).

Solution :

Applying the law of conservation of momentum, we have, $mv = (m + M)v_1$

$$v_1 = \left(\frac{mv}{m+M}\right)$$

$$\text{Loss of K.E.} = \frac{1}{2}mv^2 - \frac{1}{2}(m+M)v_1^2$$

$$= \frac{1}{2}mv^2 - \frac{1}{2}(m+M)\left(\frac{mv}{M+m}\right)^2$$

$$= \frac{1}{2}mv^2\left[1 - \frac{m}{m+M}\right] = \frac{1}{2}mv^2\left[\frac{M}{m+M}\right]$$

$$\text{Fraction of K.E. dissipated} = \frac{\text{Loss of K.E.}}{\text{Initial K.E.}} = \left(\frac{M}{m+M}\right)$$

Example 10.

A smooth sphere of mass 0.5 kg moving with horizontal speed 3 m/s strikes at right angles a vertical wall and bounces off the wall with horizontal speed 2 m/s. Find the coefficient of restitution between the sphere and the wall and the impulses exerted on the wall at impact.

Solution :

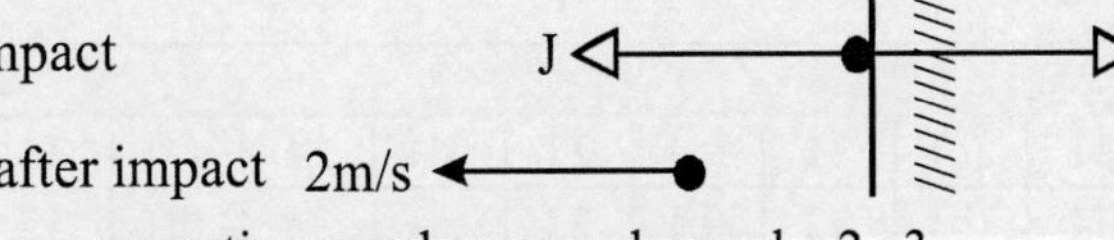

e = separation speed : approach speed = 2 : 3

Therefore the coefficient of restitution is 2/3.

Using impulse = change in momentum for the sphere we have : $= 0.5 \times 2 - 0.5(-3) = 2.5$

The equal and opposite impulse acting on the wall is therefore 2.5 N s.

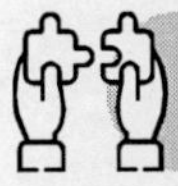

6.3 Concept Practice Problems

CPP

21. In case of elastic collision, at the time of impact
(a) total K.E. of colliding bodies is conserved.
(b) total K.E. of colliding bodies increases
(c) total K.E. of colliding bodies decreases
(d) total momentum of colliding bodies decreases.

22. A ball projected from ground at a certain angle collides a smooth inclined plane at the highest point of its trajectory. If the collision is perfectly inelastic then after the collision, ball will
(a) come to rest
(b) move along the incline
(c) retrace its path.
(d) none of the above

23. A ball is dropped from a height h. If the coefficient of restitution be e, then to what height will it rise after jumping twice from the ground?
(a) e h/2 (b) 2 e h (c) e h (d) e^4 h

24. A ball of mass m moving with a constant velocity strikes against a ball of same mass at rest. If e = coefficient of restitution, then what will be the ratio of velocity of two balls after collision?

(a) $\frac{1-e}{1+e}$ (b) $\frac{e-1}{e+1}$ (c) $\frac{1+e}{1-e}$ (d) $\frac{2+e}{e-1}$

25. A particle of mass m_1 moving with velocity v collides with a mass m_2 at rest, then they get embedded. Just after collision, velocity of the system

(a) increases (b) decreases
(c) remains constant (d) becomes zero

26. A mass m_1 moves with a great velocity. It strikes another mass m_2 at rest in a head on collision. It comes back along its path with low speed, after collision. Then

(a) $m_1 > m_2$ (b) $m_1 < m_2$
(c) $m_1 = m_2$ (d) cannot say

27. Two solid rubber balls A and B having masses 200 & 400 gm respectively are moving in opposite direction with velocity of A equal to 0.3 m/sec. After collision the two balls come to rest when the velocity of B is

(a) 0.15 m/sec (b) 1.5 m/sec
(c) –0.15 m/sec (d) None of these

28. A bomb of mass 9 kg explodes into the pieces of masses 3 kg and 6 kg. The velocity of mass 3 kg is 16 m/s. The kinetic energy of mass 6 kg in joule is

(a) 96 (b) 384 (c) 192 (d) 768

29. A body of mass 5 kg initially at rest explodes into 3 fragments with mass ratio 3 : 1 : 1. Two of fragments each of mass 'm' are found to move with a speed 60 m/s in mutually perpendicular directions. The velocity of third fragment is

(a) $60\sqrt{2}$ (b) $20\sqrt{3}$ (c) $10\sqrt{2}$ (d) $20\sqrt{2}$

30. A body is dropped from a height of 20m and rebounds to a height 10m. The loss of energy is

(a) 10% (b) 45% (c) 50% (d) 75%

31. Hail storms are observed to strike the surface of the frozen lake at 30^0 with the vertical and rebound at 60^0 with the vertical. Assume contact to be smooth, the coefficient of restitution is

(a) $e = \frac{1}{\sqrt{3}}$ (b) $e = \frac{1}{3}$ (c) $e = \sqrt{3}$ (d) $e = 3$

32. A bomb of mass 16kg at rest explodes into two pieces of masses 4 kg and 12 kg. The velolcity of the 12 kg mass is $4ms^{-1}$. The kinetic energy of the other mass is

(a) 144 J (b) 288 J (c) 192 J (d) 96 J

33. A shell is fired from a cannon with a velocity V at an angle θ with the horizontal direction. At the highest point in its path, it explodes into two pieces of equal masses. One of the pieces retraces its path to the cannon. The speed of the other piece immediately after the explosion is

(a) $3 V \cos\theta$ (b) $2 V \cos\theta$ (c) $\frac{3}{2} V \cos\theta$ (d) $V \cos\theta$

34. A rubber ball is dropped from a height of 5m on a plane, where the acceleration due to gravity is not shown. On bouncing it rises to 1.8 m. The ball loses its velocity on bouncing by a factor of

(a) $\frac{16}{25}$ (b) $\frac{2}{5}$ (c) $\frac{3}{5}$ (d) $\frac{9}{25}$

35. A stationary particle explodes into two particles of masses m_1 and m_2 which move in opposite directions with velocities v_1 and v_2. The ratio of their kinetic energies E_1/E_2 is

(a) m_1v_2/m_2v_1 (b) m_2/m_1
(c) m_1/m_2 (d) 1

ANSWER KEY

21	(c)	22	(b)	23	(d)	24	(a)	25	(b)	26	(b)	27	(a)	28	(c)	29	(d)	30	(c)
31	(b)	32	(b)	33	(a)	34	(b)	35	(b)										

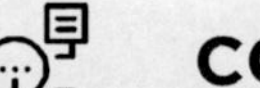

CONCEPT MAP

Positive work
When force (F) and displacement (s) are in same direction
$W_{Positive}$ when $0 < \theta < \pi/2$

Negative work
When force (F) and displacement (s) are in opposite direction
$W_{(Negative)}$ when $\pi/2 < \theta < \pi$

Zero work
When force and displacement (s) perpendicular to each other
W_{Zero} when $\theta = \pi/2$

Coefficient of restitution
$$e = \frac{v_2 - v_1}{u_1 - u_2} = \frac{\text{velocity of separation}}{\text{velocity of approach}}$$

Types of work

Perfectly elastic collision
Total mechanical/kinetic energy conserved
Momentum conserved, $e = 1$

Perfectly inelastic collision
Total energy and linear momentum conserved. Kinetic energy not conserved, coefficient of restitution $e = 0$

Conservative force
If work done by the force is path independent and depends on position only e.g., spring force

Work (W)
Work done by a constant force
$W = Fs\cos\theta = \vec{F}.\vec{s}$
Work done by a variable force
$W = \int_{s_1}^{s_2} Fds\cos\theta = \int_{s_1}^{s_2} \vec{F}.\overrightarrow{ds}$

Types of Collision

Non-conservative force
If the work done by the force is path dependent e.g., force of friction, drag force, etc.

Collision
When exchange of momentum takes place between two physical bodies due to their mutual interaction

WORK, ENERGY AND POWER

Law of Conservation of Energy
It can neither be created nor destroyed only be transformed from one form to another

Power (P) $= \dfrac{\text{work (w)}}{\text{time }(t)}$
Instantaneous power
$P_{inst} = \vec{F}.\dfrac{d\vec{s}}{dt} = \vec{F}.\vec{v} = Fv\cos\theta$
1 hp = 746 watt
1 kilowatt hour (1 kw h) = 3.6×10^6 J

Energy
Capacity of doing work

Work-energy theorem
Change in kinetic energy
= work done by net force on the body
i.e., $\frac{1}{2}mv^2 - \frac{1}{2}mu^2 = W$

Types of mechanical energy

Kinetic energy
$E_K = \frac{1}{2}mv^2 = \frac{p^2}{2m}$

Potential energy
$E_P = mgh$

Potential energy of a spring $U = \frac{1}{2}kx^2$
K = spring or force constant

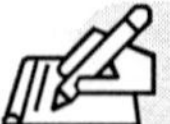

Exercise 1 - Chapter Revision Problems

CRP

1. Which of the following force(s) is/are non-conservative?
(a) Frictional force (b) Spring force
(c) Elastic force (d) All of these

2. A body of mass m accelerates uniformly from rest to v_1 in time t_1. As a function of t, the instantaneous power delivered to the body is
(a) $\frac{m v_1 t}{t_2}$ (b) $\frac{m v_1^2 t}{t_1}$ (c) $\frac{m v_1 t^2}{t_1}$ (d) $\frac{m v_1^2 t}{t_1^2}$

3. A motor cycle is moving along a straight horizontal road with a speed v_0. If the coefficient of friction between the tyres and the road is μ, the shortest distance in which the car can be stopped is
(a) $\frac{v_0^2}{2\mu g}$ (b) $\frac{v^2}{\mu}$ (c) $\left(\frac{v_0}{\mu g}\right)^2$ (d) $\frac{v_0}{\mu g}$

4. Consider the following two statement:
I. Linear momentum of a system of particles is zero.
II. Kinetic energy of a system of particles is zero.
Then
(a) I implies II but II does not imply I.
(b) I does not imply II but II implies I.
(c) I implies II and II implies I.
(d) I does not imply II and II does not imply I.

5. Which of the following must be known in order to determine the power output of an automobile?
(a) Final velocity and height
(b) Mass and amount of work performed
(c) Force exerted and distance of motion
(d) Work performed and elapsed time of work

6. The work done in stretching a spring of force constant k from length ℓ_1 and ℓ_2 is
(a) $k(\ell_2^2 - \ell_1^2)$ (b) $\frac{1}{2}k(\ell_2^2 - \ell_1^2)$
(c) $k(\ell_2 - \ell_1)$ (d) $\frac{k}{2}(\ell_2 + \ell_1)$

7. The engine of a truck moving along a straight road delivers constant power. The distance travelled by the truck in time t is proportional to
(a) t (b) t^2 (c) $\sqrt{t}$ (d) $t^{3/2}$

8. A bullet of mass 'a' and velocity 'b' is fired into a large block of wood of mass 'c'. The bullet gets embedded into the block of wood. The final velocity of the system is
(a) $\frac{b}{a+b} \times c$ (b) $\frac{a+b}{c} \times a$ (c) $\frac{a}{a+c} \times b$ (d) $\frac{a+c}{a} \times b$

9. Which one of the following physical quantities is represented by the shaded area in the given graph?

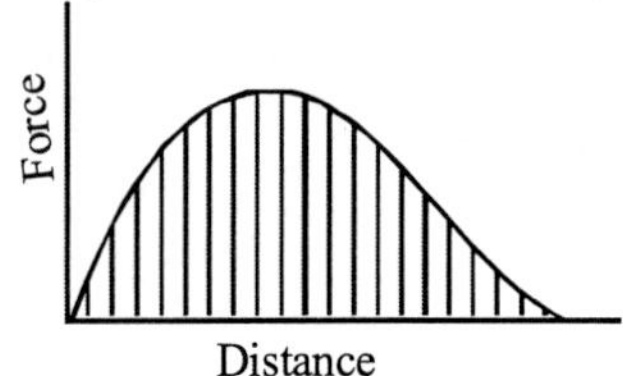

(a) Torque (b) Impulse
(c) Power (d) Work done

10. A motor of 100 H.P. moves a load with a uniform speed of 72 km/hr. The forward thrust applied by the engine on the car is
(a) 1111N (b) 3550N (c) 2222N (d) 3730N

11. Two bodies A and B having masses in the ratio of 3 : 1 possess the same kinetic energy. The ratio of linear momentum of B to A is
(a) 1 : 3 (b) 3 : 1 (c) $1:\sqrt{3}$ (d) $\sqrt{3}:1$

12. When a U^{238} nucleus, originally at rest, decays by emitting an α-particle, say with speed of v m/sec, the recoil speed of the residual nucleus is (in m/sec.)
(a) – 4 v/234 (b) – 4 v/238
(c) 4 v/238 (d) – v/4

13. A spring of force constant 800 N/m has an extension of 5 cm. The work done in extending it from 5 cm to 15 cm is
(a) 16 J (b) 8 J (c) 32 J (d) 24 J.

14. A cord is used to lower vertically a block of mass M, through a distance d at a constant downward acceleration of g/8. Then the work done by the cord on the block is
(a) Mg d/8 (b) 3 Mg d/8
(c) Mg d (d) – 7 mg d/8

15. A spring of spring constant 5×10^3 N/m is stretched initially by 5 cm from the unstretched position. Then the work required to stretch it further by another 5 cm is
(a) 18.75 J (b) 25.00 J (c) 6.25 J (d) 12.50 J

16. When the kinetic energy of a body is increased to three times, then the momentum increases
(a) 6 times (b) 1.732 times
(c) $\sqrt{2}$ times (d) 2 times

17. A machine, which is 75% efficient, uses 12 J of energy in lifting up a 1 kg mass through a certain distance. The mass is then allowed to fall through that distance. The velocity at the end of its fall is (in m/s)
(a) $\sqrt{24}$ (b) $\sqrt{12}$ (c) $\sqrt{18}$ (d) $\sqrt{9}$

18. A machine gun fires a bullet of mass 40 g with a velocity 1200 ms^{-1}. The man holding it can exert a maximum force of 144 N on the gun. How many bullets can he fire per second at the most?
(a) 2 (b) 4 (c) 1 (d) 3

19. In figure, a carriage P is pulled up from A to B. The relevant coefficient of friction is 0.40. The work done will be
(a) 10 kJ
(b) 23 kJ
(c) 25 kJ
(d) 28 kJ

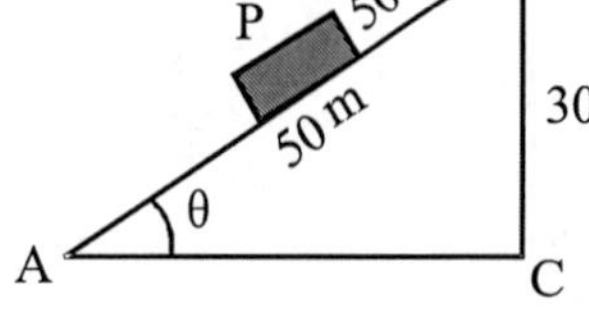

20. A neutron with velocity v strikes a stationary deuterium atom, its K.E. changes by a factor of

(a) $\frac{15}{16}$ (b) $\frac{1}{2}$

(c) $\frac{2}{1}$ (d) None of these

21. Johnny and his sister Jane race up a hill. Johnny weighs twice as much as jane and takes twice as long as jane to reach the top . Compared to Jane
(a) Johnny did more work and delivered more power.
(b) Johnny did more work and delivered the same amount of power.
(c) Johnny did more work and delivered less power
(d) Johnny did less work and johnny delivered less power.

22. A body of mass m moving with velocity v makes a head on elastic collision with another body of mass 2m which in initially at rest. The loss of kinetic energy of the colliding body (mass m) is

(a) $\frac{1}{2}$ of its initial kinetic energy

(b) $\frac{1}{9}$ of its initial kinetic energy

(c) $\frac{8}{9}$ of its initial kinetic energy

(d) $\frac{1}{4}$ of its initial kinetic energy

23. In the non-relativistic regime, if the momentum, is increase by 100% , the percentage increase in kinetic energy is
(a) 100 (b) 200 (c) 300 (d) 400

24. The rest energy of an electron is 0.511 MeV. The electron is accelerated from rest to a velocity 0.5 c. The change in its energy will be
(a) 0.026 MeV (b) 0.051 MeV
(c) 0.08 MeV (d) 0.105 MeV

25. A body starts from rest and acquires a velocity V in time T. The work done on the body in time t will be proportional to

(a) $\frac{V}{T}t$ (b) $\frac{V^2}{T}t^2$ (c) $\frac{V^2}{T^2}t$ (d) $\frac{V^2}{T^2}t^2$

26. A ball is allowed to fall from a height of 10 m. If there is 40% loss of energy due to impact, then after one impact ball will go up to
(a) 10m (b) 8m (c) 4m (d) 6m

27. The potential energy of a conservative system is given by $U = ay^2 - by$, where y represents the position of the particle and a as well as b are constants. What is the force acting on the system ?
(a) $-ay$ (b) $-by$ (c) $2ay - b$ (d) $b - 2ay$

28. A bullet fired into a fixed target loses half of its velocity after penetrating 3 cm. How much further it will penetrate before coming to rest assuming that it faces constant resistance to motion ?
(a) 2.0 cm (b) 3.0 cm (c) 1.0 cm (d) 1.5 cm

29. Given that a force $\hat{F}$ acts on a body for time t, and displaces the body by $\hat{d}$. In which of the following cases, the speed of the body must not increase?
(a) $F > d$ (b) $F < d$ (c) $\hat{F} = \hat{d}$ (d) $\hat{F} \perp \hat{d}$

30. A bag of mass M hangs by a long thread and a bullet (mass m) comes horizontally with velocity V and gets caught in the bag. Then for the combined (bag + bullet) system

(a) momentum $= \frac{mvM}{M+m}$

(b) kinetic energy $= \frac{mV^2}{2}$

(c) momentum $= \frac{mV(M+m)}{M}$

(d) kinetic energy $= \frac{m^2 v^2}{2(M+m)}$

31. A particle, initially at rest on a frictionless horizontal surface, is acted upon by a horizontal force which is constant in magnitude and direction. A graph is plotted of the work done on the particle W, against the speed of the particle v. If there are no other horizontal forces acting on the particle, the graph would look like

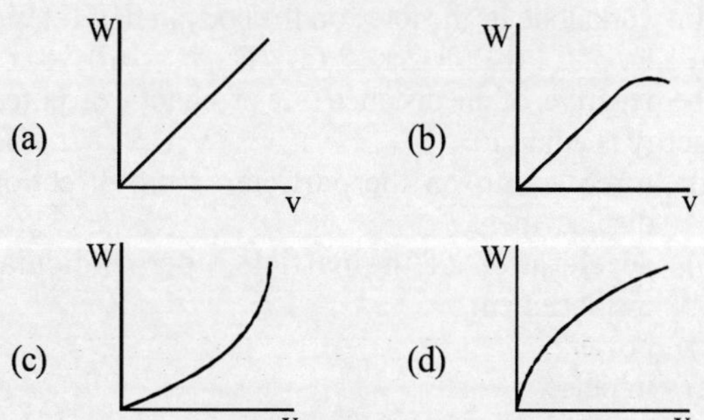

32. A small block of mass m is kept on a rough inclined surface of inclination θ fixed in an elevator. The elevator goes up with a uniform velocity v and the block does not slide on the wedge. The work done by the force of friction on the block in time t as seen by the observer on the inclined p lane will be
(a) zero (b) $mgvt \cos^2\theta$
(c) $mgvt \sin^2\theta$ (d) $mgvt \sin 2\theta$

33. A particle moves in a straight line with retardation proportional to its displacement. Its loss of kinetic energy for any displacement x is proportional to
(a) x (b) e^x (c) x^2 (d) $\log_e x$

34. A mass *m* is moving with velocity v collides inelastically with a bob of simple pendulum of mass m and gets embedded into it. The total height to which the masses will rise after collision is

(a) $\frac{v^2}{8g}$ (b) $\frac{v^2}{4g}$ (c) $\frac{v^2}{2g}$ (d) $\frac{2v^2}{g}$

35. A motor drives a body along a straight line with a constant force. The power P developed by the motor must vary with time t according to

(a) 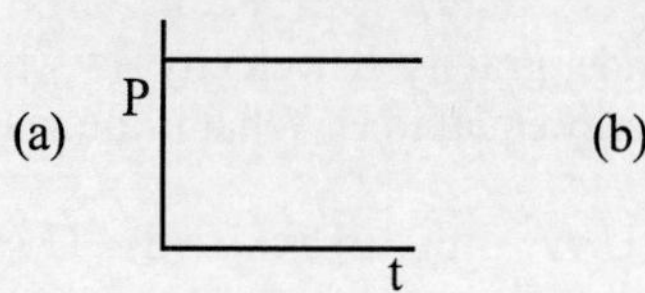

(b) 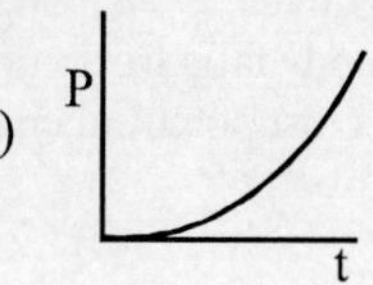

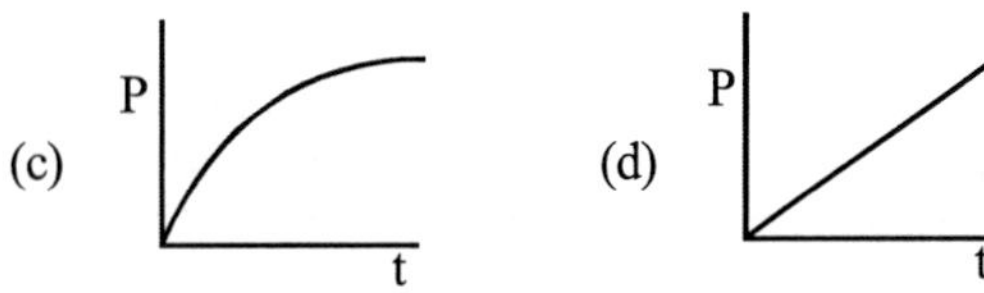

36. A smooth sphere of mass M moving with velocity u directly collides elastically with another sphere of mass m at rest. After collision, their final velocities are V and v respectively. The value of v is

(a) $\frac{2uM}{m}$ (b) $\frac{2um}{M}$ (c) $\frac{2u}{1+\frac{m}{M}}$ (d) $\frac{2u}{1+\frac{M}{m}}$

37. The kinetic energy of particle moving along a circle of radius R depends upon the distance covered S and is given by K = aS where a is a constant. Then the force acting on the particle is

(a) $\frac{aS}{R}$ (b) $\frac{2(aS)^2}{R}$ (c) $\frac{aS^2}{R^2}$ (d) $\frac{2aS}{R}$

38. The force F acting on a body moving in a circle of radius r is always perpendicular to the instantaneous velocity v. The work done by the force on the body in half rotation is

(a) Fv (b) $F\cdot 2\pi r$ (c) Fr (d) 0

39. The negative of the distance rate of change of potential energy is equal to

(a) force acting on the particle in the direction of displacement
(b) acceleration of the particle, perpendicular to displacement
(c) power
(d) impulse.

40. A horse drinks water from a cubical container of side 1 m. The level of the stomach of horse is at 2 m from the ground. Assume that all the water drunk by the horse is at a level of 2m from the ground. Then minimum work done by the horse in drinking the entire water of the container is

(Take $\rho_{water} = 1000$ kg/m^3 and $g = 10$ m/s^2) –

(a) 10 kJ
(b) 15 kJ
(c) 20 kJ
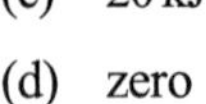
(d) zero

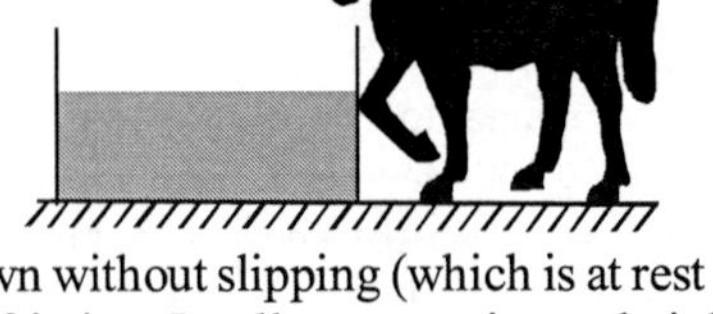

41. The ball rolls down without slipping (which is at rest at a) along ab having friction. It rolls to a maximum height h_c where bc has no friction. K_a, K_b and K_c are kinetic energies at a, b and c.
Which of the following is correct ?

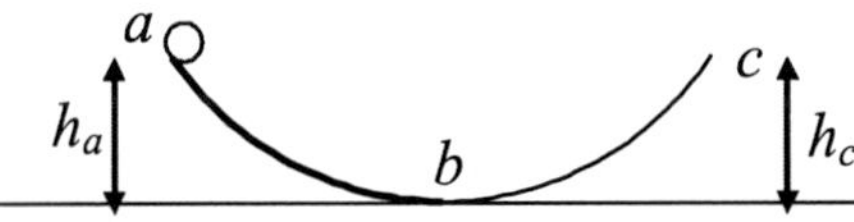

(a) $K_a = K_c, h_a = h_c$ (b) $K_b > K_c, h_a = h_c$
(c) $K_b > K_c, h_a < h_c$ (d) $K_b > K_c, h_a > h_c$

42. A body falls freely under gravity. Its velocity is v when it has lost potential energy equal to U. What is the mass of the body ?

(a) U^2/v^2 (b) $2U^2/v^2$ (c) $2U/v^2$ (d) U/v^2

43. If v be the instantaneous velocity of the body dropped from the top of a tower, when it is located at height h, then which of the following remains constant ?

(a) $gh + v^2$ (b) $gh + \frac{v^2}{2}$ (c) $gh - \frac{v^2}{2}$ (d) $gh - v^2$

44. A particle moves in the X–Y plane under the influence of a force $\vec{F}$ such that its instantaneous momentum is $\vec{p} = \hat{i}2\cos t + \hat{j}2\sin t$.
What is the angle between the force and instantaneous momentum ?

(a) 0° (b) 45° (c) 90° (d) 180°

45. A particle of mass 10 kg moving eastwards with a speed 5 ms^{-1} collides with another particle of the same mass moving north-wards with the same speed 5 ms^{-1}. The two particles coalesce on collision. The new particle of mass 20 kg will move in the north-east direction with velocity

(a) 10 ms^{-1} (b) 5 ms^{-1}
(c) $(5/\sqrt{2})$ms^{-1} (d) none of these

46. A metal ball of mass 2 kg moving with a velocity of 36 km/h has a head on collision with a stationary ball of mass 3 kg. If after the collision, the two balls move together, the loss in kinetic energy due to collision is

(a) 140 J (b) 100 J (c) 60 J (d) 40 J

47. A 3 kg ball strikes a heavy rigid wall with a speed of 10 m/s at an angle of 60°. It gets reflected with the same speed and angle as shown here. If the ball is in contact with the wall for 0.20s, what is the average force exerted on the ball by the wall?

(a) 150N
(b) Zero
(c) $150\sqrt{3}$N
(d) 300N

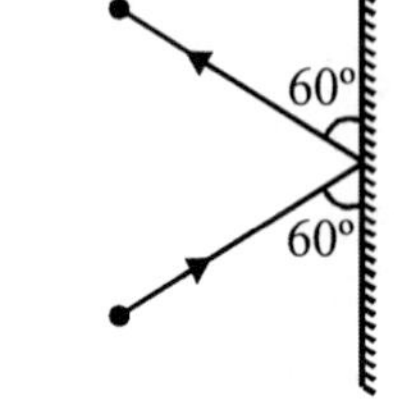

48. In a simple pendulum of length l the bob is pulled aside from its equilibrium position through an angle θ and then released. The bob passes through the equilibrium position with speed

(a) $\sqrt{2g\ell(1+\cos\theta)}$ (b) $\sqrt{2g\ell\sin\theta}$
(c) $\sqrt{2g\ell}$ (d) $\sqrt{2g\ell(1-\cos\theta)}$

49. A ball moving with velocity 2 m/s collides head on with another stationary ball of double the mass. If the coefficient of restitution is 0.5, then their velocities (in m/s) after collision will be

(a) 0, 1 (b) 1, 1 (c) 1, 0.5 (d) 0, 2

50. A body projected vertically from the earth reaches a height equal to earth's radius before returning to the earth. The power exerted by the gravitational force is greatest

(a) at the highest position of the body
(b) at the instant just before the body hits the earth
(c) it remains constant all through
(d) at the instant just after the body is projected

51. A mass m moving horizontally (along the x-axis) with velocity v collides and sticks to mass of 3m moving vertically upward (along the y-axis) with velocity 2v. The final velocity of the combination is

(a) $\frac{1}{4}v\hat{i}+\frac{3}{2}v\hat{j}$ (b) $\frac{1}{3}v\hat{i}+\frac{2}{3}v\hat{j}$

(c) $\frac{2}{3}v\hat{i}+\frac{1}{3}v\hat{j}$ (d) $\frac{3}{2}v\hat{i}+\frac{1}{4}v\hat{j}$

52. The potential energy of particle in a force field is $U=\frac{A}{r^2}-\frac{B}{r}$, where A and B are positive constants and r is the distance of particle from the centre of the field. For stable equilibrium, the distance of the particle is

(a) $B/2A$ (b) $2A/B$ (c) A/B (d) B/A

53. An explosion breaks a rock into three parts in a horizontal plane. Two of them go off at right angles to each other. The first part of mass 1 kg moves with a speed of 12 ms^{-1} and the second part of mass 2 kg moves with speed 8 ms^{-1}. If the third part flies off with speed 4 ms^{-1} then its mass is

(a) 5 kg (b) 7 kg (c) 17 kg (d) 3 kg

54. If the mass of the body is halved and velocity gets doubled then final kinetic energy would be ....of initial.

(a) same (b) four times
(c) double (d) eight times

55. A train of weight 10^7 N is running on a level track with uniform speed of 36 km h^{-1}. The frictional force is 0.5 kg per quintal. If g = 10 m/s^2, then power of engine is

(a) 500 kW (b) 50 kW (c) 5 kW (d) 0.5 kW

56. A person pushes a box on a rough horizontal platform surface. He applies a force of 200 N over a distance of 15 m. Thereafter, he gets progressively tired and his applied force reduces linearly with distance to 100 N. The total distance through which the box has been moved is 30 m. What is the work done by the person during the total movement of the box ?

(a) 3280 J (b) 2780 J (c) 5690 J (d) 5250 J

57. Consider a force $\vec{F}=-x\hat{i}+y\hat{j}$. The work done by this force in moving a particle from point A(1, 0) to B(0, 1) along the line segment is: (all quantities are in SI units)

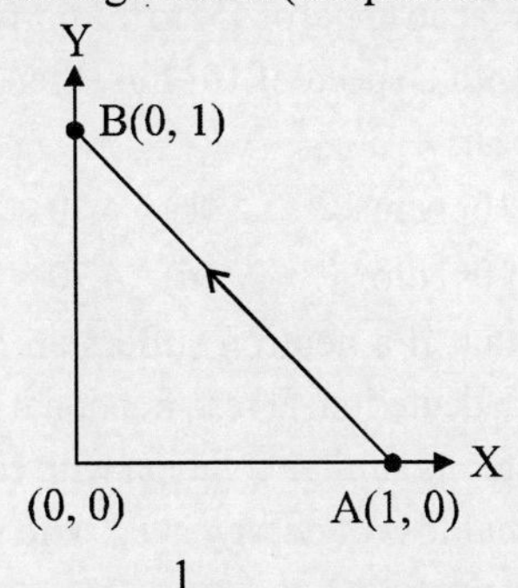

(a) 2J (b) $\frac{1}{2}$J (c) 1J (d) $\frac{3}{2}$J

58. A particle moves in one dimension from rest under the influence of a force that varies with the distance travelled by the particle as shown in the figure. The kinetic energy of the particle after it has travelled 3 m is :

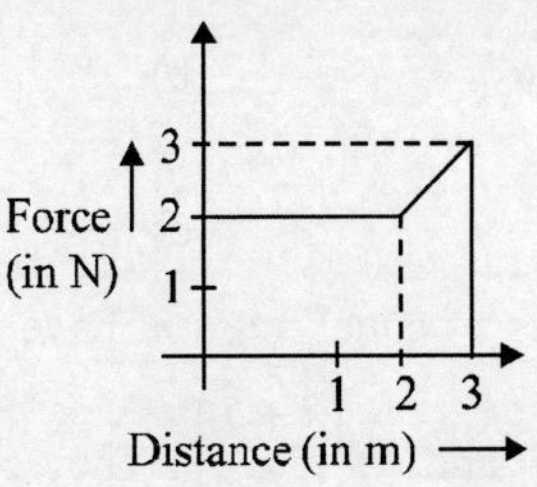

(a) 4 J (b) 2.5 J (c) 6.5 J (d) 5 J

59. A spring whose unstretched length is l has a force constant k. The spring is cut into two pieces of unstretched lengths l_1 and l_2 where, $l_1 = nl_2$ and n is an integer. The ratio k_1/k_2 of the corresponding force constants, k_1 and k_2 will be:

(a) n (b) $\frac{1}{n^2}$ (c) $\frac{1}{n}$ (d) n^2

60. A body of mass 1 kg falls freely from a height of 100m, on a platform of mass 3 kg which is mounted on a spring having spring constant k = 1.25 × 10^6 N/m. The body sticks to the platform and the spring's maximum compression is found to be x. Given that g = 10 ms^{-2}, the value of x will be close to :

(a) 40 cm (b) 4 cm (c) 80 cm (d) 8 cm

61. A force acts on a 2 kg object so that its position is given as a function of time as $x = 3t^2 + 5$. What is the work done by this force in first 5 seconds?

(a) 850 J (b) 950 J (c) 875 J (d) 900 J

62. A particle is moving in a circular path of radius a under the action of an attractive potential $U=-\frac{k}{2r^2}$. Its total energy is:

(a) $-\frac{k}{4a^2}$ (b) $\frac{k}{2a^2}$ (c) zero (d) $-\frac{3}{2}\frac{k}{a^2}$

63. A particle is moving unidirectionally on a horizontal plane under the action of a constant power supplying energy source. The displacement (s) - time (t) graph that describes the motion of the particle is (graphs are drawn schematically and are not to scale) :

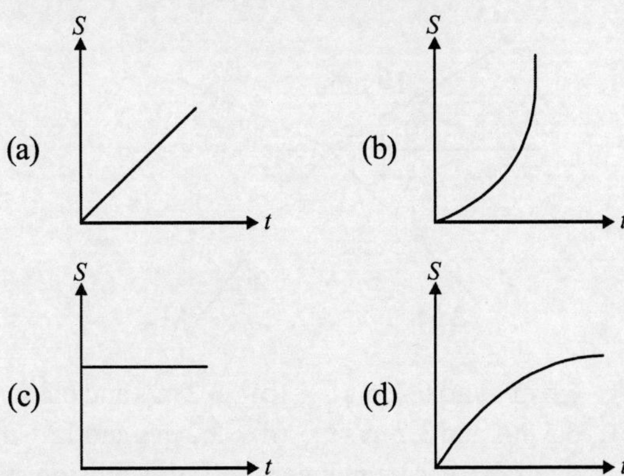

64. A particle of mass m with an initial velocity $u\hat{i}$ collides perfectly elastically with a mass 3 m at rest. It moves with a velocity $v\hat{j}$ after collision, then, v is given by :

(a) $v=\sqrt{\frac{2}{3}}u$ (b) $v=\frac{u}{\sqrt{3}}$

(c) $v=\frac{u}{\sqrt{2}}$ (d) $v=\frac{1}{\sqrt{6}}u$

65. Two particles of equal mass m have respective initial velocities $u\hat{i}$ and $u\left(\frac{\hat{i}+\hat{j}}{2}\right)$. They collide completely inelastically. The energy lost in the process is:

(a) $\frac{1}{3}$ mu² (b) $\frac{1}{8}$ mu² (c) $\frac{3}{4}$ mu² (d) $\sqrt{\frac{2}{3}}$ mu²

66. A particle of mass m is dropped from a height h above the ground. At the same time another particle of the same mass is thrown vertically upwards from the ground with a speed of $\sqrt{2gh}$. If they collide head-on completely inelastically, the time taken for the combined mass to reach the ground, in units of $\sqrt{\frac{h}{g}}$ is:

(a) $\sqrt{\frac{1}{2}}$ (b) $\sqrt{\frac{3}{4}}$ (c) $\frac{1}{2}$ (d) $\sqrt{\frac{3}{2}}$

67. A man (mass = 50 kg) and his son (mass = 20 kg) are standing on a frictionless surface facing each other. The man pushes his son so that he starts moving at a speed of 0.70 ms^{-1} with respect to the man. The speed of the man with respect to the surface is :

(a) 0.28 ms^{-1} (b) 0.20 ms^{-1}

(c) 0.47 ms^{-1} (d) 0.14 ms^{-1}

68. Two particles, of masses M and 2M, moving, as shown, with speeds of 10 m/s and 5 m/s, collide elastically at the origin. After the collision, they move along the indicated directions with speeds v_1 and v_2, respectively. The values of v_1 and v_2 are nearly :

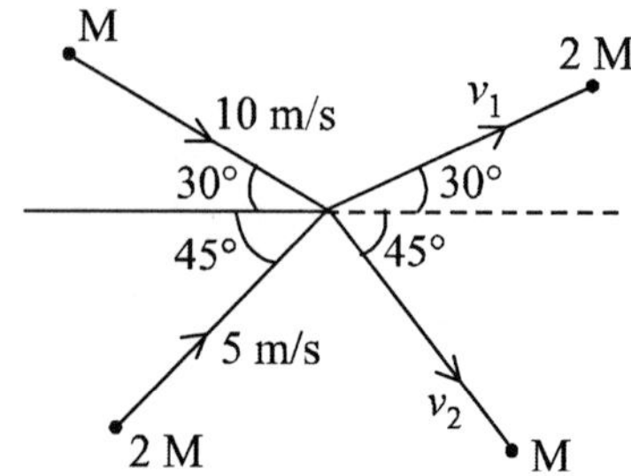

(a) 6.5 m/s and 6.3 m/s (b) 3.2 m/s and 6.3 m/s

(c) 6.5 m/s and 3.2 m/s (d) 3.2 m/s and 12.6 m/s

69. A body of mass 2 kg makes an elastic collision with a second body at rest and continues to move in the original direction but with one fourth of its original speed. What is the mass of the second body?

(a) 1.0 kg (b) 1.5 kg (c) 1.8 kg (d) 1.2 kg

70. A particle of mass 'm' is moving with speed '$2v$' and collides with a mass '$2m$' moving with speed 'v' in the same direction. After collision, the first mass is stopped completely while the second one splits into two particles each of mass 'm', which move at angle 45° with respect to the original direction.

The speed of each of the moving particle will be:

(a) $\sqrt{2}\ v$ (b) $2\sqrt{2}\ v$

(c) $v/(2\sqrt{2})$ (d) $v/\sqrt{2}$

71. A body of mass m_1 moving with an unknown velocity of $v_1\hat{i}$, undergoes a collinear collision with a body of mass m_2 moving with a velocity $v_2\hat{i}$. After collision, m_1 and m_2 move with velocities of $v_3\hat{i}$ and $v_4\hat{i}$, respectively.

If $m_2 = 0.5\ m_1$ and $v_3 = 0.5\ v_1$, then v_1 is :

(a) $v_4 - \frac{v_2}{2}$ (b) $v_4 - v_2$ (c) $v_4 - \frac{v_2}{4}$ (d) $v_4 + v_2$

72. An alpha-particle of mass m suffers 1-dimensional elastic collision with a nucleus at rest of unknown mass. It is scattered directly backwards losing, 64% of its initial kinetic energy. The mass of the nucleus is :

(a) 2m (b) 3.5m (c) 1.5m (d) 4m

73. In a collinear collision, a particle with an initial speed v_0 strikes a stationary particle of the same mass. If the final total kinetic energy is 50% greater than the original kinetic energy, the magnitude of the relative velocity between the two particles, after collision, is:

(a) $\frac{v_0}{4}$ (b) $\sqrt{2}v_0$ (c) $\frac{v_0}{2}$ (d) $\frac{v_0}{\sqrt{2}}$

74. The mass of a hydrogen molecule is 3.32×10^{-27} kg. If 10^{23} hydrogen molecules strike, per second, a fixed wall of area 2 cm² at an angle of 45° to the normal, and rebound elastically with a speed of 10^3 m/s, then the pressure on the wall is nearly:

(a) 2.35×10^3 N/m² (b) 4.70×10^3 N/m²

(c) 2.35×10^2 N/m² (d) 4.70×10^2 N/m²

75. It is found that if a neutron suffers an elastic collinear collision with deuterium at rest, fractional loss of its energy is p_d; while for its similar collision with carbon nucleus at rest, fractional loss of energy is P_c. The values of P_d and P_c are respectively:

(a) (·89,·28) (b) (·28,·89)

(c) (0, 0) (d) (0, 1)

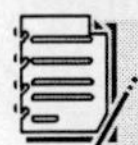

Exercise 2 - Exemplar & Past Year Questions

E&PYQs

Exemplar Questions

1. An electron and a proton are moving under the influence of mutual forces. In calculating the change in the kinetic energy of the system during motion, one ignores the magnetic force of one on another. This is, because
   (a) the two magnetic forces are equal and opposite, so they produce no net effect
   (b) the magnetic forces do not work on each particle
   (c) the magnetic forces do equal and opposite (but non-zero) work on each particle
   (d) the magnetic forces are necessarily negligible

2. A proton is kept at rest. A positively charged particle is released from rest at a distance *d* in its field. Consider two experiments; one in which the charged particle is also a proton and in another, a positron. In the same time *t*, the work done on the two moving charged particles is
   (a) same as the same force law is involved in the two experiments
   (b) less for the case of a positron, as the positron moves away more rapidly and the force on it weakens
   (c) more for the case of a positron, as the positron moves away a larger distance
   (d) same as the work done by charged particle on the stationary proton.

3. A man squatting on the ground gets straight up and stand. The force of reaction of ground on the man during the process is
   (a) constant and equal to *mg* in magnitude
   (b) constant and greater than *mg* in magnitude
   (c) variable but always greater than *mg*
   (d) at first greater than *mg* and later becomes equal to *mg*

4. A bicyclist comes to a skidding stop in 10 m. During this process, the force on the bicycle due to the road is 200N and is directly opposed to the motion. The work done by the cycle on the road is
   (a) +2000 J (b) −200 J
   (c) zero (d) −20,000 J

5. A body is falling freely under the action of gravity alone in vaccum. Which of the following quantities remain constant during the fall?
   (a) Kinetic energy
   (b) Potential energy
   (c) Total mechanical energy
   (d) Total linear momentum

6. During inelastic collision between two bodies, which of the following quantities always remain conserved?
   (a) Total kinetic energy
   (b) Total mechanical energy
   (c) Total linear momentum
   (d) Speed of each body

7. Two inclined frictionless tracks, one gradual and the other steep meet at *A* from where two stones are allowed to slide down from rest, one on each track as shown in figure. Which of the following statement is correct?

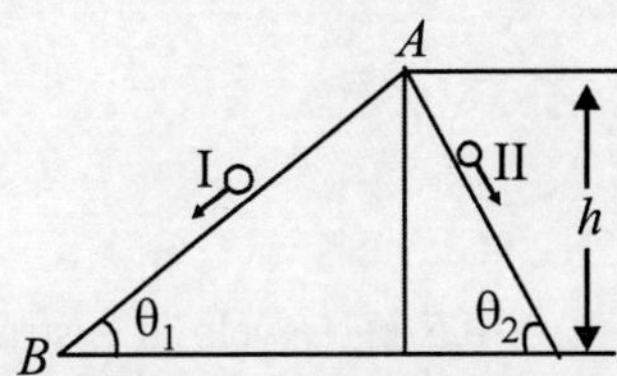

   (a) Both the stones reach the bottom at the same time but not with the same speed
   (b) Both the stones reach the bottom with the same speed and stone I reaches the bottom earlier than stone II
   (c) Both the stones reach the bottom with the same speed and stone II reaches the bottom earlier than stone I
   (d) Both the stones reach the bottom at different times and with different speeds

8. The potential energy function for a particle executing linear SHM is given by $V(x) = \frac{1}{2}kx^2$ where k is the force constant of the oscillator (Fig.). For $k = 0.5$ N/m, the graph of $V(x)$ versus x is shown in the figure. A particle of total energy E turns back when it reaches $x = \pm x_m$. If V and K indicate the PE and KE, respectively of the particle at $x = +x_m$, then which of the following is correct?

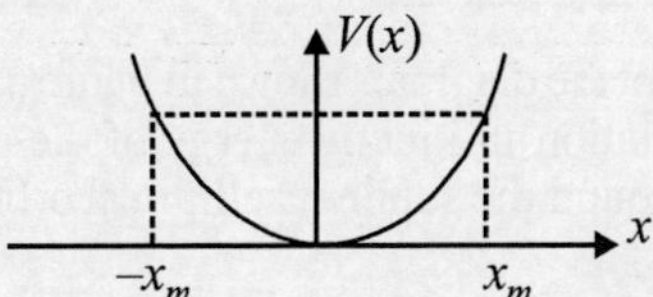

   (a) $V = O, K = E$ (b) $V = E, K = O$
   (c) $V < E, K = O$ (d) $V = O, K < E$

9. Two identical ball bearings in contact with each other and resting on a frictionless table are hit head-on by another ball bearing of the same mass moving initially with a speed v as shown in figure.

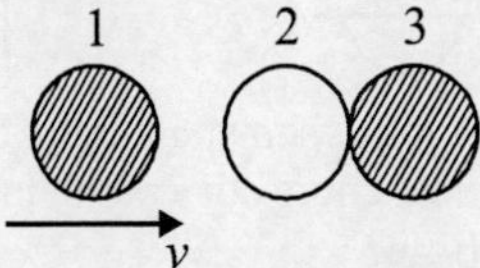

If the collision is elastic, which of the following (figure) is a possible result after collision?

(a)

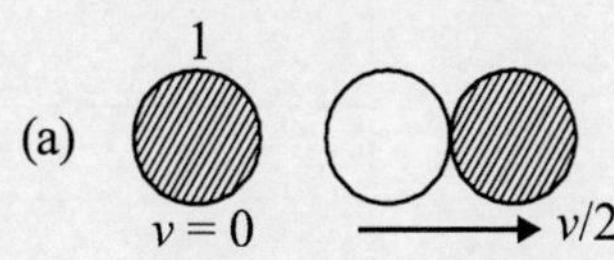

(b)

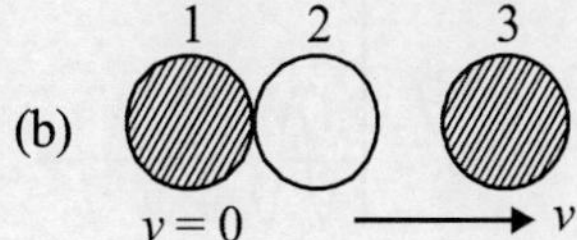

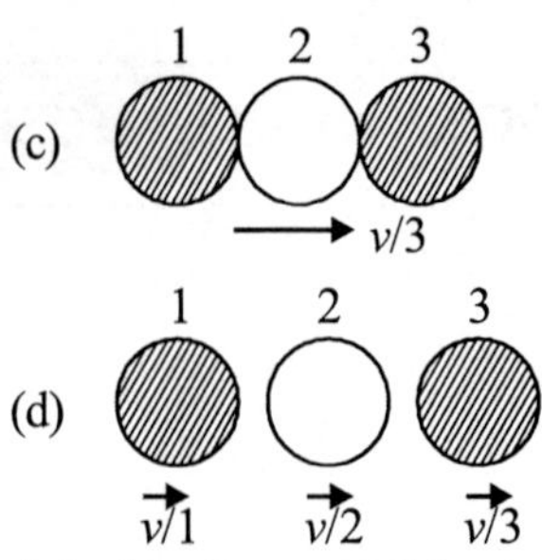

10. A body of mass 0.5 kg travels in a straight line with velocity $v = a\,x^{3/2}$ where $a = 5\ m^{-1/2}s^{-1}$. The work done by the net force during its displacement from $x = 0$ to $x = 2$ m is

(a) 15 J (b) 50 J (c) 10 J (d) 100 J

11. A body is moving unidirectionally under the influence of a source of constant power supplying energy. Which of the diagrams shown in figure correctly shown the displacement-time curve for its motion?

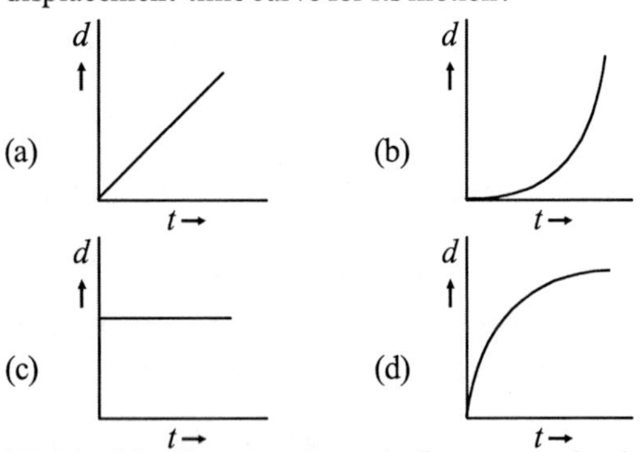

12. Which of the diagrams shown in figure most closely shows the variation in kinetic energy of the earth as it moves once around the sun in its elliptical orbit?

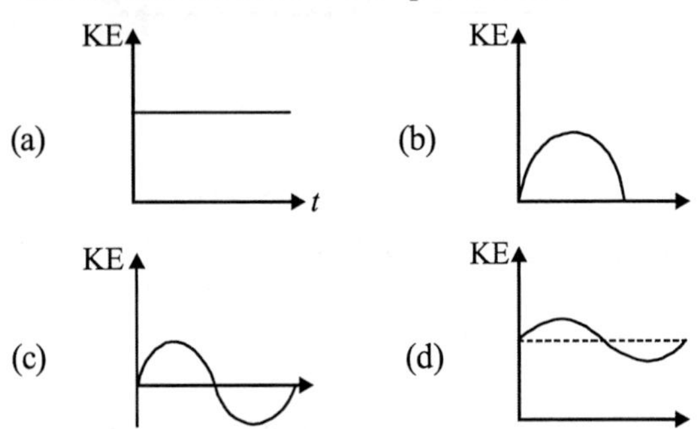

13. Which of the diagrams shown in figure represents variation of total mechanical energy of a pendulum oscillating in air as function of time?

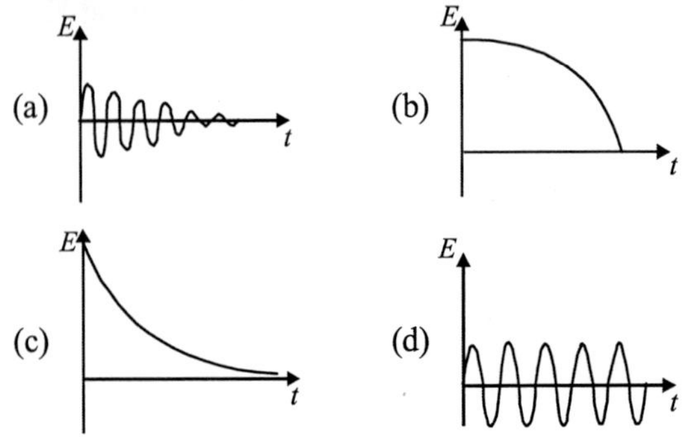

14. A mass of 5 kg is moving along a circular path of radius 1 m. If the mass moves with 300 rev/min, its kinetic energy would be

(a) $250\,\pi^2$ (b) $100\,\pi^2$ (c) $5\,\pi^2$ (d) 0

15. A raindrop falling from a height h above ground, attains a near terminal velocity when it has fallen through a height $(3/4)h$. Which of the diagrams shown in figure correctly shows the change in kinetic and potential energy of the drop during its fall up to the ground?

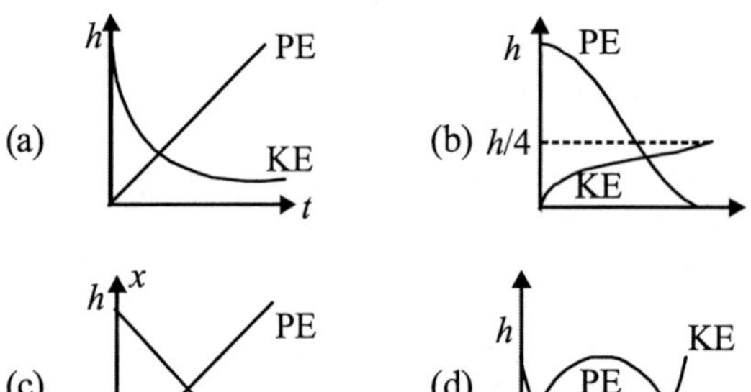

16. In a shotput event an athlete throws the shotput of mass 10 kg with an initial speed of 1 m s^{-1} at 45° from a height 1.5 m above ground. Assuming air resistance to be negligible and acceleration due to gravity to be 10 m s^{-2}, the kinetic energy of the shotput when it just reaches the ground will be

(a) 2.5 J (b) 5.0 J (c) 52.5 J (d) 155.0 J

17. Which of the diagrams in figure correctly shows the change in kinetic energy of an iron sphere falling freely in a lake having sufficient depth to impart it a terminal velocity?

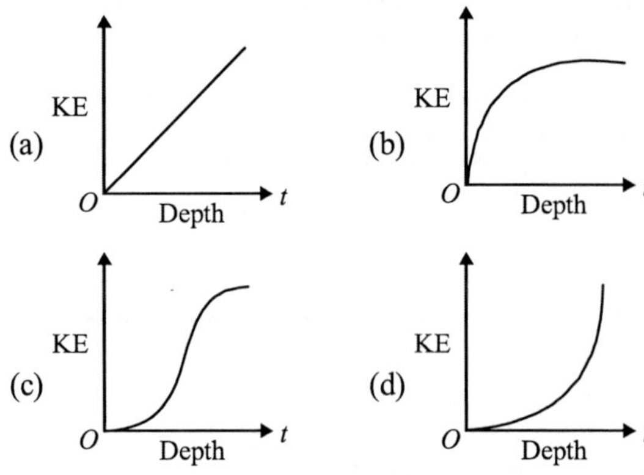

18. A cricket ball of mass 150 g moving with a speed of 126 km/h hits at the middle of the bat, held firmly at its position by the batsman. The ball moves straight back to the bowler after hitting the bat. Assuming that collision between ball and bat is completely elastic and the two remain in contact for 0.001s, the force that the batsman had to apply to hold the bat firmly at its place would be

(a) 10.5N (b) 21 N
(c) 1.05×10^4 N (d) 2.1×10^4 N

NEET/AIPMT (2013-2020) Questions

19. A uniform force of $(3\hat{i} + \hat{j})$ newton acts on a particle of mass 2 kg. The particle is displaced from position $(2\hat{i} + \hat{k})$ meter to position $(4\hat{i} + 3\hat{j} - \hat{k})$ meter. The work done by the force on the particle is *[2013]*

(a) 6 J (b) 13 J (c) 15 J (d) 9 J

20. The upper half of an inclined plane of inclination θ is perfectly smooth while lower half is rough. A block starting from rest at the top of the plane will again come to rest at the bottom, if the coefficient of friction between the block and lower half of the plane is given by *[2013]*

(a) $\mu = \frac{2}{\tan\theta}$ (b) $\mu = 2\tan\theta$

(c) $\mu = \tan\theta$ (d) $\mu = \frac{1}{\tan\theta}$

21. An explosion breaks a rock into three parts in a horizontal plane. Two of them go off at right angles to each other. The first part of mass 1 kg moves with a speed of 12 ms^{-1} and the second part of mass 2 kg moves with speed 8 ms^{-1}. If the third part flies off with speed 4 ms^{-1} then its mass is *[2013]*

(a) 5 kg (b) 7 kg (c) 17 kg (d) 3 kg

22. A person holding a rifle (mass of person and rifle together is 100 kg) stands on a smooth surface and fires 10 shots horizontally, in 5 s. Each bullet has a mass of 10 g with a muzzle velocity of 800 ms^{-1}. The final velocity acquired by the person and the average force exerted on the person are *[NEET Kar. 2013]*

(a) $-1.6\ ms^{-1}$; 8 N (b) $-0.08\ ms^{-1}$; 16 N
(c) $-0.8\ ms^{-1}$; 8 N (d) $-1.6\ ms^{-1}$; 16 N

23. A particle with total energy *E* is moving in a potential energy region *U*(*x*). Motion of the particle is restricted to the region when *[NEET Kar. 2013]*

(a) $U(x) > E$ (b) $U(x) < E$ (c) $U(x) = O$ (d) $U(x) \le E$

24. One coolie takes 1 minute to raise a suitcase through a height of 2 m but the second coolie takes 30 s to raise the same suitcase to the same height. The powers of two coolies are in the ratio of *[NEET Kar. 2013]*

(a) 1 : 2 (b) 1 : 3 (c) 2 : 1 (d) 3 : 1

25. A body of mass (4m) is lying in x-y plane at rest. It suddenly explodes into three pieces. Two pieces, each of mass (m) move perpendicular to each other with equal speeds (v). The total kinetic energy generated due to explosion is: *[2014]*

(a) mv^2 (b) $\frac{3}{2}mv^2$ (c) $2\ mv^2$ (d) $4\ mv^2$

26. The heart of man pumps 5 litres of blood through the arteries per minute at a pressure of 150 mm of mercury. If the density of mercury be $13.6 \times 10^3\ kg/m^3$ and $g = 10 m/s^2$ then the power of heart in watt is : *[2015 RS]*

(a) 2.35 (b) 3.0 (c) 1.50 (d) 1.70

27. A ball is thrown vertically downwards from a height of 20 m with an initial velocity v_0. It collides with the ground loses 50 percent of its energy in collision and rebounds to the same height. The initial velocity v_0 is : *[2015 RS]*
(Take $g = 10\ ms^{-2}$)

(a) 20 ms^{-1} (b) 28 ms^{-1} (c) 10 ms^{-1} (d) 14 ms^{-1}

28. On a frictionless surface a block of mass M moving at speed v collides elastically with another block of same mass M which is initially at rest. After collision the first block moves at an angle θ to its initial direction and has a speed $\frac{v}{3}$. The second block's speed after the collision is: *[2015 RS]*

(a) $\frac{3}{4}v$ (b) $\frac{3}{\sqrt{2}}v$ (c) $\frac{\sqrt{3}}{2}v$ (d) $\frac{2\sqrt{2}}{3}v$

29. Two particles A and B, move with constant velocities $\vec{v}_1$ and $\vec{v}_2$. At the initial moment their position vectors are $\vec{r}_1$ and $\vec{r}_2$ respectively. The condition for particles A and B for their collision is: *[2015 RS]*

(a) $\vec{r}_1 \cdot \vec{v}_1 = \vec{r}_2 \cdot \vec{v}_2$ (b) $\vec{r}_1 \times \vec{v}_1 = \vec{r}_2 \times \vec{v}_2$

(c) $\vec{r}_1 - \vec{r}_2 = \vec{v}_1 - \vec{v}_2$ (d) $\frac{\vec{r}_1 - \vec{r}_2}{|\vec{r}_1 - \vec{r}_2|} = \frac{\vec{v}_2 - \vec{v}_1}{|\vec{v}_2 - \vec{v}_1|}$

30. A particle of mass m is driven by a machine that delivers a constant power of k watts. If the particle starts from rest the force on the particle at time t is *[2015]*

(a) $\sqrt{mk}\ t^{-1/2}$ (b) $\sqrt{2mk}\ t^{-1/2}$

(c) $\frac{1}{2}\sqrt{mk}\ t^{-1/2}$ (d) $\sqrt{\frac{mk}{2}}t^{-1/2}$

31. Two similar springs P and Q have spring constants K_P and K_Q, such that $K_P > K_Q$. They are stretched, first by the same amount (case a,) then by the same force (case b). The work done by the springs W_P and W_Q are related as, in case (a) and case (b), respectively *[2015]*

(a) $W_P = W_Q$; $W_P = W_Q$
(b) $W_P > W_Q$; $W_Q > W_P$
(c) $W_P < W_Q$; $W_Q < W_P$
(d) $W_P = W_Q$; $W_P > W_Q$

32. A block of mass 10 kg, moving in x direction with a constant speed of 10 ms^{-1}, is subject to a retarding force $F = 0.1 \times$ J/m during its travel from x = 20 m to 30 m. Its final KE will be: *[2015]*

(a) 450 J (b) 275 J (c) 250 J (d) 475 J

33. A body of mass 1 kg begins to move under the action of a time dependent force $\vec{F} = (2t\hat{i} + 3t^2\hat{j})$ N, where $\hat{i}$ and $\hat{j}$ are unit vectors alogn x and y axis. What power will be developed by the force at the time t? *[2016]*

(a) $(2t^2 + 3t^3)$W (b) $(2t^2 + 4t^4)$W
(c) $(2t^3 + 3t^4)$ W (d) $(2t^3 + 3t^5)$W

34. A particle of mass 10 g moves along a circle of radius 6.4 cm with a constant tangential acceleration. What is the magnitude of this acceleration if the kinetic energy of the particle becomes equal to 8×10^{-4} J by the end of the second revolution after the beginning of the motion? *[2016]*

(a) 0.1 m/s^2 (b) 0.15 m/s^2
(c) 0.18 m/s^2 (d) 0.2 m/s^2

35. Consider a drop of rain water having mass 1 g falling from a height of 1 km. It hits the ground with a speed of 50 m/s. Take 'g' constant with a value 10 m/s^2.
The work done by the (i) gravitational force and the (ii) resistive force of air is *[2017]*
(a) (i) 1.25 J (ii) –8.25 J
(b) (i) 100 J (ii) 8.75 J
(c) (i) 10 J (ii) – 8.75 J
(d) (i) – 10 J (ii) –8.25 J

36. A moving block having mass m, collides with another stationary block having mass 4m. The lighter block comes to rest after collision. When the initial velocity of the lighter block is v, then the value of coefficient of restitution (e) will be *[2018]*
(a) 0.5 (b) 0.25 (c) 0.4 (d) 0.8

37. A force F = 20 + 10y acts on a particle in y-direction where F is in newton and y in meter. Work done by this force to move the particle from y = 0 to y = 1 m is : *[2019]*
(a) 30 J (b) 5 J (c) 25 J (d) 20 J

38. An object of mass 500 g, initially at rest, is acted upon by a variable force whose X-component varies with X in the manner shown. The velocities of the object at the points X = 8 m and X = 12 m, would have the respective values of (nearly) *[NEET Odisha 2019]*

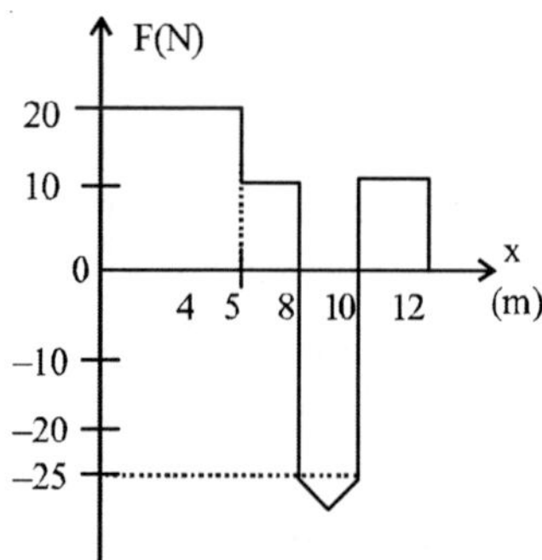

(a) 18 m/s and 20.6 m/s (b) 18 m/s and 24.4 m/s
(c) 23 m/s and 24.4 m/s (d) 23 m/s and 20.6 m/s

39. Body A of mass 4m moving with speed u collides with another body B of mass 2m, at rest. The collision is head on and elastic in nature. After the collision the fraction of energy lost by the colliding body A is : *[2019]*
(a) $\frac{1}{9}$ (b) $\frac{8}{9}$ (c) $\frac{4}{9}$ (d) $\frac{5}{9}$

40. An object flying in air with velocity $\left(20\hat{i}+25\hat{j}-12\hat{k}\right)$ suddenly breaks into two pieces whose masses are in the ratio 1 : 5. The smaller mass flies off with a velocity $\left(100\hat{i}+35\hat{j}+8\hat{k}\right)$. The velocity of the larger piece will be *[NEET Odisha 2019]*
(a) $-20\hat{i}-15\hat{j}-80\hat{k}$ (b) $4\hat{i}+23\hat{j}-16\hat{k}$
(c) $-100\hat{i}-35\hat{j}-8\hat{k}$ (d) $20\hat{i}+15\hat{j}-80\hat{k}$

41. Two bullets are fired horizontally and simultaneously towards each other from roof tops of two buildings 100 m apart of same height of 200 m, with the same velocity of 25 m/s. When and where will the two bullets collide? (g = 10 m/s^2) *[NEET Odisha 2019]*
(a) They will not collide
(b) After 2 s at a height of 180 m
(c) After 2 s at a height of 20 m
(d) After 4 s at a height of 120 m

42. A particle of mass 5 m at rest suddenly breaks on its own into three fragments. Two fragments of mass m each move along mutually perpendicular direction with speed v each. The energy released during the process is, *[NEET Odisha 2019]*
(a) $\frac{4}{3}mv^2$ (b) $\frac{3}{5}mv^2$ (c) $\frac{5}{3}mv^2$ (d) $\frac{3}{2}mv^2$

Exercise 3 - Concept Application Problems — CAP

1. Two bodies of masses 2 m and m have their KE in the ratio 8 : 1. What is the ratio of their momenta ?
(a) 8 : 1 (b) 4 : 1 (c) 2 : 1 (d) 1 : 1

2. A body accelerates uniformly from rest to a velocity of 1 ms^{-1} in 15 seconds. The kinetic energy of the body will be $\frac{2}{9}$ J when 't' is equal to [Take mass of body as 1 kg]
(a) 4s (b) 8s (c) 10s (d) 12s

3. A crane is used to lift 1000 kg of coal from a mine 100 m deep. The time taken by the crane is 1 hour. The efficiency of the crane is 80%. If g = 10 ms^{-2}, then the power of the crane is
(a) 10^4 W (b) 10^5 W
(c) $\frac{10^4}{36\times8}$W (d) $\frac{10^5}{36\times8}$W

4. A body moves a distance of 10 m along a straight line under the action of a force of 5 newtons. If the work done is 25 joules, the angle which the force makes with the direction of motion of body is
(a) 0° (b) 30° (c) 60° (d) 90°

5. A sphere of mass 8m collides elastically (in one dimension) with a block of mass 2m. If the initial energy of sphere is E. What is the final energy of sphere?
(a) 0.8 E (b) 0.36 E (c) 0.08 E (d) 0.64 E

6. A moving body with a mass m_1 and velocity u strikes a stationary body of mass m_2. The masses m_1 and m_2 should be in the ratio m_1/m_2 so as to decrease the velocity of the first body to 2u/3 and giving a velocity of u to m_2 assuming a perfectly elastic impact. Then the ratio m_1/m_2 is
(a) 5 (b) 1/5 (c) 1/25 (d) 25.

7. A body of mass m is suspended from a massless spring of natural length ℓ. It stretches the spring through a vertical distance y. The potential energy of the stretched spring is

(a) $mg(\ell + y)$ (b) $\frac{1}{2}mg(\ell + y)$

(c) $\frac{1}{2}mgy$ (d) mgy

8. Figure here shows the frictional force versus displacement for a particle in motion. The loss of kinetic energy in travelling over s = 0 to 20 m will be

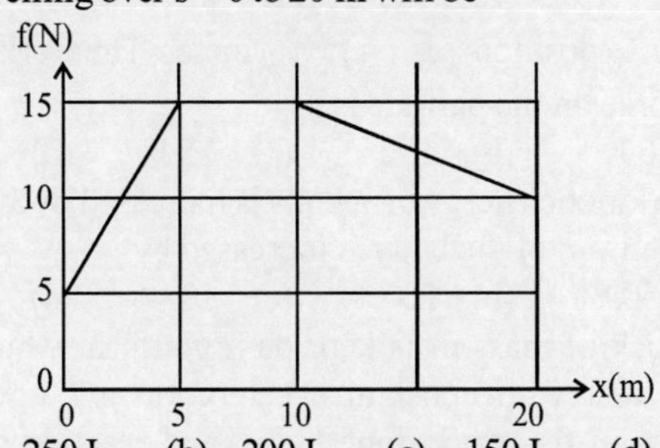

(a) 250 J (b) 200 J (c) 150 J (d) 10 J

9. Ten litre of water per second is lifted from a well through 10 m and delivered with a velocity of 10 ms^{-1}. If $g = 10\ ms^{-2}$, then the power of the motor is

(a) 1 kW (b) 1.5 kW (c) 2 kW (d) 2.5 kW

10. A nucleus ruptures into two nuclear parts which have their velocity ratio equal to $2:1$. The ratio of their respective nuclear sizes (nuclear radii)is

(a) $1:2$ (b) $1:\sqrt{2}$ (c) $1:2^{1/3}$ (d) $1:8$

11. A one-ton car moves with a constant velocity of 15 ms^{-1} on a rough horizontal road. The total resistance to the motion of the car is 12% of the weight of the car. The power required to keep the car moving with the same constant velocity of $15 ms^{-1}$ is
[Take $g = 10\ ms^{-2}$]

(a) 9 kW (b) 18 kW (c) 24 kW (d) 36 kW

12. An automobile engine of mass M accelerates and a constant power p is applied by the engine. The instantaneous speed of the engine will be

(a) $[Pt/M]^{1/2}$ (b) $[2Pt/M]^{1/2}$

(c) $[Pt/2M]^{1/2}$ (d) $[Pt/4M]^{1/2}$

13. A body is attached to the lower end of a vertical helical spring and it is gradually lowered to its equilibrium position. This stretches the spring by a length x. If the same body attached to the same spring is allowed to fall suddenly, what would be the maximum stretching in this case?

(a) x (b) 2x (c) 3x (d) x/2

14. A particle of mass m moving eastward with a speed v collides with another particle of the same mass moving northwards with the same speed. If two particles coalesce on collision, the new particle of mass 2 m will move in the north-east direction with a velocity

(a) $v/2$ (b) $v\sqrt{2}$

(c) $v/\sqrt{2}$ (d) None of these

15. A nucleus moving with a velocity $\vec{v}$ emits an α-particle. Let the velocities of the α-particle and the remaining nucleus be $\vec{v}_1$ and $\vec{v}_2$ and their masses be m_1 and m_2.

(a) $\vec{v}$, $\vec{v}_1$ and $\vec{v}_2$ must be parallel to each other

(b) None of the two of $\vec{v}$, $\vec{v}_1$ and $\vec{v}_2$ should be parallel to each other

(c) $m_1\vec{v}_1 + m_2\vec{v}_2$ must be parallel to $(m_1 + m_2)\vec{v}$.

(d) None of these

16. The bob A of a simple pendulum is released when the string makes an angle of 45° with the vertical. It hits another bob B of the same material and same mass kept at rest on the table. If the collision is elastic

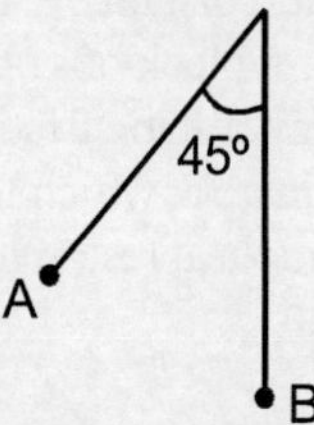

(a) both A and B rise to the same height

(b) both A and B come to rest at B

(c) both A and B move with the velocity of A

(d) A comes to rest and B moves with the velocity of A

17. Two masses m_a and m_b moving with velocities v_a and v_b in opposite direction collide elastically and after the collision m_a and m_b move with velocities V_b and V_a respectively. Then the ratio m_a/m_b is

(a) $\frac{V_a - V_b}{V_a + V_b}$ (b) $\frac{m_a + m_b}{m_a}$

(c) 1 (d) $\frac{1}{2}$

18. A particle of mass m_1 moving with velocity v strikes with a mass m_2 at rest, then the condition for maximum transfer of kinetic energy is

(a) $m_1 >> m_2$ (b) $m_2 >> m_2$

(c) $m_1 = m_2$ (d) $m_1 = 2m_2$

19. Two blocks of masses 10 kg and 4 kg are connected by a spring of negligible mass and placed on a frictionless horizontal surface. An impulse gives a velocity of 14 m/s to the heavier block in the direction of the lighter block. The velocity of the centre of mass is

(a) 30 m/s (b) 20 m/s (c) 10 m/s (d) 5 m/s

20. A glass marble dropped from a certain height above the horizontal surface reaches the surface in time t and then continues to bounce up and down. The time in which the marble finally comes to rest is

(a) $e^n t$ (b) $e^2 t$

(c) $t\left[\frac{1+e}{1-e}\right]$ (d) $t\left[\frac{1-e}{1+e}\right]$

21. A weight suspended from the free end of a vertically hanging spring produces an extension of 3 cm. The spring is cut into two parts so that the length of the longer part is $\frac{2}{3}$ of the original length, If the same weight is now suspended from the longer part of the spring, the extension produced will be

(a) 0.1 cm (b) 0.5 cm (c) 1 cm (d) 2 cm

22. A 10 m long iron chain of linear mass density 0.8 kg m^{-1} is hanging freely from a rigid support. If g = 10 ms^{-2}, then the power required to left the chain upto the point of support in 10 second

(a) 10 W (b) 20W (c) 30 W (d) 40 W

23. A ramp is constructed in parabolic shape such that the height y of any point on its surface is given in terms of the point's horizontal distance x from the bottom of the ramp be $y = x^2/2L$. A block of granite is to be set on the ramp; the coefficient of static friction is 0.80. What is the maximum x coordinate at which the block can be placed on the ramp and remain at rest, if L = 10 m?

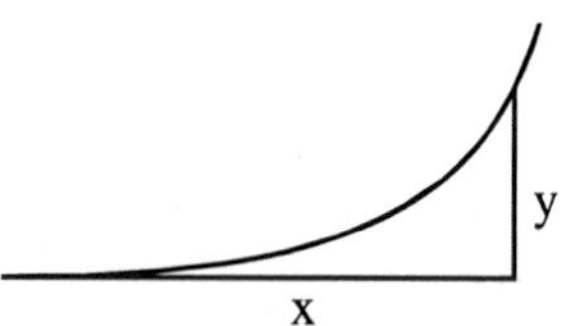

(a) 8m (b) 8.4m (c) 9m (d) 9.4m

24. n small balls each of mass m impinge elastically each second on a surface with velocity v. The force experienced by the surface will be

(a) $\frac{1}{2}$mnv (b) 2 mnv (c) mnv (d) 2 mnv

25. The coefficient of friction between the tyres and the road is μ. A car is moving with momentum p. What will be the stopping distance due to friction alone ? The mass of the car is m.

(a) $p^2/2\mu g$ (b) $p^2/2m\mu g$
(c) $p^2/2m^2\mu g$ (d) $p^2/2mg$

26. A force acts on a 30 gm particle in such a way that the position of the particle as a function of time is given by $x = 3t - 4t^2 + t^3$, where x is in metres and t is in seconds. The work done during the first 4 seconds is

(a) 576mJ (b) 450mJ (c) 490mJ (d) 530mJ

27. A bomb of mass 1 kg is thrown vertically upwards with a speed of 100 m/s. After 5 seconds it explodes into two fragments. One fragment of mass 400 gm is found to go down with a speed of 25 m/s. What will happen to the second fragment just after the explosion? ($g = 10\ m/s^2$)

(a) It will go upward with speed 40 m/s
(b) It will go upward with speed 100 m/s
(c) It will go upward with speed 60 m/s
(d) It will also go downward with speed 40m/s

28. A mass of 0.5 kg moving with a speed of 1.5 m/s on a horizontal smooth surface, collides with a nearly weightless spring of force constant k = 50 N/m. The maximum compression of the spring would be

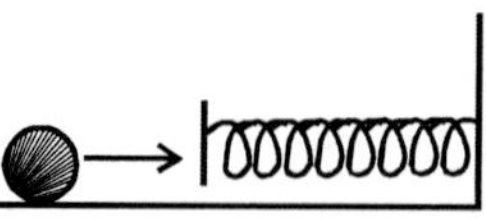

(a) 0.5m (b) 0.15m (c) 0.12m (d) 1.5m

29. A uniform force of $(3\hat{i} + \hat{j})$ newton acts on a particle of mass 2 kg. The particle is displaced from position $(2\hat{i} + \hat{k})$ meter to position $(4\hat{i} + 3\hat{j} - \hat{k})$ meter. The work done by the force on the particle is

(a) 6 J (b) 13 J (c) 15 J (d) 9 J

30. If the kinetic energy of a body is increased by 300%, the momentum of the body is increased by

(a) 300% (b) 200% (c) 100% (d) 50%

31. A block of mass m is kept on a platform which starts from rest with constant acceleration g/2 upward, as shown in fig. work done by normal reaction on block in time t is:

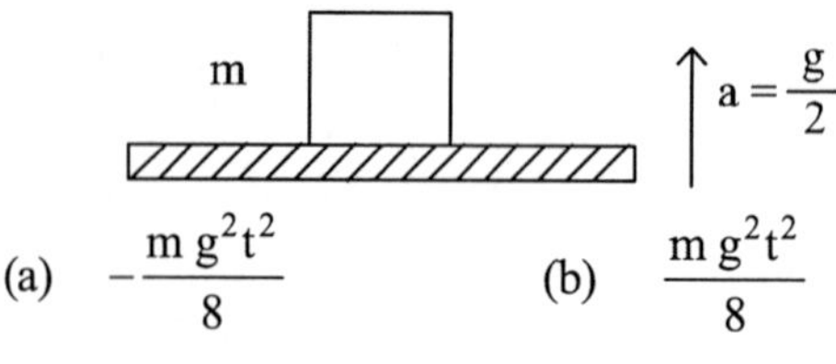

(a) $-\frac{mg^2t^2}{8}$ (b) $\frac{mg^2t^2}{8}$

(c) 0 (d) $\frac{3mg^2t^2}{8}$

32. A body of mass starts moving from rest along x-axis so that its velocity varies as $v = a\sqrt{s}$ where a is a constant s and is the distance covered by the body. The total work done by all the forces acting on the body in the first second after the start of the motion is:

(a) $\frac{1}{8}ma^4t^2$ (b) $4ma^4t^2$

(c) $8ma^4t^2$ (d) $\frac{1}{4}ma^4t^2$

33. A uniform cable of mass 'M' and length 'L' is placed on a horizontal surface such that its $\left(\frac{1}{n}\right)^{th}$ part is hanging below the edge of the surface. To lift the hanging part of the cable upto the surface, the work done should be:

(a) $\frac{MgL}{2n^2}$ (b) $\frac{MgL}{n^2}$ (c) $\frac{2MgL}{n^2}$ (d) nMgL

34. A wedge of mass M = 4m lies on a frictionless plane. A particle of mass *m* approaches the wedge with speed *v*. There is no friction between the particle and the plane or between the particle and the wedge. The maximum height climbed by the particle on the wedge is given by:

(a) $\frac{v^2}{g}$ (b) $\frac{2v^2}{7g}$ (c) $\frac{2v^2}{5g}$ (d) $\frac{v^2}{2g}$

35. A particle moves in one dimension from rest under the influence of a force that varies with the distance travelled by the particle as shown in the figure. The kinetic energy of the particle after it has travelled 3 m is :

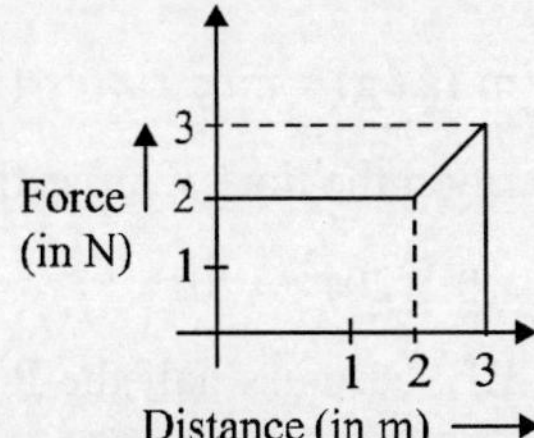

(a) 4 J (b) 2.5 J (c) 6.5 J (d) 5 J

36. A particle which is experiencing a force, given by $\vec{F} = 3\vec{i} - 12\vec{j}$, undergoes a displacement of $\vec{d} = 4\vec{i}$. If the particle had a kinetic energy of 3 J at the beginning of the displacement, what is its kinetic energy at the end of the displacement?

(a) 9 J (b) 12 J (c) 10 J (d) 15 J

37. A block of mass m, lying on a smooth horizontal surface, is attached to a spring (of negligible mass) of spring constant k. The other end of the spring is fixed, as shown in the figure. The block is initally at rest in its equilibrium position. If now the block is pulled with a constant force F, the maximum speed of the block is:

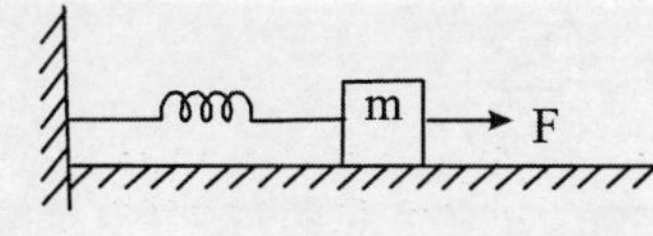

(a) $\frac{2F}{\sqrt{mk}}$ (b) $\frac{F}{\pi\sqrt{mk}}$ (c) $\frac{\pi F}{\sqrt{mk}}$ (d) $\frac{F}{\sqrt{mk}}$

38. Two particles of the same mass m are moving in circular orbits because of force, given by $F(r) = \frac{-16}{r} - r^3$

The first particle is at a distance r = 1, and the second, at r = 4. The best estimate for the ratio of kinetic energies of the first and the second particle is closest to

(a) 10^{-1} (b) 6×10^{-2} (c) 6×10^{2} (d) 3×10^{-3}

39. A 60 HP electric motor lifts an elevator having a maximum total load capacity of 2000 kg. If the frictional force on the elevator is 4000 N, the speed of the elevator at full load is close to: (1 HP = 746 W, g = 10 ms^{-2})

(a) 1.7 ms^{-1} (b) 1.9 ms^{-1} (c) 1.5 ms^{-1} (d) 2.0 ms^{-1}

40. Particle A of mass m_1 moving with velocity $(\sqrt{3}\hat{i} + \hat{j})\, ms^{-1}$ collides with another particle B of mass m_2 which is at rest initially. Let $\vec{V_1}$ and $\vec{V_2}$ be the velocities of particles A and B after collision respectively. If $m_1 = 2m_2$ and after collision $\vec{V_1} = (\hat{i} + \sqrt{3}\hat{j})\, ms^{-1}$, the angle between $\vec{V_1}$ and $\vec{V_2}$ is :

(a) 15° (b) 60° (c) −45° (d) 105°

41. Blocks of masses *m*, 2*m*, 4*m* and 8*m* are arranged in a line on a frictionless floor. Another block of mass *m*, moving with speed *v* along the same line (see figure) collides with mass *m* in perfectly inelastic manner. All the subsequent collisions are also perfectly inelastic. By the time the last block of mass 8*m* starts moving the total energy loss is *p*% of the original energy. Value of '*p*' is close to :

(a) 77 (b) 94 (c) 37 (d) 87

42. A block of mass 1.9 kg is at rest at the edge of a table, of height 1 m. A bullet of mass 0.1 kg collides with the block and sticks to it. If the velocity of the bullet is 20 m/s in the horizontal direction just before the collision then the kinetic energy just before the combined system strikes the floor, is [Take g = 10 m/s². Assume there is no rotational motion and losss of energy after the collision is negligiable.]

(a) 20 J (b) 21 J (c) 19 J (d) 23 J

43. A piece of wood of mass 0.03 kg is dropped from the top of a 100 m height building. At the same time, a bullet of mass 0.02 kg is fired vertically upward, with a velocity 100 ms^{-1}, from the ground. The bullet gets embedded in the wood. Then the maximum height to which the combined system reaches above the top of the building before falling below is: (g = 10 ms^{-2})

(a) 20m (b) 30m (c) 40m (d) 10m

44. There block A, B and C are lying on a smooth horizontal surface, as shown in the figure. A and B have equal masses, m while C has mass M. Block A is given an inital speed *v* towards B due to which it collides with B perfectly inelastically. The combined mass collides with C, also perfectly inelastically $\frac{5}{6}$th of the initial kinetic energy is lost in whole process. What is value of M/m?

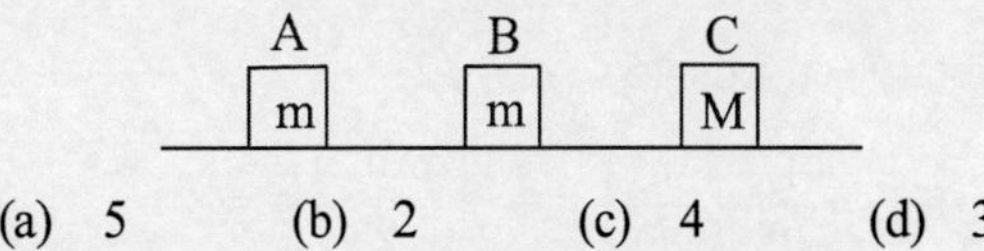

(a) 5 (b) 2 (c) 4 (d) 3

45. A proton of mass m collides elastically with a particle of unknown mass at rest. After the collision, the proton and the unknown particle are seen moving at an angle of 90° with respect to each other. The mass of unknown particle is:

(a) $\frac{m}{\sqrt{3}}$ (b) $\frac{m}{2}$ (c) 2m (d) m

Hints & Solutions

6.1 Concept Practice Problems

CPP

1. (a) The magnitude of work done by a force depends on frame of refrance.
2. (b)
3. (b) Because water enters into the vessel A, it becomes heavier. Gravity helps it sink. External work required for immersing A is obviously less than that for immersing B.
4. (d) $W = F \times s$

   $W \propto \frac{1}{x}(x) \therefore W \propto x^0$
5. (a) $W = F s \cos 90° = \text{zero}$
6. (c) As the cord is trying to hold the motion of the block, work done by the cord is negative.

   $W = -M(g-a)d = -M\left(g - \frac{g}{4}\right)d = \frac{-3Mgd}{4}$
7. (c) $W = F s \cos\theta = 10 \times 2 \cos 60° = 10$ J.
8. (c) $W = \vec{F}.\vec{s} = (5\hat{i} + 2\hat{j}).(2\hat{i} + 3\hat{j}) = 10 + 6 = 16$ J.
9. (b) $W = \int_0^{x_1} F\,dx = \int_0^{x_1} cx\,dx = \left[\frac{1}{2}cx^2\right]_0^{x_1}$

   $= \frac{1}{2}c(x_1^2 - 0) = \frac{1}{2}cx_1^2$
10. (b)

    $W = \vec{F}.\vec{x} = (5\hat{i} + 3\hat{j} + 2\hat{k}).(2\hat{i} - \hat{j}) = 10 - 3 = 7$ joules

6.2 Concept Practice Problems

CPP

11. (c) $P.E_A = P.E_B$ at the highest point of their trajectories
12. (a)
13. (c) Weight Mg moves the centre of gravity of the spring through a distance $\frac{(0+\ell)}{2} = \ell/2$

    $\therefore$ Mechanical energy stored = Work done = Mg ℓ/2.
14. (d)
15. (b) At the top of flight, horizontal component of velocity = $u \cos 45° = u/\sqrt{2}$

    $\therefore$ K.E. $= \frac{1}{2}m\left(\frac{u}{\sqrt{2}}\right)^2 = \frac{1}{2}\left(\frac{mu^2}{2}\right) = \frac{1}{2}K.$
16. (b) $F \propto \frac{1}{v}$ (given)

    Then $W = E_k = F.s$

    Become = $E_k \propto \frac{s}{v} \Rightarrow E_k \propto \frac{s}{s/t}$

    $\Rightarrow E_k \propto t$
17. (c) From horizontal position to lowest position, height through which the bob falls = ℓ

    $\therefore$ At lowest position, $v = \sqrt{2\ell g}$

    K.E. at lowest point

    $= \frac{1}{2}mv^2 = \frac{1}{2}m(2\ell g) = m\ell g = 10 \times 1 \times 9.8 = 98$ J.
18. (b) Total energy at the time of projection

    $= \frac{1}{2}mv^2 = \frac{1}{2} \times 0.1(20)^2 = 20$J

    Half way up, P.E. becomes half the P.E. at the top i.e.

    P.E. $= \frac{20}{2} = 10$J $\quad \therefore$ K.E. $= 20 - 10 = 10$J.
19. (d) As $E = \frac{p^2}{2m} \quad \therefore \frac{dE}{E} = 2\left(\frac{dp}{p}\right) = 2 \times 5\% = 10\%$
20. (d) $V = \frac{1}{2}k(x)^2 = \frac{1}{2}k(2)^2$ or $k = \frac{2V}{4} = \frac{V}{2}$

    $V' = \frac{1}{2}k(10)^2 = \frac{1}{2} \times \left(\frac{V}{2}\right)(10)^2 = 25V$

6.3 Concept Practice Problems

CPP

21. (c) At the point of impact, in case of elastic collision total K.E. of colliding bodies decreases.
22. (b)
23. (d) As $e^n = \left(\frac{h_n}{h_0}\right)^{1/2}$

    $\therefore h_n = e^{2n}h_0 = e^{2\times2}h = e^4 h.$
24. (a) As $u_2 = 0$ and $m_1 = m_2$, therefore from $m_1 u_1 + m_2 u_2 = m_1 v_1 + m_2 v_2$ we get $u_1 = v_1 + v_2$

    Also, $e = \frac{v_2 - v_1}{u_1} = \frac{v_2 - v_1}{v_2 + v_1} = \frac{1 - v_1/v_2}{1 + v_1/v_2}$,

    which gives $\frac{v_1}{v_2} = \frac{1-e}{1+e}$
25. (b)

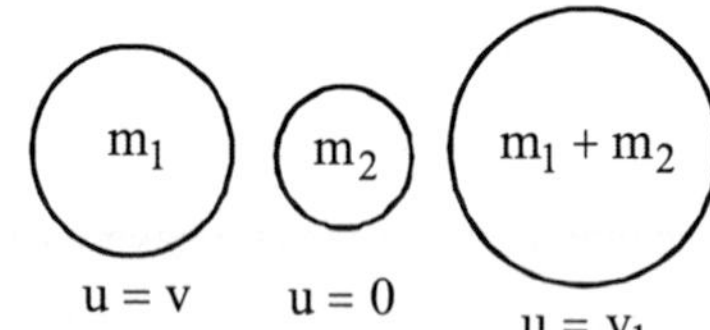

applying conservation of momentum

$m_1 v + m_2(0) = (m_1 + m_2)v_1 \Rightarrow v_1 = \frac{m_1}{(m_1 + m_2)}v$

as $m_1 < (m_1 + m_2)$ so velocity decreases.

26. (b) $v_1 = \frac{(m_1 - m_2)u_1}{m_1 + m_2}$ As v_1 is negative and less than u_1, therefore, $m_1 < m_2$.
27. (a) $m_1 = 0.2$ kg, $m_2 = 0.4$kg, $v_1 = 0.3$m/s, $v_2 = ?$

    Applying law of conservation of momentum

    $m_1v_1 - m_2v_2 = \frac{0.2 \times 0.3}{0.4} = 0.15$ m/s.

28. (c) $v_2 = \frac{-m_1 v_1}{m_2} = \frac{-3}{6} \times 16 = -8\,m/s$

$E_2 = \frac{1}{2} m_2 v_2^2 = \frac{1}{2} \times 6(-8)^2 = 192\,J.$

29. (d) Applying the principle of conservation of linear momentum, we get

$3m \times v = \sqrt{(m \times 60)^2 + (m \times 60)^2} = m \times 60\sqrt{2}$

$v = 20\sqrt{2}\,m/s$

30. (c) Since the new height gained is half, therefore there is 50% loss of energy.

31. (b) Components of velocity before and after collision parallel to the plane are equal, So

$v \sin 60° = u \sin 30°$ ....(1)

Components of velocity normal to the plane are related to each other

$v \cos 60° = e\,u\,(\cos 30°)$ ....(2)

$\Rightarrow \quad \cot 60° = e \cot 30° \Rightarrow e = \frac{\cos 60°}{\cot 30°}$

$\Rightarrow \quad e = \frac{\frac{1}{\sqrt{3}}}{\sqrt{3}} \Rightarrow e = \frac{1}{3}.$

32. (b) Let the velocity and mass of 4 kg piece be v_1 and m_1 and that of 12 kg piece be v_2 and m_2.

Applying conservation of linear momentum

$m_2 v_2 = m_1 v_1$

$\Rightarrow v_1 = \frac{12 \times 4}{4} = 12\ ms^{-1}$

$\therefore K.E._1 = \frac{1}{2} m_1 v_1^2 = \frac{1}{2} \times 4 \times 144 = 288\ J$

33. (a) Let M be the mass of shell. Applying law of conservation of linear momentum

$MV \cos\theta = \left(-\frac{MV}{2}\cos\theta\right) + \frac{M}{2} v$

ie, $MV \cos\theta + \frac{M}{2} V\cos\theta = \frac{M}{2} v$

or $v = 3V\cos\theta$.

34. (b) According to principle of conservation of energy Potential energy = kinetic energy

$\Rightarrow mgh = \frac{1}{2} mv^2 \Rightarrow v = \sqrt{2gh}$

If h_1 and h_2 are initial and final heights, then

$\Rightarrow v_1 = \sqrt{2gh_1}, v_2 = \sqrt{2gh_2}$

Loss in velocity, $\Delta v = v_1 - v_2 = \sqrt{2gh_1} - \sqrt{2gh_2}$

$\therefore$ fractional loss in velocity

$= \frac{\Delta v}{v_1} = \frac{\sqrt{2gh_1} - \sqrt{2gh_2}}{\sqrt{2gh_1}} = 1 - \sqrt{\frac{h_2}{h_1}}$

$= 1 - \sqrt{\frac{1.8}{5}} = 1 - \sqrt{0.36} = 1 - 0.6 = 0.4 = \frac{2}{5}$

35. (b) From law of conservation of momentum, before collision and after collision linear momentum (p) will be same.

or initial momentum = final momentum.

$E = \frac{p^2}{2m}$

According to question,

$\frac{E_1}{E_2} = \frac{p_1^2}{2m_1} \times \frac{2m_2}{p_2^2} \Rightarrow \frac{E_1}{E_2} = \frac{m_2}{m_1} \quad [p_1 = p_2]$

Exercise 1 - Chapter Revision Problems CRP

1. (a) Spring force and elastic force are conservative.

2. (d) From $v = u + at$, $v_1 = 0 + at_1$

$\therefore \quad a = \frac{v_1}{t_1}$

$F = ma = m\,v_1 / t_1$

Velocity acquired in t sec = $at = \frac{v_1}{t_1} t$

Power $= F \times v = \frac{m v_1}{t_1} \times \frac{v_1 t}{t_1} = \frac{m v_1^2 t}{t_1^2}$

3. (a) From $v^2 - u^2 = 2as$

$0 - v_0^2 = 2(\mu g)s \qquad \therefore\ s = \frac{v_0^2}{2\mu g}$

4. (b) If $\vec{L} = 0 \Rightarrow$ K.E may or may not be zero.

If K.E = 0 $\Rightarrow \vec{L} = 0$.

5. (d) Power is defined as the rate of doing work. For the automobile, the power output is the amount of work done (overcoming friction) divided by the length of time in which the work was done.

6. (b) $W = \frac{1}{2} k\ell_2^2 - \frac{1}{2} k\ell_1^2 = \frac{1}{2} k(\ell_2^2 - \ell_1^2)$

7. (d) $\frac{mv^2}{t} = \frac{ms^2}{t^3}$

since both P and m are constants

$\therefore \quad \frac{s^2}{t^3}$ = constant

8. (c) $v = \frac{m_1 v_1 + m_2 v_2}{m_1 + m_2} = \frac{a \times b + 0}{a + c} = \frac{a(b)}{a + c}.$

9. (d) Work done = $\int F dx$

10. (d) Forward thrust, $F = \frac{P}{v} = \frac{100 \times 746}{20} = 3730\,N.$

11. (c) As $\frac{1}{2} m_A v_A^2 = \frac{1}{2} m_B v_B^2$

$\frac{v_A}{v_B} = \sqrt{\frac{m_B}{m_A}}$;

$\frac{P_B}{P_A} = \frac{m_B v_B}{m_A v_A} = \frac{m_B}{m_A}\sqrt{\frac{m_A}{m_B}} = \sqrt{\frac{m_B}{m_A}} = \frac{1}{\sqrt{3}}$

12. (a) From $m_1 v_1 + m_2 v_2 = 0$,

$$v_2 = \frac{-m_1 v_1}{m_2} = -\frac{4}{234}$$

13. (b) Workdone, $W = \frac{1}{2}k\left(x_2^2 - x_1^2\right)$

$$= \frac{1}{2}k\left[(0.15)^2 - (0.05)^2\right]$$

$$= \frac{1}{2} \times 800 \times 0.02 = 8J$$

14. (d) $T = M(g - g/8) = \frac{7}{8}Mg$

Work done by the cord = T × d cos 180°

$$= \frac{7}{8}Mgd(-1) = -7Mgd/8.$$

15. (a) $W_1 = \frac{1}{2} \times 5 \times 10^3 (0.05)^2$

$$\Rightarrow W_2 = \frac{1}{2} \times 5 \times 10^3 (0.10)^2$$

$$\therefore \Delta W = \frac{1}{2} \times 5 \times 10^3 \times 0.15 \times 0.05 = 18.75J.$$

16. (b) If P = momentum, K = kinetic energy, then

$P_1^2 = 2mK_1$, $P_2^2 = 2mK_2$

$$\therefore \left(\frac{P_2}{P_1}\right)^2 = \frac{K_2}{K_1} = \frac{3K_1}{K_1} = 3 \;\therefore \frac{P_2}{P_1} = \sqrt{\frac{3}{1}} = 1.732$$

17. (c) Energy stored (E) $= \frac{75}{100} \times (12) = 9\,J$

As $E = \frac{1}{2}mv^2$

$$v = \sqrt{\frac{2E}{m}} = \sqrt{\frac{2 \times 9}{1}} = \sqrt{18}\ m/sec$$

18. (d) Let n be the number of bullets that the man can fire in one second.

$\therefore$ change in momentum per second $= n \times mv = F$
[m= mass of bullet, v = velocity] ($\because$ F is the force)

$$\therefore n = \frac{F}{mv} = \frac{144 \times 1000}{40 \times 1200} = 3$$

19. (b) Work done against gravity
$W_g = 50 \times 10 \times 30 = 15$ kJ
Work done against friction

$$W_f = \mu mg\cos\theta \times s = 0.4 \times 50 \times 10 \times \frac{4}{5} \times 50 = 8\,kJ$$

Total work done $= W_g + W_f = 15\ kJ + 8\ kJ = 23\ kJ$

20. (d)
21. (b) The work is done against gravity so it is equal to the change in potential energy. $W = E_p = mgh$
For a fixed height, work is proportional to weight lifted. Since Johnny weighs twice as much as Jane he works twice as hard to get up the hill.

Power is work done per unit time. For Johnny this is W/Δt. Jane did half the work in half the time, (1/2 W)/(1/2 Δt) = W/Δt which is the same power delivered by Johnny.

22. (c) Fraction of energy transferred $= \frac{4 \times 2}{(1+2)^2} = \frac{8}{9}$

23. (c) $E = \frac{p^2}{2m} \Rightarrow \frac{E_1}{E_2} = \frac{p_1^2}{p_2^2} \Rightarrow E_2 = E_1 \times 4$

$\therefore E_2 - E_1 = 3E_1$

24. (c) $mc^2 = \frac{m_0}{\sqrt{1 - \frac{v^2}{c^2}}}c^2 = \frac{m_0}{\sqrt{1 - \frac{(0.5c)^2}{c^2}}}c^2$

$$= \frac{m_0}{\sqrt{1 - 0.25}}c^2 = \frac{m_0}{\sqrt{0.75}}c^2 = 1.15m_0c^2$$

Change in energy $= 1.15\ m_0c^2 - m_0c^2$
$= 0.15 \times 9.1 \times 10^{-31} \times (3 \times 10^8)^2$
$= 12.285 \times 10^{-15}$ J

$$= \frac{12.285 \times 10^{-15}}{1.6 \times 10^{-13}}\,MeV$$
= 0.07678 MeV

25. (d) Work done on the body is gain in the kinetic energy. Acceleration of the body is a = V/T.

Velocity acquired in time t is $v = at = \frac{V}{T}t$

K.E. acquired $\propto v^2$. That is work done $\propto \frac{V^2t^2}{T^2}$

26. (d) Kinetic energy of ball when reaching the ground = mgh = mg × 10
Kinetic energy after the impact

$$= \frac{60}{100} \times mg \times 10 = 6mg$$

If the ball rises to a height h, then mgh = 6 mg.
Hence, h = 6 m.

27. (d) $F = -\frac{dU}{dy} = b - 2ay$

28. (c)
29. (d) Velocity will increase when force is along the direction of displacement i.e. $\hat{F} = \hat{d}$.
30. (d) If V is velocity of combination (bag + bullet), then from principle of conservation of linear momentum

$$(m+M)V = mv \text{ or } V = \frac{mv}{(m+M)}$$

$$K.E. = \frac{1}{2}(m+M)V^2 = \frac{m^2v^2}{2(m+M)}$$

31. (c) Workdone W = $[ML^2T^{-2}]$

It shows that $W \propto (LT^{-1})^2$ i.e. $W \propto v^2$.

$\therefore$ graph between W & v is a parabola.

Alternatively:
According to work energy theorem

$W = \frac{1}{2}mv^2 - \frac{1}{2}mu^2 = \frac{1}{2}mv^2 \; (\because u = 0)$

$\Rightarrow W \propto v^2$

32. (a) Since block does not slide on wedge so displacement is zero & hence work done by force is zero.

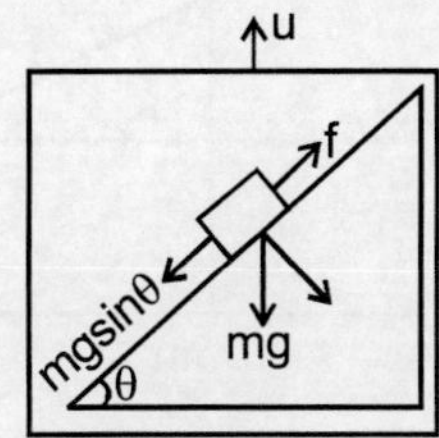

33. (c) $a = -kx \Rightarrow \frac{dv}{dt} = -kx$

Also $\frac{dx}{dt} = v$ or $dt = \frac{dx}{dv}$

$\therefore \frac{vdv}{dx} = -kx \Rightarrow \int_{v_1}^{v_2} v\,dv = -\int_0^x kxdx$

$\left(v_2^2 - v_1^2\right) = -\frac{kx^2}{2} \Rightarrow \frac{1}{2}m\left(v_2^2 - v_1^2\right) = \frac{1}{2}m\left(\frac{-kx^2}{2}\right)$

$\therefore \Delta K \; \alpha \; x^2$

34. (a) For inelastic collision, linear momentum is conserved

$\Rightarrow mv_1 = 2mv_2 \Rightarrow v_2 = \frac{v_1}{2}$

Loss in K.E. = Gain in P.E.

$= \frac{1}{2}mv_1^2 - \frac{1}{2}(2m)v_2^2 = 2mgh$

$\Rightarrow 4\,mgh = mv_1^2 - \frac{mv_1^2}{2} = \frac{mv_1^2}{2} = \frac{mv^2}{2}$

$\Rightarrow h = \frac{v^2}{8g}$

35. (d) $P = F \times v \Rightarrow P = F\,a\,t \therefore P \propto t$

36. (c) By law of conservation of momentum,

$Mu = MV + mv$ ....(i)

Also $e = \frac{|v_1 - v_2|}{|u_1 - u_2|} \Rightarrow Mu = Mv - MV$ ....(ii)

From (i) and (ii), $2Mu = (M + m)v$

$\Rightarrow v = \frac{2uM}{M + m} \Rightarrow v = \frac{2u}{1 + \frac{m}{M}}$

37. (d) Centripetal force $= \frac{mv^2}{R}$

$= \left(\frac{1}{2}mv^2\right)\frac{2}{R} = \frac{2K}{R} = \frac{2aS}{R}$

38. (d) Work done by centripetal force is zero.

39. (a) $F = -\frac{dU}{dx}$

40. (d)

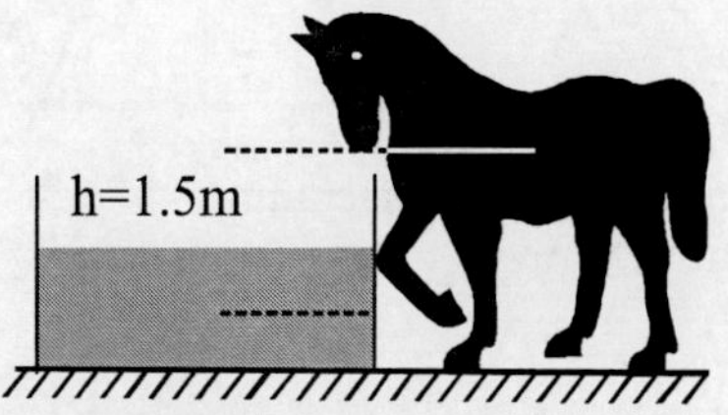

The mass of water is $m = 1 \times 10^3$ kg

$\therefore$ The increase in potential energy of water is $= mgh = (1 \times 10^3)(10)(1.5) = 15$ kJ

41. (d)

42. (c) $U = (1/2)Mv^2$

43. (b) P. E + K.E = constant, mass being constant
$gh + v^2/2 =$ constant

44. (c) $\vec{F} = \frac{d\vec{p}}{dt} = -\hat{i}2\sin t + \hat{j}2\cot t$

Hence $\vec{F}.\vec{p} = 0$, hence angle between $\vec{F}$ and $\vec{p}$ is 90°

45. (c) Here $\hat{i}mv + \hat{j}mv = 2m\vec{V}$

That is $\vec{V} = \frac{v}{2}(\hat{i} + \hat{j})$

Hence $V = \frac{v}{2} \times \sqrt{2} = \frac{v}{\sqrt{2}}$. Hence $v = 5\ ms^{-1}$

46. (c) Apply conservation of momentum,

$m_1v_1 = (m_1 + m_2)v$

$v = \frac{m_1 v_1}{(m_1 + m_2)}$

Here $v_1 = 36$ km/hr = 10 m/s,
$m_1 = 2$ kg, $m_2 = 3$ kg

$v = \frac{10 \times 2}{5} = 4\ m/s$

K.E. (initial) $= \frac{1}{2} \times 2 \times (10)^2 = 100\,J$

K.E. (Final) $= \frac{1}{2} \times (3 + 2) \times (4)^2 = 40$ J

Loss in K.E. = 100 – 40 = 60 J

Alternatively use the formula

$-\Delta E_k = \frac{1}{2}\frac{m_1m_2}{(m_1 + m_2)}(u_1 - u_2)^2$

47. (c) Change in momentum along the wall
= mv cos60° – mv cos 60° = 0
Change in momentum perpendicular to the wall
= mv sin60° – (– mv sin60°) = 2mv sin60°

$\therefore$ Applied force $= \frac{\text{Change in momentum}}{\text{Time}}$

$= \frac{2\ mv\sin 60°}{0.20} = \frac{2 \times 3 \times 10 \times \sqrt{3}}{2 \times 0.20}$

$= 50 \times 3\sqrt{3} = 150\sqrt{3}$ newton

48. (d)

49. (a) Clearly $v_1 = 2\ ms^{-1}, v_2 = 0$
$m_1 = m$ (say), $m_2 = 2m$
$v_1' = ?, v'_2 = ?$

$$e = \frac{v_1' - v_2'}{v_2 - v_1} \quad ....(i)$$

By conservation of momentum,

$$2m = mv_1' + 2mv_2' \quad ...(ii)$$

From (i), $0.5 = \frac{v_2' - v_1'}{2}$

$\therefore \quad v_2' = 1 + v_1'$

From (ii), $2 = v_1' + 2 + 2v_1'$

$\Rightarrow \quad v_1 = 0$ and $v_2 = 1\ ms^{-1}$

50. (b) Power exerted by a force is given by
$P = F.v$
When the body is just above the earth's surface, its velocity is greatest. At this instant, gravitational force is also maximum. Hence, the power exerted by the gravitational force is greatest at the instant just before the body hits the earth.

51. (a) As the two masses stick together after collision, hence it is inelastic collision. Therefore, only momentum is conserved.

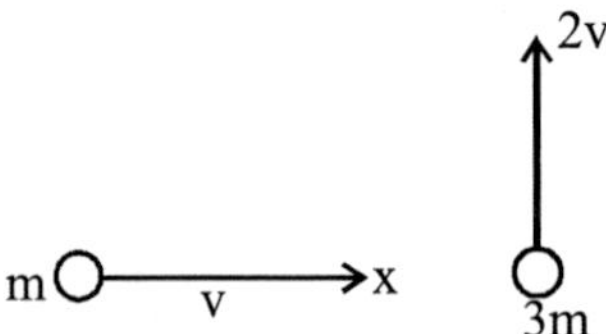

$\therefore mv\hat{i} + 3m(2v)\hat{j} = (4m)\vec{v}$

$$\vec{v} = \frac{v}{4}\hat{i} + \frac{6}{4}v\hat{j} = \frac{v}{4}\hat{i} + \frac{3}{2}v\hat{j}$$

52. (b) For equilibrium

$$\frac{dU}{dr} = 0 \Rightarrow \frac{-2A}{r^3} + \frac{B}{r^2} = 0 \Rightarrow r = \frac{2A}{B}$$

for stable equilibrium

$\frac{d^2U}{dr^2}$ should be positive for the value of r.

here $\frac{d^2U}{dr^2} = \frac{6A}{r^4} - \frac{2B}{r^3}$ is +ve value for

$r = \frac{2A}{B}$ So

53. (a)

54. (c) Let m and v be the mass and the velocity of the body. Then initial K.E.,

$$K_i = \frac{1}{2}mv^2$$

Now, mass $= \frac{m}{2}$
velocity $= 2v$

$$\therefore \quad \text{Final K.E.} = \frac{1}{2}\left(\frac{m}{2}\right)(2v)^2$$

$$= \frac{1}{2}(2mv^2) = 2\left(\frac{1}{2}mv^2\right) = 2K_i$$

55. (a)

56. (d) The given situation can be drawn graphically as shown in figure.
Work done = Area under F-x graph
= Area of rectangle $ABCD$ + Area of trapezium $BCFE$

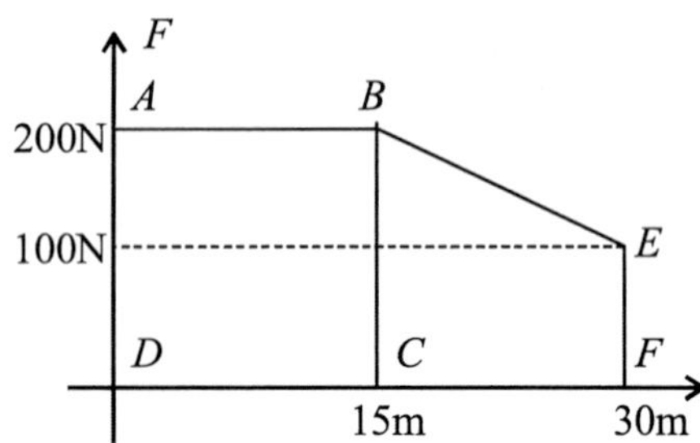

$$W = (200 \times 15) + \frac{1}{2}(100 + 200) \times 15 = 3000 + 2250$$

$$\Rightarrow W = 5250\ J$$

57. (c) Work done, $W = \int \vec{F} \cdot \vec{ds}$

$$= \left(-x\hat{i} + y\hat{j}\right) \cdot \left(d \times \hat{i} + dy\hat{j}\right) \Rightarrow W = -\int_1^0 x dx + \int_0^1 y dy$$

$$= \left(0 + \frac{1}{2}\right) + \frac{1}{2} = 1J$$

58. (c) We know area under F-x graph gives the work done by the body

$$\therefore W = \frac{1}{2} \times (3+2) \times (3-2) + 2 \times 2 = 2.5 + 4 = 6.5\ J$$

Using work energy theorem,
Δ K.E = work done
$\therefore \Delta$K.E = 6.5 J

59. (c) $l_1 + l_2 = l$ and $l_1 = nl_2$

$$\therefore \quad l_1 = \frac{nl}{n+1} \text{ and } l_2 = \frac{l}{n+1}$$

As $k \propto \frac{1}{l}$,

$$\therefore \quad \frac{k_1}{k_2} = \frac{l/(n+1)}{(nl)/(n+1)} = \frac{1}{n}$$

60. (b) Velocity of 1 kg block just before it collides with 3 kg block $= \sqrt{2gh} = \sqrt{2000}$ m/s
Using principle of conservation of linear momentum just before and just after collision, we get

$$1 \times \sqrt{2000} = 4v \Rightarrow v = \frac{\sqrt{2000}}{4} \text{ m/s}$$

Initial compression of spring
$1.25 \times 10^6 x_0 = 30 \Rightarrow x_0 \approx 0$
using work energy theorem,
$W_g + W_{sp} = \Delta KE$

$$\Rightarrow 40 \times x + \frac{1}{2} \times 1.25 \times 10^6 (0^2 - x^2)$$

$$= 0 - \frac{1}{2} \times 4 \times v^2$$

solving $x \approx 4$ cm

61. (d) Position, $x = 3t^2 + 5$

$\therefore$ Velocity, $v = \frac{dx}{dt} \Rightarrow v = \frac{d(3t^2+5)}{dt}$

$\Rightarrow v = 6t + 0$

At $t = 0$ $v = 0$

And, at $t = 5$ sec $\quad v = 30$ m/s

According to work-energy theorem, $w = \Delta KE$

or, $W = \frac{1}{2}mv^2 - 0 = \frac{1}{2}(2)(30)^2 = 900J$

62. (c) $F = -\frac{\partial u}{\partial r}\hat{r} = \frac{K}{r^3}\hat{r}$

Since particle is moving in circular path

$$F = \frac{mv^2}{r} = \frac{K}{r^3} \Rightarrow mv^2 = \frac{K}{r^2}$$

$$\therefore \text{ K.E.} = \frac{1}{2}mv^2 = \frac{K}{2r^2}$$

Total energy = P.E. + K.E.

$$= -\frac{K}{2r^2} + \frac{K}{2r^2} = \text{Zero} \qquad (\because \text{P.E.} = -\frac{K}{2r^2} \text{ given})$$

63. (b) We know that

Power, $P = Fv$

But $F = mav = m\frac{dv}{dt}v$

$\therefore P = mv\frac{dv}{dt} \Rightarrow P\,dt = mv\,dv$

Integrating both sides $\int_0^t P\,dt = m\int_0^v v\,dv$

$$P.\,t = \frac{1}{2}mv^2 \Rightarrow v = \left(\sqrt{\frac{2P}{m}}\right)t^{1/2}$$

$$\text{Distance, } s = \int_0^t v\,dt = \sqrt{\frac{2P}{m}}\int_0^t t^{1/2}\,dt = \sqrt{\frac{2P}{m}} \cdot \frac{t^{3/2}}{3/2}$$

$$\Rightarrow s = \sqrt{\frac{8P}{9m}} \cdot t^{3/2} \Rightarrow s \propto t^{3/2}$$

So, graph (b) is correct.

64. (c) From conservation of linear momentum

$mu\hat{i} + 0 = mv\hat{j} + 3m\vec{v'}$

$\vec{v'} = \frac{u}{3}\hat{i} - \frac{v}{3}\hat{j}$

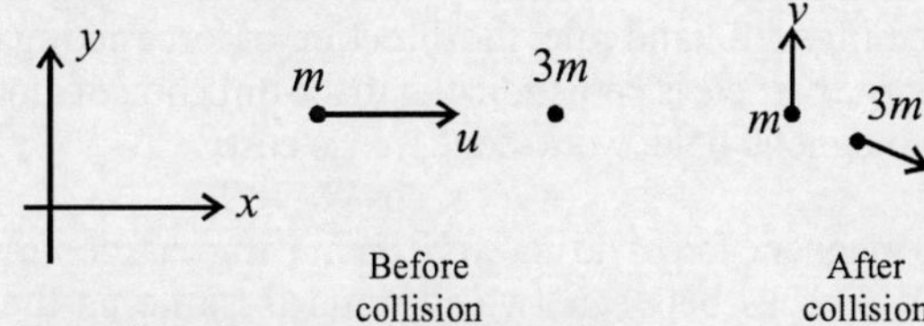

From kinetic energy conservation,

$$\frac{1}{2}mu^2 = \frac{1}{2}mv^2 + \frac{1}{2}(3m)\left(\left(\frac{u}{3}\right)^2 + \left(\frac{v}{3}\right)^2\right)$$

or, $mu^2 = mv^2 + \frac{mu^2}{3} + \frac{mv^2}{3} \qquad \therefore v = \frac{u}{\sqrt{2}}$

65. (b)

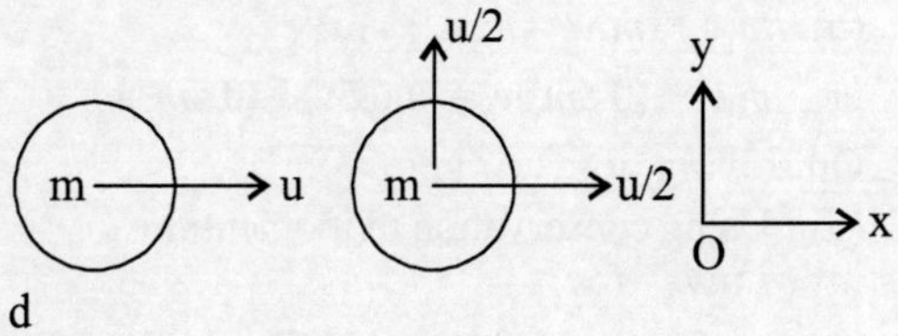

x-direction

$$mu + \frac{mu}{2} = 2mv_x' \Rightarrow V_x' = \frac{3u}{4}$$

$$\text{y-direction } 0 + \frac{mu}{2} = 2mv_y' \Rightarrow v_y' = \frac{u}{4}$$

$$K.E._i = \frac{1}{2}m\,u^2 + \frac{1}{2}m\left[\left(\frac{u}{2}\right)^2 + \left(\frac{u}{2}\right)^2\right]$$

$$= \frac{1}{2}mu^2 + \frac{mu^2}{4} = \frac{3mu^2}{4}$$

$$K.E._f = \frac{1}{2}(2m)\left(v_x'\right)^2 + \frac{1}{2}(2m)\left(v_y'\right)^2$$

$$= \frac{1}{2}2m\left[\left(\frac{3u}{4}\right)^2 + \left(\frac{u}{4}\right)^2\right] = \frac{5}{8}mu^2$$

$\therefore$ Loss in $KE = KE_f - KE_i$

$$= mu^2\left(\frac{6}{8} - \frac{5}{8}\right) = \frac{mu^2}{8}$$

66. (d)

67. (b) $P_i = P_f$

or $\quad 0 = 20(0.7 - v) = 50v$

or $\quad v = 0.2$ m/s

68. (a) Apply concervation of linear momentum in X and Y direction for the system then

M (10cos30°) + 2M (5cos45°) = 2M ($v_1$cos30°) + M($v_2$cos45°)

$$5\sqrt{3} + 5\sqrt{2} = \sqrt{3}\,v_1 + \frac{v_2}{\sqrt{2}} \qquad ....(1)$$

Also

2M(5sin45°) – M(10sin30°) = 2M$v_1$sin30° – M$v_2$sin45°

$$5\sqrt{2} - 5 = v_1 - \frac{v_2}{\sqrt{2}} \qquad ....(2)$$

Solving equation (1) and (2)

$$\left(\sqrt{3}+1\right)v_1 = 5\sqrt{3} + 10\sqrt{2} - 5 \Rightarrow v_1 = 6.5\text{m/s}$$

$v_2 = 6.3$ m/s

69. (b) $2u + 0 = 2\left(\frac{u}{4}\right) + mv_2$

and $\frac{1}{2} \times 2 \times u^2 + 0 = \frac{1}{2} \times 2 \times \left(\frac{u}{4}\right)^2 + \frac{1}{2}mv_2^2$

On solving, we get

m = 1.5 kg

70. (b) $m(2v)+2mv=0+2mv'\cos 45°$
or $v'=2\sqrt{2}v$

71. (b) $m_1v_1+m_2v_2=m_1v_2+m_2v_1$
or $m_1v_1+(0.5m_1)v_2=m_1 0.5v_1+(0.5m_1)v_4$
On solving, $v_1=v_4-v_2$

72. (d) Using conservation of momentum,
$mv_0=mv_2-mv_1$

α ⟶ V_0 (M)

After collision

← α (M) ⟶ V_2
V_1

$\frac{1}{2}mv_1^2=0.36\times\frac{1}{2}mv_0^2 \Rightarrow v_1=0.6v_0$
The collision is elastic. So,

$\frac{1}{2}MV_2^2=0.64\times\frac{1}{2}mv_0^2$ [∴ M = mass of nucleus]

$\Rightarrow V_2=\sqrt{\frac{m}{M}}\times 0.8V_0$

$mV_0=\sqrt{mM}\times 0.8V_0-m\times 0.6V_0$

$\Rightarrow 1.6m=0.8\sqrt{mM} \Rightarrow 4m^2=mM$

$\therefore M=4m$

73. (b) Before Collision After Collision

(m) ⟶ V_0 (m) ⇒ (m) ⟶ V_1 (m) ⟶ V_2
Stationary

$\frac{1}{2}mv_1^2+\frac{1}{2}mv_2^2=\frac{3}{2}\left(\frac{1}{2}mv_0^2\right)$

$\Rightarrow v_1^2+v_2^2=\frac{3}{2}v_0^2$ ....(i)

From momentum conservation
$mv_0=m(v_1+v_2)$ ....(ii)
Squarring both sides,
$(v_1+v_2)^2=v_0^2 \Rightarrow v_1^2+v_2^2+2v_1v_2=v_0^2$

$2v_1v_2=-\frac{v_0^2}{2}$

$(v_1-v_2)^2=v_1^2+v_2^2-2v_1v_2=\frac{3}{2}v_0^2+\frac{v_0^2}{2}$

Solving we get relative velocity between the two particles
$v_1-v_2=\sqrt{2}v_0$

74. (a) Change in momentum

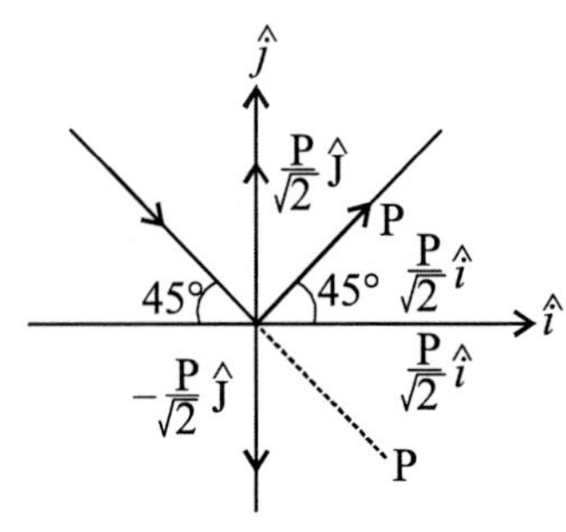

$\Delta P=\frac{P}{\sqrt{2}}\hat{j}+\frac{P}{\sqrt{2}}\hat{j}+\frac{P}{\sqrt{2}}\hat{i}-\frac{P}{\sqrt{2}}\hat{i}$

$\Delta P=\frac{2P}{\sqrt{2}}\hat{j}=I_H$ molecule

$\Rightarrow I_{wall}=-\frac{2P}{\sqrt{2}}\hat{j}$

Pressure, P

$=\frac{F}{A}=\frac{\sqrt{2}P}{A}n$ (∵ n = no. of particles)

$=\frac{\sqrt{2}\times 3.32\times 10^{-27}\times 10^3\times 10^{23}}{2\times 10^{-4}}=2.35\times 10^3 N/m^2$

75. (a) For collision of neutron with deuterium:

m ⟶ v, 2m (stationary); after: m ⟶ v_1, 2m ⟶ v_2

Applying conservation of momentum :
$mv+0=mv_1+2mv_2$ .....(i)
$v_2-v_1=v$ .....(ii)
∵ Collision is elastic, e = 1

From eqn (i) and eqn (ii) $v_1=-\frac{v}{3}$

$P_d=\frac{\frac{1}{2}mv^2-\frac{1}{2}mv_1^2}{\frac{1}{2}mv^2}=\frac{8}{9}=0.89$

Now, For collision of neutron with carbon nucleus

m ⟶ v, 12m (stationary); after: m ⟶ v_1, 12m ⟶ v_2

Applying Conservation of momentum
$mv+0=mv_1+12mv_2$ ....(iii)
$v=v_2-v_1$ ....(iv)
From eqn (iii) and eqn (iv)

$v_1=-\frac{11}{13}v$

$P_c=\frac{\frac{1}{2}mv^2-\frac{1}{2}m\left(\frac{11}{13}v\right)^2}{\frac{1}{2}mv^2}=\frac{48}{169}\approx 0.28$

Exercise 2 - Exemplar & Past Year Questions E&PYQs

Exemplar Questions

1. (b) When electron and proton are moving under influence of their mutual forces, then according to the flemings left hand rule, the direction of force acting on a charge particle is perpendicular to the direction of motion.
In magnetic field, work-done = $F.s.\cos\theta$
$=F.s.\cos 90° = 0.$
So magnetic forces do not work on moving charge particle.

2. (c) Forces between two protons is same as that of between proton and a positron.
As positron is much lighter than proton, it moves away through much larger distance compared to proton.
Work done = Force × Distance

As forces are same in case of proton and positron but distance moved by positron is larger, hence, work done on positron will be more than proton.

3. (d) When the man squatting on the ground he is tilted somewhat, hence he also has to apply frictional force besides his weight.
R (reactional force) = friction force $(f) + mg$
i.e. $R > mg$
When the man does not squat and gets straight up in that case friction $(f) \approx 0$
R (Reactional force) $\approx mg$
Hence, the reaction force (R) is larger when squatting and become equal to mg when no squatting.

4. (c) According to the question, work done by the frictional force on the cycle is :
$= 200 \times 10 = -2000$ J
As the road is not moving, hence work done by the cycle on the road is zero.

5. (c) As the body is falling freely under gravity and no external force act on body in vaccum so law of conservation, the potential energy decreases and kinetic energy increases because total mechanical energy (PE + KE) of the body and earth system will be remain constant.

6. (c) According to the question, consider the two bodies as system, the total external force on the system will be zero. Hence, in an inelastic collision KE does not conserved but total linear momentum of the system remain conserved.

7. (c) As the (inclined surface) are frictionless, hence, mechanical energy will be conserved. As both the tracks having common height, h (and no external force acts on system).
KE & PE of stone I at top = KE + PE at bottom of I.
From conservation of mechanical energy,

$$0 + \frac{1}{2}mv_1^2 = mgh + 0$$

$$\Rightarrow v_1 = \sqrt{2gh} \text{ similarly } v_2 = \sqrt{2gh}$$

Hence, speed is same for both stones.
For stone I, acceleration along inclined plane $a_1 = g \sin \theta_1$
Similarly, for stone II $a_2 = g \sin \theta_2$
$\sin \theta_1 < \sin \theta_2$ Thus, $\theta_2 > \theta_1$ hence $a_2 > a_1$.
a_2 is greater than a_1 and both length for track II is also less hence, stone II reaches earlier than stone I.

8. (b) Total Mechanical energy is E = PE + KE at any instant.
When particle is at $x = x_m$ i.e., at extreme position, partical returns back and its velocity become zero for an instant.
Hence, at $x = x_m$; $x = 0$, K.E. = 0.
From Eq. (i),

$$E = \text{PE} + 0 = \text{PE} = V(x_m) = \frac{1}{2}kx_m^2$$

but at mean position at origin $V(x_m) = 0$.

9. (b) If two bodies of equal masses collides elastically, their velocities are interchanged.
When ball 1 collides with ball-2, then velocity of ball-1, v_1 becomes zero and velocity of ball-2, v_2 becomes v, i.e., similarly then its own all momentum is mV.
So, $v_1 = 0 \Rightarrow v_2 = v,\ P_1 = 0,\ P_2 = mV$
Now ball 2 collides to ball 3 and its transfer it's momentum is mV to ball 3 and itself comes in rest.
So, $v_2 = 0 \Rightarrow v_3 = v,\ P_2 = 0,\ P_3 = mV$
So, ball 1 and ball 2, become in rest and ball 3 move with velocity v in forward direction.

10. (b) As we know that,

$$\text{W.D.} = \int_{x_1}^{x_2} \vec{F} \cdot \overrightarrow{dx} = \int_{x_1}^{x_2} m\vec{a}_0 \cdot \overrightarrow{dx}$$

As given that,
$m = 0.5$ kg, $a = 5\ \text{m}^{-1/2}\ \text{s}^{-1}$,
work done $(W) = ?$
$v = ax^{3/2}$
We also know that,
Acceleration,

$$a_0 = \frac{dv}{dt} = v \cdot \frac{dv}{dx} = ax^{3/2}\frac{d}{dx}(ax^{3/2})$$

$$= ax^{3/2} \times a \times \frac{3}{2} \times x^{1/2} = \frac{3}{2}a^2x^2$$

Now, Force $= ma_0 = m\frac{3}{2}a^2x^2$
From (i),

$$\text{Work done} = \int_{x=0}^{x=2} F dx$$

$$= \int_0^2 \left[\frac{3}{2}ma^2x^2\right] dx = \frac{3}{2}ma^2 \times \left(\frac{x^3}{3}\right)_0^2$$

$$= \frac{1}{2}ma^2 \times 8 = \frac{1}{2} \times (0.5) \times (25) \times 8 = 50 \text{ J}$$

11. (b) As given that power = constant
As we know that power (P)

$$P = \frac{dW}{dt} = \frac{\vec{F} \cdot \overrightarrow{dx}}{dt} = \frac{F\,dx}{dt}$$

As the body is moving unidirectionally.
Hence, $F \cdot dx = Fdx \cos 0° = Fdx$

$$P = \frac{Fdx}{dt} = \text{constant} \quad (\because P = \text{ constant by question})$$

Now, by dimensional formula
$F \cdot v = 0$
$[F]\,[v]$ = constant
$[\text{MLT}^{-2}]\,[\text{LT}^{-1}]$ = constant
$[\text{ML}^2\text{T}^{-3}]$ = constant

$$\text{L}^2 = \frac{\text{T}^3}{\text{M}}$$

(As mass of body constant)

$$\text{L}^2 \propto \text{T}^3 \Rightarrow \text{L} \propto \text{T}^{3/2} \Rightarrow \text{Displacement } (d) \propto t^{3/2}$$

Verifies the graph (b).

12. (d) The speed of earth around the sun can never be zero or negative, so the kinetic energy of earth cannot be zero and negative.
So, option (b) and (c) represents wrongly the variation in kinetic energy of earth.

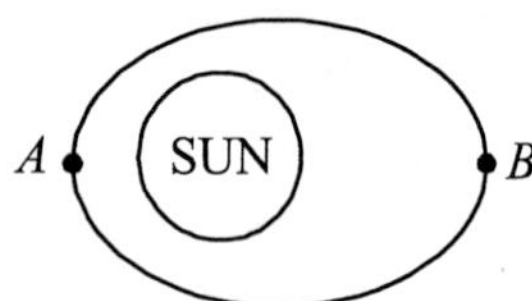

When the earth is closest to the sun, speed of the earth is maximum, hence, KE is maximum. When the earth is farthest from the sun speed is minimum hence, KE is minimum. So, K.E. of earth increases (B to A) and then decrease, variation is correctly represented by option (d).

13. (c) When a pendulum oscillates in air, due to air resistance the force of friction acts between bob of pendulum and air, so it will lose energy continuously in overcoming. Therefore, total mechanical energy (KE + PE) of the pendulum decreases continuously with time and finally becomes zero.
Sum of KE and PE can never be negative. So, option (a) and (d) are incorrect. Hence option (c) is verifies.

14. (a) As given that, mass $(m) = 5$ kg,
$n = 300$ revolution
Radius $(R) = 1$ m
$t = 60$ sec

$$\omega = \left(\frac{2\pi n}{t}\right) = (300 \times 2 \times \pi)\text{ rad} / 60\text{s}$$

$$= \frac{600 \times \pi}{60}\text{ rad/s} = 10\ \pi\text{ rad/s}$$

linear speed $(v) = \omega R = (10\pi \times 1)$
$v = 10\pi$ m/s

$$\text{KE} = \frac{1}{2}mv^2$$

$$= \frac{1}{2} \times 5 \times (10\pi)^2$$

$$= 100\pi^2 \times 5 \times \frac{1}{2}$$

$$= 250\pi^2\text{J}$$

So, verifies the option (a).

15. (b) P.E. is maximum when drop start falling at $t = 0$ as it fall is P.E. decrease gradually to zero. So, it rejects the graph (a), (c) and (d).
K.E. at $t = 0$ is zero as drop falls with zero velocity, its velocity increases (gradually), hence, first KE also increases. After sometime speed (velocity) is constant this is called terminal velocity, so, KE also become constant. It happens when it falls $\left(\frac{3}{4}\right)$ height or remains at $\left(\frac{4}{4}\right)$ from ground, then PE decreases continuously as the drop is falling continuously.
The variation in PE and KE is best represented by (b).

16. (d) As given that, $h = 1.5$ m, $v = 1$ m/s, $m = 10$ kg, $g = 10\text{ ms}^{-2}$
By the law of conservation of mechanical energy as no force acts on shotput after thrown.

$$(\text{PE})_i + (\text{KE})_i = (\text{PE})_f + (\text{KE})_f$$

$$mgh_i + \frac{1}{2}mv_i^2 = 0 + (\text{KE})_f$$

$$(\text{KE})_f = mgh_i + \frac{1}{2}mv_i^2$$

Total energy when it reaches ground, so

$$(\text{KE})_f = 10 \times 10 \times 1.5 + \frac{1}{2} \times 10 \times (1)^2$$

$E = 150 + 5 = 155$ J.

17. (b) First velocity of the iron sphere
$V = \sqrt{2gh}$ after sometime its velocity becomes constant, called terminal velocity. Hence, according first KE increases and then becomes constant due to resistance of sphere and water which is represented by (b).

18. (c) As given that,

$$m = 150\text{ g} = \frac{150}{1000}\text{ kg} = 0.15\text{ kg}$$

Δt = time of contact = 0.001 s

$$u = 126\text{ km/h} = \frac{126 \times 1000}{60 \times 60}\text{ m/s}$$

$$= 126 \times \frac{5}{18} = 35\text{ m/s}$$

$$v = -126\text{ km/h} = -126 \times \frac{5}{18} = -35\text{ m/s}$$

So, final velocity is acc. to initial force applied by batsman.
So, change in momentum of the ball

$$\Delta p = m(v - u) = \frac{3}{20}(-35 - 35)\text{ kg-m/s}$$

$$= \frac{3}{20}(-70) = -\frac{21}{2}$$

As we know that, force

$$F = \frac{\Delta p}{\Delta t} = \frac{-21/2}{0.001}\text{ N} = -1.05 \times 10^4\text{ N}$$

Hence negative sign shown that direction of force will be opposite to initial velocity which taken positive direction. Hence verify the option (c).

NEET/AIPMT (2013-2020) Questions

19. (d) Given : $\vec{F} = 3\hat{i} + \hat{j}$

$$\vec{r_1} = \left(2\hat{i} + \hat{k}\right),\ \vec{r_2} = \left(4\hat{i} + 3\hat{j} - \hat{k}\right)$$

$$\vec{r} = \vec{r_2} - \vec{r_1} = \left(4\hat{i} + 3\hat{j} - \hat{k}\right) - \left(2\hat{i} + \hat{k}\right)$$

or $\vec{r} = 2\hat{i} + 3\hat{j} - 2\hat{k}$

So work done by the given force w = $\vec{f}.\vec{r}$

$$= \left(3\hat{i} + \hat{j}\right).\left(2\hat{i} + 3\hat{j} - 2\hat{k}\right) = 6 + 3 = 9\text{J}$$

20. (b)

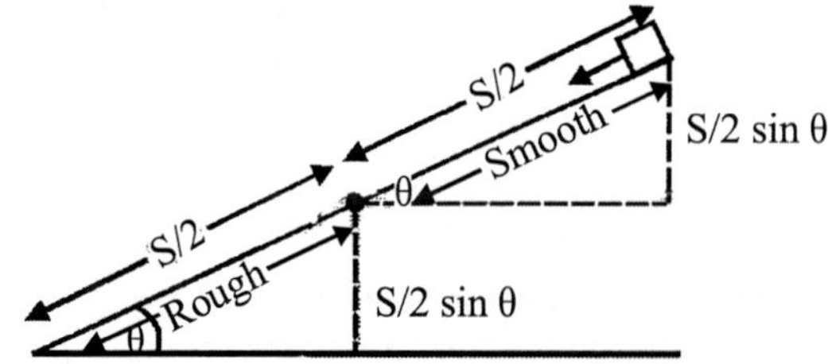

For upper half of inclined plane
$v^2 = u^2 + 2a\ S/2 = 2\ (g \sin\theta)\ S/2 = gS \sin\theta$
For lower half of inclined plane
$0 = u^2 + 2\ g\ (\sin\theta - \mu \cos\theta)\ S/2$

$\Rightarrow -gS\sin\theta = gS(\sin\theta - \mu\cos\theta)$

$\Rightarrow 2\sin\theta = \mu\cos\theta$

$\Rightarrow \mu = \dfrac{2\sin\theta}{\cos\theta} = 2\tan\theta$

21. (a)

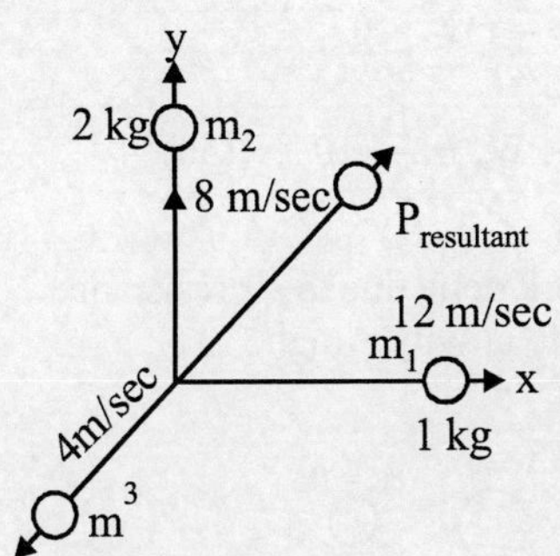

$P_{resultant} = \sqrt{12^2 + 16^2}$

$= \sqrt{144+256} = 20$

$m_3v_3 = 20$ (momentum of third part)

or, $m_3 = \dfrac{20}{4} = 5\text{ kg}$

22. (c) According to law of conservation of momentum

$MV + mnv = 0$

$\Rightarrow V = \dfrac{-mNv}{M} = \dfrac{-0.01\text{ kg}\times 10\times 800\text{ m/s}}{100} \Rightarrow -0.8\text{ m/s}$

According to work energy theorem,
Average work done = Change in average kinetic energy

i.e., $F_{av}\times S_{av} = \dfrac{1}{2}mV_{rms}^2$

$\Rightarrow \dfrac{F_{av}V_{max}t}{2} = \dfrac{1}{2}m\dfrac{V_{rms}^2}{2} \Rightarrow F_{av} = 8\text{ N}$

23. (d) As the particle is moving in a potential energy region.

$\therefore$ Kinetic energy ≥ 0

And, total energy E = K.E. + P.E.

$\Rightarrow U(x) \leq E$

24. (a) $\because$ Power $P = \dfrac{W}{t}$

$\Rightarrow \dfrac{P_1}{P_2} = \dfrac{t_2}{t_1} = \dfrac{30s}{1\text{ minute}} = \dfrac{30s}{60s} = \dfrac{1}{2}$

($t_1 = 1$ minute; $t_2 = 30$ second given)

25. (b) By conservation of linear momentum

$2mv_1 = \sqrt{2}mv \Rightarrow v_1 = \dfrac{v}{\sqrt{2}}$

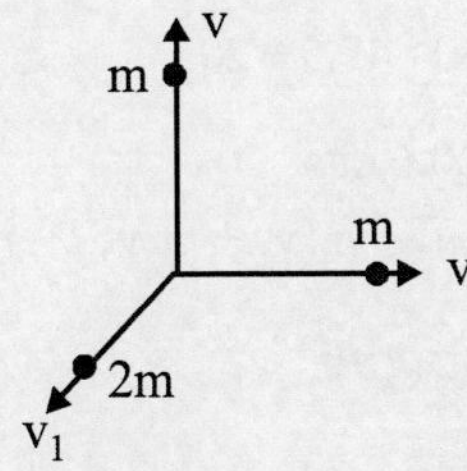

As two masses of each of mass m move perpendicular to each other.
Total KE generated

$= \dfrac{1}{2}mv^2 + \dfrac{1}{2}mv^2 + \dfrac{1}{2}(2m)v_1^2$

$= mv^2 + \dfrac{mv^2}{2} = \dfrac{3}{2}mv^2$

26. (d) Power $\vec{F}.\vec{V} = PA\vec{V} = \rho ghAV$

$\left[\because P = \dfrac{F}{A} \text{ and } P = \rho gh\right]$

$= 13.6\times 10^3\times 10\times 150\times 10^{-3}\times 0.5\times 10^{-3}/60$

$= \dfrac{102}{60} = 1.70$ watt

27. (a) When ball collides with the ground it loses its 50% of energy

$\therefore \dfrac{KE_f}{KE_i} = \dfrac{1}{2} \Rightarrow \dfrac{\frac{1}{2}mV_f^2}{\frac{1}{2}mV_i^2} = \dfrac{1}{2}$

or $\dfrac{V_f}{V_i} = \dfrac{1}{\sqrt{2}}$

or, $\dfrac{\sqrt{2gh}}{\sqrt{V_0^2 + 2gh}} = \dfrac{1}{\sqrt{2}}$

or, $4gh = V_0^2 + 2gh$

$\therefore V_0 = 20\text{ms}^{-1}$

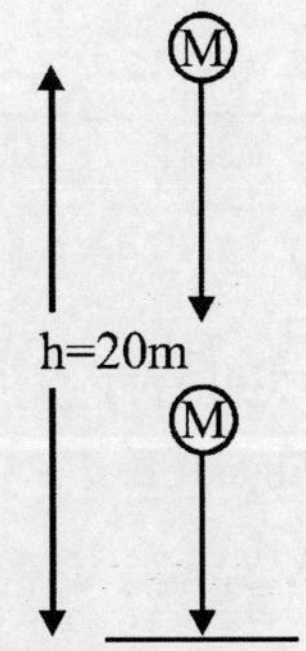

28. (d)

29. (d) For collision $\vec{V}_{B/A}$ should be along

$\overline{B\rightarrow A}(\vec{r}_{A/B})$

So, $\dfrac{\vec{V}_2 - \vec{V}_1}{|\vec{V}_2 - \vec{V}_1|} = \dfrac{\vec{r}_1 - \vec{r}_2}{|\vec{r}_1 - \vec{r}_2|}$

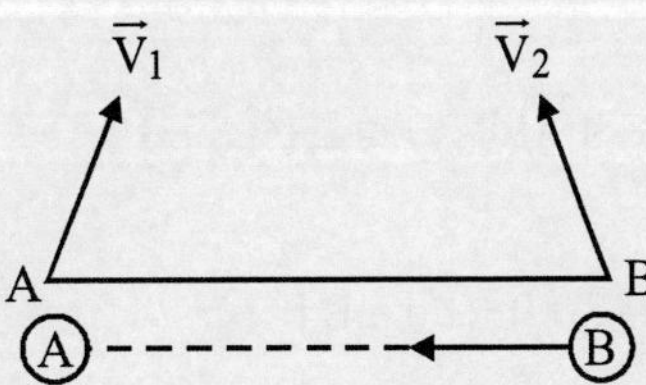

30. (d) As we know power $P = \dfrac{dw}{dt}$

$\Rightarrow w = Pt = \dfrac{1}{2}mV^2$

So, $v = \sqrt{\dfrac{2Pt}{m}}$

Hence, acceleration $a = \dfrac{dV}{dt} = \sqrt{\dfrac{2P}{m}}\cdot\dfrac{1}{2\sqrt{t}}$

Therefore, force on the particle at time 't'

$= ma = \sqrt{\dfrac{2Km^2}{m}}\cdot\dfrac{1}{2\sqrt{t}} = \sqrt{\dfrac{Km}{2t}} = \sqrt{\dfrac{mK}{2}}\,t^{-1/2}$

31. (b) As we know work done in stretching spring

$$w = \frac{1}{2}kx^2$$

where k = spring constant
x = extension

Case (a) If extension (x) is same,

$$W = \frac{1}{2}K x^2$$

So, $W_P > W_Q$ $(\because K_P > K_Q)$

Case (b) If spring force (F) is same $W = \frac{F^2}{2K}$

So, $W_Q > W_P$

32. (d) From, F = ma

$$a = \frac{F}{m} = \frac{0.1x}{10} = 0.01x = V\frac{dV}{dx}$$

So, $\int_{v_1}^{v_2} v dV = \int_{20}^{30} \frac{x}{100} dx$

$$-\frac{V^2}{2}\Big|_{V_1}^{V_2} = \frac{x^2}{200}\Big|_{20}^{30} = \frac{30 \times 30}{200} - \frac{20 \times 20}{200}$$

$= 4.5 - 2 = 2.5$

$$\frac{1}{2}m\left(V_2^2 - V_1^2\right) = 10 \times 2.5 \text{ J} = -25\text{J}$$

Final K.E.

$$= \frac{1}{2}mv_2^2 = \frac{1}{2}mv_1^2 - 25 = \frac{1}{2} \times 10 \times 10 \times 10 - 25$$

$= 500 - 25 = 475$ J

33. (d) Given force $\vec{F} = 2t\hat{i} + 3t^2\hat{j}$

According to Newton's second law of motion,

$$m\frac{d\vec{v}}{dt} = 2t\hat{i} + 3t^2\hat{j} \quad (m = 1 \text{ kg})$$

$$\Rightarrow \int_0^{\vec{v}} d\vec{v} = \int_0^t \left(2t\hat{i} + 3t^2\hat{j}\right)dt \Rightarrow \vec{v} = t^2\hat{i} + t^3\hat{j}$$

Power P = $\vec{F} \cdot \vec{v}$ $(2t\hat{i} + 3t^2\hat{j}) \cdot (t^2\hat{i} + t^3\hat{j})$

$= (2t^3 + 3t^5)$W

34. (a) Given: Mass of particle, M = 10g = $\frac{10}{1000}$kg

radius of circle R = 6.4 cm

Kinetic energy E of particle = 8×10^{-4}J

acceleration a_t = ?

$$\frac{1}{2}mv^2 = E \Rightarrow \frac{1}{2}\left(\frac{10}{1000}\right)v^2 = 8 \times 10^{-4}$$

$\Rightarrow v^2 = 16 \times 10^{-2} \Rightarrow v = 4 \times 10^{-1} = 0.4$ m/s

Now, using

$v^2 = u^2 + 2a_t s$ $(s = 4\pi R)$

$$(0.4)^2 = 0^2 + 2a_t\left(4 \times \frac{22}{7} \times \frac{6.4}{100}\right)$$

$$\Rightarrow a_t = (0.4)^2 \times \frac{7 \times 100}{8 \times 22 \times 6.4} = 0.1 \text{ m/s}^2$$

35. (c) From work-energy theorem,

$W_g + W_a = \Delta$K.E

or, $mgh + W_a = \frac{1}{2}mv^2 - 0$

$$10^{-3} \times 10 \times 10^3 + W_a = \frac{1}{2} \times 10^{-3} \times (50)^2$$

$\Rightarrow W_a = -8.75$ J

which is the work done due to air resistance

Work done due to gravity = mgh

$= 10^{-3} \times 10 \times 10^3 = 10$ J

36. (b) [Figure: Before Collision — m moving with v, 4m with v = 0; After Collision — m with v = 0, 4m moving with v′]

Before Collision After Collision

According to law of conservation of linear momentum,

$$mv + 4m \times 0 = 4mv' + 0 \Rightarrow v' = \frac{v}{4}$$

Coefficient of restitution,

$$e = \frac{\text{Relative velocity of separation}}{\text{Relative velocity of approach}}$$

$$= \frac{\frac{v}{4}}{v} \text{ or, } e = \frac{1}{4} = 0.25$$

37. (c) Work done by variable force

Work done, $W = \int_{y_i}^{y_f} F dy \Rightarrow \int_{y=0}^{y_f=1} F \cdot dy$

where, $F = 20 + 10y$

$$\therefore W = \int_0^1 (20 + 10y)dy$$

$$= \left[20y + \frac{10y^2}{2}\right]_0^1 = 25\,J$$

38. (d) Using work-energy theorem, ΔK = work = area under $F - x$ graph

From $x = 0$ to $x = 8$ m

$$\frac{1}{2}mv^2 = 100 + 30$$

$\therefore v = \sqrt{520} = 23$ m/s

From $x = 0$ to $x = 12$ m

$$\frac{1}{2}mv^2 = 100 + 30 - 47.5 + 20$$

$\therefore v = \sqrt{410} = 20.6$ m/s

39. (b) $m_1u_1 + m_2u_2 = m_1v_1 + m_2v_2$

Also, $\frac{1}{2}m_1u_1^2 + \frac{1}{2}m_2u_2^2$

$$= \frac{1}{2}m_1v_1^2 + \frac{1}{2}m_2v_2^2$$

For elastic collision

$v_2 = \frac{2m_1u_1}{m_1+m_2}$

as $u_2 = 0; u_1 = u$

$m_1 = 4m$ and $m_2 = 2m$

so, $v_2 = \frac{4}{3}u$

$\frac{\Delta KE}{KE} = \frac{1}{2}\times 2m \times \left(\frac{4}{3}u\right)^2$

$= \frac{1}{2}\times 2 \times \frac{16}{9}$

40. (b) $\vec{P}_i = \vec{P}_f$

$m\vec{v}_i = \left(\frac{m}{6}\vec{v}_1 + \frac{5m}{6}\vec{v}_2\right)$

$\vec{v}_i = \left(\frac{\vec{v}_1}{6} + \frac{5}{6}\vec{v}_2\right)$

$20\hat{i} + 25\hat{j} - 12\hat{k} = \frac{(100\hat{i} + 35\hat{j} + 8\hat{k})}{6} + \frac{5\vec{v}_2}{6}$

$\vec{v}_2 = \frac{20\hat{i} + 115\hat{j} - 80\hat{k}}{5}$

$\therefore \quad \vec{v}_2 = 4\hat{i} + 23\hat{j} - 16\hat{k}$

41. (b)

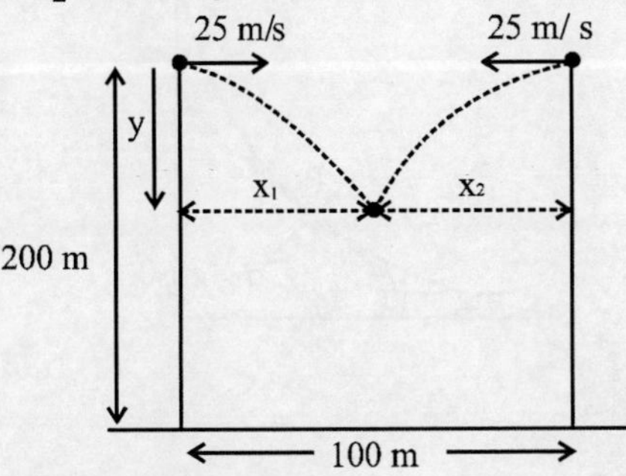

Bullets collide at time t

$x_1 + x_2 = 100$ m

$25t + 25t = 100$

$t = 2s$

$y = \frac{1}{2}gt^2 = \frac{1}{2}\times 10 \times 2^2 = 20$ m

$h = 200 - 20 = 180$ m

42. (a) From conservation of linear momentum.

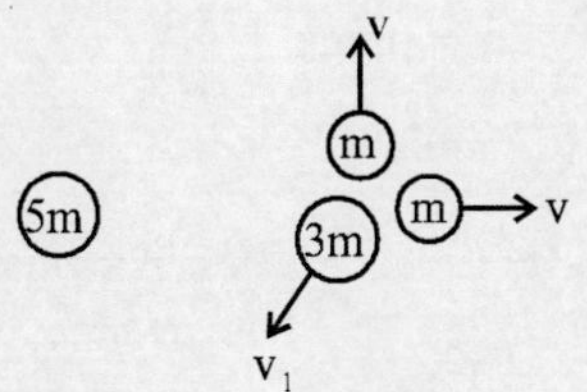

$0 = mv\hat{j} + mv\hat{i} + 3m\vec{v}_1$

$\vec{v}_1 = -\frac{v}{3}(\hat{i} + \hat{j})$

$v_1 = \frac{\sqrt{2}}{3}v$

$K_f = \frac{1}{2}mv^2 + \frac{1}{2}mv^2 + \frac{1}{2}(3m)\left(\frac{\sqrt{2}}{3}\right)^2 v^2$

$= mv^2 + \frac{mv^2}{3} = \frac{4}{3}mv^2$

$\Delta KE = K_f - K_i = \frac{4}{3}mv^2$

Exercise 3 - Concept Application Problems CAP

1. (b) $\frac{p_1}{p_2} = \sqrt{\frac{2m_1K_1}{2m_2K_2}}$

2. (c) The uniform acceleration is $a = \frac{1-0}{15} = \frac{1}{15}$ ms^{-2}

Let v be the velocity at kinetic energy $\frac{2}{9}$J

therefore $\frac{1}{2}\times 1\times v^2 = \frac{2}{9}$ or $v = \frac{2}{3}$ ms^{-1}

Using $v = u + at$

$\frac{2}{3} = 0 + \frac{1}{15}\times t \Rightarrow t = 10s$

3. (d) Power supplied $= \frac{mgh}{t}$

Power used by crane $= \frac{mgh}{t}\times\frac{100}{80}$

$= \frac{1000\times 10\times 100}{3600}\times\frac{100}{80} = \frac{10^5}{36\times 8}$ W

4. (c) $W = F s \cos\theta$, $\cos\theta = \frac{W}{Fs} = \frac{25}{5\times 10} = \frac{1}{2}$, $\theta = 60°$.

5. (b) For elastic collision in one dimension

$v_1 = \frac{2m_2u_2}{m_1+m_2} + \frac{(m_1-m_2)u_1}{(m_1+m_2)}$

As mass 2m, is at rest, So $u_2 = 0$

$\Rightarrow \quad v_1 = \frac{(8m-2m)u}{8m+2m} = \frac{3}{5}u$

Final energy of sphere = $(K.E.)_f$

$= \frac{1}{2}(8m)\left(\frac{3u}{5}\right)^2 = \frac{1}{2}(8m)u^2\times\left(\frac{3}{5}\right)^2 = \frac{9}{25}E = 0.36\,E$

6. (a) $m_1u = m_1\frac{2u}{3} + m_2u$ (By condition of linear momentum)

$\Rightarrow \quad \frac{1}{3}m_1u = m_2v$ ...... (i)

Also $e = \frac{|v_1 - v_2|}{|u_2 - u_1|}$

$\Rightarrow \quad v - \frac{2u}{3} = u \Rightarrow v = \frac{5}{3}u$ ...... (ii)

From (i) and (ii), $\frac{1}{3}m_1u = \frac{5}{3}m_2u \Rightarrow \frac{m_1}{m_2} = 5$

7. (c) At Equilibrium, $ky = mg \Rightarrow k = \frac{mg}{y}$

$$U = \frac{1}{2}\left(\frac{mg}{y}\right)y^2 = \frac{1}{2}mgy$$

8. (a) Loss in K.E = Area under the curve

9. (b) In this case, $P = \frac{mgh + \frac{1}{2}mv^2}{t}$

$$\Rightarrow P = \frac{m}{t}\left[gh + \frac{v^2}{2}\right]$$

$$\Rightarrow P = \frac{10}{1}\left[10\times10 + \frac{10\times10}{2}\right]W = 1500W$$

10. (c) By conservation of linear momentum, $\frac{m_1}{m_2} = \frac{v_2}{v_1}$

or $\frac{\rho \times \frac{4}{3}\pi r_1^3}{\rho \times \frac{4}{3}\pi r_2^3} = \frac{1}{2} \Rightarrow \frac{r_1}{r_2} = \frac{1}{2^{1/3}}$

11. (b) $F = \frac{12}{100}\times 1000\times 10\ N = 1200\ N$
$P = Fv = 1200\ N \times 15\ ms^{-1} = 18\ kW$.

12. (b) $Fv = P$. or $M\frac{dv}{dt}v = P$

That is $\int v\,dv = \int \frac{P}{M}dt$

Hence $v = [2Pt/M]^{1/2}$

13. (b) When body is lowered gradually, its weight acts at C.G. of the spring. When same body is allowed to fall freely, the same weight acts at lower end of the spring. In the latter case, original length (L) of spring is double. As $\Delta L \propto L$, therefore, ΔL becomes twice in second case i.e. 2x.

14. (c) Applying principle of conservation of linear momentum $(2m)V = \sqrt{(mv)^2 + (mv)^2} = mv\sqrt{2}$

$$\therefore\ V = \frac{v\sqrt{2}}{2} = \frac{v}{\sqrt{2}}$$

15. (c) If mass of nucleus is m, mass of α particle is m_1 & mass of remaining nucleus is m_2, then from the law of conservation of momentum.

$$\underset{\text{initial momentum of nucleus}}{m\vec{v}} = \underset{\text{momentum of }\alpha\text{ particle}}{m_1\vec{v}_1} + \underset{\text{momentum of remaining nucleus}}{m_2\vec{v}_2}$$

16. (d) As bob B is of same material and same mass as the bob A, therefore, on elastic collision, their velocities are exchanged. Bob A comes to rest and B moves with the velocity of A.

17. (c) As velocities are exchanged on perfectly elastic collision, therefore masses of two objects must be equal.

$$\therefore\ \frac{m_a}{m_b} = 1 \text{ or } m_a = m_b.$$

18. (c)

19. (c) $V_c = \frac{10\times14 + 4\times0}{10+4} = 10m/s$; since spring force is internal force.

20. (c)

21. (d) Initially, $3k = mg$ or $k = \frac{mg}{3}$
New force constant of longer part
$k' = \frac{3}{2}k = \frac{3}{2}\times\frac{mg}{3} = \frac{mg}{2}$
Finally, $k'y = mg$

$$y = \frac{mg}{k'} = \frac{mg}{mg}\times 2 = 2cm$$

22. (d) $m = 10\times0.8kg = 8kg$
height of iron chain = 5m

$$P = \frac{mgh}{t} = \frac{8\times10\times5}{10}W = 40W$$

23. (a) As the block is at rest at P.
$mg\sin\theta = \mu mg\cos\theta$

$$\mu = \tan\theta = \text{slope} = \frac{dy}{dx} = \frac{d}{dx}\left(\frac{x^2}{2L}\right) = \frac{x}{L}$$

$\therefore \frac{x}{L} = 0.8$
$\Rightarrow x = 0.8 \times 10 = 8\,m$

24. (c) The change in momentum in the ball after the collision with surface is $m(0-v) = -mv$
Since n balls impinge elastically each second on the surface, then rate of change of momentum of ball per second is
mvn (consider magnitude only)
Now According to Newton's second law
rate of change of momentum per second of ball = force experienced by surface.

25. (c) $K = p^2/2m = \mu mgx$

Hence, $x = p^2/2m^2\mu g$.

26. (a) $x = 3t - 4t^2 + t^3$ $\quad \frac{dx}{dt} = 3 - 8t + 3t^2$

Acceleration $= \frac{d^2x}{dt^2} = -8 + 6t$
Acceleration after 4 sec $= -8 + 6\times4 = 16$
Displacement in 4 sec $= 3\times4 - 4\times4^2 + 4^3 = 12\,m$
$\therefore$ Work = Force × displacement
= Mass × acc. × disp. $= 3\times10^{-3}\times16\times12 = 576\ mJ$

27. (b) Speed of bomb after 5 second,
$v = u - gt = 100 - 10\times5 = 50\text{m/s}$
Momentum of 400 g fragment
$= \frac{400}{1000}\times(-25)$ (downward)
Momentum of 600g fragment $= \frac{600}{1000}v$
Momentum of bomb just before explosion
$= 1\times50 = 50$
From conservation of momentum
Total momentum just before collision = Total momentum just after collision
$\Rightarrow 50 = -\frac{400}{1000}\times25 + \frac{600}{1000}v$
$\Rightarrow v = 100$ m/s (upward)

28. (b) $\frac{1}{2}mv^2 = \frac{1}{2}kx^2 \Rightarrow mv^2 = kx^2$ or $0.5\times(1.5)^2 = 50\times x^2$
$\therefore x = 0.15\,m$

29. (d) Given : $\vec{F} = 3\hat{i}+\hat{j}$
$\vec{r_1} = (2\hat{i}+\hat{k}),\ \vec{r_2} = (4\hat{i}+3\hat{j}-\hat{k})$
$\vec{r} = \vec{r_2}-\vec{r_1} = (4\hat{i}+3\hat{j}-\hat{k}) - (2\hat{i}+\hat{k})$
or $\vec{r} = 2\hat{i}+3\hat{j}-2\hat{k}$
So work done by the given force $w = \vec{f}.\vec{r}$
$= (3\hat{i}+\hat{j}).(2\hat{i}+3\hat{j}-2\hat{k}) = 6+3 = 9J$

30. (c) $p = \sqrt{2mK}$
$p' = \sqrt{2m[K+3K]} = 2p$
$\frac{\Delta p\times100}{p} = \frac{2p-p}{p}\times100 = 100\%$

31. (d) Here, $N - mg = ma = \frac{mg}{2} \Rightarrow N = \frac{3mg}{2}$
N = normal reaction
Now, work done by normal reaction 'N' on block in time t, $W = \vec{N}\vec{S} = \left(\frac{3mg}{2}\right)\left(\frac{1}{2}g/_2 t^2\right)$
or, $W = \frac{3mg^2t^2}{8}$

32. (a) From question, $v = a\sqrt{s} = \frac{ds}{dt}$
or, $2\sqrt{s} = at \Rightarrow S = \frac{a^2t^2}{4}$
$F = m\times\frac{a^2}{2}$
Work done $= \frac{ma^2}{2}\times\frac{a^2t^2}{4} = \frac{1}{8}ma^4t^2$

33. (a) $W = u_f - u_i$
$= 0 - \left(-\frac{mg}{n}\times\frac{L}{2n}\right) = \frac{MgL}{2n^2}.$

34. (c) $mv = (m+M)V'$
or $v = \frac{mv}{m+M} = \frac{mv}{m+4m} = \frac{v}{5}$
Using conservation of ME, we have
$\frac{1}{2}mv^2 = \frac{1}{2}(m+4m)\left(\frac{v}{5}\right)^2 + mgh$ or $h = \frac{2}{5}\frac{v^2}{g}$

35. (c) We know area under F-x graph gives the work done by the body
$\therefore W = \frac{1}{2}\times(3+2)\times(3-2)+2\times2$
$= 2.5+4 = 6.5\,J$
Using work energy theorem,
Δ K.E = work done
$\therefore \Delta K.E = 6.5\,J$

36. (d) Work done $= \vec{F}.\vec{d} = (3\vec{i}-12\vec{j}).(4\vec{i}) = 12J$
From work energy theorem,
$w_{net} = \Delta K.E. = k_f - k_i \Rightarrow 12 = k_f - 3$
$\therefore K_f = 15J$

37. (d) Maximum speed is at mean position or equilibrium
At equilibrium Position
$F = kx \Rightarrow x = \frac{F}{k}$
From work-energy theorem,
$W_F + W_{sp} = \Delta KE$
$F(x) - \frac{1}{2}kx^2 = \frac{1}{2}mv^2 - 0$
$F\left(\frac{F}{k}\right) - \frac{1}{2}k\left(\frac{F}{k}\right)^2 = \frac{1}{2}mv^2 \Rightarrow \frac{1}{2}\frac{F^2}{K} = \frac{1}{2}mv^2$
or, $v_{max} = \frac{F}{\sqrt{mk}}$

38. (b) As the particles moving in circular orbits, So
$\frac{mv^2}{r} = \frac{16}{r} + r^2$
Kinetic energy, $KE_0 = \frac{1}{2}mv^2 = \frac{1}{2}[16+r^4]$
For first particle, r = 1, $K_1 = \frac{1}{2}m(16+1)$
Similarly, for second particle, r = 4, $K_2 = \frac{1}{2}m(16+256)$
$\therefore \frac{K_1}{K_2} = \frac{\frac{16+1}{2}}{\frac{16+256}{2}} = \frac{17}{272} \approx 6\times10^{-2}$

39. (b) Total force required to lift maximum load capacity against frictional force = 400 *N*
$F_{total} = Mg +$ friction
$= 2000\times10 + 4000 = 20{,}000 + 4000 = 24000\,N$
Using power, $P = F\times v$
$60\times746 = 24000\times v \Rightarrow v = 1.86$ m/s $\approx 1.9\,m/s$
Hence speed of the elevator at full load is close to 1.9 ms^{-1}

40. (d)

41. (b) According to the question, all collisions are perfectly inelastic, so after the final collision, all blocks are moving together.

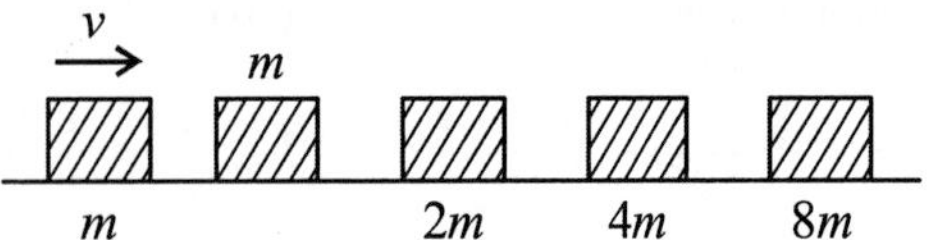

Let the final velocity be v', using momentum conservation

$$mv = 16mv' \Rightarrow v' = \frac{v}{16}$$

Now initial energy $E_i = \frac{1}{2}mv^2$

Final energy: $E_f = \frac{1}{2} \times 16m \times \left(\frac{v}{16}\right)^2 = \frac{1}{2}\frac{mv^2}{16}$

Energy loss : $E_i - E_f = \frac{1}{2}mv^2 - \frac{1}{2}m\frac{v^2}{16}$

$$\Rightarrow \frac{1}{2}mv^2\left[1 - \frac{1}{16}\right] \Rightarrow \frac{1}{2}mv^2\left[\frac{15}{16}\right]$$

The total energy loss is P% of the original energy.

$$\therefore \ \%P = \frac{\text{Energy loss}}{\text{Original energy}} \times 100$$

$$= \frac{\frac{1}{2}mv^2\left[\frac{15}{16}\right]}{\frac{1}{2}mv^2} \times 100 = 93.75\%$$

Hence, value of P is close to 94.

42. (b) Given,
Mass of block, $m_1 = 1.9$ kg
Mass of bullet, $m_2 = 0.1$ kg
Velocity of bullet, $v_2 = 20$ m/s
Let v be the velocity of the combined system. It is an inelastic collision.
Using conservation of linear momentum

$$m_1 \times 0 + m_2 \times v_2 = (m_1 + m_2)v$$

$$\Rightarrow 0.1 \times 20 = (0.1 + 1.9) \times v \Rightarrow v = 1 \text{ m/s}$$

Using work energy theorem
Work done = Change in Kinetic energy
Let K be the Kinetic energy of combined system.

$$(m_1 + m_2)gh = K - \frac{1}{2}(m_1 + m_2)V^2$$

$$\Rightarrow 2 \times g \times 1 = K - \frac{1}{2} \times 2 \times 1^2 \Rightarrow K = 21 \text{ J}$$

43. (c)

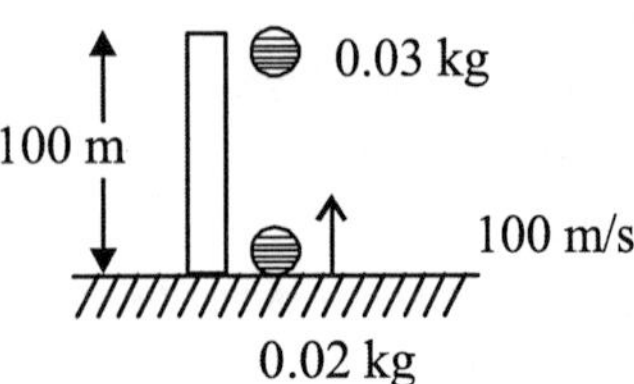

Time taken for the particles to collide,

$$t = \frac{d}{V_{rel}} = \frac{100}{100} = 1 \text{ sec}$$

Speed of wood just before collision = gt = 10 m/s and speed of bullet just before collision = v – gt
= 100 – 10 = 90 m/s

$$S = 100 \times 1 - \frac{1}{2} \times 10 \times 1 = 95 \text{ m}$$

Now, using conservation of linear momentum just before and after the collision

$$-(0.03)(10) + (0.02)(90) = (0.05)v$$

$$\Rightarrow 150 = 5v \qquad \therefore \ v = 30 \text{ m/s}$$

Max. height reached by body

$$h = \frac{30 \times 30}{2 \times 10} = 45 \text{ m}$$

Before	After
0.03 kg ↓ 10 m/s	↑ v
↑ 90 m/s 0.02 kg	0.05 kg

$\therefore$ Height above tower = 40 m

44. (c) Kinetic energy of block A

$$k_1 = \frac{1}{2}mv_0^2$$

$\therefore$ From principle of linear momentum conservation

$$mv_0 = (2m + M)v_f \Rightarrow v_f = \frac{mv_0}{2m + M}$$

According to question, of $\frac{5}{6}$th the initial kinetic energy is lost in whole process.

$$\therefore \ \frac{k_i}{k_f} = 6 \Rightarrow \frac{\frac{1}{2}mv_0^2}{\frac{1}{2}(2m + M)\left(\frac{mv_0}{2m + M}\right)^2} = 6$$

$$\Rightarrow \frac{2m + M}{m} = 6 \ \therefore \ \frac{M}{m} = 4$$

45. (d) Apply principle of conservation of momentum along x-direction,

$$mu = mv_1 \cos 45° + Mv_2 \cos 45°$$

$$mu = \frac{1}{\sqrt{2}}(mv_1 + Mv_2) \qquad \text{..... (i)}$$

Along y-direction,

$$o = mv_1 \sin 45° - Mv_2 \sin 45°$$

$$o = (mv_1 - Mv_2)\frac{1}{\sqrt{2}} \qquad \text{..... (ii)}$$

$m, u_1 = u$ (Proton) $\qquad$ $M, u_2 = 0$ (Unknown mass)

Before collision

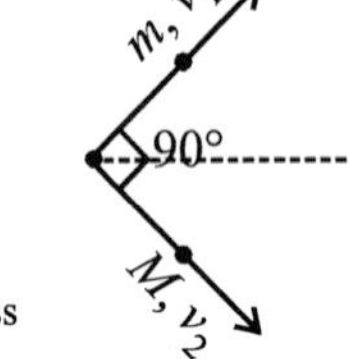

After collision

Coefficient of restution $e = 1 = \frac{v_2 - v_1 \cos 90}{u \cos 45}$

($\because$ Collision is elastic)

$$\Rightarrow \frac{v_2}{\frac{u}{\sqrt{2}}} = 1$$

$$\Rightarrow u = \sqrt{2}v_2 \qquad \text{..... (iii)}$$

Solving eqs (i), (ii), & (iii), we get mass of unknown particle, $M = m$

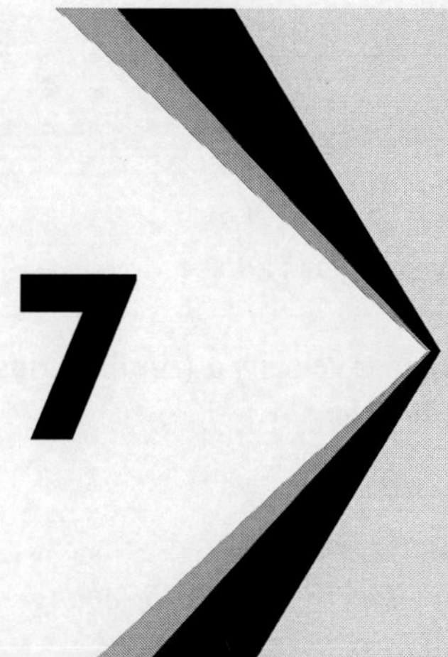

7 System of Particles and Rotational Motion

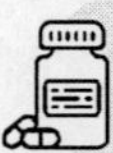

Topic 7.1 : Centre of Mass, Angular Velocity & Acceleration

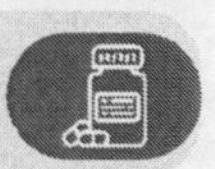

CENTRE OF MASS

Centre of mass for a system of particles is defined as that point where the entire mass of the system is imagined to be concentrated.

If $\vec{r_1}, \vec{r_2}, \vec{r_3}$ .... be the position vectors of masses m_1, m_2, m_3 .... respectively from the origin O,

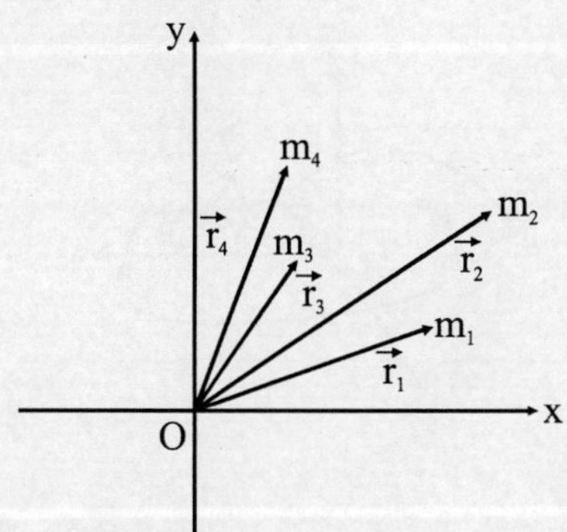

then the centre of mass of the system is

$$\overrightarrow{r_{cm}} = \frac{(m_1\vec{r_1} + m_2\vec{r_2} + m_3\vec{r_3} + ...)}{(m_1 + m_2 + m_3 + ...)} = \frac{1}{M}\sum_{i=1}^{n} m_i\ \vec{r_i}$$

where M is the total mass of the system of particles. The product of mass of the particles and its position vector w.r.t. the reference point is called **moment of mass**

i.e., *moment of mass* $= m \times \vec{r}$

Motion of Centre of Mass

The **motion of the centre of mass** is governed by the equation

$$M\vec{A}_{cm} = \vec{F}_{ext} \text{ where } \vec{A}_{cm} = \frac{d^2(\vec{r}cm)}{dt^2}$$

Momentum conservation of a system of particles :

In the absence of external forces, the velocity of the centre of mass remains constant.

We have, $MA_{cm} = F_{ext}$

If $F_{ext} = 0$

$$M\frac{d}{dt}(v_{cm}) = 0$$

$\therefore \quad v_{cm} = \text{constant}.$

Hence, momentum (Mv_{cm} = constant) of the centre of mass system is conserved.

Rigid Bodies

If a body does not undergo any change in shape by the action of a force, it is said to be rigid.

If such body undergoes some displacement, every particle in it undergoes the same displacement. No real body can be perfectly rigid.

Rotatory Motion

A body rotating about a fixed axis then every particle of the body moves in a circle and the centres of all these circles lie on axis of rotation. The motion of the body is said to possess rotational motion.

Problem Solving Tips

1. The centre of mass of a system of two identical particles lies in between them on the line joining the particles.
2. If $m_1 = m_2$
$$\vec{r}_{cm} = \frac{(m_1\vec{r_1} + m_2\vec{r_2})}{(m_1 + m_2)} = \frac{(\vec{r_1} + \vec{r_2})}{2}$$
so, for particles of equal masses the centre of mass is located at the **mean position vector** of the particles.
3. The position of centre of mass remains unchanged in pure rotatory motion. But it changes with time in translatory motion or rolling motion.
4. The position of centre of mass of a body is independent of the choice of co-ordinate system.
5. If we take the centre of mass at the origin, then the sum of the moments of the masses at of the system about the origin $\Sigma m_i\ \vec{r}_i$ is zero.
6. In pure rotatory motion, the axis of rotation passes through the centre of mass.
7. If external force is zero then the velocity of the centre of mass of a body remains constant.

8. The centre of mass and centre of gravity of a body coincide, if the value of g is same throughout the dimension of the body.
9. In kinematics and dynamics, whole of the mass of a body can be assumed to be concentrated at the centre of mass.
10. The location of the centre of mass depends on the shape and nature of distribution of mass of the body.
    (a) The position of centre of mass of continuous bodies can be found using integration as

$$X_{cm} = \frac{1}{M}\int x\,dm,\ Y_{cm} = \frac{1}{M}\int y\,dm,\ Z_{cm} = \frac{1}{M}\int z\,dm$$

    where, x, y and z are the co-ordinates of small mass dm and M is the total mass of the system.
    (b) The C.M. of a uniform rod of length L is at its middle point.
    (c) Centre of mass of a uniform semicircular wire is at $\left(0, \frac{2R}{\pi}\right)$, where R is the radius of the semicircular wire. It does not depend on mass.

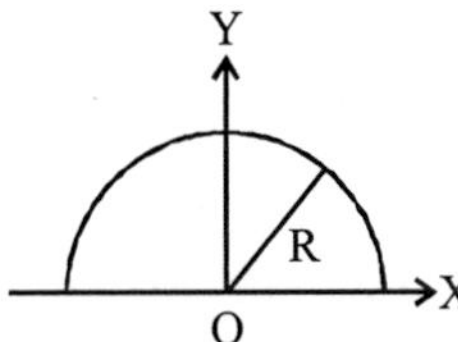

    (d) For symmetrical bodies of uniform mass distribution, the C. M. lies at the geometrical centre

ANGULAR VELOCITY AND ANGULAR ACCELERATION

The angular velocity is defined as the angle covered by the radius vector per unit time. It is denoted by ω.

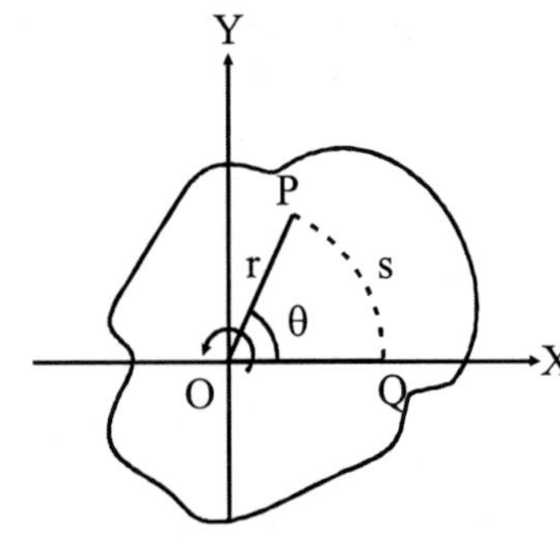

Average angular velocity $\bar{\omega} = \frac{\Delta\theta}{\Delta t}$

The unit of angular velocity is **rad/sec.**

The instantaneous angular velocity ω (similar to instantaneous linear velocity) is defined as

$$\omega = \lim_{\Delta t \to o} \frac{\Delta\theta}{\Delta t} = \frac{d\theta}{dt}$$

The angular acceleration is the rate of change of angular velocity. It is denoted by α.

The average angular acceleration $\alpha_{avg.}$ of a rotating body is

$$\alpha_{avg.} = \frac{\omega_2 - \omega_1}{t_2 - t_1} = \frac{\Delta\omega}{\Delta t}$$

In analogy to linear acceleration $\vec{a}$, the instantaneous angular acceleration is defined as

$$\alpha = \lim_{\delta t \to o} \frac{\Delta\omega}{\Delta t} = \frac{d\omega}{dt}$$

The unit of angular acceleration is **rad/sec^2**.

Relationship between angular velocity and linear velocity:

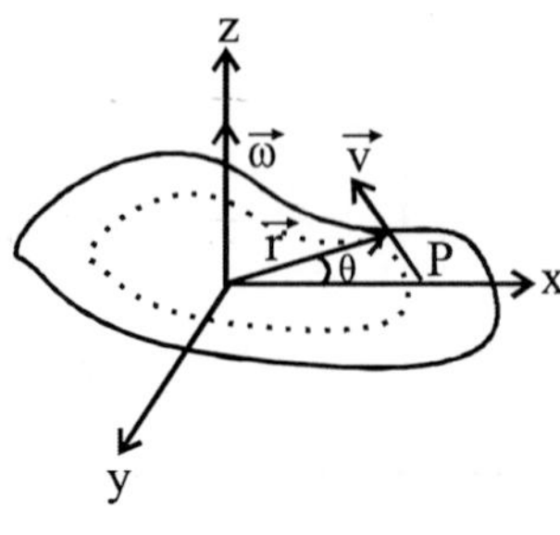

$$\vec{v} = \vec{\omega} \times \vec{r}$$

$$\Rightarrow v = rw \sin q$$

where θ is the angle between ω & r.

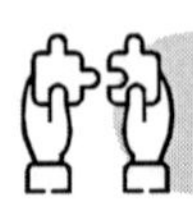
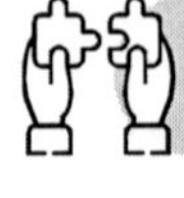

7.1 Concept Practice Problems

CPP

1. Centre of mass of the earth and the moon system lies
   (a) closer to the earth
   (b) closer to the moon
   (c) at the mid-point of line joining the earth and the moon
   (d) cannot be predicted
2. Four particles of masses m_1, m_2, m_3 and m_4 are placed at the vertices *A,B,C* and *D* as respectively of a square shown. The COM of the system will lie at diagonal *AC* if
   (a) $m_1 = m_3$
   (b) $m_2 = m_4$
   (c) $m_1 = m_2$
   (d) $m_3 = m_4$

A m_1 B m_2 m_4 D m_3 C

3. Two spheres *A* and *B* of masses *m* and 2*m* and radii 2*R* and *R* respectively are placed in contact as shown. The COM of the system lies

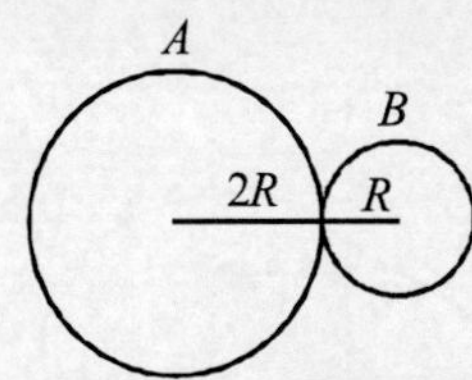

(a) inside A (b) inside B
(c) at the point of contact (d) None of these

4. Two particles A and B, initially at rest, moves towards each other under a mutual force of attraction. At the instant when the speed of A is v and the speed of B is 2 v, the speed of centre of mass is
(a) zero (b) v (c) 1.5 v (d) 3 v

5. A small disc of radius 2 cm is cut from a disc of radius 6 cm. If the distance between their centres is 3.2 cm, what is the shift in the centre of mass of the disc?
(a) 0.4 cm (b) 2.4 cm (c) 1.8 cm (d) 1.2 cm

6. Five masses are placed in a plane as shown in figure. The coordinates of the centre of mass are nearest to

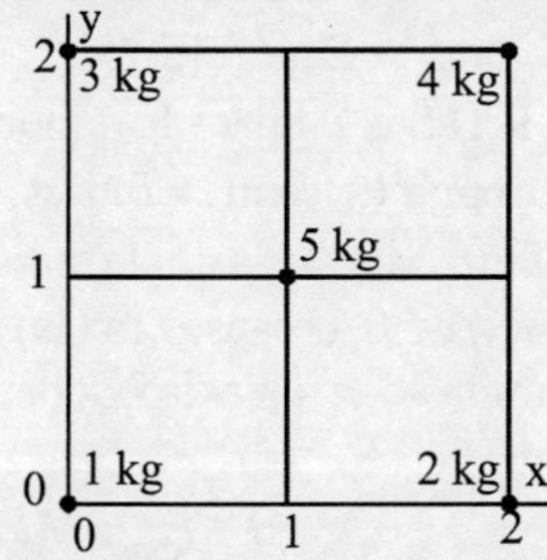

(a) 1.2, 1.4 (b) 1.3, 1.1 (c) 1.1, 1.3 (d) 1.0, 1.0

7. A boy and a man carry a uniform rod of length L, horizontally in such a way that the boy gets 1/4th load. If the boy is at one end of the rod, the distance of the man from the other end is
(a) L/3 (b) L/4 (c) 2 L/3 (d) 3 L/4

8. A solid sphere of mass M and radius R is pulled horizontally on a sufficiently rough surface as shown in the figure.

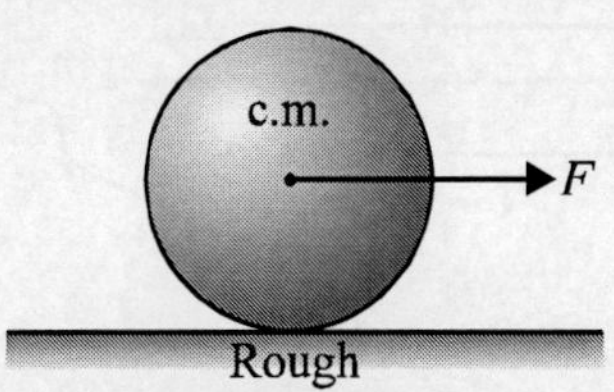

Choose the correct alternative.
(a) The acceleration of the centre of mass is F/M
(b) The acceleration of the centre of mass is $\frac{2}{3}\frac{F}{M}$
(c) The friction force on the sphere acts forward
(d) The magnitude of the friction force is F/3

9. Three identical particles each of mass 1 kg are placed touching one another with their centres on a straight line. Their centres are marked A, B and C respectively. The distance of centre of mass of the system from A is
(a) $\frac{AB+AC+BC}{3}$ (b) $\frac{AB+AC}{3}$
(c) $\frac{AB+BC}{3}$ (d) $\frac{AC+BC}{3}$

10. Three masses are placed on the x-axis : 300 g at origin, 500 g at $x = 40$ cm and 400 g at $x = 70$ cm. The distance of the centre of mass from the origin is
(a) 40 cm (b) 45 cm (c) 50 cm (d) 30 cm

ANSWER KEY

1	(a)	2	(b)	3	(c)	4	(a)	5	(a)	6	(c)	7	(a)	8	(b)	9	(b)	10	(a)

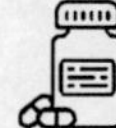

Topic 7.2 : Moment of Inertia, Radius of Gyration & Theorems on Moment of Inertia

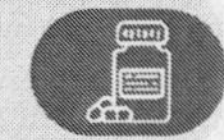

MOMENT OF INERTIA AND RADIUS OF GYRATION

A rigid body having constituent particles of masses m_1, m_2, ...m_n and r_1, r_2 ... r_n be their respective distances from the axis of rotation then **moment of inertia** is given by,

$$I = m_1 r_1^2 + m_2 r_2^2 + ... + m_n r_n^2 = \sum_{i=1}^{n} m_i r_i^2$$

The moment of inertia of continuous mass distribution is given by

$$I = \int r^2 \, dm$$

where r is the perpendicular distance of the small mass dm from the axis of rotation.

Its **SI unit** is kgm^2. It is a **tensor**.

Radius of gyration :

The radius of gyration of a body about its axis of rotation may be defined as the distance from the axis of rotation at which, if the entire mass of the body were concentrated, its moment of inertia about the given axis would be same as with its actual distribution of mass.

Radius of gyration k is given by,

$$I = MK^2$$

$$\text{or} \quad K = \left[\frac{I}{M}\right]^{\frac{1}{2}} = \left[\frac{\sum_{i}^{n} m_i r_i^2}{\sum m_i}\right]^{\frac{1}{2}}$$

where, $M = \Sigma m_i$

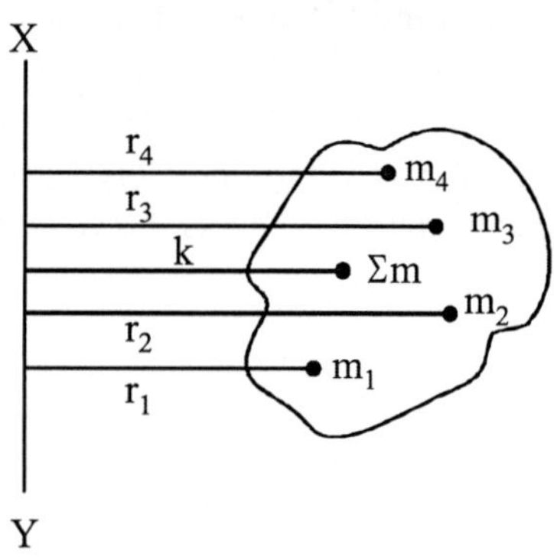

Also, $k = \sqrt{\dfrac{r_1^2 + r_2^2 + r_3^2 + ...r_n^2}{n}}$

Therefore, radius of gyration (k) equals the root mean square of the distances of particles from the axis of rotation.

GENERAL THEOREMS ON MOMENT OF INERTIA

Theorem of perpendicular axis :

According to this theorem " the moment of inertia of a plane lamina (a plane lamina is a 2-dimensional body. Its third dimension is so small that it can be neglected.) *about an axis, perpendicular to the plane of lamina is equal to the sum of the moment of inertia of the lamina about two axes perpendicular to each other, in its own plane and intersecting each other at the point, where the perpendicular axes passes through it.*

If I_x and I_y be the moment of inertia of a plane lamina (or 2D rigid body) about the perpendicular axis OX and OY respectively, which lie in plane of lamina and intersect each other at O, then moment of inertia (I_z) about an axis passing through (OZ) and perpendicular to its plane is given by

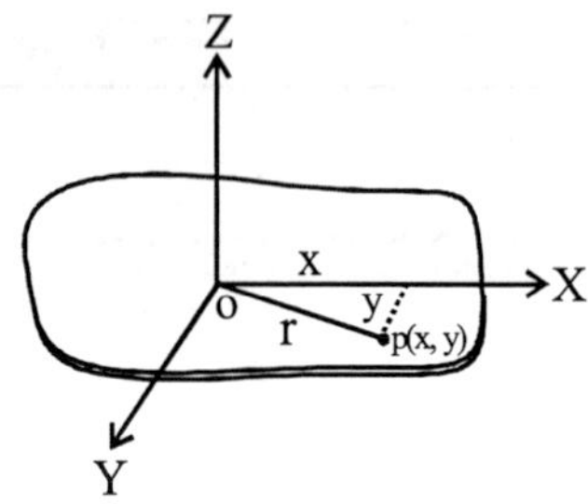

$$I_x + I_y = I_z$$

Let us consider a particle of mass m at point P distance r from origin O, where $r = \sqrt{x^2 + y^2}$

so $I_x + I_y = \Sigma my^2 + \Sigma mx^2 = \Sigma mr^2$

i.e., $I_z = I_x + I_y$

Theorem of parallel axes :

(Derived by Steiner) This theorem is true for both plane laminar body and thin 3D body. It states that *"the moment of inertia of a body about any axis is equal to its moment of inertia about a parallel axis through its centre of mass plus the product of the mass of the body and the square of the distance between two axes.*

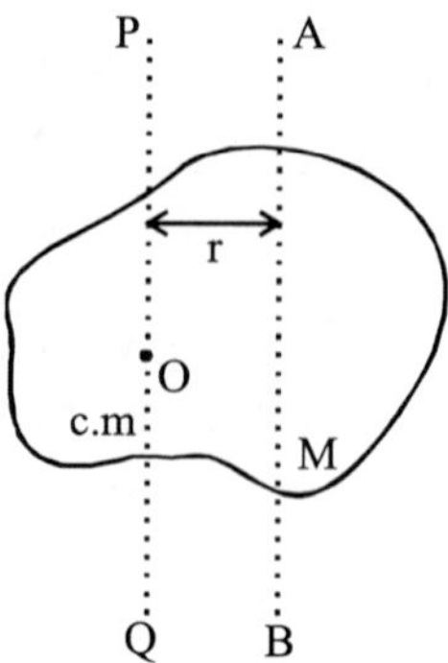

Let AB be the axis in plane of paper about which, the moment of inertia (I) of plane lamina is to be determined and PQ an axis parallel to AB, passing through centre of mass O of lamina is at a distance 'r' from AB.

Consider a mass element m of lamina at point P distant x from PQ.

Now the moment of inertia of the element about AB= m $(x+r)^2$

so moment of inertia of whole lamina about AB is

$$I = \Sigma m(x+r)^2 = \Sigma mx^2 + \Sigma mr^2 + 2\Sigma mxr$$

Where first term on R.H.S is $\Sigma\, mx^2 = I_{c.m.}$ moment of inertia of lamina about PQ through its centre of mass, second term on R.H.S. is $\Sigma mr^2 = r^2\Sigma m = Mr^2$, M is whole mass of lamina, third term on R.H.S is $(\Sigma mx)\, r = 0$, because Σmx is equal to moments of all particles of lamina about an axis PQ, passing through its centre of mass. Hence

$$I = I_{c.m.} + M.r^2$$

i.e., the moment of inertia of lamina about AB = its moment of inertia about a parallel axis PQ passing through its centre of mass + mass of lamina×(distance between two axes)^2

Example 1.

Three rings each of mass P and radius Q are arranged as shown in fig. What will be the moment of inertia of the arrangement about YY'?

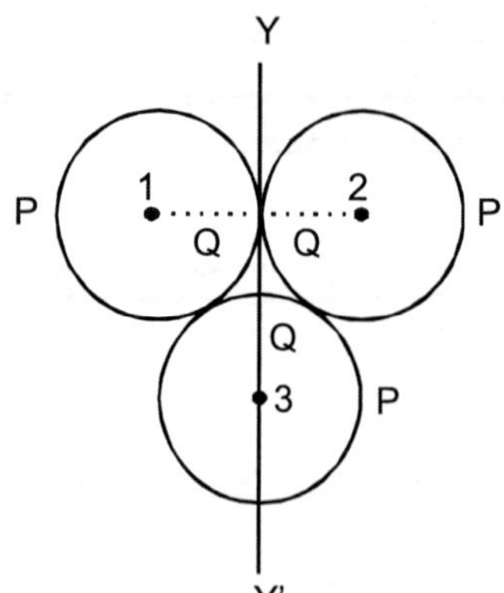

Solution :

Moment of inertia of each ring about its diameter = $\frac{1}{2}PQ^2$.

So total moment of inertia of all three rings about Y Y' is

$I_{total} = I_1 + I_2 + I_3$

Using theorem of parallel axes (for rings 1 and 2), we get

$$I_{total} = \left(\frac{1}{2}PQ^2 + PQ^2\right) + \left(\frac{1}{2}PQ^2 + PQ^2\right) + \frac{1}{2}PQ^2 = \frac{7}{2}PQ^2$$

Example 2.

Four particles each of mass m are lying symmetrically on the rim of a disc of mass M and radius R. Find MI of this system about an axis passing through one of the particles and perpendicular to plane of disc.

Solution :

According to the theorem of parallel axes, MI of disc about an axis passing through K and perpendicular to plane of disc, is

$$= \frac{1}{2}MR^2 + MR^2 = \frac{3}{2}MR^2$$

Particle 2
Particle 1 O R K Particle 3
Particle 4

Total MI of the system =

$$\frac{3}{2}MR^2 + m(2R)^2 + m(\sqrt{2}R)^2 + m(\sqrt{2}R)^2 = 19\frac{MR^2}{2}$$

Example 3.

Three identical rods, each of length ℓ, are joined to from a rigid equilateral triangle. Find its radius of gyration about an axis passing through a corner and perpendicular to the plane of the triangle.

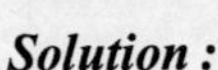

Solution :

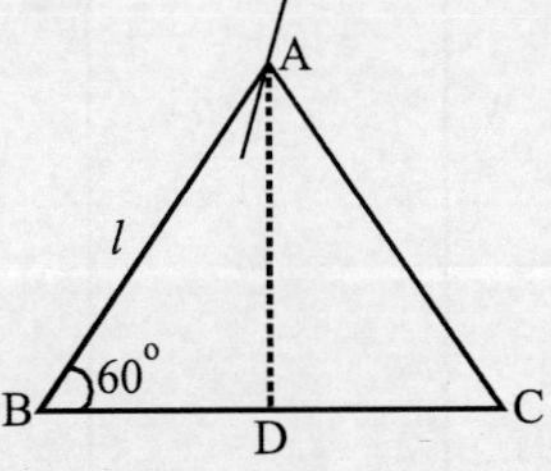

$$I = I_{AB} + I_{AC} + I_{BC} = \frac{ml^2}{3} + \frac{ml^2}{3} + (I_D + mh^2)$$

$$= \frac{2}{3}ml^2 + \frac{ml^2}{12} + m(l\sin 60)^2 = ml^2\left[\frac{2}{3} + \frac{1}{12} + \frac{3}{4}\right]$$

$$= \frac{3}{2}ml^2 = (3m)k^2 \text{ or } k = \frac{\ell}{\sqrt{2}}$$

Example 4.

A uniform rod of mass m and length ℓ makes a constant angle θ with the axis of rotation which passes through one end of the rod. Determine its moment of inertia about this axis.

Solution :

Mass of element of uniform rod $= \left(\frac{m}{\ell}\right)dx$

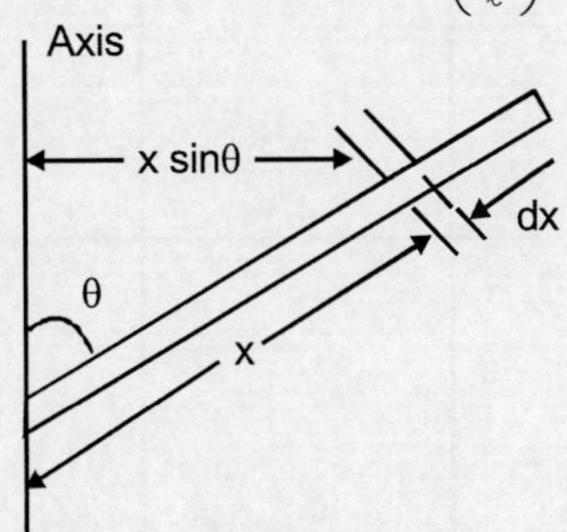

Moment of inertia of the element about the axis

$$= \left(\frac{m}{\ell}dx\right)(x\sin\theta)^2.$$

$$I = \frac{m}{\ell}\sin^2\theta.\int_0^{\ell} x^2dx = \frac{m\ell^2}{3}\sin^2\theta$$

Example 5.

A circular plate of uniform thickness has a diameter of 56 cm. A circular portion of diameter 42 cm is removed from one edge of the plate as shown. Find the position of centre of mass of the remaining portion.

Solution :

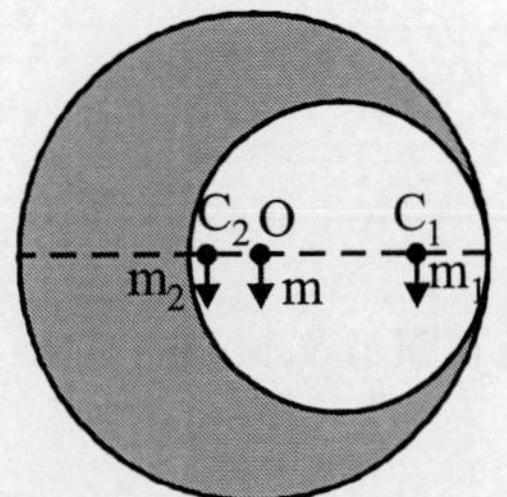

Area of whole plate = $\pi(56/2)^2 = 784\pi$ sq. cm.
Area of cut portion = $\pi(42/2)^2 = 441\pi$ sq. cm. ;
Area of remaining portion = $784\pi - 441\pi = 343\pi\,cm^2$;
As mass $\propto$ area.

$$\therefore \frac{\text{Mass of cut portion}}{\text{Mass of remaining portion}} = \frac{m_1}{m_2} = \frac{441\pi}{343\pi} = \frac{9}{7}$$

Let C_2 be centre of mass of remaining portion and C_1 be centre of mass of cut portion.
O is centre of mass of the whole disc.;
$OC_1 = r_1 = 28 - 21 = 7$ cm.
$OC_2 = r_2 = ?$;
Equating moments of masses about O,

we get $m_2 \times r_2 = m_1 \times r_1 \Rightarrow r_2 = \frac{m_1}{m_2} \times r_1 = \frac{9}{7} \times 7 = 9$

$\therefore$ Centre of mass of remaining portion is at 9 cm to the left of centre of disc.

Example 6.

Show that the centre of mass of a rod of mass M and length L lies midway between its ends, assuming the rod has a uniform mass per unit length.

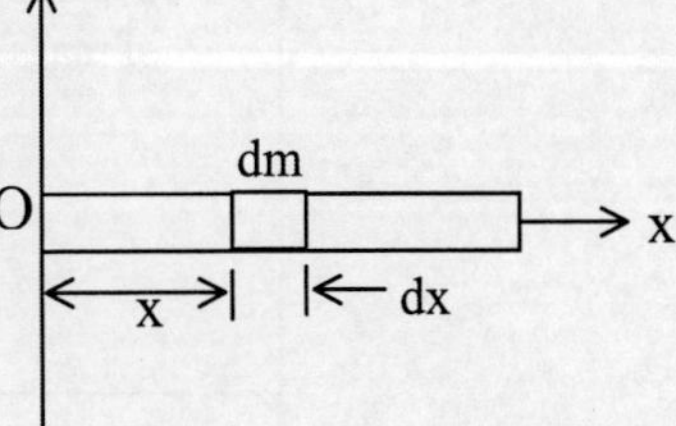

Solution :

By symmetry, we see that $y_{CM} = z_{CM} = 0$ if the rod is placed along the x axis. Furthermore, if we call the mass per unit length λ (the linear mass density), then λ = M/L for a uniform rod. If we divide the rod into elements of length dx, then the mass of each element is dm = λ dx. Since an arbitrary element of each element is at a distance x from the origin, equation gives

$$x_{CM} = \frac{1}{M}\int_0^L x\,dm = \frac{1}{M}\int_0^L x\lambda dx = \frac{\lambda L^2}{2M}$$

Because λ = M/L, this reduces to $x_{CM} = \frac{L^2}{2M}\left(\frac{M}{L}\right) = \frac{L}{2}$

One can also argue that by symmetry, $x_{CM} = L/2$.

MOMENT OF INERTIA AND RADIUS OF GYRATION OF DIFFERENT OBJECTS

Shape of body	Rotational axis	Figure	Moment of inertia	Radius of gyration
(1) Ring M = mass R = radius	(a) Perpendicular to plane passing through centre of mass	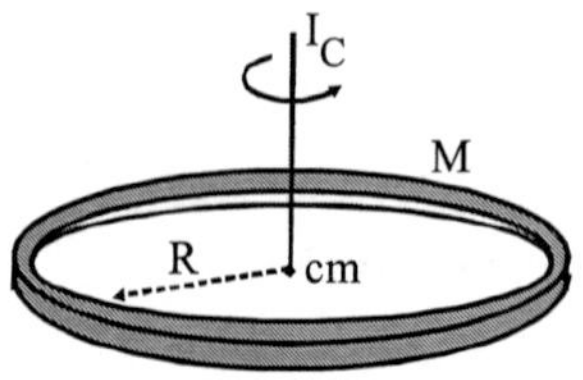 I_C, M, R, cm	MR^2	R
	(b) Diameter in the plane	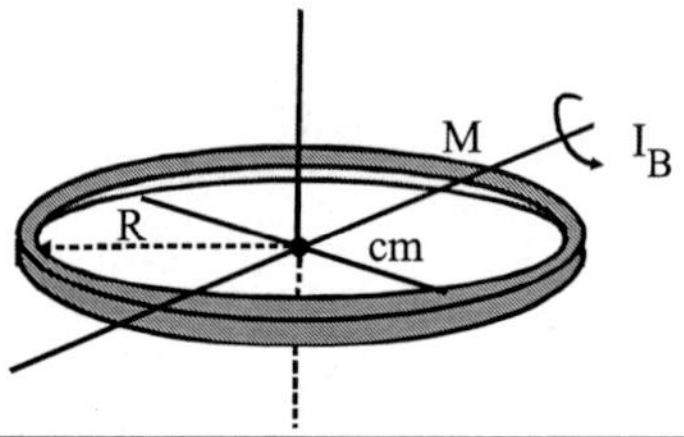 M, I_B, R, cm	$\frac{1}{2}MR^2$	$\frac{R}{\sqrt{2}}$
	(c) Tangent perpendicular to plane	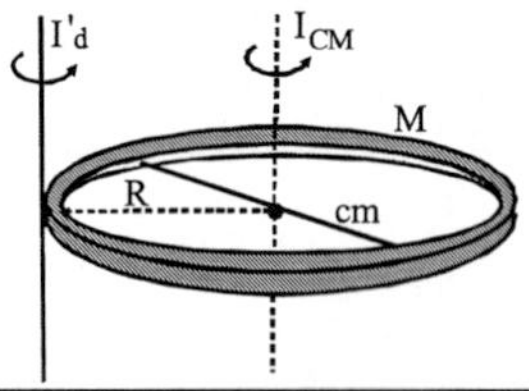 I'_d, I_{CM}, M, R, cm	$2MR^2$	$\sqrt{2}R$
	(d) Tangent in the plane	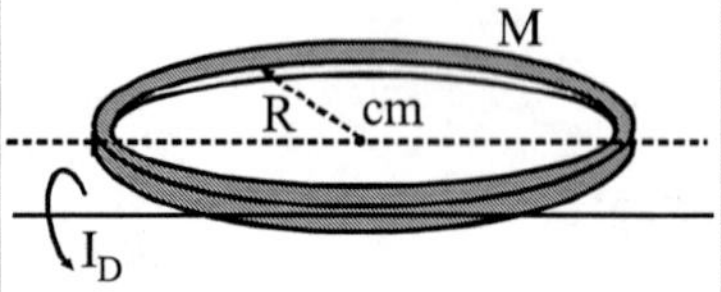 M, R, cm, I_D	$\frac{3}{2}MR^2$	$\sqrt{\frac{3}{2}}R$
(2) Disc	(a) Perpendicular to plane passing through centre of mass	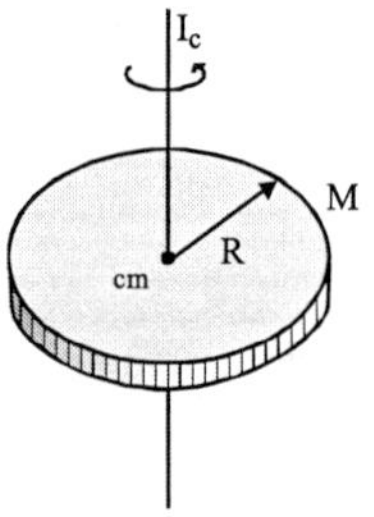 I_c, M, R, cm	$\frac{1}{2}MR^2$	$\frac{R}{\sqrt{2}}$
	(b) Diameter in the plane	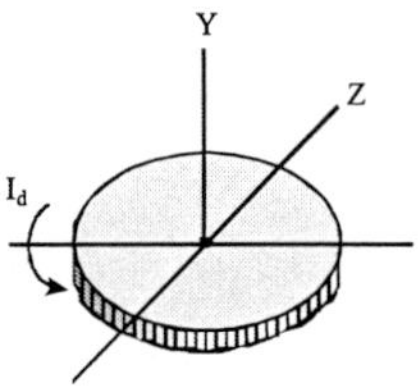 Y, Z, I_d	$\frac{MR^2}{4}$	$\frac{R}{2}$
	(c) Tangent in the plane	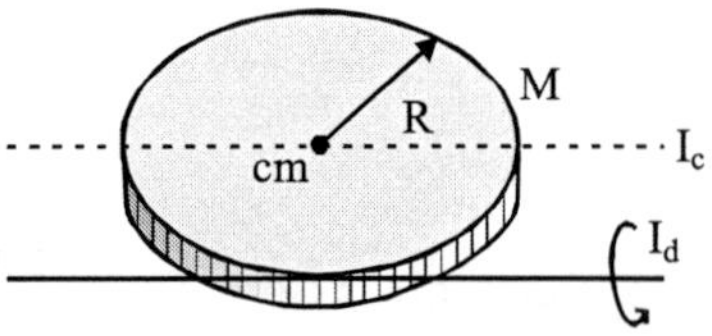 M, R, cm, I_c, I_d	$\frac{5}{4}MR^2$	$\frac{\sqrt{5}}{2}R$

	(d) Tangent perpendicular to plane	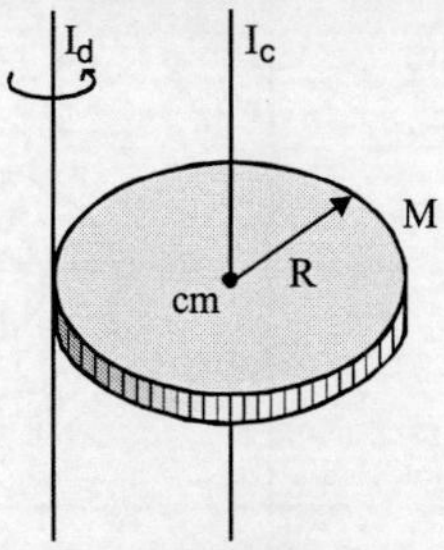	$\frac{3}{2}MR^2$	$\sqrt{\frac{3}{2}}R$
(3) Thin walled cylinder	(a) Geometrical axis	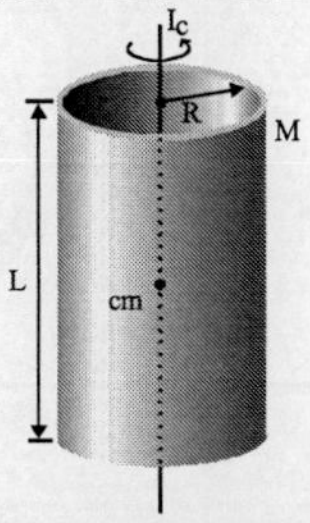	MR^2	R
	(b) Perpendicular to length passing through centre of mass	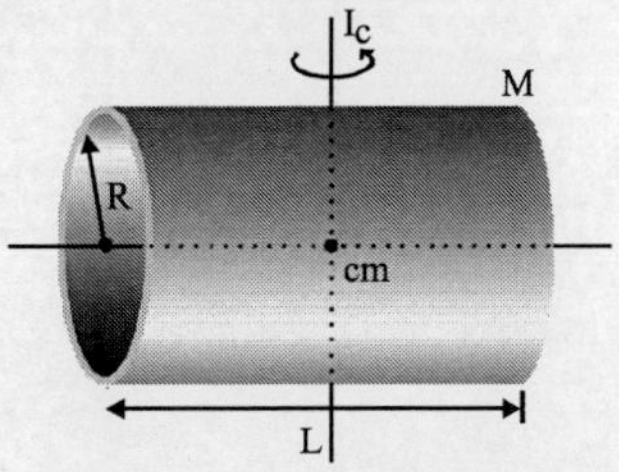	$M\left(\frac{R^2}{2}+\frac{L^2}{12}\right)$	$\sqrt{\frac{R^2}{2}+\frac{L^2}{12}}$
	(c) Perpendicular to length passing through one end	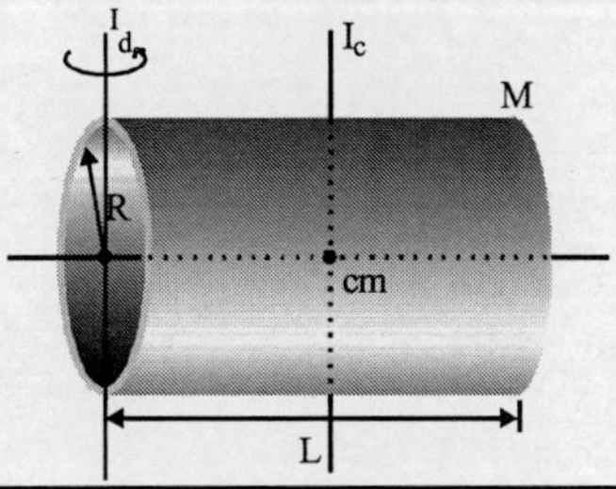	$M\left(\frac{R^2}{2}+\frac{L^2}{3}\right)$	$\sqrt{\frac{R^2}{2}+\frac{L^2}{3}}$
(4) Solid cylinder	(a) Geometrical axis	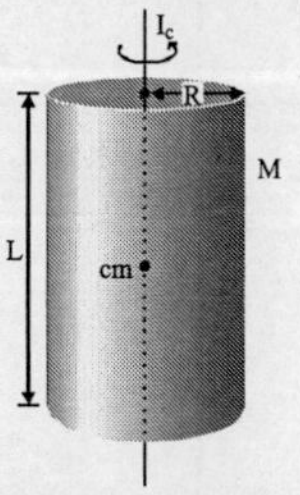	$\frac{MR^2}{2}$	$\frac{R}{\sqrt{2}}$
	(b) Perpendicular to length passing through centre of mass	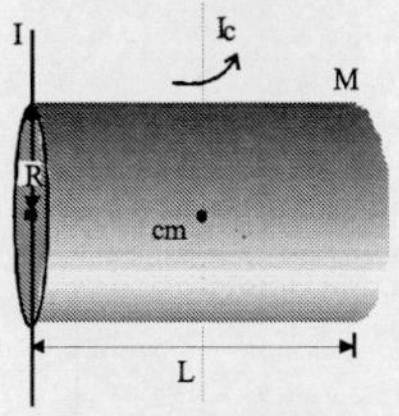	$M\left(\frac{R^2}{4}+\frac{L^2}{12}\right)$	$\sqrt{\frac{R^2}{4}+\frac{L^2}{12}}$
	(c) Perpendicular to length passing through one end	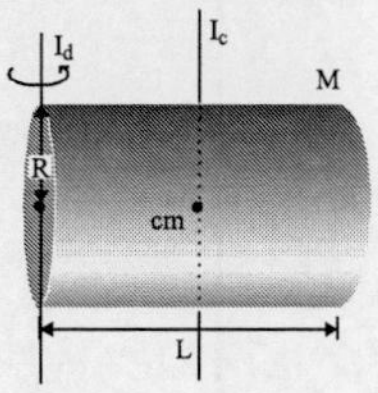	$M\left[\frac{R^2}{4}+\frac{L^2}{3}\right]$	$\sqrt{\frac{R^2}{4}+\frac{L^2}{3}}$

(5) Annular disc	(a) Perpendicular to plane passing through centre of mass	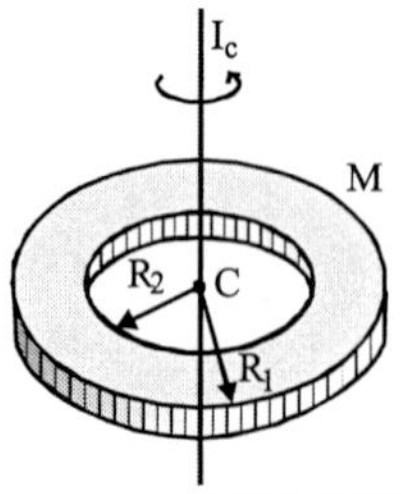	$\frac{M}{2}[R_1^2+R_2^2]$	$\sqrt{\frac{R_1^2+R_2^2}{2}}$
	(b) Diameter in the plane	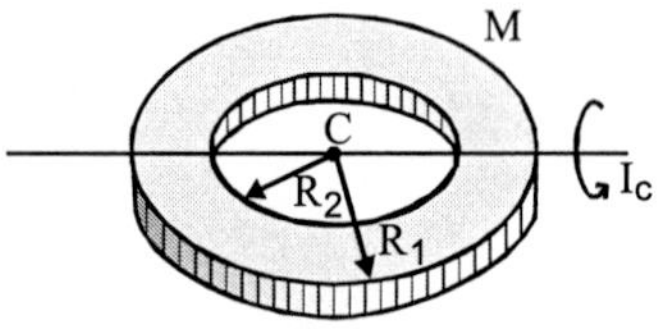	$\frac{M[R_1^2+R_2^2]}{4}$	$\sqrt{\frac{R_1^2+R_2^2}{4}}$
(6) Hollow cylinder	(a) Geometrical axis	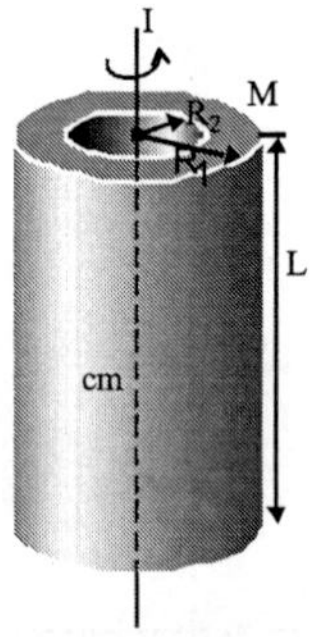	$M\left[\frac{R_1^2+R_2^2}{2}\right]$	$\sqrt{\frac{R_1^2+R_2^2}{2}}$
	(b) Perpendicular to length passing through centre of mass	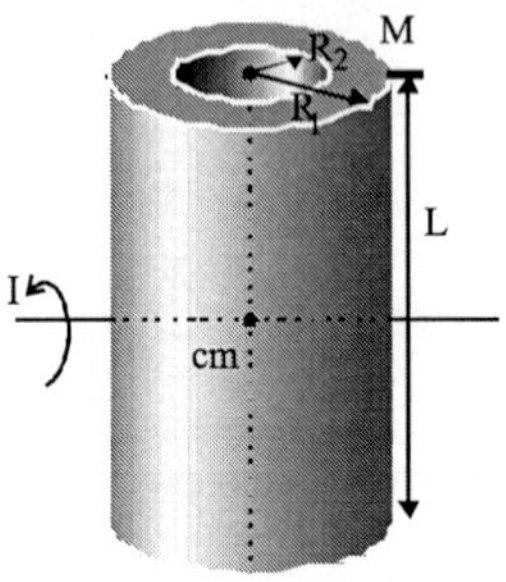	$M\left[\frac{L^2}{12}+\frac{(R_1^2+R_2^2)}{4}\right]$	$\sqrt{\frac{L^2}{12}+\frac{R_1^2+R_2^2}{4}}$
(7) Solid sphere	(a) Along the diameter	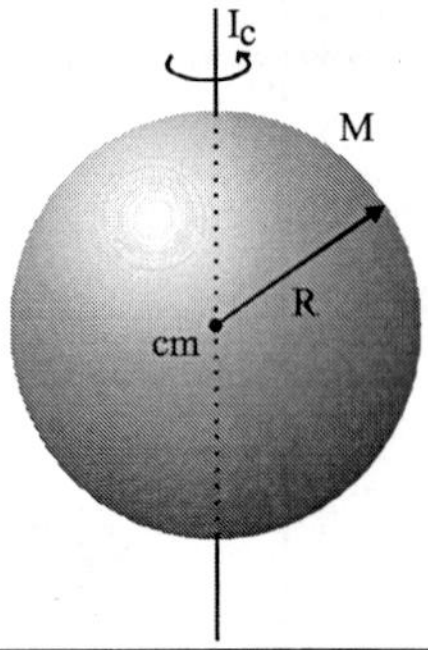	$\frac{2}{5}MR^2$	$\sqrt{\frac{2}{5}}R$
	(b) Along the tangent	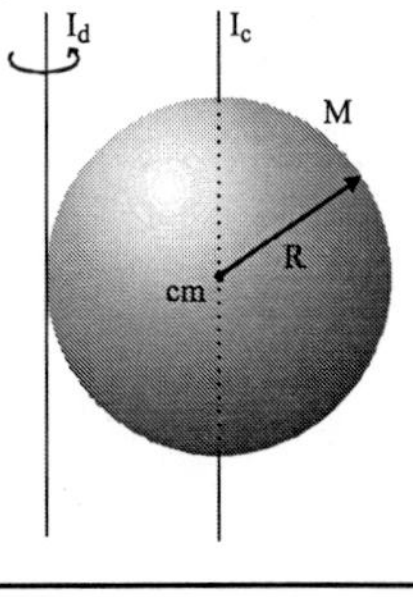	$\frac{7}{5}MR^2$	$\sqrt{\frac{7}{5}}R$

(8) Thin spherical shell	(a) Along the diameter	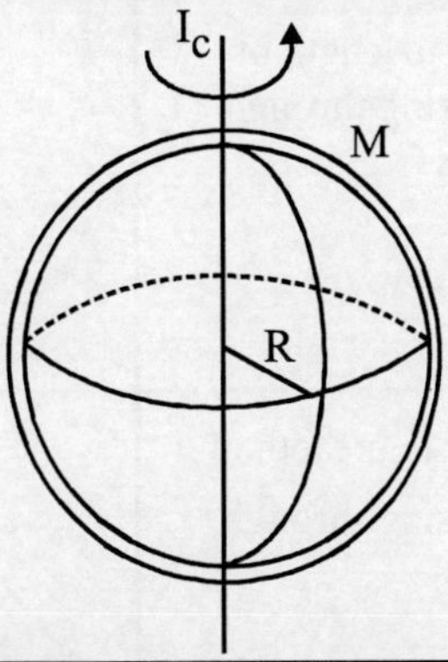	$\frac{2}{3}MR^2$	$\sqrt{\frac{2}{3}}R$
	(b) Along the tangent	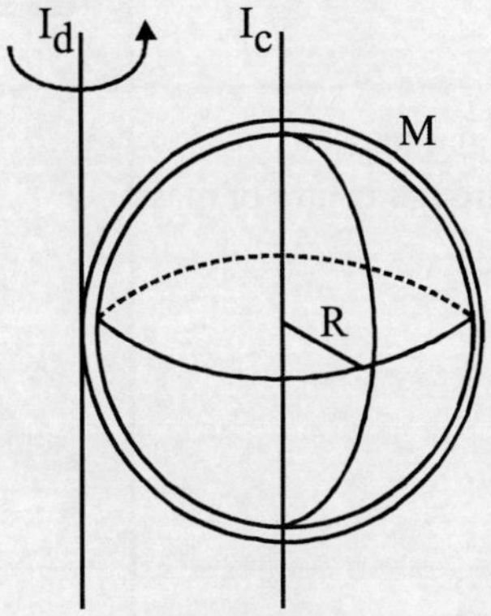	$\frac{5}{3}MR^2$	$\sqrt{\frac{5}{3}}R$
(9) Hollow sphere $\sqrt{\frac{2}{5}\frac{(R^5-r^5)}{(R^3-r^3)}}$	Along the diameter	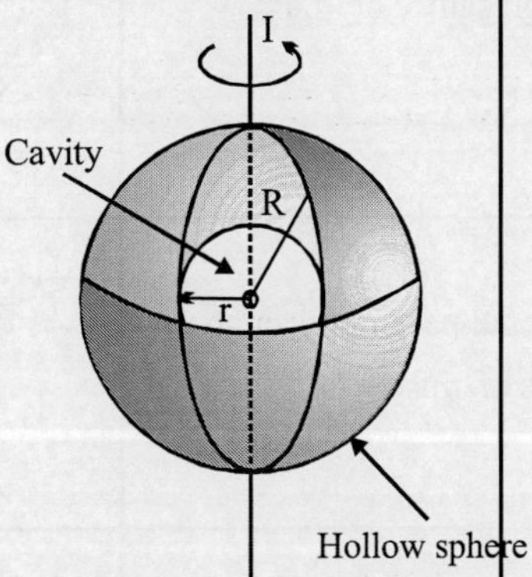	$\frac{2}{5}M\left[\frac{R^5-r^5}{R^3-r^3}\right]$	
(10) Thin rod	(a) Perpendicular to length passing through centre of mass	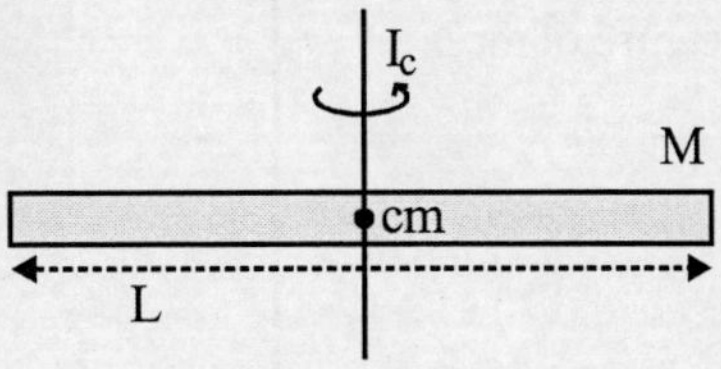	$\frac{ML^2}{12}$	$\frac{L}{2\sqrt{3}}$
	(b) Perpendicular to length passing through one end	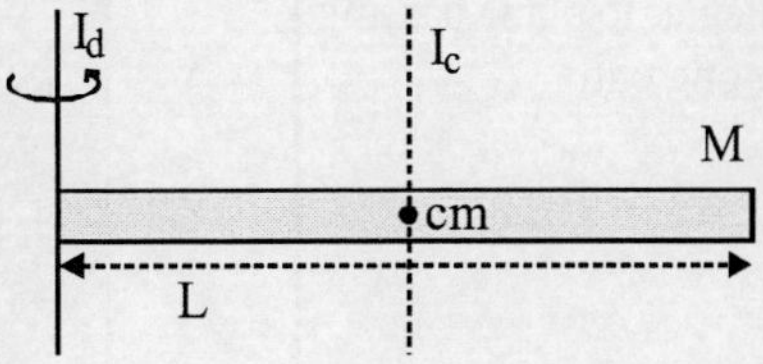	$\frac{ML^2}{3}$	$\frac{L}{\sqrt{3}}$

(11) Rectangular plate	(a) Perpendicular to length in the plane passing through centre of mass	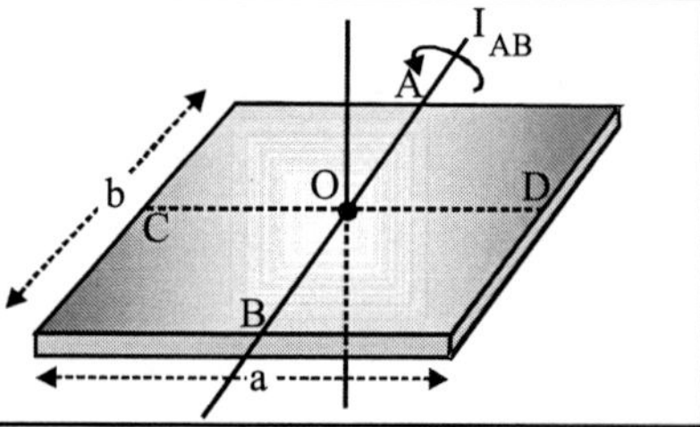	$\frac{Ma^2}{12}$	$\frac{a}{2\sqrt{3}}$
	(b) Perpendicular to breadth in the plane passing through centre of mass	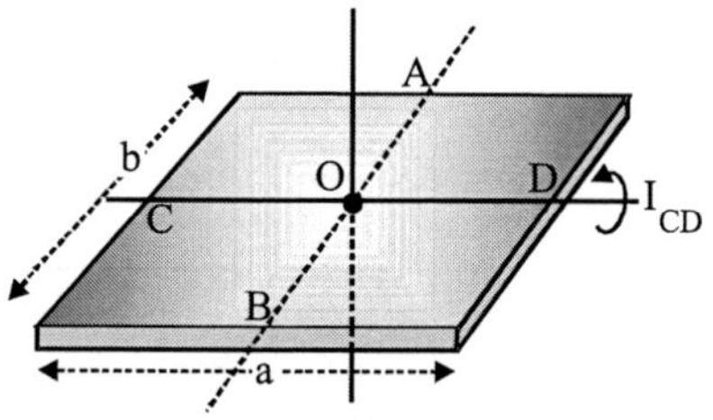	$\frac{Mb^2}{12}$	$\frac{b}{2\sqrt{3}}$
	(c) Perpendicular to plane passing through centre of mass	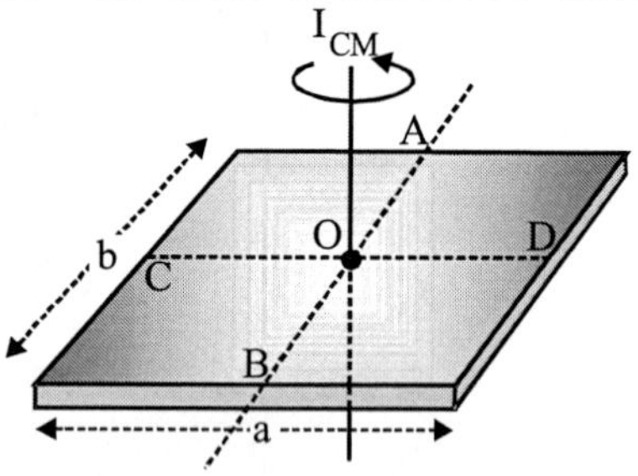	$\frac{M(a^2+b^2)}{12}$	$\frac{\sqrt{a^2+b^2}}{2\sqrt{3}}$
(12) Square Plate	(a) Perpendicular to plane passing through centre of mass	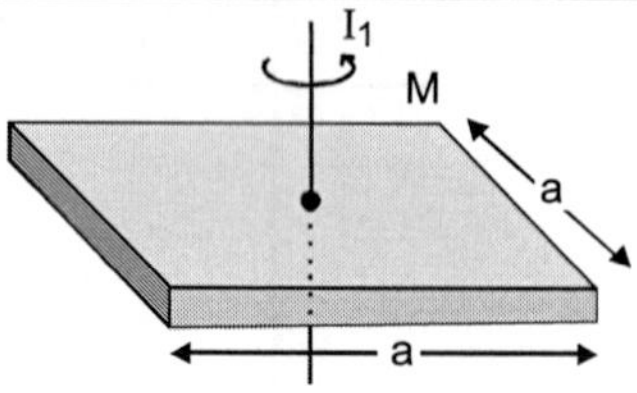	$I_1 = \frac{Ma^2}{6}$	$\frac{a}{\sqrt{6}}$
	(b) Diagonal passing through centre of mass	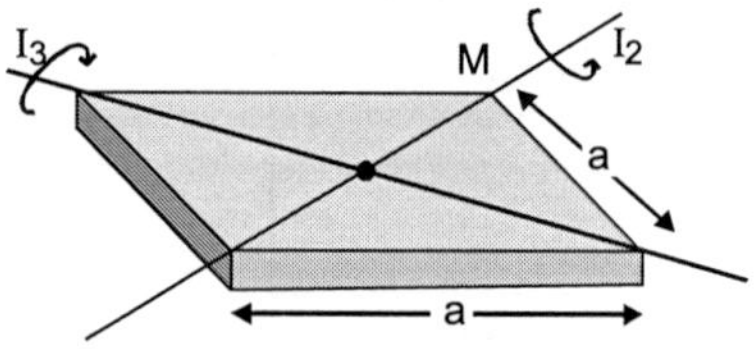	$I_2 = I_3 \frac{Ma^2}{12}$	$\frac{a}{2\sqrt{3}}$
(13) Cube	(a) Perpendicular to plane passing through centre of mass	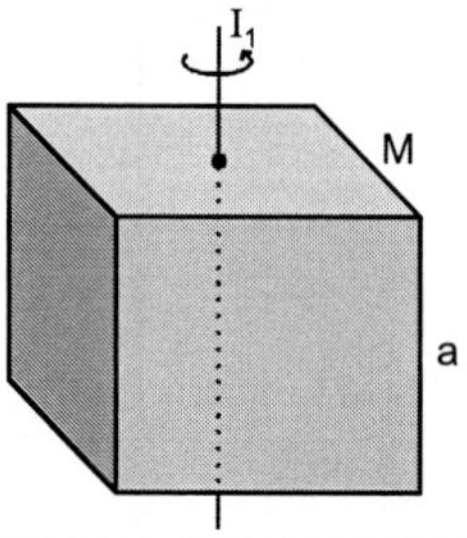	$I_1 = \frac{Ma^2}{6}$	$\frac{a}{\sqrt{6}}$
	(b) Perpendicular to plane passing through one end	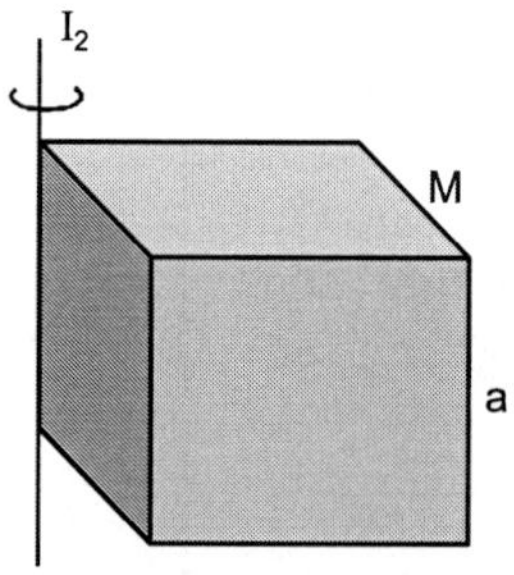	$I_2 = \frac{2Ma^2}{3}$	$\sqrt{\frac{2}{3}}\, a$

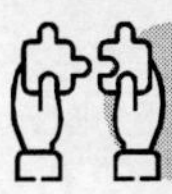

7.2 Concept Practice Problems CPP

11. Moment of inertia does not depend upon
(a) distribution of mass
(b) axis of rotation
(c) point of application of force
(d) None of these

12. Moment of inertia of a circular wire of mass *M* and radius *R* about its diameter is
(a) $MR^2/2$ (b) MR^2
(c) $2MR^2$ (d) $MR^2/4$.

13. One solid sphere A and another hollow sphere B are of same mass and same outer radii. Their moment of inertia about their diameters are respectively I_A and I_B Such that
(a) $I_A < I_B$ (b) $I_A > I_B$
(c) $I_A = I_B$ (d) $\frac{I_A}{I_B} = \frac{d_A}{d_B}$
where d_A and d_B are their densities.

14. Point masses 1, 2, 3 and 4 kg are lying at the points (0, 0, 0), (2, 0, 0), (0, 3, 0) and (–2, –2, 0) respectively. The moment of inertia of this system about X-axis will be
(a) 43 kg–m^2 (b) 34 kg–m^2
(c) 27 kg – m^2 (d) 72 kg – m^2

15. The ratio of moment of inertia of circular ring & circular disc having the same mass & radii about on axis passing the c.m & perpendicular to plane is
(a) 1 : 1 (b) 2 : 1
(c) 1 : 2 (d) 4 : 1

16. A circular disc X of radius R is made from an iron plate of thickness t, and another disc Y of radius 4R is made from an iron plate of thickness $\frac{t}{4}$. Then the relation between the moment of inertia I_X and I_Y is
(a) $I_Y = 32 I_X$ (b) $I_Y = 16 I_X$
(c) $I_Y = I_X$ (d) $I_Y = 64 I_X$

17. Two rings of radius R and nR made up of same material have the ratio of moment of inertia about an axis passing through centre as 1 : 8. The value of n is
(a) 2 (b) $2\sqrt{2}$
(c) 4 (d) $\frac{1}{2}$

18. ABC is a triangular plate of uniform thickness. The sides are in the ratio shown in the figure. I_{AB}, I_{BC} and I_{CA} are the moments of inertia of the plate about AB, BC and CA as axes respectively. Which one of the following relations is correct?
(a) $I_{AB} > I_{BC}$
(b) $I_{BC} > I_{AB}$
(c) $I_{AB} + I_{BC} = I_{CA}$
(d) I_{CA} is maximum

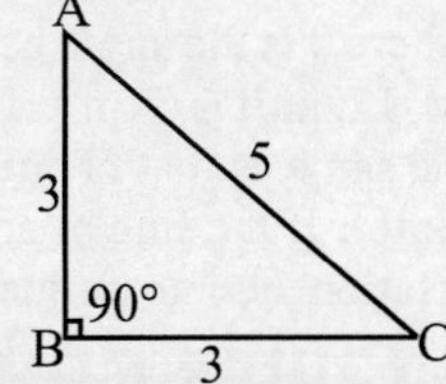

19. The moment of inertia of a disc of mass M and radius R about an axis, which is tangential to the circumference of the disc and parallel to its diameter, is
(a) $\frac{3}{2}MR^2$ (b) $\frac{2}{3}MR^2$
(c) $\frac{5}{4}MR^2$ (d) $\frac{4}{5}MR^2$

20. Three particles, each of mass m gram, are situated at the vertices of an equilateral triangle ABC of side/cm (as shown in the figure). The moment of inertia of the system about a line AX perpendicular to AB and in the plane of ABC, in gram-cm^2 units will be
(a) $\frac{3}{2}m\ell^2$
(b) $\frac{3}{4}m\ell^2$
(c) $2m\ell^2$
(d) $\frac{5}{4}m\ell^2$

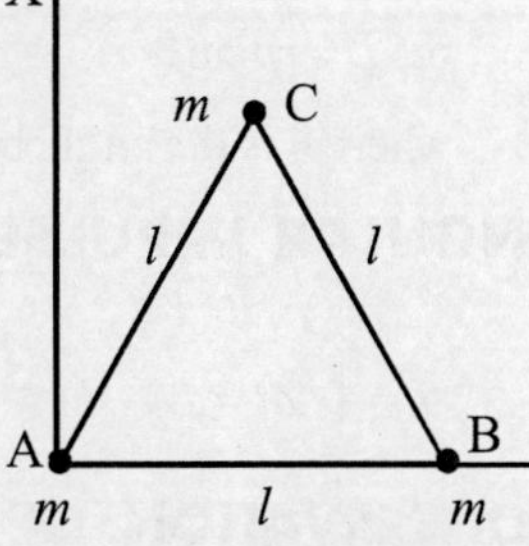

ANSWER KEY

11	(c)	12	(a)	13	(a)	14	(a)	15	(b)	16	(d)	17	(a)	18	(b)	19	(c)	20	(d)

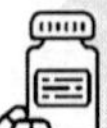

Topic 7.3 : Torque, Angular Momentum, Conservation of Angular Momentum, Rotational K.E. & Rolling Motion

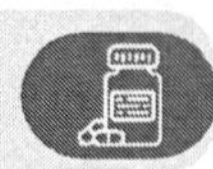

TORQUE

The moment of force is called torque. *It is defined as the product of force and the perpendicular distance of the force from the axis of rotation.*

i.e., $\vec{\tau} = \vec{r} \times \vec{F}$

or, $\tau = rF \sin\theta$

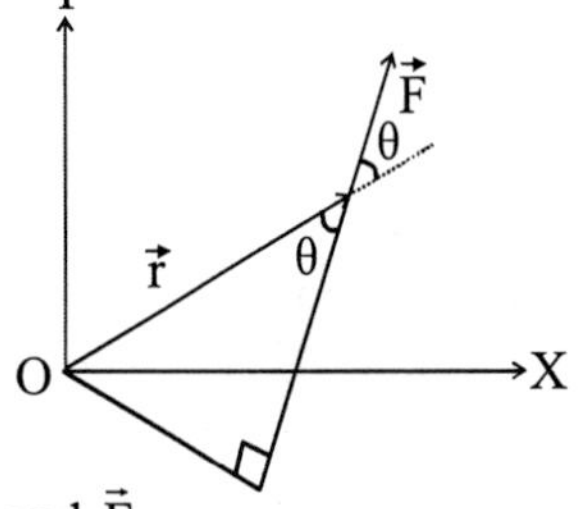

where θ is the angle between $\vec{r}$ and $\vec{F}$.

Its **S.I. unit** is (N-m). The **dimensions** of torque $[ML^2T^{-2}]$ are the same as that of energy but it is not energy.

Note : If the line of action of a force passes through axis of rotation then no torque will be formed.

ANGULAR MOMENTUM

The angular momentum of a particle about an arbitrry point 'O' is the moment of linear momentum taken about that point.

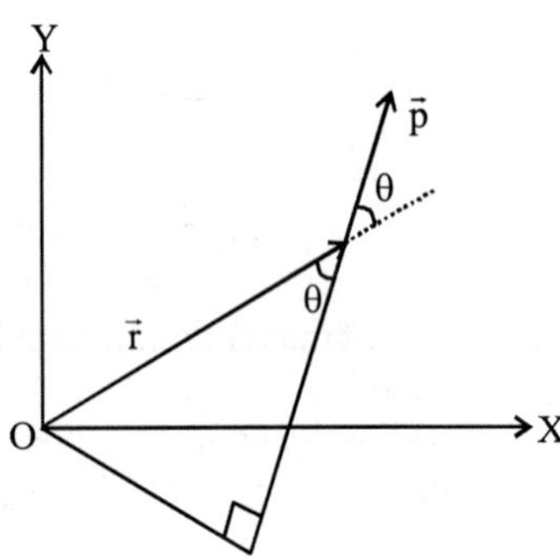

It is given as $\vec{L} = \vec{r} \times \vec{p}$

or, $L = rp\sin\theta$

where θ is the angle between $\vec{r}$ and $\vec{F}$.

ANGULAR IMPULSE

$$J = \int_{t_1}^{t_2} \tau dt = L_2 - L_1 \quad (= \text{Change in angular momentum})$$

CONSERVATION OF ANGULAR MOMENTUM

From equation $\vec{\tau}_{ext} = \frac{d\vec{L}}{dt}$.

If $\vec{\tau}_{ext} = 0 \Rightarrow \vec{L} = \text{constant}$ ...(i)

This is called law of **conservation of angular momentum.**

According to this "*if resultant external torque $\vec{\tau}_{ext}$ acting on the system is zero then total angular momentum of the system is constant.*

The magnitude of angular momentum for a system is given by

$$|\vec{L}| = \sum_{i=1}^{n}(m_i r_i)v_i = \sum_{i=1}^{n}(m_i r_i^2)\omega \quad [\because v = r\omega]$$

$$\Rightarrow \quad |\vec{L}| = \sum_{i=1}^{n}(I_i \times \omega) = I\omega \quad ...(ii)$$

Where I_i is the moment of inertia of the ith particle of that system and I is total moment of inertia of the system

$$I = \sum_{i=1}^{n} I_i = I_1 + I_2 + I_3 + ... + I_n$$

or $$I = m_1 r_1^2 + m_2 r_2^2 + ... + m_n r_n^2 \quad ...(iii)$$

So if a system undergoes a redistribution of its mass, then its moment of inertia changes but since no external torque is applied on the system so total angular momentum is constant before and after the distribution of mass, even if moment of inertia of the system is changed.

$$\vec{L}_{Initial} = \vec{L}_{Final} \quad ...(iv)$$

or, $I_1\omega_1 = I_2\omega_2$ ...(v)

where L initial denote the state previous to the redistribution of mass and final denote the state after the redistribution of mass in that system.

A comparison of useful relations in rotational and translational or linear motion :

Rotational motion about a fixed axis	*Linear motion*
Angular velocity $\omega = \frac{d\theta}{dt}$	Linear velocity $v = \frac{dx}{dt}$
Angular acceleration $\alpha = \frac{d\omega}{dt}$	Linear acceleration $a = \frac{dv}{dt}$
Resultant torque $\tau = I\alpha$	Resultant force $F = ma$
Equations of rotational motion	Equations of linear motion
α = constant then $\begin{cases} \omega = \omega_0 + \alpha t \\ \theta - \theta_0 = \omega_0 t + ½\alpha t^2 \\ \omega^2 = \omega_0^2 + 2\alpha(\theta - \theta_0) \end{cases}$	a = constant then $\begin{cases} v = u + at \\ s = ut + \frac{1}{2}at^2 \\ v^2 - u^2 = 2as \end{cases}$ where $(s = x - x_0)$
Work $W = \int_{\theta_o}^{\theta} \vec{\tau} d\vec{\theta}$	work $W = \int_{x_o}^{x} \vec{F} d\vec{x}$
Kinetic energy $E_k = ½ I\omega^2$	Kinetic energy $E_k = ½ mv^2$
Power $P = \tau\omega$	Power $P = \vec{F}\vec{v}$
Angular momentum $L = \vec{I}\vec{\omega}$	Linear momentum $p = mv$
Torque $\tau = \frac{dL}{dt}$	Force $F = \frac{dp}{dt}$

Work Energy Theorem in Rotational Motion :
According to this theorem "*the work done by external forces in rotating a rigid body about a fixed axis is equal to the change in rotational kinetic energy of the body*."
Since, we can express the torque as

$$\tau = I\alpha = I\frac{d\omega}{dt} = I\frac{d\omega}{d\theta}\cdot\frac{d\theta}{dt}$$

$$\tau = I\omega\frac{d\omega}{d\theta} \quad \text{but } \tau d\theta = dW$$

$$\Rightarrow \quad \tau d\theta = dW = I\omega d\omega$$

By integrating the above expression, we get total work done by all external force on the body, which is written as

$$W = \int_{\theta_1}^{\theta_2} \tau d\theta = \int_{\omega_1}^{\omega_2} I\omega d\omega = \frac{1}{2}I\omega_2^2 - \frac{1}{2}I\omega_1^2$$

where the angular velocity of the body changes from ω_1 to ω_2 as the angular displacement changes from θ_1 to θ_2 due to external force $\vec{F}_{ext.}$ on the body.

Rotational Kinetic Energy :
Let us consider a rigid body (collection of small particles) of high symmetry which is purely rotating about z-axis with an angular velocity ω. Each particle has some energy, determined by m_i and v_i. The kinetic energy of m_i particle is

$$(E_k)_i = \frac{1}{2}m_i v_i^2 \qquad \text{... (i)}$$

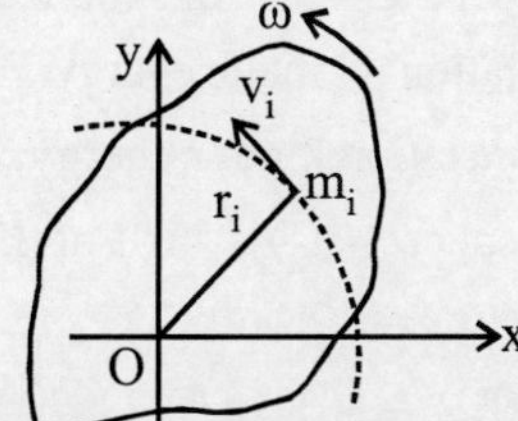

Fig. The total kinetic energy of the body is ½Iω².

Now we know that in rigid body every particle moves with same angular velocity, the individual linear velocities depends on the distance r_i from the axis of rotation according to the expression ($v_i = r_i\omega$). Hence the total kinetic energy of rotating rigid body is equal to the sum of kinetic energies of individual particles.

$$E_k = \Sigma(E_k)_i = \Sigma\frac{1}{2}m_i v_i^2 = (\Sigma m_i r_i^2)\frac{\omega^2}{2}$$

$$E_k = \frac{1}{2}I\omega^2 \qquad \text{... (ii)}$$

where $I = \Sigma m_i r_i^2$ is moment of inertia of the rigid body.

Now consider a rigid body which is rolling without slipping. In this case it possesses simultaneous translatory motion and rotatory motion and the total kinetic energy of the rigid body $K.E_{Total}$ = rotation K.E. + translational K.E. of C.M.

$$E_k = (E_k)_{rotational} + (E_k)_{translational} \qquad \text{... (iii)}$$

$$E_k = \frac{1}{2}I\omega^2 + \frac{1}{2}Mv_{cm}^2 \qquad \text{... (iv)}$$

$$E_k = \frac{1}{2}Mv_{cm}^2(1 + K^2/r^2) = \frac{1}{2}I\omega^2(1 + r^2/K^2) \quad \text{... (v)}$$

where,
v_{cm} = linear velocity of the centre of mass of the rigid body
K = radius of gyration ($I = MK^2 = \Sigma M_i r_i^2$)
r = radius of moving rigid body
I = moment of inertia of the rigid body about centre of mass
$\frac{1}{2}I\omega^2$ = rotational kinetic energy about the centre of mass.
Hence it is clear from the expression that total kinetic energy of rolling body is equal to the sum of rotational kinetic energy about centre of mass (C.M.) and translational kinetic energy of the centre of mass of body.

Body Rolling without Slipping on an Inclined Plane :
When a body performed translatory as well as rotatory motion then we can say that the body is in rolling motion.

Acceleration for body rolling down an inclined plane without slipping.
Let M is the mass of the body, R is its radius and I is the moment of inertia about the centre of mass and K is the radius of gyration.

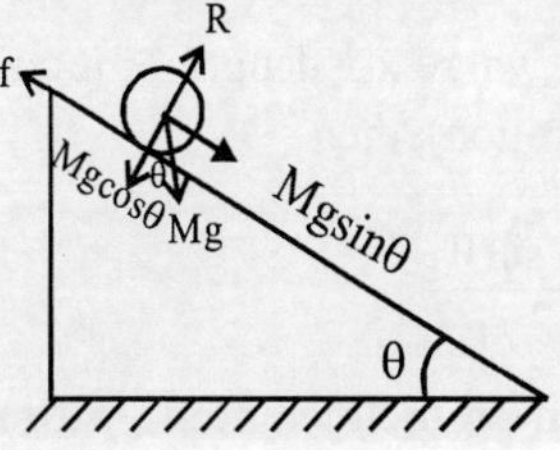

Force equation, $Mg\sin\theta - f = Ma$ ...(1)

Torque equation, $fR = I\alpha$ ...(2)

Also, $I = MK^2$ ...(3)

$$\Rightarrow \quad f = \frac{MK^2\alpha}{R} \qquad \text{...(4)}$$

Adding, eqn. (1) & (4)

$$Mg\sin\theta = M\left(\frac{K^2\alpha}{R} + a\right) \quad \alpha = \frac{a}{R} \ (\because \text{Motion is pure rolling})$$

$$Mg\sin\theta = M\left(\frac{K^2a}{R^2} + a\right) \Rightarrow a = \frac{g\sin\theta}{1 + \frac{K^2}{R^2}}$$

Now assume in fig. that a body (which has high symmetry such as cylinder, sphere etc.) is rolling down an incline plane without slipping. This is possible only if friction is present between object and incline plane, because it provides net torque to the body for rotating about the centre of mass (since the line of action of the other forces such as mg and R pass through the centre of mass of rigid body, hence they do not produce torque in a body about the centre of mass).

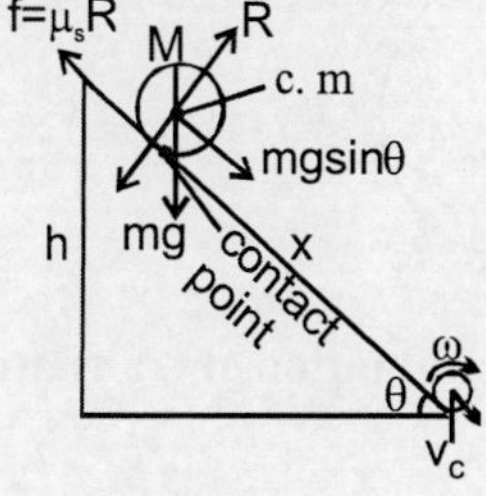

A round object rolling down an incline, mechanical energy is conserved if no slipping occurs.

But mechanical energy of the body remains constant despite of friction because the contact point is at rest relative to the surface at any instant.

For pure rolling motion $v_c = r\omega$

so $E_k = ½I(v_c/r)^2 + ½Mv_c^2$

$$E_k = \frac{1}{2}\left(\frac{I_c}{r^2} + M\right)v_c^2 \quad ...(i)$$

As body rolls down an incline, it loses potential energy Mgh (h is the height of incline). Since body starts from rest at top, hence its total kinetic energy at bottom given by eqn.(i) must be equal to Mgh at top i.e.,

$$\frac{1}{2}\left(\frac{I_c}{r^2} + M\right)v_c^2 = Mgh \Rightarrow v_c = \left(\frac{2gh}{1 + I_c/MR^2}\right)^{1/2} \quad ...(ii)$$

since h = x sin θ, where x is length of incline and $I_c = MK^2$ (K is radius of gyration), then

$$v_c = \left[\frac{2gx\sin\theta}{1 + K^2/R^2}\right]^{½} \quad ....(iii)$$

For rolling down an inclined plane without slipping, the essential condition is :

$\mu_s \geq \frac{I_{cm}}{MR^2 + I_{cm}}\tan\theta$; μ_s is the coefficient of static friction

where I_{cm} is moment of inertia of the body about its C.M.

DIFFERENT TYPES OF MOTION

Pure translational motion : In this case the velocities at all three points : (i) top most point P, (ii) C.M. and (iii) contact point O are same.

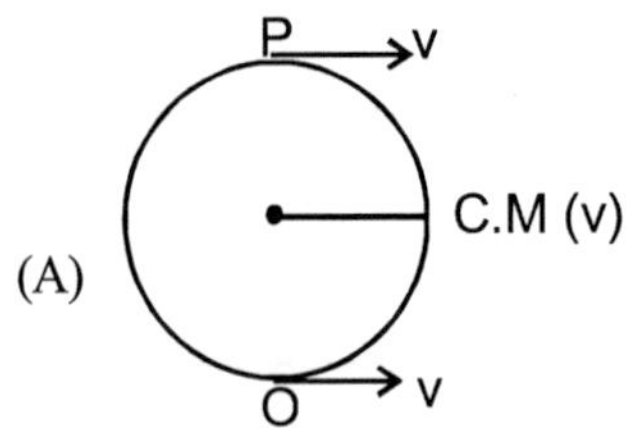

Pure rotational motion : In this case the velocity of

(i) top most point P is Rω

(ii) C.M. is zero

(iii) contact point O is – Rω

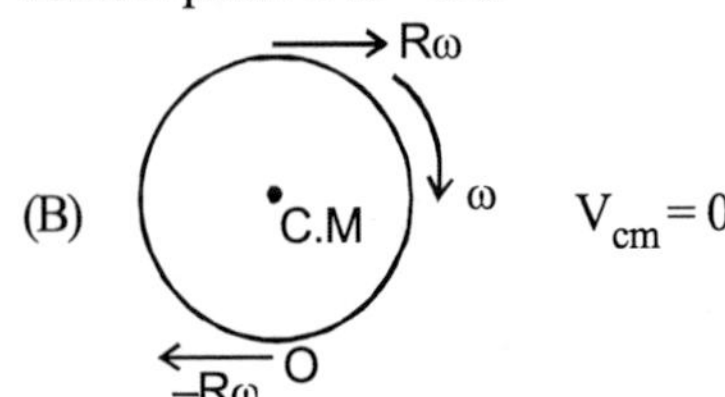

Rolling Motin Combination of translatory and rotatory motion :

(i) In pure rolling motion, the contact point O remains at rest.

(ii) In pure rolling, the velocity of top most point is, $V = V_{cm} + \omega R = 2V_{cm}$

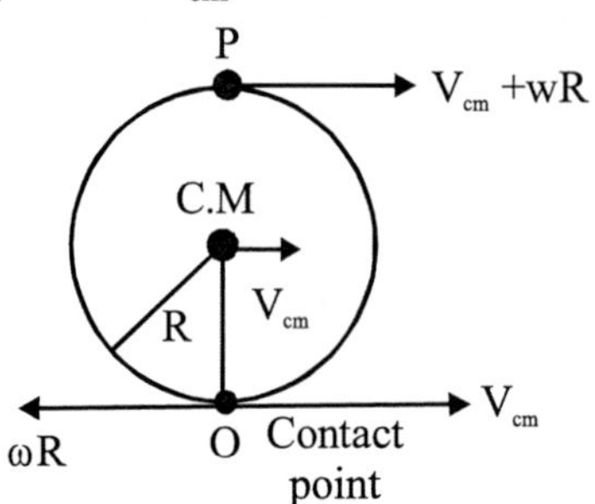

(iii) In rolling without slipping $V_{cm} = \omega R$.

$2\omega R = 2V_{cm}$

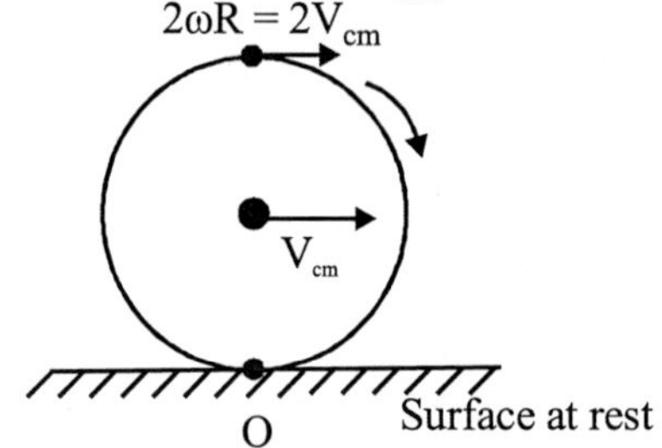

Problem Solving Tips

1. The axis of the rolling body is parallel to the plane on which the body rolls in case of sphere, disc, ring.
2. Let $(E_k)_r$ = rotational kinetic energy
   $(E_k)_t$ = translation kinetic energy
   (a) For solid sphere, $(E_k)_r = 40\%$ of $(E_k)_t$
   (b) For shell $(E_k)_r = 66\%$ of $(E_k)_t$
   (c) For disc, $(E_k)_r = 50\%$ of $(E_k)_t$
   (d) For ring, $(E_k)_r = (E_k)_t$
3. Translational kinetic energy is same for rolling bodies having same M, R and ω irrespective of their shape.
4. Total energy is minimum for solid sphere and maximum for ring having same mass and radius.
5. Rotational kinetic energy is maximum for ring and minimum for solid sphere of same mass and radius.
6. (i) The acceleration down the inclined plane for different shapes of bodies of same mass and radius are as follows :
   Sphere > disc > shell > ring
   (ii) The velocity down the plane is related as follows: Sphere > disc > shell > ring
   (iii) The time taken to reach the bottom of the inclined plane is related as follows :
   Ring > shell > disc > sphere.

This is because

(i) For ring $\frac{K^2}{R^2} = 1$

(ii) For disc $\frac{K^2}{R^2} = \frac{1}{2}$

(iii) For sphere $\frac{K^2}{R^2} = \frac{2}{5}$

(iv) For shell $\frac{K^2}{R^2} = \frac{2}{3}$

7. The angular speed of all particles of a rotating/revolving rigid body is same, although their linear velocities may be different.

8. (i) Two particles moving with angular speed ω_1 and ω_2 on the same circular path and both in anti-clockwise direction then their relative angular speed will be $\omega_r = \omega_1 - \omega_2$.

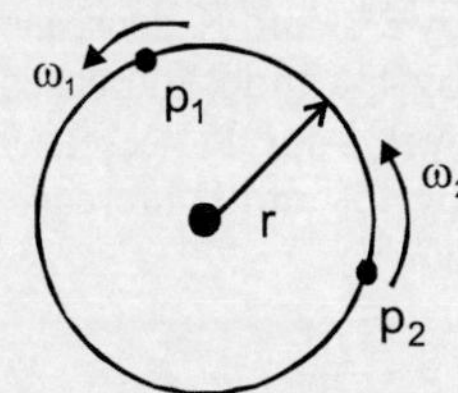

(ii) In the above case one particle will complete one revolution more or less as compared to the other in time

$$T = \frac{2\pi}{\omega_r} = \frac{2\pi}{\omega_1 - \omega_2} = \frac{T_1 T_2}{T_1 - T_2} \text{ or } \frac{1}{T} = \frac{1}{T_2} - \frac{1}{T_1}$$

9. Let two particles move on concentric circles having radius r_1 and r_2 and their linear speeds v_1, v_2 both along anti-clockwise direction then their relative angular speed will be $\omega_r = \frac{|\vec{v}_1 - \vec{v}_2|}{|\vec{r}_1 - \vec{r}_2|}$

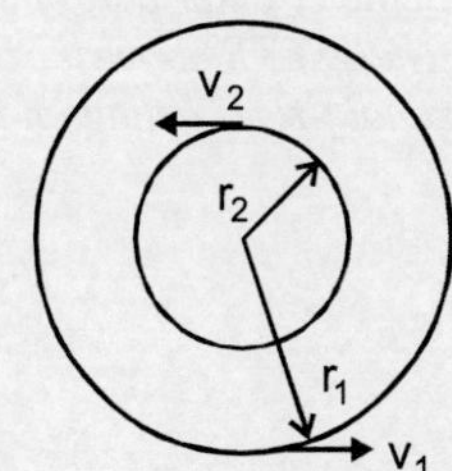

10. As $I \propto K^2$ and $I = MK^2$, hence graph between I and K will be a **parabola**. However graph between log I and log K will be straight line.

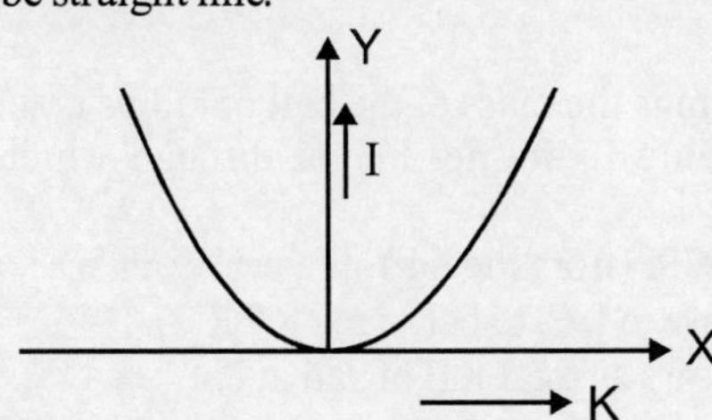

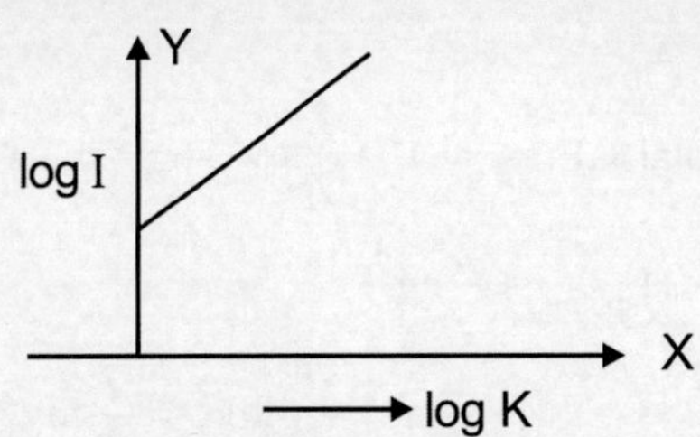

11. Rotational KE, $(E_k)_r = \frac{1}{2} I\omega^2 \quad \therefore E_r \propto \omega^2$

$\therefore$ graph between $(E_k)_r$ and ω will be as below

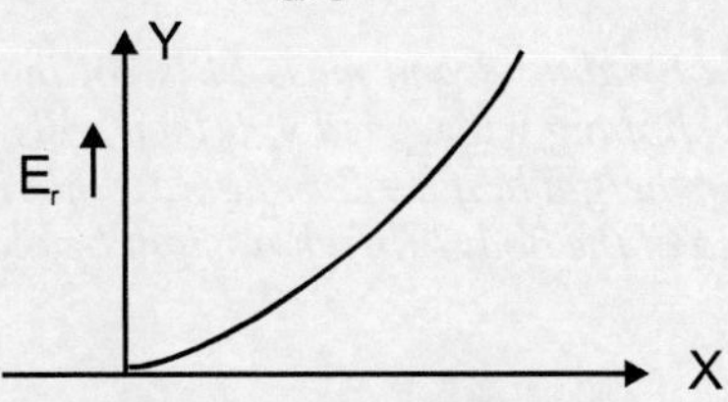

12. Angular momentum $L = I\omega$, hence $L \propto \omega$.
$\therefore$ Graph between L and ω is a straight line.

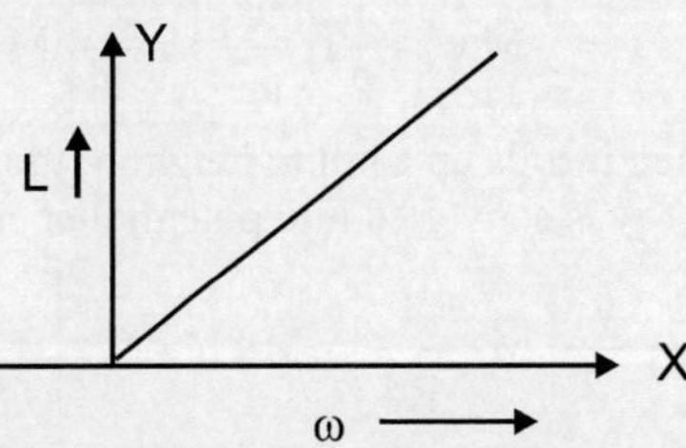

13. The moment of inertia is not a vector quantity because clockwise or anti-clockwise, direction is not associated with it. It is a tensor.

14. When a spherical/circular/cylindrical body is given a push, it only slips when the friction is absent, It may roll with slipping if friction is less than a particular value and it may roll without slipping if the friction is sufficient. (i.e. $\mu_s \geq \frac{I_{cm} \tan\theta}{(MR^2 + I_{cm}})$)

15. When a body rolls without slipping no work is done against friction.

Example 7.

A thin circular ring of mass M and radius R rotating about its axis with a constant angular speed ω. Two blocks, each of mass, m are attached gently to opposite ends of a diameter of the ring. Find the angular speed of the ring.

Solution :

As $L = I\omega$ = constant. Therefore,

$$I_2\omega_2 = I_1\omega_1 \text{ or } \omega_2 = \frac{I_1\omega_1}{I_2} = \frac{MK^2\omega}{(M + 2m)K^2} = \frac{M\omega}{M + 2m}$$

Example 8

A solid sphere of mass 500 g and radius 10 cm rolls without slipping with a velocity of 20 cm/s. Find the total K.E. of the sphere.

Solution :

$$\text{Total K.E.} = \frac{1}{2}I\omega^2 + \frac{1}{2}mv^2 = \frac{1}{2}\times\frac{2}{5}mr^2\omega^2 + \frac{1}{2}mv^2$$

$$\text{As, } I_{sphere} = \frac{2}{5}mr^2$$

$$= \frac{1}{5}mv^2 + \frac{1}{2}mv^2 = \frac{7}{10}mv^2$$

$$= \frac{7}{10}\times\frac{500}{1000}\times\left(\frac{1}{5}\right)^2 = 0.014\text{ J}.$$

Example 9.

A body of radius R and mass M is rolling horizontally without slipping with speed v, it then rolls up a hill to a maximum height h. If $h = 3v^2/4\,g$, (a) what is the moment of inertia of the body? (b) what might be the shape of the body?

Solution :

(a) $$K_{total} = K_{trans.} + K_{rot.} = \frac{1}{2}Mv^2 + \frac{1}{2}I\omega^2$$

$$= \frac{1}{2}Mv^2 + \frac{1}{2}I\left(\frac{v^2}{R^2}\right) = \frac{v^2}{2}\left[M + \frac{I}{R^2}\right]$$

When it rolls up a hill to height h, the entire kinetic energy is converted into potential energy M g h

$$\text{Thus } \frac{v^2}{2}\left[M + \frac{I}{R^2}\right] = Mgh = Mg\left[3\frac{v^2}{4g}\right]$$

$$\text{or } \left[M + \frac{I}{R^2}\right] = \frac{3}{2}M \quad \therefore \quad I = \frac{MR^2}{2}$$

(b) The body may be a circular disc or a solid cylinder.

Example 10.

The angular velocity of a body changes from ω_1 to ω_2 without applying torque but by changing moment of inertia. What will be the ratio of initial radius of gyration to the final radius of gyration?

Solution :

$$\text{Since } I_1\omega_1 = I_2\omega_2 \text{ or } MK_1^2\omega_1 = MK_2^2\omega_2$$

$$\Rightarrow \frac{K_1}{K_2} = \sqrt{\left(\frac{\omega_2}{\omega_1}\right)}$$

Example 11.

A rod of mass M and length ℓ is suspended freely from its end and it can oscillate in the vertical plane about the point of suspension. It is pulled to one side and then released. It passes through the equilibrium position with angular speed ω. What is the kinetic energy while passing through the mean position?

Solution :

$$\text{K.E, } = \frac{1}{2}I\omega^2 \text{ and } I = (M\ell^2/12) + M(\ell/2)^2 = \frac{M\ell^2}{3}$$

$$\therefore K = \frac{1}{2}\left[\frac{M\ell^2}{3}\right]\omega^2 = \frac{1}{6}M\ell^2\omega^2$$

Example 12.

A cord is wound round the circumference of wheel of radius r. The axis of the wheel is horizontal and moment of inertia about it is I. A weight mg is attached to the end of the cord and falls from rest. After falling through a distance h, what will be the angular velocity of the wheel?

Solution :

$$mgh = \frac{1}{2}I\omega^2 + \frac{1}{2}mv^2 = \frac{1}{2}I\omega^2 + \frac{1}{2}mr^2\omega^2$$

$$\text{or } 2mgh = (I + mr^2)\omega^2 \quad \therefore \quad \omega = \left[\frac{2mgh}{I + mr^2}\right]^{1/2}$$

Example 13.

Let g be the acceleration due to gravity at earth's surface and K be the rotational kinetic energy of the earth. Suppose the earth's radius decrease by 2%, keeping all other quantities same, then

(a) g decreases by 2% and K decreases by 4%
(b) g decreases by 4% and k increases by 2%
(c) g increases by 4% and K decreases by 4%
(d) g decreases by 4% and K increases by 4%

***Solution :* (c)**

$$\text{We know that, } g = \frac{GM}{R^2}$$

$$\text{Differentiating, } \frac{dg}{g} = -\left(\frac{2dR}{R}\right) \quad ....(1)$$

$$\text{Further, } K = \frac{1}{2}I\omega^2 = \frac{1}{2}\left[\frac{3}{5}MR^2\right]\omega^2$$

$$\text{or } \frac{dK}{K} = \frac{3}{10}M\omega^2 \times \left(\frac{2dR}{R}\right) \quad ....(2)$$

When radius decreases by 2%, then g increases by 4% and K decreases by 4%.

Example 14.

A small solid ball rolls without slipping along the track shown in fig. The radius of the circular part of track is R. If the ball starts from rest at a height 8 R above the bottom, what are the horizontal and vertical forces acting on it at P?

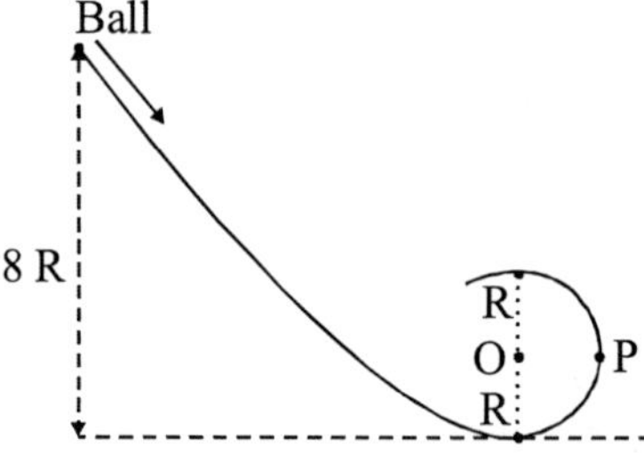

Solution :

Suppose m is the mass of the ball of radius r.

On reaching P, the net height through which the ball descends is

8 R – R = 7R, (from the fig.)

∴ decrease in P.E. of ball = mg × 7 R

This appears as total KE of ball at P.

Thus mg × 7R = KE of translation + KE of rotational

$$= \frac{1}{2}mv^2 + \frac{1}{2}I\omega^2$$

$$= \frac{1}{2}mv^2 + \frac{1}{2}\times\left(\frac{2}{5}mr^2\right)\omega^2 = \frac{7}{10}mv^2$$

$\therefore\ v^2 = 10\,gR$

(where v = rω and r is radius of solid ball)

The horizontal force acting on the ball,

F_h = centripetal force towards O

$$= \frac{mv^2}{R} = \frac{m(10gR)}{R} = 10\,mg$$

Vertical force on the ball, F_v = weight of the ball = mg.

Example 15.

A solid cylinder first rolls and then slides from rest down a smooth inclined plane. Compare the velocities in the two cases when the cylinder reaches the bottom of the incline.

Solution :

(i) We know that acc. of a body rolling down an inclined plane is $a_1 = \dfrac{g\sin\theta}{1+K^2/R^2}$

For a solid cylinder $K^2 = \dfrac{R^2}{2}$;

$a_1 = \dfrac{g\sin\theta}{(1+1/2)} = \dfrac{2}{3}g\sin\theta$; From $v^2 = u^2 + 2as$

$$v_1^2 = 0 + 2\left(\frac{2}{3}g\sin\theta\right)\times\ell = \frac{4}{3}g\sin\theta\times\ell \quad \text{...(i)}$$

(ii) Acc. of the sliding cylinder, $a_2 = g\sin\theta$

From $v^2 = u^2 + 2as$; $v_2^2 = 0 + 2g\sin\theta\times\ell$ ...(ii)

$$\therefore\ \frac{v_1^2}{v_2^2} = \frac{4g\sin\theta\times\ell}{3\times 2g\sin\theta\times\ell} = \frac{2}{3};\ \frac{v_1}{v_2} = \sqrt{2/3}.$$

Example 16.

A disc of mass M and radius R is rolling with angular speed ω on a horizontal plane (fig.). Determine the magnitude of angular momentum of the disc about the origin O.

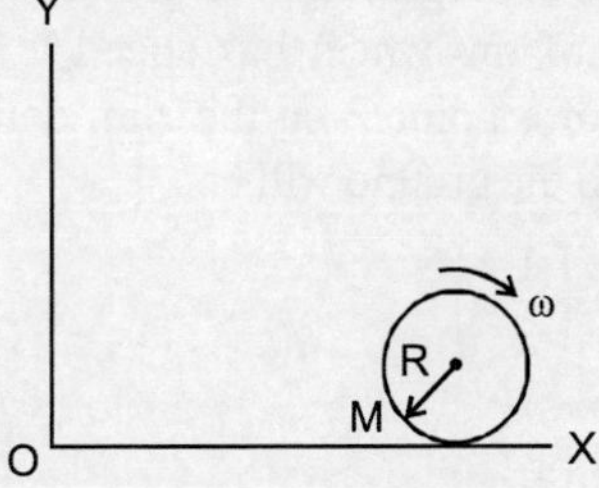

Solution :

The angular momentum L is given by

$$L = I_{cm}\omega + MvR = \left(\frac{1}{2}MR^2\right)\omega + M(\omega R)R = \frac{3}{2}MR^2\omega$$

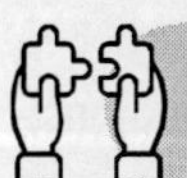

7.3 Concept Practice Problems

CPP

21. Angular momentum of a system of a particles changes, when
(a) force acts on a body
(b) torque acts on a body
(c) direction of velocity changes
(d) None of these

22. A solid sphere is rotating in free space. If the radius of the sphere is increased keeping mass same which one of the following will not be affected ?
(a) Angular velocity
(b) Angular momentum
(c) Moment of inertia
(d) Rotational kinetic energy

23. The angular momentum of a system of particle is conserved
(a) when no external force acts upon the system
(b) when no external torque acts upon the system
(c) when no external impulse acts upon the system
(d) when axis of rotation remains same

24. A solid cylinder of mass 20 kg rotates about its axis with angular speed 100 rad/s. The radius of the cylinder is 0.25 m. The K.E. associated with the rotation of the cylinder is
(a) 3025 J (b) 3225 J (c) 3250 J (d) 3125 J

25. A particles performing uniform circular motion. Its angular frequency is doubled and its kinetic energy halved, then the new angular momentum is
(a) $\dfrac{L}{4}$ (b) 2L (c) 4L (d) $\dfrac{L}{2}$

26. A mass m is moving with a constant velocity along a line parallel to the x-axis, away from the origin. Its angular momentum with respect to the origin
(a) is zero (b) remains constant
(c) goes on increasing (d) goes on decreasing.

27. A uniform bar of mass M and length L is horizontally suspended from the ceiling by two vertical light cables as shown. Cable A is connected 1/4th distance from the left end of the bar. Cable B is attached at the far right end of the bar. What is the tension in cable A?

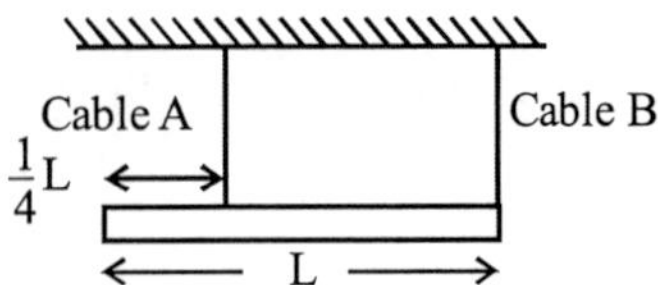

(a) 1/4 Mg (b) 1/3 Mg
(c) 2/3 Mg (d) 3/4 Mg

28. Two fly wheels A and B are mounted side by side with frictionless bearings on a common shaft. Their moments of inertia about the shaft are 5.0 kg m^2 and 20.0 kg m^2 respectively. Wheel A is made to rotate at 10 revolution per second. Wheel B, initially stationary, is now coupled to A with the help of a clutch. The rotation speed of the wheels will become

(a) $2\sqrt{5}$ rps (b) 0.5 rps
(c) 2 rps (d) None of these

29. A wheel is rolling straight on ground without slipping. If the axis of the wheel has speed v, the instantenous velocity of a point P on the rim, defined by angle θ, relative to the ground will be

(a) $v\cos\left(\frac{1}{2}\theta\right)$
(b) $2v\cos\left(\frac{1}{2}\theta\right)$
(c) $v(1+\sin\theta)$
(d) $v(1+\cos\theta)$

30. If the earth is treated as a sphere of radius R and mass M, its angular momentum about the axis of its diurnal rotation with period T is

(a) $\frac{4\pi MR^2}{5T}$ (b) $\frac{2\pi MR^2}{5T}$
(c) $\frac{MR^2T}{T}$ (d) $\frac{\pi MR^3}{T}$

31. A toy car rolls down the inclined plane as shown in the fig. It loops at the bottom. What is the relation between H and h?

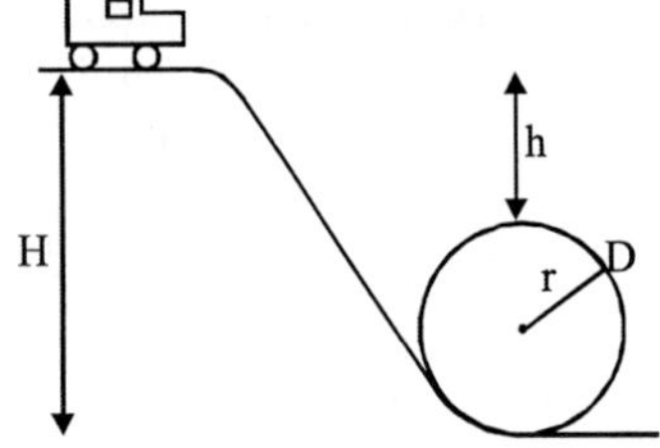

(a) $\frac{H}{h}=2$
(b) $\frac{H}{h}=3$
(c) $\frac{H}{h}=4$
(d) $\frac{H}{h}=5$

32. A sphere rolls down on an inclined plane of inclination θ. What is the acceleration as the sphere reaches bottom?

(a) $\frac{5}{7}g\sin\theta$ (b) $\frac{3}{5}g\sin\theta$
(c) $\frac{2}{7}g\sin\theta$ (d) $\frac{2}{5}g\sin\theta$

33. A wheel having moment of inertia 2 kg-m^2 about its vertical axis, rotates at the rate of 60 rpm about this axis, The torque which can stop the wheel's rotation in one minute would be

(a) $\frac{\pi}{18}$Nm (b) $\frac{2\pi}{15}$Nm
(c) $\frac{\pi}{12}$Nm (d) $\frac{\pi}{15}$Nm

34. A round disc of moment of inertia I_2 about its axis perpendicular to its plane and passing through its centre is placed over another disc of moment of inertia I_1 rotating with an angular velocity ω about the same axis. The final angular velocity of the combination of discs is

(a) $\frac{(I_1+I_2)\omega}{I_1}$ (b) $\frac{I_2\omega}{I_1+I_2}$
(c) ω (d) $\frac{I_1\omega}{I_1+I_2}$

35. A circular disk of moment of inertia I_t is rotating in a horizontal plane, its symmetry axis, with a constant angular speed ω_i. Another disk of moment of inertia I_b is dropped coaxially onto the rotating disk. Initially the second disk has zero angular speed. Eventually both the disks rotate with a constant angular speed ω_f. The energy lost by the initially rotating disk to friction is

(a) $\frac{1}{2}\frac{I_b^2}{(I_t+I_b)}\omega_i^2$ (b) $\frac{I_t^2}{(I_t+I_b)}\omega_i^2$
(c) $\frac{I_b-I_t}{(I_t+I_b)}\omega_i^2$ (d) $\frac{1}{2}\frac{I_bI_t}{(I_t+I_b)}\omega_i^2$

ANSWER KEY

21	(b)	22	(b)	23	(b)	24	(d)	25	(a)	26	(b)	27	(c)	28	(c)	29	(b)	30	(a)
31	(d)	32	(a)	33	(d)	34	(d)	35	(d)										

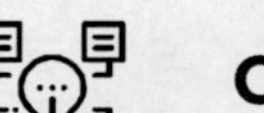

CONCEPT MAP

SYSTEM OF PARTICLES AND ROTATIONAL MOTION

Centre of mass
The point where whole mass of the system is supposed to be concentrated

Position of centre of mass of the system

$$r_{cm} = \frac{\sum_{i=1}^{n} m_i r_i}{\sum m_i}$$

Position of centre of mass of an object changes in translatory motion but remains unchanged in rotatory motion

Velocity of centre of mass of the system

$$v_{cm} = \frac{\sum_{i=1}^{n} m_i v_i}{\sum m_i}$$

Acceleration of centre of mass of the system

$$a_{cm} = \frac{\sum_{i=1}^{n} m_i a_i}{\sum m_i}$$

Position of centre of mass depends upon, shape, size distribution of mass of the body

Centre of mass for rigid bodies is independent of the state i.e, rest or motion of the body

Rigid body
A body with a perfectly definite and unchanging shape

Moment of inertia
Inertia of rotational motion

M.I., $I = \sum_{i=1}^{n} m_i r_i^2$

Radius of gyration

$$K = \sqrt{\frac{r_1^2 + r_2^2 + \ldots + r_n^2}{n}}$$

$$K = \sqrt{\frac{I}{M}}$$

Theorems of moment of inertia

Theorem of perpendicular axes $I_z = I_x + I_y$
I_x, I_y and I_z moments of inertia about perpendicular axes x, y and z respectively.

Theorem of parallel axes
$I = I_{cm} + mr^2$
I_{cm} = M.I. about the parallel axis through the centre of mass

Moment of inertia of some regular shaped body
(1) Rod $I_{cm} = Ml^2/12$
$I_{one\ edge} = Ml^2/3$
(2) Ring $I_{cm} = MR^2$
$I_{diameter} = MR^2/2$
(3) Disc $I_{cm} = MR^2/2$
$I_{diameter} = MR^2/4$
(4) Solid sphere $I_{diameter} = 2/5\ MR^2$

Equations of rotational motion
(i) $\omega_2 = \omega_1 + \alpha t$
(ii) $\theta = \omega_0 t + \frac{1}{2}\alpha t^2$
(iii) $\omega_2^2 = \omega_1^2 + 2\alpha\theta$

***Torque or couple* or moment of force**
$\tau = r \times F = rF \sin\theta\ \hat{n}$
$\tau_{rotational} = I\alpha$

Angular momentum
$L = I\omega = mvr = r \times mv$
$L = r \times P = rP \sin\theta$

Kinetic energy
$K.E._{rotational} = \frac{1}{2} I\omega^2$
$K.E._{rolling} = \frac{1}{2} mv^2 + \frac{1}{2} I\omega^2$

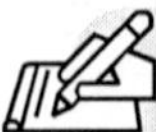

Exercise 1 - Chapter Revision Problems

CRP

1. A disc is given a linear velocity on a rough horizontal surface then its angular momentum is
(a) conserved about COM only
(b) conserved about the point of contact only
(c) conserved about all the points
(d) not conserved about any point.

2. A body cannot roll without slipping on a
(a) rough horizontal surface
(b) smooth horizontal surface
(c) rough inclined surface
(d) smooth inclined surface

3. A body is projected from ground with some angle to the horizontal. The angular momentum about the initial position will
(a) decrease (b) increase
(c) remains same (d) first increase then decrease

4. A ball tied to a string is swung in a vertical circle. Which of the following remains constant?
(a) tension in the string (b) speed of the ball
(c) centripetal force (d) earth's pull on the ball

5. Angular momentum is
(a) a polar vector (b) an axial vector
(c) a scalar (d) None of these

6. If a running boy jumps on a rotating table, which of the following is conserved?
(a) Linear momentum (b) K.E
(c) Angular momentum (d) None of these

7. Angular momentum is
(a) moment of momentum
(b) product of mass and angular velocity
(c) product of M.I. and velocity
(d) moment of angular motion

8. Analogue of mass in rotational motion is
(a) moment of inertia (b) angular momentum
(c) gyration (d) None of these

9. Moment of inertia does not depend upon
(a) angular velocity of body (b) shape and size
(c) mass (d) position of axis of rotation

10. A hollow sphere is held suspended. Sand is now poured into it in stages.

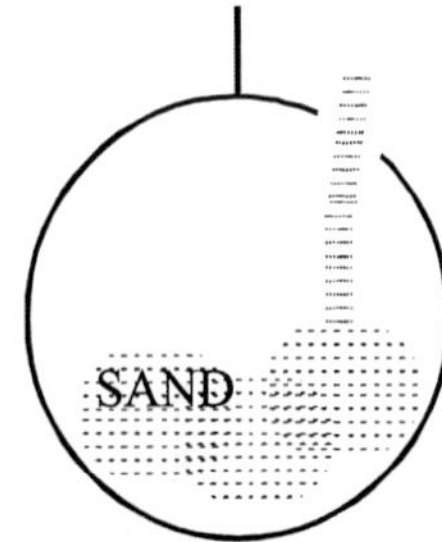

The centre of gravity of the sphere with the sand
(a) rises continuously
(b) remains unchanged in the process
(c) First rises and then falls to the original position
(d) First falls and then rises to the original position

11. A block Q of mass M is placed on a horizontal frictionless surface AB and a body P of mass m is released on its frictionless slope. As P slides by a length L on this slope of inclination θ, the block Q would slide by a distance

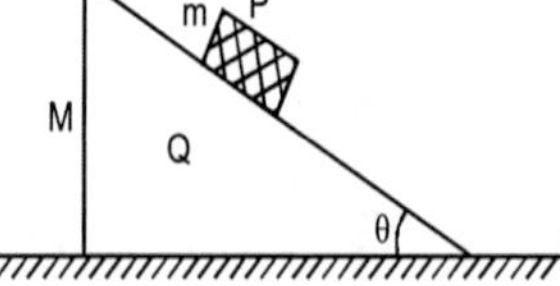

(a) $(m/M)\, L \cos\theta$
(b) $mL/(M+m)$
(c) $(M+m)/(mL\cos\theta)$
(d) $(mL\cos\theta)/(m+M)$

12. A solid sphere and a hollow sphere of the same material and of same size can be distinguished without weighing
(a) by determining their moments of inertia about their coaxial axes
(b) by rolling them simultaneously on an inclined plane
(c) by rotating them about a common axis of rotation
(d) by applying equal torque on them

13. A stick of length L and mass M lies on a frictionless horizontal surface on which it is free to move in any way. A ball of mass m moving with speed v collides elastically with the stick as shown in fig.

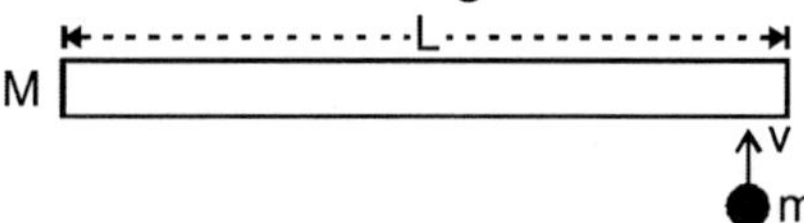

If after the collision ball comes to rest, then what should be the mass of the ball?
(a) $m = 2M$ (b) $m = M$ (c) $m = M/2$ (d) $m = M/4$

14. A raw egg and a hard boiled egg are made to spin on a table with the same angular momentum about the same axis. The ratio of the time taken by the two to stop is
(a) $=1$ (b) <1
(c) >1 (d) None of these

15. A body having moment of inertia about its axis of rotation equal to 3 kg-m^2 is rotating with angular velocity equal to 3 rad/s. Kinetic energy of this rotating body is the same as that of a body of mass 27 kg moving with a speed of
(a) 1.0 m/s (b) 0.5 m/s (c) 1.5 m/s (d) 2.0 m/s

16. A particle moves in a circle of radius 0.25 m at two revolutions per second. The acceleration of the particle in metre per second^2 is
(a) π^2 (b) $8\pi^2$ (c) $4\pi^2$ (d) $2\pi^2$

17. A particle of mass m is moving in a plane along a circular path of radius r. Its angular momentum about the axis of rotation is L. The centripetal force acting on the particle is
(a) L^2/mr (b) L^2m/r (c) L^2/mr^3 (d) L^2/mr^2

18. A solid cylinder of mass m & radius R rolls down inclined plane without slipping. The speed of its C.M. when it reaches the bottom is
(a) $\sqrt{2gh}$
(b) $\sqrt{4gh/3}$
(c) $\sqrt{3/4gh}$
(d) $\sqrt{4gh}$

19. A rod of length L is pivoted at one end and is rotated with a uniform angular velocity in a horizontal plane. Let T_1 and T_2 be the tensions at the points L/4 and 3L/4 away from the pivoted end. Then

(a) $T_1 > T_2$ (b) $T_2 > T_1$
(c) $T_1 - T_2$
(d) the relation between T_1 and T_2 depends on whether the rod rotates clockwise and anticlockwise.

20. A particle of mass m is observed from an inertial frame of reference and is found to move in a circle of radius r with a uniform speed v. The centrifugal force on it is

(a) $\frac{mv^2}{r}$ towards the centre
(b) $\frac{mv^2}{r}$ away from the centre
(c) $\frac{mv^2}{r}$ along the tangent through the particle
(d) zero

21. A simple pendulum is vibrating with angular amplitude of 90° as shown in figure.

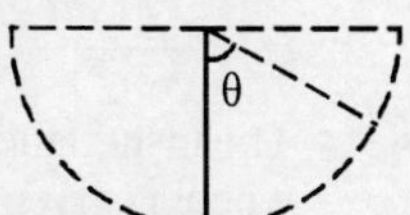

For what value of θ is the acceleration directed
(i) vertically upwards
(ii) horizontally
(iii) vertically downwards

(a) $0°, \cos^{-1}\frac{1}{\sqrt{3}}, 90°$ (b) $\cos^{-1}\frac{1}{\sqrt{3}}, 0°, 90°$
(c) $90°, \cos^{-1}\frac{1}{\sqrt{3}}, 0°$ (d) $\cos^{-1}\frac{1}{\sqrt{3}}, 90°, 0°$

22. A mass is tied to a string and rotated in a vertical circle, the minimum velocity of the body at the top is

(a) $\sqrt{gr}$ (b) g/r (c) $\left(\frac{g}{r}\right)^{3/2}$ (d) gr

23. A couple is acting on a two particle systems. The resultant motion will be
(a) purely rotational motion (b) purely linear motion
(c) both a and b (d) None of these

24. A smooth sphere A is moving on a frictionless horizontal plane with angular speed ω and centre of mass velocity v. It collides elastically and head on with an identical sphere B at rest. Neglect friction everywhere. After the collision, their angular speeds are ω_A and ω_B, respectively. Then
(a) $\omega_A < \omega_B$ (b) $\omega_A = \omega_B$ (c) $\omega_A = \omega$ (d) $\omega_B = \omega$

25. A particle moves in a circle of radius 4 cm clockwise at constant speed 2 cm s^{-1}. If $\hat{x}$ and $\hat{y}$ are unit acceleration vectors along X and Y respectively (in cm s^{-2}), the acceleration of the particle at the instant half way between P and Q is given by

(a) $-4(\hat{x} + \hat{y})$
(b) $4(\hat{x} + \hat{y})$
(c) $-(\hat{x} + \hat{y})/\sqrt{2}$
(d) $(\hat{x} - \hat{y})/4$

26. A weightless ladder 20 ft long rests against a frictionless wall at an angle of 60° from the horizontal. A 150 pound man is 4 ft from the top of the ladder. A horizontal force is needed to keep it from slipping. Choose the correct magnitude from the following.

(a) 175 lb (b) 100 lb (c) 120 lb (d) 17.3 lb

27. A tube one metre long is filled with liquid of mass 1 kg. The tube is closed at both the ends and is revolved about one end in a horizontal plane at 2 rev/s. The force experienced by the lid at the other end is
(a) $4\pi^2$N (b) $8\pi^2$N (c) $16\pi^2$N (d) 9.8 N

28. If the linear density (mass per unit length) of a rod of length 3m is proportional to x, where x is the distance from one end of the rod, the distance of the centre of gravity of the rod from this end is
(a) 2.5 m (b) 1 m (c) 1.5 m (d) 2 m

29. When a bucket containing water is rotated fast in a vertical circle of radius R, the water in the bucket doesn't spill provided
(a) the bucket is whirled with a maximum speed of $\sqrt{2gR}$
(b) the bucket is whirled around with a minimum speed of $\sqrt{[(1/2)gR]}$
(c) the bucket is having a rpm of $\sqrt{900g/(\pi^2R)}$
(d) the bucket is having a rpm of $\sqrt{3600g/(\pi^2R)}$

30. A coin placed on a gramophone record rotating at 33 rpm flies off the record, if it is placed at a distance of more than 16 cm from the axis of rotation. If the record is revolving at 66 rpm, the coin will fly off if it is placed at a distance not less than
(a) 1 cm (b) 2 cm (c) 3 cm (d) 4 cm

31. A certain bicycle can go up a gentle incline with constant speed when the frictional force of ground pushing the rear wheel is $F_2 = 4$ N. With what force F_1 must the chain pull on the sprocket wheel if $R_1 = 5$ cm and $R_2 = 30$ cm?

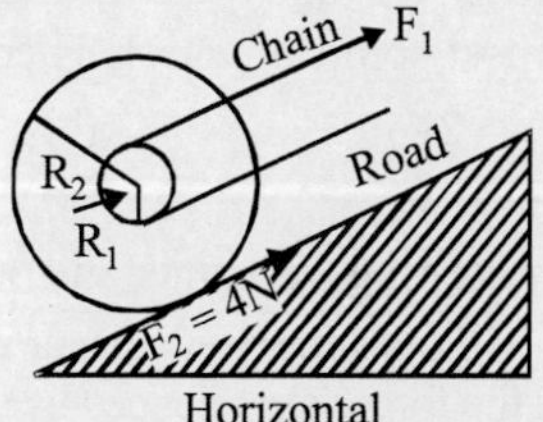

(a) 4 N
(b) 24 N
(c) 140 N
(d) $\frac{35}{4}$ N

32. A uniform rod of length l is free to rotate in a vertical plane about a fixed horizontal axis through O. The rod begins rotating from rest from its unstable equilibrium position. When it has turned through an angle θ, its angular velocity ω is given as

(a) 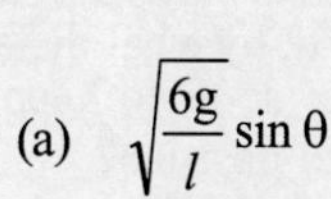 $\sqrt{\frac{6g}{l}}\sin\theta$ (b) 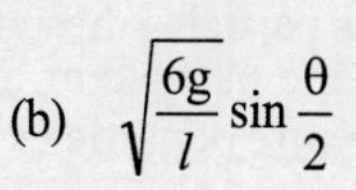 $\sqrt{\frac{6g}{l}}\sin\frac{\theta}{2}$
(c) $\sqrt{\frac{6g}{l}}\cos\frac{\theta}{2}$ (d) $\sqrt{\frac{6g}{l}}\cos\theta$

33. A solid sphere of mass 1 kg rolls on a table with linear speed 1 ms^{-1}. Its total kinetic energy is
(a) 1 J (b) 0.5 J (c) 0.7 J (d) 1.4 J

34. M.I of a circular loop of radius R about the axis in figure is

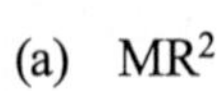

(a) MR^2

(b) $(3/4)\,MR^2$

(c) $MR^2/2$

(d) $2MR^2$

35. Four masses are fixed on a massless rod as shown in the adjoining figure. The moment of inertia about the dotted axis is about

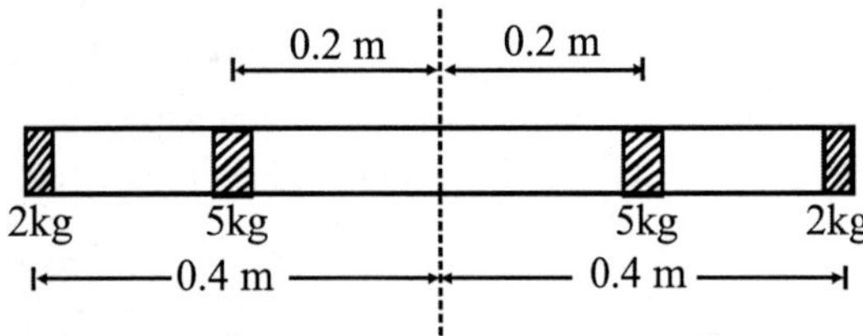

(a) $2\,kg \times m^2$ (b) $1\,kg \times m^2$
(c) $0.5\,kg \times m^2$ (d) $0.3\,kg \times m^2$

36. Fig. shows a disc rolling on a horizontal plane with linear velocity v. Its linear velocity is v and angular velocity is ω. Which of the following gives the velocity of the particle P on the rim of the disc

(a) $v(1 + \cos\theta)$
(b) $v(1 - \cos\theta)$
(c) $v(1 + \sin\theta)$
(d) $v(1 - \sin\theta)$

37. In a bicycle, the radius of rear wheel is twice the radius of front wheel. If r_F and r_F are the radii, v_r and v_r are the speed of top most points of wheel. Then

(a) $v_r = 2v_F$ (b) $v_F = 2v_r$
(c) $v_F = v_r$ (d) $v_F > v_r$

38. An annular ring with inner and outer radii R_1 and R_2 is rolling without slipping with a uniform angular speed. The ratio of the forces experienced by the two particles situated on the inner and outer parts of the ring, $\frac{F_1}{F_2}$ is

(a) $\left(\frac{R_1}{R_2}\right)^2$ (b) $\frac{R_2}{R_1}$ (c) $\frac{R_1}{R_2}$ (d) 1

39. Consider a system of two particles having masses m_1 and m_2. If the particle of mass m_1 is pushed towards the centre of mass particles through a distance d, by what distance would the particle of mass m_2 move so as to keep the mass centre of particles at the original position?

(a) $\frac{m_2}{m_1}d$ (b) $\frac{m_1}{m_1+m_2}d$
(c) $\frac{m_1}{m_2}d$ (d) d

40. The ratio of the radii of gyration of a circular disc about a tangential axis in the plane of the disc and of a circular ring of the same radius about a tangential axis in the plane of the ring is

(a) $1:\sqrt{2}$ (b) $1:3$ (c) $2:1$ (d) $\sqrt{5}:\sqrt{6}$

41. A drum of radius R and mass M, rolls down without slipping along an inclined plane of angle θ. The frictional force

(a) dissipates energy as heat.
(b) decreases the rotational motion.
(c) decreases the rotational and translational motion.
(d) converts translational energy to rotational energy

42. A tube of length L is filled completely with an incompressible liquid of mass M and closed at both ends. The tube is then rotated in a horizontal plane about one of its ends with uniform angular speed ω. What is the force exerted by the liquid at the other end?

(a) $\frac{ML\omega^2}{2}$ (b) $ML\omega^2$ (c) $\frac{ML\omega^2}{4}$ (d) $\frac{ML\omega^2}{8}$

43. The instantaneous angular position of a point on a rotating wheel is given by the equation $\theta(t) = 2t^3 - 6t^2$. The torque on the wheel becomes zero at

(a) t = 1 s (b) t = 0.5 s
(c) t = 0.25 s (d) t = 2s

44. The moment of inertia of a uniform circular disc is maximum about an axis perpendicular to the disc and passing through

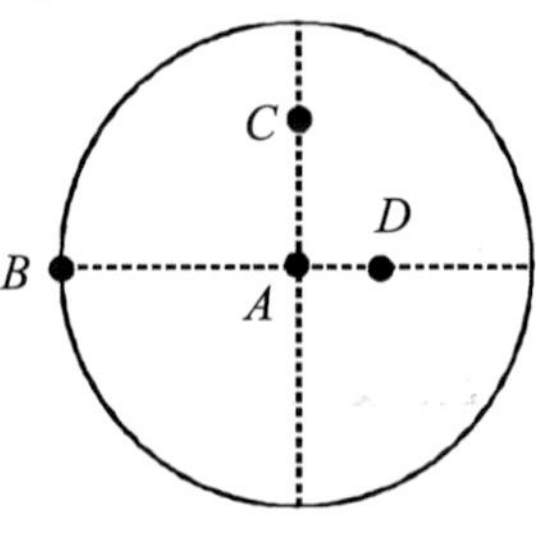

(a) *B* (b) *C* (c) *D* (d) *A*

45. If the angular velocity of a body rotating about an axis is doubled and its moment of inertia halved, the rotational kinetic energy will change by a factor of :

(a) 4 (b) 2 (c) 1 (d) $\frac{1}{2}$

46. One quarter sector is cut from a uniform circular disc of radius R. This sector has mass M. It is made to rotate about a line perpendicular to its plane and passing through the centre of the original disc. Its moment of inertia about the axis of rotation is

(a) $\frac{1}{2}mR^2$ (b) $\frac{1}{4}mR^2$ (c) $\frac{1}{8}mR^2$ (d) $\sqrt{2}mR^2$

47. The coordinates of centre of mass of a uniform flag shaped lamina (thin flat plale) of mass 4 kg. (The coordinates of the same are shown in figure) are:

(a) (1.25 m, 1.50 m)

(b) (0.75 m, 1.75 m)

(c) (0.75 m, 0.75 m)

(d) (1 m, 1.75 m)

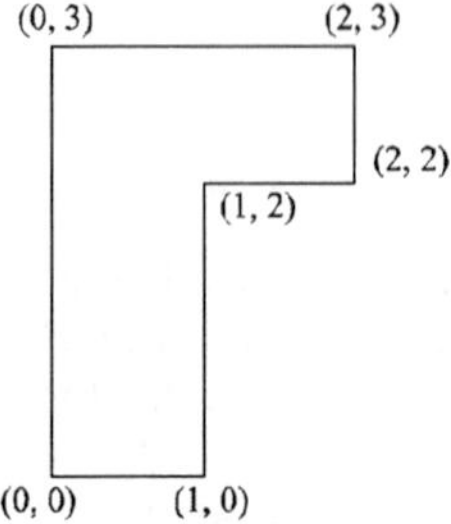

48. As shown in fig. when a spherical cavity (centred at O) of radius 1 is cut out of a uniform sphere of radius R (centred at C), the centre of mass of remaining (shaded) part of sphere is at G, i.e on the surface of the cavity. R can be determined by the equation:

(a) $(R^2+R+1)(2-R)=1$

(b) $(R^2-R-1)(2-R)=1$

(c) $(R^2-R+1)(2-R)=1$

(d) $(R^2+R-1)(2-R)=1$

49. A uniform rectangular thin sheet ABCD of mass M has length a and breadth b, as shown in the figure. If the shaded portion HBGO is cut-off, the coordinates of the centre of mass of the remaining portion will be :

(a) $\left(\frac{3a}{4}, \frac{3b}{4}\right)$

(b) $\left(\frac{5a}{3}, \frac{5b}{3}\right)$

(c) $\left(\frac{2a}{3}, \frac{2b}{3}\right)$

(d) $\left(\frac{5a}{12}, \frac{5b}{12}\right)$

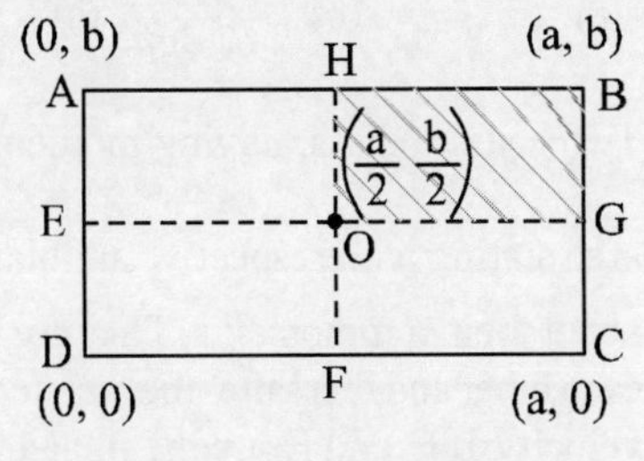

50. A force of 40 N acts on a point B at the end of an L-shaped object, as shown in the figure. The angle θ that will produce maximum moment of the force about point A is given by:

(a) $\tan\theta = \frac{1}{4}$

(b) $\tan\theta = 2$

(c) $\tan\theta = \frac{1}{2}$

(d) $\tan\theta = 4$

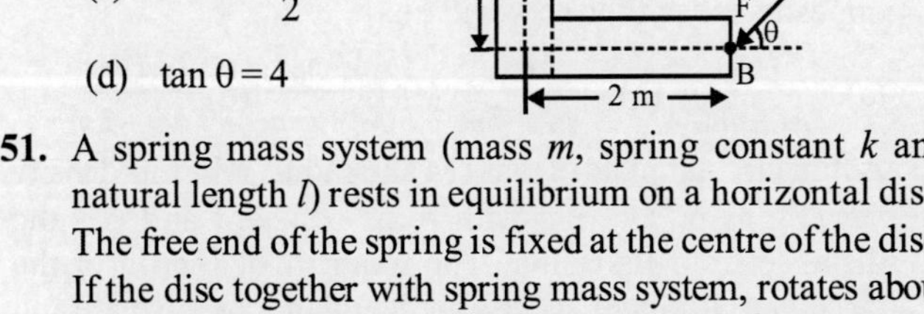

51. A spring mass system (mass m, spring constant k and natural length l) rests in equilibrium on a horizontal disc. The free end of the spring is fixed at the centre of the disc. If the disc together with spring mass system, rotates about it's axis with an angular velocity ω, ($k >> m\omega^2$) the relative change in the length of the spring is best given by the option:

(a) $\sqrt{\frac{2}{3}}\left(\frac{m\omega^2}{k}\right)$ (b) $\frac{2m\omega^2}{k}$ (c) $\frac{m\omega^2}{k}$ (d) $\frac{m\omega^2}{3k}$

52. A particle is moving with a uniform speed in a circular orbit of radius R in a central force inversely proportional to the nth power of R. If the period of rotation of the particle is T, then:

(a) $T \propto R^{3/2}$ for any n. (b) $T \propto R^{n/2+1}$

(c) $T \propto R^{(n+1)/2}$ (d) $T \propto R^{n/2}$

53. Four point masses, each of mass m, are fixed at the corners of a square of side l. The square is rotating with angular frequency ω, about an axis passing through one of the corners of the square and parallel to its diagonal, as shown in the figure. The angular momentum of the square about this axis is :

(a) $ml^2\omega$

(b) $4ml^2\omega$

(c) $3ml^2\omega$

(d) $2ml^2\omega$

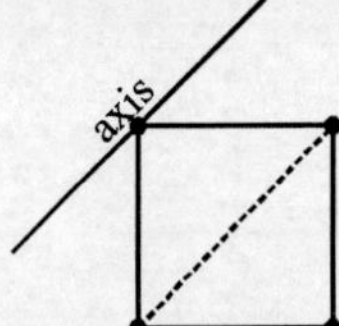

54. A uniform cylinder of mass M and radius R is to be pulled over a step of height a ($a < R$) by applying a force F at its centre 'O' perpendicular to the plane through the axes of the cylinder on the edge of the step (see figure). The minimum value of F required is :

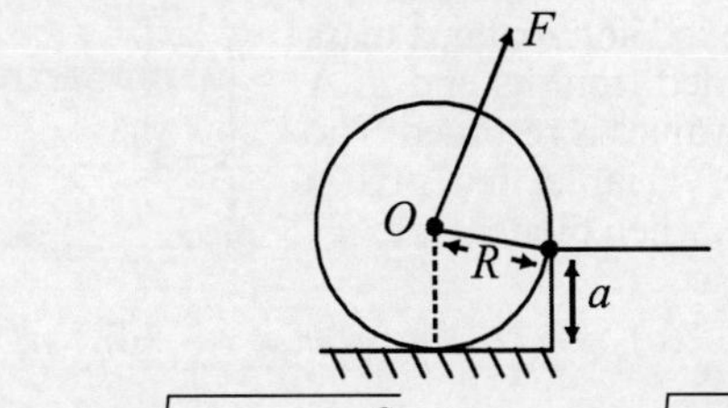

(a) $Mg\sqrt{1-\left(\frac{R-a}{R}\right)^2}$ (b) $Mg\sqrt{\left(\frac{R}{R-a}\right)^2-1}$

(c) $Mg\frac{a}{R}$ (d) $Mg\sqrt{1-\frac{a^2}{R^2}}$

55. Consider *a* uniform rod of mass $M = 4$m and length l pivoted about its centre. *A* mass m moving with velocity v making angle $\theta = \frac{\pi}{4}$ to the rod's long axis collides with one end of the rod and sticks to it. The angular speed of the rod-mass system just after the collision is:

(a) $\frac{3}{7\sqrt{2}}\frac{v}{l}$ (b) $\frac{3}{7}\frac{v}{l}$ (c) $\frac{3\sqrt{2}}{7}\frac{v}{l}$ (d) $\frac{4}{7}\frac{v}{l}$

56. A rectangular solid box of length 0.3 m is held horizontally, with one of its sides on the edge of a platform of height 5m. When released, it slips off the table in a very short time τ = 0.01 s, remaining essentially horizontal. The angle by which it would rotate when it hits the ground will be (in radians) close to :

(a) 0.5

(b) 0.3

(c) 0.02

(d) 0.28

57. To mop-clean a floor, a cleaning machine presses a circular mop of radius R vertically down with a total force F and rotates it with a constant angular speed about its axis. If the force F is distributed uniformly over the mop and if coefficient of friction between the mop and the floor is μ, the torque, applied by the machine on the mop is:

(a) μFR/3 (b) μFR/6 (c) μFR/2 (d) $\frac{2}{3}$μ μFR

58. An L-shaped object, made of thin rods of uniform mass density, is suspended with a string as shown in figure. If AB = BC, and the angle made by AB with downward vertical is θ, then:

(a) $\tan\theta = \frac{1}{2\sqrt{3}}$

(b) $\tan\theta = \frac{1}{2}$

(c) $\tan\theta = \frac{2}{\sqrt{3}}$

(d) $\tan\theta = \frac{1}{3}$

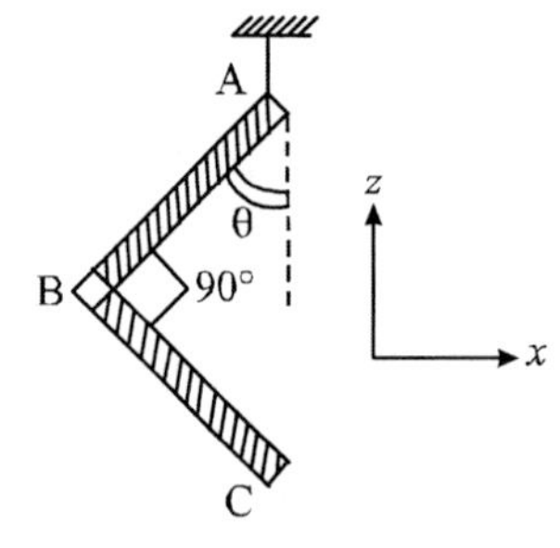

59. A uniform rod AB is suspended from a point X, at a variable distance from x from A, as shown. To make the rod horizontal, a mass m is suspended from its end A. A set of (m, x) values is recorded. The appropriate variable that give a straight line, when plotted, are:

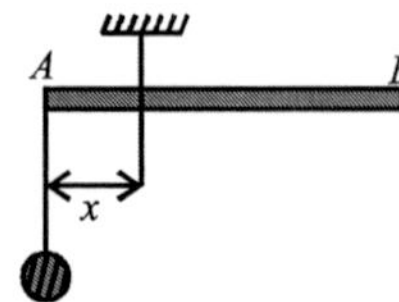

(a) $m, \frac{1}{x}$ (b) $m, \frac{1}{x^2}$ (c) m, x (d) m, x^2

60. A thin uniform bar of length L and mass 8m lies on a smooth horizontal table. Two point masses m and 2m moving in the same horizontal plane from opposite sides of the bar with speeds 2v and v respectively. The masses stick to the bar after collision at a distance $\frac{L}{3}$ and $\frac{L}{6}$ respectively from the centre of the bar. If the bar starts rotating about its center of mass as a result of collision, the angular speed of the bar will be:

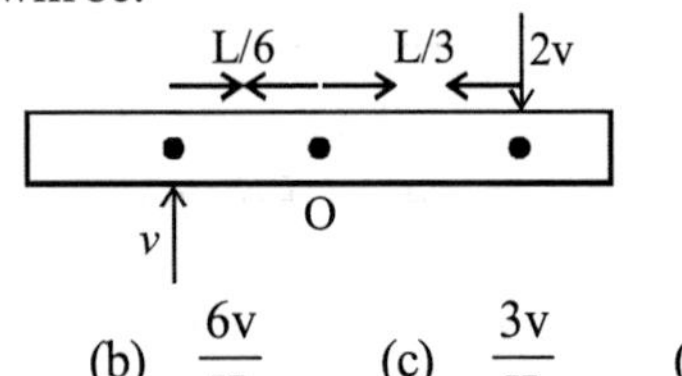

(a) $\frac{v}{6L}$ (b) $\frac{6v}{5L}$ (c) $\frac{3v}{5L}$ (d) $\frac{v}{5L}$

61. A wheel is rotating freely with an angular speed ω on a shaft. The moment of inertia of the wheel is I and the moment of inertia of the shaft is negligible. Another wheel of moment of inertia 3I initially at rest is suddenly coupled to the same shaft. The resultant fractional loss in the kinetic energy of the system is :

(a) $\frac{5}{6}$ (b) $\frac{1}{4}$ (c) 0 (d) $\frac{3}{4}$

62. For a uniform rectangular sheet shown in the figure, the ratio of moments of inertia about the axes perpendicular to the sheet and passing through O (the centre of mass) and O' (corner point) is :

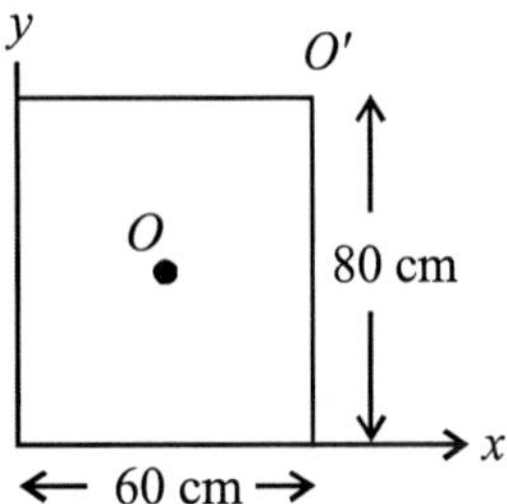

(a) 2/3 (b) 1/4 (c) 1/8 (d) 1/2

63. Moment of inertia of a cylinder of mass M, length L and radius R about an axis passing through its centre and perpendicular to the axis of the cylinder is $I = M\left(\frac{R^2}{4}+\frac{L^2}{12}\right)$. If such a cylinder is to be made for a given mass of a material, the ratio L/R for it to have minimum possible I is :

(a) $\frac{2}{3}$ (b) $\frac{3}{2}$ (c) $\sqrt{\frac{3}{2}}$ (d) $\sqrt{\frac{2}{3}}$

64. As shown in the figure, a bob of mass m is tied by a massless string whose other end portion is wound on a fly wheel (disc) of radius r and mass m. When released from rest the bob starts falling vertically. When it has covered a distance of h, the angular speed of the wheel will be:

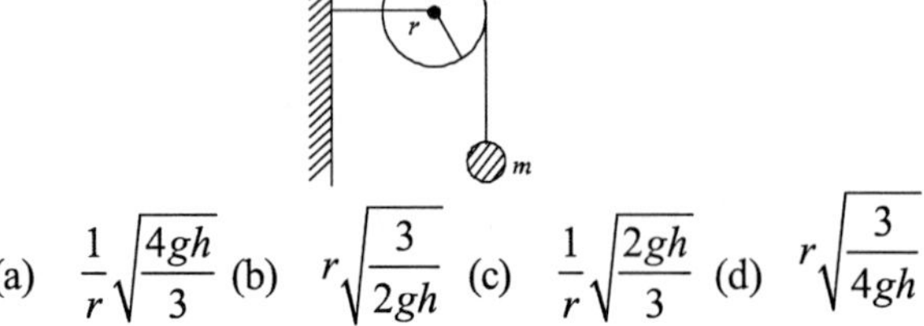

(a) $\frac{1}{r}\sqrt{\frac{4gh}{3}}$ (b) $r\sqrt{\frac{3}{2gh}}$ (c) $\frac{1}{r}\sqrt{\frac{2gh}{3}}$ (d) $r\sqrt{\frac{3}{4gh}}$

65. Two coaxial discs, having moments of inertia I_1 and $\frac{I_1}{2}$, are rotating with respective angular velocities ω_1 and $\frac{\omega_1}{2}$, about their common axis. They are brought in contact with each other and thereafter they rotate with a common angular velocity. If E_f and E_i are the final and initial total energies, then $(E_f - E_i)$ is :

(a) $-\frac{I_1\omega_1^2}{12}$ (b) $\frac{I_1\omega_1^2}{6}$ (c) $\frac{3}{8}I_1\omega_1^2$ (d) $-\frac{I_1\omega_1^2}{24}$

66. A thin smooth rod of length L and mass M is rotating freely with angular speed w_0 about an axis perpendicular to the rod and passing through its center. Two beads of mass m and negligible size are at the center of the rod initially. The beads are free to slide along the rod. The angular speed of the system, when the beads reach the opposite ends of the rod, will be:

(a) $\frac{M\omega_0}{M+m}$ (b) $\frac{M\omega_0}{M+3m}$ (c) $\frac{M\omega_0}{M+6m}$ (d) $\frac{M\omega_0}{M+2m}$

67. A thin circular plate of mass M and radius R has its density varying as $\rho(r) = \rho_0 r$ with ρ_0 as constant and r is the distance from its center. The moment of Inertia of the circular plate about an axis perpendicular to the plate and passing through its edge is $I = a\,MR^2$. The value of the coefficient a is:

(a) $1/2$ (b) $3/5$ (c) $8/5$ (d) $3/2$

68. An equilateral triangle ABC is cut from a thin solid sheet of wood. (See figure) D, E and F are the mid-points of its sides as shown and G is the centre of the triangle. The moment of inertia of the triangle about an axis passing through G and perpendicular to the plane of the triangle is I_0. If the smaller triangle DEF is removed from ABC, the moment of inertia of the remaining figure about the same axis is I. Then :

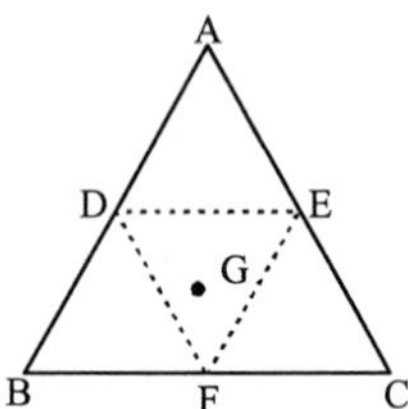

(a) $I = \frac{15}{16}I_0$ (b) $I = \frac{3}{4}I_0$ (c) $I = \frac{9}{16}I_0$ (d) $I = \frac{I_0}{4}$

69. A rod of length 50 cm is pivoted at one end. It is raised such that if makes an angle of 30° from the horizontal as shown and released from rest. Its angular speed when it passes through the horizontal (in rads^{-1}) will be (g = 10 ms^{-2})

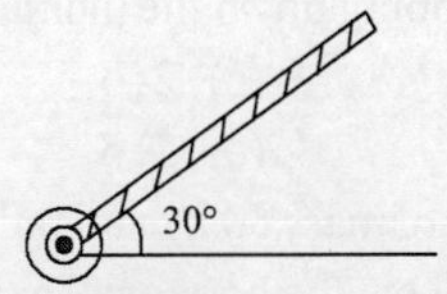

(a) $\sqrt{\frac{30}{7}}$ (b) $\sqrt{30}$ (c) $\sqrt{\frac{20}{3}}$ (d) $\sqrt{\frac{30}{2}}$

70. Seven identical circular planar disks, each of mass M and radius R are welded symmetrically as shown. The moment of inertia of the arrangement about the axis normal to the plane and passing through the point P is:

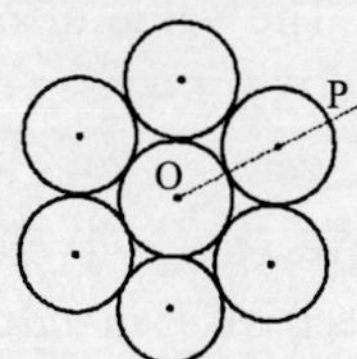

(a) $\frac{19}{2}MR^2$ (b) $\frac{55}{2}MR^2$ (c) $\frac{73}{2}MR^2$ (d) $\frac{181}{2}MR^2$

71. From a uniform circular disc of radius R and mass 9 M, a small disc of radius $\frac{R}{3}$ is removed as shown in the figure. The moment of inertia of the remaining disc about an axis perpendicular to the plane of the disc and passing, through centre of disc is :

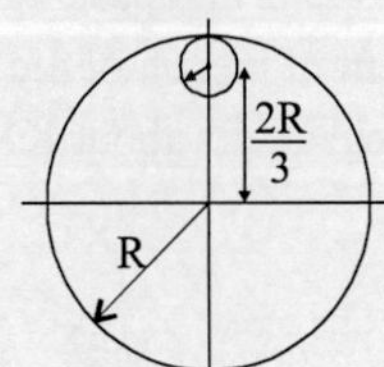

(a) $4\,MR^2$ (b) $\frac{40}{9}MR^2$ (c) $10\,MR^2$ (d) $\frac{37}{9}MR^2$

72. A uniform sphere of mass 500 g rolls without slipping on a plane horizontal surface with its centre moving at a speed of 5.00 cm/s. Its kinetic energy is:

(a) 8.75×10^{-4} J (b) 8.75×10^{-3} J
(c) 6.25×10^{-4} J (d) 1.13×10^{-3} J

73. A solid sphere and solid cylinder of identical radii approach an incline with the same linear velocity (see figure). Both roll without slipping all throughout. The two climb maximum heights h_{sph} and h_{cyl} on the incline. The ratio $\frac{h_{sph}}{h_{cyl}}$ is given by :

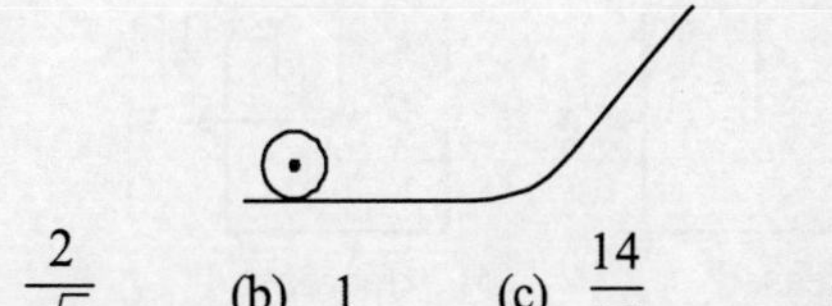

(a) $\frac{2}{\sqrt{5}}$ (b) 1 (c) $\frac{14}{15}$ (d) $\frac{4}{5}$

74. The following bodies are made to roll up (without slipping) the same inclined plane from a horizontal plane: (i) a ring of radius R, (ii) a solid cylinder of radius $\frac{R}{2}$ and (iii) a solid sphere of radius $\frac{R}{4}$. If, in each case, the speed of the center of mass at the bottom of the incline is same, the ratio of the maximum heights they climb is:

(a) 4:3:2 (b) 10:15:7
(c) 14:15:20 (d) 2:3:4

75. A roller is made by joining together two cones at their vertices O. It is kept on two rails AB and CD, which are placed asymmetrically (see figure), with its axis perpendicular to CD and its centre O at the centre of line joining AB and Cd (see figure). It is given a light push so that it starts rolling with its centre O moving parallel to CD in the direction shown. As it moves, the roller will tend to:

(a) go straight.
(b) turn left and right alternately.
(c) turn left.
(d) turn right.

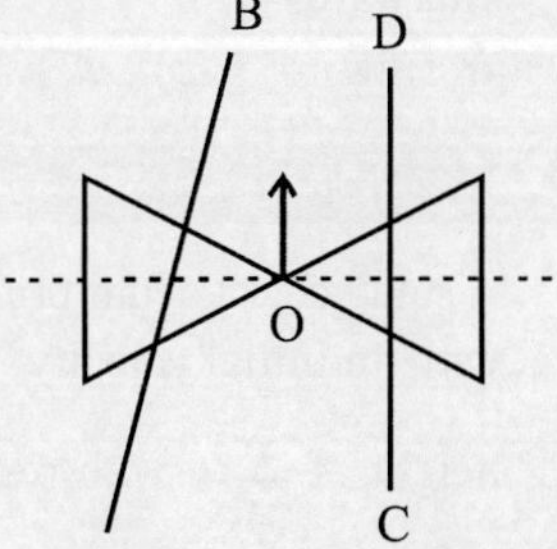

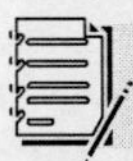

Exercise 2 - Exemplar & Past Year Questions

E&PYQs

Exemplar Questions

1. For which of the following does the centre of mass lie outside the body?
(a) A pencil (b) A shotput
(c) A dice (d) A bangle

2. Which of the following points is the likely position of the centre of mass of the system shown in figure?

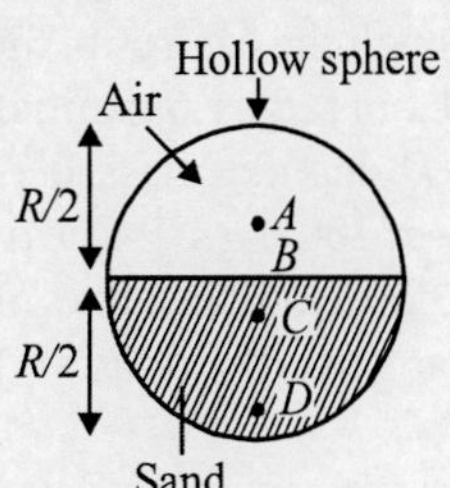

(a) A (b) B (c) C (d) D

3. When a disc rotates with uniform angular velocity, which of the following is not true?
(a) The sense of rotation remains same
(b) The orientation of the axis of rotation remains same
(c) The speed of rotation is non-zero and remains same
(d) The angular acceleration is non-zero and remains same

4. A uniform square plate has a small piece Q of an irregular shape removed and glued to the centre of the plate leaving a hole behind in figure. The moment of inertia about the z-axis is then,

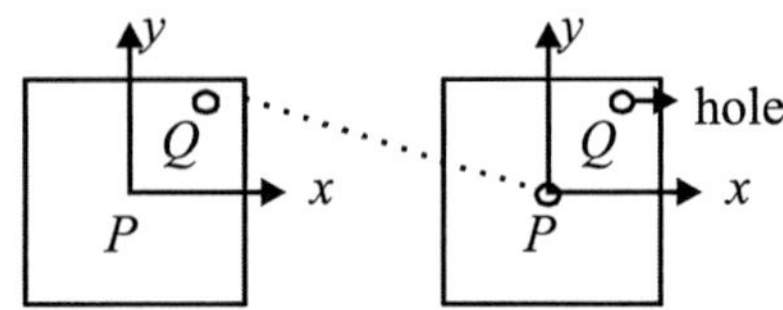

(a) increased (b) decreased
(c) the same
(d) changed in unpredicted manner

5. In problem-5, the CM of the plate is now in the following quadrant of x-y plane.
(a) I (b) II (c) III (d) IV

6. The density of a non-uniform rod of length 1 m is given by $\rho(x) = a\,(1 + bx^2)$ where, a and b are constants and $0 \le x \le 1$. The centre of mass of the rod will be at
(a) $\frac{3(2+b)}{4(3+b)}$ (b) $\frac{4(2+b)}{3(3+b)}$
(c) $\frac{3(3+b)}{4(2+b)}$ (d) $\frac{4(3+b)}{3(2+b)}$

7. A merry-go-round, made of a ring-like platform of radius R and mass M, is revolving with angular speed ω. A person of mass M is standing on it. At one instant, the person jumps off the round, radially away from the centre of the round (as seen from the round). The speed of the round of afterwards is
(a) 2w (b) w (c) $\frac{\omega}{2}$ (d) 0

NEET/AIPMT (2013-2020) Questions

8. A small object of uniform density rolls up a curved surface with an initial velocity 'v'. It reaches upto a maximum height of $\frac{3v^2}{4g}$ with respect to the initial position. The object is a **[2013]**
(a) solid sphere (b) hollow sphere
(c) disc (d) ring

9. Two discs are rotating about their axes, normal to the discs and passing through the centres of the discs. Disc D_1 has 2 kg mass and 0.2 m radius and initial angular velocity of 50 rad s^{-1}. Disc D_2 has 4kg mass, 0.1 m radius and initial angular velocity of 200 rad s^{-1}. The two discs are brought in contact face to face, with their axes of rotation coincident. The final angular velocity (in rad s^{-1}) of the system is **[NEET Kar. 2013]**
(a) 40 (b) 60 (c) 100 (d) 120

10. The ratio of radii of gyration of a circular ring and a circular disc, of the same mass and radius, about an axis passing through their centres and perpendicular to their planes are
(a) $\sqrt{2}:1$ (b) $1:\sqrt{2}$ **[NEET Kar. 2013]**
(c) $3:2$ (d) $2:1$

11. The ratio of the accelerations for a solid sphere (mass 'm' and radius 'R') rolling down an incline of angle 'θ' without slipping and slipping down the incline without rolling is :
(a) $5:7$ (b) $2:3$ **[2014]**
(c) $2:5$ (d) $7:5$

12. A solid cylinder of mass 50 kg and radius 0.5 m is free to rotate about the horizontal axis. A massless string is wound round the cylinder with one end attached to it and other hanging freely. Tension in the string required to produce an angular acceleration of 2 revolutions s^{-2} is :
(a) 25 N (b) 50 N **[2014]**
(c) 78.5 N (d) 157 N

13. A force $\vec{F} = \alpha\hat{i} + 3\hat{j} + 6\hat{k}$ is acting at a point $\vec{r} = 2\hat{i} - 6\hat{j} - 12\hat{k}$. The value of α for which angular momentum about origin is conserved is : **[2015 RS]**
(a) 2 (b) zero (c) 1 (d) –1

14. An automobile moves on a road with a speed of 54 km h^{-1}. The radius of its wheels is 0.45 m and the moment of inertia of the wheel about its axis of rotation is 3 kg m^2. If the vehicle is brought to rest in 15s, the magnitude of average torque transmitted by its brakes to the wheel is : **[2015 RS]**
(a) 8.58 kg m^2 s^{-2} (b) 10.86 kg m^2 s^{-2}
(c) 2.86 kg m^2 s^{-2} (d) 6.66 kg m^2 s^{-2}

15. Three identical spherical shells, each of mass m and radius r are placed as shown in figure. Consider an axis XX' which is touching to two shells and passing through diameter of third shell. Moment of inertia of the system consisting of these three spherical shells about XX' axis is **[2015]**
(a) $3mr^2$
(b) $\frac{16}{5}mr^2$
(c) $4mr^2$
(d) $\frac{11}{5}mr^2$

X
X'

16. A rod of weight W is supported by two parallel knife edges A and B and is in equilibrium in a horizontal position. The knives are at a distance d from each other. The centre of mass of the rod is at distance x from A. The normal reaction on A is **[2015]**
(a) $\frac{Wd}{x}$ (b) $\frac{W(d-x)}{x}$
(c) $\frac{W(d-x)}{d}$ (d) $\frac{Wx}{d}$

17. A uniform circular disc of radius 50 cm at rest is free to turn about an axis which is perpendicular to its plane and passes through its centre. It is subjected to a torque which produces a constant angular acceleration of 2.0 rad s^{-2}. Its net acceleration in ms^{-2} at the end of 2.0s is approximately: *[2016]*
(a) 8.0 (b) 7.0 (c) 6.0 (d) 3.0

18. From a disc of radius R and mass M, a circular hole of diameter R, whose rim passes through the centre is cut. What is the moment of inertia of the remaining part of the disc about a perpendicular axis, passing through the centre ? *[2016]*
(a) $15 MR^2/32$ (b) $13 MR^2/32$
(c) $11 MR^2/32$ (d) $9 MR^2/32$

19. A rope is wound around a hollow cylinder of mass 3 kg and radius 40 cm. What is the angular acceleration of the cylinder if the rope is pulled with a force of 30 N ? *[2017]*
(a) 0.25 rad/s^2 (b) 25 rad/s^2
(c) 5 m/s^2 (d) 25 m/s^2

20. A solid sphere is rotating freely about its symmetry axis in free space. The radius of the sphere is increased keeping its mass same. Which of the following physical quantities would remain constant for the sphere? *[2018]*
(a) Angular velocity (b) Moment of inertia
(c) Angular momentum (d) Rotational kinetic energy

21. A solid sphere is in rolling motion. In rolling motion a body possesses translational kinetic energy (K_t) as well as rotational kinetic energy (K_r) simultaneously. The ratio $K_t : (K_t + K_r)$ for the sphere is *[2018]*
(a) 7 : 10 (b) 5 : 7 (c) 2 : 5 (d) 10 : 7

22. Two particles A and B are moving in uniform circular motion in concentric circles of radii r_A and r_B with speed υ_A and υ_B respectively. Their time period of rotation is the same. The ratio of angular speed of A to that of B will be : *[2019]*
(a) $r_A : r_B$ (b) $\upsilon_A : \upsilon_B$ (c) $r_B : r_A$ (d) 1 : 1

23. A solid cylinder of mass 2 kg and radius 4 cm is rotating about its axis at the rate of 3 rpm. The torque required to stop after 2π revolutions is : *[2019]*
(a) 2×10^{-6} N m (b) 2×10^{-3} N m
(c) 12×10^{-4} N m (d) 2×10^{6} N m

24. A disc of radius 2 m and mass 100 kg rolls on a horizontal floor. Its centre of mass has speed of 20 cm/s. How much work is needed to stop it ? *[2019]*
(a) 3 J (b) 30 kJ (c) 2 J (d) 1J

25. A solid cylinder of mass 2 kg and radius 50 cm rolls up an inclined plane of angle of inclination 30°. The centre of mass of the cylinder has speed of 4 m/s. The distance travelled by the cylinder on the inclined surface will be, [take g = 10 m/s^2] *[NEET Odisha 2019]*
(a) 2.4m (b) 2.2m (c) 1.6m (d) 1.2m

26. Two particles of mass 5 kg and 10 kg respectively are attached to the two ends of a rigid rod of length 1 m with negligible mass. The centre of mass of the system from the 5 kg particle is nearly at a distance of: *[2020]*
(a) 50 cm (b) 67 cm (c) 80 cm (d) 33 cm

27. Find the torque about the origin when a force of $3\hat{j}$ N acts on a particle whose position vector is $2\hat{k}$ m. *[2020]*
(a) $6\hat{j}$ Nm (b) $-6\hat{i}$ Nm (c) $6\hat{k}$ Nm (d) $6\hat{i}$ Nm

Exercise 3 - Concept Application Problems CAP

1. A gymnast takes turns with her arms & legs stretched. When she pulls her arms & legs in
(a) the angular velocity decreases
(b) the moment of inertia decreases
(c) the angular velocity stays constant
(d) the angular momentum increases

2. A flywheel rotates about an axis. Due to friction at the axis, it experiences an angular retardation proportional to its angular velocity. If its angular velocity falls to half while it makes n rotations, how many more rotations will it make before coming to rest?
(a) 2n (b) n (c) n/2 (d) n/3

3. What is the moment of inertia of a solid sphere of density ρ and radius R about its diameter?
(a) $\frac{105}{176}R^5\rho$ (b) $\frac{105}{176}R^2\rho$ (c) $\frac{176}{105}R^5\rho$ (d) $\frac{176}{105}R^2\rho$

4. The radius of gyration of a body about an axis at a distance 6 cm from its centre of mass is 10 cm. Then, its radius of gyration about a parallel axis through its centre of mass will be
(a) 80 cm (b) 8 cm (c) 0.8 cm (d) 80 m

5. A particle is confined to rotate in a circular path decreasing linear speed, then which of the following is correct?
(a) $\vec{L}$ (angular momentum) is conserved about the centre
(b) only direction of angular momentum $\vec{L}$ is conserved
(c) It spirals towards the centre
(d) its acceleration is towards the centre.

6. A cylinder rolls down an inclined plane of inclination 30°, the acceleration of cylinder is
(a) $\frac{g}{3}$ (b) g (c) $\frac{g}{2}$ (d) $\frac{2g}{3}$

7. In carbon monoxide molecule, the carbon and the oxygen atoms are separated by a distance 1.12×10^{-10} m. The distance of the centre of mass, from the carbon atom is
(a) 0.64×10^{-10} m (b) 0.56×10^{-10} m
(c) 0.51×10^{-10} m (d) 0.48×10^{-10} m

8. A composite disc is to be made using equal masses of aluminium and iron so that it has as high a moment of inertia as possible. This is possible when

(a) the surfaces of the disc are made of iron with aluminium inside
(b) the whole of aluminium is kept in the core and the iron at the outer rim of the disc
(c) the whole of the iron is kept in the core and the aluminium at the outer rim of the disc
(d) the whole disc is made with thin alternate sheets of iron and aluminium

9. A ball rolls without slipping. The radius of gyration of the ball about an axis passing through its centre of mass is K. If radius of the ball be R, then the fraction of total energy associated with its rotational energy will be

(a) $\frac{R^2}{K^2+R^2}$ (b) $\frac{K^2+R^2}{R^2}$ (c) $\frac{K^2}{R^2}$ (d) $\frac{K^2}{K^2+R^2}$

10. A sphere of mass 2000 g and radius 5 cm is rotating at the rate of 300 rpm .Then the torque required to stop it in 2π revolutions, is
(a) 1.6×10^2 dyne cm (b) 1.6×10^3 dyne cm
(c) 2.5×10^4 dyne cm (d) 2.5×10^5 dyne cm

11. The wheel of a car is rotating at the rate of 1200 revolutions per minute. On pressing the accelerator for 10 seconds it starts rotating at 4500 revolutions per minute. The angular acceleration of the wheel is
(a) 30 radian / second^2 (b) 1880 degrees/ second^2
(c) 40 radian / second^2 (d) 1980 degree/second^2

12. The moment of inertia of a body about a given axis is 1.2 kg m^2. Initially, the body is at rest . In order to produce a rotational kinetic energy of 1500 J, an angular acceleration of 25 rad s^{-2} must be applied about that axis for a duration of
(a) 4 s (b) 2 s (c) 8 s (d) 10 s

13. The moment of inertia of a uniform circular disc of radius 'R' and mass 'M' about an axis passing from the edge of the disc and normal to the disc is

(a) MR^2 (b) $\frac{1}{2}MR^2$ (c) $\frac{3}{2}MR^2$ (d) $\frac{7}{2}MR^2$

14. Two bodies have their moments of inertia I and 2I respectively about their axis of rotation. If their kinetic energies of rotation are equal, their angular momenta will be in the ratio
(a) $2:1$ (b) $1:2$ (c) $\sqrt{2}:1$ (d) $1:\sqrt{2}$

15. The moment of inertia of a thin uniform rod of mass M and length L about an axis passing through its midpoint and perpendicular to its length is I_0. Its moment of inertia about an axis passing through one of its ends and perpendicular to its length is
(a) $I_0 + ML^2/2$ (b) $I_0 + ML^2/4$
(c) $I_0 + 2ML^2$ (d) $I_0 + ML^2$

16. A rod of length L has non-uniform linear mass density given by $\rho(x) = a + b\left(\frac{x}{L}\right)^2$, where a and b are constants and $0 \le x \le L$. The value of x for the centre of mass of the rod is at:

(a) $\frac{3}{2}\left(\frac{a+b}{2a+b}\right)L$ (b) $\frac{3}{4}\left(\frac{2a+b}{3a+b}\right)L$

(c) $\frac{4}{3}\left(\frac{a+b}{2a+3b}\right)L$ (d) $\frac{3}{2}\left(\frac{2a+b}{3a+b}\right)L$

17. Three point particles of masses 1.0 kg, 1.5 kg and 2.5 kg are placed at three corners of a right angle triangle of sides 4.0 cm, 3.0 cm and 5.0 cm as shown in the figure. The center of mass of the system is at a point:

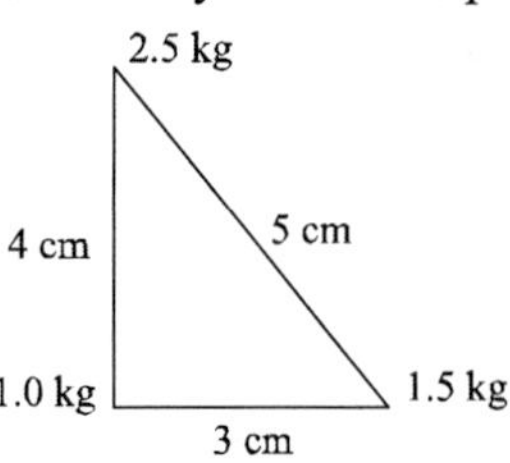

(a) 0.6 cm right and 2.0 cm above 1 kg mass
(b) 1.5 cm right and 1.2 cm above 1 kg mass
(c) 2.0 cm right and 0.9 cm above 1 kg mass
(d) 0.9 cm right and 2.0 cm above 1 kg mass

18. Four particles A, B, C and D with masses $m_A = m$, $m_B = 2m$, $m_C = 3m$ and $m_D = 4m$ are at the corners of a square. They have accelerations of equal magnitude with directions as shown. The acceleration of the centre of mass of the particles is :

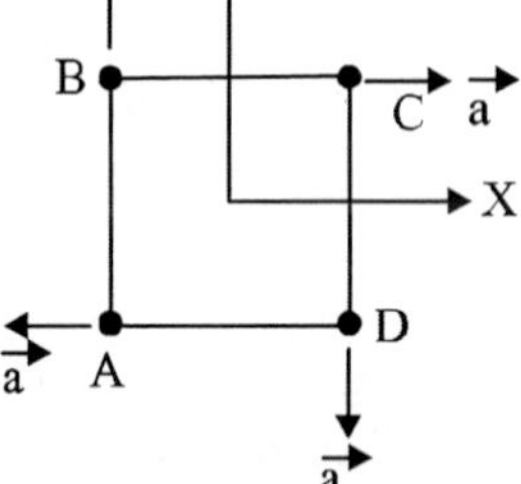

(a) $\frac{a}{5}(\hat{i}-\hat{j})$
(b) a
(c) Zero
(d) $\frac{a}{5}(\hat{i}+\hat{j})$

19. A bead of mass m stays at point $P(a, b)$ on a wire bent in the shape of a parabola $y = 4Cx^2$ and rotating with angular speed ω (see figure). The value of ω is (neglect friction) :

(a) $2\sqrt{2gC}$
(b) $2\sqrt{gC}$
(c) $\sqrt{\frac{2gC}{ab}}$
(d) $\sqrt{\frac{2g}{C}}$

20. A particle of mass m is fixed to one end of a light spring having force constant k and unstretched length l. The other end is fixed. The system is given an angular speed ω about the fixed end of the spring such that it rotates in a circle in gravity free space. Then the stretch in the spring is:

(a) $\frac{ml\omega^2}{k-\omega m}$ (b) $\frac{ml\omega^2}{k-m\omega^2}$ (c) $\frac{ml\omega^2}{k+m\omega^2}$ (d) $\frac{ml\omega^2}{k+m\omega}$

21. A long cylindrical vessel is half filled with a liquid. When the vessel is rotated about its own vertical axis, the liquid rises up near the wall. If the radius of vessel is 5 cm and its rotational speed is 2 rotations per second, then the difference in the heights between the centre and the sides, in cm, will be :
(a) 2.0 (b) 0.1 (c) 0.4 (d) 1.2

22. 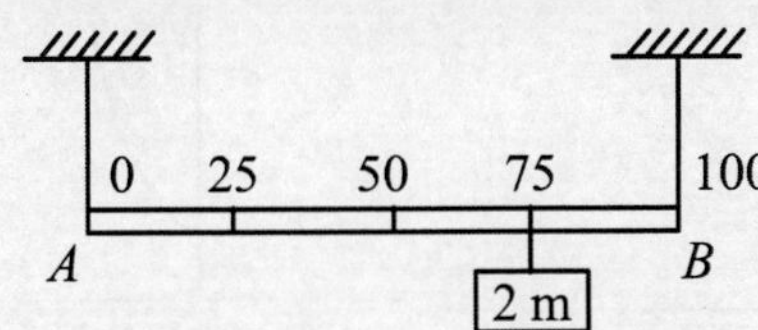

Shown in the figure is rigid and uniform one meter long rod AB held in horizontal position by two strings tied to its ends and attached to the ceiling. The rod is of mass 'm' and has another weight of mass 2 m hung at a distance of 75 cm from A. The tension in the string at A is :

(a) 0.5 mg (b) 2 mg (c) 0.75 mg (d) 1 mg

23. A particle of mass m is moving along a trajectory given by

$x = x_0 + a\cos\omega_1 t$

$y = y_0 + b\cos\omega_2 t$

The torque, acting on the particle about the origin, at $t = 0$ is:

(a) $m(-x_0 b + y_0 a)\omega_1^2\hat{k}$ (b) $+my_0 a\omega_1^2\hat{k}$

(c) zero (d) $-m(x_0 b\omega_2^2 - y_0 a\omega_1^2)\hat{k}$

24. The time dependence of the position of a particle of mass $m = 2$ is given by $\vec{r}(t) = 2t\hat{i} - 3t^2\hat{j}$. Its angular momentum, with respect to the origin, at time t = 2 is :

(a) $48(\hat{i}+\hat{j})$ (b) $36\hat{k}$ (c) $-34(\hat{k}-\hat{i})$ (d) $-48\hat{k}$

25. A metal coin of mass 5 g and radius 1 cm is fixed to a thin stick AB of negligible mass as shown in the figure The system is initially at rest. The constant torque, that will make the system rotate about AB at 25 rotations per second in 5s, is close to :

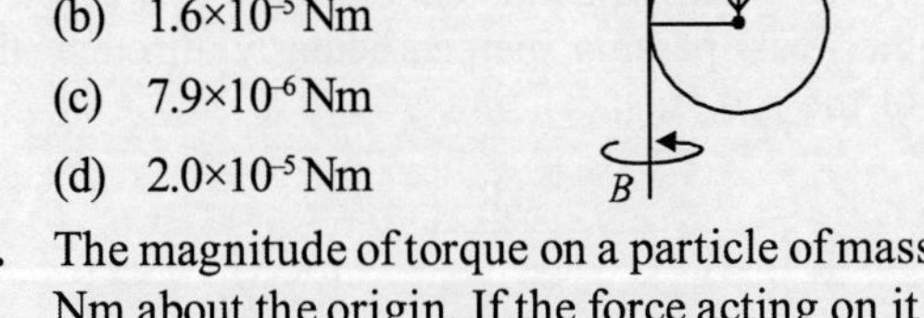

(a) 4.0×10^{-6} Nm

(b) 1.6×10^{-5} Nm

(c) 7.9×10^{-6} Nm

(d) 2.0×10^{-5} Nm

26. The magnitude of torque on a particle of mass 1 kg is 2.5 Nm about the origin. If the force acting on it is 1 N, and the distance of the particle from the origin is 5m, the angle between the force and the position vector is (in radians):

(a) $\frac{\pi}{6}$ (b) $\frac{\pi}{3}$ (c) $\frac{\pi}{8}$ (d) $\frac{\pi}{4}$

27. A rigid massless rod of length $3l$ has two masses attached at each end as shown in the figure. The rod is pivoted at point P on the horizontal axis (see figure). When released from initial horizontal position, its instantaneous angular acceleration will be:

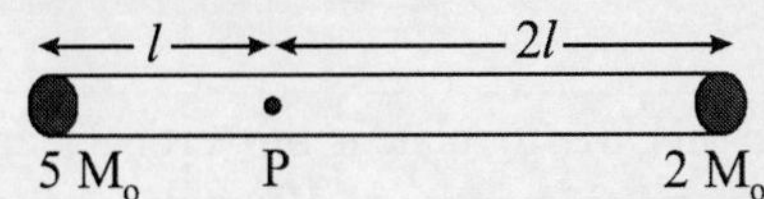

(a) $\frac{g}{13l}$ (b) $\frac{g}{3l}$ (c) $\frac{g}{2l}$ (d) $\frac{7g}{3l}$

28. Shown in the figure is a hollow icecream cone (it is open at the top). If its mass is M, radius of its top, R and height, H, then its moment of inertia about its axis is :

(a) $\frac{MR^2}{2}$

(b) $\frac{M(R^2+H^2)}{4}$

(c) $\frac{MH^2}{3}$

(d) $\frac{MR^2}{3}$

29. The linear mass density of a thin rod AB of length L varies from A to B as $\lambda(x) = \lambda_0\left(1+\frac{x}{L}\right)$, where x is the distance from A. If M is the mass of the rod then its moment of inertia about an axis passing through A and perpendicular to the rod is :

(a) $\frac{5}{12}ML^2$ (b) $\frac{7}{18}ML^2$ (c) $\frac{2}{5}ML^2$ (d) $\frac{3}{7}ML^2$

30. Consider two uniform discs of the same thickness and different radii $R_1 = R$ and $R_2 = \alpha R$ made of the same material. If the ratio of their moments of inertia I_1 and I_2, respectively, about their axes is $I_1 : I_2 = 1 : 16$ then the value of α is :

(a) $2\sqrt{2}$ (b) $\sqrt{2}$ (c) 2 (d) 4

31. Three solid spheres each of mass m and diameter d are stuck together such that the lines connecting the centres form an equilateral triangle of side of length d. The ratio $\frac{I_0}{I_A}$ of moment of inertia I_0 of the system about an axis passing the centroid and about center of any of the spheres I_A and perpendicular to the plane of the triangle is:

(a) $\frac{13}{23}$

(b) $\frac{15}{13}$

(c) $\frac{23}{13}$

(d) $\frac{13}{15}$

32. The radius of gyration of a uniform rod of length l, about an axis passing through a point $\frac{l}{4}$ away from the centre of the rod, and perpendicular to it, is:

(a) $\frac{1}{4}l$ (b) $\frac{1}{8}l$ (c) $\sqrt{\frac{7}{48}}l$ (d) $\sqrt{\frac{3}{8}}l$

33. Mass per unit area of a circular disc of radius a depends on the distance r from its centre as $\sigma(r) = A + Br$. The moment of inertia of the disc about the axis, perpendicular to the plane and passing through its centre is:

(a) $2\pi a^4\left(\frac{A}{4}+\frac{aB}{5}\right)$ (b) $2\pi a^4\left(\frac{aA}{4}+\frac{B}{5}\right)$

(c) $\pi a^4\left(\frac{A}{4}+\frac{aB}{5}\right)$ (d) $2\pi a^4\left(\frac{A}{4}+\frac{B}{5}\right)$

34. A circular disc of radius b has a hole of radius a at its centre (see figure). If the mass per unit area of the disc varies as $\left(\frac{\sigma_0}{r}\right)$, then the radius of gyration of the disc about its axis passing through the centre is :

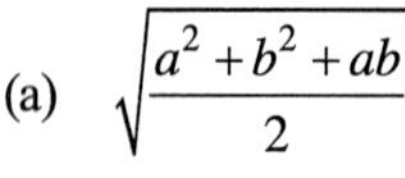

(a) $\sqrt{\frac{a^2+b^2+ab}{2}}$

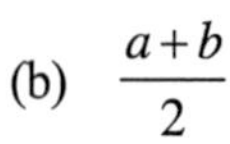

(b) $\frac{a+b}{2}$

(c) $\sqrt{\frac{a^2+b^2+ab}{3}}$ (d) $\frac{a+b}{3}$

35. A thin disc of mass M and radius R has mass per unit area $\sigma(r) = kr^2$ where r is the distance from its centre. Its moment of inertia about an axis going through its centre of mass and perpendicular to its plane is :

(a) $\frac{MR^2}{3}$ (b) $\frac{2MR^2}{3}$ (c) $\frac{MR^2}{6}$ (d) $\frac{MR^2}{2}$

36. A solid sphere of mass M and radius R is divided into two unequal parts. The first part has a mass of $\frac{7M}{8}$ and is converted into a uniform disc of radius 2R. The second part is converted into a uniform solid sphere. Let I_1 be the moment of inertia of the new sphere about its axis. The ratio I_1/I_2 is given by :

(a) 185 (b) 140 (c) 285 (d) 65

37. A stationary horizontal disc is free to rotate about its axis. When a torque is applied on it, its kinetic energy as a function of θ, where θ is the angle by which it has rotated, is given as $k\theta^2$. If its moment of inertia is I then the angular acceleration of the disc is:

(a) $\frac{k}{4I}\theta$ (b) $\frac{k}{I}\theta$ (c) $\frac{k}{2I}\theta$ (d) $\frac{2k}{I}\theta$

38. Moment of inertia of a body about a given axis is 1.5 kg m^2. Initially the body is at rest. In order to produce a rotational kinetic energy of 1200 J, the angular acceleration of 20 rad/s^2 must be applied about the axis for a duration of:

(a) 2.5s (b) 2s (c) 5s (d) 3s

39. Let the moment of inertia of a hollow cylinder of length 30 cm (inner radius 10 cm and outer radius 20 cm), about its axis be 1. The radius of a thin cylinder of the same mass such that its moment of inertia about its axis is also I, is:

(a) 12 cm (b) 16 cm (c) 14 cm (d) 18 cm

40. The moment of inertia of a solid sphere, about an axis parallel to its diameter and at a distance of x from it, is '$I(x)$'. Which one of the graphs represents the variation of $I(x)$ with x correctly?

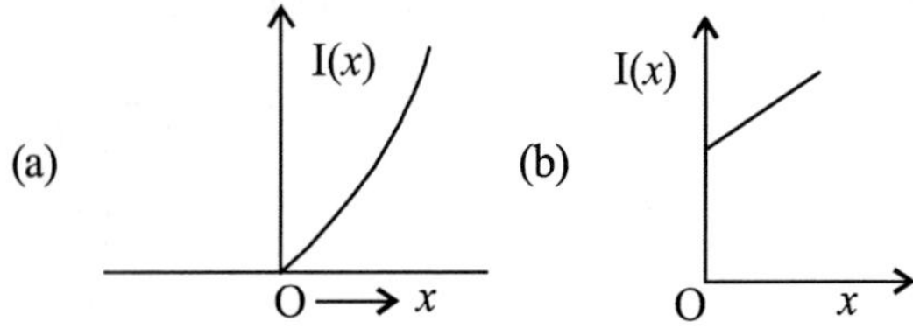

(c) (d)

41. a string is wound around a hollow cylinder of mass 5 kg and radius 0.5 m. If the string is now pulled with a horizontal force of 40 N, and the cylinder is rolling without slipping on a horizontal surface (see figure), then the angular acceleration of the cylinder will be (Neglect the mass and thickness of the string)

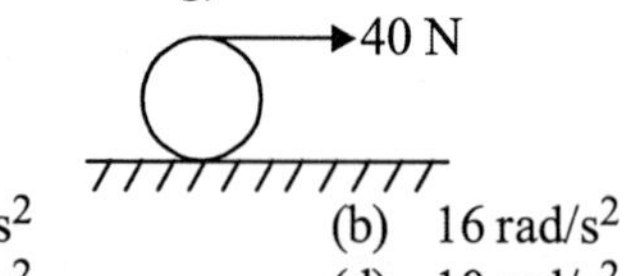

(a) 20 rad/s^2 (b) 16 rad/s^2
(c) 12 rad/s^2 (d) 10 rad/s^2

42. A circular disc D_1 of mass M and radius R has two identical discs D_2 and D_3 of the same mass M and radius R attached rigidly at its opposite ends (see figure). The moment of inertia of the system about the axis OO', passing through the centre of D_1, as shown in the figure, will be :

(a) MR^2
(b) $3MR^2$
(c) $\frac{4}{5}MR^2$
(d) $\frac{2}{3}MR^2$

43. Two identical spherical balls of mass M and radius R each are stuck on two ends of a rod of length 2R and mass M (see figure). The moment of inertia of the system about the axis passing perpendicularly through the centre of the rod is:

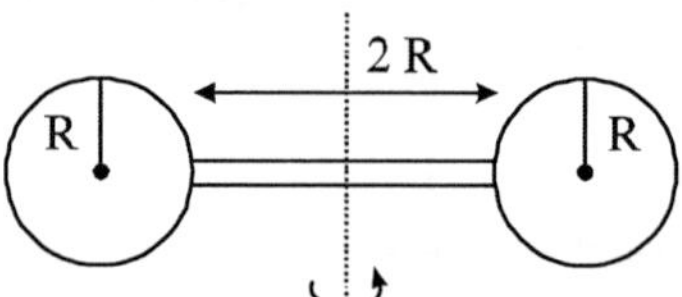

(a) $\frac{137}{15}MR^2$ (b) $\frac{17}{15}MR^2$ (c) $\frac{209}{15}MR^2$ (d) $\frac{152}{15}MR^2$

44. A thin circular disk is in the xy plane as shown in the figure. The ratio of its moment of inertia about z and z' axes will be

(a) 1 : 2
(b) 1 : 4
(c) 1 : 3
(d) 1 : 5

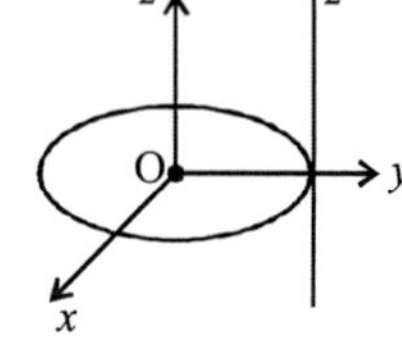

45. A thin rod MN, free to rotate in the vertical plane about the fixed end N, is held horizontal. When the end M is released the speed of this end, when the rod makes an angle α with the horizontal, will be proportional to: (see figure)

(a) $\sqrt{\cos\alpha}$ (b) $\cos\alpha$
(c) $\sin\alpha$ (d) $\sqrt{\sin\alpha}$

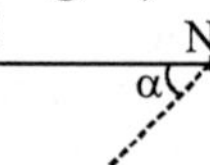
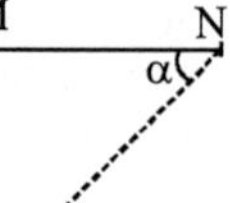

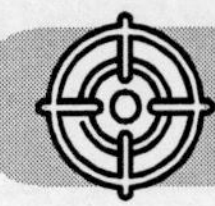

Hints & Solutions

7.1 Concept Practice Problems

1. (a) Earth is heavier than moon.
2. (b) 3. (c)
4. (a) If we consider the two masses in a system then no external force is acting on the system. Mutual forces are internal forces. Since the centre of mass is initially at rest, it well remain at rest
5. (a) The situation can be shown as : Let radius of complete disc is a and that of small disc is b. Also let centre of mass now shifts to O_2 at a distance x_2 from original centre.

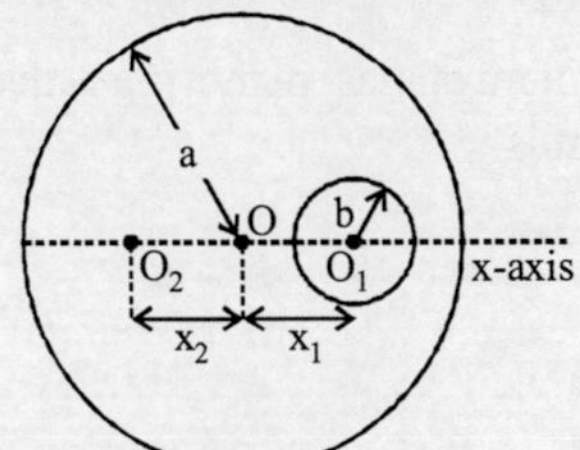

The position of new centre of mass is given by

$$X_{CM} = \frac{-\sigma .\pi b^2 .x_1}{\sigma .\pi a^2 - \sigma .\pi b^2}$$

Here, a = 6 cm, b = 2 cm, x_1 = 3.2 cm

$$\text{Hence, } X_{CM} = \frac{-\sigma \times \pi (2)^2 \times 3.2}{\sigma \times \pi \times (6)^2 - \sigma \times \pi \times (2)^2} = \frac{12.8\pi}{32\pi} = -0.4 \text{cm.}$$

6. (c) $X_{C.M.} = \dfrac{1\times 0 + 2\times 2 + 3\times 0 + 4\times 2 + 5\times 1}{1+2+3+4+5}$

$$= \frac{4+8+5}{15} = \frac{17}{15} = 1.1$$

$$Y_{C.M} = \frac{1\times 0 + 2\times 0 + 3\times 2 + 4\times 2 + 5\times 1}{1+2+3+4+5} = \frac{6+8+5}{15} = 1.3$$

7. (a) So couple about the C.M must be zero for rotational equilibrium, It means that

$$\frac{W}{4}\times\frac{L}{2} = \frac{3W}{4}\times x \Rightarrow x = \frac{L}{6}$$

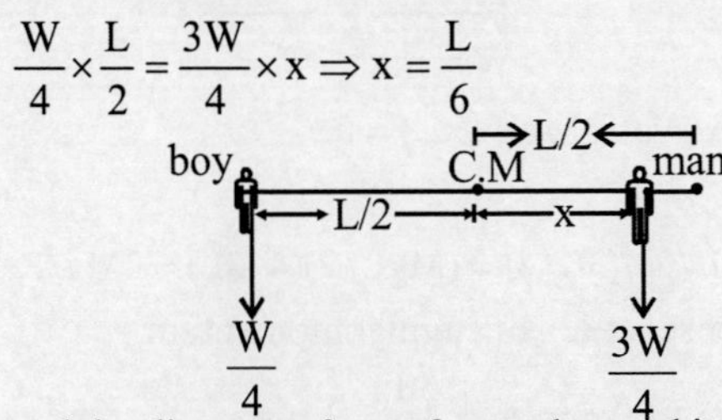

and the distance of man from other end is

$$\frac{L}{2} - x = \frac{L}{2} - \frac{L}{6} = \frac{L}{3}$$

8. (b)
9. (b) Position of C.M w.r. to A

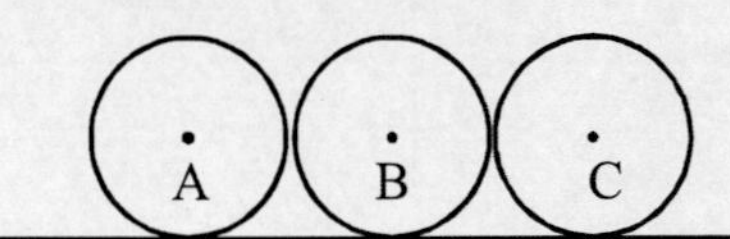

$$= \frac{1\times 0 + 1\times AB + 1\times AC}{1+1+1} = \frac{AB + AC}{3}$$

10. (a) $X_{cm} = \dfrac{m_1x_1 + m_2x_2 + m_3x_3}{m_1 + m_2 + m_3}$

$$X_{cm} = \frac{300\times(0) + 500(40) + 400\times 70}{300 + 500 + 400}$$

$$X_{cm} = \frac{500\times 40 + 400\times 70}{1200}$$

$$X_{cm} = \frac{50+70}{3} = \frac{120}{3} = 40 \text{ cm}$$

7.2 Concept Practice Problems

11. (c) Moment of inertia is independent of application of force.
12. (a)
13. (a) $I_B = MR^2 \quad I_A = \frac{1}{2}MR^2 \quad \therefore I_A < I_B$
14. (a) Moment of inertia of the whole system about the axis of rotation will be equal to the sum of the moments of inertia of all the particles.

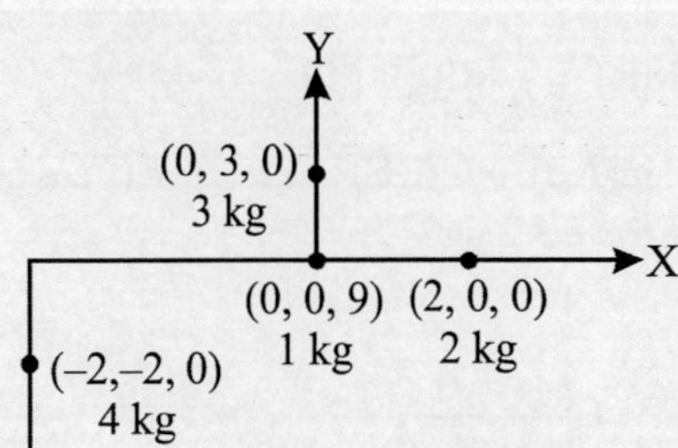

$\therefore \quad I = I_1 + I_2 + I_3 + I_4 = 0 + 0 + 27 + 16 = 43 \text{ kg m}^2$

15. (b) Moment of inertia (M.I) of circular ring $I_1 = mr^2$ moment of inertia (M.I) of circular disc $I_2 = ½mr^2$

$$\Rightarrow \frac{I_1}{I_2} = \frac{2}{1}$$

16. (d) $I = \frac{1}{2}mR^2$

$$M \propto t \propto R^2$$

For disc X, $I_X = \frac{1}{2}(m)(R)^2 = \frac{1}{2}(\pi r^2 t).(R)^2$

for disc Y, $I_Y = \frac{1}{2}[\pi(4R)^2.t/4][4R]^2$

$$\Rightarrow \frac{I_X}{I_Y} = \frac{1}{(4)^3} \Rightarrow I_Y = 64\, I_X$$

17. (a) The moment of inertia (I) of circular ring whose axis of rotation is passing through its center, $I_1 = m_1R^2$

Also, $I_2 = m_2(nR)^2$

Since both rings have same density,

$$\Rightarrow \frac{m_2}{2\pi(nR)\times A_2}=\frac{m_1}{2\pi R\times A_1}$$

Where A is cross-section of ring,

$A_1 = A_2$ (Given) $\therefore m_2 = nm_1$

Given $\frac{I_1}{I_2}=\frac{1}{8}=\frac{m_1R^2}{m_2(nR)^2}=\frac{m_1R^2}{nm_1(nR)^2}$

$\Rightarrow \frac{1}{8}=\frac{1}{n^3}$ or $n=2$

18. (b) The intersection of medians is the centre of mass of the triangle. Since distances of centre of mass from the sides are related as : $x_{BC}<x_{AB}<x_{AC}$ therefore $I_{BC}>I_{AB}>I_{AC}$ or $I_{BC}>I_{AB}$.

19. (c) Moment of inertia of disc about its diameter is $I_d=\frac{1}{4}MR^2$

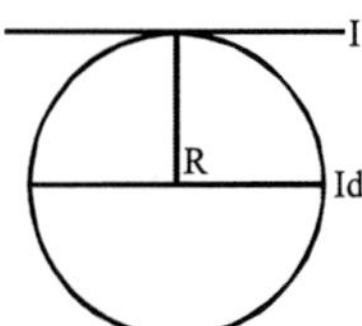

MI of disc about a tangent passing through rim and in the plane of disc is

$$I=I_G+MR^2=\frac{1}{4}MR^2+MR^2=\frac{5}{4}MR^2$$

20. (d) $I_{AX}=m(AB)^2+m(OC)^2=m\ell^2+m(\ell\cos 60^\circ)^2$
$=m\ell^2+m\ell^2/4=5/4\,m\ell^2$

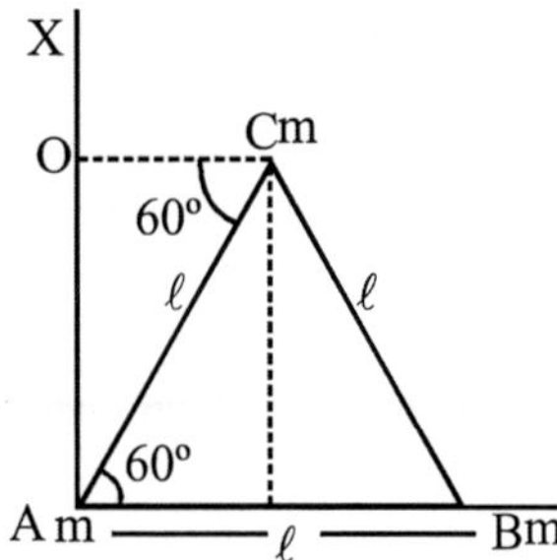

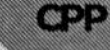

7.3 Concept Practice Problems

CPP

21. (b) If we apply a torque on a body, then angular momentum of the body changes according to the relation

$$\vec{\tau}=\frac{d\vec{L}}{dt}\Rightarrow \text{if } \vec{\tau}=0 \text{ then, } \vec{L}=\text{constant}$$

22. (b) Angular momentum will remain the same since external torque is zero.

23. (b) We know that $\tau_{ext}=\frac{dL}{dt}$
if angular momentum is conserved, it means change in angular momentum $=0$

or, $dL=0$, $\frac{dL}{dt}=0\Rightarrow \tau_{ext}=0$

Thus total external torque $=0$.

24. (d) K.E. of rotation $=\frac{1}{2}I\omega^2$

$=\frac{1}{2}\times\left(\frac{1}{2}mr^2\right)\omega^2$

$=\frac{1}{4}\times 20\times(0.25)^2\times 100\times 100=3125$ J

25. (a) Angular momentum $\propto \frac{1}{\text{Angular frequency}}$
$\propto$ Kinetic energy

$\Rightarrow \vec{L}=\frac{K.E.}{\omega}$

$\frac{L_1}{L_2}=\left(\frac{K.E_1}{\omega_1}\right)\times\frac{\omega_2}{K.E_2}=4 \Rightarrow L_2=\frac{L}{4}$

26. (b) Angular momentum of mass m moving with a constant velocity about origin is

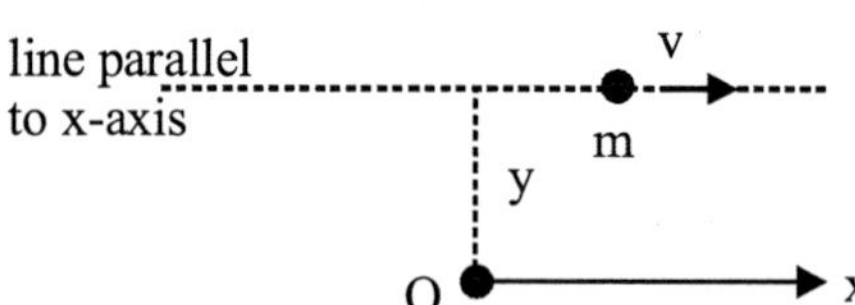

L = momentum × perpendicular distance of line of action of momentum from origin

$L = mv\times y$

In the given condition mvy is a constant. Therefore angular momentum is constant.

27. (c) This is a torque problem. While the fulcrum can be placed anywhere, placing it at the far right end of the bar eliminated cable B from the calculation. There are now only two forces acting on the bar ; the weight that produces a counterclockwise rotation and the tension in cable A that produces a clockwise rotation. Since the bar is in equilibrium, these two torques must sum to zero.

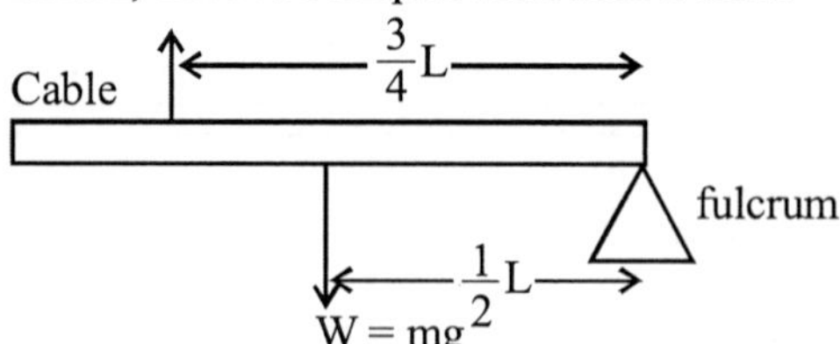

$\Sigma\tau=T_A(3/4L)-Mg(1/2L)=0$

Therefore

$T_A=(MgL/2)/(3L/4)=(MgL/2)(4/3L)=2Mg/3$

28. (c) By conservation of angular momentum,

$5\times 10=5\omega+20\omega\Rightarrow \omega=\frac{50}{25}=2$ rps

29. (b)

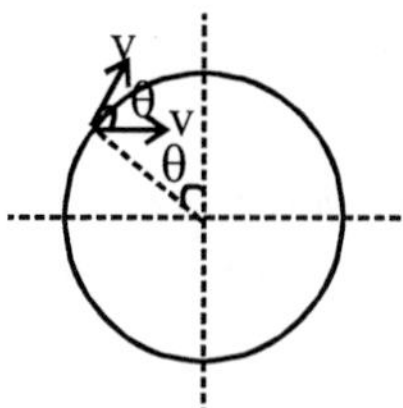

$v_R = \sqrt{v^2 + v^2 + 2v^2 \cos\theta} = \sqrt{2v^2(1+\cos\theta)}$

$= 2v\cos\frac{\theta}{2}$

30. (a) Angular momentum $= I\omega = \frac{2}{5}MR^2.\frac{2\pi}{T} = \frac{4\pi MR^2}{5T}$

31. (d) Velocity at the bottom and top of the circle is $\sqrt{5gr}$ and $\sqrt{gr}$. Therefore $(1/2)M(5gr) = MgH$ and $(1/2)M(gr) = Mgh$.

32. (a) Acceleration of a body rolling down an inclined plane is given by, $a = \frac{g\sin\theta}{1+\frac{K^2}{R^2}}$

In case of a solid sphere, we have

$\frac{K^2}{R^2} = \frac{[(I/M)]}{R^2} = \frac{I}{MR^2} = \frac{(2/5)MR^2}{MR^2} = \frac{2}{5}$

Substituting $\frac{K^2}{R^2} = \frac{2}{5}$ in equation (1) we get

$a = \frac{5}{7}g\sin\theta$

33. (d) $\tau \times \Delta t = L_0$ $\{\because \text{since } L_f = 0\}$

$\Rightarrow \tau \times \Delta t = I\omega$

or $\tau \times 60 = 2 \times 2 \times 60\pi/60$

$\left(\because f = 60\text{rpm} \therefore \omega = 2\pi f = 2\pi \times \frac{60}{60}\right)$

$\tau = \frac{\pi}{15}\text{N}-\text{m}$

34. (d) Angular momentum will be conserved

$I_1\omega = I_1\omega' + I_2\omega' \Rightarrow \omega' = \frac{I_1\omega}{I_1 + I_2}$

35. (d) By conservation of angular momentum, $I_t\omega_i = (I_t + I_b)\,\omega_f$

where ω_f is the final angular velocity of disks

$\therefore \quad \omega_f = \left(\frac{I_t}{I_t + I_b}\right)\omega_i$

Loss in K.E., ΔK = Initial K.E. – Final K.E.

$= \frac{1}{2}I_t\omega_i^2 - \frac{1}{2}(I_t + I_b)\omega_f^2$

$\Rightarrow \Delta K = \frac{1}{2}I_t\omega_i^2 - \frac{1}{2}(I_t + I_b)\frac{I_t^2}{(I_t + I_b)^2}\omega_i^2$

$= \frac{1}{2}\omega_i^2\frac{I_t}{I_t + I_b}(I_t + I_b - I_t) = \frac{1}{2}\omega_i^2\frac{I_t I_b}{I_t + I_b}$

Exercise 1 - Chapter Revision Problems CRP

1. (b) When a disc is given a linear velocity on a rough horizontal surface then L conserved about the point of contact only.

2. (d) 3. (b)

4. (d) The pull of earth changes only when the body moves so that g changes. It is an exceptional case and should not be considered unless otherwise mentioned.

5. (b) Angular momentum $\vec{L}$ is defined as $\vec{L} = \vec{r} \times m(\vec{v})$ so $\vec{L}$ is, an axial vector.

6. (c) The boy does not exert a torque to rotating table by jumping, so angular momentum is conserved i.e., $\frac{d\vec{L}}{dt} = 0 \Rightarrow \vec{L} = \text{constant}$

7. (a) Angular momentum $= \vec{r} \times (\text{linear momentum})$

8. (a) Analogue of mass in rotational motion is moment of inertia. It plays the same role as mass plays in translational motion.

9. (a) Basic equation of moment of inertia is given by $I = \sum_{i=1}^{n} m_i r_i^2$

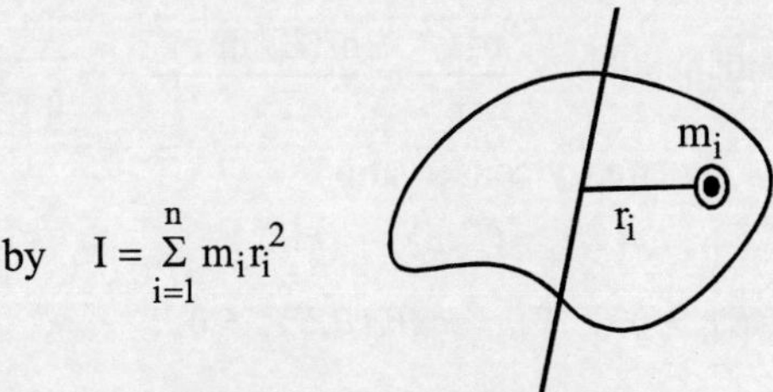

where m_i is the mass of ith particle at a distance of r_i from axis of rotation.

Thus it does not depend on angular velocity.

10. (d) Initially centre of gravity is at the centre. When sand is poured it will fall and again after a limit, centre of gravity will rise.

11. (d) Here, the centre of mass of the system remains unchanged. in the horizontal direction. When the mass m moved forward by a distance $L\cos\theta$, let the mass $(m + M)$ moves by a distance x in the backward direction. hence $(M + m)x - mL\cos\theta = 0$

$\therefore x = (mL\cos\theta)/(m + M)$

12. (b) Acceleration of solid sphere is more than that of hollow sphere, it rolls faster, and reaches the bottom of the inclined plane earlier.

Hence, solid sphere and hollow sphere can be distinguished by rolling them simultaneously on an inclined plane.

13. (d) Applying the law of conservation of momentum

$mv = MV$ ...(1)

By conservation of angular momentum

$mv(L/2) = \left(\frac{ML^2}{12}\right)\omega$ ...(2)

As the collision is elastic, we have

$\frac{1}{2}mv^2 = \frac{1}{2}MV^2 + \frac{1}{2}I\omega^2$ ...(3)

Substituting the values, we get $m = M/4$

14. (b) So raw egg is like a spherical shell & hard bioled egg is like solid sphere. Let I_1, I_2 be M. I. of raw egg and boiled egg respectively.

Given that angular momentum L, is same

$\therefore I_1\omega_1 = I_2\omega_2 \Rightarrow \omega_2 > \omega_1 \because I_1 > I_2$

Now from first equation of angular motion ($\omega_f = \omega_i + \alpha t$) here α is retarding decceleration for both cases & $\omega_f = 0$ for both case.

So $\frac{t_1(\text{raw egg})}{t_2(\text{hard egg})} = \frac{\omega_1/\alpha}{\omega_2/\alpha} \Rightarrow \frac{t_1}{t_2} < 1$

15. (a) $E_r = \frac{1}{2}I\omega^2 = \frac{1}{2}\times 3\times(3)^3 = 13.5\,J$

$K.E. = \frac{1}{2}mv^2 = \frac{1}{2}\times 27\times v^2 = 13.5$

$v = 1\ m/s$

16. (c) Centripetal acceleration

$a_c = 4\pi^2 v^2 r = 4\pi^2\times 2\times 2\times 0.25 = 4\pi^2 ms^{-2}$

17. (c) $L = mvr$ or $v = L/mr$

Centripetal force $\frac{mv^2}{r} = \frac{m(L/mr)^2}{r} = \frac{L^2}{mr^3}$

18. (b) By energy conservation

$(K.E)_i + (P.E)_i = (K.E)_f + (P.E)_f$

$(K.E)_i = 0, (P.E)_i = mgh, (P.E)_f = 0$

$(K.E)_f = ½I\omega^2 + ½mv_{cm}^2$

Where I (moment of inertia) = ½mR²
(for solid cylinder)

so $mgh = ½(½mR^2)\left(\frac{v_{cm}^2}{R^2}\right) + ½mv_{cm}^2 \Rightarrow v_{cm} = \sqrt{4gh/3}$

19. (a) Tension provides the necessary centripetal force for the rest of rod.

20. (d) Centrifugal force is observed when the observer is in a frame undergoing circular motion.

21. (a) When $\theta = 0°$, the net force is directed vertically upwards.

22. (a)

23. (a) A couple consists of two equal and opposite forces whose lines of action are parallel and laterally separated by same distance. Therefore, net force (or resultant) of a couple is null vector, hence no translatory motion will be produced and only rotational motion will be produced.

24. (c) Since the spheres are smooth, there will be no transfer of angular momentum from the sphere A to sphere B. The sphere A only transfers its linear velocity v to the sphere B and will continue to rotate with the same angular speed ω.

25. (c) $\hat{n} = \frac{-(\hat{x}+\hat{y})}{\sqrt{2}}$

$-a\cos 45°\,\hat{x}$, $45°$, $\vec{a}$, $-a\sin 45°\,\hat{y}$

$\vec{a} = \frac{v^2}{r}\hat{n}$

$= \frac{4}{4}\times\frac{-(\hat{x}+\hat{y})}{\sqrt{2}}$

26. (d)

27. (b) $F = mr\omega^2 = 1\times\frac{1}{2}\times 4\pi^2\times 2\times 2 = 8\pi^2 N$

28. (d)

29. (c) At the highest point

$mg = mR4\pi^2 v^2 \Rightarrow v = \sqrt{\frac{g}{4\pi^2 R}}$

Revolution per minute $= 60v = \sqrt{\frac{900\,g}{\pi^2 R}}$

30. (d) $\mu mg = mr4\pi^2 v^2$

$\Rightarrow r_2 v_2^2 = r_1 v_1^2 \Rightarrow r_2 = \frac{r_1 v_1^2}{v_2^2} = \frac{r_1 v_1^2}{4v_1^2}$

$r_2 = \frac{r_1}{4} = 4\ cm$

31. (b) For no angular acceleration $\tau_{net} = 0$

$\Rightarrow F_1\times 5 = F_2\times 30$ (given $F_2 = 4N$) $\Rightarrow F_1 = 24N$

32. (c) $\frac{1}{2}I\omega^2$ = Loss of gravitational potental energy

$\frac{1}{2}\times\frac{ml^2}{3}\omega^2 = \frac{mgl}{2}(1+\cos\theta)$

$\Rightarrow \omega^2 = \frac{3g}{l}\left(2\cos^2\frac{\theta}{2}\right) \Rightarrow \omega = \sqrt{\frac{6g}{l}}\cos\frac{\theta}{2}$

33. (c) $E = \frac{1}{2}Mv^2 + \frac{1}{2}I\omega^2$

$= \frac{1}{2}Mv^2 + \frac{1}{2}\times\frac{2}{5}MR^2\times\frac{v^2}{R^2} = \frac{7}{10}Mv^2 = 0.7\ J$

34. (b) Use theorem of parallel axes.

35. (b) $I = 2\times 5\times(0.2)^2 + 2\times 2\times(0.4)^2 = 1kg\times m^2$

36. (c) Velocity of $P = (NP)\omega = (NM + MP)\omega$

$= r(r + \sin\theta)\omega = v(1+\sin\theta)$

37. (c) The velocity of the top point of the wheel is twice that of centre of mass. And the speed of centre of mass is same for both the wheels.

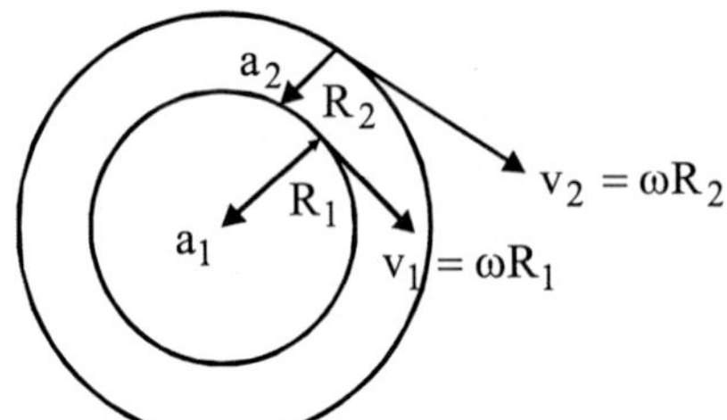

38. (c) $a_1 = \frac{v_1^2}{R_1} = \frac{\omega^2 R_1^2}{R_1} = \omega^2 R_1$

$a_2 = \frac{v_2^2}{R_2} = \omega^2 R_2$

Taking particle masses equal

$\frac{F_1}{F_2} = \frac{ma_1}{ma_2} = \frac{a_1}{a_2} = \frac{R_1}{R_2}$

39. (c) $m_1 d = m_2 d_2 \Rightarrow d_2 = \dfrac{m_1 d}{m_2}$

40. (d)

41. (d) Net work done by frictional force when drum rolls down without slipping is zero.

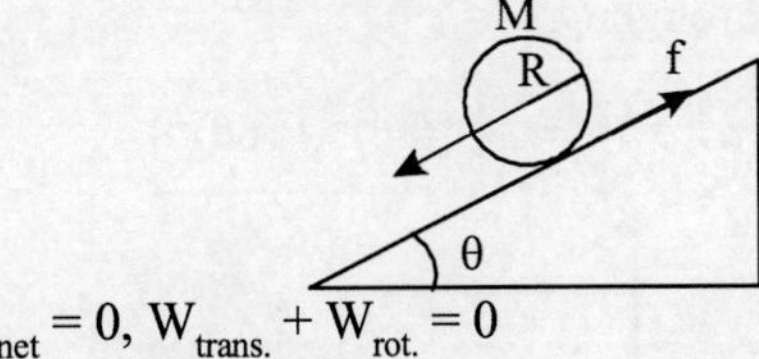

$W_{net} = 0,\ W_{trans.} + W_{rot.} = 0$
$\Delta K_{trans.} + \Delta K_{rot.} = 0$
$\Delta K_{trans} = -\Delta K_{rot}.$
i.e., converts translation energy to rotational energy.

42. (a) Tube may be treated as a particle of mass M at distance L/2 from one end.

Centripetal force $= Mr\omega^2 = \dfrac{ML}{2}\omega^2$

43. (a) When angular acceleration (α) is zero then torque on the wheel becomes zero.
$\theta(t) = 2t^3 - 6t^2$

$\Rightarrow \dfrac{d\theta}{dt} = 6t^2 - 12t \Rightarrow \alpha = \dfrac{d^2\theta}{dt^2} = 12t - 12 = 0$

$\therefore t = 1$ sec.

44. (a) According to parallel axis theorem of the moment of Inertia
$I = I_{cm} + md^2$
d is maximum for point B so I_{max} about B.

45. (b) $K = \dfrac{1}{2}I\omega^2 \Rightarrow K' = \dfrac{1}{2}\left(\dfrac{1}{2}\right)(2\omega)^2 = 2K$

46. (a) For complete disc with mass '4M', M.I. about given axis $= (4M)(R^2/2) = 2\,MR^2$

Hence, by symmetry, for the given quarter of the disc

M.I. $= 2\,MR^2/4 = \dfrac{1}{2}MR^2$

47. (b)

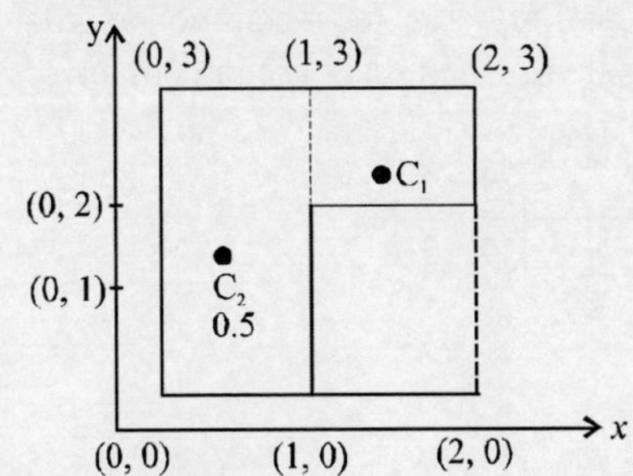

For given Lamina

$\quad\quad x\ \ y$
$m_1 = 1,\ C_1 = (1.5, 2.5)$
$m_2 = 3,\ C_2 = (0.5, 1.5)$

$X_{cm} = \dfrac{m_1x_1 + m_2x_2}{m_1 + m_2} = \dfrac{1.5 + 1.5}{4} = 0.75$

$Y_{cm} = \dfrac{m_1y_1 + m_2y_2}{m_1 + m_2} = \dfrac{2.5 + 4.5}{4} = 1.75$

$\therefore$ Coordinate of centre of mass of flag shaped lamina (0.75, 1.75)

48. (a) 49. (d)

50. (c) To produce maximum moment of force line of action of force must be perpendicular to line AB.

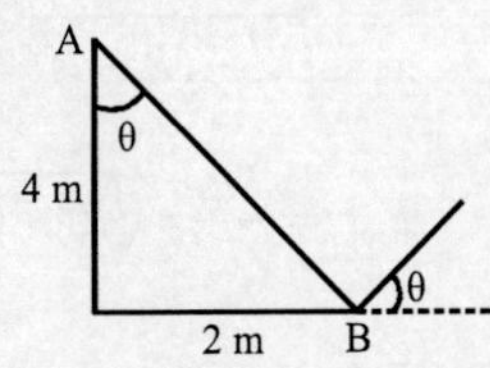

$\therefore \tan\theta = \dfrac{2}{4} = \dfrac{1}{2}$

51. (c) Free body diagram in the frame of disc

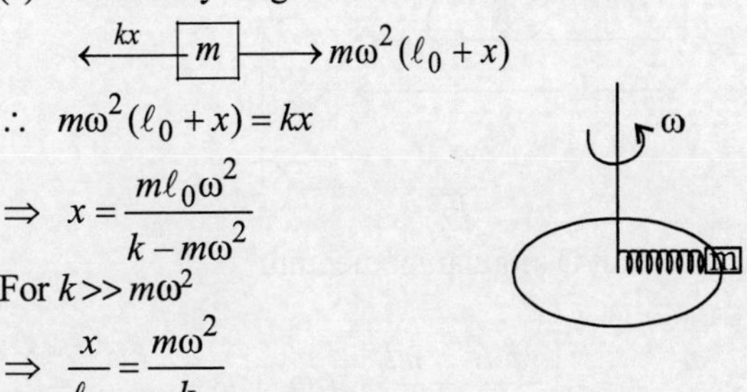

$\longleftarrow kx\ \boxed{m} \longrightarrow m\omega^2(\ell_0 + x)$

$\therefore\ m\omega^2(\ell_0 + x) = kx$

$\Rightarrow x = \dfrac{m\ell_0\omega^2}{k - m\omega^2}$

For $k >> m\omega^2$

$\Rightarrow \dfrac{x}{\ell_0} = \dfrac{m\omega^2}{k}$

52. (c) $m\omega^2R = \text{Force} \propto \dfrac{1}{R^n}$ (Force $= \dfrac{mv^2}{R}$)

$\Rightarrow \omega^2 \propto \dfrac{1}{R^{n+1}} \Rightarrow \omega \propto \dfrac{1}{R^{\frac{n+1}{2}}}$

Time period $T = \dfrac{2\pi}{\omega}$

Time period, $T \propto R^{\frac{n+1}{2}}$

53. (c) Angular momentum, $L = I\omega$

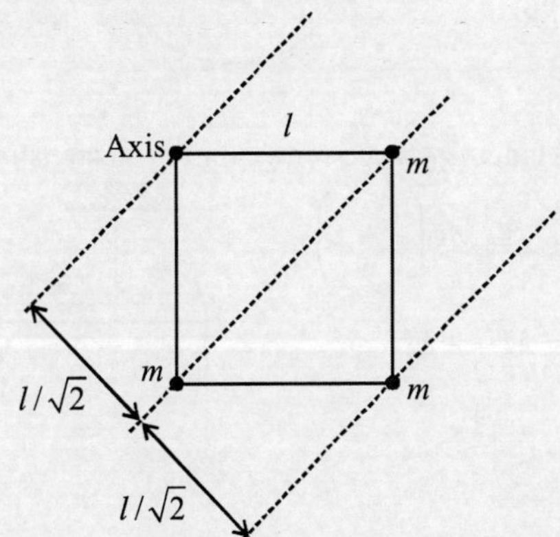

$I = m(0)^2 + m\left(\dfrac{l}{\sqrt{2}}\right)^2 \times 2 + m(\sqrt{2}l)^2$

$= \dfrac{2ml^2}{2} + 2ml^2 = 3ml^2$

Angular momentum $L = I\omega = 3ml^2\omega$

54. (a)

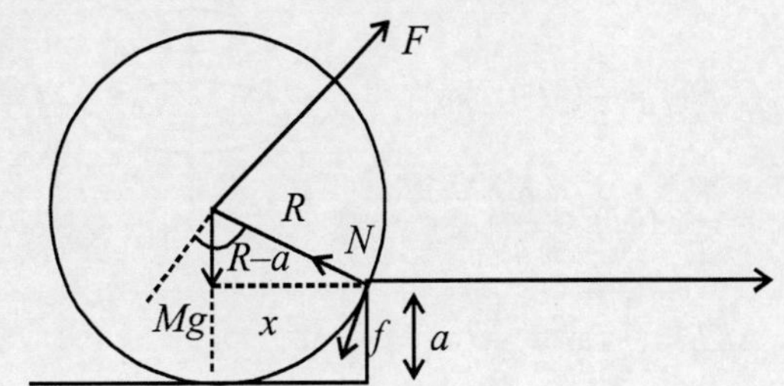

For step up, $F \times R \geq Mg \times x$

$x = \sqrt{R^2 - (R-a)^2}$ from figure

$$F_{\min} = \frac{Mg}{R} \times \sqrt{R^2 - (R-a)^2} = Mg\sqrt{1 - \left(\frac{R-a}{R}\right)^2}$$

55. (c)

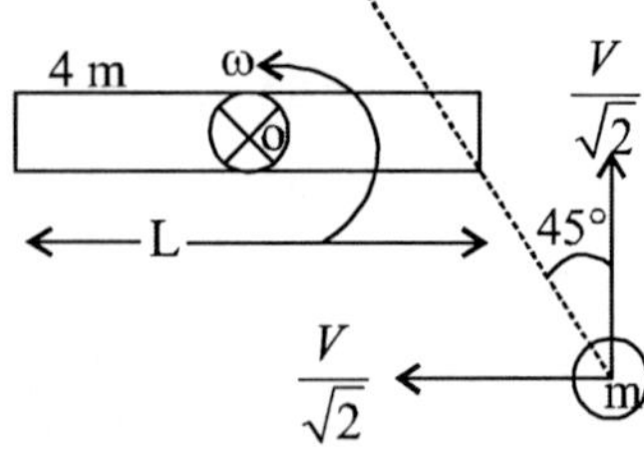

About point O angular momentum

$L_{\text{initial}} = L_{\text{final}}$

$$\Rightarrow \frac{mV}{\sqrt{2}} \times \frac{1}{2} = \left[\frac{4mL^2}{12} + \frac{mL^2}{4}\right] \times \omega \quad \therefore \omega = \frac{6V}{7\sqrt{2L}} = \frac{3\sqrt{2}V}{7L}$$

56. (a)

57. (d) Consider a strip of radius x and thickness dx,
Torque due to friction on this strip
Net torque = Σ Torque on ring

$$\int d\tau = \int_0^R \frac{\mu F.2\pi x dx}{\pi R^2}$$

$$\Rightarrow \tau = \frac{2\mu F}{R^2} \cdot \frac{R^3}{3}$$

$$\tau = \frac{2\mu FR}{3}$$

58. (d)

59. (a) Balancing torque w.r.t. point of suspension

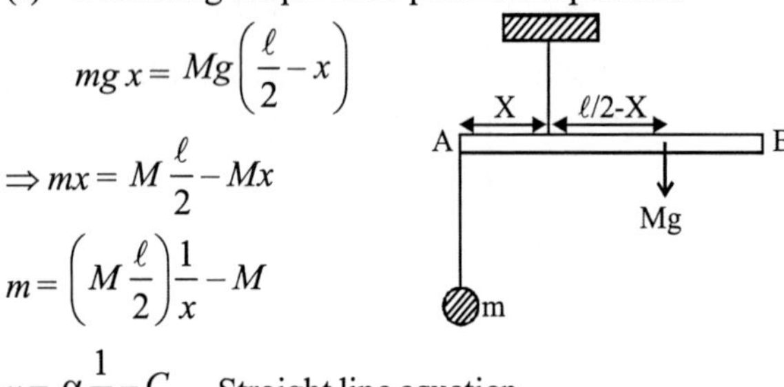

$$mg\,x = Mg\left(\frac{\ell}{2} - x\right)$$

$$\Rightarrow mx = M\frac{\ell}{2} - Mx$$

$$m = \left(M\frac{\ell}{2}\right)\frac{1}{x} - M$$

$y = \alpha\frac{1}{x} - C$ Straight line equation.

60. (a)

61. (d) By angular momentum conservation, $L_c = L_f$

$$\omega I + 3I \times 0 = 4I\omega' \Rightarrow \omega' = \frac{\omega}{4}$$

$$(KE)_i = \frac{1}{2}I\omega^2$$

$$(KE)_f = \frac{1}{2}(3I + I)\omega'^2$$

$$= \frac{1}{2} \times (4I) \times \left(\frac{\omega}{4}\right)^2 = \frac{I\omega^2}{8}$$

$$\Delta KE = \frac{1}{2}I\omega^2 - \frac{1}{8}I\omega^2 = \frac{3}{8}I\omega^2$$

$$\therefore \text{Fractional loss in K.E.} = \frac{\Delta KE}{KE_{I_i}} = \frac{\frac{3}{8}I\omega^2}{\frac{1}{2}I\omega^2} = \frac{3}{4}.$$

62. (b) Moment of inertia of rectangular sheet about an axis passing through O,

$$I_O = \frac{M}{12}(a^2 + b^2) = \frac{M}{12}[(80)^2 + (60)^2]$$

From the parallel axis theorem, moment of inertia about O',

$$I_{O'} = I_O + M(50)^2$$

$$\frac{I_O}{I_{O'}} = \frac{\frac{M}{12}(80^2 + 60^2)}{\frac{M}{12}(80^2 + 60^2) + M(50)^2} = \frac{1}{4}$$

63. (c)

64. (a) When the bob covered a distance 'h'

Using $mgh = \frac{1}{2}mv^2 + \frac{1}{2}I\omega^2$

$$= \frac{1}{2}m(\omega r)^2 + \frac{1}{2} \times \frac{mr^2}{2} \times \omega^2 \quad (\because v = \omega r \textit{ no slipping})$$

$$\Rightarrow \quad mgh = \frac{3}{4}m\omega^2 r^2 \Rightarrow \omega = \sqrt{\frac{4gh}{3r^2}} = \frac{1}{r}\sqrt{\frac{4gh}{3}}$$

65. (d) As no external torque is acting so angular momentum should be conserved
$(I_1 + I_2)\,\omega = I_1\omega_1 + I_2\omega_2$ [ω_c = common angular velocity of the system, when discs are in contact]

$$\omega_c = \frac{I_1\omega_1 + \frac{I_1\omega_1}{4}}{I_1 + \frac{I_1}{2}}\left(\frac{5}{4} \times \frac{2}{3}\right)\omega_1$$

$$\omega_c = \frac{5\omega_1}{6}$$

$$E_f - E_i = \frac{1}{2}(I_1 + I_2)\,\omega_c^2 - \frac{1}{2}I_1\omega_1^2 - \frac{1}{2}I_2\omega_2^2$$

Put $I_2 = I_1/2$ and $\omega_c = \frac{5\omega_1}{6}$ $5\omega_1/6$

We get :

$$E_f - E_i = -\frac{I_1\omega_1^2}{24}$$

66. (c) $I_i\omega_i = I_f\omega_f$

$$\text{or} \quad \left(\frac{ML^2}{12}\right)\omega_0 = \left(\frac{ML^2}{12} + 2m\left(\frac{L}{2}\right)^2\right)\omega_f$$

$\therefore \omega_f = \left(\frac{M\omega_0}{M+6m}\right)$

67. (c) Taking a circular ring of radius r and thickness dr as a mass element, so total mass,

$$M = \int_0^R \rho_0 r \times 2\pi r dr = \frac{2\pi\rho_0 R^3}{3}$$

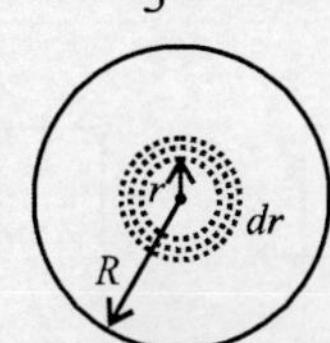

$$I_C = \int_0^R \rho_0 r \times 2\pi r dr \times r^2 = \frac{2\pi\rho_0 R^5}{5}$$

Using parallel axis theorem

$$\therefore\ I = I_C + MR^2 = 2\pi\rho_0 R^5\left(\frac{1}{3}+\frac{1}{5}\right) = \frac{16\pi\rho_0 R^5}{15}$$

$$= \frac{8}{5}\left[\frac{2}{3}\pi\rho_0 R^3\right]R^2 = \frac{8}{5}MR^2$$

68. (a) Let mass of the larger triangle = M

Side of larger triangle = ℓ

Moment of inertia of larger triangle = ma^2

Mass of smaller triangle = $\frac{M}{4}$

Length of smaller triangle = $\frac{\ell}{2}$

Moment of inertia of removed triangle

$$= \frac{M}{4}\left(\frac{a}{2}\right)^2 \qquad \therefore \frac{I_{removed}}{I_{original}} = \frac{\frac{M}{4}\cdot\left(\frac{a}{2}\right)^2}{M\cdot(a)^2}$$

$$I_{removed} = \frac{I_0}{16}$$

$$\text{So, } I = I_0 - \frac{I_0}{16} = \frac{15I_0}{16}$$

69. (d)

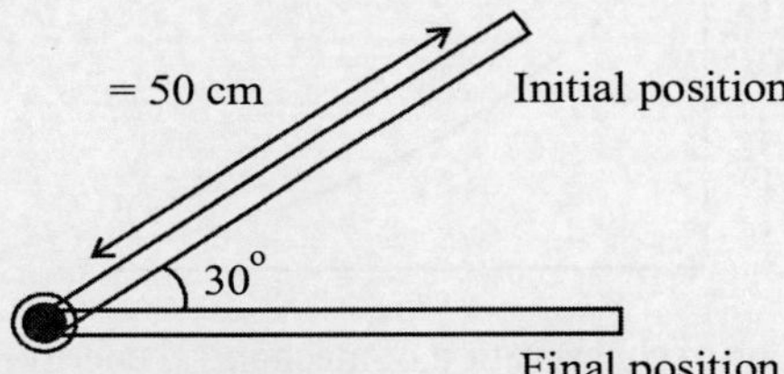

By the low of conservation of energy,

P.E. of rod = Rotational K.E.

$$mg\,\frac{\ell}{2}\,\text{Sin}\,\theta = \frac{1}{2}\,I\omega^2$$

$$\Rightarrow mg\frac{\ell}{2}\,\text{Sin}\,30° = \frac{1}{2}\,\frac{m\ell^2}{3}\omega^2 \quad \Rightarrow mg\frac{\ell}{2}\times\frac{1}{2} = \frac{1}{2}\frac{m\ell^2}{3}\omega^2$$

For complete length of rod,

$$\omega = \sqrt{3g/2(2\ell)} = \sqrt{\frac{30}{2}}\ \text{rod s}^{-1}$$

70. (d) Using parallel axes theorem, moment of inertia about 'O'

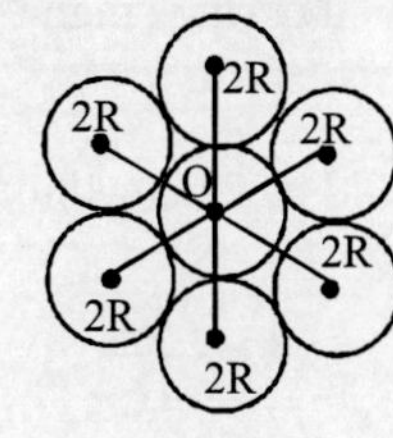

$$I_o = I_{cm} + md^2$$

$$= \frac{7MR^2}{2} + 6(M\times(2R)^2) = \frac{55MR^2}{2}$$

Again, moment of inertia about point P, $I_p = I_o + md^2$

$$= \frac{55MR^2}{2} + 7M(3R)^2 = \frac{181}{2}MR^2$$

71. (a)

72. (a) $K.E$ of the sphere = translational $K.E$ + rotational $K.E$

$$= \frac{1}{2}mv^2 + \frac{1}{2}I\omega^2$$

Where, I = moment of inertia,

ω = Angular, velocity of rotation

m = mass of the sphere

v = linear velocity of centre of mass of sphere

$\because$ Moment of inertia of sphere $I = \frac{2}{5}mR^2$

$$\therefore\ K.E = \frac{1}{2}mv^2 + \frac{1}{2}\times\frac{2}{5}mR^2\times\omega^2$$

$$\Rightarrow K.E = \frac{1}{2}mv^2 + \frac{1}{2}\times\frac{2}{5}mR^2\times\left(\frac{v}{R}\right)^2 \left(\because \omega = \frac{v}{R}\right)$$

$$\Rightarrow KE = \frac{1}{2}\left(\frac{2}{5}mR^2 + mR^2\right)\left(\frac{v}{R}\right)^2$$

$$\Rightarrow KE = \frac{1}{2}mR^2\times\frac{7}{5}\times\frac{v^2}{R^2} = \frac{7}{10}\times\frac{1}{2}\times\frac{25}{10^4}$$

$$\Rightarrow KE = \frac{35}{4}\times 10^{-4}\ \text{joule}$$

$\Rightarrow$ KE = 8.75×10^{-4} joule

73. (c) For sphere,

$$\frac{1}{2}mv^2 + \text{Iw}^2 = \frac{1}{2}mgh$$

$$\text{or}\quad \frac{1}{2}mv^2 + \frac{1}{2}\left(\frac{2}{5}mR^2\right)\frac{v^2}{R^2} = mgh \text{ or } h = \frac{7v^2}{10g}$$

For cylinder

$$\frac{1}{2}mv^2 + \frac{1}{2}\left(\frac{mR^2}{2}\right) = mgh'$$

$$\text{or}\quad h' = \frac{3v^2}{4g} \qquad \therefore \frac{h}{h'} = \frac{7v^2/10g}{3v^2/4g} = \frac{14}{15}$$

74. (Bonus) $mgh = \frac{1}{2}mv_{cm}^2 + \frac{1}{2}I_{cm}\omega^2$

$$= \frac{1}{2}mv_{cm}^2 + \frac{1}{2}I_{cm}\left(\frac{v_{cm}}{R}\right)^2 = \frac{1}{2}\left(m + \frac{I_{cm}}{R^2}\right)v_{cm}^2$$

For ring : mgh $=\frac{1}{2}\left(m+\frac{mR^2}{R^2}\right)v_{cm}^2 \therefore h=\frac{v_{cm}^2}{g}$.

For solid cylinder, $mgh=\frac{1}{2}\left(m+\frac{mR^2}{2R^2}\right)v_{cm}^2$

$\therefore h=\frac{3v_{cm}^2}{4g}$

For sphere, $mgh=\frac{1}{2}\left(m+\frac{2}{5}\frac{mR^2}{R^2}\right)v_{cm}^2$

$\therefore h=\frac{7v_{cm}^2}{10g}$

Ratio of heights $1:\frac{3}{4}:\frac{7}{10} \Rightarrow 20:15:14$

75. (c) As shown in the diagram, the normal reaction of AB on roller will shift towards O.
This will lead to tending of the system of cones to turn left.

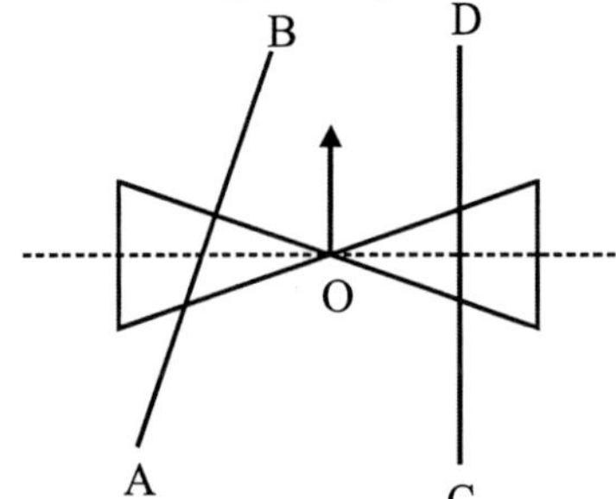

 Exercise 2 - Exemplar & Past Year Questions 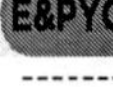

Exemplar Questions

1. (d) A bangle is in the form of a ring as shown in figure. The centre of mass of the ring lies at its centre, which is outside the ring or bangle.

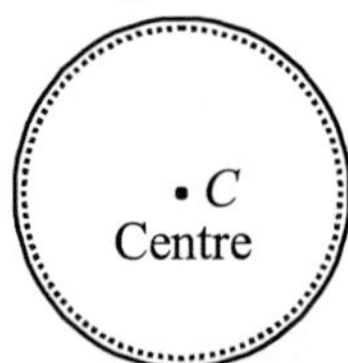

2. (c) Centre of mass of a system lies towards the part of the system, having bigger mass. In the above diagram, lower part is heavier, hence *CM* of the system lies below the horizontal diameter at C point.

3. (d) Angular acceleration $\alpha=\frac{d\omega}{dt}$
where ω is angular velocity of the disc and is uniform or constant.
$$\alpha=\frac{d\omega}{dt}=0$$
Hence, angular acceleration is zero.

4. (b) According to the question, when the small piece Q removed it is stick at P through axis of rotation passes, but axis of rotation does not passes through Q and It is glued to the centre of the plate, the mass comes closer to the z-axis, hence, moment of inertia decreases.

5. (c) Let us consider the diagram of problem 5, there is a line shown in the figure drawn along the diagonal. First, centre of mass of the system was on the dotted line and was shifted towards Q from the centre (1st quadrant).

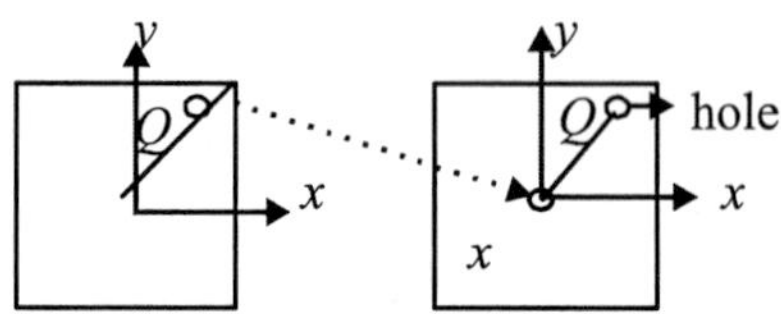

When the mass Q is decrease, it will be on the same line but shifted towards other side of Q on the line joining QPor away from the centre so, new CM will lies in IIIrd quadrant in x-y plane.

6. (a)

7. (a) As there is external torque acting on the system, angular momentum should be conserved.
Hence $I\omega$ = constant ...(i)
where, I is moment of inertia of the system and ω is angular velocity of the system.
From Eq. (i),
$I_1\omega_1=I_2\omega_2$
where ω_1 and ω_2 are angular velocities before and after jumping.
$(\because I=mr^2)$ So, given that,
$m_1=2M, m_2=M, \omega_1=\omega, \omega_2=?$
$r_1=r_2=R \quad m_1r_1^2\omega_1=m_2r_2^2\omega_2$
$2MR^2\omega=MR^2\omega_2$
as mass reduced to half, hence, moment of inertia also reduced to half.
$\omega_2=2\omega$

NEET/AIPMT (2013-2020) Questions

8. (c)

$\frac{3V^2}{4g}$ V

From law of conservation of mechanical energy

$$\frac{1}{2}I\omega^2+0+\frac{1}{2}mv^2=mg\times\frac{3v^2}{4g}$$

$$\Rightarrow \frac{1}{2}I\omega^2=\frac{3}{4}mv^2-\frac{1}{2}mv^2=\frac{mv^2}{2}\left(\frac{3}{2}-1\right)$$

or, $\frac{1}{2}I\frac{V^2}{R^2}=\frac{mv^2}{4}$ or, $I=\frac{1}{2}mR^2$

Hence, object is a disc.

9. (c) Given: $m_1 = 2\text{ kg}$ $m_2 = 4\text{ kg}$
$r_1 = 0.2\text{ m}$ $r_2 = 0.1\text{ m}$
$w_1 = 50\text{ rad s}^{-1}$ $w_2 = 200\text{ rad s}^{-1}$
As, $I_1W_1 = I_2W_2 = \text{Constant}$

$$\therefore W_f = \frac{I_1W_1 + I_2W_2}{I_1 + I_2} = \frac{\frac{1}{2}m_1r_1^2w_1 + \frac{1}{2}m_2r_2^2w_2}{\frac{1}{2}m_1r_1^2 + \frac{1}{2}m_2r_2^2}$$

By putting the value of m_1, m_2, r_1, r_2 and solving we get = 100 rad s^{-1}

10. (a) $\because I = MK^2 \therefore K = \sqrt{\frac{I}{M}}$

$I_{ring} = MR^2$ and $I_{disc} = \frac{1}{2}MR^2$

$$\frac{K_1}{K_2} = \sqrt{\frac{I_1}{I_2}} = \sqrt{\frac{MR^2}{\left(\frac{MR^2}{2}\right)}} = \sqrt{2}:1$$

11. (a) For solid sphere rolling without slipping on inclined plane, acceleration

$$a_1 = \frac{g\sin\theta}{1 + \frac{K^2}{R^2}}$$

For solid sphere slipping on inclined plane without rolling, acceleration
$a_2 = g\sin\theta$

Therefore required ratio $= \frac{a_1}{a_2}$

$$= \frac{1}{1 + \frac{K^2}{R^2}} = \frac{1}{1 + \frac{2}{5}} = \frac{5}{7}$$

12. (d) Here $\alpha = 2$ revolutions/s^2 $= 4\pi$ rad/s^2 (given)

$$I_{cylinder} = \frac{1}{2}MR^2 = \frac{1}{2}(50)(0.5)^2$$

$$= \frac{25}{4}\text{ Kg-m}^2$$

As $\tau = I\alpha$ so $TR = I\alpha$

$$\Rightarrow T = \frac{I\alpha}{R} = \frac{\left(\frac{25}{4}\right)(4\pi)}{(0.5)}\text{N} = 50\pi\text{N} = 157\text{ N}$$

13. (d) From Newton's second law for rotational motion,

$$\vec{\tau} = \frac{d\vec{L}}{dt}, \text{ if } \vec{L} = \text{constant then } \vec{\tau} = 0$$

So, $\vec{\tau} = \vec{r}\times\vec{F} = 0$

$$(2\hat{i} - 6\hat{j} - 12\hat{k})\times(\alpha\hat{i} + 3\hat{j} + 6\hat{k}) = 0$$

Solving we get $\alpha = -1$

14. (d) **Given :** Speed $V = 54\text{ kmh}^{-1} = 15\text{ ms}^{-1}$
Moment of inertia, $I = 3\text{ kgm}^2$
Time $t = 15s$

$$\omega_i = \frac{V}{r} = \frac{15}{0.45} = \frac{100}{3} \quad \omega_f = 0$$

$\omega_f = \omega_i + \alpha t$

$$0 = \frac{100}{3} + (-\alpha)(15) \Rightarrow \alpha = \frac{100}{45}$$

Average torque transmitted by brakes to the wheel

$$\tau = (I)(\alpha) = 3\times\frac{100}{45} = 6.66\text{ kgm}^2\text{s}^{-2}$$

15. (c) Moment of inertia of shell 1 along diameter

$$I_{diameter} = \frac{2}{3}MR^2$$

Moment of inertia of shell 2 = m. i of shell 3

$$= I_{tangential} = \frac{2}{3}MR^2 + MR^2 = \frac{5}{3}MR^2$$

So, I of the system along xx^1

$= I_{diameter} + (I_{tangential})\times 2$

$$\text{or,} \quad I_{total} = \frac{2}{3}MR^2 + \left(\frac{5}{3}MR^2\right)\times 2$$

$$= \frac{12}{3}MR^2 = 4MR^2$$

X
1
2 3
X′

16. (c)

17. (a) **Given:** Radius of disc, R = 50 cm
angular acceleration $\alpha = 2.0\text{ rads}^{-2}$; time t = 2s
Particle at periphery (assume) will have both radial (one) and tangential acceleration
$a_t = R\alpha = 0.5\times 2 = 1\text{ m/s}^2$
From equation,
$\omega = \omega_0 + \alpha t$
$\omega = 0 + 2\times 2 = 4$ rad/sec
$a_c = \omega^2R = (4)^2\times 0.5 = 16\times 0.5 = 8\text{m/s}^2$
Net acceleration,

$$a_{total} = \sqrt{a_t^2 + a_c^2} = \sqrt{1^2 + 8^2} \approx 8\text{ m/s}^2$$

18. (b)

19. (b) Given, mass of cylinder m = 3kg
R = 40 cm = 0.4 m
F = 30 N; α = ?
As we know, torque $\tau = I\alpha$
$F\times R = MR^2\alpha$

$$\alpha = \frac{F\times R}{MR^2}$$

$$\alpha = \frac{30\times(0.4)}{3\times(0.4)^2} \quad \text{or, } \alpha = 25\text{rad/s}^2$$

40 cm
F = 30 N

20. (c) Angular momentum, remains conserved until the torque acting on sphere remains zero. $\tau_{ex} = 0$

$$\text{So,} \quad \frac{dL}{dt} = 0$$

i.e., angular momentum L = constant.

21. (b) In rolling motion, rotational kinetic energy.

$K_t = \frac{1}{2}mv^2$

And, $K_t + K_r = \frac{1}{2}mv^2 + \frac{1}{2}I\omega^2$

$= \frac{1}{2}mv^2 + \frac{1}{2}\left(\frac{2}{5}mr^2\right)\left(\frac{v}{r}\right)^2 = \frac{7}{10}mv^2$

$\therefore \quad \frac{K_t}{K_t + K_r} = \frac{\frac{1}{2}mv^2}{\frac{7}{10}mv^2} = \frac{5}{7}$

22. (d) Let T_A and T_B are the time periods of particle A and B respectively. According to question,

$T_A = T_B = T$

If ω_A and ω_B are their angular speeds, then

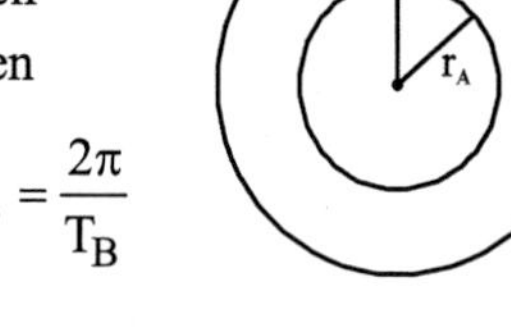

$\omega_A = \frac{2\pi}{T_A}$ and $\omega_B = \frac{2\pi}{T_B}$

$\therefore \quad \frac{\omega_A}{\omega_B} = \frac{T_B}{TA} = \frac{T}{T} = 1:1$

23. (a) According to the Work-energy theorem,

$W = \frac{1}{2}I\left(\omega_f^2 - \omega_i^2\right)$

Given that,

$\theta = 2\pi$ revolution/minute

$\theta = 2\pi \times 2\pi = 4\pi^2$ rad

$\omega_i = 3 \times \frac{2\pi}{60}$ rad / s

$\omega_f = 0$ rad/s

Putting the values of ω_f and ω_i we get

$\Rightarrow \; -\tau\theta = \frac{1}{2} \times \frac{1}{2}mr^2\left(0^2 - \omega_i^2\right)$

$\Rightarrow \; -\tau = \frac{\frac{1}{2} \times \frac{1}{2} \times 2 \times \left(4 \times 10^{-2}\right)\left(-3 \times \frac{2\pi}{60}\right)^2}{4\pi^2}$

$\Rightarrow \tau = 2 \times 10^{-6}$ N-m

24. (a) Work done to stop the disc = change in total kinetic energy of disc

Final KE = 0

Initial KE = Translational K.E. + Rotational K.E.

$= \frac{1}{2}mv^2 + \frac{1}{2}I\omega^2$

$= \frac{1}{2}mv^2 + \frac{1}{2} \times \frac{mR^2}{2} \times \left(\frac{v}{R}\right)^2 = \frac{1}{2}mv^2 + \frac{1}{4}mv^2 = \frac{3}{4}mv^2$

$= \frac{3}{4} \times 100 \times (20 \times 10^{-2})^2 = 3J$

$|\Delta KE| = 3J$

25. (a) Kinetic energy at the bottom

$= \frac{1}{2}mv_0^2 + \frac{1}{2}I\omega^2 = \frac{3}{4}mv_0^2$

As $I_{\text{solid cylinder}} = \frac{1}{2}MR^2$ and $V = R\omega$

From work – energy theorem

$\frac{3}{4}mv_0^2 = mgh = mgd\sin\theta$

$d = \frac{\frac{3}{4}mv_0^2}{mg\sin\theta}$

$\Rightarrow d = \frac{3}{4}\frac{v_0^2}{g\sin\theta} = \frac{3}{4} \cdot \frac{16}{10 \times 1/2} = 2.4$ m

26. (b)

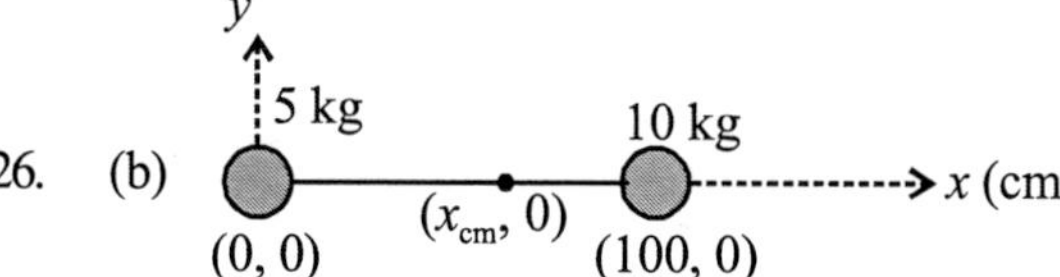

Centre of mass of a system of two particles of masses m_1 and m_2 having position vectors $\overrightarrow{x_1}$ and $\overrightarrow{x_2}$ is

$x_{cm} = \frac{m_1x_1 + m_2x_2}{m_1 + m_2}$

Taking particle of mass 5 kg at origin.

$\Rightarrow x_{cm} = \frac{5 \times 0 + 100 \times 10}{5 + 10} = \frac{200}{3} = 66.66$ cm

$\Rightarrow x_{cm} = 67$ cm

27. (b) Given :

Force, $\vec{F} = 3\hat{j}$ N

Position vector, $\vec{r} = 2\hat{k}$ m

Torque, $\vec{\tau} = \vec{r} \times \vec{F} = 2\hat{k} \times 3\hat{j} = 6(\hat{k} \times \hat{j}) = 6(-\hat{i})$

$\Rightarrow \vec{\tau} = -6\hat{i}$ Nm

Exercise 3 - Concept Application Problems CAP

1. (b) Since no external torque act on gymnast, so angular momentum (L=I ω) is conserved. After pulling her arms & legs, the angular velocity increases but moment of inertia of gymnast, decreases in, such a way that angular momentum remains constant.

2. (b) α is propotional to ω

Let $\alpha = k\omega$ $\quad$ ($\because$ k is a constant)

$\frac{d\omega}{dt} = k\omega$ $\quad$ [also $\frac{d\theta}{dt} = \omega \Rightarrow dt = \frac{d\theta}{\omega}$]

$\therefore \frac{\omega d\omega}{d\theta} = k\omega \Rightarrow d\omega = kd\theta$

Now $\int_{\omega}^{\omega/2} d\omega = k\int d\theta$

$\int_{\omega/2}^{0} d\omega = k\int_0^{\theta} d\theta \Rightarrow -\frac{\omega}{2} = k\theta \Rightarrow -\frac{\omega}{2} = k\theta_1$

($\because \theta_1 = 2\pi n$)

$\therefore\ \theta = \theta_1$ or $2\pi n_1 = 2\pi n$

$n_1 = n$

3. (c) For solid sphere

$$I = \frac{2}{5}MR^2 = \frac{2}{5}\left(\frac{4}{3}\pi R^3 \rho\right)R^2$$

$$= \frac{8}{15} \times \frac{22}{7} R^5 \rho = \frac{176}{105} R^5 \rho$$

4. (b) From the theorem of parallel axes, the moment of inertia $I = I_{CM} + Ma^2$
where I_{CM} is moment of inertia about centre of mass and a is the distance of axis from centre.
$mk^2 = m(k^1)^2 + m(6)^2$
($\because I = mk^2$ where k is radius of gyration)
or, $k^2 = (k^1)^2 + 36$
or, $100 = (k^1)^2 + 36 \Rightarrow (k^1)^2 = 64$ cm $\quad \therefore k^1 = 8$ cm

5. (b) Since v is changing (decreasing), L is not conserved in magnitude. Since it is given that a particle is confined to rotate in a circular path, it can not have spiral path. Since the particle has two accelerations a_c and a_t therefore the net acceleration is not towards the centre.

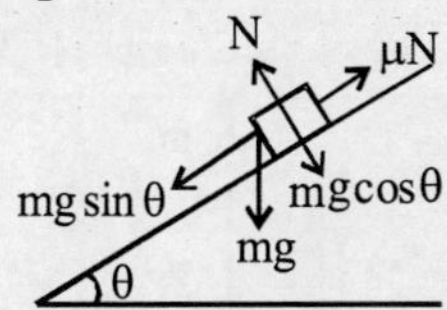

The direction of $\vec{L}$ remains same even when the speed decreases.

6. (a) Remember that acceleration of a cylinder down a smooth inclined plane is

N μN mg sin θ mgcosθ mg θ

$$a = \frac{g\sin\theta}{\left(1 + \frac{I}{mR^2}\right)} \text{ where } I = \frac{mR^2}{2} \text{ is the moment of Inertia}$$

for cylinder

$$a = \frac{g \sin 30°}{\left(1 + \frac{mR^2}{2} \times \frac{1}{mR^2}\right)} = \frac{g \times \frac{1}{2}}{1 + \frac{1}{2}} = \frac{g}{3}$$

7. (a) (12 amu) ← 1.12×10^{-10} → (16 amu)
C c.m. O
← d → ← $1.12\times10^{-10} - d$ →

From definition of centre of mass.

$$d = \frac{16 \times 1.12 \times 10^{-10} + 12 \times 0}{16 + 12} = \frac{16 \times 1.12 \times 10^{-10}}{28}$$

$= 0.64 \times 10^{-10}$ m.

8. (b) Density of iron > density of aluminium

moment of inertia $= \int r^2 dm$.

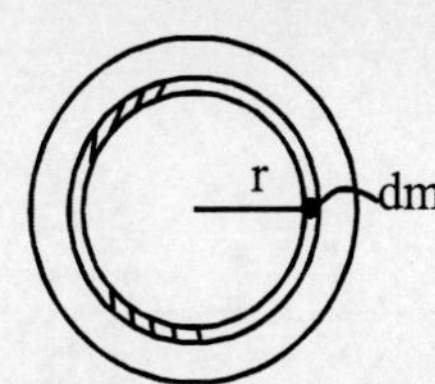

$\therefore$ Since $\rho_{iron} > \rho_{aluminium}$
so whole of aluminium is kept in the core and the iron at the outer rim of the disc.

9. (d) Rotational energy $= \frac{1}{2}I(\omega)^2 = \frac{1}{2}(mK^2)\omega^2$

Linear kinetic energy $= \frac{1}{2}m\omega^2R^2$

$\therefore$ Required fraction

$$= \frac{\frac{1}{2}(mK^2)\omega^2}{\frac{1}{2}(mK^2)\omega^2 + \frac{1}{2}m\omega^2R^2} = \frac{K^2}{K^2 + R^2}$$

10. (d) Use $\tau = I\alpha$

and $\omega^2 - \omega_0^2 = 2\alpha\theta$ Here $I = \frac{2}{5}MR^2$

Given $M = 2000g = 2kg$
$R = 5cm = 5 \times 10^{-2}m$
$\theta = 2\pi \times 2\pi$ radians
$n = 300$ rpm $= 5$ rps

$$\therefore\ \tau = I\alpha = = \left(\frac{2}{5}MR^2\right)\left(\frac{\omega^2 - \omega_0^2}{2\theta}\right)$$

$$= \frac{2}{5} \times 2 \times \left(5 \times 10^{-2}\right)^2 \frac{4\pi^2\left(5^2 - 0^2\right)}{2 \times 4\pi^2}$$

$= 0.025$ N – m. $= 2.5 \times 10^5$ dyne cm.

11. (d) $\alpha = \frac{\omega_2 - \omega_1}{t_2 - t_1}$

$$\omega_1 = \frac{2\pi \times 1200}{60} = 40\pi\ ;\ \omega_2 = \frac{2\pi \times 4500}{60} = 150\pi$$

$$\alpha = \frac{110\pi}{10} \text{ rad/sec}^2$$

Now, π radian $= 180°$

$$\therefore\ 1 \text{ rad} = \frac{180}{\pi} \text{ degree}$$

$$\therefore\ \alpha = \frac{11\pi \times 180}{\pi} \text{ degree/sec}^2 = 1980 \text{ degree/sec}^2$$

12. (b) $E = 1500 = 1/2 \times 1.2\,\omega^2$

$$\omega^2 = \frac{3000}{1.2} = 2500$$

$\omega = 50$ rad/sec

$$t = \frac{\omega}{\alpha} = \frac{50}{25} = 2 \text{ sec}$$

13. (c) M.I. of a uniform circular disc of radius 'R' and mass 'M' about an axis passing through C.M. and normal to the disc is

$I_{C.M.} = \frac{1}{2} MR^2$

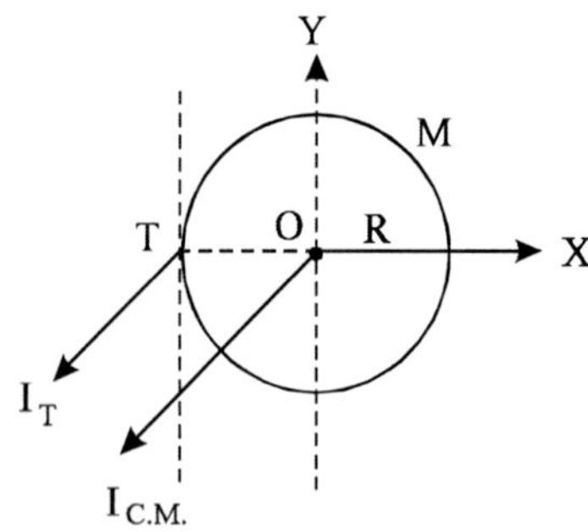

From parallel axis theorem

$I_T = I_{C.M.} + MR^2 = \frac{1}{2}MR^2 + MR^2 = \frac{3}{2}MR^2$

14. (d) $K = \frac{L^2}{2I} \Rightarrow L^2 = 2KI \Rightarrow L = \sqrt{2KI}$

$\frac{L_1}{L_2} = \sqrt{\frac{K_1}{K_2} \cdot \frac{I_1}{I_2}} = \sqrt{\frac{K}{K} \cdot \frac{I}{2I}} = \frac{1}{\sqrt{2}}$

$L_1 : L_2 = 1 : \sqrt{2}$

15. (b) By theorem of parallel axes,
$I = I_{cm} + Md^2$
$I = I_0 + M(L/2)^2 = I_0 + ML^2/4$

16. (b)

17. (d)

2.5 kg (0, 4); 4 cm; 5 cm; 1.0 kg (0, 0); 3 cm; 1.5 kg (3, 0)

$$X_{cm} = \frac{m_1x_1 + m_2x_2 + m_3x_3}{m_1 + m_2 + m_3}$$

$$X_{cm} = \frac{1\times 0 + 1.5\times 3 + 2.5\times 0}{1 + 1.5 + 2.5} = \frac{1.5\times 3}{5} = 0.9cm$$

$$Y_{cm} = \frac{m_1y_1 + m_2y_2 + m_3y_3}{m_1 + m_2 + m_3}$$

$$Y_{cm} = \frac{1\times 0 + 1.5\times 0 + 2.5\times 4}{1 + 1.5 + 2.5} = \frac{2.5\times 4}{5} = 2cm$$

Hence, centre of mass of system is at point (0.9, 2)

18. (a) Acceleration of centre of mass (a_{cm}) is given by

$$\therefore \vec{a}_{cm} = \frac{m_1\vec{a}_1 + m_2\vec{a}_2 + ...}{m_1 + m_2 + ...}$$

$$= \frac{(2m)a\hat{j} + 3m\times a\hat{i} + ma(-\hat{i}) + 4m\times a(-\hat{j})}{2m + 3m + 4m + m}$$

$$= \frac{2a\hat{i} - 2a\hat{j}}{10} = \frac{a}{5}(\hat{i} - \hat{j})$$

19. (a) $y = 4Cx^2 \Rightarrow \frac{dy}{dx} = \tan\theta = 8Cx$

At P, $\tan\theta = 8Ca$

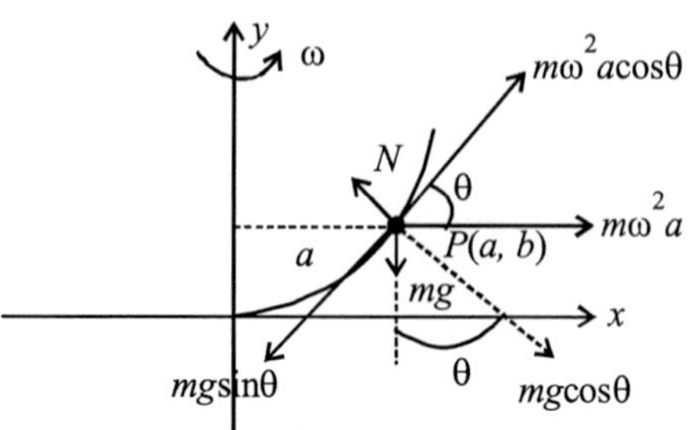

For steady circular motion

$m\omega^2 a\cos\theta = mg\sin\theta$

$\Rightarrow \omega = \sqrt{\frac{g\tan\theta}{a}}$ $\therefore \omega = \sqrt{\frac{g\times 8aC}{a}} = 2\sqrt{2gC}$

20. (b) At elongated position (x),

$F_{radial} = \frac{mv^2}{r} = mr\omega^2$

$\therefore kx = m(\ell + x)\omega^2$

$(\because r = \ell + x$ here)

ω; kx; m; $(\ell + x)$

$kx = m\ell\omega^2 + mx\omega^2$ $\therefore x = \frac{m\ell\omega^2}{k - m\omega^2}$

21. (a) Using $v^2 = u^2 + 2gy$ $[\therefore u = 0$ at $(0,0)]$
$v^2 = 2gy$ $[\therefore v = \omega x]$

Y; ω; ⇒; y; X; (0,0)

$$\Rightarrow y = \frac{\omega^2x^2}{2g} = \frac{(2\times 2\pi)^2\times(0.05)^2}{20} \simeq 2cm$$

22. (d) Net torque, τ_{net} about B is zero at equilibrium

$\therefore T_A \times 100 - mg\times 50 - 2mg\times 25 = 0$

$\Rightarrow T_A \times 100 = 100mg$

$\Rightarrow T_A = 1mg$ (Tension in the string at A)

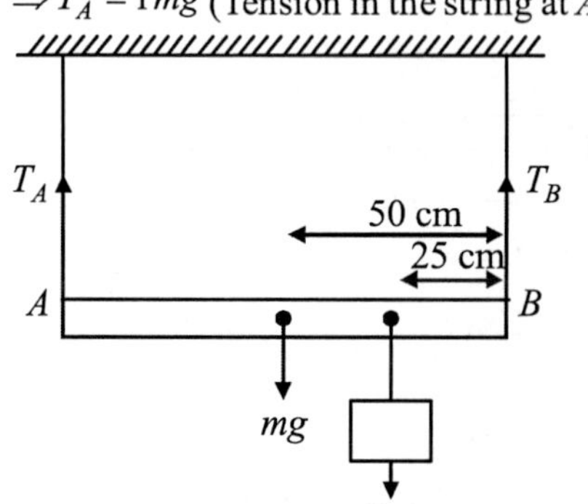

23. (b) Given that, $x = x_0 + a\cos\omega_1 t$
$y = y_0 + b\sin\omega_2 t$

$\frac{dx}{dt} = V_x$

$\Rightarrow v_x = -a\omega_1 \sin(\omega_1 t)$, and $\frac{dy}{dt} = v_y = b\omega_2 \cos(\omega_2 t)$

$\frac{dv_x}{dt} = a_x = -a\omega_1^2 \cos(\omega_1 t)$, $\frac{dv_y}{dt} = a_y = -b\omega_2^2 \sin(\omega_2 t)$

At $t = 0$, $x = x_0 + a$, $y = y_0$

$a_x = -a\omega_1^2$, $a_y = 0$

Now, $\vec{\tau} = \vec{r} \times \vec{F} = m(\vec{r} \times \vec{a})$

$= [(x_0 + a)\hat{i} + y_0\hat{j}] \times m(-a\omega_1^2\hat{i}) = +my_0 a\omega_1^2\hat{k}$

24. (d) We have given $\vec{r} = 2t\hat{i} - 3t^2\hat{j}$

$\vec{r}(\text{at } t = 2) = 4\hat{i} - 12\hat{j}$

Velocity, $\vec{v} = \frac{d\vec{r}}{dt} = 2\hat{i} - 6t\hat{j}$

$\vec{v}(\text{at } t = 2) = 2\hat{i} - 12\hat{j}$

$\vec{L} = mvr\sin\theta\hat{n} = m(\vec{r} \times \vec{v})$

$= 2(4\hat{i} - 12\hat{j}) \times (2\hat{i} - 12\hat{j}) = -48\hat{k}$

25. (d) Angular acceleration,

$$\alpha = \frac{\omega - \omega_0}{t} = \frac{25 \times 2\pi - 0}{5} = 10\,\pi\,\text{rad/s}^2$$

$\tau = I\alpha$

$$\Rightarrow \tau = \left(\frac{5}{4}mR^2\right)\alpha \approx \left(\frac{5}{4}\right)(5 \times 10^{-3})(10^{-4})10\pi$$

$= 2.0 \times 10^{-5}$ Nm

26. (a) Torque about the origin = $\vec{\tau} = \vec{r} \times \vec{F}$

$= r\,F\sin\theta \Rightarrow 2.5 = 1 \times 5\sin\theta$

$\sin\theta = 0.5 = \frac{1}{2} \Rightarrow \theta = \frac{\pi}{6}$

27. (a) Applying torque equation about point P.

$\tau = I\alpha = [2M_0(2\ell)^2 + 5M_0\ell^2]\alpha$

$\Rightarrow 5M_0 g\ell - 4M_0 g\ell = [2M_0(2\ell)^2 + 5M_0\ell^2]\alpha$

$\Rightarrow M_0 g\ell = (13M_0 g\ell^2)\alpha$

$\therefore \alpha = \frac{g}{13\ell}$

28. (d) 29. (b)

30. (c) Let p be the density of the discs and t is the thickness of discs.

Moment of inertia of disc is given by

$$I = \frac{MR^2}{2} = \frac{[\rho(\pi R^2)t]R^2}{2}$$

$I \propto R^4$ (As ρ and t are same)

$$\frac{I_2}{I_1} = \left(\frac{R_2}{R_1}\right)^4 \Rightarrow \frac{16}{1} = \alpha^4 \Rightarrow \alpha = 2$$

31. (a)

32. (c) Moment inertia of the rod passing through a point $\frac{\ell}{4}$ away from the centre of the rod

$I = Ig + m\ell^2$

$$\Rightarrow I = \frac{MI^2}{12} + M \times \left(\frac{I^2}{16}\right) = \frac{7MI^2}{48}$$

Using $I = MK^2 = \frac{7MI^2}{48}$ (K = radius of gyration)

$\Rightarrow K = \sqrt{\frac{7}{48}}I$

33. (a) Given,

mass per unit area of circular disc, $\sigma = A + Br$

Area of the ring = $2\,\pi r dr$

Mass of the ring, $dm = \sigma 2\pi r dr$

Moment of inertia,

$I = \int dmr^2 = \int \sigma 2\pi r dr.r^2$

$$\Rightarrow I = 2\pi\int_0^a (A + Br)r^3 dr = 2\pi\left[\frac{Aa^4}{4} + \frac{Ba^5}{5}\right]$$

$$\Rightarrow I = 2\pi a^4\left[\frac{A}{4} + \frac{Ba}{5}\right]$$

34. (c) $I = \int_a^b (dm)r^2$

$$= \int_a^b \left(\frac{\sigma_0}{r} \times 2\pi r\,dr\right)r^2 = \frac{2\pi\sigma_0}{3}|\,r^3\,|_a^b$$

$$= \frac{2\pi\sigma_0}{3}(b^3 - a^3)$$

Mass of the disc,

$$m = \int_a^b \frac{\sigma_0}{r} \times 2\pi r\,dr = 2\pi\sigma_0(b - a)$$

Radius of gyration,

$$k = \sqrt{\frac{I}{m}} = \sqrt{\frac{(2\pi\sigma_0/3)(b^3 - a^3)}{2\pi\sigma_0(b - a)}} = \sqrt{\frac{a^2 + b^2 + ab}{3}}$$

35. (b) As from the question density $(\sigma) = kr^2$

$$\text{Mass of disc } M = \int_0^R (kr^2)2\pi r dr = 2\pi k\frac{R^4}{4} = \frac{\pi kR^4}{2}$$

$$\Rightarrow k = \frac{2M}{\pi R^4} \quad \text{....(i)}$$

$\therefore$ Moment of inertia about the axis of the disc.

$I = \int dI = \int (dm)r^2 = \int \sigma dAr^2$

$= \int (kr^2)(2\pi r dr)r^2$

$$= \int_0^R 2\pi k\, r^5 dr = \frac{\pi k R^6}{3} = \frac{\pi \times \left(\frac{2M}{\pi R^4}\right) \times R^6}{3} = \frac{2}{3} MR^2$$

[putting value of k from eqn ....(i)]

36. (b)

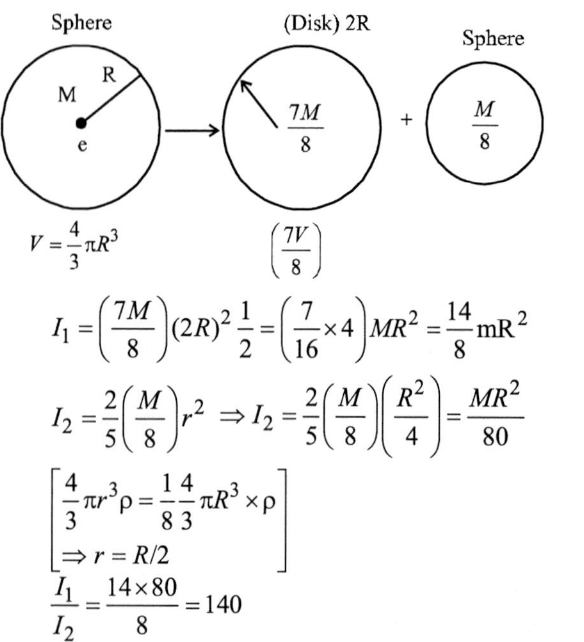

$$I_1 = \left(\frac{7M}{8}\right)(2R)^2 \frac{1}{2} = \left(\frac{7}{16} \times 4\right) MR^2 = \frac{14}{8} mR^2$$

$$I_2 = \frac{2}{5}\left(\frac{M}{8}\right) r^2 \Rightarrow I_2 = \frac{2}{5}\left(\frac{M}{8}\right)\left(\frac{R^2}{4}\right) = \frac{MR^2}{80}$$

$$\left[\begin{array}{l} \frac{4}{3}\pi r^3 \rho = \frac{1}{8}\frac{4}{3}\pi R^3 \times \rho \\ \Rightarrow r = R/2 \end{array}\right]$$

$$\frac{I_1}{I_2} = \frac{14 \times 80}{8} = 140$$

37. (d) $\frac{1}{2} I\omega^2 = kQ^2$

or $\omega = \left(\sqrt{\frac{2k}{I}}\right) Q$ or $\alpha = \frac{d\omega}{\pi} = \sqrt{\frac{2K}{I}}\left(\frac{dQ}{dt}\right) = \left(\sqrt{\frac{2k}{I}}\right)\omega$

$$= \left(\sqrt{\frac{2k}{I}}\right)\left(\sqrt{\frac{2k}{I}}\right)\theta = \frac{2k\theta}{I}$$

38. (b) $\omega = \alpha t = 20t$

Given, $\frac{1}{2} I\omega^2 = 1200$

or $\frac{1}{2} \times 1.5 \times (20t)^2 = 1200$ or $t = 2$ s

39. (b)

40. (d) According to parallel axes theorem

$$I = \frac{2}{5} mR^2 + mx^2$$

Hence graph (d) correctly depicts I vs x.

41. (b)

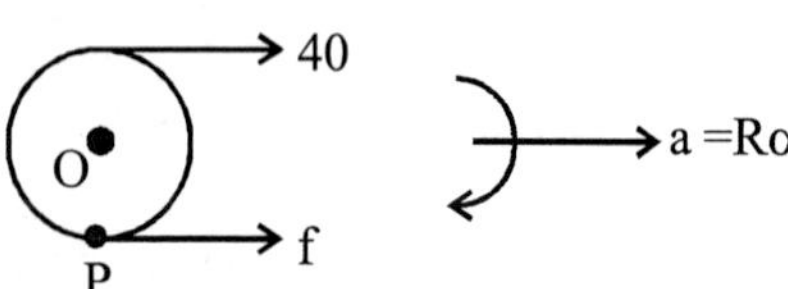

From newton's second law

$40 + f = m(R\alpha)$ .....(i)

Taking torque about 0 we get

$40 \times R - f \times R = I\alpha$

$40 \times R - f \times R = mR^2 \alpha$

$40 - f = mR\alpha$ ...(ii)

Solving equation (i) and (ii)

$$\alpha = \frac{40}{mR} = 16 \text{ rad/s}^2$$

42. (b) Moment of inertia of disc D_1 about $OO' = I_1 = \frac{MR^2}{2}$

M.O.I of D_2 about OO'

$$= I_2 = \frac{1}{2}\left(\frac{MR^2}{2}\right) + MR^2 = \frac{MR^2}{4} + MR^2$$

M.O.I of D_3 about OO'

$$= I_3 = \frac{1}{2}\left(\frac{MR^2}{2}\right) + MR^2 = \frac{MR^2}{4} + MR^2$$

so, resultant M.O.I about OO' is $I = I_1 + I_2 + I_3$

$$\Rightarrow I = \frac{MR^2}{2} + 2\left(\frac{MR^2}{4} + MR^2\right)$$

$$= \frac{MR^2}{2} + \frac{MR^2}{2} + 2MR^2 = 3\,MR^2$$

43. (a) For Ball

using parallel axes theorem, for ball moment of inertaia,

$$I_{ball} = \frac{2}{5} MR^2 + M(2R)^2 = \frac{22}{5} MR^2$$

For two balls $I_{balls} = 2 \times \frac{22}{5} MR^2$=and,

$$Irod = \frac{M(2R)^2}{12} = \frac{MR^2}{3}$$

$$I_{system} = I_{balls} + I_{rod}$$

$$= \frac{44}{5} MR^2 + \frac{MR^2}{3} = \frac{137}{15} MR^2$$

44. (c) As we know, moment of inertia of a disc about an axis passing through C.G. and perpendicular to its plane,

$$I_z = \frac{mR^2}{2}$$

Moment of inertia of a disc about a tangential axis perpendicular to its own plane,

$$I_z' = \frac{3}{2} mR^2$$

q q r

$$\therefore \quad I_z / I_z' = \frac{mR^2}{2} \Big/ \frac{3mR^2}{2} = 1/3$$

45. (a) When the rod makes an angle α

Displacement of centre of mass $= \frac{l}{2}\cos\alpha$

$$mg\frac{l}{2}\cos\alpha = \frac{1}{2} I\omega^2$$

$mg\frac{l}{2}\cos\alpha = \frac{ml^2}{6}\omega^2$ ($\because$ M.I. of thin uniform rod about an axis passing through its centre of mass and perpendicular to the rod $I = \frac{ml^2}{12}$)

$$\Rightarrow \quad \omega = \sqrt{\frac{3g\cos\alpha}{l}}$$

Speed of end $= \omega \times l = \sqrt{3g\cos\alpha l}$

i.e., Speed of end, $\omega \propto \sqrt{\cos\alpha}$

8 Gravitation

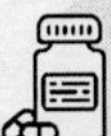

Topic 8.1 : Newton's Universal Law of Gravitation and Acceleration due to Gravity

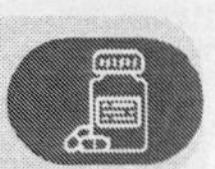

NEWTON'S UNIVERSAL LAW OF GRAVITATION

Gravitational force is an attractive force between any two point masses M_1 and M_2 separated by any distance r.

It is given by $F = G\left(\frac{M_1M_2}{r^2}\right)$

where G is the **universal gravitational constant.**

Its value, $G = 6.67 \times 10^{-11}\ Nm^2\ kg^{-2}$

Dimensions of G are $[M^{-1} L^3 T^{-2}]$

(a) The gravitational force is the central force and follows inverse square law. It acts along the line joining the particles.

(b) Since the work done by the gravitational force is independent of the path followed and hence it is a conservative force.

(c) It is the weakest force in nature. It is 10^{38} times smaller than nuclear force and 10^{36} times smaller than electric force. Strongest force being nuclear force (for small range) followed by electric force.

(d) Gravitation is independent of the presence of other bodies around it.

ACCELERATION DUE TO GRAVITY (g)

The force of attraction exerted by earth on a body of mass m is the force of gravity.

So the force of gravity from Newton's gravitational law is

$$F = \frac{GM_e m}{r^2} \quad ......(i)$$

where M_e = mass of earth

r = distance of the body from the centre of earth.

The force of gravity can be written as F = mg ......(ii)

where g is called the **acceleration due to gravity.**

From the expression (i) and (ii), we get

$$g = \frac{GM_e}{r^2} \quad ...(iii)$$

If body is located at the surface of earth i.e., r = R_e (radius of earth) then

$$g = \frac{GM_e}{R_e^2} = \frac{G(4/3\pi R_e^3 \rho)}{R_e^2} = \frac{4}{3}\pi\rho G R_e \quad ...(iv)$$

where ρ is the density of earth.

This is the relation between universal gravitational constant 'G' and acceleration due to gravity 'g'.

Change in the Value of Acceleration due to Gravity (g)

(i) ***Due to rotation or latitude of earth :*** Let us consider a particle P at rest on the surface of earth at a latitude ϕ.

$$g(\phi) = g - R_e\omega^2 \cos^2 \phi$$

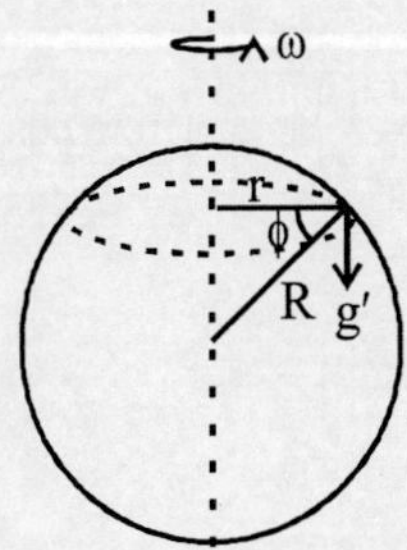

At poles ϕ = 90°, so g(ϕ) = g ...(v)

At equator ϕ = 0° so g(ϕ) = g – $\omega^2 R_e$ ...(vi)

(ii) ***Due to shape of earth :*** The shape of the earth is not perfectly spherical. It is flattened at poles. The polar radius is 21 km less than the equatorial radius. Hence acceleration due to gravity at poles is greater than at the equator.

$g_p = 9.83\ ms^{-2}$ = *value of g at poles*

$g_e = 9.78\ ms^{-2}$ = *values of g at equator*

i.e. $g_p > g_e$

(iii) ***At a depth 'd' below the earth surface :*** The acceleration due to gravity at the surface of earth.

$$g = \frac{GM_e}{R_e^2} = \left[\left(\frac{4}{3}\right)\pi R_e \rho\right] G \text{ (from eq}^n\text{. iv)} \qquad ...(vii)$$

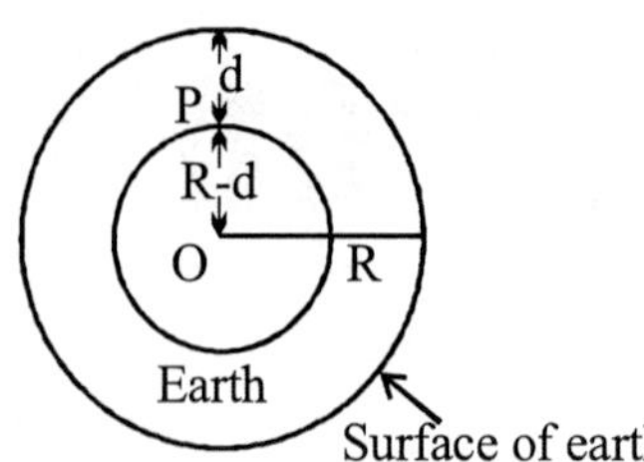

If a body is taken at a depth d below the earth surface, then the body is attracted by inner core of mass M' of earth radius (R_e– d). Then acceleration due to gravity at point P is

$$g' = \frac{GM'}{(R_e - d)^2} = \frac{G\left[(4/3)\pi(R_e - d)^3 \rho\right]}{(R_e - d)^2}$$

$$= G((4/3)\pi(R_e - d)\rho) \qquad ...(viii)$$

From eq^{ns}. (vii) and (viii) we have

$$g' = g\left(\frac{R_e - d}{R_e}\right) = g\left(1 - \frac{d}{R_e}\right) \qquad ...(ix)$$

The value of acceleration due to gravity at the centre of the earth is zero.

(iv) ***At a height 'h' above the earth surface :*** The acceleration due to gravity at the surface of earth from expression (iv) is defined as

$$g = \frac{GM_e}{R_e^2}$$

At a height h above the earth surface, the acceleration due to gravity is

$$g' = \frac{GM_e}{(R_e + h)^2} = \frac{GM_e}{r^2} \qquad ...(x)$$

$$\Rightarrow \quad g' = g\left(\frac{R_e + h}{R_e}\right)^{-2} \quad \text{[from eqs. (ix) \& (x)]}$$

If $h << R_e$

$$g' \approx g\left(1 - \frac{2h}{R_e}\right) \qquad ...(xi)$$

Problem Solving Tips

1. The value of the acceleration due to gravity on the moon is about one sixth of that on the earth and on the sun is about 27 times that on the earth.

$$\left(g_s = 27 g_E \text{ and } g_M = \frac{g_E}{6}\right)$$

2. The value of g is minimum on the mercury, among all planets.
3. For h<<R, the rate of decrease of the acceleration due to gravity with height is twice as compared to that with depth.
4. The value of g increases with the increase in latitude. Its value at latitude θ is given by : $g_\theta = g - R\omega^2 \cos^2\theta$.
5. Rotation of the earth about its own axis is responsible for decrease in the value of g with latitude.
6. The weight of the body varies along with the value of g (i.e. W = mg)
7. ***Inertial mass and gravitational mass-***
   (a) Inertial mass (M_i) defined by Newton's law of motion

$$M_i = F/a = \frac{\text{External force applied on the body}}{\text{Acceleration produced in it}}$$

$$\frac{(M_i)_1}{(M_i)_2} = \frac{a_2}{a_1}$$

(ff applied force on $(M_i)_1$ and $(M_i)_2$ is same.)

   (b) Gravitational mass M_g defined by Newton's law of gravitation

$$M_g = \frac{F_g}{g} = \frac{W}{g} = \frac{\text{Weight of body}}{\text{Accelerati on due to gravity}}$$

8. If two spheres of same material, mass and radius are put in contact, the gravitational attraction between them is directly proportional to the fourth power of the radius.

$$F = \frac{1}{4}G\left(\frac{4}{3}\pi\sigma\right)^2 R^4$$

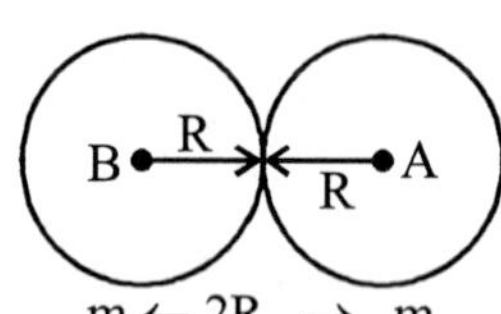

This system may be considered to be made up of two mass each separated by 2R distance.

9. If the earth stops rotating about its axis, the value of g at the equator will increase by about 0.35%, but that at the poles will remain unchanged.
   If the earth starts rotating at the angular speed of about 17 times the present value, there will be weightlessness on equator, but g at the poles will remain unchanged. In such a case, the duration of the day will be about 84 min.
10. If the radius of planet decreases by n%, keeping the mass unchanged, the acceleration due to gravity on its surface increases by 2n%. i.e., $\frac{\Delta g}{g} = \frac{-2\Delta R}{R}$
11. If the mass of the planet increases by m% keeping the radius constant, the acceleration due to gravity on its surface increases by m% i.e., $\frac{\Delta g}{g} = \frac{\Delta M}{M}$ where R = constant.
12. If the density of planet decreases by ρ % keeping the radius constant, the acceleration due to gravity decreases by ρ%.
13. If the radius of the planet decreases by r% keeping the density constant, the acceleration due to gravity decreases by r%.

Example 1.

What will be the acceleration due to gravity on the surface of the moon with its radius as 1/4th the radius of the earth and its mass as 1/80th the mass of earth?

Solution :

$$g=\frac{GM_e}{R_e^{\,2}} \text{ and } g'=\frac{GM_m}{R_m^{\,2}};$$

$$\therefore \quad \frac{g'}{g}=\frac{M_m}{M_e}\left(\frac{R_e}{R_m}\right)^2=\frac{1}{80}\times\left(\frac{4}{1}\right)^2=\frac{1}{5}; \quad \therefore\ g'=g/5$$

Example 2.

A mass M splits into two parts m and (M–m), which are then separated by a certain distance. What will be the ratio m/M which maximizes the gravitational force between the two parts?

Solution :

$$F=\frac{Gm\,(M-m)}{x^2}; \text{For maxima,}$$

$$\frac{dF}{dm}=\frac{G}{x^2}(M-2m)=0 \text{ or } \frac{m}{M}=\frac{1}{2}$$

Example 3.

Identical point masses each equal to m are placed at x = 0, x = 1, x = 2, x = 4, ... The total gravitational force on mass m at x = 0 due to all other masses is

(a) infinite (b) (4/3) Gm^2

(c) (4/3 GM^2) (d) zero

***Solution :* (c)**

O m m m
x=0 x=1 x=2 x=4

$$F_0=\frac{Gm^2}{1^2}+\frac{Gm^2}{2^2}+\frac{Gm^2}{4^2}+....$$

$$F_0=Gm^2\left[\frac{1}{1^2}+\frac{1}{2^2}+\frac{1}{4^2}+...\right]$$

It is a G.P. with common ratio 1/4.

$$\therefore \quad F_0=Gm^2\left[\frac{1}{1-1/4}\right] \quad F_0=\frac{4Gm^2}{3}$$

Example 4.

Four identical point masses each equal to m are placed at the corners of a square of side a. The force on a point mass m' placed at the point of intersection of the two diagonals is

(a) $(4Gmm')/a^2$ (b) $(2Gmm')/a^2$

(c) $(Gmm')/a^2$ (d) zero

***Solution :* (d)**

The forces acting on the mass m′ placed at the point of intersection of diagonals are balanced by each other as shown in figure. Therefore net force is zero.

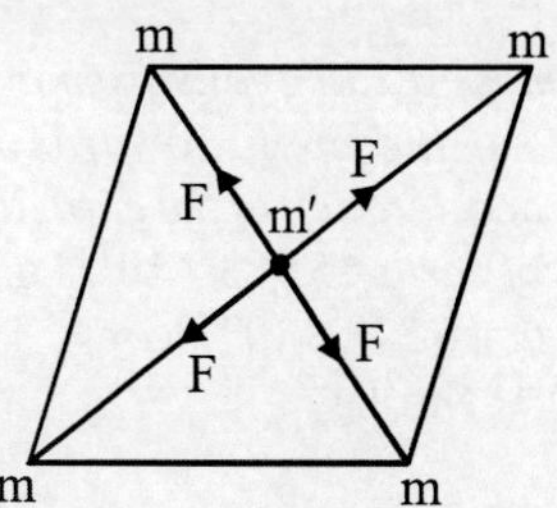

Example 5.

A tunnel is dug along the diameter of the earth. Determine the force on a particle of mass m placed in the tunnel at a distance x from the centre.

Solution :

Force on a mass m placed at a distance x from the centre is equal to the force of gravity due to a mass of spherical volume of earth of radius x.

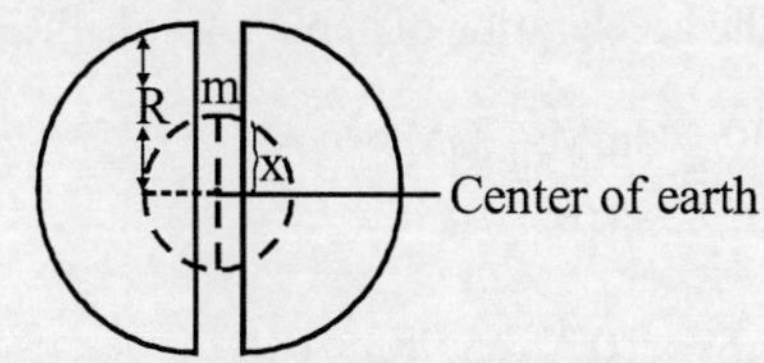

$$\therefore F=\frac{G\left(\frac{4\pi x^3}{3}d\right)m}{x^2}$$

$$\text{where } d=\text{density of earth}=\frac{3M}{4\pi R^3};$$

$$\therefore F=\frac{GMm}{R^3}.x \text{ [M is total mass of earth]}$$

Example 6.

If the radius of the earth were to shrink by two per cent, its mass remaining the same, the acceleration due to gravity on the earth's surface would

(a) decrease by 2% (b) increase by 2%

(c) increase by 4% (d) decrease by 4%

Solution : (c)

As $g=\frac{GM}{R^2}$; So, if R decreases then g increases.

Taking logarithm of both the sides;

log g = log G + log M – 2 log R

Differentiating it, we get $\frac{dg}{g}=0+0-\frac{2dR}{R}$;

$$\therefore \frac{dg}{g}=-2\left(\frac{-2}{100}\right)=\frac{4}{100}$$

$$\therefore \% \text{ increase in } g=\frac{dg}{g}\times 100=\frac{4}{100}\times 100=4\%$$

Example 7.

An apple of mass 0.25 kg falls from a tree. What is the acceleration of the apple towards the earth? Also calculate the acceleration of the earth towards the apple. Given : Mass of earth = 5.983 × 10^{24} kg, Radius of earth = 6.378 × 10^6 metre, G = 6.67 × 10^{-11} Nm^{2}kg^{-2}.

Solution :

Mass of apple, m = 0.25 kg,
Mass of earth, M = 5.983 × 10^{24} kg,
Radius of earth, R = 6.378 × 10^6 metre
Gravitational constant, G = 6.67 × 10^{-11} Nm^{2}kg^{-2}
Let F be the gravitational force of attraction between the apple and earth.

Then, $$F=\frac{GmM}{R^2}$$

Let a be the acceleration of apple towards the earth.

$$a=\frac{F}{m}=\frac{GmM}{mR^2}=\frac{GM}{R^2}$$

$$\Rightarrow a=\frac{6.67\times10^{-11}\times5.983\times10^{24}}{(6.378\times10^6)^2}ms^{-2}=9.810\,ms^{-2}$$

Let a′ be the acceleration of the earth towards the apple.

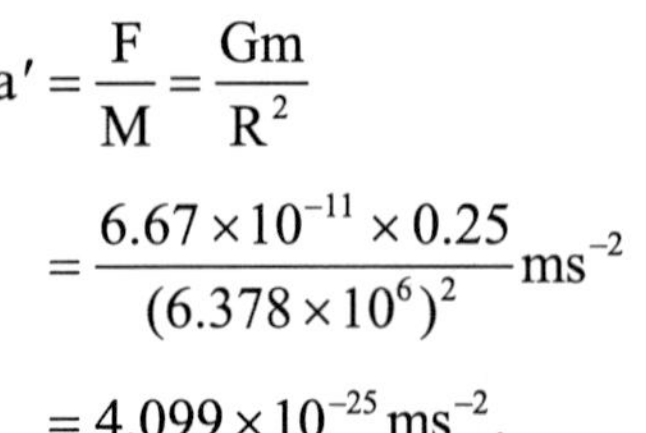

$$a'=\frac{F}{M}=\frac{Gm}{R^2}$$

$$=\frac{6.67\times10^{-11}\times0.25}{(6.378\times10^6)^2}ms^{-2}$$

$$=4.099\times10^{-25}\,ms^{-2}.$$

Example 8.

The acceleration due to gravity at the moon's surface is 1.67 ms^{-2}. If the radius of the moon is 1.74 × 10^6 m, calculate the mass of the moon. Use the known value of G.

Solution :

$$g=\frac{GM}{R^2}\text{ or }M=\frac{gR^2}{G}$$

This relation is true not only for earth but for any heavenly body which is assumed to be spherical.

Here, $g=1.67ms^{-2}$, $R=1.74\times10^6$ m and

$$G=6.67\times10^{-11}Nm^2kg^{-2}$$

∴ Mass of moon,

$$M=\frac{1.67\times(1.74\times10^6)^2}{6.67\times10^{-11}}kg=7.58\times10^{22}kg$$

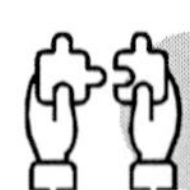

8.1 Concept Practice Problems

CPP

1. Due to rotation of the earth the acceleration due to gravity g is
   (a) maximum at the equator and minimum at the poles
   (b) minimum at the equator and maximum at the poles
   (c) same at both places
   (d) None of these
2. Two point masses each equal to 1 kg attract one another with a force of 10^{-10} N. The distance between the two point masses is (G = 6.6 × 10^{-11} MKS units)
   (a) 8 cm (b) 0.8 cm (c) 80 cm (d) 0.08 cm
3. A planet of mass 3 × 10^{29} gm moves around a star with a constant speed of 2 × 10^6 ms^{-1} in a circle of radii 1.5 × 10^{14} cm. The gravitational force exerted on the planet by the star is
   (a) 6.67 × 10^{22} dyne (d) 8 × 10^{27} Newton
   (c) 8 × 10^{26} N (d) 6.67 × 10^{19} dyne
4. If the mass of earth is eighty times the mass of a planet and diameter of the planet is one fourth that of earth, then acceleration due to gravity on the planet would be
   (a) 7.8 m/s^2 (b) 9.8 m/s^2 (c) 6.8 m/s^2 (d) 2.0 m/s^2
5. The radii of two planets are respectively R_1 and R_2 and their densities are respectively ρ_1 and ρ_2. The ratio of the accelerations due to gravity at their surfaces is
   (a) $g_1:g_2=\frac{\rho_1}{R_1^2}:\frac{\rho_2}{R_2^2}$ (b) $g_1:g_2=R_1R_2:\rho_1\rho_2$
   (c) $g_1:g_2=R_1\rho_2:R_2\rho_1$ (d) $g_1:g_2=R_1\rho_1:R_2\rho_2$
6. If earth is supposed to be a sphere of radius R, if g_{30} is value of acceleration due to gravity at lattitude of 30° and g at the equator, the value of $g-g_{30}$ is
   (a) $\frac{1}{4}\omega^2R$ (b) $\frac{3}{4}\omega^2R$ (c) ω^2R (d) $\frac{1}{2}\omega^2R$
7. A man of mass m starts falling towards a planet of mass M and radius R. As he reaches near to the surface, he realizes that he will pass through a small hole in the planet. As he enters the hole, he sees that the planet is really made of two pieces a spherical shell of negligible thickness of mass 2M/3 and a point mass M/3 at the centre. Change in the force of gravity experienced by the man is
   (a) $\frac{2}{3}\frac{GMm}{R^2}$ (b) 0
   (c) $\frac{1}{3}\frac{GMm}{R^2}$ (d) $\frac{4}{3}\frac{GMm}{R^2}$
8. If g_E and g_M are the accelerations due to gravity on the surfaces of the earth and the moon respectively and if Millikan's oil drop experiment could be performed on the two surfaces, one will find the ratio
   $\frac{\text{electronic charge on the moon}}{\text{electronic charge on the earth}}$ to be

(a) g_M / g_E (b) 1
(c) 0 (d) g_E / g_M

9. The density of a newly discovered planet is twice that of earth. The acceleration due to gravity at the surface of the planet is equal to that at the surface of the earth. If the radius of the earth is R, the radius of the planet would be
(a) ½R (b) 2R (c) 4R (d) 1/4R

10. Imagine a new planet having the same density as that of earth but it is 3 times bigger than the earth in size. If the acceleration due to gravity on the surface of earth is g and that on the surface of the new planet is g', then
(a) g' = g/9 (b) g' = 27g (c) g'=9g (d) g'=3g

ANSWER KEY

1	(b)	2	(c)	3	(c)	4	(d)	5	(d)	6	(b)	7	(a)	8	(b)	9	(a)	10	(d)

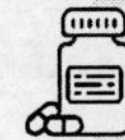

Topic 8.2 : Gravitational-Field, Potential & Gravitational Potential Energy

GRAVITATIONAL FIELD

(or Gravitational Field Intensity)

The region or space around a body in which its gravitational influence is experienced by other bodies is the gravitational field of that body.

The gravitational field strength E_g, produced by a mass M at any point P is defined as the force exerted on the unit mass placed at that point P. Then

$$E_g = \frac{F}{m} = \left(\frac{GMm}{r^2}\right) \Big/ m = \frac{GM}{r^2} \quad ...(i)$$

where m = test mass

r = distance between M and m

(i) The direction of E_g always points towards the mass producing it.

(ii) The gravitational field can be represented by gravitational lines of force.

(iii) The S.I **unit** of E_g is newton/kg. Its **dimensions** are $[M^0LT^{-2}]$.

Gravitational intensity (E_g) for spherical shell

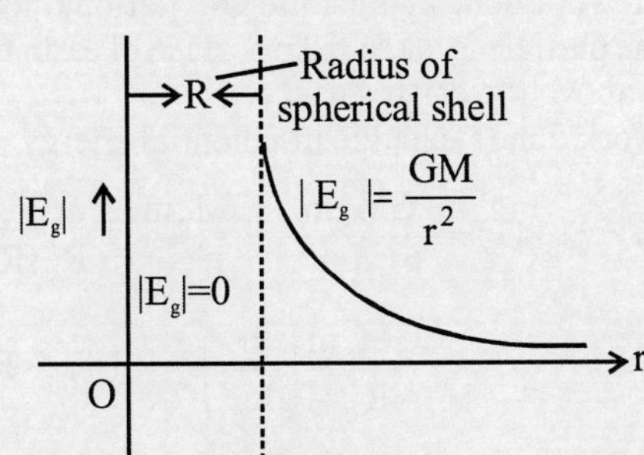

(i) $|E_g| = 0$ at points inside the spherical shell (i.e. r < R)

(ii) $|E_g| = \left|\frac{-GM}{R^2}\right|$ at the surface of shell (i.e. r = R)

(iii) $|E_g| = \left|\frac{-GM}{r^2}\right|$ for outside the spherical shell (r > R).

It is clear that as r increases, E_g decreases.

Gravitational intensity for solid sphere :

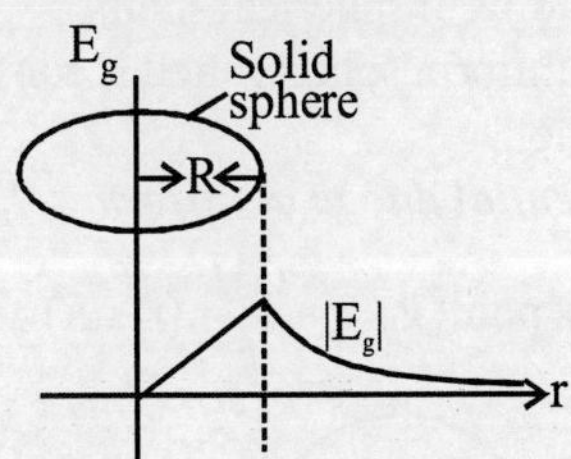

(i) $|E_g| = \left|-\frac{GM.r}{R^3}\right|$ for points inside the solid sphere (r<R)

(ii) At the surface of solid sphere (r = R) $|E_g| = \left|-\frac{GM}{R^2}\right|$

(iii) Outside the solid sphere $|E_g| = \left|-\frac{GM}{r^2}\right|$ $(r > R)$

GRAVITATIONAL POTENTIAL

Gravitational potential at any point is the work done by gravitational force in carrying a body of unit mass from infinity to that point in gravitational influence of source.

i.e., $V_A = \frac{W}{m_0} = \frac{-GM}{r}$

where r is the distance of point from source mass M.

The **S.I. unit** of V is joule/kg. Its **dimensions** are $[M^0L^2T^{-2}]$. It is a scalar quantity.

Gravitational potential at the earth surface is

$$V_A = \frac{-GM_e}{R_e} = -gR_e$$

Gravitational potential due to a uniform ring at a point on its axis

$$V_g = -\frac{GM}{\sqrt{a^2 + r^2}}$$

Gravitational potential due to a uniform thin spherical shell

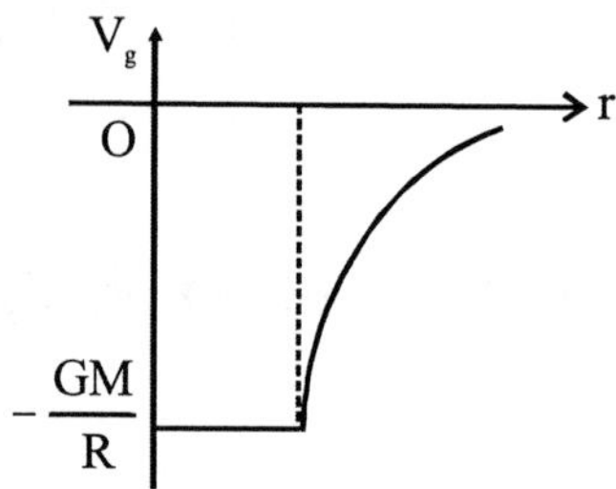

(i) at a point outside the shell, $V_g = \frac{-GM}{r}$ (r > R)

(ii) at a point inside the shell, $V_g = -\frac{GM}{R}$ (r < R)

where R = radius of spherical shell.

Potential due to a uniform spheral shell is constant throughout the cavity of the shell.

Gravitational potential due to a uniform solid sphere

(i) at an external point $V_g = -\frac{GM}{r}$ $(r \geq R)$

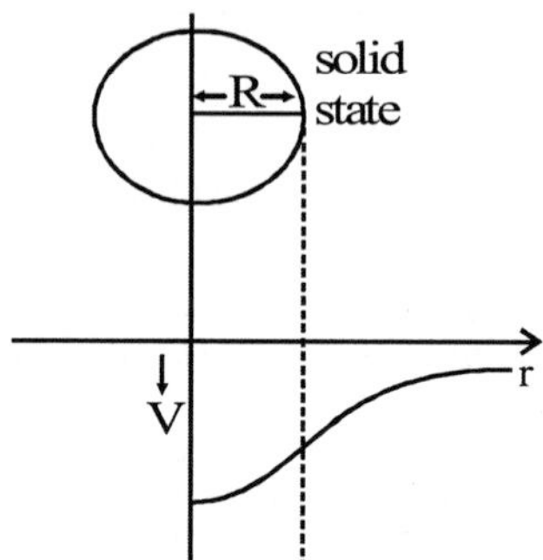

(ii) at an internal point $V_g = -\frac{GM}{2R^3}(3R^2 - r^2)$ $(r < R)$

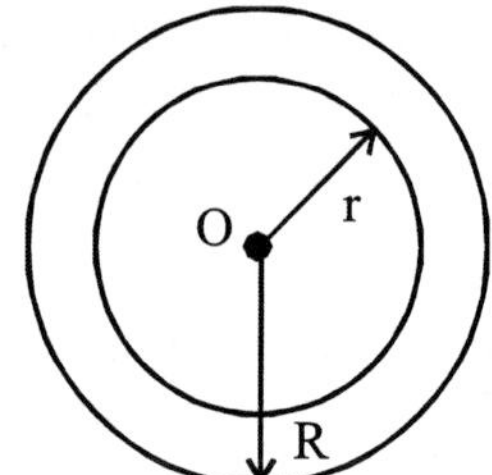

(iii) *Potential at the centre of solid sphere is* $V = \frac{-3GM}{2R}$

GRAVITATIONAL POTENTIAL ENERGY

Let V_g be the gravitational potential at a point. If we place a mass m at that point, then we say that the gravitational potential energy possessed by the mass is

$$U_g = V_g \times m \Rightarrow U_g = -\frac{GM}{r} \times m \quad \left[\therefore V_g = -\frac{GM}{r}\right]$$

We can also therefore say that the gravitational potential energy of a system containing two masses m_1 and m_2 placed such that the centre to centre distance between them is r then

$$U_g = -\frac{Gm_1m_2}{r}$$

This formula is valid taking into consideration the fact that we have taken the gravitational potential of few at infinity. Please remember that unless otherwise stated it is understood that the gravitational potential is taken to be zero at infinity.

Relation between gravitational potential energy and gravitational potential.

Gravitational potential energy = gravitational potential × mass

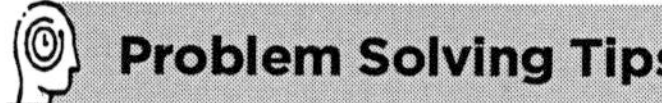

1. The gravitational potential energy of a mass m at a point above the surface of the earth at a height h is given by

$U_g = \frac{-GMm}{R + h}$. The –ve sign shows that if h increases, the gravitational PE decreases and becomes zero at infinity.

2. (a) If we take reference level to be at the surface of earth (not at infinity) i.e., we assume that the gravitational P.E of a mass m is zero at the surface of earth, then the gravitational potential energy at a height h above the surface of earth is (mgh), where h << R_e (radius of earth)

(b) The gravitational P.E of mass m on the earth's surface is

$$U_g = \frac{-GM_em}{R_e} = -mgR$$

If we assume that gravitational P.E of mass m is zero at infinity i.e., we take reference level at infinity then P.E. of any mass m at a height h above the earth surface

$$U_h = \frac{-GM_em}{(R_e + h)}$$

So work done against the gravitational force, when the particle is taken from surface of earth to a height h above the earth surface

Work done = change in potential energy

$$\Rightarrow U_h - U_g = \frac{-GM_em}{R_e + h} + \frac{GM_em}{R_e} \cong \frac{GM_em \times h}{R_e(R_e + h)}$$

$$\approx \frac{GM_em}{R_e}\left(\frac{h}{R_e}\right) \quad \text{(if h<<R)}$$

$$= m\left(\frac{GM_e}{R_e^2}\right)h$$

So, work done = mgh is stored in the particle as particle potenital energy, when kept at height 'h'.

Example 9.

Four particles each of mass 1 kg are at the four corners of a square of side 1m. Find the work done to remove one of the particles to infinity.

Solution :

The gravitational potential energy associated with any pair of particle of mass m_1 and m_2 separated by a distance r is $U = \frac{-Gm_1m_2}{r}$

Initial P.E. of system, $-U_1 = 4.\frac{G\times1\times1}{1} + \frac{2G\times1\times1}{\sqrt{2}}$

or $U_1 = -G\left[\frac{4\sqrt{2}+2}{\sqrt{2}}\right]$

1 Kg 1m 1 Kg
√2m
1m 1m
√2m
1 Kg 1m 1 Kg

When one mass is removed, then

$$P.E. = U_2 = -\left[2.\frac{G\times1\times1}{\sqrt{1}} + \frac{G\times1\times1}{\sqrt{2}}\right]$$

$$U_2 = -\left[\frac{2\sqrt{2}+1}{\sqrt{2}}\right]G;$$

$$\therefore \text{Work done} = G\left[\frac{4\sqrt{2}+2-2\sqrt{2}-1}{\sqrt{2}}\right]$$

$$= G\left[\frac{2\sqrt{2}+1}{\sqrt{2}}\right]$$

[$\because$ Work done = change in P.E. $= -U_2-[-U_1] = U_1-U_2$]

Example 10.

A solid sphere of uniform density and mass M has a radius of 4m. Its centre is at the origin of coordinate system. Two spheres of radii 1m are taken out so that their centres are at P(0, –2, 0) and Q(0, 2, 0) respectively. This leaves two spherical cavities. What is the gravitational field at the centre of each cavity?

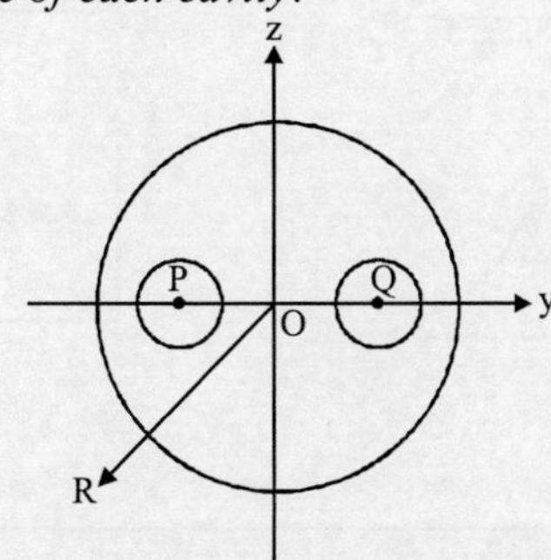

Solution :

If the cavities are not made, then the intensity at the point P (or Q), due to whole sphere

$$I = \frac{GM}{R^3}.x = \frac{GM}{64}\times2 = \frac{GM}{32} \quad \text{where } \vec{I} = \vec{I}_P + \vec{I}_Q + \vec{I}_R$$

$$\therefore \vec{I}_R = \vec{I} - \vec{I}_P - \vec{I}_Q \qquad ......(i)$$

Where I_R is the intensity of gravitational field at a point, distance x from O due to remainder sphere (exclude cavity)

Mass of big sphere $M = \frac{4\pi\times(4)^3 d}{3}$

Mass of small sphere P or Q, $m = \frac{4\pi\times(1)^3 d}{3}$ $\therefore$ $m = \frac{M}{64}$

At P, $I_p = 0$, $I_Q = \frac{Gm}{r^2} = \frac{G}{4^2}.\left(\frac{M}{64}\right)$

$\therefore I_R = \frac{GM}{32} - \frac{GM}{1024}$ [From eq (i)]

$$\therefore I_R = \frac{31GM}{1024}$$

Example 11.

Find the gravitational potential energy of a system of four particles, each having mass m, placed at the vertices of a square of side l. Also obtain the gravitational potential at the centre of the square.

Solution :

The system has four pairs with distance ℓ and two diagonal pairs with distance $\sqrt{2}\,\ell$.

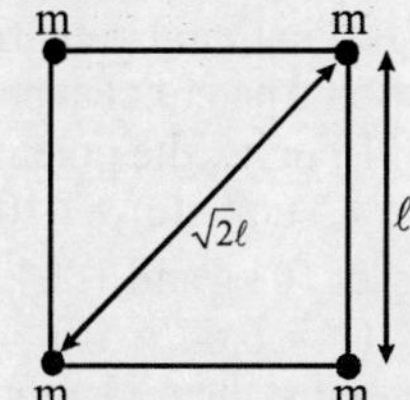

$$\therefore \quad U = -4\frac{Gm^2}{\ell} - 2\frac{Gm^2}{\sqrt{2}\ell} = -\frac{2Gm^2}{\ell}\left(2+\frac{1}{\sqrt{2}}\right) = -5.41\frac{Gm^2}{\ell}$$

The gravitational potential at the centre of the square is $\left(r = \sqrt{2}\ell/2\right)$

V = Algebraic sum of potential due to each particle

$$\Rightarrow \; V = -\frac{4\sqrt{2}Gm}{\ell}$$

Example 12.

The radius of earth is R. Find the work done in raising a body of mass m from the surface of earth to a height R/2.

Solution :

If a body of mass m is placed at a distance x from the centre of earth, the gravitational force of attraction F between the body and the earth is $F = \frac{GM\,m}{x^2}$

Small amount of work done in raising a body through a small distance dx is given by

$$dW = F\,dx = \frac{GM\,m}{x^2}dx$$

Total work done in raising the body from the surface of earth to a height R/2 is given by

$$W = \int_{R}^{R+R/2} \frac{GM\,m}{x^2}dx$$

$$= GMm \int_{R}^{3R/2} x^{-2}\,dx = -GMm\left(\frac{1}{x}\right)_{R}^{3R/2}$$

$$= -GMm\left[\frac{2}{3R} - \frac{1}{R}\right] = \frac{GM\,m}{3R} = \frac{gR^2m}{3R}$$

$$= \frac{1}{3}mg\,R\ [\therefore GM = gR^2]$$

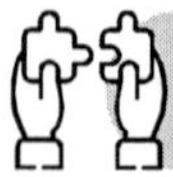

8.2 Concept Practice Problems

CPP

11. If the gravitational force had varied as $r^{-5/2}$ instead of r^{-2}; the potential energy of a particle at a distance 'r' from the centre of the earth would be proportional to

(a) r^{-1} (b) r^{-2} (c) $r^{-3/2}$ (d) $r^{-5/2}$

12. Energy required to move a body of mass m from an orbit of radius 2R to 3R is

(a) $GMm/12R^2$ (b) $GMm/3R^2$
(c) $GMm/8R$ (d) $GMm/6R$

13. There are two bodies of masses 10^3 kg and 10^5 kg separated by a distance of 1 km. At what distance from the smaller body, the intensity of gravitational field will be zero

(a) 1/9 km (b) 1/10 km (c) 1/11 km (d) 10/11 km

14. Taking the gravitational potential at a point infinte distance away as zero, the gravitational potential at a point A is –5 unit. If the gravitational potential at point infinite distance away is taken as + 10 units, the potential at point A is

(a) – 5 unit (b) + 5 unit (c) + 10 unit (d) + 15 unit

15. Two bodies of masses 10 kg and 100 kg are separated by a distance of 2m ($G = 6.67 \times 10^{-11}$ $Nm^2\ kg^{-2}$). The gravitational potential at the mid point on the line joining the two is

(a) 7.3×10^{-7} J/kg (b) 7.3×10^{-9} J/kg
(c) -7.3×10^{-9} J/kg (d) 7.3×10^{-6} J/kg

16. Consider Earth to be a homogeneous sphere. Scientist A goes deep down in a mine and scientist B goes high up in a balloon. The gravitational field measured by

(a) A goes on decreasing and that by B goes on increasing
(b) B goes on decreasing and that by A goes on increasing
(c) each decreases at the same rate
(d) each decreases at different rates

17. The gravitational potential difference between the surface of a planet and a point 20 m above the surface is 2 joule/kg. If the gravitational field is uniform, then the work done in carrying a 5 kg body to a height of 4 m above the surface is

(a) 2 J (b) 20 J (c) 40 J (d) 10 J

18. The amount of work done in lifting a mass 'm' from the surface of the earth to a height 2R is

(a) 2mgR (b) 3mgR (c) $\frac{3}{2}$mgR (d) $\frac{2}{3}$mgR

19. In a region of only gravitational field of mass 'M' a particle is shifted from A to B via three different paths in the figure. The work done in different paths are W_1, W_2, W_3 respectively then

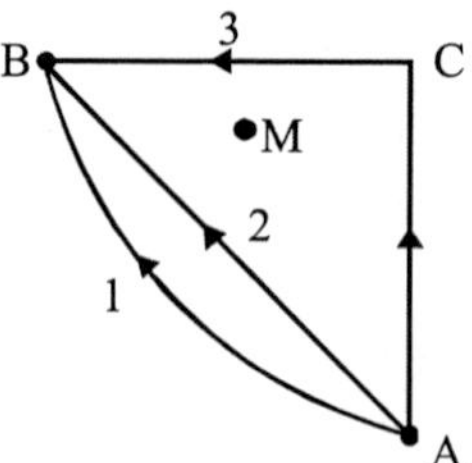

(a) $W_1 = W_2 = W_3$ (b) $W_1 > W_2 > W_3$
(c) $W_1 = W_2 > W_3$ (d) $W_1 < W_2 < W_3$

20. Which one of the following graphs represents correctly the variation of the gravitational field intensity (I) with the distance (r) from the centre of a spherical shell of mass M and radius a ?

(a)
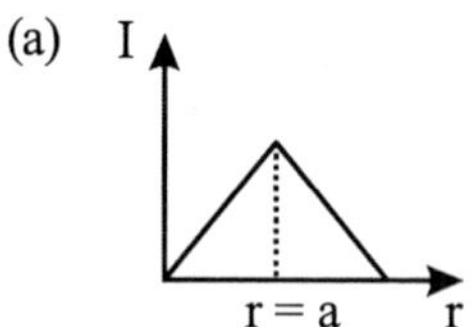

(b)
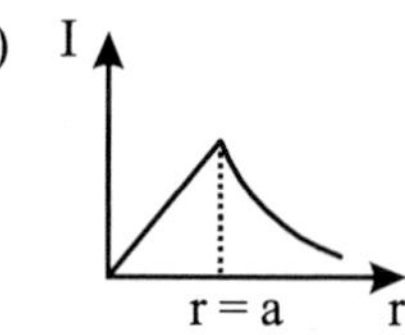

(c)
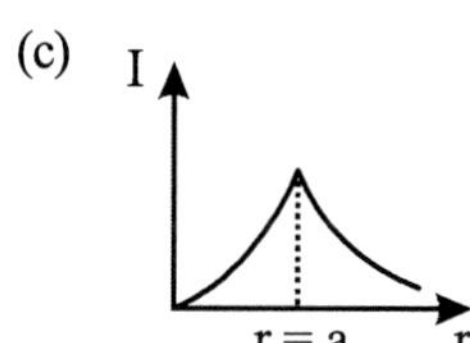

(d)
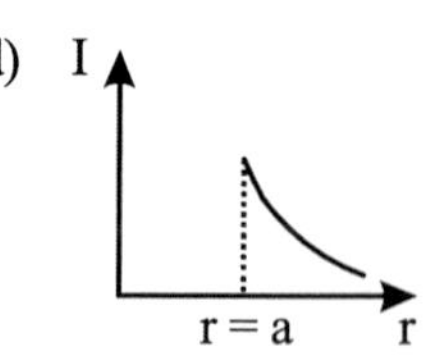

ANSWER KEY

11	(c)	12	(d)	13	(c)	14	(b)	15	(c)	16	(d)	17	(a)	18	(d)	19	(a)	20	(d)

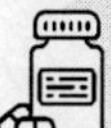

Topic 8.3 : Satellites-Geostationary & Polar; Orbital & Escape Speed; Kepler's Laws of Planetary Motion and Weightlessness

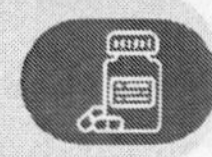

SATELLITES

A **satellite** *is any body revolving around a large body under the gravitational influence of the latter.*

The period of motion T of an artificial satellite of earth at a distance h above the surface of the earth is given by,

$$T = 2\pi\sqrt{\frac{(R_e+h)^3}{gR_e^2}}$$

where, R_e = radius of the earth

g = acceleration due to gravity on the surface of the earth.

If $R_e >> h$, then $T = 2\pi\sqrt{\frac{R_e}{g}}$; $R_e = 6.4 \times 10^6$ m;

$g = 9.8\ ms^{-2}$

i.e. $T \simeq 84.58$ minutes ≈ 5075 sec

Assuming $R_e + h = r$, the distance of the satellite from the centre of the earth, $T \propto (r)^{3/2}$

Orbital velocity (v_0)

Let a satellite of mass m revolve around the earth in circular orbit of radius r with speed v_0. The gravitational pull between satellite and earth provides the necessary centripetal force.

Centripetal force required for the motion $= \frac{mv_0^2}{r}$

Gravitational force $= \frac{GMm}{r^2}$

$$\frac{mv_0^2}{r} = \frac{GMm}{r^2} \quad \text{or} \quad v_0^2 = \frac{GM}{r}$$

$$\text{or } v_0 = \sqrt{\frac{GM}{r}} \quad \text{..........(1)}$$

$$\text{or} \quad v_0 = R\sqrt{\frac{g}{R+h}} \quad \left[\because g = \frac{GM}{R^2} \text{ and } r = (R+h)\right]$$

Orbital velocity, $Vo = \sqrt{\frac{GM_e}{R_e}} = \sqrt{gR_e}$

(i) Value of orbital velocity does not depend on the mass of the satellite.

(ii) Around the earth the value of orbital velocity is **7.92 km/sec**.

(iii) Greater is the height of the satellite, smaller is the orbital velocity.

(iv) The direction of orbital velocity is along the tangent to the path.

(v) The work done by the satellite in a complete orbit is zero.

***Angular momentum (L)*:** For satellite motion, angular momentum will be given by

$$L = mvr = mr\sqrt{\frac{GM}{r}} \quad \text{i.e., } L = [m^2GMr]^{1/2}$$

Angular momentum of a satellite depends on both, the mass of orbiting and central body. It also depends on the radius of the orbit.

Energy of a satellite

Total energy of satellite revolving in an orbit of radius r around the earth can be calculated as follows :

(i) The **gravitational potential energy** of a satellite of mass m is $U_g = -\frac{GMm}{r}$, where r is the radius of the orbit.

(ii) **Kinetic energy** of the satellite is $E_k = \frac{1}{2}mv_0{}^2 = \frac{GMm}{2r}$

(iii) So, **total energy** of the satellite $E = U_g + E_k = -\frac{GMm}{2r}$

The negative sign shows that satellite cannot leave the orbit itself. It requires an energy equal to $\frac{GMm}{2R}$, which is called **Binding Energy (B.E.)** of satellite.

(iv) Total energy of a satellite at a height equal to the radius of the earth

$$= -\frac{GMm}{2(R+R)} = -\frac{GMm}{4R} = \frac{1}{4}mgR$$

GEO-STATIONARY SATELLITE

A satelite which appears to be stationary for a person on the surface of the earth is called geostationary satellite.

It is also known as **parking satellite** or **synchronous satellite.**

(i) The orbit of the satellite must be circular and in the equatorial plane of the earth.

(ii) The angular velocity of the satellite must be in the same direction as the angular velocity of rotation of the earth i.e., from west to east.

(iii) The period of revolution of the satellite must be equal to the period of rotation of earth about its axis.

i.e. 24 hours = 24 × 60 × 60 = 86400 sec.

$$T^2 = \frac{4\pi^2}{GM} r^3 \text{ or}$$

$$r = \left(\frac{GMT^2}{4\pi^2}\right)^{\frac{1}{3}} = \left(\frac{GM}{R^2} \times \frac{R^2T^2}{4\pi^2}\right)^{\frac{1}{3}}$$

$$= \left[9.8 \times (6.38 \times 10^6)^2 \times \frac{(86400)^2}{4\pi^2}\right]^{\frac{1}{3}}$$

$= 42237 \times 10^3$ m = 42,237 km. ≈ 42000 km.

h = r – R = 42000 – 6400 = 35600 km.

(a) Height of geostationary satellite from the surface of the earth is nearly 35600 km.

(b) The orbital velocity of this satellite is nearly 3.08 km/sec.

(c) The relative velocity of geostationary satellite with respect to earth is zero.

This type of satellite is used for communication purposes. The orbit of a geostationary satellite is called 'Parking Orbit'.

Polar Satellite :

Polar satellites travel around the earth in an orbit that travels around the earth over the poles. The earth rotates on its axis as the satellite goes around the earth. Thus over a period of many orbits it looks down on every part of the earth.

Different orbital shapes corresponding to different velocities of a satellite :

[1] When $v < v_0$

(i) The path is spiral. The satellite finally falls on the earth

(ii) Kinetic energy is less then potential energy

(iii) Total energy is negative

[2] When $v = v_0$

(i) The path is circular

(ii) Eccentricity is zero

(iii) Kinetic energy is less than potential energy

(iv) Total energy is negative

[3] When $v_0 < v < v_e$

(i) The path is elliptical

(ii) Eccentricity < 1

(iii) Kinetic energy is less than potential energy

(iv) Total energy is negative

[4] When $v = v_e$

(i) The path is a parabola

(ii) Eccentricity = 1

(iii) Kinetic energy is equal to potential energy

(iv) Total energy is zero

[5] When $v > v_e$

(i) The path is a hyperbola

(ii) Eccentricity > 1

(iii) Kinetic energy is greater than potential energy

(iv) Total energy is positive

If the orbit of a satellite is elliptical

(1) The energy $E = -\dfrac{GMm}{2a}$ = const. with 'a' as semi-major axis;

(2) KE will be maximum when the satellite is closest to the central body (at perigee) and minimum when it is farthest from the central body (at apogee) [as for a given orbit L = const., i.e., mvr = const., i.e., $v \propto 1/r$]

(3) PE = (E – KE) will be minimum when KE = max, i.e., the satellite is closest to the central body (at perigee) and maximum when KE = min, i.e., the satellite is farthest from the central body (at apogee).

ESCAPE SPEED (V_e)

It is the minimum speed with which a body should be projected from the surface of a planet so as to reach at infinity i.e., beyond the gravitational field of the planet.

If a body of mass m is projected with speed v from the surface of a planet of mass M and radius R, then

$$\text{as } K = \frac{1}{2}mv^2 \text{ and } U = -\frac{GMm}{R},\ E_S = \frac{1}{2}mv^2 - \frac{GMm}{R}$$

Now if v' is the speed of body at ∞, then

$$E_\infty = \frac{1}{2}m(v')^2 + 0 = \frac{1}{2}m(v')^2 \quad [\text{as } U_\infty = 0]$$

So by conservation of energy

$$= \frac{1}{2}mv^2 - \frac{GMm}{R} = \frac{1}{2}m(v')^2$$

$$\text{i.e. } \frac{1}{2}mv^2 = \frac{GMm}{R} + \frac{1}{2}m(v')^2$$

so v will be minimum when $v' \to 0$,

$$\text{i.e. } v_e = v_{\min} = \sqrt{\frac{2GM}{R}} = \sqrt{2gR} \qquad \left[\text{as } g = \frac{GM}{R^2}\right]$$

- The value of escape velocity does not depend upon the mass of the projected body, instead it depends on the mass and radius of the planet from which it is being projected.
- The value of escape velocity does not depend on the angle and direction of projection.
- The value of escape velocity from the surface of the earth is **11.2** km/sec.
- The minimum energy needed for escape is = GMm/R.
- If the velocity of a satellite orbiting near the surface of the earth is increased by 41.4%, then it will escape away from the gravitational field of the earth.
- If a body falls freely from infinite distance, then it will reach the surface of earth with a velocity of 11.2 km/sec.

Relation between orbital velocity (V_0) and escape speed (V_e)

$$V_e = \sqrt{2gR} = \sqrt{2}\, V_0$$

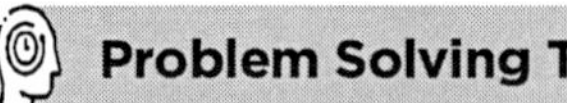

Problem Solving Tips

1. The escape velocity on moon is low $\left(as\ g_m = \dfrac{g_E}{6}\right)$ hence there is no atmosphere on moon.
2. If the orbital radius of the earth around the sun be one fourth of the present value, then the duration of the year will be one eighth of the present value.
3. The satellites revolve around the earth in a plane that coincides with the great circle around the earth.

KEPLER'S LAWS OF PLANETARY MOTION

1. **The law of orbits :** *Each planet revolves about the sun in an elliptical orbit with the sun at one of the foci of the ellipse.*

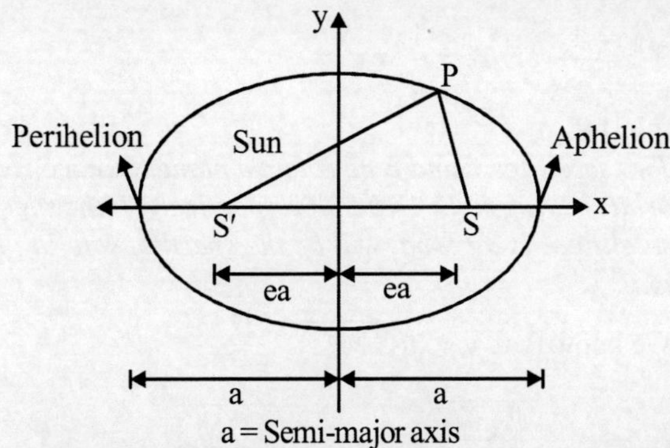

a = Semi-major axis

A planet of mass m moving in an elliptical orbit around the sun. The sun of mass M, is at one focus S′ of the ellipse. The other focus is S, which is located in empty space. Each focus is at distance ‘ea’ from the ellipse’s centre, with ‘e’ being the **eccentricity** of the ellipse and ‘a’ semimajor axis of the ellipse, the perihelion (nearest to the sun) distance $r_{min.}$, and the aphelion (farthest from the sun) distance $r_{max.}$ are also shown.

$r_{max} = a + e\,a = (1 + e)\,a$

$r_{min} = a - e\,a = (1 - e)\,a$

The distance of each focus from the centre of ellipse is ea, where e is the dimensionless number between 0 to 1 called the eccentricity. If e = 0, the ellipse is a circle.

For earth e = 0.017.

2. ***Law of areas :*** *An imaginary line that connects a planet to the sun sweeps out equal areas in the plane of the planet's orbit in equal times;*

i.e., the rate dA/dt at which it sweeps out area A is constant.

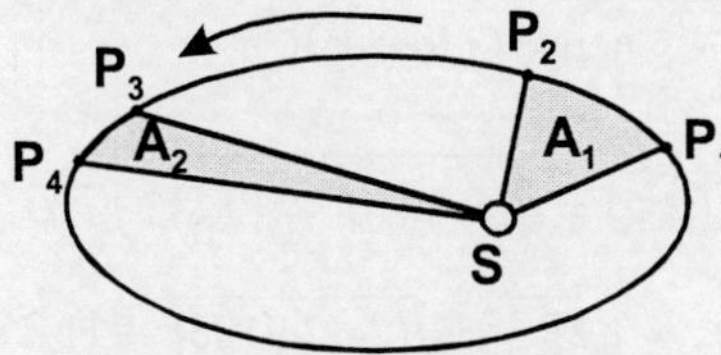

If $t_{P_1P_2} = t_{P_3P_4}$ then $A_1 = A_2$

$$\frac{dA}{dt} = \frac{1}{2}\frac{(r)(v\,dt)}{dt} = \frac{1}{2}rv \text{ and as } L = mvr$$

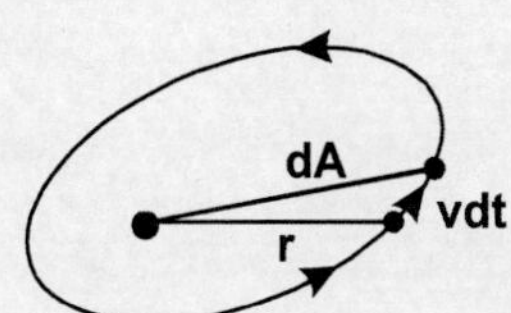

$$\text{so } \frac{dA}{dt} = \frac{L}{2m} \qquad ....(1)$$

But as L = constt., (force is central, so torque = 0 and hence angular momentum of the planet is conserved)

areal velocity (dA/dt) = constant which is Kepler's IInd law, i.e., Kepler's IInd law or constancy of areal velocity is a consequence of conservation of angular momentum.

3. ***Law of periods :*** *The square of the period of revolution of any planet is proportional to the cube of the semi-major axis of the orbit,*

i.e., $T^2 \propto r^3$.

or, $$\frac{T_1^2}{T_2^2} = \frac{r_1^3}{r_2^3}$$

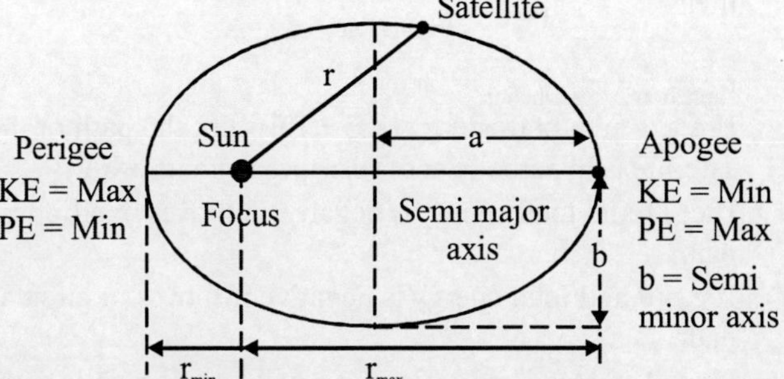

WEIGHTLESSNESS

The “weightlessness” you may feel in an aircraft occurs any time the aircraft is accelerating downward with acceleration g. It is possible to experience weightlessness for a considerable length of time by turning the nose of the craft upward and cutting power so that it travels in a ballistic trajectory. A ballistic trajectory is the common type of trajectory you get by throwing a rock or a baseball, neglecting air friction. At every point on the trajectory, the acceleration is equal to g downward since there is no support. A considerable amount of experimentation has been done with such ballistic trajectories to practice for orbital missions where you experience weightlessness all the time.

The satellite is moving in a circular orbit, it has a radial acceleration

$$a = \frac{v_0^2}{r} = \frac{GM}{r^2} \qquad \left[\text{as } v_0 = \sqrt{\left(\frac{GM}{r}\right)}\right]$$

i.e., it is falling towards earth's centre with acceleration a, so apparent weight of the body in it $W_{ap} = m(g' - a)$ where g′ is the acceleration due to gravity of earth at the position (height) of satellite, i.e. $g' = (GM/r^2)$, so that

$$W_{ap} = m\left[\frac{GM}{r^2} - \frac{GM}{r^2}\right] = 0$$

i.e., the apparent weight of a body in a satellite is zero and is independent of the radius of the orbit.

Problem Solving Tips

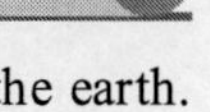

1. The moon takes 27.3 days to revolve around the earth. The radius of its orbit is 3.85×10^5 km.
2. Kepler's second law is based on conservation of angular momentum.
3. Perihelion distance is the shortest distance between the sun and the planet.

4. Aphelion distance is the largest distance between the Sun and the planet.

$$\frac{\text{Vaphelion}}{\text{Vperihelion}} = \frac{r_{perihelion}}{r_{aphelion}}$$

5. If e is the eccentricity of the orbit

then $$\frac{1+e}{1-e} = \frac{r_{aphelion}}{r_{perihelion}}$$

$r_{aphelion} + r_{perihelion} = 2r$

6. If e > 1 and total energy (KE + PE) > 0, the path of the satellite is hyperbolic and it escapes from its orbit.
7. If e < 1 and total energy is negative it moves in elliptical path.
8. If e = 0 and total energy is negative it moves in circular path.
9. If e = 0 and total energy is zero it will take parabolic path.
10. The path of the projectiles thrown to lower heights is parabolic and thrown to greater heights is elliptical.
11. Kepler's laws may be applied to natural and artificial satellites as well.
12. Gravitational force does not depend upon medium so no medium can shield it or block it.
13. The escape velocity and the orbital velocity are independent of the mass of the body being escaped or put into the orbit.

Example 13.

If the earth is at 1/4 of its present distance from the sun, what would be the duration of the year?

Solution :

We know that, $$\frac{T_1^2}{T_2^2} = \frac{R_1^3}{R_2^3}$$

Substituting the given values, we get

$$\frac{(1)^2}{T_2^2} = \frac{R^3}{\left(\frac{R}{4}\right)^3} \text{ or } \frac{1}{T_2^2} = (4)^3 = 64$$

$$T_2^2 = \frac{1}{64} \text{ or } T_2 = \frac{1}{8} \text{ year.}$$

Example 14.

Two satellites A and B go round a planet P in a circular orbits having radii 4R and R respectively. If the speed of satellite A is 3v, what will be the speed of satellite B?

Solution :

We know that $v = \sqrt{(GM/r)}$

Here $3v = \sqrt{\left(\frac{GM}{4R}\right)}$ and $v' = \sqrt{\left(\frac{GM}{R}\right)}$;

$$\therefore \frac{v'}{3v} = \sqrt{\left(\frac{GM}{R}\right)} \times \sqrt{\left(\frac{4R}{GM}\right)} = 2;\ v' = 6v$$

Example 15.

A spaceship is launched into a circular orbit close to earth's surface. What additional velocity has now to be imparted to the spaceship in the orbit to overcome the gravitational pull? Radius of earth = 6400 km and g = 9.8 m/s².

Solution :

The orbital velocity of spaceship in circular orbit

$$v_0 = \sqrt{\frac{GM}{r}} = \sqrt{\frac{GM}{R}}$$

($\because$ spaceship is very close to earth, r = R)

As $g = \frac{GM}{R^2}$ hence $GM = gR^2$

$$\therefore v_0 = \sqrt{(Rg)} = \sqrt{(6.4 \times 10^6) \times (9.8)} = 7.9195 \text{ km/s}$$

Further, $v_e = \sqrt{2Rg} = \sqrt{(2 \times 7.9195)} = 11.2 \text{ km/s}$

(where v_e is escape velocity)

Additional velocity required = 11.2000 – 7.0195
= 3.2805 km/s

So the velocity 3.2805 km/s must be added to orbital velocity of spaceship.

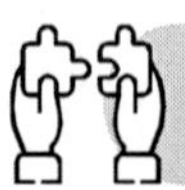

8.3 Concept Practice Problems

CPP

21. Which of the following graphs represents the motion of a planet moving about the sun ?

(a)

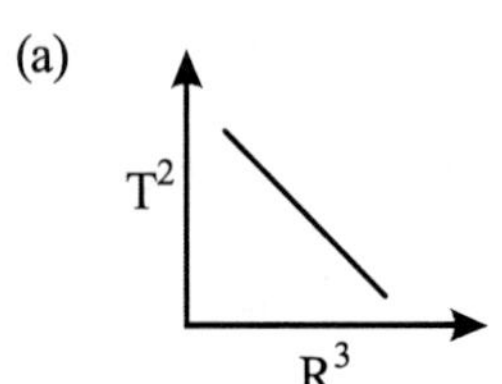

(b)

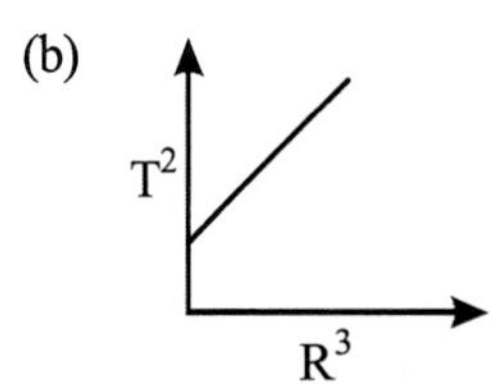

(c) (d)

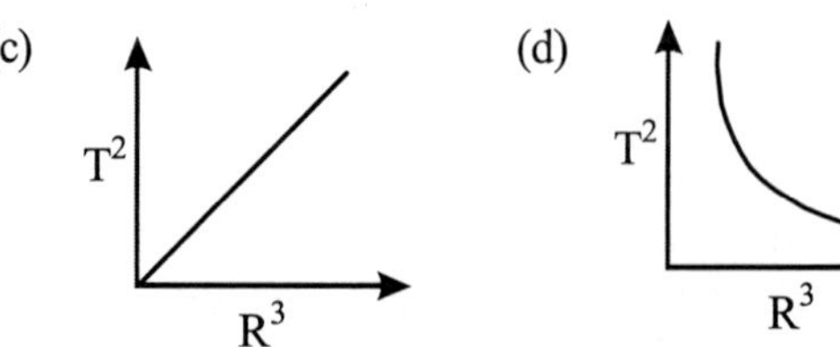

22. The ratio of the radii of the planets R_1 and R_2 is k. The ratio of the acceleration due to gravity is r. The ratio of the escape velocities from them will be

(a) kr (b) $\sqrt{kr}$ (c) $\sqrt{(k/r)}$ (d) $\sqrt{(r/k)}$

23. If v_e and v_0 represent the escape velocity and orbital velocity of a satellite corresponding to a circular orbit of radius R, then

(a) $v_e = v_o$

(b) $v_e = \sqrt{2}\, v_o$

(c) $v_e = (1/\sqrt{2})\, v_o$

(d) v_e and v_o are not related

24. The orbital velocity of an artificial satellite in a circular orbit very close to Earth is v. The velocity of a geosynchronous satellite orbiting in a circular orbit at an altitude of 6R from Earth's surface will be

(a) $\frac{v}{\sqrt{7}}$ (b) $\frac{v}{\sqrt{6}}$ (c) v (d) $\sqrt{6}v$

25. The mass of the moon is 1/81 of earth's mass and its radius 1/4 that of the earth. If the escape velocity from the earth's surface is 11.2 km/sec, its value from the surface of the moon will be

(a) $0.14\ kms^{-1}$ (b) $0.5\ kms^{-1}$

(c) $2.5\ kms^{-1}$ (d) $5.0\ kms^{-1}$

26. The distance of neptune and saturn from the sun is nearly 10^{13} and 10^{12} meter respectively. Assuming that they move in circular orbits, their periodic times will be in the ratio

(a) 10 (b) 100 (c) $10\sqrt{10}$ (d) 1000

27. A geostationary satellite is orbiting the earth at a height of 5*R* above that surface of the earth, *R* being the radius of the earth. The time period of another satellite in hours at a height of 2*R* from the surface of the earth is

(a) 5 (b) 10 (c) $6\sqrt{2}$ (d) $\frac{6}{\sqrt{2}}$

28. A satellite of mass m revolves around the earth of radius R at a height 'x' from its surface. If g is the acceleration due to gravity on the surface of the earth, the orbital speed of the satellite is

(a) $\frac{gR^2}{R+x}$ (b) $\frac{gR}{R-x}$

(c) gx (d) $\left(\frac{gR^2}{R+x}\right)^{1/2}$

29. An earth satellite of mass m revolves in a circular orbit at a height h from the surface of the earth. R is the radius of the earth and g is acceleration due to gravity at the surface of the earth. The velocity of the satellite in the orbit is given by

(a) $gR^2/(R+h)$ (b) gR

(c) $gR/(R-h)$ (d) $\sqrt{[gR^2/(R+h)]}$

30. A satellite of mass 'm', moving around the earth in a circular orbit of radius R, has angular momentum L. The areal velocity of satellite is (M_e = mass of earth)

(a) L/2m (b) L/m (c) 2L/m (d) $2L/M_e$

31. The largest and the shortest distance of the earth from the sun are r_1 and r_2. Its distance from the sun when it is at perpendicular to the major-axis of the orbit drawn from the sun

(a) $(r_1+r_2)/4$ (b) $(r_1+r_2)/(r_1-r_2)$

(c) $2r_1r_2/(r_1+r_2)$ (d) $(r_1+r_2)/3$

32. The orbital velocity of an artificial satellite in a circular orbit just above the centre's surface is υ. For a satellite orbiting at an altitude of half of the earth's radius, the orbital velocity is

(a) $\left(\sqrt{\left(\frac{2}{3}\right)}\right)v_0$ (b) $\frac{2}{3}v_0$

(c) $\frac{3}{2}v_0$ (d) $\sqrt{\left(\frac{3}{2}\right)}v_0$

33. Two identical geostationary satellites are moving with equal speeds in the same orbit but their sense of rotation brings them on a collision course. The debris will

(a) fall down

(b) move up

(c) begin to move from east to west in the same orbit

(d) begin to move from west to east in the same orbit

34. The escape velocity from a planet is v_e. A tunnel is dug along a diameter of the planet and a small body is dropped into it at the surface. When the body reaches the centre of the planet, its speed will be

(a) v_e (b) $v_e/\sqrt{2}$ (c) $v_e/2$ (d) zero

35. Four equal masses (each of mass M) are placed at the corners of a square of side a. The escape velocity of a body from the centre O of the square is

(a) $4\sqrt{\frac{2CM}{a}}$ (b) $\sqrt{\frac{8\sqrt{2}GM}{a}}$

(c) $\frac{4GM}{a}$ (d) $\sqrt{\frac{4\sqrt{2}GM}{a}}$

ANSWER KEY

21	(c)	22	(b)	23	(b)	24	(a)	25	(c)	26	(c)	27	(c)	28	(d)	29	(d)	30	(b)
31	(c)	32	(a)	33	(a)	34	(b)	35	(b)										

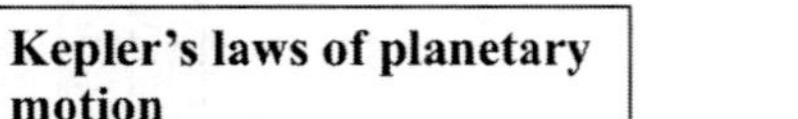

CONCEPT MAP

GRAVITATION
Force of attraction between any two bodies

Kepler's laws of planetary motion

(i) **Law of orbit :** Every planet revolve around the Sun in an elliptical orbit and Sun is at its one focus

(ii) **Law of area :** The radius vector drawn from the Sun to a planet sweeps out equal areas in equal intervals of time

i.e., $\frac{dA}{dt} = \frac{L}{2m}$ = Constant

(iii) **Law of periods :** Time period, $T^2 \propto a^3$
a = semi-major axis

Gravitational field intensity

$I = \frac{GM}{r^2}$

Gravitational potential

$V_g = \frac{\text{work done}}{\text{mass}} = \frac{-GM}{r}$

Gravitational Potential energy

$U = \frac{-GMm}{r}$

Characteristics of Gravitational force

(i) Weakest force in nature
(ii) Central as well as conservative
(iii) Always attractive nature
(iv) Applicable for all bodies irrespective of their size, shape and position

Newton's universal law of Gravitation

$F = \frac{Gm_1m_2}{r^2}, G = 6.67 \times 10^{-11} Nm^2kg^{-2}$

Satellite : A heavenly object revolves around a planet

Geostationary satellite :
Height from earth's surface = 36000 km
Radius of orbit = 42,400 km
Time period = 24 hours
Orbital velocity = 3.1 km/s

Polar satellite
Height from earth's surface = 880 km
Time period T = 84 min
Orbital velocity = 7.92 km/s

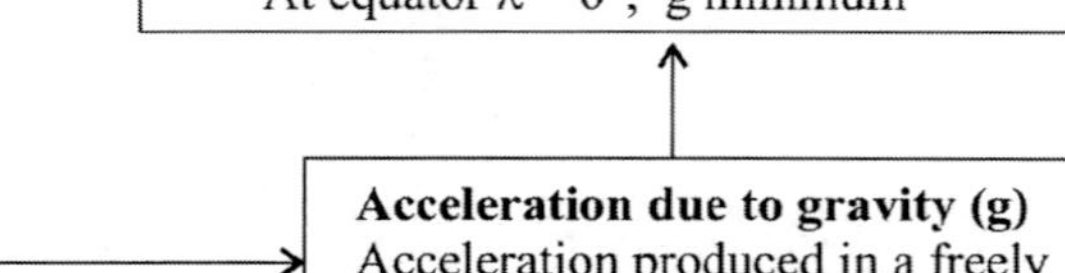

Acceleration due to gravity (g)
Acceleration produced in a freely falling object due to earth's gravitational pull. $g = \frac{gM_E}{R_E^2}$

Variation in acceleration due to gravity (g)

(i) with height $g' = g\left(1 - \frac{2h}{R_E}\right)$

i.e., g decreases with height

(ii) with depth $g' = g\left(1 - \frac{d}{R_E}\right)$

i.e., g decreases with depth

(iii) With rotation of earth about its own axis

$g' = g - R\omega^2 \cos^2 \lambda$

At poles $\lambda = 90°$, g maximum
At equator $\lambda = 0°$, g minimum

Escape speed $V_{esc} = \sqrt{2GM/R} = \sqrt{2gR}$
At earth V_{esc} = 11.2 km/s

Orbital speed $V_{orb} = \sqrt{gR} = \frac{V_e}{\sqrt{2}}$

Total energy of a satellite
E = KE + PE
$= \left(\frac{GMm}{2r}\right) + \left(\frac{-GMm}{r}\right)$

Weightlessness
During freely falling under gravity inside a spacecraft or satellite a body is weightless i.e., effective weight becomes zero

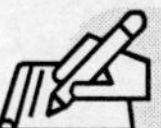

Exercise 1 - Chapter Revision Problems

CRP

1. The weight of an object in the coal mine, sea level and at the top of the mountain, are respectively W_1, W_2 and W_3 then
(a) $W_1 < W_2 > W_3$ (b) $W_1 = W_2 = W_3$
(c) $W_1 < W_2 < W_3$ (d) $W_1 > W_2 > W_3$

2. The maximum kinetic energy of a planet moving around the sun is at a position

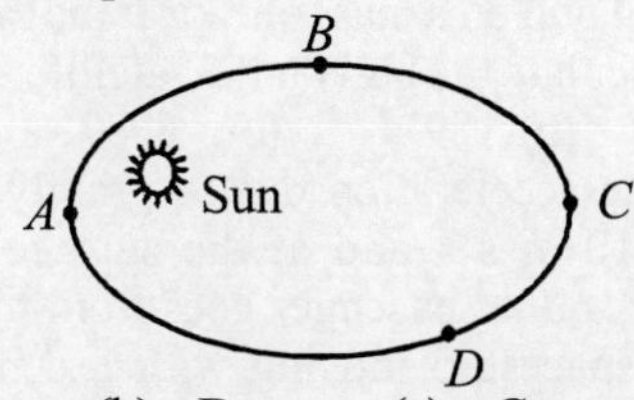

(a) A (b) B (c) C (d) D

3. A man waves his arms while walking. This is to
(a) keep constant velocity
(b) ease the tension
(c) increase the velocity
(d) balance the effect of earth's gravity

4. A missile is launched with a velocity less than escape velocity. The sum of its kinetic and potential energies is
(a) zero (b) negative (c) positive
(d) may be positive, negative or zero.

5. A planet moves around the sun. At a point P it is closest from the sun at a distance d_1 and has a speed v_1. At another point Q, when it is farthest from the sun at a distnace d_2 its speed will be
(a) $d_1^2 v_1 / d_2^2$ (b) $d_2 v_1 / d_1$
(c) $d_1 v_1 / d_2$ (d) $d_2^2 v_1 / d_1^2$

6. A satellite is orbiting around the earth near its surface. If its kinetic energy is doubled, then
(a) it will remain in the same orbit.
(b) it will fall on the earth.
(c) it will revolve with greater speed.
(d) it will escape out of the gravitational field of the earth.

7. What would be the length of a sec. pendulum at a planet (where acc. due to gravity is g/4) if it's length on earth is ℓ
(a) $\ell/2$ (b) 2ℓ (c) $\ell/4$ (d) 4ℓ

8. Time period of a simple pendulum inside a satellite orbiting earth is
(a) zero (b) ∞ (c) T (d) 2T

9. The kinetic energy needed to project a body of mass *m* from the earth surface (radius *R*) to infinity is
(a) mgR/2 (b) 2mgR (c) mgR (d) mgR/4.

10. The escape velocity of a body depends upon mass as
(a) m^0 (b) m^1 (c) m^2 (d) m^3.

11. Two satellites revolve round the earth with orbital radii 4R and 16R, if the time period of first satellite is T then that of the other is
(a) 4T (b) $4^{2/3}$ T
(c) 8T (d) None of these

12. A planet revolves in an elliptical orbit around the sun. The semi-major and semi-minor axes are a and b. Then the square of time period, T is directly proportional to
(a) a^3 (b) b^3
(c) $\left(\frac{a+b}{2}\right)^3$ (d) $\left(\frac{a-b}{2}\right)^3$

13. Which of the following quantities do not depend upon the orbital radius of the satellite ?
(a) $\frac{T}{R}$ (b) $\frac{T^2}{R}$ (b) $\frac{T^2}{R^2}$ (d) $\frac{T^2}{R^3}$

14. Escape velocity when a body of mass m is thrown vertically from the surface of the earth is v, what will be the escape velocity of another body of mass 4 m is thrown vertically
(a) v (b) 2v
(c) 4v (d) None of these

15. The escape velocity from the earth's surface is 11 km/s. The escape velocity from a planet having twice the radius and same mean density as that of earth is
(a) 5.5 km/s (b) 11 km/s
(c) 22 km/s (d) None of these

16. At sea level, a body will have minimum weight at
(a) pole (b) equator
(c) 42° south latitude (d) 37° north latitude

17. The escape velocity for a body projected vertically upwards from the surface of earth is 11 km/s. If the body is projected at an angle of 45º with the vertical, the escape velocity will be
(a) 22 km/s (b) 11 km/s
(c) $\frac{11}{\sqrt{2}}$ km/s (d) $11\sqrt{2}$ km/s

18. The kinetic energy of a satellite in its orbit around the earth is E. What should be the kinetic energy of the satellite so as to enable it to escape from the gravitational pull of the earth?
(a) 4E (b) 2E (c) $\sqrt{2}$E (d) E

19. If the change in the value of g at the height h above the surface of the earth is the same as at a depth 'x' below it, then (both x and h being much smaller than the radius of the earth)
(a) x=h (b) x=2h (c) x=h/2 (d) $x=h^2$

20. There are ______ gravitational lines of force inside a spherically symmetric shell.
(a) infinitely many
(b) zero
(c) varying number depending upon surface area
(d) varying number depending upon volume

21. A uniform ring of mass m and radius r is placed directly above a uniform sphere of mass M and of equal radius. The centre of the ring is directly above the centre of the sphere at a distance $r\sqrt{3}$ as shown in the figure.

The gravitational force exerted by the sphere on the ring will be

(a) $\frac{GMm}{8r^2}$

(b) $\frac{GMm}{4r^2}$

(c) $\sqrt{3}\frac{GMm}{8r^2}$

(d) $\frac{GMm}{8r^3\sqrt{3}}$

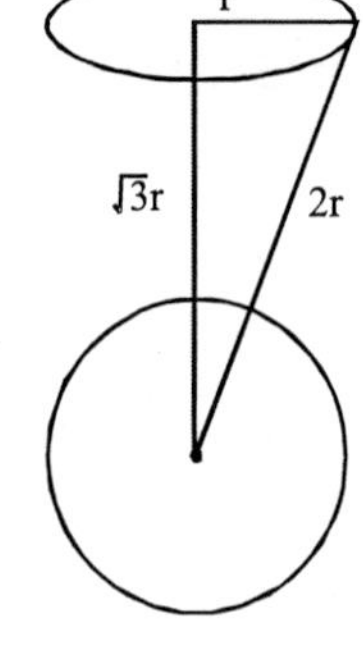

22. If value of acceleration due to gravity changes from one place to another, which of the following forces will undergo a change ?
(a) Viscous force (b) Buoyant force
(c) Magnetic force (d) All of the above

23. The radius of the earth is 4 times that of the moon and its mass is 80 times that of the moon. If the acceleration due to gravity on the surface of the earth is 10 m/s^2, then on the surface of the moon its value will be
(a) 1 ms^{-2} (b) 2 ms^{-2} (c) 3 ms^{-2} (d) 4 ms^{-2}

24. A solid sphere of uniform density and radius R applies a gravitational force of attraction equal to F_1 on a particle placed at A, distance 2R from the centre of the sphere.

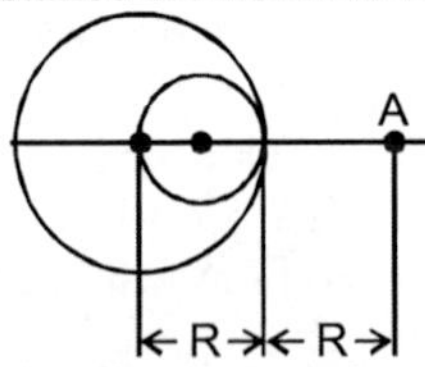

A spherical cavity of radius R/2 is now made in the sphere as shown in the figure. The sphere with cavity now applies a gravitational force F_2 on the same particle placed at A. The ratio F_2/F_1 will be
(a) 1/2 (b) 3 (c) 7 (d) 1/9

25. A planet is revolving around the sun in an elliptical orbit. Its closests distance from the sun is r_{min}. The farthest distance from the sun is r_{max}. If the orbital angular velocity of the planet when it is nearest to the sun is ω, then the orbital angular velocity at the point when it is at the farthest distance from the sun is
(a) $\sqrt{(r_{min}/r_{max})}\,\omega$ (b) $\sqrt{(r_{max}/r_{min})}\,\omega$
(c) $(r_{max}^2/r_{min}^2)\,\omega$ (d) $(r_{min}^2/r_{max}^2)\,\omega$

26. If there were a small gravitational effect, then which of the following forces will undergo a change?
(a) Viscous force (b) Electrostatic force
(c) Magnetic force (d) Archimedes' uplift

27. The gravitational force of attraction between a uniform sphere of mass M and a uniform rod of length l and mass m oriented as shown is

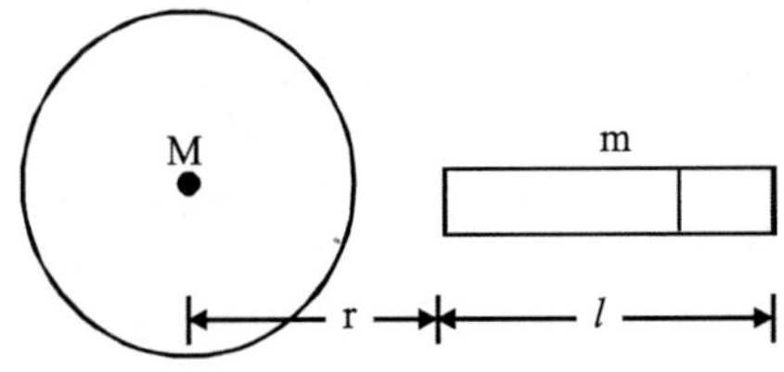

(a) $\frac{GMm}{r(r+l)}$ (b) $\frac{GM}{r^2}$
(c) Mmr^2+l (d) $(r^2+l)mM$

28. Explorer 38, a radio-astronomy satellite of mass 200 kg, circles the Earth in an orbit of average radius $\frac{3R}{2}$ where R is the radius of the Earth. Assuming the gravitational pull on a mass of 1 kg at the earth's surface to be 10 N, calculate the pull on the satellite
(a) 889 N (b) 89 N (c) 8889 N (d) 8.9 N

29. Suppose, the acceleration due to gravity at the Earth's surface is 10 m s^{-2} and at the surface of Mars it is 4.0 m s^{-2}. A 60 kg pasenger goes from the Earth to the Mars in a spaceship moving with a constant velocity. Neglect all other objects in the sky. Which part of figure best represents the weight (net gravitational force) of the passenger as a function of time?

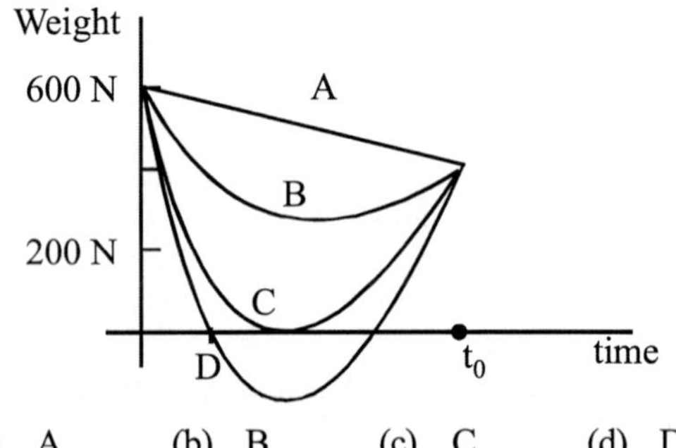

(a) A (b) B (c) C (d) D

30. Four similar particles of mass m are orbiting in a circle of radius r in the same angular direction because of their mutual gravitational attractive force. Velocity of a particle is given by

(a) $\left[\frac{GM}{r}\left(\frac{1+2\sqrt{2}}{4}\right)\right]^{1/2}$

(b) $\sqrt[3]{\frac{GM}{r}}$

(c) $\sqrt{\frac{GM}{r}(1+2\sqrt{2})}$

(d) $\left[\frac{1}{2}\frac{GM}{r}\left(\frac{1+\sqrt{2}}{2}\right)\right]^{1/2}$

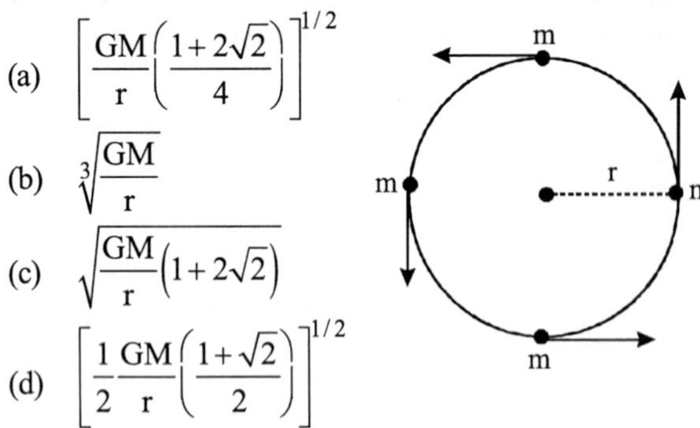

31. A satellite is revolving round the earth in an orbit of radius r with time period T. If the satellite is revolving round the earth in an orbit of radius r + Δr (Δr << r) with time period T + Δ T then,
(a) $\frac{\Delta T}{T}=\frac{3}{2}\frac{\Delta r}{r}$ (b) $\frac{\Delta T}{T}=\frac{2}{3}\frac{\Delta r}{r}$
(c) $\frac{\Delta T}{T}=\frac{\Delta r}{r}$ (d) $\frac{\Delta T}{T}=-\frac{\Delta r}{r}$

32. A cavity of radius R/2 is made inside a solid sphere of radius R. The centre of the cavity is located at a distance R/2 from the centre of the sphere. The gravitational force

on a particle of mass 'm' at a distance R/2 from the centre of the sphere on the line joining both the centres of sphere and cavity is – (opposite to the centre of gravity)
[Here $g = GM/R^2$, where M is the mass of the sphere]

(a) $\frac{mg}{2}$ (b) $\frac{3mg}{8}$

(c) $\frac{mg}{16}$ (d) None of these

33. A (nonrotating) star collapses onto itself from an initial radius R_i with its mass remaining unchanged. Which curve in figure best gives the gravitational acceleration a_g on the surface of the star as a function of the radius of the star during the collapse

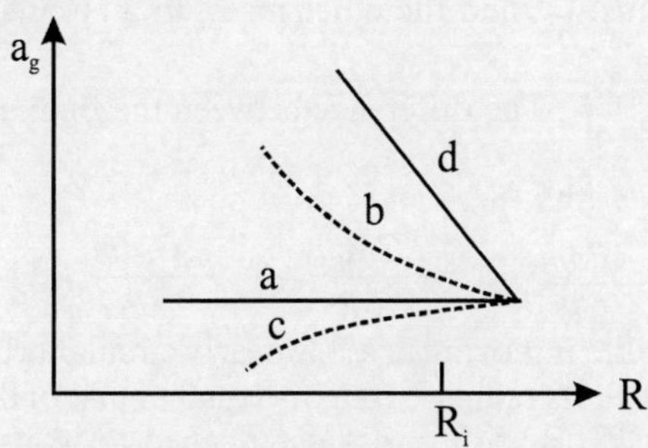

(a) a (b) b (c) c (d) d

34. The earth is assumed to be sphere of radius R. A platform is arranged at a height R from the surface of Earth. The escape velocity of a body from this platform is kv, where v is its escape velocity from the surface of the earth. The value of k is

(a) $\frac{1}{\sqrt{2}}$ (b) $\frac{1}{3}$ (c) $\frac{1}{2}$ (d) $\sqrt{2}$

35. The change in potential energy, when a body of mass m is raised to a height nR from the earth's surface is (R = radius of earth)

(a) $mgR\left(\frac{n}{n-1}\right)$ (b) nmgR

(c) $mgR\left(\frac{n^2}{n^2+1}\right)$ (d) $mgR\left(\frac{n}{n+1}\right)$

36. A satellite is launched into a circular orbit of radius R around the earth. A second satellite is launched into an orbit of radius 1.01 R. The period of second satellite is larger than the first one by approximately

(a) 0.5% (b) 1.0% (c) 1.5% (d) 3.0%

37. For a satellite moving in an orbit around the earth, the ratio of kinetic energy to potential energy is

(a) $\frac{1}{2}$ (b) $\frac{1}{\sqrt{2}}$ (c) 2 (d) $\sqrt{2}$

38. The figure shows elliptical orbit of a planet m about the sun S. The shaded area SCD is twice the shaded area SAB. If t_1 is the time for the planet to move from C to D and t_2 is the time to move from A to B then :

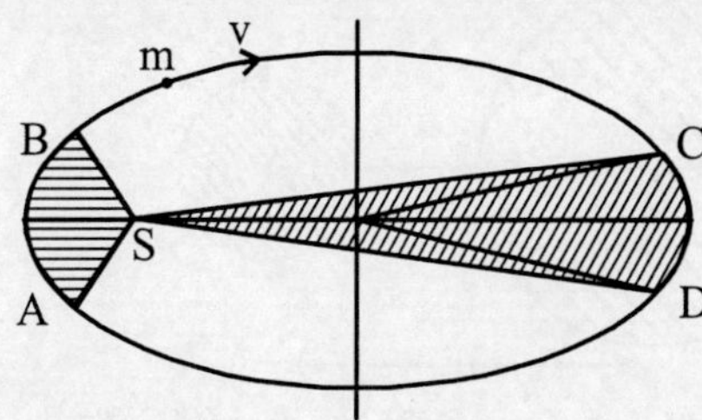

(a) $t_1 = 4t_2$ (b) $t_1 = 2t_2$ (c) $t_1 = t_2$ (d) $t_1 > t_2$

39. The radii of circular orbits of two satellites A and B of the earth, are 4R and R, respectively. If the speed of satellite A is 3 V, then the speed of satellite B will be

(a) 3 V/4 (b) 6V (c) 12V (d) 3 V/2

40. A particle of mass m is thrown upwards from the surface of the earth, with a velocity u. The mass and the radius of the earth are, respectively, M and R. G is gravitational constant and g is acceleration due to gravity on the surface of the earth. The minimum value of u so that the particle does not return back to earth, is

(a) $\sqrt{\frac{2GM}{R}}$ (b) $\sqrt{\frac{2GM}{R^2}}$ (c) $\sqrt{2gR^2}$ (d) $\sqrt{\frac{2GM}{R^2}}$

41. India's Mangalyan was sent to the Mars by launching it into a transfer orbit EOM around the sun. It leaves the earth at E and meets Mars at M. If the semi-major axis of Earth's orbit is $a_e = 1.5 \times 10^{11}$ m, that of Mars orbit $a_m = 2.28 \times 10^{11}$ m, taken Kepler's laws give the estimate of time for Mangalyan to reach Mars from Earth to be close to:

(a) 500 days

(b) 320 days

(c) 260 days

(d) 220 days

Mars orbit

O

a_m a_e

M E

Sun

Earth's orbit

42. A straight rod of length L extends from $x = a$ to $x = L + a$. The gravitational force it exerts on point mass 'm' at $x = 0$, if the mass per unit length of the rod is $A + Bx^2$, is given by:

(a) $Gm\left[A\left(\frac{1}{a+L}-\frac{1}{a}\right)-BL\right]$

(b) $Gm\left[A\left(\frac{1}{a}-\frac{1}{a+L}\right)-BL\right]$

(c) $Gm\left[A\left(\frac{1}{a+L}-\frac{1}{a}\right)+BL\right]$

(d) $Gm\left[A\left(\frac{1}{a}-\frac{1}{a+L}\right)+BL\right]$

43. From a sphere of mass M and radius R, a smaller sphere of radius $\frac{R}{2}$ is carved out such that the cavity made in the original sphere is between its centre and the periphery (See figure). For the configuration in the figure where the distance between the centre of the original sphere and the removed sphere is 3R, the gravitational force between the two sphere is:

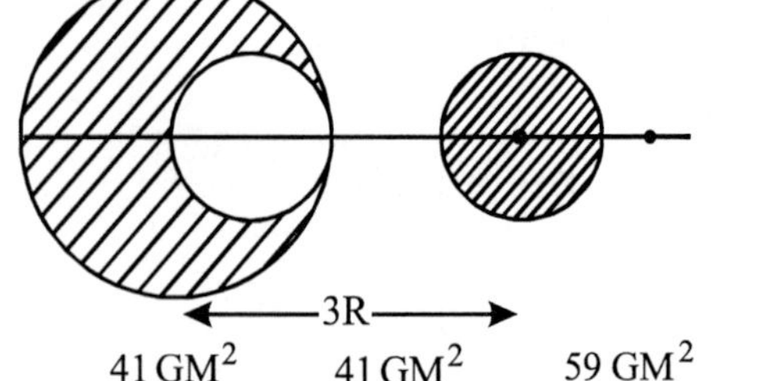

(a) $\frac{41\,GM^2}{3600\,R^2}$ (b) $\frac{41\,GM^2}{450\,R^2}$ (c) $\frac{59\,GM^2}{450\,R^2}$ (d) $\frac{GM^2}{225\,R^2}$

44. The acceleration due to gravity on the earth's surface at the poles is g and angular velocity of the earth about the axis passing through the pole is ω. An object is weighed at the equator and at a height h above the poles by using a spring balance. If the weights are found to be same, then h is : ($h<<R$, where R is the radius of the earth)

(a) $\frac{R^2\omega^2}{2g}$ (b) $\frac{R^2\omega^2}{g}$ (c) $\frac{R^2\omega^2}{4g}$ (d) $\frac{R^2\omega^2}{8g}$

45. The ratio of the weights of a body on the Earth's surface to that on the surface of a planet is 9:4. The mass of the planet is $\frac{1}{9}$th of that of the Earth. If 'R' is the radius of the Earth, what is the radius of the planet ? (Take the planets to have the same mass density).

(a) $\frac{R}{3}$ (b) $\frac{R}{4}$ (c) $\frac{R}{9}$ (d) $\frac{R}{2}$

46. Suppose that the angular velocity of rotation of earth is increased. Then, as a consequence.

(a) There will be no change in weight anywhere on the earth
(b) Weight of the object, everywhere on the earth, wild decrease
(c) Weight of the object, everywhere on the earth, will increase
(d) Except at poles, weight of the object on the earth will decrease

47. The change in the value of acceleration of earth towards sun, when the moon comes from the position of solar eclipse to the position on the other side of earth in line with sun is:

(mass of the moon = 7.36×10^{22} kg, radius of the moon's orbit = 3.8×10^8 m).

(a) 6.73×10^{-5} m/s^2 (b) 6.73×10^{-3} m/s^2
(c) 6.73×10^{-2} m/s^2 (d) 6.73×10^{-4} m/s^2

48. Two planets have masses M and $16\,M$ and their radii are a and $2a$, respectively. The separation between the centres of the planets is $10a$. A body of mass m is fired from the surface of the larger planet towards the smaller planet along the line joining their centres. For the body to be able to reach the surface of smaller planet, the minimum firing speed needed is :

(a) $2\sqrt{\frac{GM}{a}}$ (b) $4\sqrt{\frac{GM}{a}}$

(c) $\sqrt{\frac{GM^2}{ma}}$ (d) $\frac{3}{2}\sqrt{\frac{5GM}{a}}$

49. On the x-axis and at a distance x from the origin, the gravitational field due to a mass distribution is given by $\frac{Ax}{(x^2+a^2)^{3/2}}$ in the x-direction. The magnitude of gravitational potential on the x-axis at a distance x, taking its value to be zero at infinity, is :

(a) $\frac{A}{(x^2+a^2)^{1/2}}$ (b) $\frac{A}{(x^2+a^2)^{3/2}}$

(c) $A(x^2+a^2)^{1/2}$ (d) $A(x^2+a^2)^{3/2}$

50. A body of mass m is moving in a circular orbit of radius R about a planet of mass M. At some instant, it splits into two equal masses. The first mass moves in a circular orbit of radius $\frac{R}{2}$, and the other mass, in a circular orbit of radius $\frac{3R}{2}$. The difference between the final and initial total energies is:

(a) $-\frac{GMm}{2R}$ (b) $+\frac{GMm}{6R}$ (c) $-\frac{GMm}{6R}$ (d) $\frac{GMm}{2R}$

51. A satellite is moving in a low nearly circular orbit around the earth. Its radius is roughly equal to that of the earth's radius R_e. By firing rockets attached to it, its speed is instantaneously increased in the direction of its motion so that it become $\sqrt{\frac{3}{2}}$ times larger. Due to this the farthest distance from the centre of the earth that the satellite reaches is R. Value of R is :

(a) $4R_e$ (b) $2.5R_e$ (c) $3R_e$ (d) $2R_e$

52. A body A of mass m is moving in a circular orbit of radius R about a planet. Another body B of mass $\frac{m}{2}$ collides with A with a velocity which is half $\left(\frac{\vec{v}}{2}\right)$ the instantaneous velocity $\vec{v}$ or A. The collision is completely inelastic. Then, the combined body:

(a) continues to move in a circular orbit
(b) Escapes from the Planet's Gravitational field
(c) Falls vertically downwards towards the planet
(d) starts moving in an elliptical orbit around the planet

53. A rocket has to be launched from earth in such a way that it never returns. If E is the minimum energy delivered by the rocket launcher, what should be the minimum energy that the launcher should have if the same rocket is to be launched from the surface of the moon? Assume that the density of the earth and the moon are equal and that the earth's volume is 64 times the volume of the moon.

(a) $\frac{E}{64}$ (b) $\frac{E}{32}$ (c) $\frac{E}{4}$ (d) $\frac{E}{16}$

54. Two satellites, A and B, have masses m and 2m respectively. A is in a circular orbit of radius R, and B is in a circular orbit of radius 2R around the earth. The ratio of their kinetic energies, T_A/T_B, is :

(a) $\frac{1}{2}$ (b) 1 (c) 2 (d) $\sqrt{\frac{1}{2}}$

55. A satellite is revolving in a circular orbit at a height h from the earth surface, such that h << R where R is the radius of the earth. Assuming that the effect of earth's atmosphere can be neglected the minimum increase in the speed required so that the satellite could escape from the gravitational field of earth is:

(a) $\sqrt{2gR}$ (b) $\sqrt{gR}$

(c) $\sqrt{\frac{gR}{2}}$ (d) $\sqrt{gR}\left(\sqrt{2}-1\right)$

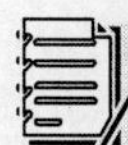

Exercise 2 - Exemplar & Past Year Questions

E&PYQs

Exemplar Questions

1. The earth is an approximate sphere. If the interior contained matter which is not of the same density everywhere, then on the surface of the earth, the acceleration due to gravity
   (a) will be directed towards the centre but not the same everywhere
   (b) will have the same value everywhere but not directed towards the centre
   (c) will be same everywhere in magnitude directed towards the centre
   (d) cannot be zero at any point
2. As observed from the earth, the sun appears to move in an approximate circular orbit. For the motion of another planet like mercury as observed from the earth, this would
   (a) be similarly true
   (b) not be true because the force between the earth and mercury is not inverse square law
   (c) not be true because the major gravitational force on mercury is due to the sun
   (d) not be true because mercury is influenced by forces other than gravitational force
3. Different points in the earth are at slightly different distances from the sun and hence experience different forces due to gravitation. For a rigid body, we know that if various forces act at various points in it, the resultant motion is as if a net force acts on the CM (centre of mass) causing translation and a net torque at the CM causing rotation around an axis through the CM. For the earth-sun system (approximating the earth as a uniform density sphere).
   (a) the torque is zero
   (b) the torque causes the earth to spin
   (c) the rigid body result is not applicable since the earth is not even approximately a rigid body
   (d) the torque causes the earth to move around the sun
4. Satellites orbitting the earth have finite life and sometimes debris of satellites fall to the earth. This is because
   (a) the solar cells and batteries in satellites run out
   (b) the laws of gravitation predict a trajectory spiralling inwards
   (c) of viscous forces causing the speed of satellite and hence height to gradually decrease
   (d) of collisions with other satellites
5. Both the earth and the moon are subject to the gravitational force of the sun. As observed from the sun, the orbit of the moon
   (a) will be elliptical
   (b) will not be strictly elliptical because the total gravitational force on it is not central
   (c) is not elliptical but will necessarily be a closed curve
   (d) deviates considerably from being elliptical due to influence of planets other than the earth
6. In our solar system, the inter-planetary region has chunks of matter (much smaller in size compared to planets) called asteroids. They
   (a) will not move around the sun, since they have very small masses compared to the sun
   (b) will move in an irregular way because of their small masses and will drift away into outer space
   (c) will move around the sun in closed orbits but not obey Kepler's laws
   (d) will move in orbits like planets and obey Kepler's laws
7. Choose the wrong option.
   (a) Inertial mass is a measure of difficulty of accelerating a body by an external force whereas the gravitational mass is relevant in determining the gravitational force on it by an external mass
   (b) That the gravitational mass and inertial mass are equal is an experimental result
   (c) That the acceleration due to gravity on the earth is the same for all bodies is due to the equality of gravitational mass and inertial mass
   (d) Gravitational mass of a particle like proton can depend on the presence of neighbouring heavy objects but the inertial mass cannot
8. Particles of masses $2M$, m and M are respectively at points A, B and C with $AB = \frac{1}{2}(BC) \cdot m$ is much-much smaller than M and at time $t = 0$, they are all at rest as given in figure.

   At subsequent times before any collision takes place.

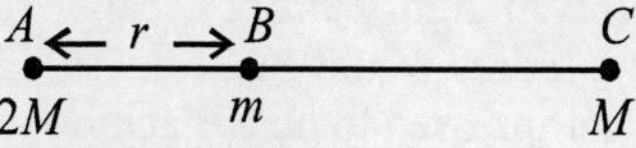

   (a) m will remain at rest
   (b) m will move towards M
   (c) m will move towards $2M$
   (d) m will have oscillatory motion

NEET/AIPMT (2013-2020) Questions

9. A body of mass 'm' is taken from the earth's surface to the height equal to twice the radius (R) of the earth. The change in potential energy of body will be **[2013]**

   (a) $\frac{2}{3}$ mgR (b) 3 mgR (c) $\frac{1}{3}$ mgR (d) mg2R

10. Infinite number of bodies, each of mass 2 kg are situated on x-axis at distances 1m, 2m, 4m, 8m, ... respectively, from the origin. The resulting gravitational potential due to this system at the origin will be *[2013]*

(a) $-\frac{8}{3}G$ (b) $-\frac{4}{3}G$ (c) $-4G$ (d) $-G$

11. The radius of a planet is twice the radius of earth. Both have almost equal average mass-densities. If V_P and V_E are escape velocities of the planet and the earth, respectively, then *[NEET Kar. 2013]*

(a) $V_E = 1.5V_P$ (b) $V_P = 1.5V_E$
(c) $V_P = 2V_E$ (d) $V_E = 3V_P$

12. A particle of mass '*m*' is kept at rest at a height 3*R* from the surface of earth, where '*R*' is radius of earth and '*M*' is mass of earth. The minimum speed with which it should be projected, so that it does not return back, is (*g* is acceleration due to gravity on the surface of earth) *[NEET Kar. 2013]*

(a) $\left(\frac{GM}{R}\right)^{\frac{1}{2}}$ (b) $\left(\frac{GM}{2R}\right)^{\frac{1}{2}}$ (c) $\left(\frac{gR}{4}\right)^{\frac{1}{2}}$ (d) $\left(\frac{2g}{4}\right)^{\frac{1}{2}}$

13. A projectile is fired from the surface of the earth with a velocity of 5 ms^{-1} and angle θ with the horizontal. Another projectile fired from another planet with a velocity of 3 ms^{-1} at the same angle follows a trajectory which is identical with the trajectory of the projectile fired from the earth. The value of the acceleration due to gravity on the planet is (in ms^{-2}) given g = 9.8 m/s^2 *[2014]*

(a) 3.5 (b) 5.9 (c) 16.3 (d) 110.8

14. Dependence of intensity of gravitational field (E) of earth with distance (r) from centre of earth is correctly represented by: *[2014]*

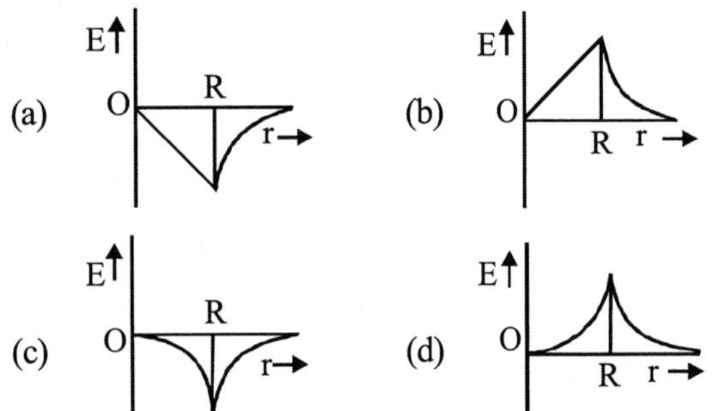

15. A black hole is an object whose gravitational field is so strong that even light cannot escape from it. To what approximate radius would earth (mass = 5.98×10^{24} kg) have to be compressed to be a black hole? *[2014]*

(a) 10^{-9} m (b) 10^{-6} m (c) 10^{-2} m (d) 100 m

16. A remote - sensing satellite of earth revolves in a circular orbit at a height of 0.25×10^6 m above the surface of earth. If earth's radius is 6.38×10^6 m and g = 9.8 ms^{-2}, then the orbital speed of the satellite is: *[2015 RS]*

(a) 8.56 km s^{-1} (b) 9.13 km s^{-1}
(c) 6.67 km s^{-1} (d) 7.76 km s^{-1}

17. Two spherical bodies of mass M and 5 M and radii R and 2 R released in free space with initial separation between their centres equal to 12 R. If they attract each other due to gravitational force only, then the distance covered by the smaller body before collision is *[2015]*

(a) 4.5R (b) 7.5R (c) 1.5R (d) 2.5R

18. The ratio of escape velocity at earth (v_e) to the escape velocity at a planet (v_p) whose radius and mean density are twice as that of earth is : *[2016]*

(a) 1 : 2 (b) 1 : 2 $\sqrt{2}$ (c) 1 : 4 (d) 1 : 2

19. At what height from the surface of earth the gravitational potential and the value of g are -5.4×10^7 J kg^{-1} and 6.0 ms^{-2} respectively ?
Take the radius of earth as 6400 km : *[2016]*

(a) 2600 km (b) 1600 km (c) 1400 km (d) 2000 km

20. Two astronauts are floating in gravitation free space after having lost contact with their spaceship. The two will *[2017]*

(a) move towards each other.
(b) move away from each other.
(c) become stationary
(d) keep floating at the same distance between them.

21. The acceleration due to gravity at a height 1 km above the earth is the same as at a depth d below the surface of earth. Then *[2017]*

(a) d = 1 km (b) d = $\frac{3}{2}$ km
(c) d = 2 km (d) d = $\frac{1}{2}$ km

22. The kinetic energies of a planet in an elliptical orbit about the Sun, at positions A, B and C are K_A, K_B and K_C, respectively. AC is the major axis and SB is perpendicular to AC at the position of the Sun S as shown in the figure. Then *[2018]*

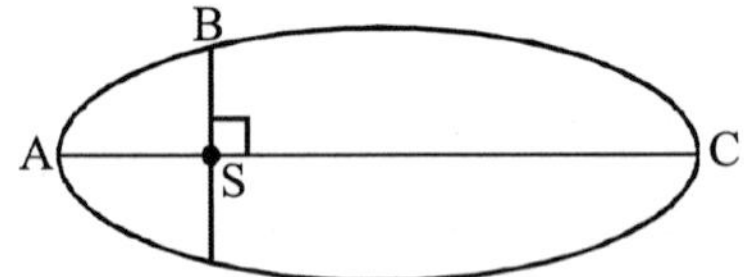

(a) $K_A < K_B < K_C$ (b) $K_A > K_B > K_C$
(c) $K_B > K_A > K_C$ (d) $K_B < K_A < K_C$

23. The work done to raise a mass m from the surface of the earth to a height *h*, which is equal to the radius of the earth, is : *[2019]*

(a) mgR (b) 2mgR (c) $\frac{1}{2}$mgR (d) $\frac{3}{2}$mgR

24. Assuming that the gravitational potential energy of an object at infinity is zero, the change in potential energy (final – initial) of an object of mass *m*, when taken to a height *h* from the surface of earth (of radius *R*), is given by, *[NEET Odisha 2019]*

(a) $\frac{GMm}{R+h}$ (b) $-\frac{GMm}{R+h}$ (c) $\frac{GMmh}{R(R+h)}$ (d) *mgh*

25. The time period of a geostationary satellite is 24 *h*, at a height $6R_E$ (R_E is radius of earth) from surface of earth. The time period of another satellite whose height is 2.5 R_E from surface will be, *[NEET Odisha 2019]*

(a) $\frac{12}{2.5}h$ (b) $6\sqrt{2}\,h$ (c) $12\sqrt{2}\,h$ (d) $\frac{24}{2.5}h$

26. A body weighs 72 N on the surface of the earth. What is the gravitational force on it, at a height equal to half the radius of the earth? *[2020]*

(a) 32 N (b) 30 N (c) 24 N (d) 48 N

Exercise 3 - Concept Application Problems

CAP

1. There is no atmosphere on the moon because
   (a) it is closer to the earth and also it has the inactive inert gases in it.
   (b) it is too for from the sun and has very low pressure in its outer surface.
   (c) escape velocity of gas molecules is greater than their root mean square velocity.
   (d) escape velocity of gas molecules is less than their root mean square velocity.
2. Two planets of radii r_1 and r_2 are made from the same material. The ratio of the acceleration due to gravity g_1/g_2 at the surfaces of the two planets is
   (a) r_1/r_2 (b) r_2/r_1 (c) $(r_1/r_2)^2$ (d) $(r_2/r_1)^2$
3. The radius of a planet is $1/4^{th}$ of R_e and its acc. due to gravity is 2g. What would be the value of escape velocity on the planet, if escape velocity on earth is v_e.
   (a) $\frac{v_e}{\sqrt{2}}$ (b) $v_e\sqrt{2}$ (c) $2\,v_e$ (d) $\frac{v_e}{2}$
4. The potential energy of a satellite of mass m and revolving at a height R_e above the surface of earth where R_e = radius of earth, is
   (a) $-mgR_e$ (b) $\frac{-mgR_e}{2}$
   (c) $\frac{-mgR_e}{3}$ (d) $\frac{-mgR_e}{4}$
5. The time period of a satellite of earth is 5 hours. If the separation between the earth and the satellite is increased to 4 times the previous value, the new time period will become
   (a) 10 hours (b) 80 hours
   (c) 40 hours (d) 20 hours
6. If the length of a simple pendulum is increased by 2%, then the time period
   (a) increases by 2% (b) decreases by 2%
   (c) increases by 1% (d) decreases by 1%
7. The time period of a satellite in a circular orbit of radius R is T, the period of another satellite in a circular orbit of radius 4 R is
   (a) 4 T (b) T/4 (c) 8 T (d) T/8
8. The time period of an earth satellite in circular orbit is independent of
   (a) both the mass and radius of the orbit
   (b) radius of its orbit
   (c) the mass of the satellite
   (d) neither the mass of the satellite nor the radius of its orbit.
9. Suppose the gravitational force varies inversely as the nth power of distance. Then the time period of a planet in circular orbit of radius 'R' around the sun will be proportional to
   (a) R^n (b) $R^{\left(\frac{n-1}{2}\right)}$ (c) $R^{\left(\frac{n+1}{2}\right)}$ (d) $R^{\left(\frac{n-2}{2}\right)}$
10. Mass of the Earth has been determined through
   (a) use of Kepler's $\frac{T^2}{R^3}$ constancy law and Moon's period
   (b) sampling the density of Earth's crust and using Earth's radius
   (c) Cavendish's determination of G and using Earth radius and g at its surface
   (d) use of periods of satellites at different heights above Earth's surface and known radius of Earth
11. The ratio of the kinetic energy required to be given to a satellite so that it escapes the gravitational field of Earth to the kinetic energy required to put the satellite in a circular orbit just above the free surface of Earth is
   (a) 1 (b) 2 (c) 3 (d) 9
12. An artificial satellite moving in a circular orbit around the earth has a total (K.E. + P.E.) is E_0. Its potential energy is –
   (a) $-E_0$ (b) $1.5\,E_0$ (c) $2E_0$ (d) E_0
13. A body starts from rest from a point distance R_0 from the centre of the earth. The velocity acquired by the body when it reaches the surface of the earth will be (R represents radius of the earth).
   (a) $2GM\left(\frac{1}{R}-\frac{1}{R_0}\right)$ (b) $\sqrt{2GM\left(\frac{1}{R_0}-\frac{1}{R}\right)}$
   (c) $GM\left(\frac{1}{R}-\frac{1}{R_0}\right)$ (d) $2GM\sqrt{\left(\frac{1}{R}-\frac{1}{R_0}\right)}$
14. Two spherical bodies of mass M and 5M and radii R and 2R respectively are released in free space with initial separation between their centres equal to 12 R. If they attract each other due to gravitational force only, then the distance covered by the smaller body just before collision is
   (a) 2.5 R (b) 4.5 R (c) 7.5 R (d) 1.5 R
15. If the radius of the earth were to shrink by one per cent, its mass remaining the same, the acceleration due to gravity on the earth's surface would
   (a) decrease (b) remain unchanged
   (c) increase (d) None of these
16. A ball is dropped from a satellite revolving around the earth at height of 120 km. The ball will
   (a) continue to move with same speed along a straight line tangentially to the satellite at that time
   (b) continue to move with same speed along the original orbit of satellite.
   (c) fall down to earth gradually
   (d) go far away in space
17. A projectile is fired vertically from the Earth with a velocity kv_e where v_e is the escape velocity and k is a constant less than unity. The maximum height to which projectile rises, as measured from the centre of Earth, is
   (a) $\frac{R}{k}$ (b) $\frac{R}{k-1}$ (c) $\frac{R}{1-k^2}$ (d) $\frac{R}{1+k^2}$
18. A diametrical tunnel is dug across the Earth. A ball is dropped into the tunnel from one side. The velocity of the ball when it reaches the centre of the Earth is .... (Given : gravitational potential at the centre of Earth = $-\frac{3}{2}\frac{GM}{R}$)

(a) $\sqrt{R}$ (b) $\sqrt{gR}$

(c) $\sqrt{2.5gR}$ (d) $\sqrt{7.1gR}$

19. The percentage change in the acceleration of the earth towards the sun from a total eclipse of the sun to the point where the moon is on a side of earth directly opposite to the sun is

(a) $\frac{M_s}{M_m}\frac{r_2}{r_1}\times 100$ (b) $\frac{M_s}{M_m}\left(\frac{r_2}{r_1}\right)^2\times 100$

(c) $2\left(\frac{r_1}{r_2}\right)^2\frac{M_m}{M_s}\times 100$ (d) $\left(\frac{r_1}{r_2}\right)^2\frac{M_s}{M_m}\times 100$

20. A spherical uniform planet is rotating about its axis. The velocity of a point on its equator is V. Due to the rotation of planet about its axis the acceleration due to gravity g at equator is 1/2 of g at poles. The escape velocity of a particle on the pole of planet in terms of V is

(a) $V_e=2V$ (b) $V_e=V$

(c) $V_e=V/2$ (d) $V_e=\sqrt{3}V$

21. A planet of mass m moves around the sun of mass M in an elliptical orbit. The maximum and minimum distance of the planet from the sun are r_1 and r_2 respectively. The time period of planet is proportional to

(a) $r_1^{2/5}$ (b) $(r_1+r_2)^{3/2}$

(c) $(r_1-r_2)^{3/2}$ (d) $r^{3/2}$

22. A particle of mass M is situated at the centre of a spherical shell of same mass and radius a. The gravitational potential at a point situated at $\frac{a}{2}$ distance from the centre, will be

(a) $-\frac{3GM}{a}$ (b) $-\frac{2GM}{a}$ (c) $-\frac{GM}{a}$ (d) $-\frac{4GM}{a}$

23. A planet moving along an elliptical orbit is closest to the sun at a distance r_1 and farthest away at a distance of r_2. If v_1 and v_2 are the linear velocities at these points respectively, then the ratio $\frac{v_1}{v_2}$ is

(a) $(r_1/r_2)^2$ (b) r_2/r_1 (c) $(r_2/r_1)^2$ (d) r_1/r_2

24. If the angular momentum of a planet of mass m, moving around the Sun in a circular orbit is L, about the center of the Sun, its areal velocity is:

(a) $\frac{L}{m}$ (b) $\frac{4L}{m}$ (c) $\frac{L}{2m}$ (d) $\frac{2L}{m}$

25. Take the mean distance of the moon and the sun from the earth to be 0.4×10^6 km and 150×10^6 km respectively. Their masses are 8×10^{22} kg and 2×10^{30} kg respectively. The radius of the earth is 6400 km. Let ΔF_1 be the difference in the forces exerted by the moon at the nearest and farthest points on the earth and ΔF_2 be the difference in the force exerted by the sun at the nearest and farthest points on the earth. Then, the number closest to $\frac{\Delta F_1}{\Delta F_2}$ is:

(a) 2 (b) 6 (c) 10^{-2} (d) 0.6

26. The value of acceleration due to gravity is g_1 at a height $h=\frac{R}{2}$ (R = radius of the earth) from the surface of the earth. It is again equal to g_1 and a depth d below the surface of the earth. The ratio $\left(\frac{d}{R}\right)$ equals :

(a) $\frac{4}{9}$ (b) $\frac{5}{9}$ (c) $\frac{1}{3}$ (d) $\frac{7}{9}$

27. The height 'h' at which the weight of a body will be the same as that at the same depth 'h' from the surface of the earth is (Radius of the earth is R and effect of the rotation of the earth is neglected) :

(a) $\frac{\sqrt{5}}{2}R-R$ (b) $\frac{R}{2}$

(c) $\frac{\sqrt{5}R-R}{2}$ (d) $\frac{\sqrt{3}R-R}{2}$

28. A box weighs 196 N on a spring balance at the north pole. Its weight recorded on the same balance if it is shifted to the equator is close to (Take $g = 10\ ms^{-2}$ at the north pole and the radius of the earth = 6400 km):

(a) 195.66N (b) 194.32N

(c) 194.66N (d) 195.32N

29. The value of acceleration due to gravity at Earth's surface is 9.8 ms^{-2}. The altitude above its surface at which the acceleration due to gravity decreases to 4.9 ms^{-2}, is close to : (Radius of earth = 6.4×10^6 m)

(a) 2.6×10^6 m (b) 6.4×10^6 m

(c) 9.0×10^6 m (d) 1.6×10^6 m

30. If the Earth has no rotational motion, the weight of a person on the equator is W. Determine the speed with which the earth would have to rotate about its axis so that the person at the equator will weight $\frac{3}{4}$W. Radius of the Earth is 6400 km and g=10 m/s^2.

(a) 1.1×10^{-3} rad/s (b) 0.83×10^{-3} rad/s

(c) 0.63×10^{-3} rad/s (d) 0.28×10^{-3} rad/s

31. Assuming the earth to be a sphere of uniform density, the acceleration due to gravity inside the earth at a distance of r from the centre is proportional to

(a) r (b) r^{-1} (c) r^2 (d) r^{-2}

32. The mass density of a planet of radius R varies with the distance r from its centre as $\rho(r)=\rho_0\left(1-\frac{r^2}{R^2}\right)$. Then the gravitational field is maximum at :

(a) $r=\sqrt{\frac{3}{4}}R$ (b) $r=R$

(c) $r=\frac{1}{\sqrt{3}}R$ (d) $r=\sqrt{\frac{5}{9}}R$

33. A solid sphere of mass 'M' and radius 'a' is surrounded by a uniform concentric spherical shell of thickness 2a and mass 2M. The gravitational field at distance '3a' from the centre will be:

(a) $\frac{2GM}{9a^2}$ (b) $\frac{GM}{9a^2}$ (c) $\frac{GM}{3a^2}$ (d) $\frac{2GM}{3a^2}$

34. Four identical particles of mass M are located at the corners of a square of side 'a'. What should be their speed if each of them revolves under the influence of others' gravitational field in a circular orbit circumscribing the square ?

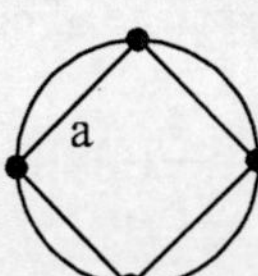

(a) $1.35\sqrt{\frac{GM}{a}}$ (b) $1.16\sqrt{\frac{GM}{a}}$

(c) $1.21\sqrt{\frac{GM}{a}}$ (d) $1.41\sqrt{\frac{GM}{a}}$

35. A test particle is moving in circular orbit in the gravitational field produced by a mass density $r(r) = \frac{K}{r^2}$. Identify the correct relation between the radius R of the particle's orbit and its period T:

(a) T/R is a constant (b) T^2/R^3 is a constant

(c) T/R^2 is a constant (d) TR is a constant

36. From a solid sphere of mass M and radius R, a spherical portion of radius R/2 is removed, as shown in the figure. Taking gravitational potential V = 0 at r = ∞, the potential at the centre of the cavity thus formed is :
(*G = gravitational constant*)

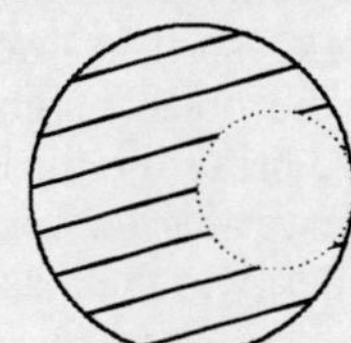

(a) $\frac{-2GM}{3R}$ (b) $\frac{-2GM}{R}$ (c) $\frac{-GM}{2R}$ (d) $\frac{-GM}{R}$

37. The gravitational field in a region is given by $\vec{g} = 5N/kg\hat{i} + 12N/kg\hat{j}$. The change in the gravitational potential energy of a particle of mass 1 kg when it is taken from the origin to a point (7 m, – 3 m) is:

(a) 71 J (b) $13\sqrt{58}$J (c) –71 J (d) 1 J

38. A satellite is in an elliptical orbit around a planet P. It is observed that the velocity of the satellite when it is farthest from the planet is 6 times less than that when it is closest to the planet. The ratio of distances between the satellite and the planet at closest and farthest points is :

(a) 1 : 6 (b) 1 : 3 (c) 1 : 2 (d) 3 : 4

39. A body is moving in a low circular orbit about a planet of mass *M* and radius *R*. The radius of the orbit can be taken to be *R* itself. Then the ratio of the speed of this body in the orbit to the escape velocity from the planet is :

(a) $\frac{1}{\sqrt{2}}$ (b) 2 (c) 1 (d) $\sqrt{2}$

40. The mass density of a spherical galaxy varies as $\frac{K}{r}$ over a large distance '*r*' from its centre. In that region, a small star is in a circular orbit of radius *R*. Then the period of revolution, *T* depends on *R* as :

(a) $T^2 \propto R$ (b) $T^2 \propto R^3$ (c) $T^2 \propto \frac{1}{R^3}$ (d) $T \propto R$

41. The energy required to take a satellite to a height 'h' above Earth surface (radius of Eareth = 6.4×10^3 km) is E_1 and kinetic energy required for the satellite to be in a circular orbit at this height is E_2. The value of h for which E_1 and E_2 are equal, is:

(a) 1.6×10^3 km (b) 3.2×10^3 km

(c) 6.4×10^3 km (d) 28×10^4 km

42. Planet A has mass M and radius R. Planet B has half the mass and half the radius of Planet A. If the escape velocities from the Planets A and B are v_A and v_B, respectively, then $\frac{v_A}{v_B} = \frac{n}{4}$. The value of *n* is :

(a) 4 (b) 1 (c) 2 (d) 3

43. A spaceship orbits around a planet at a height of 20 km from its surface. Assuming that only gravitational field of the planet acts on the spaceship, what will be the number of complete revolutions made by the spaceship in 24 hours around the planet ? [Given : Mass of Planet = 8×10^{22} kg, Radius of planet = 2×10^6 m, Gravitational constant $G = 6.67 \times 10^{-11} Nm^2/kg^2$]

(a) 9 (b) 17 (c) 13 (d) 11

44. A satellite of mass M is in a circular orbit of radius R about the centre of the earth. A meteorite of the same mass, falling towards the earth collides with the satellite completely in elastically. The speeds of the satellite and the meteorite are the same, Just before the collision. The subsequent motion of the combined body will be

(a) such that it escape to infinity
(b) In an elliptical orbit
(c) in the same circular orbit of radius R
(d) in a circular orbit of a different radius

45. A satellite is moving with a constant speed *v* in circular orbit around the earth. An object of mass 'm' is ejected from the satellite such that it just escapes from the gravitational pull of the earth. At the time of ejection, the kinetic energy of the object is:

(a) $2mv^2$ (b) mv^2 (c) $\frac{1}{2}mv^2$ (d) $\frac{3}{2}mv^2$

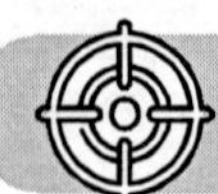

Hints & Solutions

8.1 Concept Practice Problems CPP

1. (b) $g' = g - R\omega^2\cos^2\lambda$
2. (c) According to Newton's Gravitation Law

$F_g = \frac{GM_1M_2}{r^2}$ here $F_g = 10^{-10}$ Newton,

$m_1 = m_2 = 1kg$,
$G = 6.6 \times 10^{-11}$

So $r^2 = \frac{GM_1M_2}{F_g} = \frac{6.6 \times 10^{-11} \times 1 \times 1}{10^{-10}} = 0.66$

or $r = 0.8125$ metre $= 81.25$ cm ≈ 80cm

3. (c) Gravitational force supplies centripetal force

$\therefore F = \frac{mv^2}{r} = \frac{3 \times 10^{29} \times (2 \times 10^8)^2}{1.5 \times 10^{14}}$ dynes

$= 8 \times 10^{31}$ dyne $= 8 \times 10^{26}$ N ($\because$ 1N $= 10^5$ dyne.)

4. (d) Since gravitational acceleration on earth is defined

as $g_e = \frac{GM_e}{R_e^{\,2}}$ ......(i)

mass of planet is $M_P = \frac{M_e}{80}$ & radius $R_P = \frac{R_e}{4}$

So $g_P = \frac{GM_P}{R_P^2}$ ......(ii)

From (i) & (ii), we get

$g_P = g_e \frac{M_P}{R_P^2} \times \frac{R_e^{\,2}}{M_e} = \frac{g_e}{5} = 2\text{m/sec}^2$

(as $g = 10\text{m/sec}^2$)

5. (d) $g \propto \rho R$
6. (b) Acceleration due to gravity at lattitude' λ ' is given

by $g_\lambda = g_e - R_e\omega^2\cos^2\lambda$

At equator, $\lambda = 90° \Rightarrow \cos\lambda = \cos 90° = 0$

or $g_\lambda = g_e = g$ (as given in question)

At 30°, $g_{30} = g - R\omega^2\cos^2 30 = g - \frac{3}{4}R\omega^2$

or, $g - g_{30} = \frac{3}{4}R\omega^2$

7. (a) Change in force of gravity

$= \frac{GMm}{R^2} - \frac{G\frac{M}{3}m}{R^2}$ (only due to mass M/3 due to shell gravitational field is zero (inside the shell))

$= \frac{2GMm}{3R^2}$

8. (b) Electronic charge does not depend on acceleration due to gravity as it is a universal constant.

So, electronic charge on earth
= electronic charge on moon
$\therefore$ Required ratio = 1.

9. (a) $g = \frac{GM}{R^2}$ also $M = d \times \frac{4}{3}\pi R^3$

$\therefore g = \frac{4}{3}d\pi R$ at the surface of planet

$g_p = \frac{4}{3}(2d)\pi R'$, $g_e = \frac{4}{3}(d)\pi R$

$g_e = g_p \Rightarrow dR = 2d\,R'$
$\Rightarrow R' = R/2$

10. (d) We know that

$g = \frac{GM}{R^2} = \frac{G\left(\frac{4}{3}\pi R^3\right)\rho}{R^2} = \frac{4}{3}\pi G R\rho$

$\frac{g'}{g} = \frac{R'}{R} = \frac{3R}{R} = 3 \quad \therefore g' = 3g$

8.2 Concept Practice Problems

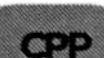

11. (c) The potential energy for a conservative force is defined as

$F = \frac{-dU}{dr}$ or $U = -\int_{\infty}^{r} \vec{F}.\vec{dr}$ ......(i)

or $U_r = \int_{\infty}^{r} \frac{GM_1M_2}{r^2}dr = \frac{-GM_1M_2}{r}$ ......(ii)

($\because U_\infty = 0$)

If we bring the mass from the infinity to the centre of earth, then we obtain work, 'so it has negative (gravitational force do work on the object) sign & potential energy decreases. But if we bring the mass from the surface of earth to infinite, then we must do work against gravitational force & potential energy of the mass increases.

Now in equation (i) if $F = \frac{GM_1M_2}{r^{5/2}}$ instead of

$F = \frac{GM_1M_2}{r^2}$ then

$U_r = \int_{\infty}^{r} \frac{GM_1M_2}{r^{5/2}}dr = \frac{-2}{3}\frac{GM_1M_2}{r^{3/2}} \Rightarrow U_r \propto \frac{1}{r^{+3/2}}$

12. (d) Energy required to move a body of mass m from an orbit of radius 2R to 3R is

$\Delta U = -\frac{GMm}{3R} - \frac{-GMm}{2R} = \frac{GMm}{2R} - \frac{GMm}{3R} = \frac{GMm}{6R}$

13. (c) $\frac{G \times 10^3}{(r)^2} = \frac{G \times 10^5}{(1-r)^2}$

$\frac{1}{r^2} = \frac{10^2}{(1-r)^2}$

$\frac{1}{r} = \frac{10}{1-r} \Rightarrow 10r = 1 - r$

$\therefore r = \frac{1}{11}$ km

14. (b)

15. (c) $V_g = \frac{-6.67\times10^{-11}\times10}{1} - \frac{6.67\times10^{-11}\times100}{1}$

$= -6.67\times10^{-10} - 6.67\times10^{-9}$

$= -6.67\times10^{-10}\times11 = -7.3\times10^{-9}$ J/kg

16. (d) Both decreases but variation are different.

17. (a) For uniform gravitational field

$E_g = -\frac{V}{r} = -\frac{-2}{20} = \frac{1}{10}\ ms^{-2}$

Now, $W = mgh = 5\times\frac{1}{10}\times4 = 2J$

18. (d) Work done $= U_f - U_i$

$= -\frac{GMm}{2R+R} - \left(-\frac{Gmm}{R}\right) = \frac{2}{3}\frac{GmM}{R} = \frac{2}{3}mgR$

19. (a)

20. (d) Intensity will be zero inside the spherical shell.

$I = 0$ upto $r = a$ and $I \propto \frac{1}{r^2}$ when $r > a$

8.3 Concept Practice Problems CPP

21. (c) $T^2 \propto R^3$

22. (b) We know that, $v_e = \sqrt{(2gR)}$

$\therefore \frac{(v_e)_{P_1}}{(v_e)_{P_2}} = \frac{\sqrt{(2g_1R_1)}}{\sqrt{(2g_2R_2)}} = \sqrt{\left(\frac{g_1}{g_2}\right)}\times\sqrt{\left(\frac{R_1}{R_2}\right)} = \sqrt{kr}$

23. (b) $v_e = \sqrt{2}v_o$ where v_e and v_o are the escape velocity and orbital velocity respectively.

24. (a) $v_1 \propto \frac{1}{\sqrt{R}},\ v_2 \propto \frac{1}{\sqrt{7R}}$

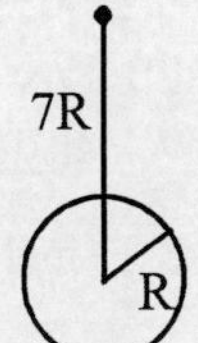

$\frac{v_2}{v_1} = \frac{1}{\sqrt{7}} \Rightarrow v_2 = \frac{v_1}{\sqrt{7}} = \frac{v}{\sqrt{7}}$

25. (c) $v_e = \sqrt{\frac{2GM_e}{R_e}};\quad v_m = \sqrt{\frac{2G\frac{M_e}{81}}{\frac{R_e}{4}}} = \frac{2}{9}v_e$

$= 2/9\times11.2\ kms^{-1} = 2.5\ kms^{-1}$

26. (c) $T^2 \propto R^3$ (According to Kepler's law)

$T_1^2 \propto (10^{13})^3$ and $T_2^2 \propto (10^{12})^3$

$\therefore \frac{T_1^2}{T_2^2} = (10)^3$ or $\frac{T_1}{T_2} = 10\sqrt{10}$.

27. (c) According to Kepler's law of period $T^2 \propto R^3$

$\frac{T_1^2}{T_2^2} = \frac{R_1^3}{R_2^3} = \frac{(6R)^3}{(3R)^3} = 8$

$\frac{24\times24}{T_2^2} = 8$

$T_2^2 = \frac{24\times24}{8} = 72 = 36\times2$

$T_2 = 6\sqrt{2}$

28. (d) $\frac{mv^2}{(R+x)} = \frac{GmM}{(R+x)^2}$ also $g = \frac{GM}{R^2}$

$\therefore \frac{mv^2}{(R+x)} = m\left(\frac{GM}{R^2}\right)\frac{R^2}{(R+x)^2}$

$\therefore \frac{mv^2}{(R+x)} = mg\frac{R^2}{(R+x)^2}$

$\therefore v^2 = \frac{gR^2}{R+x} \Rightarrow v = \left(\frac{gR^2}{R+x}\right)^{1/2}$

29. (d) According to Newton gravitational force

$\frac{GM_em}{R_e^2} = mg$ & $\frac{GM_em}{(R_e+h)^2} = mg'$

$\Rightarrow g' = g\frac{1}{(1+h/R_e)^2} = \frac{gR_e^2}{(R_e+h)^2}$

where M_e is mass of earth, G is gravitational constant, R_e is radius & earth, h is height of satellite above the surface of earth, g is value at the surface of earth, g' is value at height h above the surface of earth.

so $\frac{mv^2}{(R_e+h)} = \frac{mgR_e^2}{(R_e+h)^2} = mg' \Rightarrow v = \sqrt{\frac{gR_e^2}{R_e+h}}$

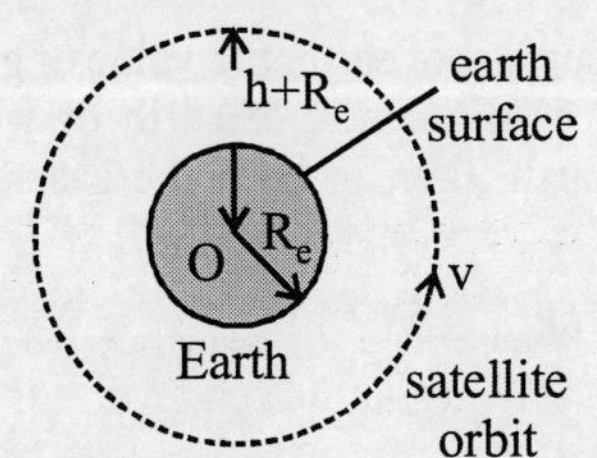

30. (a)

31. (c) Applying the properties of ellipse, we have

$\frac{2}{R} = \frac{1}{r_1} + \frac{1}{r_2} = \frac{r_1+r_2}{r_1r_2}$

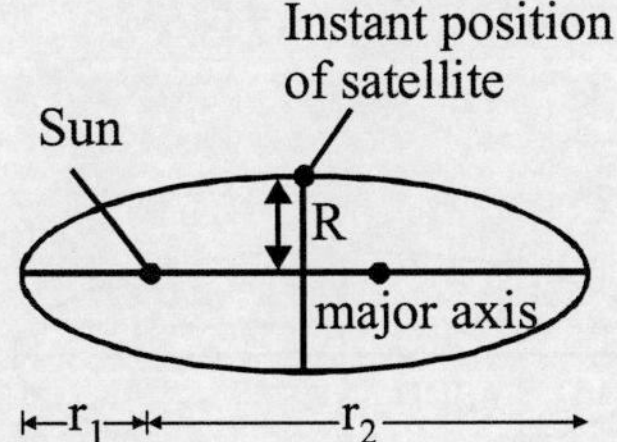

$R = \frac{2r_1r_2}{r_1+r_2}$

32. (a) $v = \sqrt{\left(\frac{GM}{r}\right)}$ where r is radius of the orbit of the satellite.

here $r = R_e + h = R_e + \frac{R_e}{2} = \frac{3}{2}R_e$

So, $v = \sqrt{\frac{2GM}{3R_e}} = v_0\sqrt{\frac{2}{3}}$,

where v_0 is the orbital velocity of the satellite, which is moving in circular orbit of radius, $r = R_e$

33. (a) The total momentum will be zero and hence velocity will be zero just after collisiion. The pull of earth will make it fall down.

34. (b) $\frac{1}{2}mv_e^2 = \frac{GMm}{R}$; $v_e = \sqrt{\frac{GMm}{R}} = \sqrt{2gR}$

In tunnel body will perform SHM at centre

$V_{max} = A\omega$ (see chapter on SHM)

$$= \frac{R2\pi}{2\pi\sqrt{R/g}} = \sqrt{gR} = \frac{v_e}{\sqrt{2}}$$

35. (b) Potential energy of particle at the centre of square

$$= -4\left(\frac{GMm}{\frac{a}{\sqrt{2}}}\right)$$

$$\therefore -4\left(\frac{GMm}{a/\sqrt{2}}\right) + \frac{1}{2}mv^2 = 0 \Rightarrow v^2 = \frac{8\sqrt{2}GM}{a}$$

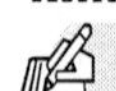

Exercise 1 - Chapter Revision Problems

1. (a) At the surface of earth, the value of $g = 9.8 m/sec^2$. If we go towards the centre of earth or we go above the surface of earth, then in both the cases the value of g decreases.

Hence $W_1 = mg_{mine}$, $W_2 = mg_{sea\ level}$, $W_3 = mg_{moun}$

So $W_1 < W_2 > W_3$ (g at the sea level = g at the suface of earth)

2. (a) 3. (d) 4. (b)

5. (c) In planetary motion $\vec{\tau}_{ext.} = 0 \Rightarrow \vec{L} =$ constant

$\vec{L} = \vec{r} \times \vec{p}(= m\vec{v}) = mrv$ ($\because \theta = 90°$)

So $m_1 d_1 v_1 = m_2 d_2 v_2$ (here r = d)

$$\Rightarrow v_2 = \frac{v_1 d_1}{d_2}$$

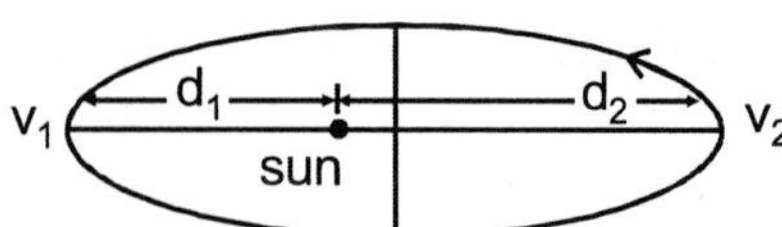

6. (d)

7. (c) Since $T(\text{time period}) = 2\pi\sqrt{\frac{l}{g}}$

for second pendulum T=2sec

Now on the planet the value of acceleration due to gravity is g/4.

So for the planet, the length of sec. pendulam l' is

$$\frac{2\sec}{2\sec} = \sqrt{\frac{l}{g} \times \frac{g/4}{l'}} \Rightarrow l' = l/4$$

8. (b) Since $T = 2\pi\sqrt{\frac{l}{g}}$

but inside the satellite $g = 0$

So $T = \infty$

9. (c) $KE = \frac{1}{2}mv_{esc}^2 = \frac{1}{2}m(\sqrt{2gR})^2 = mgR$.

10. (a) $v_{esc} = \sqrt{2gR}$, where R is radius of the planet. Hence escape velocity is independent of m.

11. (c) $\frac{T_1}{T_2} = \left(\frac{R_1}{R_2}\right)^{3/2} \Rightarrow \frac{T}{T_2} = \left(\frac{4R}{16R}\right)^{3/2}$

$\Rightarrow T_2 = 8T$

12. (a) $T^2 \propto (\text{major axis})^3 \Rightarrow T^2 \alpha a^3$

13. (d) According to 3rd law of Kepler

$T^2 \propto R^3$

$\Rightarrow T^2 = KR^3$

where K is a constant

Thus $\frac{T^2}{R^3}$ does not depends on radius.

14. (a) Escape velocity does not depend upon the mass of the body.

15. (c)

16. (b) At poles, the effect of rotation is zero and also the distance from the centre of earth is least.

17. (b) Since escape velocity $\left(v_e = \sqrt{2gR_e}\right)$ is independent of angle of projection, so it will not change.

18. (b) We know that $v_e = \sqrt{2}\,v_0$, where v_0 is orbital velocity.

K.E. in the orbit, $E = \frac{1}{2}M v_0^2$

K.E. to escape $E = \frac{1}{2}M v_e^2 = \frac{1}{2}M(2v_0^2)$

$$= \frac{1}{2}M v_0^2 \times 2 = 2E$$

19. (b) $g_h = g\left(1 - \frac{2h}{R}\right)$

$g_x = g\left(1 - \frac{x}{R}\right)$

Given that, $g_h = g_x$

$\therefore x = 2h$

20. (b) There is no gravitational field in the shell.

21. (c) The gravitational field due to the ring at a distance $\sqrt{3}r$ is given by

$$E = \frac{Gm(\sqrt{3}r)}{[r^2 + (\sqrt{3}r)^2]^{3/2}} \Rightarrow E = \frac{\sqrt{3}Gm}{8r^2}$$

Attractive force $= \frac{\sqrt{3}GmM}{8r^2}$

22. (b) As buoyant force involves 'g' in it.
23. (b)
24. (d) The gravitational force due to the whole sphere at A point is

$F_1 = \frac{GM_e m_o}{(2R)^2}$, where m_0 is the assumed rest mass at point A.

In the second case, when we made a cavity of radius (R/2), then gravitational force at point A is

$F_2 = \frac{GM_e m_o}{(R+R/2)^2}$ $\therefore F_2/F_1 = 1/9$

25. (d) $v_1 r_1 = v_2 r_2$ or $r_1^2 \omega_1 = r_2^2 \omega_2$ ($\because$ L=mrv= constant)

or $r_{min}^2 \omega = r_{max}^2 \omega'$

$\therefore \omega' = (r_{min}^2 / r_{max}^2)\omega$

26. (d) Weight of liquid displaced = mg.
27. (a)
28. (a) $g_h = g\left(1-\frac{2h}{R}\right) = \frac{4g}{h}\left(\text{since } h = R+\frac{3R}{2}\right)$

Force on the satellite = $mg_h = \frac{4}{9}$ mg

$=\frac{4}{9}\times 200\times 10 \approx 889$ N

29. (c) $g \propto \frac{1}{R^2}$ so we will not get a straight line.

Also F = 0 at a point where Force due to Earth = Force due to mars

30. (a)
31. (a) Since, $T^2 = kr^3$

Differentiating the above equation

$\Rightarrow 2\frac{\Delta T}{T} = 3\frac{\Delta r}{r} \Rightarrow \frac{\Delta T}{T} = \frac{3}{2}\frac{\Delta r}{r}$

32. (b)
33. (b) $g \propto \frac{1}{R^2}$

R decreasing g increase hence, curve b represents correct variation.

34. (a) Here, $v = \sqrt{\frac{2GM}{R}}$ and $kv = \sqrt{\frac{2GM}{R+R}}$.

Solving $k = \frac{1}{\sqrt{2}}$

35. (d) $\Delta U = U_f - U_i = -\frac{GMm}{nR+h} - \left(-\frac{GMm}{R}\right)$

$= \frac{n}{n+1}.\frac{GMm}{R} = \frac{n}{n+1}mgR$

36. (c) $T = 2\pi\sqrt{\frac{(R+h)^3}{GM}}$

$T_1 = 2\pi\sqrt{\frac{R^3}{GM}}$, $T_2 = 2\pi\sqrt{\frac{(1.01R)^3}{GM}}$

$\frac{T_2 - T_1}{T_1}\times 100 = 1.5\%$

37. (a) K.E. of satellite moving in an orbit around the earth is

$K = \frac{1}{2}mv^2 = \frac{1}{2}m\left(\sqrt{\frac{GM}{r}}\right)^2 = \frac{GMm}{2r}$

P.E. of satellite and earth system is

$U = \frac{GMm}{r} \Rightarrow \frac{K}{U} = \frac{\frac{GMm}{2r}}{\frac{GMm}{r}} = \frac{1}{2}$

38. (b) According to Kepler's law, the areal velocity of a planet around the sun always remains constant.

SCD : $A_1 - t_1$ (areal velocity constant)

SAB : $A_2 - t_2$

$\frac{A_1}{t_1} = \frac{A_2}{t_2}$,

$t_1 = t_2 \cdot \frac{A_1}{A_2}$, (given $A_1 = 2A_2$)

$= t_2 \cdot \frac{2A_2}{A_2}$

$\therefore$ $t_1 = 2t_2$

39. (b) Orbital velocity of a satellite in a circular orbit of radius a is given by

$v = \sqrt{\frac{GM}{a}} \Rightarrow v \alpha \sqrt{\frac{1}{a}} \Rightarrow \frac{v_2}{v_1} = \sqrt{\frac{a_1}{a_2}}$

$\therefore$ $v_2 = v_1\sqrt{\frac{4R}{R}} = 2v_1 = 6V$

40. (a) The velocity u should be equal to the escape velocity. That is, $u = \sqrt{2gR}$

But $g = \frac{GM}{R^2}$

$\therefore u = \sqrt{2\cdot\frac{GM}{R^2}\cdot R}$ Þ $\sqrt{\frac{2GM}{R}}$

41. (b)
42. (d) Given $\lambda = (A+Bx^2)$,

Taking small element dm of length dx at a distance x from x = 0

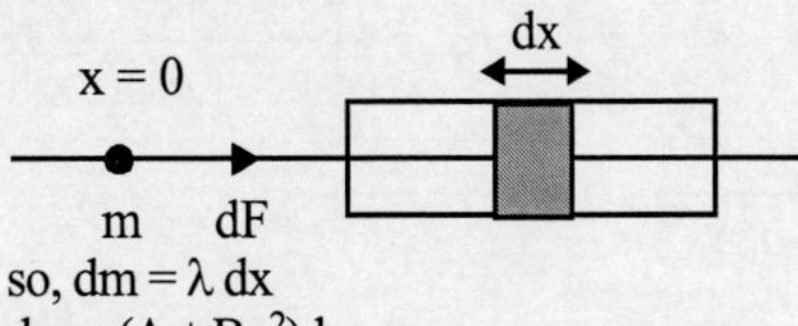

so, $dm = \lambda\, dx$

$dm = (A+Bx^2)dx$

$dF = \frac{Gmdm}{x^2} \Rightarrow F = \int_a^{a+L}\frac{Gm}{x^2}(A+Bx^2)dx$

$= Gm\left[-\frac{A}{x}+Bx\right]_a^{a+L} = Gm\left[A\left(\frac{1}{a}-\frac{1}{a+L}\right)+BL\right]$

43. (a) Volume of removed sphere

$V_{remo} = \frac{4}{3}\pi\left(\frac{R}{2}\right)^3 = \frac{4}{3}\pi R^3\left(\frac{1}{8}\right)$

Volume of the sphere (remaining)

$$V_{\text{remain}} = \frac{4}{3}\pi R^3 - \frac{4}{3}\pi R^3\left(\frac{1}{8}\right) = \frac{4}{3}\pi R^3\left(\frac{7}{8}\right)$$

Therefore mass of sphere carved and remaining sphere are at respectively $\frac{1}{8}$ M and $\frac{7}{8}$M.

Therefore, gravitational force between these two sphere,

$$F = \frac{GMm}{r^2} = \frac{G\frac{7M}{8}\times\frac{1}{8}M}{(3R)^2} = \frac{7}{64\times 9}\frac{GM^2}{R^2}$$

$$\simeq \frac{41}{3600}\frac{GM^2}{R^2}$$

44. (b) Value of g at equator, $g_A = g\cdot - R\omega^2$

Value of g at height h above the pole,

$$g_B = g\cdot\left(1-\frac{2h}{R}\right)$$

As object is weighed equally at the equator and poles, it means g is same at these places.

$$g_A = g_B$$

$$\Rightarrow g - R\omega^2 = g\left(1-\frac{2h}{R}\right) \Rightarrow R\omega^2 = \frac{2gh}{R} \Rightarrow h = \frac{R^2\omega^2}{2g}$$

45. (d) $\frac{W_e}{W_p} = \frac{mg_e}{mg_p} = \frac{9}{4}$ or $\frac{g_e}{g_p} = \frac{9}{4}$

or $\frac{GM/R^2}{G(M/9)/R_p^2} = \frac{9}{4}$ $\therefore R_p = \frac{R}{2}$

46. (d) With rotation of earth or latitude, acceleration due to gravity vary as $g' = g - \omega^2 R\cos^2\phi$

Where ϕ is latitude, there will be no change in gravity at poles as $\phi = 90°$

At all other points as ω increases g' will decreases hence, weight, W = mg decreases.

47. (a) 48. (d)

49. (a) Given : Gravitational field,

$$E_G = \frac{Ax}{(x^2+a^2)^{3/2}},\ V_\infty = 0$$

$$\int_{V_\infty}^{V_x} dV = -\int_\infty^x \vec{E}_G\cdot\vec{d}_x \Rightarrow V_x - V_\infty = -\int_\infty^x \frac{Ax}{(x^2+a^2)^{3/2}}dx$$

$$\therefore V_x = \frac{A}{(x^2+a^2)^{1/2}} - 0 = \frac{A}{(x^2+a^2)^{1/2}}$$

50. (c) Initial gravitational potential energy, $E_i = -\frac{GMm}{2R}$

Final gravitational potential energy,

$$E_f = -\frac{GMm/2}{2\left(\frac{R}{2}\right)} - \frac{GMm/2}{2\left(\frac{3R}{2}\right)} = -\frac{GMm}{2R} - \frac{GMm}{6R}$$

$$= -\frac{4GMm}{6R} = -\frac{2GMm}{3R}$$

$\therefore$ Difference between initial and final energy,

$$E_f - E_i = \frac{GMm}{R}\left(-\frac{2}{3}+\frac{1}{2}\right) = -\frac{GMm}{6R}$$

51. (c)

52. (d) From law of conservation of momentum, $\vec{p}_i = \vec{p}_f$

$$m_1u_1 + m_2u_2 = MV_f$$

$$\Rightarrow v_f = \frac{\left(mv+\frac{mv}{4}\right)}{\frac{3m}{2}} = \frac{5v}{6}$$

Clearly, $v_f < v_i$ $\therefore$ Path will be elliptical

53. (d) Escape velocity,

$$v_e = \sqrt{\frac{2GM}{R}} = \sqrt{\frac{2G\rho V}{R}}$$

$$= \sqrt{\frac{2GS\times 4\pi R^3}{R}} = \sqrt{\frac{8}{3}\pi\rho GR^2}$$

For moon, $v_e' = \sqrt{\frac{8}{3}\pi\rho GR_m^2}$

Given, $\frac{4}{3}\pi R^3 = 64\times\frac{4}{3}\pi R_m^3$ or $R_m = \frac{R}{4}$

$$\therefore\quad v_e' = \sqrt{\frac{8}{3}\pi\rho G\left(\frac{R}{4}\right)^2} = \frac{v_e}{4}$$

$$\frac{E}{E'} = \frac{\frac{1}{2}mv_e^2}{\frac{1}{2}mv_e'^2} = \frac{v_e^2}{v_e'^2} = \frac{v_e}{\left(\frac{v_e}{4}\right)} = 16$$

or $E' = \frac{E}{16}$

54. (b) Orbital, velocity, $v = \sqrt{\frac{GM}{r}}$

Kinetic energy of satellite A,

$$T_A = \frac{1}{2}m_A V_A^2$$

Kinetic energy of satellite B,

$$T_B = \frac{1}{2}m_B V_B^2 \Rightarrow \frac{T_A}{T_B} = \frac{m\times\frac{GM}{R}}{2m\times\frac{GM}{2R}} = 1$$

55. (d) For a satellite orbiting close to the earth, orbital velocity is given by

$$v_0 = \sqrt{g(R+h)} \approx \sqrt{gR}$$

Escape velocity (v_e) is

$$v_e = \sqrt{2g(R+h)} \approx \sqrt{2gR} \qquad [\because h << R]$$

$$\Delta v = v_e - v_0 = (\sqrt{2}-1)\sqrt{gR}$$

Exercise 2 - Exemplar & Past Year Questions E&PYQs

Exemplar Questions

1. (d) Let the density of earth as a sphere is uniform, then it can be treated as point mass placed at its centre then acceleration due to gravity g = 0, at the centre. But if the density of earth is considered as a sphere of non-uniform then value of 'g' will be different at different points $\left(\because g = \frac{4}{3}\pi\rho GR\right)$. So g cannot be zero at any point.

2. (c) Force of attraction between any two objects obeys the inverse square law.
As observed from the earth, the sun appears to move in an approximate circular orbit. The gravitational force of attraction between the earth and the sun always follows inverse square law.
Due to relative motion between the earth and mercury, the orbit of mercury, as observed from the earth will not be approximately circular, since the major gravitational force on mercury is due to the sun is very large than due to earth and due to the relative motion to sun and earth with mercury.

3. (a) As we know that, the torque on earth due to gravitational attractive force on earth is zero.
As the earth is revolving around the sun in a circular motion due to gravitational attraction. The force of attraction will be of radial nature i.e., angle between position vector r and force F is also, zero.
So, torque $= |\tau| = |r \times F| = rF \sin 0° = 0$

4. (c) As the total (P.E.) of the earth satellite orbiting in orbit is negative $\left(\frac{-GM}{2r}\right)$, where r is radius of the satellite and M is mass of the earth.
Due to the viscous force acting on satellite, energy decreases continuously and radius of the orbit or height decreases gradually.

5. (b) The major force acting on moon is due to gravitational force of attraction by sun and earth and moon is not always in line of joining sun and earth.
As observed from the sun, two types of forces are acting on the moon one is due to gravitational attraction between the sun and the moon and the other is due to gravitational attraction between the earth and the moon. So these two force have different lines of action and it will not be strictly elliptical because total force on the moon is not central.

6. (d) Asteroids are also being acted upon by central gravitational forces, hence Asteroid will move in circular orbits like planets and obey Kepler's laws.

7. (d) Gravitational mass of proton is equivalent to its inertial mass and is independent of presence of neighbouring heavy objects so verifies the option (d).

8. (c) Force of Gravitation, $F_g = \frac{GMm}{r^2}$
Let $AB = r$
So, force on B due to A

$= F_{BA} = \frac{G(2Mm)}{(AB)^2}$ towards BA.

$= \frac{G(2Mm)}{r^2} = 2F_g$

and force on B due to C

$= F_{BC} = \frac{GMm}{(BC)^2}$ towards BC

As, $(BC) = 2AB$

$\Rightarrow F_{BC} = \frac{GMm}{(2AB)^2} = \frac{GMm}{4(AB)^2} = \frac{GMm}{4r^2} = \frac{F_g}{4}$

As $F_{BA} > F_{BC}$,
hence, m will move towards (BA) i.e., $(2M)$.

NEET/AIPMT (2013-2020) Questions

9. (a) Initial P. E., $U_i = \frac{-GMm}{R}$,

Final P.E., $U_f = \frac{-GMm}{3R}$ $[\because R' = R + 2R = 3R]$

$\therefore$ Change in potential energy,

$\Delta U = \frac{-GMm}{3R} + \frac{GMm}{R}$

$= \frac{GMm}{R}\left(1 - \frac{1}{3}\right) = \frac{2}{3}\frac{GMm}{R} = \frac{2}{3}mgR$

$\left(\because \frac{GMm}{R} = mgR\right)$

10. (c) [number line: 2 kg at 1, 2 kg at 2, 2 kg at 4; marks 0 1 2 3 4 5 6 7 8 m]

Gravitational potential $V = \frac{-Gm}{r}$

$V_0 = -\frac{G\times 2}{1} - \frac{G\times 2}{2} - \frac{G\times 2}{4} - \frac{G\times 2}{8}$

$-2G\left[1 + \frac{1}{2} + \frac{1}{4} + \frac{1}{8} + ...\infty\right]$

$= -2G \times \frac{1}{1 - \frac{1}{2}} = -2G \times \frac{1}{\frac{1}{2}} = -4G$

11. (c) Escape velocity, $V_e = R\sqrt{\frac{8}{3}\pi GP}$

$\Rightarrow V_e \propto R \Rightarrow \frac{V_P}{V_E} = \frac{R_P}{R_E} = 2 \Rightarrow V_P = 2V_E$.

12. (b) As we know, the minimum speed with which a body is projected so that it does not return back is called escape speed.

$V_e = \sqrt{\frac{2GM}{r}} = \sqrt{\frac{2GM}{R+h}} = \sqrt{\frac{2GM}{4R}}$

$= \left(\frac{GM}{2R}\right)^{\frac{1}{2}}$ $(\because h = 3R)$

13. (a) Horizontal range $= \frac{u^2 \sin 2\theta}{g}$ so g µ u²

or $\frac{g_{planet}}{g_{earth}} = \frac{(u_{planet})^2}{(u_{earth})^2}$

Therefore $g_{planet} = \left(\frac{3}{5}\right)^2 (9.8\ m/s^2) = 3.5\ m/s^2$

14. (b) First when $(r < R)$ $E \propto r$ and then when $r > R$ $E \propto \frac{1}{r^2}$.
Hence graph (b) correctly dipicts.

15. (c) From question,
Escape velocity

$= \sqrt{\frac{2GM}{R}} = c =$ speed of light

$\Rightarrow R = \frac{2GM}{c^2}$

$= \frac{2 \times 6.6 \times 10^{-11} \times 5.98 \times 10^{24}}{(3 \times 10^8)^2} m = 10^{-2} m$

16. (d) **Given:** Height of the satellite from the earth's surface $h = 0.25 \times 10^6$m
Radius of the earth $R = 6.38 \times 10^6$m
Acceleration due to gravity $g = 9.8$ m/s^2
Orbital velocity, $V_0 = ?$

$$V_0 = \sqrt{\frac{GM}{(R+h)}} = \sqrt{\frac{GM}{R^2} \cdot \frac{R^2}{(R+h)}} = \sqrt{\frac{9.8 \times 6.38 \times 6.38}{6.63 \times 10^6}}$$

$$= 7.76 \text{ km/s} \qquad \left[\because \frac{GM}{R^2} = g\right]$$

17. (b)

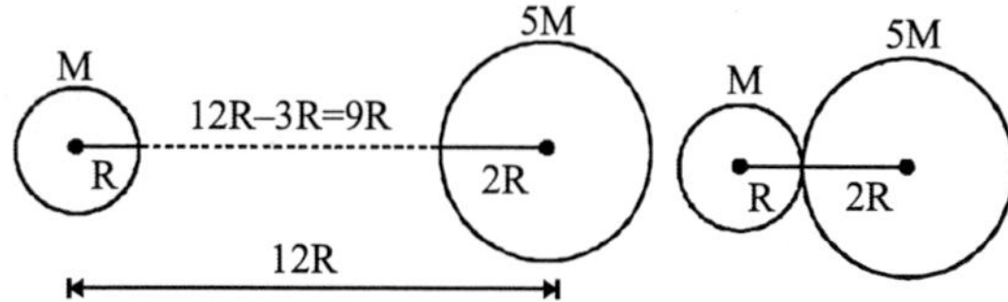

Let the distance moved by spherical body of mass M is x_1 and by spherical body of mass 5m is x_2
As their C.M. will remain stationary
So, $(M)(x_1) = (5M)(x_2)$ or, $x_1 = 5x_2$
and for tauching $x_1 + x_2 = 9R$
So, $x_1 = 7.5R$

18. (b) As we know, escape velocity,

$$V_e = \sqrt{\frac{2GM}{R}} = \sqrt{\frac{2G}{R} \cdot \left(\frac{4}{3}\pi R^3 \rho\right)} \propto R\sqrt{\rho}$$

$$\therefore \quad \frac{V_e}{V_p} = \frac{R_e}{R_p}\sqrt{\frac{\rho_e}{\rho_p}} \Rightarrow \frac{V_e}{V_p} = \frac{R_e}{2R_e}\sqrt{\frac{\rho_e}{2\rho_e}}$$

$$\therefore \quad \text{Ratio } \frac{V_e}{V_p} = 1 : 2\sqrt{2}$$

19. (a) As we know, gravitational potential (v) and acceleration due to gravity (g) with height

$$V = \frac{-GM}{R+h} = -5.4 \times 10^7 \qquad \ldots(1)$$

$$\text{and } g = \frac{GM}{(R+h)^2} = 6 \qquad \ldots(2)$$

Dividing (1) by (2)

$$\frac{\frac{-GM}{R+h}}{\frac{GM}{(R+h)^2}} = \frac{-5.4 \times 10^7}{6} \Rightarrow \frac{5.4 \times 10^7}{(R+h)} = 6$$

$\Rightarrow$ R + h = 9000 km so, h = 2600 km

20. (a) Both the astronauts are in the condition of weightlessness. Gravitational force between them pulls towards each other. Hence Astronauts move towards each other under mutual gravitional force.

21. (c) Above earth surface Below earth surface

$$g_h = g\left(1 - \frac{2h}{R_e}\right) \qquad g_d = g\left(1 - \frac{d}{R_e}\right)$$

According to question, $g_h = g_d$

$$g\left(1 - \frac{2h}{R_e}\right) = g\left(1 - \frac{d}{R_e}\right)$$

Clearly,
d = 2h = 2 km

22. (b) Speed of the planet will be maximum when its distance from the sun is minimum as mvr = constant.

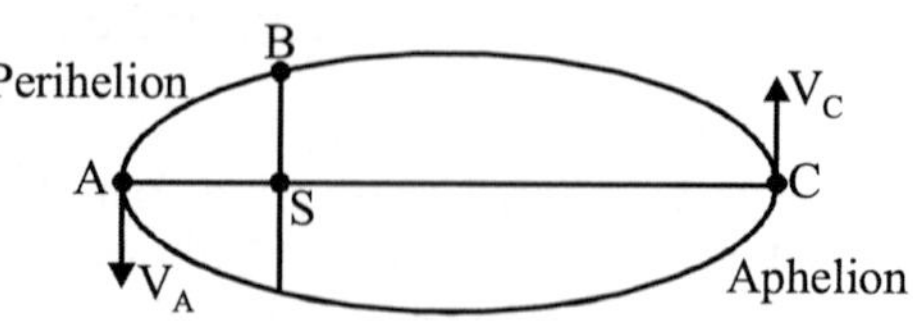

Point A is perihelion and C is aphelion.
Clearly, $V_A > V_B > V_C$
So, $K_A > K_B > K_C$

23. (c)

24. (c) As $U = -\frac{GMm}{r}$

$$\therefore \quad (P.E)_A = -\frac{GMm}{R}; (P.E)_B = -\frac{GMm}{R+h}$$

$$\therefore \quad \Delta U = (P.E)_B - (P.E)_A$$

$$= -\frac{GMm}{R+h} + \frac{GMm}{R} = \frac{GMmh}{(R)(R+h)}$$

25. (b) $T^2 \propto r^3$
$T^2 \propto (R_E + h)^3$

$$\frac{T_1^2}{T_2^2} = \frac{(R_E + 6R_E)^3}{(R_E + 2.5R_E)^3} \Rightarrow \frac{T_1^2}{T_2^2} = \frac{7^3}{\left(\frac{7}{2}\right)^3}$$

$$T_2 = 6\sqrt{2}\, h$$

26. (a) Weight of a body on the surface of the earth, $W_S = mgs = 72$ N
Acceleration due to gravity, g varies with height,

$h = \frac{R}{2}$ (given)

$$W_h = \frac{mgs}{\left(1 + \frac{h}{R}\right)^2} = \frac{72}{\left(1 + \frac{R/2}{R}\right)^2} = \frac{72}{(3/2)^2}$$

$$= \frac{4}{9} \times 72 = 32 \text{ N}$$

Exercise 3 - Concept Application Problems CAP

1. (d) On the moon escape velocity of gas molecules is less than their rms velocity.

2. (a) According to Gravitational Law

$$F = \frac{GM_1M_2}{r^2} \qquad \ldots\ldots(i)$$

Where M_1 is mass of planet & m_2 is the mass of any body. Now according to Newton's second law, body of mass m_2 feels gravitational acceleration g which is
$F = m_2 g \qquad \ldots\ldots(ii)$

So from (i) & (ii), we get $g = \frac{GM_1}{r^2}$

So the ratio of gravitational acceleration due to two planets is

$$\frac{g_1}{g_2} = \frac{M_1}{r_1^2} \times \frac{r_2^2}{M_2} = \frac{(4/3)\pi r_1^3 \times \rho}{r_1^2} \times \frac{r_2^2}{(4/3)\pi r_2^3 \times \rho}$$

$\frac{g_1}{g_2} = \left(\frac{r_1}{r_2}\right)$ (both planet have same material, so density is same)

3. (a) The escape velocity on the earth is defined as

$v_e = \sqrt{2g_eR_e}$

Where R_e & g_e are the radius & acceleration due to gravity of earth.

Now for planet $g_P=2g_e$, $R_P=R_e/4$

So $v_P = \sqrt{2g_PR_P} = \sqrt{2\times 2g_e \times R_e/4} = \frac{v_e}{\sqrt{2}}$

4. (b) At a height h above the surface of earth the gravitational potential energy of the particle of mass m is

$U_h = -\frac{GM_em}{R_e+h}$

Where M_e & R_e are the mass & radius of earth respectively. In this question, since $h = R_e$

So $U_{h=R_e} = -\frac{GM_em}{2R_e} = \frac{-mgR_e}{2}$

5. (c) $T^2 \propto R^3$

$\Rightarrow \left(\frac{T_1}{T_2}\right)^2 = \left(\frac{R_1}{R_2}\right)^3 \Rightarrow \left(\frac{T_1}{T_2}\right) = \left(\frac{R_1}{R_2}\right)^{3/2} = \left(\frac{1}{4}\right)^{3/2}$

$\Rightarrow \frac{T_2}{T_1} = (4)^{3/2} = 8 \Rightarrow T_2 = 8\times T_1 = 8\times 5 = 40$ hours

6. (c) Given that $\ell_2 = 1.02\,\ell_1$

We know that $T = 2\pi\sqrt{\left(\frac{\ell}{g}\right)}$ or $T \propto \sqrt{\ell}$

$\therefore \frac{T_2}{T_1} = \sqrt{\left(\frac{\ell_2}{\ell_1}\right)} = \sqrt{\frac{(1.02\ell_1)}{\ell_1}} = 101$

Thus time period increases by 1%.

7. (c) $T = \frac{2\pi}{R}\left[\frac{(R+h)^3}{g}\right]^{1/2}$

Here (R + h) changes from R to 4 R. Hence period of revolution changes from T to $(4^3)^{1/2}$ T = 8 T.

8. (c) $\frac{mv^2}{R+x} = \frac{GmM}{(R+x)^2}$

x = height of satellite from earth surface

m = mass of satellite

$\Rightarrow v^2 = \frac{GM}{(R+x)}$ or $v = \sqrt{\frac{GM}{R+x}}$

$T = \frac{2\pi(R+x)}{v} = \frac{2\pi(R+x)}{\sqrt{\frac{GM}{R+x}}}$

which is independent of mass of satellite

9. (c) $F = KR^{-n} = MR\omega^2 \Rightarrow \omega^2 = KR^{-(n+1)}$

or $\omega = K'R^{\frac{-(n+1)}{2}}$ [where $K' = K^{1/2}$, a constant]

$\frac{2\pi}{T} \alpha R^{\frac{-(n+1)}{2}}$

$\therefore T \alpha R^{\frac{(n+1)}{2}}$

10. (c)

11. (b) $E_1 = \frac{1}{2}mv_e^2$, $E_2 = \frac{1}{2}mv_0^2$

$\therefore \frac{E_1}{E_2} = \left(\frac{v_e}{v_0}\right)^2 = 2 \quad \because v_e = \sqrt{2}v_0$

12. (c)

13. (b) $P.E. = \int_{R_0}^{R}\frac{GMm}{r^2}dr = -GMm\left[\frac{1}{R}-\frac{1}{R_0}\right]$

The K.E. acquired by the body at the surface $= \frac{1}{2}m\,v^2$

$\therefore \frac{1}{2}mv^2 = -GMm\left[\frac{1}{R}-\frac{1}{R_0}\right]$

$v = \sqrt{2GM\left(\frac{1}{R_0}-\frac{1}{R}\right)}$

14. (c) Distance between the surface of the spherical bodies = 12R – R – 2R = 9R

Force ∝ Mass

Acceleration ∝ Mass

Distance ∝ Acceleration

$\Rightarrow \frac{a_1}{a_2} = \frac{M}{5M} = \frac{1}{5} \Rightarrow \frac{S_1}{S_2} = \frac{1}{5} \Rightarrow S_2 = 5S_1$

$S_1 + S_2 = 9 \Rightarrow 6S_1 = 9 \Rightarrow S_1 = \frac{9}{6} = 1.5$

$S_2 = 1.5\times 5 = 7.5$

Note: Maximum distance will be travelled by smaller bodies due to the greater acceleration caused by the same gravitational force

15. (c) $g = \frac{GM}{R^2}$; $g' = \frac{GM}{(0.99R)^2}$

$\therefore \frac{g'}{g} = \left(\frac{R^2}{0.99R^2}\right) \Rightarrow g' > g$

16. (b) The orbital speed of satellite is independent of mass of satellite, so ball will behave as a satellite & will continue to move with same speed in original orbit.

17. (c) Applying conservation of energy principle, we get

$\frac{1}{2}mk^2v_e^2 - \frac{GMm}{R} = -\frac{GMm}{r}$

$\Rightarrow \frac{1}{2}mk^2\frac{2GM}{R} - \frac{GMm}{R} = -\frac{GMm}{r}$

$\Rightarrow \frac{k^2}{R} - \frac{1}{R} = -\frac{1}{r} \Rightarrow \frac{1}{r} = \frac{1}{R} - \frac{k^2}{R}$

$\Rightarrow \frac{1}{r} = \frac{1}{R}(1-k^2) \Rightarrow r = \frac{R}{1-k^2}$

18. (b) Loss in potential energy = Gain in kinetic energy

$-\frac{GMm}{R} - \left(-\frac{3}{2}\frac{GMm}{R}\right) = \frac{1}{2}mv^2$

$\Rightarrow \frac{GMm}{2R} = \frac{1}{2}mv^2 \Rightarrow v = \sqrt{\frac{GM}{R}} = \sqrt{gR}$

19. (c)

20. (a) $V = \omega R$

$g = g_0 - \omega^2 R$ [g = at equator, g_0 = at poles]

$\frac{g_0}{2} = g_0 - \omega^2 R$; $\omega^2 R = \frac{g_0}{2}$; $V^2 = \frac{g_0 R}{2}$

$V_e = \sqrt{2g_0 R} = \sqrt{4V^2} = 2V$

21. (b) $T^2 \alpha r^3$, where r = mean radius $= \frac{r_1 + r_2}{2}$

22. (a) Potential at the given point = Potential at the point due to the shell + Potential due to the particle

$= -\frac{GM}{a} - \frac{2GM}{a} = -\frac{3GM}{a}$

23. (b) Angular momentum is conserved

$\therefore L_1 = L_2$

$\Rightarrow mr_1v_1 = mr_2v_2 \Rightarrow r_1v_1 = r_2v_2 \Rightarrow \frac{v_1}{v_2} = \frac{r_2}{r_1}$

24. (c) Areal velocity; $\frac{dA}{dt}$

$dA = \frac{1}{2}r^2 d\theta \Rightarrow \frac{dA}{dt} = \frac{1}{2}r^2 \frac{d\theta}{dt} = \frac{1}{2}r^2\omega$

Also, $L = mvr = mr^2\omega$

$\therefore \frac{dA}{dt} = \frac{1}{2}\frac{L}{m}$

25. (a)

26. (b) According to question, $g_h = g_d = g_1$

$g_h = \frac{GM}{\left(R + \frac{R}{2}\right)^2}$ and $g_d = \frac{GM(R-d)}{R^3}$

h = R/2

d

(R-d)

$\frac{GM}{\left(\frac{3R}{2}\right)^2} = \frac{GM(R-d)}{R^3} \Rightarrow \frac{4}{9} = \frac{(R-d)}{R}$

$\Rightarrow 4R = 9R - 9d \Rightarrow 5R = 9d \quad \therefore \frac{d}{R} = \frac{5}{9}$

27. (c)

28. (d) Weight at pole, $w = mg = 196\ N$

$\Rightarrow m = 19.6$ kg

Weight at equator, $w' = mg' = m(g - \omega^2 R)$

$= 19.6\left[10 - \left(\frac{2\pi}{24 \times 3600}\right)^2 \times 6400 \times 10^3\right] N \quad \left(\because \omega = \frac{2\pi}{T}\right)$

$= 19.6\,[10 - 0.034] = 195.33\ N$

29. (a) Given acceleration due to gravity at a height h from earth's surface is

$g_h = g\left(1 + \frac{h}{R_e}\right)^{-2} \Rightarrow 4.9 = 9.8\left(1 + \frac{h}{R_e}\right)^{-2}$

$\frac{1}{\sqrt{2}} = \left(1 - \frac{h}{R_e}\right)$ [as $h <<< R_e$]

$h = R_e\left(\sqrt{2} - 1\right)$

$h = 6400 \times 0.414$ km $= 2.6 \times 10^6$ m

30. (c) We know, $g' = g - \omega^2 R \cos^2\theta$

$\frac{3g}{4} = g - \omega^2 R$ Given, $g' = \frac{3}{4}g$

$\omega^2 R = \frac{g}{4}$

$\omega = \sqrt{\frac{g}{4R}} = \sqrt{\frac{10}{4 \times 6400 \times 10^3}}$

$= \frac{1}{2 \times 8 \times 100} = 0.6 \times 10^{-3}$ rad/s

31. (a) Acceleration due to gravity at depth d from the surface of the earth or at a distance r from the centre 'O' of the earth

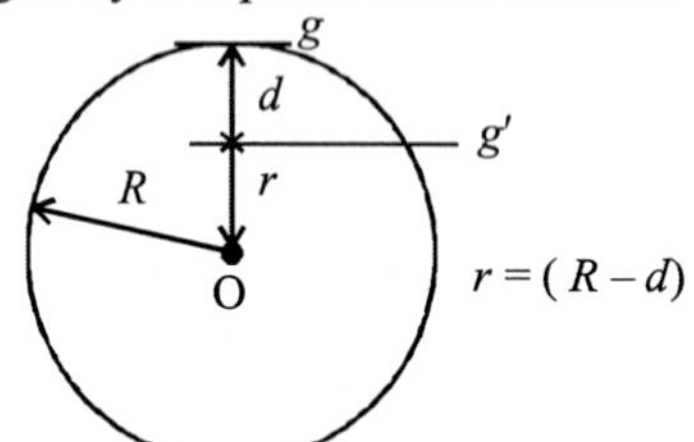

$g' = \frac{4}{3}\pi\rho G r$

Hence $g' \propto r$

32. (d)

33. (c) $E_g = \frac{GM}{(3a)^2} + \frac{G(2M)}{(3a)^2} = \frac{GM}{3a^2}$

34. (b) $AC = a\sqrt{2} \quad \because r = \frac{AC}{2} = \frac{a\sqrt{2}}{2} = \frac{a}{\sqrt{2}}$

Resultant force on the body

$B = \frac{GM^2}{a^2}\hat{i} + \frac{GM^2}{a^2}\hat{j} + \frac{GM^2}{(a\sqrt{2})^2}(\cos 45°\hat{i} + \sin 45°\hat{j})$

$\Rightarrow |F| = \frac{GM^2}{a^2}(\sqrt{2}) + \frac{GM^2}{2a^2}$

$\frac{Mv^2}{r}$ = Resultant force towards centre

$\therefore \frac{Mv^2}{\left(\frac{a}{\sqrt{2}}\right)} = \frac{GM^2}{a^2}\left(\sqrt{2} + \frac{1}{2}\right)$

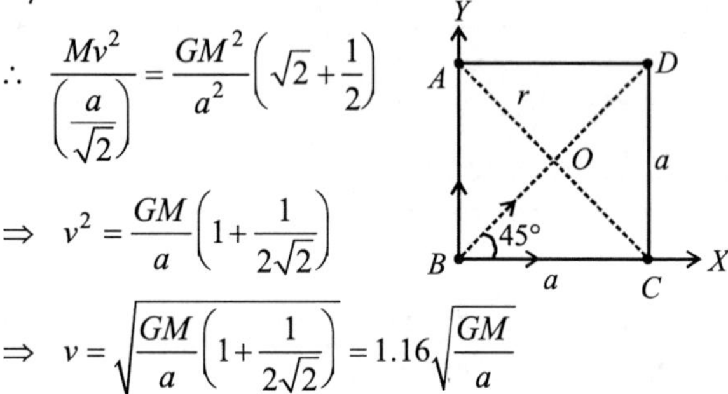

$\Rightarrow v^2 = \frac{GM}{a}\left(1 + \frac{1}{2\sqrt{2}}\right)$

$\Rightarrow v = \sqrt{\frac{GM}{a}\left(1 + \frac{1}{2\sqrt{2}}\right)} = 1.16\sqrt{\frac{GM}{a}}$

35. (a)

36. (d) Due to complete solid sphere, potential at point P

$V_{sphere} = \frac{-GM}{2R^3}\left[3R^2 - \left(\frac{R}{2}\right)^2\right]$

$= \frac{-GM}{2R^3}\left(\frac{11R^2}{4}\right) = -11\frac{GM}{8R}$

Solid sphere

P

Cavity

Due to cavity part potential at point P

$V_{cavity} = -\frac{3}{2}\frac{\frac{GM}{8}}{\frac{R}{2}} = -\frac{3GM}{8R}$

So potential at the centre of cavity

$= V_{sphere} - V_{cavity}$

$= -\frac{11GM}{8R} - \left(-\frac{3}{8}\frac{GM}{R}\right) = \frac{-GM}{R}$

37. (d) Gravitational field, $I = (5\hat{i} + 12\hat{j})$ N/kg

$I = -\frac{dv}{dr} \Rightarrow v = -\left[\int_0^x I_x dx + \int_0^y I_y dy\right]$

$= -\left[I_x.x + I_y.y\right] = -\left[5(7-0) + 12(-3-0)\right]$

$= -\left[35 + (-36)\right] = 1\text{ J/kg}$

i.e., change in gravitational potential 1 J/kg.
Hence change in gravitational potential energy 1 J

38. (a) By angular momentum conservation

$r_{min} v_{max} = m r_{max} v_{min}$

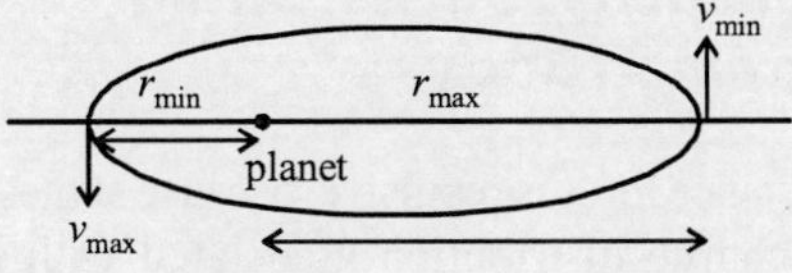

Given, $v_{min} = \frac{v_{max}}{6}$ $\therefore \frac{r_{min}}{r_{max}} = \frac{v_{min}}{v_{max}} = \frac{1}{6}$

39. (a) Orbital speed of the body when it revolves very close to the surface of planet

$V_0 = \sqrt{\frac{GM}{R}}$ ...(i)

Here, G = gravitational constant
Escape speed from the surface of planet

$V_e = \sqrt{\frac{2GM}{R}}$ ...(ii)

Dividing (i) by (ii), we have

$\frac{V_0}{V_e} = \frac{\sqrt{\frac{GM}{R}}}{\sqrt{\frac{2GM}{R}}} = \frac{1}{\sqrt{2}}$

40. (a)

41. (b) K.E. of satellite is zero at earth surface and at height h from energy conservation

$U_{surface} + E_1 = U_h$

$-\frac{GM_e m}{R_e} + E_1 = -\frac{GM_e m}{(Re+h)}$

$\Rightarrow E_1 = GM_e m\left(\frac{1}{R_e} - \frac{1}{R_e+h}\right) \Rightarrow E_1 = \frac{GM_e m}{(R_e+h)} \times \frac{h}{R_e}$

Gravitational attraction

$F_G = ma_c = \frac{mv^2}{(R_e+h)} = \frac{GM_e m}{(R_e+h)^2}$

$mv^2 = \frac{GM_e m}{(R_e+h)}$

$E_2 = \frac{mv^2}{2} = \frac{GM_e m}{2(R_e+h)}$

$E_1 = E_2$

Clearly, $\frac{h}{R_e} = \frac{1}{2} \Rightarrow h = \frac{R_e}{2} = 3200\text{km}$

42. (a) Escape velocity of the planet A is $V_A = \sqrt{\frac{2GM_A}{R_A}}$

where M_A and R_A be the mass and radius of the planet A.
According to given problem

$M_B = \frac{M_A}{2}, \ R_B = \frac{R_A}{2}$

$\therefore V_B = \sqrt{\frac{2G\frac{M_A}{2}}{\frac{R_A}{2}}}$ $\therefore \frac{V_A}{V_B} = \sqrt{\frac{\frac{2GM_A}{R_A}}{\frac{2GM_A/2}{R_A/2}}} = \frac{n}{4} = 1$

$\Rightarrow n = 4$

43. (d) Time period of revolution of satellite,

$T = \frac{2\pi r}{v}$

$v = \sqrt{\frac{GM}{r}}$ $\therefore T = 2\pi r\sqrt{\frac{r}{GM}} = 2\pi\sqrt{\frac{r^3}{GM}}$

Substituting the values, we get

$T = 2\pi\sqrt{\frac{(202)^3 \times 10^{12}}{6.67 \times 10^{-11} \times 8 \times 10^{22}}}$ sec

$T = 7812.2$ s

$T \simeq 2.17$ hr $\Rightarrow$ 11 revolutions.

44. (b) $mv\hat{i} + mv\hat{j} = 2m\vec{v}$

$\Rightarrow \vec{v} = \frac{v}{2}\hat{i} + \frac{v}{2}\hat{j}$

$\Rightarrow \vec{v} = \sqrt{\left(\frac{v}{2}\right)^2 + \left(\frac{v}{2}\right)^2} = \frac{v}{\sqrt{2}}$

$= \frac{1}{\sqrt{2}} \times \sqrt{\frac{GM}{R}}$

45. (b) At height r from center of earth, orbital velocity

$v = \sqrt{\frac{GM}{r}}$

By principle of energy conservation

KE of 'm' $+ \left(-\frac{GMm}{r}\right) = 0 + 0$

($\because$ At infinity, PE = KE = 0)

or KE of 'm' $= \frac{GMm}{r} = \left(\sqrt{\frac{GM}{r}}\right)^2 m = mv^2$

9 Mechanical Properties of Solids

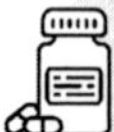

Topic 9.1 : Interatomic & Intermolecular Force, Elasticity, Stress, Strain Hooke's Law and Energy Stored in a Strained Body

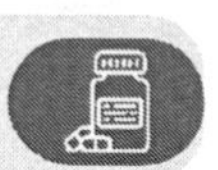

INTERATOMIC AND INTERMOLECULAR FORCE

The force between atoms of an element is called **interatomic force**. The force between molecules of a compound (or element) is called **intermolecular force**. These forces are electrical in nature. Depending on the distance between the atoms, this force may be attractive or repulsive in nature. These forces are responsible for the definite size or shape of a solid.

Detailed calculations as well as deductions from experiment show that the interaction between any isolated pairs of atoms or molecules may be represented by a curve that shows how the potential energy varies with separation between them as shown in the figure.

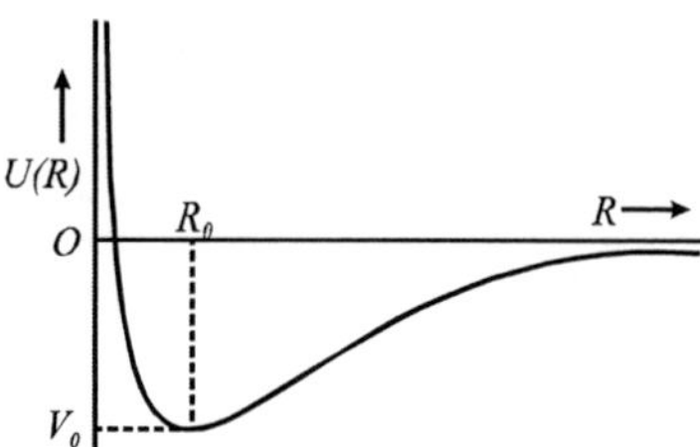

This curve describes the interatomic potential. The force between the atoms can be found from the potential energy by using the relation

$$F = -\frac{dU}{dr}$$

The resulting interatomic force curve is shown in figure.

Force is along the line joining the atoms or molecules, and is shown negative for attraction and positive for repulsion.

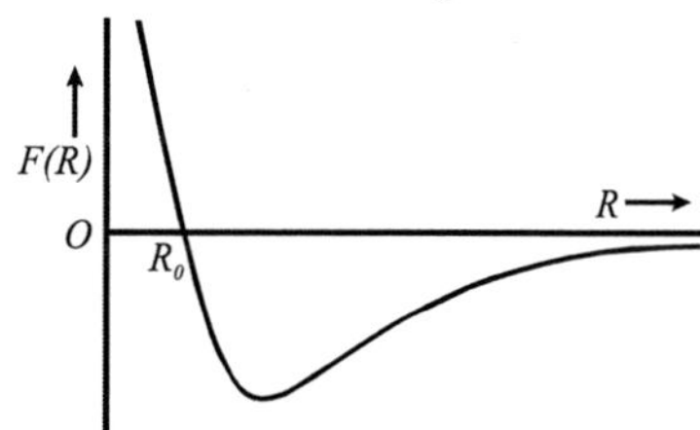

We see that as the distance decreases, the attractive force first increases and then decreases to zero at a separation where the potential energy is minimum.

For smaller distance force is repulsive, because at these distance the negative charge distribution associated with one atom begins to over lap with that associated with the neighboring atom.

The force of attraction between molecules may be written as

$$F_a = -\frac{a}{r^7}$$

The negative sign shows that F_a is a force of attraction and 'a' is a constant which depends on the kind of attractive force between the molecules and the structure of the molecules. The force of attraction results from the creation of induced dipole moment in one molecule by the neighbouring molecule.

When the molecules are brought closer there is a force of repulsion between them. It can be shown that the repulsive force is

$$F_r = +\frac{b}{r^9},$$

where b is a constant like a. The force of repulsion varies very rapidly. F_r is inversely proportional to the ninth power of distance between the molecules. The resultant force acting on the molecules is

$$F = -\frac{a}{r^7} + \frac{b}{r^9}$$

The distance between the molecules decides the sign of the resultant force.

ELASTICITY

The property of the body by virtue of which it tends to regain its original shape and size after removing the deforming force is called ***elasticity***. If the body regains its original shape and size completely, after the removal of deforming forces, then the body is said to be **perfectly elastic**.

- *The property of the body by virtue of which it tends to retain its deformed state after removing the deforming force is called* ***plasticity***. If the body does not have any tendency to recover its original shape and size, it is called **perfectly plastic**.

STRESS AND STRAIN

Stress :

When a deforming force is applied to a body, an internal restoring force comes into play.

*The restoring force per unit area is called **stress**.*

$$Stress = \frac{Restoring\ force}{Area}$$

Its **S.I. Unit** is Nm^{-2}

Stress is a **tensor** as its value changes when direction changes.

Types of Stress :

Longitudinal stress or tensile stress, volumetric stress and tangential stress are the types of stress.

Strain :

It is defined as the ratio of the change in shape or size to the original shape or size of the body.

$$Strain = \frac{Change\ in\ dimension}{Original\ dimension}$$

Strain has **no units or dimensions.**

Types of Strain :

Longitudinal strain : It is defined as the ratio of the change in length to the original length.

$$Longitudinal\ strain = \frac{\Delta\ell}{\ell}$$

Volume strain : It is the ratio of the change in volume to the original volume.

$$Volume\ strain = \frac{\Delta V}{V}$$

Shearing strain : It is the angular deformation produced in a body.

$$Shearing\ strain\ (\theta) = \frac{\Delta x}{h}$$

HOOKE'S LAW

It is the fundamental law of elasticity given by Robert Hooke in 1679. *It states that "the stress is directly proportional to strain provided the strain is small ".*

i.e. $Stress \propto strain \Rightarrow \frac{stress}{strain} = \text{constant} = E$

This proportionality constant is called **modulus of elasticity** (name given by Thomas Young) or **coefficient of elasticity (E)**. Since stress has same dimensions as that of pressure and strain is dimensionless. So the **dimensions** of E is same as, that of stress or pressure i.e. $[ML^{-1}T^{-2}]$

The modulus of elasticity depends on the material and on the nature of deformation. There are three type of deformations and therefore three **types of modulus of elasticity**.

(i) ***Young's modulus (Y) :*** It measures the resistance of a solid to elongation.

(ii) ***Shear modulus*** (η) ***or modulus of rigidity :*** It measures the resistance to motion of the plane of a solid sliding part on each other.

(iii) ***Bulk modulus (B) :*** It measure the resistance that solid or liquid offer to their volume change.

The stress under which the system breaks is called breaking stress.

(i) **Young's modulus (Y) :** Let us consider a long bar (shown in fig.) of cross-sectional area A and length ℓ_o, which is clamped at one end. When we apply external force F_ℓ longitudinally along the bar, internal forces in bar resist distortion, but bar attains equilibrium in which its length is greater and in which external force is exactly balanced by internal forces. The bar is said to be stressed in this condition.

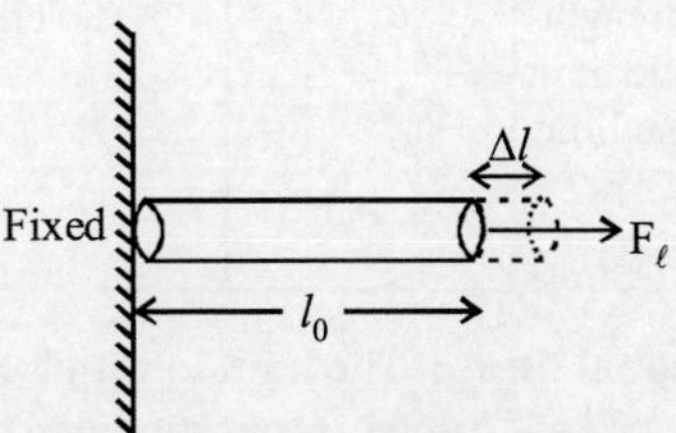

Now if the solid bar obey the Hooke' law, the Young's modulus, Y is defined as

$$Y = \frac{Tensile\ stress}{Tensile\ strain} = \frac{F_\ell / A}{\Delta\ell / \ell}$$

Where Δl is change in the length of bar, when we apply F_ℓ.

(ii) **Shear modulus (η) :** Shear modulus or modulus of rigidity η is

$$\eta = \frac{Shearing\ stress}{Shearing\ strain} = \frac{F_t / A}{\Delta x / h}$$

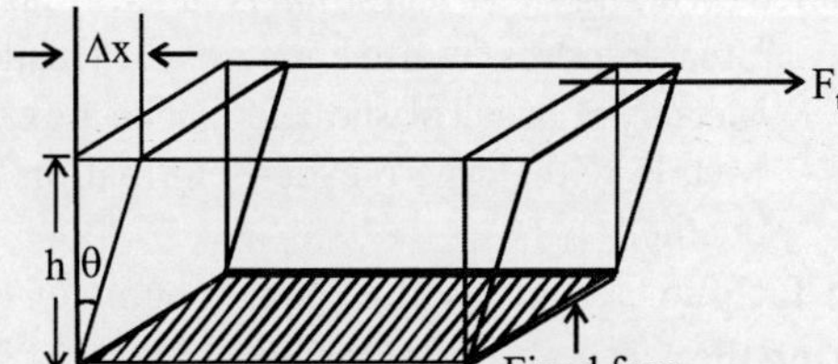

(a) As we see, there is no change in volume under this deformation, but shape changes.

(b) $\frac{\Delta x}{h} = \tan\theta \approx \theta$ (see the figure), where θ is shear angle.

(iii) **Bulk modulus (B) :** The Bulk modulus B is defined as

$$B = \frac{Volume\ stress}{Volume\ stain} = \frac{F_n / A}{\Delta V / V} = \frac{-\Delta P}{\Delta V / V}$$

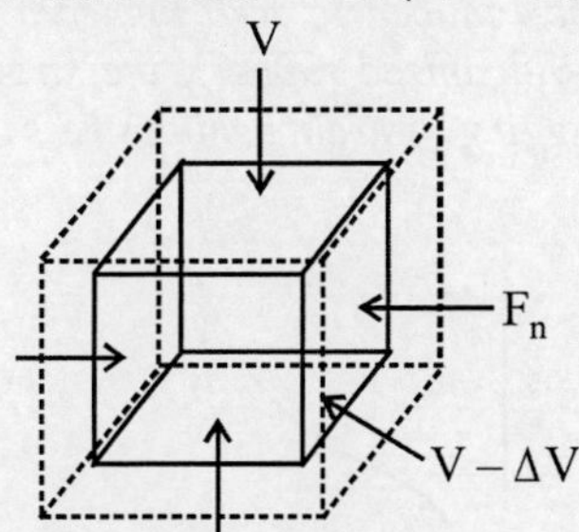

Negative sign comes to make B positive, because with the increase of pressure, the volume of body decreases or vice versa.

The reciprocal of the Bulk modulus is called compressibility of material

i.e., $Compressibility = 1/B$.

Poisson's Ratio (σ) :

Lateral strain/longitudinal strain = Poisson's ratio (σ).

The theoretical value of σ lies between –1 and 0.5 and practical value of σ lies between 0 and 0.5.

STRESS-STRAIN CURVE

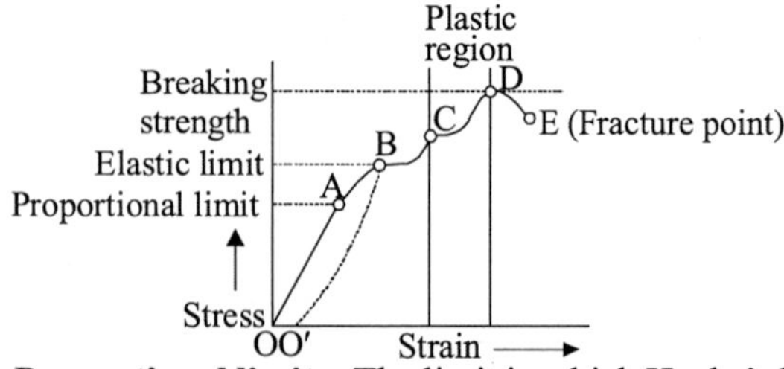

(i) **Proportional limit :** The limit in which Hooke's law is valid i.e, stress is directly proportional to strain is called proportion limit. **Stress ∝ strain**

(ii) **Elastic limit :** It is a maximum stress upto which the body completely recovers its original state after the removal of the deforming forces.

(iii) **Yield point :** The point beyond elastic limit, at which the length of wire starts increasing without increasing stress, is defined as the yield point.

(iv) **Breaking point :** The position when the strain becomes so large that the wire breaks down at last, is called breaking point. At this position the stress acting in that wire is called breaking stress and strain is called breaking strain.

- Breaking stress is also known as the tensile strength.
- Metals with small plastic deformation are called brittle.
- Metals with large plastic deformation are called ductile.

Elastic fatigue : This is the phenomenon of a delay in recovering the original configuration by a body, if it had been subjected to stress for a longer time the body looses the property of elasticity temporarily.

Elastic relaxation time : It is the time delay in regaining the original shape after removal of deforming forces. Elastic relaxation time for gold, silver and phosphor bronze is negligible.

Elastic Hysteresis

*When the stress applied on a body, is decreased to zero, the strain will not be reduced to zero immediately. For some substances (e.g.-vulcanized rubber), the strain lags behind the stress. This lagging of strain behind stress is called **elastic hysteresis**.*

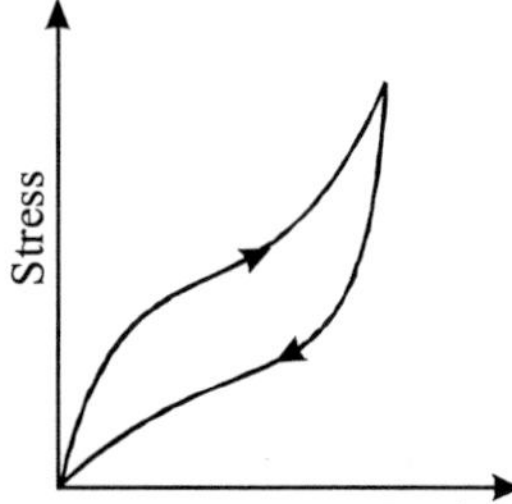

The stress-strain graph for increasing and decreasing load encloses a loop, as shown in figure. The area of the loop gives the energy dissipated during its deformation.

Problem Solving Tips

1. Thermal stress $=\frac{F}{A}=Y\alpha\Delta T$, where α is the coefficient of linear expansion and ΔT is the change in temperature.

2. (i) The modulus of rigidity (η) for liquids is zero.

   (ii) For a given tensile force, the increase in length is inversely proportional to square of its diameter.

   (iii) The pressure required to stop volume expansion of a piece of metal is

   $$P = B\gamma dT,$$

   where γ = coefficient of volume expansion = 3α

   (iv) To compare elasticities of different materials, their identical small balls are made and they are dropped from same height on a hard floor. The ball which rises maximum after striking the floor, is most elastic. The order of elasticity of different materials on this basis is as follows :

   $$Y_{ivory} > Y_{steel} > Y_{rubber} > Y_{clay}$$

   (v) For the construction of rails, bridges, girders and machines, materials with high Young's modulus are used so that they may not get permanently deformed.

   For a spring, $F=\frac{YA\Delta L}{L}=kx.$

   Hence spring constant $k=\frac{YA}{L}$. Here ΔL = x.

3. When equal force is applied on identical wires of different materials then the wire in which minimum elongation is produced is more elastic. For the same load, more elongation is produced in rubber than in steel wire, hence steel is more elastic than rubber.

Relation between Y, B, η and σ

(i) $Y=3B(1-2\sigma)$ (ii) $Y=2\eta(1+\sigma)$

(iii) $\sigma=\frac{3B-2\eta}{6B+2\eta}$ (iv) $\frac{9}{Y}=\frac{3}{\eta}+\frac{1}{B}$

ENERGY STORED PER UNIT VOLUME IN A STRAINED BODY

Energy per unit volume $=\frac{1}{2}$ *stress × strain*

$=\frac{1}{2}$ modulus of elasticity × (strain)^2

$=\frac{1}{2}$ (stress)^2 /modulus of elasticity.

Work done in stretching a wire or work done per unit volume

$$=\frac{1}{2}\times stress \times strain = \frac{1}{2}\times load \times extension$$

Torsional rigidity of a cylinder :

(i) The torsional rigidity C of a cylinder is given by,

$$C=\frac{\pi\eta R^4}{2\ell}$$

where η = modulus of rigidity of material of cylinder, R = radius of cylinder, ℓ = length of cylinder

(ii) Restoring couple, $\tau = C\phi = \dfrac{\pi\eta R^4\phi}{2\ell}$

(iii) Work done in twisting the cylinder through an angle

$$\phi,\ W = \frac{\pi\eta R^4\phi^2}{4\ell}\ \text{joule} = \frac{1}{2}C\phi^2$$

Cantilever :

A beam fixed at one end and loaded at the other end is called a cantilever.

(i) The depression y at a distance x from the fixed end is (when the weight of cantilever is ineffective)

$$y = \frac{mg}{YI}\left(\frac{\ell x^2}{2} - \frac{x^3}{6}\right)$$

where mg = load applied, ℓ = length of cantilever, I = geometrical moment of inertia of its cross section.

(ii) Maximum depression at free end of cantilever,

$$y_{max} = \delta = \frac{mg\ell^3}{3YI}$$

(a) For rectangular beam, $I = \dfrac{bd^3}{12}$

(b) For a circular cross section beam of radius r, $I = \dfrac{\pi r^4}{4}$

(iv) Depression produced in a beam supported at two ends and loaded at the middle, $\delta = \dfrac{mg\ell^3}{48YI}$

For rectangular beam, $\delta = \dfrac{mgl^3}{4Ybd^3}$

and for circular beam, $\delta = \dfrac{mgl^3}{12\pi r^4 Y}$

Problem Solving Tips

1. Wound spring possess elastic potential energy.
2. A material which can be drawn into wires is called **ductile** and a material which can be hammered into sheet is called **malleable.**
3. Ductility, brittleness, malleability, etc., are not elastic properties.
4. The substance which breaks just beyond the elastic limit is called **brittle.**
5. (i) Breaking force of a wire = breaking stress × area of cross section
   (ii) Breaking stress does not depend on the length of wire
   (iii) Breaking stress depends on the material of wire.

Example 1.

A uniform rod of mass m, length L, area of cross section A and Young's modulus Y hangs from a ceiling. Its elongation under its own weight will be

(a) $\dfrac{2mgL}{AY}$ (b) $\dfrac{mgL}{AY}$ (c) $\dfrac{mgL}{2AY}$ (d) zero

***Solution* (c)**

Mass of section BC of wire $= \dfrac{m}{L}(L-x)$;

Tension at B, $T = \dfrac{m}{L}(L-x)g$

Elongation of element dx at B,

$$d\ell = \frac{T\,dx}{AY} = \frac{m(L-x)g}{LAY}dx$$

Total elongation $= \int d\ell = \dfrac{mg}{LAY}\displaystyle\int_0^L (L-x)dx = \dfrac{mgL}{2YA}$

Example 2.

If the potential energy of the molecule is given by $U = \dfrac{A}{r^6} - \dfrac{B}{r^{12}}$. Then at equilibrium position its potential energy is equal to

(a) $-A^2/4B$ (b) $A^2/4B$ (c) $2A/B$ (d) $A/2B$

***Solution :* (b)**

$$F = -\frac{dU}{dr} = -\frac{d}{dr}\left[\frac{A}{r^6} - \frac{B}{r^{12}}\right] = \left[\frac{-A\times 6}{r^7} + \frac{12B}{r^{13}}\right]$$

In equilibrium position F = 0.

so, $\dfrac{6A}{r^7} = \dfrac{12B}{r^{13}}$ or $r^6 = \dfrac{2B}{A}$

∴ Potential energy at equilibrium position

$$U = \frac{A}{(2B/A)} - \frac{B}{(2B/A)^2} = \frac{A^2}{2B} - \frac{A^2}{4B} = \frac{A^2}{4B}$$

Example 3.

The normal density of gold is ρ and its bulk modulus is K. The increase in density of a lump of gold when a pressure P is applied uniformly on all sides is

(a) K/ρP (b) P/ρK (c) ρP/K (d) ρK/P

***Solution :* (a)**

$$K = \frac{p}{\Delta V/V} \text{ or } \frac{\Delta V}{V} = \frac{p}{K};$$

Also $\rho = \dfrac{M}{V}$ and $\rho' = \dfrac{M}{V-\Delta V}$;

$$\therefore\ \frac{\rho'}{\rho} = \frac{V}{(V-\Delta V)} = \frac{1}{(1-\Delta V/V)} = \left(1 - \frac{\Delta V}{V}\right)^{-1}$$

$$\approx \left(1 + \frac{\Delta V}{V}\right) = 1 + \frac{p}{K} \text{ or } \frac{\rho'}{\rho} - 1 = \frac{p}{K}$$

or $\rho' - \rho = \dfrac{p\rho}{K}$ $\quad (\because \Delta V << V)$

Example 4.

A wire 3 m in length and 1 mm in diameter at 30°C and kept in a low temperature at –170°C and is stretched by hanging a weight of 10 kg at one end. Calculate the change in the length of the wire. Given $\alpha = 1.2\times10^{-5}$/°C and $Y = 2\times10^{11}$ N/m². Take g = 10 m/s².

Solution :

We know that,

$$\ell = \frac{FL}{YA} = \frac{10\times10\times3}{2\times10^{11}\times0.785\times10^{-6}} = 1.91\times10^{-3}$$

(where $A = \pi r^2$) $= 0.785\times10^{-6}$ m²

Contraction in length $= -\alpha L \Delta T$

$= -(1.2 \times 10^{-5})(3)(-170-30)$

$= 7.2 \times 10^{-3}$ m

The resultant change in length

$= 7.2 \times 10^{-3} - 1.91 \times 10^{-3} = 5.29$ mm

Example 5.

A material has Poisson's ratio 0.5. If a uniform rod of it suffers a longitudinal strain of 2×10^{-3}, what is the percentage increase in volume?

Solution :

Here

$$\frac{\Delta V}{V} = \frac{\Delta(\pi r^2 \ell)}{\pi r^2 \ell} = \frac{r^2 \Delta\ell + 2r\ell\Delta r}{r^2 \ell} \text{ or } \frac{\Delta V}{V} = \frac{\Delta\ell}{\ell} + 2\frac{\Delta r}{r}$$

Now $\sigma = -\frac{\Delta r / r}{\Delta\ell / \ell}$ or $\frac{\Delta r}{r} = -\sigma\frac{\Delta\ell}{\ell}$;

$\therefore \frac{\Delta r}{r} = -0.5 \times (2 \times 10^{-3}) = -1 \times 10^{-3}$

Further, $\frac{\Delta V}{V} = (2 \times 10^{-3}) - 2 \times (1 \times 10^{-3}) = 0$

$\therefore$ % increase in volume is 0.

Example 6.

(a) *A heavy machine is to be installed in a factory. To absorb vibrations of the machine, a block of rubber is placed between the machine and floor, which of the two rubbers A and B would you prefer to use for the purpose ? Why ?*

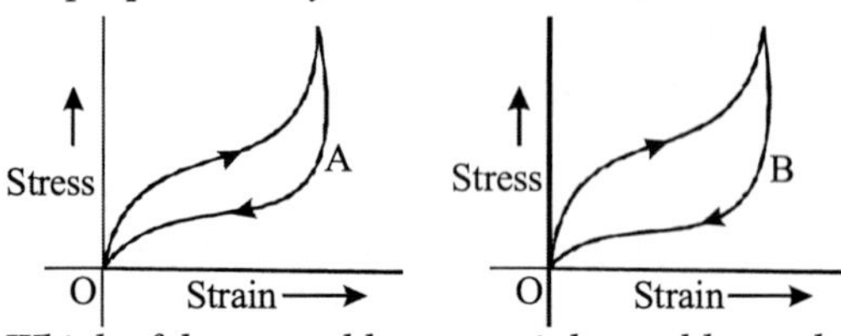

(b) *Which of the two rubber materials would you choose for a car tyre ?*

Solution :

(a) Rubber B is preferred. The area of the hysteresis loop measures the amount of heat energy dissipated by the material. The area of loop B is more than A. So B can absorb more vibrations.

(b) To avoid excessive heating of car tyre, rubber A would be preferred over rubber B.

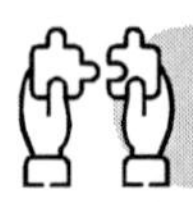

9.1 Concept Practice Problems

CPP

1. The length of a metal is ℓ_1 when the tension in it is T_1 and is ℓ_2 when the tension is T_2. The original length of the wire is

(a) $\frac{\ell_1 + \ell_2}{2}$ (b) $\frac{\ell_1 T_2 + \ell_2 T_1}{T_1 + T_2}$

(c) $\frac{\ell_1 T_2 - \ell_2 T_1}{T_2 - T_1}$ (d) $\sqrt{T_1 T_2 \ell_1 \ell_2}$

2. According to Hooke's law of elasticity, if stress is increased, then the ratio of stress to strain

(a) becomes zero (b) remains constant

(c) decreases (d) increases

3. The length of an iron wire is L and area of corss-section is A. The increase in length is l on applying the force F on its two ends. Which of the statement is correct?

(a) Increase in length is inversely proportional to its length

(b) Increase in length is proportional to area of cross-section

(c) Increase in length is inversely proportional to area of cross-section

(d) Increase in length is proportional to Young's modulus

4. For a constant hydraulic stress on an object, the fractional change in the object volume $\left(\frac{\Delta V}{V}\right)$ and its bulk modulus (B) are related as

(a) $\frac{\Delta V}{V} \propto B$ (b) $\frac{\Delta V}{V} \propto \frac{1}{B}$ (c) $\frac{\Delta V}{V} \propto B^2$ (d) $\frac{\Delta V}{V} \propto B^{-2}$

5. When an elastic material with Young's modulus Y is subjected to stretching stress S, elastic energy stored per unit volume of the material is

(a) $YS/2$ (b) $S^2Y/2$ (c) $S^2/2Y$ (d) $S/2Y$

6. A force of 10^3 newton, stretches the length of a hanging wire by 1 millimetre. The force required to stretch a wire of same material and length but having four times the diameter by 1 millimetre is

(a) 4×10^3 N (b) 16×10^3 N (c) $\frac{1}{4} \times 10^3$ N (d) $\frac{1}{16} \times 10^3$ N

7. There are two wire of same material and same length while the diameter of second wire is two times the diameter of first wire, then the ratio of extension produced in the wires by applying same load will be

(a) 1 : 1 (b) 2 : 1 (c) 1 : 2 (d) 4 : 1

8. An iron rod of length 2m and cross-sectional area of 50 mm^2 stretched by 0.5 mm, when a mass of 250 kg is hung from its lower end. Young's modulus of iron rod is

(a) 19.6×10^{20} N/m^2 (b) 19.6×10^{18} N/m^2

(c) 19.6×10^{10} N/m^2 (d) 19.6×10^{15} N/m^2

9. The diagram below shows the change in the length X of a thin uniform wire caused by the application of stress F at two different temperatures T_1 and T_2. The variation shown suggests that

(a) $T_1 > T_2$

(b) $T_1 < T_2$

(c) $T_2 > T_1$

(d) $T_1 \geq T_2$

F, T_2, T_1, X

10. Two wires are made of the same material and have the same volume. However wire 1 has cross-sectional area A and wire 2 has cross-sectional area $3A$. If the length of wire 1 increases by Δx on applying force F, how much force is needed to stretch wire 2 by the same amount?

(a) $4F$ (b) $6F$ (c) $9F$ (d) F

ANSWER KEY

1	(c)	2	(b)	3	(c)	4	(b)	5	(c)	6	(b)	7	(d)	8	(c)	9	(a)	10	(c)

CONCEPT MAP

MECHANICAL PROPERTIES OF SOLIDS

Elasticity
Property of materials by virtue of which it regain its original configuration after the removal of deforming force.

Hooke's laws
Within the elastic limit stress is directly proportional to strain i.e. stress $\propto$ strain
or, stress = E × strain

Types of modulus of elasticity

Young's modulus of elasticity
$Y = \frac{\text{longitudinal stress}}{\text{longitudinal strain}} = \frac{F\Delta\ell}{A\ell} = \frac{Mg\Delta\ell}{\pi r^2 \ell}$

Bulk modulus or volume modulus of elasticity
$B = \frac{\text{hydraulic stress}}{\text{volume strain}}$
$B = -\frac{\Delta P}{\Delta V / V}; \frac{1}{B} =$ compressibility

Rigidity or shear modulus of elasticity
$\eta = \frac{\text{tangential stress}}{\text{shearing strain}}$
$\eta = \frac{\sigma_s}{\varepsilon_s} = \frac{F/A}{\theta}$

Stress
Restoring force per unit area i.e., stress $= \frac{F}{A}$

Types of stress

(i) Longitudinal stress
$= \frac{\text{deforming force applied normal}}{\text{area}}$
$= \frac{F_n}{A}$

(ii) Volumetric stress
$= \frac{\text{force changing volume}}{\text{area}} = \frac{F_v}{A}$

(iii) Shearing or tangential stress
$= \frac{\text{tangential force}}{\text{area}} = \frac{F_t}{A}$

Elastic potential energy in a stretched wire
$= \frac{1}{2}$ stress × strain × volume of the wire

Strain
Ratio of change in configuration to the original configuration
$\text{Strain} = \frac{\text{change in configuration}}{\text{original configuration}}$

Types of strain

(i) Longitudinal strain $= \frac{\text{change in length}}{\text{original length}} = \frac{\Delta l}{l_0}$

(ii) Volumetric strain $\varepsilon_v = \frac{\text{change in volume}}{\text{original volume}} = \frac{\Delta V}{V_0}$

(iii) Shearing strain = angular displacement of the plane perpendicular to the fixed surface

Relation between Y, B, η and σ
(i) $Y = 3B(1 - 2\sigma)$
(ii) $Y = 2\eta(1 + \sigma)$
(iii) $\sigma = \frac{3B - 2\eta}{2\eta + 6B}$
(iv) $\frac{9}{Y} = \frac{1}{B} + \frac{3}{\eta}$ or $Y = \frac{9B\eta}{\eta + 3B}$

Poisson's ratio (σ)
$= \frac{\text{lateral strain } (\beta)}{\text{longitudinal strain } (\alpha)} = \frac{\Delta d / d}{\Delta \ell / \ell}$
Value of σ lies between 0 and 0.5

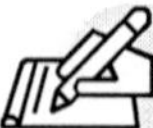

Exercise 1 - Chapter Revision Problems

CRP

1. Elastomers are the materials which
(a) are not elastic at all
(b) have very small elastic range
(c) do not obey Hooke's law
(d) None of these

2. Which of the following affects the elasticity of a substance?
(a) hammering and annealing
(b) change in temperature
(c) impurity in substance
(d) All of these

3. Which of the following has no dimensions ?
(a) strain (b) angular velocity
(c) momentum (d) angular momentum

4. Minimum and maximum values of Possion's ratio for a metal lies between
(a) $-\infty$ to $+\infty$ (b) 0 to 1
(c) $-\infty$ to 1 (d) 0 to 0.5

5. In solids interatomic forces are
(a) totally repulsive (b) totally attractive
(c) both (a) and (b) (d) None of these

6. Which one of the following is not a unit of Young's modulus ?
(a) Nm^{-1} (b) Nm^{-2}
(d) dyne cm^{-2} (d) mega pascal

7. The value of tan (90 – θ) in the graph gives

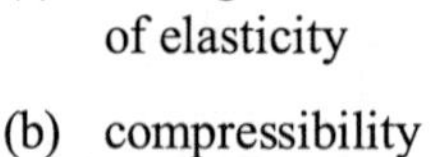

(a) Young's modulus of elasticity
(b) compressibility
(c) shear strain
(d) tensile strength

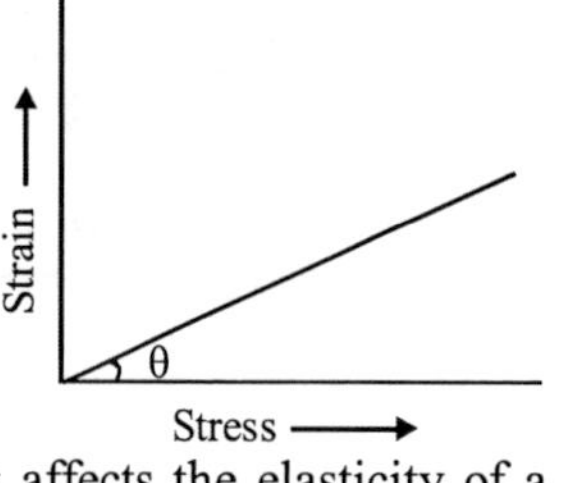

8. Which one of the following affects the elasticity of a substance ?
(a) Change in temperature
(b) Hammering and annealing
(c) Impurity in substance
(d) All of the above

9. A and B are two wires. The radius of A is twice that of B. They are stretched by the same load. Then the stress on B is
(a) equal to that on A (b) four times that on A
(c) two times that on A (d) half that on A

10. Cooking gas containers are kept in a lorry moving with uniform speed. The temperature of the gas molecules inside will
(a) increase
(b) decrease
(c) remain same
(d) decrease for some, while increase for others

11. The diagram shown below represents the applied forces per unit area with the corresponding change X (per unit length) produced in a thin wire of uniform cross section in the curve shown. The region in which the wire behaves like a liquid is
(a) ab
(b) bc
(c) cd
(d) Oa

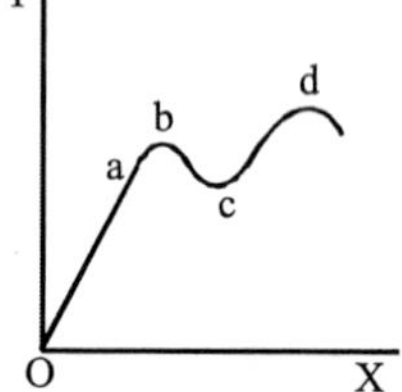

12. A steel wire is suspended vertically from a rigid support. When loaded with a weight in air, it extends by ℓ_a and when the weight is immersed completely in water, the extension is reduced to ℓ_w. Then the relative density of material of the weight is
(a) ℓ_a / ℓ_w (b) $\frac{\ell_a}{\ell_a - \ell_w}$
(c) $\ell_w / (\ell_a - \ell_w)$ (d) ℓ_w / ℓ_a

13. The ratio of shearing stress to the corresponding shearing strain is called
(a) bulk modulus (b) Young's modulus
(c) modulus of rigidity (d) None of these

14. Two wires of same material and length but cross-sections in the ratio 1 : 2 are used to suspend the same loads. The extensions in them will be in the ratio
(a) 1:2 (b) 2:1 (c) 4:1 (d) 1:4

15. A body of mass 10 kg is attached to a wire of radius 3 cm. It's breaking stress is 4.8×10^7 Nm^{-2}, the area of cross-section of the wire is 10^{-6} m^2. What is the maximum angular velocity with which it can be rotated in the horizontal circle ?
(a) 1 rad sec^{-1} (b) 2 rad sec^{-1}
(c) 4 rad sec^{-1} (d) 8 rad sec^{-1}

16. A cube is subjected to a uniform volume compression. If the side of the cube decreases by 2% the bulk strain is
(a) 0.02 (b) 0.03 (c) 0.04 (d) 0.06

17. A 2 m long rod of radius 1 cm which is fixed from one end is given a twist of 0.8 radian. The shear strain developed will be
(a) 0.002 (b) 0.004 (c) 0.008 (d) 0.016

18. For a given material, the Young's modulus is 2. 4 times that of rigidity modulus. Its Poisson's ratio is
(a) 2.4 (b) 1.2 (c) 0.4 (d) 0.2

19. From a steel wire of density ρ is suspended a brass block of density ρ_b. The extension of steel wire comes to e. If the brass block is now fully immersed in a liquid of density ρ_l, the extension becomes e'. The ratio $\frac{e}{e'}$ will be
(a) $\frac{\rho_b}{\rho_b - \rho_l}$ (b) $\frac{\rho_b - \rho_l}{\rho_b}$ (c) $\frac{\rho_b - \rho}{\rho_l - \rho}$ (d) $\frac{\rho_l}{\rho_b - \rho_l}$

20. A wire fixed at the upper end stretches by length ℓ by applying a force F. The work done in stretching is

(a) $2F\ell$ (b) $F\ell$ (c) $\frac{F}{2\ell}$ (d) $\frac{F\ell}{2}$

21. A metalic rod of length l and cross-sectional area A is made of a material of Young modulus Y. If the rod is elongated by an amount y, then the work done is proportional to

(a) y (b) $\frac{1}{y}$ (c) y^2 (d) $\frac{1}{y^2}$

22. What per cent of length of wire increases by applying a stress of 1 kg weight/mm^2 on it?
($Y = 1 \times 10^{11}$ N/m^2 and 1 kg weight = 9.8 newton)
(a) 0.0067% (b) 0.0098% (c) 0.0088% (d) 0.0078%

23. If a rubber ball is taken at the depth of 200 m in a pool, its volume decreases by 0.1%. If the density of the water is 1×10^3 kg/m^3 and g = 10m/s^2, then the volume elasticity in *N/m^2* will be
(a) 10^8 (b) 2×10^8 (c) 10^9 (d) 2×10^9

24. A 5 metre long wire is fixed to the ceiling. A weight of 10 kg is hung at the lower end and is 1 metre above the floor. The wire was elongated by 1 mm. The energy stored in the wire due to stretching is
(a) zero (b) 0.05 joule
(c) 100 joule (d) 500 joule

25. Two wires A and B are of the same material. Their lengths are in the ratio of 1 : 2 and the diameter are in the ratio 2 : 1. If they are pulled by the same force, then increase in length will be in the ratio of
(a) 2 : 1 (b) 1 : 4 (c) 1 : 8 (d) 8 : 1

26. The potential energy U between two atoms in a diatomic molecules as a function of the distance x between atoms has been shown in the figure. The atoms are

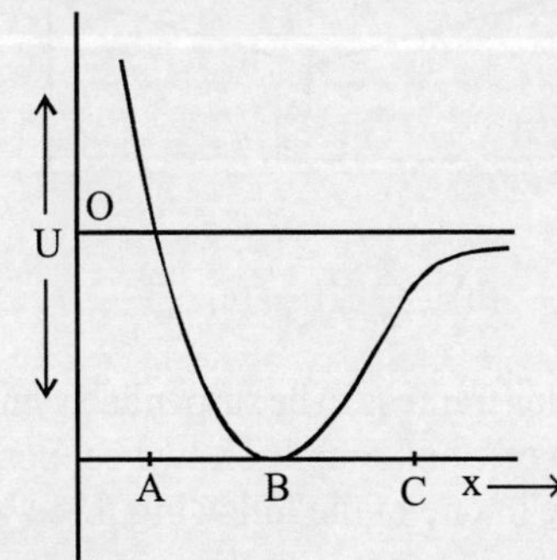

(a) attracted when x lies between A and B and are repelled when x lies between B and C
(b) attracted when x lies between B and C and are repelled when x lies between A and B
(c) are attracted when they reach B from C
(d) are repelled when they reach B from A

27. To break a wire, a force of 10^6 N/m^2 is required. If the density of the material is 3×10^3 kg/m^3, then the length of the wire which will break by its own weight will be
(a) 34m (b) 30m (c) 300m (d) 3m

28. The upper end of a wire of diameter 12mm and length 1m is clamped and its other end is twisted through an angle of 30°. The angle of shear is
(a) 18° (b) 0.18° (c) 36° (d) 0.36°

29. A uniform cube is subjected to volume compression. If each side is decreased by 1%, then bulk strain is
(a) 0.01 (b) 0.06 (c) 0.02 (d) 0.03

30. When a 4 kg mass is hung vertically on a light spring that obeys Hooke's law, the spring stretches by 2 cms. The work required to be done by an external agent in stretching this spring by 5 cms will be (g = 9.8 m/sec^2)
(a) 4.900 joule (b) 2.450 joule
(c) 0.495 joule (d) 0.245 joule

31. If the potential energy between two molecules is given by $U = -\frac{A}{r^6} + \frac{B}{r^{12}}$, then at equilibrium, separation between molecules, and the potential energy are:

(a) $\left(\frac{B}{2A}\right)^{\frac{1}{6}}, -\frac{A^2}{2B}$ (b) $\left(\frac{B}{A}\right)^{\frac{1}{6}}, 0$

(c) $\left(\frac{2B}{A}\right)^{\frac{1}{6}}, -\frac{A^2}{4B}$ (d) $\left(\frac{2B}{A}\right)^{\frac{1}{6}}, -\frac{A^2}{2B}$

32. A steel wire having a radius of 2.0 mm, carrying a load of 4kg, is hanging from a ceiling. Given that g = 3.1 À ms^{-2}, what will be the tensile stress that would be developed in the wire?
(a) 6.2×10^6 Nm^{-2} (b) 5.2×10^6 Nm^{-2}
(c) 3.1×10^6 Nm^{-2} (d) 4.8×10^6 Nm^{-2}

33. A steel wire having a radius of 2.0 mm, carrying a load of 4kg, is hanging from a ceiling. Given that g = 3.1 À ms^{-2}, what will be the tensile stress that would be developed in the wire?
(a) 6.2×10^6 Nm^{-2} (b) 5.2×10^6 Nm^{-2}
(c) 3.1×10^6 Nm^{-2} (d) 4.8×10^6 Nm^{-2}

34. Young's moduli of two wires A and B are in the ratio 7 : 4. Wire A is 2 m long and has radius R. Wire B is 1.5 m long and has radius 2 mm. If the two wires stretch by the same length for a given load, then the value of R is close to :
(a) 1.5 mm (b) 1.9 mm (c) 1.7 mm (d) 1.3 mm

35. As shown in the figure, forces of 10^5N each are applied in opposite directions, on the upper and lower faces of a cube of side 10cm, shifting the upper face parallel to itself by 0.5cm. If the side of another cube of the same material is, 20cm, then under similar conditions as above, the displacement will be:

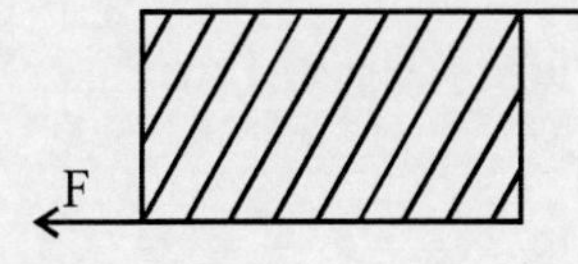

(a) 1.00cm
(b) 0.25cm
(c) 0.37cm
(d) 0.75cm

36. A thin 1 m long rod has a radius of 5 mm. A force of 50 πkN is applied at one end to determine its Young's modulus. Assume that the force is exactly known. If the least count in the measurement of all lengths is 0.01 mm, which of the following statements is false ?
(a) The maximum value of Y that can be determined is $2 \times 10^{14} N/m^2$.
(b) $\frac{\Delta Y}{Y}$ gets minimum contribution from the uncertainty in the length
(c) $\frac{\Delta Y}{Y}$ gets its maximum contribution from the uncertainty in strain
(d) The figure of merit is the largest for the length of the rod.

37. A copper wire of length 1.0 m and a steel wire of length 0.5 m having equal cross-sectional areas are joined end to end. The composite wire is stretched by a certain load which stretches the copper wire by 1 mm. If the Young's moduli of copper and steel are respectively 1.0×10^{11} Nm^{-2} and 2.0×10^{11} Nm^{-2}, the total extension of the composite wire is :
(a) 1.75 mm (b) 2.0 mm (c) 1.50 mm (d) 1.25 mm

38. A wire elongates by l mm when a load W is hanged from it. If the wire goes over a pulley and two weights W each are hung at the two ends, the elongation of the wire will be (in mm)
(a) l (b) $2l$ (c) zero (d) $l/2$

39. Steel ruptures when a shear of 3.5×10^8 N m^{-2} is applied. The force needed to punch a 1 cm diameter hole in a steel sheet 0.3 cm thick is nearly:
(a) 1.4×10^4 N (b) 2.7×10^4 N
(c) 3.3×10^4 N (d) 1.1×10^4 N

40. The bulk moduli of ethanol, mercury and water are given as 0.9, 25 and 2.2 respectively in units of 10^9 Nm^{-2}. For a given value of pressure, the fractional compression in volume is $\frac{\Delta V}{V}$. Which of the following statements about $\frac{\Delta V}{V}$ for these three liquids is correct ?
(a) Ethanol > Water > Mercury
(b) Water > Ethanol > Mercury
(c) Mercury > Ethanol > Water
(d) Ethanol > Mercury > Water

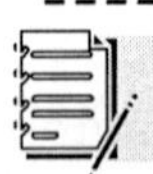

Exercise 2 - Exemplar & Past Year Questions

E&PYQs

Exemplar Questions

1. Modulus of rigidity of ideal liquids is
(a) infinity (b) zero (c) unity
(d) some finite small non-zero constant value

2. The maximum load a wire can withstand without breaking, when its length is reduced to half of its original length, will
(a) be double (b) be half
(c) be four times (d) remain same

3. The temperature of a wire is doubled. The Young's modulus of elasticity
(a) will also double (b) will become four times
(c) will remain same (d) will decrease

4. A spring is stretched by applying a load to its free end. The strain produced in the spring is
(a) volumetric (b) shear
(c) longitudinal and shear (d) longitudinal

5. A rigid bar of mass M is supported symmetrically by three wires each of length l. Those at each end are of copper and the middle one is of iron. The ratio of their diameters, if each is to have the same tension, is equal to
(a) Y_{copper} / Y_{iron} (b) $\sqrt{\frac{Y_{iron}}{Y_{copper}}}$
(c) $\frac{Y_{iron}^2}{Y_{copper}^2}$ (d) $\frac{Y_{iron}}{Y_{copper}}$

6. A mild steel wire of length $2L$ and cross-sectional area A is stretched, well within elastic limit, horizontally between two pillars (figure). A mass m is suspended from the mid-point of the wire. Strain in the wire is

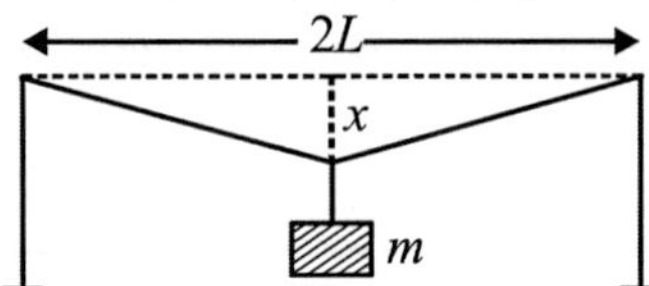

(a) $\frac{x^2}{2L^2}$ (b) $\frac{x}{L}$ (c) $\frac{x^2}{L}$ (d) $\frac{x^2}{2L}$

7. A rectangular frame is to be suspended symmetrically by two strings of equal length on two supports (figure). It can be done in one of the following three ways;

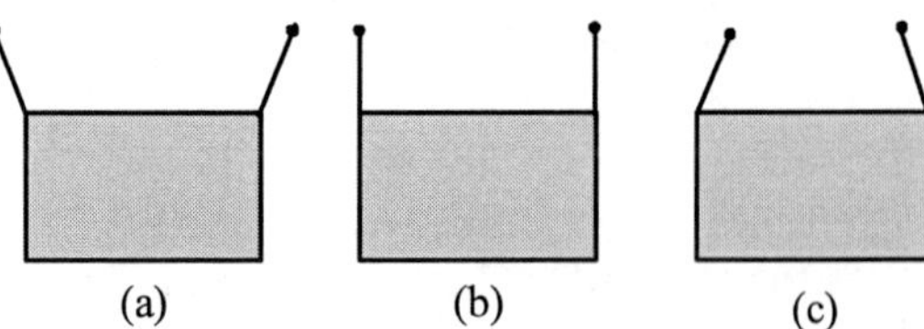

The tension in the strings will be
(a) the same in all cases (b) least in (a)
(c) least in (b) (d) least in (c)

8. Consider two cylindrical rods of identical dimensions, one of rubber and the other of steel. Both the rods are fixed rigidly at one end to the roof. A mass M is attached to each of the free ends at the centre of the rods.

(a) Both the rods will elongate but there shall be no perceptible change in shape

(b) The steel rod will elongate and change shape but the rubber rod will only elongate

(c) The steel rod will elongate without any perceptible change in shape, but the rubber rod will elongate and the shape of the bottom edge will change to an ellipse

(d) The steel rod will elongate, without any perceptible change in shape, but the rubber rod will elongate with the shape of the bottom edge tapered to a tip at the centre

NEET/AIPMT (2013-2020) Questions

9. The following four wires are made of the same material. Which of these will have the largest extension when the same tension is applied ? ***[2013]***

(a) Length = 100 cm, diameter = 1 mm

(b) Length = 200 cm, diameter = 2 mm

(c) Length = 300 cm, diameter = 3 mm

(d) Length = 50 cm, diameter = 0.5 mm

10. If the ratio of diameters, lengths and Young's modulus of steel and copper wires shown in the figure are p, q and s respectively, then the corresponding ratio of increase in their lengths would be ***[NEET Kar. 2013]***

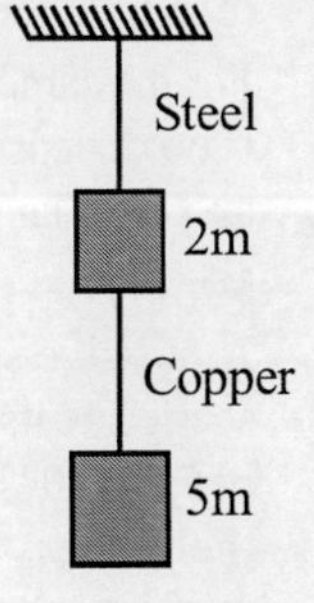

(a) $\frac{7q}{(5sp)}$

(b) $\frac{5q}{(7sp^2)}$

(c) $\frac{7q}{(5sp^2)}$

(d) $\frac{2q}{(5sp)}$

11. Copper of fixed volume 'V; is drawn into wire of length 'l'. When this wire is subjected to a constant force 'F', the extension produced in the wire is 'Δl'. Which of the following graphs is a straight line? ***[2014]***

(a) Δl versus $\frac{1}{l}$ (b) Δl versus l^2

(c) Δl versus $\frac{1}{l^2}$ (d) Δl versus l

12. The Young's modulus of steel is twice that of brass. Two wires of same length and of same area of cross section, one of steel and another of brass are suspended from the same roof. If we want the lower ends of the wires to be at the same level, then the weights added to the steel and brass wires must be in the ratio of : ***[2015 RS]***

(a) 2 : 1 (b) 4 : 1 (c) 1 : 1 (d) 1 : 2

13. The approximate depth of an ocean is 2700 m. The compressibility of water is 45.4×10^{-11} Pa^{-1} and density of water is 10^3 kg/m^3. What fractional compression of water will be obtained at the bottom of the ocean ? ***[2015]***

(a) 1.0×10^{-2} (b) 1.2×10^{-2}

(c) 1.4×10^{-2} (d) 0.8×10^{-2}

14. The bulk modulus of a spherical object is 'B'. If it is subjected to uniform pressure 'p', the fractional decrease in radius is ***[2017]***

(a) $\frac{B}{3p}$ (b) $\frac{3p}{B}$ (c) $\frac{p}{3B}$ (d) $\frac{p}{B}$

15. Two wires are made of the same material and have the same volume. The first wire has cross-sectional area A and the second wire has cross-sectional area 3A. If the length of the first wire is increased by $\Delta \ell$ on applying a force F, how much force is needed to stretch the second wire by the same amount? ***[2018]***

(a) 9F (b) 6F (c) F (d) 4F

16. The stress-strain curves are drawn for two different materials X and Y. It is observed that the ultimate strength point and the fracture point are close to each other for material X but are far apart for material Y.

We can say that materials X and Y are likely to be (respectively), ***[NEET Odisha 2019]***

(a) Plastic and ductile (b) Ductile and brittle

(c) Brittle and ductile (d) Brittle and plastic

17. When a block of mass M is suspended by a long wire of length L, the length of the wire becomes (L + l). The elastic potential energy stored in the extended wire is : ***[2019]***

(a) Mgl (b) MgL (c) $\frac{1}{2}$Mgl (d) $\frac{1}{2}$MgL

18. A wire of length L, area of cross section A is hanging from a fixed support. The length of the wire changes to L_1 when mass M is suspended from its free end. The expression for Young's modulus is : ***[2020]***

(a) $\frac{Mg(L_1 - L)}{AL}$ (b) $\frac{MgL}{AL_1}$

(c) $\frac{MgL}{A(L_1 - L)}$ (d) $\frac{MgL_1}{AL}$

Exercise 3 - Concept Application Problems

CAP

1. The load versus elongation graph for four wires is shown. The thinnest wire is

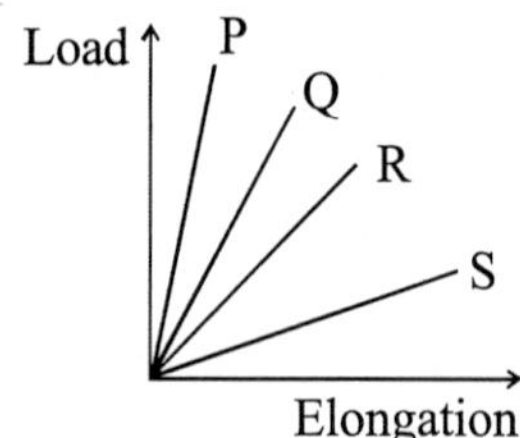

(a) P (b) Q (c) R (d) S

2. Two rods A and B of the same material and length have their radii r_1 and r_2 respectively. When they are rigidly fixed at one end and twisted by the same couple applied at the other end, the ratio

$$\left(\frac{\text{Angle of twist at the end of A}}{\text{Angle of twist at the end of B}}\right) \text{ is}$$

(a) r_1^2/r_2^2 (b) r_1^3/r_2^3 (c) r_2^4/r_1^4 (d) r_1^4/r_2^4

3. Uniform rod of mass m, length ℓ, area of cross-section A has Young's modulus Y. If it is hanged vertically, elongation under its own weight will be

(a) $\frac{mg\ell}{2AY}$ (b) $\frac{2mg\ell}{AY}$ (c) $\frac{mg\ell}{AY}$ (d) $\frac{mgY}{A\ell}$

4. In case of steel wire (or a metal wire), the limit is reached when
   (a) the wire just break
   (b) the load is more than the weight of wire
   (c) elongation is inversely proportional to the tension
   (d) None of these

5. A steel ring of radius r and cross sectional area A is fitted onto a wooden disc of radius R (R > r). If the Young's modulus of steel is Y, then the force with which the steel ring is expanded is
   (a) AY (R/r) (b) AY (R−r)/r
   (c) (Y/A)[(R−r)/r] (d) Yr/AR

6. Which of the following relation is true ?

(a) $3Y = K(1-\sigma)$ (b) $K = \frac{9\eta Y}{Y+\eta}$

(c) $\sigma = (6K+\eta)Y$ (d) $\sigma = \frac{05.Y-\eta}{\eta}$

7. The Young's modulus of a perfectly rigid body is
   (a) unity (b) zero (c) infinity
   (d) some finite non-zero constant

8. The Young's modulus of brass and steel are respectively 10^{10} N/m^2. and 2×10^{10} N/m^2. A brass wire and a steel wire of the same length are extended by 1 mm under the same force, the radii of brass and steel wires are R_B and R_S respectively. Then

(a) $R_S = \sqrt{2}\,R_B$ (b) $R_S = R_B/\sqrt{2}$
(c) $R_S = 4R_B$ (d) $R_S = R_B/4$

9. A steel wire of length 20 cm and uniform cross-section 1 mm^2 is tied rigidly at both the ends. The temperature of the wire is altered from 40°C to 20°C. Coefficient of linear expansion for steel $\alpha = 1.1 \times 10^{-5}$/°C and Y for steel is 2.0×10^{11} N/m^2. The change in tension of the wire is
   (a) 2.2×10^6 newton (b) 16 newton
   (c) 8 newton (d) 44 newton

10. A wire suspended vertically from one of its ends is stretched by attaching a weight of 200N to the lower end. The weight stretches the wire by 1 mm. Then the elastic energy stored in the wire is
    (a) 0.2 J (b) 10 J (c) 20 J (d) 0.1 J

11. A metal rod of Young's modulus 2×10^{10} N m^{-2} undergoes an elastic strain of 0.06%. The energy per unit volume stored in J m^{-3} is
    (a) 3600 (b) 7200 (c) 10800 (d) 14400

12. A cube at temperature 0°C is compressed equally from all sides by an external pressure P. By what amount should its temperature be raised to bring it back to the size it had before the external pressure was applied. The bulk modulus of the material of the cube is B and the coefficient of linear expansion is α.
    (a) $P/B\alpha$ (b) $P/3B\alpha$ (c) $3\pi\alpha/B$ (d) $3B/P$

13. The compressibility of water is 4×10^{-5} per unit atmospheric pressure. The decrease in volume of 100 cm^3 of water under a pressure of 100 atmosphere will be
    (a) 0.4 cm^3 (b) 4×10^{-5} cm^3
    (c) 0.025 cm^3 (d) 0.004 cm^3

14. For the same cross-sectional area and for a given load, the ratio of depressions for the beam of a square cross-section and circular cross-section is
    (a) $3:\pi$ (b) $\pi:3$ (c) $1:\pi$ (d) $\pi:1$

15. A massive stone pillar 20 m high and of uniform cross-section rests on a rigid base and supports a vertical load of 5.0×10^5 N at its upper end. If the compressive stress in the pillar is not to exceed 1.6×10^6 N m^{-2}, what is the minimum cross-sectional area of the pillar? Density of the stone = 2.5×10^3 kg m^{-3}. (Take g = 10 N kg^{-1})
    (a) 0.15 m^2 (b) 0.25 m^2 (c) 0.35 m^2 (d) 0.45 m^2

16. A circular tube of mean radius 8 cm and thickness 0.04 cm is melted up and recast into a solid rod of the same length. The ratio of the torsional rigidities of the circular tube and the solid rod is

(a) $\frac{(8.02)^4-(7.98)^4}{(0.8)^4}$ (b) $\frac{(8.02)^2-(7.98)^2}{(0.8)^2}$

(c) $\frac{(0.8)^2}{(8.02)^4-(7.98)^4}$ (d) $\frac{(0.8)^2}{(8.02)^3-(7.98)^2}$

17. One end of a uniform wire of length L and of weight W is attached rigidly to a point in the roof and W_1 weight is suspended from looser end. If A is area of cross-section of the wire, the stress in the wire at a height $\frac{L}{4}$ from the upper end is

(a) $\frac{W_1 + W}{a}$ (b) $\frac{W_1 + 3W/4}{a}$

(c) $\frac{W_1 + W/4}{a}$ (d) $\frac{4W_1 + 3W}{a}$

18. A beam of metal supported at the two edges is loaded at the centre. The depression at the centre is proportional to

(a) Y^2 (b) Y (c) 1/Y (d) $1/Y^2$

19. On stretching a wire, the elastic energy stored per unit volume is

(a) *Fl/2AL* (b) *FA/2L* (c) *FL/2A* (d) *FL/2*

20. When a pressure of 100 atmosphere is applied on a spherical ball, then its volume reduces to 0.01%. The bulk modulus of the material of the rubber in dyne/cm^2 is

(a) 10×10^{12} (b) 100×10^{12}

(c) 1×10^{12} (d) 10×10^{12}

21. K is the force constant of a spring. The work done in increasing its extension from l_1 to l_2 will be

(a) $K(l_2 - l_1)$ (b) $\frac{K}{2}(l_2 + l_1)$

(c) $K(l_2^2 - l_1^2)$ (d) $\frac{K}{2}(l_2^2 - l_1^2)$

22. A material has poisson's ratio 0.50. If a uniform rod of it suffers a longitudinal strain of 2×10^{-3}, then the percentage change in volume is

(a) 0.6 (b) 0.4 (c) 0.2 (d) Zero

23. A rubber cord catapult has cross-sectional area 25 mm^2 and initial length of rubber cord is 10 cm. It is stretched to 5 cm and then released to project a missile of mass 5 gm. Taking $Y_{rubber} = 5 \times 10^8$ N/m^2. Velocity of projected missile is

(a) 20 ms^{-1} (b) 100 ms^{-1} (c) 250 ms^{-1} (d) 200 ms^{-1}

24. The diagram shows a force - extension graph for a rubber band. Consider the following statements :

I. It will be easier to compress this rubber than expand it

II. Rubber does not return to its original length after it is stretched

III. The rubber band will get heated if it is stretched and released

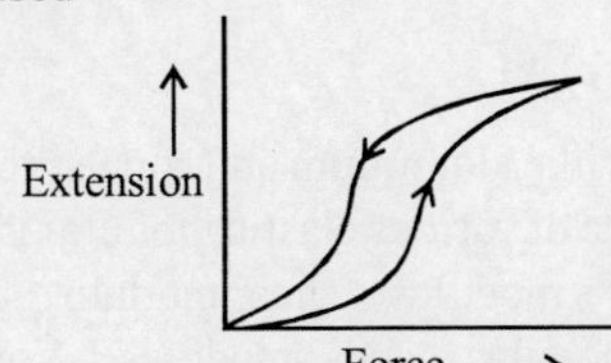

Which of these can be deduced from the graph?

(a) III only (b) II and III (c) I and III (d) I only

25. A rod of length *l* and radius *r* is joined to a rod of length *l*/2 and radius *r*/2 of same material. The free end of small rod is fixed to a rigid base and the free end of larger rod is given a twist of θ°, the twist angle at the joint will be

(a) θ/4 (b) θ/2 (c) 5θ/6 (d) 8θ/48

26. A steel wire of uniform cross-section of 1mm^2 is heated upto 50°C and clamped rigidly at its ends. If temperature of wire falls to 40°C, change in tension in the wire is (coefficient of linear expansion of steel is 1.1×10^{-5}/°C and Young's modulus of elasticity of steel is 2×10^{11} N/m^2)

(a) 22 N (b) 44 N

(c) 88 N (d) 88×10^6 N

27. In Searle's experiment to find Young's modulus the diameter of wire is measured as d = 0.05cm, length of wire is ℓ = 125cm and when a weight, m = 20.0 kg is put, extension in wire was found to be 0.100 cm. Find maximum permissible error in Young's modulus (Y). Use : $Y = \frac{mg\ell}{(\pi/4)\, d^2 x}$.

(a) 6.3% (b) 5.3% (c) 2.3% (d) 1%

28. If the ratio of lengths, radii and Young's modulus of steel and brass wires shown in the figure are a, b, and c, respectively. The ratio between the increase in lengths of brass and steel wires would be

(a) $\frac{b^2 a}{2c}$

(b) $\frac{bc}{2a^2}$

(c) $\frac{ba^2}{2c}$

(d) $\frac{a}{2b^2 c}$

29. The following four wires are made of the same material. Which of these will have the largest extension when the same tension is applied ?

(a) Length = 100 cm, diameter = 1 mm

(b) Length = 200 cm, diameter = 2 mm

(c) Length = 300 cm, diameter = 3 mm

(d) Length = 50 cm, diameter = 0.5 mm

30. A steel rod of radius R = 10 mm and length L = 100 cm is stretched along its length by a force F = 6.28 $\times 10^4$ N. If the Young's modulus of steel is $Y = 2 \times 10^{11}$ N/m^2, the percentage elongation in the length of the rod is :

(a) 0.100 (b) 0.314 (c) 2.015 (d) 1.549

31. A body of mass m = 10 kg is attached to one end of a wire of length 0.3 m. The maximum angular speed (in rad s^{-1}) with which it can be rotated about its other end in space station is (Breaking stress of wire = 4.8×10^7 Nm^{-2} and area of cross-section of the wire = 10^{-2} cm^2) is _______.

32. A uniform cylindrical rod of length L and radius r, is made from a material whose Young's modulus of Elasticity equals Y. When this rod is heated by temperature T and simultaneously subjected to a net longitudinal compressional force F, its length remains unchanged. The coefficient of volume expansion, of the material of the rod, is (nearly) equal to :

(a) $9F/(\pi r^2 YT)$ (b) $6F/(\pi r^2 YT$
(c) $3F/(\pi r^2 YT)$ (d) $F/(3\pi r^2 YT)$

33. In an environment, brass and steel wires of length 1 m each with areas of cross section 1 mm^2 are used. The wires are connected in series and one end of the combined wire is connected to a rigid support and other end is subjected to elongation. The stress required to produce a net elongation of 0.2 mm is,
[Given, the Young's modulus for steel and brass are, respectively, 120×10^9N/m^2 and 60×10^9N/m^2]

(a) 1.2×10^6N/m^2 (b) 4.0×10^6N/m^2
(c) 1.8×10^6N/m^2 (d) 0.2×10^6N/m^2

34. The elastic limit of brass is 379 MPa. What should be the minimum diameter of a brass rod if it is to support a 400 N load without exceeding its elastic limit?

(a) 1.00 mm (b) 1.16mm (c) 0.90 mm (d) 1.36 mm

35. A uniformly tapering conical wire is made from a material of Young's modulus Y and has a normal, unextended length L. The radii, at the upper and lower ends of this conical wire, have values R and 3R, respectively. The upper end of the wire is fixed to a rigid support and a mass M is suspended from its lower end. The equilibrium extended length, of this wire, would equal :

(a) $L\left(1+\frac{2}{9}\frac{Mg}{\pi YR^2}\right)$ (b) $L\left(1+\frac{1}{9}\frac{Mg}{\pi YR^2}\right)$

(c) $L\left(1+\frac{1}{3}\frac{Mg}{\pi YR^2}\right)$ (d) $L\left(1+\frac{2}{3}\frac{Mg}{\pi YR^2}\right)$

36. The pressure that has to be applied to the ends of a steel wire of length 10 cm to keep its length constant when its temperature is raised by 100°C is:
(For steel Young's modulus is $2\times10^{11}\text{Nm}^{-2}$ and coefficient of thermal expansion is $1.1\times10^{-5}\text{K}^{-1}$)

(a) 2.2×10^8 Pa (b) 2.2×10^9 Pa
(c) 2.2×10^7 Pa (d) 2.2×10^6 Pa

37. Two blocks of masses m and M are connected by means of a metal wire of cross-sectional area A passing over a frictionless fixed pulley as shown in the figure. The system is then released. If M = 2 m, then the stress produced in the wire is :

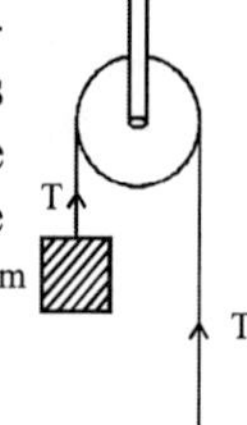

(a) $\frac{2mg}{3A}$ (b) $\frac{4mg}{3A}$
(c) $\frac{mg}{A}$ (d) $\frac{3mg}{4A}$

38. A uniform wire (Young's modulus 2×10^{11} Nm^{-2}) is subjected to longitudinal tensile stress of 5×10^7 Nm^{-2}. If the overall volume change in the wire is 0.02%, the fractional decrease in the radius of the wire is close to :

(a) 1.0×10^{-4} (b) 1.5×10^{-4}
(c) 0.25×10^{-4} (d) 5×10^{-4}

39. A steel wire can sustain 100 kg weight without breaking. If the wire is cut into two equal parts, each part can sustain a weight of

(a) 50 kg (b) 400 kg (c) 100 kg (d) 200 kg

40. A structural steel rod has a radius of 10 mm and length of 1.0 m. A 100 kN force stretches it along its length. Young's modulus of structural steel is 2×10^{11} Nm^{-2}. The percentage strain is about

(a) 0.16% (b) 0.32% (c) 0.08% (d) 0.24%

41. Two steel wires having same length are suspended from a ceiling under the same load. If the ratio of their energy stored per unit volume is 1 : 4, the ratio of their diameters is:

(a) $\sqrt{2}:1$ (b) $1:2$ (c) $2:1$ (d) $1:\sqrt{2}$

42. A boy's catapult is made of rubber cord which is 42 cm long, with 6 mm diameter of cross-section and of negligible mass. The boy keeps a stone weighing 0.02 kg on it and stretches the cord by 20 cm by applying a constant force. When released, the stone flies off with a velocity of 20 ms^{-1}. Neglect the change in the area of cross-section of the cord while stretched. The Young's modulus of rubber is closest to :

(a) 10^6 N/m^{-2} (b) 10^4 N/m^{-2}
(c) 10^8 N/m^{-2} (d) 10^3 N/m^{-2}

43. A solid sphere of radius r made of a soft material of bulk modulus K is surrounded by a liquid in a cylindrical container. A massless piston of area a floats on the surface of the liquid, covering entire cross-section of cylindrical container. When a mass m is placed on the surface of the piston to compress the liquid, the fractional decrement in the radius of the sphere $\left(\frac{dr}{r}\right)$, is :

(a) $\frac{Ka}{mg}$ (b) $\frac{Ka}{3mg}$ (c) $\frac{mg}{3Ka}$ (d) $\frac{mg}{Ka}$

44. A bottle has an opening of radius a and length b. A cork of length b and radius (a + Δa) where (Δa < < a) is compressed to fit into the opening completely (see figure). If the bulk modulus of cork is B and frictional coefficient between the bottle and cork is μ then the force needed to push the cork into the bottle is :

(a) $(\pi\mu B b)$ a
(b) $(2\pi\mu Bb)\,\Delta a$
(c) $(\pi\mu B b)\,\Delta a$
(d) $(4\pi\mu B b)\,\Delta a$

45. In materials like aluminium and copper, the correct order of magnitude of various elastic modului is:

(a) Young's modulus < shear modulus < bulk modulus.
(b) Bulk modulus < shear modulus < Young's modulus
(c) Shear modulus < Young's modulus < bulk modulus.
(d) Bulk modulus < Young's modulus < shear modulus.

Hints & Solutions

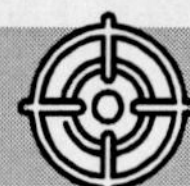

9.1 Concept Practice Problems

CPP

1. (c) If ℓ is the original length of wire, then change in length of first wire, $\Delta\ell_1 = (\ell_1 - \ell)$

change in length of second wire, $\Delta\ell_2 = (\ell_2 - \ell)$

Now, $Y = \frac{T_1}{A} \times \frac{\ell}{\Delta\ell_1} = \frac{T_2}{A} \times \frac{\ell}{\Delta\ell_2}$

or $\frac{T_1}{\Delta\ell_1} = \frac{T_2}{\Delta\ell_2}$ or $\frac{T_1}{\ell_1 - \ell} = \frac{T_2}{\ell_2 - \ell}$

or $T_1\ell_2 - T_1\ell = T_2\ell_1 - \ell T_2$ or $\ell = \frac{T_2\ell_1 - T_1\ell_2}{T_2 - T_1}$

2. (b) The ratio of stress to strain is always constant. If stress is increased, strain will also increase so that their ratio remains constant.

3. (c) $l = \frac{FL}{YA} \Rightarrow l \propto \frac{1}{A}$

4. (b) $B = \frac{\Delta p}{\Delta V / V} \Rightarrow \frac{1}{B} \propto \frac{\Delta V}{V}$ [Δp = constant]

5. (c) Energy stored per unit volume

$= \frac{1}{2} \times \text{stress} \times \text{strain}$

$= \frac{1}{2} \times \text{stress} \times (\text{stress / Young's modulus})$

$= \frac{1}{2} \times (\text{stress})^2 / (\text{Young's modulus}) = \frac{S^2}{2Y}$

6. (b) $F = Y \times A \times \frac{l}{L} \Rightarrow F \propto r^2$ (Y, l and and L are constant)

If diameter is made four times then force required will be 16 times, i.e., 16×10^3 N

7. (d) ∵ Both wires are same materials so both will have same Young's modulus, and let it be Y.

$Y = \frac{\text{stress}}{\text{strain}} = \frac{F}{A.(\Delta L/L)}$, F = applied force

A = area of cross-section of wire

Now, $Y_1 = Y_2 \Rightarrow \frac{FL}{(A_1)(\Delta L_1)} = \frac{FL}{(A_2)(\Delta L_2)}$

Since load and length are same for both

$\Rightarrow r_1^2 \Delta L_1 = r_2^2 \Delta L_2$, $\left(\frac{\Delta L_1}{\Delta L_2}\right) = \left(\frac{r_2}{r_1}\right)^2 = 4$

$\Delta L_1 : \Delta L_2 = 4:1$

8. (c) $Y = \frac{F/A}{\Delta\ell/\ell} = \frac{\frac{250 \times 9.8}{50 \times 10^{-6}}}{\frac{0.5 \times 10^{-3}}{2}} = \frac{250 \times 9.8}{50 \times 10^{-6}} \times \frac{2}{0.5 \times 10^{-3}}$

$\Rightarrow 19.6 \times 10^{10}\ \text{N/m}^2$

9. (a) When same stress is applied at two different temperatures, the increase in length is more at higher temperature. Thus $T_1 > T_2$.

10. (c)

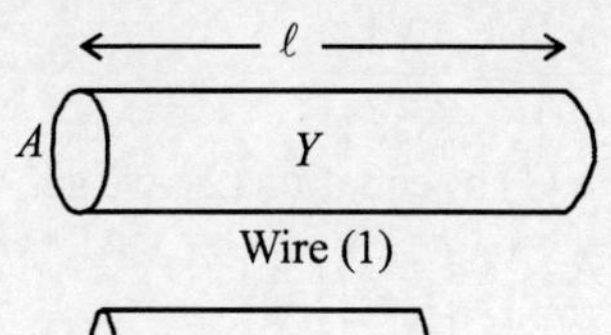

Wire (1)

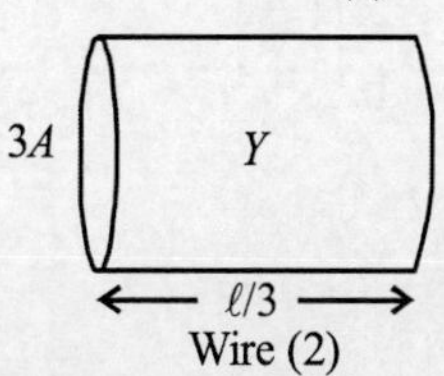

Wire (2)

As shown in the figure, the wires will have the same Young's modulus (same material) and the length of the wire of area of cross-section $3A$ will be $\ell/3$ (same volume as wire 1).

For wire 1, $Y = \frac{F/A}{\Delta x/\ell}$ ...(i)

For wire 2, $Y = \frac{F'/3A}{\Delta x/(\ell/3)}$ ...(ii)

From (i) and (ii), $\frac{F}{A} \times \frac{\ell}{\Delta x} = \frac{F'}{3A} \times \frac{\ell}{3\Delta x} \Rightarrow F' = 9F$

Exercise 1 - Chapter Revision Problems

CRP

1. (c) Elastomers do not obey Hooke's law.
2. (d) 3. (a) 4. (d) 5. (c) 6. (a)
7. (a) $\tan(90 - \theta) = \frac{\text{stress}}{\text{strain}}$
8. (d) The elasticity of a material depends upon the temperature of the material. Hammering & annealing reduces elastic property of a substance.
9. (b) $\text{Stress} = \frac{\text{Force}}{\text{Area}}$ ∴ $\text{Stress} \propto \frac{1}{\pi r^2}$

$\frac{S_B}{S_A} = \left(\frac{r_A}{r_B}\right)^2 = (2)^2 \Rightarrow S_B = 4S_A$

10. (c)
11. (b) The wire starts behaving like a liquid at point b. It behaves like a viscous liquid in the region bc of the graph.
12. (b) Let V be the volume of the load and ρ its relative density

So, $Y = \frac{FL}{A\ell_a} = \frac{V\rho g L}{A\ell_a}$ .....(1)

When the load is immersed in the liquid, then

$Y = \frac{F'L}{A\ell_w} = \frac{(V\rho g - V \times 1 \times g)L}{A\ell_w}$ ....(2)

(∵ Now net weight = weight – upthrust)

From eqs. (1) and (2), we get

$\frac{\rho}{\ell_a} = \frac{(\rho - 1)}{\ell_w}$ or $\rho = \frac{\ell_a}{(\ell_a - \ell_w)}$

13. (c)

14. (b) Let W newton be the load suspended. Then

$$Y=\frac{(W/A_1)}{(\ell_1/L)}=\frac{WL}{A_1\ell_1} \quad ...(1)$$

and $$Y=\frac{(W/A_2)}{(\ell_2/L)}=\frac{WL}{A_2\ell_2} \quad ....(2)$$

Dividing equation (1) by equation (2), we get

$$1=\left(\frac{\ell_2}{\ell_1}\right)\left(\frac{A_2}{A_1}\right)=\left(\frac{\ell_2}{\ell_1}\right)\left(\frac{2}{1}\right)$$

$\therefore \quad \frac{\ell_1}{\ell_2}=\frac{2}{1}$ or $\ell_1:\ell_2=2:1$

15. (c) Given that $F/A=4.8\times10^7\ Nm^{-2}$

$\therefore \quad F=4.8\times10^7\times A$

or $$\frac{mv^2}{r}=4.8\times10^7\times10^{-6}=48$$

or $$\frac{mr^2\omega^2}{r}=48 \text{ or } \omega^2=\frac{48}{mr}$$

$$\omega=\sqrt{\left(\frac{48}{10\times0.3}\right)}=\sqrt{16}=4\text{ rad/sec}$$

16. (d)

17. (b) $\phi=\frac{r\theta}{\ell}=\frac{1}{100}\times\frac{0.8}{2}=0.004$ radian

18. (d) $Y=2\eta(1+\sigma)$

$2.4\eta=2\eta(1+\sigma)\Rightarrow1.2=1+\sigma\Rightarrow\sigma=0.2$

19. (a) Weights without and with liquid proportional to ρ_b and $\rho_b-\rho_l$.

20. (d) Work done by constant force in displacing the object by a distance ℓ.

= change in potential energy

$=\frac{1}{2}\times$ stress $\times$ strain $\times$volume

$$=\frac{1}{2}\times\frac{F}{A}\times\frac{\ell}{L}\times A\times L=\frac{F\ell}{2}$$

21. (c) Volume V = cross sectional $A\times$ length l or $V=Al$

$$\text{Strain}=\frac{\text{Elongation}}{\text{Original length}}=\frac{Y}{l}$$

$$\text{Young's modulus } Y=\frac{\text{Stress}}{\text{Strain}}$$

Work done, W = $\frac{1}{2}\times$ stress $\times$ strain $\times$ volume

$$W=\frac{1}{2}\times Y\times(\text{strain})^2\times Al$$

$$=\frac{1}{2}\times Y\times\left(\frac{y}{l}\right)^2\times Al=\frac{1}{2}\left(\frac{YA}{l}\right)y^2\Rightarrow W\propto y^2$$

22. (b) Stress $=1$ kg wt/mm$^2=9.8$ N/mm^2
$=9.8\times10^6$ N/m^2.

$$Y=1\times10^{11}N/m^2,\ \frac{\Delta\ell}{\ell}\times100=?$$

$$Y=\frac{\text{Stress}}{\text{Strain}}=\frac{\text{Stress}}{\Delta\ell/\ell}$$

$$\therefore \frac{\Delta\ell}{\ell}=\frac{\text{Stress}}{Y}=\frac{9.8\times10^6}{1\times10^{11}}$$

$$\frac{\Delta\ell}{\ell}\times100=9.8\times10^{-11}\times100\times10^6$$

$$=9.8\times10^{-3}=0.0098\ \%$$

23. (d) $K=\frac{\Delta P}{\Delta V/V}=\frac{h\rho g}{\Delta V/V}=\frac{200\times10^3\times10}{0.1/100}=2\times10^9$

24. (b) $W=\frac{1}{2}\times F\times l=\frac{1}{2}mgl$

$$=\frac{1}{2}\times10\times10\times1\times10^{-3}=0.05J$$

25. (c) We know that Young's modulus

$$Y=\frac{F}{\pi r^2}\times\frac{L}{\ell}$$

Since Y, F are same for both the wires, we have,

$$\frac{1}{r_1^2}\frac{L_1}{\ell_1}=\frac{1}{r_2^2}\frac{L_2}{\ell_2} \text{ or, } \frac{\ell_1}{\ell_2}=\frac{r_2^2\times L_1}{r_1^2\times L_2}=\frac{(D_2/2)^2\times L_1}{(D_1/2)^2\times L_2}$$

$$\text{or, } \frac{\ell_1}{\ell_2}=\frac{D_2^2\times L_1}{D_1^2\times L_2}=\frac{D_2^2}{(2D_2)^2}\times\frac{L_2}{2L_2}=\frac{1}{8}$$

So, $\ell_1:\ell_2=1:8$

26. (b) The atoms when brought from infinity are attracted due to interatomic electrostatic force of attraction. At point B, the potential energy is minimum and force of attraction is maximum. But if we bring atoms closer than x = B, force of repulsion between two nuclei starts and P.E. increases.

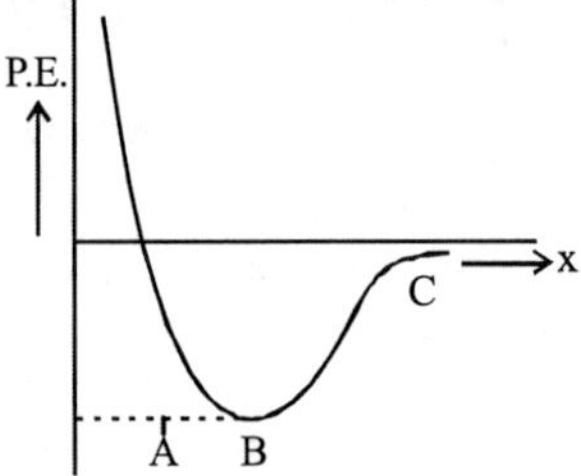

27. (a) $L=\frac{S}{dg}=\frac{10^6}{3\times10^3\times10}=\frac{100}{3}=34\,m$

28. (b) $r\theta=\ell\phi\Rightarrow\phi=\frac{r\theta}{\ell}=\frac{6\text{mm}\times30°}{1\text{m}}=0.18°$

29. (d) If side of the cube is L then $V=L^3\Rightarrow\frac{dV}{V}=3\frac{dL}{L}$

$\therefore$ % change in volume = 3 × (% change in length)
= 3 × 1% = 3%

$\therefore$ Bulk strain $\frac{\Delta V}{V}=0.03$

30. (b) $K=\frac{F}{x}=\frac{4\times9.8}{2\times10^{-2}}=19.6\times10^2$

Work done $=\frac{1}{2}19.6\times10^2\times(0.05)^2=2.45J$

31. (c) Given : $U = \frac{-A}{r^6} + \frac{B}{r^{12}}$

For equilibrium,

$$F = \frac{dU}{dr} = -(A(-6r^{-7})) + B(-12r^{-13}) = 0$$

$$\Rightarrow 0 = \frac{6A}{r^7} - \frac{12B}{r^{13}} \Rightarrow \frac{6A}{12B} = \frac{1}{r^6}$$

$\therefore$ Separation between molecules, $r = \left(\frac{2B}{A}\right)^{1/6}$

Potential energy,

$$U\left(r = \left(\frac{2B}{A}\right)^{1/6}\right) = -\frac{A}{2B/A} + \frac{B}{4B^2/A^2}$$

$$= \frac{-A^2}{2B} + \frac{A^2}{4B} = \frac{-A^2}{4B}$$

32. (c) Given, Radius of wire, $r = 2$ mm

Mass of the load m = 4 kg

$$\text{Stress} = \frac{F}{A} = \frac{mg}{\pi(r)^2}$$

$$= \frac{4 \times 3.1\pi}{\pi \times (2 \times 10^{-3})^2} = 3.1 \times 10^6 \text{ N/m}^2$$

33. (c) Given,

Radius of wire, $r = 2$ mm

Mass of the load m = 4 kg

$$\text{Stress} = \frac{F}{A} = \frac{mg}{\pi(r)^2} = \frac{4 \times 3.1\pi}{\pi \times (2 \times 10^{-3})^2} = 3.1 \times 10^6 \text{ N/m}^2$$

34. (c) $\Delta_1 = \Delta_2$

or $\frac{Fl_1}{\pi r_1^2 y_1} = \frac{Fl_2}{\pi r_2^2 y_2}$ or $\frac{2}{R^2 \times 7} = \frac{1.5}{2^2 \times 4}$

$\therefore R = 1.75$ mm

35. (b) For same material the ratio of stress to strain is same

For first cube

$$\text{Stress}_1 = \frac{\text{force}_1}{\text{area}_1} = \frac{10^5}{(0.1^2)}$$

$$\text{Strain}_1 = \frac{\text{change in length}_1}{\text{original length}_1} = \frac{0.5 \times 10^{-2}}{0.1}$$

For second block,

$$\text{stress}_2 = \frac{\text{force}_2}{\text{area}_2} = \frac{10^5}{(0.2^2)}$$

$$\text{strain}_2 = \frac{\text{change in length}_2}{\text{original length}_2} = \frac{x}{0.2}$$

x is the displacement for second block.

For same material, $\frac{\text{stress}_1}{\text{strain}_1} = \frac{\text{stress}_2}{\text{strain}_2}$

$$\text{or, } \frac{\frac{10.5}{(0.1)^2}}{\frac{0.5 \times 10^{-2}}{0.1}} = \frac{\frac{10^5}{(0.2)^2}}{\frac{x}{0.2}}$$

Solving we get, $x = 0.25$ cm

36. (a) Young's modulus $Y = \frac{F}{A} / \frac{\Delta\ell}{\ell}$

$$Y = \frac{F\ell}{pr^2 D\ell}$$

Given, radius r = 5mm, force F = 50πk N,

$$\frac{\ell}{D\ell} = 0.01 \text{ mm}$$

$$\therefore Y = \frac{F}{\pi r^2} \frac{\ell}{\Delta\ell} = 2 \times 10^{14} \text{ N/m}^2.$$

37. (d) $Y_c \times (\Delta L_c / L_c) = Y_s \times (\Delta L_s / L_s)$

$$\Rightarrow 1 \times 10^{11} \times \left(\frac{1 \times 10^{-3}}{1}\right) = 2 \times 10^{11} \times \left(\frac{\Delta L_s}{0.5}\right)$$

$$\therefore \Delta L_s = \frac{0.5 \times 10^{-3}}{2} = 0.25 \text{ mm}$$

Therefore, total extension of the composite wire

$= \Delta L_c + \Delta L_s$

$= 1 \text{ mm} + 0.25 \text{ m} = 1.25 \text{ m}$

38. (a) Case (i)

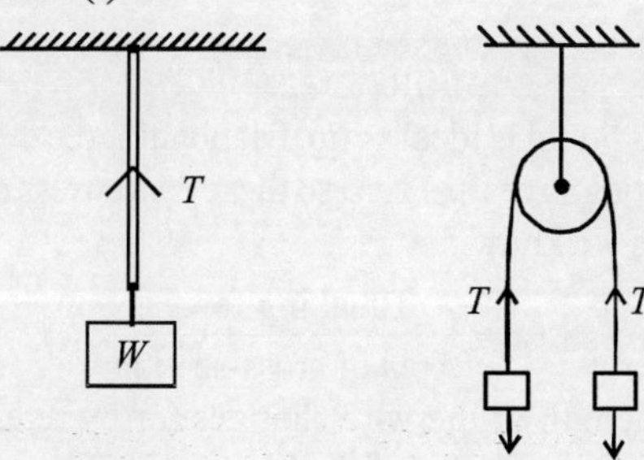

At equilibrium, $T = W$

Young's modules, $Y = \frac{W/A}{\ell/L}$ .....(1)

Elongation, $\ell = \frac{W}{A} \times \frac{L}{Y}$

Case (ii) At equilibrium $T = W$

$\therefore$ Young's moduls, $Y = \frac{W/A}{\frac{\ell/2}{L/2}}$

$$\Rightarrow Y = \frac{W/A}{\ell/L} \Rightarrow \ell = \frac{W}{A} \times \frac{L}{Y}$$

$\Rightarrow$ Elongation is the same.

39. (c)

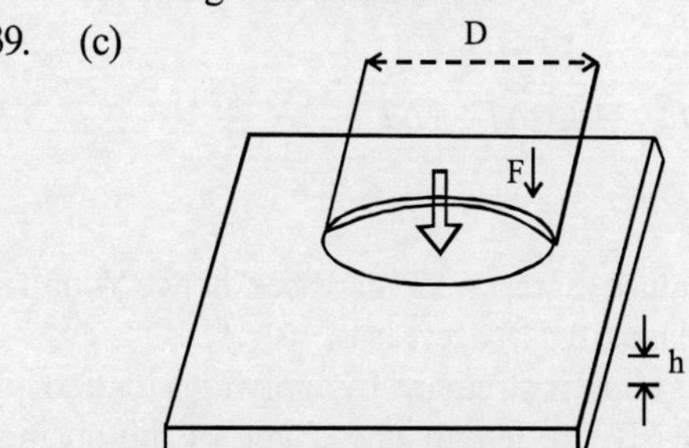

Shearing strain is created along the side surface of the punched disk. Note that the forces exerted on the disk are exerted along the circumference of the disk, and the total force exerted on its center only.

Let us assume that the shearing stress along the side surface of the disk is uniform, then

$$F = \int_{surface} dF_{max} = \int_{surface} \sigma_{max} dA = \sigma_{max} \int_{surface} dA$$

$$= \int \sigma_{max} . A = \sigma_{max} . 2\pi\left(\frac{D}{2}\right)h$$

$$= 3.5\times10^{8}\times\left(\frac{1}{2}\times10^{-2}\right)\times0.3\times10^{-2}\times2\pi$$

$$= 3.297\times10^{4} \simeq 3.3\times10^{4}\,N$$

40. (a) Compressibility $= \frac{1}{\text{Bulk modulus}}$

As bulk modulus is least for ethanol (0.9) and maximum for mercury (25) among ehtanol, mercury and water. Hence compression in volume $\frac{\Delta V}{V}$

Ethanol > Water > Mercury

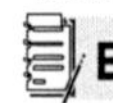

Exercise 2 - Exemplar & Past Year Questions

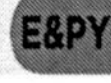

Exemplar Questions

1. (b) As liquid is ideal so no. frictional force exists hence, tangential forces are zero so there is no stress developed.
2. (d) As we know that,

Breaking stress $= \frac{\text{Breaking force}}{\text{Area of cross-section}}$ ..(i)

When length of the wire changes (or by reducing half) area of cross-section remains same.

Hence, breaking force will be same because breaking stress does not depend on length.

3. (d) As we know that, length of a wire when the temperature increased

$$L_t = L_0(1+\alpha\Delta T)$$

where ΔT is change in the temperature.

L_0 is original length,

α is coefficient of linear expansion and

L_t is length at temperature T.

Now, $\Delta L = L_t - L_0 = L_0\alpha\Delta T$

Now, Young's modulus $(Y) = \frac{\text{Stress}}{\text{Strain}}$

$$= \frac{FL_0}{A\times\Delta L} = \frac{FL_0}{AL_0\alpha\Delta T} \propto \frac{1}{\Delta T}$$

As, $Y \propto \frac{1}{\Delta T}$

So, if temperature increass ΔT increases, hence Young's modulus of elasticity (Y) decreases.

4. (c) When a spring is stretched by applying a load to its free end. Clearly the length and shape of the spring changes. So strain produced when change in length corresponds to longitudinal strain and change in shape corresponds to shearing strain.

5. (b) As we know that,

The Young's modulus

$$Y = \frac{\text{Stress}}{\text{Strain}} = \frac{F/A}{\Delta L/L} = \frac{F}{A}\times\frac{L}{\Delta L}$$

$$= \frac{F}{\pi(D/2)^2}\times\frac{L}{\Delta L} = \frac{4FL}{\pi D^2\Delta L}$$

$$D^2 = \frac{4FL}{\pi\Delta LY} \Rightarrow D = \sqrt{\frac{4FL}{\pi\Delta LY}}$$

If F and $\frac{L}{\Delta L}$ are constants.

So, $D \propto \sqrt{\frac{1}{Y}}$

Hence, we can find ratio as

$$\frac{D_{copper}}{D_{iron}} = \sqrt{\frac{Y_{iron}}{Y_{copper}}}$$

6. (a) Consider the given diagram

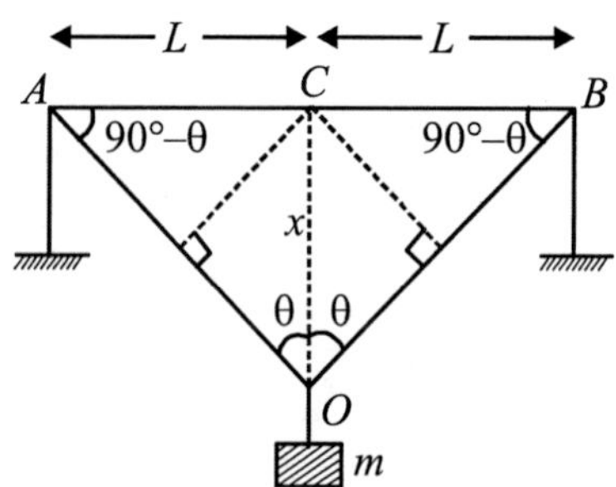

So, change in length

$$\Delta L = (A_0 + B_0) - (AC + CB)$$

$$= 2BO - 2AC$$

$$= 2[BO - AC] \quad (\because AO = BO, AC = CB)$$

$$= 2[(x^2 + L^2)^{1/2} - L]$$

$$= 2L\left[\left(1+\frac{x^2}{L^2}\right)^{1/2} - 1\right]$$

$$\Delta L \approx 2L\left[1+\frac{1}{2}\frac{x^2}{L^2} - 1\right] = \frac{x^2}{L} \qquad [\because x << L]$$

$$\text{Strain} = \frac{\Delta L}{2L} = \frac{x^2/L}{2L} = \frac{x^2}{2L^2}$$

7. (c) Let us consider the free body diagram of the rectangular frame

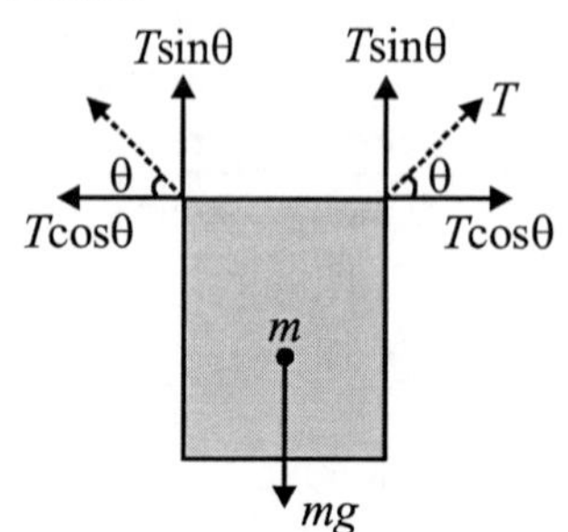

Net forces acting on frame will be zero.

So, Balancing vertical forces

$2T\sin\theta - mg = 0$ [T is tension in the string]

$2T\sin\theta = mg$ ...(i)

Total horizontal force

$= T\cos\theta - T\cos\theta = 0$

Now from Eq. (i), $T = \frac{mg}{2\sin\theta}$

$T_{max} = \frac{mg}{2\sin\theta_{min}}$

As mg is constant then

$T \propto \frac{1}{\sin\theta}$

$\sin\theta_{min} = 0 \Rightarrow \theta_{min} = 0$

No option matches with $\theta = 0°$

$T_{min} = \frac{mg}{2\sin\theta_{max}}$ (since, $\sin\theta_{max} = 1$)

$\sin\theta_{max} = 1 \Rightarrow \theta = 90°$

So tension is all three cases are different rejects option (a)

For minimum tension θ must be 90° i.e. $\sin\theta = 1$

Hence, tension is the least for the case (b).

8. (d) A mass M is attached at the centre or midpoint of rod of rubber and steel. As the mass is attached to both the rods, both rod will be elongated as shown in figures but due to different elastic properties of material rubber changes shape also.

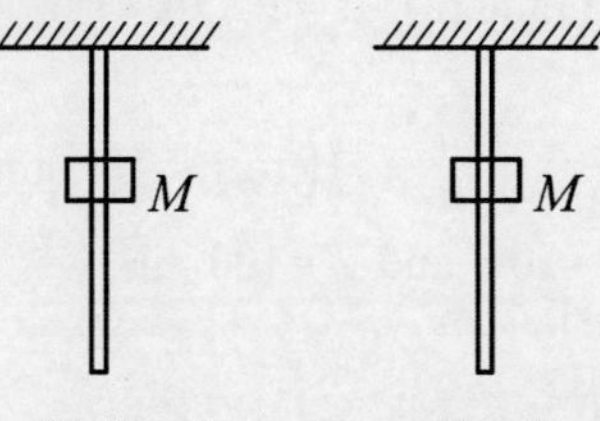

As the Young's modulus of rigidity for steel, is larger than rubber, so strain $\frac{\Delta L}{L}$ for rubber is larger than steel for same stress.

NEET/AIPMT (2013-2020) Questions

9. (d) $F = \frac{YA}{L} \times \ell$ So, extension, $\ell \propto \frac{L}{A} \propto \frac{L}{D^2}$

[$\because$ F and Y are constant]

$\ell_1 \propto \frac{100}{1^2} \propto 100$ and $\ell_2 \propto \frac{200}{2^2} \propto 50$

$\ell_3 \propto \frac{300}{3^2} \propto \frac{100}{3}$ and $\ell_4 \propto \frac{50}{\frac{1}{4}} \propto 200$

The ratio of $\frac{L}{D^2}$ is maximum for case (d).

Hence, option (d) is correct.

10. (c) From formula,

Increase in length $\Delta L = \frac{FL}{AY} = \frac{4FL}{\pi D^2 Y}$

$\frac{\Delta L_S}{\Delta L_C} = \frac{F_S}{F_C}\left(\frac{D_C}{D_S}\right)^2 \frac{Y_C}{Y_S}\frac{L_S}{L_C} = \frac{7}{5} \times \left(\frac{1}{p}\right)^2 \left(\frac{1}{s}\right) q$

$= \frac{7q}{(5sp^2)}$

11. (b) As $Y = \frac{\frac{F}{A}}{\frac{\Delta l}{l}} \Rightarrow \Delta l = \frac{Fl}{AY}$

But $V = Al$ so $A = \frac{V}{l}$

Therefore $\Delta l = \frac{Fl^2}{VY} \propto l^2$

Hence graph of Δl versus l^2 will give a straight line.

12. (a) Young's modulus $Y = \frac{W}{A}\cdot\frac{l}{\Delta l}$

$\frac{W_1}{Y_1} = \frac{W_2}{Y_2}$ [$\because$ A, l, Δl same for both brass and steel]

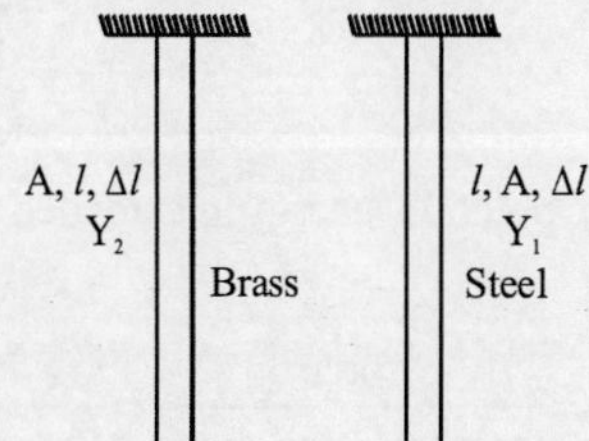

$\frac{W_1}{W_2} = \frac{Y_1}{Y_2} = 2$ [$Y_{steel}/Y_{brass} = 2$ given]

13. (b) Compressibility of water,

$K = 45.4 \times 10^{-11}\ Pa^{-1}$

density of water $P = 10^3\ kg/m^3$

depth of ocean, $h = 2700$ m

We have to find $\frac{\Delta V}{V} = ?$

As we know, compressibility,

$K = \frac{1}{B} = \frac{(\Delta V/V)}{P}$ $(P = \rho g h)$

So, $(\Delta V/V) = K\rho g h$

$= 45.4 \times 10^{-11} \times 10^3 \times 10 \times 2700 = 1.2258 \times 10^{-2}$

14. (c) Bulk modulus is given by

$B = \frac{P}{\left(\frac{\Delta V}{V}\right)}$ or $\frac{\Delta V}{V} = \frac{P}{B}$

$3\frac{\Delta R}{R} = \frac{P}{B}$ (here, $\frac{\Delta R}{R}$ = fractional decreases in radius)

$\Rightarrow \frac{\Delta R}{R} = \frac{P}{3B}$

15. (a) Wire 1: F (A, 3ℓ)

$\Delta\ell = \left(\frac{F}{AY}\right)3\ell$ ...(i)

Wire 2: F′ (3A, ℓ)

$\Delta\ell = \left(\frac{F'}{3AY}\right)\ell$ ...(ii)

From equation (i) & (ii),

$\Delta\ell = \left(\frac{F}{AY}\right)3\ell = \left(\frac{F'}{3AY}\right)\ell$ or, $F' = 9F$

16. (c) Fracture point and ultimate strength point is close for material *X*, hence *X* is brittle in nature and both points are far apart for material *Y* hence it is ductile.

17. (c) Here,

$Kx_0 = Mg$

where K = force constant

$\Delta E = \frac{1}{2}Kx_0^2$

$= \frac{1}{2}\frac{Mg}{x_0}x_0^2$

$= \frac{1}{2}Mgx_0$

L, ℓ, Mg

Stored elastic potential energy in extended wire, $= \frac{1}{2}Mg\ell$

[here $x_0 = \ell$]

18. (c) Stress $= \frac{\text{force}}{\text{cross-section area}} = \frac{Mg}{A}$

Strain $= \frac{\text{change in length}}{\text{original length}} = \frac{\Delta L}{L} = \frac{L_1 - L}{L}$

Young's modulus, $Y = \frac{\text{stress}}{\text{strain}} = \frac{MgL}{A(L_1 - L)}$

Exercise 3 - Concept Application Problems CAP

1. (b) According to Hooke's law stress $\propto$ strain

2. (c) Couple per unit angle of twist, $C = \frac{\pi\eta r^4}{2\ell}$

$\therefore$ Couple $\tau = C\theta = \frac{\pi\eta r^4\theta}{2\ell}$

Here η, ℓ, C & τ are same. So, $r^4\theta$ = constant

$\therefore \frac{\theta_1}{\theta_2} = \left(\frac{r_2^4}{r_1^4}\right)$

3. (c) $Y = \frac{F\ell}{A\Delta\ell} \Rightarrow \Delta\ell = \frac{F\ell}{YA} = \frac{mg\ell}{YA}$

4. (d) According to Hooke's Law, within the elastic limits stress is directly proportional to strain.

5. (b) Let T be the tension in the ring, then

$Y = \frac{T.2\pi r}{A.2\pi(R-r)} = \frac{Tr}{A(R-r)} \therefore T = \frac{YA(R-r)}{r}$

6. (d) $Y = 2\eta(1+\sigma) \Rightarrow \sigma = \frac{0.5Y - \eta}{\eta}$

7. (c) For a perfectly rigid body strain produced is zero for the given force applied, so

Y = stress/strain = ∞

8. (b) We know that $Y = FL/\pi r^2 \ell$ or $r^2 = FL/(Y\pi\ell)$

$\therefore$ $R_B^2 = FL/(Y_B\pi\ell)$ and $R_S^2 = FL/(Y_S\pi\ell)$

or $\frac{R_B^2}{R_S^2} = \frac{Y_S}{Y_B} = \frac{2\times10^{10}}{10^{10}} = 2$

or $R_B^2 = 2R_S^2$ or $R_B = \sqrt{2}\,R_S$ $\therefore R_S = R_B/\sqrt{2}$

9. (d) $F = YA\alpha t = (2.0\times10^{11})(10^{-6})(1.1\times10^{-5})(20)$
= 44 newton

10. (d) Elastic energy $= \frac{1}{2}\times F\times x$

$F = 200$ N, $x = 1$ mm $= 10^{-3}$ m

$\therefore E = \frac{1}{2}\times200\times1\times10^{-3} = 0.1$ J

11. (a) $U/\text{volume} = \frac{1}{2}Y\times\text{strain}^2 = 3600\ \text{J m}^{-3}$

[Strain $= 0.06\times10^{-2}$]

12. (b) Bulk modulus $B = \frac{-P}{(\Delta V/V)} = \frac{-PV}{\Delta V}$ ....(1)

and $\Delta V = \gamma V\Delta T = 3\alpha.V.T$ or $\frac{-V}{\Delta V} = \frac{1}{3\alpha.T.}$ ...(2)

From eqs. (1) and (2), $B = P/(3\alpha.T)$ or $T = \frac{P}{3\alpha B}$

13. (a) $K = \frac{1}{B} = \frac{\Delta V/V}{P}$. Here, P = 100 atm,

$K = 4\times10^{-5}$ and $V = 100\ \text{cm}^3$.

Hence, $\Delta V = 0.4\ \text{cm}^3$

14. (a) $\delta = \frac{W\ell^3}{3YI}$, where W = load, ℓ = length of beam and I is geometrical moment of inertia for rectangular beam,

$I = \frac{bd^3}{12}$ where b = breadth and d = depth

For square beam b = d

$\therefore I_1 = \frac{b^4}{12}$

For a beam of circular cross-section, $I_2 = \left(\frac{\pi r^4}{4}\right)$

$\therefore \delta_1 = \frac{W\ell^3\times12}{3Yb^4} = \frac{4W\ell^3}{Yb^4}$ (for sq. cross section)

and $\delta_2 = \frac{W\ell^3}{3Y(\pi r^4/4)} = \frac{4W\ell^3}{3Y(\pi r^4)}$

(for circular cross-section)

Now $\frac{\delta_1}{\delta_2} = \frac{3\pi r^4}{b^4} = \frac{3\pi r^4}{(\pi r^2)^2} = \frac{3}{\pi}$

($\because b^2 = \pi r^2$ i.e., they have same cross-sectional area)

15. (d) $\frac{\text{Weight of load + Weight of puller}}{\text{area}} = \text{Compressive stress}$

$$\Rightarrow \frac{20A \times d \times 10 + 5 \times 10^5}{\text{area}} = 1.6 \times 10^6$$

Where d is the density.

$$\frac{20A \times 2.5 \times 10^3 \times 10 + 5 \times 10^5}{A} = 1.6 \times 10^6$$

ie, $5 \times 10^5 = 1.1 \times 10^6 A$ or $A = 0.45 m^2$

16. (a) $C_1 = \frac{\pi\eta(r_2^4 - r_1^4)}{2\ell}, C_2 = \frac{\pi\eta r^4}{2\ell}$

Initial volume = Final volume

$$\therefore \pi[r_2^2 - r_1^2]\ell\rho = \pi r^2 \ell\rho$$

$$\Rightarrow r^2 = r_2^2 - r_1^2 \Rightarrow r^2 = (r_2 + r_1)(r_2 - r_1)$$

$$\Rightarrow r^2 = (8.02 + 7.98)(8.02 - 7.98)$$

$$\Rightarrow r^2 = 16 \times 0.04 = 0.64 \text{ cm} \Rightarrow r = 0.8 \text{ cm}$$

$$\therefore \frac{C_1}{C_2} = \frac{r_2^4 - r_1^4}{r^4} = \frac{[8.02]^4 - [7.98]^4}{[0.8]^4}$$

17. (b)

18. (c)

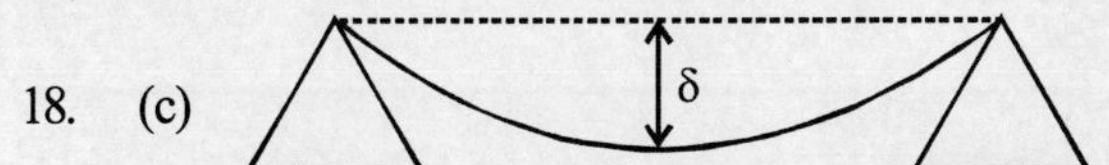

For a beam, the depression at the centre is given by,

$$\delta = \left(\frac{f L}{4Ybd^3}\right)$$

[f, L, b, d are constants for a particular beam]

i.e. $\delta \propto \frac{1}{Y}$

19. (a) Energy stored per unit volume $= \frac{1}{2}\left(\frac{F}{A}\right)\left(\frac{l}{L}\right) = -\frac{Fl}{2AL}$

20. (c) $K = \frac{100}{0.01/100} = 10^6$ atm

$= 10^{11} N/m^2 = 10^{12}$ dyne/cm^2

21. (d) At extension l_1, the stored energy $= \frac{1}{2}Kl_1^2$

At extension l_2, the stored energy $= \frac{1}{2}Kl_2^2$

Work done in increasing its extension from l_1 to l_2

$$= \frac{1}{2}K(l_2^2 - l_1^2)$$

22. (d)

23. (c) Young's modulus of rubber, Y_{rubber}

$$= \frac{F}{A} \times \frac{\ell}{\Delta\ell} \Rightarrow F = YA.\frac{\Delta\ell}{\ell}$$

On putting the values from question,

$$F = \frac{5 \times 10^8 \times 25 \times 10^{-6} \times 5 \times 10^{-2}}{10 \times 10^{-2}}$$

$$= 25 \times 25 \times 10^{2-1} = 6250N$$

kinetic energy = potential energy of rubber

$$\frac{1}{2}mv^2 = \frac{1}{2}F\Delta\ell$$

$$v = \sqrt{\frac{F\Delta\ell}{m}} = \sqrt{\frac{6250 \times 5 \times 10^{-2}}{5 \times 10^{-3}}} = \sqrt{62500}$$

$= 25 \times 10 = 250$ m/s

24. (c)

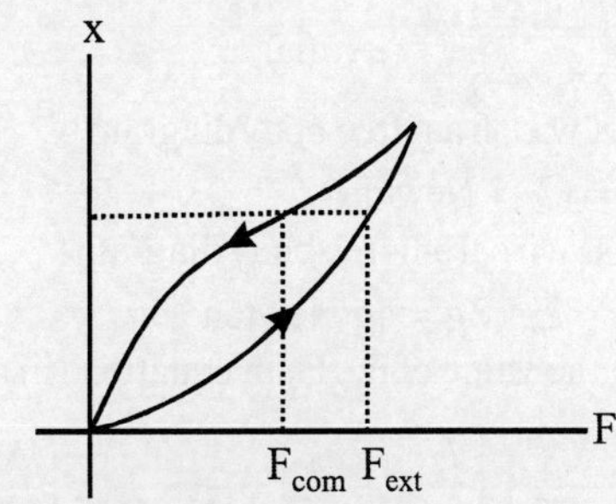

From the figure, it is clear that

$F_{com} < F_{ext}$.

25. (d) $r = C.\theta = \frac{\pi\eta r^4\theta}{2L} = \text{Constant}$

$$\Rightarrow \frac{\pi\eta r^4(\theta - \theta_0)}{2l} = \frac{\pi\eta(r/2)^4(\theta_0 - \theta')}{2(l/2)}$$

$$\Rightarrow \frac{(\theta - \theta_0)}{2} = \frac{\theta_0}{16} \Rightarrow \theta_0 = \frac{8}{9}\theta$$

θ′ = 0
l/2
θ₀
l
θ

26. (a) $F = YA\frac{\Delta\ell}{\ell} = YA\alpha\Delta\theta$

$= 2 \times 10^{11} \times (1 \times 10^{-6}) \times 1.1 \times 10^{-5} \times (10) = 22$ N

27. (a) $Y = \frac{mg\ell}{(\pi/4)d^2x}$ ....(1)

$$\left(\frac{dY}{Y}\right)_{max} = \frac{\Delta m}{m} + \frac{\Delta\ell}{\ell} + 2\frac{\Delta d}{d} + \frac{\Delta x}{x}$$

m = 20.0 kg ⇒ Δm = 0.1 kg

ℓ = 125cm ⇒ Δℓ = 1 cm.

d = 0.050 cm. ⇒ Δd = 0.001 cm

x = 0.100 cm. ⇒ Δx = 0.001 cm.

$$\left(\frac{dY}{Y}\right)_{max} = \left(\begin{array}{c}\frac{0.1kg}{20.0kg} + \frac{1cm}{125cm} \\ +2 \times \frac{0.001cm}{0.05cm} + \frac{0.001cm}{0.100cm}\end{array}\right) \times 100\% = 6.3\%$$

28. (d) Given, $\frac{l_1}{l_2} = a, \frac{r_1}{r_2} = b, \frac{Y_1}{Y_2} = c$

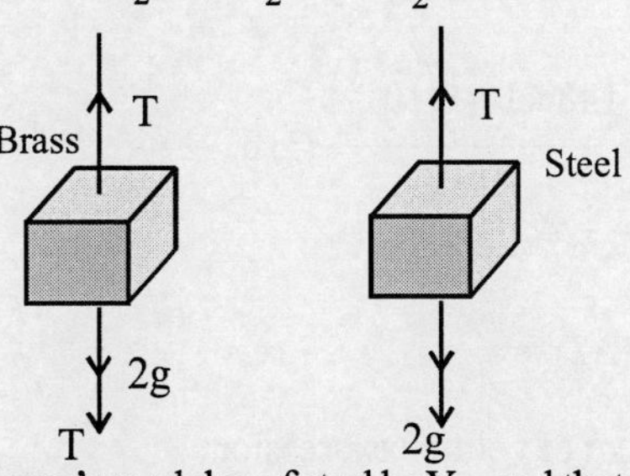

Let Young's modulus of steel be Y_1, and that of brass be Y_2

$$\therefore Y_1 = \frac{F_1 l_1}{A_1 \Delta l_1} \quad ...(i)$$

and $Y_2 = \frac{F_2 l_2}{A_2 \Delta l_2}$ ...(ii)

Dividing equation (i) by equation (ii), we get

$$\frac{Y_1}{Y_2} = \frac{F_1 A_2 l_1 \Delta l_2}{F_2 A_1 l_2 \Delta l_1} \quad ...(iii)$$

Force on steel wire from free body diagram

$T = F_1 = (2g)$ Newton

Force on brass wire from free body diagram

$F_2 = T_1 = T + 2g = 4g$ Newton

Now putting the value of F_1, F_2 in equation (iii), we get

$$\frac{Y_1}{Y_2} = \left(\frac{2g}{4g}\right)\left(\frac{\pi r_2^2}{\pi r_1^2}\right)\cdot\left[\frac{l_1}{l_2}\right]\cdot\left(\frac{\Delta l_2}{\Delta l_1}\right) = \frac{1}{2}\left(\frac{1}{b^2}\right).a\left(\frac{\Delta l_2}{\Delta l_1}\right)$$

29. (d) $F = \frac{YA}{L} \times \ell$

So, extension, $\ell \propto \frac{L}{A} \propto \frac{L}{D^2}$ [$\because$ F and Y are constant]

$\ell_1 \propto \frac{100}{1^2} \propto 100$ and $\ell_2 \propto \frac{200}{2^2} \propto 50$

$\ell_3 \propto \frac{300}{3^2} \propto \frac{100}{3}$ and $\ell_4 \propto \frac{50}{\frac{1}{4}} \propto 200$

The ratio of $\frac{L}{D^2}$ is maximum for case (d).

Hence, option (d) is correct.

30. (a) Percentage elongation in the wire $= \frac{F\ell}{AY}$

$$= \frac{6.28 \times 10^4 \times (1)}{\pi(0.01)^2 \times 2 \times 10^{11}} = \frac{1}{1000}$$

31. (4) Given : Wire length, $l = 0.3$ m

Mass of the body, m = 10 kg

Breaking stress, $\sigma = 4.8 \times 10^7$ Nm^{-2}

Area of cross-section, a = 10^{-2} cm^2

Maximum angular speed ω = ?

$T = Ml\omega^2$

$$\sigma = \frac{T}{A} = \frac{ml\omega^2}{A}$$

$$\frac{ml\omega^2}{A} \le 48 \times 10^7 \Rightarrow \omega^2 \le \frac{(48 \times 10^7)A}{ml}$$

$$\Rightarrow \omega^2 \le \frac{(48 \times 10^7)(10^{-6})}{10 \times 3} = 16 \Rightarrow \omega_{max} = 4 \text{ rad/s}$$

32. (c) $\Delta_{temp} = \Delta_{force}$

or $L\alpha(\Delta T) = \frac{FL}{AY}$ $\therefore$ $\alpha = \frac{FL}{AYT} = \frac{F}{\pi r^2 YT}$

Coefficient of volume expression

$$r = 3\alpha = \frac{3F}{\pi r^2 YT}.$$

33. (Bonus)

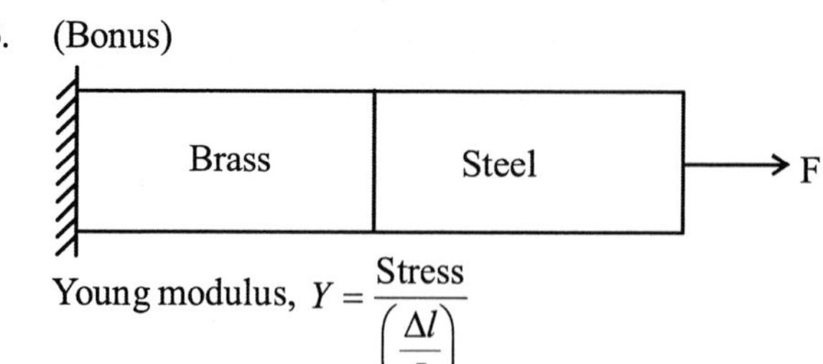

Young modulus, $Y = \frac{\text{Stress}}{\left(\frac{\Delta l}{L}\right)}$

Let σ be the stress

Total elongation $\Delta l_{net} = \frac{\sigma L_1}{Y_1} + \frac{\sigma L_2}{Y_2}$

$$\Delta l_{net} = \sigma\left[\frac{1}{Y_1} + \frac{1}{Y_2}\right] \quad [\because L_1 = L_2 = 1\text{m}]$$

$$\sigma = \Delta l\left(\frac{Y_1 Y_2}{Y_1 + Y_2}\right)$$

$$= 0.2 \times 10^{-3} \times \left(\frac{120 \times 60}{180}\right) \times 10^9 = 8 \times 10^6 \frac{N}{m^2}$$

34. (b) Stress $= \frac{F}{A} = \frac{400 \times 4}{\pi d^2} = 379 \times 10^6$ N/m^2

$$\Rightarrow d^2 = \frac{400 \times 4}{379 \times 10^6 \pi}$$

$d = 1.15$ mm

35. (c) Consider a small element dx of radius r,

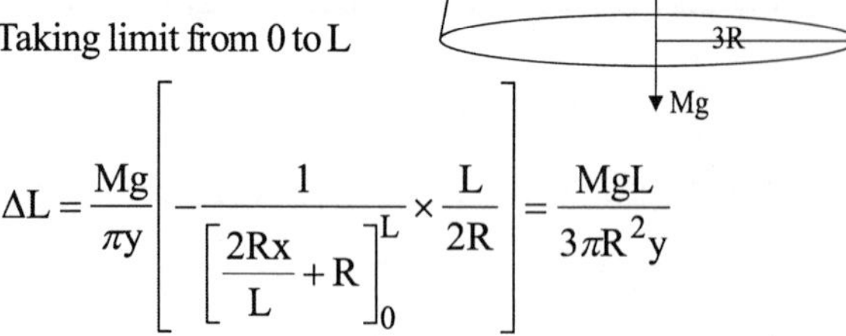

$$r = \frac{2R}{L}x + R$$

At equilibrium change in length of the wire

$$\int_0^1 dL = \int \frac{Mg\,dx}{\pi\left[\frac{2R}{L}x + R\right]^2 y}$$

Taking limit from 0 to L

$$\Delta L = \frac{Mg}{\pi y}\left[-\frac{1}{\left[\frac{2Rx}{L} + R\right]_0^L} \times \frac{L}{2R}\right] = \frac{MgL}{3\pi R^2 y}$$

The equilibrium extended length of wire = L + ΔL

$$= L + \frac{MgL}{3\pi R^2 Y} = L\left(1 + \frac{1}{3}\frac{Mg}{\pi Y R^2}\right)$$

36. (a) Young's modulus $Y = \frac{\text{stress}}{\text{strain}}$

stress = Y × strain

Stress in steel wire = Applied pressure

Pressure = stress = Y × strain

Strain $= \frac{\Delta L}{L} = \alpha \Delta T$ (As length is constant)

$= 2 \times 10^{11} \times 1.1 \times 10^{-5} \times 100 = 2.2 \times 10^8$ Pa

37. (b) Tension in the wire, $T = \left(\frac{2mM}{m+M}\right)g$

$$\text{Stress} = \frac{\text{Force / Tension}}{\text{Area}} = \frac{2mM}{A(m+M)}g$$

$$= \frac{2(m \times 2m)g}{A(m+2m)} \quad (M = 2\,m \text{ given})$$

$$= \frac{4m^2}{3mA}g = \frac{4mg}{3A}$$

38. (c) Given, $y = 2\times10^{11}\,Nm^{-2}$

$$\text{Stress}\left(\frac{F}{A}\right) = 5\times10^7\,Nm^{-2}$$

$\Delta V = 0.02\% = 2\times10^{-4}\,m^3$

$$\frac{\Delta r}{r} = ?$$

$$\gamma = \frac{\text{stress}}{\text{strain}} \Rightarrow \text{strain}\left(\frac{\Delta\ell}{\ell_0}\right) = \frac{\gamma}{\text{stress}} \quad \ldots(i)$$

$$\Delta V = 2\pi r\ell_0\Delta r - \pi r^2\Delta\ell \quad \ldots(ii)$$

From eqns (i) and (ii) putting the value of $\Delta\ell$, ℓ_0 and ΔV and solving we get

$$\frac{\Delta r}{r} = 0.25\times10^{-4}$$

39. (c) Breaking force α area of cross section of wire
Load hold by wire is independent of length of the wire.

40. (a) Given: $F = 100\,kN = 10^5\,N$
$Y = 2\times10^{11}\,Nm^{-2}$
$\ell_0 = 1.0\,m$
radius $r = 10\,mm = 10^{-2}\,m$

From formula, $Y = \frac{\text{Stress}}{\text{Strain}}$

$$\Rightarrow \quad \text{Strain} = \frac{\text{Stress}}{Y} = \frac{F}{AY}$$

$$= \frac{10^5}{\pi r^2 Y} = \frac{10^5}{3.14\times10^{-4}\times2\times10^{11}} = \frac{1}{628}$$

$$\text{Therefore \% strain} = \frac{1}{628}\times100 = 0.16\%$$

41. (a) If force F acts along the length L of the wire of cross-section A, then energy stored in unit volume of wire is given by

$$\text{Energy density} = \frac{1}{2}\,\text{stress}\times\text{strain}$$

$$= \frac{1}{2}\times\frac{F}{A}\times\frac{F}{AY} \quad \left(\because \text{ stress} = \frac{F}{A} \text{ and strain} = \frac{X}{AY}\right)$$

$$= \frac{1}{2}\frac{F^2}{A^2Y} = \frac{1}{2}\frac{F^2\times16}{(\pi d^2)^2Y} = \frac{1}{2}\frac{F^2\times16}{\pi d^4 Y}$$

If u_1 and u_2 are the densities of two wires, then

$$\frac{u_1}{u_2} = \left(\frac{d_2}{d_1}\right)^4 \Rightarrow \frac{d_1}{d_2} = (4)^{1/4} \Rightarrow \frac{d_1}{d_2} = \sqrt{2}:1$$

42. (a) When a catapult is stretched up to length l, then the stored energy in it = Δk. E $\Rightarrow \frac{1}{2}\cdot\left(\frac{YA}{L}\right)(\Delta l)^2 = \frac{1}{2}mv^2$

$$\Rightarrow y = \frac{mv^2L}{A(\Delta l)^2}$$

$m = 0.02\,kg$
$v = 20\,ms^{-1}$
$L = 0.42\,m$
$A = (\pi d^2)/(4)$
$d = 6\times10^{-3}\,m$
$\Delta l = 0.2\,m$

$$y = \frac{0.02\times400\times0.42\times4}{\pi\times36\times10^{-6}\times0.04} = 2.3\times10^6\,N/m^2$$

So, order is 10^6.

43. (c) Bulk modulus, $K = \frac{\text{volumetric stress}}{\text{volumetric strain}}$

$$K = \frac{mg}{a\left(\frac{dV}{V}\right)}$$

$$\Rightarrow \quad \frac{dV}{V} = \frac{mg}{Ka} \quad \ldots(i)$$

volume of sphere, $V = \frac{4}{3}\pi R^3$

$$\text{Fractional change in volume } \frac{dV}{V} = \frac{3dr}{r} \quad \ldots(ii)$$

$$\text{Using eq. (i) \& (ii) } \frac{3dr}{r} = \frac{mg}{Ka}$$

$$\therefore \quad \frac{dr}{r} = \frac{mg}{3Ka} \text{ (fractional decrement in radius)}$$

44. (d) $\text{Stress} = \frac{\text{Normal force}}{\text{Area}} = \frac{N}{A} = \frac{N}{(2pa)b}$

Stress = B×strain

$$\frac{N}{(2pa)b} = B\frac{2paDa'\,b}{pa^2b}$$

$$\Rightarrow N = B\frac{(2\pi a)^2\Delta ab^2}{\pi a^2 b}$$

Force needed to push the cork.

f = mN = m4pbDaB = (4πμBb)Δa

45. (c) Poisson's ratio, $\sigma = \frac{\text{lateral strain }(\beta)}{\text{longitudinal strain }(\alpha)}$

For material like copper, $\sigma = 0.33$
And, $Y = 3k(1-2\sigma)$

Also, $\frac{9}{Y} = \frac{1}{k} + \frac{3}{\eta}$

$Y = 2\eta(1+\sigma)$
Hence, $\eta < Y < k$

10 Mechanical Properties of Fluids

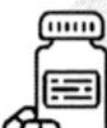

Topic 10.1 : Fluids, Pascal's Law & Its Applications, Atmospheric, Hydrostatic, Guage Pressure, Buoyancy and Archimedes' Principle

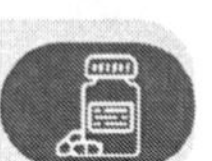

FLUIDS

Fluid is something that can flow. All liquids and gases are fluids. *The force exerted normally at a unit area of the surface of a fluid is called* **fluid pressure**.

$$\text{i.e., } P=\frac{F}{a}$$

Its **S.I. unit** is Nm^{-2} or Pascal. Its **dimensions** are $[ML^{-1}T^{-2}]$.

PASCAL'S LAW AND ITS APPLICATIONS

Pascal's law : *Pressure in a fluid in equilibrium is the same everywhere, if the effect of gravity is neglected.*

Another form of Pascal's law : *The excess pressure, applied anywhere in a mass of confined incompressible fluid is transmitted by the fluid in all directions without being diminished in magnitude.*

Applications of Pascal's Law

Hydraulic lift : Its working is based on Pascal's law. A piston of small cross-sectional area (a) exerts a force (f) on the liquid.

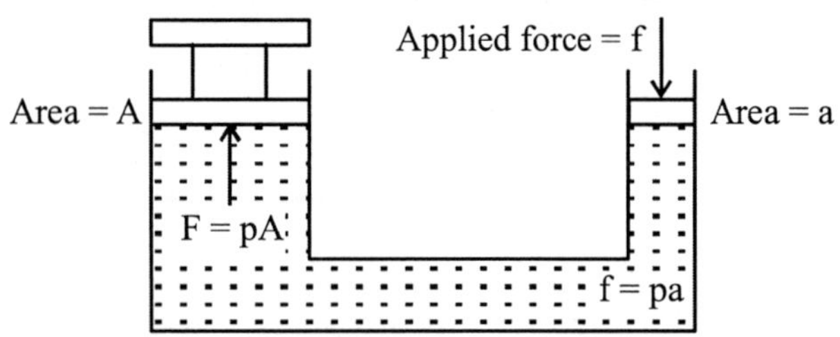

The pressure is transmitted undiminished to the larger cylinder of cross-sectional area A.

$$P=\frac{f}{a}=\frac{F}{A} \Rightarrow F=\frac{A}{a}f$$

Hydraulic brakes also work on pascal's law.

ATMOSPHERIC, HYDROSTATIC AND GUAGE PRESSURE

Atmospheric pressure : The atmosphere exerts pressure on the earth's surface. The atmospheric pressure at sea level is given by

$$P_0 = 1.01 \times 10^5\, Pa$$

Hydrostatic pressure : The hydrostatic pressure at a depth h below the surface of a fluid is given by

$$P = h\rho g$$

where ρ is the density of the fluid, g acceleration due to gravity and h is the depth of the liquid column.

Gauge pressure : The pressure at any point in a fluid is equal to the sum of the atmospheric pressure acting on its surface and the hydrostatic pressure due to the weight of the fluid above that point which is at a depth h below the surface of the fluid.

The gauge pressure is given by

$$P = P_0 + h\rho g$$

or, $$P - P_0 = h\rho g$$

BUOYANCY AND ARCHIMEDES' PRINCIPLE

Buoyancy

If a body is partially or wholly immersed in a fluid, it experiences an upward force due to the fluid surrounding it. The phenomenon of force exerted by fluid on the body called **buoyancy** and the force is called **buoyant force** or **upthrust**.

A body experiences buoyant force whether it floats or sinks, under its own weight or due to other forces applied on it.

Archimedes' Principle

When any body is immersed (totally or partially) in a liquid it appears to lose part of its weight and the apparent loss of weight is equal to the weight of liquid displaced.

Let a body of weight W is immersed in a fluid and W' is upthrust on it then

(i) if $W > W'$, then body will sink.

(ii) if $W = W'$, then the body floats with whole or some part of its volume inside the fluid.

Let V be the volume of a body of density d and V' be the volume of liquid of density ρ displaced. If the body floats then $Vd = V'\rho$

$\therefore \frac{d}{\rho}=\frac{V'}{V}$ gives the fraction of the volume inside the liquid in which the body floats.

Also, body immersed in a fluid experiences an upward buoyant force equivalent to the weight of the fluid displaced by it.

The proof of this principle is very simple. Imagine a body of arbitrary shape completely immersed in a liquid of density ρ as shown in the figure (a). A body is being acted upon by the forces from all directions. Let us consider a vertical element of height h and cross-sectional area dA (as shown in the figure (b)).

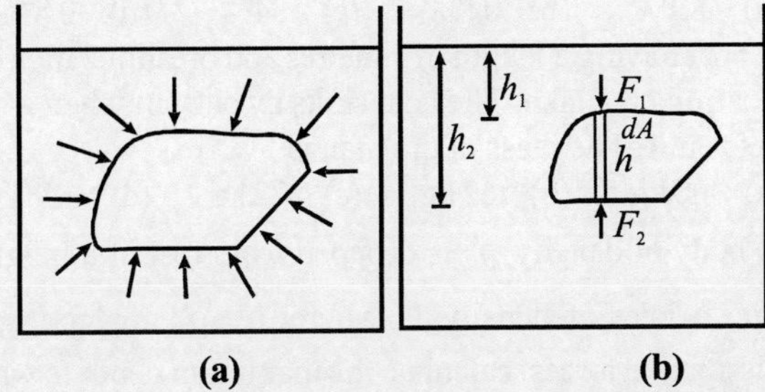

(a) (b)

The force acting on the upper surface of the element is F_1 (downward) and that on the lower surface is F_2 (upward). Since $F_2 > F_1$, therefore, the net upward force acting on the element is $dF = F_2 - F_1$

It can be easily seen from the figure (b), that

$F_1 = (\rho g h_1)dA$ and $F_2 = (\rho g h_2)dA$ so $dF = \rho g(h)dA$

Also, $h_2 - h_1 = h$ and $d(dA) = dV$

∴ The net upward force is $F = \int \rho g dV = \rho V g$

Hence, for the entire body, the buoyant force is the weight of the volume of the fluid displaced.

The buoyant force acts through the centre of gravity of the displaced fluid.

Problem Solving Tips

1. The pressure is perpendicular to the surface of the fluid.
2. The upthrust on a body immersed in a liquid does not depend on the mass, density or shape of the body. It only depends on the volume of the body.
3. The weight of the plastic bag full of air is same as that of the empty bag because the upthrust is equal to the weight of the air enclosed.
4. The cross-section of the water stream from a top decreases as it goes down in accordance with the equation of continuity.
5. We cannot sip a drink with a straw on the moon, because there is no atmosphere on the moon.
6. The line joining the centre of gravity and centre of buoyancy is called **central line**.
7. **Metacenter** - is a point where the vertical line passing through the centre of buoyancy intersects the central line.
8. The floating body is in **stable equilibrium** when the metacenter is **above** the centre of gravity (centre of gravity is below the centre of buoyancy).
9. The floating body is in the **unstable equilibrium** when the metacenter lies **below** the centre of gravity (centre of gravity is above the centre of buoyancy).
10. The floating body is in the **neutral equilibrium** when centre of gravity coincides with the metacenter (centre of gravity coincides with the centre of buoyancy).
11. The wooden rod cannot float vertically in a pond of water because centre of gravity lies above the metacenter.
12. (i) If a body just floats in a liquid (density of the body is equal to the density of liquid) then the body sinks if it is pushed downwards.
    (ii) If two bodies have equal upthrust when just immersed in a liquid, both will have the same volume.
    (iii) If a person floats on his back on the surface of water, the apparent weight of person is zero.
13. The hydrometer can be used to measure density of the liquid or fluid.

Relative Density (or Specific Gravity)

Liquids may be treated as incompressible. Hence their density may be assumed to be constant throughout.

$$\text{Relative density} = \frac{\textit{Weight of substance in air}}{\textit{Weight of equal volume of water}}$$

$$= \frac{\textit{Weight of substance in air}}{\textit{Loss of weight in water}}$$

$$= \frac{\textit{Density of substance}}{\textit{Density of water at } 4^\circ C}$$

Density in SI system = 1000 × density in the cgs system.

(i) The density of liquid of bulk modulus B at a depth h is given by $\rho_h = \rho_0\left(1 + \frac{\rho g h}{B}\right)$ where ρ_0 is the density of liquid on its surface and ρ is the average density of liquid.

(ii) The density of liquid changes with pressure as

$$P_h = P_0\left(1 + \frac{\Delta P}{B}\right)$$

where ΔP = change in pressure and B = bulk modulus of liquid.

(iii) If two liquids of masses m_1, m_2 and densities ρ_1, ρ_2 are mixed together, then the density of the mixture is given by

$$\rho = \frac{m_1 + m_2}{\frac{m_1}{\rho_1} + \frac{m_2}{\rho_2}}$$

And if $m_1 = m_2$ but different densities are mixed together, then the density of the mixture is harmonic mean of the densities.

$$\text{i.e., } \rho = \frac{2\rho_1\rho_2}{\rho_1 + \rho_2} \text{ or } \frac{1}{\rho} = \frac{1}{2}\left[\frac{1}{\rho_1} + \frac{1}{\rho_2}\right]$$

(iv) If two drops of same volume but different densities are mixed together, then the density of the mixture is the arithmetic mean of the densities.

$$\text{i.e., } \rho = \frac{\rho_1 + \rho_2}{2} \quad \left(\textit{as } \rho = \frac{\rho_1 V_0 + \rho_2 V_0}{V_0 + V_0}\right)$$

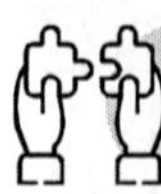

10.1 Concept Practice Problems

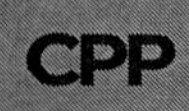

1. A beaker containing a liquid of density ρ moves up with an acceleration a. The pressure due to the liquid at a depth h below the free surface of the liquid is
(a) $h\rho g$ (b) $h\rho(g-a)$
(c) $h\rho(g+a)$ (d) $2h\rho g\left(\frac{g+a}{g-a}\right)$

2. The density of ice is x gram/litre and that of water is y gram/litre. What is the change in volume when m gram of ice melts?
(a) $mxy(x-y)$ (b) $m/(y-x)$
(c) $m\left(\frac{1}{y}-\frac{1}{x}\right)$ (d) $(y-x)/x$

3. Consider a 1 c.c. sample of air at absolute temperature T_0 at sea level and another 1 c.c. sample of air at a height where the pressure is one-third atmosphere. The absolute temperature T of the sample at the height is
(a) equal to $T_0/3$
(b) equal to $3/T_0$
(c) equal to T_0
(d) cannot be determined in terms of T_0 from the above data

4. A man is sitting in a boat which is floating in pond. If the man drinks some water from the pond, the level of water in the pond will
(a) rise a little (b) fall a little
(c) remain stationary (d) none of these

5. The reading of spring balance when a block is suspended from it in air is 60 newton. This reading is changed to 40 newton when the block is submerged in water. The specific gravity of the block must be therefore
(a) 3 (b) 2 (c) 6 (d) 3/2

6. An ice-berg floating partly immersed in sea water of density 1.03 g/cm^3. The density of ice is 0.92 g/cm^3. The fraction of the total volume of the iceberg above the level of sea water is
(a) 8.1% (b) 11% (c) 34% (d) 0.8%

7. A boat having a length of 3 metres and breadth 2 metres is floating on a lake. The boat sinks by one cm when a man gets on it. The mass of the man is
(a) 60 kg (b) 62 kg (c) 72 kg (d) 128 kg

8. A body of density ρ' is dropped from rest at a height h into a lake of density ρ where $\rho > \rho'$ neglecting all dissipative forces, calculate the maximum depth to which the body sinks before returning to float on the surface :
(a) $\frac{h}{\rho-\rho'}$ (b) $\frac{h\rho'}{\rho}$ (c) $\frac{h\rho'}{\rho-\rho'}$ (d) $\frac{h\rho}{\rho-\rho'}$

9. Two pieces of metals are suspended from the arms of a balance and are found to be in equilibrium when kept immersed in water. The mass of one piece is 32 g and its density 8 g cm^{-3}. The density of the other is 5 g per cm^3. Then the mass of the other is
(a) 28 g (b) 35 g (c) 21 g (d) 33.6 g

10. Two vessels A and B of cross-sections as shown in figure contain a liquid up to the same height. As the temperature rises, the liquid pressure at the bottom (neglecting expansion of the vessels) will

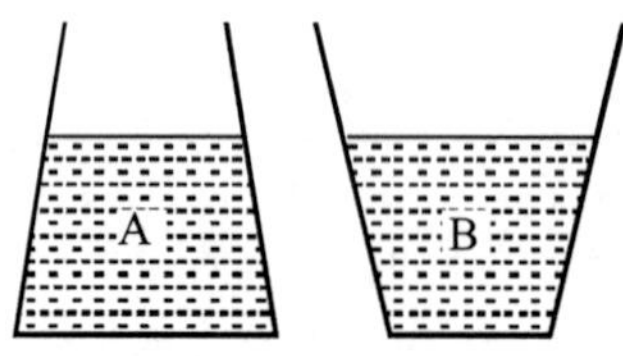

(a) increase in A, decrease in B
(b) increase in B, decrease in A
(c) increase in both A and B
(d) decrease in both A and B

ANSWER KEY																			
1	(c)	2	(c)	3	(a)	4	(c)	5	(a)	6	(b)	7	(a)	8	(c)	9	(b)	10	(a)

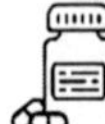

Topic 10.2 : Surface Tension, Angle of Contact, Capillarity, Shape of Liquid Meniscus

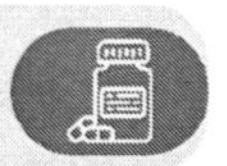

SURFACE TENSION

It is defined as the force per unit length acting at right angles on either side of an imaginary line drawn on the free surface of the liquid.

i.e., $S=\frac{F}{\ell}$

The surface tension is also defined as the work required to increase unit area of that liquid film.

Its **SI unit** is N/m or J/m^2 and **dimensions** are [ML^0T^{-2}].

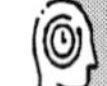

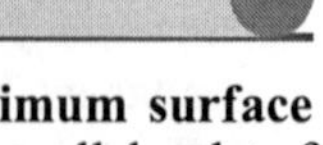

Problem Solving Tips

1. The liquid surface always acquires **minimum surface area** due to **surface tension (ST)**. So, the small droplet of any liquid is always spherical.
2. The ST is a molecular phenomenon as ST is due to 'cohesion' between the molecules of a liquid.
3. The force of attraction between the molecules of the same substance is called a **cohesive force** and that between molecules of different substance is called **adhesive force**.

4. The molecular range is the maximum distance (10^{-9} m) upto which the molecules attract each other.
5. In general the ST of liquids decreases with increase in temperature but the ST of molten Cadmium and Copper increases with increase in temperature.
6. If the impurity is completely soluble then on mixing it in the liquid, its surface tension increases. For example on dissolving ionic salts in small quantities in a liquid, its surface tension increases. On dissolving salt in water, its surface tension increases.
7. If the impurity is partially soluble in a liquid, then its surface tension decreases. For example on mixing detergent or phenol in water its surface tension decreases.
8. On increasing temperature surface tension decreases. At critical temperature and boiling point it becomes zero. Surface tension of water is maximum at 4°C.

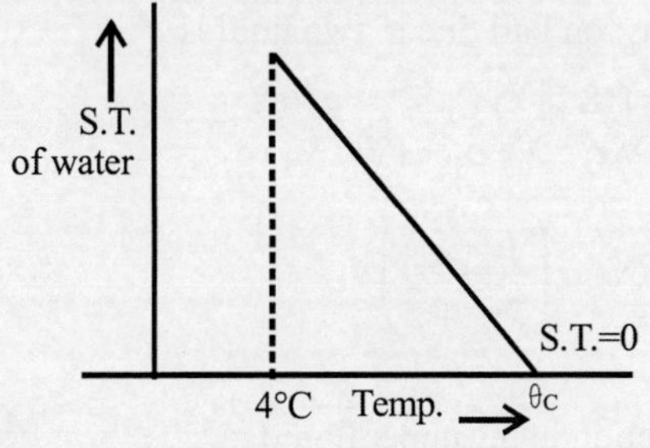

ANGLE OF CONTACT

The angle between the tangent to the liquid surface and the tangent to the solid surface at the point of contact (inside the liquid) is known as angle of contact.

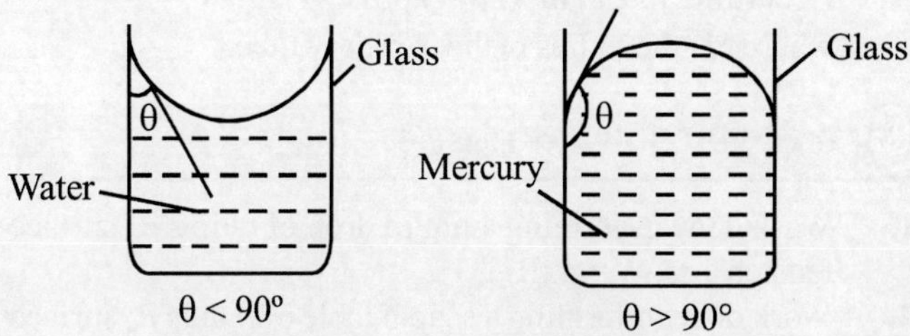

Some values of angle of contact of solid and liquid :

Pair of surface	Angle of contact
Pure water and glass	0°
Silver and glass	90°
Alcohol and glass	138°
Normal water & glass	8°
Mercury & glass	135°

Adhesion > cohesion	Adhesion = cohesion	Adhesion < cohesion
1. Liquid will wet the solid	Critical	Liquid will not wet the solid
2. Meniscus is concave	Meniscus is plane	Meniscus is convex
3. Angle of contact is acute ($\theta < 90°$)	Angle of contact is 90°	Angle of contact is obtuse ($\theta > 90°$)
4. Pressure below the menisucs is lesser than above it by (2T/r), i.e. $p = p_0 - \frac{2T}{r}$	Pressure below the meniscus is same as above it, i.e. $p = p_0$	Pressure below the meniscus is more then above it by (2T/r), i.e., $p = p_0 + \frac{2T}{r}$
5. In capillary tube liquid will ascend.	No capillary rise	In capillary tube liquid will descend.

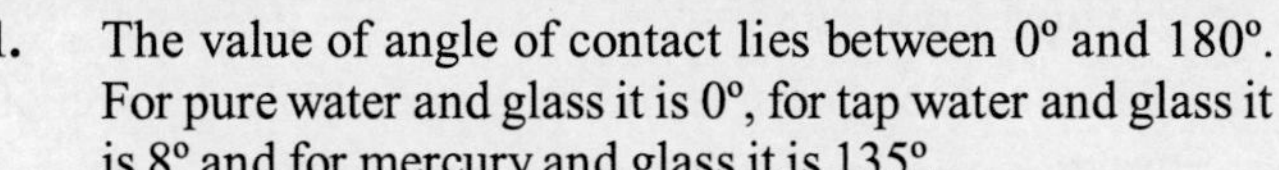

Problem Solving Tips

1. The value of angle of contact lies between 0° and 180°. For pure water and glass it is 0°, for tap water and glass it is 8° and for mercury and glass it is 135°.
2. For all those liquids which wet the solid surface and which rise up in a capillary tube, the angle of contact is an acute angle ($\theta < 90°$), e.g. water and glass.
3. For all those liquids which do not wet a solid surface and which depress in a capillary tube, the angle of contact is an obtuse angle ($\theta > 90°$), e.g. glass and mercury.
4. For all those liquids which neither rise nor get depressed in a capillary tube, the angle of contact is right angle ($\theta = 90°$), e.g. silver and water.
5. Angle of contact depends on impurities, water proofing agent, surface in contact and temperature. Angle of contact $\theta_C \propto T$ where T is the temperature.

CAPILLARITY

The phenomenon of rise or fall of liquids in capillary tube is known as capillarity.

The rise or fall of a liquid in a capillary tube is given by

$$h = \frac{2T\cos\theta}{r\rho g} = \frac{2T}{R\rho g}$$

$$\Rightarrow h\rho g = \frac{2T}{R}$$

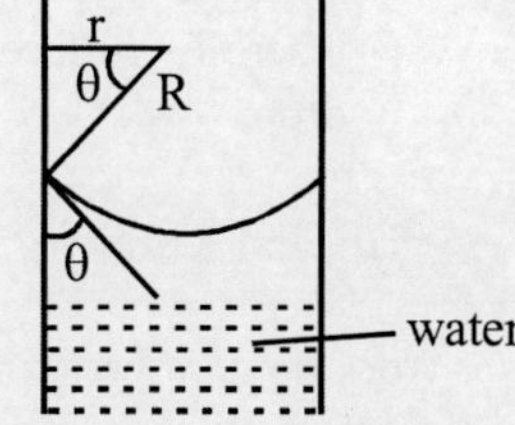

where T = surface tension, θ = angle of contact, ρ = density of liquid, r = radius of capillary tube, R = radius of meniscus.

(i) If capillary tube is of insufficient length ℓ (i.e. $\ell < h$), then the liquid rises to a full height h with radius R' such that $hR = \ell R'$

(ii) When the capillary tube is tilted from vertical by an angle α, then the vertical height h of liquid column remains the same. The length of liquid in capillary increases such that

$$\cos\alpha = \frac{h}{h'} \text{ or } h' = \frac{h}{\cos\alpha}.$$

According to **Zurin's law** capillary rise $h \propto \frac{1}{r}$ where r is the radius of the capillary tube.

Problem Solving Tips

1. Work done in forming a liquid drop of radius R, surface tension T is, $W = 4\pi R^2 T$.
2. Work done in forming a soap bubble of radius R, surface tension T is, $W = 2\times4\pi R^2 T = 8\pi R^2 T$.
3. When n no. of smaller drops of liquid, each of radius r, surface tension T are combined to form a bigger drop of radius R then $R = n^{1/3} r$.
4. The surface area of bigger drop $= 4\pi R^2 = 4\pi n^{2/3} r^2$. It is less than the area of n smaller drops.

SHAPE OF LIQUID MENISCUS :

The pressure on the concave side is always greater than the pressure on the convex side.

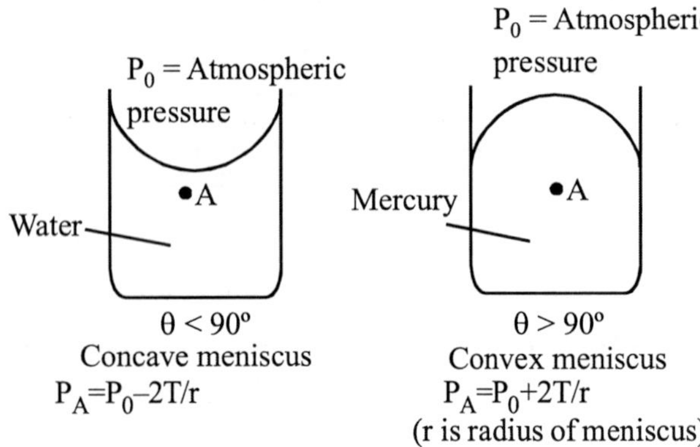

Excess pressure of liquid drop and soap bubble :

(i) Excess of pressure for spherical soap bubble is $p = 4T/r$ and excess of pressure for liquid drop and air bubble in a liquid is $p = 2T/r$.

(ii) (a) Excess of pressure within a cylindrical liquid drop $p = T/R$

(b) Excess of pressure within a cylindrical soap bubble $p = 2T/R$

where T = surface tension, R = radius of the cylindrical drop.

Problem Solving Tips

1. Work done in breaking a liquid drop of radius R into n equal small drops $= 4\pi R^2 (n^{1/3} - 1)T$; where T = surface tension.
2. Work done in breaking a soap bubble of radius R into n equal small drops $= 8\pi R^2 (n^{1/3} - 1)T$; where T = surface tension.

Example 1.

A solid uniform ball having volume V and density ρ floats at the interface of two unmixable liquids as shown in fig. The densities of the upper and the lower liquids are ρ_1 and ρ_2 respectively, such that $\rho_1 < \rho < \rho_2$. What fraction of the volume of the ball will be in the lower liquid ?

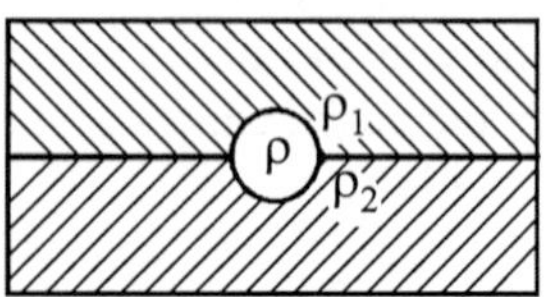

Solution :

Let V_1 and V_2 be the volumes of the ball in the upper and lower liquids respectively. So $V_1 + V_2 = V$.

As ball is floating in the two liquids ; weight of the ball = upthrust on ball due to two liquids

i.e., $V\rho g = V_1\rho_1 g + V_2\rho_2 g$;

or $V\rho = V_1\rho_1 + (V - V_1)\rho_2$;

or $V_1 = \left(\frac{\rho - \rho_2}{\rho_1 - \rho_2}\right)V$

$\therefore$ Fraction in the upper liquid $= \frac{V_1}{V} = \frac{\rho - \rho_2}{\rho_1 - \rho_2}$

Fraction in the lower liquid $= 1 - \frac{V_1}{V}$

$$= 1 - \frac{\rho - \rho_2}{\rho_1 - \rho_2} = \frac{\rho_1 - \rho}{\rho_1 - \rho_2}$$

Example 2.

A piece of cork is embedded inside of block of ice which floats on water. What will happen to the level of water when all the ice melts?

Solution :

Let , M = mass of the block of ice, m = mass of piece of cork and V = Volume of water displaced.

Now $(M + m) = V \times 1 = V$ ...(1)

When the ice melts, let it be converted into V' c.c. of water.

Also $M = V' \times 1 = V'$

The piece of cork floats on the surface of water when all ice melts. Let the cork displaces a volume V'' c.c. of water. Then $m = V'' \times 1 = V''$

If V_1 be the volume of water displaced by melted ice and cork, then

$(M + m) = V' + V'' = V_1$ ...(2)

From eqns. (1) and (2), $V = V_1$

Hence, no change in the level of water.

Example 3.

Two substances of densities ρ_1 and ρ_2 are mixed in equal volume and the relative density of mixture is 4. When they are mixed in equal masses, the relative density of the mixture is 3. Determine the values of ρ_1 and ρ_2.

Solution :

When the substances are mixed in equal volumes, then

$$V\rho_1 + V\rho_2 = 2V \times 4 \quad \text{... (1)}$$

When the two substances are mixed in equal masses, then

$$\frac{m}{\rho_1} + \frac{m}{\rho_2} = \frac{2m}{3} \quad \text{...(2)}$$

From eq. (1), $\rho_1 + \rho_2 = 8$ ... (3)

From eqn. (2) $\frac{1}{\rho_1} + \frac{1}{\rho_2} = \frac{2}{3}$ or $\frac{\rho_1 + \rho_2}{\rho_1 \rho_2} = \frac{2}{3}$

or $\frac{8}{\rho_1 \rho_2} = \frac{2}{3}$ or $\rho_1 \rho_2 = 12$ ...(4)

Now $\rho_1 - \rho_2 = [(\rho_1 + \rho_2)^2 - 4\rho_1\rho_2]^{1/2}$

$= [64 - 48]^{1/2} = 4$ ...(5)

Solving eqns. (3) and (5), we get $\rho_1 = 6$ and $\rho_2 = 2$]

Example 4.

A sealed tank containing a liquid of density ρ moves with a horizontal acceleration a, as shown in fig. Find the difference in pressure between the points A and B.

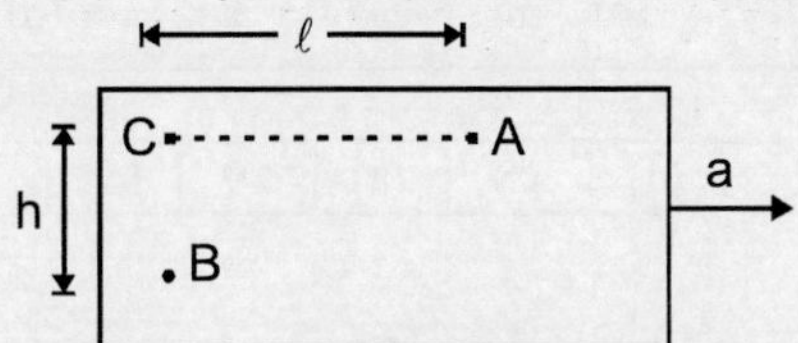

Solution :

Since points A and C are in the same horizontal line but separated by distance ℓ and liquid tank is moving horizontally with acceleration a, hence

$P_C - P_A = \ell\rho a$ or $P_C = P_A + \ell\rho a$

Points B and C are vertically separated by h

$\therefore \quad P_B - P_C = h\rho g$

or $\quad P_B - (P_A + \ell\rho a) = h\rho g$

or $\quad P_B - P_A = h\rho g + \ell\rho a$

Example 5.

Calculate the excess pressure within a bubble of air of radius 0.1 mm in water. If the bubble had been formed 10 cm below the water surface when the atmospheric pressure was 1.013×10^5 Pa, then what would have been the total pressure inside the bubble?

Solution :

Excess pressure within air bubble

$$= \frac{2T}{r} = \frac{2 \times 73 \times 10^{-3}}{0.1 \times 10^{-3}} = 1460 \text{ Pa}$$

The pressure at a depth d, in liquid P = hdg. Therefore, the total pressure inside the air bubble is

$$P_{in} = P_{atm} + hdg + \frac{2T}{r}$$

or $P_{in} = 1.013 \times 10^5 + 10 \times 10^{-2} \times 10^3 \times 9.8 + 1460$

$= 101300 + 980 + 1460$

$= 103740 = 1.037 \times 10^5$ Pa.

Example 6.

A capillary of the shape as shown is dipped in a liquid. Contact angle between the liquid and the capillary is 0° and effect of liquid inside the meniscus is to be neglected. T is the surface tension of the liquid, r is radius of the meniscus, g is acceleration due to gravity and ρ is density of the liquid then determine the height h in equilibrium.

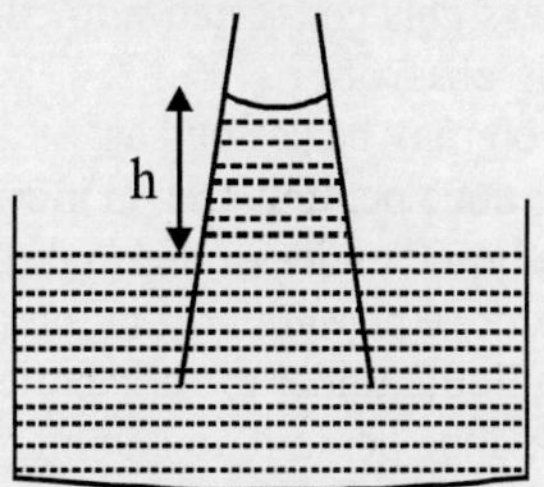

Solution :

As weight of liquid in capillary is balanced by surface tension, then $T \times 2\pi r = \pi r^2 h_1 \rho g$ (for a tube of uniform radius r)

$$h_1 = \frac{2T}{r\rho g}$$

But weight of liquid in tapered tube is more than uniform tube of radius r, then in order to balance $h < h_1$.

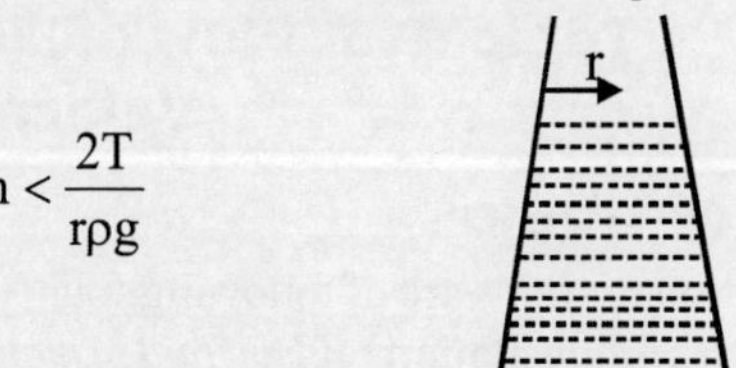

$$h < \frac{2T}{r\rho g}$$

Example 7.

A hydraulic automobile lift is designed to lift car with a maximum mass of 3000 kg. The area of cross-section of the piston carrying the load is 425 cm². What maximum pressure would the smaller piston have to bear ?

Solution :

Here mass of car = 3000 kg.

Area of cross section of larger piston

$= 425 \text{ cm}^2 = 425 \times 10^{-4} \text{ m}^2$.

$\therefore$ The maximum pressure that the smaller piston would have to bear

$$= \frac{\text{Weight of car}}{\text{Area of cross-section}} = \frac{3000 \times 9.8}{425 \times 10^{-4}}$$

$= 6.92 \times 10^5 \text{ Nm}^{-2}$

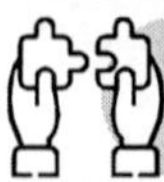

10.2 Concept Practice Problems

CPP

11. At the boiling point of a liquid, surface tension
(a) is zero
(b) is infinite
(c) is same as that at any other temperature
(d) cannot be determined

12. The surface energy of a liquid drop of radius r is proportional to
(a) r^3 (b) r^2 (c) r (d) $\frac{1}{r}$

13. Two liquids drops coalesce to form a large drop. Now,
(a) energy is liberated
(b) energy is neither liberated nor absorbed
(c) some mass gets converted into energy
(d) energy is absorbed

14. Surface tension may be defined as
(a) the work done per unit area in increasing the surface area of a liquid under isothermal condition
(b) the work done per unit area in increasing the surface area of a liquid under the adiabatic condition
(c) the work done per unit area in increasing the surface area of liquid under both isothermal and adiabatic condition
(d) free surface energy per unit volume

15. A liquid does not wet the sides of a solid, if the angle of contact is
(a) Zero (b) Obtuse (more than 90°)
(c) Acute (less than 90°) (d) 90° (right angle)

16. Fevicol is added to paint to be painted on the walls, because
(a) it increases adhesive force between paint and wall.
(b) it decreases adhesive force between paint and wall molecules.
(c) it decreases cohesive force between paint molecules.
(d) None of these

17. A liquid is contained in a vessel. The liquid-solid adhesive force is very weak as compared to the cohesive force in the liquid. The shape of the liquid surface will be
(a) horizontal (b) vertical
(c) concave (d) convex

18. The excess of pressure inside a soap bubble is twice the excess pressure inside a second soap bubble. The volume of the first bubble is n times the volume of the second where n is
(a) 0.125 (b) 0.250 (c) 1 (d) 2

19. One drop of soap bubble of diameter D breaks into 27 drops having surface tension σ. The change in surface energy is
(a) $2\pi\sigma D^2$ (b) $4\pi\sigma D^2$
(c) $\pi\sigma D^2$ (d) $8\pi\sigma D^2$

20. A capillary tube of radius r is immersed in a liquid. The liquid rises to a height h. The corresponding mass is m. What mass of water shall rise in the capillary if the radius of the tube is doubled?
(a) m (b) 2m (c) 3m (d) 4m

ANSWER KEY

11	(a)	12	(b)	13	(a)	14	(a)	15	(b)	16	(a)	17	(d)	18	(a)	19	(d)	20	(b)

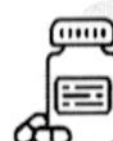

Topic 10.3 : Flow of Liquids, Viscosity, Bernoulli's Theorem, Stoke's Law, Velocity of Efflux and Torricelli's Theorem

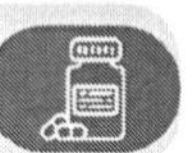

FLOW OF LIQUIDS

The motion of fluids are of following four types :

(i) Streamline motion : *When fluid in motion, if fluid particles preceeding or succeeding a fluid particle follow the same path, then the path is called streamline and the motion of the fluid is called streamline motion.* This type of motion takes place in non-viscous fluids having very small speed.

Principle of continuity : *When incompressible, non-viscous liquid flows in non-uniform tube then in streamline flow product of area and velocity at any section remains same.*

The mass of liquid flowing in equals the mass flowing out.

i.e., $m_1 = m_2$

or, $v_1 A_1 \rho_1 \Delta t = v_2 A_2 \rho_2 \Delta t$ ..... (1)

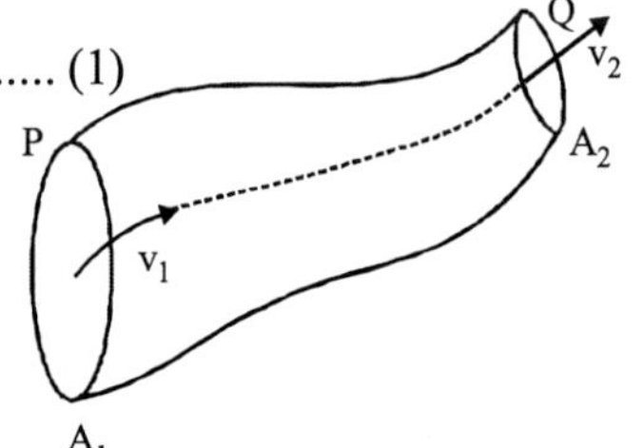

As we have considered the fluid incompressible thus,

$v_1 A_1 = v_2 A_2$

or $Av = constant$ ....(2)

(Since $\rho_1 = \rho_2$)

Equations (1) and (2) are said to be as **equation of continuity**.

(ii) Steady state motion : *In a liquid in motion, when liquid particles, crossing a point, cross it with same velocity, then the motion of the liquid is called steady state motion.* This type of motion takes place in non-viscous liquids having very small speed.

(iii) Laminar motion : *Viscous liquids flow in bounded region or in a pipe, in layers and when viscous liquid is in motion, different layers have different velocities. The layers in contact with the fixed surface has least velocity and the velocity of other parallel layers increases uniformly and continuously with the distance from the fixed surface to the free surface of the liquid. This is called laminar motion of the liquid.*

(iv) Turbulent motion : *When the velocity of a liquid is irregular, haphazard and large, i.e. Beyond a limiting value called critical velocity the flow of liquid loses steadiness then the motion of the liquid is called turbulent motion.*

Critical velocity $V_c = \frac{K\eta}{\rho r}$

Here η is called coefficient of viscosity.

VISCOSITY

The internal friction of the fluid, which tends to oppose relative motion between different layers of the fluid is called viscosity. The viscous force between two layers of a fluid of area A having a velocity gradient $\frac{dv}{dx}$ is given by $F = -\eta A \frac{dv}{dx}$

where η is called the **coefficient of viscosity.**

Its **S.I. unit** is poiseuille or decapoise. The **C.G.S. unit** is called poise.

1 decapoise = 10 poise.

Effects on Viscosity :

(1) Effect of temperature : On increasing temperature viscosity of a liquid decreases.

(2) Effect of pressure : On increasing pressure viscosity of a liquid increases but viscosity of water decreases.

Problem Solving Tips

1. The viscosity of gases increases with increase of temperature, the rate of diffusion increases.
2. The viscosity of liquids decrease with increase of temperature, because the cohesive force between the liquid molecules decreases with increase of temperature.

Critical Velocity :

It is the maximum velocity of a fluid above which a stream line flow changes to a turbulent flow, i.e. it is the maximum velocity of a liquid below which its flow remains streamline.

(i) Reynold's formula for critical velocity is

$$V_c = \frac{N\eta}{\rho r} \quad \text{or} \quad N = \frac{V_c \rho r}{\eta}$$

where N = Reynold's no., η = coefficient of viscosity, ρ = density of liquid; r = radius of tube, N = 1000 for narrow tube.

(ii) (a) If $0 < N < 2000$ then the flow is laminar

(b) If $2000 < N < 3000$ then flow of liquid is unstable and may change from laminar to turbulent

(c) If $N > 3000$, then the flow is turbulent.

(iii) When velocity of fluid is less than its critical velocity then the flow of liquid is determined by its viscosity, its density has no effect on its flow.

(iv) When the velocity of liquid is more than its critical velocity then its flow is determined by its density, where viscosity has little effect on its flow. For example lava from volcano is highly thick, despite that it comes out with high speed.

(v) When $V \le V_c$ the flow of liquid is streamline and when $V > V_c$ then the flow of liquid is turbulent.

$\frac{V_{c_1}}{V_{c_2}} = \frac{r_2}{r_1}$ for same liquid, which is flowing in two tubes of radii r_1 and r_2 respectively.

(vi) The critical velocity of a liquid with high viscosity and smaller radius is higher than that of a liquid with low viscosity and greater radius.

Reynold's Number (N) :

It is pure number which determines the nature of flow of liquid through a pipe.

$$N = \frac{V_c dr}{\eta} = \frac{V_c^2}{\left(\frac{\eta V_c}{r}\right)} = \frac{\textit{Inertial force/area}}{\textit{Viscous force/area}}$$

N is a dimensionless quantity and carries no unit.

BERNOULLI'S THEOREM

For non-viscous, incompressible, streamline flow of fluids the sum of pressure per unit volume, potential energy per unit volume and Kinetic energy per unit volume remain constant.

i.e., $\frac{p}{\rho} + gh + \frac{1}{2}v^2 = constant$

where ρ = density of fluid.

When h = 0 then $\frac{p}{\rho} + \frac{1}{2}v^2$ = constant

Bernoulli's theorem is strictly applicable for an ideal fluid. An ideal fluid is one which is (a) incompressible (b) streamline (c) irrotational and (d) non-viscous.

Applications of Bernoulli's Principle

Dynamic lift :

(i) ***Wings of aeroplane :*** The wings of the aeroplane are having tapering. Due to this specific shape of wings when the aeroplane runs, air passes at higher speed over it as compared to its lower surface. This difference of air speeds above and below the wings, in accordance with Bernoulli's principle, creates a pressure difference, due to which an upward force called 'dynamic lift' (= pressure difference area of wing) acts on the plane. If this force becomes greater than the weight of the plane, the plane will rise up.

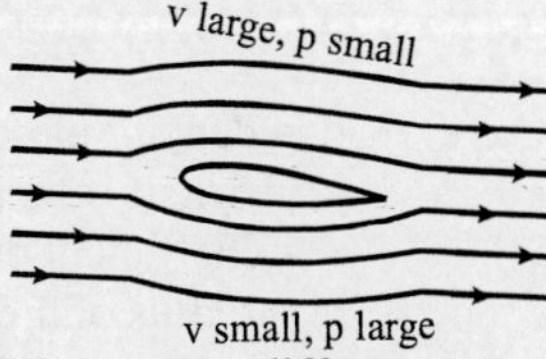

(ii) ***Ball moving without spin:*** The velocity of fluid (air) above and below the ball at corresponding points is the same resulting in zero pressure difference. The air therefore, exerts no upward or downward force on the ball.

(iii) ***Ball moving with spin:*** A ball which is spinning drags air along with it. If the surface is rough more air will be dragged. The streamlines of air for a ball which is moving and spinning at the same time. The ball is moving forward and relative to it the air is moving backwards. Therefore, the velocity of air above the ball relative to it is larger and below it is smaller. The stream lines thus get crowded above and rarified below.

This difference in the velocities of air results in the pressure difference between the lower and upper faces and their is a net upward force on the ball. This dynamic lift due to spinning is called **Magnus effect.**

Some other applications of Bernoulli's principle :

(i) The action of carburator, sprayer or atomizer based on Bernoulli's principle.

(ii) The action of bunsen burner, exhaust pump etc.

(iii) Air foil or lift on aircraft wing works on Bernoulli's principle.

(iv) Motion of a spinning ball i.e., magnus effect.

(v) Blowing of roofs by wind storms etc. based on Bernoullis principle.

STOKE'S LAW

When a solid moves through a viscous medium, its motion is opposed by a viscous force depending on the velocity and shape and size of the body. The energy of the body continuously decreases in overcoming the viscous resistance of the medium. This is why cars, aeroplanes etc. are shaped streamline to minimize the viscous resistance on them.

The viscous drag on a spherical body of radius r, moving with velocity v, in a viscous medium of viscosity η is given by

$$F_{viscous} = 6\pi\eta rv$$

This relation is called Stokes' law.

Importance of Stoke's law :

(i) It is used in the determination of electronic charge with the help of milikan's experiment.

(ii) It accounts the formation of clouds.

(iii) It accounts why the speed of rain drops is less than that of a body falling freely with a constant velocity from the height of clouds.

(iv) It helps a man coming down with the help of a parachute.

Terminal Velocity :

When a spherical body is allowed to fall through viscous medium, its velocity increases till the viscous drag plus upthrust is equal to the weight of the body. After that body moves with constant velocity, called terminal velocity.

The terminal velocity is given by $v = \frac{2R^2}{9\eta}(d-\sigma)g$

where d = density of body,
σ = density of medium,
η = coefficient of viscosity of medium,
R = radius of the spherical body.

From terminal velocity, $V \alpha \frac{1}{\eta}$, i.e. greater the viscosity, smaller is the terminal speed.

Flow of liquid through tube /pipe :

(i) Poiseuille's equation is $Q = \frac{\pi pr^4}{8\eta\ell}$, where p is the pressure difference between the two ends of the tubes, r is the radius, ℓ is the length of the tube and η is the coefficient of viscosity, Q = rate of flow of liquid.

Equivalent liquid resistance $= \frac{8\eta\ell_1}{\pi r_1^4} + \frac{8\eta\ell_2^2}{\pi r_2^4}$, *when tube are joined* **in series**.

It means that liquid flow through capillary tube is similar to flow of electric current through a conductor i.e., Q (rate of liquid flow) corresponds to I (rate of flow of charge), pressure difference similar to potential difference.

(ii) When two tubes are joined in series then the volume of fluid flowing through the two tubes is the same but the pressure difference across the two tubes is different. The total pressure difference, $P = P_1 + P_2$.

(iii) If two tubes are joined in **parallel** then the pressure difference across the two tubes is the same but the volume of fluid flowing through the two tubes is different. The total volume of the fluid flowing through the tube in one second is $Q = Q_1 + Q_2$.

VELOCITY OF EFFLUX AND TORRICELLI'S THEOREM

(i) **Torricelli's theorem :** For liquid filled in a tank upto a height H having a hole O at a depth h from free level of liquid through which the liquid is coming out, *velocity of efflux of liquid* $v = \sqrt{2gh}$.

(ii) *Time taken by the liquid in falling from hole to ground level*

$$t = \sqrt{\frac{2(H-h)}{g}}$$

(iii) *The horizontal range covered by the liquid*

x = horizontal velocity (v) × time (t)

$$= \sqrt{2gh} \times \sqrt{\frac{2(H-h)}{g}} = 2\sqrt{h(H-h)}.$$

For maximum horizontal range, differentiating both side w.r.t. h and we get h = H/2, the range is maximum.

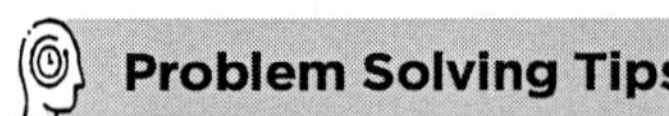

Problem Solving Tips

1. The cross-section of the water stream from a top decreases as it goes down in accordance with the equation of continuity.
2. When a hale blows over a roof, the force on the roof is upwards.
3. Sudden fall in atmospheric pressure predicts possibility of a storm.
4. **Venturimeter** is a device used for the measurement of the rate of flow of incompressible fluid through a tube. Its working is based on Bernoulli's principle.

Example 8.

The vessel of area of cross-section A has liquid to a height H. There is a hole at the bottom of vessel having area of cross-section a. Find the time taken to decrease the level from H_1 to H_2.

Solution :

The average velocity of efflux, $v = \frac{\sqrt{2gH_1} + \sqrt{2gH_2}}{2}$

Let t be the time taken to empty the tank from level H_1 to H_2.

Then, $\frac{\sqrt{2gH_1} + \sqrt{2gH_2}}{2} \times a \times t = A\,[H_1 - H_2]$

or t $= \frac{A}{a} \times \sqrt{\left(\frac{2}{g}\right)} \times \left[\frac{(H_1 - H_2) \times \left(\sqrt{H_1} - \sqrt{H_2}\right)}{\left(\sqrt{H_1} + \sqrt{H_2}\right)\left(\sqrt{H_1} - \sqrt{H_2}\right)}\right]$

$$= \frac{A}{a} \times \sqrt{\left(\frac{2}{g}\right)} \times \left(\sqrt{H_1} - \sqrt{H_2}\right) = \frac{A}{a} \times \sqrt{\left(\frac{2}{g}\right)} \times \left(\sqrt{H_1} - \sqrt{H_2}\right)$$

Example 9.

In a test experiment on a model aeroplane in a wind tunnel, the flow speeds on the upper and lower surfaces of the wing are 70 m/s and 63 m/s respectively. What is the lift on the wing if its area is 2.5 m^2 ? Take the density of air to be 1.3 kg m^{-3}.

Solution :

Let v_1 be the speed and P_1 be the pressure on the upper surface of the wing, and corresponding values on the lower surface be v_2 and P_2 respectively.

$\therefore$ $v_1 = 70$ m/s, $v_2 = 63$ m/s, $A = 2.5\ m^2$,
$P = 1.3\ kg\ m^{-3}$.

According to Bernoulli's theorem

$$P_1 + \frac{1}{2}\rho v_1^2 = P_2 + \frac{1}{2}\rho v_2^2$$

$$P_2 - P_1 = \frac{1}{2}\rho(v_1^2 - v_2^2) = P_2 - P_1 = \frac{1}{2} \times 3 \times (70^2 - 63^2)$$

Force (lift) on the wing $= A(P_2 - P_1)$

$$= 2.5 \times \frac{1}{2} \times 1.3 \times (70^2 - 63^2)$$

$$= 2.5 \times \frac{1}{2} \times 1.3 \times 133 \times 7$$

$$= 1.5 \times 10^3 N$$

Example 10.

In Millikan's oil drop experiment, what is the terminal speed of an uncharged drop of radius 2.0×10^{-5} m and density $1.2 \times 10^3\ kg\ m^{-3}$. Take the viscosity of air at the temperature of the experiment to be 1.8×10^{-5} Pa s. How much is the viscous force on the drop at that speed ? Neglect buoyancy of the drop due to air.

Solution :

Here, $r = 2.0 \times 10^{-5}$ m, $\rho = 1.2 \times 10^3\ kg\ m^{-3}$,
$\eta = 1.8 \times 10^{-5}$ Pa s.

From formula, terminal velocity

$$V = \frac{2}{9}\frac{r^2(\rho - \sigma)g}{\eta}$$

$$\Rightarrow V = \frac{2 \times (2 \times 10^{-5})^2 (1.2 \times 10^3 - 0) \times 9.8}{9 \times 1.8 \times 10^{-5}} = 5.8 \times 10^{-2}\ ms^{-1}$$

Now viscous force on the drop

$F = 6\pi\eta rv$

$$\Rightarrow F = 6 \times \frac{22}{7} \times (1.8 \times 10^{-5}) \times (2 \times 10^{-5}) \times 5.8 \times 10^{-2}$$

$$= 3.93 \times 10^{-19} N$$

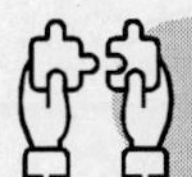

10.3 Concept Practice Problems

CPP

21. The difference between viscosity and solid friction is/are
(a) viscosity depends on area while solid friction does not
(b) viscosity depends on nature of material but solid friction does not
(c) both (a) and (b)
(d) neither (a) nor (b)

22. Water is flowing through a horizontal pipe having a restriction, then
(a) pressure will be greater at the restriction.
(b) pressure will be greater in the wider portion.
(c) pressure will be same throughout the length of the pipe.
(d) None of these

23. A cylinder is filled with non-viscous liquid of density d to a height h_0 and a hole is made at a height h_1 from the bottom of the cylinder. The velocity of the liquid issuing out of the hole is
(a) $\sqrt{2gh_0}$ (b) $\sqrt{2g(h_0 - h_1)}$
(c) $\sqrt{dgh_1}$ (d) $\sqrt{dgh_0}$

24. The velocity of efflux of a liquid through an orifice in the bottom of the tank does not depend upon
(a) size of orifice
(b) height of liquid
(c) acceleration due to gravity
(d) density of liquid

25. The lift of an air plane is based on
(a) Torricelli's theorem
(b) Bernoulli's theorem
(c) Law of gravitation
(d) conservation of linear momentum

26. The level of water in a tank is 5m high. A hole of area 1 cm^2 is made in the bottom of the tank. The rate of leakage of water from the hole ($g = 10\ m/s^2$) is
(a) $10^{-2}\ m^3/s$ (b) $10^{-3}\ m^3/s$
(c) $10^{-4}\ m^3/s$ (d) $10^3\ m^3/s$

27. A cylinder of height 20m is completely filled with water. The velocity of efflux of water (in ms^{-1}) through a small hole on the side wall or the cylinder near its bottom is
(a) 10 m/s (b) 20 m/s (c) 25.5 m/s (d) 5 m/s

28. Water flows in a stream line manner through a capillary tube of radius a, the pressure difference being P and the rate flow Q. If the radius is reduced to $\frac{a}{2}$ and the pressure is increased to 2P, the rate of flow becomes
(a) 4Q (b) Q (c) $\frac{Q}{2}$ (d) $\frac{Q}{8}$

29. Horizontal tube of non-uniform cross-section has radii of 0.1 m and 0.05 m respectively at M and N for a streamline flow of liquid the rate of liquid flow is
(a) continuously changes with time
(b) greater at M than at N
(c) greater at N than at M
(d) same at M and N

30. There is a hole in the bottom of tank having water. If total pressure at bottom is 3 atm (1 atm = $10^5\ N/m^2$) then the velocity of water flowing from hole is
(a) $\sqrt{400}$ m/s (b) $\sqrt{600}$ m/s
(c) $\sqrt{60}$ m/s (d) None of these

ANSWER KEY

21	(a)	22	(b)	23	(b)	24	(a)	25	(b)	26	(b)	27	(b)	28	(d)	29	(d)	30	(a)

CONCEPT MAP

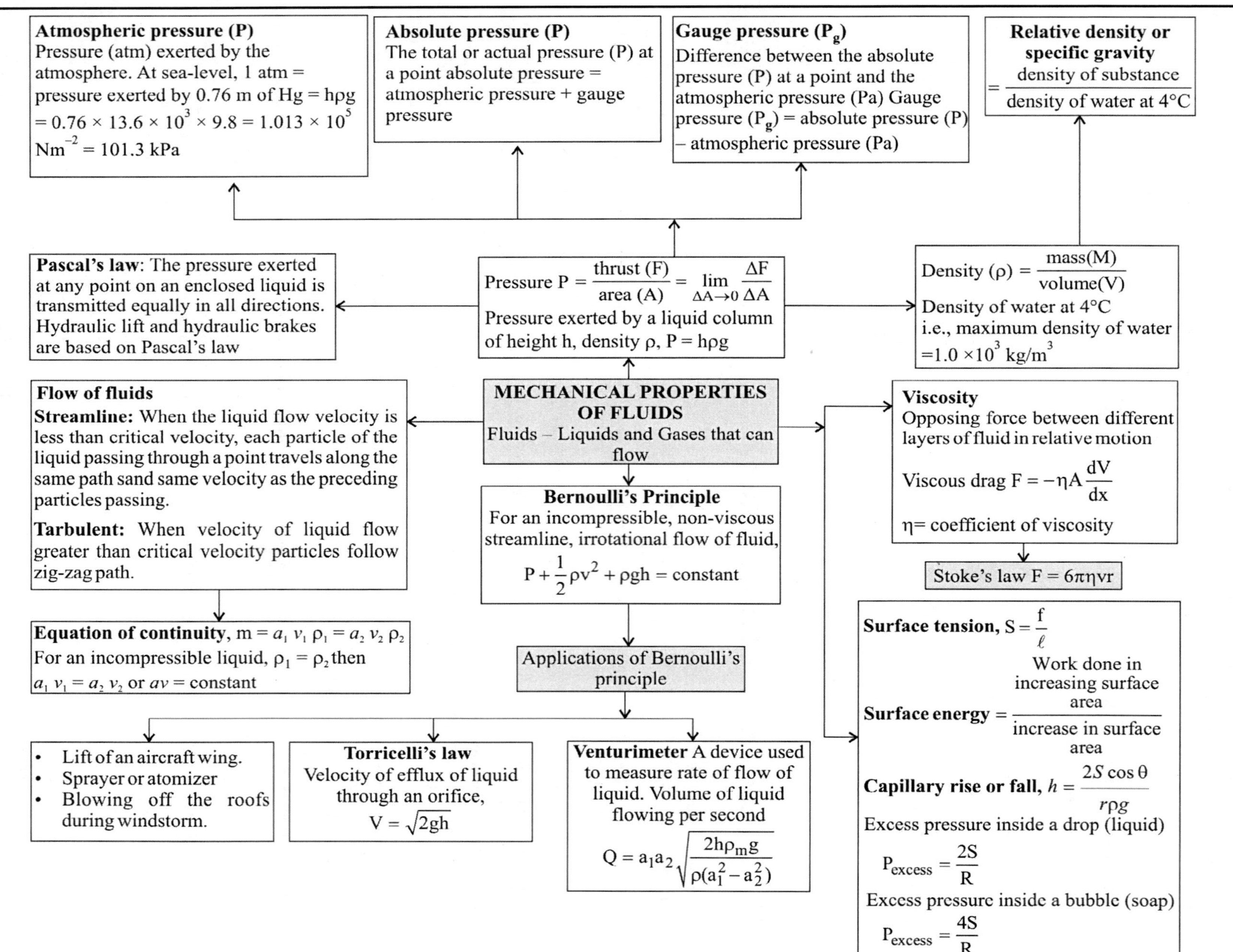
Atmospheric pressure (P)
Pressure (atm) exerted by the atmosphere. At sea-level, 1 atm = pressure exerted by 0.76 m of Hg = hρg = 0.76 × 13.6 × 10³ × 9.8 = 1.013 × 10⁵ Nm⁻² = 101.3 kPa
Absolute pressure (P)
The total or actual pressure (P) at a point absolute pressure = atmospheric pressure + gauge pressure
Gauge pressure (Pg)
Difference between the absolute pressure (P) at a point and the atmospheric pressure (Pa) Gauge pressure (Pg) = absolute pressure (P) – atmospheric pressure (Pa)
Relative density or specific gravity
= density of substance / density of water at 4°C
Pascal's law: The pressure exerted at any point on an enclosed liquid is transmitted equally in all directions. Hydraulic lift and hydraulic brakes are based on Pascal's law
Pressure P = thrust (F) / area (A) = lim ΔA→0 ΔF/ΔA
Pressure exerted by a liquid column of height h, density ρ, P = hρg
Density (ρ) = mass(M) / volume(V)
Density of water at 4°C
i.e., maximum density of water
=1.0 ×10³ kg/m³
Flow of fluids
Streamline: When the liquid flow velocity is less than critical velocity, each particle of the liquid passing through a point travels along the same path sand same velocity as the preceding particles passing.
Tarbulent: When velocity of liquid flow greater than critical velocity particles follow zig-zag path.
MECHANICAL PROPERTIES OF FLUIDS
Fluids – Liquids and Gases that can flow
Viscosity
Opposing force between different layers of fluid in relative motion
Viscous drag F = −ηA dV/dx
η= coefficient of viscosity
Bernoulli's Principle
For an incompressible, non-viscous streamline, irrotational flow of fluid,
P + ½ρv² + ρgh = constant
Stoke's law F = 6πηvr
Equation of continuity, m = a₁ v₁ ρ₁ = a₂ v₂ ρ₂
For an incompressible liquid, ρ₁ = ρ₂ then
a₁ v₁ = a₂ v₂ or av = constant
Applications of Bernoulli's principle
Surface tension, S = f/ℓ
Surface energy = Work done in increasing surface area / increase in surface area
Capillary rise or fall, h = 2S cos θ / rρg
Excess pressure inside a drop (liquid)
P_excess = 2S/R
Excess pressure inside a bubble (soap)
P_excess = 4S/R
• Lift of an aircraft wing.
• Sprayer or atomizer
• Blowing off the roofs during windstorm.
Torricelli's law
Velocity of efflux of liquid through an orifice,
V = √2gh
Venturimeter A device used to measure rate of flow of liquid. Volume of liquid flowing per second
Q = a₁a₂ √(2hρₘg / ρ(a₁² − a₂²))

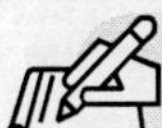

Exercise 1 - Chapter Revision Problems

CRP

1. The terminal velocity depends upon

(a) $\frac{1}{r}$ (b) $\frac{1}{r^2}$ (c) $\frac{1}{r^3}$ (d) r^2

2. Water is not used in thermometer because

(a) it sticks to glass

(b) its shows anamalous expansion

(c) both (a) and (b)

(d) neither (a) nor (b)

3. Gases do not posses

(a) density (b) surface tension

(c) volume (d) viscosity

4. A small ball (menu) falling under graivty in a viscous medium experiences a drag force proportional to the instantaneous speed u such that $F_{drag} = Ku$. Then the terminal speed of the ball within the viscous medium is

(a) $\frac{K}{mg}$ (b) $\frac{mg}{K}$ (c) $\sqrt{\frac{mg}{K}}$ (d) $\left(\frac{mg}{K}\right)^2$

5. The constant velocity attained by a body while falling through a viscous medium is termed as

(a) critical velocity (b) terminal velocity

(c) threshold velocity (d) None of these

6. A liquid is allowed to flow into a tube of truncated cone shape. Identify the correct statement from the following.

(a) The speed is high at the wider end and high at the narrow end.

(b) The speed is low at the wider end and high at the narrow end.

(c) The speed is same at both ends in a stream line flow.

(d) The liquid flows with uniform velocity in the tube.

7. A spherical ball of iron of radius 2 mm is falling through a column of glycerine. If densities of glycerine and iron are respectively 1.3×10^3 kg/m^3 and 8×10^3 kg/m^3. η for glycerine = 0.83 Nm^{-2} sec, then the terminal velocity is

(a) 0.7 m/s (b) 0.07 m/s

(c) 0.007 m/s (d) 0.0007 m/s

8. 8 mercury drops coalesce to form one mercury drop, the energy changes by a factor of

(a) 1 (b) 2 (c) 4 (d) 6

9. Water rises to a height of 10 cm in capillary tube and mercury falls to a depth of 3.1 cm in the same capillary tube. If the density of mercury is 13.6 and the angle of contact for mercury is 135°, the approximate ratio of surface tensions of water and mercury is

(a) 1 : 0.15 (b) 1 : 3 (c) 1 : 6 (d) 1.5 : 1

10. A vessel with water is placed on a weighing pan and it reads 600 g. Now a ball of mass 40 g and density 0.80 g cm^{-3} is sunk into the water with a pin of negligible volume, as shown in figure keeping it sunk. The weighting pan will show a reading

(a) 600 g

(b) 550 g

(c) 650 g

(d) 632 g

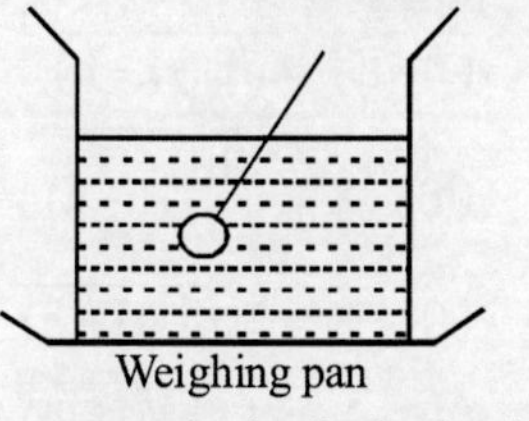

11. A rain drop of radius 0.3 mm has a terminal velocity in air = 1 m/s. The viscosity of air is 8×10^{-5} poise. The viscous force on it is

(a) 45.2×10^{-4} dyne (b) 101.73×10^{-5} dyne

(c) 16.95×10^{-4} dyne (d) 16.95×10^{-5} dyne

12. 1 m^3 water is brought inside the lake upto 200 metres depth from the surface of the lake. What will be change in the volume when the bulk modulus of elastically of water is 22000 atmosphere?

(density of water is 1×10^3 kg/m^3 atmosphere pressure = 10^5 N/m^2 and g = 10 m/s^2)

(a) 8.9×10^{-3} m^3 (b) 7.8×10^{-3} m^3

(c) 9.1×10^{-4} m^3 (d) 8.7×10^{-4} m^3

13. In the figure, the velocity V_3 will be

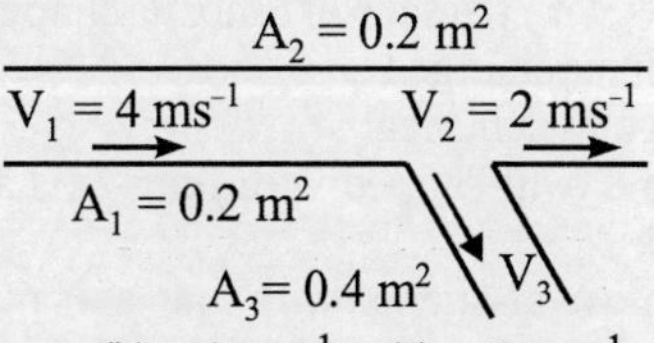

(a) Zero (b) 4 ms^{-1} (c) 1 ms^{-1} (d) 3 ms^{-1}

14. 1 centipoise is equal to

(a) 1 kg m^{-1} s^{-1} (b) 1000 kg m^{-1} s^{-1}

(c) 0.1 kg m^{-1} s^{-1} (d) 0.001 kg m^{-1} s^{-1}

15. If a water drop is kept between two glass plates, then its shape is

(a) 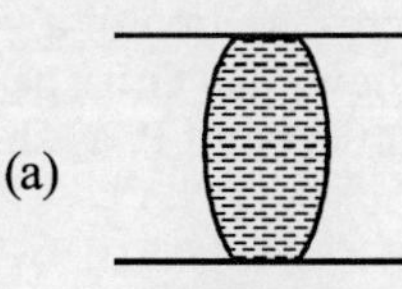 (b) 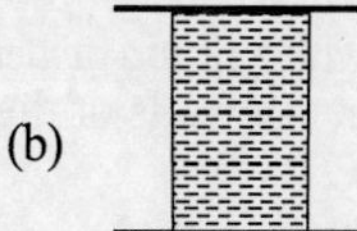

(c) 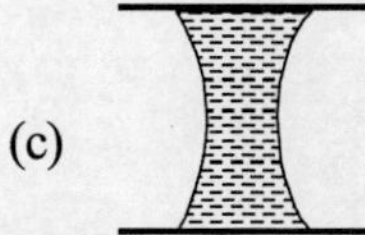 (d) None of these

16. The fraction of a floating object of volume V_0 and density d_0 above the surface of liquid of density d will be

(a) $\frac{d_0}{d - d_0}$ (b) $\frac{d - d_0}{d}$ (c) $\frac{d_0}{d}$ (d) $\frac{d_0 d}{d + d_0}$

17. Two drops of the same radius are falling through air with a steady velocity of 5 cm per sec. If the two drops coalesce, the terminal velocity would be

(a) 10 cm per sec (b) 2.5 cm per sec

(c) $5 \times (4)^{1/3}$ cm per sec (d) $5 \times \sqrt{3}$ cm per sec

18. A tank is filled with water upto a height H. Water is allowed to come out of a hole P in one of the walls at a depth h below the surface of water (see fig.) Express the horizontal distance X in terms H and h.

(a) $X=\sqrt{h(H-h)}$

(b) $X=\sqrt{\frac{h}{2}(H-h)}$

(c) $X=2\sqrt{h(H-h)}$

(d) $X=4\sqrt{h(H-h)}$

19. In case A, when an 80 kg skydiver falls with arms and legs fully extended to maximize his surface area, his terminal velocity is 60 m/s. In Case B, when the same skydiver falls with arms and legs pulled in and body angled downward to minimize his surface area, his terminal velocity increases to 80 m/s. In going from Case A to Case B, which of the following statements most accurately describes what the skydiver experiences?

(a) $F_{air\ resistance}$ increases and pressure P increases
(b) $F_{air\ resistance}$ increases and pressure P decreases
(c) $F_{air\ resistance}$ decreases and pressure P increases
(d) $F_{air\ resistance}$ remains the same and pressure P increases

20. In a satellite moving round any planet, the gravitational force is effectively balanced. If an ice cube exists there, and it melts with passage of time, its shape will

(a) remain unchanged
(b) change to spherical
(c) become oval-shaped with long-axis along the orbit plane
(d) become oval-shaped with long axis perpendicular to orbit plane

21. An egg when placed in ordinary water sinks but floats when placed in brine. This is because

(a) density of brine is less than that of ordinary water
(b) density of brine is equal to that of ordinary water
(c) density of brine is greater than that of ordinary water
(d) None of these

22. Figure here shows the vertical cross section of a vessel filled with a liquid of density ρ. The normal thrust per unit area on the walls of the vessel at the point P, as shown, will be

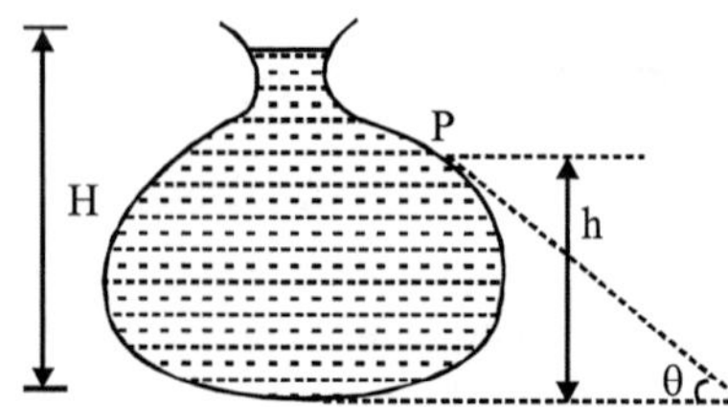

(a) $h\rho g$ (b) $H\rho g$
(c) $(H-h)\rho g$ (d) $(H-h)\rho g\cos\theta$

23. The pressure energy per unit volume of a liquid is

(a) $\frac{P}{\rho}$ (b) P (c) $P\times\rho$ (d) $\frac{\rho}{P}$

24. A fast train goes past way side station platform at high speed. A person standing at the edge of the platform is

(a) attracted to train
(b) repelled from train
(c) unaffected by outgoing train
(d) affected only if the train's speed is more than the speed of sound

25. Figure shows a capillary rise H. If the air is blown through the horizontal tube in the direction as shown then rise in capillary tube will be

(a) =H
(b) >H
(c) <H
(d) zero

26. Two liquids of densities d_1 and d_2 are flowing in identical capillary tubes uder the same pressure difference. If t_1 and t_2 are time taken for the flow of equal quantities (mass) of liquids, then the ratio of coefficient of viscosity of liquids must be

(a) $\frac{d_1t_1}{d_2t_2}$ (b) $\frac{t_1}{t_2}$ (c) $\frac{d_2}{d_1}\frac{t_2}{t_1}$ (d) $\sqrt{\frac{d_1t_1}{d_2t_2}}$

27. A tank has a small hole at its botom of area of cross-section a. Liquid is being poured in the tank at the rate Vm^3/s, the maximum level of liquid in the container will be (Area of tank A)

(a) $\frac{V}{gaA}$ (b) $\frac{V^2}{2gAa}$ (c) $\frac{V^2}{gAa}$ (d) $\frac{V}{2gaA}$

28. A hollow spherical shell at outer radius *R* floats just submerged under the water surface. The inner radius of the shell is *r*. If the specific gravity of the shell material is $\frac{27}{8}$ w.r.t water, the value of *r* is :

(a) $\frac{8}{9}R$ (b) $\frac{4}{9}R$ (c) $\frac{2}{3}R$ (d) $\frac{1}{3}R$

29. An air bubble of radius 1 cm in water has an upward acceleration 9.8 cm s^{-2}. The density of water is 1 gm cm^{-3} and water offers negligible drag force on the bubble. The mass of the bubble is ($g = 980\ cm/s^2$)

(a) 4.51 gm (b) 3.15 gm (c) 4.15 gm (d) 1.52 gm

30. A submarine experiences a pressure of 5.05×10^6 Pa at depth of d_1 in a sea. When it goes further to a depth of d_2, it experiences a pressure of 8.08×10^6 Pa. Then $d_1 - d_1$ is approximately (density of water $=10^3$ kg/m^3 and acceleration due to gravity = 10 ms^{-2}):

(a) 300 m (b) 400 m (c) 600 m (d) 500 m

31. A wooden block floating in a bucket of water has $\frac{4}{5}$ of its volume submerged. When certain amount of an oil poured into the bucket, it is found that the block is just under the oil surface with half of its volume under water and half in oil. The density of oil relative to that of water is:

(a) 0.5 (b) 0.8 (c) 0.6 (c) 0.7

32. A soap bubble, blown by a mechanical pump at the mouth of a tube, increases in volume, with time, at a constant rate. The graph that correctly depicts the time dependence of pressure inside the bubble is given by:

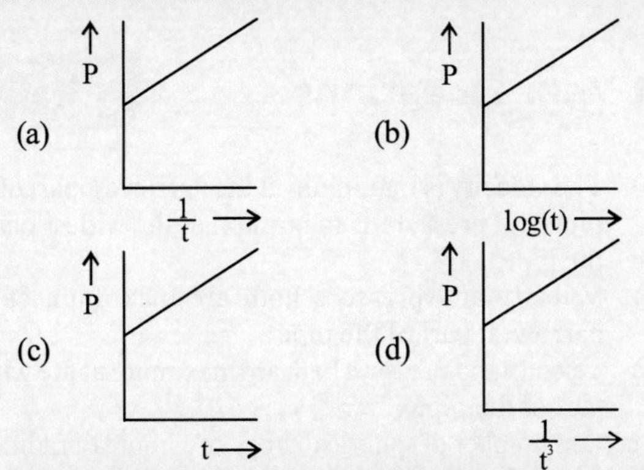

33. A jar is filled with two non-mixing liquids 1 and 2 having densities ρ_1 and, ρ_2 respectively. A solid ball, made of a material of density ρ_3, is dropped in the jar. It comes to equilibrium in the position shown in the figure. Which of the following is true for ρ_1, ρ_2 and ρ_3?

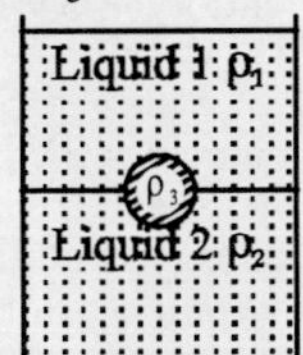

(a) $\rho_3 < \rho_1 < \rho_2$
(b) $\rho_1 > \rho_3 > \rho_2$
(c) $\rho_1 < \rho_2 < \rho_3$
(d) $\rho_1 < \rho_3 < \rho_2$

34. A liquid rises in a capillary tube if the angle of contact is
(a) obtuse (b) acute (c) π (d) $\pi/2$

35. A fluid is flowing through a horizontal pipe of varying cross-section, with speed v ms^{-1} at a point where the pressure is P Pascal. At another point where pressure is $\frac{P}{2}$ Pascal its speed is V ms^{-1}. If the density of the fluid is ρ kg m^{-3} and the flow is streamline, then V is equal to :

(a) $\sqrt{\frac{P}{\rho}+v}$ (b) $\sqrt{\frac{2P}{\rho}+v^2}$ (c) $\sqrt{\frac{P}{2\rho}+v^2}$ (d) $\sqrt{\frac{P}{\rho}+v^2}$

36. Water from a pipe is coming at a rate of 100 liters per minute. If the radius of the pipe is 5 cm, the Reynolds number for the flow is of the order of : (density of water = 1000 kg/m^3, coefficient of viscosity of water = 1 mPa *s*)
(a) 10^3 (b) 10^4 (c) 10^2 (d) 10^6

37. Water flows into a large tank with flat bottom at the rate of 10^{-4} m^3 s$^{-(}$1) Water is also leaking out of a hole of area 1 cm^2 at its bottom. If the height of the water in the tank remains steady, then this height is:
(a) 5.1 cm (b) 7 cm (c) 4 cm (d) 9 cm

38. If it takes 5 minutes to fill a 15 litre bucket from a water tap of diameter $\frac{2}{\sqrt{\pi}}$ cm then the Reynolds number for the flow is (density of water = 10^3 kg/m^3) and viscosity of water = 10^{-3} Pa.s) close to :
(a) 1100 (b) 11,000 (c) 550 (d) 5500

39. Water is flowing at a speed of 1.5 ms^{-1} through horizontal tube of cross-sectional area 10^{-2} m^2 and you are trying to stop the flow by your palm. Assuming that the water stops immediately after hitting the palm, the minimum force that you must exert should be
(density of water = 10^3 kgm^{-3})
(a) 15 N (b) 22.5 N (c) 33.7 N (d) 45 N

40. Air of density 1.2 kg m^{-3} is blowing across the horizontal wings of an aeroplane in such a way that its speeds above and below the wings are 150 ms^{-1} and 100 ms^{-1}, respectively. The pressure difference between the upper and lower sides of the wings, is :
(a) 60 Nm^{-2} (b) 180 Nm^{-2}
(c) 7500 Nm^{-2} (d) 12500 Nm^{-2}

41. Water is flowing continuously from a tap having an internal diameter 8×10^{-3} m. The water velocity as it leaves the tap is 0.4 ms^{-1}. The diameter of the water stream at a distance 2×10^{-1} m below the tap is close to:
(a) 7.5×10^{-3} m (b) 9.6×10^{-3} m
(c) 3.6×10^{-3} m (d) 5.0×10^{-3} m

42. In an experiment to verify Stokes law, a small spherical ball of radius r and density ρ falls under gravity through a distance h in air before entering a tank of water. If the terminal velocity of the ball inside water is same as its velocity just before entering the water surface, then the value of h is proportional to : (ignore viscosity of air)
(a) r^4 (b) r (c) r^3 (d) r^2

43. At which of the following temperature the value of surface tension of water is minimum?
(a) 4°C (b) 25°C (c) 75°C (d) 50°C

44. The terminal velocity of a small sphere of radius a in a viscous liquid is proportional to
(a) a^2 (b) a^3 (c) a (d) a^{-1}

45. Spherical balls of radius 'R' are falling in a viscous fluid of viscosity 'η' with a velocity 'v'. The retarding viscous force acting on the spherical ball is
(a) inversely proportional to both radius 'R' and velocity 'v'
(b) directly proportional to both radius 'R' and velocity 'v'
(c) directly proportional to 'R' but inversely proportional to 'v'
(d) inversely proportional to 'R' but directly proportional to velocity 'v'

46. Pressure inside two soap bubbles are 1.01 and 1.02 atmosphere, respectively. The ratio of their volumes is :
(a) 4 : 1 (b) 0.8 : 1 (c) 8 : 1 (d) 2 : 1

47. If 'M' is the mass of water that rises in a capillary tube of radius 'r', then mass of water which will rise in a capillary tube of radius '2r' is :
(a) M (b) $\frac{M}{2}$ (c) 4 M (d) 2 M

48. Wax is coated on the inner wall of a capillary tube and the tube is then dipped in water. Then, compared to the unwaxed capillary, the angle of contact θ and the height h upto which water rises change. These changes are :
(a) θ increases and h also increases
(b) θ decreases and h also decreases
(c) θ increases and h decreases
(d) θ decreases and h increases

49. Work done in increasing the size of a soap bubble from a radius of 3 cm to 5 cm is nearly (Surface tension of soap solution = 0.03 Nm^{-1})
(a) 0.2πmJ (b) 2πmJ (c) 0.4πmJ (d) 4πmJ

50. Two mercury drops (each of radius 'r') merge to form bigger drop. The surface energy of the bigger drop, if T is the surface tension, is :
(a) $4\pi r^2 T$ (b) $2\pi r^2 T$ (c) $2^{8/3}\pi r^2 T$ (d) $2^{5/3}\pi r^2 T$

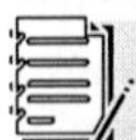

Exercise 2 - Exemplar & Past Year Questions

E&PYQs

Exemplar Questions

1. Which of the following diagrams does not represent a streamline flow?

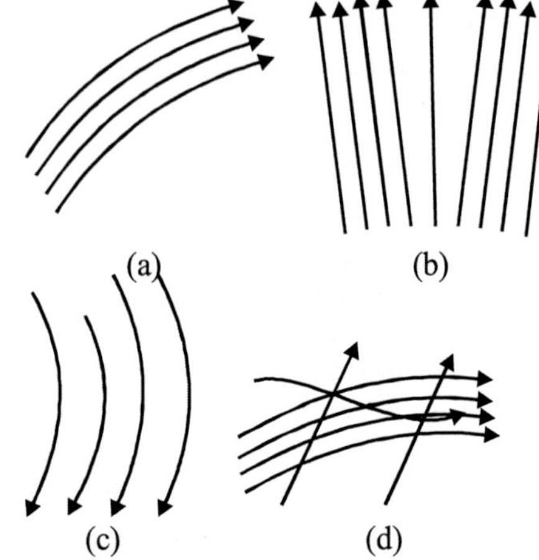

2. Along a streamline,
   (a) the velocity of a fluid particle remains constant
   (b) the velocity of all fluid particles crossing a given position is constant
   (c) the velocity of all fluid particles at a given instant is constant
   (d) the speed of a fluid particle remains constant

3. An ideal fluid flows through a pipe of circular cross-section made of two sections with diameters 2.5 cm and 3.75 cm. The ratio of the velocities in the two pipes is

   (a) $9:4$ (b) $3:2$ (c) $\sqrt{3}:\sqrt{2}$ (d) $\sqrt{2}:\sqrt{3}$

4. The angle of contact at the interface of water-glass is 0°, ethyl alcohol-glass is 0°, mercury-glass is 140° and methyliodide-glass is 30°. A glass capillary is put in a trough containing one of these four liquids. It is observed that the meniscus is convex. The liquid in the trough is
   (a) water (b) ethylalcohol
   (c) mercury (d) methyliodide

NEET/AIPMT (2013-2020) Questions

5. The wetability of a surface by a liquid depends primarily on *[2013]*
   (a) surface tension
   (b) density
   (c) angle of contact between the surface and the liquid
   (d) viscosity

6. A fluid is in streamline flow across a horizontal pipe of variable area of cross section. For this which of the following statements is correct? *[NEET Kar. 2013]*
   (a) The velocity is minimum at the narrowest part of the pipe and the pressure is minimum at the widest part of the pipe
   (b) The velocity is maximum at the narrowest part of the pipe and pressure is maximum at the widest part of the pipe
   (c) Velocity and pressure both are maximum at the narrowest part of the pipe
   (d) Velocity and pressure both are maximum at the widest part of the pipe

7. A certain number of spherical drops of a liquid of radius 'r' coalesce to form a single drop of radius 'R' and volume 'V'. If 'T' is the surface tension of the liquid, then : *[2014]*

   (a) energy $= 4VT\left(\frac{1}{r}-\frac{1}{R}\right)$ is released

   (b) energy $= 3VT\left(\frac{1}{r}+\frac{1}{R}\right)$ is absorbed

   (c) energy $= 3VT\left(\frac{1}{r}-\frac{1}{R}\right)$ is released

   (d) energy is neither released nor absorbed

8. The cylindrical tube of a spray pump has radius, R, one end of which has n fine holes, each of radius r. If the speed of the liquid in the tube is V, the speed of the ejection of the liquid through the holes is : *[2015 RS]*

   (a) $\frac{VR^2}{nr^2}$ (b) $\frac{VR^2}{n^3r^2}$ (c) $\frac{V^2R}{nr}$ (d) $\frac{VR^2}{n^2r^2}$

9. A wind with speed 40 m/s blows parallel to the roof of a house. The area of the roof is 250 m^2. Assuming that the pressure inside the house is atmospheric pressure, the force exerted by the wind on the roof and the direction of the force will be $(\rho_{air} = 1.2\ kg/m^3)$ *[2015]*
   (a) 4.8×10^5 N, upwards
   (b) 2.4×10^5 N, upwards
   (c) 2.4×10^5 N, downwards
   (d) 4.8×10^5 N, downwards

10. Two non-mixing liquids of densities ρ and $n\rho (n > 1)$ are put in a container. The height of each liquid is h. A solid cylinder of length L and density d is put in this container. The cylinder floats with its axis vertical and length $pL (p < 1)$ in the denser liquid. The density d is equal to : *[2016]*
    (a) $\{1+(n+1)p\}\rho$ (b) $\{2+(n+1)p\}\rho$
    (c) $\{2+(n-1)p\}\rho$ (d) $\{1+(n-1)p\}\rho$

11. A small sphere of radius 'r' falls from rest in a viscous liquid. As a result, heat is produced due to viscous force. The rate of production of heat when the sphere attains its terminal velocity, is proportional to *[2018]*
    (a) r^3 (b) r^2 (c) r^4 (d) r^5

12. A small hole of area of cross-section 2 mm^2 is present near the bottom of a fully filled open tank of height 2 m. Taking $g = 10\ m/s^2$, the rate of flow of water through the open hole would be nearly: *[2019]*
    (a) $12.6\ 10^{-6}\ m^3/s$ (b) $8.9\ 10^{-6} m^3/s$
    (c) $2.23\ 10^{-6}\ m^3/s$ (d) $6.4\ 10^{-6}\ m^3/s$

13. Two small spherical metal balls, having equal masses, are made from materials of densities ρ_1 and ρ_2 $(\rho_1 = 8\rho_2)$ and have radii of 1 mm and 2 mm, respectively, they are made to

fall vertically (from rest) in a viscous medium whose coefficient of viscosity equals η and whose density is $0.1\rho_2$. The ratio of their terminal velocities would be,
[NEET Odisha 2019]

(a) $\frac{79}{36}$ (b) $\frac{79}{72}$ (c) $\frac{19}{36}$ (d) $\frac{39}{72}$

14. A soap bubble, having radius of 1 mm, is blown from a detergent solution having a surface tension of 2.5 10–2 N/m. The pressure inside the bubble equals at a point Z_0 below the free surface of water in a container. Taking $g = 10\ m/s^2$, density of water = $10_3\ kg/m_3$, the value of Z_0 is : *[2019]*

(a) 100 cm (b) 10 cm (c) 1 cm (d) 0.5 cm

15. A capillary tube of radius r is immersed in water and water rises in it to a height h. The mass of the water in the capillary is 5 g. Another capillary tube of radius 2r is immersed in water. The mass of water that will rise in this tube is : *[2020]*

(a) 5.0 g (b) 10.0 g (c) 20.0 g (d) 2.5 g

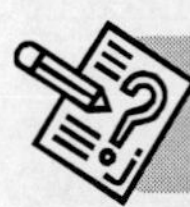

Exercise 3 - Concept Application Problems

CAP

1. A water tank of height 10m, completely filled with water is placed on a level ground. It has two holes one at 3 m and the other at 7 m from its base. The water ejecting from

(a) both the holes will fall at the same spot
(b) upper hole will fall farther than that from the lower hole
(c) upper hole will fall closer than that from the lower hole
(d) more information is required

2. Paint-gun is based on

(a) Bernoulli's theorem (b) Archimedes' principle
(c) Boyle's law (d) Pascal's law

3. The rain drops falling from the sky neither injure us nor make holes on the ground because they move with

(a) constant acceleration
(b) variable acceleration
(c) variable speed
(d) constant terminal velocity

4. A big drop of radius R is formed by 1000 small droplets of water. The radius of small drop is

(a) $\frac{R}{10}$ (b) $\frac{R}{100}$ (c) $\frac{R}{500}$ (d) $\frac{R}{1000}$

5. An open vessel containing water is given a constant acceleration a in the horizontal direction. Then the free surface of water gets sloped with the horizontal at an angle θ, given by

(a) $\theta = \cos^{-1}\frac{g}{a}$ (b) $\theta = \tan^{-1}\frac{a}{g}$

(c) $\theta = \sin^{-1}\frac{a}{g}$ (d) $\theta = \tan^{-1}\frac{g}{a}$

6. Two capillary of length L and 2L and of radius R and 2R are connected in series. The net rate of flow of fluid through them will be (given rate to the flow through single capillary, $X = \frac{\pi PR^4}{8\eta L}$)

(a) $\frac{8}{9}X$ (b) $\frac{9}{8}X$ (c) $\frac{5}{7}X$ (d) $\frac{7}{5}X$

7. A ring is cut from a platinum tube 8.5 cm internal and 8.7 cm external diameter. It is supported horizontally from the pan of a balance, so that it comes in contact with the water in a glass vessel. If an extra 3.97. If is required to pull it away from water, the surface tension of water is

(a) 72 dyne cm^{-1} (b) 70.80 dyne cm^{-1}
(c) 63.35 dyne cm^{-1} (d) 60 dyne cm^{-1}

8. Figure shows a weigh-bridge, with a beaker P with water on one pan and a balancing weight R on the other. A solid ball Q is hanging with a thread outside water. It has volume 40 cm^3 and weighs 80 g. If this solid is lowered to sink fully in water, but not touching the beaker anywhere, the balancing weight R' will be

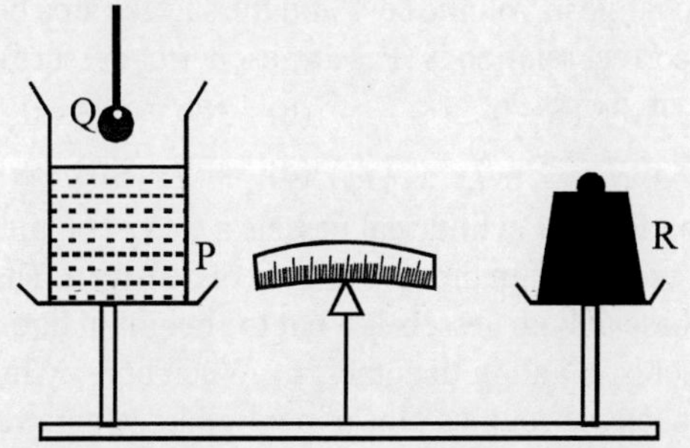

(a) same as R (b) 40 g less than R
(c) 40 g more than R (d) 80 g more than R

9. A beaker with a liquid of density 1.4 g cm^{-3} is in balance over one pan of a weighing machine. If a solid of mass 10 g and density 8 g cm^{-3} is now hung from the top of that pan with a thread and sinking fully in the liquid without touching the bottom, the extra weight to be put on the other pan for balance will be

(a) 10.0 g
(b) 8.25 g
(c) 11.75 g
(d) –1.75 g

10. Toricelli's theorem is used to find

(a) the velocity of efflux through an orifice.
(b) the velocity of flow of liquid through a pipe.
(c) terminal velocity
(d) critical velocity

11. Three tubes X, Y and Z are connected to a horizontal pipe in which ideal liquid is flowing. The radii of the tubes X, Y and Z at the junction are respectively 3 cm, 1 cm and 3 cm. It can be said

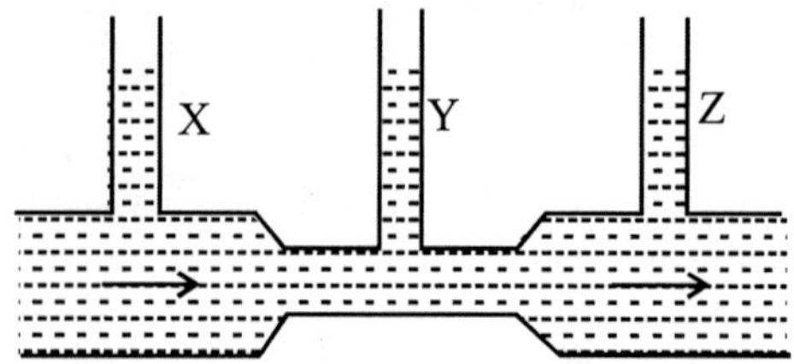

(a) the height of the liquid in the tube A is maximum.
(b) the height of liquid in the tubes Aand B is same.
(c) the height liquid in the tubes A,B and C is same.
(d) the height of the liquid in the tubes A and C is the same.

12. A sphere of brass released in a long liquid column attains a terminial speed v_0. If the terminal speed attained by sphere of marble of the same radius and released in the same liquid is nv_0, then the value of n will be (Given : The specific gravities of brass, marbles and the liquid are 8.5, 2.5 and 0.8 respectively.)

(a) $\frac{5}{17}$ (b) $\frac{17}{77}$ (c) $\frac{11}{31}$ (d) $\frac{17}{5}$

13. Two soap bubbles (surface tension T) coalesce to form a big bubble under isothermal condition. If in this process the change in volume be V and the surface area be S, then the correct relation is (P is atmospheric pressure)

(a) $PV+TS=0$ (b) $3PV+4TS=0$
(c) $3PV+TS=0$ (d) $4PV+3TS=0$

14. Two identical cylindrical vessels are kept on the ground and each contain the same liquid of density *d*. The area of the base of both vessels is *S* but the height of liquid in one vessel is x_1 and in the other, x_2. When both cylinders are connected through a pipe of negligible volume very close to the bottom, the liquid flows from one vessel to the other until it comes to equilibrium at a new height. The change in energy of the system in the process is :

(a) $gdS(x_2^2+x_1^2)$ (b) $gdS(x_2+x_1)^2$

(c) $\frac{3}{4}gdS(x_2-x_1)^2$ (d) $\frac{1}{4}gdS(x_2-x_1)^2$

15. A leak proof cylinder of length 1 m, made of a metal which has very low coefficient of expansion is floating vertically in water at 0°C such that its height above the water surface is 20 cm. When the temperature of water is increased to 4°C, the height of the cylinder above the water surface becomes 21 cm. The density of water at $T = 4°C$, relative to the density at $T = 0°C$ is close to:

(a) 1.26 (b) 1.04 (c) 1.01 (d) 1.03

16. Consider a solid sphere of radius *R* and mass density

$\rho(r)=\rho_0\left(1-\frac{r^2}{R^2}\right), 0<r\leq R$. The minimum density of a liquid in which it will float is:

(a) $\frac{\rho_0}{3}$ (b) $\frac{\rho_0}{5}$ (c) $\frac{2\rho_0}{5}$ (d) $\frac{2\rho_0}{3}$

17.

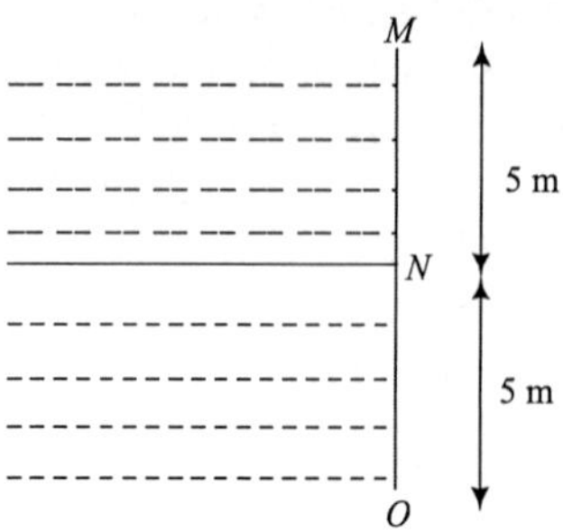

Two liquids of densities ρ_1 and $\rho_2(\rho_2 = 2\rho_1)$ are filled up behind a square wall of side 10 m as shown in figure. Each liquid has a height of 5 m. The ratio of the forces due to these liquids exerted on upper part *MN* to that at the lower part *NO* is (Assume that the liquids are not mixing):

(a) 1/3 (b) 2/3 (c) 1/2 (d) 1/4

18. A cubical block of side 0.5 m floats on water with 30% of its volume under water. What is the maximum weight that can be put on the block without fully submerging it under water? [Take, density of water = 10^3 kg/m^3]

(a) 46.3 kg (b) 87.5 kg (c) 65.4 kg (d) 30.1 kg

19. A load of mass M kg is suspended from a steel wire of length 2 m and radius 1.0 mm in Searle's apparatus experiment. The increase in length produced in the wire is 4.0 mm. Now the load is fully immersed in a liquid of relative density 2. The relative density of the material of load is 8. The new value of increase in length of the steel wire is :

(a) 3.0 mm (b) 4.0 mm (c) 5.0 mm (d) Zero

20. Water flows in a horizontal tube (see figure). The pressure of water changes by 700 Nm^{-2} between A and B where the area of cross section are 40 cm^2 and 20 cm^2, respectively. Find the rate of flow of water through the tube. (density of water = 1000 kgm^{-3})

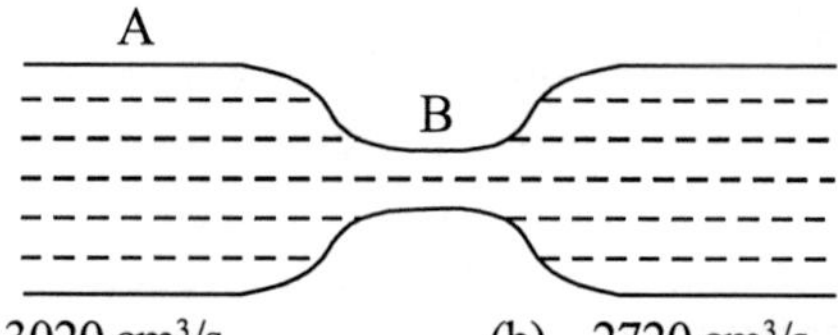

(a) 3020 cm^3/s (b) 2720 cm^3/s
(c) 2420 cm^3/s (d) 1810 cm^3/s

21. An ideal fluid flows (laminar flow) through a pipe of non-uniform diameter. The maximum and minimum diameters of the pipes are 6.4 cm and 4.8 cm, respectively. The ratio of the minimum and the maximum velocities of fluid in this pipe is:

(a) $\frac{9}{16}$ (b) $\frac{\sqrt{3}}{2}$ (c) $\frac{3}{4}$ (d) $\frac{81}{256}$

22. Water from a tap emerges vertically downwards with an initial speed of 1.0 ms^{-1}. The cross-sectional area of the tap is 10^{-4} m^2. Assume that the pressure is constant throughout the stream of water and that the flow is streamlined. The cross-sectional area of the stream, 0.15 m below the tap would be : [Take g = 10 ms^{-2})

(a) 2×10^{-5} m^2 (b) 5×10^{-5} m^2
(c) 5×10^{-4} m^2 (d) 1×10^{-5} m^2

23. A liquid of density ρ is coming out of a hose pipe of radius a with horizontal speed v and hits a mesh. 50% of the liquid passes through the mesh unaffected. 25% looses all of its momentum and 25% comes back with the same speed. The resultant pressure on the mesh will be:

(a) $\frac{1}{4}\rho v^2$ (b) $\frac{3}{4}\rho v^2$ (c) $\frac{1}{2}\rho v^2$ (d) ρv^2

24. A thin uniform tube is bent into a circle of radius r in the vertical plane. Equal volumes of two immiscible liquids, whose densities are ρ_1 and ρ_1 $(\rho_1 > \rho_2)$ fill half the circle. The angle θ between the radius vector passing through the common interface and the vertical is

(a) $\theta = \tan^{-1}\left[\frac{\pi}{2}\left(\frac{\rho_1-\rho_2}{\rho_1+\rho_2}\right)\right]$ (b) $\theta = \tan^{-1}\frac{\pi}{2}\left(\frac{\rho_1-\rho_2}{\rho_1+\rho_2}\right)$

(c) $\theta = \tan^{-1}\pi\left(\frac{\rho_1}{\rho_2}\right)$ (d) None of above

25. There is a circular tube in a vertical plane. Two liquids which do not mix and of densities d_1 and d_2 are filled in the tube. Each liquid subtends 90° angle at centre. Radius joining their interface makes an angle α with vertical. Ratio $\frac{d_1}{d_2}$ is:

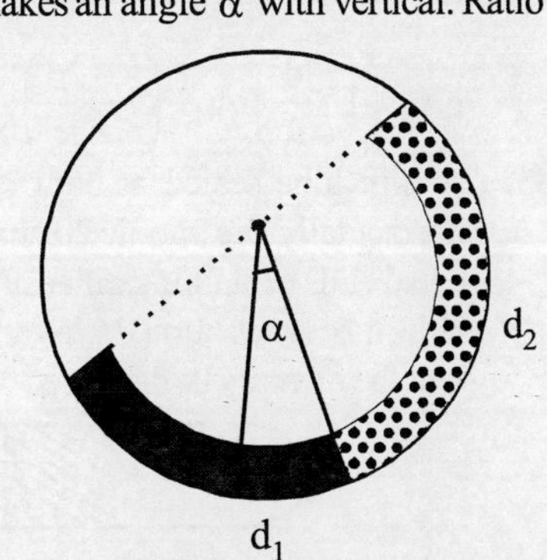

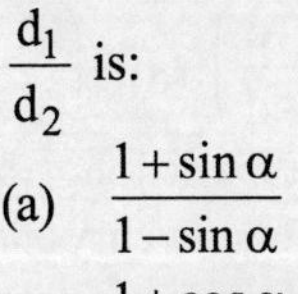
(a) $\frac{1+\sin\alpha}{1-\sin\alpha}$

(b) $\frac{1+\cos\alpha}{1-\cos\alpha}$

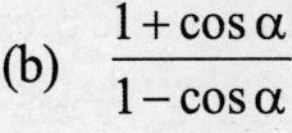
(c) $\frac{1+\tan\alpha}{1-\tan\alpha}$

(d) $\frac{1+\sin\alpha}{1-\cos\alpha}$

26. The top of a water tank is open to air and its water lavel is maintained. It is giving out $0.74 m^3$ water per minute through a circular opening of 2 cm radius in its wall. The depth of the centre of the opening from the level of water in the tank is close to:

(a) 6.0 m (b) 4.8 m (c) 9.6 m (d) 2.9 m

27. When an air bubble of radius r rises from the bottom to the surface of a lake, its radius becomes $\frac{5r}{4}$. Taking the atmospheric pressure to be equal to 10m height of water column, the depth of the lake would approximately be (ignore the surface tension and the effect of temperature):

(a) 10.5m (b) 8.7m (c) 11.2m (d) 9.5m

28. A uniform cylinder of length L and mass M having cross-sectional area A is suspended, with its length vertical, from a fixed point by a massless spring such that it is half submerged in a liquid of density σ at equilibrium position. The extension x_0 of the spring when it is in equilibrium is:

(a) $\frac{Mg}{k}$ (b) $\frac{Mg}{k}\left(1-\frac{LA\sigma}{M}\right)$

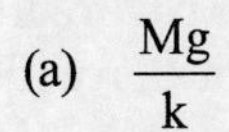
(c) $\frac{Mg}{k}\left(1-\frac{LA\sigma}{2M}\right)$ (d) $\frac{Mg}{k}\left(1+\frac{LA\sigma}{M}\right)$

29. Two identical charged spheres are suspended by strings of equal lengths. The strings make an angle of 30° with each other. When suspended in a liquid of density $0.8 g\ cm^{-3}$, the angle remains the same. If density of the material of the sphere is $1.6\ g\ cm^{-3}$, the dielectric constant of the liquid is

(a) 4 (b) 3 (c) 2 (d) 1

30. An open glass tube is immersed in mercury in such a way that a length of 8 cm extends above the mercury level. The open end of the tube is then closed and sealed and the tube is raised vertically up by additional 46 cm. What will be length of the air column above mercury in the tube now? (Atmospheric pressure = 76 cm of Hg)

(a) 16 cm (b) 22 cm (c) 38 cm (d) 6 cm

31. A cylindrical vessel of cross-section A contains water to a height h. There is a hole in the bottom of radius 'a'. The time in which it will be emptied is:

(a) $\frac{2A}{\pi a^2}\sqrt{\frac{h}{g}}$ (b) $\frac{\sqrt{2}A}{\pi a^2}\sqrt{\frac{h}{g}}$

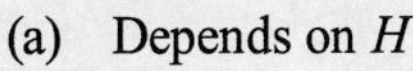
(c) $\frac{2\sqrt{2}A}{\pi a^2}\sqrt{\frac{h}{g}}$ (d) $\frac{A}{\sqrt{2}\pi a^2}\sqrt{\frac{h}{g}}$

32. In a cylindrical water tank, there are two small holes A and B on the wall at a depth of h_1, from the surface of water and at a height of h_2 from the bottom of water tank. Surface of water is at heigh H from the bottom of water tank. Water coming out from both holes strikes the ground at the same point S. Find the ratio of h_1 and h_2

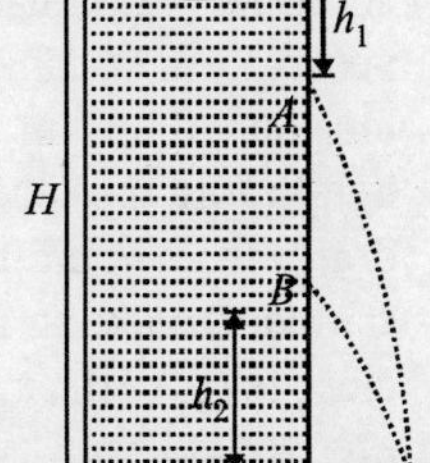

(a) Depends on H

(b) 1:1

(c) 2:2

(d) 1:2

33. Water is flowing through a horizontal tube having cross-sectional areas of its two ends being A and A' such that the ratio A/A' is 5. If the pressure difference of water between the two ends is $3 \times 10^5\ N\ m^{-2}$, the velocity of water with which it enters the tube will be (neglect gravity effects)

(a) $5\ m\ s^{-1}$ (b) $10\ m\ s^{-1}$

(c) $25\ m\ s^{-1}$ (d) $50\sqrt{10}\ m\ s^{-1}$

34. A square hole of side length ℓ is made at a depth of h and a circular hole of radius r is made at a depth of 4h from the surface of water in a water tank kept on a horizontal surface. If $\ell << h$, $r << h$ and the rate of water flow from the holes is the same, then r is equal to

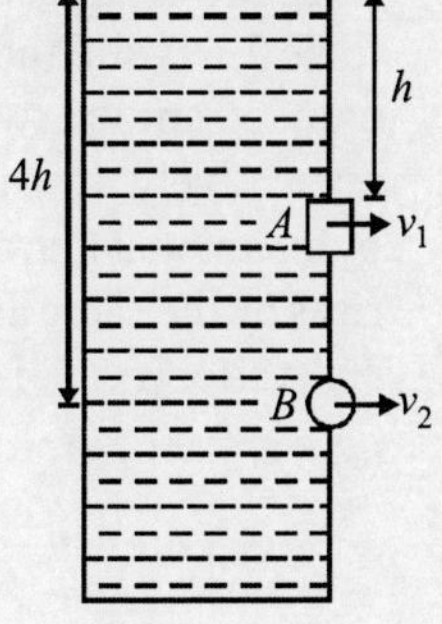

(a) $\frac{\ell}{\sqrt{2\pi}}$

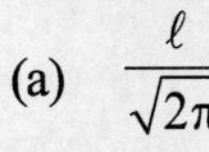
(b) $\frac{\ell}{\sqrt{3\pi}}$

(c) $\frac{\ell}{3\pi}$

(d) $\frac{\ell}{2\pi}$

35. A solid sphere, of radius R acquires a terminal velocity v_1 when falling (due to gravity) through a viscous fluid having a coefficient of viscosity $\hbar$. The sphere is broken into 27 identical solid spheres. If each of these spheres acquires a terminal velocity, v_2, when falling through the same fluid, the ratio (v_1/v_2) equals:

(a) 9 (b) 1/27 (c) 1/9 (d) 27

36. The velocity of water in a river is 18 km/hr near the surface. If the river is 5 m deep, find the shearing stress between the horizontal layers of water. The co-efficient of viscosity of water = 10^{-2} poise.

(a) 10^{-1} N/m^2 (b) 10^{-2} N/m^2
(c) 10^{-3} N/m^2 (d) 10^{-4} N/m^2

37. A spherical solid ball of volume V is made of a material of density ρ_1. It is falling through a liquid of density ρ_1 $(\rho_2 < \rho_1)$. Assume that the liquid applies a viscous force on the ball that is proportional to the square of its speed v, i.e., $F_{viscous} = -kv^2$ $(k > 0)$. The terminal speed of the ball is

(a) $\sqrt{\frac{Vg(\rho_1 - \rho_2)}{k}}$ (b) $\frac{Vg\rho_1}{k}$

(c) $\sqrt{\frac{Vg\rho_1}{k}}$ (d) $\frac{Vg(\rho_1 - \rho_2)}{k}$

38. A capillary tube made of glass of radius 0.15 mm is dipped vertically in a beaker filled with methylene iodide (surface tension = 0.05 Nm^{-1}, density = 667 kg m^{-3}) which rises to height h in the tube. It is observed that the two tangents drawn from liquid-glass interfaces (from opp. sides of the capillary) make an angle of 60° with one another. Then h is close to (g = 10 ms^{-2}).

(a) 0.049m (b) 0.087m (c) 0.137m (d) 0.172m

39. A small spherical droplet of density d is floating exactly half immersed in a liquid of density ρ and surface tension T. The radius of the droplet is (take note that the surface tension applies an upward force on the droplet):

(a) $r = \sqrt{\frac{2T}{3(d+\rho)g}}$ (b) $r = \sqrt{\frac{T}{(d-\rho)g}}$

(c) $r = \sqrt{\frac{T}{(d+\rho)g}}$ (d) $r = \sqrt{\frac{3T}{(2d-\rho)g}}$

40. The ratio of surface tensions of mercury and water is given to be 7.5 while the ratio of their densities is 13.6. Their contact angles, with glass, are close to 135° and 0°, respectively. It is observed that mercury gets depressed by an amount h in a capillary tube of radius r_1, while water rises by the same amount h in a capillary tube of radius r_2. The ratio, (r_1/r_2), is then close to :

(a) 4/5 (b) 2/5 (c) 3/5 (d) 2/3

41. On heating water, bubbles being formed at the bottom of the vessel detach and rise. Take the bubbles to be spheres of radius R and making a circular contact of radius r with the bottom of the vessel. If $r \ll R$ and the surface tension of water is T, value of r just before bubbles detach is: (density of water is ρ_w)

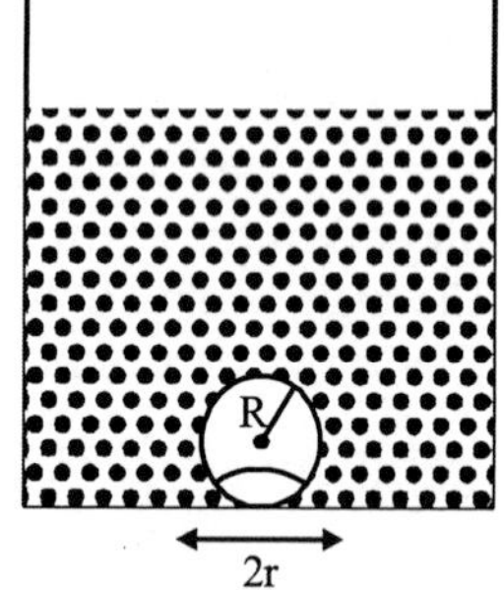

(a) $R^2\sqrt{\frac{2\rho_w g}{3T}}$

(b) $R^2\sqrt{\frac{\rho_w g}{6T}}$

(c) $R^2\sqrt{\frac{\rho_w g}{T}}$

(d) $R^2\sqrt{\frac{3\rho_w g}{T}}$

42. A capillary tube is immersed vertically in water and the height of the water column is x. When this arrangement is taken into a mine of depth d, the height of the water column is y. If R is the radius of earth, the ratio $\frac{x}{y}$ is:

(a) $\left(1-\frac{d}{R}\right)$ (b) $\left(1-\frac{2d}{R}\right)$ (c) $\left(\frac{R-d}{R+d}\right)$ (d) $\left(\frac{R+d}{R-d}\right)$

43. A thin tube sealed at both ends is 100 cm long. It lies horizontally, the middle 20 cm containing mercury and two equal ends containing air at standard atmospheric pressure. If the tube is now turned to a vertical position, by what amount will the mercury be displaced ?

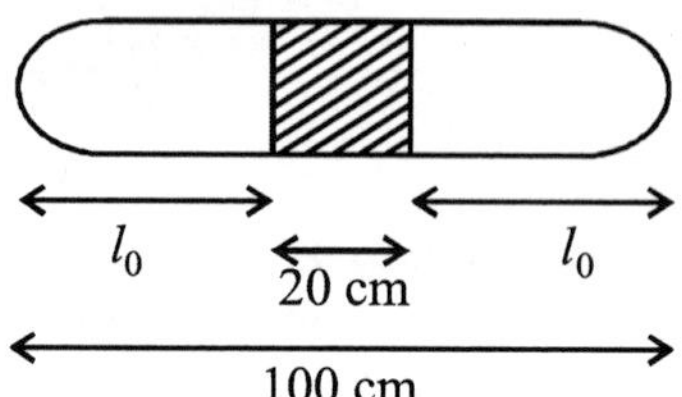

(Given : cross-section of the tube can be assumed to be uniform)

(a) 2.95 cm (b) 5.18 cm (c) 8.65 cm (d) 0.0 cm

44. A thin liquid film formed between a U-shaped wire and a light slider supports a weight of 1.5×10^{-2} N (see figure). The length of the slider is 30 cm and its weight is negligible. The surface tension of the liquid film is

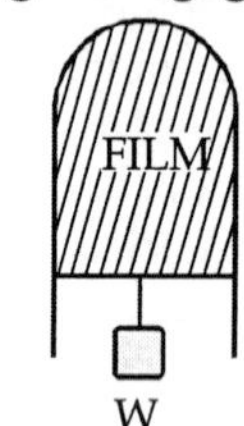

(a) 0.0125 Nm^{-1}

(b) 0.1 Nm^{-1}

(c) 0.05 Nm^{-1}

(d) 0.025 Nm^{-1}

45. A 20 cm long capillary tube is dipped in water. The water rises up to 8 cm. If the entire arrangement is put in a freely falling elevator the length of water column in the capillary tube will be

(a) 10 cm (b) 8 cm (c) 20 cm (d) 4 cm

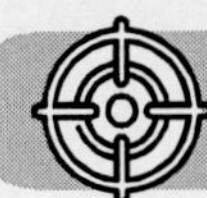

Hints & Solutions

10.1 Concept Practice Problems

1. (c) When a beaker containing a liquid of density ρ moves up with an acceleration a, it will work as a lift moving upward with acceleration a. The effective acceleration due to gravity in lift = (a + g)
   ∴ Pressure of liquid of height h = h ρ (a + g)
2. (c) Volume of m g of ice = m/x and volume of m g of water = m/y. So change in volume
   $$= \frac{m}{y} - \frac{m}{x} = m\left(\frac{1}{y} - \frac{1}{x}\right)$$
3. (a) $P \propto T$
4. (c)
5. (a) Specific gravity of block $= \frac{\text{weight of block in air}}{\text{loss of weight in water}}$
   $$= \frac{60}{60-40} = 3$$
6. (b) Let v be the volume of the ice-berg outside the sea water and V be the total volume of ice-berg. Then as per question
   0.92 V = 1.03 (V – v) or v/V = 1 – 0.92/1.03 = 11/103
   ∴ (v/V) × 100 = 11 × 100 / 103 ≅ 11%
7. (a) Weight of a man = wt. of water displaced
   $= \text{volume} \times \text{density} = 3 \times 2 \times \frac{1}{100} \times 10^3 = 60 \text{ kg}$
8. (c) The effective acceleration of the body $g' = \left(1 - \frac{\rho}{\rho'}\right)g$

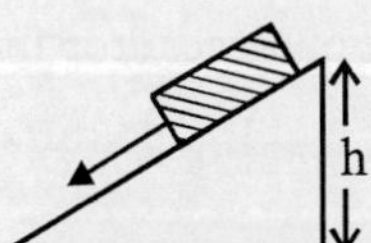

Now, the depth to which the body sinks

$$h' = \left(\frac{u^2}{2g'}\right) = \frac{2gh}{2g'} = \frac{gh}{g'} = \frac{h \times \rho'}{\rho - \rho'}$$

9. (b) Volume of first piece of metal $= \frac{32}{8} = 4 \text{ cm}^3$
   Upthrust = 4 gf
   Effective weight = (32 – 4) gf = 28 gf
   If m be the mass of second body, volume of second body is $\frac{m}{5}$
   Now, $28 = m - \frac{m}{5} \Rightarrow m = 35$ g
10. (a) As temperature rises, the density decreases, height increases. In A, the top cross-section is smaller. Therefore $h_A > h_B$.

10.2 Concept Practice Problems

11. (a) Surface tension of the liquid at boiling point is zero.
12. (b) Surface energy ∝ surface area $= \pi r^2$
13. (a) When liquid drops coalesce, there is a decrease of surface area and therefore decrease of surface energy. Hence, energy is liberated.
14. (a) In Isothermal conditons $T = \frac{W}{\Delta A}$
    where, T = surface tension, W = work done, ΔA = change in area.
15. (b)
16. (a)
17. (d)
18. (a) Given, $\frac{4T}{r_1} = 2 \times \frac{4T}{r_2}$ or $r_2 = 2r_1$
    $$\frac{4}{3}\pi r_1^3 = n \times \frac{4}{3}\pi r_2^3 = n \times \frac{4}{3}\pi(2r_1)^3 \text{ or } n = \frac{1}{8} = 0.125$$
19. (d) Volume of bigger bubble = volume of 27 smaller bubbles
    $$\Rightarrow \frac{4}{3}\pi D^3 = 27 \times \frac{4}{3}\pi d^3 \Rightarrow d = \frac{D}{3}$$
    Initial surface energy $S_i = 4\pi D^2 \sigma$
    Final surface energy $S_f = 27 \times 4\pi d^2 \sigma$
    $\Delta S = S_f - S_i$ and using $d = \frac{D}{3}$
    $$\Delta S = \sigma \times 4\pi\left[27 \times \frac{D^2}{9} - D^2\right]$$
    $$= 2D^2 \times 4\pi \times \sigma = 8\pi\sigma D^2$$
20. (b) Mass of liquid which rises in the capillary,
    $$m = (\pi r^2)h\rho = \pi r^2 \times \frac{2\sigma\cos\theta}{r\rho g} \times \rho$$
    $\Rightarrow m \propto r$

10.3 Concept Practice Problems

21. (a) Viscosity depends on area.
22. (b)
23. (b) Velocity of liquid flowing out of hole $= \sqrt{2gh}$.
    Here $h = (h_0 - h_1)$
24. (a) v = velocity of efflux through an orifice $= \sqrt{2gH}$

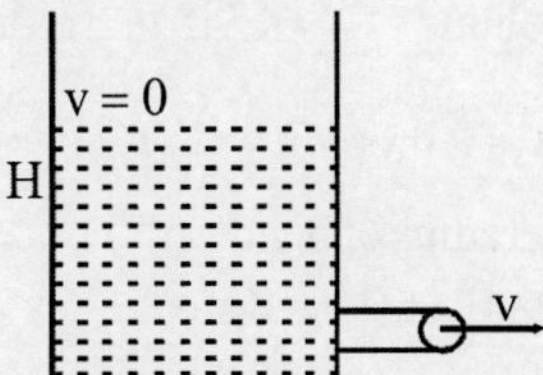

It is independent of the size of orifice.

25. (b) Apply Bernoulli's theorem.

26. (b) Velocity of efflux, $v = \sqrt{2gh}$;
volume of liquid flowing out per sec
$= v \times A = \sqrt{2gh} \times A = \sqrt{2 \times 10 \times 5} \times 10^{-4} = 10^{-3}\ m^3/s$

27. (b) P.E. = K.E.
$mgh = \frac{1}{2}mv^2$
$v = \sqrt{2gh} = \sqrt{2 \times 10 \times 20}$
(Here $g = 10\ m/s^2$)
$= 20\ m/s$

20 m = h
v

28. (d) $Q' = \dfrac{\pi(2P)\left(\frac{a}{2}\right)^4}{8\eta\ell} = \dfrac{Q}{8}$ $\left[\because Q = \dfrac{\pi P a^4}{8\eta\ell}\right]$

29. (d) According to principle of continuity, for a streamline flow of fluid through a tube of non-uniform cross-section the rate of flow of fluid (Q) is same at every point in the tube.
i.e., Av = constant $\Rightarrow A_1v_1 = A_2v_2$
Therefore, the rate of flow of fluid is same at M and N.

30. (a) Pressure at the bottom of tank $P = h\rho g = 3 \times 10^5 \dfrac{N}{m^2}$
Pressure due to liquid column
$P_1 = 3 \times 10^5 - 1 \times 10^5 = 2 \times 10^5$
and velocity of water $v = \sqrt{2gh}$
$\therefore\ v = \sqrt{\dfrac{2P_1}{\rho}} = \sqrt{\dfrac{2 \times 2 \times 10^5}{10^3}} = \sqrt{400}\ m/s$

Exercise 1 - Chapter Revision Problems CRP

1. (d) Terminal velocity, $v_T = \dfrac{2r^2g}{9\eta}(\rho - \sigma)$, $v_T \propto r^2$

2. (c) 3. (b) 4. (b) 5. (b)

6. (b) The theorem of continuity is valid.
$\therefore A_1v_1\rho = A_2v_2\rho$ as the density of the liquid can be taken as uniform.
$\therefore\ A_1v_1 = A_2v_2$
$\Rightarrow$ Smaller the area, greater the velocity.

A_1 A_2

7. (b) Terminal velocity, $v_0 = \dfrac{2\,r^2(\rho - \rho_0)g}{9\eta}$
$= \dfrac{2 \times (2 \times 10^{-3})^2 \times (8 - 1.3) \times 10^3 \times 9.8}{9 \times 0.83} = 0.07\ ms^{-1}$

8. (c) Surface energy = suface tension × area of surface
For 1 drop, volume $= \frac{4}{3}\pi R^3$ if R = radius of drop.
Total volume of 8 drops $= 8.\frac{4}{3}\pi R^3 = \frac{4}{3}\pi(2R)^3$
R' = 2R, new radius of big drop
New area $= 4\pi 4R^2 = 4 \times$ old area
Energy ∝ area
$E_1 = 4\pi R^2$ .....(1)
$E_2 = 4.4\pi R^2$ .....(2)
From equation (1) and (2) we get, $E_2 = 4E_1$

9. (c) $h = \dfrac{2\sigma\cos\theta}{r\rho g} \Rightarrow \sigma \propto \dfrac{h\rho}{\cos\theta}$
$\Rightarrow \dfrac{\sigma_w}{\sigma_m} = \dfrac{h_w\rho_w}{\cos\theta_w} \times \dfrac{\cos\theta_m}{h_m\rho_m} = \dfrac{10 \times 1}{\cos 0^\circ} \times \dfrac{\cos 135^\circ}{-3.1 \times 13.6}$
$= \dfrac{10 \times (-0.707)}{-3.1 \times 13.6} \approx \dfrac{1}{6}$

10. (c) Volume of ball $= \dfrac{40}{0.8} = 50\ cm^3$
Downthrust on water = 50 g.
Therefore reading is 650 g.

11. (a) $F = 6\pi\eta r v$
$= 6 \times 3.14 \times (8 \times 10^{-5}) \times 0.03 \times 100 = 4.52 \times 10^{-3}$ dyne

12. (c) $K = \dfrac{P}{\Delta V / V}$ $\therefore\ \Delta V = \dfrac{PV}{K}$
$P = h\rho g = 200 \times 10^3 \times 10\ N/m^2$
$K = 22000\ atm = 22000 \times 10^5\ N/m^2$
$V = 1m^3$
$\Delta V = \dfrac{200 \times 10^3 \times 10 \times 1}{22000 \times 10^5} = 9.1 \times 10^{-4} m^3$

13. (c) According to equation of continuity
$A_1V_1 = A_2V_2 + A_3V_3$
$\Rightarrow\ 4 \times 0.2 = 2 \times 0.2 + 0.4 \times V_3 \Rightarrow V_3 = 1\ m/s.$

14. (d) 1 centipoise $= 10^{-2}\ gcm^{-1}\ s^{-1} = 0.001\ kg\ m^{-1}s^{-1}$

15. (c) Angle of contact is acute.

16. (b) Let x be the fraction of volume of object floating above the surface of the liquid.
As weight of liquid displaced = weight of object
$\therefore\ (V_0 - x\,V_0)d\,g = V_0\,d_0\,g$
$(1 - x)d = d_0$ or $x = 1 - \dfrac{d_0}{d} = \dfrac{d - d_0}{d}$

17. (c) If R is radius of bigger drop formed, then
$\frac{4}{3}\pi R^3 = 2 \times \frac{4}{3}\pi r^3$ or $R = 2^{1/3} r$
As $v_0 \propto r^2$
$\therefore\ \dfrac{v_{01}}{v_0} = \dfrac{R^2}{r^2} = \dfrac{(2^{1/3}r)^2}{r^2} = 2^{2/3}$
or $v_{01} = v_0 \times 2^{2/3} = 5 \times (4)^{1/3}$

18. (c) Vertical distance covered by water before striking ground = (H – h). Time taken is, $t = \sqrt{2(H - h)/g}$
: Horizontal velocity of water coming out of hole at P, $u = \sqrt{2gh}$
∴ Horizontal range $= ut = \sqrt{2gh} \times \sqrt{2(H - h)/g}$
$= 2\sqrt{h(H - h)}$

19. (d) For the first part of the question, remember that terminal velocity means the acceleration experienced becomes zero.
Since $a = 0\ m/s^2$, then, $\Sigma F_y = F_{air\ resistance} - F_w = 0$
$F_{air\ resistance} = F_w mg$

For the second part of the question, while the velocity is higher, the acceleration is still zero. Therefore, the $F_{\text{air resistance}}$ is still equal to the skydiver's weight.

$$F_{\text{air resistance Case A}} = F_{\text{air resistance Case B}}$$

What has changed is the surface area of the skydiver. Since pressure is P = F/A, as A decreases, the pressure experienced increases.

$$P_A A_A = P_B A_B = mg$$

Since $A_A > A_B$, then $P_A < P_B$

20. (b) Because of surface tension.
21. (c) Brine due to its high density exerts an upthrust which can balance the weight of the egg.
22. (c) Pressure is proportional to depth from the free surface and is same in all directions.
23. (b) Bernoulli's theorem.
24. (a) Apply Bernoulli's theorem.
25. (b) Due to increase in velocity, pressure will be low above the surface of water.
26. (a) 27. (b)
28. (a) In equilibrium, $mg = F_e$

$F_B = V\rho_0 g$ and mass = volume × density

$$\frac{4}{3}\pi(R^3 - r^3)\rho_0 g = \frac{4}{3}\pi R^3 \rho_w g$$

Given, relative density, $\frac{\rho_0}{\rho_w} = \frac{27}{8}$

$$\Rightarrow \left[1 - \left(\frac{r}{R}\right)^3\right]\frac{27}{8}\rho_w = \rho_w$$

$$\Rightarrow 1 - \frac{r^3}{R^3} = \frac{9}{27} \Rightarrow 1 - \frac{1}{3} = \frac{r^3}{R^3} \Rightarrow \frac{2}{3} = \frac{r^3}{R^3}$$

$$\Rightarrow \frac{r}{R} = \left(\frac{2}{3}\right)^{1/3} \quad \Rightarrow 1 - \frac{r^3}{R^3} = \frac{8}{27} \Rightarrow \frac{r^3}{R^3} = 1 - \frac{8}{27} = \frac{19}{27}$$

$$\therefore r = 0.89R = \frac{8}{9}R.$$

29. (c) Given:

Radius of air bubble = 1 cm,

Upward acceleration of bubble, $a = 9.8$ cm/s^2,

$\rho_{water} = 1$ g cm^{-3}

Volume $V = \frac{4\pi}{3}r^3 = \frac{4\pi}{3}\times(1)^3 = 4.19$ cm^3

$$F_{buoyant} - mg = ma \Rightarrow m = \frac{F_{buoyant}}{g+a}$$

$$\therefore m = \frac{(V\rho_\omega g)}{g+a} = \frac{V\rho_\omega}{1+\frac{a}{g}} = \frac{(4.19)\times 1}{1+\frac{9.8}{980}} = \frac{4.19}{1.01} = 4.15\,\text{g}$$

F buoyant, a, mg

30. (a) $P_1 = P_0 + {}_-gd_1$

$P_2 = P_0 + {}_-gd_2$

$\Delta P = P_2 - P_1 = \rho g \Delta d$

$3.03 \times 10^6 = 10^3 \times 10 \times \Delta d \Rightarrow \Delta d \simeq 300$ m

31. (c) $Mg = \left(\frac{4V}{5}\right)\rho\omega g$

or $\left(\frac{M}{V}\right) = \frac{4\rho\omega}{5}$ or $\rho = \frac{4\rho\omega}{5}$

When block floats fully in water and oil, then

$$Mg = F_{b_1} + F_{b_2}$$

$$(\rho V)g = \left(\frac{V}{2}\right)\rho_{oil}\, g + \frac{V}{2}\rho\omega g$$

or $_{\rightarrow oil} = \frac{3}{5}\rho\omega = 0.6\rho\omega$

32. (d) $V = ct$ or, $\frac{4}{3}\pi r^3 = ct \Rightarrow r = kt^{\frac{1}{3}}$

$$P = P_0 + \frac{4T}{kt^{1/3}} \Rightarrow P = P_0 + c\left(\frac{1}{t^{1/3}}\right)$$

33. (d) As liquid 1 floats over liquid 2. The lighter liquid floats over heavier liquid. So, $\rho_1 < \rho_2$

Also $\rho_3 < \rho_2$ because the ball of density ρ_3 does not sink to the bottom of the jar.

Also $\rho_3 > \rho_1$ otherwise the ball would have floated in liquid 1. we conclude that

$\rho_1 < \rho_3 < \rho_2$.

34. (b)
35. (d) Using Bernoulli's equation

$$P_1 + \frac{1}{2}\rho\upsilon_1^2 + \rho g h_1 = P_2 + \frac{1}{2}\rho\upsilon_2^2 + \rho g h_2$$

For horizontal pipe, $h_1 = 0$ and $h_2 = 0$ and taking

$P_1 = P, P_2 = \frac{P}{2}$, we get

$$\Rightarrow P + \frac{1}{2}\rho\upsilon^2 = \frac{P}{2} + \frac{1}{2}\rho V^2 \Rightarrow \frac{P}{2} + \frac{1}{2}\rho\upsilon^2 = \frac{1}{2}\rho V^2$$

$$\Rightarrow V = \sqrt{\upsilon^2 + \frac{P}{\rho}}$$

36. (b) Rate of flow of water $(V) = 100$ lit/min

$$= \frac{100\times 10^{-3}}{60} \times \frac{5}{3}\times 10^{-3}\,\text{m}^3$$

$\therefore$ Velocity of flow of water $(v) = \frac{V}{A} = \frac{5\times 10^{-3}}{3\times\times(5\times 10^{-2})^2}$

$$= \frac{10}{15\pi} = \frac{2}{3\pi}\,\text{m/s} = 0.2\,\text{m/s}$$

$\therefore$ Reynold number $(N_R) = \frac{Dv\rho}{\eta}$

$$= \frac{(10\times 10^{-2})\times\frac{2}{3\pi}\times 1000}{1} = 2\times 10^4$$

Order of $N_R = 10^4$

37. (a)
38. (d) Given: Diameter of water tap $= \frac{2}{\sqrt{\pi}}$ cm

$\therefore$ Radius, $r = \frac{1}{\sqrt{\pi}}\times 10^{-2}$ m

$$\frac{dm}{dt} = \rho AV$$

$$\frac{15}{5\times 60} = 10^3 \times \pi\left(\frac{1}{\sqrt{\pi}}\right)^2 \times 10^{-4} V \Rightarrow V = 0.05\text{ m/s}$$

Reynold's number, $R_e = \frac{\rho Vr}{n}$

$$= \frac{10^3\times 0.5\times\frac{2}{\sqrt{\pi}}10^{-2}}{10^{-3}} \cong 5500$$

39. (a) For 1 m length of horizontal tube
Mass of water M = density × volume
$= 10^3 \times$ area × length
$= 10^3 \times 10^{-2} \times 1 = 10$ kg

Therefore minimum force $= \frac{\Delta p}{\Delta t}$ (rate of change of momentum)
$= 10 \times 1.5 = 15\,N$

40. (c) Pressure difference

$$P_2 - P_1 = \frac{1}{2}\rho\left(v_2^2 - v_1^2\right) \quad = \frac{1}{2}\times 1.2\left((150)^2 - (100)^2\right)$$

$$= \frac{1}{2}\times 1.2(22500 - 10000)$$

$= 7500$ Nm^{-2}

41. (c) Using Bernoulli's theorem, for horizontal flow

$$P_0 + \frac{1}{2}\rho v_1^2 + \rho gh = P_0 + \frac{1}{2}\rho v_2^2 + 0$$

$$v_2 = \sqrt{v_1^2 + 2gh} = \sqrt{0.16 + 2\times 10\times 0.2} = 2.03 \text{ m/s}$$

According to equation of continuity
$A_2 v_2 = A_1 v_1$

$$\pi\frac{D_2^2}{4}\times v_2 = \pi\frac{D_1^2}{4}v_1$$

$$\Rightarrow D_2 = D_1\sqrt{\frac{v_1}{v_2}} = 3.55\times 10^{-3}\text{ m}$$

42. (a) Using, $v^2 - u^2 = 2gh$

$$\Rightarrow v^2 - 0^2 = 2gh \Rightarrow v = \sqrt{2gh}$$

Terminal velocity,

$$V_T = \frac{2}{9}\frac{r^2(\rho - \sigma)g}{\eta}$$

After falling through h the velocity should be equal to terminal velocity

$$\therefore \sqrt{2gh} = \frac{2}{9}\frac{r^2(\rho-\sigma)g}{\eta}$$

$$\Rightarrow 2gh = \frac{4}{81}\frac{r^4 g^2(\rho-\sigma)^2}{\eta^2} \Rightarrow h = \frac{2r^4 g(\rho-\sigma)^2}{81\eta^2} \Rightarrow h \propto r^4$$

43. (c)

44. (a) Terminal velocity in a viscous medium is given by:

$$V_T = \frac{2a^2(\rho-\sigma)g}{9\eta}$$

$\therefore V_T \propto a^2$

45. (b) From Stoke's law, force of viscosity acting on a spherical body is
$F = 6\pi\eta rv$
hence F is directly proportional to radius & velocity.

46. (c) According to question, pressure inside, 1st soap bubble,

$$\Delta P_1 = P_1 - P_0 = 0.01 = \frac{4T}{R_1} \quad ...(i)$$

$$\text{And } \Delta P_2 = P_2 - P_0 = 0.02 = \frac{4T}{R_2} \quad ...(ii)$$

Dividing, equation (ii) by (i),

$$\frac{1}{2} = \frac{R_2}{R_1} \Rightarrow R_1 = 2R_2$$

Volume $V = \frac{4}{3}\pi R^3$

$$\therefore \frac{V_1}{V_2} = \frac{R_1^3}{R_2^3} = \frac{8R_2^3}{R_2^3} = \frac{8}{1}$$

47. (d) We have, $h = \frac{2T\cos\theta}{r\rho g}$
Mass of the water in the capillary

$$m = \rho V = \rho\times\pi r^2 h = \rho\times\pi r^2\times\frac{2T\cos\theta}{r\rho g}$$

$\Rightarrow m \propto r$

$$\therefore \frac{m_1}{m_2} = \frac{r}{2r} \text{ or } m_2 = 2m_1 = 2m.$$

48. (c) Angle of contact θ

$$\cos\theta = \frac{T_{SA} - T_{SL}}{T_{LA}}$$

when water is on a waxy or oily surface
$T_{SA} < T_{SL}$ cos θ is negative i.e.,
$90° < \theta < 180°$
i.e., angle of contact θ increases
And for $\theta > 90°$ liquid level in capillary tube fall. i.e., h decreases

49. (c) Work done = increase in surface area × surface tension
$\Rightarrow W = 2T4\pi[(5^2) - (3)^2]\times 10^{-4}$
$= 2\times 0.03\times 4\pi[25 - 9]\times 10^{-4}$ J
$= 0.4\pi\times 10^{-3}$ J $= 0.4\pi$ mJ

50. (c) As volume remains constant
∴ Sum of volumes of 2 smaller drops
= Volume of the bigger drop

$$2.\frac{4}{3}\pi r^3 = \frac{4}{3}\pi R^3 \Rightarrow R = 2^{1/3}\,r$$

Surface energy = Surface tension × Surface area $= T.4\pi R^2$

$$= T4\pi 2^{2/3} r^2 = T.2^{8/3}\pi r^2.$$

Exercise 2 - Exemplar & Past Year Questions E&PYQs

Exemplar Questions

1. (d) In a streamline flow the velocity of fluid particles remaines constant across any cross-sectional area, then a point on the area cannot have different velocities at the same time, hence two streamlines flow layers do not cross each other.

2. (b) In streamline flow, the speed of liquid of each particle at a point in a particular cross-section is constant, between two cross-section of a tube of flow because AV = constant (law of continuity).

3. (a)

4. (c) We observed that meniscus of liquid is convex shape as shown in figure which is possible if only, the angle of contact is obtuse. Hence, the combination will be of case of mercury-glass (140°). Hence verifies the option (c).

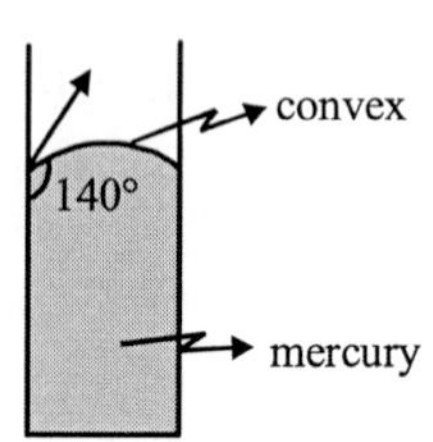

NEET/AIPMT (2013-2020) Questions

5. (c) Wetability of a surface by a liquid primarily depends on angle of contact between the surface and liquid. If angle of contact is acute liquids wet the solid and vice-versa.

6. (b) According to Bernoulli's theorem,

$$P+\frac{1}{2}\rho v^2 = \text{constant and } Av = \text{constant}$$

If A is minimum, v is maximum, P is minimum.

7. (c) As surface area decreases so energy is released.
Energy released $= 4\pi R^2 T[n^{1/3}-1]$
where $R = n^{1/3} r$

$$= 4\pi R^3 T\left[\frac{1}{r}-\frac{1}{R}\right] = 3VT\left[\frac{1}{r}-\frac{1}{R}\right]$$

8. (a) Inflow rate of volume of the liquid = Outflow rate of volume of the liquid

$$\pi R^2 V = n\pi r^2 (v) \Rightarrow v = \frac{\pi R^2 V}{n\pi r^2} = \frac{VR^2}{nr^2}$$

9. (b) According to Bernoulli's theorem,

$$P + \frac{1}{2}\rho v^2 = P_0 + 0$$

So, $\Delta P = \frac{1}{2}\rho v^2$

$$F = \Delta PA = \frac{1}{2}\rho v^2 A$$

$$= \frac{1}{2}\times 1.2 \times 40 \times 40 \times 250$$

$= 2.4\times 10^5$ N (upwards)

10. (d) As we know,
Pressure $P = Vdg$
Here, $LAdg = (pL)A(n\rho)g + (1-p)LA\rho g$
$\Rightarrow d = (1-p)\rho + pn\rho$
$= [1+(n-1)p]\rho$

11. (d) Power = rate of production of heat = F.V
$= 6\pi\eta r V_T \cdot V_T = 6\pi\eta r V_T^2$ $(\because F = 6\pi\eta V_T r$ stoke's formula)
$V_T \propto r^2$

$$\because\ V_T = \frac{2}{9}\frac{r^2(\rho-\sigma)}{\eta}g$$

$\therefore$ Power $\propto r^5$

12. (a) Volumetric flow rate of liquid

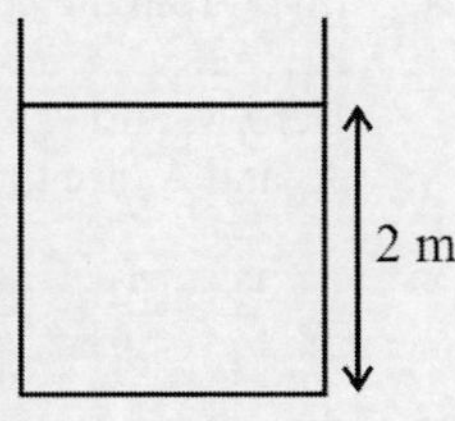

$$Q = au = a\sqrt{2gh}$$

$$= 2\times 10^{-6}\,\text{m}^2 \times \sqrt{2\times 10\times 2}\ \text{m/s}$$

$= 2\times 2\times 3.14\times 10^{-6}\,\text{m}^3/\text{s}$
$= 12.56\times 10^{-6}\,\text{m}^3/\text{s}$
$= 12.6\times 10^{-6}\,\text{m}^3/\text{s}$

13. (a) Terminal velocity $V_T = (\rho-\sigma)g$

$$V_{T_1} = \frac{2\times(1)^2}{9\eta}(\rho_1 - 0.1\rho_2)g$$

$$V_{T_1} = \frac{2\times 1}{9\eta}(8\rho_2 - 0.1\rho_2)g \Rightarrow V_{T_2} = \frac{2\times(2)^2}{9\eta}(\rho_2 - 0.1\rho_2)g$$

$$\therefore\ \frac{V_{T_1}}{V_{T_2}} = \frac{7.9}{4(0.9)} = \frac{79}{36}$$

14. (c) Pressure inside the soap bubble

$$= P_0 + \frac{4T}{R}$$

And pressure at a point below the surface of water $= \rho g Z_0 + P_0$ [where P_0 = atmospheric pressure]
By equating these pressure we get,

$$P_0 + \frac{4T}{R} = P_0 + rgZ_0$$

$$Z_0 = \frac{4T}{R\times\rho g} \Rightarrow Z_0 = \frac{4\times 2.5\times 10^{-2}}{10^{-3}\times 1000\times 10}\text{m}$$

$Z_0 = 1$ cm

15. (b) Force of surface tension balances the weight of water in capillary tube.

$$F_S = 2\pi r T\cos\theta = mg$$

Here, T and θ are constant.
So, $m \propto r$
Let m_1 and m_2 be the mass of water in two capillary tube.

$$\therefore\ \frac{m_2}{m_1} = \frac{r_2}{r_1} \Rightarrow \frac{m_2}{5.0} = \frac{2r}{r} \quad (\because r_2 = 2r) \Rightarrow m_2 = 10.0\text{ g}$$

Exercise 3 - Concept Application Problems CAP

1. (a) Velocity of water from hole A
$= v_1 = \sqrt{2gh}$
Velocity of water from hole B
$= v_2 = \sqrt{2g(H_0 - h)}$
Time of reaching the ground from hole B
$= t_1 = \sqrt{2(H_0-h)/g}$
Time of reaching the ground from hole A
$= t_2 = \sqrt{2h/g}$

2. (a) 3. (b) 4. (a)

5. (d) $\tan\theta = \frac{mg}{ma} = \frac{g}{a}$ or $\theta = \tan^{-1} g/a$

6. (a) Fluid resistance is given by $R = \frac{8\eta L}{\pi r^4}$

When two capillary tubes of same size are joined in parallel, then equivalent fluid resistance is

$$R_S = R_1 + R_2 = \frac{8\eta L}{\pi R^4} + \frac{8\eta\times 2L}{\pi(2R)^4} = \left(\frac{8\eta L}{\pi R^4}\right)\times\frac{9}{8}$$

$$\text{Rate of flow} = \frac{P}{R_S} = \frac{\pi P R^4}{8\eta L}\times\frac{8}{9} = \frac{8}{9}X \quad \left[\text{as } X = \frac{\pi P R^4}{8\eta L}\right]$$

7. (a) $(2\pi r_1 + 2\pi r_2)\sigma = mg$

$$\left[2\pi\times\frac{8.7}{2}+2\pi\times\frac{8.5}{2}\right]\sigma = 3.97\times 980$$

$\Rightarrow \sigma = 72$ dyne cm^{-1}

8. (c) Upthrust = weight of 40 cm^3 of water
= 40 g = down thrust on water

9. (a) 10g is the force on water = extra wt. on other pan.

10. (a)

11. (d) Use the equation of continuity and Bernoulli's theorem.

12. (b) For the same radius, terminal velocity is directly proportional to density difference.

13. (b) 14. (d)

15. (c) When cylinder is floating in water at 0°C

Net thrust $= A(h_2 - h_1)\rho_{0°c}g$

$= A(100-80)\rho_{0°c}g$

When cylinder is floating in water at 4° C

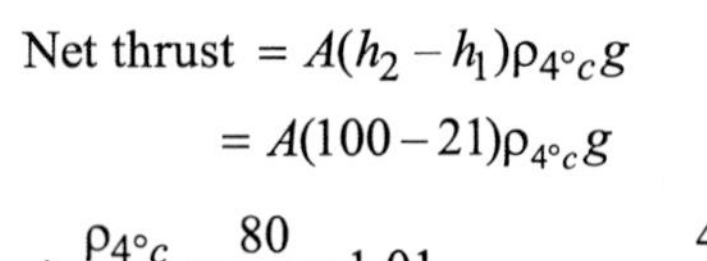

Net thrust $= A(h_2 - h_1)\rho_{4°c}g$

$= A(100-21)\rho_{4°c}g$

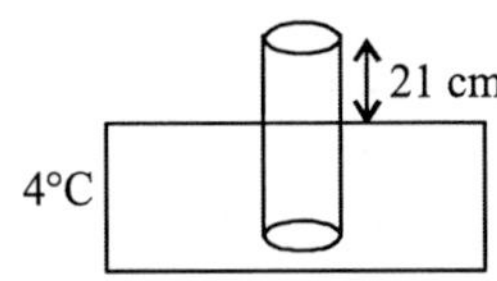

$$\therefore \frac{\rho_{4°c}}{\rho_{0°c}} = \frac{80}{79} = 1.01$$

16. (c) For minimum density of liquid, solid sphere has to float (completely immersed) in the liquid.

$mg = F_B$ (also $V_{immersed} = V_{total}$)

$$\text{or} \int \rho dV = \frac{4}{3}\pi R^3 \rho_\ell$$

$$\left[\rho(r) = \rho_0\left(1-\frac{r^2}{R^2}\right) 0 < r \le R \text{ given}\right]$$

$$\Rightarrow \int_0^R \rho_0 4\pi\left(1-\frac{r^2}{R^2}\right).r^2 dr = \frac{4}{3}\pi R^3\rho_\ell$$

$$\Rightarrow 4\pi\rho_0\left[\frac{r^3}{3}-\frac{r^5}{5R^2}\right]_0^R = \frac{4}{3}\pi R^3\rho_\ell$$

$$\frac{4\pi\rho_0 R^3}{3}\times\frac{2}{5} = \frac{4}{3}\pi R^3\rho_\ell$$

$$\therefore \rho_\ell = \frac{2\rho_0}{5}$$

17. (d) Let P_1, P_2 and P_3 be the pressure at points M, N and O respectively.

Pressure is given by $P = \rho gh$

Now, $P_1 = 0$ ($\because h = 0$)

$P_2 = \rho g(5)$

$P_3 = \rho g(15)$

$= 15\ \rho g$

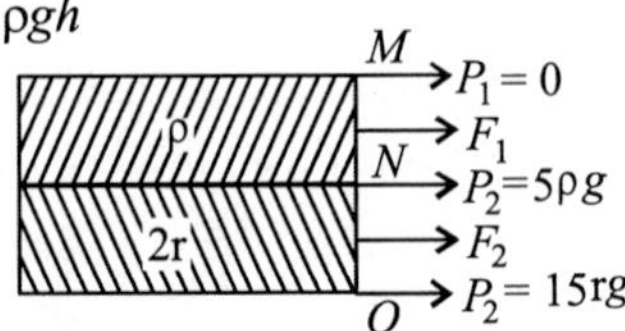

Force on upper part, $F_1 = \frac{(P_1 + P_2)}{2}A$

Force on lower part, $F_2 = \frac{(P_2 + P_3)}{2}A$

$$\therefore \frac{F_1}{F_2} = \frac{5\rho g}{20\rho g} = \frac{5}{20} = \frac{1}{4}$$

18. (b) When a body floats then the weight of the body = upthrust

$$\therefore (50)^3 \times \frac{30}{100}\times(1)\times g = M_{cube}g \quad ...(i)$$

Let m mass should be placed, then

$$(50)^3\times(1)\times g = (M_{cube} + m)g \quad ...(ii)$$

Subtracting equation (i) from equation (ii), we get

$\Rightarrow mg = (50)^3 \times g(1-0.3) = 125\times 0.7\times 10^3 g$

$\Rightarrow m = 87.5$ kg

19. (a) Using $\frac{F}{A} = Y\cdot\frac{\Delta\ell}{\ell}$

$\Rightarrow \Delta\ell \propto F$ ...(i)

$T = Mg$

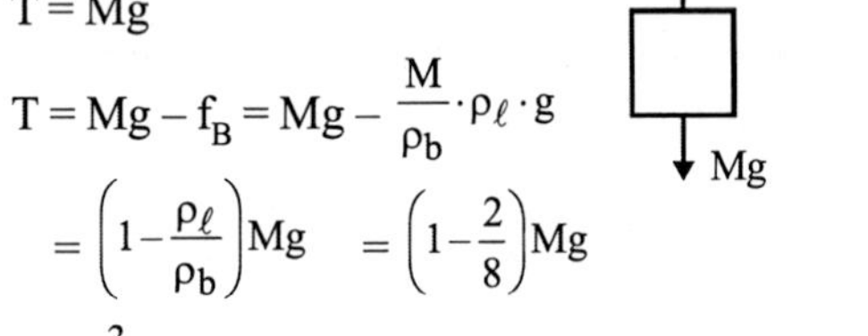

$$T = Mg - f_B = Mg - \frac{M}{\rho_b}\cdot\rho_\ell\cdot g$$

$$= \left(1-\frac{\rho_\ell}{\rho_b}\right)Mg = \left(1-\frac{2}{8}\right)Mg$$

$$T = \frac{3}{4}Mg$$

From eqn (i)

$$\frac{\Delta\ell'}{\Delta\ell} = \frac{T'}{T} = \frac{3}{4} \quad [\text{Given: } \Delta\ell = 4\text{ mm}]$$

$$\therefore \Delta\ell' = \frac{3}{4}\cdot\Delta\ell = \frac{3}{4}\times 4 = 3\text{ mm}$$

20. (b) According to question, area of cross-section at A, $aA = 40\ cm^2$ and at B, $aB = 20\ cm^2$

Let velocity of liquid flow at A, $= V_A$ and at B, $= V_B$

Using equation of continuity $a_A V_A = a_B V_B$

$40V_A = 20V_B$

$\Rightarrow 2V_A = V_B$

Now, using Bernoulli's equation

$$P_A + \frac{1}{2}\rho V_A^2 = P_B + \frac{1}{2}\rho V_B^2 \Rightarrow P_A - P_B = \frac{1}{2}\rho\left(V_B^2 - V_A^2\right)$$

$$\Rightarrow \Delta P = \frac{1}{2}1000\left(V_B^2 - \frac{V_B^2}{4}\right) \Rightarrow \Delta P = 500\times\frac{3V_B^2}{4}$$

$$\Rightarrow V_B = \sqrt{\frac{(\Delta P)\times 4}{1500}} = \sqrt{\frac{(700)\times 4}{1500}}\text{m/s} = 1.37\times 10^2\text{ cm/s}$$

Volume flow rate $Q = a_B \times v_B$

$= 20\times 100\times V_B = 2732\ cm^3/s \approx 2720\ cm^3/s$

21. (a) From the equation of continuity

$A_1 v_1 = A_2 v_2$

Here, v_1 and v_2 are the velocities at two ends of pipe. A_1 and A_2 are the area of pipe at two ends

$$\Rightarrow \frac{v_1}{v_2} = \frac{A_2}{A_1} = \frac{\pi(4.8)^2}{\pi(6.4)^2} = \frac{9}{16}$$

22. (b) Using Bernoullie's equation

$$P + \frac{1}{2}(v_1^2 - v_2^2) + \rho gh = P$$

$$\Rightarrow v_2^2 = v_1^2 + 2gh \Rightarrow v_2 = \sqrt{v_1^2 + 2gh}$$

Equation of continuity

$A_1v_1 = A_2v_2$

$(1\ cm^2)(1\ m/s) = (A_2)\left(\sqrt{(1)^2 + 2\times 10\times \frac{15}{100}}\right)$

$10^{-4}\times 1 = A_2 \times 2$

$\therefore\ A_2 = \frac{10^{-4}}{2} = 5\times 10^{-5}\ m^2$

23. (b) Mass per unit time of the liquid = ρav
Momentum per second carried by liquid
= ρav × v
Net force due to bounced back liquid,

$F_1 = 2\times\left[\frac{1}{4}\rho a v^2\right]$

Net force due to stopped liquid, $F_2 = \frac{1}{4}\rho a v^2$

Total force,

$F = F_1 + F_2 = \frac{1}{2}\rho a v^2 + \frac{1}{4}\rho a v^2 = \frac{3}{4}\rho a v^2$

Net pressure $= \frac{3}{4}\rho v^2$

24. (d) Pressure at interface A must be same from both the sides to be in equilibrium.

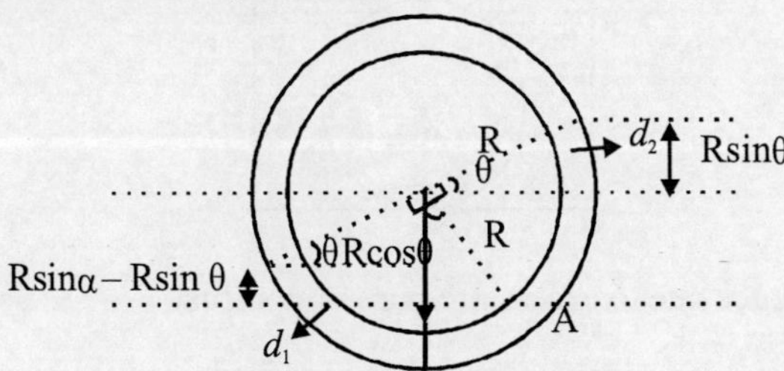

$\therefore\quad (R\cos\theta + R\sin\theta)\rho_2 g = (R\cos\theta - R\sin\theta)\rho_1 g$

$\Rightarrow\quad \frac{d_1}{d_2} = \frac{\cos\theta + \sin\theta}{\cos\theta - \sin\theta} = \frac{1+\tan\theta}{1-\tan\theta}$

$\Rightarrow\quad \rho_1 - \rho_1\tan\theta = \rho_2 + \rho_2\tan\theta$

$\Rightarrow\quad (\rho_1 + \rho_2)\tan\theta = \rho_1 - \rho_2$

$\therefore\quad \theta = \tan^{-1}\left(\frac{\rho_1 - \rho_2}{\rho_1 + \rho_2}\right)$

25. (c) Pressure at interface A must be same from both the sides to be in equilibrium.

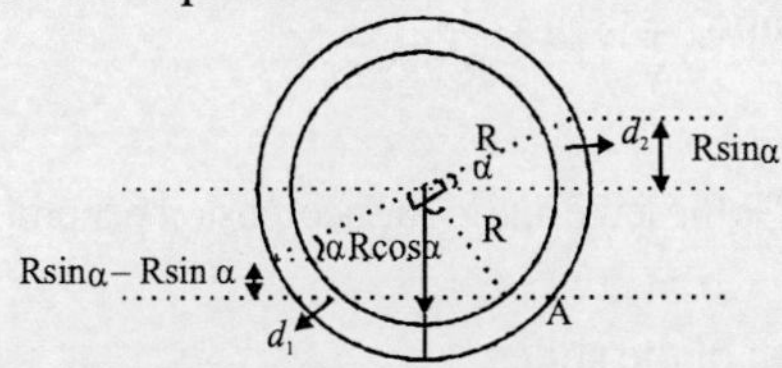

$\therefore\ (R\cos\alpha + R\sin\alpha)d_2 g = (R\cos\alpha - R\sin\alpha)d_1 g$

$\Rightarrow\ \frac{d_1}{d_2} = \frac{\cos\alpha + \sin\alpha}{\cos\alpha - \sin\alpha} = \frac{1+\tan\alpha}{1-\tan\alpha}$

26. (b) Here, volume tric flow rate

$= \frac{0.74}{60} = \pi r^2 v = (\pi\times 4\times 10^{-4})\times\sqrt{2gh}$

$\Rightarrow \sqrt{2gh} = \frac{74\times 100}{240\pi} \Rightarrow \sqrt{2gh} = \frac{740}{24\pi}$

$\Rightarrow 2gh = \frac{740\times 740}{24\times 24\times 10}\ (\because \pi^2 = 10)$

$\Rightarrow h = \frac{74\times 74}{2\times 24\times 24} \approx 4.8\,m$

i.e., The depth of the centre of the opening from the level of water in the tank is close to 4.8 m

27. (d) Using $P_1V_1 = P_2V_2$

$(P_1)\frac{4}{3}\pi r^3 = (P_2)\frac{4}{3}\pi\frac{125 r^3}{64}$

$\frac{\rho g(10) + \rho g h}{\rho g(10)} = \frac{125}{64}$

$640 + 64h = 1250$

On solving we get $h = 9.5$ m

28. (c) From figure, $kx_0 + F_B = Mg$

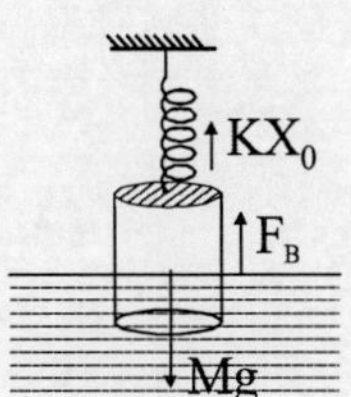

$kx_0 + \sigma\frac{L}{2}Ag = Mg$

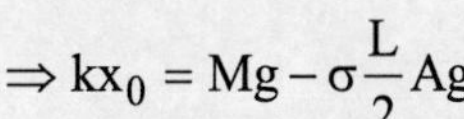
[∵ mass = density × volume]

$\Rightarrow kx_0 = Mg - \sigma\frac{L}{2}Ag$

$\Rightarrow x_0 = \frac{Mg - \frac{\sigma LAg}{2}}{k} = \frac{Mg}{k}\left(1 - \frac{LA\sigma}{2M}\right)$

Hence, extension of the spring when it is in equilibrium is,

$x_0 = \frac{Mg}{k}\left(1 - \frac{LA\sigma}{2M}\right)$

29. (c)

30. (a) Length of the air column above mercury in the tube is,

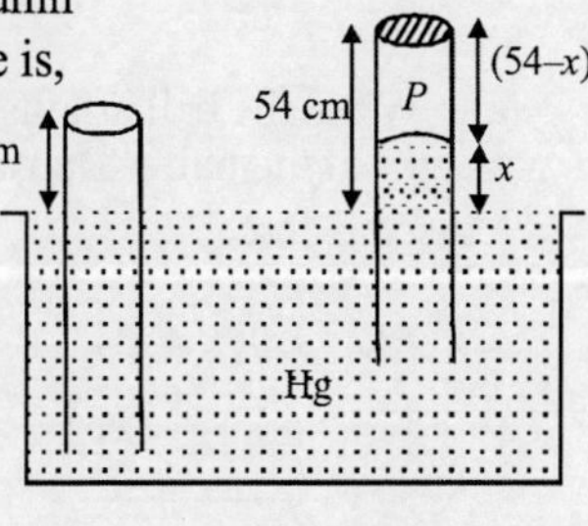

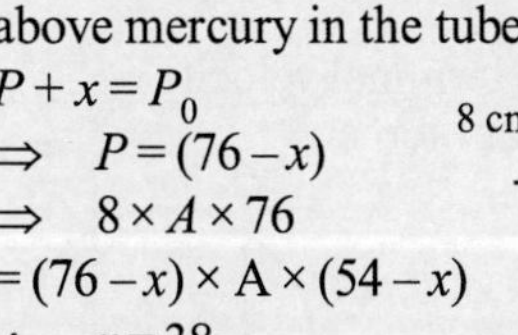
$P + x = P_0$

$\Rightarrow\ P = (76 - x)$

$\Rightarrow\ 8\times A\times 76$

$= (76 - x)\times A\times(54 - x)$

$\therefore\ x = 38$

Thus, length of air column
= 54 – 38 = 16 cm.

31. (b) Let the rate of falling water level be $-\frac{dh}{dt}$

Initially at $t = 0;\ h = h$

$t = t;\ h = 0$

Then, $A\left(-\frac{dh}{dt}\right) = \pi a^2.v$

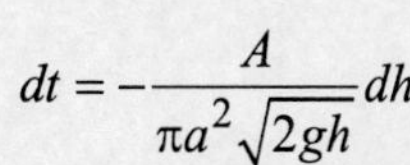
$dt = -\frac{A}{\pi a^2\sqrt{2gh}}dh$

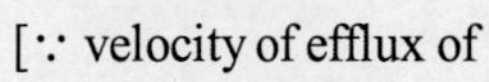
[∵ velocity of efflux of

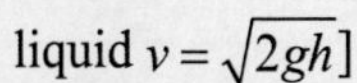
liquid $v = \sqrt{2gh}$]

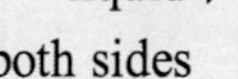
Integrating both sides

$\int_0^t dt = -\frac{A}{\sqrt{2g}\pi a^2}\int_h^0 h^{-1/2}dh$

$$[t]_0^t = -\frac{A}{\sqrt{2g}\pi a^2}\cdot\left[\frac{h^{1/2}}{1/2}\right]_h^0$$

$$t = \frac{\sqrt{2}A}{\pi a^2}\sqrt{\frac{h}{g}}$$

32. (b) 33. (a)

34. (a) As $A_1v_1 = A_2v_2$ (Principle of continuity)

or, $\ell^2\sqrt{2gh} = \pi r^2\sqrt{2g\times 4h}$ (Efflux velocity= $\sqrt{2gh}$)

$\therefore \quad r^2 = \frac{\ell^2}{2\pi}$ or $r = \sqrt{\frac{\ell^2}{2\pi}} = \frac{\ell}{\sqrt{2\pi}}$

35. (a) $27\times\frac{4}{3}\pi r^3 = \frac{4}{3}\pi r^3$ or $r = \frac{R}{3}$.

Terminal velocity, $v \propto r^2$

$\therefore \frac{v_1}{v_2} = \frac{r_1^2}{r_2^2}$

or $v_2 = \left(\frac{r_2}{r_1}\right)^2 v_1 = \left(\frac{R/3}{R}\right)^2 v_1 = \frac{1}{9}$ or $\frac{v_1}{v_2} = 9$.

36. (b) $\eta = 10^{-2}$ poise

$v = 18$ km/h $= \frac{18000}{3600} = 5$ m/s

$l = 5$ m

Strain rate $= \frac{v}{l}$

Coefficient of viscosity, $\eta = \frac{\text{shearing stress}}{\text{strain rate}}$

$\therefore$ Shearing stress $= \eta \times$ strain rate

$= 10^{-2}\times\frac{5}{5} = 10^{-2}$ Nm^{-2}

37. (a) When the ball attains terminal velocity

Weight of the ball = Buoyant force + Viscous force

$\therefore V\rho_1 g = V\rho_2 g + kv_t^2$

$\Rightarrow Vg(\rho_1 - \rho_2)g = kv_t^2$

$\Rightarrow v_t = \sqrt{\frac{Vg(\rho_1-\rho_2)}{k}}$

F_v $B = V\rho_2 g$ $W = V\rho_1 g$

38. (b) Given,

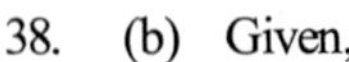

Angle of contact $\theta = 30°$

Surface tension, $T = 0.05$ Nm^{-1}

Radius of capillary tube, $r = 0.15$ mm $= 0.15\times 10^{-3}$m

Density of methylene iodide,

$\rho = 667$ kg m^{-3}

Capillary rise, $h = \frac{2T\cos\theta}{\rho g r}$

$$= \frac{2\times 0.05\times\frac{\sqrt{3}}{2}}{667\times 10\times 0.15\times 10^{-3}}$$

$= 0.087$ m

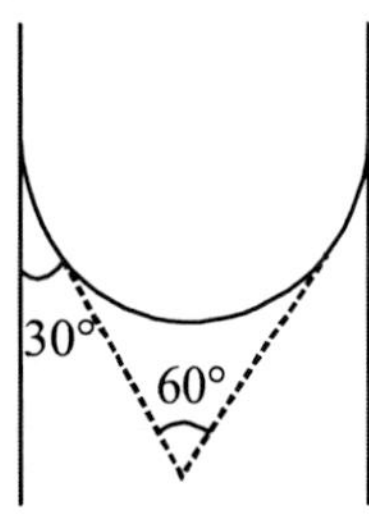

39. (d) For the drops to be in equilibrium upward force on drop = downward force on drop

$$T.2\pi R = \frac{4}{3}\pi R^3 dg - \frac{2}{3}\pi R^3\rho g$$

$$\Rightarrow \quad T(2\pi R) = \frac{2}{3}\pi R^3(2d-\rho)g$$

$$\Rightarrow \quad T = \frac{R^2}{3}(2d-\rho)g \;\Rightarrow\; R = \sqrt{\frac{3T}{(2d-\rho)g}}$$

40. (b) As we know that

$$\frac{2T\cos\theta}{r\rho g} = \text{R h} \Rightarrow \frac{T_{Hg}}{T_{Water}} = 7.5$$

$$\frac{\rho_{Hg}}{\rho_W} = 13.6\,\&\,\frac{\cos\theta_{Hg}}{\cos\theta_W} = \frac{\cos 135°}{\cos 0°} = \frac{1}{\sqrt{2}}$$

$$\frac{R_{Hg}}{R_{Water}} = \left(\frac{T_{Hg}}{T_W}\right)\left(\frac{\rho_W}{\rho_{Hg}}\right)\left(\frac{\cos\theta_{Hg}}{\cos\theta_W}\right)$$

$$= 7.5\times\frac{1}{13.6}\times\frac{1}{\sqrt{2}} = 0.4 = \frac{2}{5}$$

41. (a) When the bubble gets detached,

Buoyant force = force due to surface tension

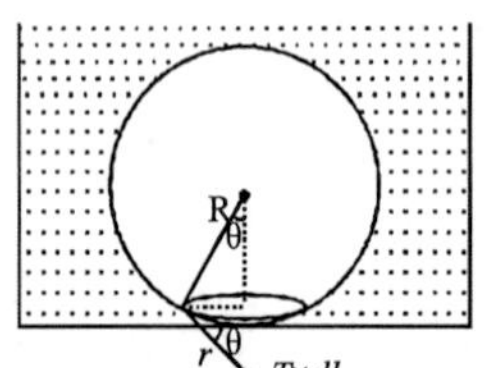

Force due to excess pressure = upthrust

Access pressure in air bubble $= \frac{2T}{R}$

$$\frac{2T}{R}(\pi r^2) = \frac{4\pi R^3}{3T}\rho_w g$$

$$\Rightarrow r^2 = \frac{2R^4\rho_w g}{3T} \Rightarrow r = R^2\sqrt{\frac{2\rho_w g}{3T}}$$

42. (a) Acceleration due to gravity changes with the depth,

$$g' = g\left(1 - \frac{d}{R}\right)$$

Pressure, P = ρgh

Hence ratio, $\frac{x}{y}$ is $\left(1 - \frac{d}{R}\right)$

43. (b)

44. (d) Let T is the force due to surface tension per unit length, then

$F = 2lT$

l = length of the slider.

At equilibrium, $F = W$

$\therefore 2Tl = mg$

$$\Rightarrow T = \frac{mg}{2l} = \frac{1.5\times 10^{-2}}{2\times 30\times 10^{-2}} = \frac{1.5}{60} = 0.025\,\text{Nm}^{-1}$$

45. (c) Water fills the tube entirely in gravityless condition i.e., 20 cm.

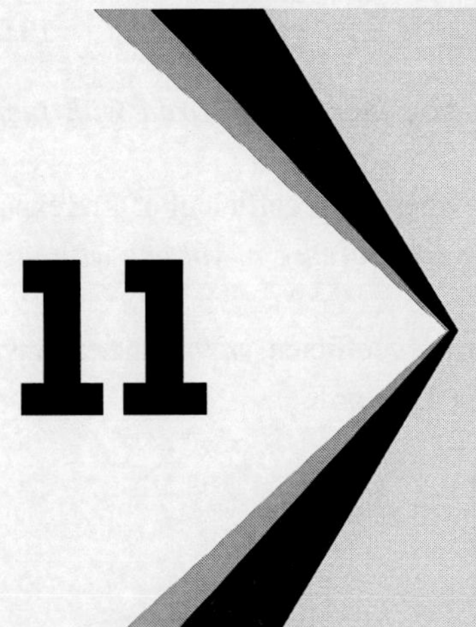

11 Thermal Properties of Matter

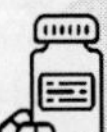

Topic 11.1 : Temperature, Ideal Gas Equation & Absolute Temperature and Thermal Expansion

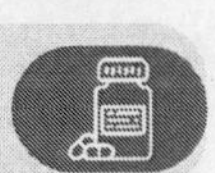

TEMPERATURE

The temperature of a body is that physical quantity which indicates how much hot or cold the body is? So *temperature indicates the hotness or coldness of a body.*

The flow of heat is always from higher temperature to lower temperature. Temperature is a macroscopic concept.

Two bodies are said to be in **thermal equilibrium** with each other, when no heat flows from one body to the other, that is when both the bodies are at the same temperature.

Temperature measuring device :

Thermometer is a device to measure the temperature. Thermometers used for measuring very high temperatures are called **pyrometers.**

Different types of temperature scales

Name of the scale	*Symbol for each degree*	*Lower fixed point*	*Upper fixed point*	*No. of divisions on the scale*
Reaumur	°R	0°R	80°R	80
Celsius	°C	0°C	100°C	100
Fahrenheit	°F	32°F	212°F	180
Rankine	Ra	460Ra	672Ra	212
Kelvin	K	273K	373K	100

* Lower fixed point (LFP) is the freezing point of water.

* Upper fixed point (UFP) is the boiling point of water.
$T°K = (t°C + 273)$ or $t°C = (TK - 273)$

Relationship between different temperature scales

$$\frac{R}{80} = \frac{C}{100} = \frac{F-32}{180} = \frac{Ra-460}{212} = \frac{K-273}{100}$$

The zero of the Kelvin scale is called ***absolute zero***. The Kelvin scale is often termed as the absolute scale. In common use the absolute zero corresponds to –273°C. However, its exact value is –273.16°C.

IDEAL GAS EQUATION AND ABSOLUTE TEMPERATURE

The equation, $PV = nRT$

where, n = number of moles in the sample of gas

R = universal gas constant; (its value is 8.31 J mol^{-1} K^{-1}), is known as **ideal-gas equation**

It is the combination of following three laws :

(i) **Boyle's law :** *When temperature is held constant, the pressure is inversely proportional to volume.*
i.e., $P \propto \frac{1}{V}$ (at constant temperature)

(ii) **Charle's law :** *When the pressure is held constant, the volume of the gas is directly porportional to the absolute temperature.*
i.e., $V \propto T$ (at constant pressure)

(iii) **Avogadro's law :** *When the pressure and temperature are kept constant, the volume is directly proportional to the number of moles of the ideal gas in the container.*
i.e., $V \propto n$ (at constant pressure and temperature)

Absolute Temperature

The lowest temperature of –273.16 °C at which a gas is supposed to have zero volume and zero pressure and at which entire molecular motion stops is called absolute zero temperature. A new scale of temperature starting with –273.16°C by Lord Kelvin as zero. This is called Kelvin scale or absolute scale of temperature.

T(K) = t°C + 273.16

Thermometric property : It is the property used to measure the temperature. Any physical quantity such as length of mercury (in a glass capillary), pressure of a gas (at constant volume), electrical resistance (of a metal wire), thermo emf (thermo-couple thermometer) which changes with a change in temperature can be used to measure temperature.

The unknown temperature t on a scale by utilising a general property X of the substance is given by

$$t = \left(\frac{X_t - X_0}{X_{100} - X_0}\right) \times 100° C$$

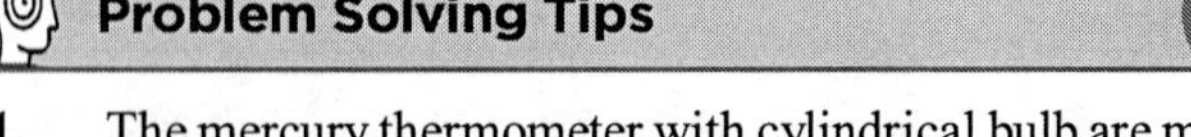

1. The mercury thermometer with cylindrical bulb are more sensitive than those with spherical bulb.
2. Alcohol thermometer is preferred to the mercury thermometer due to the larger value of the coefficient of cubical expansion.
3. **Properties that make mercury the ideal thermometric substance are :**
   (i) It does not stick to the glass walls
   (ii) Available in pure form
   (iii) Low thermal conductivity and low specific heat
   (iv) Vapour Pressure is low
   (v) Coefficient of expansion is uniform
   (vi) It shines
4. Gas thermometer is more sensitive than the mercury thermometer, because its coefficient of cubical expansion is much larger.
5. At the following temperatures **different temperature scales have the same reading :**
   (i) Fahreinheit and Reaumur at –25.6°F = –25.6°R
   (ii) Reaumur and Celsius at 0°R = 0°C
   (iii) Celsius and Fahrenheit at –40°C = –40°F
   (iv) Fahrenheit and Kelvin at 574.25°F = 574.25K
6. The Celsius scale and the Kelvin cannot have the same reading at any temperature.
7. Six's thermometer measures minimum and maximum temperature during a day. It uses mercury as well as alcohol as the thermometric substances.
8. Normal human body temperature is 37°C = 98.6°F.
9. Clinical thermometers are much shorter than the laboratory thermometers because they are used to measure a limited range (96° F to 100° F) of temperature.
10. Rapidly changing temperature is measured by using thermo electric thermometer.
11. The temperature inside a motor engine is measured using platinum resistance thermometer.
12. The radiation thermometers can measure temperature from a distance.
13. Adiabatic demagnetisation can be used to measure temperature very near to the absolute zero.
14. The Rankine is the smallest temperature range among all the scales of temperature.
15. When a substance is heated it expands along each dimension in the same proportion. (if it is uniform)

THERMAL EXPANSION

Thermal Expansion of Substances

Linear expansion : *i.e., increase in length with increase in temperature*

$$\Delta l = \alpha l_0 \Delta T$$

or $$l - l_0 = \alpha l_0 \Delta T \Rightarrow l = l_0(1 + \alpha \Delta T)$$

where l_0 is the initial length, l = final length, ΔT = change in temperature, α = coefficient of linear expansion.

Areal expansion : *i.e., increase in area with increase in temperature.*

$$\Delta A = \beta A_0 \Delta T \text{ where } \beta = \text{coefficient of area expansion}$$

Volume expansion : *i.e. increase in volume with increase in temperature.*

$\Delta V = \gamma V_0 \Delta T$ where γ = coefficient of volume expansion. The units of α, β and γ is $(°C)^{-1}$ or K^{-1}.

Graph of α_v versus T :

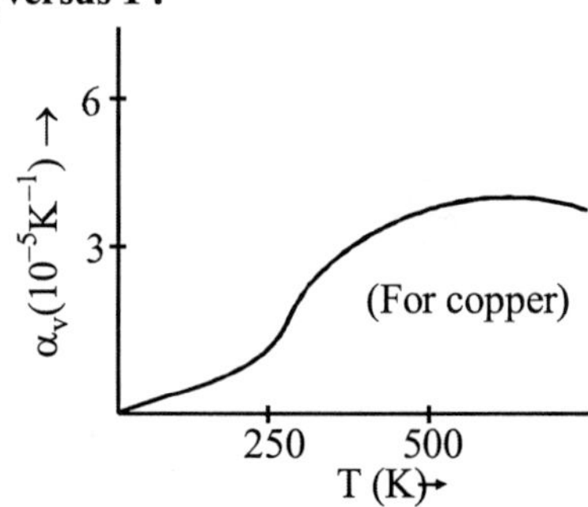

Problem Solving Tips

1. During change in temperature, the mass does not change but the density decreases due to increase in volume. Therefore

$$\rho = \frac{\rho_0}{1 + \gamma \Delta T}$$

2. **Relation between α, β and γ**

$$\gamma = 3\alpha \text{ and } \beta = 2\alpha$$

3. Water has negative coefficient of volume expansion for temperature range (0°C – 4°C). Therefore water contracts when the temperature rises from 0°C to 4°C and then expands as the temperature increases further.
   Density of water reaches a maximum value of 1000 kg m^{-3} at 4°C. This is the **anomalous behaviour of water.**

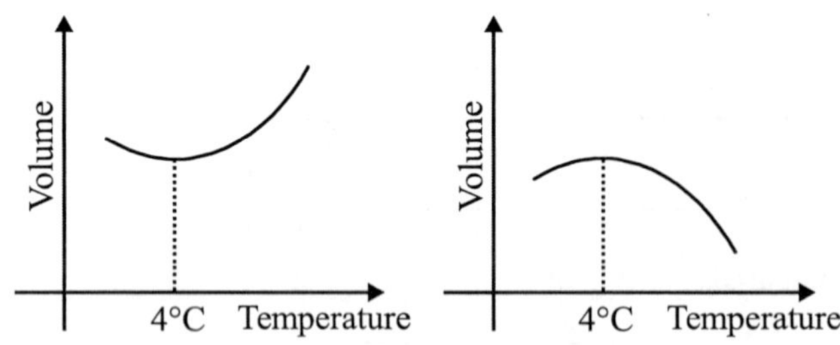

Thermal Expansion of Liquid (which is heated in a vessel)

$$\Delta V_{app} = V(\gamma - 3\alpha)\Delta T$$

where ΔV_{app} = apparent change in volume
V = volume of the liquid initially
γ = coefficient of volume expansion of liquid
α = coefficient of linear expansion of vessel

It is clear from the formula that if $\gamma = 3\alpha$, $\Delta V_{app} = 0$ but if $\gamma > 3\alpha$, ΔV_{app} is positive and the liquid rises in the vessel and if $\gamma < 3\alpha$, ΔV_{app} is negative and liquid falls in vessel.

Change in density of solids and liquids with temperature.
The density at t°C is given by

$$\rho_t = \frac{\rho_0}{(1+\gamma t)}$$

where ρ_0 is the density at 0°C. If ρ_1 and ρ_2 are the densities at temperature t_1 and t_2 respectively, then

$$\gamma = \frac{\rho_1 - \rho_2}{\rho_2(t_2 - t_1)}$$

Thermal Stress

If a rod fixed at two ends is heated or cooled, then stress are produced in the rod.

$$\text{Thermal stress} = Y \times \alpha\Delta T \quad \left(\frac{\Delta l}{l_0} = \alpha\Delta T = \text{strain}\right)$$

Effect of Temperature on Pendulum Clock

A Pendulum clock consists of a metal bar attached with a bob at one end and fixed at the other end. Let pendulum clock read correct time when its length is ℓ_0. The time period

$$t_0 = 2\pi\sqrt{\frac{\ell_0}{g}}$$

Suppose that the temperature is raised by ΔT, then new time period is

$$t = 2\pi\sqrt{\frac{\ell}{g}} \Rightarrow \frac{t}{t_0} = \sqrt{\frac{\ell}{\ell_0}} \quad .....(i)$$

We have $\ell = \ell_0(1+\alpha\Delta t)$

$$\Rightarrow \frac{\ell}{\ell_0} = (1+\alpha\Delta t) \quad .....(ii)$$

From equations (i) and (ii),

$$\frac{t}{t_0} = (1+\alpha\Delta t)^{\frac{1}{2}}$$

$$= 1 + \frac{1}{2}\alpha\Delta t \quad (\text{since } \alpha \text{ is very small})$$

$$\Rightarrow \frac{t}{t_0} - 1 = \frac{1}{2}\alpha\Delta t \Rightarrow \frac{t - t_0}{t_0} = \frac{1}{2}\alpha\Delta t$$

so, fractional change in time

$$\frac{\Delta t}{t_0} = \frac{1}{2}\alpha\Delta T$$

$$\text{Loss of time per day} = \frac{1}{2}\alpha\Delta T \times 86400 \text{ second}.$$

($\because$ no. of seconds in one day = 86400 sec.)

When temperature increases (during summer), the length of the pendulum increases due to which the time period increases and the clock loses time. On the other hand, when temperature decreases (during winter season), the length decreases and the time period decrease, the clock in this case, gains time.

Error in scale reading :

As the temperature changes, the length of the metal scale changes so is the difference in graduation

$$R_a = R_m(1+\alpha\Delta T)$$

where R_a = actual reading, R_m = measured reading

Isothermal and adiabatic elasticities :

(i) Isothermal elasticity, $E_{iso} \equiv \dfrac{dP}{-\left(\dfrac{dV}{V}\right)} = P.$

(since PV = RT = constant, $\dfrac{dP}{dV} = -\dfrac{P}{V}$)

(ii) Adiabatic elasticity,

$$E_{adia} = \frac{dP}{-\left(\dfrac{dV}{V}\right)} = \gamma P; \text{ where } \gamma = \frac{C_p}{C_v}$$

(iii) $E_{adia} = \gamma E_{iso}$

Expansion of Gases

There are two coefficients of expansion of gases.

(a) Pressure coefficient of expansion of gas (γ_P)

$$\gamma_P = \frac{P_t - P_0}{P_0 t}$$

where P_0 = Pressure at 0°C, P_t = Pressure at t°C

(b) Volume coefficient of expansion of gas (γ_v)

$$\gamma_v = \frac{V_t - V_0}{V_0 t}$$

where V_0 = Volume at 0°C, V_t = Volume at t°C

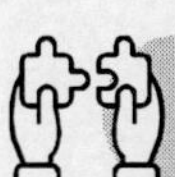

11.1 Concept Practice Problems CPP

1. A vessel completely filled with a liquid is heated. If α and γ represent coefficient of linear expansion of material of vessel and coefficient of cubical expansion of liquid respectively, then the liquid will not overflow if
(a) $\gamma = 3\alpha$ (b) $\gamma > 3\alpha$ (c) $\gamma < 3\alpha$ (d) $\gamma \le 3\alpha$

2. Two straight metallic strips each of thickness t and length ℓ are rivetted together. Their coefficients of linear expansions are α_1 and α_2. If they are heated through temperature ΔT, the bimetallic strip will bend to form an arc of radius
(a) $t/\{(\alpha_1 + \alpha_2)\Delta T\}$ (b) $t/\{(\alpha_2 - \alpha_1)\Delta T\}$
(c) $t(\alpha_1 - \alpha_2)\Delta T$ (d) $t(\alpha_2 - \alpha_1)\Delta T$

3. For the construction of a thermometer, one of the essential requirements is a thermometric substance which
(a) remains liquid over the entire range of temperatures to be meaured.
(b) has property that varies linearly with temperature
(c) has a property that varies with temperature
(d) obey Boyle's law

4. The temperature of an iron block is 140°F. Its temperature on the Celsius scale is
(a) 60° (b) 160° (c) 140° (d) 132°

5. A metallic bar is heated from 0°C to 100°C. The coeficient of linear expansion is 10^{-5} K^{-1}. What will be the percentage increase in length?
(a) 0.01% (b) 0.1% (c) 1% (d) 10%

6. A mountain climber finds that water boils at 80°C. The temperature of this boiling water is...... Fahrenheit
(a) 50° (b) 150° (c) 176° (d) 200°

7. A metal cube of length 10.0 mm at 0°C (273K) is heated to 200°C (473K). Given : its coefficient of linear expansion is 2×10^{-5} K^{-1}. The percent change of its volume is
(a) 0.1 (b) 0.2 (c) 0.4 (d) 1.2

8. A crystal has a coefficient of expansion 13×10^{-7} in one direction and 231×10^{-7} in every direction at right angles to it. Then the cubical coefficient of expansion is
(a) 462×10^{-7} (b) 244×10^{-7}
(c) 475×10^{-7} (d) 257×10^{-7}

9. A rectangular block is heated from 0°C to 100°C. The percentage increase in its length is 0.10%. What will be the percentage increase in its volume?
(a) 0.03% (b) 0.10%
(c) 0.30% (d) None of these

10. Which of the following temperatures is the highest?
(a) 100K (b) –13°F (c) –20°C (d) –23°C.

ANSWER KEY

1	(d)	2	(b)	3	(c)	4	(a)	5	(b)	6	(c)	7	(d)	8	(a)	9	(c)	10	(b)

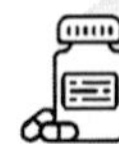

Topic 11.2 : Heat, Specific Heat Capacity, Thermal Capacity Latent Heat, Heat Transfer & Newton's Law of Cooling

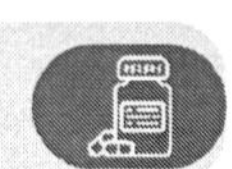

HEAT

Heat is the form of energy which is transferred from one body to another body due to temperature difference between two bodies. Thermal energy of a body is the sum of kinetic energy of random motion of the molecules/atoms and the potential energy due to the interatomic forces.

Calorimeter is an instrument used to measure the heat.

The **SI unit** of heat is joule and its **dimensions** are $[ML^2 T^{-2}]$.

Other units of heat are :

(i) **Calorie:** It is the amount of heat required to raise the temperature of 1g of water from 14.5°C to 15.5°C.
1 calorie = 4.2 joule. Calorie is the unit of heat in **CGS system.**

(ii) **Kilocalorie,** 1Kcal = 1000 cal

(iii) **British Thermal Unit (BTU):** It is the fps unit of heat = 252 cal = amount of heat required to raise the temperature of 1 lb of water through 1°F (from 63°F to 64°F).

SPECIFIC HEAT CAPACITY

It is the amount of heat required to raise the temperature of unit mass of substance through 1 degree.

$$\textit{Specific heat capacity, } c = \frac{Q}{m \times \Delta t}$$

Its **SI unit** is J kg^{-1}K^{-1}

CGS unit cal g^{-1}°C^{-1}

It **dimensions** are $[M^0L^2T^{-2}\theta^{-1}]$

For gases : During the **isothermal** process

$\Delta t = 0 \Rightarrow c = \infty$ (infinite)

and during the **adiabatic** process

$Q = 0 \Rightarrow c = 0$ (zero)

Specific heat of gas : The specific heat of a gas varies from zero to infinity. It may have any positive or negative value.

Following of two specific heats of gas are more significant.

(a) **Molar specific heat at constant volume** (C_V) : It is the amount of heat required to raise the temperature of 1 mole of a gas through 1K or 1°C at constant volume.

$$C_V = \frac{1}{n}\left(\frac{dQ}{dT}\right)$$

(b) **Molar specific heat at constant pressure** (C_P) : It is the amount of heat required to raise the temperature of 1 mole of a gas through 1K or 1°C at constant pressure.

$$C_P = \frac{1}{n}\left(\frac{dQ}{dT}\right)$$

Mayer's relation : $C_P - C_V = R$

[where R is a gas constant. (R = 8.314 Jmol^{-1}K^{-1})]

Why C_P is greater than C_V ?

When heat is supplied to a gas at constant volume entirely used to raise its temperature. When a gas is heated at constant pressure, some work is done in expansion of gas which is in addition to raise its temperature and hence $C_P > C_V$.

THERMAL CAPACITY OR HEAT CAPACITY

It is the amount of heat required to raise the temperature of substance through 1°C or 1K.

Thermal capacity = mass × specific heat.

This is the relation between sp. heat capacity and heat capacity. Its **SI unit** is JK^{-1} **CGS unit** cal/°C. Its **dimensions** are $[ML^2T^{-2}\theta^{-1}]$

Water Equivalent

It is the mass of water in gram which would require the same amount of heat to raise its temperature through 1°C as the body when heated through the same temperature. It is measured in gram. Hence

Water equivalent of a body = mass of the body × specific heat

Principle of Heat (or Calorimetry)

When two bodies at different temperatures are placed in contact with each other then heat will flow from the body at higher temperature to the body at lower temperature until both reach to a common temperature.

i.e. *Heat lost by hot body = heat gained by cold body.*

It follows the law of conservation of energy.

LATENT HEAT

It is defined as the amount of heat absorbed or given out by a body during the change of state while its temperature remaining constant.

It is of two types :

(i) **Latent heat of fusion :** It is the quantity of heat required to change unit mass of the solid into liquid at its melting point.

Latent heat of fusion of ice is 80 cal/g.

(ii) **Latent heat of vaporisation :** It is the quantity of heat required to convert unit mass of liquid into vapour at its boiling point.

Latent heat of vaporisation of water is 536 cal/g.

Latent heat increases the intermolecular potential energy of the molecules while kinetic energy remains constant.

Different Processes of Phase Change or State Change

(i) **Sublimation :** It is the process of conversion of solids to gaseous state on heating. On cooling the vapours get converted back into solids.

(ii) **Condensation :** It is the process of conversion of gases/vapours to liquid state on cooling. On heating, these liquids are converted into vapours/gases.

(iii) **Boiling :** It is the process of conversion of liquid to gaseous state on heating. It is a cooling process.

(iv) **Melting :** It is the process in which solid gets converted into liquid on heating.

(v) **Evaporation :** Conversion of liquid into gaseous state at all temperatures is called evaporation. It is a phenomenon that occurs at the surface of the liquid.

Melting and boiling occur at definite temperature called melting point and boiling point respectively. The *liquid boils at a temperature, at which its **vapour pressure is equal to the atmospheric pressure.***

How evaporation is different from boiling?

Evaporation is a slow process occurring at all the temperature at the surface of liquid while boiling is a fast process involving whole of the liquid heated to a particular temperature called boiling point of the liquid.

Problem Solving Tips

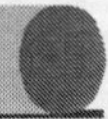

1. The heat capacity or thermal capacity depends on nature of the substance (specific heat capacity) and mass of quantity of matter of the body.
2. In case of melting and boiling, the temperature does not change, only intermolecular potential energy of the system changes.
3. System are in thermal equilibrium when their temperature are same or average kinetic energy per molecule is same.
4. Internal energy is the sum of all energies in a system which includes energy of translational, rotational as well as vibrational motion of the molecules.
5. The molar specific heat capacity depends on the molecular weight of the substance.
6. The temperature, volume or pressure of a system may remain constant when it absorbs heat.
7. When we press two block of ice together such that after releasing the pressure two block join this phenomenon is called **regelation**.

Phase Diagram

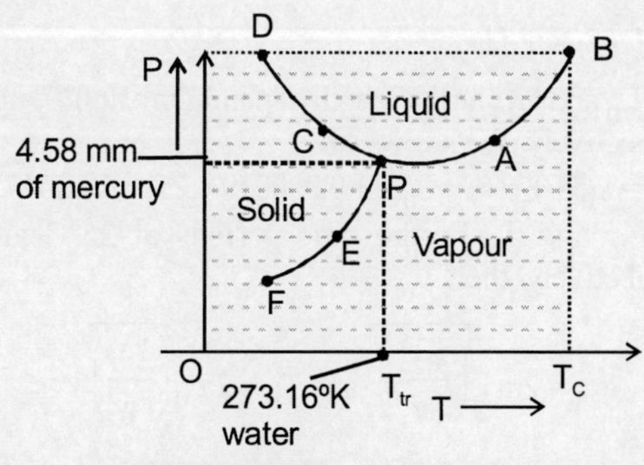

(i) The diagram shows vaporisation curve (AB), fusion curve (CD), sublimation curve (EF).

(ii) For water, AB is called steam line, CD is called ice line and EF is called hoar-frost line.

(iii) The temperature at which all the three states of matter (solid, liquid, gas) are mutually in thermal equilibrium is called the triple point (point P in diagram) of the substance.

(iv) The temperature upto which a gas can be liquified under pressure alone is called the **critical temperature** (T_c).

Example 1.

A solid material is supplied with heat at a constant rate. The temperature of the material is changing with the heat input as shown in Fig. Study the graph carefully and answer the following :

(i) What is represented by horizontal regions AB & CD?

(ii) If CD = 2 AB. What do you infer?

Solution :

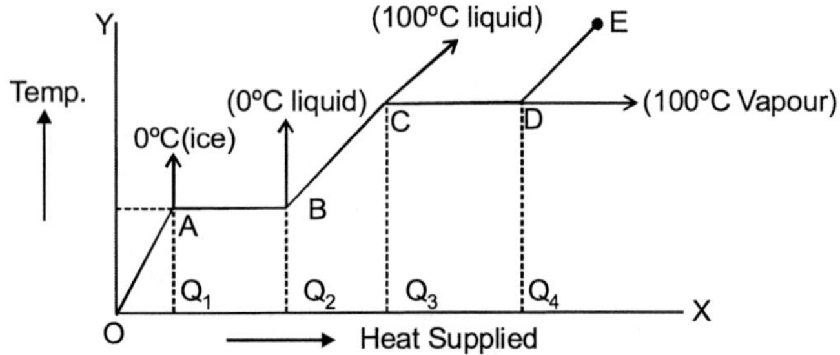

(i) In the horizontal regions AB and CD heat is supplied but temp. remains constant. Therefore, they represent change of state. The graph AB represents change from solid state to liquid state, at constant temp. = melting point of solid.
AB = latent heat of fusion.
Again CD represents change of state from liquid to vapour at boiling point of the liquid.
CD = latent heat of vaporisation.

(ii) As CD = 2 AB
∴ Latent heat of vaporisation is twice the latent heat of fusion.

Example 2.

A clock which keeps correct time at 25°C has a pendulum made of brass whose coefficient of linear expansion is 0.000019. How many seconds a day will it gain if the temperature fall to 0°C?

Solution :

Let L_0 and L_{25} be the length of pendulum at 0°C and 25°C respectively. We know that

$L_{25} = L_0(1+\alpha T) = L_0(1+0.000019\times 25) = 1.000475\, L_0$

If T_{25} and T_0 be the time periods at 25°C and 0°C respectively, then

$$T_{25} = 2\pi\sqrt{\left(\frac{L_{25}}{g}\right)} \text{ and } T_0 = 2\pi\sqrt{\left(\frac{L_0}{g}\right)}$$

$$\therefore \quad \frac{T_{25}}{T_0} = \sqrt{\left(\frac{L_{25}}{L_0}\right)} = \sqrt{\left(\frac{1.000475 L_0}{L_0}\right)}$$

$$= \sqrt{(1.000475)} = 1.000237$$

$$\text{Now } \frac{T_{25}-T_0}{T_0} = 0.000237$$

∴ Gain in time for one vibration = 2 × 0.000237 sec.

$$\text{Number of vibration in one day} = \frac{24\times 60\times 60}{2}$$

(T = 2 sec.)

Hence the gain in time in one day

$$= 2\times 0.000237\times \frac{24\times 60\times 60}{2} = 20.52 \text{sec.}$$

Example 3.

A circular hole in an aluminium plate is 2.54 cm in diameter at 0°C. What is the diameter when the temperature of the plate is raised to 100°C ? Given $\alpha_A = 2.3\times 10^{-5}\,(°C)^{-1}$

Solution :

Let D_0 and D_t be diameters of hole at 0°C and t°C respectively.

Circumference of hole at 0°C

$\ell_0 = 2\pi r_0 = \pi D_0$

Circumference of hole at t = 100°C

$\ell_t = 2\pi r_t = \pi D_t$

From relation $\ell_t = \ell_0(1+\alpha.t)$, we get

$\pi D_t = \pi D_0 (1 + 2.3\times 10^{-5}\times 100)$

$D_t = 2.54(1+0.0023) = 2.5458$ cm

Example 4.

If the volume of a block of a metal changes by 0.12% when it is heated through 20°C, what is the coefficient of linear expansion of metal ?

Solution :

Coefficient of cubical expansion of metal is given by

$$\gamma = \frac{\Delta V}{Vt}$$

$$\text{Here } \gamma = \frac{\Delta V}{Vt} = \frac{0.12}{100t}, \ t = 20°C$$

$$\therefore \gamma = \frac{0.12}{100\times 20} = 6.0\times 10^{-5} \text{ per °C}$$

Coefficient of linear expansion

$$\alpha = \frac{\gamma}{3} = \frac{6.0\times 10^{-5}}{3} = 2.0\times 10^{-5} \text{ Per °C}$$

Example 5.

From what height must a block of ice be dropped into a well of water so that 5% of it may melt? Given : both ice and water are at 0°C, L = 80 cal g^{-1}, J = 4.2 J cal^{-1} and g = 980 cm s^{-2}.

Solution :

Let m be the mass of ice. Let h be the height from which block of ice is dropped. Work done,

W = mgh = m × 980 × h erg

$$\text{Mass of ice to be melted} = \frac{5}{100}\times m$$

$$\text{Heat required, } Q = \frac{5}{100}\times m\times 80 \text{ cal or } Q = 4m \text{ cal}$$

$[\because L = 80 \text{ cal } g^{-1}]\,[\because W = JQ]$

Now, m × 980 × h = J × 4 m

$$h = \frac{4.2 \times 10^7 \times 4m}{m \times 980} \text{ cm} = 1714.3 \text{ m}$$
$$[\because J = 4.2 \times 10^7 \text{ erg cal}^{-1}]$$

Saturated and Unsaturated Air

The air is said to be **saturated** when the maximum possible amount of water vapours are present in it. The pressure of the water vapours in the saturated air is **called saturation vapour pressure.**

If the air contains vapours less than the maximum possible amount possible in the air, then it (air) is said to be **unsaturated.**

Vapour Pressure

A vapour differs from a gas in that the former can be liqufied by pressure alone, wheras the latter cannot be liqufied unless it is first cooled.

If a liquid is kept in a closed vessel, the space above the liquid becomes saturated with vapour. The pressure exerted by this vapour is called saturated vapour pressure. Its value depends only on temperature. It is independent of any external pressure.

Humidity

The **humidity** shows the presence of water vapours in the atmosphere. The amount of water vapours present per unit volume of the air is called **absolute humidity**.

Relative humidity (*RH*) *is defined as the ratio of the mass of water vapour (m) actually present in the given volume of air to the mass of water vapour (M) required to saturate the same volume at the same temperature.* Normally RH is expressed in percentage

i.e., $\%RH = \frac{m}{M} \times 100\%$

RH is also defined as the ratio of actual pressure (p) of water vapour to the saturated vapour pressure (P) of the water at the same temperature

i.e., $\%RH = \frac{p}{P} \times 100\%$

Also,

$$RH = \frac{\text{Saturated vapour pressure of water at dew point}}{\text{Saturated vapour pressure of water at room temperature}}$$

Dew Point :

It is the temperature at which the amount of water vapours actually present in a certain volume of the air which is sufficient to saturate that volume of air.

At the dew point the actual vapour pressure becomes the saturated vapour pressure.

It means that vapour pressure at room temperature = saturated vapour pressure(S.V.P) at dew point

If room teperature = dew point

then Relative humidity (R.H.) = 100%

Problem Solving Tips

1. **Hygrometry** is the branch of thermal physics that deals with the measurement of amount of water vapours present in the atmosphere.
2. **Hygrometer** is an instrument used to determine dew point and relative humidity.
3. Relative humidity is low when the air is dry.
4. Saturated vapours do not obey (except Dalton's law) gas laws, while unsaturated vapours obey them. The S.V.P. varies linearly with temperature (keeping volume constant) and equal to one atmospheric pressure at boiling point.(shown in fig.(a)) S.V.P. constant at constant temperature on increasing or decreasing volume fig. (b).

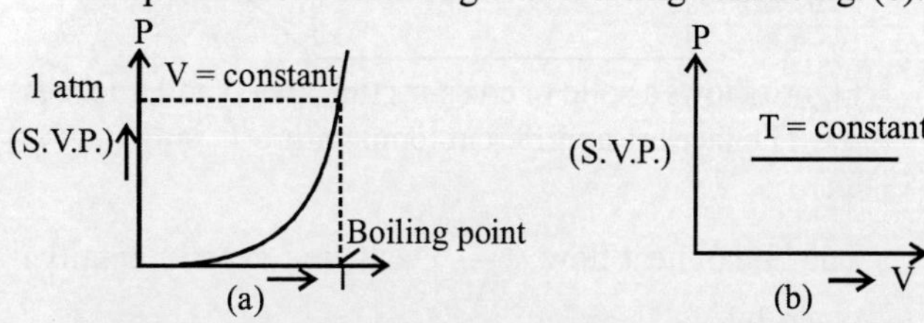

5. At 0°C, the saturation vapour pessure is 4.6 mm of Hg. Therefore, water vapours are always present around the ice. It increases with the increase in temperature.
6. The **relative humidity** is 100% when the temperature of the atmosphere is equal to the dew point.
7. **Cryogenics** is the study of low temperature.
8. As RH is expressed in percentage, hence the maximum value of RH may be 100%.
9. The saturation vapour pressure of water at 100°C is 760 mm of Hg at sea level.
10. As the temperature rises, the absolute humidity may increase and the relative humidity may remain constant or may even decrease.
11. If the relative humidity is high then at the same temperatue one feels hotter.
12. If the air is absolutley dry, the dew point is not observed.
13. The relative humidity decreases with the increase in temperature.
14. If water is sprinkled in the room, both relative humidity as well as the dew point increase.
15. Dew appears on the leaves of the trees etc. due to the condensation of saturated vapours.
16. The mist or fog is the small droplets of water formed due to the condensation of water vapours near the surface of earth.
17. Mist or fog formed much higher above the surface of earth is called cloud.
18. The Relative humidity between 50% and 60% gives comfortable feeling to human beings.
19. When the relative humidity is 100%, the reading of the dry and wet bulbs is same.
20. Smaller the difference in the temperature of dry and wet bulbs, larger is the relative humidity.
21. Water vapours are always seen around the ice, because the temperature around it is less than the dew point.

HEAT TRANSFER

Three modes of transmission of heat :

(a) **Conduction** (b) **Convection** and (c) **Radiation**

(a) ***Conduction :*** *In thermal conduction particles of body at higher temperature transmit heat to the particles at lower* *temperature by mutual contact (collision) only and not by the movement of the particles.* All solids are heated by conduction. Conduction cannot take place in vacuum.

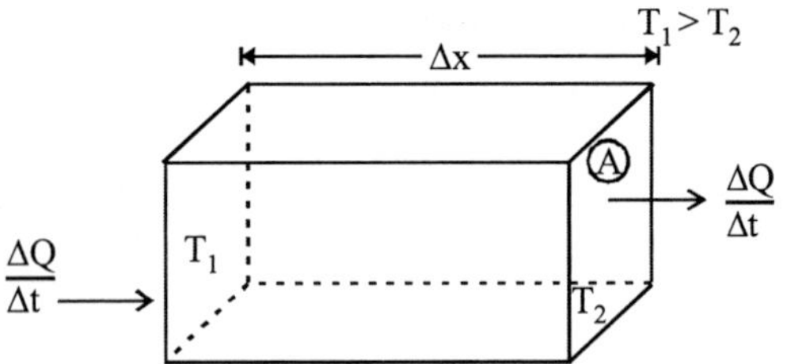

Figure shows a solid of cross-section area A and thickness Δx. The face are at different temperature T_1 and T_2 ($T_1 > T_2$)

The rate of heat flow $\left(\frac{\Delta Q}{\Delta t}\right)$ as found experimentally is given by

$$\frac{\Delta Q}{\Delta t} \propto A\left(\frac{\Delta T}{\Delta x}\right) \qquad \text{where } \Delta T = T_1 - T_2$$

$$\Rightarrow \quad \frac{\Delta Q}{\Delta t} = KA\left(\frac{\Delta T}{\Delta x}\right) \qquad \ldots(1)$$

where K is proportionality constant called **thermal conductivity.**

It is a measure of how quickly heat energy can conduct through the substance.

Coefficient of thermal conductivity (K) : The coefficient of thermal conductivity, K, of a material is defined as *the amount of heat that flowing per second through a rod of that material having unit length and unit area of cross-section in the steady state, when the difference of temperature between two ends of the rod is 1 ºC and flow of heat is perpendicular to the end faces of the rod.*

Unit of coefficient of thermal conductivity in **SI system** is watt/m-K

Dimensions : $[M L T^{-3} \theta^{-1}]$

For a perfect conductor thermal conductivity K is infinite and for a perfect insulator K is zero.

In general, solids are better conductors than liquids and liquids are better conductors than gases. (Heat transfer through the process of conduction is possible in liquids and gases also, if they are heated from the top.) Metals are much better conductors than non-metals.

A good conductor of heat is also a good conductor of electricity The conduction of both heat and electricity is due to the movement of free electrons.

(b) ***Convection :*** *It is the process by which heat is transferred from one place to another in a medium by the movement of particles of the medium.* It occurs due to density difference. This phenomenon occurs in fluids.

(c) ***Radiation :*** *It is the process by which heat is transferred from one place to another without any intervening medium.* The light reaches from Sun to Earth by radiation process.

Problem Solving Tips

1. The equation $\frac{\Delta Q}{\Delta t} = KA\left(\frac{\Delta T}{\Delta x}\right)$ is valid for steady state condition. The condition is said to occur when no part of heat is used up in raising the temperature of any part of cross-section of the solid.
2. On comparing equation (1) with the following equation used for flowing of charge on account of potential difference.

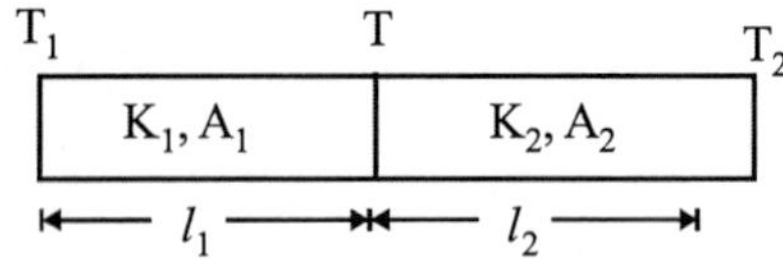

We find : $\frac{\Delta q}{\Delta t} = \sigma A \frac{\Delta V}{l}$

The role of resistance (thermal resistance) is played by $\frac{\Delta x}{KA}$

3. **Series combination of conductors**

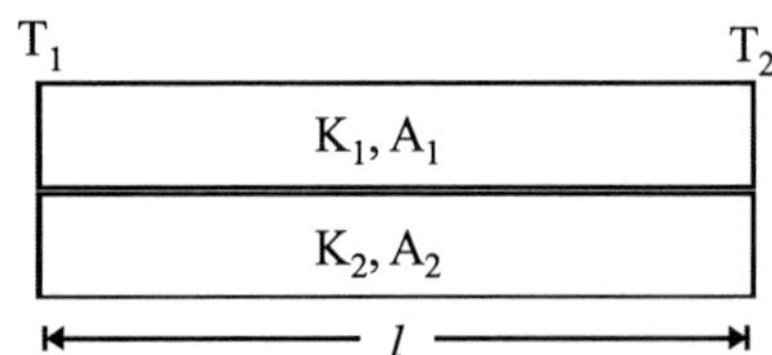

Equivalent thermal conductivity :

$$K_{eq} = \frac{2K_1K_2}{K_1 + K_2} \text{ and } H = \frac{A(T_1 - T_2)}{\frac{l_1}{K_1} + \frac{l_2}{K_2}}$$

where H = heat flow per second

4. **Parallel combination of conductors**

T_1 T_2

K_1, A_1
K_2, A_2

l

Equivalent thermal conductivity :

$$K_{eq} = \frac{K_1A_1 + K_2A_2}{A_2 + A_2} \text{ and } H = \frac{\frac{K_1}{l_1}T_1 + \frac{K_2}{l_2}T_2}{\frac{K_1}{l_1} + \frac{K_2}{l_2}}$$

5. Davy's safety lamp is based on the conduction. It is used in mines to know the ignition temperature of gases. Danger of explosion can be avoided.
6. (i) Principle of chimney used in a kitchen or a factory is based on the convection.
   (ii) Land and sea breezes are due ot the convection.
   (iii) Temperature of the upper part of the flame is more than the temperature on the sides, because the currents of air carry the heat upwards.
   (iv) Radiation can be detected by differential air thermometer, Bolometer, thermopile, etc.

Example 6.

Two plates of same area are placed in contact. Their thickness as well as thermal conductivities are in the ratio 2 : 3. The outer surface of one plate is maintained at 10°C and that of other at 0°C. What is the temp. of the common surface?

Solution :

Let θ be the temp. of common surface.

As $\left(\frac{\Delta Q}{\Delta t}\right)_1 = \left(\frac{\Delta Q}{\Delta t}\right)_2$

$$K_1 A_1 \frac{(10-\theta)}{x_1} = K_2 A_2 \frac{(\theta - 0)}{x_2} \quad \text{or} \quad \frac{K_1}{K_2}(10-\theta) = \frac{x_1}{x_2}\theta$$

Plate 1 Plate 2

K_1 K_2

10°C 8°C 0°C

x_1 x_2

Now,

$$A_1 = A_2; \quad \frac{x_1}{x_2} = \frac{K_1}{K_2} = \frac{2}{3}; \quad \frac{2}{3}(10-\theta) = \frac{2}{3}\theta \text{ or } \theta = 5°C.$$

Example 7.

A slab consists of two parallel layers of two different materials of same thickness and thermal conductivities K_1 and K_2. Find the equivalent thermal conductivity of the slab.

Solution :

Rate of flow of heat through each layer of slab is same, because slabs are in series.

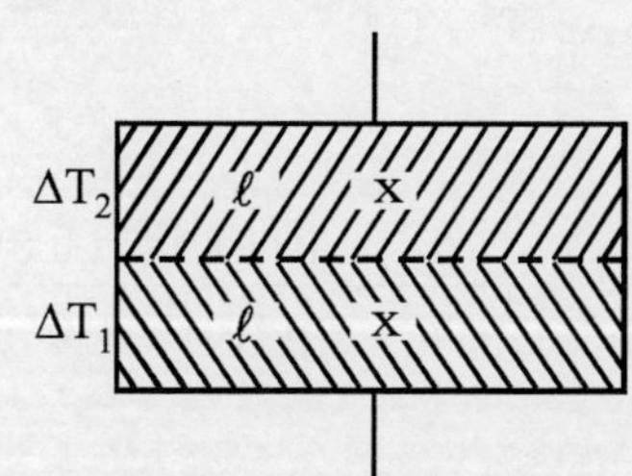

$$K_1 A \frac{\Delta T_1}{\ell} = K_2 A \frac{\Delta T_2}{\ell} = \frac{K(\Delta T_1 + \Delta T_2)A}{2\ell}$$

$$\text{or} \quad K_1 \Delta T_1 = K_2 \Delta T_2 = \frac{K(\Delta T_1 + \Delta T_2)}{2} = C\text{, say}$$

$$\therefore \quad \Delta T_1 = \frac{C}{K_1}, \ \Delta T_2 = \frac{C}{K_2}, \ \Delta T_1 + \Delta T_2 = \frac{2C}{K}$$

$$\text{or} \quad \frac{C}{K_1} + \frac{C}{K_2} = \frac{2C}{K} \quad \text{or} \quad K = \frac{2K_1 K_2}{K_1 + K_2}$$

Example 8.

Two walls of thickness d_1 and d_2 and thermal conductivities K_1 and K_2 are in contact. In the steady state, if the temperatures at the outer surfaces are T_1 and T_2 then find the temperature at the common wall.

Solution :

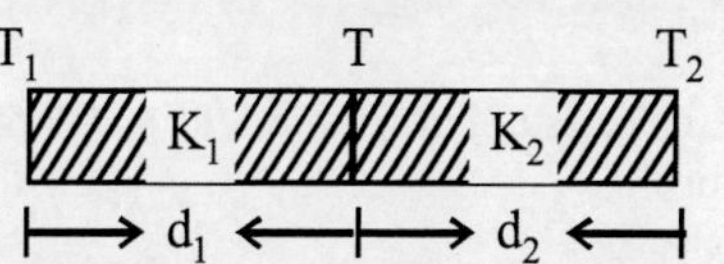

Let the temperature of common wall be T. Then

$$\frac{K_1 A (T_1 - T)t}{d_1} = \frac{K_2 A (T - T_2)t}{d_2}$$

$$\text{or,} \quad \frac{K_1 (T_1 - T)t}{d_1} = \frac{K_2 (T - T_2)t}{d_2}$$

or, $d_2 [K_1 (T_1 - T)] = d_1 [K_2 (T - T_2)]$

or, $K_1 T_1 d_2 - K_1 d_2 T = d_1 K_2 T - d_1 K_2 T_2$

or, $K_1 T_1 d_2 - K_2 d_1 T_2 = T[K_1 d_2 + d_1 K_2]$

$$\therefore \quad T = \left[\frac{K_1 T_1 d_2 - K_2 d_1 T_2}{K_1 d_2 + K_2 d_1}\right]$$

Stefan's Law:

This law is also called Stefan Boltzmann law. This law states that *the power radiated for overall wavelength from a black body is proportional to the fourth power of thermodynamic temperature T.*

$$E \propto T^4 \Rightarrow E = \sigma T^4 \text{ for perfectly black body} \quad ....(1)$$

where E is energy emitted per second from unit sruface area of the black body, T is temperature and σ is Stefan's constant, and $\sigma = 5.67 \times 10^{-8}\ Wm^{-2}K^{-4}$.

If body is not perfectly black body, then

$$E = e\sigma T^4 \quad ....(2)$$

where *e* is emissivity. Then energy radiated per second by a body of area A is

$$E_1 = e\sigma T^4 \quad ....(3)$$

If the body temperature is T and surrounding temperature is T_0, then net rate of loss of energy by body through radiation from equation (3) is

$$E_1' = eA\sigma(T^4 - T_0^4) \quad ....(4)$$

Now rate of loss of energy in terms of specific heat *c* is

$$\frac{dQ}{dt} = mc\frac{dT}{dt} = E_1' \quad ....(5)$$

$$\text{and} \quad \frac{dT}{dt} = \frac{eA\sigma}{mc}(T^4 - T_0^4) \quad ....(6)$$

(T- temperature, t - time in second)

So body cools by radiation and rate of cooling depends on *e* (emissivity of body), A (area of cross-section of body), *m* (mass of body) and *c* (specific heat capacity of body).

A black body is defined as a body which completely absorbs all the heat radiation falling on it without reflecting and transmitting any of it.

Weins Law :

$\lambda_m T = b$,

where b is the Weins constant and $b = 2.898 \times 10^{-3}$mK and T = temperature.

Graph of λ_m versus T

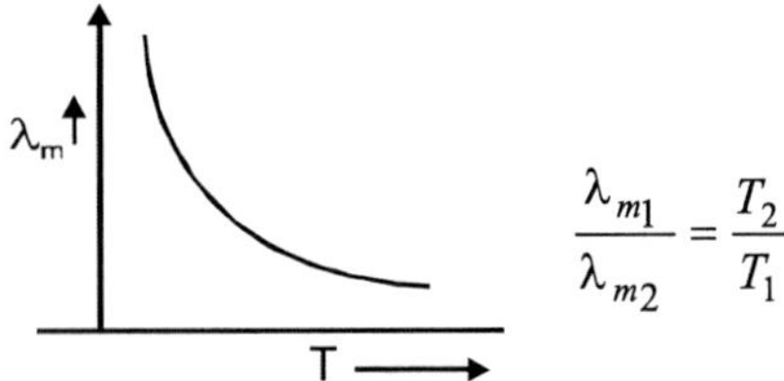

$$\frac{\lambda_{m1}}{\lambda_{m2}} = \frac{T_2}{T_1}$$

Hence on increasing temperature of a body, its colour changes gradually from red to orange → yellow → green → blue → violet. Thus the temperature of violet star is maximum and temperature of red star is minimum. Sun is a medium category star with $\lambda_m = 4753$A° (yellow colour) and temperature 6000K.

Kirchhoff's Law

According to this law, *the ratio of emissive power to absorptive power is same for all surfaces at the same temperature and is equal to the emissive power of a perfectly black body at the same temperature.*

i.e. $E = \frac{e}{a} A$

where e = emissive power of a given surface
a = absorptive power of a given surface
E = emissive power of a perfect black body
A = absorptive power of a perfect black body

(i) For a perfect black body, $A = 1$, $\therefore E = \frac{e}{a}$

(ii) If emissive and absorptive power are considered for a particular wavelenth λ then $E_\lambda = \frac{e_\lambda}{a_\lambda}$

(iii) Since E_λ is constant at a given temperature, according to this law if a surface is good absorber of a particular wavelength then it is also a good emitter of that wavelength.

Fraunhoffer's Line

(i) Fraunhoffer lines are the dark lines in the spectrum of sun and are explained on the basis of Kirchoff's law. When white light emitted from central core of sun (photosphere) passes through its atmosphere (chromosphere) radiation of those wavelength will be absorbed by the gases present there, which they usually emit (as good emitter is a good absorber) resulting dark lines in the spectrum of sun.

(ii) On the basis of Kirchoff's law, Fraunhoffer identified some of the elements present in the chromosphere. They are hydrogen, helium, sodium, iron, calcium, etc. Fraunhoffer had observed about 600 darklines in the spectrum of sun.

NEWTON'S LAW OF COOLING

The rate of loss of heat of a body is directly proportional to the temperature difference between the body and the surroundings.

i.e. $\frac{dT}{dt} = -K(T - T_0)$

where T = temperature of body, T_0 = temperature of surrounding.

and $K = \frac{eA\sigma}{mc}$ where, e = emissivity of body, A = area of surface of body, σ = Stefan's constant, m = mass of body, c = specific heat of body.

It is a special case of Stefan's law and above relation is applicable only when the temperature of body is not much different from the temperature of surroundings.

Solar constant : *Solar constant is the solar radiation incident normally per second on one square metre at the mean distance of the earth from the sun in free space.*

It is given by $S = 1.34 \times 10^9$ $Jm^{-2}s^{-1}$.

Temperature of sun is given $T^4 = S/\sigma(R/r)^2$, where R is mean distance of the earth from the sun and r is the radius of the sun.

Problem Solving Tips

1. Good absorber is a good emitter.
2. Cooking utensils are provided with wooden or ebonite handles, since wood or ebonite is a bad conductor of heat.
3. Good conductor of heat are good conductors of electricity, Mica is an exception which being a good conductor of heat is a bad conductor of electricity.

Example 9.

Compare the rate of loss of heat from a metal sphere of temperature 827°C, with the rate of loss of heat from the same sphere at 427 °C, if the temperature of surroundings is 27°C.

Solution :

Given : $T_1 = 827\,°C = 1100$ K, $T_2 = 427\,°C = 700$ K
and $T_0 = 27\,°C = 300$ K

According to Steafan Boltzmann law of radiation,

$$\frac{dQ}{dt} = \sigma A\varepsilon (T^4 - T_0^4)$$

$$\therefore \frac{\left(\frac{dQ}{dt}\right)_1}{\left(\frac{dQ}{dt}\right)_2} = \frac{(T_1^4 - T_0^4)}{(T_2^4 - T_0^4)} = \frac{[(1100)^4 - (300)^4]}{[(700)^4 - (300)^4]} = 6.276$$

$$\text{or} \quad \left(\frac{dQ}{dt}\right)_1 : \left(\frac{dQ}{dt}\right)_2 = 6.276 : 1$$

Example 10.

The filament of an evacuated light bulb has a length 10 cm, diameter 0.2 mm and emissivity 0.2, calculate the power it radiates at 2000 K. ($\sigma = 5.67 \times 10^{-8}$ $W/m^2 K^4$)

Solution :

$\ell = 10$ cm $= 0.1$ m, $d = 0.2$ mm $= 2 \times 10^{-4}$ m
$r = 0.1$ mm $= 1 \times 10^{-4}$ m,
$\varepsilon = 0.2$, $T = 2000$ K, $\sigma = 5.67 \times 10^{-8}$ $W/m^2 K^4$

According to stefan's law of radiation, rate of emission of heat for an ordinary body,

$E = \sigma A \varepsilon T^4 = \sigma(2\pi r \ell)\varepsilon T^4$ $[\because A = 2\pi r\ell]$
$= 5.67 \times 10^{-8} \times 2 \times 3.14 \times 1 \times 10^{-4} \times 0.1 \times 0.2 \times (2000)^4$
$= 11.4$ W

∴ Power radiated by the filament = 11.4 W

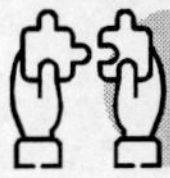

11.2 Concept Practice Problems

CPP

11. The coefficient of thermal conductivity depends upon
    (a) temperature difference between the two surfaces.
    (b) area
    (c) material
    (d) All of these
12. The wavelength of radiation emitted by a body depends upon
    (a) the nature of its surface
    (b) the area of its surface
    (c) the temperature of its surface
    (d) All of the above
13. The fastest mode of transfer of heat is
    (a) conduction (b) convection
    (c) radiation (d) None of these
14. In order that the heat flows from one part of a solid to another part, what is required?
    (a) Uniform density
    (b) Temperature gradient
    (c) Density gradient
    (d) Uniform temperature
15. The sprinkling of water slightly reduces the temperature of a closed room because
    (a) temperature of water is less than that of the room
    (b) specific heat of water is high
    (c) water has large latent heat of vaporisation
    (d) water is a bad conductor of heat
16. Which of the following is not close to a black body?
    (a) Black board paint (b) Green leaves
    (c) Black holes (d) Red roses
17. According to Newton's law of cooling, the rate of cooling of a body is proportional to $(\Delta\theta)^n$, where $\Delta\theta$ is the difference of the temperature of the body and the surroundings, and n is equal to
    (a) two (b) three
    (c) four (d) one
18. The temperature of stars is determined by
    (a) Stefan's law
    (b) Wien's displacement law
    (c) Kirchhoff's law
    (d) Ohm's law
19. At a certain temperature for given wave length , the ratio of emissive power of a body to emissive power of black body in same circumstances is known as
    (a) relative emissivity (b) emissivity
    (c) absorption coefficient (d) coefficient of reflection
20. If a liquid is heated in weightlessness, the heat is transmitted through
    (a) conduction
    (b) convection
    (c) radiation
    (d) None of these, because the liquid cannot be heated in weightlessness.

ANSWER KEY

11	(c)	12	(d)	13	(c)	14	(b)	15	(c)	16	(a)	17	(d)	18	(b)	19	(c)	20	(a)

CONCEPT MAP

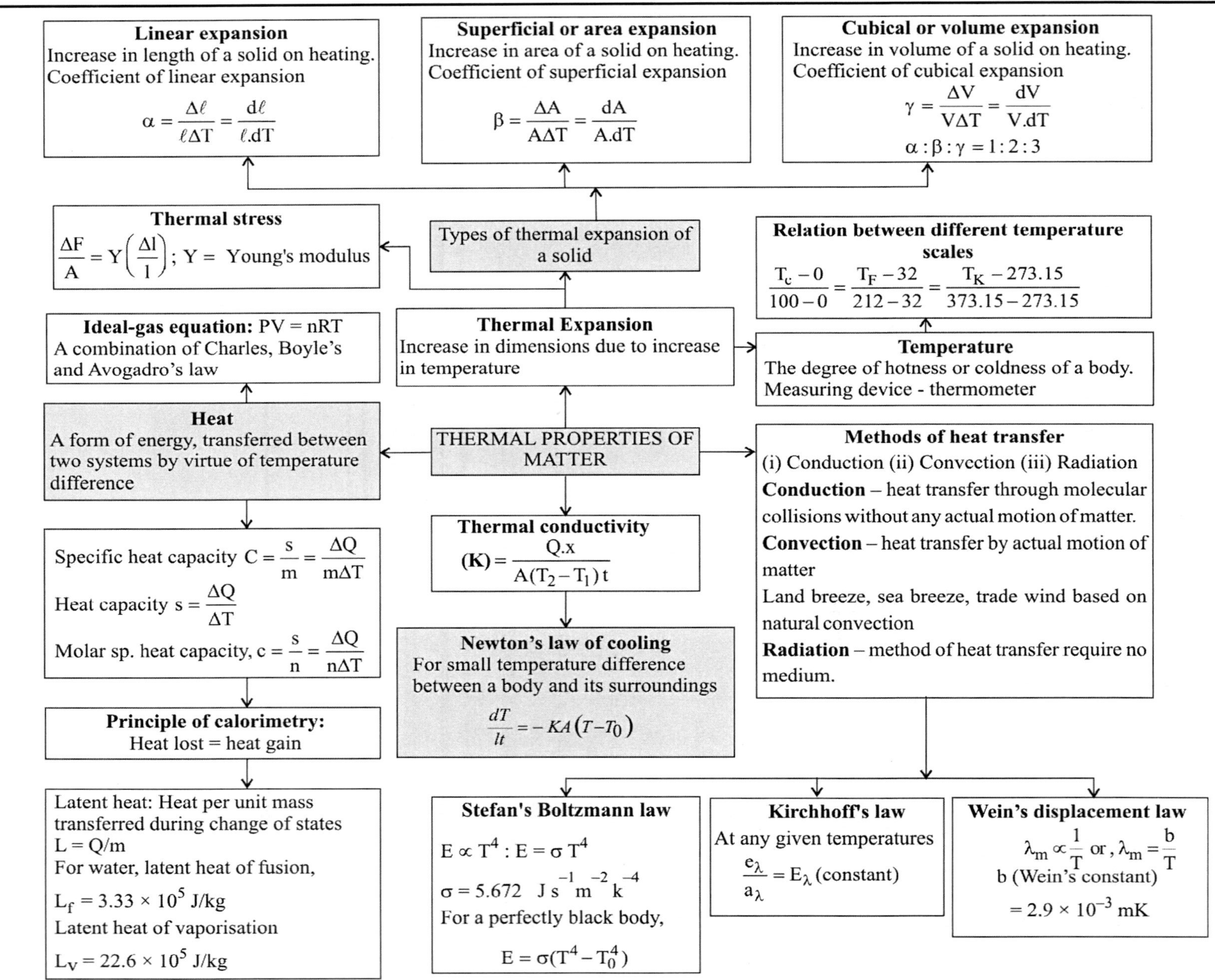
Linear expansion
Increase in length of a solid on heating.
Coefficient of linear expansion
$\alpha = \frac{\Delta\ell}{\ell\Delta T} = \frac{d\ell}{\ell.dT}$
Superficial or area expansion
Increase in area of a solid on heating.
Coefficient of superficial expansion
$\beta = \frac{\Delta A}{A\Delta T} = \frac{dA}{A.dT}$
Cubical or volume expansion
Increase in volume of a solid on heating.
Coefficient of cubical expansion
$\gamma = \frac{\Delta V}{V\Delta T} = \frac{dV}{V.dT}$
$\alpha : \beta : \gamma = 1 : 2 : 3$
Thermal stress
$\frac{\Delta F}{A} = Y\left(\frac{\Delta l}{l}\right)$; Y = Young's modulus
Types of thermal expansion of a solid
Relation between different temperature scales
$\frac{T_c - 0}{100 - 0} = \frac{T_F - 32}{212 - 32} = \frac{T_K - 273.15}{373.15 - 273.15}$
Ideal-gas equation: PV = nRT
A combination of Charles, Boyle's and Avogadro's law
Thermal Expansion
Increase in dimensions due to increase in temperature
Temperature
The degree of hotness or coldness of a body.
Measuring device - thermometer
Heat
A form of energy, transferred between two systems by virtue of temperature difference
THERMAL PROPERTIES OF MATTER
Methods of heat transfer
(i) Conduction (ii) Convection (iii) Radiation
Conduction – heat transfer through molecular collisions without any actual motion of matter.
Convection – heat transfer by actual motion of matter
Land breeze, sea breeze, trade wind based on natural convection
Radiation – method of heat transfer require no medium.
Specific heat capacity $C = \frac{s}{m} = \frac{\Delta Q}{m\Delta T}$
Heat capacity $s = \frac{\Delta Q}{\Delta T}$
Molar sp. heat capacity, $c = \frac{s}{n} = \frac{\Delta Q}{n\Delta T}$
Thermal conductivity
$(K) = \frac{Q.x}{A(T_2 - T_1)t}$
Newton's law of cooling
For small temperature difference between a body and its surroundings
$\frac{dT}{lt} = -KA(T - T_0)$
Principle of calorimetry:
Heat lost = heat gain
Latent heat: Heat per unit mass transferred during change of states
L = Q/m
For water, latent heat of fusion,
$L_f = 3.33 \times 10^5$ J/kg
Latent heat of vaporisation
$L_V = 22.6 \times 10^5$ J/kg
Stefan's Boltzmann law
$E \propto T^4 : E = \sigma T^4$
$\sigma = 5.672 \ J s^{-1} m^{-2} k^{-4}$
For a perfectly black body,
$E = \sigma(T^4 - T_0^4)$
Kirchhoff's law
At any given temperatures
$\frac{e_\lambda}{a_\lambda} = E_\lambda$ (constant)
Wein's displacement law
$\lambda_m \propto \frac{1}{T}$ or, $\lambda_m = \frac{b}{T}$
b (Wein's constant)
$= 2.9 \times 10^{-3}$ mK

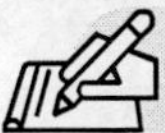

Exercise 1 - Chapter Revision Problems

CRP

1. A metallic rod ℓ cm long, A square cm in cross-section is heated through t°C. If Young's modulus of elasticity of the metal is E and the mean coefficient of linear expansion is α per degree celsius, then the compressional force required to prevent the rod from expanding along its length is
(a) $EA\alpha t$ (b) $EA\alpha t/(1+\alpha t)$
(c) $EA\alpha t/(1-\alpha t)$ (d) $E\ell\alpha t$

2. A black body rediates energy at the rate of E watt per metre^2 at a high temperature T K. when the temperature is reduced to (T/2) K, the radiant energy will be
(a) E/16 (b) E/4 (c) E/2 (d) 2E

3. The tempearture of an isolated black body falls from T_1 to T_2 in time t, then t is (Let c be a constant)
(a) $t = c\left(\frac{1}{T_2} - \frac{1}{T_1}\right)$ (b) $t = c\left(\frac{1}{T_2^2} - \frac{1}{T_1^2}\right)$
(c) $t = c\left(\frac{1}{T_2^3} - \frac{1}{T_1^3}\right)$ (d) $t = c\left(\frac{1}{T_2^4} - \frac{1}{T_1^4}\right)$

4. Two solid spheres, of radii R_1 and R_2 are made of the same material and have similar surfaces. The spheres are raised to the same temperature and then allowed to cool under identical conditions. Assuming spheres to be perfect conductors of heat, their initial rates of loss of heat are
(a) R_1^2/R_2^2 (b) R_1/R_2 (c) R_2/R_1 (d) R_2^2/R_1^2

5. A radiation of energy E falls normally on a perfectly reflecting surface. The momentum transferred to the surface is
(a) Ec (b) 2E/c (c) E/c (d) E/c^2

6. Which of the following graph correctly represents the relation between $\ln E$ and $\ln T$ where E is the amount of radiation emitted per unit time from unit area of body and T is the absolute temperature

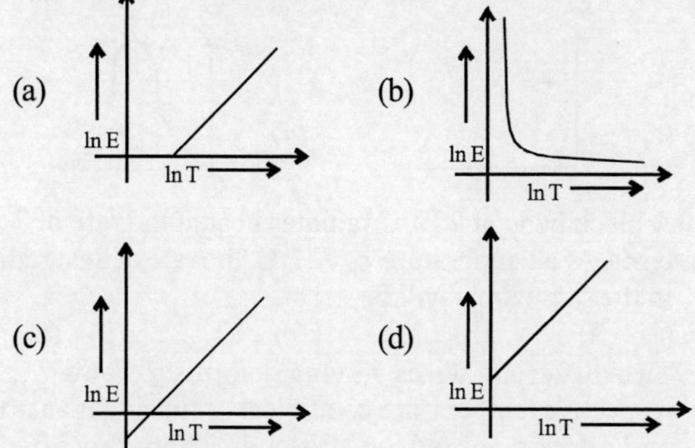

7. The temperature of the Sun is measured with
(a) platinum thermometer
(b) gas thermometer
(c) pyrometer
(d) vapour pressure thermometer.

8. Which of the following circular rods, (given radius r and length l) each made of the same material and whose ends are maintained at the same temperature will conduct most heat?
(a) $r = 2r_0; l = 2l_0$ (b) $r = 2r_0; l = l_0$
(c) $r = r_0; l = 2l_0$ (d) $r = r_0; l = l_0$

9. When a body is heated, which colour corresponds to high temperature
(a) red (b) yellow
(c) white (d) orange

10. The two ends of a rod of length L and a uniform cross-sectional area A are kept at two temperatures T_1 and T_2 $(T_1 > T_2)$. The rate of heat transfer, $\frac{dQ}{dt}$ through the rod in a steady state is given by
(a) $\frac{dQ}{dt} = \frac{k(T_1 - T_2)}{LA}$ (b) $\frac{dQ}{dt} = kLA(T_1 - T_2)$
(c) $\frac{dQ}{dt} = \frac{kA(T_1 - T_2)}{L}$ (d) $\frac{dQ}{dt} = \frac{kL(T_1 - T_2)}{A}$

11. The resistance of a resistance thermometer has values 2.71 and 3.70 ohms at 10°C and 100°C respectively. The temperature at which the resistance is 3.26 ohm is
(a) 40°C (b) 50°C (c) 60°C (d) 70°C

12. A pendulum clock is 5 seconds fast at temperature of 15°C and 10 seconds slow at a temperature of 30°C. At what temperature does it give the correct time? (take time interval = 24 hours)
(a) 18°C (b) 20°C (c) 22°C (d) 25°C

13. Steam is passed into 22 gm of water at 20°C. The mass of water that will be present when the water acquires a temperatue of 90°C (Latent heat of steam is 540 cal/g) is
(a) 24.83 gm (b) 24 gm (c) 36.6 gm (d) 30 gm

14. A cylindrical rod of aluminium is of length 20 cms and radius 2 cms. The two ends are maintained at temperatures of 0°C and 50°C the coefficient of thermal conductivity is $\frac{0.5 \text{ cal}}{\text{cm} \times \text{sec} \times {}^\circ\text{C}}$. Then the thermal resistance of the rod in $\frac{\text{cal}}{\text{sec} \times {}^\circ\text{C}}$ is
(a) 318 (b) 31.8 (c) 3.18 (d) 0.318

15. The rate of radiation of a black body at 0°C is E joule per sec. Then the rate of radiation of this black body at 273°c will be
(a) 16E (b) 8E (c) 4E (d) E

16. A bucket full of hot water is kept in a room and it cools from 75°C to 70°C in T_1 minutes, from 70°C to 65°C in T_2 minutes and from 65°C to 60°C in T_3 minutes. Then
(a) $T_1 = T_2 = T_3$ (b) $T_1 < T_2 < T_3$
(c) $T_1 > T_2 > T_3$ (d) $T_1 < T_2 > T_3$

17. The temperature of a furnace is 2324°C and the intensity is maximum in its radiation spectrum nearly at 12000 Å. If the intensity in the spectrum of a star is maximum nearly at 4800Å, then the surface temperature of the star is
(a) 8400°C (b) 7200°C (c) 6492.5°K (d) 5900°C

18. No other thermometer is suitable as a platinum resistance thermometer to measure temperatures in the entire range of

(a) –50ºC to + 350ºC (b) –200ºC to + 600ºC
(c) 0ºC to 100ºC (d) 100ºC to 1500ºC

19. Calculate the surface temperature of the planet, if the energy radiated by unit area in unit time is 5.67×10^4 watt.

(a) 1273ºC (b) 1000ºC (c) 727ºC (d) 727K

20. In a surrounding medium of temperature 10°C, a body takes 7 min for a fall of temperature from 60°C to 40°C. In what time the temperature of the body will fall from 40°C to 28°C?

(a) 7 min (b) 11 min (c) 14 min (d) 21 min

21. Two rods P and Q of same length and same diameter having thermal conductivity ratio 2 : 3 joined end to end. If temperature at one end of P is 100°C and at one and of Q 0°C, then the temperature of the interface is

(a) 40ºC (b) 50ºC (c) 60ºC (d) 70ºC

22. 100 g of ice is mixed with 100 g of water at 100ºC. What will be the final temperature of the mixture ?

(a) 13.33ºC (b) 20ºC (c) 23.33ºC (d) 40ºC

23. The coefficient of apparent expansion of mercury in a glass vessel is 153×10^{-6}/ºC and in a steel vessel is 144×10^{-6}/ ºC. If α for steel is 12×10^{-6}/ºC, then, that of glass is

(a) 9×10^{-6}/ºC (b) 6×10^{-6}/ºC
(c) 36×10^{-6}/ºC (d) 27×10^{-6}/ºC

24. Steam at 100°C is passed into 1.1 kg of water contained in a calorimeter of water equivalent 0.02 kg at 15ºC till the temperature of the calorimeter and its contents rises to 80ºC.The mass of the steam condensed in kg is

(a) 0.130 (b) 0.065 (c) 0.260 (d) 0.135

25. A body of mass 5 kg falls from a height of 20 metres on the ground and it rebounds to a height of 0.2 m. If the loss in potential energy is used up by the body, then what will be the temperature rise?

(specific heat of material = 0.09 cal gm^{-1} $°C^{-1}$)

(a) 0ºC (b) 4ºC (c) 8ºC (d) None of these

26. 80 g of water at 30ºC are poured on a large block of ice at 0ºC. The mass of ice that melts is

(a) 1600 g (b) 30 g (c) 150 g (d) 80 g

27. The spectral energy distribution of the sun (temperature 6050 K) is maximum at 4753 Å. The temperature of a star for which this maximum is at 9506 Å is

(a) 6050 K (b) 3025 K (c) 12100 K (d) 24200 K

28. Two bodies A and B are placed in an evacuated vessel maintained at a temperature of 27ºC. The temperature of A is 327ºC and that of B is 227ºC. The ratio of heat loss from A and B is about

(a) 2 : 1 (b) 1 : 2 (c) 4 : 1 (d) 1 : 4

29. The thermal capacity of 40g of aluminium (specific heat = 0.2 cal g^{-1} $°C^{-1}$) is

(a) 40 cal $°C^{-1}$ (b) 160 cal $°C^{-1}$
(c) 200 cal $°C^{-1}$ (d) 8 cal $°C^{-1}$

30. 5 kg of water at 10°C is added to 10 kg of water at 40°C. Neglecting heat capacity of vessel and other losses, the equilibrium temperature will be

(a) 30ºC (b) 25ºC (c) 35ºC (d) 33ºC

31. A beaker contains 200 g of water. The heat capacity of beaker is equal to that 20 g of water. The initial temperature of water in the beaker is 20°C . If 440 g of hot water at 92°C is poured in, the final temperature, neglecting radiation loss, will be

(a) 58ºC (b) 68ºC (c) 73ºC (d) 78ºC

32. The rectangular surface of area 8 cm × 4 cm of a black body at temperature 127°C emits energy E per second. If the length and breadth are reduced to half of the initial value and the temperature is raised to 327°C, the rate of emission of energy becomes

(a) $\frac{3}{8}E$ (b) $\frac{81}{16}E$ (c) $\frac{9}{16}E$ (d) $\frac{81}{64}E$

33. Two rods of same length and transfer a given amount of heat 12 second, when they are joined as shown in figure (i). But when they are joined as shwon in figure (ii), then they will transfer same heat in same conditions in

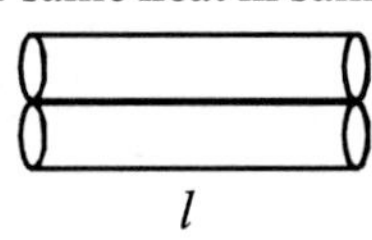

Fig. (i)

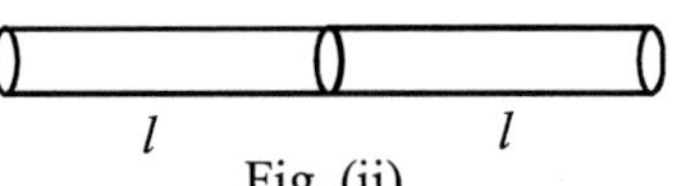

Fig. (ii)

(a) 24 s (b) 13 s (c) 15 s (d) 48 s

34. Three identical rods A, B and C of equal lengths and equal diameters are joined in series as shown in figure. Their thermal conductivities are 2k, k and k/2 respectively. The temperatures at two junction points are

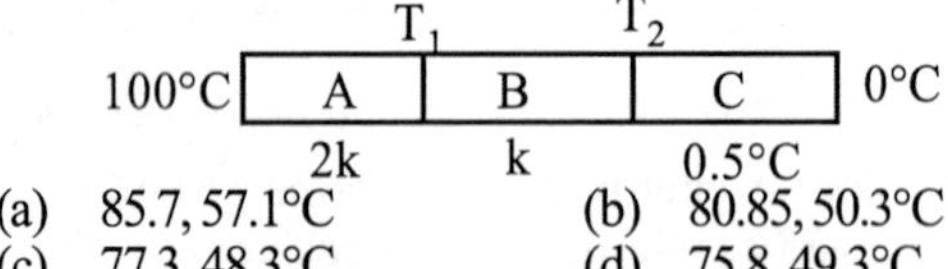

(a) 85.7, 57.1°C (b) 80.85, 50.3°C
(c) 77.3, 48.3°C (d) 75.8, 49.3°C

35. Which one of the following graphs best represents the ways in which the total power P radiated by a black body depends upon the thermodynamic temperature T of the body?

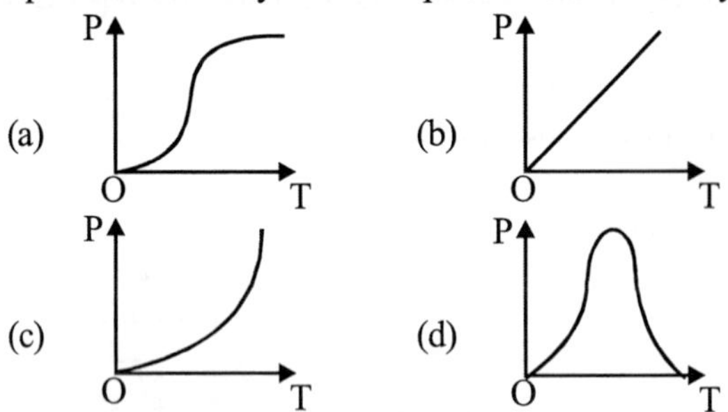

36. A black body at 227°C radiates heat at the rate of 7 cals/ cm^2s. At a temperature of 727°C, the rate of heat radiated in the same units will be

(a) 50 (b) 112 (c) 80 (d) 60

37. Two different wires having lengths L_1 and L_2, and respective temperature coefficient of linear expansion α_1 and α_2, are joined end-to-end. Then the effective temperature coefficient of linear expansion is :

(a) $\frac{\alpha_1 L_1 + \alpha_2 L_2}{L_1 + L_2}$ (b) $2\sqrt{\alpha_1 \alpha_2}$

(c) $\frac{\alpha_1 + \alpha_2}{2}$ (d) $4\frac{\alpha_1 \alpha_2}{\alpha_1 + \alpha_2}\frac{L_2 L_1}{(L_2 + L_1)^2}$

38. When the temperature of a metal wire is increased from 0°C to 10°C, its length increased by 0.02%. The percentage change in its mass density will be closest to :
(a) 0.06 (b) 2.3 (c) 0.008 (d) 0.8

39. A steel rail of length 5 m and area of cross-section 40 cm^2 is prevented from expanding along its length while the temperature rises by 10°C. If coefficient of linear expansion and Young's modulus of steel are $1.2 \times 10^{-5}\,K^{-1}$ and $2 \times 10^{11}\,Nm^{-2}$ respectively, the force developed in the rail is approximately:
(a) 2×10^7 N (b) 1×10^5 N (c) 2×10^9 N (d) 3×10^{-5} N

40. On a linear temperature scale Y, water freezes at – 160° Y and boils at – 50° Y. On this Y scale, a temperature of 340 K would be read as : (water freezes at 273 K and boils at 373 K)
(a) –73.7° Y (b) –233.7° Y (c) –86.3° Y (d) – 106.3° Y

41. When M_1 gram of ice at –10 °C (Specific heat = 0.5 cal g^{-1}°C^{-1}) is added to M_2 gram of water at 50°C, finally no ice is left and the water is at 0°C. The value of latent heat of ice, in cal g^{-1} is:
(a) $\frac{50M_2}{M_1} - 5$ (b) $\frac{5M_1}{M_2} - 50$ (c) $\frac{50M_2}{M_1}$ (d) $\frac{5M_2}{M_1} - 5$

42. Ice at –20°C is added to 50 g of water at 40°C, When the temperature of the mixture reaches 0°C, it is found that 20 g of ice is still unmelted. The amount of ice added to the water was close to
(Specific heat of water = 4.2J/g/°C
Specific heat of Ice = 2.1 J/g/°C
Heat of fusion of water at 0°C = 334J/g)
(a) 50g (b) 100 g (c) 60 g (d) 40 g

43. When 100 g of a liquid A at 100°C is added to 50 g of a liquid B at temperature 75°C, the temperature of the mixture becomes 90°C. The temperature of the mixture, if 100 g of liquid A at 100°C is added to 50 g of liquid B at 50°C, will be:
(a) 85°C (b) 60°C (c) 80°C (d) 70°C

44. A heat source at T = 10^3 K is connected to another heat reservoir at T = 10^2 K by a copper slab which is 1 m thick. Given that the thermal conductivity of copper is 0.1 $WK^{-1}\,m^{-1}$, the energy flux through it in the steady state is:
(a) 90 Wm^{-2} (b) 120 Wm^{-2} (c) 65 Wm^{-2} (d) s200 Wm^{-2}

45. If the temperature of the sun were to increase from T to $2T$ and its radius from R to $2R$, then the ratio of the radiant energy received on earth to what it was previously will be
(a) 32 (b) 16 (c) 4 (d) 64

46. A metallic sphere cools from 50°C to 40°C in 300 s. If atmospheric temperature around is 20°C, then the sphere's temperature after the next 5 minutes will be close to :
(a) 31°C (b) 33°C (c) 28°C (d) 35°C

47. A body takes 10 minutes to cool from 60°C to 50°C. The temperature of surroundings is constant at 25°C. Then, the temperature of the body after next 10 minutes will be approximately
(a) 43°C (b) 47°C (c) 41°C (d) 45°C

48. Two rods A and B of identical dimensions are at temperature 30°C. If A is heated upto 180°C and B upto T°C, then the new lengths are the same. If the ratio of the coefficients of linear expansion of A and B is 4 : 3, then the value of T is :
(a) 230°C (b) 270°C (c) 200°C (d) 250°C

49. A calorimter of water equivalent 20 g contains 180 g of water at 25°C. 'm' grams of steam at 100°C is mixed in it till the temperature of the mixture is 31°C. The value of 'm' is close to (Latent heat of water = 540 cal g^{-1}, specific heat of water = 1 cal g^{-1} °C^{-1})
(a) 2 (b) 4 (c) 3.2 (d) 2.6

50. The specific heat of water = 4200 J $kg^{-1}\,K^{-1}$ and the latent heat of ice = 3.4×10^5 J kg^{-1}. 100 grams of ice at 0°C is placed in 200 g of water at 25°C. The amount of ice that will melt as the temperature of water reaches 0°C is close to (in grams) :
(a) 61.7 (b) 63.8 (c) 69.3 (d) 64.6

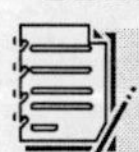

Exercise 2 - Exemplar & Past Year Questions

E&PYQs

Exemplar Questions

1. A bimetallic strip is made of aluminium and steel ($\alpha_{Al} > \alpha_{steel}$). On heating, the strip will
(a) remain straight
(b) get twisted
(c) will bend with aluminium on concave side
(d) will bend with steel on concave side

2. A uniform metallic rod rotates about its perpendicular bisector with constant angular speed. If it is heated uniformly to raise its temperature slightly
(a) its speed of rotation increases
(b) its speed of rotation decreases
(c) its speed of rotation remains same
(d) its speed increases because its moment of inertia increases

3. An aluminium sphere is dipped into water. Which of the following is true?
(a) Buoyancy will be less in water at 0°C than that in water at 4°C
(b) Buoyancy will be more in water at 0°C than that in water at 4°C
(c) Buoyancy in water at 0°C will be same as that in water at 4°C
(d) Buoyancy may be more or less in water at 4°C depending on the radius of the sphere

4. As the temperature is increased, the period of a pendulum
(a) increases as its effective length increases even though its centre of mass still remains at the centre of the bob
(b) decreases as its effective length increases even though its centre of mass still remains at the centre of the bob
(c) increases as its effective length increases due to shifting to centre of mass below the centre of the bob
(d) decreases as its effective length remains same but the centre of mass shifts above the centre of the bob

5. Heat is associated with
(a) kinetic energy of random motion of molecules
(b) kinetic energy of orderly motion of molecules

(c) total kinetic energy of random and orderly motion of molecules
(d) kinetic energy of random motion in some cases and kinetic energy of orderly motion in other

6. The radius of a metal sphere at room temperature T is R and the coefficient of linear expansion of the metal is α. The sphere heated a little by a temperature ΔT so that its new temperature is $T + \Delta T$. The increase in the volume of the sphere is approximately.

(a) $2\pi R\alpha\Delta T$ (b) $\pi R^2\alpha\Delta T$
(c) $4\pi R^3\alpha\Delta T/3$ (d) $4\pi R^3\alpha\Delta T$

7. A sphere, a cube and a thin circular plate, all of same material and same mass are initially heated to same high temperature.
(a) Plate will cool fastest and cube the slowest
(b) Sphere will cool fastest and cube the slowest
(c) Plate will cool fastest and sphere the slowest
(d) Cube will cool fastest and plate the slowest

Past Years (2013-2020) NEET/AIPMT Questions

8. A piece of iron is heated in a flame. It first becomes dull red then becomes reddish yellow and finally turns to white hot. The correct explanation for the above observation is possible by using ***[2013]***
(a) Wien's displacement law
(b) Kirchoff's law
(c) Newton's law of cooling
(d) Stefan's law

9. The molar specific heats of an ideal gas at constant pressure and volume are denoted by C_p and C_v, respectively. If $\gamma = \dfrac{C_p}{C_v}$ and R is the universal gas constant, then C_v is equal to ***[2013]***

(a) $\dfrac{R}{(\gamma-1)}$ (b) $\dfrac{(\gamma-1)}{R}$ (c) γR (d) $\dfrac{1+\gamma}{1-\gamma}$

10. The density of water at 20°C is 998 kg/m^3 and at 40°C 992 kg/m^3. The coefficient of volume expansion of water is ***[NEET Kar. 2013]***
(a) 10^{-4}/°C (b) 3×10^{-4}/°C
(c) 2×10^{-4}/°C (d) 6×10^{-4}/°C

11. Two metal rods 1 and 2 of same lengths have same temperature difference between their ends. Their thermal conductivities are K_1 and K_2 and cross sectional areas A_1 and A_2, respectively. If the rate of heat conduction in rod 1 is four times that in rod 2, then ***[NEET Kar. 2013]***
(a) $K_1A_1 = K_2A_2$ (b) $K_1A_1 = 4K_2A_2$
(c) $K_1A_1 = 2K_2A_2$ (d) $4K_1A_1 = K_2A_2$

12. Certain quantity of water cools from 70°C to 60°C in the first 5 minutes and to 54°C in the next 5 minutes. The temperature of the surroundings is: ***[2014]***
(a) 45°C (b) 20°C (c) 42°C (d) 10°C

13. Steam at 100°C is passed into 20 g of water at 10°C. When water acquires a temperature of 80°C, the mass of water present will be: ***[2014]***
[Take specific heat of water = 1 cal g^{-1} °C^{-1} and latent heat of steam = 540 cal g^{-1}]
(a) 24 g (b) 31.5 g (c) 42.5 g (d) 22.5 g

14. The value of coefficient of volume expansion of glycerine is 5×10^{-4} K^{-1}. The fractional change in the density of glycerine for a rise of 40°C in its temperature, is: ***[2015 RS]***
(a) 0.020 (b) 0.025 (c) 0.010 (d) 0.015

15. The two ends of a metal rod are maintained at temperatures 100°C and 110°C. The rate of heat flow in the rod is found to be 4.0 J/s. If the ends are maintained at temperatures 200°C and 210°C, the rate of heat flow will be ***[2015]***
(a) 16.8 J/s (b) 8.0 J/s (c) 4.0 J/s (d) 44.0 J/s

16. A piece of ice falls from a height h so that it melts completely. Only one-quarter of the heat produced is absorbed by the ice and all energy of ice gets converted into heat during its fall. The value of h is : ***[2016]***
[Latent heat of ice is 3.4×10^5 J/kg and g = 10 N/kg]
(a) 34 km (b) 544 km (c) 136 km (d) 68 km

17. A black body is at a temperature of 5760 K. The energy of radiation emitted by the body at wavelength 250 nm is U_1, at wavelength 500 nm is U_2 and that at 1000 nm is U_3. Wien's constant, b = 2.88×10^6 nmK. Which of the following is correct ? ***[2016]***
(a) $U_1 = 0$ (b) $U_3 = 0$ (c) $U_1 > U_2$ (d) $U_2 > U_1$

18. A spherical black body with a radius of 12 cm radiates 450 watt power at 500 K. If the radius were halved and the temperature doubled, the power radiated in watt would be: ***[2017]***
(a) 450 (b) 1000 (c) 1800 (d) 225

19. The power radiated by a black body is P and it radiates maximum energy at wavelength, λ_0. If the temperature of the black body is now changed so that it radiates maximum energy at wavelength $\dfrac{3}{4}\lambda_0$, the power radiated by it becomes nP. The value of n is ***[2018]***

(a) $\dfrac{3}{4}$ (b) $\dfrac{4}{3}$ (c) $\dfrac{81}{256}$ (d) $\dfrac{256}{81}$

20. A copper rod of 88 cm and an aluminium rod of unknown length have their increase in length independent of increase in temperature. The length of aluminium rod is : ($\alpha_{Cu} = 1.7 \times 10^{-5}$ K^{-1} and $\alpha_{Al} = 2.2 \times 10^{-5}$K^{-1}) ***[2019]***
(a) 6.8 cm (b) 113.9 cm (c) 88 cm (d) 68 cm

21. An object kept in a large room having air temperature of 25°C takes 12 minutes to cool from 80°C to 70°C.
The time taken to cool for the same object from 70°C to 60°C would be nearly. ***[NEET Odisha 2019]***
(a) 15 min (b) 10 min (c) 12 min (d) 20 min

Exercise 3 - Concept Application Problems

CAP

1. The rate of heat flow through the cross-section of the rod shown in figure is ($T_2 > T_1$ and thermal conductivity of the material of the rod is K)

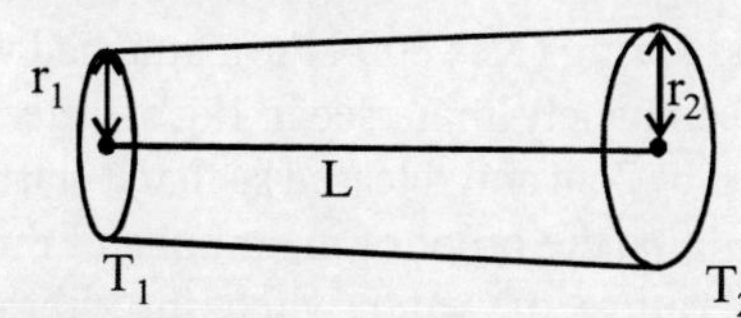

(a) $\frac{K\pi r_1 r_2(T_2-T_1)}{L}$ (b) $\frac{K\pi(r_1+r_2)^2(T_2-T_1)}{4L}$

(c) $\frac{K\pi(r_1+r_1)^2(T_2-T_1)}{L}$ (d) $\frac{K\pi(r_1+r_1)^2(T_2-T_1)}{2L}$

2. Two rods of the same length and areas of cross-section A_1 and A_2 have their ends at the same temperature. K_1 and K_2 are the thremal conductivities of the two rods. The rate of flow of heat is same in both rods if

(a) $\frac{A_1}{A_2}=\frac{K_1}{K_2}$ (b) $\frac{A_1}{A_2}=\frac{K_2}{K_1}$

(c) $A_1A_2=K_1K_2$ (d) $A_1 K_1{}^2 = A_2 K_2{}^2$

3. If a bar is made of copper whose coefficient of linear expansion is one and a half times that of iron, the ratio of force developed in the copper bar to the iron bar of identical lengths and cross-sections, when heated through the same temperature range (Young's modulus of copper may be taken to be equal to that of iron) is
(a) 3/2 (b) 2/3 (c) 9/4 (d) 4/9

4. A metal ball of surface area 200 square cm, temperature 527°C is surrounded by a vessel at 27°C. If the emissivity of the metal is 0.4, then the rate of loss of heat from the ball is approximately $\sigma = 5.67\times10^{-8}\frac{\text{joule}}{m^2\times\sec\times K^2}$
(a) 108 joule (b) 168 joule (c) 182 joule (d) 192 joule

5. Solar radiation emitted by sun resembles that emitted by a black body at a temperature of 6000 K. Maximum intensity is emitted at wavelength of about 4800 Å. If the sun were to cool down from 6000 K to 3000 K, then the peak intensity would occur at a wavelength
(a) 4800 Å (b) 9600 Å (c) 2400 Å (d) 19200 Å

6. The maximum energy in the thermal radiation from a hot source occurs at a wavelength of 11×10^{-5} cm. According to Wien's law, the temperature of this source (on Kelvin scale) will be n times the temperature of another source (on Kelvin scale) for which the wavelength at maximum energy is 5.5×10^{-5} cm. The value n is
(a) 2 (b) 4 (c) 1/2 (d) 1

7. In a thermocouple, the temperature of the cold junction and the neutral temperature are –40°C and 275°C respectively. If the cold junction temperature is increased by 60°C, the neutral temperature and temperature of inversion respectively become
(a) 275°C, 530°C (b) 355°C, 530°C
(c) 375°C, 590°C (d) 355°C, 590°C

8. A glass flask of volume 1 litre is fully filled with mercury at 0°C. Both the flask and mercury are now heated to 100°C. If the coefficient of volume expansion of mercury is 1.82×10^{-4}/°C, volume coefficient of linear expansion of glass is 10×10^{-6}/°C, the amount of mercury which is spilted out is
(a) 15.2 ml (b) 17.2 ml (c) 19.2 ml (d) 21.2 ml

9. A beaker contains 200 gm of water. The heat capacity of the beaker is equal to that of 20 gm of water. The initial temperatue of water in the beaker is 20°C. If 440 gm of hot water at 92°C is poured in it, the final temperature, neglecting radiation loss, will be nearest to
(a) 58°C (b) 68°C (c) 73°C (d) 78°C

10. Ice starts forming in a lake with water at 0°C when the atomspheric temperature is –10°C. If the time taken for the first 1 cm of ice to be formed is 7 hours, then the time taken for the thickness of ice to change from 1 cm to 2 cm is
(a) 7 hours (b) 14 hours (c) 21 hours (d) 3.5 hours

11. Two identical rods of copper and iron are coated with wax uniformly. When one end of each is kept at temperature of boiling water, the length upto which wax melts are 8.4 cm amd 4.2 cm, respectively. If thermal conductivity of copper is 0.92, then thermal conductivity of iron is
(a) 0.23 (b) 0.46 (c) 0.115 (d) 0.69

12. Two vessels of different materials are similar in size in every respect. The same quantity of ice filled in them gets melted in 20 min and 35 min, respectivley. The ratio of coefficients of thermal conduction of the metals is
(a) 4 : 7 (b) 7 : 4 (c) 25 : 16 (d) 16 : 25

13. A partition wall has two layers A and B, in contact, each made of a different material. They have the same thickness but the thermal conductivity of layer A is twice that of layer B. If the steady state temperature difference across the wall is 60 K, then the corresponding difference across the layer A is
(a) 10 K (b) 20 K (c) 30 K (d) 40 K

14. A slab consists of two parallel layers of copper and brass of the same thickness and having thermal conductivities in the ratio 1 : 4. If the free face of brass is at 100°C and that of copper at 0°C, the temperature of interface is
(a) 80°C (b) 20°C (c) 60°C (d) 40°C

15. 540 g of ice at 0°C is mixed with 540 g of water at 80°C. The final temperature of mixture is
(a) 0°C (b) 40°C
(c) 80°C (d) less than 0°C

16. The top of an insulated cylindrical container is covered by a disc having emissivity 0.6 and conductivity 0.167 $WK^{-1}m^{-1}$ and thickness 1 cm. The temperature is maintained by circulating oil as shown in figure. Find the radiation loss to the surrounding in $Jm^{-2}s^{-1}$ if temperature of the upper surface of the disc is 27°C and temperature of the surrounding is 27°C.

(a) 595 $Jm^{-2}s^{-1}$
(b) 545 $Jm^{-2}s^{-1}$
(c) 495 $Jm^{-2}s^{-1}$
(d) None of these

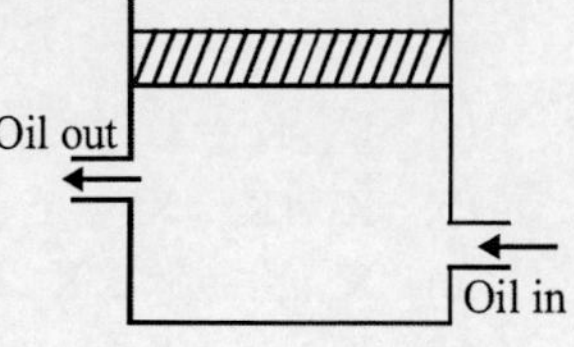

17. Two marks on a glass rod 10 cm apart are found to increase their distance by 0.08 mm when the rod is heated from 0°C to 100°C. A flask made of the same glass as that of rod measures a volume of 1000 cc at 0°C. The volume it measures at 100°C in cc is

(a) 1002.4 (b) 1004.2 (c) 1006.4 (d) 1008.2

18. At 40°C, a brass wire of 1 mm radius is hung from the ceiling. A small mass, M is hung from the free end of the wire. When the wire is cooled down from 40°C to 20°C it regains its original length of 0.2 m. The value of M is close to: (Coefficient of linear expansion and Young's modulus of brass are 10^{-5}/°C and 10^{11} N/m^2, respectively; $g = 10$ ms^{-2})

(a) 9 kg (b) 0.5 kg (c) 1.5 kg (d) 0.9 kg

19. A thermometer graduated according to a linear scale reads a value x_0 when in contact with boiling water, and $x_0/3$ when in contact with ice. What is the temperature of an object in °C, if this thermometer in the contact with the object reads $x_0/2$?

(a) 25 (b) 60 (c) 40 (d) 35

20. A rod, of length L at room temperature and uniform area of cross section A, is made of a metal having coefficient of linear expansion α/°C. It is observed that an external compressive force F, is applied on each of its ends, prevents any change in the length of the rod, when its temperature rises by ΔT K. Young's modulus, Y, for this metal is:

(a) $\frac{F}{A\alpha\Delta T}$ (b) $\frac{F}{A\alpha(\Delta T - 273)}$

(c) $\frac{F}{2A\alpha\Delta T}$ (d) $\frac{2F}{A\alpha\Delta T}$

21. An external pressure P is applied on a cube at 0°C so that it is equally compressed from all sides. K is the bulk modulus of the material of the cube and α is its coefficient of linear expansion. Suppose we want to bring the cube to its original size by heating. The temperature should be raised by :

(a) $\frac{3\alpha}{PK}$ (b) $3PK\alpha$ (c) $\frac{P}{3\alpha K}$ (d) $\frac{P}{\alpha K}$

22. Three rods of identical cross-section and lengths are made of three different materials of thermal conductivity K_1, K_2 and K_3, respectively. They are joined together at their ends to make a long rod (see figure). One end of the long rod is maintained at 100°C and the other at 0°C (see figure). If the joints of the rod are at 70°C and 20°C in steady state and there is no loss of energy from the surface of the rod, the correct relationship between K_1, K_2 and K_3 is:

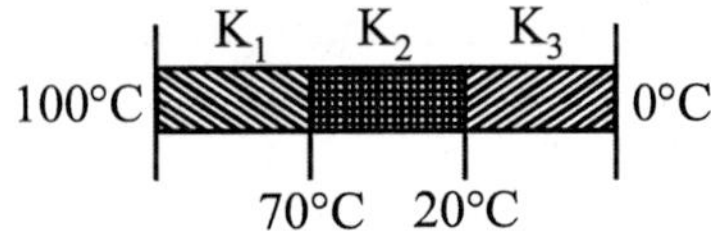

(a) $K_1 : K_3 = 2 : 3, K_1 < K_3 = 2 : 5$

(b) $K_1 < K_2 < K_3$

(c) $K_1 : K_2 = 5 : 2, K_1 : K_3 = 3 : 5$

(d) $K_1 > K_2 > K_3$

23. A bullet of mass 5 g, travelling with a speed of 210 m/s, strikes a fixed wooden target. One half of its kinetics energy is converted into heat in the bullet while the other half is converted into heat in the wood. The rise of temperature of the bullet if the specific heat of its material is 0.030 cal/(g – °C) (1 cal = 4.2 × 10^7 ergs) close to :

(a) 87.5°C (b) 83.3°C (c) 119.2°C (d) 38.4°C

24. A massless spring (K = 800 N/m), attached with a mass (500 g) is completely immersed in 1kg of water. The spring is stretched by 2cm and released so that it starts vibrating. What would be the order of magnitude of the change in the temperature of water when the vibrations stop completely? (Assume that the water container and spring receive negligible heat and specific heat of mass = 400 J/kg K, specific heat of water = 4184 J/kg K)

(a) 10^{-4} K (b) 10^{-5} K (c) 10^{-1} K (d) 10^{-3} K

25. Two materials having coefficients of thermal conductivity '3K' and 'K' and thickness 'd' and '3d', respectively, are joined to form a slab as shown in the figure. The temperatures of the outer surfaces are 'θ_2' and 'θ_1' respectively, ($\theta_2 > \theta_1$). The temperature at the interface is:

	d	3d	
θ_2	3K	K	θ_1

(a) $\frac{\theta_1}{10} + \frac{9\theta_2}{10}$ (b) $\frac{\theta_2 + \theta_1}{2}$

(c) $\frac{\theta_1}{6} + \frac{5\theta_2}{6}$ (d) $\frac{\theta_1}{3} + \frac{2\theta_2}{3}$

26. A cylinder of radius R is surrounded by a cylindrical shell of inner radius R and outer radius 2R. The thermal conductivity of the material of the inner cylinder is K_1 and that of the outer cylinder is K_2. Assuming no loss of heat, the effective thermal conductivity of the system for heat flowing along the length of the cylinder is:

(a) $\frac{K_1 + K_2}{2}$ (b) $K_1 + K_2$

(c) $\frac{2K_1 + 3K_2}{5}$ (d) $\frac{K_1 + 3K_2}{4}$

27. A metal ball of mass 0.1 kg is heated upto 500°C and dropped into a vessel of heat capacity 800 JK^{-1} and containing 0.5 kg water. The initial temperature of water and vessel is 30°C. What is the approximate percentage increment in the temperature of the water? [Specific Heat Capacities of water and metal are, respectively, 4200 Jkg^{-1}K^{-1} and 400 Jkg^{-1} K^{-1}]

(a) 15% (b) 30% (c) 25% (d) 20%

28. An unknown metal of mass 192 g heated to a temperature of 100°C was immersed into a brass calorimeter of mass 128 g containing 240 g of water at a temperature of 8.4°C. Calculate the specific heat of the unknown metal if water temperature stablizes at 21.5°C. (Specific heat of brass is 394 J kg^{-1} K^{-1})

(a) 458 J kg^{-1} K^{-1} (b) 1232 J kg^{-1} K^{-1}

(c) 916 J kg^{-1} K^{-1} (d) 654 J kg^{-1} K^{-1}

29. Temperature difference of 120°C is maintained between two ends of a uniform rod AB of length 2L. Another bent rod PQ, of same cross-section as AB and length $\frac{3L}{2}$, is connected across AB (See figure). In steady state, temperature difference between P and Q will be close to:

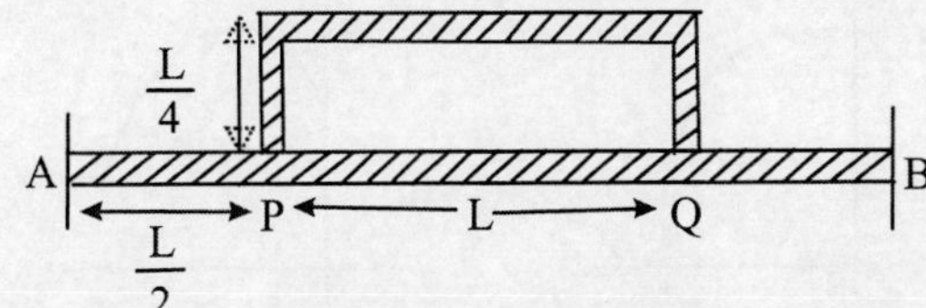

(a) 45°C (b) 75°C (c) 60°C (d) 35°C

30. One end of a thermally insulated rod is kept at a temperature T_1 and the other at T_2. The rod is composed of two sections of length l_1 and l_2 and thermal conductivities K_1 and K_2 respectively. The temperature at the interface of the two section is

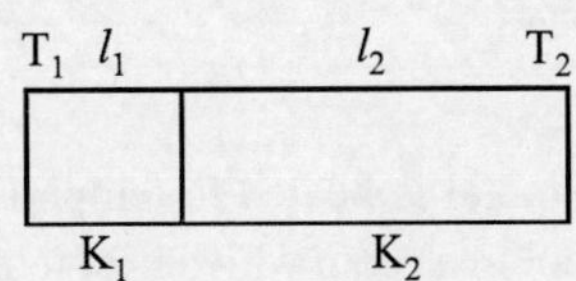

(a) $\frac{(K_1 l_1 T_1 + K_2 l_2 T_2)}{(K_1 l_1 + K_2 l_2)}$ (b) $\frac{(K_2 l_2 T_1 + K_1 l_1 T_2)}{(K_1 l_1 + K_2 l_2)}$

(c) $\frac{(K_2 l_1 T_1 + K_1 l_2 T_2)}{(K_2 l_1 + K_1 l_2)}$ (d) $\frac{(K_1 l_2 T_1 + K_2 l_1 T_2)}{(K_1 l_2 + K_2 l_1)}$

31. Two identical beakers A and B contain equal volumes of two different liquids at 60°C each and left to cool down. Liquid in A has density of 8×10^2 kg/m^3 and specific heat of 2000 J kg^{-1} K^{-1} while liquid in B has density of 10^3 kg m^{-3} and specific heat of 4000 J kg^{-1} K^{-1}. Which of the following best describes their temperature versus time graph schematically ? (assume the emissivity of both the beakers to be the same)

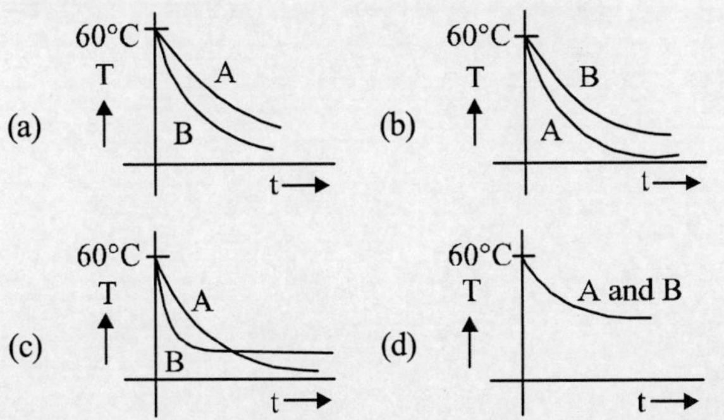

32. The ratio of the coefficient of volume expansion of a glass container to that of a viscous liquid kept inside the container is 1 : 4. What fraction of the inner volume of the container should the liquid occupy so that the volume of the remaining vacant space will be same at all temperatures ?

(a) 2:5 (b) 1:4

(c) 1:64 (d) 1:8

33. An experiment takes 10 minutes to raise the temperature of water in a container from 0ºC to 100ºC and another 55 minutes to convert it totally into steam by a heater supplying heat at a uniform rate. Neglecting the specific heat of the container and taking specific heat of water to be 1 cal / g ºC, the heat of vapourization according to this experiment will come out to be :

(a) 560 cal/ g (b) 550 cal/ g

(c) 540 cal/ g (d) 530 cal/ g

34. Three rods of Copper, Brass and Steel are welded together to form a Y shaped structure. Area of cross - section of each rod = 4 cm^2. End of copper rod is maintained at 100ºC where as ends of brass and steel are kept at 0ºC. Lengths of the copper, brass and steel rods are 46, 13 and 12 cms respectively. The rods are thermally insulated from surroundings excepts at ends. Thermal conductivities of copper, brass and steel are 0.92, 0.26 and 0.12 CGS units respectively. Rate of heat flow through copper rod is:

(a) 1.2 cal/s (b) 2.4 cal/s

(c) 4.8 cal/s (d) 6.0 cal/s

35. A black coloured solid sphere of radius R and mass M is inside a cavity with vacuum inside. The walls of the cavity are maintained at temperature T_0. The initial temperature of the sphere is $3T_0$. If the specific heat of the material of the sphere varies as αT^3 per unit mass with the temperature T of the sphere, where α is a constant, then the time taken for the sphere to cool down to temperature $2T_0$ will be (σ is Stefan Boltzmann constant)

(a) $\frac{M\alpha}{4\pi R^2 \sigma} \text{In}\left(\frac{3}{2}\right)$ (b) $\frac{M\alpha}{4\pi R^2 \sigma} \text{In}\left(\frac{16}{3}\right)$

(c) $\frac{M\alpha}{16\pi R^2 \sigma} \text{In}\left(\frac{16}{3}\right)$ (d) $\frac{M\alpha}{16\pi R^2 \sigma} \text{In}\left(\frac{3}{2}\right)$

36. Water of volume 2 L in a closed container is heated with a coil of 1 kW. While water is heated, the container loses energy at a rate of 160 J/s. In how much time will the temperature of water rise from 27°C to 77°C? (Specific heat of water is 4.2 kJ/kg and that of the container is negligible).

(a) 8 min 20 s (b) 6 min 2 s

(c) 7 min (d) 14 min

37. Assume that a drop of liquid evaporates by decrease in its surface energy, so that its temperature remains unchanged. What should be the minimum radius of the drop for this to be possible? The surface tension is T, density of liquid is ρ and L is its latent heat of vaporization.

(a) $\rho L/T$ (b) $\sqrt{T/\rho L}$

(c) $T/\rho L$ (d) $2T/\rho L$

38. A mass of 50g of water in a closed vessel, with surroundings at a constant temperature takes 2 minutes to cool from 30°C to 25°C. A mass of 100g of another liquid in an identical vessel with identical surroundings takes the same time to cool from 30° C to 25° C. The specific heat of the liquid is :
(The water equivalent of the vessel is 30g.)
(a) 2.0 kcal/kg (b) 7 kcal/kg
(c) 3 kcal/kg (d) 0.5 kcal/kg

39. 500 g of water and 100 g of ice at 0°C are in a calorimeter whose water equivalent is 40 g. 10 g of steam at 100°C is added to it. Then water in the calorimeter is : (Latent heat of ice = 80 cal/g, Latent heat of steam = 540 cal/ g)
(a) 580 g (b) 590 g (c) 600 g (d) 610 g

40. Given that 1 g of water in liquid phase has volume 1 cm^3 and in vapour phase 1671 cm^3 at atmospheric pressure and the latent heat of vaporization of water is 2256 J/g; the change in the internal energy in joules for 1 g of water at 373 K when it changes from liquid phase to vapour phase at the same temperature is:
(a) 2256 (b) 167 (c) 2089 (d) 1

41. A large cylindrical rod of length L is made by joining two identical rods of copper and steel of length $\left(\frac{L}{2}\right)$ each. The rods are completely insulated from the surroundings. If the free end of copper rod is maintained at 100°C and that of steel at 0°C then the temperature of junction is (Thermal conductivity of copper is 9 times that of steel)
(a) 90°C (b) 50°C (c) 10°C (d) 67°C

42. 100g of water is heated from 30°C to 50°C. Ignoring the slight expansion of the water, the change in its internal energy is (specific heat of water is 4184 J/kg/K):
(a) 8.4 kJ (b) 84 kJ (c) 2.1 kJ (d) 4.2 kJ

43. A long metallic bar is carrying heat from one of its ends to the other end under steady–state. The variation of temperature θ along the length x of the bar from its hot end is best described by which of the following figures?

(a) 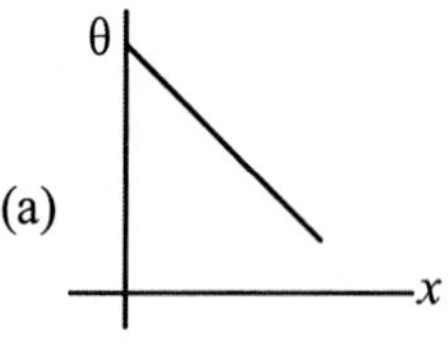

(b) 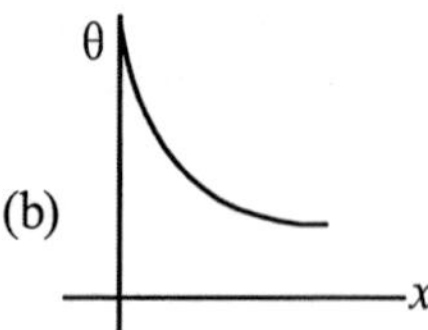

(c) 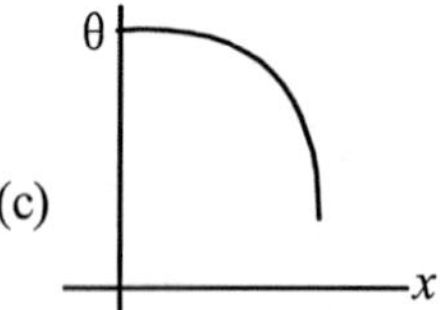

(d) 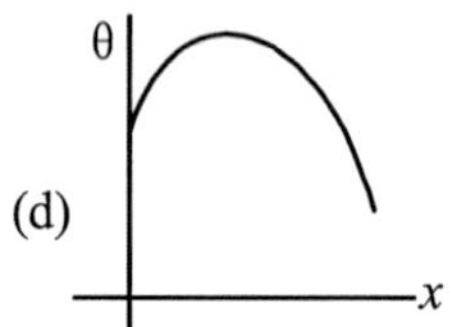

44. Assuming the Sun to be a spherical body of radius R at a temperature of TK, evaluate the total radiant powerd incident of Earth at a distance r from the Sun

(a) $4\pi r_0^2 R^2 \sigma \frac{T^4}{r^2}$ (b) $\pi r_0^2 R^2 \sigma \frac{T^4}{r^2}$

(c) $r_0^2 R^2 \sigma \frac{T^4}{4\pi r^2}$ (d) $R^2 \sigma \frac{T^4}{r^2}$

45. If a piece of metal is heated to temperature θ and then allowed to cool in a room which is at temperature θ_0, the graph between the temperature T of the metal and time t will be closest to

(a) 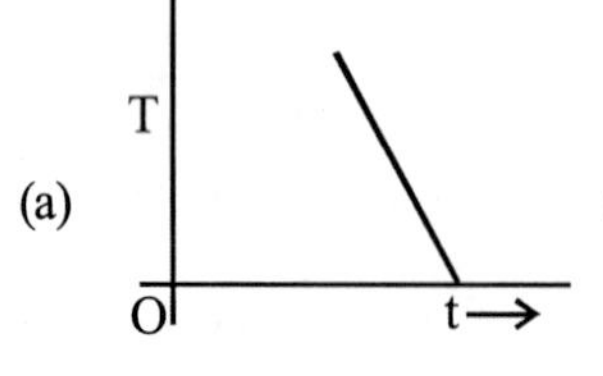

(b) 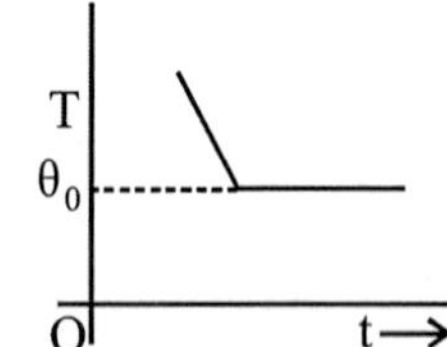

(c) 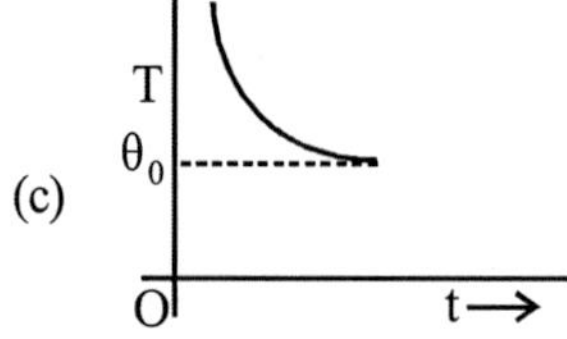

(d) 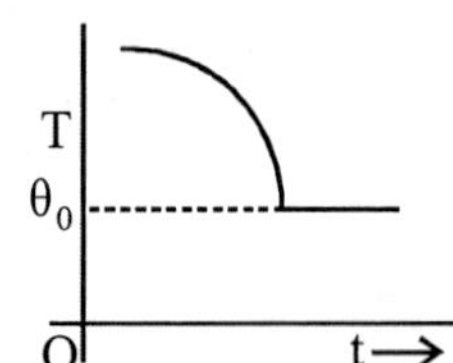

Hints & Solutions

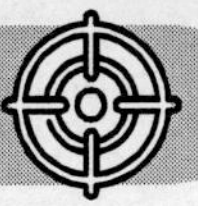

11.1 Concept Practice Problems

CPP

1. (d) Liquid will not flow if $\gamma \le 3\alpha$
2. (b) Let the angle subtended by the arc formed be θ. Then

$\theta = \frac{\ell}{r}$ or $\theta = \frac{\Delta\ell}{\Delta r} = \frac{\ell_2 - \ell_1}{r_1 - r_2}$

$\therefore\ \theta = \frac{\ell(\alpha_2 - \alpha_1)\Delta T}{t}$ or $\frac{\ell}{r} = \frac{\ell(\alpha_2 - \alpha_1)\Delta T}{t}$

So, $r = \frac{t}{(\alpha_2 - \alpha_1)\Delta T}$

3. (c) The temperature is measured by the value of the thermodynamic property of a substance i.e., the property which varies linearly with the temperature.
4. (a) $\frac{140 - 32}{9} = \frac{C}{5}$ or $\frac{700 - 160}{9} = C$ or $C = 60°C$
5. (b) $\frac{\Delta\ell}{\ell} = \alpha\Delta T = 10^{-5} \times 100 = 10^{-3}$

$\frac{\Delta\ell}{\ell} \times 100\% = 10^{-3} \times 100 = 10^{-1} = 0.1\%$

6. (c) $\frac{F - 32}{9} = \frac{80}{5}$

$F - 32 = 144$ or $F = 176°F$.

7. (d) Percentage change in volume $= \gamma t \times 100$

$= 3\alpha t \times 100 = 300\alpha t = 300 \times 2 \times 10^{-5} \times 200 = 1.2$

8. (a) $\gamma = \alpha_1 + \alpha_2 + \alpha_3$

$= 13 \times 10^{-7} + 231 \times 10^{-7} + 231 \times 10^{-7} = 475 \times 10^{-7}$

9. (c) Given $\Delta\ell/\ell = 0.10\% = 0.001$ and $\Delta T = 100°C$

Now $\frac{\Delta\ell}{\ell} = \alpha\Delta T$

or $0.001 = \alpha \times 100$ or $\alpha = 10^{-5}\ /°C$

Further $\gamma = 3\alpha = 3 \times 10^{-5}/°C$

$\therefore\ \frac{\Delta V}{V} \times 100 = (3 \times 10^{-3})(100) = 0.30\%$

10. (b) $-13°F$ is $(13 + 32)°$ below ice point on F scale.

11.2 Concept Practice Problems

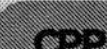

11. (c) Coefficient of thermal conductivity depends upon the material.
12. (d) 13.(c) 14. (b) 15. (c) 16. (a) 17. (d)
18. (b) Temperature of stars can be determined by Wein's displacement law

$\lambda_m =$ constant

19. (c)
20. (a) In condition of weightlessness, convection is not possible.

Exercise 1 - Chapter Revision Problems

CRP

1. (a) $E = \frac{F/A}{\Delta l/l} = \frac{\text{stress}}{\text{strain}}$ where $\Delta l = (l' - l) = l\alpha t$ so $F = EA\alpha t$
2. (a) 3. (c)
4. (a) Initial rate of loss of heat $= \frac{\sigma T^4 \times A_1 \times e}{\sigma T^4 \times A_2 \times e} = \frac{R_1^2}{R_2^2}$
5. (b) Momentum of photon $= \frac{E}{c}$

Change in momentum $= \frac{2E}{c}$

= momentum transferred to the surface

(the photon will reflect with same magnitude of momentum in opposite direction).

6. (c) 7. (c) 8. (b)
9. (c) When a body is heated then relation between colours and temperature is according to Prevost's theory of radiation which states that everybody emitting radiant energy in all directions at a rate depending only on the nature of its surface and its temperature e.g., when a body is placed in an enclosure (furnace) it would acquire the temperature of furnace and seem white means radiate white light. So it becomes first dark and then white.
10. (c) $\frac{dQ}{dt} = \frac{kA\,(T_1 - T_2)}{L}$

$[(T_1 - T_2)$ is the temperature difference$]$

11. (c) $R_t = R_0(1 + \alpha t)$

$2.71 = R_0(1 + \alpha \times 10)$ ...(1)

$3.70 = R_0(1 + \alpha \times 100)$ ...(2)

$3.26 = R_0(1 + \alpha t)$ ...(3)

Solve these equations to obtain the value of t.

12. (c) $\Delta t = \frac{1}{2}\alpha\Delta T \times t$

$\therefore\ 5 = \frac{1}{2}\alpha(T - 15) \times 86400$

and $10 = \frac{1}{2}\alpha(30 - T) \times 86400$

13. (a) Let m be the mass of steam condensed. Then $m \times 540 + m \times 10/2 = 22 \times 70$

$\therefore\ m = 2.83$ gm

Now, total mass $= 22 + 2.83 = 24.83$ gm

14. (d) Thermal resistance $R = l/KA$

Where $l = 20$cm. & A(cylindrical rod) $= \pi r^2 = 40\pi cm^2$

So $R = \frac{20}{0.5 \times 40\pi} = 0.318 \frac{\text{cal}}{\sec \times °C}$

15. (a) According to Stefan's Law

energy radiated per sec $E = \sigma A T^4$

(here e = 1 for black body)

for first case $E = \sigma A(273)^4$

for second case $E_1 = \sigma A(546)^4$ so $E_1 = 16E$

16. (b) The time of cooling increases as the difference between the temperature of body & surrounding is reduced. So $T_1 < T_2 < T_3$ (according to Newton's Law of cooling).
17. (c) 18. (b)

19. (c) According to Stefan's Boltzmann law, the energy radiated per unit time E = σAT^4.
$\therefore\ 5.67\times10^4 = 5.67\times10^{-8}\times1\times T^4\ \ (\because A = 1\ m^2)$

or, $T = \left(\dfrac{5.67\times10^4}{5.67\times10^{-8}}\right)^{1/4} = 1000K$

or, $T = 1000 - 273 = 727°C$.

20. (a) According to Newton's law of cooling,

$$\frac{\theta_1-\theta_2}{t} = K\left[\frac{\theta_1+\theta_2}{2}-\theta_0\right]$$

where θ_0 is the surrounding temperature.

$$\therefore\ \frac{60-40}{7} = K\left(\frac{60+40}{2}-10\right) \Rightarrow \frac{20}{7} = 40K \Rightarrow K = \frac{1}{14}$$

$$\therefore\ \frac{40-28}{t} = K\left[\frac{40+28}{2}-10\right] \Rightarrow \frac{12}{t} = 24K$$

or $t = \dfrac{12}{24K} = \dfrac{12\times14}{24} = 7\ \text{min}$

21. (a) Let θ be temperature of interface.

$$\therefore\ \frac{K_PA(100-\theta)}{\ell} = \frac{K_QA(\theta-0)}{\ell}$$

$$\therefore\ \frac{K_P}{K_Q} = \frac{\theta}{100-\theta} \Rightarrow \frac{2}{3} = \frac{\theta}{100-\theta}$$

or, $200 - 2\theta = 3\theta$ or, $5\theta = 200$ or, $\theta = 40°C$

22. (a) Let the final temperature of mixture be T.
Then $100\times80 + 100(T-0)\times½$
(as specific heat of ice is 0.5 cal/g C° and specific heat of water is 1 cal/gC°)
$= 100\times1\times(100-T)$
Solving, we get $T = 13.33°C$.

23. (a)

24. (a) $mL + m(100-80)$
$= 1.1\times1\times(80-15) + 0.02\times(80-15)$
$m\times540 + 20m = 71.5 + 1.30$
$560m = 72.80\ \ \therefore\ m = 0.130$

25. (d) $W = W_1 - W_2 = mgh - mgh' = mg(h-h')$
$= 5\times10\ (20-0.2) = 5\times10\times19.8$
$= 5\times198 = 990$ joule
This energy is converted into heat when the ball strikes the earth. Heat produced is

$Q = \dfrac{990}{4.2}$ calorie

$$\Delta T = \frac{Q}{mc} = \frac{99\times100}{42\times5000\times0.09} = \frac{11}{32}\ °C$$

26. (b) $80\times1\times30 = m\times80 \Rightarrow m = 30$ gm.

27. (b) $\lambda_1T_1 = \lambda_2T_2$
$6050\times4753 = 9506.T_2$
$T_2 = 3025$ K

28. (a) $\dfrac{E_1}{E_2} = \dfrac{\sigma(T_1^4-T_0^4)}{\sigma(T_2^4-T_0^4)} = \dfrac{(600)^4-(300)^4}{(500)^4-(300)^4}$

29. (d) Thermal capacity $= 40\times0.2 = 8$ cal $°C^{-1}$

30. (a) Mass ratio 1 : 2; hence ΔT ratio 2 : 1. Therefore equilibrium temp is 30°C.

31. (b) Heat capacity of cold : hot = 1 : 2
So final temp. is $\dfrac{1}{3}\times(2\times92+1\times20) = 68°C$.

32. (d) $E = \sigma\times\text{area}\times T^4$; T increases by a factor $\dfrac{3}{2}$.
Area increases by a factor $\dfrac{1}{4}$.

33. (d) $t \propto \dfrac{\ell}{A},\ t' \propto \dfrac{2\ell}{A/2}$

34. (a)

35. (c) The total power radiated by a black body of area A at temperature TK is given by $P = A\sigma T^4$
Where σ = Stefan's constant
$= 5.7\times10^{-8}\ W\,m^{-2}\,K^{-4}$
Which is best represented in graph. (c)

36. (b) According to Stefan's law $E = \sigma T^4$,
$T_1 = 500$ K
$T_2 = 1000$ K

$$\frac{E_2}{E_1} = \left(\frac{T_2}{T_1}\right)^4 = \left(\frac{1000}{500}\right)^4 = 16$$

$\therefore\ E_2 = 16\times7 = 112\ \text{cal/cm}^2\text{s}$

37. (a) Let L_1' and L_2' be the lengths of the wire when temperature is changed by $\Delta T°C$.
At $T°C$,
$L_{eq} = L_1 + L_2$
At $T + \Delta°C$
$L_{eq}' = L_1' + L_2'$
$\therefore\ L_{eq}(1+\alpha_{eq}\Delta T) = L_1(1+\alpha_1\Delta T) + L_2(1+\alpha_2\Delta T)$
$[\because L' = L(1+\alpha\Delta T)]$
$\Rightarrow (L_1+L_2)(1+\alpha_{eq}\Delta T) = L_1 + L_2 + L_1\alpha_1\Delta T + L_2\alpha_2\Delta T$

$$\Rightarrow \alpha_{eq} = \frac{\alpha_1L_1+\alpha_2L_2}{L_1+L_2}$$

38. (a) Change in length of the metal wire (Δl) when its temperature is changed by ΔT is given by
$\Delta l = l\alpha\Delta T$
Here, α = Coefficient of linear expansion
Here, $\Delta l = 0.02\%$, $\Delta T = 10°C$

$$\therefore \alpha = \frac{\Delta l}{l\Delta T} = \frac{0.02}{100\times10} \Rightarrow \alpha = 2\times10^{-5}$$

Volume coefficient of expansion, $\gamma = 3\alpha = 6\times10^{-5}$

$\because \rho = \dfrac{M}{V}$

$\dfrac{\Delta V}{V}\times100 = \gamma\Delta T = (6\times10^{-5}\times10\times100) = 6\times10^{-2}$

Volume increase by 0.06% therefore density decrease by 0.06%.

39. (b) Young's modulus $= \dfrac{\text{Thermal stress}}{\text{Strain}} = \dfrac{F/A}{\Delta L/L}$

$Y = \frac{F}{A.\alpha.\Delta\theta}$ $\left(\because \frac{\Delta L}{L} = \alpha\Delta\theta\right)$

Force developed in the rail $F = YA\alpha\Delta t$
$= 2\times10^{11}\times40\times10^{-4}\times1.2\times10^{-5}\times10$
$= 9.6\times10^4 = 1\times10^5$ N

40. (c) $\frac{\text{Reading on any scale} - \text{LFP}}{\text{UFP} - \text{LFP}}$
= constant for all scales

$\frac{340-273}{373-273} = \frac{°Y-(-160)}{-50-(-160)} \Rightarrow \frac{67}{100} = \frac{y+160}{110}$

$\therefore$ Y = – 86.3° Y

41. (a) $M_1C_{ice}\times(10) + M_1L = M_2C_\omega(50)$
or $M_1\times C_{ice}(=0.5)\times10 + M_1L = M_2\times1\times50$
$\Rightarrow L = \frac{50M_2}{M_1} - 5$

42. (d) Let m gram of ice is added.
From principal of calorimeter
heat gained (by ice) = heat lost (by water)
$\therefore 20\times2.1\times m + (m-20)\times334$
$= 50\times4.2\times40$
$376m = 8400 + 6680$
$m = 40.1$

43. (c) Heat loss = Heat gain = $mS\Delta\theta$
So, $m_AS_A\Delta\theta_A = m_BS_B\Delta\theta_B$
$\Rightarrow 100\times S_A\times(100-90) = 50\times S_B\times(90-75)$
$2S_A = 1.5S_B \Rightarrow S_A = \frac{3}{4}S_B$
Now, $100\times S_A\times(100-\theta) = 50\times S_B\times(\theta-50)$
$2\times\left(\frac{3}{4}\right)\times(100-\theta) = (\theta-50)$
$300-3\theta = 2\theta-100$
$400 = 5\theta \Rightarrow \theta = 80°C$

44. (a)

Temp. of heat source — Temp. of heat reservoir

10^3K ←1 m→ 10^2K

$\left(\frac{dQ}{dt}\right) = \frac{kA\Delta T}{\ell}$

Energy flux, $\frac{1}{A}\left(\frac{dQ}{dt}\right) = \frac{k\Delta T}{\ell} = \frac{(0.1)(900)}{1} = 90\ \text{W/m}^2$

45. (d) From stefan's law, energy radiated by sun per second
$E = \sigma AT^4$;
$\therefore A \propto R^2$
$\therefore E \propto R^2T^4$ $\therefore \frac{E_2}{E_1} = \frac{R_2^2T_2^4}{R_1^2T_1^4}$
put $R_2 = 2R, R_1 = R; T_2 = 2T, T_1 = T$
$\Rightarrow \frac{E_2}{E_1} = \frac{(2R)^2(2T)^4}{R^2T^4} = 64$

46. (b)

47. (a) According to Newton's law of cooling,
$\left(\frac{\theta_1-\theta_2}{t}\right) = K\left(\frac{\theta_1+\theta_2}{2} - \theta_0\right)$

$\left(\frac{60-50}{10}\right) = K\left(\frac{60+50}{2} - 25\right)$ ..... (i)

and, $\left(\frac{50-\theta}{10}\right) = K\left(\frac{50+\theta}{2} - 25\right)$ ..... (ii)

Dividing eq. (i) by (ii),
$\frac{10}{(50-\theta)} = \frac{60}{\theta} \Rightarrow \theta = 42.85°C \cong 43°C$

48. (a) Change in length in both rods are same i.e.
$\Delta\ell_1 = \Delta\ell_2$
$\ell\alpha_1\Delta\theta_1 = \ell\alpha_2\Delta\theta_2$
$\frac{\alpha_1}{\alpha_2} = \frac{\Delta\theta_2}{\Delta\theta_1}$ $\left[\because \frac{\alpha_1}{\alpha_2} = \frac{4}{3}\right]$
$\frac{4}{3} = \frac{\theta-30}{180-30}$
$\boxed{\theta = 230°C}$

49. (a) Heat given by water $= m_wC_w(T_{mix} - T_w)$
$= 200\times1\times(31-25)$

Heat taken by steam $= mL_{stem} + mC_w(T_s - T_{mix})$
$= m\times540 + m(1)\times(100-31)$
$= m\times540 + m(1)\times(69)$
From the principal of calorimeter,
Heat lost = Heat gained
$\therefore (200)(31-25) = m\times540 + m(1)(69)$
$\Rightarrow 1200 = m(609) \Rightarrow m \approx 2.$

50. (a) Here ice melts due to water.
Let the amount of ice melts = m_{ice}
$m_ws_w\Delta\theta = m_{ice}L_{ice}$
$\therefore m_{ice} = \frac{m_ws_w\Delta\theta}{L_{ice}}$
$= \frac{0.2\times4200\times25}{3.4\times10^5} = 0.0617\ \text{kg} = 61.7\ \text{g}$

Exercise 2 - Exemplar & Past Year Questions E&PYQs

Exemplar Questions

1. (d) If strips of aluminium and steel are fixed together on metallic strip and both are heated then ($\alpha_{Al} > \alpha_{steel}$) aluminium will exapnd more because the metallic strip with higher coefficient of linear expansion (α_{Al}) will expand more Thus it should have larger radius of curvature. Hence, aluminium will be on convex side.

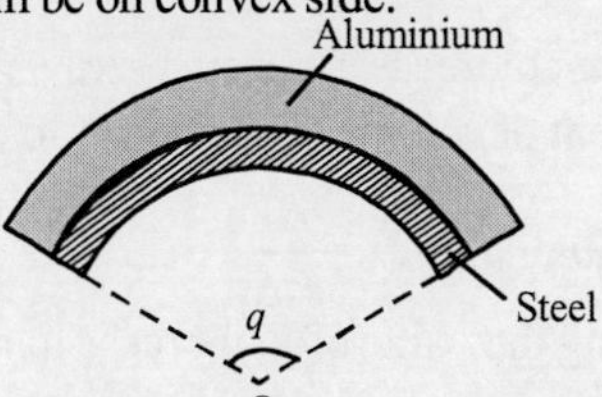

2. (b) On heating a uniform metallic rod its length will increase so moment of inertia of rod increased from I_1 to I_2.
No external torque is acting on the system so angular momentum should be conserved.

L = Angular momentum = $I\omega$ = constant

$I_1\omega_1 = I_2\omega_2$

So, $\frac{\omega_2}{\omega_1} = \frac{I_1}{I_2} < 1$

$\omega_2 < \omega_1$

($\because$ Due to expansion of the rod $I_2 > I_1$)

So, angular veloctiy decreases.

3. (a) As we know that, the Buoyant force (F) on a body volume (V) and density of (ρ), when immersed in liquid of density (ρ_l) is $= V'\rho_l g$
where V' = volume of displaced liquid by dipped body (V).
Let volume of the sphere is V and ρ is its density, then we can write buoyant force

$F = V\rho_s G$

$F \propto \rho_l$ (for liquid)

$$\frac{F_{4°C}}{F_{0°C}} = \frac{\rho_{4°C}}{\rho_{0°C}} > 1 \qquad (\because \rho_{4°C} > \rho_{0°C})$$

$F_{4°C} > F_{0°C}$

Hence, buoyancy will be less in water at 0°C than that in water at 4°C.

4. (a) As the temperature increased the length (L) of the pendulum increases due to expansion is linear.

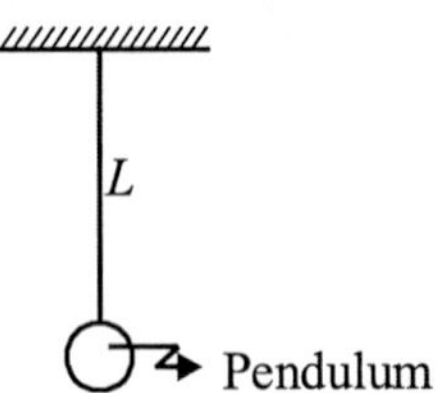

So, Time period of pendulum

$$T = 2\pi\sqrt{\frac{L}{g}} \Rightarrow T \propto \sqrt{L}$$

Hence on increasing temperature, time period (T) also increases.

5. (a) As we know that when the temperature increases vibration of molecules about their mean position increases hence the kinetic energy associated with random motion of molecules increases.

6. (d) Let the radius of the sphere is R. As the temperature increases radius of the sphere increases as shown.

Original volume $V = \frac{4}{3}\pi R^3$

Coefficient of linear expansion = α

Coefficient of volume expansion = 3α

As we know that $Y = \frac{\Delta V}{V\Delta t}$

By putting the value of V, increase in the volume

$\Rightarrow \Delta V = 3V\alpha\Delta t = 4\pi R^3\alpha\Delta t$

$\therefore 3\alpha = \frac{\Delta V}{V\Delta t}$

7. (c)

Past Years (2013-2020) NEET/AIPMT Questions

8. (a) Wein's displacement law
According to this law

$$\lambda_{max} \propto \frac{1}{T}$$

or, $\lambda_{max} \times T$ = constant

So, as the temperature increases λ decreases.

9. (a) $C_p - C_v = R \Rightarrow C_p = C_v + R$

$$\because \gamma = \frac{C_p}{C_v} = \frac{C_v + R}{C_v} = \frac{C_v}{C_v} + \frac{R}{C_v}$$

$$\Rightarrow \gamma = 1 + \frac{R}{C_v} \Rightarrow \frac{R}{C_v} = \gamma - 1 \Rightarrow C_v = \frac{R}{\gamma - 1}$$

10. (b) From question,

$\Delta\rho = (998 - 992)\ kg/m^3 = 6\ kg/m^3$

$\rho = \frac{998 + 992}{2}\ kg/m^3 = 995\ kg/m^3$

$$\rho = \frac{m}{V} \Rightarrow \frac{\Delta\rho}{\rho} = -\frac{\Delta V}{V} \Rightarrow \left|\frac{\Delta\rho}{\rho}\right| = \left|\frac{\Delta V}{V}\right|$$

$\therefore$ Coefficient of volume expansion of water,

$$\frac{1}{V}\frac{\Delta V}{\Delta t} = \frac{1}{\rho}\frac{\Delta\rho}{\Delta t} = \frac{6}{995 \times 20} \approx 3 \times 10^{-4}/°C$$

11. (b) $Q_1 = 4Q_2$ (Given)

$$\Rightarrow \frac{K_1A_1\Delta t}{L} = 4\frac{K_2A_2\Delta t}{L} \Rightarrow K_1A_1 = 4K_2A_2.$$

12. (a) Let the temperature of surroundings be θ_0
By Newton's law of cooling

$$\frac{\theta_1 - \theta_2}{t} = k\left[\frac{\theta_1 + \theta_2}{2} - \theta_0\right]$$

$$\Rightarrow \frac{70 - 60}{5} = k\left[\frac{70 + 60}{2} - \theta_0\right]$$

$$\Rightarrow 2 = k[65 - \theta_0] \quad ...(i)$$

Similarly, $\frac{60 - 54}{5} = k\left[\frac{60 + 54}{2} - \theta_0\right]$

$$\Rightarrow \frac{6}{5} = k[57 - \theta_0] \quad ...(ii)$$

By dividing (i) by (ii) we have

$$\frac{10}{6} = \frac{65 - \theta_0}{57 - \theta_0} \Rightarrow \theta_0 = 45°$$

13. (d) According to the principle of calorimetry.
Heat lost = Heat gained

$mL_v + ms_w\Delta\theta = m_w s_w\Delta\theta \Rightarrow m \times 540 + m \times 1 \times (100 - 80) = 20 \times 1 \times (80 - 10) \Rightarrow m = 2.5\ g$

Therefore total mass of water at 80°C = (20 + 2.5) g = 22.5 g

14. (a) From question,
Rise in temperature Δt = 40°C

Fractional change in the density $\frac{\Delta\rho}{\rho_0}$ = ?

Coefficient of volume expansion

$\gamma = 5 \times 10^{-4} K^{-1}$

$\rho = \rho_0(1-\gamma\Delta t) \Rightarrow \frac{\Delta\rho}{\rho_0} = \gamma\Delta T = (5\times10^{-4})(40) = 0.02$

15. (c) As the temperature difference $\Delta T = 10°C$ as well as the thermal resistance is same for both the cases, so thermal current or rate of heat flow will also be same for both the cases.

16. (c) According to question only one-quarter of the heat produced by falling piece of ice is absorbed in the melting of ice.

i.e., $\frac{mgh}{4} = mL \Rightarrow h = \frac{4L}{g} = \frac{4\times3.4\times10^5}{10} = 136$ km.

17. (d) According to wein's displacement law, maximum amount of emitted radiation corresponding to $\lambda_m = \frac{b}{T}$

$\lambda_m = \frac{2.88\times10^6 \text{ nmK}}{5760\text{K}} = 500$ nm

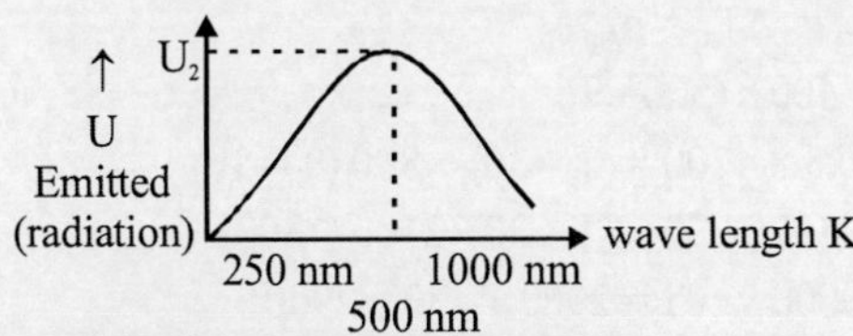

From the graph $U_1 < U_2 > U_3$

18. (c) Given $r_1 = 12$ cm, $r_2 = 6$ cm
$T_1 = 500$ K and $T_2 = 2\times500 = 1000$ K
$P_1 = 450$ watt
Rate of power loss $P \propto r^2T^4$

$\frac{P_1}{P_2} = \frac{r_1^2T_1^4}{r_2^2T_2^4} \Rightarrow P_2 = P_1\frac{r_2^2T_2^4}{r_1^2T_1^4}$

Solving we get, $P_2 = 1800$ watt

19. (d) From Wien's law
λ_{max} T = constant
i.e., $\lambda_{max_1} T_1 = \lambda_{max_2} T_2$

$\Rightarrow \lambda_0 T = \frac{3\lambda_0}{4}T' \Rightarrow T' = \frac{4}{3}T$

Power radiated $P \propto T^4$

So, $\frac{P_2}{P_1} = n = \left(\frac{T'}{T}\right)^4 = \left(\frac{4}{3}\right)^4 = \frac{256}{81}$

20. (d) $l'_{Cu} = l_{Cu}(1+\alpha_{Cu}\Delta T)$
$\Delta l_{Cu} = l_{Cu}\alpha_{Cu}\Delta T$
$l'_{Al} = l_{Al}(1+\alpha_{Al}\Delta T) \Rightarrow \Delta l_{Al} = l_{Al}\alpha_{Al}\Delta T$
Since, change in length is independent of temperature
$\therefore \alpha_{Cu}l_{Cu} = \alpha_{Al}l_{Al}$
$\Rightarrow 1.7\times10^{-5}\times88 \text{ cm} = 2.2\times10^{-5}\times l_{Al}$

$\Rightarrow l_{Al} = \frac{1.7\times88}{2.2} = 68$ cm

21. (a) According to Newton's law of cooling

$\frac{(T_1-T_2)}{t} = K\left(\frac{T_1+T_2}{2} - T_0\right)$

$\frac{(80-70)}{12} = K(75-25)$ ...(i)

$\frac{(70-60)}{t'} = K(65-25)$ ...(ii)

$\Rightarrow t' = 12\times = 15$ min

Exercise 3 - Concept Application Problems CAP

1. (a) $r_{eff} = \sqrt{r_1r_2}$

$\frac{dQ}{dt} = \frac{KA(T_2-T_1)}{L} = \frac{K\pi r_1r_2(T_2-T_1)}{L}$

2. (b)

3. (a) $F = Y\alpha tA$ or $F \propto \alpha$
($\because$ Y t A is same for both copper and iron)

or $F_C \propto \alpha_C$ and $F_I \propto \alpha_I$ $\therefore \frac{F_C}{F_I} = \frac{3/2}{1} = \frac{3}{2}$

4. (c) According to Stefan's Law, the rate of loss of heat is

$\frac{Q}{t} = \sigma A(T_1^4 - T_2^4)\times e$

here $\sigma = 5.67\times10^{-8}$ J/m² × sec.K²,
$T_1 = 527+273 = 800$K,
$T_2 = 27+273 = 300$K & $A = 200\times10^{-4}$m²

So. $\frac{Q}{t} = 5.67\times10^{-8}\times2\times10^{-2}[(800)^4 - (300)^4]\times0.4$
$\cong 182$ joule

5. (b) According to Wein's displacement law, $\lambda_m T = b$.
where $b = 2.884\times10^{-3}$ mK.
So $\lambda_{m_1}T_1 = \lambda_{m_2}T_2$
or $4800\times6000 = \lambda_{m_2}\times3000$ or $\lambda_{m_2} = 9600$A°

6. (c) $11.0\times10^{-5}T_1 = 5.5\times10^{-5}T_2$

$\frac{T_1}{T_2} = \frac{1}{2}$

7. (a) When the temperature of cold junction is increased, the neutral temperature remains constant for a given thermocouple and it is independent of the temperature of the cold junction.
$\therefore \theta_n = 275°C$, $\theta_i - \theta_n = \theta_n - \theta_c \therefore \theta_i = 2\theta_n - \theta_c = 530°C$.

8. (a) $\Delta V = V_0(\gamma_m - \gamma_g)\Delta T$
$= 1[1.82\times10^{-4} - 3\times(10\times10^{-6})]\,100$
$= 1[1.82\times10^{-4} - 0.3\times10^{-4})]\,100 = 15.2$ ml

9. (b) Let the final temperature be T.
Then $200\times1\times(T-20) + 20\times(T-20) = 440(92-T)$
Solving it, we get T = 68°C.

10. (c)

11. (a) Use $\frac{K_1}{K_2} = \frac{\ell_1^2}{\ell_2^2}$

12. (b) Here flow of heat, area of vessels & temperature gradient are same so

$Q = K_1A\frac{dT}{dx}t_1 = K_2A\frac{dT}{dx}t_2$

so $\frac{K_1}{K_2} = \frac{t_2}{t_1} = \frac{35}{20} = \frac{7}{4}$

13. (b)

14. (a) $4K(100-\theta) = K(\theta-0) \Rightarrow 400 - 4\theta = \theta \Rightarrow \theta = 80°C$

15. (a) $540 \times 80 + 540\,\theta = 540\,(80 - \theta)$
$\Rightarrow 80 + \theta = 80 - \theta \Rightarrow 2\theta = 0 \Rightarrow \theta = 0°$

16. (a) The rate of heat loss per unit area due to radiation
$= \epsilon\sigma\,(T^4 - T_0^{\,4})$
$= 0.6 \times 5.67 \times 10^{-8}\,[(400)^4 - (300)^4] = 595\ Jm^{-2}s^{-1}$.

17. (a) $\gamma = \dfrac{V_2 - V_1}{V_1(T_2 - T_1)};\ \alpha = \dfrac{\ell_2 - \ell_1}{\ell_1(T_2 - T_1)}$
$T_1 = 0°C,\ T_2 = 100°C$
$\gamma = \dfrac{V_2 - V_1}{100V_1};\ \alpha = \dfrac{\ell_2 - \ell_1}{100\ell_1}$
$\ell_1 = 10$ cm; $\ell_2 - \ell_1 = 0.08$ mm $= 0.008$ cm
$\alpha = \dfrac{0.008}{10 \times 100} = 8 \times 10^{-6}\,/°C;\ \gamma = 3\alpha = 24 \times 10^{-6}\,/°C$
$\therefore\ 24 \times 10^{-6} = \dfrac{V_2 - 1000}{1000 \times 100}$
$V_2 - 1000 = 24 \times 10^{-6} \times 10^5 = 2.4\ \therefore\ V_2 = 1002.4$ cc

18. (Bonus) $\Delta_{temp} = \Delta_{load}$ and $A = \pi r^2 = \pi(10^{-3})^2 = \pi \times 10^{-6}$
$L\,\alpha\,\Delta T = \dfrac{FL}{AY}$
or $0.2 \times 10^{-5} \times 20 = \dfrac{F \times 0.2}{(\pi \times 10^{-6}) \times 10^{11}}$
$\therefore\ F = 20\pi N\ \therefore m = \dfrac{f}{g} = 2\pi = 6.28$ kg

19. (a)

20. (a) Young's modulus $Y = \dfrac{\text{stress}}{\text{strain}} = \dfrac{F/A}{A(\Delta\ell/\ell)}$
Using, coefficient of linear expansion,
$\alpha = \dfrac{\Delta\ell}{\ell\Delta T} \Rightarrow \dfrac{\Delta\ell}{\ell} = \alpha\Delta T \qquad \therefore Y = \dfrac{F}{A(\alpha\Delta T)}$

21. (c) As we know, Bulk modulus
$K = \dfrac{\Delta P}{\left(\dfrac{-\Delta V}{V}\right)} \quad \Rightarrow \dfrac{\Delta V}{V} = \dfrac{P}{K}$

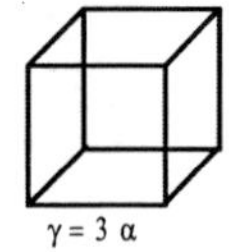

$V = V_0(1 + \gamma\Delta t)$
$\dfrac{\Delta V}{V_0} = \gamma\Delta t \quad \therefore\ \dfrac{P}{K} = \gamma\Delta t \Rightarrow \Delta t = \dfrac{P}{\gamma K} = \dfrac{P}{3\alpha K}$

22. (a)

23. (a) According to question, one half of its kinetic energy is converted into heat in the wood.
$\dfrac{1}{2}mv^2 \times \dfrac{1}{2} = ms\Delta T$
$\Rightarrow \Delta T = \dfrac{v^2}{4 \times s} = \dfrac{210 \times 210}{4 \times 4.2 \times 0.3 \times 1000} = 87.5°C$

24. (b) $\dfrac{1}{2}.kx^2 = mC(\Delta T) + m_\omega C_\omega \Delta T$
or $\dfrac{1}{2} \times 800 \times 0.02^2 = 0.5 \times 400 \times \Delta T + 1 \times 4184 \times \Delta T$
$\therefore \Delta T = 1 \times 10^{-5}\,K$

25. (a) $H_1 = H_2$ θ_2 [3k | k] θ_1 (lengths d, $3d$; interface temperature θ)
or $(3k)A\left(\dfrac{\theta_2 - \theta}{d}\right) = kA\left(\dfrac{\theta - \theta_1}{3d}\right)$ or $\theta = \left(\dfrac{\theta_1 + 9\theta_2}{10}\right)$

26. (d) Effective thermal conductivity of system
$K_{eq} = \dfrac{K_1A_1 + K_2A_2}{A_1 + A_2}$
$= \dfrac{K_1\pi R^2 + K_2[\pi(2R)^2 - \pi R^2]}{\pi(2R)^2}$
$= \dfrac{K_1(\pi R^2) + K_2(3\pi R^2)}{4\pi R^2} = \dfrac{K_1 + 3K_2}{4}$

27. (d) Assume final temperature = T°C
Heat lass = Heat gain = $ms\Delta T$
$\Rightarrow m_B\,s_B\,\Delta T_B = m_w\,s_w\Delta T_w$
$0.1 \times 400 \times (500 - T)$
$= 0.5 \times 4200 \times (T - 30) + 800\,(T - 30)$
$\Rightarrow 40\,(500 - T) = (T - 30)\,(2100 + 800)$
$\Rightarrow 20000 - 40T = 2900\,T - 30 \times 2900$
$\Rightarrow 20000 + 30 \times 2900 = T(2940)$
$T = 30.4°C$
$\dfrac{\Delta T}{T} \times 100 = \dfrac{6.4}{30} \times 100 = 21\%$,
so the closest answer is 20%.

28. (c) Let specific heat of unknown metal be 's' According to principle of calorimetry, Heat lost
= Heat gain $m \times s\Delta\theta = m_1 s_{brass}\,(\Delta\theta_1 + m_2\,s_{water} + \Delta\theta_2)$
$\Rightarrow 192 \times S \times (100 - 21.5) = 128 \times 394 \times (21.5 - 8.4)$
Solving we get,+ $240 \times 4200 \times (21.5 - 8.4)$
$S = 916\ Jkg^{-1}k^{-1}$

29. (a) $\dfrac{\Delta T_{AB}}{R_{AB}} = \dfrac{120}{\frac{8}{5}R} = \dfrac{120 \times 5}{8R}$

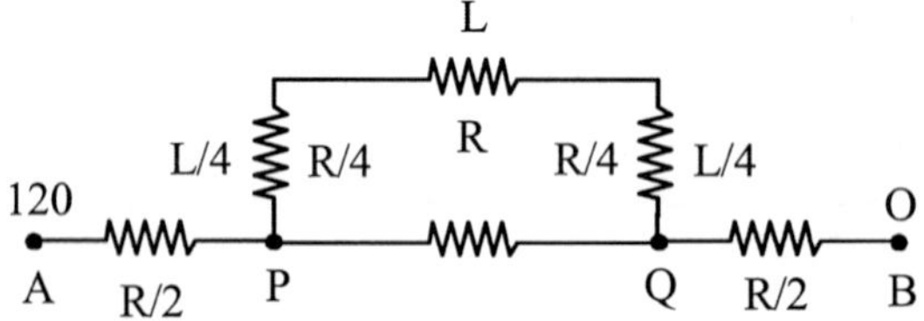

In steady state temperature difference between P and Q,
$\Delta T_{PQ} = \dfrac{120 \times 5}{8R} \times \dfrac{3}{5}R = \dfrac{360}{8} = 45°C$

30. (d) Let T be the temperature of the interface. In the steady state, $Q_1 = Q_2$

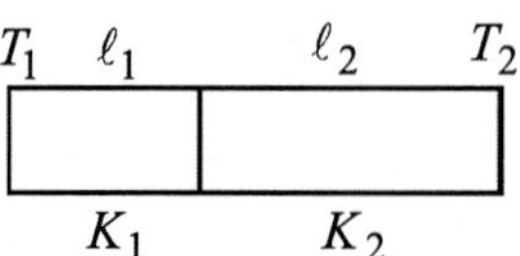

$\therefore\ \dfrac{K_1A(T_1 - T)}{\ell_1} = \dfrac{K_2A(T - T_2)}{\ell_2}$, where A is the area of cross-section.

$\Rightarrow \quad K_1A(T_1-T)\ell_2 = K_2A(T-T_2)\ell_1$

$\Rightarrow \quad K_1T_1\ell_2 - K_1T\ell_2 = K_2T\ell_1 - K_2T_2\ell_1$

$\Rightarrow \quad (K_2\ell_1 + K_1\ell_2)T = K_1T_1\ell_2 + K_2T_2\ell_1$

$\Rightarrow \quad T = \dfrac{K_1T_1\ell_2 + K_2T_2\ell_1}{K_2\ell_1 + K_1\ell_2} = \dfrac{K_1\ell_2T_1 + K_2\ell_1T_2}{K_1\ell_2 + K_2\ell_1}.$

31. (b) Rate of Heat loss $= mS\left(\dfrac{dT}{dt}\right) = e\sigma AT^4$

$-\dfrac{dT}{dt} = \dfrac{e\sigma \times A \times T^4}{\rho \times Vol. \times S} \Rightarrow -\dfrac{dT}{dt} \propto \dfrac{1}{\rho S}$

$\dfrac{\left(-\dfrac{dT}{dt}\right)_A}{\left(-\dfrac{dT}{dt}\right)_B} = \dfrac{\rho_B}{\rho_A} \times \dfrac{S_B}{S_A} = \dfrac{10^3}{8\times10^2} \times \dfrac{4000}{2000}$

$\Rightarrow \left(-\dfrac{dT}{dt}\right)_A > \left(-\dfrac{dT}{dt}\right)_B$

So, A cools down at faster rate.

32. (b) When there is no change in liquid level in vessel then $\gamma'_{real} = \gamma'_{vessel}$

Change in volume in liquid relative to vessel

$\Delta V_{app} = V\gamma'_{app}\Delta\theta = V(\gamma'_{real} - \gamma'_{vessel})$

33. (b) As $Pt = mC\Delta T$

So, $P \times 10 \times 60 = mC\,100$ ...(i)

and $P \times 55 \times 60 = mL$ ...(ii)

Dividing equation (i) by (ii) we get

$\dfrac{10}{55} = \dfrac{C\times100}{L} \qquad \therefore L = 550$ cal./g.

34. (c) 35. (c)

36. (a) From question,

In 1 sec heat gained by water

= 1 KW – 160 J/s = 1000 J/s – 160 J/s = 840 J/s

Total heat required to raise the temperature of water (volume 2L) from 27°c to 77°c

$= m_{water} \times$ sp. ht $\times \Delta\theta$

$= 2 \times 10^3 \times 4.2 \times 50$ [$\because$ mass = density × volume]

And, $840 \times t = 2 \times 10^3 \times 4.2 \times 50$

or, $t = \dfrac{2\times10^3\times4.2\times50}{840} = 500\,s = 8$ min 20s

37. (d) When radius is decrease by ΔR,

$4\pi R^2\Delta R\rho L = 4\pi T[R^2 - (R-\Delta R)^2]$

$\Rightarrow \rho R^2\Delta RL = T[R^2 - R^2 + 2R\Delta R - \Delta R^2]$

$\Rightarrow \rho R^2\Delta RL = T2R\Delta R$ [ΔR is very small]

$\Rightarrow R = \dfrac{2T}{\rho L}$

38. (d) As the surrounding is identical, vessel is identical time taken to cool both water and liquid (from 30°C to 25°C) is same 2 minutes, therefore

$\left(\dfrac{dQ}{dt}\right)_{water} = \left(\dfrac{dQ}{dt}\right)_{liquid}$

or, $\dfrac{(m_WC_W + W)\Delta T}{t} = \dfrac{(m_\ell C_\ell + W)\Delta T}{t}$

(W = water equivalent of the vessel)

or, $m_WC_W = m_\ell C_\ell$

$\therefore$ Specific heat of liquid, $C_\ell = \dfrac{m_WC_W}{m_\ell}$

$= \dfrac{50\times1}{100} = 0.5$ kcal / kg

39. (b) As 1g of steam at 100°C melts 8g of ice at 0°C.

10 g of steam will melt 8× 10 g of ice at 0°C

Water in calorimeter = 500 + 80 + 10g = 590g

40. (c) 41. (a)

42. (a) $\Delta U = \Delta Q = mc\Delta T = \dfrac{100}{1000} \times 4184\,(50-30) \approx 8.4$ kJ

43. (a) Let Q be the temperature at a distance x from hot end of bar. Let Q is the temperature of hot end.

The heat flow rate is given by

$\dfrac{dQ}{dt} = \dfrac{kA(\theta_1 - \theta)}{x}$

$\Rightarrow \theta_1 - \theta = \dfrac{x}{kA}\dfrac{dQ}{dt} \quad \Rightarrow \theta = \theta_1 - \dfrac{x}{kA}\dfrac{dQ}{dt}$

Thus, the graph of Q versus x is a straight line with a positive intercept and a negative slope.

The above equation can be graphically represented by option (a).

44. (b) From stefan's law, total power radiated by Sun,

$E = \sigma T^4 \times 4\pi R^2$

The intensity of power Per unit area incident on earth's surface

$= \dfrac{\sigma T^4 \times 4\pi R^2}{4\pi r^2}$

Total power received by Earth

$E' = \dfrac{E}{4\pi r^2} \times$ Cross – Section area of earth facing the sun

$= \dfrac{\sigma T^4 R^2}{r^2}(\pi r_0^2)$

45. (c) According to Newton's law of cooling, the temperature goes on decreasing with time non-linearly.

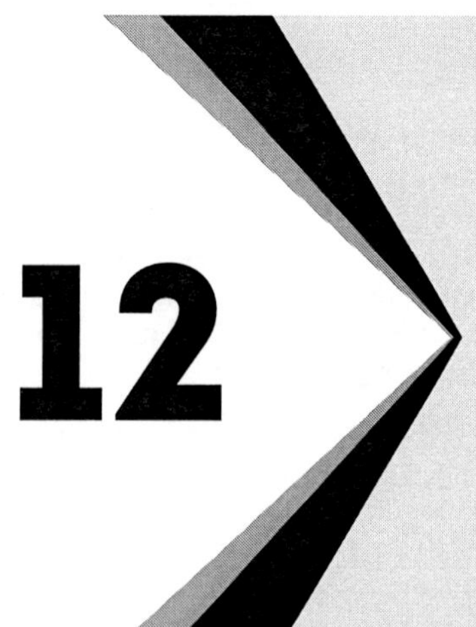

12 Thermodynamics

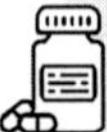

Topic 12.1 : Thermal Equilibrium, Zeroth & First Law of Thermodynamics and Thermodynamic Processes

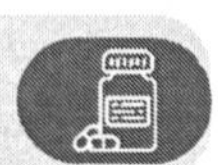

THERMAL EQUILIBRIUM AND ZEROTH LAW OF THERMODYNAMICS

Thermal Equilibrium

Two systems are said to be in thermal equilibrium with each other if they have the same temperature.

Zeroth Law of Thermodynamics

If objects A and B are separately in thermal equilibrium with a third object C then objects A and B are in thermal equilibrium with each other.

FIRST LAW OF THERMODYNAMICS

First law of thermodynamics gives a relationship between heat, work and internal energy.

(a) **Heat :** *It is the energy which is transferred from a system to surrounding or vice-versa due to temperature difference between system and surroundings.*

(i) It is a macroscopic quantity.

(ii) It is path dependent i.e., it is not point function.

(iii) If system liberates heat, then by sign convention it is taken negative, If system absorbs heat, it is positive.

(b) **Work :** *It is the energy that is transmitted from one system to another by a force moving its points of application.* The expression of work done on a gas or by a gas is

$$W = \int dW = \int_{V_1}^{V_2} PdV$$

where V_1 is volume of gas in initial state and V_2 in final state.

(i) It is also macroscopic and path dependent function.

(ii) By sign convention it is +ive if system does work (i.e., expands against surrounding) and it is – ive, if work is done on system (i.e., contracts).

(iii) In cyclic process the work done is equal to area under the cycle and is negative if cycle is anti-clockwise and +ive if cycle is clockwise (shown in fig.(a) and (b)).

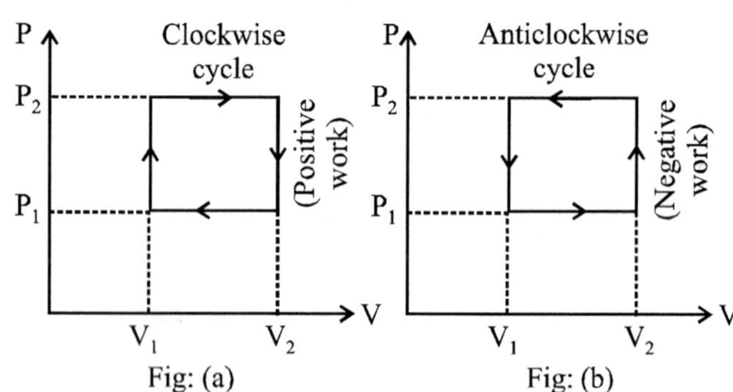

Fig: (a) Fig: (b)

(c) **Internal energy :** *The internal energy of a gas is sum of internal energy due to moleculer motion (called internal kinetic energy U_K) and internal energy due to molecular configuration (called internal potential energy $U_{P.E.}$)*

i.e., $U = U_K + U_{P.E.}$ ......(1)

(i) In ideal gas, as there is no intermolecular attraction, hence

$$U = U_K = \frac{3n}{2}RT \qquad ......(2)$$

(for n mole of ideal gas)

(ii) Internal energy is path independent i.e., point function.

(iii) In cyclic process, there is no change in internal energy (shown in fig.)

i.e., $dU = U_f - U_i = 0$

$\Rightarrow$ $U_f = U_i$

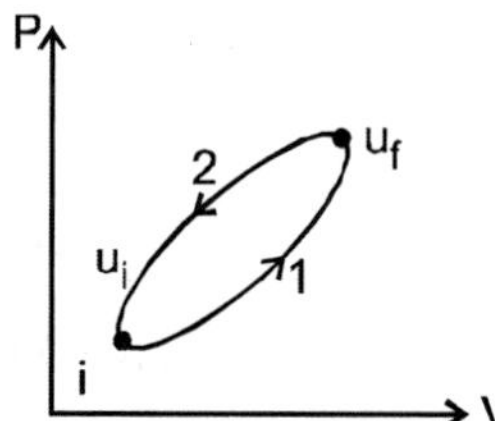

(iv) Internal energy of an ideal gas depends only on temperature eq.(2).

First law of thermodynamics is a generalisation of the law of conservation of energy that includes possible change in internal energy.

First law of thermodynamics *"If certain quantity of heat dQ is added to a system, a part of it is used in increasing the internal energy by dU and a part is use in performing external work done dW*

$$i.e.,\ dQ = dU + dW \Rightarrow dU = dQ - dW$$

The quantity dU (i.e., $dQ - dW$) is path independent but dQ and dW individually are not path independent.

Applications of First Law of Thermodynamics

(i) In **isobaric process** P is constant

$$\text{so } dW = \int_{V_1}^{V_2} PdV = P(V_2 - V_1)$$

so $dQ = dU + dW = n\, C_P\, dT$

(ii) In **cyclic process** heat given to the system is equal to work done (area of cycle).

(iii) In **isothermal process** temperature T is constant and work done is

$$dW = \int_{V_1}^{V_2} PdV = nRT\,\text{Log}_e \frac{V_2}{V_1}$$

Since, T = constant so for ideal gas dU = 0

Hence, $dQ = dW = nRT\ \text{Log}_e \dfrac{V_2}{V_1}$ (for ideal gas)

(iv) In **isochoric process** W = 0 as V = constant

It means that heat given to system is used in increasing internal energy of the gas.

(v) In **adiabatic process** heat given or taken by system from surrounding is zero i.e., dQ = 0

$$dU = -dW = -\left[\frac{nR}{\gamma - 1}(T_1 - T_2)\right] = \left[\frac{(P_1V_1 - P_2V_2)}{\gamma - 1}\right]$$

It means that if system expands dW is +ive and dU is –ive (i.e., temperature decrease) and if system contracts dW is –ive and dU is +ive (i.e., temperature increase).

THERMODYNAMIC PROCESSES

(i) ***Isothermal process :** If a thermodynamic system is perfectly conducting to surroundings and undergoes a physical change in such a way that temperature remains constant throughout, then process is said to be isothermal process.*

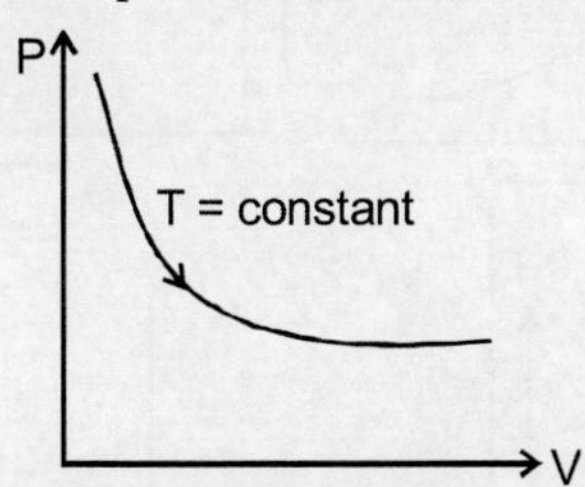

For isothermal process, the equation of state is

$PV = nRT = constant$, where n is no. of moles.

For ideal gas, since internal energy depends only on temperature.

$$dU = 0 \Rightarrow dQ = dW = \int_{V_1}^{V_2} PdV = nRT\int_{V_1}^{V_2} \frac{dV}{V}$$

$$\text{or } dQ = nRT \log_e \frac{V_2}{V_1} = 2.303nRT \log_{10} \frac{V_2}{V_1}$$

(ii) ***Adiabatic process :** If system is completely isolated from the surroundings so that no heat flows in or out of it, then any change that the system undergoes is called an adiabatic process.*

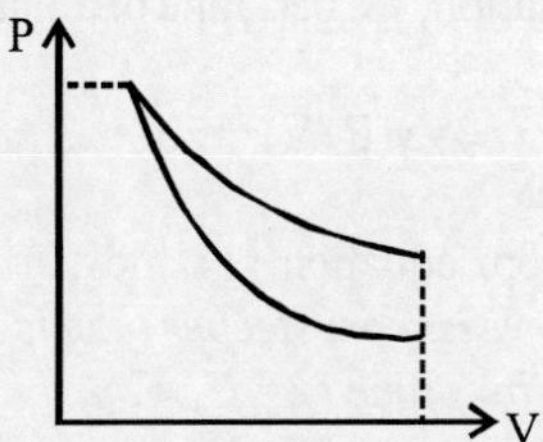

For ideal gas, dQ = 0

$dU = \mu C_V dT$ (for any process)

$$dW = \int_{V_1}^{V_2} PdV = \int_{V_1}^{V_2} \frac{K}{V^\gamma} dV$$

(where $PV^\gamma = K$ = constant)

$$= \frac{K}{1-\gamma}\left(\frac{1}{V_2^{\gamma-1}} - \frac{1}{V_1^{\gamma-1}}\right) = \frac{(P_2V_2 - P_1V_1)}{1-\gamma}$$

where PV^γ = constant is applicable only in adiabatic process. Adiabatic process is called isoentropic process (in these process entropy is constant).

(iii) ***Isobaric process :** A process taking place at constant pressure is called an isobaric process.* In this process $dQ = n\, C_p dT$, $dU = n\, C_V dT$ and $dW = P(V_2 - V_1)$

(iv) ***Isochoric process :** A process taking place at constant volume is called isochoric process.*

In this process, $dQ = dU = n\, C_V dT$ and dW = 0

(v) ***Cyclic process :** In this process the inital state and final state after traversing a cycle (shown in fig.) are same.*

In cyclic process, $dU = 0 = U_f - U_i$ and dW = area of cycle = area (abcd)

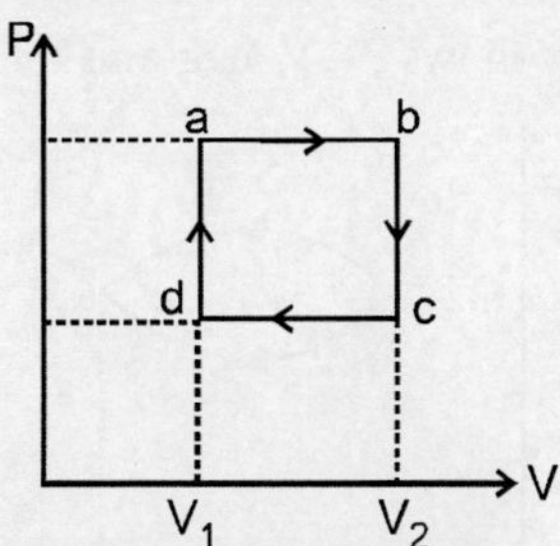

Slope of adiabatic and isothermal curve :

For isothermal process PV = constant

On differentiating, we get PdV + VdP = 0

And slope of isothermal curves

$$\left(\frac{dP}{dV}\right)_{\text{isothermal}} = -\frac{P}{V} \quad ...(1)$$

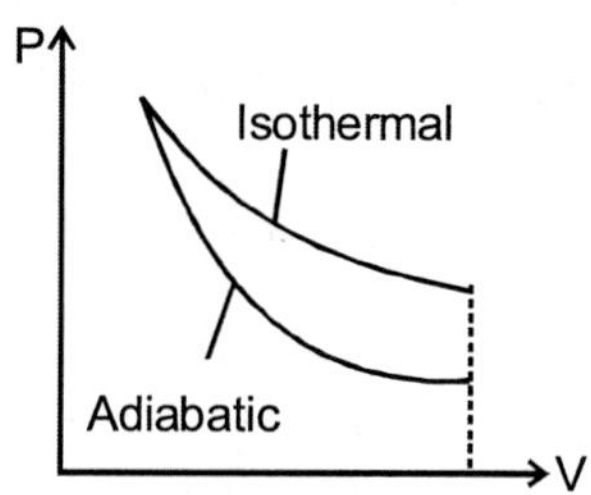

For adiabatic process PV^{γ} = constant

On differentiation, we get slope of adiabatic curve

$$\left(\frac{dP}{dV}\right)_{adiabatic} = -\gamma(P/V) \quad \text{.... (2)}$$

It is clear from equation (1) and (2) that *the slope of adiabatic curve is more steeper than isothermal curve as shown by fig by γ time ($\gamma = C_P/C_V$)*

Graphs of thermodynamic processes :

1. In the figure (i) P–V graph the process ab is isothermal, bc is isobaric and ca is isochoric.

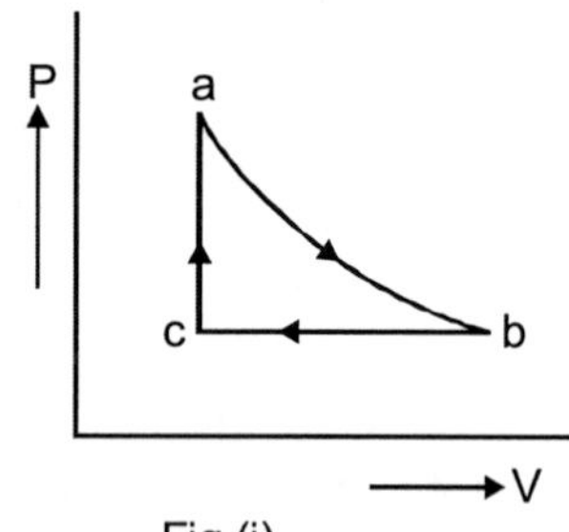

Fig (i)

The fig (ii) is the P–T diagram of fig (i)

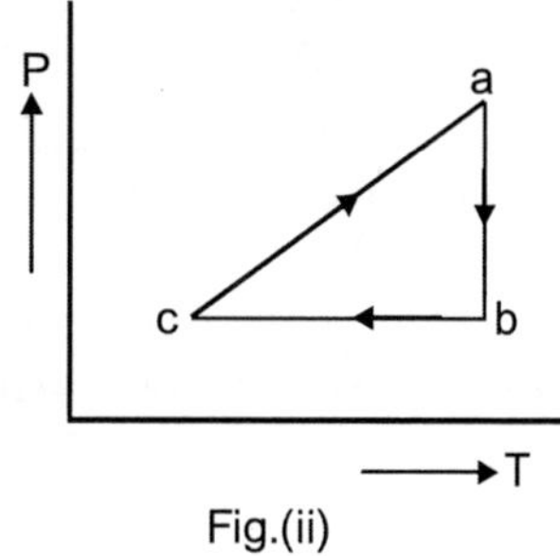

Fig.(ii)

2. Figure below shows P – V diagrams for two processes.

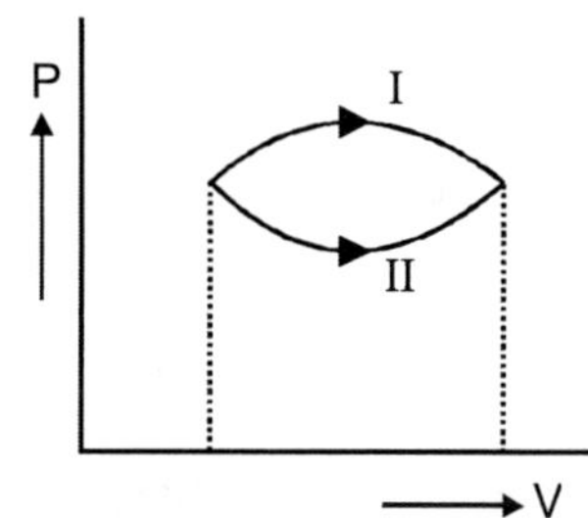

The heat absorbed in process I is more than that in II. Because, area under process I is also more than area under process II. The work done in the process I is more than that in II. Also, the change in internal energy is same in both cases.

3. The P–V and corresponding V–T diagram for a cyclic process abca on a sample of constant mass of ideal gas are shown below:

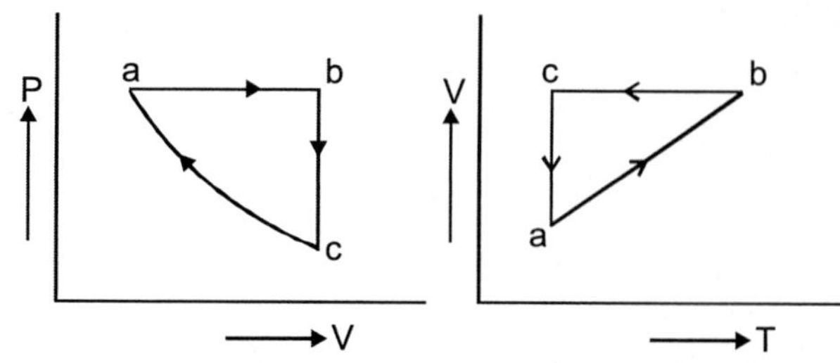

4. For isochoric process, the P–V, V–T and P–T graphs :

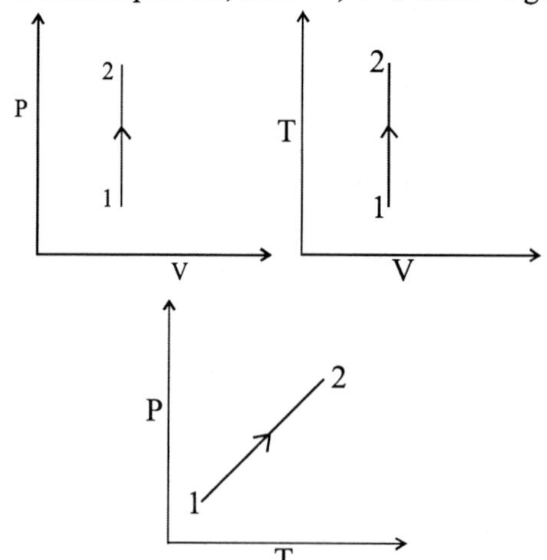

5. For isobaric process, the P – V, P – T and V – T graphs :

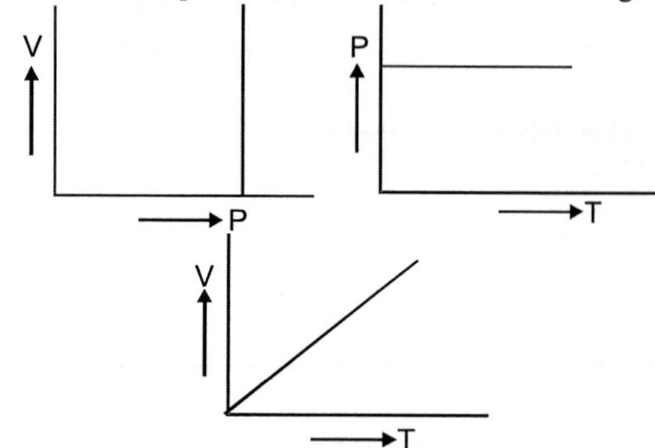

6. For isothermal process, the P – V, V – T and P – T graphs :

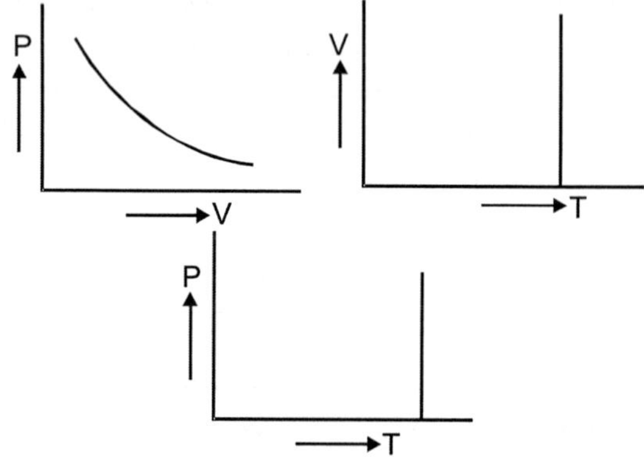

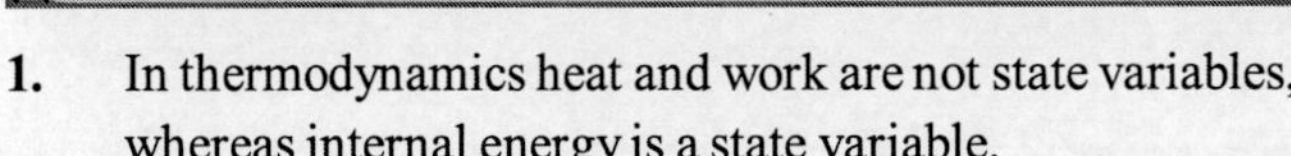

1. In thermodynamics heat and work are not state variables, whereas internal energy is a state variable.
2. For ideal-gas
   (i) *relation between P and V is* PV^γ = *constant*
   (ii) *relation between V and T is* $TV^{\gamma-1}$ = *constant*
   (iii) *relation between P and T is* $T^\gamma P^{1-\gamma}$ = *constant*
3. A quasi-static process is an infinitely slow process such that system remains in thermal and mechanical equilibrium with the surroundings throughout.
4. Pressure, volume, temperature and mass are state variables. Heat and work are not state variables.
5. A graphical representation of the state of a system with the help of two thermodynamical variables is called **indicator diagram**.

Example 1.

A cyclic process is shown in fig. Work done during isobaric expansion is

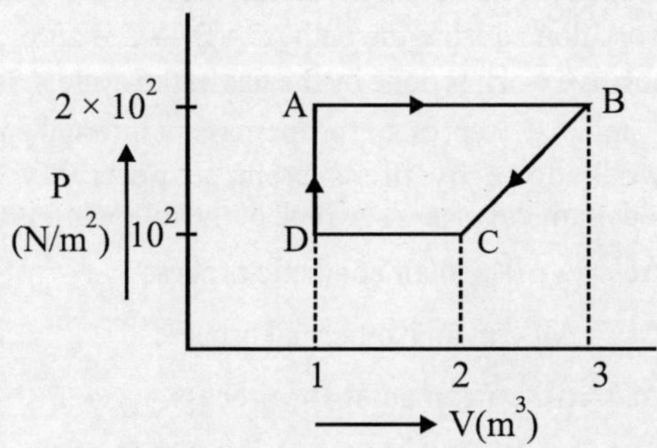

(a) 1600 J (b) 100 J (c) 400 J (d) 600 J

***Solution :* (c)**

Isobaric expansion is represented by curve AB;

Work done = area under AB

$= 2 \times 10^2 \times (3-1) = 4 \times 10^2 = 400$ J.

Example 2.

When a system is taken from state a to state b, in fig. along the path a → c → b, 60 J of heat flow into the system, and 30 J of work are done :

(i) How much heat flows into the system along the path a → d → b if the work is 10 J.

(ii) When the system is returned from b to a along the curved path, the work done by the system is –20 J. Does the system absorb or liberate heat, and how much?

(iii) If, $U_a = 0$ *and* $U_d = 22$ *J, find the heat absorbed in the process a → d and d → b.*

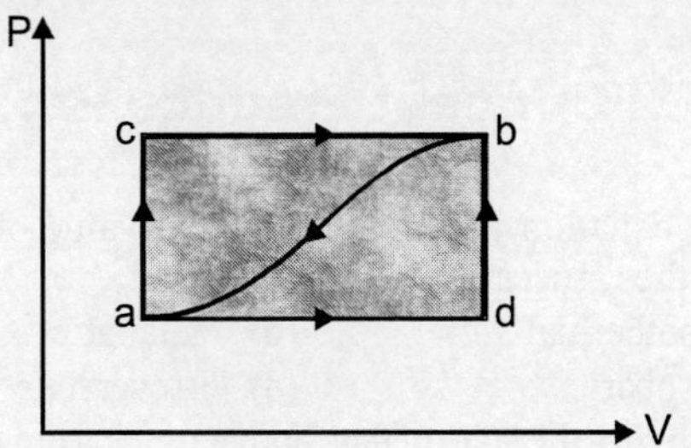

Solution :

For the path $a \to c \to b$

$dU = dQ - dW = 60 - 30 = 30$ J or $U_b - U_a = 30$ J

(i) Along the path $a \to d \to b$

$dQ = dU + dW = 30 + 10 = 40$ J

(ii) Along the curved path b – a

$dQ = (U_a - U_b) + W = (-30) + (-20) = -50$ J,

heat flows out the system

(iii) $Q_{ad} = 32$ J; $Q_{db} = 8$ J

Example 3.

Two samples of a gas initially at same temperature and pressure are compressed from a volume V to V/2. One sample is compressed isothermally and the other adiabatically. In which sample is the pressure greater?

Solution :

Let initial volume, $V_1 = V$ and final volume, $V_2 = V/2$

Initial pressure, $P_1 = P$; final pressure, $P_2 = ?$

For isothermal compression

$$P_2V_2 = P_1V_1 \text{ or } P_2 = \frac{P_1V_1}{V_2} = \frac{PV}{V/2} = 2P$$

For adiabatic compression

$$P_2'V_2^\gamma = P_1V_1^\gamma \text{ or } P_2' = P_1\left(\frac{V_1}{V_2}\right)^\gamma = P\left(\frac{V}{V/2}\right)^\gamma$$

or $P_2' = 2^\gamma P$

Since $\gamma > 1$ $\therefore 2^\gamma > 2 \therefore P_2' > P_2$

Pressure during adiabatic compression is greater than the pressure during isothermal compression.

Example 4.

An ideal gas heat engine operates in carnot cycle between 227°C and 127°C. It absorbs 6 × 10⁴ cal of heat at higher temp. Amount of heat converted into work is

(a) 1.2×10^4 cal (b) 2.4×10^4 cal
(c) 6×10^4 cal (d) 4.8×10^4 cal

***Solution :* (a)**

$$\text{As } \frac{Q_2}{Q_1} = \frac{T_2}{T_1};$$

$$\therefore \frac{Q_2}{6 \times 10^4} = \frac{127+273}{227+273} = \frac{400}{500} \quad \left(\text{As } \eta = 1 - \frac{Q_2}{Q_1} = 1 - \frac{T_2}{T_1}\right)$$

$$Q_2 = \frac{4}{5} \times 6 \times 10^4 = 4.8 \times 10^4 \text{ cal}$$

$$\therefore W = Q_1 - Q_2 = 6 \times 10^4 - 4.8 \times 10^4 = 1.2 \times 10^4 \text{ cal.}$$

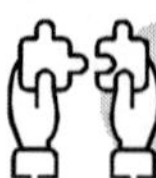

12.1 Concept Practice Problems

CPP

1. In the equation PV^{γ} = constant, the value of γ is unity. Then the process is
   (a) isothermal (b) adiabatic
   (c) isobaric (d) irreversible
2. In changing the state of thermodynamics from A to B state, the heat required is Q and the work done by the system is W. The change in its internal energy is
   (a) $Q+W$ (b) $Q-W$ (c) Q (d) $\frac{Q-W}{2}$
3. A gas has pressure P and volume V. It is now compressed adiabatically to 1/32 times the original volume. Given that $(32)^{1.4} = 128$, the final pressure is ($\gamma = 1.4$)
   (a) P/128 (b) P/32 (c) 32P (d) 128P
4. An ideal gas heat engine operates in Carnot cycle between 227°C and 127°C. It absorbs 6×10^4 cals of heat at higher temperature. Amount of heat converted to work is
   (a) 4.8×10^4 cal (b) 6×10^4 cal
   (c) 2.4×10^4 cal (d) 1.2×10^4 cal
5. 1 gm of water at a pressure of 1.01×10^5 Pa is converted into steam without any change of temperature. The volume of 1 g of steam is 1671 cc and the latent heat of evaporation is 540 cal. The change in internal energy due to evaporation of 1 gm of water is
   (a) ≈ 167 cal (b) ≈ 500 cal
   (c) 540 cal (d) 581 cal
6. During an adiabatic process an object does 100J of work and its temperature decreases by 5K. During another process it does 25J of work and its temperature decreases by 5K. Its heat capacity for 2nd process is
   (a) 20 J/K (b) 24 J/K (c) 15 J/K (d) 100 J/K
7. The internal energy change in a system that has absorbed 2 kcals of heat and done 500 J of work is
   (a) 6400 J (b) 5400 J (c) 7900 J (d) 8900 J
8. In an adiabatic process, the pressure is increased by $\frac{2}{3}\%$. If $\gamma = \frac{3}{2}$, then the volume decreases by nearly
   (a) $\frac{4}{9}\%$ (b) $\frac{2}{3}\%$ (c) 1% (d) $\frac{9}{4}\%$
9. The figure shows the P-V plot of an ideal gas taken through a cycle *ABCDA*. The part *ABC* is a semi-circle and *CDA* is half of an ellipse. Then,

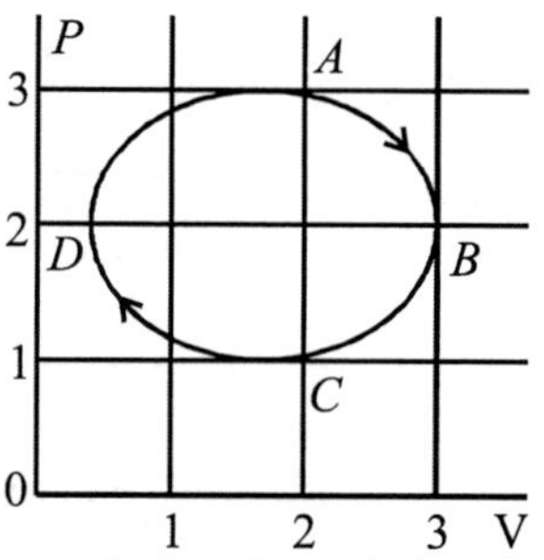

   (a) the process during the path $A \rightarrow B$ is isothermal
   (b) heat flows out of the gas during the path $B \rightarrow C \rightarrow D$
   (c) work done during the path $A \rightarrow B \rightarrow C$ is zero
   (d) positive work is done by the gas in the cycle *ABCDA*
10. If ΔU and ΔW represent the increase in internal energy and work done by the system respectively in a thermodynamical process, which of the following is true?
   (a) $\Delta U = -\Delta W$, in an adiabatic process
   (b) $\Delta U = \Delta W$, in an isothermal process
   (c) $\Delta U = \Delta W$, in an adiabatic process
   (d) $\Delta U = -\Delta W$, in an isothermal process

ANSWER KEY

1	(a)	2	(b)	3	(d)	4	(d)	5	(b)	6	(c)	7	(c)	8	(a)	9	(b, d)	10	(a)

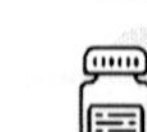

Topic 12.2 : Reversible & Irreversible Process, Heat Engine, Refrigerator, Heat Pump, Carnot Engine and Second Law of Thermodynamics

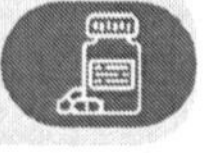

REVERSIBLE AND IRREVERSIBLE PROCESS

Reversible Process :

A process which can proceed in opposite direction in such a way that the system passes through the same states as in direct process and finally the system and the surroundings acquire the intial conditions.

Conditions for a process to be reversible :

(a) The process must be extremely slow.

(b) There should no loss of energy due to conduction, or radiation. The dissipating forces should not be in the system.

(c) The system must always be in thermal and chemical equilibrium with the surroundings.

Examples : Fusion of ice, vaporisation of water, etc.

Irreversible Process :

The process which cannot be traced back in the opposite direction is defined as irreversible process.

Examples : Work done against friction, magnetic hysteresis.

- In nature all process are irreversible, because no natural process can fulfil the requirement of a reversible process.

HEAT ENGINE

A heat engine is a device which converts heat energy into mechanical energy.

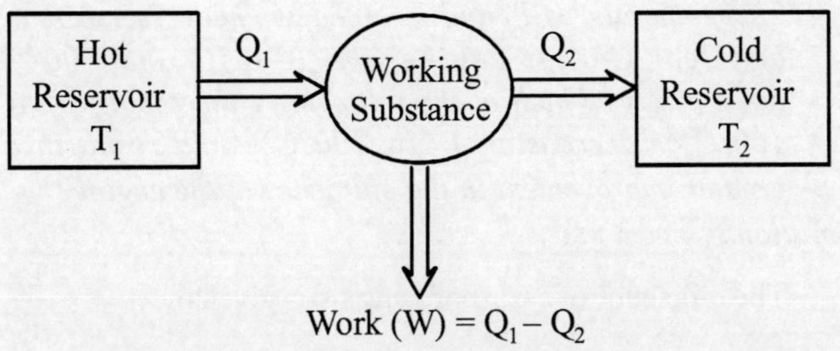

Efficiency of heat engine is given by

$$\textit{Efficiency}\ \eta = \frac{\textit{Work done}\ (W)}{\textit{Heat taken from source}\ (T_1)}$$

$$= 1 - \frac{Q_2}{Q_1} = 1 - \frac{T_2}{T_1}$$

where Q_2 = amount of heat rejected per cycle to the sink (of temp T_2)

Q_1 = amount of heat energy absorbed per cycle from the source (of temp T_1).

The efficiency of heat engine η is never greater than unity, $\eta = 1$ only for ideal engine & for practical heat engine $\eta < 1$.

REFRIGERATOR AND HEAT PUMP :

Refrigerator or heat pump is a heat engine running in backward direction i.e. working substance (a gas) takes heat from a cold body and gives out to a hotter body with the use of external energy i.e. electrical energy. A heat pump is the same as a refrigerator.

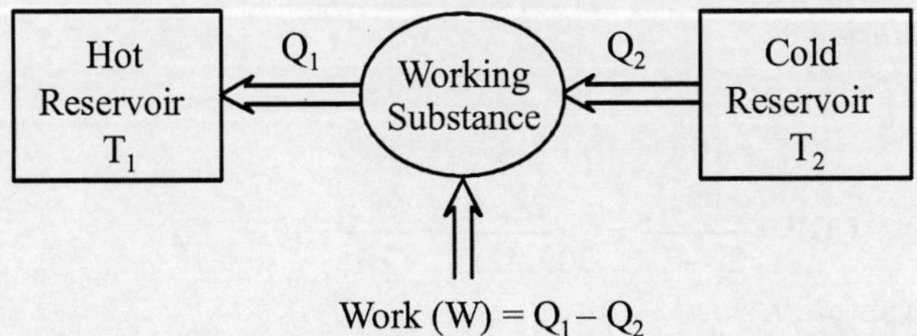

The coefficient of performance of refrigerator or heat pump is

$$\beta = \frac{\text{Heat extracted from cold reservoir}}{\text{Work done on refrigerator}} = \frac{Q_2}{Q_1 - Q_2} = \frac{T_2}{T_1 - T_2},$$

where T_2 is temperature of cold body and T_1 is temperature of hot body.

CARNOT ENGINE

Carnot devised an ideal engine which is based on a reversible cycle of four operations in succession : *isothermal expansion, adiabatic expansion, isothermal compression and adiabatic compression.*

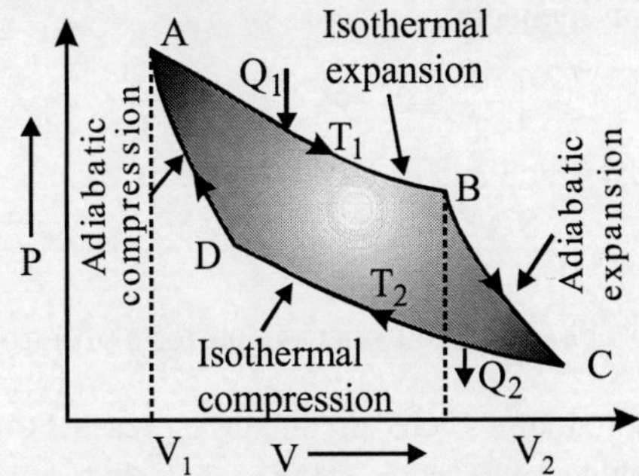

Efficiency of Carnot engine,

$$\eta = \frac{W}{Q_1} = \frac{\mu RT_1\ In\left(\frac{V_2}{V_1}\right) + \mu RT_2\ In\left(\frac{V_4}{V_3}\right)}{\mu RT_1\ In\left(\frac{V_2}{V_1}\right)}$$

The points B and C are connected by an adiabatic path as are the points D and A. Hence, using this eq^n. and the adiabatic gas eq^n.

$T_1V_2^{(\gamma-1)} = T_2\,V_3^{(\gamma-1)}$ and $T_1V_1^{(\gamma-1)} = T_2\,V_4^{(\gamma-1)}$.

Combination of the above eq^ns. gives $\frac{V_2}{V_1} = \frac{V_3}{V_4}$, and,

$$\eta = \frac{T_1 - T_2}{T_1} = \frac{Q_1 - Q_2}{Q_1}$$

or, $\eta = 1 - \frac{Q_2}{Q_1} = 1 - \frac{T_2}{T_1}$.

The percentage efficiency of Carnot's engine,

$$\eta = \frac{T_1 - T_2}{T_1} \times 100\% \text{ or, } \eta = \frac{Q_1 - Q_2}{Q_1} \times 100\%$$

The efficiency of a Carnot engine is never 100% because it is 100% only if temperature of sink $T_2 = 0$ which is impossible.

In a Carnot cycle, $\frac{Q_2}{Q_1} = \frac{T_2}{T_1}$ or $\frac{Q_1}{T_1} = \frac{Q_2}{T_2}$.

Carnot Theorem : *No irreversible engine (I) can have efficiency greater than Carnot reversible engine (R) working between same hot and cold reservoirs.*

i.e., $\eta_R > \eta_I$ or $1 - \frac{T_2}{T_1} > 1 - \frac{Q_2}{Q_1}$

SECOND LAW OF THERMODYNAMICS

It states that *it is impossible for a self acting machine unaided by any external agency, to transfer heat from a body at a lower temperature to a body at higher temperature.*

It is deduced from this law that the efficiency of any heat engine can never be 100%.

Entropy :

Entropy is a measure of disorder of the molecular motion of a system. The greater the disorder, the greater is the entropy. The change in entropy is given by

$$\Delta S = \frac{\textit{Heat absorbed by the system}\ (dQ)}{\textit{Absolute temperature}\ (T)}$$

$$S_1 - S_2 = \int \frac{dQ}{T} \text{ (here T is not differentiable)}$$

Clausius inequality

$$\oint \frac{dQ}{T} \le 0 \quad \text{or,} \quad dS \ge \int \frac{dQ}{T}$$

or, $dQ = TdS \ge dU + PdV$

Also, $S = K \log_e \omega$

$\Delta S = K \log_e \frac{\omega_2}{\omega_1}$ is the microscopic form of entropy, where K is Boltzmann's constant and ω respresents the number of possible microscopic states.

Energy entering a body increases disorder.

Energy leaving a body decreases disorder.

When a hot body is brought into thermal contact with a cold body for a short time, then :

(i) Each body will experience a change in the entropy of its particle.

(ii) The hot body experiences a decrease in entropy (a negative change) of magnitude

$$\Delta S_1 = \frac{\Delta Q}{T_1}$$

(iii) The cold body experiences an increase in entropy (a positive change) of magnitude

$$\Delta S_2 = \frac{\Delta Q}{T_2}$$

(iv) The net change in entropy

$$\Delta S = \Delta S_1 + \Delta S_2$$

The effect of naturally occurring processes is always to increase the total entropy (or disorder) of the universe.

Example 5.

An ideal carnot engine whose efficiency is 40% receives heat at 500 K. If its efficiency were 50%, then what would be intake temp. for same exhaust temp ?

Solution :

From, $\eta = 1 - \frac{T_2}{T_1}$; $\frac{T_2}{T_1} = 1 - \eta = 1 - \frac{40}{100} = \frac{3}{5}$;

$\therefore \; T_2 = \frac{3}{5} T_1 = \frac{3}{5} \times 500 = 300\,K$

Again $\frac{T_2}{T_1'} = 1 - \eta'$ or $\frac{300}{T_1'} = 1 - \frac{50}{100} = \frac{1}{2}$

or $T_1' = 600\,K$

Example 6.

A Carnot engine working between 300 K and 600 K has a work output of 800 J per cycle. What is the amount of heat energy supplied to the engine from source per cycle?

Solution :

$W = 800\,J, T_1 = 600\,K, T_2 = 300\,K$

$$\therefore \; \eta = 1 - \frac{T_1}{T_2} = \frac{W}{Q_1} = 1 - \frac{300}{600} = \frac{800}{Q_1} \text{ or } 0.5 = \frac{800}{Q_1}$$

Heat energy supplied by source,

$$Q = \frac{800}{0.5} = 1600 \text{ joule per cycle}$$

Example 7.

The temperatures T_1 and T_2 of the two heat reservoirs in an ideal Carnot engine are 1500°C and 500°C respectively. Which of the following : increasing T_1 by 100°C or decreasing T_2 by 100°C would result in a greater improvement in the efficiency of the engine?

Solution :

The efficiency of a Carnot's engine is given by $\eta = 1 - \frac{T_2}{T_1}$

Given $T_1 = 1500°C = 1500 + 273 = 1773$ K and

$T_2 = 500°C = 500 + 273 = 773$ K.

When the temperature of the source is increased by 100°C, keeping T_2 unchanged, the new temperature of the source is $T'_1 = 1500 + 100 = 1600°C = 1873$ K. The efficiency becomes

$$\eta' = 1 - \frac{T_2}{T'_1} = 1 - \frac{773}{1873} = 0.59$$

On the other hand, if the temperature of the sink is decreased by 100°C, keeping T_1 unchanged, the new temperature of the sink is $T'_2 = 500 - 100 = 400°C = 673$ K. The efficiency now becomes

$$\eta'' = 1 - \frac{T'_2}{T_1} = 1 - \frac{673}{1773} = 0.62$$

Since η'' is greater than η', decreasing the temperature of the sink by 100°C results in a greater efficiency than increasing the temperature of the source by 100°C.

Example 8.

A refrigerator is to maintain eatables kept inside at 90C. If room temperature is 360C, calculate the coefficient of performance.

Solution :

Here, $T_1 = 36°C = 36 + 273 = 309$ K,

$T_2 = 10°C = 10 + 273 = 283$ K

$$COP = \frac{T_2}{T_1 - T_2} = \frac{283}{309 - 283} = \frac{283}{26} = 10.9$$

Example 9.

A Carnot's heat engine works with an ideal monatomic gas, and an adiabatic expansion ratio 2. Determine its efficiency.

Solution :

Given, $\rho = \frac{V_3}{V_2} = 2$ and γ for a monatomic gas = 5/3.

Using, $\eta = 1 - \left(\frac{1}{\rho}\right)^{\gamma - 1}$

we have, the required efficiency

$$\eta = 1 - \left(\frac{1}{2}\right)^{\frac{5}{3} - 1} = 1 - 0.63 = 0.37 \text{ or } 37\%$$

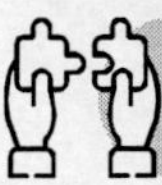

12.2 Concept Practice Problems

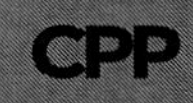

11. The efficiency of carnot engine when source temperature is T_1 and sink temperature is T_2 will be

(a) $\frac{T_1 - T_2}{T_1}$ (b) $\frac{T_2 - T_1}{T_2}$ (c) $\frac{T_1 - T_2}{T_2}$ (d) $\frac{T_1}{T_2}$

12. Which of the following processes is reversible?

(a) Transfer of heat by conduction

(b) Transfer of heat by radiation

(c) Isothermal compression

(d) Electrical heating of a nichrome wire

13. A refrigerator works between 0°C and 27°C. Heat is to be removed from the refrigerated space at the rate of 50 kcal/minute, the power of the motor of the refrigerator is

(a) 0.346 kW (b) 3.46 kW

(c) 34.6 kW (d) 346 kW

14. The efficiency of a Carnot engine operating with reservoir temperatures of 100°C and –23°C will be

(a) $\frac{100+23}{100}$ (b) $\frac{100-23}{100}$

(c) $\frac{100+23}{373}$ (d) $\frac{100-23}{373}$

15. A carnot's engine takes 300 calories of heat at 500 K and rejects 150 calories of heat to the sink. The temperature of the sink is

(a) 1000 K (b) 750 K (c) 250 K (d) 125 K

16. The source and sink temperatures of a Carnot engine are 400 K and 300 K, respectively. What is its efficiency?

(a) 100% (b) 75% (c) 33.3% (d) 25%

17. A Carnot's engine works as a refrigerator between 250 K and 300 K. If it receives 750 calories of heat from the reservoir at the lower temperature, the amount of heat rejected at the higher temperature is

(a) 900 calories (b) 625 calories

(c) 750 calories (d) 1000 calories

18. A Carnot engine is working between 127°C and 27°C. The increase in efficiency will be maximum when the temperature of

(a) the source is increased by 50°C

(b) the sink is decreased by 50°C

(c) source is increased by 25°C and that of sink is decreased by 25°C

(d) both source and sink are decreased by 25°C each.

19. A gas is taken through the cycle $A \rightarrow B \rightarrow C \rightarrow A$, as shown in figure. What is the net work done by the gas ?

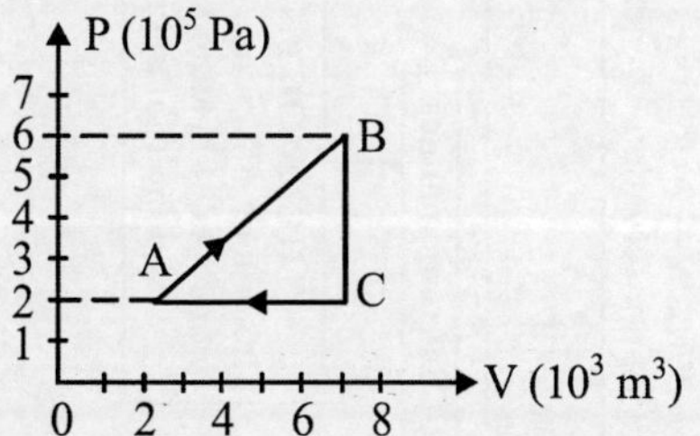

(a) 1000 J (b) zero (c) –2000 J (d) 2000 J

20. In a Carnot engine efficiency is 40% at hot reservoir temperature T. For efficiency 50%, what will be the temperature of hot reservoir?

(a) T (b) $\frac{2}{3}$T (c) $\frac{4}{5}$T (d) $\frac{6}{5}$T

ANSWER KEY

11	(a)	12	(c)	13	(a)	14	(c)	15	(c)	16	(d)	17	(a)	18	(b)	19	(d)	20	(d)

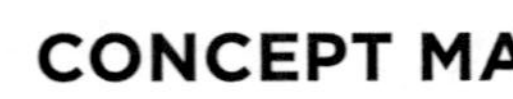

CONCEPT MAP

THERMODYNAMICS
The branch of science deals with the concepts of heat and temperature and their interconversion

Laws of thermodynamics

Zeroth law of thermodynamics
Two systems A and B are in thermal equilibrium with a third system C, then A and B are in thermal equilibrium with each other.

First law of thermodynamics
$\Delta Q = \Delta U + \Delta W$ ($\Delta W = P\Delta V$) It is a statement of law of conservation of energy

Second law of thermodynamics
It is impossible for an engine working between a cyclic process to extract heat from a reservoir and convert completely into work.

Entropy(S) – A measure of molecular disorder of a system.
Change in entropy $\delta S = \frac{\delta Q}{T}$

Thermal equilibrium
Two systems are in thermal equilibrium with each other if they have the same temperature.

Thermodynamic state variable
(i) Extensive - indicate the size of the system e.g. U, volume, total mass
(ii) Intensive - do not indicate size of the system e.g., pressure and temperature

Specific heat capacity
$C = \frac{\Delta Q}{m(\Delta T)}$
$C_P - C_V = R$ **(Mayer's formula)**

Thermodynamic processes

Quasi – static process
Infinitely slow process such that system remains in thermal and mechanical equilibrium with the surroundings throughout

In Quasi – static process,
The pressure (P) and temperature (T) of the environment can differ from those of the system only infinitesimally

Reversible and Irreversible process
Any process made to proceed in the reverse direction by variation in its conditions – Reversible process.
Any process that cannot be retraced in the reverse direction exactly – Irreversible process.

Carnot's Engine
An Ideal engine works on a reversible cycle of four operations in succession –
(i) isothermal expansion, (ii) adiabatic expansion, (iii) isothermal compression and (iv) adiabatic compression.
Efficiency of carnot's engine $\eta = 1 - \frac{Q_2}{Q_1} = 1 - \frac{T_2}{T_1}$

Isothermal process
Temperature = Constant
PV = Constant = n RT
$W = \int_{V_1}^{V_2} \frac{nRT}{V} dV$

Adiabatic process
A thermally insulated system, neither gains nor loses heat
PV^{γ} = constant
$TV^{\gamma-1}$ = constant
$\frac{P^{\gamma-1}}{T^{\gamma}}$ = constant $C_p/C_v = \gamma$

Isochoric process
Volume remains constant
$\frac{P}{T}$ = constant
$\frac{P_1}{T_1} = \frac{P_2}{T_2}$

Isobaric process
Pressure remains constatnt
$\frac{V}{T}$ = constant
$\frac{V_1}{T_1} = \frac{V_2}{T_2}$

Cyclic Process
In this process, system returns to initial state
For a cyclic process $\Delta U = 0$

Heat engine
Converts continuously heat into mechanical energy in cyclic process. Efficiency
$\eta = \frac{W}{Q} = 1 - \frac{Q_2}{Q_1} = 1 - \frac{T_2}{T_1}$

Refrigerator and Heat pump
Refrigerator is a heat engine working in the reverse direction. Coefficient of performance,
$\beta = \frac{Q_2}{W} = \frac{Q_2}{Q_1 - Q_2} = \frac{T_2}{T_1 - T_2}$

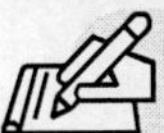

Exercise 1 - Chapter Revision Problems

CRP

1. Which of the following is incorrect regarding first law of thermodynamics?
   (a) It is a restatement of principle of conservation of energy.
   (b) It is applicable to cyclic processes
   (c) It introduces the concept of entropy
   (d) It introduces the concept of internal energy
2. Choose the incorrect statement related to an isobaric process.
   (a) $\frac{V}{T}$ = constant
   (b) $W = P\Delta V$
   (c) Heat given to a system is used up in raising the temperature only.
   (d) $\Delta Q > W$
3. The internal energy of an ideal gas does not depend upon
   (a) temperature of the gas
   (b) pressure of the gas
   (c) atomicity of the gas
   (d) number of moles of the gas.
4. During isothermal expansion, the slope of *P-V* graph
   (a) decreases
   (b) increases
   (c) remains same
   (d) may increase or decrease
5. During melting of ice, its entropy
   (a) increases (b) decreases
   (c) remains same (d) cannot say
6. Which of the following processes is adiabatic ?
   (a) Melting of ice
   (b) Bursting of tyre
   (c) Motion of piston of an engine with constant speed
   (d) None of these
7. At a given temperature the internal energy of a substance
   (a) in liquid state is equal to that in gaseous state.
   (b) in liquid state is less than that in gaseous state.
   (c) in liquid state is more than that in gaseous state.
   (d) is equal for the three states of matter.
8. Air conditioner is based on the principle of
   (a) Carnot cycle
   (b) refrigerator
   (c) first low of thermodynamics
   (d) None of these
9. A mass of ideal gas at pressure P is expanded isothermally to four times the original volume and then slowly compressed adiabatically to its original volume. Assuming γ to be 1.5, the new pressure of the gas is
   (a) 2P (b) P (c) 4P (d) P/2
10. One mole of an ideal gas at temperature T was cooled isochorically till the gas pressure fell from P to $\frac{P}{n}$. Then, by an isobaric process, the gas was restored to the initial temperature. The net amount of heat absorbed by the gas in the process is
    (a) nRT (b) $\frac{RT}{n}$
    (c) $RT(1-n^{-1})$ (d) $RT(n-1)$
11. Ice contained in a beaker starts melting when
    (a) the specific heat of the system is zero
    (b) internal energy of the system remains constant
    (c) temperature remains constant
    (d) entropy remains constant
12. A uniform sphere is supplied heat electrically at the centre at a constant rate. In the steady state, steady temperatures are established at all radial locations *r*, heat flows outwards radial and is ultimately radiated out by the outer surface isotropically. In this steady state, the temperature gradient varies with radial distance r according to
    (a) r^{-1} (b) r^{-2} (c) r^{-3} (d) $r^{-3/2}$
13. For an ideal gas graph is shown for three processes. Process 1, 2 and 3 are respectively.

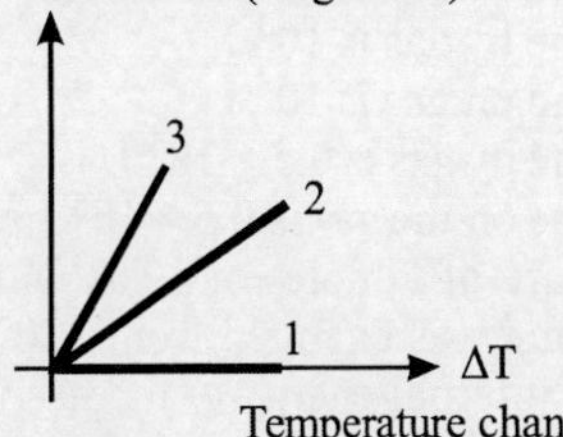

    (a) Isobaric, adiabatic, isochoric
    (b) Adiabatic, isobaric, isochoric
    (c) Isochoric, adiabatic, isobaric
    (d) Isochoric, isobaric, adiabatic
14. The gas law $\frac{PV}{T}$ = constant is true for
    (a) isothermal changes only
    (b) adiabatic changes only
    (c) both isothermal and adiabatic changes
    (d) neither isothermal nor adiabatic change
15. If ΔQ and ΔW represent the heat supplied to the system and the work done on the system respectively, then the first law of thermodynamics can be written as
    (a) $\Delta Q = \Delta U + \Delta W$ (b) $\Delta Q = \Delta U - \Delta W$
    (c) $\Delta Q = \Delta W - \Delta U$ (d) $\Delta Q = -\Delta W - \Delta U$
16. Monatomic, diatomic and polyatomic ideal gases each undergo slow adiabatic expansions from the same initial volume and same initial pressure to the same final volume. The magnitude of the work done by the environment on the gas is
    (a) the greatest for the polyatomic gas
    (b) the greatest for the monatomic gas
    (c) the greatest for the diatomic gas
    (d) the question is irrelevant, there is no meaning of slow adiabatic expansion
17. A gas at 27°C and pressure of 30 atm. is allowed to expand to atmospheric pressure and volume 15 times larger. The final temperature of the gas is
    (a) −123°C (b) +123°C (c) 273°C (d) 373°C
18. A system changes from the state (P_1, V_1) to (P_2, V_2) as shown in the figure. What is the work done by the system?

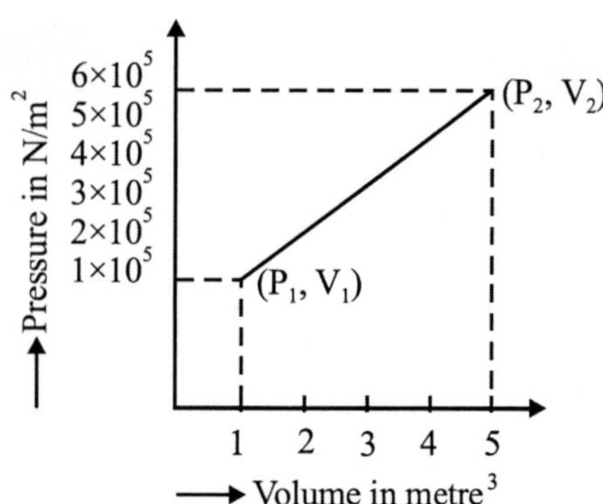

(a) 7.5×10^5 joule (b) 7.5×10^5 erg
(c) 12×10^5 joule (d) 6×10^5 joule

19. A perfect gas goes from a state A to another state B by absorbing 8×10^5 J of heat and doing 6.5×10^5 J of external work. It is now transferred between the same two states in another process in which it absorbs 10^5 J of heat. In the second process
(a) work done by gas is 10^5 J
(b) work done on gas is 10^5 J
(c) work done by gas is 0.5×10^5 J
(d) work done on the gas is 0.5×10^5 J

20. The temperature of 5 moles of a gas which was held at constant volume was changed from 100° to 120°C. The change in the internal energy of the gas was found to be 80 joule, the total heat capacity of the gas at constant volume will be equal to
(a) 8 joule per K (b) 0.8 joule per K
(c) 4.0 joule per K (d) 0.4 joule per K

21. By what percentage should the pressure of a given mass of a gas be increased so as to decrease its volume by 10% at a constant temperature?
(a) 8.1% (b) 9.1% (c) 10.1% (d) 11.1%

22. A diatomic gas initally at 18°C is compressed adiabatically to one eighth of its original volume. The temperature after compression will be
(a) 18°C (b) 887°C
(c) 327°C (d) None of these

23. Absolute zero is obtained from
(a) P–V graph (b) $P - \frac{1}{V}$ graph
(c) P–T graph (d) V–T graph

24. Three moles of an ideal gas kept at a constant temperature at 300 K are compressed from a volume of 4 litre to 1 litre. The work done in the process is
(a) – 10368 J (b) –110368 J (c) 12000 J (d) 120368 J

25. The temperature at which speed of sound in air becomes double of its value at 27° C is
(a) 54°C (b) 327°C
(c) 927°C (d) None of these

26. An ideal refrigerator has a freezer at a temperature of 13°C. The coefficient of performance of the engine is 5. The temperature of the air (to which heat is rejected) is
(a) 320°C (b) 39°C (c) 325 K (d) 325°C

27. The volume of a gas is reduced adiabatically to 1/4 of its volume at 27°C. If $\gamma = 1.4$ the new temperature is
(a) $(300)\,2^{0.4}$ K (b) $(300)\,2^{1.4}$ K
(c) $300\,(4)^{0.4}$ K (d) $300\,(2)^{1.4}$ K

28. In pressure-volume diagram, the isochoric, isothermal, isobaric and iso-entropic parts respectively, are

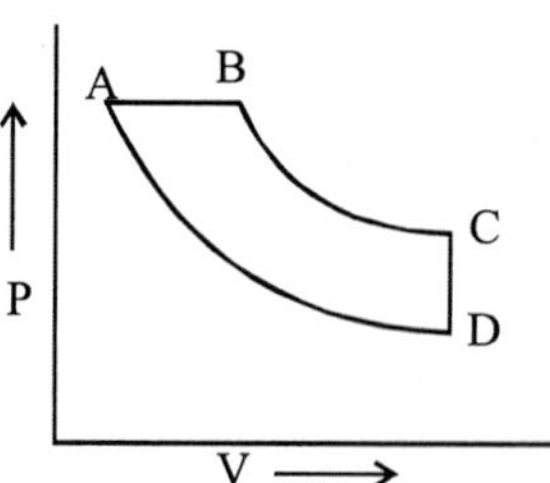

(a) BA, AD, DC, CB (b) DC, CB, BA, AD
(c) AB, BC, CD, DA (d) CD, DA, AB, BC

29. A Carnot engine works first between 200°C and 0°C and then between 0°C and –200°C. The ratio of its efficiency in the two cases is
(a) 1.0 (b) 0.577 (c) 0.34 (d) 0.68

30. A closed gas cylinder is divided into two parts by a piston held tight. The pressure and volume of gas in two parts respectively are (P, 5V) and (10P, V). If now the piston is left free and the system undergoes isothermal process, then the volumes of the gas in two parts respectively are
(a) 2V, 4V (b) 3V, 3V
(c) 5V, V (d) $\frac{10}{11}V, \frac{20}{11}V$

31. Figure shows the variation of internal energy (U) with the pressure (P) of 2.0 mole gas in cyclic process abcda. The temperature of gas at c and d are 300 K and 500 K. Calculate the heat absorbed by the gas during the process.

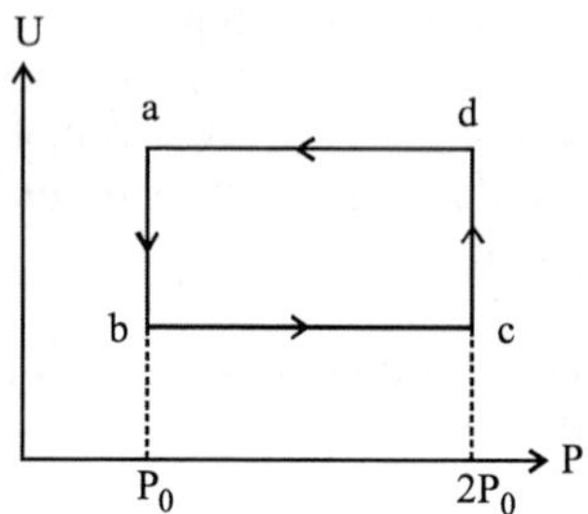

(a) 400 R ln 2 (b) 200 R ln 2
(c) 100 R ln 2 (d) 300 R ln 2

32. A mass of diatomic gas ($\gamma = 1.4$) at a pressure of 2 atmospheres is compressed adiabatically so that its temperature rises from 27°C to 927°C. The pressure of the gas in final state is
(a) 28 atm (b) 68.7 atm (c) 256 atm (d) 8 atm

33. A thermodynamic system is taken through the cycle *ABCD* as shown in figure. Heat rejected by the gas during the cycle is

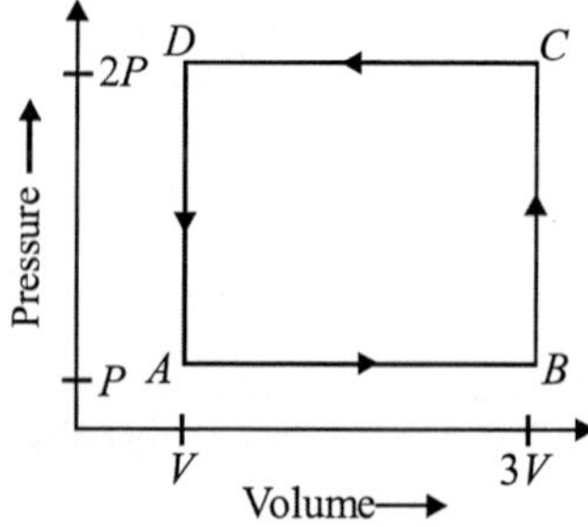

(a) 2PV (b) 4PV (c) $\frac{1}{2}$PV (d) PV

34. An ideal gas goes from state A to state B via three different processes as indicated in the P-V diagram :

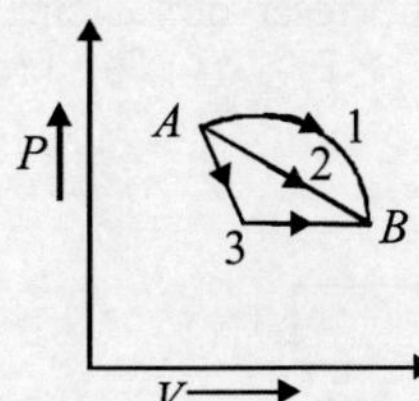

If Q_1, Q_2, Q_3 indicate the heat a absorbed by the gas along the three processes and ΔU_1, ΔU_2, ΔU_3 indicate the change in internal energy along the three processes respectively, then

(a) $Q_1 > Q_2 > Q_3$ and $\Delta U_1 = \Delta U_2 = \Delta U_3$
(b) $Q_3 > Q_2 > Q_1$ and $\Delta U_1 = \Delta U_2 = \Delta U_3$
(c) $Q_1 = Q_2 = Q_3$ and $\Delta U_1 > \Delta U_2 > \Delta U_3$
(d) $Q_3 > Q_2 > Q_1$ and $\Delta U_1 > \Delta U_2 > \Delta U_3$

35. In the given (V – T) diagram, what is the relation between pressure P_1 and P_2 ?

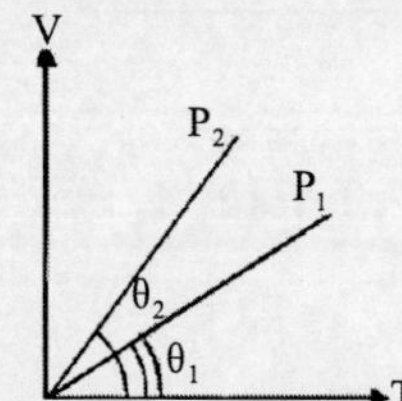

(a) $P_2 > P_1$ (b) $P_2 < P_1$
(c) $P_2 = P_1$ (d) Cannot be predicted

36. A system goes from A to B via two processes I and II as shown in figure. If ΔU_1 and ΔU_2 are the changes in internal energies in the processes I and II respectively, then

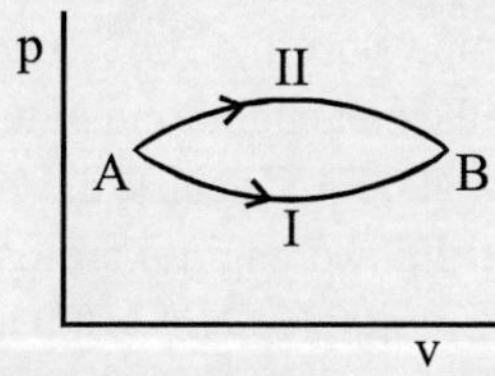

(a) relation between ΔU_1 and ΔU_2 can not be determined
(b) $\Delta U_1 = \Delta U_2$
(c) $\Delta U_1 < \Delta U_2$
(d) $\Delta U_1 > \Delta U_2$

37. A gas can be taken from A to B via two different processes ACB and ADB.

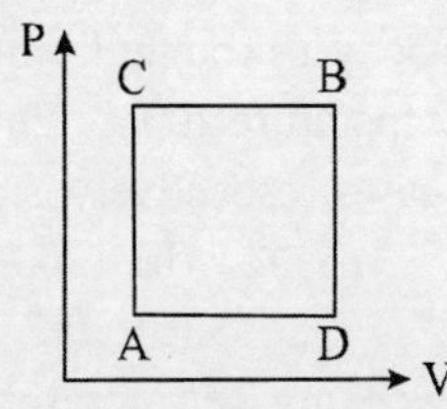

When path ACB is used 60 J of heat flows into the system and 30J of work is done by the system. If path ADB is used work done by the system is 10 J. The heat Flow into the system in path ADB is :

(a) 40 J (b) 80 J (c) 100 J (d) 20 J

38. Three different processes that can occur in an ideal monoatomic gas are shown in the P vs V diagram. The paths are lebelled as $A \rightarrow B$, $A \rightarrow C$ and $A \rightarrow D$. The change in internal energies during these process are taken as E_{AB}, E_{AC} and E_{AD} and the workdone as W_{AB}, W_{AC} and W_{AD}. The correct relation between these parameters are :

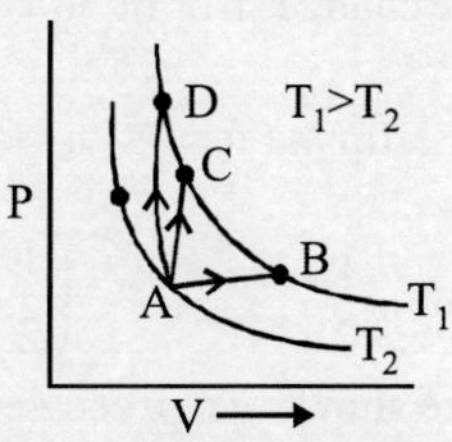

(a) $E_{AB} = E_{AC} < E_{AD}$, $W_{AB} > 0$, $W_{AC} = 0$, $W_{AD} < 0$
(b) $E_{AB} = E_{AC} = E_{AD}$, $W_{AB} > 0$, $W_{AC} = 0$, $W_{AD} > 0$
(c) $E_{AB} < E_{AC} < E_{AD}$, $W_{AB} > 0$, $W_{AC} > W_{AD}$
(d) $E_{AB} > E_{AC} > E_{AD}$, $W_{AB} < W_{AC} < W_{AD}$

39. Match the thermodynamic processes taking place in a system with the correct conditions. In the table : ΔQ is the heat supplied, ΔW is the work done and ΔU is change in internal energy of the system.

Process	Condition
(I) Adiabatic	(A) $\Delta W = 0$
(II) Isothermal	(B) $\Delta Q = 0$
(III) Isochoric	(C) $\Delta U \neq 0, \Delta W \neq 0, \Delta Q \neq 0$
(IV) Isobaric	(D) $\Delta U = 0$

(a) (I)-(A), (II)-(B), (III)-(D), (IV)-(D)
(b) (I)-(B), (II)-(A), (III)-(D), (IV)-(C)
(c) (I)-(A), (II)-(A), (III)-(B), (IV)-(C)
(d) (I)-(B), (II)-(D), (III)-(A), (IV)-(C)

40. Which of the following is an equivalent cyclic process corresponding to the thermodynamic cyclic given in the figure? where, $1 \rightarrow 2$ is adiabatic.
(Graphs are schematic and are not to scale)

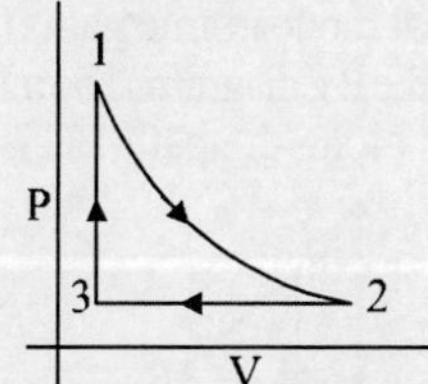

(a)
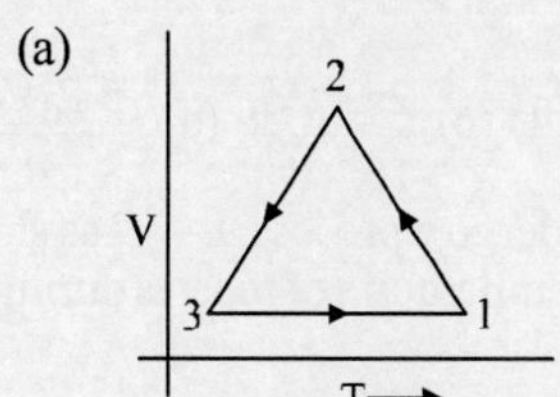

(b)
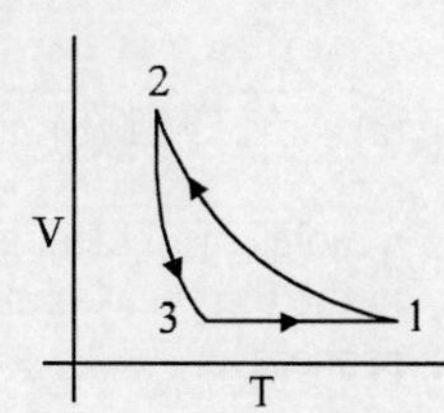

(c)
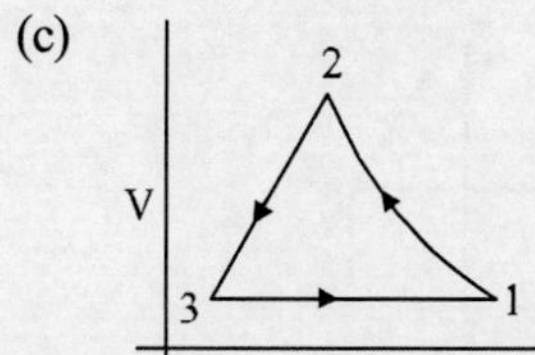

(d)
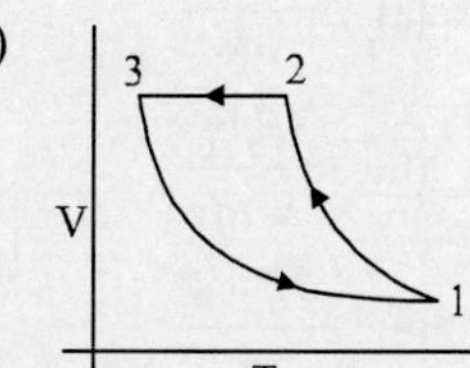

41. A litre of dry air at STP expands adiabatically to a volume of 3 litres. If $\gamma = 1.40$, the work done by air is: ($3^{1.4} = 4.6555$) [Take air to be an ideal gas]

(a) 60.7 J (b) 90.5 J (c) 100.8 J (d) 48 J

42. Under an adiabatic process, the volume of an ideal gas gets doubled. Consequently the mean collision time between the gas molecule changes from τ_1 to τ_2. If $\frac{C_p}{C_v} = \gamma$ for this gas then a good estimate for $\frac{\tau_2}{\tau_1}$ is given by:

(a) 2 (b) $\frac{1}{2}$ (c) $\left(\frac{1}{2}\right)^{\gamma}$ (d) $\left(\frac{1}{2}\right)^{\frac{\gamma+1}{2}}$

43. Following figure shows two processes A and B for a gas. If ΔQ_A and ΔQ_B are the amount of heat absorbed by the system in two cases, and ΔU_A and ΔU_B are changes in internal energies, respectively, then:

(a) $\Delta Q_A < \Delta Q_B, \Delta U_A < \Delta U_B$

(b) $\Delta Q_A > \Delta Q_B, \Delta U_A > \Delta U_B$

(c) $\Delta Q_A > \Delta Q_B, \Delta U_A = \Delta U_B$

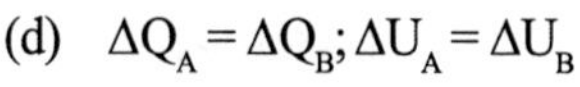

(d) $\Delta Q_A = \Delta Q_B; \Delta U_A = \Delta U_B$

44. For the given cyclic process CAB as shown for gas, the work done is:

(a) 30 J

(b) 10 J

(c) 1 J

(d) 5 J

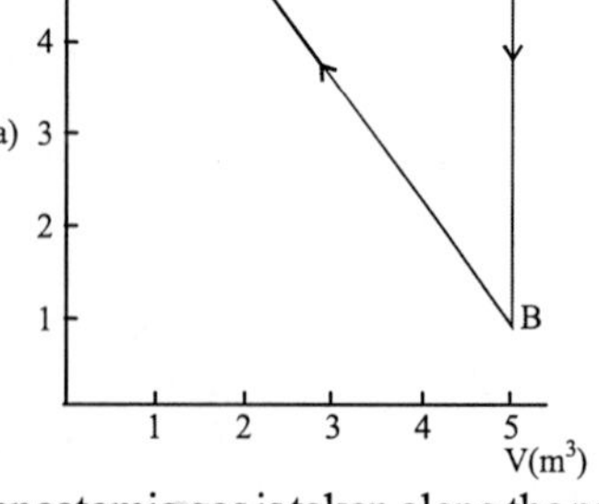

45. One mole of an ideal monoatomic gas is taken along the path ABCA as shown in the PV diagram. The maximum temperature attained by the gas along the path BC is given by

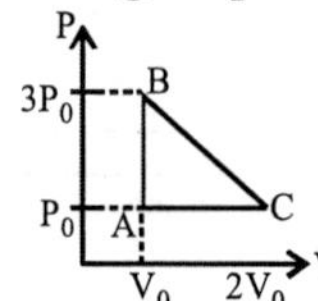

(a) $\frac{25}{8}\frac{P_0V_0}{R}$ (b) $\frac{25}{4}\frac{P_0V_0}{R}$ (c) $\frac{25}{16}\frac{P_0V_0}{R}$ (d) $\frac{5}{8}\frac{P_0V_0}{R}$

46. *n* moles of an ideal gas undergo a process $A \to B$ as shown in the figure. Maximum temperature of the gas during the process is

(a) $\frac{9P_0V_0}{nR}$

(b) $\frac{3P_0V_0}{2nR}$

(c) $\frac{9P_0V_0}{2nR}$

(d) $\frac{9P_0V_0}{4nR}$

47. Three Carnot engines operate in series between a heat source at a temperature T_1 and a heat sink at temperature T_4 (see figure). There are two other reservoirs at temperature T_2 and T_3, as shown, with $T_1 > T_2 > T_3 > T(4)$ The three engines are equally efficient if:

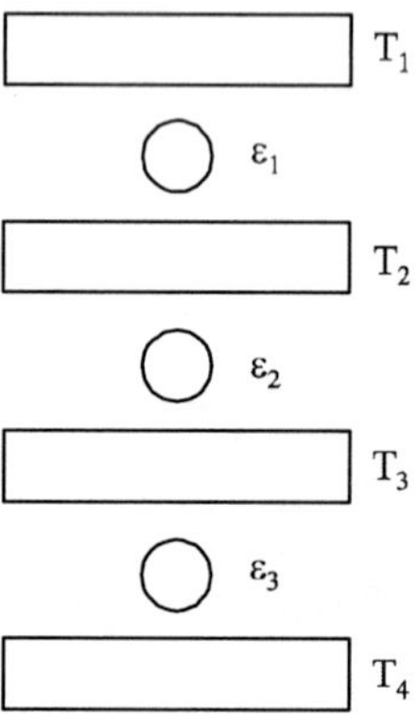

(a) $T_2 = (T_1T_4)^{1/2}; T_3 = (T_1^2T_4)^{1/3}$

(b) $T_2 = (T_1^2T_4)^{1/3}; T_3 = (T_1T_4^2)^{1/3}$

(c) $T_2 = (T_1T_4^2)^{1/3}; T_3 = (T_1^2T_4)^{1/3}$

(d) $T_2 = (T_1^3T_4)^{1/4}; T_3 = (T_1T_4^3)^{1/4}$

48. Two Carnot engines A and B are operated in series. The first one, A receives heat at T_1 (= 600 K) and rejects to a reservoir at temperature T_2. The second engine B receives heat rejected by the first engine and in turn, rejects to a heat reservoir at T_3 (= 400 K). Calculate the temperature T_2 if the work outputs of the two engines are equal:

(a) 600 K (b) 400 K (c) 300 K (d) 500 K

49. A solid body of constant heat capacity 1 J/°C is being heated by keeping it in contact with reservoirs in two ways :

(i) Sequentially keeping in contact with 2 reservoirs such that each reservoir supplies same amount of heat.

(ii) Sequentially keeping in contact with 8 reservoirs such that each reservoir supplies same amount of heat.

In both the cases body is brought from initial temperature 100°C to final temperature 200°C. Entropy change of the body in the two cases respectively is :

(a) *ln2, 2ln2* (b) *2ln2, 8ln2*

(c) *ln2, 4ln2* (d) *ln2, ln2*

50. The door of a working refrigerator is left open in a well insulated room. The temperature of air in the room will

(a) decrease

(b) increase in winters and decrease in summers

(c) remain the same

(d) increase

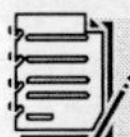

Exercise 2 - Exemplar & Past Year Questions

E&PYQs

Exemplar Questions

1. An ideal gas undergoes four different processes from the same initial state (figure). Four processes are adiabatic, isothermal, isobaric and isochoric. Out of 1, 2, 3 and 4 which one is adiabatic?

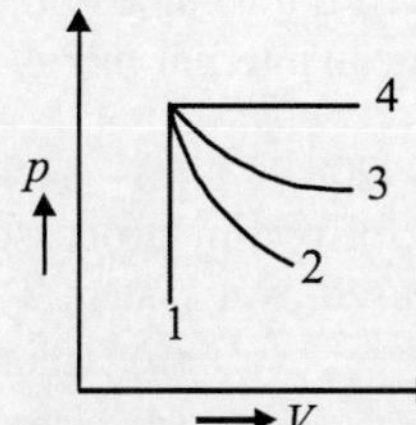

(a) 4 (b) 3 (c) 2 (d) 1

2. If an average person jogs, he produces 14.5×10^3 cal/min. This is removed by the evaporation of sweat. The amount of sweat evaporated per minute (assuming 1 kg requires 580×10^3 cal for evaporation) is

(a) 0.025 kg (b) 2.25 kg (c) 0.05 kg (d) 0.20 kg

3. An ideal gas undergoes cyclic process *ABCDA* as shown in given *p-V* diagram. The amount of work done by the gas is

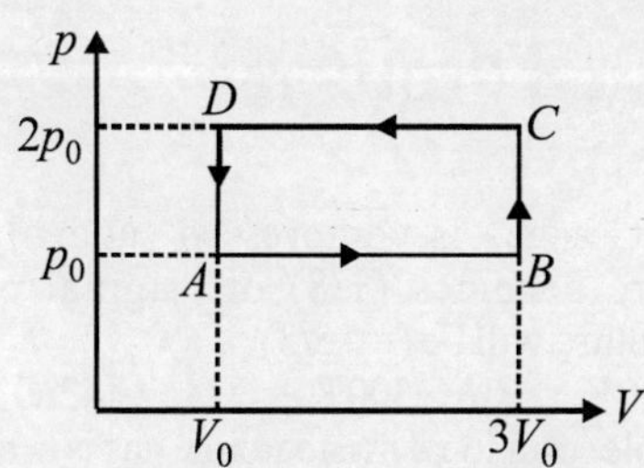

(a) $6p_0V_0$ (b) $-2p_0V_0$ (c) $+2p_0V_0$ (d) $+4p_0V_0$

4. Consider two containers *A* and *B* containing identical gases at the same pressure, volume and temperature. The gas in container *A* is compressed to half of its original volume isothermally while the gas in container *B* is compressed to half of its original value adiabatically. The ratio of final pressure of gas in *B* to that of gas in *A* is

(a) $2^{\gamma-1}$ (b) $\left(\frac{1}{2}\right)^{\gamma-1}$ (c) $\left(\frac{1}{1-\gamma}\right)^2$ (d) $\left(\frac{1}{\gamma-1}\right)^2$

NEET/AIPMT (2013-2020) Questions

5. During an adiabatic process, the pressure of a gas is found to be proportional to the cube of its temperature. The ratio of $\frac{C_p}{C_v}$ for the gas is **[2013]**

(a) 2 (b) $\frac{5}{3}$ (c) $\frac{3}{2}$ (d) $\frac{4}{3}$

6. Which of the following relations does not give the equation of an adiabatic process, where terms have their usual meaning? **[NEET Kar. 2013]**

(a) $P^{\gamma}T^{1-\gamma}$ = constant (b) $P^{1-\gamma}T^{\gamma}$ = constant
(c) PV^{γ} = constant (d) $TV^{\gamma-1}$ = constant

7. Two Carnot engines *A* and *B* are operated in series. The engine *A* receives heat from the source at temperature T_1 and rejects the heat to the sink at temperature *T*. The second engine *B* receives the heat at temperature *T* and rejects to its sink at temperature T_2. For what value of *T* the efficiencies of the two engines are equal? **[NEET Kar. 2013]**

(a) $\frac{T_1+T_2}{2}$ (b) $\frac{T_1-T_2}{2}$ (c) T_1T_2 (d) $\sqrt{T_1T_2}$

8. A thermodynamic system undergoes cyclic process ABCDA as shown in fig. The work done by the system in the cycle is : **[2014]**

(a) P_0V_0
(b) $2P_0V_0$
(c) $\frac{P_0V_0}{2}$
(d) Zero

9. A monoatomic gas at a pressure P, having a volume V expands isothermally to a volume 2V and then adiabatically to a volume 16V. The final pressure of the gas is : (take $\gamma = \frac{5}{3}$) **[2014]**

(a) 64P (b) 32P (c) $\frac{P}{64}$ (d) 16P

10. The coefficient of performance of a refrigerator is 5. If the inside temperature of freezer is –20°C, then the temperature of the surroundings to which it rejects heat is **[2015 RS]**

(a) 41°C (b) 11°C (c) 21°C (d) 31°C

11. An ideal gas is compressed to half its initial volume by means of several processes. Which of the process results in the maximum work done on the gas? **[2015 RS]**

(a) Isobaric (b) Isochoric
(c) Isothermal (d) Adiabatic

12. A gas is compressed isothermally to half its initial volume. The same gas is compressed separately through an adiabatic process until its volume is again reduced to half. Then : **[2016]**

(a) Compressing the gas isothermally will require more work to be done.
(b) Compressing the gas through adiabatic process will require more work to be done.
(c) Compressing the gas isothermally or adiabatically will require the same amount of work.
(d) Which of the case (whether compression through isothermal or through adiabatic process) requires more work will depend upon the atomicity of the gas.

13. A refrigerator works between 4°C and 30°C. It is required to remove 600 calories of heat every second in order to keep the temperature of the refrigerated space constant. The power required is: (Take 1 cal = 4.2 joules) **[2016]**

(a) 2.365 W (b) 23.65 W (c) 236.5 W (d) 2365 W

14. A carnot engine having an efficiency of $\frac{1}{10}$ as heat engine, is used as a refrigerator. If the work done on the system is 10 J, the amount of energy absorbed from the reservoir at lower temperature is :- *[2017, 2015]*

(a) 90 J (b) 99 J (c) 100 J (d) 1 J

15. The efficiency of an ideal heat engine working between the freezing point and boiling point of water, is *[2018]*

(a) 26.8% (b) 20% (c) 12.5% (d) 6.25%

16. The volume (V) of a monatomic gas varies with its temperature (T), as shown in the graph. The ratio of work done by the gas, to the heat absorbed by it, when it undergoes a change from state A to state B, is *[2018]*

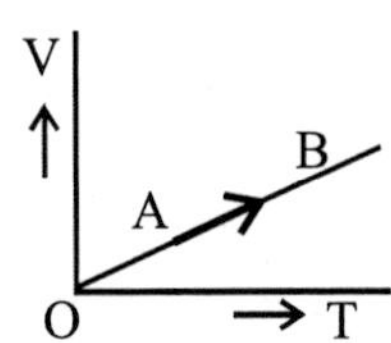

(a) $\frac{2}{5}$ (b) $\frac{2}{3}$ (c) $\frac{2}{7}$ (d) $\frac{1}{3}$

17. 1 g of water, of volume 1 cm3 at 100°C, is converted into steam at same temperature under normal atmospheric pressure (» 1×10^5 Pa). The volume of steam formed equals 1671 cm^3. If the specific latent heat of vaporisation of water is 2256 J/g, the change in internal energy is, *[NEET Odisha 2019]*

(a) 2256 J (b) 2423 J (c) 2089 J (d) 167 J

18. A sample of 0.1 g of water at 100°C and normal pressure ($1.013 \times 10^5 \, Nm^{-2}$) requires 54 cal of heat energy to convert to steam at 100°C. If the volume of the steam produced is 167.1 cc, the change in internal energy of the sample, is *[2019]*

(a) 104.3 J (b) 208.7 J (c) 84.5 J (d) 42.2 J

19. In which of the following processes, heat is neither absorbed nor released by a system ? *[2019]*

(a) isothermal (b) adiabatic
(c) isobaric (d) isochoric

20. Two cylinders A and B of equal capacity are connected to each other via a stop cock. A contains an ideal gas at standard temperature and pressure. B is completely evacuated. The entire system is thermally insulated. The stop cock is suddenly opened. The process is : *[2020]*

(a) adiabatic (b) isochoric
(c) isobaric (d) isothermal

Exercise 3 - Concept Application Problems CAP

1. For adiabatic processes (Letters have usual meanings)

(a) $P^{\gamma}V$ = constant (b) $T^{\gamma}V$ = constant
(c) $TV^{\gamma-1}$ = constant (d) TV^{γ} = constant

2. When heat is given to a gas in an isothermal change, the result will be

(a) external work done
(b) rise in temperature
(c) increase in internal energy
(d) external work done and also rise in temperature

3. Volume of one mole gas changes according to the V = a/T. If temperature change is ΔT, then work done will be

(a) $R\Delta T$ (b) $-R\Delta T$ (c) $\frac{R}{\gamma-1}\Delta T$ (d) $R(\gamma-1)\Delta T$

4. The work done in which of the following processes is equal to the internal energy of the system?

(a) Adiabatic process (b) Isothermal process
(c) Isochoric process (d) None of these

5. In thermodynamic processes which of the following statements is not true?

(a) In an isochoric process pressure remains constant
(b) In an isothermal process the temperature remains constant
(c) In an adiabatic process PV^{γ} = constant
(d) In an adiabatic process the system is insulated from the surroundings

6. A polyatomic gas ($\gamma = 4/3$) is compressed to 1/8th of its volume adiabatically. If its initial pressure is P_0, its new pressure will be

(a) $8P_0$ (b) $16P_0$ (c) $6P_0$ (d) $2P_0$

7. At 27°C a gas is compressed suddenly such that its pressure becomes (1/8) of original pressure. Final temperature will be ($\gamma = 5/3$)

(a) 450 K (b) 300 K (c) –142°C (d) 327°C

8. One mole of an ideal monoatomic gas is heated at a constant pressure of one atmosphere from 0°C to 100°C. Then the work done by the gas is

(a) 6.56 joule (b) 8.32×10^2 joule
(c) 12.48×10^2 joule (d) 20.8×10^2 joule

9. The pressure inside a tyre is 4 times that of atmosphere. If the tyre bursts suddenly at temperature 300 K, what will be the new temperature?

(a) $300\,(4)^{7/2}$ (b) $300\,(4)^{2/7}$
(c) $300\,(2)^{7/2}$ (d) $300\,(4)^{-2/7}$

10. A monatomic ideal gas expands at constant pressure, with heat Q supplied. The fraction of Q which goes as work done by the gas is

(a) 1 (b) $\frac{2}{3}$ (c) $\frac{3}{5}$ (d) $\frac{2}{5}$

11. Two cylinders fitted with pistons contain equal amount of an ideal diatomic gas at 300 K. The piston of A is free to move, while that of B is held fixed. The same amount of heat is given to the gas in each cylinder. If the rise in temperature of the gas in A is 30 K, then the rise in temperature of gas in B is

(a) 30 K (b) 18 K (c) 50 K (d) 42 K

12. A thermodynamic system goes from states (i) P_1, V to $2P_1, V$ (ii) P, V_1 to $P, 2V_1$. Then work done in the two cases is

(a) zero, zero (b) zero, PV_1
(c) PV_1, zero (d) PV_1, P_1V_1

13. For an isothermal expansion of a perfect gas, the value of $\frac{\Delta P}{P}$ is equal to

(a) $-\gamma^{1/2}\frac{\Delta V}{V}$ (b) $-\frac{\Delta V}{V}$ (c) $-\gamma\frac{\Delta V}{V}$ (d) $-\gamma^2\frac{\Delta V}{V}$

14. One mole of an ideal gas at an initial temperature of T K does 6R joules of work adiabatically. If the ratio of specific heats of this gas at constant pressure and at constant volume is 5/3, the final temperature of gas will be

(a) (T – 4) K (b) (T + 2.4) K
(c) (T – 2.4) K (d) (T + 4) K

15. During an isothermal expansion, a confined ideal gas does –150 J of work against its surroundings. This implies that

(a) 150 J heat has been removed from the gas
(b) 300 J of heat has been added to the gas
(c) no heat is transferred because the process is isothermal
(d) 150 J of heat has been added to the gas

16. When 1 kg of ice at 0°C melts to water at 0°C, the resulting change in its entropy, taking latent heat of ice to be 80 cal/°C, is

(a) 273 cal/K (b) 8 × 104 cal/K
(c) 80 cal/K (d) 293 cal/K

17. Which of the following statements about a thermodynamic process is wrong ?

(a) For an adiabatic process $\Delta E_{int} = -W$
(b) For a constant volume process $\Delta E_{int} = +Q$
(c) For a cyclic process $\Delta E_{int} = 0$
(d) For free expansion of a gas $\Delta E_{int} > 0$

18. 200g water is heated from 40°C to 60°C. Ignoring the slight expansion of water, the change in its internal energy is close to (Given specific heat of water = 4184 J/kgK):

(a) 167.4 kJ (b) 8.4 kJ (c) 4.2 kJ (d) 16.7 kJ

19. A gas is compressed from a volume of $2m^3$ to a volume of $1m^3$ at a constant pressure of 100 N/m^2. Then it is heated at constant volume by supplying 150 J of energy. As a result, the internal energy of the gas:

(a) increases by 250 J (b) decreases by 250 J
(c) increases by 50 J (d) decreases by 50 J

20. In an adiabatic process, the density of a diatomic gas becomes 32 times its initial value. The final pressure of the gas is found to be *n* times the initial pressure. The value of *n* is :

(a) 32 (b) 326 (c) 128 (d) $\frac{1}{32}$

21. A balloon filled with helium (32°C and 1.7 atm.) bursts. Immediately afterwards the expansion of helium can be considered as :

(a) irreversible isothermal (b) irreversible adiabatic
(c) reversible adiabatic (d) reversible isothermal

22. The coefficient of performance of a Carnot refrigerator working between 30°C and 0°C is

(a) 10 (b) (1) (c) 9 (d) 0

23. A sample of an ideal gas is taken through the cyclic process abca as shown in the figure. The change in the internal energy of the gas along the path ca is – 180 J, The gas absorbs 250 J of heat along the path ab and 60 J along the path bc. The work down by the gas along the path abc is:

(a) 120 J
(b) 130 J
(c) 100 J
(d) 140 J

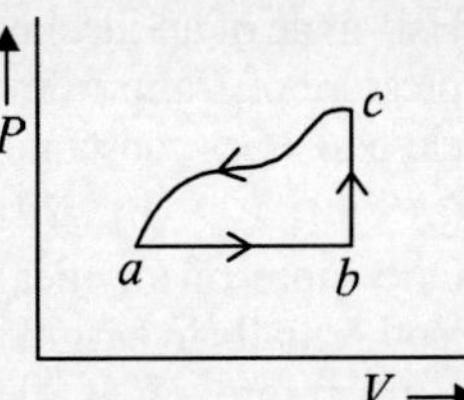

24. A cylinder with fixed capacity of 67.2 lit contains helium gas at STP. The amount of heat needed to raise the temperature of the gas by 20°C is : [Given that R = 8.31 J $mol^{-1}K^{-1}$]

(a) 350 J (b) 374 J (c) 748 J (d) 700 J

25. n moles of an ideal gas with constant volume heat capacity C_V undergo an isobaric expansion by certain volume. The ratio of the work done in the process, to the heat supplied is:

(a) $\frac{nR}{C_V + nR}$ (b) $\frac{nR}{C_V - nR}$

(c) $\frac{4nR}{C_V - nR}$ (d) $\frac{4nR}{C_V + nR}$

26. One mole of an ideal gas passes through a process where pressure and volume obey the relation $P = P_0\left[1 - \frac{1}{2}\left(\frac{V_0}{V}\right)^2\right]$.

Here P_o and V_o are constants. Calculate the charge in the temperature of the gas if its volume changes from V_o to $2V_o$.

(a) $\frac{1}{2}\frac{P_oV_o}{R}$ (b) $\frac{5}{4}\frac{P_oV_o}{R}$

(c) $\frac{3}{4}\frac{P_oV_o}{R}$ (d) $\frac{1}{4}\frac{P_oV_o}{R}$

27. A thermally insulted vessel contains 150 g of water at 0°C. Then the air from the vessel is pumped out adiabatically. A fraction of water turns into ice and the rest evaporates at 0°C itself. The mass of evaporated water will be closed to:

(Latent heat of vaporization of water = 2.10×10^6 J kg^{-1} and Latent heat of Fusion of water = 3.36×10^5 J kg^{-1})

(a) 150 g (b) 20 g (c) 130 g (d) 35 g

28. The given diagram shows four processes *i.e.*, isochoric, isobaric, isothermal and adiabatic. The correct assignment of the processes, in the same order is given by :

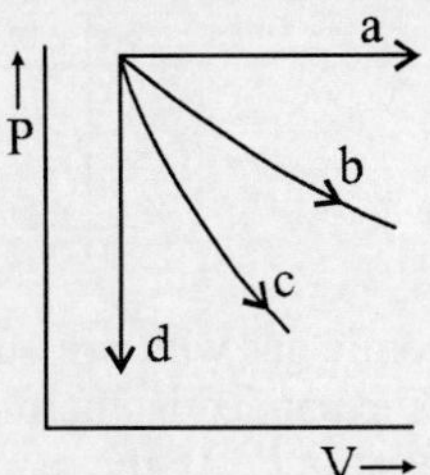

(a) a d b c (b) d a c b (c) a d c b (d) d a b c

29. A rigid diatomic ideal gas undergoes an adiabatic process at room temperature. The relation between temperature and volume for this process is TV^x = constant, then x is:

(a) $\frac{3}{5}$ (b) $\frac{2}{5}$ (c) $\frac{2}{3}$ (d) $\frac{5}{3}$

30. Half mole of an ideal monoatomic gas is heated at constant pressure of 1 atm from 20°C to 90°C. Work done by gas is close to: (Gas constant R = 8.31 J/mol-K)
(a) 581 J (b) 291 J (c) 146 J (d) 73 J

31. One mole of an ideal monoatomic gas is compressed isothermally in a rigid vessel to double its pressure at room temperature, 27°C. The work done on the gas will be:
(a) 300R ln 6 (b) 300R
(c) 300R ln 7 (d) 300R ln 2

32. The ratio of work done by an ideal monoatomic gas to the heat supplied to it in an isobaric process is :
(a) $\frac{2}{5}$ (b) $\frac{3}{2}$ (c) $\frac{3}{5}$ (d) $\frac{2}{3}$

33. Consider an ideal gas confined in an isolated closed chamber. As the gas undergoes an adiabatic expansion, the average time of collision between molecules increases as V^q, where V is the volume of the gas. The value of q is : $\left(\gamma = \frac{C_p}{C_v}\right)$
(a) $\frac{\gamma+1}{2}$ (b) $\frac{\gamma-1}{2}$ (c) $\frac{3\gamma+5}{6}$ (d) $\frac{3\gamma-5}{6}$

34. During an adiabatic compression, 830 J of work is done on 2 moles of a diatomic ideal gas to reduce its volume by 50%. The change in its temperature is nearly: ($R = 8.3\ JK^{-1}\ mol^{-1}$)
(a) 40 K (b) 33 K (c) 20 K (d) 14 K

35. The equation of state for a gas is given by $PV = nRT + \alpha V$, where n is the number of moles and α is a positive constant. The initial temperature and pressure of one mole of the gas contained in a cylinder are T_o and P_o respectively. The work done by the gas when its temperature doubles isobarically will be:
(a) $\frac{P_oT_oR}{P_o - \alpha}$ (b) $\frac{P_oT_oR}{P_o + \alpha}$
(c) $P_oT_oR \ln 2$ (d) P_oT_oR

36. Helium gas goes through a cycle ABCDA (consisting of two isochoric and isobaric lines) as shown in figure. The efficiency of this cycle is nearly : (Assume the gas to be close to ideal gas)
(a) 15.4%
(b) 9.1%
(c) 10.5%
(d) 12.5%

37. An ideal monatomic gas with pressure P, volume V and temperature T is expanded isothermally to a volume $2V$ and a final pressure P_i. If the same gas is expanded adiabatically to a volume $2V$, the final pressure is P_a. The ratio $\frac{P_a}{P_i}$ is
(a) $2^{-1/3}$ (b) $2^{1/3}$ (c) $2^{2/3}$ (d) $2^{-2/3}$

38. A heat engine is involved with exchange of heat of 1915 J, – 40 J, +125 J and – Q J, during one cycle achieving an efficiency of 50.0%. The value of Q is :
(a) 640 J (b) 40 J (c) 980 J (d) 400 J

39. A Carnot engine having an efficiency of $\frac{1}{10}$ is being used as a refrigerator. If the work done on the refrigerator is 10 J, the amount of heat absorbed from the reservoir at lower temperature is:
(a) 99 J (b) 100 J (c) 1 J (d) 90 J

40. Two ideal Carnot engines operate in cascade (all heat given up by one engine is used by the other engine to produce work) between temperatures, T_1 and T_2. The temperature of the hot reservoir of the first engine is T_1 and the temperature of the cold reservoir of the second engine is T_2. T is temperature of the sink of first engine which is also the source for the second engine. How is T related to T_1 and T_2, if both the engines perform equal amount of work ?
(a) $T = \frac{2T_1T_2}{T_1 + T_2}$ (b) $T = \frac{T_1 + T_2}{2}$
(c) $T = \sqrt{T_1T_2}$ (d) $T = 0$

41. A Carnot engine has an efficiency of 1/6. When the temperature of the sink is reduced by 62°C, its efficiency is doubled. The temperatures of the source and the sink are, respectively.
(a) 62°C, 124°C (b) 99°C, 37°C
(c) 124°C, 62°C (d) 37°C, 99°C

42. A Carnot's engine works as a refrigerator between 250 K and 300 K. It receives 500 cal heat from the reservoir at the lower temperature. The amount of work done in each cycle to operate the refrigerator is:
(a) 420 J (b) 2100 J (c) 772 J (d) 2520 J

43. Two Carnot engines A and B are operated in series. Engine A receives heat from a reservoir at 600K and rejects heat to a reservoir at temperature T. Engine B receives heat rejected by engine A and in turn rejects it to a reservoir at 100K. If the efficiencies of the two engines A and B are represented by η_A and η_B respectively, then what is the value of $\frac{\eta_A}{\eta_B}$
(a) $\frac{12}{7}$ (b) $\frac{12}{5}$ (c) $\frac{5}{12}$ (d) $\frac{7}{12}$

44. A Carnot freezer takes heat from water at 0°C inside it and rejects it to the room at a temperature of 27°C. The latent heat of ice is $336 \times 10^3\ J\ kg^{-1}$. If 5 kg of water at 0°C is converted into ice at 0°C by the freezer, then the energy consumed by the freezer is close to :
(a) 1.51×10^5 J (b) 1.68×10^6 J
(c) 1.71×10^7 J (d) 1.67×10^5 J

45. A Carnot engine absorbs 1000 J of heat energy from a reservoir at 127°C and rejects 600 J of heat energy during each cycle. The efficiency of engine and temperature of sink will be:
(a) 20% and – 43°C (b) 40% and – 33°C
(c) 50% and – 20°C (d) 70% and – 10°C

Hints & Solutions

12.1 Concept Practice Problems

CPP

1. (a) PV = constant, represents isothermal process.
2. (b) $\Delta Q = \Delta U + \Delta W$

$\Rightarrow \Delta U = \Delta Q - \Delta W = Q - W$ (using proper sign)

3. (d) $PV^{\gamma} = P_1\left(\frac{V}{32}\right)^{\gamma}$

or $P_1 = (32)^{\gamma}$, $P = (32)^{1.4}$, $P = 128P$

4. (d)
5. (b) $dW = P\Delta V = 1.01 \times 10^5 [1671 - 1] \times 10^{-6}$ Joule

$= \frac{1.01 \times 167}{4.2}$ cal. $= 40$ cal. nearly

$\Delta Q = mL = 1 \times 540,$

$\Delta Q = \Delta W + \Delta U$

or $\Delta U = 540 - 40 = 500$ cal.

6. (c) For adiabatic process, $dU = -100$ J which remains same for other processes also. Let C be the heat capacity of 2nd process then

$-(C)5 = dU + dW$

$= -100 + 25 = -75$

$\therefore C = 15$ J/K

7. (c) According to first law of thermodynamics

$Q = \Delta U + W$

$\Delta U = Q - W$

$= 2 \times 4.2 \times 1000 - 500$

$= 8400 - 500 = 7900$ J

8. (a) $PV^{3/2} = K$

$\log P + \frac{3}{2}\log V = \log K$

$\frac{\Delta P}{P} + \frac{3}{2}\frac{\Delta V}{V} = 0 \Rightarrow \frac{\Delta V}{V} = -\frac{2}{3}\frac{\Delta P}{P}$

or $\frac{\Delta V}{V} = \left(-\frac{2}{3}\right)\left(\frac{2}{3}\right) = -\frac{4}{9}$

9. (b,d) (a) Process is not isothermal.
(b) Volume decreases and temperature decreases ΔU = negative,
So, ΔQ = negative
(c) Work done in process $A \to B \to C$ is positve
(d) Cycle is clockwise, so work done by the gas is positive
10. (a) By first law of thermodynamics,

$\Delta Q = \Delta U + \Delta W$

In adiabatic process, $\Delta Q = 0$

$\therefore \Delta U = -\Delta W$

In isothermal process, $\Delta U = 0$

$\therefore \Delta Q = \Delta W$

12.2 Concept Practice Problems

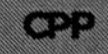

11. (a) Efficiency of carnot engine $= \eta = \frac{T_1 - T_2}{T_1}$

where T_1 = source temperature

T_2 = sink temperature.

12. (c) For process to be reversible it must be quasi-static. For quasi static process all changes take place infinitely slowly. Isothermal process occur very slowly so it is quasi-static and hence it is reversible.
13. (a) $\frac{T_2}{T_1 - T_2} = \frac{Q_2}{W}$

$\frac{273}{300 - 273} = \frac{50,000}{W}$

$W = \frac{27 \times 50,000}{273}$ cal/min

$P = \frac{W}{t} = \frac{4.2 \times 27 \times 50,000}{60 \times 273}$ Joule/sec

$= 346$ watt $= 0.346$ kW

14. (c) $\eta = 1 - \frac{T_2}{T_1} \Rightarrow \eta = 1 - \frac{250}{373} = \frac{123}{373} = \frac{100 + 23}{373}$
15. (c) $\eta = 1 - \frac{Q_2}{Q_1} = 1 - \frac{T_2}{T_1} \Rightarrow \frac{Q_2}{Q_1} = \frac{T_2}{T_1}$

So $T_2 = \frac{Q_2 \times T_1}{Q_1} = \frac{150 \times 500}{300} = 250$K

16. (d) Efficiency, $\eta = 1 - \frac{T_2}{T_1}$

T_1 (source temp.) = 400 K

T_2 (sink temp.) = 300 K

$\therefore \eta = 1 - \frac{300}{400} = \frac{1}{4} = 25\%$

17. (a) $\frac{750}{W} = \frac{250}{300 - 250}$

Heat rejected = 750 + 150 = 900 cal.

18. (b) $\frac{T_1 - T_2}{T_1}$ is maximum in case (b).
19. (d) Efficiency $\eta = \frac{W}{\theta_1}$ and $W = \theta_1 - \theta_2$

$\therefore \eta = \frac{\theta_1 - \theta_2}{\theta} = 1 - \frac{\theta_2}{\theta_1}$

20. (d)

Exercise 1 - Chapter Revision Problems CRP

1. (c) Second law of thermodynamics introduces the concepts of entropy
2. (c) 3. (b) 4. (a) 5. (a) 6. (b) 7. (b) 8. (b)
9. (a) Let P and V be the initial pressure and volume of ideal gas. After isothermal expansion, pressure is P/4. So volume is 4 V. Let P_1 be the pressure after adiabatic compression. Then $P_1 V^{\gamma} = (P/4)(4V)^{\gamma}$ $P_1 = (P/4)(4)^{3/2} = 2P$
10. (c)
11. (c) During melting temperature remains constant
12. (b) Flow rate $\propto$ gradient $\times r^2$. When flow rate is constant, gradient $\propto r^{-2}$.
13. (d) Isochoric proceess $dV = 0$ $W = 0$ proceess 1
Isobaric : $W = P\Delta V = nR\Delta T$
Adiabatic $|W| = \dfrac{nR\Delta T}{\gamma - 1}$ $0 < \gamma - 1 < 1$
As workdone in case of adiabatic process is more so process 3 is adiabatic and process 2 is isobaric.
14. (c)
15. (b) From FLOT $\Delta Q = \Delta U + \Delta W$
$\because$ Heat supplied to the system so $\Delta Q \rightarrow$ Positive and work is done on the system so $\Delta W \rightarrow$ Negative
Hence $+\Delta Q = \Delta U - \Delta W$
16. (a) $W = \dfrac{nRdT}{\gamma - 1}$ γ is minimum for a polyatomic gas
Hence, W is greatest for polyatomic gas
17. (a) We know that $\dfrac{P_1 V_1}{T_1} = \dfrac{P_2 V_2}{T_2}$ $\therefore$ $T_2 = \dfrac{P_2 V_2 T_1}{P_1 V_1}$
Here $P_1 = 30$ atm., $P_2 = 1$ atm, $V_1 = V$ (say), $V_2 = 15\,V$, $T_1 = 27°C = 27 + 273 = 300°K$ and $T_2 = ?$
Substituting these values, we get $T_2 = 150°K$
$\therefore$ $T_2 = 150°K = 150 - 273 = -123°C$.
18. (c) $W = \dfrac{(1\times10^5 + 6\times10^5)(5-1)}{2}$
$= \dfrac{6\times10^5\times4}{2} = 12\times10^5$ joule
19. (d) $dU = dQ - dW = (8\times10^5 - 6.5\times10^5) = 1.5\times10^5$ J
$dW = dQ - dU == 10^5 - 1.5\times10^5 = -0.5\times10^5\, J$
– ve sign indicates that work done on the gas is 0.5×10^5 J.
20. (c) $dU = nC_v\,dT$ or $80 = 5\times C_v(120 - 100)$
$C_v = 4.0$ joule/K
21. (d) $\dfrac{PV}{T} = \dfrac{P'(90/100)V}{T}$
or $\dfrac{P'}{P} = \dfrac{100}{90} = 1 + \dfrac{10}{90}$ or $\dfrac{P' - P}{P} = \dfrac{10}{90} = 11.1\%$
22. (d) $T_1 = 18°C = (273 + 18) = 291$ K
and $V_2 = V_1/8$
We know that $TV^{\gamma-1} = $ constant
or, $T_2 V_2^{\gamma-1} = T_1 V_1^{\gamma-1}$
$\therefore$ $T_2 = T_1\left(\dfrac{V_1}{V_2}\right)^{\gamma-1} = 291\times(8)^{1.4-1}$
$= 668.5\,K = 395.5°C$
23. (c) $P \propto T$ if V is constant, where P is pressure of certain amount of gas and T is absolute zero temperature.
24. (a) Work done in an isothermal process is given by
$W = 2.3026nRT\log_{10}\dfrac{V_2}{V_1}$
Here, $n = 3$, $R = 8.31$ J mol^{-1} degree^{-1}
$T = 300$ K, $V_1 = 4$ litre, $V_2 = 1$ litre.
Hence, $W = 2.3026\times3\times8.31\times300\times\log_{10}\dfrac{1}{4}$
$= 17221.15(-2\log_{10}2)$
$= -17221.15\times2\times0.3010 = -10368$ J.
25. (c) The speed of sound in air, $v \propto \sqrt{T}$
$\dfrac{v_1}{v_2} = \sqrt{\dfrac{T_1}{T_2}} \Rightarrow \dfrac{v_1}{2v_1} = \sqrt{\dfrac{(27+273)}{T_2}}$
$\dfrac{1}{2} = \sqrt{\dfrac{300}{T_2}}$
$T_2 = 1200\,K = (1200 - 273)°C = 927°C$
26. (b) $T_2 = 273 - 13 = 260$,
$K = \dfrac{T_2}{T_1 - T_2} \Rightarrow 5 = \dfrac{260}{T_1 - 260}$ or $T_1 - 260 = 52$
$T_1 = 312\,K$,
$T_2 = 312 - 273 = 39°C$
27. (c) $(300)\,V^{(1.4-1)} = T_2.\left(\dfrac{V}{4}\right)^{(1.4-1)}$
$T_2 = (300)(4)^{0.4}$
28. (d) From C to D, V is constant. So process is isochoric. From D to A, the curve represents constant temperature. So the process is isothermal.
From A to B, pressure is constant. So, the process is isobaric. BC represents constant entropy.
29. (b)
30. (a) The volume on both sides will be so adjusted that the original pressure × volume is kept constant as the piston moves slowly (isothermal change)
P5V = P'V' ....(1)
10PV = P'V" ....(2)
From (1) and (2), V" = 2V'
and from V' + V" = 6V
V' = 2V, V" = 4V
31. (a) 32. (c)
33. (a) $\because$ Internal ensergy is the state function.
$\therefore$ In cyclie process; $\Delta U = 0$
According to 1st law of thermodynamics
$$\boxed{\Delta Q = \Delta U + W}$$

So heat absorbed

$\Delta Q = W =$ Area under the curve

$= -(2V)(P) = -2PV$

So heat rejected $= 2PV$

34. (a) Initial and final condition is same for all process

$\Delta U_1 = \Delta U_2 = \Delta U_3$

from first law of thermodynamics

$\Delta Q = \Delta U + \Delta W$

Work done

$\Delta W_1 > \Delta W_2 > \Delta W_3$ (Area of P.V. graph)

So $\Delta Q_1 > \Delta Q_2 > \Delta Q_3$

35. (b) $P_1 > P_2$

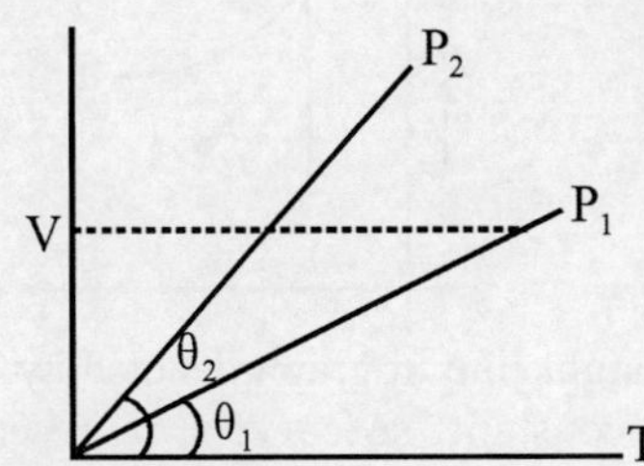

As V = constant $\Rightarrow P \propto T$

Hence from V–T graph $P_1 > P_2$

36. (b) Change in internal energy do not depend upon the path followed by the process. It only depends on initial and final states i.e.,

$$\Delta U_1 = \Delta U_2$$

37. (a)

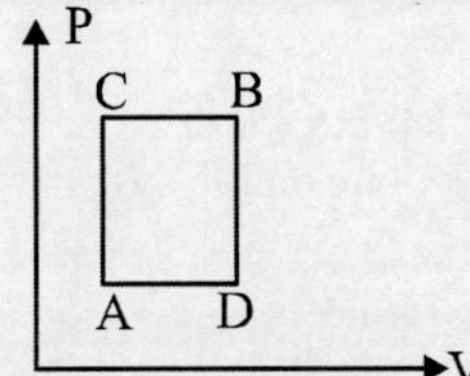

ΔU remains same for both paths ACB and ADB

$\Delta Q_{ACB} = \Delta W_{ACB} + \Delta U_{ACB}$

$\Rightarrow 60\,J = 30\,J + \Delta U_{ACB} \Rightarrow U_{ACB} = 30\,J$

$\therefore \Delta U_{ADB} = \Delta U_{ACB} = 30\,J$

$\Delta Q_{ADB} = \Delta U_{ADB} + \Delta W_{ADB}$

$= 10\,J + 30\,J = 40\,J$

38. (b) Temperature change ΔT is same for all three processes

$A \to B$; $A \to C$ and $A \to D$

$\Delta U = nC_v\Delta T =$ same

$E_{AB} = E_{AC} = E_{AD}$

Work done, $W = P \times \Delta V$

$AB \to$ volume is increasing $\Rightarrow W_{AB} > 0$

$AD \to$ volume is decreasing $\Rightarrow W_{AD} < 0$

$AC \to$ volume is constant $\Rightarrow W_{AC} = 0$

39. (d)

(I) **Adiabatic process :** No exchange of heat takes place with surroundings.

$\Rightarrow \Delta Q = 0$

(II) **Isothermal process :** Temperature remains constant

$\therefore \Delta T = 0 \Rightarrow \Delta U = \frac{f}{2}nR\Delta T \Rightarrow \Delta U = 0$

No change in internal energy $[\Delta U = 0]$.

(III) Isochoric process volume remains constant

$\Delta V = 0 \Rightarrow W = \int P \cdot dV = 0$

Hence work done is zero.

(IV) In isobaric process pressure remains constant.

$W = P \cdot \Delta V \neq 0$

$\Delta U = \frac{f}{2}nR\Delta T = \frac{f}{2}[P\Delta V] \neq 0$

$\therefore \Delta Q = nC_p\Delta T \neq 0$

40. (c) For process $3 \to 1$ volume is constant

$\therefore$ Graph given in option (d) is wrong.

And process $1 \to 2$ is adiabatic $\therefore$ graph in option (1) is wrong

$\because$ $v =$ constant

$P\uparrow, T\uparrow$

For Process $2 \to 3$ Pressure constant *i.e.*, $P =$ constant

$\therefore$ $V\downarrow T\downarrow$

Hence graph (c) is the correct $V - T$ graph of given $P - V$ graph

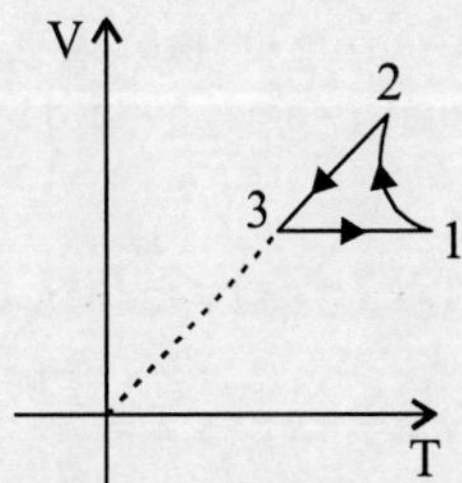

41. (b) Given, $V_1 = 1$ litre, $P_1 = 1$ atm

$V_2 = 3$ litre, $\gamma = 1.40$,

Using, $PV^\gamma =$ constant $\Rightarrow P_1V_1^\gamma = P_2V_2^\gamma$

$$\Rightarrow P_2 = P_1 \times \left(\frac{1}{3}\right)^{1.4} = \frac{1}{4.6555}\,atm$$

$$\therefore \text{Work done, } W = \frac{P_1V_1 - P_2V_2}{\gamma - 1}$$

$$= \frac{\left(1 \times 1 - \frac{1}{4.6555} \times 3\right)1.01325 \times 10^5 \times 10^{-3}}{0.4} = 90.1\,J$$

Closest value of $W = 90.5\,J$

42. (Bonus) We know that Relaxation time,

$T \propto \frac{V}{\sqrt{T}}$ ...(i)

Equation of adiabatic process is

$TV^{\gamma-1} =$ constant

$$\Rightarrow \quad T \propto \frac{1}{V^{\gamma-1}} \Rightarrow T \propto V^{1+\frac{\gamma-1}{2}} \quad \text{using (i)}$$

$$\Rightarrow \quad T \propto V^{\frac{1+\gamma}{2}} \Rightarrow \frac{T_f}{T_i} = \left(\frac{2V}{V}\right)^{\frac{1+\gamma}{2}} = (2)^{\frac{1+\gamma}{2}}$$

43. (c) Internal energy depends only on initial and final state
So, $\Delta U_A = \Delta U_B$
Also $\Delta Q = \Delta U + W$
As $W_A > W_B \Rightarrow \Delta Q_A > \Delta Q_B$

44. (b) Total work done by the gas during the cycle is equal to area of triangle ABC.
$\therefore\ \Delta W = \frac{1}{2} \times 4 \times 5 = 10\text{ J}$

45. (a) Equation of the BC
$$P = P_0 - \frac{2P_0}{V_0}(V - 2V_0)$$
using PV = nRT
$$\text{Temperature, } T = \frac{P_0 V - \frac{2P_0 V^2}{V_0} + 4P_0 V}{1 \times R}$$
($\because$ n = 1 mole given)
$$T = \frac{P_0}{F}\left[5V - \frac{2V^2}{V_0}\right]$$
$$\frac{dT}{dV} = 0 \Rightarrow 5 - \frac{4V}{V_0} = 0 \Rightarrow V = \frac{5}{4}V_0$$
$$T = \frac{P_0}{R}\left[5 \times \frac{5V_0}{4} - \frac{2}{V_0} \times \frac{25}{16}V_0^2\right] = \frac{25}{8}\frac{P_0 V_0}{R}$$

46. (b) Work done during the process $A \to B$
= Area of trapezium (= area bounded by indicator diagram with V-axis)
$$= \frac{1}{2}(2P_0 + P_0)(2V_0 - V_0) = \frac{3}{2}P_0 V_0$$
Ideal gas eqn : $PV = nRT \Rightarrow T = \frac{PV}{nR} = \frac{3P_0V_0}{2nR}$

47. (b) According to question, $\eta_1 = \eta_2 = \eta_3$
$$\therefore 1 - \frac{T_2}{T_1} = 1 - \frac{T_3}{T_2} = 1 - \frac{T_4}{T_3}$$
[$\because$ Three engines are equally efficient]
$$\Rightarrow \frac{T_2}{T_1} = \frac{T_3}{T_2} = \frac{T_4}{T_3}$$
$$\Rightarrow T_2 = \sqrt{T_1 T_3} \quad ...(i)$$
$$T_3 = \sqrt{T_2 T_4} \quad ...(ii)$$
From (i) and (ii)
$$T_2 = (T_1^2 T_4)^{1/3}$$
$$T_3 = (T_1 T_4^2)^{1/3}$$

48. (d) $\eta_A = \frac{T_1 - T_2}{T_1} = \frac{W_A}{Q_1}$ and, $\eta_B = \frac{T_2 - T_3}{T_2} = \frac{W_B}{Q_2}$
According to question,
$W_A = W_B$
$$\therefore \frac{Q_1}{Q_2} = \frac{T_1}{T_2} \times \frac{T_2 - T_3}{T_1 - T_2} = \frac{T_1}{T_2}$$
$$\therefore T_2 = \frac{T_1 + T_3}{2} = \frac{600 + 400}{2} = 500\text{K}$$

49. (d) The entropy change of the body in the two cases is same as entropy is a state function.

50. (d) In a refrigerator, the heat dissipated in the atmosphere is more than that taken from the cooling chamber, therefore the room is heated. If the door of a refrigerator is kept open.

Exercise 2 - Exemplar & Past Year Questions E&PYQs

Exemplar Questions

1. (c) For the straight line in the graph denoted by 4, that shows pressure is constant, so curve 4 represents an isobaric process.

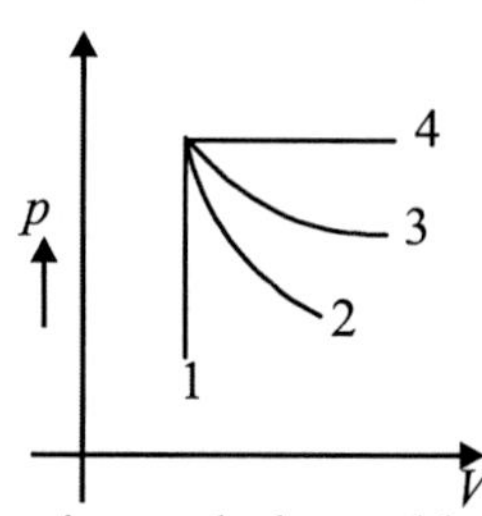

For the straight line in graph denoted by 1, that shows volume is constant, so curve 1 represents isochoric process. Out of curves 3 and 2, curve 2 is steeper. Hence, curve 2 is adiabatic and curve 3 is isothermal.

2. (a)

3. (b) According to the given p-V diagram.
Work done in the process $ABCD$
$= (AB) \times BC = (3V_0 - V_0) \times (2p_0 - p_0)$
$= 2V_0 \times p_0 = 2p_0V_0$
Here the direction of arrow is anti-clockwise, so work done is negative.
Hence, work done by the gas $= -2p_0V_0$
That shows external work done on the system.

4. (a)

NEET/AIPMT (2013-2020) Questions

5. (c) According to question $P \propto T^3$
But as we know for an adiabatic process the pressure P
$\propto T^{\frac{\gamma}{\gamma-1}}$. So, $\frac{\gamma}{\gamma - 1} = 3 \Rightarrow \gamma = \frac{3}{2}$ or, $\frac{C_p}{C_v} = \frac{3}{2}$

6. (a) Adiabatic equations of state are
PV^γ = constant
$TV^{\gamma-1}$ = constant
$P^{1-\gamma}T^\gamma$ = constant.

7. (d) Efficiency of engine A, $\eta_1 = 1 - \frac{T}{T_1}$,
Efficiency of engine B, $\eta_2 = 1 - \frac{T_2}{T}$
Here, $\eta_1 = \eta_2$
$$\therefore \frac{T}{T_1} = \frac{T_2}{T} \Rightarrow T = \sqrt{T_1 T_2}$$

8. (d)

9. (c) For isothermal process $P_1V_1 = P_2V_2$
$$\Rightarrow PV = P_2(2V) \Rightarrow P_2 = \frac{P}{2}$$

For adiabatic process

$$P_2V_2^\gamma = P_3V_3^\gamma \Rightarrow \left(\frac{P}{2}\right)(2v)^\gamma = P_3 16v)^\gamma$$

$$\Rightarrow P_3 = \frac{3}{2}\left(\frac{1}{8}\right)^{5/3} = \frac{P}{64}$$

10. (d) Coefficient of performance,

$$Cop = \frac{T_2}{T_1 - T_2}$$

$$5 = \frac{273-20}{T_1-(273-20)} = \frac{253}{T_1-253}$$

$$5T_1 - (5\times 253) = 253$$

$$5T_1 = 253 + (5\times 253) = 1518 \ \therefore T_1 = \frac{1518}{5} = 303.6$$

or, $T_1 = 303.6 - 273 = 30.6 \cong 31°C$

11. (d) Since area under the curve is maximum for adiabatic process so, work done (W = PdV) on the gas will be maximum for adiabatic process

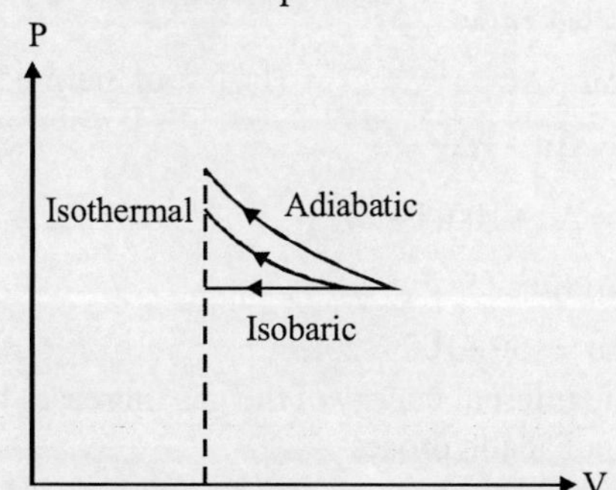

12. (b) W_{ext} = negative of area with volume-axis
W(adiabatic) > W(isothermal)

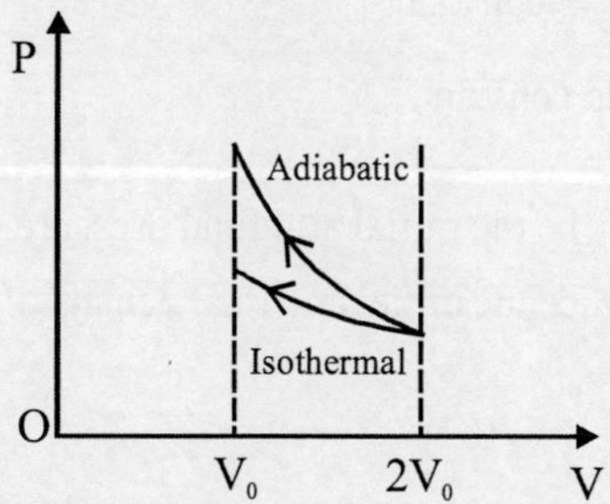

13. (c) Coefficient of performance of a refrigerator,

$$\beta = \frac{Q_2}{W} = \frac{T_2}{T_1 - T_2} \quad \text{(Where } Q_2 \text{ is heat removed)}$$

Given: $T_2 = 4°C = 4 + 273 = 277\,k$

$T_1 = 30°C = 30 + 273 = 303\,k$

$$\therefore \ \beta = \frac{600\times 4.2}{W} = \frac{277}{303-277}$$

$\Rightarrow$ W = 236.5 joule

$$\text{Power } P = \frac{W}{t} = \frac{236.5\,\text{joule}}{1\,\text{sec}} = 236.5 \text{ watt.}$$

14. (a) Given, efficiency of engine, $\eta = \frac{1}{10}$

work done on system W = 10J

Coefficient of performance of refrigerator

$$\beta = \frac{Q_2}{W} = \frac{1-\eta}{\eta} = \frac{1-\frac{1}{10}}{\frac{1}{10}} = \frac{\frac{9}{10}}{\frac{1}{10}} = 9$$

Energy absorbed from reservoir

$Q_2 = \beta w$

$Q_2 = 9 \times 10 = 90$ J

15. (a) Efficiency of ideal heat engine, $\eta = \left(1 - \frac{T_2}{T_1}\right)$

Sink temperature, $T_2 = 100°C = 100 + 273 = 373$ K

Source temperature, $T_1 = 0°C = 0 + 273 = 273$ K

$$\text{Percentage efficiency, } \%\eta = \left(1 - \frac{T_2}{T_1}\right)\times 100$$

$$= \left(1 - \frac{273}{373}\right)\times 100 = \left(\frac{100}{373}\right)\times 100 = 26.8\%$$

16. (a) Gas is monatomic, so $C_p = \frac{5}{2}R$

Given process is isobaric

$\therefore \ dQ = n\,C_p\,dT$

$$\Rightarrow dQ = n\left(\frac{5}{2}R\right)dT$$

$dW = P\,dV = n\,RdT$

$$\therefore \ \text{Required ratio} = \frac{dW}{dQ} = \frac{nRdT}{n\left(\frac{5}{2}R\right)dT} = \frac{2}{5}$$

17. (c) $\Delta Q = 2256 \times 1 = 2256$ J

$\Delta W = P[V_{steam} - V_{water}]$ $[\because dw = pdv]$

$= 1 \times 105[1671 - 1] \times 106 = 167$ J

As $\Delta Q = \Delta U + \Delta W$

$2256 = \Delta U + 167 \Rightarrow \Delta U = 2089$ J

18. (b) Using first law of thermodynamics equation,

$\Delta Q = \Delta U + \Delta W \Rightarrow 54 \times 4.18$

$= \Delta U + 1.013 \times 10^5(167.1 \times 10^{-6} - 0)$ $(\because \Delta W = P\Delta V)$

$\Rightarrow \ \Delta U = 208.7$ J

19. (b) In adiabatic process, there is no exchange of heat, with the surroundings.

20. (a) Entire system is thermally insulated. So, no heat exchange with surrounding will take place. Hence, process will be adiabatic.

Exercise 3 - Concept Application Problems CAP

1. (c) For adiabatic process, $TV^{\gamma-1}$ = constant
2. (a)
3. (b) PV = RT ;

$$P = \frac{RT}{V} = \frac{RT^2}{a}$$

$$V = \frac{a}{T} \quad \therefore dV = -\frac{a}{T^2}dT$$

$$W = \int P\,dV = \int \frac{RT^2}{a}\left(-\frac{a}{T^2}dT\right)$$

$W = -R\,\Delta T$

4. (a) In adiabatic process
$\Delta Q = 0$
$\therefore \quad \Delta W = -\Delta U$

5. (a) In an isochoric process volume remains constant whereas pressure remains constant in isobaric process.

6. (b) $P_0 V^{4/3} = P_1 \left(\frac{V}{8}\right)^{4/3} \Rightarrow P_1 = P_0 8^{4/3} = 16P_o$

7. (c) $T_1^{\gamma} P_1^{1-\gamma} = T_2^{\gamma} P_2^{1-\gamma}$

8. (b) $dQ = n\ C_p dT = 1 \times \frac{5}{2} R \times 100$
$= 2077.5\ J = 20.8 \times 10^2\ J$
$dU = n C_v dT = 1 \times \frac{3}{2} R \times 100 = 1246.5\ J$
$\therefore\ dU = dQ - dU = 8.31 \times 10^2\ J$

9. (d) Under adiabatic change
$$\frac{T_2}{T_1} = \left(\frac{P_1}{P_2}\right)^{\frac{1-\gamma}{\gamma}} \text{ or } T_2 = T_1 (P_1 / P_2)^{\frac{1-\gamma}{\gamma}}$$
$$\therefore\ T_2 = 300\,(4/1)^{\frac{1-(7/5)}{(7/5)}};\ \gamma = 1.4 = 7/5 \text{ for air}$$
or $T_2 = 300\,(4)^{-2/7}$

10. (d) $Q = nC_p \Delta T$ and $W = P\Delta V = nR\Delta T$.
For monatomic gas, $C_p = \frac{5R}{2}. \Rightarrow \frac{W}{Q} = \frac{2}{5}$

11. (d) In cylinder A, heat is supplied at constant pressure while in cylinder B heat is supplied at constant volume.
$(\Delta Q)_A = nC_P (\Delta T)_A$
and $(\Delta Q)_B = nC_V (\Delta T)_B$
Given : $(\Delta Q)_A = (\Delta Q)_B$
$\therefore (\Delta T)_B = \frac{C_P}{C_V} (\Delta T)_A = 1.4 \times 30 = 42K$
[$\because$ for diatomic gas $\frac{C_P}{C_V} = 1.4$]

12. (b) (i) Case $\rightarrow$ Volume = constant $\Rightarrow \int PdV = 0$
(ii) Case $\rightarrow P =$ constant
$$\Rightarrow \int_{V_1}^{2V_1} PdV = P\int_{V_1}^{2V_1} dV = PV_1$$

13. (b) Differentiate PV = constant w.r.t V
$$\Rightarrow P\Delta V + V\Delta P = 0 \Rightarrow \frac{\Delta P}{P} = -\frac{\Delta V}{V}$$

14. (a) $W = \frac{P_1V_1 - P_2V_2}{\gamma - 1} = \frac{nRT_1 - nRT_2}{\gamma - 1} = \frac{nR(T_1 - T_2)}{\gamma - 1}$
$n = 1, T_1 = T \Rightarrow \frac{R(T - T_2)}{5/3 - 1} = 6R \Rightarrow T_f = (T - 4)K$

15. (a, d) If a process is expansion then work done is positive so answer will be (a).
But in question work done by gas is given -150J so that according to it answer will be (d).

16. (d) Change in entropy is given by
$$dS = \frac{dQ}{T} \text{ or } \Delta S = \frac{\Delta Q}{T} = \frac{mL_f}{273}$$
$$\Delta S = \frac{1000 \times 80}{273} = 293\,\text{cal/K}.$$

17. (a) For adiabatic process $Q = 0$.
By first law of thermodynamics,
$Q = \Delta E + W$
$\Rightarrow \Delta E_{int} = -W.$

18. (d) Volume of water does not change, no work is done on or by the system ($W = 0$)
According to first law of thermodynamics
$Q = DU + W$
For Isochoric process $Q = DU$
$\Delta U = \mu c dT = 2 \times 4184 \times 20 = 16.7$ kJ.

19. (a) As we know,
$\Delta Q = \Delta u + \Delta w$ (Ist law of thermodynamics)
$\Rightarrow \Delta Q = \Delta u + P\Delta v$
or $150 = \Delta u + 100(1-2)$
$= \Delta u - 100$
$\therefore \quad \Delta u = 150 + 100 = 250$J
Thus the internal energy of the gas increases by 250 J

20. (c) In adiabatic process
PV^{γ} = constant
$\therefore P\left(\frac{m}{\rho}\right)^{\gamma}$ = constant $\quad \left(\because V = \frac{m}{\rho}\right)$
As mass is constant
$\therefore P \propto \rho^{\gamma}$
If P_i and P_f be the initial and final pressure of the gas and ρ_i and ρ_f be the initial and final density of the gas. Then
$$\frac{P_f}{P_i} = \left(\frac{\rho_f}{\rho_i}\right)^{\gamma} = (32)^{7/5}$$
$$\Rightarrow \frac{nP_i}{P_i} = (2^5)^{7/5} = 2^7$$
$\Rightarrow n = 2^7 = 128.$

21. (b) Bursting of helium balloon is irreversible and in this process $\Delta Q = 0$, so adiabatic.

22. (c)

23. (b) $\Delta U_{ac} = -(\Delta U_{ca}) = -(-180) = 180$ J
$Q = 250 + 60 = 310$ J
Now $Q = \Delta U + W$
or $\quad 310 = 180 + W$
or $\quad W = 130$ J

24. (c) As the process is isochoric so,

$$Q = nc_v\Delta T = \frac{67.2}{22.4}\times\frac{3R}{2}\times 20 = 90R = 90\times 8.31 \simeq 748\text{j}.$$

25. (a) At constant volume
Work done (W) = nRΔT

Heat given $Q = C_v\Delta T + nR\Delta T$

So, $\therefore \frac{W}{Q} = \frac{nR\Delta T}{C_V\Delta T + nR\Delta T} = \frac{nR}{C_V + nR}$

26. (b) We have given,

$$P = P_0\left[1-\frac{1}{2}\left(\frac{V_0}{V}\right)^2\right]$$

When $V_1 = V_0$

$$\Rightarrow P_1 = P_0\left[1-\frac{1}{2}\right] = \frac{P_0}{2}$$

When $V_2 = 2V_0$

$$\Rightarrow P_2 = P_0\left[1-\frac{1}{2}\left(\frac{1}{4}\right)\right] = \left(\frac{7P_0}{8}\right)$$

$$\Delta T = T_2 - T_1 = \left|\frac{P_1V_1}{nR} - \frac{P_2V_2}{nR}\right| \qquad \left[\because T = \frac{PV}{nR}\right]$$

$$\Delta T = \left|\left(\frac{1}{nR}\right)(P_1V_1 - P_2V_2)\right| = \left(\frac{1}{nR}\right)\left|\left(\frac{P_0V_0}{2} - \frac{7P_0V_0}{4}\right)\right|$$

$$= \frac{5P_0V_0}{4nR} = \frac{5P_0V_0}{4R} \qquad (\because n = 1)$$

27. (b) Suppose amount of water evaporated be M gram. Then (150 – M) gram water converted into ice.
so, heat consumed in evoporation = Heat released in fusion
$M \times L_v = (150 - M) \times L_s$
$M \times 2.1 \times 10^6 = (150 - M) \times 3.36 \times 10^5$
$\Rightarrow M - 20$ g

28. (d) a → Isobasic, b → Isothermal, c → Adiabatic, d → Isochoric

29. (b) Equation of adiabatic change is
$TV^{\gamma-1}$ = constant

Put $\gamma = \frac{7}{5}$, we get: $\gamma - 1 = \frac{7}{5} - 1$

$\therefore x = \frac{2}{5}$

30. (b) Work done,

$$W = P\Delta V = nR\Delta T = \frac{1}{2}\times 8.31\times 70 \simeq 291\text{J}$$

31. (d) Work done on gas = nRT $\ell n\left(\frac{p_f}{p_1}\right)$ = R(300) ℓn(2)

$$= 300\ \text{Rln}2 \left(\because \frac{P_f}{p_i} = 2 \text{ given}\right)$$

32. (a) Efficiency of heat engine is given by

$$\eta = \frac{w}{Q} = 1 - \frac{C_V}{C_P} = \frac{R}{C_p} = \frac{R}{\frac{5R}{2}} = \frac{2}{5}$$

$(\because C_p - C_v = R)$

For monoatomic gas $C_P = \frac{5}{2}R$.

33. (a) $\tau = \frac{1}{\sqrt{2}\pi d^2\left(\frac{N}{V}\right)\sqrt{\frac{3RT}{M}}}$

$$\tau \propto \frac{V}{\sqrt{T}}$$

As, $TV^{\gamma-1} = K$
So, $\tau \propto V^{\gamma + 1/2}$

Therefore, $q = \frac{g+1}{2}$

34. (c) **Given :** work done, $W = 830$ J
No. of moles of gas, $\mu = 2$
For diatomic gas $\gamma = 1.4$
Work done during an adiabatic change

$$W = \frac{\mu R(T_1 - T_2)}{\gamma - 1}$$

$$\Rightarrow 830 = \frac{2\times 8.3(\Delta T)}{1.4 - 1} = \frac{2\times 8.3(\Delta T)}{0.4}$$

$$\Rightarrow \Delta T = \frac{830\times 0.4}{2\times 8.3} = 20\text{ K}$$

35. (a)

36. (a)

37. (d) For isothermal process :
$PV = P_i\,.2V$
$P = 2P_i$ ...(i)
For adiabatic process
$PV^{\gamma} = P_a(2V)^{\gamma}$
($\because$ for monatomic gas $\gamma = 5/3$)

or, $2P_iV^{\frac{5}{3}} = P_a(2V)^{\frac{5}{3}}$ [From (i)]

$$\Rightarrow \frac{P_a}{P_i} = \frac{2}{2^{\frac{5}{3}}} \Rightarrow \frac{P_a}{P_i} = 2^{\frac{-2}{3}}$$

38. (c) Efficiency, $\eta = \frac{\text{Work done}}{\text{Heat absorbed}} = \frac{W}{\Sigma Q}$

$$= \frac{Q_1 + Q_2 + Q_3 + Q_4}{Q_1 + Q_3} = 0.5$$

Here, $Q_1 = 1915$ J, $Q_2 = -40$ J and $Q_3 = 125$ J

$$\therefore \frac{1915-40+125+Q_4}{1915+125}=0.5$$

$$\Rightarrow 1915-40+125+Q_4=1020$$

$$\Rightarrow Q_4=1020-2000 \Rightarrow Q_4=-Q=-980 \text{ J}$$

$$\Rightarrow Q=980 \text{ J}$$

39. (d) For carnot refrigerator

$$\text{Efficiency}=\frac{Q_1-Q_2}{Q_1}$$

Where,

Q_1 = heat lost from sorrounding

Q_2 = heat absorbed from reservoir at low temperature.

$$\text{Also, } \frac{Q_1-Q_2}{Q_1}=\frac{w}{Q_1} \Rightarrow \frac{1}{10}=\frac{w}{Q_1} \Rightarrow Q_1=w\times 10=100\,J$$

So, $Q_1-Q_2=w \Rightarrow Q_2=Q_1-w \Rightarrow 100-10=Q_2=90\,J$

40. (b)

41. (b) Using, $n=1-\frac{T_2}{T_1}$

$$n=\frac{1}{6}=1-\frac{T_2}{T_1} \text{ and } \frac{T}{3}=1-\frac{T_2-62}{T_1}$$

On solving, we get

$T_1=99°C$ and $T_2=37°C$

42. (a) Given: Temperature of cold body, T_2 = 250 K temperature of hot body; T_1 = 300 K

Heat received, Q_2 = 500 cal work done, W = ?

$$\text{Efficiency}=1-\frac{T_2}{T_1}=\frac{W}{Q_2+W} \Rightarrow 1-\frac{250}{300}=\frac{W}{Q_2+W}$$

$$W=\frac{Q_2}{5}=\frac{500\times 4.2}{5}J=420 \text{ J}$$

43. (d) Efficiency of engine A, $n_A=\frac{T_1-T_2}{T_1}$

and $n_B=\frac{T_2-T_3}{T_2}$; $T_2=\frac{T_1+T_3}{2}=350\,K$

$$\text{or } \frac{n_A}{n_B}=\frac{\frac{600-350}{600}}{\frac{350-100}{350}}=\frac{7}{12}$$

44. (d) $\Delta H=mL=5\times 336\times 10^3=Q_{sink}$

$$\frac{Q_{sink}}{Q_{source}}=\frac{T_{sink}}{T_{source}}$$

$$\therefore Q_{source}=\frac{T_{source}}{T_{sink}}\times Q_{sink}$$

Energy consumed by freezer

$$\therefore w_{output}=Q_{source}-Q_{sink}=Q_{sink}\left(\frac{T_{source}}{T_{sink}}-1\right)$$

Given: T_{source} = 27°C + 273 = 300K,

T_{sink} = 0°C + 273 = 273 k

$$W_{output}=5\times 336\times 10^3\left(\frac{300}{273}-1\right)=1.67\times 10^5 \text{J}$$

45. (b) Efficiency of carnot engine,

$$\eta=\frac{W}{Q_1}\times 100\% \text{ or, } \eta=\frac{Q_2-Q_1}{Q_1}\times 100\%$$

$$\text{or, } \eta=\frac{1000-600}{1000}\times 100\%=40\%$$

Now, for carnot cycle $\frac{Q_2}{Q_1}=\frac{T_2}{T_1}$

$$\frac{600}{1000}=\frac{T_2}{400} \Rightarrow T_2=\frac{600\times 400}{1000} \quad \therefore T_2=-33°C$$

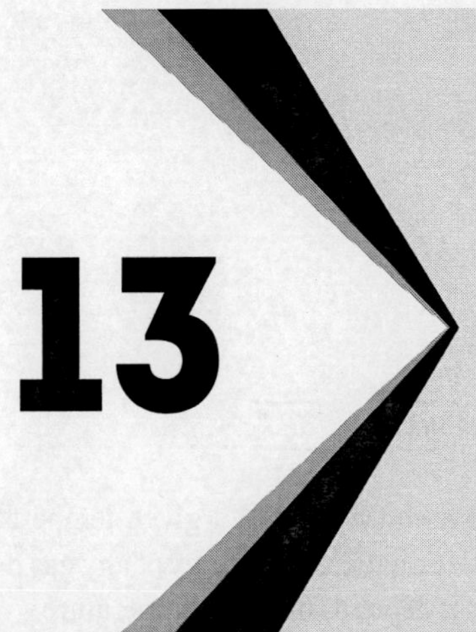

13 Kinetic Theory

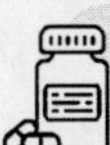

Topic 13.1 : Behaviour of Gases, Kinetic Theory of an Ideal Gas

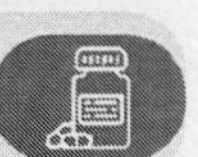

BEHAVIOUR OF GASES

Ideal gas : In an ideal gas, we assume that molecules are point masses and there is no mutual attraction between them. The ideal gas obeys following laws :

(i) **Boyle's law :** According to Boyle's law for a given mass of ideal gas, the pressure of a ideal gas is inveresly proportional to the volume at constant temperature

i.e., $P \propto \frac{1}{V} \Rightarrow PV = \text{constant}$

(ii) **Charle's law :** For a given mass, the volume of a ideal gas is proportional to temperature at a constant pressure

i.e., $V \propto T \Rightarrow \frac{V}{T} = \text{constant}$

(iii) **Gay-Lussac's law :** For a given mass of ideal gas, the pressure is proportional to temperature at constant volume

i.e., $P \propto T \ \frac{P}{T} = \text{constant}$

(iv) **Avogadro's law :** According to Avogadro's law, the number of molecules of all gases are same at same temperature, pressure and volume

i.e., $N_{A_1} = N_{A_2}$ for same P, V and T.

The value of Avagadro number is 6.02×10^{23} molecules.

(v) **Graham's law :**

(a) At constant temperature and pressure, the rms speed of diffusion of two gases is inversely proportional to the square root of the relative density

i.e., $v_{rms} \ \alpha \frac{1}{\sqrt{d}} \Rightarrow \frac{(v_{rms})_1}{(v_{rms})_2} = \sqrt{\frac{d_2}{d_1}}$

(b) According to Graham's law, the rate of diffusion of a gas is inversely proportional to the square root of its density, provided pressure and temperature are constant

$$r(\text{rate of diffusion}) \propto \frac{1}{\sqrt{\rho}}$$

(vi) **Dalton's law:** The pressure exerted by a gaseous mixture is equal to sum of partial pressure of each component gases present in the mixture,

i.e., $P = P_1 + P_2 + P_3 + \ldots\ldots\ldots\ldots P_n$

A relation connecting macroscopic properties P, V and T of a gas describing the state of the system is called **equation of state**.

The equation of state for an ideal gas of n mole is

$$\frac{PV}{T} = nR$$

where R is universal gas constant whose value is R = 8.31 J/mol K and $R = N_A k$, where k is Boltzmann's constant (N_A is Avagadro number). n is the number of moles of a gas and

$$n = \frac{m}{M} = \frac{N}{N_A}, \ N_A \text{ is Avagadro's number}$$

where m is the mass of a gas, N is the number of molecules and M is the molecular weight of a gas.

Equation of Real Gas :

The real gas follows Vander Wall's law. According to this:

$$\left(p + \frac{n^2 a}{V^2}\right)(V - nb) = nRT;$$

here a and b are Vander Wall's constant

Critical Temperature, Volume and Pressure :

(a) The temperature at or below which a gas can be liquefied by applying pressure alone is called **critical temperature**. It is given by $T_c = \frac{8a}{27\,Rb}$

(b) The volume of gas at a critical temperature T_C is called **critical volume** V_C, where $V_C = 3b$

(c) The pressure of gas at a critical temperature T_C is called **critical pressure** P_C, where $P_C = \frac{a}{27b^2}$

Gas Equation

(i) The gases found in nature are real gases.

(ii) The real gas do not obey ideal gas equation but they obey vander wall's gas equation

$$\left(P + \frac{a}{V^2}\right)(V - b) = RT$$

(a) 'a' depends upon the intermolecular force and the nature of gas.
(b) 'b' depends upon the size of the gas molecules and represents the volume occupied by the molecules of the gas.

(iii) The molecules of real gas have potential energy as well as kinetic energy.
(iv) The real gas can be liquefied and solidified.
(v) The real gases like CO_2, NH_3, SO_2 etc. obey Vander Wall's equ^n at high pressure and low temperature.

KINETIC THEORY OF AN IDEAL GAS

The basic assumptions of kinetic theory are :

(i) A gas consist of particles called molecules which move randomly in all directions.
(ii) The volume of molecule is very small in comparison to the volume occupied by gas i.e., the size of molecule is infinitesimely small.
(iii) The collision between two molecules or between a molecule and wall are perfectely elastic and collision time (duration of collision) is very small.
(iv) The molecules exert no force on each other or on the walls of containers except during collision.
(v) The total number of molecules are large and they obey Newtonian mechanics.

$$pV = \frac{1}{3} mn\,\overline{C^2} \qquad ....(i)$$

where $\overline{C^2}$ is called mean square velocity and $\sqrt{\overline{C^2}}$ is called root mean square velocity

i.e, $$\overline{C^2} = \frac{C_1^2 + C_2^2 + ...C_n^2}{n} \qquad ....(ii)$$

and $$v_{r.m.s.} = \sqrt{\overline{C^2}} \qquad ....(iii)$$

where m = mass of one molecule and n = number of molecules

$$\Rightarrow P = \frac{M}{3V}\overline{C^2} = \frac{1}{3}\rho v_{r.m.s}^2 \qquad ....(iv)$$

or $$P = \frac{2}{3}\left[\frac{1}{2}\rho v_{r.m.s}^2\right] \quad \left(\text{where } M = m \times n \text{ and } \rho = \frac{M}{V}\right)$$

or $$P = \frac{2}{3}E \qquad ....(v)$$

where E is translational kinetic energy per unit volume of the gas. It is clear that pressure of ideal gas is equal to 2/3 of translational kinetic energy per unit volume.

Kinetic interpretation of temperature : From eq^n. (iv), we get

$$PV = \frac{1}{3}M\overline{C^2}$$

For 1 mole of a gas at temperature T :

$$PV = RT \text{ so } \frac{1}{3}m\overline{C^2} = RT$$

$$\frac{1}{3}m\overline{C^2} = \frac{R}{N}T = kT \quad \left(k = \frac{R}{N} \text{ is Boltzmann constant}\right)$$

or $$\frac{1}{2}m\overline{C^2} = \frac{3}{2}kT \qquad ....(vi)$$

or $$\frac{1}{2}mv_{r.m.s}^2 = \frac{3}{2}kT$$

or $$v_{r.m.s}^2 = \frac{3kT}{m} \qquad ....(vii)$$

or $$v_{r.m.s} = \sqrt{\frac{3nkT}{nm}} = \sqrt{\frac{3RT}{M}}$$

(a) It is clear from eq.(vi) that at a given temperature, the average translational kinetic energy of any gas molecules are equal i.e., it depends only on temperature.
(b) From eq^n. (vii) It is clear that
 (a) $v_{r.m.s} \propto \sqrt{T}$
 (b) $v_{r.m.s} \propto \frac{1}{\sqrt{M}}$, where M is moleculer mass of the gas.

Example 1.

A gas cylinder of 50 litres capacity contained helium at 80 atmospheric pressure. Due to slow leakage it was found after a while that the pressure had dropped to 40 atmosphere. Find the proportion of the gas that has escaped and also the volume the escaped gas would occupy at atmospheric pressure.

Solution :

Volume of the remaining gas
= volume of cylinder = 50 l at 40 atmospheric pressure
The volume of this gas at 80 atmospheric pressure, using Boyle's law $p_1V_1 = p_2V_2$

$$= \frac{40 \times 50}{80} = 25\,l$$

Volume of the gas (at 80 atmospheric pressure) which has escaped = 50 – 25 = 25 l

$$\therefore \frac{\text{Mass of gas escaped}}{\text{Original mass of gas}} = \frac{25}{50} = \frac{1}{2}$$

Again using Boyle's law,

$$1 \times V = 80 \times 25 \text{ or } V = 2000 \text{ litre}$$

Example 2.

In Vander Wal's equation the critical pressure P_c is given by

(a) 3b (b) $\frac{a}{27b^2}$ (c) $\frac{27a}{b^2}$ (d) $\frac{b^2}{a}$

***Solution :* (b)**

The Vander Wall's equation of state is

$$\left(P + \frac{a}{V^2}\right)(V - b) = RT \text{ ; or } P = \frac{RT}{V-b} - \frac{a}{V^2}$$

At the critical point, $P = P_c$, $V = V_c$, and $T = T_c$;

$$\therefore \quad P_c = \frac{RT_c}{V_c - b} - \frac{a}{V_c^2} \qquad ... (i)$$

At the critical point on the isothermal, $\frac{dP_c}{dV_c} = 0$

$$\therefore 0 = \frac{-RT_c}{(V_c - b)^2} - \frac{2a}{V_c^3} \text{ ; or } \frac{RT_c}{(V_c - b)^2} = \frac{2a}{V_c^3} \qquad ...(ii)$$

Also at critical point, $\frac{d^2P_c}{dV_c^2} = 0$

$$\therefore\ 0 = \frac{2RT_c}{(V_c - b)^3} - \frac{6a}{V_c^4}\ ;\ \text{or}\ \frac{2RT_c}{(V_a - b)^3} = \frac{6a}{V_c^4} \quad ...(iii)$$

Dividing eq^n. (iii) by (ii), we get,

$$\frac{1}{2}(V_c - b) = \frac{1}{3}V_c \text{ or } V_c = 3b \quad ...(iv)$$

Putting this value in eq^n. (ii), we get,

$$\frac{RT}{4b^2} = \frac{2a}{27b^3} \text{ or } T_c = \frac{8a}{27bR} \quad ...(v)$$

Putting the values of V_c and T_c in eq^n. (i), we get,

$$P_c = \frac{R}{2b}\left(\frac{8a}{27bR}\right) - \frac{a}{9b^2} = \frac{a}{27b^2}$$

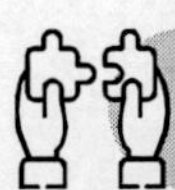
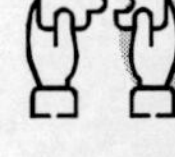

13.1 Concept Practice Problems

CPP

1. The kinetic theory of gases
   (a) explains the behaviour of an ideal gas.
   (b) describes the motion of a single atom or molecule.
   (c) relates the temperature of the gas with K.E. of atoms of the gas
   (d) All of the above
2. In kinetic theory of gases, it is assumed that molecules
   (a) have same mass but can have different volume
   (b) have same volume but mass can be different
   (c) have different mass as well as volume
   (d) have same mass but negligible volume.
3. The adjoining figure shows graph of pressure and volume of a gas at two tempertures T_1 and T_2. Which of the following inferences is correct?

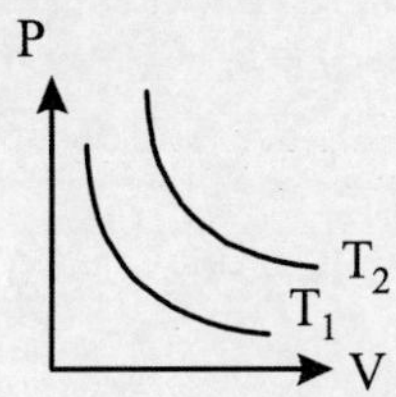

   (a) $T_1 > T_2$ (b) $T_1 = T_2$
   (c) $T_1 < T_2$ (d) None of these
4. At constant pressure, the ratio of increase in volume of an ideal gas per degree rise in kelvin temperature to its original volume is (T = absolute temperature of the gas) is
   (a) T^2 (b) T (c) $1/T$ (d) $1/T^2$
5. The value of critical temperature in terms of van der Waal's constant a and b is given by
   (a) $T_c = \frac{8a}{27Rb}$ (b) $T_c = \frac{a}{27bR}$
   (c) $T_c = \frac{a}{2Rb}$ (d) $T_c = \frac{-a}{Rb}$
6. The perfect gas equation for 4 gram of hydrogen gas is
   (a) PV = RT (b) PV = 2RT
   (c) PV = $\frac{1}{2}$RT (d) PV = 4RT
7. According to kinetic theory of gases, which one of the following statement is correct?
   (a) Real gas behave as ideal gas at high temperature and low pressure.
   (b) Liquid state of ideal gas is impossible
   (c) At any temerature and pressure, ideal gas obeys Boyle's law and charles' law
   (d) The molecules of real gas do not exert any force on one another.
8. If the critical temperature of a gas is 100°C, its Boyle temperature will be approximately
   (a) 337.5°C (b) 500°C (c) 33.3°C (d) 1000°C
9. If pressure of a gas contained in a closed vessel is increased by 0.4% when heated by 1°C, the initial temperature must be
   (a) 250 K (b) 250°C (c) 2500 K (d) 25°C
10. In Vander Waal's equation the critical pressure P_c is given by
   (a) 3 b (b) $\frac{a}{27b^2}$ (c) $\frac{27a}{b^2}$ (d) $\frac{b^2}{a}$

ANSWER KEY

1	(d)	2	(d)	3	(c)	4	(c)	5	(a)	6	(b)	7	(d)	8	(a)	9	(a)	10	(b)

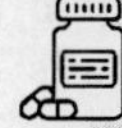

Topic 13.2 : Degree of Freedom, Mean Free Path, Law of Equipartition of Energy, Average, Root Mean Square and Most Probable Speed

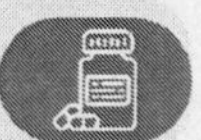

DEGREE OF FREEDOM

The degree of freedom of a particle is the number of independent modes of exchanging energy or *the number of idependent motion, which the particle can undergo.*

For **monatomic** (such as helium, argon, neon etc.) gas the molecules can have three independent motion i.e., it has *3 degree of freedom, all translational.*

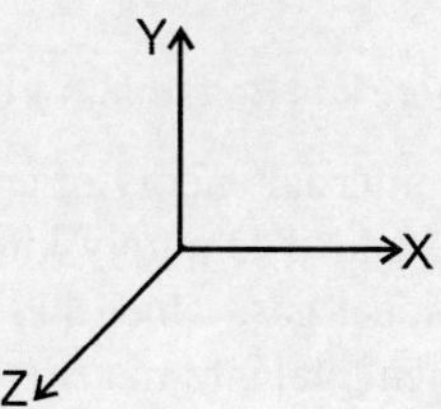

For a **diatomic gas** molecules such as H_2, O_2, N_2, etc. it has two independent rotational motion besides of three independent translational motion, so it has *5 degree of freedom.*

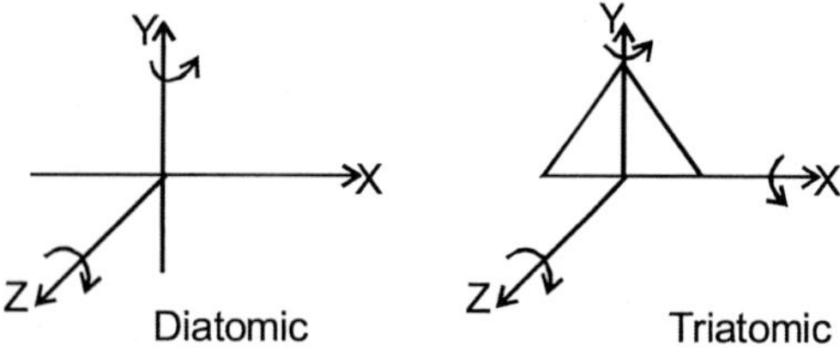

Diatomic Triatomic

In **polyatomic gas** molecules such as CO_2, it can rotate about any of three coordinate axes. It has *six degree (three translational +three rotational) of freedom.* At high temperature the molecule can vibrate also and degree of freedom due to vibration also arises, but we neglect it.

MEAN FREE PATH

The distance covered by the molecules between two successive collisions is called the **free path.**

The average distance covered by the molecules between two successive collisions is called the ***mean free path***

i.e., $\lambda = \dfrac{1}{\sqrt{2}\,.\,\pi n d^2} = \dfrac{K_B T}{\sqrt{2}\pi d^2 P}$

where, n = number of molecules per unit volume

d = diameter of each molecule

K_B = Boltzmann's constant

T = temperature

P = pressure

Mean free path depends on the diameter of molecule (d) and the number of molecules per unit volume n.

At N.T.P., λ for air molecules is 0.01 μm.

LAW OF EQUIPARTITION OF ENERGY

If we dealing with a large number of particles in thermal equilibrium to which we can apply Newtonian mechanics, the energy associated with each degree of freedom has the same average value (i.e., $\frac{1}{2}$kT*), and this average value depends on temperature.*

From the kinetic theory of monatomic ideal gas, we have

$$\frac{1}{2}m\overline{C^2} = \frac{3}{2}kT \quad ....(i)$$

or

Energy of molecule

$$= \textit{(number of degree of freedom)} \times \frac{1}{2}\text{kT} \quad ....(ii)$$

So it is clear from equation (i) and (ii) that monatomic gas has three degree of freedom and energy associated per degree of freedom is $\frac{1}{2}$kT (where k is Boltzmann's constant)

Since we know that internal energy of an ideal gas depends only on temperature and it is purely kinetic energy. Let us consider an 1 mole ideal gas, which has N molecules and f degree of freedom, then total internal energy

U = (total number of molecules)

× (degree of freedom of one molecule)

× (energy associated with each degree of freedom)

$= (N)\,(f) \times (\frac{1}{2}\text{kT})$

$$U = Nf\frac{1}{2}\text{kT} \quad ....(iii)$$

Differentiating eq.(iii) w.r.t T, at constant volume, we get,

$$\left(\frac{\partial U}{\partial T}\right)_V = \frac{NfK}{2} \quad ....(iv)$$

Now **molar, specific heat at constant volume** is defined as

$$C_V = \left(\frac{\partial Q}{\partial T}\right)_V = \left(\frac{\partial U}{\partial T}\right)_V \quad ....(v)$$

so $$C_V = \frac{NfK}{2} = \frac{fR}{2} \quad ....(vi)$$

where R is universal gas constant.

Now by **Mayer's formula,**

$$C_P - C_V = R \Rightarrow C_P = R\left(1+\frac{f}{2}\right) \quad ... (vii)$$

So ratio of specific heat $\gamma = \frac{C_P}{C_V}$ is $\gamma = 1 + \frac{2}{f} = \frac{C_P}{C_V}$ ...(viii)

where f is degree of freedom of one molecule.

(a) **For monatomic gas,** $f = 3$, $C_v = \frac{3}{2}R$, $C_p = \frac{5}{2}R$

so $\gamma = 1 + \frac{2}{3} = 1.67$

(b) **For diatomic gas,** $f = 5$, $C_v = \frac{5}{2}R$, $C_p = \frac{7}{2}R$

$\gamma = 1 + \frac{2}{5} = 1.4$

(c) **For Polyatomic gas,** $f = 6$, $C_v = 3R$, $C_p = 4R$

$\gamma = 1 + \frac{2}{6} = 1.33$

Problem Solving Tips

1. **Real gases** behave like perfect gas at **high temperature** and **low pressure.**

   In real gas, we assume that the molecules have finite size ant intermolecular attraction acts between them.

2. Real gases deviate most from the perfect gas at high pressure and low temperature.

3. Gaseous state of matter below critical temperature is called vapours. Below critical temperature gas is vapour and above critical temperature vapour is gas.

4. Random motion of the consituents of the system involving exchange of energy due to mutual collisions is called **thermal motion**.

5. Total kinetic energy or internal energy or total energy does not depend on the direction of flow of heat. It is determined by the temperature alone.

6. The internal energy of a perfect gas consists only of kinetic energy of the molecules. But in case of the real gas it consists of both the kinetic energy and potential energy of inter molecular configuration.

Distribution of Molecular Speeds :

The speed of all molecules in a gas is not same but speeds of individual molecules vary over a wide range of magnitude.

Maxwell derived the molecular distribution law (by which we can find distribution of molecules in different speeds) for sample of a gas containing N molecules, which is

$$N(v) = 4\pi N\left(\frac{m}{2\pi kT}\right)^{3/2} v^2 e^{-mv^2/2kT} \quad ...(1)$$

where N(v)dv is the number of molecules in the gas sample having speeds between v and v + dv.

where T = absolute temperature of the gas

m = mass of molecule

k = Boltzmann's constant

The total number of molecules N in the gas can be find out by integrating eqation (1) from 0 to ∞ i.e.,

$$N = \int_0^\infty N(v)dv \quad ....(2)$$

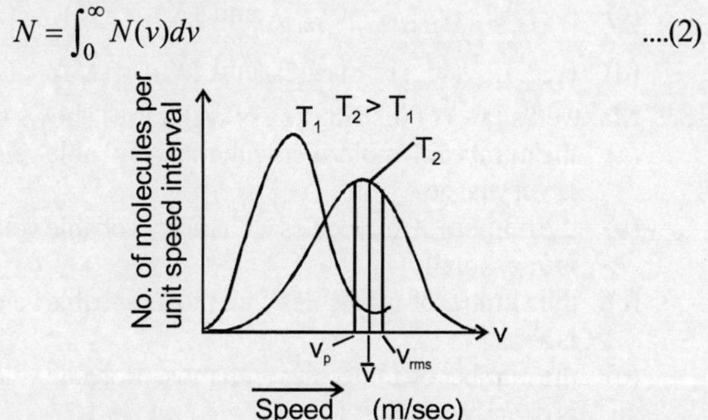

Figure shows Maxwell distribution law for molecules at two different temperature T_1 and $T_2(T_2 > T_1)$.

The number of molecules between v_1 and v_2 equals the area under the curve between the vertical lines at v_1 and v_2 and the total number of molecules as given by equation (2) is equal to area under the distribution curve.

The distribution curve is not symmetrical about most probable speed, v_P,(v_P is the speed, which is possesed in a gas by a large number of molecules) because the lowest speed must be zero, whereas there is no limit to the upper speed a molecule can attain. It is clear from fig.1 that

v_{rms}(root mean square) > $\bar{v}$ (average speed of molecules) > (most probable speed) v_P

AVERAGE, ROOT MEAN SQUARE AND MOST PROBABLE SPEED

Average speed

To find the average speed $\bar{v}$, we multiply the number of particles in each speed interval by speed v characteristic of that interval. We sum these products over all speed intervals and divide by total number of particles

i.e., $\bar{v} = \frac{\int_o^\infty N(v)vdv}{N}$ (where summation is replaced by integration because N is large)

$$h\bar{v} = \sqrt{\frac{8kT}{\pi m}} = 1.59\sqrt{\frac{kT}{m}} \quad ....(1)$$

Root Mean Square Speed

In this case we multiply the number of particles in each speed interval by v^2 characterstic of that interval; sum of these products over all speed interval and divide by N

$$\text{i.e., } \overline{v^2} = \frac{\int_o^\infty N(v)v^2dv}{N} \quad ....(2)$$

Root mean square speed is defined as

$$v_{r.m.s} = \sqrt{\overline{v^2}} = \sqrt{\frac{3kT}{m}} = 1.73\sqrt{\frac{kT}{m}}$$

Most Probable Speed

It is the speed at which N(v) has its maximum value (or possessed by large number of molecules), so

$$\frac{d}{du}[N(v)] = 0 \text{ Þ } v_p = \sqrt{\frac{2kT}{m}} = 1.41\sqrt{\frac{kT}{m}} \quad ....(3)$$

It is clear from eq^n. (1), (2) and (3)

$$v_{r.m.s} > \bar{v} > v_p$$

The root mean square velocity of a particle in thermal system is given by

$$C_{rms} = \sqrt{\frac{3RT}{M}} = \sqrt{\frac{3kT}{m}}$$

where R - universal gas constant

T - temperature of gas

m - mass of the gas

M - molecular weight of gas or mass of one mole of a gas.

The average speed of the gas molecules is given by

$$C_{av} = \sqrt{\frac{8kT}{\pi m}} = \sqrt{\frac{8RT}{\pi M}}$$

where M is the mass of one mole and m is the mass of one particle.

Most probable speed is that with which the maximum number of molecules move. It is given by

$$V_p = \sqrt{\frac{2}{3}} c_{rms} = \sqrt{\frac{2RT}{M}} = \sqrt{\frac{2kT}{m}}$$

The most probable speed, the average speed as well as root mean square speed increases with temperature.

Example 3.

The root mean square velocity of the molecules in a sample of helium is 5/7th that of the molecules in a samzple of hydrogen. If the temperature of the hydrogen gas is 0°c, then find the temperature of helium sample.

Solution :

$$\frac{(v_{r.m.s})_{He}}{(v_{r.m.s})_H} = \frac{\sqrt{(3KT_{He}/m_{He})}}{\sqrt{3KT_H/m_H}} = \sqrt{\frac{T_{He}}{T_H} \times \frac{m_H}{m_{He}}}$$

$$= \sqrt{\frac{T_{He} \times 1}{273 \times 4}} \Rightarrow \frac{5}{7} = \frac{1}{2}\sqrt{\frac{T_{He}}{273}}$$

or $T_{He} = 557.14°K = 284.14°C$

Example 4.

Let $\overline{v}$, v_{rms} and v_p *respectively denote the mean speed, r.m.s. speed, and most probable speed of the molecules in an ideal monatomic gas at absolute temperature T. The mass of a molecule is m, then which of the following is correct ?*

(a) No molecule can have a speed greater than $\sqrt{2}\,v_{max}$

(b) No molecule can have a speed less than $v_p/\sqrt{2}$

(c) $v_p < \overline{v} < v_{r.m.s.}$

(d) None of these

Solution : (c)

According to kinetic theory of gases, a molecule of a gas can have speed such that $0 < v < \infty$, so the alternatives (a) and (b) can never be correct, Since

$$v_{r.m.s.} = \sqrt{\frac{3kT}{m}};\ v_{av} = \sqrt{\frac{8kT}{3m}}\ ;\ \text{and}\ \ v_{mp} = \sqrt{\frac{2kT}{m}}$$

so $v_{r.m.s.} > v_{av} > v_p$ i.e. $v_p < \overline{v} < v_{r.m.s.}$;

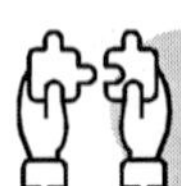

13.2 Concept Practice Problems

CPP

11. The correct statement of the law of equipartition of energy is

(a) the total energy of a gas is equally divided among all the molecules.

(b) The gas possess equal energies in all the three directions *x*,*y* and *z*-axis.

(c) the total energy of a gas is equally divided between kinetic and potential energies.

(d) the total kinetic energy of a gas molecules is equally divided among translational and rotational kinetic energies.

12. The ratio of principal molar heat capacities of a gas is maximum for

(a) a diatomic gas

(b) a monatomic gas

(c) a polyatomic gas having linear molecules.

(d) a polyatomic gas having non-linear molecules.

13. For a gas if ratio of specific heats at constant pressure and volume is γ then value of degrees of freedom is

(a) $\frac{3\gamma-1}{2\gamma-1}$ (b) $\frac{2}{\gamma-1}$ (c) $\frac{9}{2}(\gamma-1)$ (d) $\frac{25}{2}(\gamma-1)$

14. A gas mixture consists of molecules of type 1, 2 and 3, with molar masses $m_1 > m_2 > m_3$. v_{rms} and $\bar{K}$ are the r.m.s. speed and average kinetic energy of the gases. Which of the following is true?

(a) $(v_{rms})_1 < (v_{rms})_2 < (v_{rms})_3$ and $(\bar{K})_1 = (\bar{K})_2 = (\bar{K})_3$

(b) $(v_{rms})_1 = (v_{rms})_2 = (v_{rms})_3$ and $(\bar{K})_1 = (\bar{K})_2 > (\bar{K})_3$

(c) $(v_{rms})_1 > (v_{rms})_2 > (v_{rms})_3$ and $(\bar{K})_1 < (\bar{K})_2 > (\bar{K})_3$

(d) $(v_{rms})_1 > (v_{rms})_2 > (v_{rms})_3$ and $(\bar{K})_1 < (\bar{K})_2 < (\bar{K})_3$

15. Maxwell's laws of distribution of velocities shows that

(a) the number of molecules with most probable velocity is very large

(b) the number of molecules with most probable velocity is very small

(c) the number of molecules with most probable velocity is zero

(d) the number of molecules with most probable velocity is exactly equal to 1

16. For hydrogen gas $C_p - C_v = a$ and for oxygen gas $C_p - C_v = b$. So, the relation between a and b is given by

(a) a = 16 b(b) 16 a = b (c) a = 4 b (d) a = b

17. The gases are at absolute temperature 300°K and 350°K respectively. The ratio of average kinetic energy of their molecules is

(a) 7 : 6 (b) 6 : 7 (c) 36 : 49 (d) 49 : 36

18. The total degree of freedom of a CO_2 gas molecule is

(a) 3 (b) 6 (c) 5 (d) 4

19. Four molecules have speeds 2 km/sec, 3 km/sec, 4 km/sec and 5 km/sec. The root mean square speed of these molecules (in km/sec) is

(a) $\sqrt{54/4}$ (b) $\sqrt{54/2}$ (c) 3.5 (d) $3\sqrt{3}$

20. How many degrees of freedom are associated with 2 grams of He at NTP ?

(a) 3 (b) 3.01×10^{23} (c) 9.03×10^{23} (d) 6

ANSWER KEY

11	(b)	12	(b)	13	(b)	14	(a)	15	(a)	16	(d)	17	(b)	18	(c)	19	(a)	20	(c)

Problem Solving Tips

1. Brownian motion, provides a direct evidence for the existance of molecules and their motion. The zig-zag motion of gas molecules is Brownian motion.

2. Average speed $\overline{v} = \sqrt{\frac{8k_BT}{\pi m}} = \sqrt{\frac{8RT}{\pi M}} = \sqrt{\frac{8PV}{\pi M}}$

3. Root mean square speed,
$$v_{rms} = \sqrt{\frac{3k_BT}{m}} = \sqrt{\frac{3RT}{M}} = \sqrt{\frac{3PV}{M}}$$

4. Most probable speed $V_{mp} = \sqrt{\frac{2k_BT}{m}} = \sqrt{\frac{2RT}{M}} = \sqrt{\frac{2PV}{M}}$

5. $V_{rms} : \overline{V} : V_{mp} = 1.73 : 1.60 : 1.41$
$V_{rms} > \overline{V} > V_{mp}$.

CONCEPT MAP

KINETIC THEORY

Boyle's Law: $P \propto \frac{1}{V}$
PV=constant (If T=constant)
or, $P_1V_1 = P_2V_2$

Charle's Law: $V \propto T$
$\frac{V}{T}$ = constant (If P = constant)
or, $\frac{V_1}{T_1} = \frac{V_2}{T_2}$

Gay Lussac's Law: $P \propto T$
$\frac{P}{T}$ = constant (If V = constant)
or, $\frac{P_1}{T_1} = \frac{P_2}{T_2}$

Behaviour of Gases
An ideal gas satisfies, equation PV = nRT at all Pressure and temperatures
n = no. of moles, $R = N_A k_B$
universal gas constant

Dalton's Law of Partial Pressure
Total pressure of a mixture of non-reacting gases, $P = P_1 + P_2 + ... + P_n$

Avogadro's Law
Under the same condition of temperature and pressure equal volumes of all gases contain equal no. of molecules
i.e., $N_1 = N_2$

Pressure exerted by a gas
$$P = \frac{1}{3}\rho v_{rms}^2$$

Relation between Pressure (P) and Kinetic energy (E)
$$E = \frac{3}{2}PV$$

Degree of freedom (f)
For monatomic gas: f=3
For diatomic gas:
(i) at room temperature, f=5
(ii) at high temperature, f=7
For polyatomic gas:
(i) at room temperature, f=6
(ii) at high temperature, f=8

Mean free Path
$$\lambda = \frac{1}{\sqrt{2}\pi n d^2} = \frac{k_\beta T}{\sqrt{2}\pi d^2 P}$$

Assumptions of Kinetic Theory of Gases

- All the molecules of a gas are identical.
- The molecules of different gases are different.
- The molecules of gases are in a state of random motion.
- The collisions of gases molecules are perfectly elastic

Law of Equipartion of Energy
Energy associated with each degree of freedom per molecule
$$= \frac{1}{2}kT$$

Root Mean Square Speed
$$v_{rms} = \sqrt{\frac{3PV}{M}} = \sqrt{\frac{3P}{\rho}} = \sqrt{\frac{3RT}{M}}$$

Average Speed
$$v_{av} = \frac{v_1 + v_3 + v_3 + ... + v_N}{N}$$
$$v_{av} = \sqrt{\frac{8RT}{\pi M}} = \left(\sqrt{\frac{8}{3\pi}}\right) v_{rms} = 0.92\, v_{rms}$$

Most Probable speed
$$v_{mp} = \sqrt{\frac{2RT}{M}} = \left(\sqrt{\frac{2}{3}}\right) v_{rms} = 0.816\, v_{rms}$$

Specific heat capacity
for an ideal gas, $C_P - C_V = R$

for monatomic $\frac{C_P}{C_V} = \gamma = \frac{5}{3}$

for diatomic $\frac{C_P}{C_V} = \gamma = \frac{7}{5}$

for polyatomic gases, $\frac{C_P}{C_V} = \gamma = \frac{(4+f)}{(3+f)}$

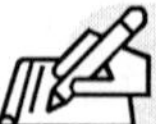

Exercise 1 - Chapter Revision Problems

CRP

1. The internal energy of an ideal gas is
   (a) the sum of total kinetic and potential energies.
   (b) the total translational kinetic energy.
   (c) the total kinetic energy of randomly moving molecules.
   (d) the total kinetic energy of gas molecules.
2. A fixed mass of gas at constant pressure occupies a volume V. The gas undergoes a rise in temperature so that the root mean square velocity of its molecules is doubled. The new volume will be
   (a) V/2 (b) $V/\sqrt{2}$ (c) 2V (d) 4V
3. Gases exert pressure on the walls of the container because the gas molecules
   (a) possess momentum (b) collide with each other
   (c) have finite volume (d) obey gas laws.
4. Let v denote the rms speed of the molecules in an ideal diatomic gas at absolute temperature T.
   The mass of a molecule is 'm' Neglecting vibrational energy terms, the false statement is
   (a) a molecule can have a speed greater than $\sqrt{2}v$
   (b) v is proportional to $\sqrt{T}$
   (c) the average rotational K.E. of a molecule is $\frac{1}{4}mv^2$
   (d) the average K.E. of a molecule is $\frac{5}{6}mv^2$
5. The K.E. of one mole of an ideal gas is E = (3/2) RT. Then C_p will be
   (a) 0.5 R (b) 0.1 R (c) 1.5 R (d) 2.5 R
6. The root mean square speed of the molecules of a diatomic gas is v. When the temperature is doubled, the molecules dissociate into two atoms. The new root mean square speed of the atom is
   (a) $\sqrt{2}$v (b) v (c) 2v (d) 4v
7. Which of the following formula is wrong?
   (a) $C_V = \frac{R}{\gamma - 1}$ (b) $C_P = \frac{\gamma R}{\gamma - 1}$
   (c) $C_p / C_V = \gamma$ (d) $C_p - C_V = 2R$
8. In the kinetic theory of gases, which of these statements is/are true ?
   (i) The pressure of a gas is proportional to the mean speed of the molecules.
   (ii) The root mean square speed of the molecules is proportional to the pressure.
   (iii) The rate of diffusion is proportional to the mean speed of the molecules.
   (iv) The mean translational kinetic energy of a gas is proportional to its kelvin temperature.
   (a) (ii) and (iii) only (b) (i),(ii)and (iv) only
   (c) (i) and (iii) only (d) (iii) and (iv) only
9. A sample of an ideal gas occupies a volume of V at a pressure P and absolute temperature. T. The mass of each molecule is m. The equation for density is
   (a) mkT (b) P/kT
   (c) P/(kTV) (d) Pm/kT
10. At room temperature, the rms speed of the molecules of a certain diatomic gas is found to be 1930 m/s. The gas is
    (a) H_2 (b) F_2 (c) O_2 (d) Cl_2
11. Two gases A and B having the same temperature T, same pressure P and same volume V are mixed. If the mixture is at the same temperature T and occupies a volume V, the pressure of the mixture is
    (a) 2P (b) P (c) P/2 (d) 4P
12. The relation between the gas pressure P and average kinetic energy per unit volume E is
    (a) $P = \frac{1}{2}E$ (b) $P = E$
    (c) $P = \frac{3}{2}E$ (d) $P = \frac{2}{3}E$
13. The r.m.s. velocity of oxygen molecule at 16°C is 474 m/sec. The r.m.s. velocity in m/s of hydrogen molecule at 127°C is
    (a) 1603 (b) 1896 (c) 2230.59 (d) 2730
14. If one mole of a monatomic gas ($\gamma = 5/3$) is mixed with one mole of a diatomic gas ($\gamma = 7/3$), the value of γ for the mixture is
    (a) 1.40 (b) 1.50 (c) 1.53 (d) 3.07
15. If masses of all molecule of a gas are halved and their speed doubled then the ratio of initial and final pressure will be
    (a) 2 : 1 (b) 1 : 2 (c) 4 : 1 (d) 1 : 4
16. The velocity of the molecules of a gas at temperature 120 K is v. At what temperature will the velocity be 2 v?
    (a) 120 K (b) 240 K (c) 480 K (d) 1120 K
17. One mole of a gas occupies 22.4 lit at N.T.P. Calculate the difference between two molar specific heats of the gas. J = 4200 J/kcal.
    (a) 1.979 k cal/kmol K (b) 2.378 k cal/kmol K
    (c) 4.569 kcal/kmol K (d) 3.028 k cal/ kmol K
18. The density of air at pressure of 10^5 Nm^{-2} is 1.2 kg m^{-3}. Under these conditions, the root mean square velocity of the air molecules in ms^{-1} is
    (a) 500 (b) 1000 (c) 1500 (d) 3000
19. At what temperature is the r.m.s. velocity of a hydrogen molecule equal to that of an oxygen molecule at 47°C
    (a) 80 K (b) –73 K (c) 3 K (d) 20 K
20. To what temperature should be the hydrogen at 327°C be cooked at constant pressure so that the root mean square velocity of its molecules becomes half of its previous value
    (a) –123°C (b) 120°C (c) –100°C (d) 0°C

21. At what temperature, pressure remaining constant, will the r.m.s. velocity of a gas be half of its value at 0°C?
(a) 0°C (b) –273°C (c) 32°C (d) –204°C

22. Graph of specific heat at constant volume for a monatomic gas is

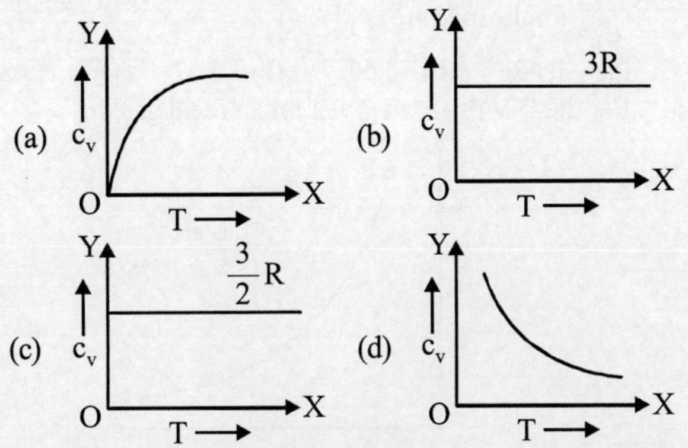

23. The order of magnitude of the number of nitrogen molecules in an air bubble of diameter 2 mm under ordinary conditions is
(a) 10^5 (b) 10^9 (c) 10^{13} (d) 10^{17}

24. 1 mole of a gas with $\gamma = 7/5$ is mixed with 1 mole of a gas with $\gamma = 5/3$, then the value of γ for the resulting mixture is
(a) 7/5 (b) 2/5 (c) 24/16 (d) 12/7

25. A gas mixture consists of 2 moles of oxygen and 4 moles of Argon at temperature T. Neglecting all vibrational moles, the total internal energy of the system is
(a) 4 RT (b) 15 RT (c) 9 RT (d) 11RT

26. The molar heat capacities of a mixture of two gases at constant volume is 13R/6. The ratio of number of moles of the first gas to the second is 1 : 2. The respective gases may be
(a) O_2 and N_2 (b) He and Ne
(c) He and N_2 (d) N_2 and He

27. A graph is plotted with PV/T on y-axis and mass of the gas along x-axis for different gases. The graph is
(a) a straight line parallel to x-axis for all the gases
(b) a straight line passing through origin with a slope having a constant value for all the gases
(c) a straight line passing through origin with a slope having different values for different gases
(d) a straight line parallel to y-axis for all the gases

28. Four mole of hydrogen, two mole of helium and one mole of water vapour form an ideal gas mixture. What is the molar specific heat at constant pressure of mixture?
(a) $\frac{16}{7}R$ (b) $\frac{7}{16}R$ (c) R (d) $\frac{23}{7}R$

29. An ideal gas is taken through a process in which the pressure and the volume are changed according to the equation P = kV. Molar heat capacity of the gas for the process is
(a) $C = C_v + R$ (b) $C = C_v + \frac{R}{2}$
(c) $C = C_v - \frac{R}{2}$ (d) $C = C_v + 2R$

30. A vessel has 6g of hydrogen at pressure P and temperature 500K. A small hole is made in it so that hydrogen leaks out. How much hydrogen leaks out if the final pressure is P/2 and temperature falls to 300 K?
(a) 2g (b) 3g (c) 4g (d) 1g

31. Which one the following graphs represents the behaviour of an ideal gas?

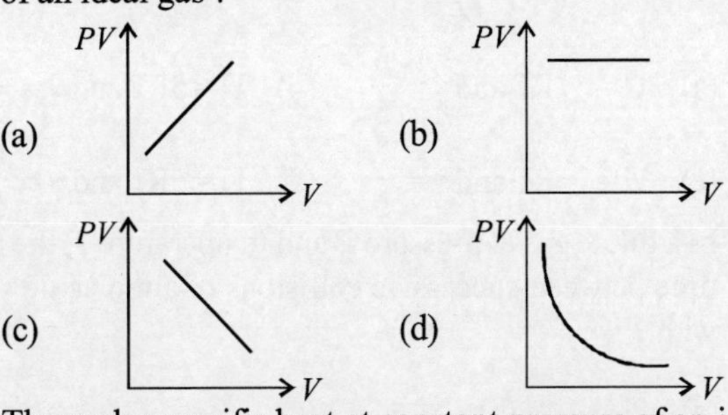

32. The molar specific heat at constant pressure of an ideal gas is (7/2)R. The ratio of specific heat at constant pressure to that at constant volume is
(a) 5/7 (b) 9/7 (c) 7/5 (d) 8/7

33. The number density of molecules of a gas depends on their distance r from the origin as, $n(r) = n_0 e^{-\alpha r^4}$. Then the total number of molecules is proportional to :
(a) $n_0\alpha^{-3/4}$ (b) $\sqrt{n_0}\,\alpha^{1/2}$ (c) $n_0\alpha^{1/4}$ (d) $n_0\alpha^{-3}$

34. A vertical closed cylinder is separated into two parts by a frictionless piston of mass m and of negligible thickness. The piston is free to move along the length of the cylinder. The length of the cylinder above the piston is l_1, and that below the piston is l_2, such that $l_1 > l_2$. Each part of the cylinder contains n moles of an ideal gas at equal temperature T. If the piston is stationary, its mass, m, will be given by: (R is universal gas constant and g is the acceleration due to gravity)
(a) $\frac{RT}{ng}\left[\frac{l_1 - 3l_2}{l_1 l_2}\right]$ (b) $\frac{RT}{g}\left[\frac{2l_1 + l_2}{l_1 l_2}\right]$
(c) $\frac{nRT}{g}\left[\frac{1}{l_2} + \frac{1}{l_1}\right]$ (d) $\frac{nRT}{g}\left[\frac{l_1 - l_2}{l_1 l_2}\right]$

35. Cooking gas containers are kept in a lorry moving with uniform speed. The temperature of the gas molecules inside will
(a) increase (b) decrease (c) remain same
(d) decrease for some, while increase for others

36. For a given gas at 1 atm pressure, rms speed of the molecules is 200 m/s at 127°C. At 2 atm pressure and at 227°C, the rms speed of the molecules will be:
(a) 100 m/s (b) $80\sqrt{5}$ m/s
(c) $100\sqrt{5}$ m/s (d) 80 m/s

37. A mixture of 2 moles of helium gas (atomic mass = 4u), and 1 mole of argon gas (atomic mass = 40u) is kept at 300 K in a container. The ratio of their rms speeds
$\left[\frac{V_{rms}(\text{helium})}{V_{rms}(\text{argon})}\right]$ is close to :
(a) 3.16 (b) 0.32 (c) 0.45 (d) 2.24

38. Molecules of an ideal gas are known to have three translational degrees of freedom and two rotational degrees of freedom. The gas is maintained at a temperature of T.
The total internal energy, U of a mole of this gas, and the value of $\gamma\left(=\frac{C_p}{C_v}\right)$ are given, respectively, by:

(a) $U=\frac{5}{2}RT$ and $\gamma=\frac{6}{5}$ (b) $U=5RT$ and $\gamma=\frac{7}{5}$
(c) $U=\frac{5}{2}RT$ and $\gamma=\frac{7}{5}$ (d) $U=5RT$ and $\gamma=\frac{6}{5}$

39. In a dilute gas at pressure *P* and temperature *T*, the mean time between successive collisions of a molecule varies with *T* is :
(a) T (b) $\frac{1}{\sqrt{T}}$ (c) $\frac{1}{T}$ (d) $\sqrt{T}$

40. To raise the temperature of a certain mass of gas by 50°C at a constant pressure, 160 calories of heat is required. When the same mass of gas is cooled by 100°C at constant volume, 240 calories of heat is released. How many degrees of freedom does each molecule of this gas have (assume gas to be ideal)?
(a) 5 (b) 6 (c) 3 (d) 7

41. An ideal gas in a closed container is slowly heated. As its temperature increases, which of the following statements are true?
(1) The mean free path of the molecules decreases
(2) The mean collision time between the molecules decreases
(3) The mean free path remains unchanged
(4) The mean collision time remains unchanged
(a) (2) and (3) (b) (1) and (2)
(c) (3) and (4) (d) (1) and (4)

42. Consider a mixture of *n* moles of helium gas and 2*n* moles of oxygen gas (molecules taken to be rigid) as an ideal gas. Its C_P/C_V value will be:
(a) 19/13 (b) 67/45 (c) 40/27 (d) 23/15

43. The plot that depicts the behavior of the mean free time τ (time between two successive collisions) for the molecules of an ideal gas, as a function of temperature (*T*), qualitatively, is: (Graphs are schematic and not drawn to scale)

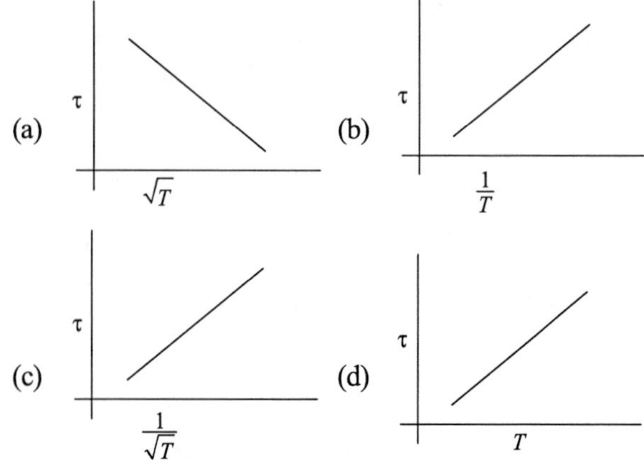

44. Two moles of an ideal gas with $\frac{C_p}{C_V}=\frac{5}{3}$ are mixed with 3 moles of another ideal gas with $\frac{C_p}{C_V}=\frac{4}{3}$. The value of $\frac{C_p}{C_V}$ for the mixture is:
(a) 1.45 (b) 1.50 (c) 1.47 (d) 1.42

45. For the P-V diagram given for an ideal gas,

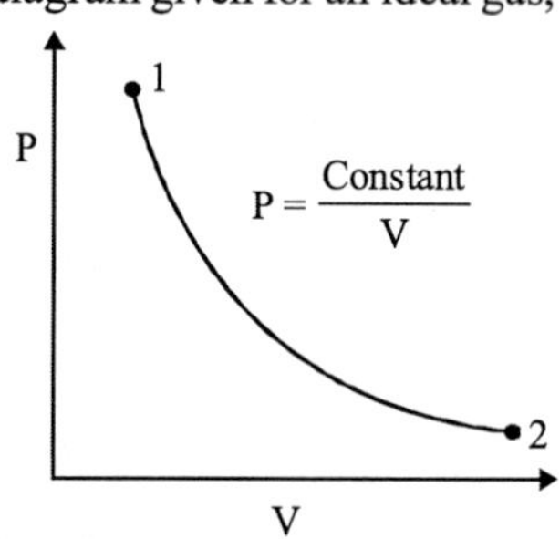

out of the following which one correctly represents the T-P diagram ?

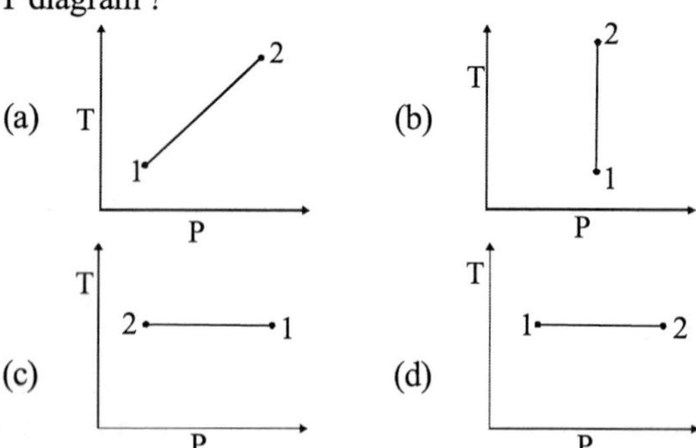

46. In the isothermal expansion of 10g of gas from volume V to 2V the work done by the gas is 575J. What is the root mean square speed of the molecules of the gas at that temperature?
(a) 398m/s (b) 520m/s (c) 499m/s (d) 532m/s

47. A perfect gas at 27°C is heated at constant pressure so as to double its volume. The final temperature of the gas will be, close to
(a) 327°C (b) 200°C (c) 54°C (d) 300°C

48. One kg of a diatomic gas is at a pressure of $8\times10^4 N/m^2$. The density of the gas is $4 kg/m^3$. What is the energy of the gas due to its thermal motion?
(a) 5×10^4 J (b) 6×10^4 J (c) 7×10^4 J (d) 3×10^4 J

49. Three perfect gases at absolute temperatures T_1, T_2 and T_3 are mixed. The masses of molecules are m_1, m_2 and m_3 and the number of molecules are n_1, n_2 and n_3 respectively. Assuming no loss of energy, the final temperature of the mixture is :

(a) $\frac{n_1T_1+n_2T_2+n_3T_3}{n_1+n_2+n_3}$ (b) $\frac{n_1T_1^2+n_2T_2^2+n_3T_3^2}{n_1T_1+n_2T_2+n_3T_3}$

(c) $\frac{n_1^2T_1^2+n_2^2T_2^2+n_3^2T_3^2}{n_1T_1+n_2T_2+n_3T_3}$ (d) $\frac{(T_1+T_2+T_3)}{3}$

50. Using equipartition of energy, the specific heat (in J kg^{-1} K^{-1}) of aluminium at room temperature can be estimated to be (atomic weight of aluminium = 27)
(a) 410 (b) 25 (c) 1850 (d) 925

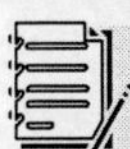

Exercise 2 - Exemplar & Past Year Questions

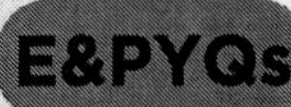

Exemplar Questions

1. A cubic vessel (with face horizontal + vertical) contains an ideal gas at NTP. The vessel is being carried by a rocket which is moving at a speed of 500 m s^{-1} in vertical direction. The pressure of the gas inside the vessel as observed by us on the ground
(a) remains the same because 500 ms^{-1} is very much smaller than v_{rms} of the gas
(b) remains the same because motion of the vessel as a whole does not affect the relative motion of the gas molecules and the walls
(c) will increase by a factor equal to $(v_{rms}^2 + (500)^2)/v_{rms}^2$ where v_{rms} was the original mean square velocity of the gas
(d) will be different on the top wall and bottom wall of the vessel

2. Boyle's law is applicable for an
(a) adiabatic process (b) isothermal process
(c) isobaric process (d) isochoric process

3. A cylinder containing an ideal gas is in vertical position and has a piston of mass M that is able to move up or down without friction (figure). If the temperature is increased
(a) both p and V of the gas will change
(b) only p will increase according to Charles' law
(c) V will change but not p
(d) p will change but not V

4. 1 mole of H_2 gas is contained in a box of volume $V = 1.00$ m^3 at T=300 K. The gas is heated to a temperature of T= 3000 K and the gas gets converted to a gas of hydrogen atoms. The final pressure would be (considering all gases to be ideal)
(a) same as the pressure initially
(b) 2 times the pressure initially
(c) 10 times the pressure initially
(d) 20 times the pressure initially

5. A vessel of volume V contains a mixture of 1 mole of hydrogen and 1 mole oxygen (both considered as ideal). Let $f_1(v)dv$, denote the fraction of molecules with speed between v and $(v + dv)$ with $f_2(v)dv$, similarly for oxygen. Then,
(a) $f_1(v) + f_2(v) = f(v)$ obeys the Maxwell's distribution law
(b) $f_1(v), f_2(v)$ will obey the Maxwell's distribution law separately
(c) neither $f_1(v)$, nor $f_2(v)$ will obey the Maxwell's distribution law
(d) $f_2(v)$ and $f_1(v)$ will be the same

6. An inflated rubber balloon contains one mole of an ideal gas, has a pressure p, volume V and temperature T. If the temperature rises to 1.1 T, and the volume is increased to 1.05 V, the final pressure will be
(a) 1.1p (b) p
(c) less than p (d) between p and 1.1

NEET/AIPMT (2013-2020) Questions

7. In the given (V – T) diagram, what is the relation between pressure P_1 and P_2 ? *[2013]*

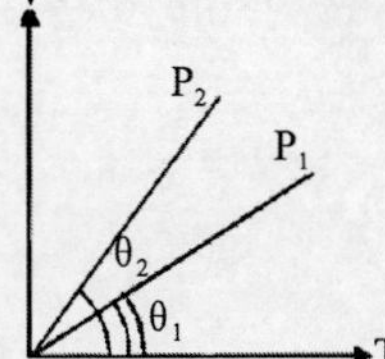

(a) $P_2 > P_1$
(b) $P_2 < P_1$
(c) Cannot be predicted
(d) $P_2 = P_1$

8. The amount of heat energy required to raise the temperature of 1g of Helium at NTP, from T_1K to T_2K is *[2013]*
(a) $\frac{3}{2}N_a k_B(T_2 - T_1)$ (b) $\frac{3}{4}N_a k_B(T_2 - T_1)$
(c) $\frac{3}{4}N_a k_B\frac{T_2}{T_1}$ (d) $\frac{3}{8}N_a k_B(T_2 - T_1)$

9. In a vessel, the gas is at a pressure P. If the mass of all the molecules is halved and their speed is doubled, then the resultant pressure will be *[NEET Kar. 2013]*
(a) 4P (b) 2P (c) P (d) P/2

10. The mean free path of molecules of a gas, (radius 'r') is inversely proportional to : *[2014]*
(a) r^3 (b) r^2 (c) r (d) $\sqrt{r}$

11. The ratio of the specific heats $\frac{C_p}{C_v} = \gamma$ in terms of degrees of freedom (n) is given by *[2015]*
(a) $\left(1+\frac{n}{3}\right)$ (b) $\left(1+\frac{2}{n}\right)$ (c) $\left(1+\frac{n}{2}\right)$ (d) $\left(1+\frac{1}{n}\right)$

12. The molecules of a given mass of a gas have r.m.s. velocity of 200 ms^{-1} at 27°C and 1.0×10^5 Nm^{-2} pressure. When the temperature and pressure of the gas are respectively, 127°C and 0.05×10^5 Nm^{-2}, the r.m.s. velocity of its molecules in ms^{-1} is : *[2016]*
(a) $100\sqrt{2}$ (b) $\frac{400}{\sqrt{3}}$ (c) $\frac{100\sqrt{2}}{3}$ (d) $\frac{100}{3}$

13. A gas mixture consists of 2 moles of O_2 and 4 moles of Ar at temperature T. Neglecting all vibrational modes, the total internal energy of the system is : *[2017]*
(a) 15 RT (b) 9 RT (c) 11 RT (d) 4 RT

14. At what temperature will the rms speed of oxygen molecules become just sufficient for escaping from the Earth's atmosphere?
(Given : Mass of oxygen molecule (m) = 2.76×10^{-26} kg
Boltzmann's constant $k_B = 1.38 \times 10^{-23}$ JK^{-1}) *[2018]*
(a) 2.508×10^4 K (b) 8.360×10^4 K
(c) 1.254×10^4 K (d) 5.016×10^4 K

15. Increase in temperature of a gas filled in a container would lead to: *[2019]*
(a) increase in its mass
(b) increase in its kinetic energy
(c) decrease in its pressure
(d) decrease in intermolecular distance

16. The value of $\gamma = \left(\dfrac{C_p}{C_v}\right)$, for hydrogen, helium and another ideal diatomic gas *X* (whose molecules are not rigid but have an additional vibrational mode), are respectively equal to, *[NEET Odisha 2019]*
(a) $\frac{7}{5},\frac{5}{3},\frac{7}{5}$ (b) $\frac{7}{5},\frac{5}{3},\frac{9}{7}$ (c) $\frac{5}{3},\frac{7}{5},\frac{9}{7}$ (d) $\frac{5}{3},\frac{7}{5},\frac{7}{5}$

17. A cylinder contains hydrogen gas at pressure of 249 kPa and temperature 27°C. *[2020]*
Its density is : (R = 8.3 J mol^{-1} K^{-1})
(a) 0.2 kg/m^3 (b) 0.1 kg/m^3
(c) 0.02 kg/m^3 (d) 0.5 kg/m^3

18. The mean free path for a gas, with molecular diameter d and number density n can be expressed as : *[2020]*
(a) $\frac{1}{\sqrt{2}n\pi d^2}$ (b) $\frac{1}{\sqrt{2}n^2\pi d^2}$ (c) $\frac{1}{\sqrt{2}n^2\pi^2 d^2}$ (d) $\frac{1}{\sqrt{2}n\pi d}$

Exercise 3 - Concept Application Problems

CAP

1. The molecules of a given mass of gas have a root mean square velocity of 200m s^{-1} at 27°C and 1.0×10^5 N m^{-2} pressure. When the temperature is 127°C and the pressure 0.5×10^5 Nm^{-2}, the root mean square velocity in ms^{-1}, is
(a) $\frac{400}{\sqrt{3}}$ (b) $100\sqrt{2}$ (c) $\frac{100\sqrt{2}}{3}$ (d) $\frac{100}{3}$

2. On a particular day, the relative humidity is 100% and the room temperature is 30°C, then the dew point is
(a) 70°C (b) 30°C (d) 100°C (d) 0°C

3. The density of a gas is 6×10^{-2} kg/m^3 and the root mean square velocity of the gas molecules is 500 m/s. The pressure exerted by the gas on the walls of the vessel is
(a) $5\times10^3\,N/m^2$ (b) $1.2\times10^{-4}\,N/m^2$
(c) $0.83\times10^{-4}\,N/m^2$ (d) $30\,N/m^2$

4. The temperature of the mixture of one mole of helium and one mole of hydrogen is increased from 0°C to 100°C at constant pressure. The amount of heat delivered will be
(a) 600 cal (b) 1200 cal (c) 1800 cal (d) 3600 cal

5. Helium gas is filled in a closed vessel (having negligible thermal expansion coefficient) when it is heated from 300 K to 600 K, then average kinetic energy of helium atom will be
(a) $\sqrt{2}$ times (b) 2 times
(c) unchanged (d) half

6. If 2 mole of an ideal monatomic gas at temperature T_0 is mixed with 4 moles of another ideal monatomic gas at temperature $2T_0$, then the temperature of the mixture is
(a) $\frac{5}{3}T_0$ (b) $\frac{3}{2}T_0$ (c) $\frac{4}{3}T_0$ (d) $\frac{5}{4}T_0$

7. The temperature at which the root mean square velocity of the gas molecules would become twice of its value at 0°C is
(a) 819°C (b) 1092°C (c) 1100°C (d) 1400°C

8. One litre of oxygen at a pressure of 1 atm, and 2 litres of nitrogen at a pressure of 0.5 atm. are introduced in the vessel of 1 litre capacity, without any change in temperature. The total pressure would be
(a) 1.5 atm. (b) 0.5 atm. (c) 2.0 atm. (d) 1.0 atm.

9. The air in a room has 15 gm of water vapours per cubic metre of its volume. However for saturation one cubic metre of volume requires 20 gm of water vapour then relative humidity is
(a) 50% (b) 75% (c) 20% (d) 25%

10. A vessel contains air at a temperature of 15°C and 60% R.H. What will be the R.H. if it is heated to 20°C? (S.V.P. at 15°C is 12.67 & at 20°C is 17.36mm of Hg respectively)
(a) 262% (b) 26.2% (c) 44.5% (d) 46.2%

11. N molecules, each of mass m, of gas A and 2 N molecules, each of mass 2 m, of gas B are contained in the same vessel which is maintained at a temperature T. The mean square of the velocity of molecules of B type is denoted by v^2 and the mean square of the X component of the velocity of A type is dentoed by ω^2, ω^2/v^2 is
(a) 2 (b) 1 (c) 1/3 (d) 2/3

12. At identical temperatures, the rms speed of hydrogen molecules is 4 times that for oxygen molecules. In a mixture of these in mass ratio $H_2 : O_2 = 1:8$, the rms speed of all molecules is n times the rms speed for O_2 molecules, where n is
(a) 3 (b) 4/3 (c) $(8/3)^{1/2}$ (d) $(11)^{1/2}$

13. N molecules, each of mass m, of gas A and 2 N molecules, each of mass 2 m, of gas B are contained in the same vessel which is maintained at a temperature T. The mean square velocity of molecules of B type is denoted by V_2 and the mean square velocity of A type is denoted by V_1, then $\frac{V_1}{V_2}$ is
(a) 2 (b) 1 (c) 1/3 (d) 2/3

14. An ideal gas is found to obey an additional law VP^2 = constant. The gas is initially at temperature T and volume V. When it expands to a volume 2 V, the temperature becomes

(a) $T/\sqrt{2}$ (b) 2T (c) $2T\sqrt{2}$ (d) 4T

15. Two monatomic ideal gases 1 and 2 of molecular masses m_1 and m_2 respectively are enclosed in separate containers kept at the same temperature. The ratio of the speed of sound in gas 1 to that in gas 2 is given by

(a) $\sqrt{\frac{m_1}{m_2}}$ (b) $\sqrt{\frac{m_2}{m_1}}$ (c) $\frac{m_1}{m_2}$ (d) $\frac{m_2}{m_1}$

16. If the potential energy of a gas molecule is $U = M/r^6 - N/r^{12}$, M and N being positive constants, then the potential energy at equilibrium must be

(a) zero (b) $M^2/4N$ (c) $N^2/4M$ (d) $MN^2/4$

17. Air is pumped into an automobile tube upto a pressure of 200 kPa in the morning when the air temperature is 22°C. During the day, temperature rises to 42°C and the tube expands by 2%. The pressure of the air in the tube at this temperature, will be approximately

(a) 212 kPa (b) 209 kPa (c) 206 kPa (d) 200 kPa

18. Work done by a system under isothermal change from a volume V_1 to V_2 for a gas which obeys Vander Waal's equation $(V-\beta n)\left(P+\frac{\alpha n^2}{V}\right) = nRT$ is

(a) $nRT\log_e\left(\frac{V_2-n\beta}{V_1-n\beta}\right)+\alpha n^2\left(\frac{V_1-V_2}{V_1V_2}\right)$

(b) $nRT\log_{10}\left(\frac{V_2-n\beta}{V_1-n\beta}\right)+\alpha n^2\left(\frac{V_1-V_2}{V_1V_2}\right)$

(c) $nRT\log_e\left(\frac{V_2-n\beta}{V_1-n\beta}\right)+\beta n^2\left(\frac{V_1-V_2}{V_1V_2}\right)$

(d) $nRT\log_e\left(\frac{V_1-n\beta}{V_2-n\beta}\right)+\alpha n^2\left(\frac{V_1V_2}{V_1-V_2}\right)$

19. Figure shows a parabolic graph between T and 1/V for a mixture of a gas undergoing an adiabatic process. What is the ratio of V_{rms} of molecules and speed of sound in mixture?

(a) $\sqrt{3/2}$

(b) $\sqrt{2}$

(c) $\sqrt{2/3}$

(d) $\sqrt{3}$

T
$2T_0$
T_0
$1/V_0$ $4/V_0$
1/V

20. Number of molecules in a volume of 4 cm^3 of a perfect monoatomic gas at some temperature T and at a pressure of 2 cm of mercury is close to? (Given, mean kinetic energy of a molecule (at T) is 4×10^{-14} erg, $g = 980$ cm/s^2, density of mercury = 13.6 g/cm^3)

(a) 4.0×10^{18} (b) 4.0×10^{16}
(c) 5.8×10^{16} (d) 5.8×10^{18}

21. If 10^{22} gas molecules each of mass 10^{-26} kg collide with a surface (perpendicular to it) elastically per second over an area 1 m^2 with a speed 10^4 m/s, the pressure exerted by the gas molecules will be of the order of :

(a) 10^4 N/m^2 (b) 10^8 N/m^2
(c) 10^3 N/m^2 (d) 10^{16} N/m^2

22. The temperature, at which the root mean square velocity of hydrogen molecules equals their escape velocity from the earth, is closest to :
[Boltzmann Constant $k_B = 1.38 \times 10^{-23}$ J/K
Avogadro Number $N_A = 6.02 \times 10^{26}$ /kg
Radius of Earth : 6.4×10^6 m
Gravitational acceleration on Earth = 10 ms^{-2}]

(a) 800 K (b) 3×10^5 K (c) 10^4 K (d) 650 K

23.

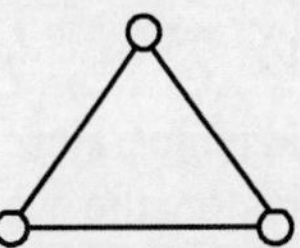

Consider a gas of triatomic molecules. The molecules are assumed to be triangular and made of massless rigid rods whose vertices are occupied by atoms. The internal energy of a mole of the gas at temperature T is :

(a) $\frac{5}{2}RT$ (b) $\frac{3}{2}RT$ (c) $\frac{9}{2}RT$ (d) $3RT$

24. A gas mixture consists of 3 moles of oxygen and 5 moles of argon at temperature T. Assuming the gases to be ideal and the oxygen bond to be rigid, the total internal energy (in units of RT) of the mixture is :

(a) 15 (b) 13 (c) 20 (d) 11

25. Consider two ideal diatomic gases A and B at some temperature T. Molecules of the gas A are rigid, and have a mass m. Molecules of the gas B have an additional vibrational mode, and have a mass $\frac{m}{4}$. The ratio of the specific heats (C_V^A and C_V^B) of gas A and B, respectively is:

(a) 7 : 9 (b) 5 : 9 (c) 3 : 5 (d) 5 : 7

26. Two gases-argon (atomic radius 0.07 nm, atomic weight 40) and xenon (atomic radius 0.1 nm, atomic weight 140) have the same number density and are at the same temperature. The ratio of their respective mean free times is closest to:

(a) 3.67 (b) 1.83 (c) 2.3 (d) 4.67

27. An ideal gas is enclosed in a cylinder at pressure of 2 atm and temperature, 300 K. The mean time between two successive collisions is 6×10^{-8} s. If the pressure is doubled and temperature is increased to 500 K, the mean time between two successive collisions wiil be close to:

(a) 2×10^{-7} s (b) 4×10^{-8} s
(c) 0.5×10^{-8} s (d) 3×10^{-6} s

28. A gas mixture consists of 3 moles of oxygen and 5 moles of argon at temperature T. Considering only translational and rotational modes, the total internal energy of the system is :
(a) 15 RT (b) 12 RT (c) 4 RT (d) 20 RT

29. Two moles of an ideal monoatomic gas occupies a volume V at 27°C. The gas expands adiabatically to a volume 2 V. Calculate (1) the final temperature of the gas and (2) change in its internal energy.
(a) (1) 189 K (2) 2.7 kJ
(b) (1) 195 K (2) –2.7 kJ
(c) (1) 189 K (2) –2.7 kJ
(d) (1) 195 K (2) 2.7 kJ

30. N moles of a diatomic gas in a cylinder are at a temperature T. Heat is supplied to the cylinder such that the temperature remains constant but n moles of the diatomic gas get converted into monoatomic gas. What is the change in the total kinetic energy of the gas ?
(a) $\frac{1}{2}$nRT (b) 0 (c) $\frac{3}{2}$nRT (d) $\frac{5}{2}$nRT

31. In an ideal gas at temperature T, the average force that a molecule applies on the walls of a closed container depends on T as T^q. A good estimate for q is:
(a) $\frac{1}{2}$ (b) 2 (c) 1 (d) $\frac{1}{4}$

32. Modern vacuum pumps can evacuate a vessel down to a pressure of 4.0×10^{-15} atm. at room temperature (300 K). Taking $R = 8.0\ JK^{-1}\ mole^{-1}$, 1 atm = 10^5 Pa and $N_{Avogadro} = 6 \times 10^{23}\ mole^{-1}$, the mean distance between molecules of gas in an evacuated vessel will be of the order of:
(a) 0.2 μm (b) 0.2 mm (c) 0.2 cm (d) 0.2 nm

33. A gas molecule of mass M at the surface of the Earth has kinetic energy equivalent to 0°C. If it were to go up straight without colliding with any other molecules, how high it would rise? Assume that the height attained is much less than radius of the earth. (k_B is Boltzmann constant).
(a) 0 (b) $\frac{273k_B}{2Mg}$ (c) $\frac{546k_B}{3Mg}$ (d) $\frac{819k_B}{2Mg}$

34. An ideal gas occupies a volume of 2 m^3 at a pressure of 3×10^6 Pa. The energy of the gas:]
(a) 9×10^6 J (b) 6×10^4 J (c) 10^8 J (d) 3×10^2 J

35. In a process, temperature and volume of one mole of an ideal monoatomic gas are varied according to the relation VT = K, where K is a constant. In this process the temperature of the gas is increased by ΔT. The amount of heat absorbed by gas is (R is gas constant) :
(a) $\frac{1}{2}R\Delta T$ (b) $\frac{1}{2}KR\Delta T$ (c) $\frac{3}{2}R\Delta T$ (d) $\frac{2K}{3}\Delta T$

36. Two kg of a monoatomic gas is at a pressure of 4×10^4 N/m^2. The density of the gas is 8 kg/m^3. What is the order of energy of the gas due to its thermal motion?
(a) 10^3 J (b) 10^5 J (c) 10^4 J (d) 10^6 J

37. A 15 g mass of nitrogen gas is enclosed in a vessel at a temperature 27°C. Amount of heat transferred to the gas, so that rms velocity of molecules is doubled, is about: [Take R = 8.3 J/K mole]
(a) 0.9 kJ (b) 6 kJ (c) 10 kJ (d) 14 kJ

38. Two moles of an ideal monoatomic gas occupies a volume V at 27°C. The gas expands adiabatically to a volume 2 V. Calculate (1) the final temperature of the gas and (2) change in its internal energy.
(a) (1) 189 K (2) 2.7 kJ
(b) (1) 195 K (2) –2.7 kJ
(c) (1) 189 K (2) –2.7 kJ
(d) (1) 195 K (2) 2.7 kJ

39. Two moles of helium are mixed with n with moles of hydrogen. If $\frac{C_P}{C_V} = \frac{3}{2}$ for the mixture, then the value of n is
(a) 3/2 (b) 2 (c) 1 (d) 3

40. The specific heats, C_p and C_v of a gas of diatomic molecules, A, are given (in units of J mol^{-1} k^{-1}) by 29 and 22, respectively. Another gas of diatomic molecules, B, has the corresponding values 30 and 21. If they are treated as ideal gases, then:
(a) A is rigid but B has a vibrational mode.
(b) A has a vibrational mode but B has none.
(c) A has one vibrational mode and B has two.
(d) Both A and B have a vibrational mode each.

41. An HCl molecule has rotational, translational and vibrational motions. If the rms velocity of HCl molecules in its gaseous phase is $\bar{v}$, m is its mass and k_B is Boltzmann constant, then its temperature will be:
(a) $\frac{m\bar{v}^2}{6k_B}$ (b) $\frac{m\bar{v}^2}{3k_B}$ (c) $\frac{m\bar{v}^2}{7k_B}$ (d) $\frac{m\bar{v}^2}{5k_B}$

42. When heat Q is supplied to a diatomic gas of rigid molecules, at constant volume its temperature increases by ΔT. The heat required to produce the same change in temperature, at a constant pressure is :
(a) $\frac{2}{3}Q$ (b) $\frac{5}{3}Q$ (c) $\frac{7}{5}Q$ (d) $\frac{3}{2}Q$

43. A 25×10^{-3} m^3 volume cylinder is filled with 1 mol of O_2 gas at room temperature (300 K). The molecular diameter of O_2, and its root mean square speed, are found to be 0.3 nm and 200 m/s, respectively. What is the average collision rate (per second) for an O_2 molecule?
(a) $\sim 10^{12}$ (b) $\sim 10^{11}$ (c) $\sim 10^{10}$ (d) $\sim 10^{13}$

44. A diatomic gas with rigid molecules does 10 J of work when expanded at constant pressure. What would be the heat energy absorbed by the gas, in this process ?
(a) 25 J (b) 35 J (c) 30 J (d) 40 J

45. Two moles of helium gas is mixed with three moles of hydrogen molecules (taken to be rigid). What is the molar specific heat of mixture at constant volume? (R = 8.3 J/mol K)
(a) 19.7 J/mol L (b) 15.7 J/mol K
(c) 17.4 J/mol K (d) 21.6 J/mol K

Hints & Solutions

13.1 Concept Practice Problems (CPP)

1. (d) 2. (d)
3. (c) For a given pressure, volume will be more if temperature is more (Charle's law)
From the graph it is clear that $V_2 > V_1 \Rightarrow T_1 > T_2$

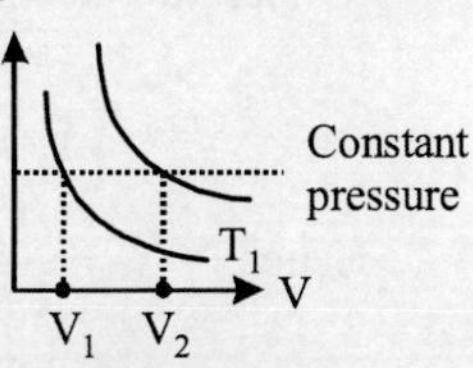

4. (c) At constant pressure $V \propto T \Rightarrow \frac{\Delta V}{V} = \frac{\Delta T}{T}$
Hence ratio of increase in volume per degree rise in kelvin temperature to it's origianl volume
$= \frac{(\Delta V / \Delta T)}{V} = \frac{1}{T}$
5. (a)
6. (b) $n = \frac{4}{2} = 2$
7. (a, b, c)
8. (a) Boyle temperature is defined as
$$T_B = \frac{a}{Rb} = \frac{27}{8}\left(\frac{8a}{27Rb}\right) = \frac{27}{8}T_c = 3.375\,T_c$$
$= 3.375 \times 100 = 337.5°C$
9. (a) $\frac{P_1V_1}{T_1}$ = constant for one mole
& $\frac{P_1}{T_1}$ = constant for constant volume
so $\frac{P_1}{T_1} = \frac{1.004P_1}{(T_1+1)} \Rightarrow T_1 = 250K$
10. (b) The Vander waal's equation of state is
$$\left(P + \frac{a}{V^2}\right)(V-b) = RT \text{ or } P = \frac{RT}{V-b} - \frac{a}{V^2}$$
At the critical point, $P = P_c$, $V = V_c$, and $T = T_c$
$$\therefore \quad P_c = \frac{RT_c}{V_c - b} - \frac{a}{V_c^2} \quad ....(i)$$
At the critical point on the isothermal, $\frac{dP_c}{dV_c} = 0$
$$\therefore \quad 0 = \frac{-RT_c}{(V_c-b)^2} + \frac{2a}{V_c^3} \text{ or } \frac{RT_c}{(V_c-b)^2} = \frac{2a}{V_c^3} \quad ....(ii)$$
Also at critical point, $\frac{d^2P_c}{dV_c^2} = 0$
$$\therefore \quad 0 = \frac{2RT_c}{(V_c-b)^3} - \frac{6a}{V_c^4} \text{ or } \frac{2RT_c}{(V_c-b)^3} = \frac{6a}{V_c^4} \quad ..(iii)$$
Dividing (ii) by (iii), we get
$$\frac{1}{2}(V_c - b) = \frac{1}{3}V_c \text{ or } V_c = 3b \quad ....(iv)$$
Putting this value in (ii), we get
$$\frac{RTc}{4b^2} = \frac{2a}{27b^3} \text{ or } T_c = \frac{8a}{27bR} \quad ...(v)$$
Putting the values of V_c and T_c in (i), we get
$$P_c = \frac{R}{2b}\left(\frac{8a}{27bR}\right) - \frac{a}{9b^2} = \frac{a}{27b^2}$$

13.2 Concept Practice Problems (CPP)

11. (b) Gas possess equal energies in x, y and z-directions.
12. (b)
13. (b) $\gamma = 1 + \frac{2}{f}, \Rightarrow \gamma - 1 = \frac{2}{f} \Rightarrow \frac{f}{2} = \frac{1}{\gamma - 1} \Rightarrow f = \frac{2}{\gamma - 1}$
14. (a) $v_{rms} \propto \frac{1}{\sqrt{M}} \Rightarrow (v_{rms})_1 < (v_{rms})_2 < (v_{rms})_3$ also in mixture temperature of each gas will be same, hence kinetic energy also remains same.
15. (a) Based on Maxwell's velocity distribution curve.
16. (d) Both are diatomic gases and $C_p - C_v = R$ for all gases.
17. (b) 18. (c)
19. (a) $v_{rms} = \left[\frac{(2)^2 + (3)^2 + (4)^2 + (5)^2}{4}\right]^{1/2} = \sqrt{\left[\frac{54}{4}\right]}$
20. (c) Moles of He $= \frac{2}{4} = \frac{1}{2}$
Molecules $= \frac{1}{2} \times 6.02 \times 10^{23} = 3.01 \times 10^{23}$
As there are 3 degrees of freedom corresponding to 1 molecule of a monatomic gas.
$\therefore$ Total degrees of freedom $= 3 \times 3.01 \times 10^{23}$
$= 9.03 \times 10^{23}$

Exercise 1 - Chapter Revision Problems (CRP)

1. (d) Total kinetic energy of gas molecules is the internal energy of an ideal gas.
2. (d) Since v_{rms} is doubled by increasing the temp. so by $v_{rms} = \sqrt{\frac{3KT}{m}}$, the temp. increase by four times.
Now for constant pressure $\frac{V_1}{T_1} = \frac{V_2}{T_2}$
$V_1 = V$, $T_1 = T°K$, $T_2 = 4T°K$, $V_2 = ?$
$V_2 = 4V$
3. (a) 4. (c)
5. (d) $C_v = dE/dT = \frac{3}{2}R$
$C_p = \frac{3}{2}R + R = \frac{5}{2}R = 2.5R$
6. (c) $v_{rms} = \sqrt{\frac{3RT}{M}}$. According to problem T will become 2T and M will becomes M/2 so the value of v_{rms} will increase by $\sqrt{4} = 2$ times i.e. new root mean square velocity will be 2v.
7. (d) The difference of C_P and C_V is equal to R, not $2R$.
8. (d)

9. (d) We know that $PV = nRT = (m/M)RT$
where M = Molecular weight.

Now $P \times \left(\frac{m}{d}\right) = \left(\frac{m}{M}\right)RT$

where d = density of the gas

$$\frac{P}{d} = \frac{RT}{M} = \frac{kN_AT}{M} \quad ...(2)$$

where $R = kN_A$, k is Boltzmann constant.

But $\frac{M}{N_A} = m$ = mass of each molecule so

$$d = \frac{P \times m}{kT}$$

10. (a) For one mole of gas $v_{rms} = \sqrt{\frac{3RT}{M}}$

$$1930 = \sqrt{\frac{3 \times 8.31 \times 300}{M}} \Rightarrow M = 2 \times 10^{-3}\text{ kg} = 2\text{ g}$$

So that di-atomic gas is hydrogen.

11. (a) Here, initially $P_1 = P, V_1 = V + V = 2V$;
Finally, $P_2 = P; V_2 = V$
As $P_1V_1 = P_2V_2$ or $P_2 = \frac{P_1V_1}{V} = \frac{P \times 2V}{V} = 2P$

12. (d) $P = \frac{2}{3}E$

13. (c) $v_{oxg.} = \sqrt{\frac{3R \times 289}{32}}$ $\left(v_{rms} = \sqrt{\frac{3RT}{M}}\right)$

$v_H = \sqrt{\frac{3R \times 400}{2}}$ so $v_H = 2230.59$ m/sec

14. (c) Let γ_1 and γ_2 denote the ratio of two specific heats of gas 1 and gas 2 respectively when they are mixed in the ratio of n_1 and n_2 mole. The resultant value of γ is the weighted mean of γ_1 and γ_2 i.e.,

$$\gamma = \frac{n_1\gamma_1 + n_2\gamma_2}{n_1 + n_2} = \frac{1(5/3) + 1(7/5)}{1+1}$$

$$= \frac{25 + 21}{15 \times 2} = \frac{46}{30} = 1.53$$

15. (b) Since $P = \frac{1}{3}\frac{mNv_{rms}^2}{V}$

since m is halved & speed is doubled so pressure become twice.

16. (c) $v \propto \sqrt{T}$ $\quad \therefore \frac{v'}{v} = \sqrt{\frac{T'}{T}}$

Given $v' = 2v$ or, $\frac{2}{1} = \sqrt{\frac{T'}{T}}$

$\therefore T' = 4T = 4 \times 120K = 480K$

17. (a) $V = 22.4$ litre $= 22.4 \times 10^{-3}\text{ m}^3$, $J = 4200$ J/kcal
by ideal gas equation for one mole of a gas,

$$R = \frac{PV}{T} = \frac{1.013 \times 10^5 \times 22.4 \times 10^{-3}}{273}$$

$$C_p - C_v = \frac{R}{J} = \frac{1.013 \times 10^5 \times 22.4}{273 \times 4200} = 1.979\text{ kcal/kmol K}$$

18. (a) $c = \sqrt{\frac{3P}{\rho}} = \sqrt{\frac{3 \times 10^5}{1.2}} = 500\text{ ms}^{-1}$

19. (d) The r.m.s. velocity of the molecule of a gas of molecular weight M at Kelvin temperature T is given by,

$$v_{r.m.s.} = \sqrt{\frac{3RT}{M}}$$

Let M_O and M_H are molecular weight of oxygen and hydrogen and T_O and T_H the corresponding Kelvin temperature at which $v_{r.m.s.}$ is same for both,

$$v_{r.m.s.} = \sqrt{\frac{3RT_O}{M_O}} = \sqrt{\frac{3RT_H}{M_H}}$$

Hence, $\frac{T_O}{M_O} = \frac{T_H}{M_H}$

$T_o = 273° + 47° = 320\text{ K}, M_o = 32, M_H = 2$

$T_H = \frac{2}{32} \times 320 = 20\text{ K}$

20. (a) $\frac{(v_{rms})_2}{(v_{rms})_1} = \sqrt{\frac{t+273}{327+273}}$ or $\frac{1}{2} = \sqrt{\frac{t+273}{600}}$

or $t = -123°C$

21. (d) $v_{rms} \propto \sqrt{T}$

At 0°C, $v_{rms} \propto \sqrt{273}$

At temp. T, $\frac{v_{rms}}{2} \propto \sqrt{T}$

$\therefore \frac{1}{2} = \frac{\sqrt{T}}{\sqrt{273}}$ or $T = \frac{273}{4} = 68.2\text{ K} \simeq 69\text{K}$

$T = 69 - 273 = -204°C$

22. (c) For a monatomic gas

$C_v = \frac{3}{2}R$

So correct graph is

23. (d) Molar volume = 22400 cm^3

Bubble volume $= \frac{4}{3}\pi\frac{d^3}{8} = \frac{4}{3}\pi 10^{-3}$

No. of molecules $= \frac{6 \times 10^{23} \times 4\pi 10^{-3}}{22400 \times 3} \approx 10^{17}$

24. (c) γ for resulting mixture should be in between 7/5 and 5/3.

25. (d) Internal energy of 2 moles of oxygen

$Uo_2 = \mu\left(\frac{5}{2}RT\right) = 2.\frac{5}{2}RT = 5RT$

Internal energy of 4 moles of Argon.

$U_{Ar} = \mu\left(\frac{3}{2}RT\right) = 4.\frac{3}{2}RT = 6RT$

$\therefore$ Total internal energy

$U = U_{O_2} + U_{Ar} = 11RT$

26. (c) $C_{v_{mix}} = \frac{n_1C_{v_1} + n_2C_{v_2}}{n_1 + n_2}$

$\Rightarrow \frac{13R}{6} = \frac{n_1C_{v_1} + 2n_1C_{v_2}}{n_1 + 2n_1}$ $\left[\because \frac{n_1}{n_2} = \frac{1}{2}\right]$

$\Rightarrow \frac{13R}{2} = C_{v_1} + 2C_{v_2}$

Possible values are, $C_{V_1} = \frac{3R}{2}$, $C_{V_2} = \frac{5R}{2}$

$\therefore$ Gases are monatomic (like He) and diatomic (like N_2)

27. (c) $\frac{PV}{T} = nR = \left(\frac{m}{M}\right) R$ or $\frac{PV}{T} = \left(\frac{R}{M}\right) m$

i.e. $\frac{PV}{T}$ versus m graph is straight line passing through origin with slope R/M, i.e. the slope depends on molecular mass of the gas M and is different for different gases.

28. (d) C_v for hydrogen $= \frac{5}{2}R$

C_v for helium $= \frac{3R}{2}$

C_v for water vapour $= \frac{6R}{2} = 3R$

$$\therefore (C_v)_{mix} = \frac{4 \times \frac{5}{2}R + 2 \times \frac{3}{2}R + 1 \times 3R}{4+2+1} = \frac{16}{7}R$$

$\therefore C_p = C_v + R$

$C_p = \frac{16}{7}R + R$ or $C_p = \frac{23}{7}R$

29. (b) $P = kV \Rightarrow PV^{-1} = k$

It is polytropic process (PV^n = constant)

So $n = -1$

So, $C = C_V + \frac{R}{1-n} = C_V + \frac{R}{2}$

30. (d) $PV = \frac{m}{M}RT$ Initially, $PV = \frac{6}{M}R \times 500$

Finally, $\frac{P}{2}V = \frac{(6-x)}{M}R \times 300$ (if x g gas leaks out)

Hence, $2 = \frac{6}{6-x} \times \frac{5}{3}$ $\therefore x = 1$ gram

31. (b) For an ideal gas PV = constant i.e. PV doesn't vary with V.

32. (c) Molar specific heat at constant pressure $C_P = \frac{7}{2}R$

Since, $C_P - C_V = R \Rightarrow C_V - C_P - R = \frac{7}{2}R - R = \frac{5}{2}R$

$\therefore \frac{C_P}{C_V} = \frac{(7/2)R}{(5/2)R} = \frac{7}{5}.$

33. (a) $N = \int \rho(dv)$

$$= \int_0^r n_0 e^{-\alpha r^4} \times 4\pi r^2 dr = 4\text{p}\, n_0 \int_0^r r^2 (e^{-\alpha r^4}) dr$$

$\propto n_0\, a^{-3/4}$

34. (d) Clearly from figure, $P_2A = P_1A + mg$

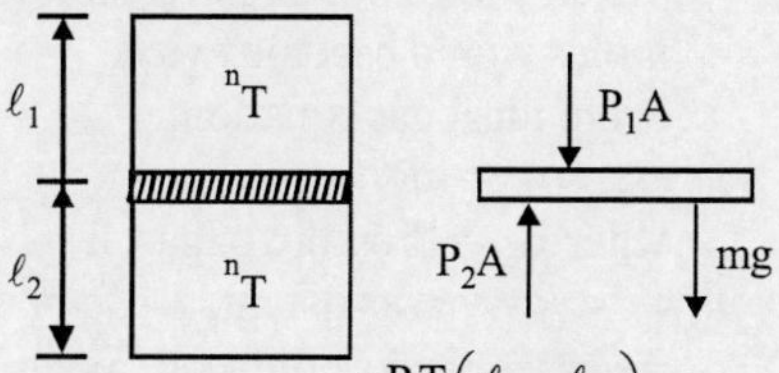

or, $\frac{nRT \cdot A}{A\ell_2}$

$= \frac{nRT \cdot A}{A\ell_1} + mg$

$\Rightarrow nRT\left(\frac{1}{\ell_2} - \frac{1}{\ell_1}\right) = mg$ $\therefore m = \frac{nRT}{g}\left(\frac{\ell_1 - \ell_2}{\ell_1 \cdot \ell_2}\right)$

35. (c) The centre of mass of gas molecules also moves with lorry with uniform speed. As there is no relative motion of gas molecule. So, kinetic energy and hence temperature remain same.

36. (c) $V_{rms} = \sqrt{\frac{3RT}{M}}$

$$\frac{v_1}{v_2} = \sqrt{\frac{T_1}{T_2}} = \frac{(273+127)}{(273+237)} = \sqrt{\frac{400}{500}} = \sqrt{\frac{4}{5}} = \frac{2}{\sqrt{5}}$$

$\therefore v_2 = \frac{\sqrt{5}}{2}v_1 = \frac{\sqrt{5}}{2} \times 200 = 100\sqrt{5}$ m/s.

37. (a) Using $\frac{V_{1rms}}{V_{2rms}} = \sqrt{\frac{M_2}{M_1}}$

$$\frac{V_{rms}(He)}{V_{rms}(Ar)} = \sqrt{\frac{M_{Ar}}{M_{He}}} = \sqrt{\frac{40}{4}} = 3.16$$

38. (c) Total degree of freedom $f = 3 + 2 = 5$

Total energy, $U = \frac{nfRT}{2} = \frac{5RT}{2}$

And $\gamma = \frac{C_p}{C_v} = 1 + \frac{2}{f} = 1 + \frac{2}{5} = \frac{7}{5}$

39. (b) Mean free path, $\lambda = \frac{1}{\sqrt{2}\pi n d^2}$

where, d = diameter of the molecule

n = number of molecules per unit volume

But, mean time of collision, $\tau = \frac{\lambda}{v_{rms}}$

But $v_{rms} = \sqrt{\frac{3kT}{R}}$ $\therefore \tau = \frac{\lambda}{\sqrt{\frac{3kT}{m}}} \Rightarrow t \propto \frac{1}{\sqrt{T}}$

40. (b) Let C_p and C_v be the specific heat capacity of the gas at constant pressure and volume.

At constant pressure, heat required

$\Delta Q_1 = nC_p \Delta T$

$\Rightarrow 160 = nC_p \cdot 50$ ...(i)

At constant volume, heat required

$\Delta Q_2 = nC_v \Delta T$

$\Rightarrow 240 = nC_v \cdot 100$ ...(ii)

Dividing (i) by (ii), we get

$$\frac{160}{240} = \frac{C_p}{C_v} \cdot \frac{50}{100} \Rightarrow \frac{C_p}{C_v} = \frac{4}{3}$$

$\gamma = \frac{C_p}{C_v} = \frac{4}{3} = 1 + \frac{2}{f}$ (Here, f = degree of freedom)

$\Rightarrow f = 6.$

41. (a) As we know mean free path

$$\lambda = \frac{1}{\sqrt{2}\left(\frac{N}{V}\right)\pi d^2}$$

Here, N = no. of molecule

V = volume of container

d = diameter of molecule

But $PV = nRT = nNKT \Rightarrow \frac{N}{V} = \frac{P}{KT} = n$

$$\lambda = \frac{1}{\sqrt{2}}\frac{KT}{\pi d^2 P}$$

For constant volume and hence constant number density n of gas molecules $\frac{P}{T}$ is constant.

So mean free path remains same.

As temperature increases no. of collision increases so relaxation time decreases.

42. (a) Helium is a monoatomic gas and Oxygen is a diatomic gas.

For helium, $C_{V_1} = \frac{3}{2}R$ and $C_{P_1} = \frac{5}{2}R$

For oxygen, $C_{V_2} = \frac{5}{2}R$ and $C_{P_2} = \frac{7}{2}R$

$$\gamma = \frac{N_1C_{P_1} + N_2C_{P_2}}{N_1C_{V_1} + N_2C_{V_2}} \Rightarrow \gamma = \frac{n.\frac{5}{2}R + 2n.\frac{7}{2}R}{n.\frac{3}{2}R + 2n.\frac{5}{2}R} = \frac{19nR \times 2}{2(13nR)}$$

$$\therefore \left(\frac{C_P}{C_V}\right)_{mixture} = \frac{19}{13}$$

43. (c) Relaxation time $(\tau) \propto \frac{\text{mean free path}}{\text{speed}} \Rightarrow \tau \propto \frac{1}{v}$

and, $v \propto \sqrt{T}$

$\therefore \tau \propto \frac{1}{\sqrt{T}}$

Hence graph between τ v/s $\frac{1}{\sqrt{T}}$ is a straight line which is correctly depicted by graph shown in option (c).

44. (d) Using, $\gamma_{\text{mixture}} = \frac{n_1C_{p_1} + n_2C_{p_2}}{n_1C_{v_1} + n_2C_{v_2}}$

$$\Rightarrow \frac{n_1}{\gamma_1 - 1} + \frac{n_2}{\gamma_2 - 1} = \frac{n_1 + n_2}{\gamma_m - 1}$$

$$\Rightarrow \frac{3}{\frac{4}{3} - 1} + \frac{2}{\frac{5}{3} - 1} = \frac{5}{\gamma_m - 1}$$

$$\Rightarrow \frac{9}{1} + \frac{2 \times 3}{2} = \frac{5}{\gamma_m - 1} \Rightarrow \gamma_m - 1 = \frac{5}{12}$$

$$\Rightarrow \gamma_m = \frac{17}{12} = 1.42$$

45. (c) From P-V graph,

$P \propto \frac{1}{V}$, T = constant and Pressure is increasing from 2 to 1 so option (3) represents correct T-P graph.

46. (c) $v_{rms} = \sqrt{\frac{3\rho v}{\text{mass of the gas}}}$

47. (a) Given, $V_1 = V$

$V_2 = 2V$

$T_1 = 27° + 273 = 300$ K

$T_2 = ?$

From charle's law

$$\frac{V_1}{T_1} = \frac{V_2}{T_2} \ (\because \text{Pressure is constant}) \text{ or, } \frac{V}{300} = \frac{2V}{T_2}$$

$\therefore \quad T_2 = 600\text{ K} = 600 - 273 = 327°\text{C}$

48. (a) Given, mass = 1 kg

Density = 4 kg m^{-3}

$$\text{Volume} = \frac{\text{mass}}{\text{density}} = \frac{1}{4}\text{ m}^3$$

Internal energy of the diatomic gas

$$= \frac{5}{2}PV = \frac{5}{2} \times 8 \times 10^4 \times \frac{1}{4} = 5 \times 10^4 J$$

49. (a) Number of moles of first gas = $\frac{n_1}{N_A}$

Number of moles of second gas = $\frac{n_2}{N_A}$

Number of moles of third gas = $\frac{n_3}{N_A}$

If there is no loss of energy then

$P_1V_1 + P_2V_2 + P_3V_3 = PV$

$$\frac{n_1}{N_A}RT_1 + \frac{n_2}{N_A}RT_2 + \frac{n_3}{N_A}RT_3$$

$$= \frac{n_1 + n_2 + n_3}{N_A}RT_{mix}$$

$$T_{mix} = \frac{n_1T_1 + n_2T_2 + n_3T_3}{n_1 + n_2 + n_3}$$

50. (d) Using equipartition of energy, we have

$$\frac{6}{2}KT = mCT$$

$$C = \frac{3 \times 1.38 \times 10^{-23} \times 6.02 \times 10^{23}}{27 \times 10^{-3}}$$

$\therefore$ C = 925 J/kgK

Exercise 2 - Exemplar & Past Year Questions E&PYQs

Exemplar Questions

1. (b) As the relative velocity of molecule with respect to the walls of container does not change in rocket, due to the mass of a molecule is negligible with respect to the mass of whole system and system of gas moves as a whole and $(g = 0)$ on molecule energy where.

Hence pressure of the gas inside the vessel, as observed by us, on the ground remain the same.

2. (b) Boyle's law is applicable at constant temperature and temperature remains constant in isothermal process.

For ideal gas, $pV = nRT$ = constant

So, pV = constant (at constant temperature)

$$p \propto \frac{1}{V}$$

So, this process can be called as isothermal process.

3. (c)

4. (d) Pressure exerted by gas is due to rate of change of momentum (p) imparted by particles to wall.

When the molecules breaks into atoms, the number of moles would become twice.

From ideal gas equation,

$$pV = nRT$$

where, p = Pressure of gas, n = Number of moles

R = Gas constant, T = temperature

As gases breaks number of moles becomes twice of initial, so $n_2 = 2n_1$

So, $p \propto nT$

or $\frac{p_2}{p_1} = \frac{n_2T_2}{n_1T_1} = \frac{(2n_1)(3000)}{n_1(300)} = 20$

So, $p_2 = 20p_1$

Hence, final pressure of the gas would be 20 times to the initial pressure.

5. (b) For a function $f_1(v)$ the number of molecules (n) which will have their speeds between v and $v + dv$.
For each function $f_1(v)$ and $f_2(v)$ number of molecules remain same 1 mole each but due to mass difference their speed will be different.
Hence both gases of each function $f_1(v)$ and $f_2(v)$ will obey the Maxwell's distribution law separately.

6. (d)

NEET/AIPMT (2013-2020) Questions

7. (b) $P_1 > P_2$

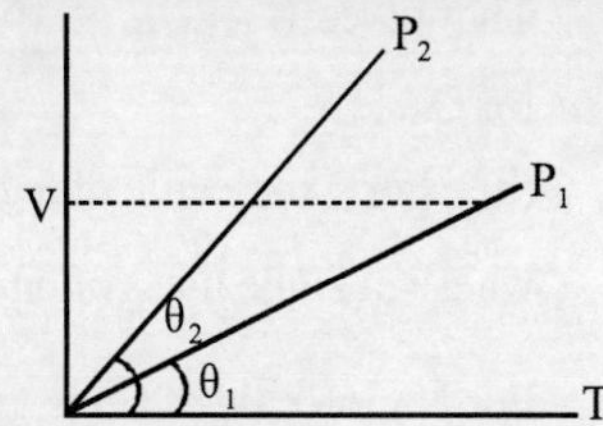

As V = constant ⇒ $P \propto T$

Hence from V–T graph $P_1 > P_2$

8. (d) From first law of thermodynamics

$$\Delta Q = \Delta U + \Delta W = \frac{3}{2} \cdot \frac{1}{4} R(T_2 - T_1) + 0$$

$$= \frac{3}{8} N_a K_B (T_2 - T_1) \ [\because K = \frac{R}{N}]$$

9. (b) $\because P = \frac{1}{3}\frac{mn}{V}V_{rms}^2$

When mass is halved and speed is doubled then

Resultant pressure, $P' = \frac{1}{3} \times \frac{m}{2} \times \frac{n}{V}(2v_{rms})^2 = 2P.$

10. (b) Mean free path $\lambda_m = \frac{1}{\sqrt{2}\pi d^2 n}$

where d = diameter of molecule and d = 2r

$\therefore \quad \lambda_m \propto \frac{1}{r^2}$

11. (b) Let 'n' be the degree of freedom

$$\gamma = \frac{C_p}{C_v} = \frac{\left(\frac{n}{2}+1\right)R}{\left(\frac{n}{2}\right)R} = \left(1 + \frac{2}{n}\right)$$

12. (b) Here $v_1 = 200$ m/s;

temperature $T_1 = 27°C = 27 + 273 = 300$ k

temperature $T_2 = 127°$ C $= 127 + 273 = 400$ k, V = ?

R.M.S. Velocity, $V \propto \sqrt{T}$

$$\Rightarrow \quad \frac{v}{200} = \sqrt{\frac{400}{300}}$$

$$\Rightarrow \quad v = \frac{200 \times 2}{\sqrt{3}} m/s \Rightarrow v = \frac{400}{\sqrt{3}} m/s$$

13. (c) Internal energy of the system is given by

$$U = \frac{f}{2} nRT$$

Degree of freedom

$F_{diatomic} = 5$

$f_{monoatomic} = 3$

and, number of moles

$n(O_2) = 2$

$n(Ar) = 4$

$$U_{total} = \frac{5}{2}(2)RT + \frac{3}{2}(4)RT = 11RT$$

14. (b) Let at temperature T rms speed of oxygen molecules become just sufficient for escaping from the Earth's atmosphere

$V_{escape} = 11200$ m/s

Also, $V_{rms} = V_{escape} = \sqrt{\frac{3k_BT}{m_{O_2}}} = 11200$ m/s

Putting value of K_B and m_{O_2} we get,

$T = 8.360 \times 10^4$ K

15. (b) $U = \frac{F}{2} nRT$

As $U \propto T$

$\therefore$ Increase in temperature would lead to the increase in kinetic energy of gas.

16. (b) For Hydrogen $f = 5$

For Helium $f = 3$

For gas X

$f = 7.$

$$\gamma = 1 + \frac{2}{f} = 1 + \frac{2}{7} = \frac{9}{7}$$

So, $\left(\frac{7}{5}, \frac{5}{3}, \frac{9}{7}\right)$

17. (a) Given : Pressure $P = 249\ kPa = 249 \times 10^3$ N/m²

Mass of hydrogen, $M = 2g = 2 \times 10^{-3}$ kg

Temperature, $T = 27 + 273 = 300$ K

Using, ideal gas equation, $PV = nRT$

$$PM = \rho RT \Rightarrow \rho = \frac{PM}{RT} \quad \left(\because \rho = \frac{M}{V}\right)$$

$$\therefore \rho = \frac{(249 \times 10^3)(2 \times 10^{-3})}{8.3 \times 300} = 0.2 \text{ kg/m}^3.$$

18. (a) Mean free path for a gas $\lambda_m = \frac{1}{\sqrt{2}n\pi d^2}$

Here, d = diameter of a gas molecule and, n = molecular density.

Exercise 3 - Concept Application Problems CAP

1. (a) $\frac{c_2}{c_1} = \sqrt{\frac{400}{300}} = \frac{2}{\sqrt{3}} \Rightarrow c_2 = \frac{2}{\sqrt{3}} \times 200 = \frac{400}{\sqrt{3}}$ ms^{-1}

2. (b) Relative humidity (R.H) $= \frac{\text{S.V.P at dew point}}{\text{S.V.P at room temp.}}$

since here R.H is 100%

⇒ room temp. = dew point = 30°C

3. (a) $P=\frac{1}{3}\rho\bar{\upsilon}^2=\frac{1}{3}\times(6\times10^{-2})\times(500)^2$

$=5\times10^3\ N/m^2$

4. (b) $(C_p)_{mix}=\frac{\mu_1C_{p_1}+\mu_2C_{p_2}}{\mu_1+\mu_2}$

$(C_{p_1}(He)=\frac{5}{2}R$ and $C_{p_2}(H_2)=\frac{7}{2}R)$

$(C_p)_{mix}=\frac{1\times\frac{5}{2}R+1\times\frac{7}{2}R}{1+1}=3R=3\times2=6$ cal/mol.°C

∴ Amount of heat needed to raise the temperature from 0°C to 100°C

$(\Delta Q)_p=\mu C_p\Delta T=2\times6\times100=1200\,cal$

5. (b) Average K.E. $=\frac{1}{2}mc^2=\frac{3}{2}kT\propto T$

$\therefore\ \frac{(Av.K.E.)_{600K}}{(Av.K.E.)_{300K}}=\frac{600}{300}=2$

∴ At 600K it will be 2 times than that at 300K.

6. (a) Let T be the temperature of the mixture, then

$U=U_1+U_2$

$\Rightarrow \frac{f}{2}(n_1+n_2)RT=\frac{f}{2}(n_1)(R)(T_0)+\frac{f}{2}(n_2)(R)(2T_0)$

$\Rightarrow (2+4)T=2T_0+8T_0\ (\because\ n_1=2,n_2=4)$

$\therefore\ T=\frac{5}{3}T_0$

7. (a) $\frac{c_t}{c_0}=\sqrt{\frac{273+t}{273}}\Rightarrow 4\times273-273=t\Rightarrow t=819°C$

8. (c) According to Dalton's Law

$P=P_1+P_2$.....................

here 1 litre of orygen at a pressure of 1atm, & 2 litre of nitrogen at a pressure of 5 atm are introduced in a vessel of 1 litre capacity.

so $P=\frac{V_1P_1+P_2V_2}{\text{volume of vessel}}=\frac{1\times1+2\times.5}{1}=2atm$

9. (b) Relative humidity $=\frac{m}{M}\times100\%$

where m is the mass of vapour actually present in certain volume of air & M is the mass required to saturate the air fully of that volume

so $R.H=\frac{15}{20}\times100=75\%$

10. (c) By definition

$\Rightarrow R.H=\frac{\text{V.P at room temp.}}{\text{S.V.P at room temp.}}\times100;\ \frac{60}{100}$

$=\frac{(V.P.)_{15}}{12.67}$

$(V.P)_{15}=7.6$mm of Hg.

Now since unsaturated vapour obeys gas equation & mass of water remains constant so

$P=\left(\frac{nRT}{V}\right)\Rightarrow P\alpha T$

$\frac{(V.P)_{15}}{(V.P)_{20}}=\frac{273+15}{273+20}\Rightarrow (V.P)_{20}=7.73$ mm of Hg

So $(R.H)_{20}=\frac{(V.P)_{20}}{(S.V.P)_{20}}\times100=44.5\%$

11. (d) Total K.E. of A type molecules $=\frac{3}{2}m\omega^2$

Total K.E. of A type of molecule is

$K.E_A=\frac{1}{2}m\left[(v_{r.ms})_x^2+(v_{r.ms})_y^2+(v_{r.ms})_z^2\right]$

but $(v_{r.ms})_x=\omega$

so $(v_{r.ms})_y=(v_{r.ms})_z=\omega$

Total K.E. of B type molecules $=\frac{1}{2}\times2\,m\,v^2=m\,v^2$

Now, $\frac{3}{2}\times m\,\omega^2=m\,v^2$ or $(\omega^2/v^2)=\frac{2}{3}$

12. (d) Molecule number ratio is $H_2:O_2=\frac{2}{3}:\frac{1}{3}$.

That gives $(c_{rms})^2=16\left(\frac{2}{3}\right)+1\left(\frac{1}{3}\right)$ times the value for O_2.

13 (b) For 1 molecule of a gas, $v_{rms}=\sqrt{\frac{3KT}{m}}$

where m is the mass of one molecule

For N molecule of a gas, $v_1=\sqrt{\frac{3KT\times N}{m}}$

For 2N molecule of a gas $v_2=\sqrt{\frac{3KI\times N}{(2m)}\times N}$

$\therefore\ \frac{v_1}{v_2}=1$

14. (a) Since $VP^2=$ constant,

$VP^2=2VP'^2\quad \therefore P'=\frac{P}{\sqrt{2}}$

As $\frac{P}{T}=$ constant or $T\alpha P$, thus T becomes $T/\sqrt{2}$

15. (a) We know that, $C_{rms}=\sqrt{\left(\frac{\gamma RT}{M}\right)}$

Here $C_{rms}\propto\sqrt{\frac{1}{M}};\ \therefore\ \frac{C_{rms_1}}{C_{rms_2}}=\sqrt{\left(\frac{m_2}{m_1}\right)}$

16. (b) $F=\frac{dU}{dr}=-\frac{d}{dr}\left[\frac{M}{r^3}-\frac{N}{R^{12}}\right]=-\left[\frac{-6M}{r^2}+\frac{12N}{r^{13}}\right]$

In equilibrium position, $F=0$

$\therefore\ \frac{6M}{r^2}-\frac{12N}{r^{13}}=0$ or, $r^6=\frac{2N}{M}$

∴ Potential energy at equilibrium position

$U=\frac{M}{(2N/M)}=\frac{N}{(2N/M)^2}=\frac{M^2}{2N}-\frac{M^2}{4N}=\frac{M^2}{4N}$

17. (b) $\frac{P_1V_1}{T_1}=\frac{P_2V_2}{T_2}$ Here, $P_1=200kPa$

$T_1=22°C=295\,K\quad T_2=42°C=315K$

$V_2=V_1+\frac{2}{100}V_1=1.02V_1$

$\therefore\ P_2=\frac{200\times315V_1}{295\times1.02V_1}=209.37kPa$

18. (a) According to given Vander Waal's equation

$$P=\frac{nRT}{V-n\beta}-\frac{\alpha n^2}{V^2}$$

Work done, $W=\int_{V_1}^{V_2} PdV = nRT\int_{V_1}^{V_2}\frac{dV}{V-n\beta}-\alpha n^2\int_{V_1}^{V_2}\frac{dV}{V^2}$

$$= nRT\left[\log_e(V-n\beta)\right]_{V_1}^{V_2}+\alpha n^2\left[\frac{1}{V}\right]_{V_1}^{V_2}$$

$$= nRT\log_e\left(\frac{V_2-n\beta}{V_1-n\beta}\right)+\alpha n^2\left[\frac{V_1-V_2}{V_1V_2}\right]$$

19. (b) From graph, $T^2V=$ const. .....(1)

As we know that $TV^{\gamma-1}=$ const

$\Rightarrow VT^{\frac{1}{\gamma-1}}=$ cons. ....(2)

On comparing (1) and (2), we get

$\Rightarrow \gamma = 3/2$

Also $v_{rms}=\sqrt{\frac{3P}{\rho}}$ and $v_{sound}=\sqrt{\frac{P\gamma}{\rho}}$

$$\Rightarrow \frac{v_{rms}}{v_{sound}}=\sqrt{\frac{3}{\gamma}}=\sqrt{2}$$

20. (c) Given : $K.E._{mean}=\frac{3}{2}kT=4\times10^{-14}$

$P=2$ cm of Hg, $V=4$ cm^3

$$N=\frac{PV}{KT}=\frac{P\rho gV}{KT}\frac{2\times13.6\times980\times4}{\frac{8}{3}\times10^{-14}}\simeq 4\times10^{18}$$

21. (Bouns) Rate of change of momentum during collision

$$=\frac{mv-(-mv)}{\Delta t}=\frac{2mv}{\Delta t}N$$

so pressure $P=\frac{N\times(2mv)}{\Delta t\times A}$

$$=\frac{10^{22}\times2\times10^{-26}\times10^4}{1\times1}=2\,N/m^2$$

22. (c) $v_{rms}=v_e$

$$\sqrt{\frac{3RT}{M}}=11.2\times10^3 \text{ or } \sqrt{\frac{3kT}{m}}=11.2\times10^3$$

or $\sqrt{\frac{3\times1.38\times10^{-23}T}{2\times10^{-3}}}=11.2\times10^3 \quad \therefore v=10^4$K

23. (d) Here degree of freedom, $f=3+3=6$ for triatomic non-linear molecule.

Internal energy of a mole of the gas at temperature T,

$$U=\frac{f}{2}nRT=\frac{6}{2}RT=3RT$$

24. (a) Total energy of the gas mixture,

$$E_{mix}=\frac{f_1n_1RT_1}{2}+\frac{f_2n_2RT_2}{2}=3\times\frac{5}{2}RT+\frac{5}{2}\times3RT=15RT$$

25. (d) Specific heat of gas at constant volume

$C_v=\frac{1}{2}fR;\ f=$ degree of freedom

For gas A (diatomic)

f = 5 (3 translational + 2 rotational)

$$\therefore C_v^A=\frac{5}{2}R$$

For gas B (diatomic) in addition to (3 translational + 2 rotational) 2 vibrational degree of freedom.

$$\therefore \quad C_v^B=\frac{7}{2}R \text{ Hence } \frac{C_v^A}{C_v^B}=\frac{\frac{5}{2}R}{\frac{7}{2}R}=\frac{5}{7}$$

26. (Bonus)

27. (b) Using, $\tau=\frac{1}{2n\pi d^2 V_{avg}}$

$$\therefore t\propto\frac{\sqrt{T}}{P}\left[\therefore n=\frac{\text{no.of molecules}}{\text{Volume}}\right]$$

or, $\frac{t_1}{6\times10^{-8}}=\frac{\sqrt{500}}{2P}\times\frac{P}{\sqrt{300}}\approx4\times10^{-8}$

28. (a) $U=\frac{f_1}{2}n_1RT+\frac{f_2}{2}n_2RT$

Considering translational and rotational modes, degrees of freedom $f_1=5$ and $f_2=3$

$$\therefore u=\frac{5}{2}(3RT)+\frac{3}{2}\times5RT$$

U = 15RT

29. (c) In an adiabatic process

$TV^{\gamma-1}=$ Constant or, $T_1V_1^{\gamma-1}=T_2V_2^{\gamma-1}$

For monoatomic gas $\gamma=\frac{5}{3}$

$(300)V^{2/3}=T_2(2V)^{2/3} \Rightarrow T_2=\frac{300}{(2)^{2/3}}$

$T_2=189$ K (final temperature)

Change in internal energy $\Delta U=n\frac{f}{2}R\ \Delta T$

$$=2\left(\frac{3}{2}\right)\left(\frac{25}{3}\right)(-111)=-2.7\text{kJ}$$

30. (a) Energy associated with N moles of diatomic gas,

$U_i=N\frac{5}{2}RT$

Energy associated with n moles of monoatomic gas

$=n\frac{3}{2}RT$

Total energy when n moles of diatomic gas converted into monoatomic $(U_f)=2n\frac{3}{2}RT+(N-n)\frac{5}{2}RT$

$$=\frac{1}{2}nRT+\frac{5}{2}NRT$$

Now, change in total kinetic energy of the gas

$$\Delta U=Q=\frac{1}{2}nRT$$

31. (c) Pressure, $P=\frac{1}{3}\frac{mN}{V}V_{rms}^2$ or, $P=\frac{(mN)T}{V}$

If the gas mass and temperature are constant then

$P\propto(V_{rms})^2\propto T$

So, force $\propto(V_{rms})^2\propto T$

i.e., Value of $q=1$

32. (b)

33. (d) Kinetic energy of each molecule,

$K.E. = \frac{3}{2}K_B T$

In the given problem,

Temperature, T = 0°C = 273 K

Height attained by the gas molecule, h = ?

$K.E. = \frac{3}{2}K_B(273) = \frac{819K_B}{2}$

K.E. = P.E.

$\Rightarrow \frac{819K_B}{2} = Mgh$ or $h = \frac{819K_B}{2Mg}$

34. (a) Energy of the gas, E

$= \frac{f}{2}nRT = \frac{f}{2}PV = \frac{f}{2}(3\times10^6)(2) = f\times3\times10^6$

Considering gas is monoatomic i.e., f = 3

Energy, E = 9×10^6 J

35. (a) According to question VT = K

we also know that PV = nRT

$\Rightarrow T = \left(\frac{PV}{nR}\right) \Rightarrow V\left(\frac{PV}{nR}\right) = k \Rightarrow PV^2 = K$

$\because C = \frac{R}{1-x} + C_V$ (For polytropic process)

$C = \frac{R}{1-2} + \frac{3R}{2} = \frac{R}{2}$ $\quad \therefore \Delta Q = nC\Delta T$

$= \frac{R}{2}\times\Delta T$ [here, n = 1 mole]

36. (c) Thermal energy of N molecule

$= N\left(\frac{3}{2}kT\right) = \frac{N}{N_A}\frac{3}{2}RT = \frac{3}{2}(nRT) = \frac{3}{2}PV$

$= \frac{3}{2}P\left(\frac{m}{\rho}\right) = \frac{3}{2}P\left(\frac{2}{8}\right)$

$= \frac{3}{2}\times4\times10^4\times\frac{2}{8} = 1.5\times10^4$ J

therefore, order = 10^4 J

37. (c) Heat transferred,

$Q = nC_v\Delta T$ as gas in closed vessel

To double the rms speed, temperature should be 4 times

i.e., $T' = 4T$ as $v_{rms} = \sqrt{3RT/M}$

$\therefore Q = \frac{15}{28}\times\frac{5\times R}{2}\times(4T - T)$

$\left[\therefore \frac{CP}{CV} = \gamma_{diatomic} = \frac{7}{5} \& C_p - C_v = R\right]$

or, Q = 10000 J = 10 kJ

38. (c) In an adiabatic process

$TV^{\gamma-1}$ = Constant $\quad$ or, $T_1V_1^{\gamma-1} = T_2V_2^{\gamma-1}$

For monoatomic gas $\gamma = \frac{5}{3}$

$(300)V^{2/3} = T_2(2V)^{2/3} \Rightarrow T_2 = \frac{300}{(2)^{2/3}}$

T_2 = 189 K (final temperature)

Change in internal energy $\Delta U = n\frac{f}{2}R\,\Delta T$

$= 2\left(\frac{3}{2}\right)\left(\frac{25}{3}\right)(-111) = -2.7$ kJ

39. (b) Using formula,

$$\gamma_{mixture} = \left(\frac{C_p}{C_v}\right)_{mix} = \frac{\frac{n_1\gamma_1}{\gamma_1-1}+\frac{n_2\gamma_2}{\gamma_2-1}}{\frac{n_1}{\gamma_1-1}+\frac{n_2}{\gamma_2-1}}$$

Putting the value of $n_1 = 2, n_2 = n, \left(\frac{C_p}{C_v}\right)_{mix} = \frac{3}{2}$

$\gamma_1 = \frac{5}{3}, \gamma_2 = \frac{7}{5}$ and solving we get, n = 2

40. (b) $\gamma_A = \frac{C_P}{C_v} = \frac{29}{22} = 1.32 < 1.4$ (diatomic)

and $\gamma_B = \frac{30}{21} = \frac{10}{7} = 1.43 > 1.4$

Gas A has more than 5-degrees of freedom.

41. (a) $\frac{1}{2}m\bar{v}^2 = 3k_BT$ or $T = \frac{m\bar{v}^2}{6k_B}$

42. (c) Amount of heat required (Q) to raise the temperature at constant volume

$Q = nC_v\Delta T$ ...(i)

Amount of heat required (Q_1) at constant pressure

$Q_1 = nC_P\Delta T$ ...(ii)

Dividing equation (ii) by (i), we get

$\therefore \frac{Q_1}{Q} = \frac{C_p}{C_v} \Rightarrow Q_1 = (Q)\left(\frac{7}{5}\right) \left(\because \gamma = \frac{C_p}{C_v} = \frac{7}{5}\right)$

43. (c) V = 25×10^{-3} m³, N = 1 mole of O_2

T = 300 K

V_{rms} = 200 m/s $\quad \therefore \lambda = \frac{1}{\sqrt{2}N\pi r^2}$

Average time $\frac{1}{\tau} = \frac{<V>}{\lambda} = 200.N\pi r^2.\sqrt{2}$

$= \frac{\sqrt{2}\times200\times6.023\times10^{23}}{25\times10^{-3}}.\pi\times10^{-18}\times0.09$

The closest value in the given option is = 10^{10}

44. (b) $F = \frac{C_v}{C_p} = \frac{1}{r} = \frac{1}{(7/5)} = \frac{5}{7}$

or $\frac{W}{Q} = 1 - \frac{5}{7} = \frac{2}{7}$

or $Q = \frac{7}{2}W = \frac{7\times10}{2} = 35$ J

45. (c) $[C_v]_{min} = \frac{n_1[C_{v_1}]+n_2[C_{v_2}]}{n_1+n_2}$

$= \left[\frac{2\times\frac{3R}{2}+3\times\frac{5R}{2}}{2+3}\right]$

= 2.1 R = 2.1 × 8.3 = 17.4 J/mol–k

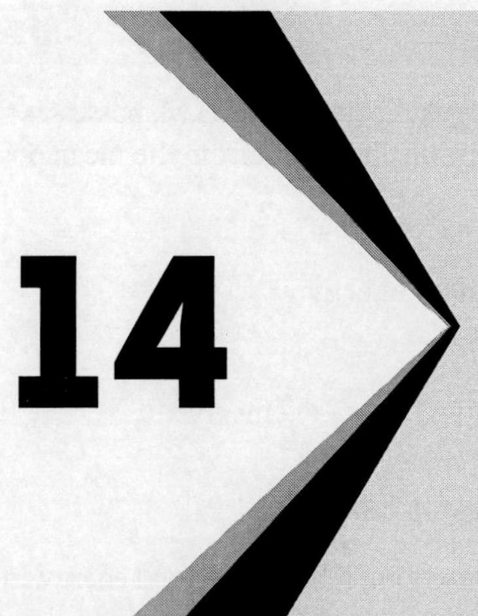

14 Oscillations

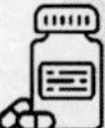

Topic 14.1 : Periodic & Oscillatory Motion, Simple Harmonic Motion, Simple, Compound and Spring Pendulum

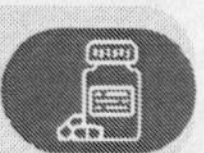

PERIODIC AND OSCILLATORY MOTION

Periodic Motion

When a body repeats its motion after regular interval of time, it is said to be in periodic motion. The path of periodic motion may be rectilinear, open/ closed curvilinear.

Example : (i) Motion of moon around earth.
(ii) Motion of a piston in a cylinder.
(iii) Motion of a simple pendulum etc.

Oscillatory Motion

If during a periodic motion, the particle moves to and fro on the same path, the motion is vibratory or oscillatory.

Example :
(i) The motion of a ball in bowl
(ii) The needle of a sewing machine
(iii) Vibrations of prongs of tuning fork etc.

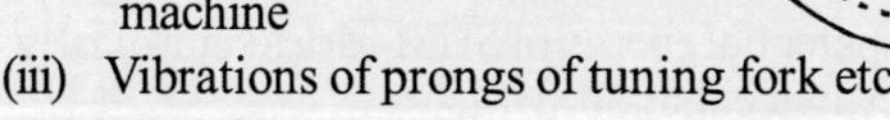

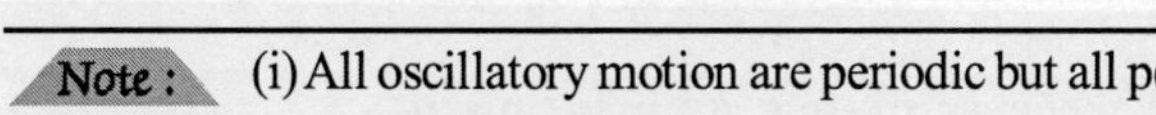

Note : (i) All oscillatory motion are periodic but all periodic motion are not oscillatory motion.
(ii) The oscillatory motion which can be expressed in terms of sine and cosine function, is said to be harmonic motion.

SIMPLE HARMONIC MOTION (S.H.M.)

"If a particle moves up and down (back and forth) about a mean position (also called equilibrium position) in such a way that a restoring force/ torque acts on particle, which is proportional to displacement from mean position, but in opposite direction from displacement, then motion of the particle is called simple harmonic motion. If displacement is linear, it is called **linear S.H.M.** and if displacement is angular, it is called an **angular S.H.M.**

Example : (i) Motion of a body suspended by spring.
(ii) Oscillations of simple pendulum.

Equations of S.H.M.

(a) ***Linear S.H.M.***
The restoring force is proportional to the displacement from mean position.

i.e., $F \propto -x$

or, $\vec{F} = -k\vec{x}$

where k is called force constant or spring constant

or, $m\dfrac{d^2\vec{x}}{dt^2} + \dfrac{k\vec{x}}{m} = 0$

(b) ***Angular S.H.M.***
The restoring torque is proporational to the angular displacement from the mean position.

$\vec{\tau} = -C\vec{\theta}$ where C is called torsional rigidity

or, $I\dfrac{d^2\vec{\theta}}{dt^2} = -C\vec{\theta}$

or, $\dfrac{d^2\vec{\theta}}{dt^2} + \dfrac{C}{I}\vec{\theta} = 0.$

Terms Related to S.H.M.

(i) **Amplitude :** The maximum displacement of the oscillating particle on either side of its mean position is called its amplitude. It is denoted by A.

(ii) **Time period :** The time taken by a oscillating particle to complete one oscillation is called its time period. It is denoted by T.

(iii) **Frequency :** It is the number of oscillations completed in one second. It is denoted by υ.

$$\upsilon = \frac{1}{T}$$

The **S.I. unit** of frequency is s^{-1} or Hz.

(iv) **Angular frequency**

$$\omega = 2\pi\upsilon = \frac{2\pi}{T}$$

The **S.I. unit** of angular frequency is rad/sec.

(v) **Phase :** The parameter, by which the position of particle from its mean position is represented, is known as phase. The phase at any instant tells the state of position & direction of motion at that instant. The phase at time t = 0 is known as the **initial phase** or **epoch (e).**

(vi) **Total phase angle :** The total angle ($\omega t + \theta$) is known as total phase angle.

Characteristics of S.H.M.

(i) **Displacement :** The displacement of a particle in S.H.M. is given by

$$y = A\sin(\omega t + \phi)$$

where A is amplitude, ω is angular frequency and **($\omega t + \phi$) is called the phase** of the particle at any instant t.

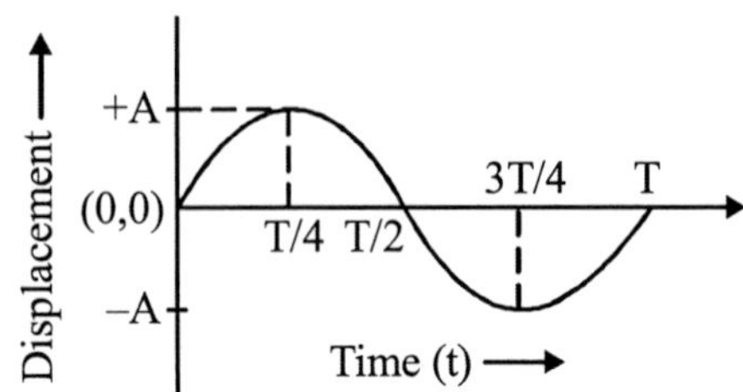

(ii) **Velocity :** The velocity of a particle in S.H.M. is given by

$$\frac{dy}{dt} = A\omega\cos(\omega t + \phi) \text{ or, } v = \omega\sqrt{A^2 - y^2}$$

At y = 0 (at mean position), $v_{max} = \omega A$

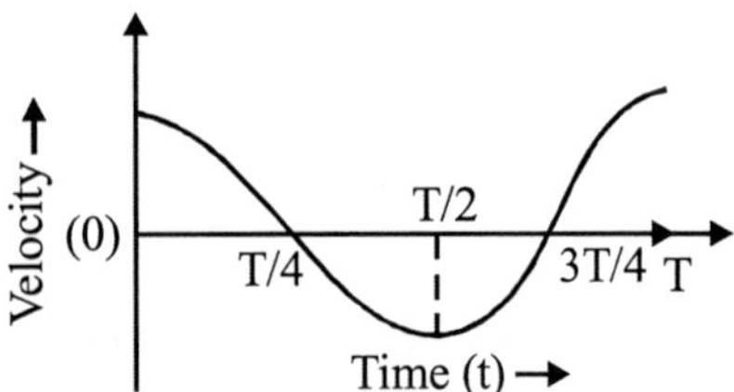

(iii) **Acceleration :** The acceleration of a particle in S.H.M. is given by

$$a = \frac{dv}{dt} = -\omega^2 A\sin(\omega t + \phi)$$

or, $a = -\omega^2 y$

The negative sign indicates that the acceleration is directed towards the mean position

At y = A (at extreme position),

$a_{max} = -\omega^2 A$

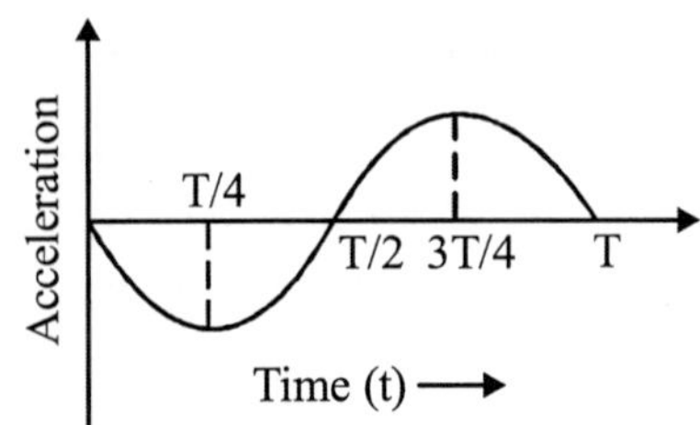

Energy in S.H.M. :

(i) **Kinetic energy :** A particle in S.H.M. possesses kinetic energy by virtue of its motion.

$$K.E. = \frac{1}{2}mv^2 = \frac{1}{2}m\omega^2(A^2 - y^2)$$

(ii) **Potential energy :** A particle in S.H.M. possesses potential energy due to its displacement from the mean position.

$$P.E. = \frac{1}{2}ky^2 = \frac{1}{2}m\omega^2 y^2$$

(iii) **Total mechanical energy**

$$E = K.E. + P.E.$$

$$= \frac{1}{2}m\omega^2(A^2 - y^2) + \frac{1}{2}m\omega^2 y^2$$

$$E = \frac{1}{2}m\omega^2 A^2 = \frac{1}{2}kA^2$$

(iv) The curves representing KE, PE and total energy are shown in figure.

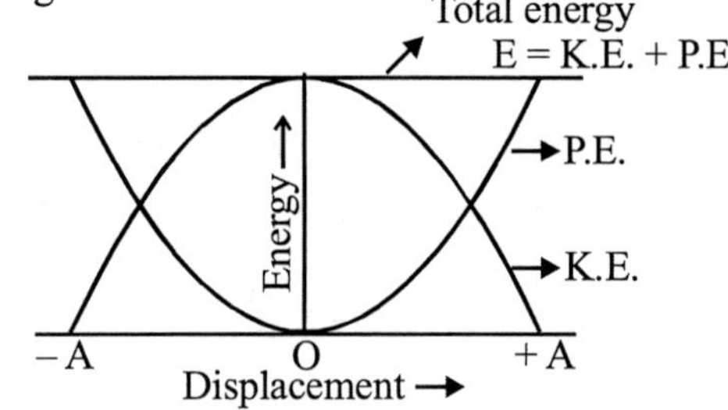

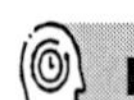

Problem Solving Tips

1. Restoring force $F = -M\omega^2 x$
2. Kinetic energy $= (1/2)\,M\omega^2(A^2 - x^2)$
3. Potential energy $= 1/2\,M\omega^2 x^2$
4. Total energy of SHM $= 1/2\,M\omega^2 A^2$

   Equation $a = -\omega^2 y$ shows that if body perform S.H.M. then acceleration of the body is proportional to displacement, but in the opposite direction of displacement. It is an essential requirement for any motion to be S.H.M.
5. The kinetic and potential energy of SHM varies sinusoidally with a frequency twice that of SHM.
6. Total energy $= \frac{1}{2}m\omega^2 A^2 = 2\pi^2 mA^2 n^2$

   where n = frequency of vibration.
7. $a = -\omega^2 x$ where ω is constant $v = \omega\sqrt{A^2 - x^2}$

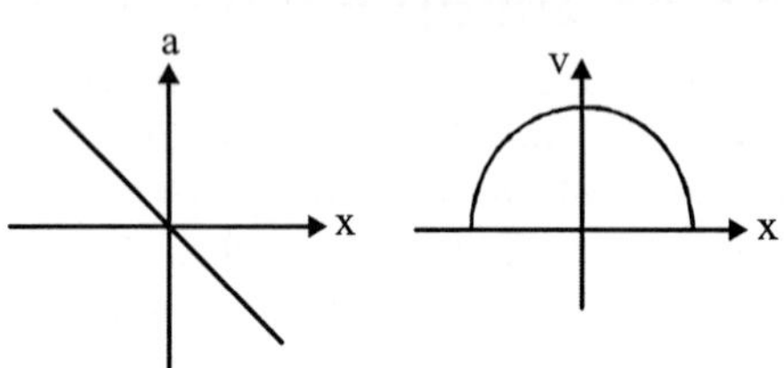

8. Geometrically the projection of the body undergoing **uniform circular motion** on the diameter of the circle is SHM.
9. In a non-inertial frame. $T = 2\pi\sqrt{\frac{l}{g_{eff}}}$

   $g_{eff} = \sqrt{(g - a_y)^2 + a_x^2}$

SOME SYSTEMS EXECUTING S.H.M.

Case 1 Spring mass system :

(i) When two springs having force constants k_1 and k_2 connected in parallel, then

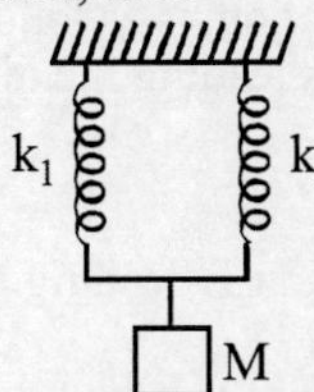

The force constant of the combination is $k = k_1 + k_2$ and hence $T = 2\pi[M/(k_1 + k_2)]^{1/2}$

(ii) When two springs of force constants k_1 and k_2 are connected in series, then

The force constant of the combination is $1/k = 1/k_1 + 1/k_2$. i.e.,

$k = k_1k_2/(k_1 + k_2)$ Hence $T = 2\pi\sqrt{\dfrac{m}{K}}$

(iii) If two mass M_1 and M_2 are connected at the two ends of the spring, then their period of oscillation is given by

$T = 2\pi[\mu/k)]^{1/2}$ where $\mu = \dfrac{M_1M_2}{M_1 + M_2}$ is the reduced mass.

(iv) When the length of spring increases, spring constant decreases. If the length of spring becomes n times, its spring constant becomes $\dfrac{1}{n}$ times and therefore time period will be increased by $\sqrt{n}$ times.

(v) If we divide the spring into n equal parts, the spring constant of each part becomes n k. Hence time period when the same mass is suspended from each part is:

$$T = 2\pi\left[\frac{M}{nk}\right]^{1/2}$$

Case 2 Simple pendulum : *A simple pendulum consists of a point mass suspended by a weightless inextensible cord from a rigid support.*

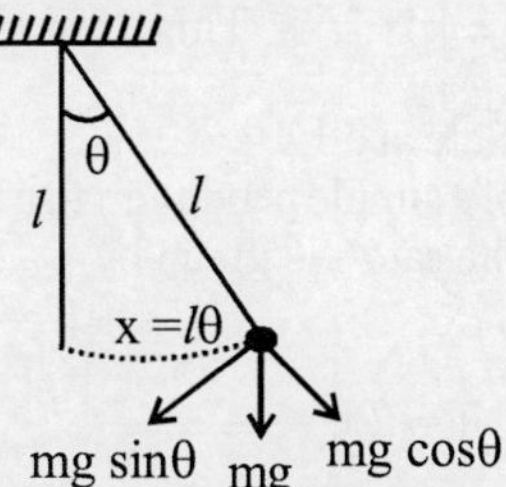

Let a bob of mass m is displaced from its, equilibrium position and released, then it oscillates in a vertical plane under gravity. Let θ be the angular displacement at any time t, then corresponding linear displacement along the arc is

$x = \ell\theta$.

It is clear from the diagram that mg sinθ, is the restoring force acting on m tending to return it to mean position. So from Newton's second law

$$F = \frac{md^2x}{dt^2} = -mg\sin\theta \qquad ...(i)$$

where negative sign indicates that restoring force mg sin θ (= F) is opposite to displacement θ. If θ is very small, then $\sin\theta \approx \theta$, so from equation (i)

$$\frac{md^2x}{dt^2} = -mg\sin\theta = -mg\frac{x}{\ell} \text{ or} \qquad ...(ii)$$

where $\omega^2 = g/\ell$.

This is the equation of S.H.M. of the bob with time period

$$T = \frac{2\pi}{\omega} = 2\pi\sqrt{\left(\frac{\ell}{g}\right)}$$

How to find the time period of a body undergoing S.H.M.?

Step 1 : First, find the equilibrium position. Equilibrium position will be one for which $\Sigma F = 0$ and $\Sigma\tau = 0$

Step 2 : Displace the body, from the equilibrium position by x.

Find the restoring force acting on the body F = –kx (for translation)

Find the restoring torque acting on the body $\tau = -k\theta$ (for rotational)

Step 3 : Since $F = ma = \dfrac{md^2x}{dt^2}$

$\therefore$ Use $\dfrac{md^2x}{dt^2} = -kx$ ... (i) for translational

$\dfrac{md^2x}{dt^2} = -k\theta$ ... (ii) for rotational

Step 4 : $T = 2\pi\sqrt{\dfrac{m}{k}}$ (for translational)

$T = 2\pi\sqrt{\dfrac{I}{k}}$ (for rotational) where, I = moment of inertia

MISCONCEPTIONS

✘ ***Incorrect.*** The time period of **spring mass-system** is dependent on the value of g.

✔ ***Correct.*** Time period of spring-mass system shifts only the equilibrium position. It does not change the time period. Because of this reason, time period of spring mass system remains same on plains / mountains / in satellites.

✘ ***Incorrect.*** The time taken to cover half the amplitude form equilibrium position is $\dfrac{T}{8}$.

✔ ***Correct.*** The actual time taken is $\dfrac{T}{12}$.

✘ ***Incorrect.*** In a spring mass system, mass oscillate about the end of a spring when the spring is in unstretched condition.

✔ ***Correct.*** The mass oscillates about the equilibrium position which may or may not be at the unstretched length.

Case 3 Liquid in U-tube : A U-tube of uniform cross-sectional area A has been set up vertically with open ends facing up.

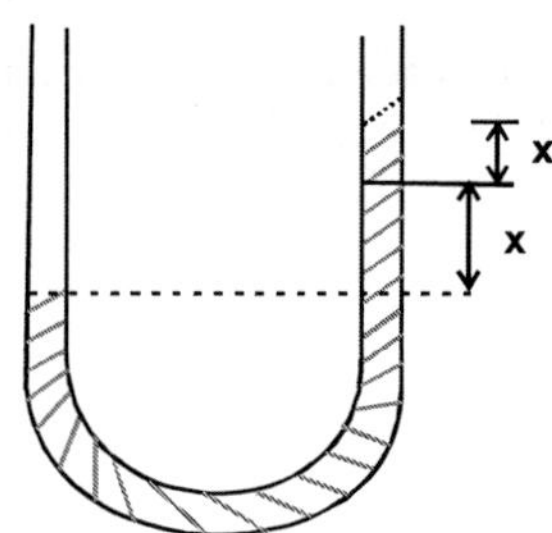

[Restoring force = –2Adg x]

If m gm of a liquid of density d is poured into it then time period of oscillation.

$$T = 2\pi\sqrt{\frac{m}{2Adg}}$$

Case 4 Rectangular block in liquid :

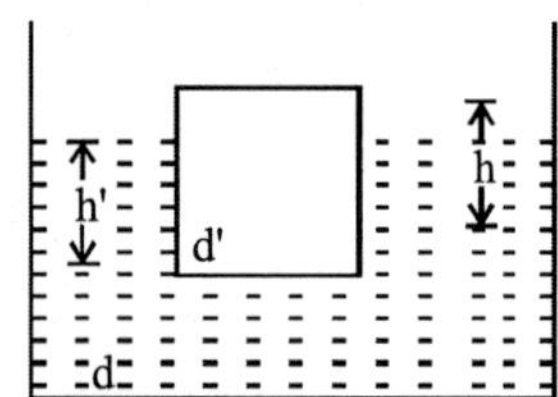

Rectangular block floating in a liquid, $T = 2\pi\sqrt{\frac{h'd'}{gd}}$; where d = density of liquid, d′ = density of block, h = height of block

Case 5 : Vibration of gas system in a cylinder with frictionless piston.

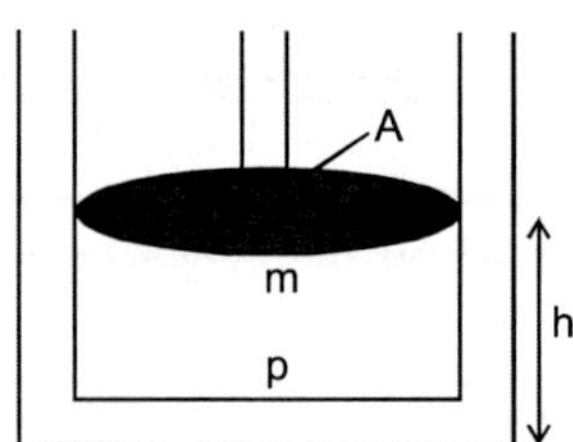

Time period, $T = 2\pi\sqrt{\frac{mh}{AP}}$

where m = mass of gas, A = cross sectional area of piston
P = pressure exerted by gas on the piston, h = height of piston

Case 6: If a tunnel is dig in the earth diametrically or along a chord then time period, $T = 2\pi\sqrt{\frac{R}{g}} = 84$ min 36 sec for a particle released in the tunnel.

Case 7: The time period of a ball oscillating in the neck of a chamber

$$T = \frac{2\pi}{A}\sqrt{\frac{mV}{B}}$$

Case 8 : If a dipole of dipole moment p is suspended in a uniform electric field E then time period of oscillation

$$T = 2\pi\sqrt{\frac{I}{PE}}$$

Problem Solving Tips

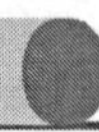

1. In S.H.M. the phase relationship between displacement, velocity and accleration, is as follows :
   (a) The velocity is leading the displacement by a phase $\frac{\pi}{2}$ radian
   (b) The acceleration is leading the displacement by a phase π radian
   (c) The acceleration is leading the velocity by a phase $\frac{\pi}{2}$ radian.
2. (a) When $x = \frac{A}{2}$, then velocity $V = 0.86V_{max}$.
   (b) When $V = V_{max}/2$, the displacement x = 0.87A.
   (c) When $x = \frac{A}{2}$, the kinetic energy of S.H.M. is 75% of the total energy and potential energy 25% of the total energy.
   (d) When the kinetic energy of S.H.M. is 50% of the total energy, the displacement is 71% of the amplitude.
3. The time period of a **simple pendulum** of length ℓ which is comparable with radius of earth.

$$T = 2\pi\left[\frac{R}{\left(1+\frac{R}{\ell}\right)g}\right]^{1/2} = 2\pi\left[\frac{\ell R}{(\ell+R)g}\right]^{1/2}$$

   where R = radius of the earth and g is the acceleration due to gravity on the surface of the earth.
   (a) When $\ell << R$, then $T = 2\pi\sqrt{\frac{\ell}{g}}$
   (b) When $\ell = R$, we find $T = 2\pi\left[\sqrt{\frac{R}{2g}}\right]^{1/2} \approx 1$ hour
   (c) When $\ell = \infty$, then $T = 2\pi\left[\sqrt{\frac{R}{g}}\right]^{1/2} = 84.6$ minutes. Thus maximum of T is 84.6 minutes.
   (d) Under weightlessness or in the freely falling lift $T = 2\pi\left[\frac{\ell}{0}\right]^{1/2} = \infty$. This means, the pendulum does not oscillate at all.
4. Time period of a simple pendulum in a train accelerating or retarding at the rate a is given by

$$T = 2\pi\left[\frac{\ell}{\sqrt{g^2+a^2}}\right]^{1/2}$$

5. If a **simple pendulum** whose bob is of density d_o is made to oscillate in a liquid of density d, then its time period of vibration in liquid will increase and is given by

$$T = 2\pi\sqrt{\frac{\ell}{\left(1-\frac{d}{d_o}\right)g}} \quad (\text{where } d_0 > d)$$

6. The time period of a simple pendulum in a vehicle moving along a circular path of radius r and with constant velocity V is given by, $T = 2\pi\left[\frac{\ell}{\sqrt{\frac{V^4}{r^2}+g^2}}\right]^{1/2}$

7. If T_1 and T_2 are the time periods of a body oscillating under the restoring force F_1 and F_2 then the time period of the body under the influence of the resultant force $\vec{F} = \vec{F}_1 + \vec{F}_2$ will be $T = \frac{T_1 T_2}{\sqrt{T_1^2 + T_2^2}}$

8. (a) The percentage change in time period of simple pendulum when its length changes is
$$\frac{\Delta T}{T}\times 100 = \frac{1}{2}\left(\frac{\Delta \ell}{\ell}\right)\times 100\%$$
(b) The percentage change in time period of simple pendulum when g changes but ℓ remains constant is
$$\frac{\Delta T}{T}\times 100 = \frac{1}{2}\left(\frac{\Delta g}{g}\right)\times 100\,\%$$
(c) The percentage change in time peirod of simple pendulum when both ℓ and g change is
$$\frac{\Delta T}{T}\times 100 = \frac{1}{2}\left(\frac{\Delta \ell}{\ell}+\frac{\Delta g}{g}\right)\times 100\%$$

9. If a wire of length ℓ, area of cross-section A, Young's modulus Y is stretched by suspending a mass m, then the mass can oscillate with time period: $T = 2\pi\sqrt{\frac{TA}{m\ell}}$

10. If a **simple pendulum** is suspended from the roof of compartment of a train moving down an inclined plane of inclination θ, then the time period of oscillations
$$T = 2\pi\left[\frac{\ell}{g\cos\theta}\right]^{1/2}$$

11. If a ball of radius r oscillates in a bowl of radius R, then its time period is given by: $T = 2\pi\left[\frac{R-r}{g}\right]^{1/2}$

12. If a disc of radius r oscillates about a point at its rim, then its time period is given by: $T = 2\pi\left[\frac{r}{g}\right]^{1/2}$
It behaves as a simple pendulum of length r.

13. The graph between the length of a simple pendulum and its time period is a **parabola**.

14. The graph between the length of a simple pendulum and the square of its time period is a **straight line**.

15. The graph between ℓ & T and between ℓ & T^2 intersect at T = 1 second.

16. The time period of the mass attached to spring does not change with the change in acceleration due to gravity.

17. If the mass m attached to a spring oscillates in a non viscous liquid density σ, then its time period is given by $T = 2\pi\left[\frac{m}{k}\left(1-\frac{\sigma}{\rho}\right)\right]^{-1/2}$
where k = force constant and ρ is density of the mass suspended from the spring.

18. The length of second pendulum (T = 2 sec) is 99 cm

Physical Pendulum

$T_{restoring} = -\,mgd\sin\theta$

If θ is small, $\sin\theta \approx \theta$

$\therefore\ T_{restoring} = -\,mgd\theta$

And $T = 2\pi\sqrt{\frac{I}{mgd}}$

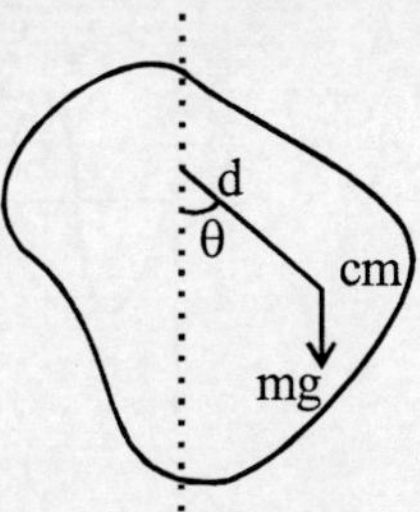

Let a test-tube of radius r, carrying lead shots of mass m is held vertically when partly immersed in liquid of density ρ. On pushing the tube little into liquid and let it executes S.H.M. of time period
$$T = 2\pi\sqrt{\frac{m}{\pi r^2 \rho g}}$$

Conical Pendulum

When the bob of a simple pendulum moves in a horizontal circle it is called as conical pendulum.

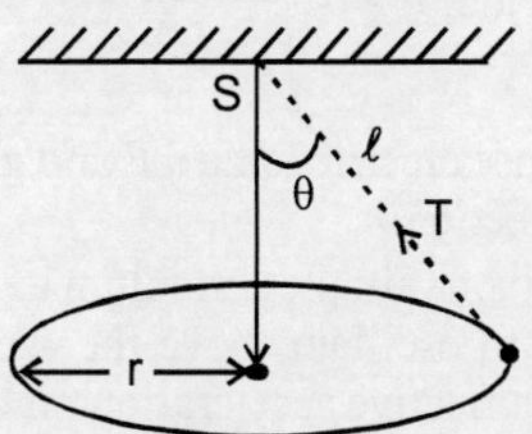

If ℓ is the length of the pendulum and the string makes an angle θ with vertical then time period, $T = 2\pi\sqrt{\frac{\ell\cos\theta}{g}}$

Torsional Pendulum

It is an arrangement which consists of a heavy mass suspended from a long thin wire whose other and is clamped to a rigid support. Time period
$$T = 2\pi\sqrt{\frac{I}{C}}$$
where I = moment of inertia of body about the suspension wire as axis of rotation.
C = restoring couple per unit thirst.

Problem Solving Tips

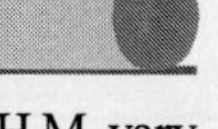

1. The displacement, velocity and acceleration of S.H.M. vary simple harmonically with the same time period and frequency.
2. The kinetic energy and potential energy vary periodically but not simple harmonically. The time period of kinetic energy or potential energy is half that of displacement, velocity and acceleration.
3. The graph between displacement, velocity or acceleration and t is a **sine curve**. But the graph between P.E. or K.E. of S.H.M. and time t is **parabola**.

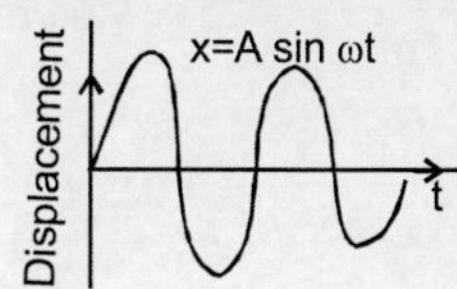

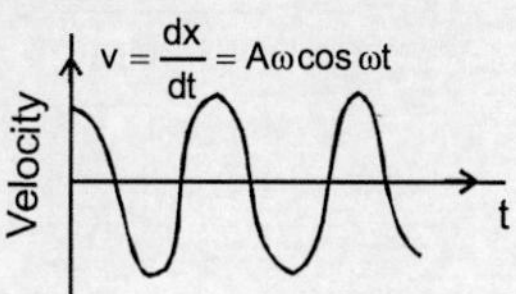

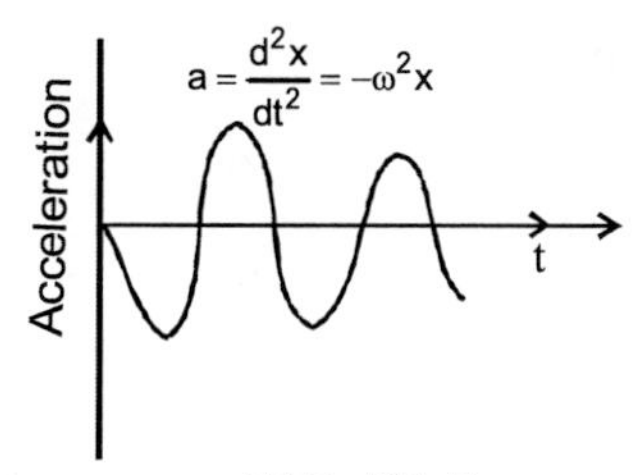

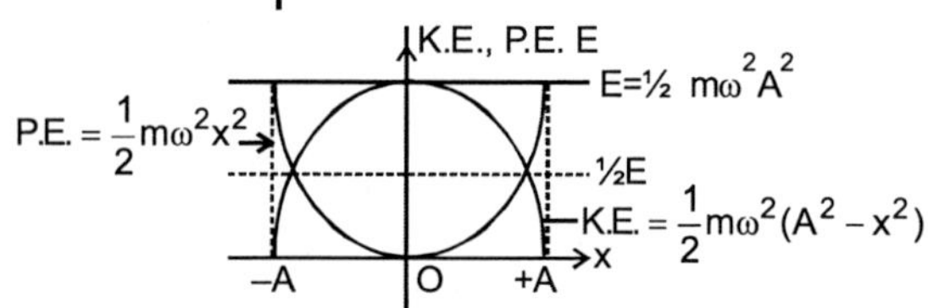

4. (a) If the bob of simple pendulum is -vely charged and a +vely charged plate is placed below it, then the effective acceleration on bob increases and consequently time period decreases.

Time period, $T = 2\pi\sqrt{\dfrac{\ell}{g+\dfrac{qE}{m}}}$

In this case electric force q E and gravity force act in same direction.

(b) If the bob of a simple pendulum is -vely charged and is made to oscillate above the -vely charged plate, then the effective acceleration on bob decreases and the time period increases. $T = 2\pi\sqrt{\dfrac{\ell}{g-\dfrac{qE}{m}}}$

In this case electric force qE and gravity force are opposite.

5. A pendulum clock slows down in summer and goes faster in winter.

6. Potential energy of a particle executing S.H.M. is equal to average force × displacement.

i.e., $U_P = \left[\dfrac{0+F}{2}\right]x = \left(\dfrac{0+m\omega^2 x}{2}\right)x = \dfrac{1}{2}m\omega^2 x^2$.

7. If the total energy of a particle executing S.H.M. is E, then its potential energy at displacement x is

$U_P = \dfrac{x^2}{A^2}E$ and kinetic energy $U_k = \left(1-\dfrac{x^2}{A^2}\right)E$

Example 1.

A spring is stretched by 0.20 metre when a mass of 0.50 kg is suspended. Calculate the period of the spring when a mass of 0.25 kg is suspended and put to oscillation. (g = 10 m/sec²).

Solution :

The force constant K of the spring is given by

$$K = \frac{F}{y} = \frac{0.5\text{ kg Wt}}{0.20\text{m}} = \frac{0.5\times 10\text{ newton}}{0.20\text{ m}} = 25\text{ newton/metre}$$

$$\text{Now } T = 2\pi\sqrt{\left(\frac{m}{K}\right)} = 2\times 3.14\sqrt{\left(\frac{0.25}{25}\right)} = 0.628\text{ s}$$

Example 2.

What will be the force constant of the spring system shown in fig?

(a) $\dfrac{k_1}{2}+k_2$

(b) $\left[\dfrac{1}{2k_1}+\dfrac{1}{k_2}\right]^{-1}$

(c) $\left[\dfrac{1}{2k_1}+\dfrac{1}{k_2}\right]$

(d) $\left[\dfrac{2}{k_1}+\dfrac{1}{k_2}\right]^{-1}$

Solution : (b)

Two springs of force constants k_1 and k_2 are in parallel. Hence

$$k' = k_1 + k_1 = 2k_1$$

The third spring is in series with spring of force constant k'.

$$\therefore \frac{1}{k} = \left[\frac{1}{2k_1}+\frac{1}{k_2}\right] \text{ or } k = \left[\frac{1}{2k_1}+\frac{1}{k_2}\right]^{-1}$$

Example 3.

A cylindrical piston of mass M slides smoothly inside a long cylinder closed at one end, enclosing a certain mass of gas. The cylinder is kept with its axis horizontal. If the piston is disturbed from its equilibrium position, it oscillates simple harmonically. The period of oscillation will be

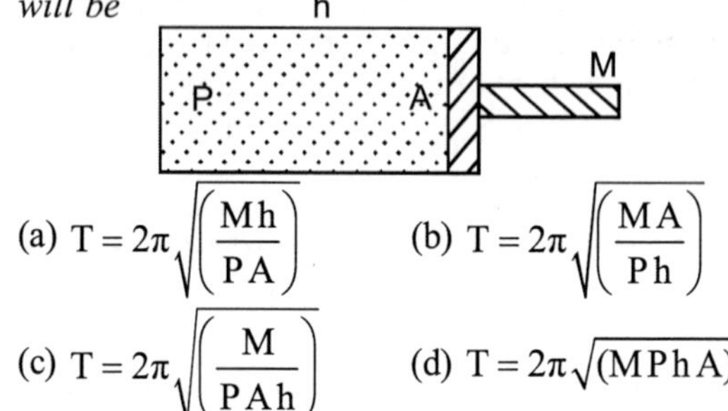

(a) $T = 2\pi\sqrt{\left(\dfrac{Mh}{PA}\right)}$ (b) $T = 2\pi\sqrt{\left(\dfrac{MA}{Ph}\right)}$

(c) $T = 2\pi\sqrt{\left(\dfrac{M}{PAh}\right)}$ (d) $T = 2\pi\sqrt{(MPhA)}$

Solution : (a)

We know that $PV = RT$

$\therefore \; V\Delta P + P\Delta V = 0$ or $\Delta P = P\,(\Delta V/V)$

or $\dfrac{F}{A} = -P\left(\dfrac{Ax}{Ah}\right) = -P\left(\dfrac{x}{h}\right)$

$F = -P\left(\dfrac{Ax}{h}\right) \therefore \; a = -P\left(\dfrac{Ax}{h}\right)\dfrac{1}{M} = -\left(\dfrac{PA}{Mh}\right)x$

This gives, $\omega^2 = \dfrac{PA}{Mh}$ or $T = \dfrac{2\pi}{\omega} = 2\pi\sqrt{\left(\dfrac{Mh}{PA}\right)}$

Example 4.

Which one of the following equations does not represent S.H.M.; where x = displacement and t = time. Parameters a, b and c are the constants of motion

(a) x = a sin bt (b) x = a cos bt + c

(c) x = a sin bt + c cos bt (d) x = a sec bt + c cosec bt

Solution : (d)

Sec bt is not defined for $bt = \pi/2$.

$$x = a \sec bt + c \operatorname{cosec} bt = \frac{a \sin bt + c \cos bt}{\sin bt \cos bt}$$

This equation cannot be modified in the form of simple equation of S.H.M.

i.e. $x = a \sin(\omega t + \phi)$.

so, it cannot represent S.H.M.

Example 5.

A small spherical steel ball is placed a little away from the centre of a large concave mirror whose radius of curvature R = 2.5 cm. When the ball is released, it begins to oscillate about the centre. Show that the motion of the ball is simple harmonic and find the period of motion. Neglect friction and take g = 10 m/sec².

Solution :

$F = -mg\sin\theta = -mg\,\theta \qquad (\because \theta \text{ is small})$

$= -mg\,(x/R)$

$\therefore\ F = -kx, \qquad \text{where } k = (mg/R)$

Now, $a = F/m = -kx/m = -\omega^2 x$

Hence, motion is simple harmonic motion and

$$T = \frac{2\pi}{\omega} = 2\pi\sqrt{\left(\frac{R}{g}\right)} = 2 \times 3.14 \times \sqrt{\left(\frac{2.5}{10}\right)} = 3.142 \text{ sec.}$$

Example 6.

A spring of stiffness constant k and natural length ℓ is cut into two parts of length $3\ell/4$ and $\ell/4$ respectively, and an arrangement is made as shown in the figure. If the mass is slightly displaced, find the time period of oscillation.

Solution :

The stiffness of a spring is inversely proportional to its length. Therefore the stiffness of each part is

$k_1 = \frac{4}{3}k$ and $k_2 = 4k$

Time period,

$$T = 2\pi\sqrt{\frac{m}{k_1 + k_2}} \text{ or } T = 2\pi\sqrt{\frac{3m}{16k}} = \frac{\pi}{2}\sqrt{\frac{3m}{k}}$$

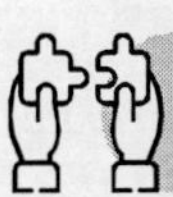

14.1 Concept Practice Problems

CPP

1. A pendulum is undergoing S.H.M. The velocity of the bob in the mean position is v. If now its amplitude is doubled, keeping the length same, its velocity in the mean position will be
(a) v/2 (b) v (c) 2 v (d) 4 v

2. The potential energy of a particle (U_x) executing S.H.M. is given by
(a) $U_x = \frac{k}{2}(x-a)^2$ (b) $U_x = k_1x + k_2x^2 + k_3x^3$
(c) $U_x = Ae^{-bx}$ (d) U_x = a constant

3. An instantaneous displacement of a simple harmonic oscillator is $x = A\cos(\omega t + \pi/4)$. Its speed will be maximum at time
(a) $\pi/4\omega$ (b) $\pi/2\omega$ (c) π/ω (d) $2\pi/\omega$

4. A mass M is suspended from a spring of negligible mass. The spring is pulled a little and then released so that the mass executes SHM of time period T. If the mass is increased by m, the time period becomes $\frac{5T}{3}$. Then the ratio of $\frac{m}{M}$ is
(a) $\frac{25}{9}$ (b) $\frac{16}{9}$ (c) $\frac{5}{3}$ (d) $\frac{3}{5}$

5. The time period of the oscillating system (see figure) is

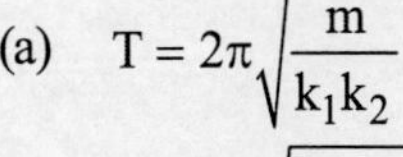

(a) $T = 2\pi\sqrt{\frac{m}{k_1k_2}}$

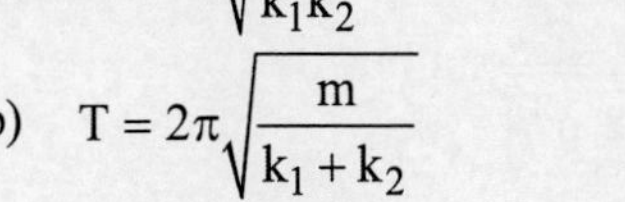

(b) $T = 2\pi\sqrt{\frac{m}{k_1+k_2}}$

(c) $T = 2\pi\sqrt{mk_1k_2}$

(d) None of these

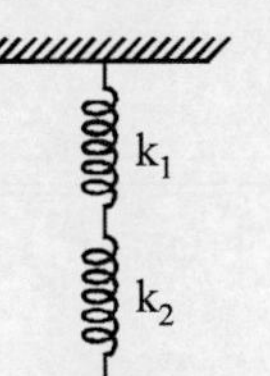

6. A boy is executing simple Harmonic Motion. At a displacement x its potential energy is E_1 and at a displacement y its potential energy is E_2. The potential energy E at displacement (x + y) is
(a) $\sqrt{E} = \sqrt{E_1} - \sqrt{E_2}$ (b) $\sqrt{E} = \sqrt{E_1} + \sqrt{E_2}$
(c) $E = E_1 + E_2$ (d) $E = E_1 - E_2$

7. A simple spring has length l and force constant K. It is cut into two springs of lengths l_1 and l_2 such that $l_1 = n\,l_2$ (n = an integer). The force constant of spring of length l_1 is
(a) K(1 + n) (b) (K/n)(1 + n)
(c) K (d) K/(n + 1)

8. A simple pendulum attached to the roof of a lift has a time period of 2s in a stationary lift. If the lift is allowed to fall freely the frequency of oscillations of pendulum will be
(a) zero (b) 2 Hz (c) 0.5 Hz (d) infinity

9. The graph shown in figure represents
(a) S.H.M.
(b) circular motion
(c) rectilinear motion
(d) uniform circular motion

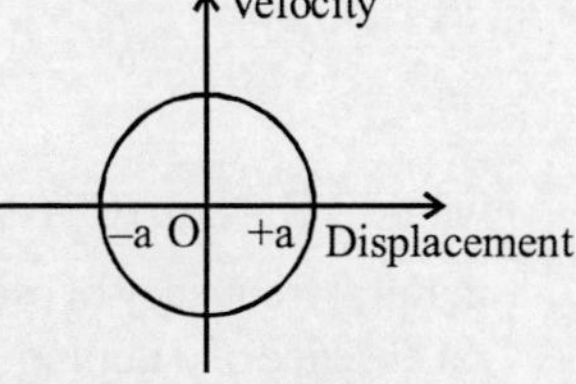

10. A circular hoop of radius R is hung over a knife edge. The period of oscillation is equal to that of a simple pendulum of length
(a) R (b) 2R (c) 3R (d) $\frac{3R}{2}$

ANSWER KEY

1	(c)	2	(a)	3	(a)	4	(b)	5	(b)	6	(b)	7	(b)	8	(a)	9	(a)	10	(b)

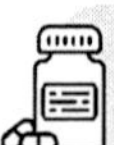

Topic 14.2 : Free, Damped, Forced Oscillations and Resonance

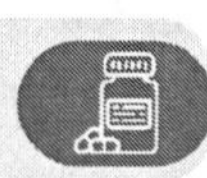

FREE OSCILLATION

If a system oscillates on its own and without any external influence then it is called as ***free oscillation.***

Frequency of free oscillation is called *natural frequency*. The equation for free S.H.M. oscillation

$$\frac{md^2x}{dt^2} = F_{restoring\,force} = -kx, \text{ where k is constant.}$$

The differential equation of harmonic motion in absence of damping and external force is

$$\frac{d^2x}{dt^2} + \omega_0^2 x = 0, \text{ where } \omega_0 \text{ is natural frequency of body.}$$

The time period is

$$T = \frac{2\pi}{\omega_0} = 2\pi\sqrt{\frac{m}{k}}$$

DAMPED OSCILLATION

Oscillation performed under the influence of frictional force is called as ***damped oscillation.***

(a) In case of damped oscillations the amplitude goes on decreasing and ultimately the system comes to a rest.

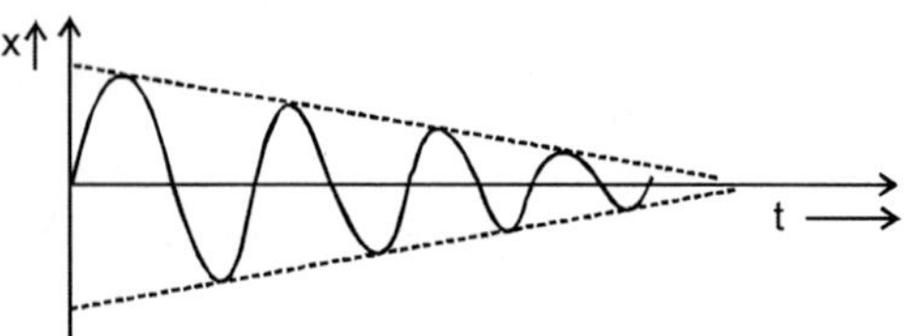

(b) The damping force ($F_{damping} \propto -v \Rightarrow F_{damping} = -bv$) is proportional to the speed of particle. Hence the equation of motion $m\frac{dV}{dt} = -kx - bv$

where b is positive constant and is called **damping coefficient**. Then the differential equation of a damped harmonic oscillation is

$$\frac{d^2x}{dt^2} + 2C\frac{dx}{dt} + \omega_0^2 x = 0 \qquad ...(i)$$

where 2 C = b/m (C is damping constant) & $\frac{k}{m} = \omega_0^2$, the natural frequency of oscillating particle i.e., its frequency in absence of damping.

In case of over damping the displacement of the particle is

$$x = A_0 \exp(-t/2\tau)\sin(\omega t + \phi) \qquad ...(ii)$$

$\Rightarrow$ $x = A\sin(\omega t + \phi)$ where A_0 = max. amplitude of the oscillator.

$$\omega = \sqrt{\omega_0^2 - c^2} \text{ and } \tau = \frac{m}{b} \text{ (relaxation time)}$$

It is clear from the fig & eq^n. (ii) that the amplitude of damped harmonic oscillator decreases with time. In this case, the motion does not repeat itself & is not periodic in usual sense of term.

However it has still a time period, $T = \frac{2\pi}{\omega} = \frac{2\pi}{\sqrt{\omega_0^2 - c^2}}$, which is the time interval between its successive passage in same direction passing the equilibrium point.

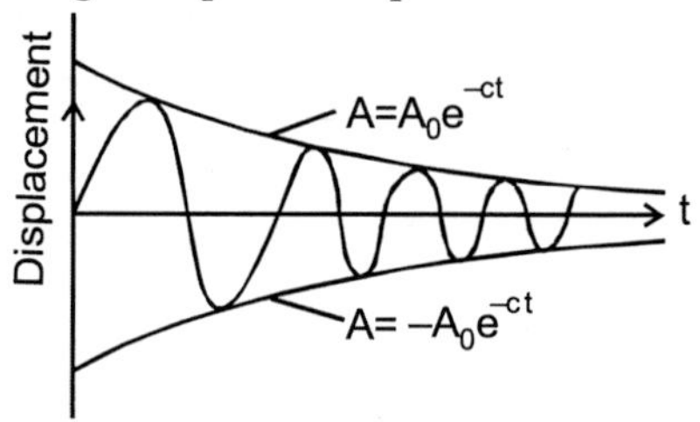

FORCED OSCILLATION AND RESONANCE :

The oscillation of a system under the action of external periodic force is called ***forced oscillation.***

External force can maintain the amplitude of damped oscillation. *When the frequency of the external periodic force is equal to the natural frequency of the system,* ***resonance*** *takes place.*

The amplitude of resonant oscillations is very very large. In the absence of damping, it may tend to infinity.

At resonance, the oscillating system continuously absorbs energy from the agent applying external periodic force.

In case of forced oscillations, the total force acting on the system is

$$F = -\underbrace{kx}_{\text{Restorting force}} - \underbrace{\frac{bdx}{dt}}_{\text{Damping force}} + \underbrace{F_0 \sin pt}_{\text{Ext periodic force}} \qquad ......(i)$$

Then by Newton's second law :

$$\Rightarrow \quad m\frac{d^2x}{dt^2} = -kx - b\frac{dx}{dt} + F_0 \sin pt$$

$$\text{or} \quad \frac{d^2x}{dt^2} + 2C\frac{dx}{dt} + \omega_0^2 x = f_0 \sin\beta t \qquad ......(ii)$$

$$\text{where } 2C = \frac{b}{m}, \omega_0^2 = \frac{k}{m}, f_0 = \frac{F_0}{m}$$

The **equation (ii) is the differential equation of motion of forced harmonic oscillator.**

The amplitude at any time t is

$$x = \frac{f_0}{\sqrt{[(\omega_0^2 - p^2) + 4c^2p^2]}}\sin(pt - \theta)$$

where $\tan\theta = \frac{2cp}{\omega^2 - p^2}$ & p is the frequency of external periodic force.

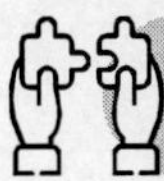

14.2 Concept Practice Problems

CPP

11. If a body oscillates at the angular frequency ω_d of the driving force, then the oscillations are called
(a) free oscillations (b) coupled oscillations
(c) forced oscillations (d) maintained oscillations

12. In case of a forced vibration, the resonance wave becomes very sharp when the
(a) quality factor is small
(b) damping force is small
(c) restoring force is small
(d) applied periodic force is small

13. What is the amplitude of simple harmonic motion at resonance in the ideal case of zero damping?
(a) Zero (b) –1 (c) 1 (d) Infinite

14. A particle oscillating under a force $\vec{F} = -k\bar{x} - b\bar{\upsilon}$ is a (k and b are constants)
(a) simple harmonic oscillator
(b) non linear oscillator
(c) damped oscillator
(d) forced oscillator

15. In case of sustained forced oscillations the amplitude of oscillations
(a) decreases linearly (b) decreases sinusoidally
(c) decreases exponentially (d) always remains constant

16. The frequency of the simple harmonic motion attained in forced oscillations, after the forced oscillation die out, is
(a) the natural frequency of the particle
(b) the frequency of the driving force
(c) double the frequency of the driving force
(d) double the natural frequency of the particle

17.

Column I	Column II
(A) $\frac{d^2y}{dt^2} = v^2 \frac{d^2y}{dx^2}$	(1) Resonant vibration
(B) $\frac{d^2y}{dt^2} + \omega^2 y = 0$	(2) Free vibration
(C) $\frac{d^2y}{dt^2} + 2k\frac{dy}{dt} + \omega^2 y = 0$	(3) Damped vibration
(D) $\frac{d^2y}{dt^2} + 2k\frac{dy}{dt} + \omega^2 y = F \sin pt$	(4) Forced vibration
	(5) Progressive wave

(a) (A) - (1), (B) - (3), (C) - (2, 4), (D) - (5)
(b) (A) - (1, 3), (B) - (2, 5), (C) - (3), (D) - (4, 5)
(c) (A) - (5), (B) - (2), (C) - (3), (D) - (1, 4)
(d) (A) - (1), (B) - (2), (C) - (3), (D) - (4)

18. Choose the false statement(s) for a forced oscillation.
I. Displacement amplitude of an oscillator is independent of the angular frequency of the driving force.
II. The amplitude tends to infinity when the driving frequency equals the natural frequency.
III. Maximum possible amplitude for a given driving frequency is governed by the driving frequency and the damping.
(a) I only (b) II only
(c) I and II (d) I, II and III

19.

Column I	Column II
(A) Motion of a satellite	(1) Damped oscillations
(B) Motion of a simple pendulum	(2) Resonant oscillations
(C) Oscillation of stretched string in air	(3) Periodic motion
(D) Flying off of a paper rider placed on the stretched string	(4) Simple harmonic motion

(a) (A) - (2), (B) - (3), (C) - (4), (D) - (1)
(b) (A) - (3), (B) - (2), (C) - (4), (D) - (1)
(c) (A) - (1), (B) - (3), (C) - (2), (D) - (4)
(d) (A) - (3), (B) - (4), (C) - (1), (D) - (2)

20. The amplitude of velocity of a particle is given by, $V_m = V_0/(a\omega^2 - b\omega + c)$ where V_0, a, b and c are positive : The condition for a single resonant frequency is
(a) $b^2 < 4ac$ (b) $b^2 = 4ac$
(c) $b^2 = 5ac$ (d) $b^2 = 7ac$

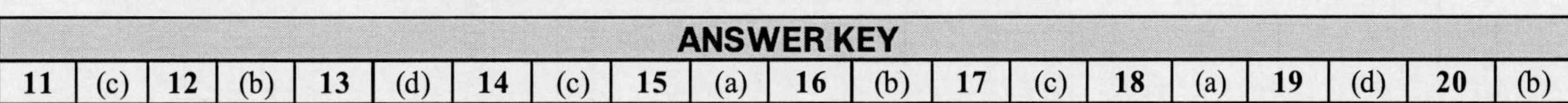

ANSWER KEY

11	(c)	12	(b)	13	(d)	14	(c)	15	(a)	16	(b)	17	(c)	18	(a)	19	(d)	20	(b)

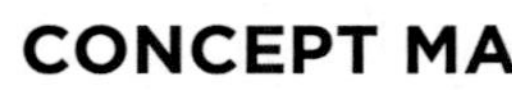

CONCEPT MAP

OSCILLATIONS
To-and-fro motion repeatedly about a fixed point in a definite interval of time

SHM
Simple Harmonic motion is the simplest form of oscillatory motion

Displacement in SHM
$x(t) = A(\cos \omega t + \phi)$
A = Amplitude i.e., Maximum displacement of particle

Phase
Time varying quantity $(\omega t + \phi)$

Phase constant or Phase angle (ϕ):
Depends on velocity (v) and displacement of particle at t = 0

Time Period (T)
The smallest interval of time after which the motion is repeated

Frequency(f)
The number of oscillations per second. i.e.,
$f = \frac{1}{T} = \frac{\omega}{2\pi}$

Simple Pendulum
Time Period
$T = 2\pi\sqrt{\frac{I}{mgl}} = 2\pi\sqrt{\frac{l}{g}}$

Oscillations due to a spring
Time period
$T = 2\pi\sqrt{\frac{m}{k}}$
$k = \frac{F}{x}$ spring constant

Velocity in SHM
$v = \frac{dx}{d(t)} = -\omega A \sin(\omega t + \phi)$
$v_{max} = \omega A$

Acceleration in SHM
$a = \frac{dv}{dt} = -\omega^2 A \cos(\omega t + \phi)$
$a_{max} = \omega^2 A$

Energy in SHM
Kinetic energy
K.E. $= 1/2\, m\omega^2 A^2 \sin^2(\omega t + \phi)$
Potential energy
P.E. $= 1/2\, m\omega^2 A^2 \cos^2(\omega t + \phi)$
Total energy T.E.= K.E. + P.E.
$= 1/2\, kA^2 [\cos^2(\omega t + \phi) + \sin^2(\omega t + \phi)]$

Force law equation for SHM
$F = -k(x),\ k = m\omega^2$
$\therefore\ \omega = \sqrt{\frac{k}{m}}$

Every oscillatory motion is periodic, but every periodic motion need not be oscillatory

Forced oscillations
Driving force $F(t) = F_0 \cos \omega_d t$
Displacement, $x(t) = A\cos(\omega_d t + \phi)$
Amplitude, $A = \frac{F_0}{\left\{m^2\left(\omega^2 - \omega_d^2\right)^2 + \omega_d^2 b^2\right\}^{\frac{1}{2}}}$
$\tan\phi = \frac{-\upsilon_0}{\omega_d x_0}$

Resonance
When frequency of external force is equal to natural frequency of oscillator

Damped Oscillation
Oscillation of a body whose amplitude goes on decreasing with time.
Damping force $F_d = -bv$
b = damping constant
Displacement of damped oscillator
$x = x_m e^{-bt/2m} \sin(\omega t + \phi)$
Amplitude decreases with time as
$x = x_m e^{-(b/2m)t}$

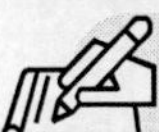

Exercise 1 - Chapter Revision Problems

CRP

1. A rectangular block of mass m and area of cross-section A floats in a liquid of density ρ. If it is given a small vertical displacement from equilibrium. It undergoes oscillations with a time period T then
(a) $T \propto m$ (b) $T \propto \rho$ (c) $T \propto 1/A$ (d) $T \propto 1/\rho$

2. The graph of time period (T) of simple pendulum versus its length (l) is

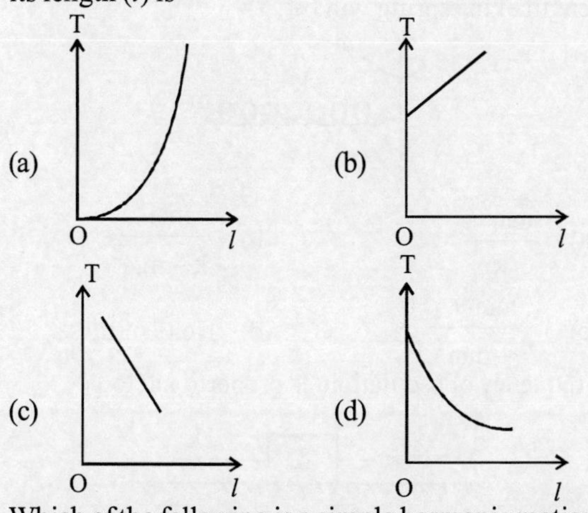

3. Which of the following is a simple harmonic motion?
(a) Particle moving through a string fixed at both ends.
(b) Wave moving through a string fixed at both ends.
(c) Earth spinning about its axis.
(d) Ball bouncing between two rigid vertical walls.

4. A rod is hinged vertically at one end and is forced to oscillate in a vertical plane with hinged end at the top, the motion of the rod:
(a) is simple harmonic
(b) is oscillatory but not simple harmonic
(c) is pericolic but not oscillatory
(d) may be simple harmonic

5. The graph plotted between the velocity and displacement from mean position of a particle executing SHM is
(a) circle (b) ellipse
(c) parabola (d) straight line

6. Acceleration of a particle executing SHM, at it's mean position is
(a) infinity (b) variable (c) maximum (d) zero

7. A vertical mass-spring system executes simple harmonic oscillations with a period of 2s. A quantity of this system which exhibits simple harmonic variation with a period of 1 s is
(a) velocity
(b) potential energy
(c) phase difference between acceleration and displacement
(d) difference between kinetic energy and potential energy

8. A simple pendulum has a metal bob, which is negatively charged. If it is allowed to oscillate above a positively charged metallic plate, then its time period will
(a) increase (b) decrease
(c) become zero (d) remain the same

9. In the fig. S1 and S2 are identical springs. The oscillation frequency of the mass m is f. If one spring is removed, the frequency will become

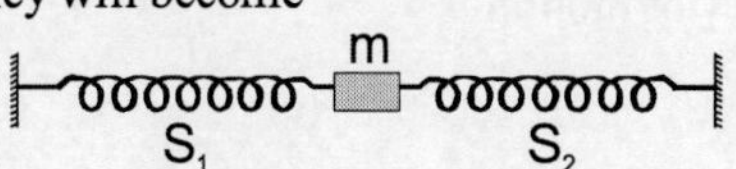

(a) f (b) $f \times 2$ (c) $f \times \sqrt{2}$ (d) $f/\sqrt{2}$

10. A particle executes S.H.M. having time period T, then the time period with which the potential energy changes is
(a) T (b) 2T (c) T/2 (d) ∞

11. The tension in the string of a simple pendulum is
(a) constant
(b) maximum in the extreme position
(c) zero in the mean position
(d) None of these

12. A child swinging on swing in sitting position stands up. The time period of the swing will
(a) increase
(b) decrease
(c) remain same
(d) increase if the child is tall and decrease if the child is short.

13. The graph shown in figure represents

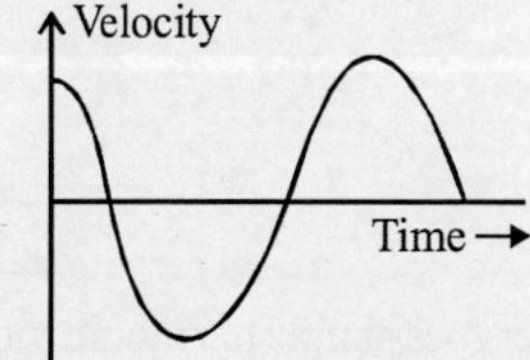

(a) motion of a simple pendulum starting from mean position
(b) motion of a simple pendulum starting from extreme position
(c) simple pendulum describing a horizontal circle
(d) None of these

14. Resonance is an example of
(a) tuning fork (b) forced vibration
(c) free vibration (d) damped vibration

15. Out of the following functions, representing motion of a particle, which represents SHM?
(A) $y = \sin\omega t - \cos\omega t$ (B) $y = \sin^3 \omega t$
(C) $y = 5\cos\left(\frac{3\pi}{4} - 3\omega t\right)$ (D) $y = 1 + \omega t + \omega^2 t^2$
(a) Only (A)
(b) Only (D) does not represent SHM
(c) Only (A) and (C)
(d) Only (A) and (B)

16. The period of oscillation of a mass M suspended from a spring of negligible mass is T. If along with it another mass M is also suspended, the period of oscillation will now be
(a) T (b) $T/\sqrt{2}$ (c) 2T (c) $\sqrt{2}$T

17. A body of mass 5 gram is executing S.H.M. about a fixed point O. With an amplitude of 10 cm, its maximum velocity is 100 cm/s. Its velocity will be 50 cm s^{-1} at a distance (in cm)
(a) 5 (b) $5\sqrt{2}$ (c) $5\sqrt{3}$ (d) $10\sqrt{2}$

18. The length of a second's pendulum at the surface of earth is 1 m. The length of second's pendulum at the surface of moon where g is 1/6th that at earth's surface is

(a) 1/6 m (b) 6 m (c) 1/36 m (d) 36 m

19. The equation of SHM of a particle is $A + 4\pi^2 x = 0$ where a is instantaneous linear acceleration at displacement x. The frequency of motion is

(a) 1 Hz (b) 4π Hz (c) $\frac{1}{4}$ Hz (d) 4 Hz

20. $y = 2\,(\text{cm}) \sin\left[\frac{\pi t}{2} + \phi\right]$ what is the maximum acceleration of the particle doing the S.H.M.

(a) $\frac{\pi}{2}$ cm/s^2 (b) $\frac{\pi^2}{2}$ cm/s^2

(c) $\frac{\pi^2}{4}$ cm/s^2 (d) $\frac{\pi}{4}$ cm/s^2

21. If the mass shown in figure is slightly displaced and then let go, then the system shall oscillate with a time period of

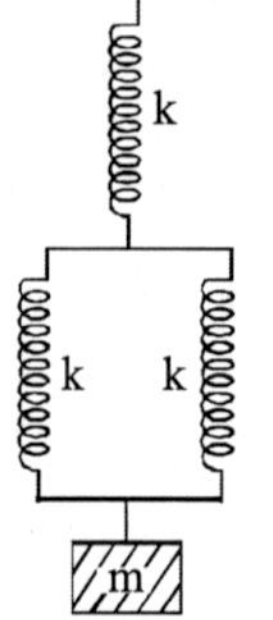

(a) $2\pi\sqrt{\frac{m}{3k}}$

(b) $2\pi\sqrt{\frac{3m}{2k}}$

(c) $2\pi\sqrt{\frac{2m}{3k}}$

(d) $2\pi\sqrt{\frac{3k}{m}}$

22. A particle undergoes simple harmonic motion having time period T. The time taken in 3/8th oscillation is

(a) $\frac{3}{8}T$ (b) $\frac{5}{8}T$ (c) $\frac{5}{12}T$ (d) $\frac{7}{12}T$

23. Lissajous figure obtained by combining $x = a \sin \omega t$ and $y = a \sin (\omega t + \pi/4)$ will be a/an

(a) ellipse (b) straight line

(c) circle (d) parabola

24. A Second's pendulum is placed in a space laboratory orbiting around the earth at a height 3 R from the earth's surface where R is earth's radius. The time period of the pendulum will be

(a) zero (b) $2\sqrt{3}$ (c) 4 sec (d) infinite

25. Two simple pendulums of length 0.5 m and 20 m respectively are given small linear displacement in one direction at the same time. They will again be in the phase when the pendulum of shorter length has completed oscillations

[$nT_1 = (n-1)T_2$, where T_1 is time period of shorter length & T_2 be time period of longer wavelength and n are no. of oscillations completed]

(a) 5 (b) 1 (c) 2 (d) 3

26. A mass is suspended separately by two different springs in successive order then time periods is t_1 and t_2 respectively. It is connected by both springs as shown in fig. then time period is t_0, the correct relation is

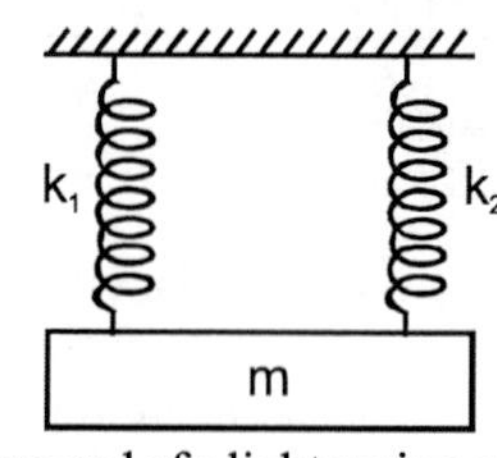

(a) $t_0^2 = t_1^2 + t_2^2$

(b) $t_0^{-2} = t_1^{-2} + t_2^{-2}$

(c) $t_0^{-1} = t_1^{-1} + t_2^{-1}$

(d) $t_0 = t_1 + t_2$

27. A particle of mass m is fixed to one end of a light spring of force constant k and unstretched length ℓ. The system is rotated about the other end of the spring with an angular velocity ω, in gravity free space. The increase in length of the spring will be

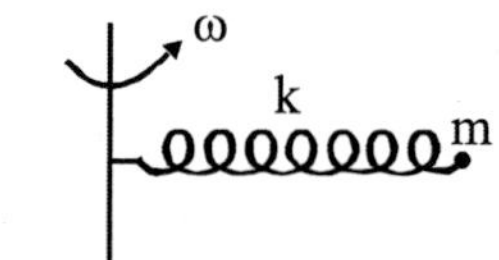

(a) $\frac{m\omega^2\ell}{k}$ (b) $\frac{m\omega^2\ell}{k - m\omega^2}$

(c) $\frac{m\omega^2\ell}{k + m\omega^2}$ (d) None of these

28. Frequency of oscillation is proportional to

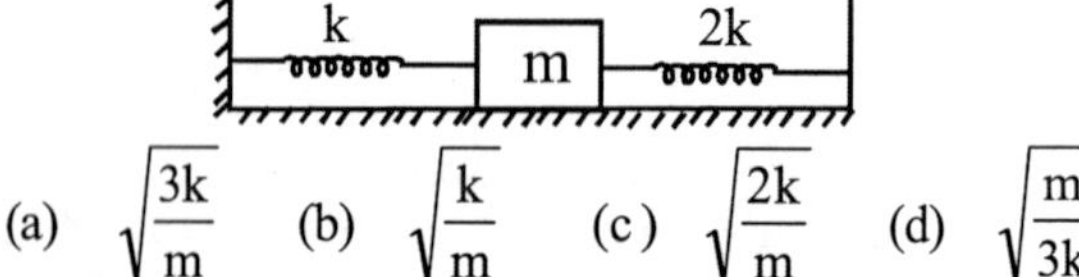

(a) $\sqrt{\frac{3k}{m}}$ (b) $\sqrt{\frac{k}{m}}$ (c) $\sqrt{\frac{2k}{m}}$ (d) $\sqrt{\frac{m}{3k}}$

29. A pendulum bob is raised to a height h and released from rest. At what height will it attain half of its maximum speed?

(a) $\frac{3h}{4}$ (b) $\frac{h}{2}$ (c) $\frac{h}{4}$ (d) 0.707h

30. The time period of a simple pendulum of infinite length is (R_e = radius of Earth)

(a) $T = 2\pi\sqrt{\frac{R_e}{g}}$ (b) $T = 2\pi\sqrt{\frac{2R_e}{g}}$

(c) $T = 2\pi\sqrt{\frac{R_e}{2g}}$ (d) $T = \infty$

31. A uniform pole of length $\ell = 2L$ is laid on smooth horizontal table as shown in figure. The mass of pole is M and it is connected to a frictionless axis at O. A spring with force constant k is connected to the other end. The pole is displaced by a small angle θ_0 from equilibrium position and released such that it performs small oscillations. Then

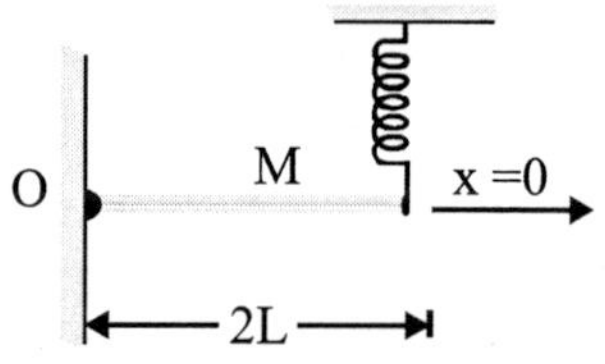

(a) $\omega_0 = \sqrt{\frac{M}{3k}}$ (b) $\omega_0 = \sqrt{\frac{k}{3M}}$

(c) $\omega_0 = \sqrt{\frac{3k}{M}}$ (d) $\omega_0 = \sqrt{\frac{k}{2M}}$

32. A body of mass m falls from a height h onto a pan (of negligible mass) of a spring balance as shown. The spring also possesses negligible mass and has spring constant k. Just after striking the pan, the body starts socillatory motion in vertical directioin of amplitude A and energy E. Then

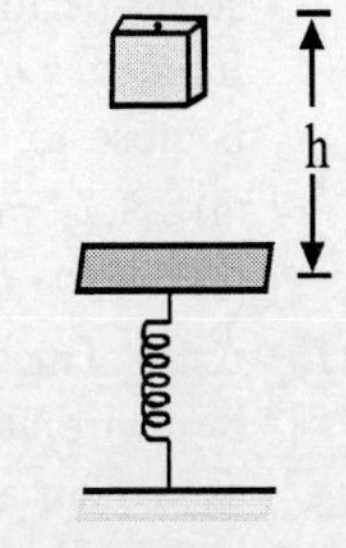

(a) $A = \frac{mg}{k}$

(b) $A = \frac{mg}{k}\sqrt{1 + \frac{2kh}{mg}}$

(c) $E = mgh + \frac{1}{2}kA^2$

(d) $E = mgh + \left(\frac{2mg}{2k}\right)^2$

33. A coin is placed on a horizontal platform which undergoes vertical simple harmonic motion of angular frequency ω. The amplitude of oscillation is gradually increased. The coin will leave contact with the platform for the first time

(a) at the mean position of the platform

(b) for an amplitude of $\frac{g}{\omega^2}$

(c) for an amplitude of $\frac{g^2}{\omega^2}$

(d) at the highest position of the platform

34. A point particle of mass 0.1 kg is executing S.H.M. of amplitude of 0.1 m. When the particle passes through the mean position, its kinetic energy is 8×10^{-3} Joule. Obtain the equation of motion of this particle if this initial phase of oscillation is 45º.

(a) $y = 0.1\sin\left(\pm 4t + \frac{\pi}{4}\right)$ (b) $y = 0.2\sin\left(\pm 4t + \frac{\pi}{4}\right)$

(c) $y = 0.1\sin\left(\pm 2t + \frac{\pi}{4}\right)$ (d) $y = 0.2\sin\left(\pm 2t + \frac{\pi}{4}\right)$

35. A forced oscillator is acted upon by a force $F = F_0 \sin \omega t$. The amplitude of oscillation is given by $\frac{55}{\sqrt{2\omega^2 - 36\omega + 9}}$.

The resonant angular frequency is

(a) 2 unit (b) 9 unit (c) 18 unit (d) 36 unit

36. Two simple harmonic motions, as shown, are at right angles. They are combined to form Lissajous figures.

$x(t) = A\sin(at + \delta)$

$y(t) = B\sin(bt)$

Identify the correct match below

(a) Parameters: A = B, a = 2b; $\delta = \frac{\pi}{2}$; Curve: Circle

(b) Parameters: A = B, a = b; $\delta = \frac{\pi}{2}$; Curve: Line

(c) Parameters: A ≠ B, a = b; $\delta = \frac{\pi}{2}$; Curve: Ellipse

(d) Parameters: A ≠ B, a = b; δ = 0; Curve: Parabola

37. x and y displacements of a particle are given as $x(t) = a \sin \omega t$ and $y(t) = a \sin 2\omega t$. Its trajectory will look like :

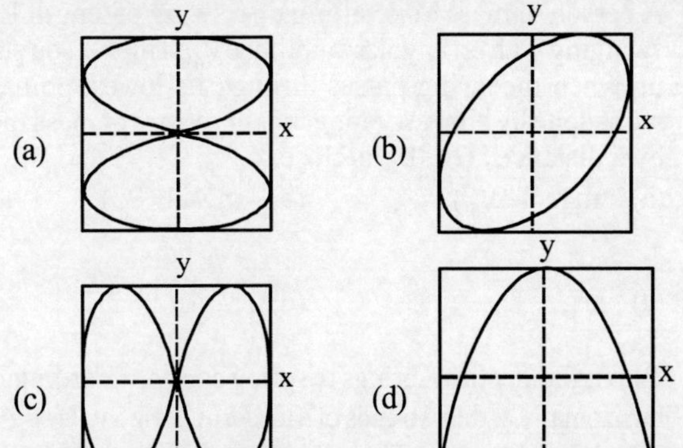

38. The displacement $y(t) = A\sin(\omega t + \phi)$ of a pendulum for $\phi = \frac{2\pi}{3}$ is correctly represented by

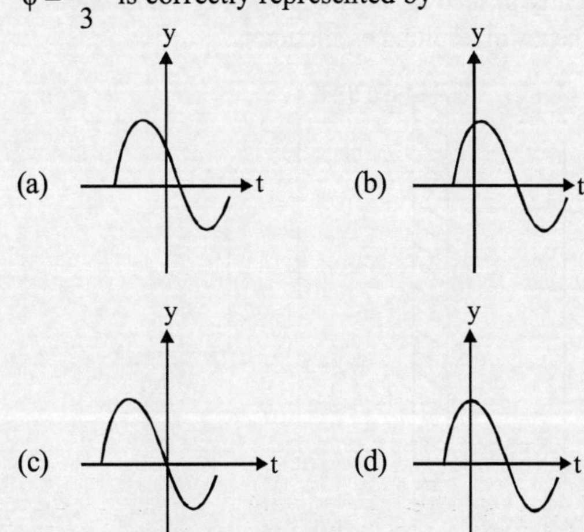

39. The displacement time graph of a particle executing S.H.M. is given in figure : (sketch is schematic and not to scale)

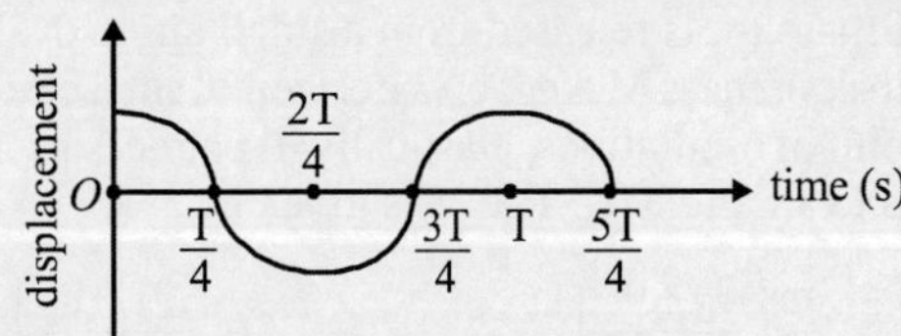

Which of the following statements is/are true for this motion?

(1) The force is zero at $t = \frac{3T}{4}$

(2) The acceleration is maximum at $t = T$

(3) The speed is maximum at $t = \frac{T}{4}$

(4) The P.E. is equal to K.E. of the oscillation at $t = \frac{T}{2}$

(a) (1), (2) and (4) (b) (2), (3) and (4)

(c) (1), (2) and (3) (d) (1) and (4)

40. A pendulum is executing simple harmonic motion and its maximum kinetic energy is K_1. If the length of the pendulum is doubled and it performs simple harmonic motion with the same amplitude as in the first case, its maximum kinetic energy is K_2.

(a) $K_2 = 2K_1$ (b) $K_2 = \frac{K_1}{2}$

(c) $K_2 = \frac{K_1}{4}$ (d) $K_2 = K_1$

41. A person of mass M is, sitting on a swing of length L and swinging with an angular amplitude θ_0. If the person stands up when the swing passes through its lowest point, the work done by him, assuming that his centre of mass moves by a distance l (l<<L), is close to :

(a) $mgl(1-\theta_0^2)$ (b) $mgl(1+\theta_0^2)$

(c) mgl (d) $Mgl\left(1+\frac{\theta_0^2}{2}\right)$

42. Two light identical springs of spring constant k are attached horizontally at the two ends of a uniform horizontal rod AB of length l and mass m. The rod is pivoted at its centre 'O' and can rotate freely in horizontal plane. The other ends of two springs are fixed to rigid supports as shown in figure. The rod is gently pushed through a small angle and released. The frequency of resulting oscillation is:

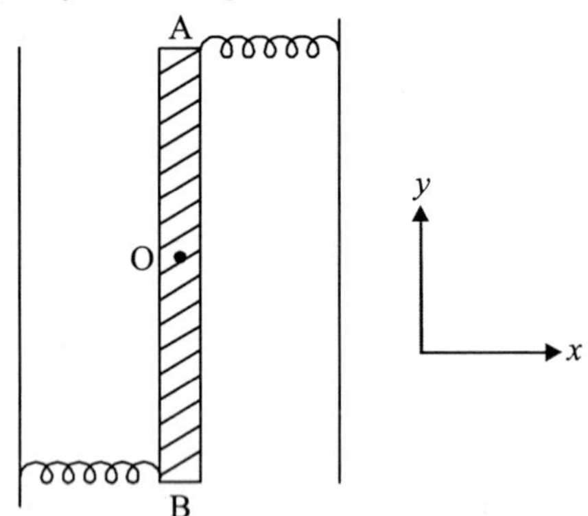

(a) $\frac{1}{2\pi}\sqrt{\frac{3k}{m}}$ (b) $\frac{1}{2\pi}\sqrt{\frac{2k}{m}}$ (c) $\frac{1}{2\pi}\sqrt{\frac{6k}{m}}$ (d) $\frac{1}{2\pi}\sqrt{\frac{k}{m}}$

43. A simple pendulum, made of a string of length l and a bob of mass m, is released from a small angle θ_0. It strikes a block of mass M, kept on a horizontal surface at its lowest point of oscillations, elastically. It bounces back and goes up to an angle θ_1. The M is given by :

(a) $\frac{m}{2}\left(\frac{\theta_0+\theta_1}{\theta_0-\theta_1}\right)$ (b) $m\left(\frac{\theta_0-\theta_1}{\theta_0+\theta_1}\right)$

(c) $m\left(\frac{\theta_0+\theta_1}{\theta_0-\theta_1}\right)$ (d) $\frac{m}{2}\left(\frac{\theta_0-\theta_1}{\theta_0+\theta_1}\right)$

44. A simple harmonic motion is represented by :

$y = 5(\sin 3\pi t + \sqrt{3}\cos 3\pi t)$ cm

The amplitude and time period of the motion are :

(a) 10 cm, $\frac{2}{3}$ s (b) 10 cm, $\frac{3}{2}$ s

(c) 5 cm, $\frac{3}{2}$ s (d) 5 cm, $\frac{2}{3}$ s

45. The mass and the diameter of a planet are three times the respective values for the Earth. The period of oscillation of a simple pendulum on the Earth is 2s. The period of oscillation of the same pendulum on the planet would be:

(a) $\frac{\sqrt{3}}{2}$ s (b) $\frac{2}{\sqrt{3}}$ s (c) $\frac{3}{2}$ s (d) $2\sqrt{3}$ s

46. A cylindrical plastic bottle of negligible mass is filled with 310 ml of water and left floating in a pond with still water. If pressed downward slightly and released, it starts performing simple harmonic motion at angular frequency ω. If the radius of the bottle is 2.5 cm then ω is close to: (density of water = 10^3 kg/m^3)

(a) 3.75 rad s^{-1} (b) 1.25 rad s^{-1}

(c) 2.50 rad s^{-1} (d) 5.00 rad s^{-1}

47. A rod of mass 'M' and length '2L' is suspended at its middle by a wire. It exhibits torsional oscillations; If two masses each of 'm' are attached at distance 'L/2' from its centre on both sides, it reduces the oscillation frequency by 20%. The value of ratio m/M is close to :

(a) 0.77 (b) 0.57 (c) 0.37 (d) 0.17

48. A particle executes simple harmonic motion and is located at x = a, b and c at times t_0, $2t_0$ and $3t_0$ respectively. The frequency of the oscillation is

(a) $\frac{1}{2\pi t_0}\cos^{-1}\left(\frac{a+b}{2c}\right)$ (b) $\frac{1}{2\pi t_0}\cos^{-1}\left(\frac{a+b}{3c}\right)$

(c) $\frac{1}{2\pi t_0}\cos^{-1}\left(\frac{2a+3c}{b}\right)$ (d) $\frac{1}{2\pi t_0}\cos^{-1}\left(\frac{a+c}{2b}\right)$

49. Two bodies of masses 1 kg and 4 kg are connected to a vertical spring, as shown in the figure. The smaller mass executes simple harmonic motion of angular frequency 25 rad/s, and amplitude 1.6 cm while the bigger mass remains stationary on the ground. The maximum force exerted by the system on the floor is (take g = 10 ms^{-2})

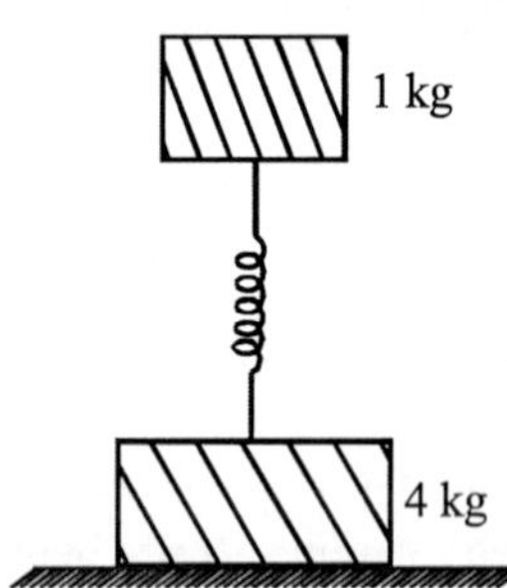

(a) 20 N (b) 10 N (c) 60 N (d) 40 N

50. An oscillator of mass M is at rest in its equilibrium position in a potential $V=\frac{1}{2}k(x-X)^2$. A particle of mass m comes from right with speed u and collides completely inelastically with M and sticks to it. This process repeats every time the oscillator crosses its equilibrium position. The amplitude of oscillations after 13 collisions is: (M = 10, m = 5, u = 1, k = 1).

(a) $\frac{1}{2}$ (b) $\frac{1}{\sqrt{3}}$ (c) $\frac{2}{3}$ (d) $\sqrt{\frac{3}{5}}$

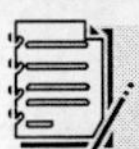

Exercise 2 - Exemplar & Past Year Questions

E&PYQs

Exemplar Questions

1. The displacement of a particle is represented by the equation $y = 3\cos\left(\frac{\pi}{4} - 2\omega t\right)$. The motion of the particle is
   (a) simple harmonic with period $2\pi/\omega$
   (b) simple harmonic with period π/ω
   (c) periodic but not simple harmonic
   (d) non-periodic
2. The displacement of a particle is represented by the equation $y = \sin^3 \omega t$. The motion is
   (a) non-periodic
   (b) periodic but not simple harmonic
   (c) simple harmonic with period $2\pi/\omega$
   (d) simple harmonic with period π/ω
3. The relation between acceleration and displacement of four particles are given below
   (a) $a_x = +2x$ (b) $a_x = +2x^2$
   (c) $a_x = -2x^2$ (d) $a_x = -2x$
   Which, one of the particle is exempting simple harmonic motion?
4. Motion of an oscillating liquid column in a U-tube is
   (a) periodic but not simple harmonic
   (b) non-periodic
   (c) simple harmonic and time period is independent of the density of the liquid
   (d) simple harmonic and time period is directly proportional to the density of the liquid
5. A particle is acted simultaneously by mutually perpendicular simple harmonic motion $x = a\cos\omega t$ and $y = a\sin\omega t$. The trajectory of motion of the particle will be
   (a) an ellipse (b) a parabola
   (c) a circle (d) a straight line
6. The displacement of a particle varies with time according to the relation $y = a\sin\omega t + b\cos\omega t$.
   (a) The motion is oscillatory but not SHM
   (b) The motion is SHM with amplitude $a + b$
   (c) The motion is SHM with amplitude $a^2 + b^2$
   (d) The motion is SHM with amplitude $\sqrt{a^2 + b^2}$
7. The equation of motion of a particle is $x = a\cos(\alpha t)_2$. The motion is
   (a) periodic but not oscillatory
   (b) periodic and oscillatory
   (c) oscillatory but not periodic
   (d) neither periodic nor oscillatory
8. A particle executing SHM maximum speed of 30 cm/s and a maximum acceleration of 60 cm/s^2. The period of oscillation is
   (a) π sec (b) $\frac{\pi}{2}$ sec (c) 2π sec (d) $\frac{\pi}{t}$ sec

Past Years (2013-2020) NEET/AIPMT Questions

9. A particle of mass m oscillates along x-axis according to equation $x = a\sin\omega t$. The nature of the graph between momentum and displacement of the particle is **[NEET Kar. 2013]**
   (a) straight line passing through origin
   (b) circle
   (c) hyperbola
   (d) ellipse
10. The oscillation of a body on a smooth horizontal surface is represented by the equation,
    $X = A\cos(\omega t)$
    where X = displacement at time t
    ω = frequency of oscillation
    Which one of the following graphs shows correctly the variation of 'a' with 't'? **[2014]**

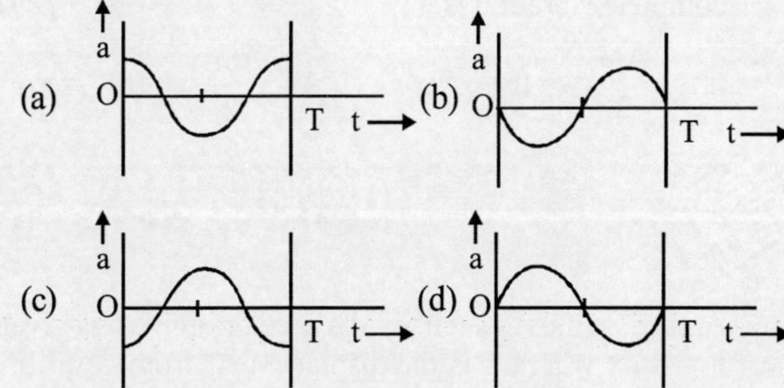

11. A particle is executing a simple harmonic motion. Its maximum acceleration is α and maximum velocity is β. Then its time period of vibration will be : **[2015 RS]**
    (a) $\frac{\alpha}{\beta}$ (b) $\frac{\beta^2}{\alpha}$ (c) $\frac{2\pi\beta}{\alpha}$ (d) $\frac{\beta^2}{\alpha^2}$
12. A particle is executing SHM along a straight line. Its velocities at distances x_1 and x_2 from the mean position are V_1 and V_2, respectively. Its time period is **[2015]**
    (a) $2\pi\sqrt{\frac{x_2^2 - x_1^2}{V_1^2 - V_2^2}}$ (b) $2\pi\sqrt{\frac{V_1^2 + V_2^2}{x_1^2 + x_2^2}}$
    (c) $2\pi\sqrt{\frac{V_1^2 - V_2^2}{x_1^2 - x_2^2}}$ (d) $2\pi\sqrt{\frac{x_1^2 - x_2^2}{V_1^2 - V_2^2}}$
13. When two displacements represented by $y_1 = a\sin(\omega t)$ and $y_2 = b\cos(\omega t)$ are superimposed the motion is: **[2015]**
    (a) simple harmonic with amplitude $\frac{a}{b}$
    (b) simple harmonic with amplitude $\sqrt{a^2 + b^2}$
    (c) simple harmonic with amplitude $\frac{(a+b)}{2}$
    (d) not a simple harmonic

14. A particle executes linear simple harmonic motion with an amplitude of 3 cm. When the particle is at 2 cm from the mean position, the magnitude of its velocity is equal to that of its acceleration. Then its time period in seconds is *[2017]*

(a) $\frac{\sqrt{5}}{2\pi}$ (b) $\frac{4\pi}{\sqrt{5}}$ (c) $\frac{2\pi}{\sqrt{3}}$ (d) $\frac{\sqrt{5}}{\pi}$

15. A spring of force constant k is cut into lengths of ratio 1 : 2 : 3. They are connected in series and the new force constant is k'. Then they are connected in parallel and force constant is k'' . Then k' : k'' is *[2017]*

(a) 1 : 9 (b) 1 : 11 (c) 1 : 14 (d) 1 : 6

16. A pendulum is hung from the roof of a sufficiently high building and is moving freely to and fro like a simple harmonic oscillator. The acceleration of the bob of the pendulum is 20 m/s^2 at a distance of 5 m from the mean position. The time period of oscillation is *[2018]*

(a) 2π s (b) π s (c) 1 s (d) 2 s

17. Average velocity of a particle executing SHM in one complete vibration is: *[2019]*

(a) $\frac{A\omega}{2}$ (b) $A\omega$ (c) $\frac{A\omega^2}{2}$ (d) zero

18. The displacement of a particle executing simple harmonic motion is given by $y = A_0 + A\sin\omega t + B\cos\omega t$. *[2019]*
Then the amplitude of its oscillation is given by:

(a) $A_0 + \sqrt{A^2 + B^2}$ (b) $\sqrt{A^2 + B^2}$

(c) $\sqrt{A_0^2 + (A+B)^2}$ (d) A+B

19. The distance covered by a particle undergoing SHM in one time period is (amplitude = A), *[NEET Odisha 2019]*

(a) 4A (b) Zero (c) A (d) 2A

20. A mass falls from a height 'h' and its time of fall 't' is recorded in terms of time period T of a simple pendulum. On the surface of earth it is found that $t = 2T$. The entire set up is taken on the surface of another planet whose mass is half of that of earth and radius the same. Same experiment is repeated and corresponding times noted as t' and T'. Then we can say *[NEET Odisha 2019]*

(a) $t' = 2T'$ (b) $t' = T'$ (c) $t' > 2T'$ (d) $t' < 2T'$

21. The phase difference between displacement and acceleration of a particle in a simple harmonic motion is : *[2020]*

(a) $\frac{3\pi}{2}$ rad (b) $\frac{\pi}{2}$ rad (c) zero (d) π rad

Exercise 3 - Concept Application Problems

CAP

1. A particle moves such that its acceleration 'a' is given by a = – bx where x is the displacement from equilibrium position and b is constant. The period of oscillation is

(a) $2\pi/b$ (b) $2\pi/\sqrt{b}$ (c) $\sqrt{2\pi/b}$ (d) $2\sqrt{\pi/b}$

2. If the magnitude of displacement is numerically equal to that of acceleration, then the time period is

(a) 1 second (b) π second (c) 2π second (d) 4π second

3. A particle executing simple harmonic motion along y-axis has its motion described by the equation $y = A\sin(\omega t) + B$. The amplitude of the simple harmonic motion is

(a) A (b) B (c) A+B (d) $\sqrt{A+B}$

4. Which one of the following equations of motion represents simple harmonic motion?

(a) Acceleration $= -k(x+a)$
(b) Acceleration $= k(x+a)$
(c) Acceleration $= kx$
(d) Acceleration $= -k_0x + k_1x^2$
where k, k_0, k_1 and a are all postive.

5. The total mechanical energy of a spring-mass system in simple harmonic motion is $E = \frac{1}{2}m\omega^2A^2$. Suppose the oscillating particle is replaced by another particle of double the mass while the amplitude A remains the same. The new mechanical energy will

(a) become 2E (b) become E/2
(c) become $\sqrt{2}$E (d) remain E

6. The displacement of aparticle along the x-axis is given by $x = a\sin^2\omega t$. The motion of the particle corresponds to:

(a) simple harmonic motion of frequency ω/π
(b) simple harmonic motion of frequency $3\omega/2\pi$
(c) non simple harmonic motion
(d) simple harmonic motion of frequency $\omega/2\pi$

7. A simple pendulum performs S.H.M. about x = 0 with an amplitude a, and time period T. The speed of the pendulum at x = a/2 will be

(a) $\pi\frac{a\sqrt{3}}{T}$ (b) $\frac{\pi a\sqrt{3}}{2T}$ (c) $\frac{\pi a}{T}$ (d) $\frac{3\pi^2 a}{T}$

8. A tunnel has been dug through the centre of the earth and a ball is released in it. It executes S.H.M. with time period

(a) 42 minutes (b) 1 day
(c) 1 hour (d) 84.6 minutes

9. A particle of mass 1 kg is moving in S.H.M. with an amplitude 0.02 and a frequency of 60 Hz. The maximum force acting on the particle is

(a) $144\pi^2$ (b) $188\pi^2$
(c) $288\pi^2$ (d) None of these

10. The displacement of a S.H.M. doing particle when K.E. = P.E. (amplitude = 4 cm) is

(a) $2\sqrt{2}$ cm (b) 2 cm (c) $\frac{1}{\sqrt{2}}$ cm (d) $\sqrt{2}$ cm

11. A simple pendulum has time period 't'. Its time period in a lift which is moving upwards with acceleration 3 ms^{-2} is

(a) $t\sqrt{\frac{9.8}{12.8}}$ (b) $t\sqrt{\frac{12.8}{9.8}}$ (c) $t\sqrt{\frac{9.8}{6.8}}$ (d) $t\sqrt{\frac{6.8}{9.8}}$

12. Two particles are oscillating along two close parallel straight lines side by side, with the same frequency and amplitudes. They pass each other, moving in opposite directions when their displacement is half of the amplitude. The mean positions of the two particles lie on a straight line perpendicular to the paths of the two particles. The phase difference is

(a) 0 (b) $2\pi/3$ (c) π (d) $\pi/6$

13. If a simple pendulum of length l has maximum angular displacement θ, then the maximum K.E. of bob of mass m is

(a) $\frac{1}{2}\,ml/g$ (b) $mg/2l$

(c) $mgl(1-\cos\theta)$ (d) $mgl\sin\theta/2$

14. Three masses of 500 g, 300 g and 100 g are suspended at the end of a spring as shown, and are in equilibrium. When the 500 g mass is removed, the system oscillates with a period of 2 second. When the 300 g mass is also removed, it will oscillate with a period of

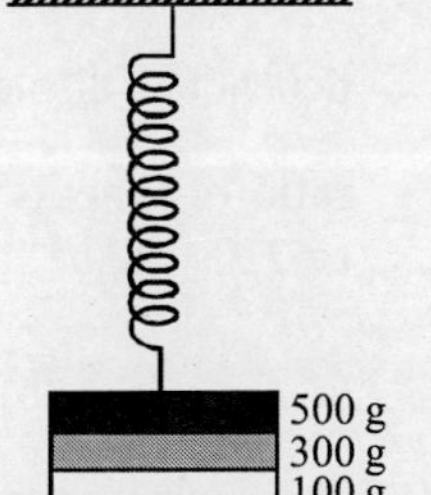

(a) 2 s

(b) 4 s

(c) 8 s

(d) 1 s

15. Two oscillators are started simultaneously in same phase. After 50 oscillations of one, they get out of phase by π, that is half oscillation. The percentage difference of frequencies of the two oscillators is nearest to

(a) 2% (b) 1% (c) 0.5% (d) 0.25%

16. Two wires are kept tight between the same pair of supports. The tensions in the wires are in the ratio 2 : 1, the radii are in the ratio 3 : 1 and the densities are in the ratio 1 : 2. The ratio of their fundamental frequencies is

(a) 2:3 (b) 2:4 (c) 2:5 (d) 2:6

17. A particle of mass 10 gm is describing S.H.M. along a straight line with period of 2 sec and amplitude of 10 cm. Its kinetic energy when it is at 5 cm from its equilibrium position is

(a) $37.5\pi^2$ *erg* (b) $3.75\pi^2$ *erg*

(c) $375\pi^2$ *erg* (d) $0.375\pi^2$ *erg*

18. Two particles are executing S.H.M. of same amplitude and frequency along the same straight line path. They pass each other when going in opposite directions, each time their displacement is half of their amplitude. What is the phase difference between them ?

(a) $5\pi/6$ (b) $2\pi/3$ (c) $\pi/3$ (d) $\pi/6$

19. The spring constant from the adjoining combination of springs is

(a) K

(b) 2K

(c) 4K

(d) 5K/2

20. A clock which keeps correct time at 20ºC, is subjected to 40ºC. If coefficient of linear expansion of the pendulum is 12×10^{-6} per ºC. How much will it gain or loose in time ?

(a) 10.3 seconds/day (b) 20.6 seconds/day

(c) 5 seconds/day (d) 20 minutes/day

21. When an oscillator completes 100 oscillations its amplitude reduces to $\frac{1}{3}$ of its initial value. What will be its amplitude, when it completes 200 oscillations ?

(a) $\frac{1}{8}$ (b) $\frac{2}{3}$ (c) $\frac{1}{6}$ (d) $\frac{1}{9}$

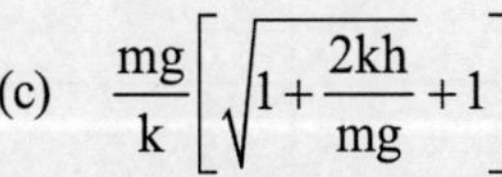

22. A mass m fall on spring of spring constant k and negligible mass from a height h. Assuming it sticks to the pan and executes simple harmonic motion, the maximum height upto which the pan will rise is

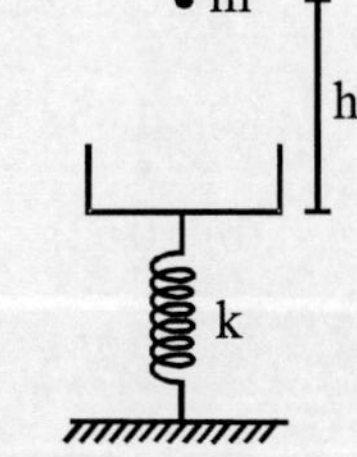

(a) $\frac{mg}{k}$

(b) $\frac{mg}{k}\left[\sqrt{1+\frac{2kh}{mg}}-1\right]$

(c) $\frac{mg}{k}\left[\sqrt{1+\frac{2kh}{mg}}+1\right]$

(d) $\frac{mg}{k}\left[\sqrt{1+\frac{kh}{mg}}-1\right]$

23. A block rests on a horizontal table which is executing SHM in the horizontal plane with an amplitude 'a'. If the coefficient of friction is 'μ', then the block just starts to slip when the frequency of oscillation is

(a) $\frac{1}{2\pi}\sqrt{\frac{\mu g}{a}}$ (b) $\sqrt{\frac{\mu g}{a}}$ (c) $2\pi\sqrt{\frac{a}{\mu g}}$ (d) $\sqrt{\frac{a}{\mu g}}$

24. On Earth, a body suspended on a spring of negligible mass causes extension L and undergoes oscillations along length of the spring with frequency f. On the Moon, the same quantities are L/n and f' respectively. The ratio f'/f is

(a) n (b) $\frac{1}{n}$ (c) $n^{-1/2}$ (d) 1

25. A particle of mass is executing oscillations about the origin on the x-axis. Its potential energy is $V(x) = k|x|^3$, where k is a positive constant. If the amplitude of oscillation is a, then its time period T is

(a) proportional to $\frac{1}{\sqrt{a}}$ (b) proportional to $\sqrt{a}$

(c) independent $a^{\frac{3}{2}}$ (d) None of these

26. In the figure shown, the spring is light and has a force constant k. The pulley is light and smooth and the strring is light . The suspended block has a mass m. On giving a slight displacement vartically to the block in the downward direction from its equilibrium position the block executes S.H.M. on being released with time period T. Then

(a) $T = 2\pi\sqrt{\frac{m}{k}}$

(b) $T = 2\pi\sqrt{\frac{m}{2k}}$

(c) $T = 2\pi\sqrt{\frac{2m}{k}}$

(d) $T = 4\pi\sqrt{\frac{m}{k}}$

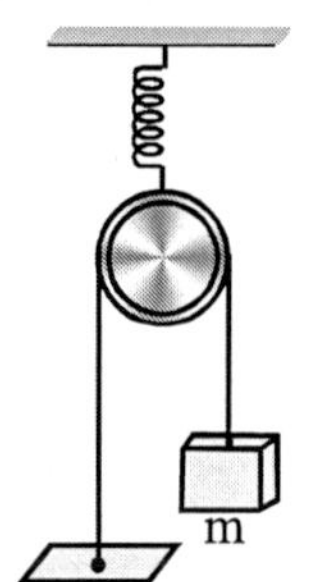

27. A body of mass 0.01 kg executes simple harmonic motion about x = 0 under the influence of a force as shown in figure. The time period of S.H.M. is

(a) 1.05 s

(b) 0.52 s

(c) 0.25 s

(d) 0.03 s

28. The position co-ordinates of a particle moving in a 3-D coordinate system is given by

$x = a\cos\omega t$

$y = a\sin\omega t$

and $z = a\omega t$

The speed of the particle is:

(a) $\sqrt{2}\,a\omega$ (b) $a\omega$ (c) $\sqrt{3}\,a\omega$ (d) $2a\omega$

29. The ratio of maximum acceleration to maximum velocity in a simple harmonic motion is $10\ s^{-1}$. At, t = 0 the displacement is 5 m. What is the maximum acceleration ? The initial phase is $\frac{\pi}{4}$

(a) $500\ m/s^2$ (b) $500\sqrt{2}\ m/s^2$

(c) $750\ m/s^2$ (d) $750\sqrt{2}\ m/s^2$

30. A simple harmonic oscillator of angular frequency 2 rad s^{-1} is acted upon by an external force $F = \sin t$ N. If the oscillator is at rest in its equilibrium position at $t = 0$, its position at later times is proportional to :

(a) $\sin t + \frac{1}{2}\cos 2t$ (b) $\cos t - \frac{1}{2}\sin 2t$

(c) $\sin t - \frac{1}{2}\sin 2t$ (d) $\sin t + \frac{1}{2}\sin 2t$

31. Which of the following expressions corresponds to simple harmonic motion along a straight line, where x is the displacement and a, b, c are positive constants?

(a) $a + bx - cx^2$ (b) bx^2

(c) $a - bx + cx^2$ (d) $-bx$

32. A point mass oscillates along the x-axis according to the law $x = x_0\cos(\omega t - \pi/4)$. If the acceleration of the particle is written as $a = A\cos(\omega t + \delta)$,then

(a) $A = x_0\omega^2,\ \delta = 3\pi/4$ (b) $A = x_0, \delta = -\pi/4$

(c) $A = x_0\omega^2,\ \delta = \pi/4$ (d) $A = x_0\omega^2,\ \delta = -\pi/4$

33. A particle undergoing simple harmonic motion has time dependent displacement given by $x(t) = A\sin\frac{\pi t}{90}$. The ratio of kinetic to potential energy of this particle at t = 210s will be :

(a) $\frac{1}{9}$ (b) 1 (c) 2 (d) $\frac{1}{3}$

34. A particle is executing simple harmonic motion (SHM) of amplitude A, along the x-axis, about $x = 0$. When its potential Energy (PE) equals kinetic energy (KE), the position of the particle will be:

(a) $\frac{A}{2}$ (b) $\frac{A}{2\sqrt{2}}$ (c) $\frac{A}{\sqrt{2}}$ (d) A

35. An object of mass m is suspended at the end of a massless wire of length L and area of cross-section, A. Young modulus of the material of the wire is Y. If the mass is pulled down slightly its frequency of oscillation along the vertical direction is:

(a) $f = \frac{1}{2\pi}\sqrt{\frac{mL}{YA}}$ (b) $f = \frac{1}{2\pi}\sqrt{\frac{YA}{mL}}$

(c) $f = \frac{1}{2\pi}\sqrt{\frac{mA}{YL}}$ (d) $f = \frac{1}{2\pi}\sqrt{\frac{YL}{mA}}$

36. When a particle of mass m is attached to a vertical spring of spring constant k and released, its motion is described by $y(t) = y_0\sin^2\omega t$, where 'y' is measured from the lower end of unstretched spring. Then ω is :

(a) $\frac{1}{2}\sqrt{\frac{g}{y_0}}$ (b) $\sqrt{\frac{g}{y_0}}$ (c) $\sqrt{\frac{g}{2y_0}}$ (d) $\sqrt{\frac{2g}{y_0}}$

37. A block of mass m attached to a massless spring is performing oscillatory motion of amplitude 'A' on a frictionless horizontal plane. If half of the mass of the block breaks off when it is passing through its equilibrium point, the amplitude of oscillation for the remaining system become fA. The value of f is :

(a) $\frac{1}{\sqrt{2}}$ (b) 1 (c) $\frac{1}{2}$ (d) $\sqrt{2}$

38. A simple pendulum oscillating in air has period T. The bob of the pendulum is completely immersed in a non-viscous liquid. The density of the liquid is $\frac{1}{16}$ th of the material of the bob. If the bob is inside liquid all the time, its period of oscillation in this liquid is :

(a) $2T\sqrt{\frac{1}{10}}$ (b) $2T\sqrt{\frac{1}{14}}$ (c) $4T\sqrt{\frac{1}{15}}$ (d) $4T\sqrt{\frac{1}{14}}$

39. A simple pendulum of length 1 m is oscillating with an angular frequency 10 rad/s. The support of the pendulum starts oscillating up and down with a small angular frequency of 1 rad/s and an amplitude of 10^{-2} m. The relative change in the angular frequency of the pendulum is best given by :

(a) 10^{-3} rad/s (b) 1 rad/s
(c) 10^{-1} rad/s (d) 10^{-5} rad/s

40. A particle executes simple harmonic motion with an amplitude of 5 cm. When the particle is at 4 cm from the mean position, the magnitude of its velocity in SI units is equal to that of its acceleration. Then, its periodic time in seconds is:

(a) $\frac{4\pi}{3}$ (b) $\frac{3}{8}\pi$ (c) $\frac{8\pi}{3}$ (d) $\frac{7}{3}\pi$

41. A silver atom in a solid oscillates in simple harmonic motion in some direction with a frequency of 10^{12}/sec. What is the force constant of the bonds connecting one atom with the other? (Mole wt. of silver = 108 and Avagadro number = 6.02×10^{23} gm mole^{-1})

(a) 6.4 N/m (b) 7.1 N/m (c) 2.2 N/m (d) 5.5 N/m

42. A pendulum clock loses 12 s a day if the temperature is 40°C and gains 4 s a day if the temperature is 20° C. The temperature at which the clock will show correct time, and the co-efficient of linear expansion (α) of the metal of the pendulum shaft are respectively :

(a) 30°C; $\alpha = 1.85 \times 10^{-3}$/°C
(b) 55°C; $\alpha = 1.85 \times 10^{-2}$/°C
(c) 25°C; $\alpha = 1.85 \times 10^{-5}$/°C
(d) 60°C; $\alpha = 1.85 \times 10^{-4}$/°C

43. In an experiment for determining the gravitational acceleration g of a place with the help of a simple pendulum, the measured time period square is plotted against the string length of the pendulum in the figure.

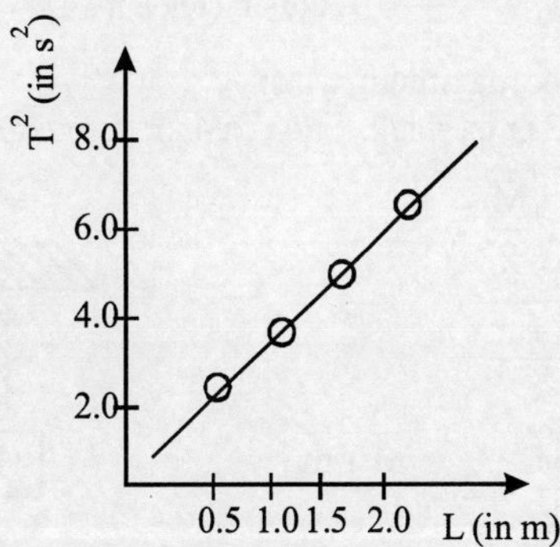

What is the value of g at the place?

(a) 9.81 m/s^2 (b) 9.87 m/s^2
(c) 9.91 m/s^2 (d) 10.0 m/s^2

44. A damped harmonic oscillator has a frequency of 5 oscillations per second. The amplitude drops to half its value for every 10 oscillations. The time it will take to drop to $\frac{1}{1000}$ of the original amplitude is close to :

(a) 50s (b) 100s (c) 20s (d) 10s

45. The displacement of a damped harmonic oscillator is given by $x(t) = e^{-0.1t}.\cos(10\pi t + \varphi)$. Here t is in seconds. The time taken for its amplitude of vibration to drop to half of its initial value is close to :

(a) 4s (b) 7s (c) 13s (d) 27s

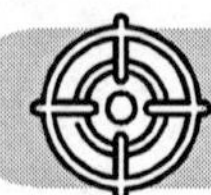

Hints & Solutions

14.1 Concept Practice Problems CPP

1. (c) $v_{max} = a\omega$; $v'_{max} = 2a\omega = 2v_{max} = 2v$ (since $v_{max} = v$)
2. (a) P.E. of body in S.H.M. at an instant,
$$U = \frac{1}{2}m\omega^2 y^2 = \frac{1}{2}ky^2$$
If the displacement, $y = (a - x)$ then
$$U = \frac{1}{2}k(a-x)^2 = \frac{1}{2}k(x-a)^2$$
3. (a) Velocity, $v = \frac{dx}{dt} = -A\omega\sin(\omega t + \pi/4)$
Velocity will be maximum, when
$\omega t + \pi/4 = \pi/2$ or $\omega t = \pi/2 - \pi/4 = \pi/4$ or $t = \pi/4\omega$
4. (b)

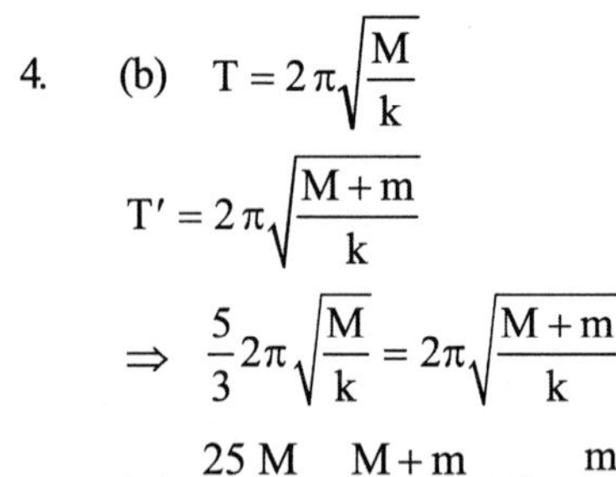

$$T = 2\pi\sqrt{\frac{M}{k}}$$
$$T' = 2\pi\sqrt{\frac{M+m}{k}}$$
$$\Rightarrow \frac{5}{3}2\pi\sqrt{\frac{M}{k}} = 2\pi\sqrt{\frac{M+m}{k}}$$
$$\Rightarrow \frac{25}{9}\frac{M}{k} = \frac{M+m}{k} \Rightarrow \frac{m}{M} = \frac{16}{9}$$

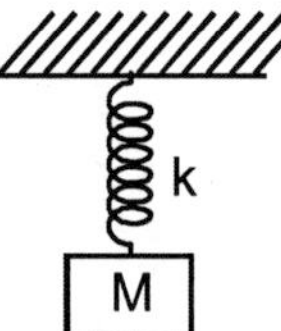

5. (b)
6. (b)
$$E_1 = \frac{1}{2}kx^2 \Rightarrow x = \sqrt{\frac{2E_1}{k}},\ E_2 = \frac{1}{2}ky^2 \Rightarrow y = \sqrt{\frac{2E_2}{k}}$$
and $E = \frac{1}{2}k(x+y)^2 \Rightarrow x + y = \sqrt{\frac{2E}{k}}$
$$\Rightarrow \sqrt{\frac{2E_1}{k}} + \sqrt{\frac{2E_2}{k}} = \sqrt{\frac{2E}{k}} \Rightarrow \sqrt{E_1} + \sqrt{E_2} = \sqrt{E}$$
7. (b) Let k be the force constant of spring of length l_2. Since $l_1 = n\,l_2$, where n is an integer, so the spring is made of (n + 1) equal parts in length each of length l_2.
$\therefore \frac{1}{K} = \frac{(n+1)}{k}$ or $k = (n+1)K$
The spring of length l_1 (= n l_2) will be equivalent to n springs connected in series where spring constant
$k' = \frac{k}{n} = (n+1)K/n$ & spring constant of length ℓ_2 is K(n+1).
8. (a) When lift is falling freely, the effective acceleration due to gravity inside the lift is zero i.e. g' = g – g = 0. Therefore time period will be infinity and frequency is zero
9. (a) t = 0, v maximum. The motion begins from mean position. So it represents S.H.M.
10. (b) $T = 2\pi\sqrt{\frac{2R}{g}} = 2\pi\sqrt{\frac{\ell}{g}}$

14.2 Concept Practice Problems CPP

11. (c) In forced oscillations, the body oscillates at the angular frequency of the driving force.
12. (b) The resonance wave becomes very sharp when damping force is small.
13. (d)
14. (c) A particle oscillating under a force $\overline{F} = -k\overline{x} - b\overline{\upsilon}$ is a damped oscillator. the first term $-k\overline{x}$ represents the restoring force and second term $-b\overline{\upsilon}$ represents the damping force.
15. (a) In case of sustained force oscillations the amplitude of oscillations decreases linearly.
16. (b) 17. (c)
18. (a) Displacement amplitude of an oscillator depends on the angular frequency of the driving force.
19. (d)
20. (b) $V_m = V_0/(a\omega^2 - b\omega + c)$
If there is a single resonant frequency, then this equation should be satisfied for only one that particular resonant frequency, hence $a\omega^2 - b\omega + c = 0$ will have equal roots therefore;
$D = 0 \Rightarrow (-b)^2 - 4ac = 0 \Rightarrow b^2 = 4ac$

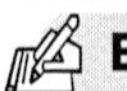

Exercise 1 - Chapter Revision Problems

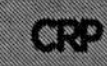

1. (a) A rectangular block of mass m and area of cross-section
A floats in a liquid of density ρ. If it is given a small vertical displacement from equilibrium. It undergoes oscillations with a time period T then : $T \propto m$.
2. (a) 3. (b) 4. (d) 5. (b)
6. (d) 7. (b) 8. (b)
9. (d) Here effective spring factor, $k_{eff} = 2\,k$;
Frequency of oscillation, $f = \frac{1}{2\pi}\sqrt{\frac{2k}{m}}$; when one spring is removed, then spring factor = k ;
New frequency of oscillation $f' = \frac{1}{2\pi}\sqrt{\frac{k}{m}} = \frac{f}{\sqrt{2}}$
10. (c) P.E. changes from zero to maximum twice in each vibration so its time period is T/2
11. (d) Tension is maximum at the mean position.
12. (b)
13. (a) At displacement ± a, the velocity is zero. At zero displacement, velocity is maximum.
14. (b)
15. (c) Only functions given in (A) & (C) represent SHM.
16. (d) $T = 2\pi\sqrt{\frac{m}{K}} \quad \therefore \frac{T_1}{T_2} = \sqrt{\frac{M_1}{M_2}}$

$\therefore \quad T_2 = T_1\sqrt{\frac{M_2}{M_1}} = T_1\sqrt{\frac{2M}{M}}$

$T_2 = T_1\sqrt{2} = \sqrt{2}\,T$ (where $T_1 = T$)

17. (c) $v_{max} = 100 = a\omega$; $\omega = 100/a = 100/10 = 10$ rad/s

$v^2 = \omega^2(a^2 - y^2)$ or 50^2
$= 10^2(10^2 - y^2)$ or $25 = 100 - y^2$

or $y = \sqrt{75} = 5\sqrt{3}$ cm.

18. (a) $T = 2\pi\sqrt{\frac{\ell}{g}}$; $2 = 2\pi\sqrt{\frac{\ell}{g}} = 2\pi\sqrt{\frac{\ell'}{(g/6)}}$

Time period will remain constant if on moon,
$\ell' = \ell/6 = 1/6$ m

19. (a) Comparing $A + \omega^2 x = 0$

$\omega^2 = 4\pi^2 \Rightarrow \omega = 2\pi$, $2\pi\nu = 2\pi$, $\nu = 1$Hz

20. (b) $y = 2\sin\left(\frac{\pi t}{2} + \phi\right)$

velocity of particle $\frac{dy}{dt} = 2 \times \frac{\pi}{2}\cos\left(\frac{\pi t}{2} + \phi\right)$

acceleration $\frac{d^2y}{dt} = -\frac{\pi^2}{2}\sin\left(\frac{\pi t}{2} + \phi\right)$

Thus $a_{max} = \frac{\pi^2}{2}$

21. (b) The equivalent situation is a series combination of two springs of spring constants k and 2k.
If k' is the equivalent spring constant, then

$k' = \frac{(k)(2k)}{3k} = \frac{2k}{3}$

$\Rightarrow T = 2\pi\sqrt{\frac{3m}{2k}}$

22. (c) Time to complete 1/4th oscillation is $\frac{T}{4}$ s. Time to complete $\frac{1}{8}$ th vibration from extreme position is obtained from

$y = \frac{a}{2} = a\cos\omega t = a\cos\frac{2\pi}{T}t$ or $t = \frac{T}{6}$ s

So time to complete 3/8th oscillation

$= \frac{T}{4} + \frac{T}{6} = \frac{5T}{12}$

23. (a) $\sin\omega t = x/a$ and

$\cos\omega t = \sqrt{1 - \sin^2\omega t} = \sqrt{1 - x^2/a^2}$

$y = \sin(\omega t + \pi/4)$
$= \sin\omega t\cos\pi/4 + \cos\omega t\sin\pi/4$

$= \frac{x}{a} \times \frac{1}{\sqrt{2}} + \left(\sqrt{1 - x^2/a^2}\right) \times \frac{1}{\sqrt{2}}$

or $\sqrt{2}\,y = x + \sqrt{a^2 - x^2}$

or $2y^2 = x^2 + (a^2 - x^2) + 2x\sqrt{a^2 - x^2}$

$= a^2 + 2x\sqrt{a^2 - x^2}$

It is an equation of an ellipse.

24. (d) The second pendulum placed in a space laboratory orbiting around the earth is in a weightlessness state. Hence $g = 0$ so $T = \infty$

25. (b) Let T_1, T_2 be the time period of shorter length and longer length pendulums respectively. As per question, n $T_1 = (n - 1)\,T_2$;

so $n\,2\pi\sqrt{\frac{0.5}{g}} = (n-1)\,2\pi\sqrt{\frac{20}{g}}$

or $n = (n-1)\sqrt{40} \approx (n-1)6$

Hence $n = 6/5 \approx 1$

26. (b) $t_1 = 2\pi\sqrt{\frac{m}{k_1}}$ or $t_1^2 = \frac{4\pi^2 m}{k_1}$ or $k_1 = \frac{4\pi^2 m}{t_1^2}$

Similarly, $k_2 = \frac{4\pi^2 m}{t_2^2}$ and $(k_1 + k_2) = \frac{4\pi^2 m}{t_0^2}$

$\therefore \quad \frac{4\pi^2 m}{t_0^2} = \frac{4\pi^2 m}{t_1^2} + \frac{4\pi^2 m}{t_2^2}$ or $\frac{1}{t_0^2} = \frac{1}{t_1^2} + \frac{1}{t_2^2}$

27. (b) Let x = the increase in the length of spring. Then the particle moves along a circular path of radius $(\ell + x)$, and the spring force = kx = centripetal force

$\therefore m\omega^2(\ell + x) = kx$ or $x = \frac{m\omega^2\ell}{k - m\omega^2}$

28. (a)

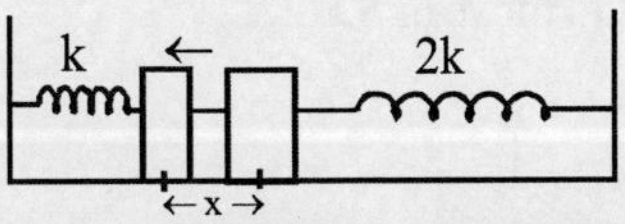

Let mass is displaced towards left by x then force on mass $= -kx - 2kx = -3kx$
[negative sign is taken because force is opposite to the direction of motion]

$\Rightarrow F = -3kx = -m\omega^2 x \Rightarrow \omega = \sqrt{\frac{3k}{m}}$.

$f = \frac{\omega}{2\pi} = \frac{1}{2\pi}\sqrt{\frac{3k}{m}}$.

Thus it is propotional to $\sqrt{3k/m}$

29. (a) Maximum velocity can be found out by energy conservation.

$mgh = \frac{1}{2}mv^2$ or $v_{max} = \sqrt{2gh}$;

$\frac{v_{max}}{2} = v' = \sqrt{\frac{gh}{2}}$

$mgh = \frac{1}{2}m(v')^2 + mgh'$;

$$mgh = \frac{1}{2}\frac{mgh}{2} + mgh'$$

$$\Rightarrow \frac{3mgh}{4} = mgh' \text{ or } h' = \frac{3h}{4}$$

30. (a)

31. (c) $I = \frac{1}{3}M(2L)^2 = \frac{4}{3}ML^2$

Force applied by the spring is $F = -kx$

$\Rightarrow F = -k(2L\theta)$

(θ is the angular displacement from the equilibrium position). Further

$$\tau = |\vec{\ell} \times \vec{F}| = 4L^2k\sin\theta = -4L^2k\theta$$

Also, $\tau = I\alpha = I\ddot{\theta} = -4L^2k\theta$

$$\Rightarrow \ddot{\theta} + \frac{3k}{M}\theta = 0 \Rightarrow \omega_0 = \sqrt{\frac{3k}{M}}$$

32. (b) $mg(h + y) = \frac{1}{2}ky^2$

$$\Rightarrow y = \frac{mg}{k} \pm \frac{mg}{k}\sqrt{1 + \frac{2kh}{mg}}$$

At equilibrium

$$mg = ky_0 \Rightarrow y_0 = \frac{mg}{k}$$

$$\Rightarrow \text{Amplitude } A = y - y_0 = \frac{mg}{k}\sqrt{1 + \frac{2kh}{mg}}$$

Energy of oscillation is

$$E = \frac{1}{2}kA^2 = mgh + \left(\frac{mg}{2k}\right)^2$$

33. (b) For block A to move in S.H.M.

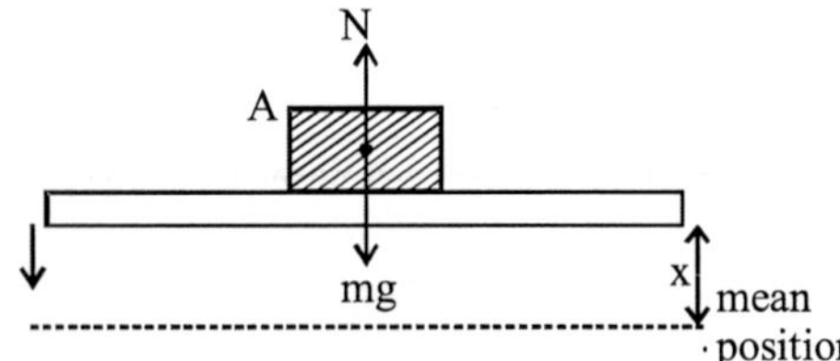

$mg - N = m\omega^2 x$

where x is the distance from mean position

For block to leave contact $N = 0$

$$\Rightarrow mg = m\omega^2 x \Rightarrow x = \frac{g}{\omega^2}$$

34. (a)

35. (b) At resonance, amplitude of oscillation is maximum

$\Rightarrow 2\omega^2 - 36\omega + 9$ is minimum

$\Rightarrow 4\omega - 36 = 0$ (derivative is zero)

$\Rightarrow \omega = 9$

36. (c) From the two mutually perpendicular S.H.M.'s, the general equation of Lissajous figure,

$$\frac{x^2}{A^2} + \frac{y^2}{B^2} - \frac{2xy}{AB}\cos\delta = \sin^2\delta$$

$x = A\sin(at + \delta)$

$y = B\sin(bt + r)$

Clearly $A \neq B$ hence ellipse.

37. (c) At $t = 0$, $x(t) = 0$; $y(t) = 0$

$x(t)$ is a sinusoidal function

At $t = \frac{\pi}{2\omega}$; $x(t) = a$ and $y(t) = 0$

Hence trajectory of particle will look like as (c).

38. (a) Displacement $y(t) = A\sin(wt + \phi)$ [Given]

For $\phi = \frac{2\pi}{3}$

at $t = 0$; $y = A\sin\phi = A\sin\frac{2\pi}{3}$

$= A\sin 120° = 0.87A$ [$\because \sin 120° \simeq 0.866$]

Graph (a) depicts $y = 0.87A$ at $t = 0$

39. (c) From graph equation of SHM

$X = A\cos\omega t$

(1) At $\frac{3T}{4}$ particle is at mean position.

$\therefore$ Acceleration = 0, Force = 0

(2) At T particle again at extreme position so acceleration is maximum.

(3) At $t = \frac{T}{4}$, particle is at mean position so velocity is maximum.

Acceleration = 0

(4) When KE = PE

$$\Rightarrow \frac{1}{2}k(A^2 - x^2) = \frac{1}{2}kx^2$$

Here, A = amplitude of SHM

x = displacement from mean position

$$\Rightarrow A^2 = 2x^2 \Rightarrow x = \frac{+A}{\sqrt{2}}$$

$$\Rightarrow \frac{A}{\sqrt{2}} = A\cos\omega t \quad \Rightarrow t = \frac{T}{2}$$

$\therefore x = -A$ which is not possible

$\therefore$ 1, 2 and 3 are correct.

40. (a) $K = \frac{1}{2}m\omega^2x^2 \Rightarrow K_{max} = \frac{1}{2}m\omega^2A^2$

$A = L\theta$

$$\omega = \sqrt{\frac{g}{L}} \Rightarrow K = \frac{1}{2}m.\frac{g}{L}.L^2\theta^2 = \frac{1}{2}mgL\theta^2$$

$$\therefore \frac{K_1}{K_2} = \frac{L}{2L} = \frac{1}{2} \Rightarrow K_2 = 2K_1$$

41. (b)

42. (c)

43. (b)

44. (a) Given : $y = 5\left[\sin(3\pi t) + \sqrt{3}\cos(3\pi t)\right]$

$$\Rightarrow y = 10\sin\left(3\pi t + \frac{\pi}{3}\right)$$

$\therefore$ Amplitude = 10 cm

Time period, $T = \frac{2\pi}{\omega} = \frac{2\pi}{3\pi} = \frac{2}{3}s$

45. (d) Acceleration due to gravity $g = \frac{GM}{R^2}$

$$\frac{g_p}{g_e} = \frac{M_p}{M_e}\left(\frac{R_e}{R_p}\right)^2 = 3\left(\frac{1}{3}\right)^2 = \frac{1}{3}$$

Also $T \propto \frac{1}{\sqrt{g}} \Rightarrow \frac{T_p}{T_e} = \sqrt{\frac{g_e}{g_p}} = \sqrt{3}$

$\Rightarrow T_p = 2\sqrt{3}$ s

46. (Bonus)

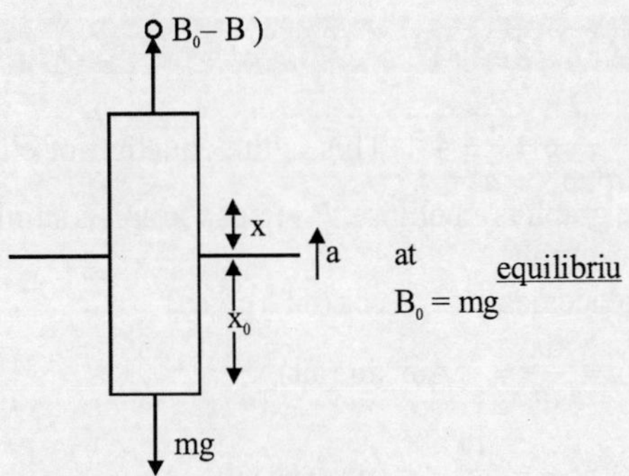

Extra boyant force = ρAxg
$B_0 + B = mg + ma$
$\therefore B = ma = \rho Axg = (\pi r^2 \rho g)x$

$a = \frac{(\pi r^2 \rho g)x}{m}$

using, $a = \omega^2 x \Rightarrow \omega = \sqrt{\frac{\pi r^2 \rho g}{m}}$ $\quad \omega = 7.95\ rads^{-1}$

47. (c)

48. (d) Using $y = A \sin \omega t$
$a = A \sin \omega t_0$
$b = A \sin 2\omega t_0$
$c = A \sin 3\omega t_0$
$a + c = A[\sin \omega t_0 + A \sin 3\omega t_0] = 2A \sin 2\omega t_0 \cos \omega t_0$

$\frac{a+c}{b} = 2\cos \omega t_0$

$\Rightarrow \omega = \frac{1}{t_0}\cos^{-1}\left(\frac{a+c}{2b}\right) \Rightarrow f = \frac{1}{2\pi t_0}\cos^{-1}\left(\frac{a+c}{2b}\right)$

49. (c) Mass of bigger body M = 4 kg
Mass of smaller body m = 1 kg
Smaller mass (m = 1 kg) executes S.H.M of angular frequency $\omega = 25$ rad/s
Amplitude $x = 1.6$ cm $= 1.6 \times 10^{-2}$
As we know,

$T = 2\pi\sqrt{\frac{m}{K}}$

or, $\frac{2\pi}{\omega} = 2\pi\sqrt{\frac{m}{K}}$

or, $\frac{1}{25} = \sqrt{\frac{1}{K}}$ $[\because m = 1kg;\ \omega = 25\ rad/s]$

or, $K = 625\ Nm^{-1}$.

The maximum force exerted by the system on the floor
$= Mg + Kx + mg$
$= 4 \times 10 + 625 \times 1.6 \times 10^{-2} + 1 \times 10$
$= 40 + 10 + 10$
$= 60$ N

50. (b) In first collision mu momentum will be imparted to system, in second collision when momentum of (M + m) is in opposite direction mu momentum of particle will make its momentum zero.

On 13th collision, $\boxed{m} \rightarrow \boxed{M+12}$; $\boxed{M+13m} \rightarrow V$

$mu = (M + 13m)v \Rightarrow v = \frac{mu}{M+13m} = \frac{u}{15}$

$v = \omega A \Rightarrow \frac{u}{15} = \sqrt{\frac{K}{M-13m}} \times A$

Putting value of M, m, u and K we get amplitude

$A = \frac{1}{15}\sqrt{\frac{75}{1}} = \frac{1}{\sqrt{3}}$

Exercise 2 - Exemplar & Past Year Questions E&PYQs

Exemplar Questions

1. (b) As given that, $y = 3\cos\left(\frac{\pi}{4} - 2\omega t\right)$

Velocity of the particle

$$v = \frac{dy}{dt} = \frac{d}{dt}\left[3\cos\left(\frac{\pi}{4} - 2\omega t\right)\right]$$

$$= 3(-2\omega)\left[-\sin\left(\frac{\pi}{4} - 2\omega t\right)\right]$$

$$= 6\omega \sin\left(\frac{\pi}{4} - 2\omega t\right)$$

So, acceleration,

$$a = \frac{dv}{dt} = \frac{d}{dt}\left[6\omega \sin\left(\frac{\pi}{4} - 2\omega t\right)\right]$$

$$= (6\omega) \times (-2\omega)\cos\left(\frac{\pi}{4} - 2\omega t\right)$$

$$= -4\omega^2\left[3\cos\left(\frac{\pi}{4} - 2\omega t\right)\right]$$

$a = -4\omega^2 y$

In simple harmonic motion acceleration (or force) is directly proportional to the negative of displacement of particle
$\Rightarrow$ as acceleration, $a \propto -y$
Hence, due to negative sign motion is simple harmonic motion (SHM.)
A simple harmonic motion is always periodic. So motion is periodic simple harmonic.
From the given equation,

$$y = 3\cos\left(\frac{\pi}{4} - 2\omega t\right)$$

Compare it by standard equation

$y = a\cos(\omega t + \phi)$

So, $\omega' = 2\omega$

$\frac{2\pi}{T'} = 2\omega \Rightarrow T' = \frac{2\pi}{2\omega} = \frac{\pi}{\omega}$

Hence, the motion is SHM with period $\frac{\pi}{\omega}$.

2. (b)
3. (d) For motion to be SHM acceleration of the particle must be opposite of restoring force and proportional to negative of displacement. So, $F = ma = m(-2x)$
i.e., $F = -2mx$, so $F \propto -x$
Hence, $a_x = -2x$
We should be clear that x has to be linear.
4. (c)
5. (c) The resultant-displacement can be find by adding x and y-components.
According to variation of x and y, trajectory will be predicted, so resultant displacement is $y' = (x + y)$
As given that,

$x = a\cos\omega t$ ...(i)

$y = a\sin\omega t$ ...(ii)

So, $y' = (a\cos\omega t + a\sin\omega t)$

$\Rightarrow y' = a(\cos\omega t + \sin\omega t)$

$y' = a\sqrt{2}\left[\frac{\cos\omega t}{\sqrt{2}} + \frac{\sin\omega t}{\sqrt{2}}\right]$

$y' = a\sqrt{2}(\cos\omega t\cos 45° + \sin\omega t\sin 45°)$

$= a\sqrt{2}\cos(\omega t - 45°)$

So, the displacement is not straight line and not parabola also.
Now, squaring and adding eqs. (i) and (ii),

$x^2 + y^2 = a^2$ $\quad [\because \cos^2\omega t + \sin^2\omega t = 1]$

This is the equation of a circle, so motion in circular (independent of time).
Clearly, the locus is a circle of constant radius a.
6. (d)
7. (c) According to the question,

$x = a\cos(\alpha t)^2$

is a cosine function, so it is an oscillatory motion.
Now, at, $t = (t + T)$. The equation of motion of particle

$x(t+T) = a\cos[\alpha(t+T)]^2$ $\quad [\because x(t) = a\cos(\alpha t)^2]$

$= a\cos[\alpha t^2 + \alpha T^2 + 2\alpha tT] \neq x(t)$

where, T is supposed as period of the function $\omega(t)$.
Hence, it is oscillatory but not periodic.
8. (a) Let us consider a equation of an SHM is represented by $y = a\sin\omega t$

$v = \frac{dy}{dt} = a\omega\cos\omega t$

$(v)_{max} = a\omega = 30$ cm/sec (given) ...(i)

Acceleration $(a) = \frac{dv}{dt} = -a\omega^2\sin\omega t$

$a_{max} = \omega^2 a = 60$ (given) ...(ii)

Eqs. (i) and (ii), we get

$\omega(\omega a) = 60 \Rightarrow \omega(30) = 60$

$\omega = 2$ rad/s

$\frac{2\pi}{T} = 2$ rad/s

$T = \pi$ sec

Past Years (2013-2020) NEET/AIPMT Questions

9. (d) As $\frac{v^2}{a^2\omega^2} + \frac{y^2}{a^2} = 1$ This is the equation of ellipse.
Hence the graph is an ellipse. P versus x graph is similar to V versus x graph.
10. (c) Displacement, $x = A\cos(\omega t)$ (given)
Velocity, $v = \frac{dx}{dt} = -A\omega\sin(\omega t)$
Acceleration, $a = \frac{dv}{dt} = -A\omega^2\cos\omega t$
Hence graph (c) correctly dipicts the variation of a with t.
11. (c) As, we know, in SHM
Maximum acceleration of the particle, $\alpha = A\omega^2$
Maximum velocity, $\beta = A\omega$

$\Rightarrow \omega = \frac{\alpha}{\beta}$

$\Rightarrow T = \frac{2\pi}{\omega} = \frac{2\pi\beta}{\alpha}$ $\quad \left[\because \omega = \frac{2\pi}{T}\right]$

12. (a)
13. (b) The two displacements equations are $y_1 = a\sin(\omega t)$

and $y_2 = b\cos(\omega t) = b\sin\left(\omega t + \frac{\pi}{2}\right)$

$y_{eq} = y_1 + y_2$

$= a\sin\omega t + b\cos\omega t = a\sin\omega t + b\sin\left(\omega t + \frac{\pi}{2}\right)$

Since the frequencies for both SHMs are same, resultant motion will be SHM.

Now $A_{eq} = \sqrt{a^2 + b^2 + 2ab\cos\frac{\pi}{2}}$

$\Rightarrow A_{eq} = \sqrt{a^2 + b^2}$

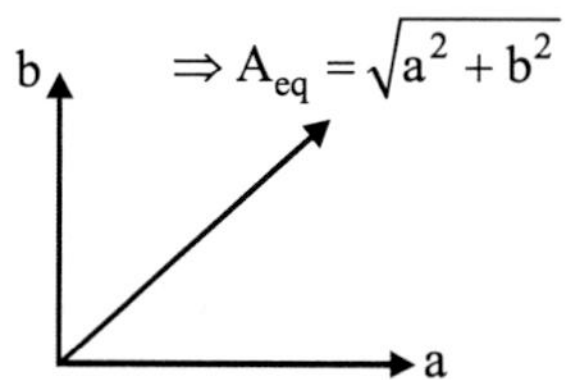

14. (b) Given, Amplitude A = 3 cm
Which particle is at x = 2 cm
According to question, magnitude of velocity = acceleration

$$\omega\sqrt{A^2 - x^2} = x\omega^2$$

$$\sqrt{(3)^2 - (2)^2} = 2\left(\frac{2\pi}{T}\right)$$

$$\sqrt{5} = \frac{4\pi}{T} \Rightarrow T = \frac{4\pi}{\sqrt{5}}$$

15. (b)

16. (b) From question, acceleration, a = 20 m/s², and displacement, y = 5m

$|a| = \omega^2 y$
$\Rightarrow 20 = \omega^2(5)$
$\Rightarrow \omega = 2$ rad/s

Time period of pendulum,

$$T = \frac{2\pi}{\omega} = \frac{2\pi}{2} = \pi \text{ s}$$

17. (d) Displacement of the particle in one complete vibration is zero, so, average velocity in one complete vibration will be

$$= \frac{\text{Displacement}}{\text{Time interval}} = \frac{y_f - y_i}{T} = 0$$

18. (b) Given equation

$y = A_0 + A\sin\omega t + B\sin\omega t$
Now assume $(y - A_0) = \gamma$
$y - A_0 = A\sin\omega t + B\sin\omega t$
$\gamma = A\sin\omega t + B\cos\omega t$

$= \sqrt{A^2 + B^2}\sin(\omega t + \phi)$
which is S.H.M.
where cos

and $\sin\phi = \dfrac{B}{\sqrt{A^2 + B^2}}$
so, resultant amplitude

$= \sqrt{A^2 + B^2}$

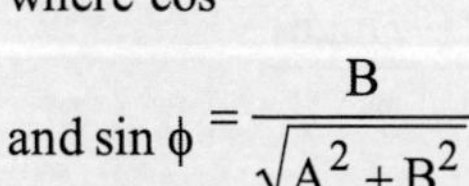

19. (a) In one time period total distance travelled by the particle is 4A.

20. (a)

21. (d) Displacement equation of a SHM

$$y = A\sin(\omega t + \phi)$$

$$\therefore \text{Velocity, } v = \frac{dy}{dt} = A\omega\cos(\omega t + \phi)$$

$$\text{Acceleration, } a = \frac{dv}{dt}$$

$$\text{or, } a = -A\omega^2\sin(\omega t + \phi)$$

$$\therefore a = A\omega^2\sin(\omega t + \phi + \pi)$$

Hence, phase difference between displacement and acceleration is π.

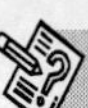

Exercise 3 - Concept Application Problems CAP

1. (b) $T = 2\pi\sqrt{\dfrac{\text{displacement}}{\text{acceleration}}} = 2\pi\sqrt{\dfrac{x}{bx}} = 2\pi/\sqrt{b}$

2. (c) $\ddot{y} = \omega^2 y,\ \omega^2 = 1,\ \dfrac{4\pi^2}{T^2} = 1$ or $T^2 = 4\pi^2$

or $T = 2\pi$ second.

3. (a) The amplitude is a maximum displacement from the mean position.

4. (a) $a = -kX, X = x + a$.
In simple harmonic motion acceleration is directly proportional to the displacement from the mean position. Also the acceleration is in the opposite direction of displacement.

5. (d) $E = \dfrac{1}{2}m\dfrac{k}{m}A^2 \Rightarrow E = \dfrac{1}{2}kA^2$

$\Rightarrow$ E does not depend on m

6. (a) $x = a\sin^2\omega t = \dfrac{a}{2}(1 - \cos 2\omega t)$

$$\frac{dx}{dt} = \frac{a}{2}\,2\omega\sin 2\omega t$$

$$\Rightarrow \frac{d^2x}{dt^2} = \frac{4\omega^2 a}{2}\cdot\cos 2\omega t$$

This represents an S. H. M. of frequency $= \dfrac{\omega}{\pi}$

7. (a) $v = \omega\sqrt{a^2 - y^2}$

At $x = 0, v = \omega\sqrt{a^2 - o^2} = \omega a$.

At $x = \dfrac{a}{2}, v' = \omega\sqrt{a^2 - \left(\dfrac{a}{2}\right)^2} = \omega\sqrt{\dfrac{3a^2}{4}}$

$$\therefore \frac{v'}{v} = \frac{\sqrt{3}}{2}$$

$$\text{or } v' = \frac{\sqrt{3}}{2}\omega a = \frac{\sqrt{3}\pi a}{2}\omega a = \frac{\sqrt{3}\pi a}{T}\left(\because \omega = \frac{2\pi}{T}\right)$$

8. (d) $T = 2\pi\sqrt{\dfrac{R}{g}} = 2\pi\sqrt{\dfrac{64\times10^6}{9.8}} = 2\times\dfrac{22}{7}\times\dfrac{8\times10^3}{7\times\sqrt{2}}$

$$= \frac{\sqrt{2}\times22\times8\times1000}{49\times60}\text{ min} = 84.6\text{ min}$$

9. (c) Max. force = mass × max. acceleration
$= m\,4\pi^2 v^2 a = 1\times4\times\pi^2\times(60)^2\times0.02 = 288\,\pi^2$

10. (a) Kinetic energy,

$$K.E = \frac{1}{2}mv^2 = \frac{1}{2}m\omega^2\left(A^2 - x^2\right)$$

Potential energy,

$$P.E = \frac{1}{2}kx^2 = \frac{1}{2}m\omega^2x^2$$

putting, K.E = P.E

$$\frac{1}{2}m\omega^2(A^2 - x^2) = \frac{1}{2}m\omega^2x^2 \quad \Rightarrow A^2 = 2x^2$$

$$x = \frac{A}{\sqrt{2}} = 2\sqrt{2}\text{cm.}$$

11. (a) $t \propto \frac{1}{\sqrt{9.8}},\ t' \propto \frac{1}{\sqrt{12.8}} \quad (\because\ g' = 9.8 + 3 = 12.8)$

$$\therefore \frac{t'}{t} = \sqrt{\frac{9.8}{12.8}} \Rightarrow t' = \sqrt{\frac{9.8}{12.8}}t$$

12. (b)

13. (c) When the bob moves from maximum angular displacement θ to mean position, then the loss of gravitational potential energy is mgh

where $h = l(1 - \cos\theta)$

14. (d) $T = 2\pi\sqrt{\frac{400}{k}},\ T' = 2\pi\sqrt{\frac{100}{k}}$

$$\therefore \frac{T'}{T} = \sqrt{\frac{100}{400}} = \frac{1}{2} \Rightarrow T' = \frac{T}{2} = \frac{2}{2} = 1\text{ s}$$

15. (b) Phase change π in 50 oscillations.
Phase change 2π in 100 oscillations.
So frequency different ~ 1 in 100.

16. (a) $\nu = \frac{1}{l(3D)}\sqrt{\frac{2T}{\pi\rho}},\ \nu' = \frac{1}{lD}\sqrt{\frac{T}{\pi(2\rho)}}$

$$\therefore \frac{\nu}{\nu'} = \frac{\sqrt{2}}{3} \times \sqrt{2} = \frac{2}{3}$$

17. (c) Kinetic energy $K = \frac{1}{2}m\omega^2(a^2 - y^2)$

$$= \frac{1}{2} \times 10 \times \left(\frac{2\pi}{2}\right)^2 [10^2 - 5^2] = 375\ \pi^2\ erg$$

18. (b) $y = a\sin(\omega t + \phi)$; when $y = a/2$,

then $\frac{a}{2} = a\sin(\omega t + \phi)$

or $\sin(\omega t + \phi) = \frac{1}{2} = \sin\frac{\pi}{6}$ or $\sin\frac{5\pi}{6}$

So phase of two particles is $\pi/6$ and $5\pi/6$ radians
Hence phase difference $= (5\pi/6) - \pi/6 = 2\pi/3$

19. (c) Here all the three springs are connected in parallel to mass m. Hence equivalent spring constant
$k = K + K + 2K = 4K$.

20. (a) $T = 2\pi\sqrt{\frac{\ell}{g}}$; $\frac{\Delta T}{T} = 2\pi \times \frac{1}{2}(\ell/g)^{-1/2} \times \Delta\ell/\ell$

$$(\because T + \Delta T = 2\pi\sqrt{\frac{\ell + \Delta\ell}{g}})$$

$$\therefore \frac{\Delta T}{T} = \frac{1}{2}\frac{\Delta\ell}{\ell} = \frac{1}{2}\alpha\,\Delta\theta$$

$$= \frac{1}{2} \times 12 \times 10^{-6} \times (40 - 20) = 12 \times 10^{-5}$$

$$\Delta T = T \times 12 \times 10^{-5} = 24 \times 60 \times 60 \times 12 \times 10^{-5}$$
$$= 10.3\text{ s/day}$$

21. (d) It is a damped oscillation, where amplitude of oscillation at time t is given by $A = a_0e^{-\gamma t}$
where a_0 = initial amplitude of oscillation
γ = damping constant.

As per question, $\frac{a_0}{3} = a_0e^{-\gamma\,100/\nu}$ ......(i)

(where ν is the frequency of oscillation)

and $A = a_0e^{-\gamma\,200/\nu}$ ......(ii)

From (i) ; $\frac{a_o}{3} = a_0e^{-\gamma \times 100/\nu}$ ......(iii)

Dividing equation (ii) by (iii), we have

$$\frac{A}{a_0(1/3)} = \frac{e^{-\gamma\,200/\nu}}{e^{-\gamma \times 100/\nu}} = e^{-\gamma \times 100/\nu} = \frac{1}{3}$$

$$\text{or } A = a_0 \times \frac{1}{3} \times \frac{1}{3} = \frac{1}{9}a_0$$

22. (b) Loss in PE of mass = gain in PE of the spring

$$\therefore \quad mg(h + x) = \frac{1}{2}kx^2$$

$$kx^2 - 2mgx - 2mgh = 0$$

$$\Rightarrow \quad x = \frac{2mg \pm \sqrt{4m^2g^2 - 4k(-2mgh)}}{2k}$$

$$\text{or} \quad x = \frac{mg}{k} \pm \sqrt{\frac{m^2g^2}{k^2} + \frac{2mgh}{k}}$$

$$x = A - \frac{mg}{k} = \sqrt{\frac{m^2g^2}{k^2} + \frac{2mgh}{k}} - \frac{mg}{k}$$

$$= \frac{mg}{k}\left[\sqrt{1 + \frac{2kh}{mg}} - 1\right]$$

23. (a) For the block is about to slip, $\mu g = \omega^2 a$

$$\text{or} \Rightarrow \omega = \sqrt{\frac{\mu g}{a}}$$

$$\Rightarrow 2\pi\nu = \sqrt{\frac{\mu g}{a}} \Rightarrow \nu = \frac{1}{2\pi}\sqrt{\frac{\mu g}{a}}$$

24. (d) Oscillations along spring length are independent of gravitation.

25. (a)

26. (d) Let the extension in the spring be x_0 at equilibrium. If F_0 be the tension in the string then $F_0 = kx_0$. Further if T_0 is the tension in the thread then $T_0 = mg$ and $2T_0 = kx_0$.
Let the mass m be displaced through a slight displacement x downwards. Let the the new tension in the string and spring be T and F respectively.

$$\Rightarrow F = \left(x_0 \frac{x}{2}\right) \text{ and } F = 2T \Rightarrow 2T = k\left(x_0 \frac{x}{2}\right)$$

$$\Rightarrow (T - T_0) = \frac{kx}{4}$$

$$\Rightarrow \text{Time period} = 2\pi\sqrt{\frac{m}{\frac{k}{4}}} = 4\pi\sqrt{\frac{m}{k}}$$

27. (d) Slope of F - x curve $= -k = -\frac{80}{0.2} \Rightarrow k = 400$ N/m,

Time period, $T = 2\pi\sqrt{\frac{m}{k}} = 0.0314$ sec.

28. (a) Here, $v_x = -a\,\omega \sin \omega t$, $v_y = a\,\omega \cos \omega t$ and $v_z = a\omega$

$$\Rightarrow v = \sqrt{v_x^2 + v_y^2 + v_z^2}$$

$$\Rightarrow v = \sqrt{(-a\omega \sin \omega t)^2 + (a\omega \cos \omega t)^2 + (a\omega)^2}$$

$v = \sqrt{2}a\omega$

29. (b) Maximum velocity in SHM, $v_{max} = a\omega$
Maximum acceleration in SHM, $A_{max} = a\omega^2$
where a and ω are maximum amplitude and angular frequency.

Given that, $\frac{A_{max}}{v_{max}} = 10$

i.e., $\omega = 10\ s^{-1}$
Displacement is given by
$x = a \sin(\omega t + \pi/4)$
at $t = 0$, $x = 5$
$5 = a \sin \pi/4$
$5 = a \sin 45° \Rightarrow a = 5\sqrt{2}$

Maximum acceleration $A_{max} = a\omega^2 = 500\sqrt{2}$ m/s²

30. (c) As we know,
$F = ma \Rightarrow a \propto F$
or, $a \propto \sin t$

$$\Rightarrow \frac{dv}{dt} \propto \sin t \Rightarrow \int_0^0 dV \propto \int_0^t \sin t\, dt$$

$V \propto -\cos t + 1$

$$\int_0^x dx = \int_0^t (-\cos t + 1)\, dt$$

$$x = \sin t - \frac{1}{2}\sin 2t$$

31. (d) In linear S.H.M., the restoring force acting on particle should always be proportional to the displacement of the particle and directed towards the equilibrium position.
i.e., $F \propto x$
or $F = -bx$ where b is a positive constant.

32. (a) Given,
Displacement, $x = x_0 \cos(\omega t - \pi/4)$

$$\therefore \text{Velocity, } v = \frac{dx}{dt} = -x_0\omega \sin\left(\omega t - \frac{\pi}{4}\right)$$

Acceleration,

$$a = \frac{dv}{dt} = -x_0\omega^2 \cos\left(\omega t - \frac{\pi}{4}\right)$$

$$= x_0\omega^2 \cos\left[\pi + \left(\omega t - \frac{\pi}{4}\right)\right]$$

$$= x_0\omega^2 \cos\left(\omega t + \frac{3\pi}{4}\right) \quad ...(1)$$

Acceleration, $a = A\cos(\omega t + \delta)$ ...(2)
Comparing the two equations, we get
$A = x_0\omega^2$ and $\delta = \frac{3\pi}{4}$.

33. (d) Kinetic energy, $k = \frac{1}{2}m\omega^2 A^2 \cos^2 \omega t$

Potential energy, $U = \frac{1}{2}m\omega^2 A^2 \sin^2 \omega t$

$$\frac{k}{U} = \cot^2 \omega t = \cot^2 \frac{\pi}{90}(210) = \frac{1}{3}$$

34. (c) Potential energy (U) $= \frac{1}{2}kx^2$

Kinetic energy (K) $= \frac{1}{2}kA^2 - \frac{1}{2}kx^2$
According to the question, U = k

$$\therefore \frac{1}{2}kx^2 = \frac{1}{2}kA^2 - \frac{1}{2}kx^2$$

$$\Rightarrow x^2 = A^2 \text{ or, } x = \pm\frac{A}{\sqrt{2}}$$

35. (b) An elastic wire can be treated as a spring and its spring constant.

$$k = \frac{YA}{L} \qquad \left[\because Y = \frac{F}{A}\bigg/\frac{\Delta l}{l_0}\right]$$

Frequency of oscillation,

$$f = \frac{1}{2\pi}\sqrt{\frac{k}{m}} = \frac{1}{2\pi}\sqrt{\frac{YA}{mL}}$$

36. (c) $y = y_0 \sin^2 \omega t$

$$\Rightarrow y = \frac{y_0}{2}(1 - \cos 2\omega t) \qquad \left(\because \sin^2 \omega t = \frac{1 - \cos 2\omega t}{2}\right)$$

$$\Rightarrow y - \frac{y_0}{2} = \frac{-y_0}{2}\cos 2\omega t \Rightarrow y = A\cos 2\omega t$$

$\therefore$ Amplitude $= \frac{y_0}{2}$

Angular velocity = 2ω

For equilibrium of mass, $\frac{ky_0}{2} = mg \Rightarrow \frac{k}{m} = \frac{2g}{y_0}$

Also, spring constant $k = m(2\omega)^2$

$$\Rightarrow 2\omega = \sqrt{\frac{k}{m}} = \sqrt{\frac{2g}{y_0}} \Rightarrow \omega = \frac{1}{2}\sqrt{\frac{2g}{y_0}} = \sqrt{\frac{g}{2y_0}}$$

37. (a) Potential energy of spring $= \frac{1}{2}kx^2$

Here, x = distance of block from mean position, k = spring constant

At mean position, potential energy $= \frac{1}{2}kA^2$

At equilibrium position, half of the mass of block breaks off, so its potential energy becomes half.

Remaining energy $= \frac{1}{2}\left(\frac{1}{2}kA^2\right) = \frac{1}{2}kA'^2$

Here, A' = New distance of block from mean position

$$\Rightarrow A' = \frac{A}{\sqrt{2}}$$

38. (c) $T = 2\pi\sqrt{\frac{l}{g}}$

When immersed non viscous liquid

$$a_{mt} = \left(g - \frac{g}{16}\right) = \frac{15g}{16}$$

Now $T' = 2\pi\sqrt{\frac{l}{0_{net}}} = 2\pi\sqrt{\frac{l}{\sqrt{\frac{15g}{16}}}} = \frac{4}{\sqrt{15}}T$

39. (a) Angular frequency of pendulum $\omega = \sqrt{\frac{g}{\ell}}$

∴ relative change in angular frequency

$\frac{\Delta\omega}{\omega} = \frac{1}{2}\frac{\Delta g}{g}$ [as length remains constant]

$\Delta g = 2A\omega_s^2$ [ω_s = angular frequency of support and, A = amplitude]

$$\frac{\Delta\omega}{\omega} = \frac{1}{2} \times \frac{2A\omega_s^2}{g}$$

$$\Delta\omega = \frac{1}{2} \times \frac{2 \times 1^2 \times 10^{-2}}{10} = 10^{-3} \text{ rad/sec.}$$

40. (c) Velocity, $v = \omega\sqrt{A^2 - x^2}$ ...(i)

acceleration, $a = -\omega^2 x$ ...(ii)

and according to question,

$|v| = |a|$

$$\Rightarrow \omega\sqrt{A^2 - x^2} = \omega^2 x$$

$$\Rightarrow A^2 - x^2 = \omega^2 x^2 \Rightarrow 5^2 - 4^2 = \omega^2(4^2)$$

$$3 = \omega \times 4 \Rightarrow \omega = \frac{3}{4}$$

$$\therefore T = 2\pi/\omega = \frac{2\pi}{3/4} = \frac{8\pi}{3}$$

41. (b) As we know, frequency in SHM

$$f = \frac{1}{2\pi}\sqrt{\frac{k}{m}} = 10^{12}$$

where m = mass of one atom

Mass of one atom of silver, $= \frac{108}{(6.02 \times 10^{23})} \times 10^{-3}$ kg

$$\frac{1}{2\pi}\sqrt{\frac{k}{108 \times 10^{-3}} \times 6.02 \times 10^{23}} = 10^{12}$$

Solving we get, spring constant,

K = 7.1N/m

42. (c) Time lost/gained per day $= \frac{1}{2} \propto \Delta\theta \times 86400$ second

$$12 = \frac{1}{2}\alpha(40 - \theta) \times 86400 \quad \text{.... (i)}$$

$$4 = \frac{1}{2}\alpha(\theta - 20) \times 86400 \quad \text{....(ii)}$$

On dividing we get, $3 = \frac{40 - \theta}{\theta - 20}$

$3\theta - 60 = 40 - \theta$

$4\theta = 100 \Rightarrow \theta = 25°C$

43. (b) From graph it is clear that when

L = 1m, $T^2 = 4s^2$

As we know,

$$T = 2\pi\sqrt{\frac{L}{g}} \Rightarrow g = \frac{4\pi^2 L}{T^2}$$

$$= 4 \times \left(\frac{22}{7}\right)^2 \times \frac{1}{4} = \left(\frac{22}{7}\right)^2$$

$$\therefore \quad g = \frac{484}{49} = 9.87 \text{m/s}^2$$

44. (c) Time of half the amplitude is = 2s

Using, $A = A_0 e^{-kt}$

$$\frac{A_0}{2} = A_e\, e^{-k \times 2} \quad \text{...(i)}$$

and $\frac{A_0}{1000} = A_e\, e^{-kt}$ ...(ii)

Dividing (i) by (ii) and solving, we get

t = 20 s

45. (b) Amplitude of vibration at time t = 0 is given by

$$A = A_0 e^{-0.1 \times 0} = 1 \times A_0 = A_0$$

also at t = t, if $A = \frac{A_0}{2}$

$$\Rightarrow \frac{1}{2} = e^{-0.1t}$$

$t = 10 \ln 2 \simeq 7$s

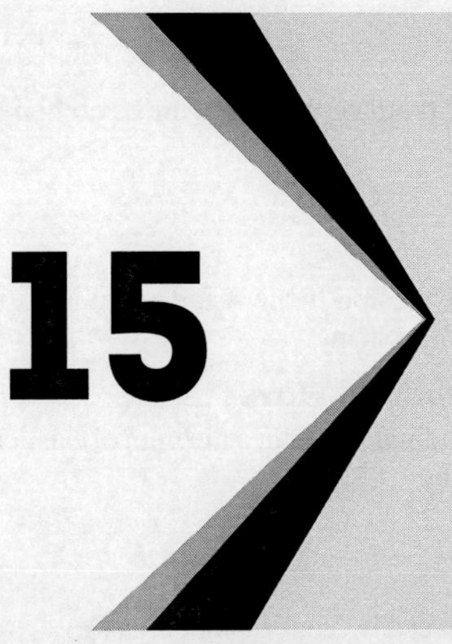

15 Waves

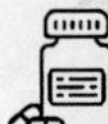

Topic 15.1 : Wave Motion, Displacement Relation for Progressive Wave & Speed of Wave Motion and Interference of Waves

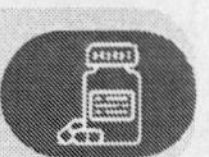

WAVE MOTION

Wave motion is a type of motion in which the disturbance travels from one point of the medium to another but the particles of the medium do not travel from one point to another.

For the propagation of wave, medium must have inertia and elasticity. These two properties of medium decide the speed of wave.

There are **two types of waves**

1. **Mechanical waves:** These waves require material medium for their propagation. For example : sound waves, waves in stretched string etc.
2. **Non-mechanical waves or electromagnetic waves :** These waves do not require any material medium for their propagation. For example : light waves, x-rays etc.

   There are **two types of mechanical waves**

   (i) **Transverse waves :** *In the transverse wave, the particles of medium oscillate in a direction perpendicular to the direction of wave propagation*. Waves in stretched string, waves on the water surface are transverse in nature.

Transverse wave can travel only in solids and surface of liquids. Transverse waves propagate in the form of crests and troughs.

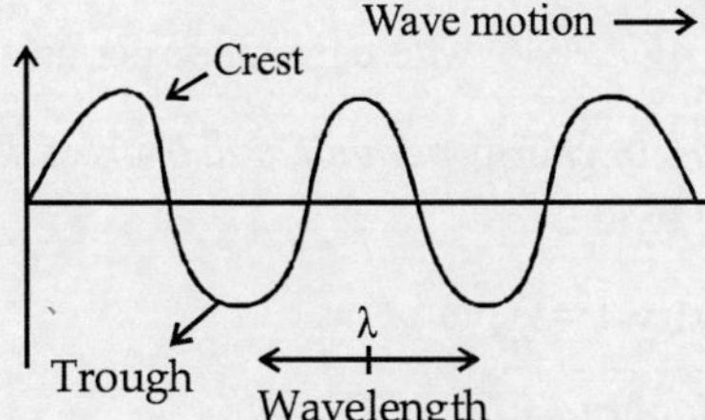

All electromagnetic waves are transverse in nature.

(ii) **Longitudinal waves :** *In longitudinal waves particles of medium oscillate about their mean position along the direction of wave propagation.*

Sound waves in air are longitudinal. These waves can travel in solids, liquids and gases.

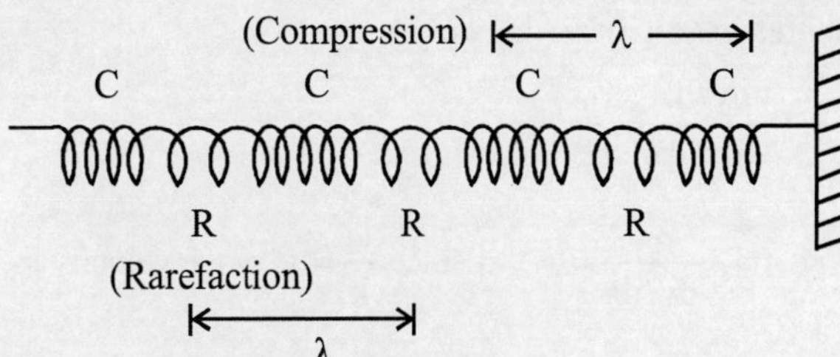

Logitudinal waves propagate through medium with the help of compressions and rarefactions.

DISPLACEMENT RELATION FOR PROGRESSIVE WAVE & SPEED OF WAVE MOTION

Equation of a Harmonic Wave or Progressive Wave

Harmonic waves are generated by sources that execute simple harmonic motion.

A harmonic wave travelling along the positive direction of x-axis is represented by

$$y = A\sin(\omega t - kx)$$

$$= A\sin\left\{2\pi\left(\frac{t}{T} - \frac{x}{\lambda}\right)\right\}$$

$$= A\sin\left\{\frac{2\pi}{\lambda}(vt - x)\right\}$$

where,

y = displacement of the particle of the medium at a location x at time t

A = amplitude of the wave

λ = wavelength

T = time period

v = $\upsilon\lambda$, wave velocity in the medium

$\omega = \frac{2\pi}{T}$, angular frequency

$k = \frac{2\pi}{\lambda}$, angular wave number or propagation constant.

If the wave is travelling along the negative direction of x-axis then

$$y = A\sin(\omega t + Kx)$$

$$= A\sin\left\{2\pi\left(\frac{t}{T}+\frac{x}{\lambda}\right)\right\}.$$

Differential equation of wave motion :

$$\frac{d^2y}{dx^2}=\frac{1}{v^2}\frac{d^2y}{dt^2}$$

Relation between wave velocity and particle velocity :

The equation of a plane progressive wave is

$$y = A\sin(\omega t - kx) \quad \text{... (i)}$$

The particle velocity

$$v_p = \frac{dy}{dt} = A\omega\cos(\omega t - kx) \quad \text{... (ii)}$$

Slope of displacement curve or strain

$$\frac{dy}{dx} = -Ak\cos(\omega t - kx) \quad \text{... (iii)}$$

Dividing eq^n. (ii) by (iii), we get

$$\frac{dy/dt}{-dy/dx}=\frac{\omega}{k}$$

$$\Rightarrow \frac{v_p}{-dy/dx} = v \quad \left(\text{since } \frac{\omega}{k} = v, \text{ wave velocity}\right)$$

$$\Rightarrow v_p = -v.\frac{dy}{dx}$$

i.e., *Particle velocity = – wave velocity × strain.*

Particle velocity changes with the time but the wave velocity is constant in a medium.

Relation between phase difference, path difference and time difference :

- Phase difference of 2π radian is equivalent to a path difference λ and a time difference of period T.
- *Phase difference* $= \frac{2\pi}{\lambda} \times$ *path difference*

$$\phi = \frac{2\pi}{\lambda}\times x \Rightarrow x = \frac{\lambda}{2\pi}\times\phi$$

- *Phase difference* $= \frac{2\pi}{T} \times$ *time difference*

$$\phi = \frac{2\pi}{T}\times t \Rightarrow t = \frac{T}{2\pi}\times\phi$$

- *Time difference* $= \frac{T}{\lambda} \times$ *path difference*

$$t = \frac{T}{\lambda}\times x \Rightarrow x = \frac{\lambda}{T}\times t$$

Speed of Transverse Waves :

(i) The **speed of transverse waves in solid** is given by

$$v = \sqrt{\frac{\eta}{\rho}}$$

where η is the modulus of rigidity of the solid and ρ is the density of material.

(ii) The **speed of transverse waves on stretched string** is given by

$$v = \sqrt{\frac{T}{\mu}}$$

where T is the tension in the string and μ is the mass per unit length of the string.

Speed of Longitudinal Waves :

The speed of longitudinal waves in a medium of elasticity E and density ρ is given by

$$v = \sqrt{\frac{E}{\rho}}$$

For solids, E is replaced by Young's modulus (Y)

$$v_{solid} = \sqrt{\frac{Y}{\rho}}$$

For liquids and gases, E is replaced by bulk modulus of elasticity (B)

$$v_{liquid/gas} = \sqrt{\frac{B}{\rho}}$$

The density of a solid is much larger than that of a gas but the elasticity is larger by a greater factor.

$$v_{solid} > v_{liquid} > v_{gas}$$

Speed of Sound in a Gas :

Newton's formula.

$$v = \sqrt{\frac{P}{\rho}}$$

where P is the atmospheric pressure and ρ is the density of air at STP.

Laplace's correction

$$v = \sqrt{\frac{\gamma P}{\rho}}$$

where γ is the ratio of two specific heats C_p and C_v

Power and Intensity of Wave Motion :

If a wave is travelling in a stretched string, energy is transmitted along the string.

Power of the wave is given by

$$P = \frac{1}{2}\mu\omega^2A^2v \quad \text{where } \mu \text{ is mass per unit length.}$$

***Intensity** is flow of energy per unit area of cross section of the string per unit time.*

$$\textbf{Intensity } I = \frac{1}{2}\rho\omega^2A^2v$$

Principle of Superposition of Waves :

If two or more waves arrive at a point simultaneously then the net displacement at that point is the algebraic sum of the displacement due to individual waves.

$$y = y_1 + y_2 + \ldots\ldots\ldots\ldots + y_n.$$

where y_1, y_2 .... y_n are the displacement due to individual waves and y is the resultant displacement.

INTERFERENCE OF WAVES

When two waves of equal frequency and nearly equal amplitude travelling in same direction having same state of polarisation in medium superimpose, then intensity is different at different points. At some points intensity is large, whereas at other points it is nearly zero.

Consider two waves

$y_1 = A_1 \sin(\omega t - kx)$ and

$y_2 = A_2 \sin(\omega t - kx + \phi)$

By principle of superposition

$y = y_1 + y_2 = A \sin(\omega t - kx + \delta)$

where, $A^2 = A_1^2 + A_2^2 + 2A_1A_2 \cos\phi$,

and $\tan\delta = \dfrac{A_2 \sin\phi}{A_1 + A_2 \cos\phi}$

As intensity $I \propto A^2$

So, *resultant intensity* $I = I_1 + I_2 + 2\sqrt{I_1 I_2}\cos\phi$

For constructive interference (maximum intensity) :

Phase difference, $\phi = 2n\pi$

and path difference $= n\lambda$

where $n = 0, 1, 2, 3, ...$

$\Rightarrow A_{max} = A_1 + A_2$ and $I_{max} = I_1 + I_2 + 2\sqrt{I_1 I_2}$

$= (\sqrt{I_1} + \sqrt{I_2})^2$

For destructive interference (minimum intensity) :

Phase difference, $\phi = (2n+1)\pi$,

and path difference $= (2n-1)\dfrac{\lambda}{2}$; where $n = 0, 1, 2, 3, ...$

$\Rightarrow A_{min} = A_1 - A_2$ *and* $I_{min} = I_1 + I_2 - 2\sqrt{I_1 I_2}$

$= (\sqrt{I_1} - \sqrt{I_2})^2$

Results :

(1) The ratio of maximum and minimum intensities in any interference wave form.

$$\frac{I_{max}}{I_{min}} = \left(\frac{\sqrt{I_1}+\sqrt{I_2}}{\sqrt{I_1}-\sqrt{I_2}}\right)^2 = \left(\frac{A_1 + A_2}{A_1 - A_2}\right)^2$$

(2) Average intensity of interference in wave form :

$$I_{av} = \frac{I_{max} + I_{min}}{2}$$

Put the value of I_{max} and I_{min}

or $I_{av} = I_1 + I_2$

If $A = A_1 = A_2$ and $I_1 = I_2 = I$

then $I_{max} = 4I$, $I_{min} = 0$ and $I_{av} = 2I$

(3) Condition of maximum contrast in interference wave form

$A_1 = A_2$ and $I_1 = I_2$

then $I_{max} = 4I$ and $I_{min} = 0$

For perfect destructive interference we have a maximum contrast in interference wave form.

Reflection of Waves :

A mechanical wave is reflected and refracted at a boundary separating two media according to the usual laws of reflection and refraction.

When sound wave is reflected from a rigid boundary or denser medium, the wave suffers a phase reversal of π but the nature does not change i.e., on reflection the compression is reflected back as compression and rarefaction as rarefaction.

When sound wave is reflected from an open boundary or rarer medium, there is no phase change but the nature of wave is changed i.e., on reflection, the compression is reflected back as rarefaction and rarefaction as compression.

Problem Solving Tips

(i) For a wave, $v = f\lambda$

(ii) The wave velocity of sound in air

$$v = \sqrt{\frac{E}{\rho}} = \sqrt{\frac{Y\rho}{\rho}} = \sqrt{\frac{\gamma RT}{M}}$$

(iii) Particle velocity is given by $v_p = \dfrac{dx}{dt}$. It changes with time. The wave velocity is the velocity with which disturbances travel in the medium and is given by $v_w = \dfrac{\omega}{k}$.

(iv) When a wave reflects from denser medium the phase change is π and when the wave reflects from rarer medium, the phase change is zero.

(v) In a tuning fork, the waves produced in the prongs is transverse whereas in the stem is longitudinal.

(vi) A medium in which the speed of wave is independent of the frequency of the waves is called non-dispersive. For example air is a non-dispersive medium for the sound waves.

(vii) Transverse waves can propagate in medium with shear modulus of elasticity e.g., solid whereas longitudinal waves need bulk modulus of elasticity hence can propagate in all media solid, liquid and gas.

Energy Transported by a Hormonic Wave Along a String :

Kinetic energy of a small element of length dx is

$$dk = \frac{1}{2}(\mu\, dx)\left(\frac{\partial y}{\partial t}\right)^2 \quad \text{where } \mu = \text{mass per unit length}$$

$$dk = \frac{1}{2}\left[\mu\,\omega^2 A^2 \cos^2(kx - \omega t)\right]dx$$

and potential energy stored

$$dU = \frac{1}{2}(T\,dx)\left(\frac{\partial y}{\partial x}\right)^2 = \frac{1}{2}\mu\,\omega^2 A^2 \cos^2(kx - \omega t)dx$$

Example 1.

The displacement y (in cm) produced by a simple harmonic wave is given by $y = (10/\pi)\sin(2000\,\pi t - \pi x/17)$. What will be the periodic time and maximum velocity of the particles in the medium?

Solution :

$$y = \frac{10}{\pi}\sin\left(2000\pi t - \frac{\pi x}{17}\right) \text{ or } y = \frac{10}{\pi}\sin 2\pi\left(1000t - \frac{x}{34}\right)$$

The standard equation of S.H.M. is,

$$y = a \sin 2\pi\left[\frac{t}{T} - \frac{x}{\lambda}\right];$$

∴ By comparison of the standard equation to above given equation,

we get $T = \frac{1}{1000} = 10^{-3}$ sec.

Particle velocity

$$= \frac{dy}{dt} = \frac{10}{\pi} \times 2000\,\pi \cos\left(2000\pi t - \frac{\pi x}{17}\right)$$

$$\Rightarrow \left(\frac{dy}{dt}\right)_{max} = 20{,}000 \text{ cm/s} = 200 \text{ m/s} \quad (\text{as } v_{max} = A\omega)$$

Example 2.

A progressive wave of frequency 500 Hz is travelling with a velocity of 360 m/s. How far apart are two points 60° out of phase?

Solution :

We known that for a wave $v = f\lambda$

so $\lambda = \frac{v}{f} = \frac{360}{500} = 0.72$ m

Now as in a wave path difference is related to phase difference by the relation.

Phase difference $\Delta\phi = 60° = (\pi/180) \times 60 = (\pi/3)$ rad

Path difference $\Delta x = \frac{\lambda}{2\pi}(\Delta\phi) = \frac{0.72}{2\pi}\frac{\pi}{3} = 0.12$ m

Example 3.

Determine the change in volume of 6 litres of alcohol if the pressure is decreased from 200 cm of Hg to 75 cm. [velocity of sound in alcohol is 1280 m/s, density of alcohol = 0.81 gm/cc, density of Hg = 13.6 gm/cc and g = 9.81 m/s²].

Solution :

For propagation of sound in liquid

$v = \sqrt{(B/\rho)}$, i.e., $B = v^2\rho$

But by definition $B = -V\frac{\Delta P}{\Delta V}$

so $-V\frac{\Delta P}{\Delta V} = v^2\rho$, i.e., $\Delta V = \frac{V(-\Delta P)}{\rho v^2}$

Here $\Delta P = H_2\rho g - H_1\rho g = (75 - 200) \times 13.6 \times 981$

$= -1.667 \times 10^6$ dyne/cm²

so $\Delta V = \frac{(6 \times 10^3)(1.667 \times 10^6)}{0.81 \times (1.280 \times 10^5)^2} = 0.75$ cc

Example 4.

(a) *Speed of sound in air is 332 m/s at NTP. What will be the speed of sound in hydrogen at NTP if the density of hydrogen at NTP is (1/16) that of air?*

(b) *Calculate the ratio of the speed of sound in neon to that in water vapour at any temperature. [Molecular weight of neon = 2.02 × 10^{-2} kg/mol and for water vapours = 1.8 × 10^{-2} kg/mol]*

Solution :

The velocity of sound in air is given by

$$v = \sqrt{\frac{E}{\rho}} = \sqrt{\frac{\gamma P}{\rho}} = \sqrt{\frac{\gamma RT}{M}}$$

(a) In terms of density and pressure

$$\frac{v_H}{v_{air}} = \sqrt{\frac{P_H}{\rho_H} \times \frac{\rho_{air}}{P_{air}}} = \sqrt{\frac{\rho_{air}}{\rho_H}} \quad [\text{as } P_{air} = P_H]$$

or $v_H = v_{air} \times \sqrt{\frac{\rho_{air}}{\rho_H}} = 332 \times \sqrt{\frac{16}{1}} = 1328$ m/s

(b) In terms of temperature and molecular weight

$$\frac{v_{Ne}}{v_W} = \sqrt{\frac{\gamma_{Ne}}{M_{Ne}} \times \frac{M_W}{\gamma_W}} \quad [\text{as } T_N = T_W]$$

Now as neon is monatomic ($\gamma = 5/3$) while water vapours polyatomic ($\gamma = 4/3$) so

$$\frac{v_{Ne}}{v_W} = \sqrt{\frac{(5/3) \times 1.8 \times 10^{-2}}{(4/3) \times 2.02 \times 10^{-2}}} = \sqrt{\frac{5}{4} \times \frac{1.8}{2.02}} = 1.05$$

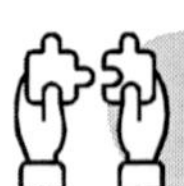

15.1 Concept Practice Problems CPP

1. The property of a medium necessary for wave propagation is
   (a) inertia (b) elasticity
   (c) low resistance (d) All of the above
2. If the intensities of two interfering waves be I_1 and I_2, the contrast between maximum and minimum intensity is maximum, when
   (a) $I_1 >> I_2$ (b) $I_1 << I_2$
   (c) $I_1 = I_2$ (d) either I_1 or I_2 is zero
3. Sound waves of length λ travelling with velocity v in a medium enter into another medium in which their velocity is 4 v. The wavelength in 2nd medium is
   (a) 4λ (b) λ (c) λ/4 (d) 16λ
4. Two periodic waves of intensities I_1 and I_2 pass through a region at the same time in the same direction. The sum of the maximum and minimum intensities is
   (a) $2(I_1 + I_2)$ (b) $I_1 + I_2$
   (c) $(\sqrt{I_1} + \sqrt{I_2})^2$ (d) $(\sqrt{I_1} - \sqrt{I_2})^2$
5. Sound waves are not transmitted to long distances because,
   (a) they are absorbed by the atmosphere
   (b) they have constant frequency
   (c) the height of antenna required, should be very high
   (d) velocity of sound waves is very less
6. Shock waves are produced by objects
   (a) carrying electric charge and vibrating
   (b) vibrating with frequency greater than 20000 Hz
   (c) vibrating with very large amplitude
   (d) moving with a speed greater than that of sound in the medium

7. The speed of sound in a medium depends on
   (a) the elastic property but not on the inertia property
   (b) the inertia property but not on the elastic property
   (c) the elastic property as well as the inertia property
   (d) neither the elastic property nor the inertia property

8. Sound waves are travelling in a medium whose adiabatic elasticity is E and isothermal elasticity E'. The velocity of sound waves is proportional to
   (a) E (b) $\sqrt{E}$ (c) $\sqrt{E'}$ (d) $\frac{E}{E'}$

9. The equation $y = a\sin\frac{2\pi}{\lambda}(vt - x)$ is expression for
   (a) stationary wave of single frequency along x-axis
   (b) a simple harmonic motion
   (c) a progressive wave of single frequency along x-axis
   (d) the resultant of two SHMs of slightly different frequencies

10. The equation $Y = 0.02\sin(500\pi t)\cos(4.5x)$ represents
   (a) progressive wave of frequency 250 Hz along x-axis
   (b) a stationary wave of wavelength 1.4 m
   (c) a transverse progressive wave of amplitude 0.02 m
   (d) progressive wave of speed of about 350 m s^{-1}

ANSWER KEY

1	(d)	2	(c)	3	(a)	4	(a)	5	(a)	6	(d)	7	(c)	8	(b)	9	(c)	10	(b)

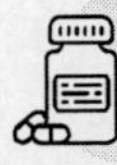

Topic 15.2 : Beats and Doppler Effect

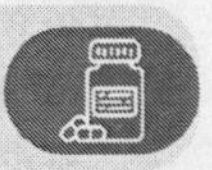

BEATS

When two wave trains slightly differing in frequencies travel along the same straight line in the same direction, then the resultant amplitude is alternately maximum and minimum at a point in the medium. This phenomenon of waxing and waning of sound is called beats.

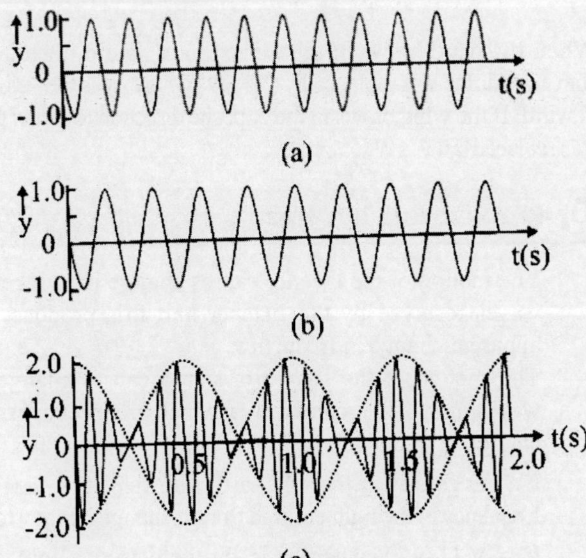

Let two sound waves of frequencies n_1 and n_2 are propagating simultaneously and in same direction. Then at x=0

$y_1 = A\sin 2\pi n_1 t$, and $y_2 = A\sin 2\pi n_2 t$,

For simplicity we take amplitude of both waves to be same. By principle of superposition, the resultant displacement at any instant is

$$y = y_1 + y_2 = 2A\cos 2\pi n_A t \sin 2\pi n_{av} t$$

where $n_{av} = \frac{n_1 + n_2}{2}$, $n_A = \frac{n_1 - n_2}{2}$

$\Rightarrow y = A_{beat}\sin 2\pi n_{av} t$ ....(i)

It is clear from the above expression (i) that

(i) $A_{beat} = 2A\cos 2\pi n_A t$, amplitude of resultant wave varies periodically as frequency

$$n_A = \left(\frac{n_1 - n_2}{2}\right)$$

A is maximum when $|\cos\theta|_{max} = 1$

$|A_{beat}|_{max} = 2A$

A is minimum when $|\cos\theta|_{min} = 0$ $\quad |A_{beat}|_{min} = 0$

(ii) Since Intensity is proportional to amplitude i.e., $I \alpha A_{beat}^2$

For I_{max} $\cos 2\pi n_A t = \pm 1$
i.e., $2\pi n_A t = 0, \pi, 2\pi$
i.e., $t = 0, 1/2n_A, 2/2n_A$

For I_{min}
$2\pi n_A t = \pi/2, 3\pi/2$
$t = 1/4n_A, 3/4n_A$.......

So time interval between two consecutive beat is

$$\Delta t = t_n - t_{n-1} = \left(\frac{1}{2n_A}\right)$$

Number of beats per sec is given by

$$n_{beat} = \frac{1}{\Delta t} = 2n_A - \frac{2(n_1 - n_2)}{2} = n_1 - n_2$$

So beat frequency is equal to the difference of frequency of two interferring waves.

To hear beats, the number of beats per second should not be more than 10. (due to hearing capabilities of human beings)

Filing/Loading a Tuning Fork

On filing the prongs of tuning fork, raises its frequency and on loading it decreases the frequency.

(i) When a tuning fork of frequency ν produces $\Delta\nu$ beats per second with a standard tuning fork of frequency ν_0, then $\qquad \nu = \nu_0 \pm \Delta\nu$

If the beat frequency decreases or reduces to zero or remains the same on filling the unknown fork, then

$$\nu = \nu_0 - \Delta\nu$$

(ii) If the beat frequency decreases or reduces to zero or remains the same on loading the unknown fork with a little wax, then $\nu = \nu_0 + \Delta\nu$

If the beat frequency increases on loading, then

$$\nu = \nu_0 - \Delta\nu$$

Example 5.

Tuning fork A has frequency 1% greater than that of standard fork B, while tuning fork C has frequency 2% smaller than that of B. When A an C are sounded together, the number of beats heard per second is 5. What is the frequency of each fork?

Solution :

Let the frequencies of forks be n_1, n_2 and n_3 respectively. Then

$n_1 = n_2(1 + 0.01) = 1.01\, n_2$ and $n_3 = n_2(1 - 0.02) = 0.98\, n_2$

Further, $n_1 - n_3 = 5$

Substituting the values, we get $(1.01\, n_2 - 0.98\, n_2) = 5$

$\therefore n_2 = 166.7$ Hz

Now $n_1 = 1.01 \times 166.7 = 168.3$ Hz

and $n_3 = 0.98 \times 166.7 = 163.3$ Hz.

Example 6.

Two tuning forks A and B sounded together give 6 beats per second. With an air resonance tube closed at one end, the two forks give resonance when the two air columns are 24 cm and 25 cm respectively. Calculate the frequencies of forks.

Solution :

Let the frequency of the first fork be f_1 and that of second be f_2.

We then have,

$$f_1 = \frac{v}{4 \times 24} \quad \text{and} \quad f_2 = \frac{v}{4 \times 25}$$

We also see that

$$f_1 > f_2$$

$$\therefore \quad f_1 - f_2 = 6 \quad \ldots(i)$$

$$\text{and} \quad \frac{f_1}{f_2} = \frac{24}{25} \quad \ldots(ii)$$

Solving eq^{ns}. (i) and (ii), we get

$f_1 = 150$ Hz and $f_2 = 144$ Hz

DOPPLER EFFECT

When a source of sound and an observer or both are in motion relative to each other there is an apparent change in frequency of sound as heard by the observer. This phenomenon is called the Doppler's effect .

Apparent change in frequency :

(a) **When source is in motion and observer at rest**

(i) *when source moving towards observer*

$$\nu_1 = \nu_0 \left(\frac{V}{V - V_S} \right)$$

(ii) *when source moving away from observer*

$$\nu_1' = \nu_0 \left(\frac{V}{V + V_S} \right)$$

Here V = velocity of sound

V_S = velocity of source

ν_0 = source frequency.

(b) **When source is at rest and observer in motion**

(i) *when observer moving towards source*

$$\nu_2 = \left(\frac{V + V_0}{V} \right) \nu_0$$

(ii) *when observer moving away from source and V_0 = velocity of observer.*

$$\nu_2' = \left(\frac{V - V_0}{V} \right) \nu_0$$

(c) **When source and observer both are in motion**

(i) *If source and observer both move away from each other.*

$$\nu_3 = \left(\frac{V - V_0}{V - V_s} \right) \nu_0$$

(ii) *If source and observer both move towards each other.*

$$\nu_3' = \left(\frac{V + V_0}{V - V_s} \right) \nu_0 ;$$

When the wind blows in the direction of sound, then in all above formulae V is replaced by (V + W) where W is the velocity of wind. If the wind blows in the opposite direction to sound then V is replaced by (V – W).

Problem Solving Tips

1. The motion of the listener causes change in number of waves received by the listener and this produces an apparent change in frequency.
2. The motion of the source of sound causes change in wavelength of the sound waves, which produces apparent change in frequency.
3. If a star goes away from the earth with velocity v, then the frequency of the light emitted from it changes from ν to ν'.

   $\nu' = \nu\,(1 - v/c)$, where c is the velocity of light and

   $\frac{\Delta\nu}{\nu} = \frac{v}{c}$ or $\frac{\Delta\lambda}{\lambda} = \frac{v}{c}$ where $\Delta\lambda$ is called **Doppler's shift.**

   If wavelength of the observed waves decreases then the object from which the waves are coming is moving towards the listener and vice versa.

Example 7.

Two engines cross each other travelling in opposite direction at 72 km/hour. One engine sounds a whistle of frequency 1088 cps. What are the frequencies as heard by an observer on the other engine before and after crossing. Take the speed of sound as 340 m/s.

Solution :

The apparent frequency before crossing,

$$n' = n\left(\frac{v+v_0}{v-v_s}\right)$$

Here $V_0 = 72$ km/hour $= 20$ m/s

$v_s = 72$ km/hour $= 20$ m/s

$$\therefore \; n' = 1088 \times \left(\frac{340+20}{340-20}\right)$$

$$= 1088 \times \frac{360}{320} = 1224 \text{ Hz}$$

The apparent frequency after crossing

$$n'' = n\left(\frac{v-v_0}{v+v_s}\right) = 1088 \times \left(\frac{340-20}{340+20}\right)$$

$$= 1088 \times \frac{32}{36} = 967.11 \text{ Hz}$$

Example 8.

A rocket is going towards moon with a speed v. The astronaut in the rocket sends signals of frequency n towards the moon and receives them back on reflection from the moon. What will be the frequency of the signal received by the astronaut? (Take v << c)

Solution :

In this case, we can assume that both the source and observer are moving towards each other with velocity v. If c be the velocity of signal, then

$$n' = \left(\frac{c+v}{c-v}\right)n \quad \text{or} \quad n' = \left(\frac{(c+v)\,(c-v)}{(c-v)^2}\right)n$$

$$\text{or } n' = \frac{(c^2-v^2)}{c^2+v^2-2cv} \Rightarrow n' = \frac{c^2}{c^2-2cv}n; \quad (\text{as } c >> v)$$

$$\therefore \; n' = \left(\frac{c}{c-2v}\right)n$$

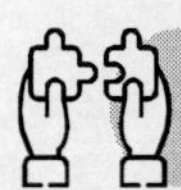

15.2 Concept Practice Problems

CPP

11. Doppler's effect is not applicable for
(a) audio waves (b) electromagnetic waves
(c) shock waves (d) None of these

12. Two sound waves of equal intensity *I* produce beats. The maximum intensity of sound produced in beats will be
(a) *I* (b) 2*I* (c) 3*I* (d) 4*I*

13. Two tones of frequencies n_1 and n_2 are sounded together. The beats can be heard distinctly when
(a) $10 < (n_1 - n_2) < 20$ (b) $5 < (n_1 - n_2) > 20$
(c) $5 < (n_1 - n_2) < 20$ (d) $0 < (n_1 - n_2) < 10$

14. There are three sources of sound of equal intensities and frequencies 400, 401 and 402 vibrations per second. The number of beats/sec is
(a) 0 (b) 1 (c) 3 (d) 2

15. A whistle of frequency 1000 Hz is sounded on a car travelling towards a cliff with velocity of 18 m s^{-1} normal to the cliff. If c = 330 m s^{-1}, then the apparent frequency of the echo as heard by the car driver is nearly
(a) 1115 Hz (b) 115 Hz (c) 67 Hz (d) 47.2 Hz

16. An organ pipe open at one end is vibrating in first overtone and is in resonance with another pipe open at both ends and vibrating in third harmonic. The ratio of length of two pipes is
(a) 1 : 2 (b) 4 : 1 (c) 8 : 3 (d) 3 : 8

17. An engine running at speed $\frac{v}{10}$ sounds a whistle of frequency 600 Hz. A passenger in a train coming from the opposite side at speed $\frac{v}{15}$ experiences this whistle to be of frequency f. If v is speed of sound in air and there is no wind, f is near to
(a) 710 Hz (b) 630 Hz (c) 580 Hz (d) 510 Hz

18. A source of sound is travelling at $\frac{100}{3}$ m s^{-1} along a road, towards a point A. When the source is 3 m away from A, a person standing at a point O on a road perpendicular to the track hears a sound of frequency ν'. The distance of O from A at that time is 4 m. If the original frequency is 640 Hz, then the value of v' is (given : velocity of sound = 340 m s^{-1})
(a) 620 Hz
(b) 680 Hz
(c) 720 Hz
(d) 840 Hz

19. A car is moving towards a high cliff. The car driver sounds a horn of frequency *f*. The reflected sound heard by the driver has as frequency 2*f*. If v be the velocity of sound, then the velocity of the car, in the same velocity units, will be
(a) v/2 (b) v/√2 (c) v/3 (d) v/4

20. A tuning fork of freqqency 512 Hz makes 4 beats per second with the vibrating string of a piano. The beat frequency decreases to 2 beats per sec when the tension in the piano string is slightly increased. The frequency of the piano string before increasing the tension was
(a) 510 *Hz* (b) 514 *Hz* (c) 516 *Hz* (d) 508 *Hz*

ANSWER KEY

11	(c)	12	(d)	13	(d)	14	(b)	15	(a)	16	(a)	17	(a)	18	(b)	19	(c)	20	(d)

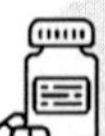

Topic 15.3 : Stationary or Standing Waves in an Organ Pipe & on a String and Characteristics of Sound

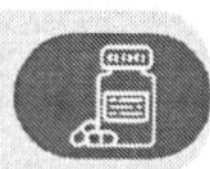

STATIONARY OR STANDING WAVES

When two progressive waves having the same amplitude, velocity and time period but travelling in opposite directions superimpose, then stationary wave is produced.

Let two waves of same amplitude and frequency travel in opposite direction at same speed, then

$y_1 = A\sin(\omega t - kx)$ and

$y_2 = A\sin(\omega t + kx)$

By principle of superposition

$y = y_1 + y_2 = (2A\cos kx)\sin\omega t$ ...(i)

$y = A_s \sin\omega t$

It is clear that amplitude of stationary wave A_s vary with position

(a) $\mathbf{A_s = 0}$, when $\cos kx = 0$ i.e., $kx = \pi/2, 3\pi/2$...........
i.e., $x = \lambda/4, 3\lambda/4$..................[as $k = 2\pi/\lambda$]
These points are called **nodes** and spacing between two nodes is $\lambda/2$.

(b) $\mathbf{A_s}$ **is maximum**, when cos kx is max
i.e., $kx = 0, \pi, 2\pi, 3\pi$ i.e., $x = 0, \lambda 1/2, 2\lambda/2$....
It is clear that **antinode** (where A_s is maximum) are also equally spaced with spacing $\lambda/2$.

(c) The distance between node and antinode is $\lambda/4$ (see figure)

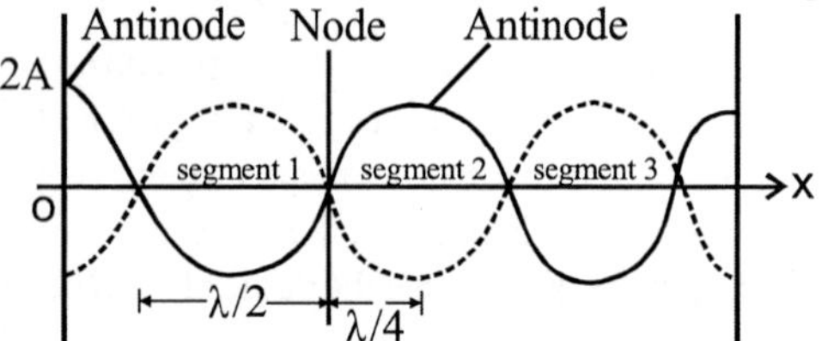

Problem Solving Tips

1. When a string vibrates in one segment, the sound produced is called **fundamental note**. The string is said to vibrate in fundamental mode.
2. The fundamental note is called first harmonic, and is given by $v_0 = \frac{v}{2\ell}$, where v = speed of wave.
3. If the fundamental frequency be v_0 then $2v_0, 3v_0, 4v_0$ ... are respectively called second third, fourth ... harmonics respectively.
4. If an instrument produces notes of frequencies v_1, v_2, v_3, v_4.... where $v_1 < v_2 < v_3 < v_4$....., then v_2 is called first overtone, v_3 is called second overtone, v_4 is called third overtone ... so on.
5. Harmonics are the integral multiples of the fundamental frequency. If v_0 be the fundamental frequency, then nv_0 is the frequency of nth harmonic.
6. Overtones are the notes of frequency higher than the fundamental frequency actually produced by the instrument.
7. In the strings all harmonics are produced.

Stationary Waves in an Organ Pipe :

In the **open organ pipe** all the harmonics are produced.

In an open organ pipe, the fundamental frequency or first harmonic is $n_0 = \frac{v}{2\ell}$, where v is velocity of sound and ℓ is the length of air column [see fig. (a)]

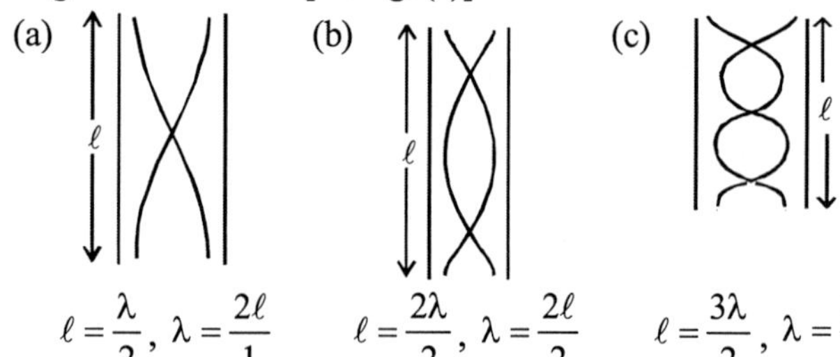

$\ell = \frac{\lambda}{2}, \lambda = \frac{2\ell}{1}$ $\quad \ell = \frac{2\lambda}{2}, \lambda = \frac{2\ell}{2}$ $\quad \ell = \frac{3\lambda}{2}, \lambda = \frac{3L}{3}$

Similarly the frequency of second harmonic or first overtone is [see fig (b)], $n_{01} = \frac{2v}{2\ell}$

Similarly the frequency of third harmonic and second overtone is, [(see fig. (c)] $n_{02} = \frac{3v}{2\ell}$

Similarly $n_{03} = \frac{4v}{2\ell}, n_{04} = \frac{5v}{2\ell}$.................

In the **closed organ pipe** only the odd harmonics are produced.

In a closed organ pipe, the fundamental frequency (or first harmonic) is (see fig. a)

$$n_c = \frac{v}{4\ell}$$

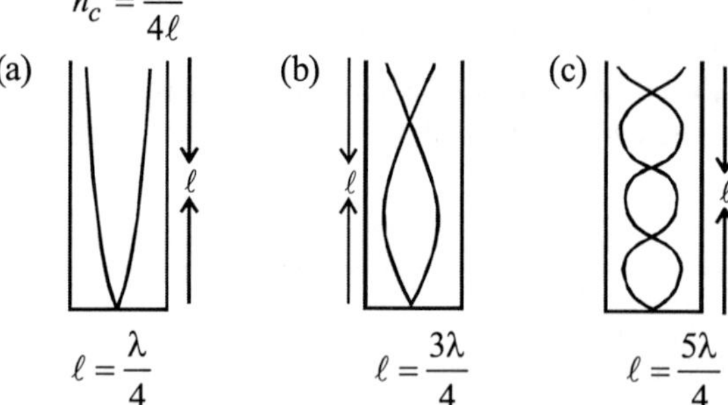

$\ell = \frac{\lambda}{4}$ $\quad \ell = \frac{3\lambda}{4}$ $\quad \ell = \frac{5\lambda}{4}$

Similarly the frequency of third harmonic or first overtone (IInd harmonic absent) is (see fig. b)

$$n_{c2} = \frac{3v}{4\ell}$$

Similarly $n_{c3} = \frac{5v}{4\ell}, n_{c4} = \frac{7v}{4\ell}$........

End Correction

It is observed that the antinode actually occurs a little above the open end. A correction is applied for this which is known as end correction and is denoted by e.

(i) For **closed organ pipe :** ℓ is replaced by $\ell + e$ where $e = 0.3D$, D is the diameter of the tube.

(ii) For **open organ pipe:** ℓ is replaced by $\ell + 2e$ where $e = 0.3D$

In **resonance tube**, *the velocity of sound in air given by* $v = 2v(l_2 - l_1)$

where ν = frequency of tuning fork, $\ell_1 = 1^{st}$ resonating length, $\ell_2 = 2^{nd}$ resonating length.

Resonance Tube :

It is used to determine velocity of sound in air with the help of a tuning fork of known frequency.

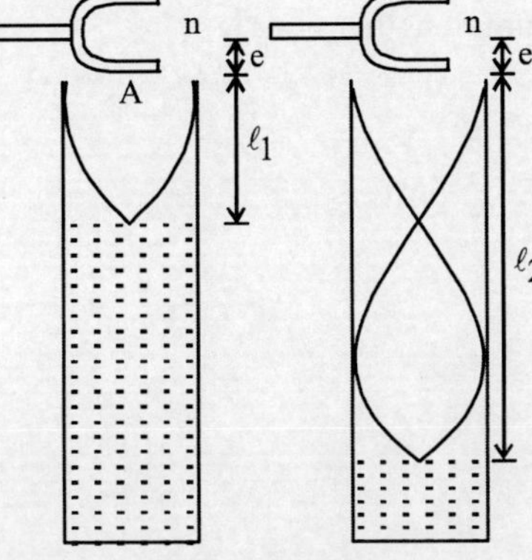

Let ℓ_1 and ℓ_2 are lengths of first and second resonances then

$$\ell_1 + e = \frac{\lambda}{4} \text{ and } \ell_2 + e = \frac{3\lambda}{4}$$

$$\Rightarrow \ell_2 - \ell_1 = \frac{\lambda}{2} \Rightarrow \lambda = 2(\ell_2 - \ell_1)$$

Speed of sound in air is

$v = \upsilon\lambda$ where υ is the frequency

$$v = 2\upsilon(\ell_2 - \ell_1)$$

For vibrating strings/ open organ pipe.

Mode of vibration	Harmonic	Tone	Frequency	Wavelength	Shape for string
First or Fundamental	First	Fundamental tone	$\nu = \frac{v}{2l}$	$2l$	N A N
Second	Second	First overtone	2ν	$\frac{2l}{2}$	N A N A N
Third	Third	Second overtone	3ν	$\frac{2l}{3}$	N A N A N A N

For closed organ pipe.

Mode of vibration	Harmonic	Tone	Frequency	Wavelength	Shape for string
First or Fundamental	First	Fundamental tone	$\nu = \frac{v}{4l}$	$4l$	
Second	Third	First overtone	3ν	$\frac{4l}{3}$	
Third	fifth	Second overtone	5ν	$\frac{4l}{5}$	

Standing Waves in Strings

Wave speed $V = \sqrt{\frac{T}{m}}$ where T = tension in string and m = mass per unit length

Fundamental mode frequency, $n_1 = \frac{1}{2\ell}\sqrt{\frac{T}{m}}$

For second mode of vibration, $n_2 = \frac{1}{\ell}\sqrt{\frac{T}{m}}$

Node position : $x = 0, \frac{\ell}{N}, \frac{2\ell}{N}, \frac{3\ell}{N}, ----$

Antinode position : $x = \frac{\ell}{2N}, \frac{3\ell}{2N}, \frac{5\ell}{2N}, ---- \frac{(2N-1)}{2N}\ell$

Comparision of Progressive (or travelling) and Stationary (or standing) Wave:

SI.	Progressive Wave	Stationary Wave
1.	The wave advances with a constant speed	The wave does not advance but remains confined in a particular region.
2.	The amplitude is the same for all the particles in the path of the wave	The amplitude varies according to position, being zero at the nodes and maximum at the antinodes.
3.	All particles within one wavelength have different phases.	Phase of all particles between two adjacent nodes is the same. Particles in adjacent segments of length $\pi/2$ have opposite phase.
4.	Energy is transmitted in the direction of propagation of the wave	Energy is associated with the wave, but there is no transfer of energy across any section of the medium.

Comparative Study of Interference, Beats and Stationary Wave:

Interference	Beats	Stationary wave
Superposition of two waves of nearly same amplitude or same amplitude having a constant phase difference (or no phase difference) travelling in the same direction and with the same wavelength show the phenomenon of interference.	Superposition of two waves of same amplitude having zero phase difference moving in the same direction having small difference in frequency (less than 10 Hz) show the phenomenon of beats.	Superposition of two waves of same amplitude having a constant phase difference (or no phase difference) moving in opposite direction having same frequency give rise to stationary waves.
Maxima and minima are fixed at their locations.	Maxima and minima vary periodically with time at every location.	Maxima and minima are fixed at their locations.

CHARACTERISTICS OF SOUND

1. A **musical sound** consists of quick, regular and periodic succession of compressions and rarefactions without a sudden change in amplitude.
2. A **noise,** consists of slow, irregular and a periodic succession of compressions and rarefactions, that may have sudden changes in amplitude.
3. **(i) Pitch, (ii) loudness** and **(iii) quality** are the characteristics of musical sound.
4. **Pitch** *depends on frequency,* **loudness** *depends on intensity and,* **quality** *depends on the number and intensity of overtones.*
5. The ratio of the frequencies of the two notes is called the **interval** between them. For example interval between two notes of frequencies 512 Hz and 1024 Hz is 1 : 2 (or 1/2).
6. Two notes are said to be in **unison** if their frequencies are equal, i.e., if the interval between them is 1 : 1.

   Some other common intervals, found useful in producing musical sound are the following:

Octave (1 : 2), majortone (8 : 9), minortone (9 : 10) and semitone (15 : 16)

7. Major diatonic scale : It consists of eight notes. The consecutive notes have either of the following three intervals. They are 8 : 9 ; 9 : 10 and 15 : 16.

Acoustics : The branch of physics that deals with the process of generation, reception and propagation of sound is called acoustics.

Acoustics may be studied under the following three subtitles.

(a) **Electro acoustics**. This branch deals with electrical sound production with music.

(b) **Musical acoustics**. This branch deals with the relationship of sound with music.

(c) **Architectural acoustics**. This branch deals with the design and construction of buildings.

Reverberation

Multiple reflections which are responsible for a series of waves falling on listener's ears, giving the impression of a persistence or prolongation of the sound are called reverberations.

The time gap between the initial direct note and the reflected note upto the minimum audibility level is called **reverberation time.**

Sabine Reverberation Formula for Time

Sabine established that the standard period of reverberation viz., the time that the sound takes to fall in intensity by 60 decibels or to one millionth of its original intensity after it was stopped, is given by $T = \dfrac{0.05V}{\Sigma \alpha_i S_i}$

where V = volume of room, $\Sigma \alpha_i S_i = \alpha_1 S_1 + \alpha_2 S_2 + ...$

S_1, S_2 .... are different kinds of surfaces of room and α_1, α_2 .... are their respective **absorption coefficient.**

The above formula was derived by Prof C. Sabine.

Shock waves : *The waves produced by a body moving with a speed greater than the speed of sound are called shock waves.* These waves carry huge amount of energy. It is due to the shock wave that we have a sudden violent sound called sonic boom when a supersonic plane passes by.

The rate of speed of the source to that of the speed of sound is called ***mach number****.*

Intensity of sound : The sound intensities that we can hear range from 10^{-12} Wm^{-2} to 10^3 Wm^{-2}. The intensity level β, measured in terms of decibel (dB) is defined as $\beta = 10 \log \dfrac{I}{I_0}$

where I = measured intensity, $I_0 = 10^{-12}$ Wm^{-1}

At the threshold $\beta = 0$

At the max $\beta = 10 \log \dfrac{1}{10^{-12}} = 120$ dB

Lissajous Figures: *when two simple harmonic waves having vibrations in mutually perpendicular directions superimpose on each other, then the resultant motion of the particle is along a closed path, called the Lissajous figures.* These figures can be of many shapes depending on

(i) ratio of frequencies or time periods of two waves

(ii) ratio of amplitude of two waves

(iii) phase difference between two waves.

Example 9.

The equation of stationary wave in stretched string is given by $y = 5 \sin \dfrac{\pi x}{3} \cos 40 \pi t$ *where x and y are in cm and t in second. Find the separation between two adjacent nodes.*

Solution :

Given that $y = 5 \sin \dfrac{\pi x}{3} \cos 40 \pi t$

We know that $y = a \sin \dfrac{2\pi}{\lambda} x \cos \dfrac{2\pi}{\lambda} vt$

$\therefore \quad \dfrac{2\pi}{\lambda} = \dfrac{\pi}{3}$ or $\lambda = 6$

Now distance between two adjacent nodes

$= \dfrac{\lambda}{2} = \dfrac{6}{2} = 3$ cm

Example 10.

For a certain organ pipe, three successive resonance frequencies are observed at 425, 595 and 765 Hz, respectively. Taking the speed of sound in the air to be 340 metre per second, (i) explain whether the pipe is closed at one end or open at both the ends and (ii) determine the fundamental frequency and the length of the pipe.

Solution :

(i) Given ratio of successive frequencies

$= 425 : 595 : 765 = 5 : 7 : 9.$

So, the harmonics are odd harmonics. Hence the pipe is closed at one end.

(ii) Fundamental frequency n is given by, $n = \dfrac{425}{5} = 85$

We known that $n = \dfrac{v}{4\ell}$ or $\ell = \dfrac{v}{4n}$ for closed organ pipe at one end.

$\therefore$ Length of the pipe $\ell = \dfrac{340}{4 \times 85} = 1$ metre

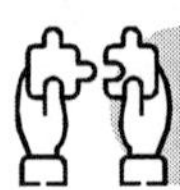

15.3 Concept Practice Problems

CPP

21. Frequencies of sound produced from an organ pipe open at both ends are
(a) only fundamental note
(b) only even harmonics
(c) only odd harmonics
(d) even and odd harmonics

22. The fundamental frequency of an organ pipe is 512 Hz. If its length is increased, then frequency will
(a) decrease (b) increase
(c) remains same (d) cannot be predicted

23. An open and closed organ pipe have the same length. The ratio of pth mode of frequency of vibration of two pipes is
(a) 1 (b) p (c) $p(2p+1)$ (d) $\frac{2p}{(2p-1)}$

24. What is the effect of increase in temperature on the frequency of sound produced by an organ pipe?
(a) increases (b) decreases
(c) no effect (d) erratic change

25. In resonance tube, the volocity of sound in air is given by
(a) $v = 2v(\ell_2 - \ell_1)$ (b) $v = v(\ell_2 - \ell_1)$
(c) $v = 2v(\ell_2 - \ell_1)$ (d) $v = \frac{v}{2}(\ell_2 - \ell_1)$

26. A closed pipe and an open pipe have their first overtones identical in frequency. Their lengths are in the ratio
(a) 1 : 2 (b) 2 : 3 (c) 3 : 4 (d) 4 : 5

27. The fundamental frequency of an open organ pipe is 300 Hz. The first overtone of this pipe has same frequency as first overtone of a closed organ pipe. If speed of sound is 330 m/s, then the length of closed organ pipe is
(a) 41 cm (b) 37 cm (c) 31 cm (d) 80 cm

28. A pipe closed at one end produces a fundamental note of 412 Hz. It is cut into two pieces of equal length. the fundamental frequencies produced by the two pieces are
(a) 206 Hz, 412 Hz (b) 824 Hz, 1648 Hz
(c) 412 Hz, 824 Hz (d) 206 Hz, 824 Hz

29. An organ pipe P_1 closed at one end vibrating in its first overtone and another pipe P_2 open at both ends vibrating in third overtone are in resonance with a given tuning fork. The ratio of the length of P_1 to that of P_2 is
(a) 8/3 (b) 3/8 (c) 1/2 (d) 1/3

30. The equation of a stationary wave is :
$y = 4\sin\left(\frac{\pi x}{15}\right)\cos(96\pi t)$. The distance between a node and its next antinode is
(a) 7.5 units (b) 1.5 units
(c) 22.5 units (d) 30 units

ANSWER KEY

21	(d)	22	(a)	23	(d)	24	(a)	25	(a)	26	(c)	27	(a)	28	(b)	29	(b)	30	(a)

CONCEPT MAP

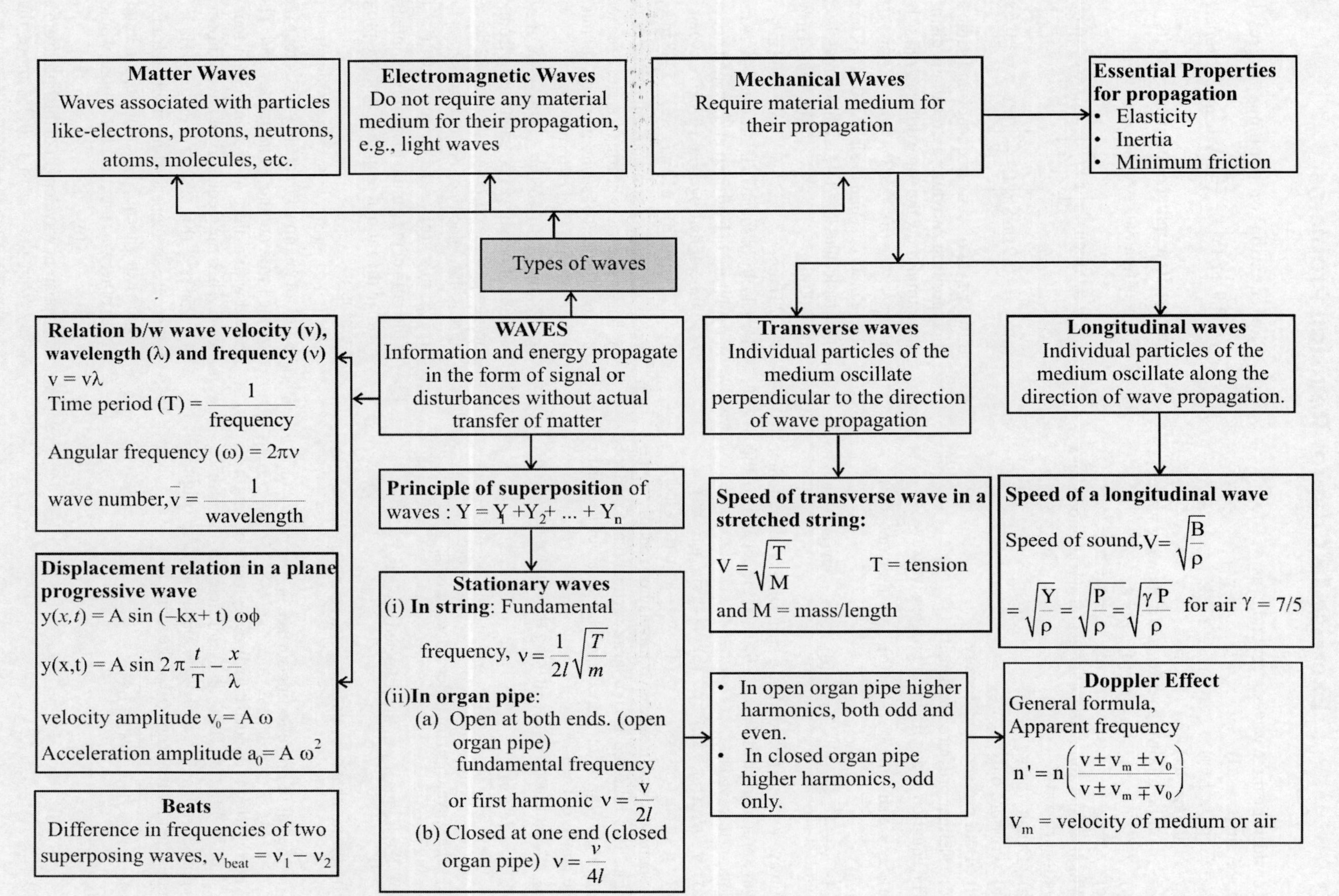
Matter Waves
Waves associated with particles like-electrons, protons, neutrons, atoms, molecules, etc.
Electromagnetic Waves
Do not require any material medium for their propagation, e.g., light waves
Mechanical Waves
Require material medium for their propagation
Essential Properties for propagation
• Elasticity
• Inertia
• Minimum friction
Types of waves
WAVES
Information and energy propagate in the form of signal or disturbances without actual transfer of matter
Transverse waves
Individual particles of the medium oscillate perpendicular to the direction of wave propagation
Longitudinal waves
Individual particles of the medium oscillate along the direction of wave propagation.
Relation b/w wave velocity (v), wavelength (λ) and frequency (ν)
$v = \nu\lambda$
Time period (T) = $\frac{1}{\text{frequency}}$
Angular frequency (ω) = 2πν
wave number, $\bar{\nu} = \frac{1}{\text{wavelength}}$
Principle of superposition of waves : $Y = Y_1 + Y_2 + \dots + Y_n$
Speed of transverse wave in a stretched string:
$V = \sqrt{\frac{T}{M}}$ T = tension
and M = mass/length
Speed of a longitudinal wave
Speed of sound, $V = \sqrt{\frac{B}{\rho}}$
$= \sqrt{\frac{Y}{\rho}} = \sqrt{\frac{P}{\rho}} = \sqrt{\frac{\gamma P}{\rho}}$ for air γ = 7/5
Displacement relation in a plane progressive wave
$y(x,t) = A \sin(-kx + t)\ \omega\phi$
$y(x,t) = A \sin 2\pi \frac{t}{T} - \frac{x}{\lambda}$
velocity amplitude $v_0 = A\omega$
Acceleration amplitude $a_0 = A\omega^2$
Stationary waves
(i) In string: Fundamental frequency, $\nu = \frac{1}{2l}\sqrt{\frac{T}{m}}$
(ii) In organ pipe:
(a) Open at both ends. (open organ pipe) fundamental frequency or first harmonic $\nu = \frac{v}{2l}$
(b) Closed at one end (closed organ pipe) $\nu = \frac{v}{4l}$
• In open organ pipe higher harmonics, both odd and even.
• In closed organ pipe higher harmonics, odd only.
Doppler Effect
General formula,
Apparent frequency
$n' = n\left(\frac{v \pm v_m \pm v_0}{v \pm v_m \mp v_0}\right)$
V_m = velocity of medium or air
Beats
Difference in frequencies of two superposing waves, $\nu_{beat} = \nu_1 - \nu_2$

Exercise 1 - Chapter Revision Problems

CRP

1. Consider the three waves z_1, z_2 and z_3 as
$z_1 = A\sin(kx - \omega t)$
$z_2 = A\sin(kx + \omega t)$
$z_3 = A\sin(ky - \omega t)$
Which of the following represents a standing wave?
(a) $z_1 + z_2$ (b) $z_2 + z_3$
(c) $z_3 + z_1$ (d) $z_1 + z_2 + z_3$

2. Which of the following changes at an antinode in a stationary wave?
(a) Density only
(b) Pressure only
(c) Both pressure and density
(d) Neither pressure nor density

3. The equation of a cylindrical progressive wave is
(a) $y = a\sin\omega t$ (b) $y = a\sin(\omega t - kr)$
(c) $y = \frac{a}{\sqrt{r}}\sin(\omega t - kr)$ (d) $y = \frac{a}{r}\sin(\omega t - kr)$

4. A wave $y = a\sin(\omega t - kx)$ on a string meets with another wave producing a node at $x = 0$. Then the equation of the unknown wave is
(a) $y = a\sin(\omega t + kx)$ (b) $y = -a\sin(\omega t + kx)$
(c) $y = a\sin(\omega t - kx)$ (d) $y = -a\sin(\omega t - kx)$

5. A sound wave of frequency f travels horizontally to the right. It is reflected from a large vertical plane surface moving to left with a speed v. The speed of sound in medium is c. Then
(a) the number of wave striking the surface per second is $f\frac{(c+v)}{c}$
(b) the wavelength of reflected wave is $\frac{c(c+v)}{f(c+v)}$
(c) the frequency of the reflected wave is $f\frac{(c-v)}{(c-v)}$
(d) the number of beats heard by a stationary listener to the left of the reflecting surface is $\frac{vf}{c-v}$

6. When a string is divided into three segments of length l_1, l_2, and l_3 the fundamental frequencies of these three segments are ν_1, ν_2 and ν_3 respectively. The original fundamental frequency (ν) of the string is
(a) $\sqrt{\nu} = \sqrt{\nu_1} + \sqrt{\nu_2} + \sqrt{\nu_3}$
(b) $\nu = \nu_1 + \nu_2 + \nu_3$
(c) $\frac{1}{\nu} = \frac{1}{\nu_1} + \frac{1}{\nu_2} + \frac{1}{\nu_3}$
(d) $\frac{1}{\sqrt{\nu}} = \frac{1}{\sqrt{\nu_1}} + \frac{1}{\sqrt{\nu_2}} + \frac{1}{\sqrt{\nu_3}}$

7. The equation of a plane progressive wave is $y = 0.9\sin 4\pi\left[t - \frac{x}{2}\right]$. When it is reflected at a rigid support, its amplitude becomes $\frac{2}{3}$ of its previous value. The equation of the reflected wave is
(a) $y = 0.6\sin 4\pi\left[t + \frac{x}{2}\right]$ (b) $y = -0.6\sin 4\pi\left[t + \frac{x}{2}\right]$
(c) $y = -0.9\sin 8\pi\left[t - \frac{x}{2}\right]$ (d) $y = -0.6\sin 4\pi\left[t + \frac{x}{2}\right]$

8. If two waves of same frequency and same amplitude, on superposition, produce a resultant disturbance of the same amplitude, the wave differ in phase by
(a) π (b) $2\pi/3$ (c) Zero (d) $\pi/3$

9. The velocity of sound in air is 330 m/s. The r.m.s. velocity of air molecules ($\gamma = 1.4$) is approximately equal to
(a) 400 m/s (b) 471.4 m/s
(c) 231 m/s (d) 462 m/s

10. The velocity of sound in hydrogen is 1224 m/s. Its velocity in a mixture of hydrogen and oxygen containing 4 parts by volume of hydrogen and 1 part oxygen is
(a) 1224 m/s (b) 612 m/s (c) 2448 m/s (d) 306 m/s

11. A person standing symmetrically between two cliffs claps his hands and starts hearing a series of echoes at intervals of 1 sec. If speed of sound in air is 340 m/s, the distance between the parallel cliffs must be
(a) 340 m (b) 680 m (c) 1020 m (d) 170 m

12. A series of ocean waves, each 5.0 m from crest to crest, moving past the observer at a rate of 2 waves per second, what is the velocity of ocean waves?
(a) 2.5 m/s (b) 5.0 m/s (c) 8.0 m/s (d) 10.0 m/s

13. If the ratio of maximum to minimum intensity in beats is 49, then the ratio of amplitudes of two progressive wave trains is
(a) 7 : 1 (b) 4 : 3 (c) 49 : 1 (d) 16 : 9

14. A fork of unknown frequency gives four beats/sec when sounded with another of frequency 256. The fork is now loaded with a piece of wax and again four beats/sec are heard. Then the frequency of the unknown fork is
(a) 256 Hz (b) 252 Hz (c) 264 Hz (d) 260 Hz

15. If there are six loops for 1 m length in transverse mode of Melde's experiment., the no. of loops in longitudinal mode under otherwise identical conditions would be
(a) 3 (b) 6 (c) 12 (d) 8

16. The apparent wavelength of the light from a star moving away from the earth is 0.2% more than its actual wavelength. Then the velocity of the star is
(a) 6×10^7 m/sec (b) 6×10^6 m/sec
(c) 6×10^5 m/sec (d) 6×10^4 m/sec

17. In a resonance column, first and second resonance are obtained at depths 22.7 cm and 70.2 cm. The third resonance will be obtained at a depth

(a) 117.7 cm (b) 92.9 cm (c) 115.5 cm (d) 113.5 cm

18. A fork of frequency 256 Hz resonates with a closed organ pipe of length 25.4 cm. If the length of pipe be increased by 2 mm, the number of beats/sec. will be

(a) 4 (b) 1 (c) 2 (d) 3

19. The speed of sound in air under ordinary conditions is around 330 m s^{-1}. The speed of sound in hydrogen under similar conditions will be (in m s^{-1}) nearest to

(a) 330 (b) 1200 (c) 600 (d) 900

20. Two waves represented by $y_1 = a\sin\omega t$ and $y_2 = a\sin(\omega t + \phi)$ with $\phi = \frac{\pi}{2}$ are superposed at any point at a particular instant. The resultant amplitude is

(a) a (b) 4a (c) $\sqrt{2}a$ (d) zero

21. If the speed of a transverse wave on a stretched string of length 1 m is 60 m/s, what is the fundamental frequency of vibration?

(a) 10 Hz (b) 30 Hz (c) 40 Hz (d) 70 Hz

22. The equation of a progressive wave is

$$y = 0.02\sin 2\pi\left[\frac{t}{0.01} - \frac{x}{0.30}\right]$$

Here x and y are in metre and t is in second. The velocity of propagation of the wave is

(a) 300 m s^{-1} (b) 30 m s^{-1}

(c) 400 m s^{-1} (d) 40 m s^{-1}

23. The intensity level of sound wave is said to be 4 decibel. If the intensity of wave is doubled, then the intensity level of sound as expressed in decibel would be

(a) 8 (b) 16 (c) 7 (d) 14

24. The equation $y = A\sin^2(kx - \omega t)$ represents a wave with

(a) amplitude A, frequency $\omega/2\pi$

(b) amplitude A/2, frequency ω/π

(c) amplitude 2A, frequency $\omega/4\pi$

(d) it does not represent a wave motion

25. When a tuning fork vibrates with 1.0 m or 1.05 m long wire of a sonometer, 5 beats per second are produced in each case. What will be the frequency of the tuning fork?

(a) 195 (b) 200 (c) 205 (d) 210

26. The speed of sound in oxygen (O_2) at a certain temperature is 460 ms^{-1}. The speed of sound in helium (He) at the same temperature will be (assume both gases to be ideal)

(a) 460 ms^{-1} (b) 500 ms^{-1}

(c) 650 ms^{-1} (d) 330 ms^{-1}

27. In expressing sound intensity, we take 10^{-12} W m^{-2} as the reference level. For ordinary conversation, the intensity level is about 10^{-6} W m^{-2}. Expressed in decibel, this is

(a) 10^6 (b) 6

(c) 60 (d) $\log_e(10^6)$

28. A uniform wire of length 20 m and weighing 5 kg hangs vertically. If g = 10 m/s^2, then the speed of transverse waves in the middle of the wire is

(a) 10 m/s (b) $10\sqrt{2}$ m/s

(c) 4 m/s (d) zero

29. The displacement of a particle varies according to the relation $x = 4(\cos\pi t + \sin\pi t)$. The amplitude of the particle is

(a) −4 m (b) 4m (c) $4\sqrt{2}$ m (d) 8m

30. Two waves of wavelengths 99 cm and 100 cm both travelling with velocity 396 m/s are made to interfere. The number of beats produced by them per second is

(a) 1 (b) 2 (c) 4 (d) 8

31. When a sound wave of frequency 300 Hz passes through a medium, the maximum displacement of a particle of the medium is 0.1 cm. The maximum velocity of the particle is equal to

(a) 60π cms^{-1} (b) 30π cms^{-1}

(c) 30 cms^{-1} 30 cm s^{-1} (d) 60 cms^{-1}

32. A source of sound produces waves of wavelength 60 cm when it is stationary. If the speed of sound in air is 320 m s^{-1} and source moves with speed 20 m s^{-1}, the wavelength of sound in the forward direction will be nearest to

(a) 56 cm (b) 60 cm (c) 64 cm (d) 68 cm

33. A longitudinal wave is represented by

$$x = x_0 \sin 2\pi\left(nt - \frac{x}{\lambda}\right)$$

The maximum particle velocity will be four times the wave velocity if

(a) $\lambda = \frac{\pi x_0}{4}$ (b) $\lambda = 2\pi x_0$

(c) $\lambda = \frac{\pi x_0}{2}$ (d) $\lambda = 4\pi x_0$

34. Two strings A and B, made of same material, are stretched by same tension. The radius of string A is double of radius of B. A transverse wave travels on A with speed v_A and on B with speed v_B. The ratio v_A / v_B is

(a) 1/2 (b) 2 (c) 1/4 (d) 4

35. A sonometer wire of length *l* vibrates in fundamental mode when excited by a tuning fork of frequency 416 Hz. If the length is doubled keeping other things same, the string will

(a) vibrate with a frequency of 416 Hz

(b) vibrate with a frequency of 208 Hz

(c) vibrate with a frequency of 832 Hz

(d) stop vibrating

36. Where should the two bridges be set in a 110cm long wire so that it is divided into three parts and the ratio of the frequencies are 3 : 2 : 1 ?
(a) 20cm from one end and 60cm from other end
(b) 30cm from one end and 70cm from other end
(c) 10cm from one end and 50cm from other end
(d) 50cm from one end and 40cm from other end

37. A source X of unknown frequency produces 8 beats per second with a source of 250 Hz and 12 beats per second with a source of 270 Hz. The frequency of the source X is
(a) 242 Hz (b) 258 Hz (c) 282 Hz (d) 262 Hz

38. A thick uniform rope of length L is hanging from a rigid support. A transverse wave of wavelength λ_0 is set up at the middle of rope as shown in figure. The wavelength of the wave as it reaches to the topmost point is

(a) $2\lambda_0$ (b) $\sqrt{2}\lambda_0$

(c) $\frac{\lambda_0}{\sqrt{2}}$ (d) λ_0

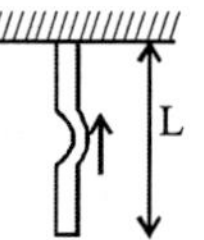

39. Wave pulse on a string shown in figure is moving to the right without changing shape. Consider two particles at positions x_1 = 1.5m and x_2 = 2.5m. Their transverse velocities at the moment shown in figure are along directions

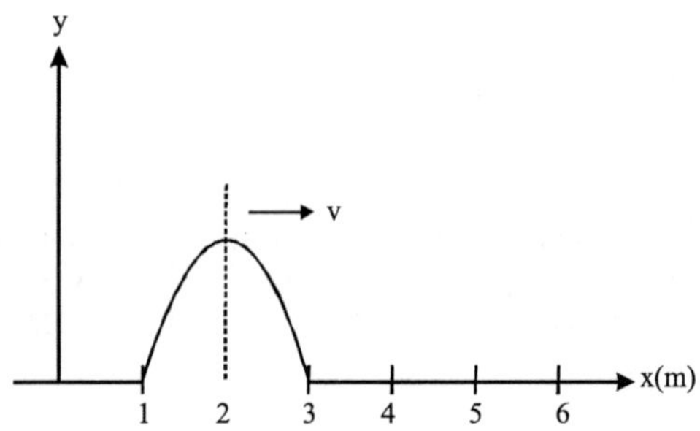

(a) positive y-axis and positive y-axis respectively
(b) negative y-axis and positive y-axis respectively
(c) positive y-axis and negative y-axis respectively
(d) negative y-axis and negative y-axis respectively

40. The transverse wave represented by the equation

$y = 4\sin\left(\frac{\pi}{6}\right)\sin(3x - 15t)$ has

(a) amplitude = 4
(b) wavelength = $4\frac{\pi}{3}$
(c) speed of propagation = 5
(d) period = $\frac{\pi}{15}$

41. Two vibrating tuning forks produce progressive waves given by $Y_1 = 4 \sin 500\, \pi t$ and $Y_2 = 2 \sin 506\, \pi t$. Number of beats produced per minute is
(a) 360 (b) 180 (c) 60 (d) 3

42. A transverse wave is represented by $y = A \sin(\omega t - kx)$. For what value of the wavelength is the wave velocity equal to the maximum particle velocity?
(a) $\frac{\pi A}{2}$ (b) πA (c) 2πA (d) A

43. Sound waves travel at 350 m/s through a warm air and at 3500 m/s through brass. The wavelength of a 700 Hz acoustic wave as it enters brass from warm air
(a) decreases by a factor 10
(b) increases by a factor 20
(c) increases by a factor 10
(d) decreases by a factor 20

44. Velocity of sound waves in air is 330 m/s. For a particular sound wave in air, a path difference of 40 cm is equivalent to phase difference of 1.6π. The frequency of this wave is
(a) 165 Hz (b) 150 Hz (c) 660 Hz (d) 330 Hz

45. Two sources of sound placed close to each other are emitting progressive waves given by $y_1 = 4 \sin 600\, \pi t$ and $y_2 = 5 \sin 608\, \pi t$. An observer located near these two sources of sound will hear
(a) 4 beats per second with intensity ratio 25 : 16 between waxing and waning.
(b) 8 beats per second with intensity ratio 25 : 16 between waxing and waning
(c) 8 beats per second with intensity ratio 81 : 1 between waxing and waning
(d) 4 beats per second with intensity ratio 81 : 1 between waxing and waning

46. A progressive wave travelling along the positive x-direction is represented by $y(x,t) = A\sin(kx - \omega t + \phi)$. Its snapshot at $t = 0$ is given in the figure.

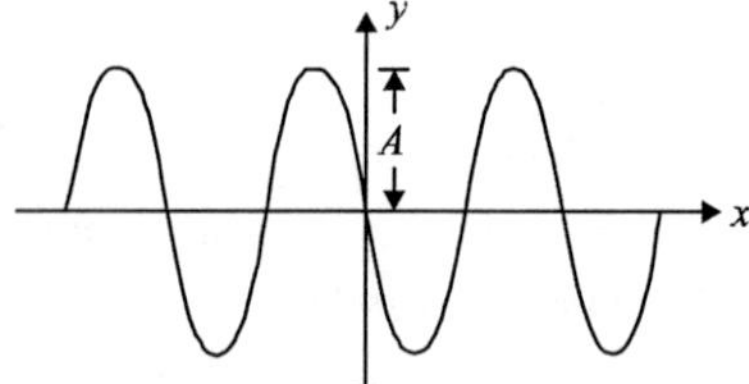

For this wave, the phase ϕ is :
(a) $-\frac{\pi}{2}$ (b) π (c) 0 (d) $\frac{\pi}{2}$

47. A travelling harmonic wave is represented by the equation $y(x, t) = 10^{-3} \sin(50t + 2x)$, where x and y are in meter and t is in seconds. Which of the following is a correct statement about the wave?
(a) The wave is propagating along the negative x-axis with speed 25 ms^{-1}.
(b) The wave is propagating along the positive x-axis with speed 100 ms^{-1}.
(c) The wave is propagating along the positive x-axis with speed 25 ms^{-1}.
(d) The wave is propagating along the negative x-axis with speed 100 ms^{-1}.

48. For a transverse wave travelling along a straight line, the distance between two peaks (crests) is 5 m, while the distance between one crest and one trough is 1.5 m. The possible wavelengths (in m) of the waves are :
(a) 1, 3, 5, ... (b) $\frac{1}{1}, \frac{1}{3}, \frac{1}{5}, ...$
(c) 1, 2, 3, ... (d) $\frac{1}{2}, \frac{1}{4}, \frac{1}{6}, ...$

49. The end correction of a resonance column is 1cm. If the shortest length resonating with the tuning fork is 10cm, the next resonating length should be
(a) 32cm (b) 40cm (c) 28cm (d) 36cm

50. A granite rod of 60 cm length is clamped at its middle point and is set into longitudinal vibrations. The density of granite is 2.7×10^3 kg/m^3 and its Young's modulus is 9.27×10^{10} Pa.
What will be the fundamental frequency of the longitudinal vibrations?
(a) 5 kHz (b) 2.5 kHz (c) 10 kHz (d) 7.5 kHz

51. A string of length 1 m and mass 5 g is fixed at both ends. The tension in the string is 8.0 N. The string is set into vibration using an external vibrator of frequency 100 Hz. The separation between successive nodes on the string is close to:
(a) 10.0 cm (b) 33.3 cm (c) 16.6 cm (d) 20.0 cm

52. A closed organ pipe has a fundamental frequency of 1.5 kHz. The number of overtones that can be distinctly heard by a person with this organ pipe will be: (Assume that the highest frequency a person can hear is 20,000 Hz)
(a) 6 (b) 4 (c) 7 (d) 5

53. A wire of length 2L, is made by joining two wires A and B of same length but different radii r and $2r$ and made of the same material. It is vibrating at a frequency such that the joint of the two wires forms a node. If the number of antinodes in wire A is p and that in B is q then the ratio $p:q$ is:

A B
← L → ← L →

(a) 3:5 (b) 4:9 (c) 1:2 (d) 1:4

54. A string is clamped at both the ends and it is vibrating in its 4th harmonic. The equation of the stationary wave is Y = 0.3 sin(0.157x) cos(200ωt). The length of the string is: (All quantities are in SI units.)
(a) 20 m (b) 80 m (c) 40 m (d) 60 m

55. A string 2.0 m long and fixed at its ends is driven by a 240 Hz vibrator. The string vibrates in its third harmonic mode. The speed of the wave and its fundamental frequency is:
(a) 180 m/s, 80 Hz (b) 320 m/s, 80 Hz
(c) 320 m/s, 120 Hz (d) 180 m/s, 120 Hz

56. A tuning fork of frequency 480 Hz is used in an experiment for measuring speed of sound (v) in air by resonance tube method. Resonance is observed to occur at two successive lengths of the air column, $l_1 = 30$ cm and $l_2 = 70$ cm. Then, v is equal to :
(a) 332 ms^{-1} (b) 384 ms^{-1}
(c) 338 ms^{-1} (d) 379 ms^{-1}

57. A wire of length L and mass per unit length 6.0×10^{-3} kgm^{-1} is put under tension of 540 N. Two consecutive frequencies that it resonates at are: 420 Hz and 490 Hz. Then L in meters is:
(a) 2.1 m (b) 1.1 m (c) 8.1 m (d) 5.1 m

58. Equation of travelling wave on a stretched string of linear density 5 g/m is y = 0.03 sin (450 t – 9x) where distance and time are measured in SI units. The tension in the string is:
(a) 10 N (b) 7.5 N (c) 12.5 N (d) 5 N

59. Two sitar strings, A and B, playing the note 'Dha' are slightly out of tune and produce beats and frequency 5 Hz. The tension of the string B is slightly increased and the beat frequency is found to decrease by 3 Hz. If the frequency of A is 425 Hz, the original frequency of B is
(a) 430 Hz (b) 428 Hz (c) 422 Hz (d) 420 Hz

60. A musician using an open flute of length 50 cm produces second harmonic sound waves. A person runs towards the musician from another end of a hall at a speed of 10 km/h. If the wave speed is 330 m/s, the frequency heard by the running person shall be close to:
(a) 666 Hz (b) 753 Hz (c) 500 Hz (d) 333 Hz

Exercise 2 - Exemplar & Past Year Questions

E&PYQs

Exemplar Questions

1. Water waves produced by a motorboat sailing in water are
(a) neither longitudinal nor transverse
(b) both longitudinal and transverse
(c) only longitudinal
(d) only transverse

2. Sound waves of wavelength λ travelling in a medium with a speed of v m/ s enter into another medium where its speed in $2v$ m/s. Wavelength of sound waves in the second medium is
(a) λ (b) $\frac{\lambda}{2}$ (c) 2λ (d) 4λ

3. Speed of sound wave in air
(a) is independent of temperature
(b) increases with pressure
(c) increases with increase in humidity
(d) decreases with increase in humidity

4. Change in temperature of the medium changes
(a) frequency of sound waves
(b) amplitude of sound waves
(c) wavelength of sound waves
(d) loudness of sound waves

5. With propagation of longitudinal waves through a medium, the quantity transmitted is
(a) matter
(b) energy
(c) energy and matter
(d) energy, matter and momentum

6. Which of the following statements are true for wave motion?
(a) Mechanical transverse waves can propagate through all mediums
(b) Longitudinal waves can propagate through solids only
(c) Mechanical transverse waves can propagate through solids only
(d) Longitudinal waves can propagate through vacuum

7. A sound wave is passing through air column in the form of compression and rarefaction. In consecutive compressions and rarefactions,
(a) density remains constant
(b) Boyle's law is obeyed
(c) bulk modulus of air oscillates
(d) there is no transfer of heat

8. A string of mass 2.5 kg is under tension of 200 N. The length of the stretched string is 20.0 m. If the transverse jerk is struck at one end of the string, the disturbance will reach the other end in

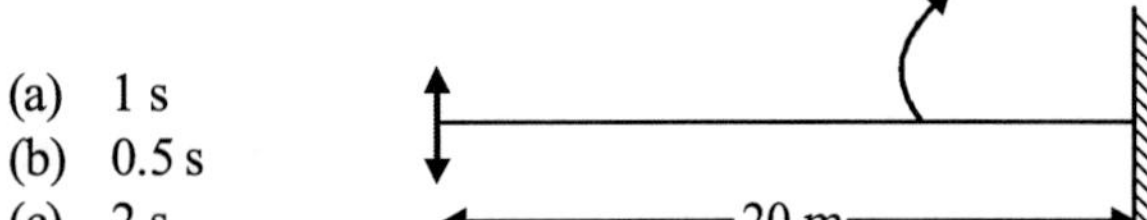

(a) 1 s
(b) 0.5 s
(c) 2 s
(d) data given is insufficient

Past Years (2013-2020) NEET/AIPMT Questions

9. If we study the vibration of a pipe open at both ends, then which of the following statements is not true ? ***[2013]***
(a) Odd harmonics of the fundamental frequency will be generated
(b) All harmonics of the fundamental frequency will be generated
(c) Pressure change will be maximum at both ends
(d) Antinode will be at open end

10. A source of unknown frequency gives 4 beats/s, when sounded with a source of known frequency 250 Hz. The second harmonic of the source of unknown frequency gives five beats per second, when sounded with a source of frequency 513 Hz. The unknown frequency is ***[2013]***
(a) 246 Hz (b) 240 Hz (c) 260 Hz (d) 254 Hz

11. A wave travelling in the +ve x-direction having displacement along y-direction as 1m, wavelength 2π m and frequency $\frac{1}{\pi}$ Hz is represented by ***[2013]***
(a) $y = \sin(2\pi x - 2\pi t)$ (b) $y = \sin(10\pi x - 20\pi t)$
(c) $y = \sin(2\pi x + 2\pi t)$ (d) $y = \sin(x - 2t)$

12. Two sources P and Q produce notes of frequency 660 Hz each. A listener moves from P to Q with a speed of 1 ms^{-1}. If the speed of sound is 330 m/s, then the number of beats heard by the listener per second will be ***[NEET Kar. 2013]***
(a) zero (b) 4 (c) 8 (d) 2

13. If n_1, n_2 and n_3 are the fundamental frequencies of three segments into which a string is divided, then the original fundamental frequency n of the string is given by : ***[2014]***
(a) $\frac{1}{n} = \frac{1}{n_1} + \frac{1}{n_2} + \frac{1}{n_3}$
(b) $\frac{1}{\sqrt{n}} = \frac{1}{\sqrt{n_1}} + \frac{1}{\sqrt{n_2}} + \frac{1}{\sqrt{n_3}}$
(c) $\sqrt{n} = \sqrt{n_1} + \sqrt{n_2} + \sqrt{n_3}$
(d) $n = n_1 + n_2 + n_3$

14. The number of possible natural oscillation of air column in a pipe closed at one end of length 85 cm whose frequencies lie below 1250 Hz are : (velocity of sound = 340 ms^{-1}) ***[2014]***
(a) 4 (b) 5 (c) 7 (d) 6

15. A speeding motorcyclist sees trafic jam ahead of him. He slows down to 36 km/hour. He finds that traffic has eased and a car moving ahead of him at 18 km/hour is honking at a frequency of 1392 Hz. If the speeds of sound is 343 m/s, the frequency of the honk as heard by him will be : ***[2014]***
(a) 1332 Hz (b) 1372 Hz (c) 1412 Hz (d) 1464 Hz

16. The fundamental frequency of a closed organ pipe of length 20 cm is equal to the second overtone of an organ pipe open at both the ends. The length of organ pipe open at both the ends is ***[2015]***
(a) 100 cm (b) 120 cm (c) 140 cm (d) 80 cm

17. A siren emitting a sound of frequency 800 Hz moves away from an observer towards a cliff at a speed of 15ms^{-1}. Then, the frequency of sound that the observer hears in the echo reflected from the cliff is : ***[2016]***
(Take velocity of sound in air = 330 ms^{-1})
(a) 765 Hz (b) 800 Hz (c) 838 Hz (b) 885 Hz

18. An air column, closed at one end and open at the other, resonates with a tuning fork when the smallest length of the column is 50 cm. The next larger length of the column resonating with the same tuning fork is : ***[2016]***
(a) 66.7 cm (b) 100 cm (c) 150 cm (d) 200 cm

19. The two nearest harmonics of a tube closed at one end and open at other end are 220 Hz and 260 Hz. What is the fundamental frequency of the system? ***[2017]***
(a) 20 Hz (b) 30 Hz (c) 40 Hz (d) 10 Hz

20. A tuning fork is used to produce resonance in a glass tube. The length of the air column in this tube can be adjusted by a variable piston. At room temperature of 27°C two successive resonances are produced at 20 cm and 73 cm of column length. If the frequency of the tuning fork is 320 Hz, the velocity of sound in air at 27°C is ***[2018]***
(a) 330 m/s (b) 339 m/s (c) 300 m/s (d) 350 m/s

21. The fundamental frequency in an open organ pipe is equal to the third harmonic of a closed organ pipe. If the length of the closed organ pipe is 20 cm, the length of the open organ pipe is ***[2018]***
(a) 13.2 cm (b) 8 cm (c) 16 cm (d) 12.5 cm

22. A tuning fork with frequency 800 Hz produces resonance in a resonance column tube with upper end open and lower end closed by water surface. Successive resonance are observed at lengths 9.75 cm, 31.25 cm and 52.75 cm. The speed of sound in air is, ***[NEET Odisha 2019]***
(a) 172 m/s (b) 500 m/s (c) 156 m/s (d) 344 m/s

23. In a guitar, two strings A and B made of same material are slightly out of tune and produce beats of frequency 6 Hz. When tension in B is slightly decreased, the beat frequency increases to 7 Hz. If the frequency of A is 530 Hz, the original frequency of B will be ***[2020]***
(a) 524 Hz (b) 536 Hz (c) 537 Hz (d) 523 Hz

Exercise 3 - Concept Application Problems

CAP

1. Two sinusoidal plane waves of same frequency having intensities I_0 and $4 I_0$ are travelling in the same direction. The resultant intensity at a point at which waves meet with a phase difference of zero radian is
(a) I_0 (b) $5 I_0$ (c) $9 I_0$ (d) $3 I_0$

2. Three transverse waves are represented by
$y_1 = A\cos(kx - \omega t)$
$y_2 = A\cos(kx + \omega t)$
$y_3 = A\cos(ky - \omega t)$
The combination of waves which can produce stationary waves is
(a) y_1 and y_2 (b) y_2 and y_3
(c) y_1 and y_3 (d) y_1, y_2 and y_3

3. A whistle S of frequency f revolves in a circle of radius R at a constant speed v. What is the ratio of largest and smallest frequency detected by a detector D at rest at a distance 2R from the centre of circle as shown in figure ? (take c as speed of sound)

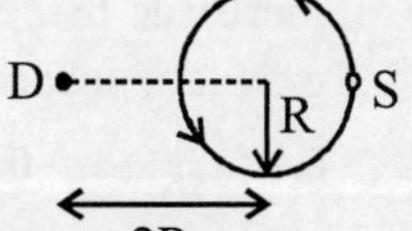

(a) $\left(\frac{c+v}{c-v}\right)$ (b) $\sqrt{2}\left(\frac{c+v}{c-v}\right)$
(c) $\sqrt{2}$ (d) $\frac{(c+v)}{c\sqrt{2}}$

4. The equation of a spherical progressive wave is
(a) $y = a\sin\omega t$ (b) $y = a\sin(\omega t - kr)$
(c) $y = \frac{a}{\sqrt{2}}\sin(\omega t - kr)$ (d) $y = \frac{a}{r}\sin(\omega t - kr)$

5. An echo repeats two syllables. If the velocity of sound is 330 m/s, then the distance of the reflecting surface is
(a) 66.0m (b) 33.0m (c) 99.0m (d) 16.5m

6. At room temperaturre, velocity of sound in air at 10 atmospheric pressure and at 1 atmospheric pressure will be in the ratio
(a) 10 : 1 (b) 1 : 10
(c) 1 : 1 (d) cannot say

7. A distant star which is moving away with a velocity of 10^6 m/sec is emitting a red line of frequency 4.5×10^{14} Hz. The observed frequency of this spectral line is
(a) 4.5×10^8 Hz (b) 4.485×10^{14} Hz
(c) 4.515×10^{14} Hz (d) 4.5×10^{14} Hz

8. A wave disturbance in a medium is described by
$y(x,t) = 0.02\cos\left(50\pi t + \frac{\pi}{2}\right)\cos(10\pi x)$ where x and y are in metre and t is in second. Which of the following is correct?
(a) A node occurs at x = 0.15 m
(b) An antinode occurs at x = 0.3 m
(c) The speed wave is 5 ms^{-1}
(d) The wavelength is 0.3 m

9. A toothed wheel is rotating at 240 rpm and a post card is held against the teeth. If the pitch of the tone is 256 Hz, then the number of teeth on the rotating wheel is
(a) 256 (b) 128 (c) 64 (d) 32

10. The threshold of hearing for the human ear is 10^{-12} W m^{-2}. This is taken as the standard level. The intensity of sound is 1 Wm^{-2}. It has intensity (in dB).
(a) 10^{12} dB (b) 12 dB (c) 240 dB (d) 120 dB

11. If two tuning forks A and B are sounded together, they produce 4 beats per sec. A is then slightly loaded with wax and same no. of beats/sec. are produced again. If frequency of A is 256, the frequency of B would be
(a) 250 (b) 262 (c) 252 (d) 260

12. A train has just completed U-curve in a track which is a semi-circle. The engine is at the forward end of the semi-circular part of the track while the last carriage is at the rear end of the semi circular track. The driver blows a whistle of frequency 200 Hz. Velocity of sound is 340 m/sec Then the apparent frequency as observed by a passenger in the middle of the train, when the speed of the train is 30 m/sec is
(a) 181 Hz (b) 200 Hz (c) 188 Hz (d) 210 Hz

13. An organ pipe, open from both end produces 5 beats per second when vibrated with a source of frequency 200 Hz. The second harmonic of the same pipes produces 10 beats per second with a source of frequency 420 Hz. The fundamental frequency of organ pipe is
(a) 195 Hz (b) 205 Hz (c) 190 Hz (d) 210 Hz

14. A progressive sound wave of frequency 500 Hz is travelling through air with a speed of 350 ms^{-1}. A compression maximum appears at a place at a given instant. The minimum time interval after which the rarefraction maximum occurs at the same point, is
(a) 200 s (b) $\frac{1}{250}$ s (c) $\frac{1}{500}$ s (d) $\frac{1}{1000}$ s

15. A person carrying a whistle emitting continuously a note of 272 Hz is running towards a reflecting surface with a speed of 18 km h^{-1}. The speed of sound in air is 345 m s^{-1}. The number of beats heard by him is
(a) 4 (b) 6 (c) 8 (d) zero

16. In the sonometer experiment, a tuning fork of frequency 256 Hz is in resonance with 0.4 m length of the wire when the iron load attached to free end of wire is 2 kg. If the load is immersed in water, the length of the wire in resonance would be (specific gravity of iron = 8)
(a) 0.37m (b) 0.43m (c) 0.31m (d) 0.2m

17. A wave travelling along the x-axis is described by the equation $y(x, t) = 0.005\cos(\alpha x - \beta t)$. If the wavelength and the time period of the wave are 0.08 m and 2.0s, respectively, then α and β in appropriate units are
(a) $\alpha = 25.00\pi, \beta = \pi$ (b) $\alpha = \frac{0.08}{\pi}, \beta = \frac{2.0}{\pi}$
(c) $\alpha = \frac{0.04}{\pi}, \beta = \frac{1.0}{\pi}$ (d) $\alpha = 12.50\pi, \beta = \frac{\pi}{2.0}$

18. An isotropic point source S of sound emits constant power. Two points A and B separated by a distance r are situated near the source as shown in figure. The difference of the intensity level of sound at the points A and B is about

r r
S A B

(a) 3 dB (b) 2 dB
(c) 6 dB (d) 12 dB

19. The phase difference between two waves, represented by $y_1 = 10^{-6}\sin\{100\,t + (x/50) + 0.5\}$ m
$y_2 = 10^{-6}\cos\{100\,t + (x/50)\}$ m
where x is expressed in metres and t is expressed in seconds, is approximately
(a) 1.5 radians (b) 1.07 radians
(c) 2.07 radians (d) 0.5 radians

20. Two waves are represented by the equations $y_1 = a\sin(\omega t + kx + 0.57)\ m$ and $y_2 = a\cos(\omega t + kx)\ m$, where x is in meter and t in sec. The phase difference between them is
(a) 1.0 radian (b) 1.25 radian
(c) 1.57 radian (d) 0.57 radian

21. Two identical piano wires kept under the same tension T have a fundamental frequency of 600 Hz. The fractional increase in the tension of one of the wires which will lead to occurrence of 6 beats/s when both the wires oscillate together would be
(a) 0.02 (b) 0.03 (c) 0.04 (d) 0.01

22. Assume that the displacement (s) of air is proportional to the pressure difference (Δp) created by a sound wave. Displacement (s) further depends on the speed of sound (v), density of air (ρ) and the frequency (f). If $\Delta p \sim 10$Pa, $v \sim 300$ m/s, $\rho \sim 1$ kg/m^3 and $f \sim 1000$ Hz, then s will be of the order of (take the multiplicative constant to be 1)
(a) $\frac{3}{100}$ mm (b) 10mm (c) $\frac{1}{10}$ mm (d) 1mm

23. A small speaker delivers 2 W of audio output. At what distance from the speaker will one detect 120 dB intensity sound ? [Given reference intensity of sound as 10^{-12}W/m^2]
(a) 40 cm (b) 20 cm (c) 10 cm (d) 30 cm

24. The pressure wave, P = 0.01 sin[1000t – 3x] Nm^{-2}, corresponds to the sound produced by a vibrating blade on a day when atmospheric temperature is 0°C. On some other day when temperature is T, the speed of sound produced by the same blade and at the same frequency is found to be 336 ms^{-1}. Approximate value of T is :
(a) 4°C (b) 11°C (c) 12°C (d) 15°C

25. In a resonance tube experiment when the tube is filled with water up to a height of 17.0 cm from bottom, it resonates with a given tuning fork. When the water level is raised the next resonance with the same tuning fork occurs at a height of 24.5 cm. If the velocity of sound in air is 330 m/s, the tuning fork frequency is :
(a) 2200 Hz (b) 550 Hz (c) 1100 Hz (d) 3300 Hz

26. A uniform thin rope of length 12 m and mass 6 kg hangs vertically from a rigid support and a block of mass 2 kg is attached to its free end. A transverse short wave-train of wavelength 6 cm is produced at the lower end of the rope. What is the wavelength of the wavetrain (in cm) when it reaches the top of the rope ?
(a) 3 (b) 6 (c) 12 (d) 9

27. Two identical strings X and Z made of same material have tension T_X and T_Z in them. If their fundamental frequencies are 450 Hz and 300 Hz, respectively, then the ratio T_X/T_Z is:
(a) 2.25 (b) 0.44 (c) 1.25 (d) 1.5

28. A transverse wave travels on a taut steel wire with a velocity of v when tension in it is 2.06×10^4 N. When the tension is changed to T, the velocity changed to $v/2$. The value of T is close to:
(a) 2.50×10^4 N (b) 5.15×10^3 N
(c) 30.5×10^4 N (d) 10.2×10^2 N

29. Speed of a transverse wave on a straight wire (mass 6.0 g, length 60 cm and area of cross-section 1.0 mm^2) is 90 ms^{-1}. If the Young's modulus of wire is 16×10^{11} Nm^{-2} the extension of wire over its natural length is:
(a) 0.03 mm (b) 0.02 mm (c) 0.04 mm (d) 0.01 mm

30. A heavy ball of mass M is suspended from the ceiling of a car by a light string of mass m (m<<M). When the car is at rest, the speeed of transverse waves in the string is 60 ms^{-1}. when the car has acceleration a, the wave-speed increases to 60.5 ms^{-1}. The value of a, in terms of gravitational acceleration g, is closest to:
(a) $\frac{g}{30}$ (b) $\frac{g}{5}$ (c) $\frac{g}{10}$ (d) $\frac{g}{20}$

31. There harmonic waves having equal frequency ν and same intensity I_0, have phase angles 0, $\frac{\pi}{4}$ and $-\frac{\pi}{4}$ respectively. When they are superimposed the intensity of the resultant wave is close to:
(a) $5.8\,I_0$ (b) $0.2\,I_0$ (c) $3\,I_0$ (d) I_0

32. The correct figure that shows, schematically, the wave pattern produced by superposition of two waves of frequencies 9 Hz and 11 Hz is :

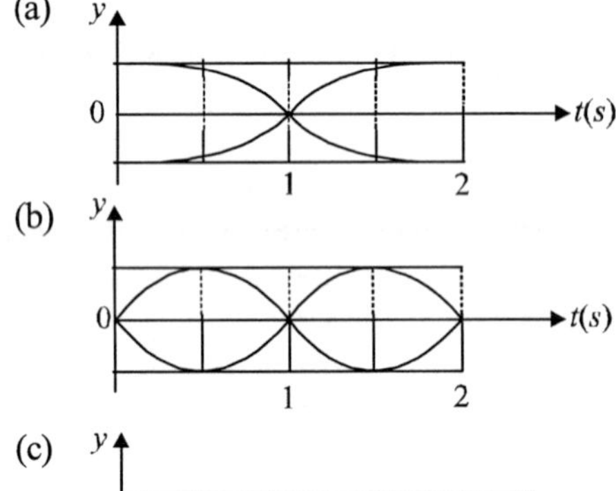

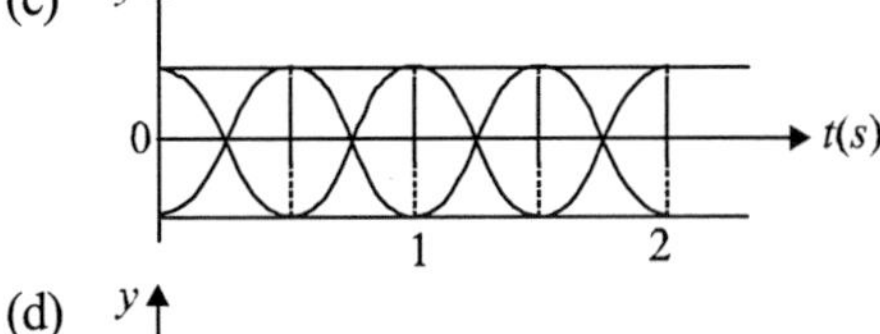

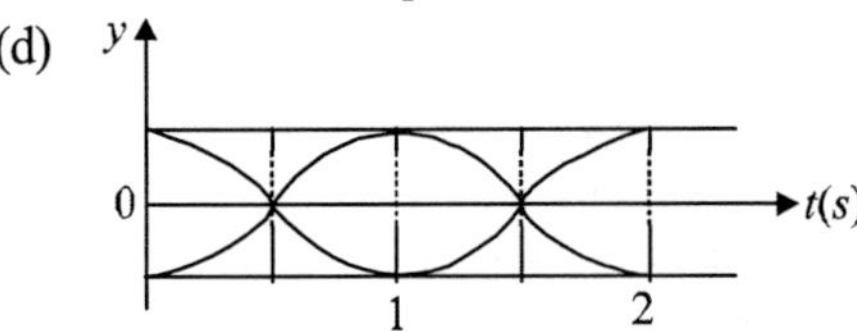

33. A resonance tube is old and has jagged end. It is still used in the laboratory to determine velocity of sound in air. A tuning fork of frequency 512 Hz produces first resonance when the tube is filled with water to a mark 11 cm below a reference mark, near the open end of the tube. The experiment is repeated with another fork of frequency 256 Hz which produces first resonance when water reaches a mark 27 cm below the reference mark. The velocity of sound in air, obtained in the experiment, is close to:

(a) 322 ms^{-1} (b) 341 ms^{-1}
(c) 335 ms^{-1} (d) 328 ms^{-1}

34. A tuning fork vibrates with frequency 256 Hz and gives one beat per second with the third normal mode of vibration of an open pipe. What is the length of the pipe? (Speed of sound of air is 340 ms^{-1})

(a) 190 cm (b) 180 cm (c) 220 cm (d) 200 cm

35. 5 beats/ second are heard when a turning fork is sounded with a sonometer wire under tension, when the length of the sonometer wire is either 0.95m or 1m. The frequency of the fork will be:

(a) 195Hz (b) 251Hz (c) 150Hz (d) 300Hz

36. A sound source *S* is moving along a straight track with speed *v*, and is emitting sound of frequency v_o (see figure). An observer is standing at a finite distance, at the point *O*, from the track. The time variation of frequency heard by the observer is best represented by:

(t_0 represents the instant when the distance between the source and observer is minimum)

(a)

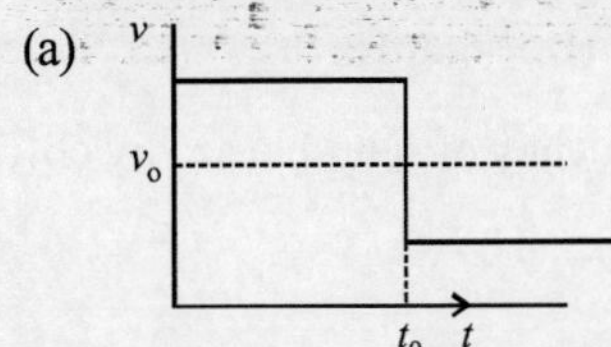

(b)

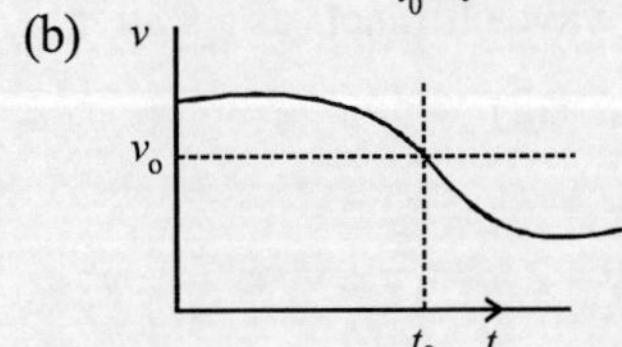

(c)

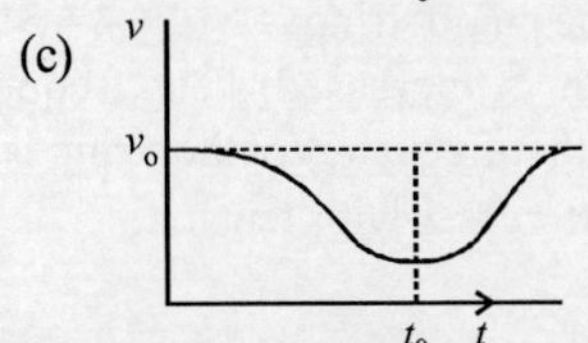

(d)

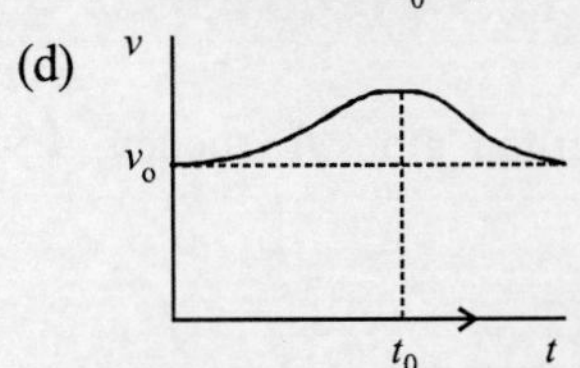

37. A driver in a car, approaching a vertical wall notices that the frequency of his car horn, has changed from 440 Hz to 480 Hz, when it gets reflected from the wall. If the speed of sound in air is 345 m/s, then the speed of the car is :

(a) 54 km/hr (b) 36 km/hr (c) 18 km/hr (d) 24 km/hr

38. The driver of a bus approaching a big wall notices that the frequency of his bus's horn changes from 420 Hz to 490 Hz when he hears it after it gets reflected from the wall. Find the speed of the bus if speed of the sound is 330 ms^{-1}.

(a) 91 kmh^{-1} (b) 81 kmh^{-1}
(c) 61 kmh^{-1} (d) 71 kmh^{-1}

39. Magnetic materials used for making permanent magnets (P) and magnets in a transformer (T) have different properties of the following, which property best matches for the type of magnet required?

(a) T : Large retentivity, small coercivity
(b) P : Small retentivity, large coercivity
(c) T : Large retentivity, large coercivity
(d) P : Large retentivity, large coercivity

40. A stationary observer receives sound from two identical tuning forks, one of which approaches and the other one recedes with the same speed (much less than the speed of sound). The observer hears 2 beats/sec. The oscillation frequency of each tuning fork is v_0 = 1400 Hz and the velocity of sound in air is 350 m/s. The speed of each tuning fork is close to:

(a) $\frac{1}{2}$ m/s (b) 1m/s (c) $\frac{1}{4}$ m/s (d) $\frac{1}{8}$ m/s

41. A submarine (A) travelling at 18 km/hr is being chased along the line of its velocity by another submarine (B) travelling at 27 km/hr. B sends a sonar signal of 500 Hz to detect A and receives a reflected sound of frequency *v*. The value of *v* is close to :

(Speed of sound in water = 1500 ms^{-1})

(a) 504 Hz (b) 507 Hz (c) 499 Hz (d) 502 Hz

42. Two sources of sound S_1 and S_2 produce sound waves of same frequency 660 Hz. A listener is moving from source S_1 towards S_2 with a constant speed *u* m/s and he hears 10 beats/s. The velocity of sound is 330 m/s. Then *u* equals:

(a) 5.5 m/s (b) 15.0 m/s (c) 2.5 m/s (d) 10.0 m/s

43. A stationary source emits sounds waves of frequency 500 Hz. Two observers moving along a line passing through the source detect sound to be of frequencies 4801 Hz and 530 Hz. Their respective speeds are, in ms^{-1}, (Given speed of sound = 300 m/s)

(a) 12, 16 (b) 12, 18 (c) 16, 14 (d) 8, 18

44. A source of sound S is moving with a velocity of 50 m/s towards a stationary observer. The observer measures the frequency of the source as 1000 Hz. What will be the apparent frequency of the source when it is moving away from the observer after crossing him? (Take velocity of sound in air 350 m/s)

(a) 750 Hz (b) 857 Hz (c) 1143 Hz (d) 807 Hz

45. Two cars A and B are moving away from each other in opposite directions. Both the cars are moving with a speed of 20 ms^{-1} with respect to the ground. If an observer in car A detects a frequency 2000 Hz of the sound coming from car B, what is the natural frequency of the sound source in car B? (speed of sound in air = 340 ms^{-1})

(a) 2250 Hz (b) 2060 Hz (c) 2300 Hz (d) 2150 Hz

Hints & Solutions

15.1 Concept Practice Problems

1. (d) For wave propagation both elasticity and inertia are necessary.
2. (c) The contrast will be maximum, when $I_1 = I_2$ i.e. $a = b$. In that event, $I_{min} = (a-b)^2 = 0$, where a and b are the amplitudes of interfering waves.
3. (a) From $v = n\lambda$, we find $\lambda \propto v$ because freq. n is constant. Therefore, new wavelength $= 4\lambda$.
4. (a) Here, $I_{max} = I_1 + I_2 + 2\sqrt{I_1 I_2}\cos 0°$

$$I_{min} = I_1 + I_2 + 2\sqrt{I_1 I_2}\cos 180°$$

$$\therefore I_{max} + I_{min} = 2(I_1 + I_2)$$

5. (a) Because they are absorbed by the atmosphere.
6. (d)
7. (c) Speed of sound is determined by elasticity and inertia.
8. (b) $v = \sqrt{\dfrac{\gamma P}{\rho}} = \sqrt{\dfrac{E}{\rho}}$
9. (c) The equation of progressive wave propagating in the positive direction of X-axis is

$$y = a\sin\frac{2\pi}{\lambda}(vt - x) \text{ or}$$

$$y = a\sin(\omega t - kx)$$

10. (b) Equation is of stationary wave. Comparing with the standard equation

$$y = 2A\sin\left(\frac{2\pi}{T}\right)t\cos\left(\frac{2\pi}{\lambda}\right)x$$

$$\frac{2\pi}{\lambda} = 4.5 \text{ or } \lambda = \frac{2\pi}{4.5} = 1.4\text{m}$$

15.2 Concept Practice Problems

11. (c) Doppler effect is not applicable for shock waves.
12. (d)
13. (d) As number of beats/sec = diff. in frequencies has to be less than 10, therefore $0 < (n_1 - n_2) < 10$
14. (b) No. of beats/sec $= 402 - 401 = 401 - 400 = 1$
15. (a) By the concept of accoustic, the observer and source are moving towards each other, each with a velocity of 18ms^{-1}.

$$\therefore v' = \frac{330+18}{330-18} \times 1000 \approx 1115 \text{ Hz}$$

16. (a) For 3rd harmonic/2nd over tone of organ pipe open at ends

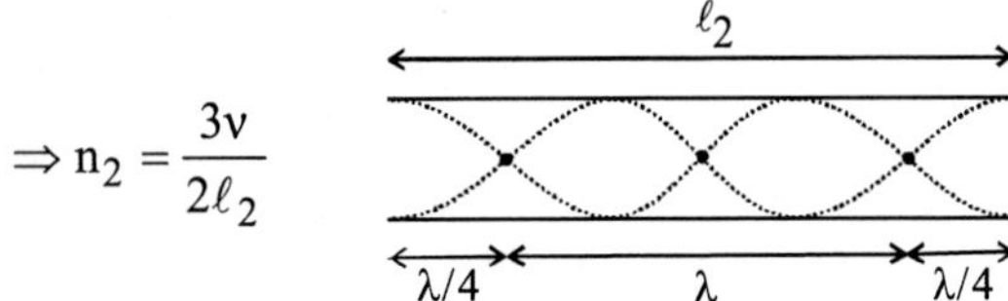

$$\Rightarrow n_2 = \frac{3v}{2\ell_2}$$

For 1st overtone of organ pipe open at one end

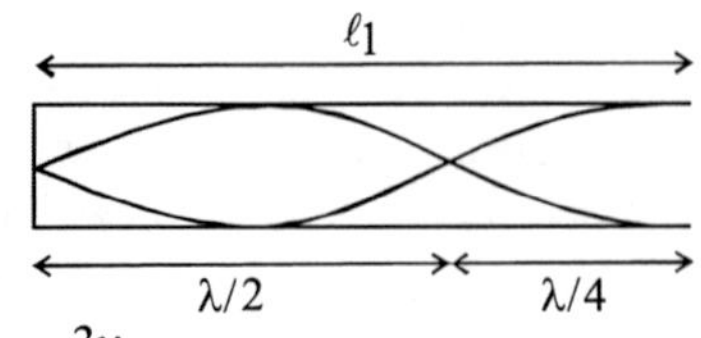

$$\Rightarrow n_1 = \frac{3v}{4\ell_1}$$

Given $n_1 = n_2 \Rightarrow \dfrac{3v}{2\ell_2} = \dfrac{3v}{4\ell_1}$ or $\dfrac{\ell_1}{\ell_2} = \dfrac{1}{2}$

17. (a) $n' = n\left[\dfrac{v+v_0}{v-v_s}\right] = 600\left[\dfrac{v+v/15}{v-v/10}\right]$

$$= 600\left[\frac{16}{15}\times\frac{10}{9}\right] = \frac{400\times 16}{9} \approx 711$$

18. (b) Effective value of velocity of source,

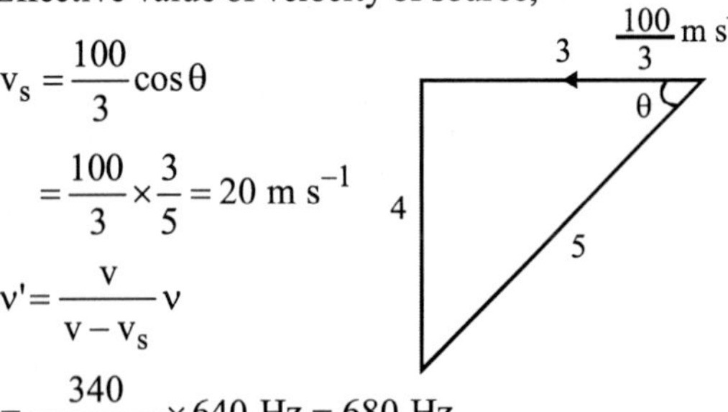

$$v_s = \frac{100}{3}\cos\theta$$

$$= \frac{100}{3}\times\frac{3}{5} = 20 \text{ m s}^{-1}$$

$$v' = \frac{v}{v - v_s}\nu$$

$$\Rightarrow v' = \frac{340}{340-20}\times 640 \text{ Hz} = 680 \text{ Hz}$$

19. (c) Let f' be the frequency of sound heard by cliff.

$$\therefore f' = \frac{vf}{v - v_c} \quad ......(1)$$

Now for the reflected wave cliff. acts as a source

$$\therefore 2f' = \frac{f'(v+v_c)}{v} \quad ......(2)$$

$$2f = \frac{(v+v_c)f}{v-v_c} \Rightarrow 2v - 2v_c = v + v_c \text{ or } \frac{v}{3} = v_c$$

20. (d) The frequency of the piano string $= 512 \pm 4 = 516$ or 508. When the tension is increased, beat frequency decreases to 2, it means that frequency of the string is 508 as frequency of string increases with tension.

15.3 Concept Practice Problems

21. (d) In case of open organ pipe, frequency, $f = \dfrac{nv}{2\ell}$ where n = 1, 2, 3, 4
22. (a)
23. (d) For open pipe, $n = p\dfrac{v}{2\ell}$

For closed pipe $n' = (2p-1)\dfrac{v}{4\ell} \quad \therefore \dfrac{n}{n'} = \dfrac{2p}{2p-1}$

24. (a) $\upsilon \propto \sqrt{T}$
25. (a) $v = 2\nu(\ell_2 - \ell_1)$

26. (c)

27. (a) For open pipe, $n = \frac{v}{2\ell}$, where n_0 is the fundamental frequency of open pipe.

$\therefore \ \ell = \frac{v}{2n} = \frac{330}{2 \times 300} = \frac{11}{20}$

As freq. of 1st overtone of open pipe = freq. of 1st overtone of closed pipe

$$2\frac{v}{2\ell} = 3\frac{v}{4\ell'} \Rightarrow \ell' = \frac{3\ell}{4} = \frac{3}{4} \times \frac{11}{20} = 41.25 \text{ cm}$$

28. (b) $\frac{v}{4\ell} = 412$, when cut into two equal pieces, frequency of closed pipe of half the length

$$= \frac{v}{4(\ell/2)} = \frac{2v}{4\ell} = 2 \times 412 = 824 \text{ Hz}$$

frequency of open pipe of half the length

$$= \frac{v}{2(\ell/2)} = 4 \times 412 = 1648 \text{Hz}$$

29. (b) $3 \times \frac{v}{4l_c} = 4 \times \frac{v}{2l_0}$ or $\frac{l_c}{l_0} = \frac{3v}{4} \times \frac{2}{4v} = \frac{3}{8}$

30. (a) $k = \frac{\pi}{15} \Rightarrow \frac{2\pi}{\lambda} = \frac{\pi}{15} \Rightarrow \lambda = 30$ units

Distance between node and next antinode

$$= \frac{\lambda}{4} = \frac{30}{4} = 7.5 \text{ units}$$

Exercise 1 - Chapter Revision Problems CRP

1. (a) Standing waves are produced when two waves propagate in opposite direction
As z_1 & z_2 are propagating in +ve x-axis & –ve x-axis so, $z_1 + z_2$ will represent a standing wave.
2. (d) 3. (c)
4. (b) Equation of a wave
$y_1 = a \sin(\omega t - kx)$ ....(i)
Let equations of another wave may be,
$y_2 = a \sin(\omega t + kx)$ ....(ii)
$y_3 = -a \sin(\omega t + kx)$ ....(iii)
If Eq. (i) propagate with Eq. (ii), we get
$y = 2a \cos kx \sin \omega t$
If Eq. (i), propagate with Eq. (iii), we get
$y = -2a \sin kx \cos \omega t$
At $x = 0, y = 0$, wave produce node
So, Eq.(iii) is the equation of unknown wave
5. (a) Frequency of reflected wave is,
$$f' = \left(\frac{c+v}{c}\right) f$$
This is the number of wave striking the surface per second.
6. (c) Fundamental frequency is given by
$$\nu = \frac{1}{2l}\sqrt{\frac{T}{\mu}} \Rightarrow \nu \propto \frac{1}{l} \Rightarrow P \propto \frac{1}{\nu}$$
Since, P divided into l_1, l_2 and l_3 segments
Here $l = l_1 + l_2 + l_3$
So $\frac{1}{\nu} = \frac{1}{\nu_1} + \frac{1}{\nu_2} + \frac{1}{\nu_3}$
7. (b) Amplitude of reflected wave $= \frac{2}{3} \times 0.9 = 0.6$
It would travel along negative direction of x-axis, and on reflection at a rigid support, there occurs a phase change of π.
8. (b) As $R^2 = a^2 + b^2 + 2ab\cos\phi$
$\therefore \ a^2 = a^2 + a^2 + 2a^2 \cos\phi$, $\cos\phi = -\frac{1}{2}$, $\phi = \frac{2\pi}{3}$
9. (b) $c_{r.m.s.} = v\sqrt{\frac{3}{\gamma}} = 330 \times \sqrt{\frac{3}{1.4}} \approx 471.4$ m/s
10. (b) If $\rho_H = 1$, then $\rho_{mix} = \frac{4 \times 1 + 1 \times 16}{(4+1)} = 4$
$$\frac{v_{mix}}{v_H} = \sqrt{\frac{\rho_H}{\rho_{mix}}} = \sqrt{\frac{1}{4}} = \frac{1}{2}$$
$$v_{mix} = \frac{v_H}{2} = \frac{1224}{2} = 612 \text{ m/s}$$
11. (a) Let x be distance of person from each cliff
$\therefore \ x + x = v \times t = 340 \times 1 = 340$
$x = 170$ m
Distance between two cliffs = 2 x 170 = 340 m
12. (d) Here, $\lambda = 5.0$ m, $n = 2$
$\therefore \ v = n\lambda = 2 \times 5.0 = 10.0$ m/s
13. (b) $\frac{I_{max}}{I_{min}} = \frac{(a+b)^2}{(a-b)^2} = 49 \quad \therefore \ \frac{a+b}{a-b} = 7$
$7a - 7b = a + b$ or $6a = 8b$ or $\frac{a}{b} = \frac{8}{6} = \frac{4}{3}$
14. (d) Freq. of unknown fork $= 256 \pm 4 = 260$ or 252
As frequency decreases on loading, therefore, orginal freq. of unknown fork = 260 Hz
15. (a) No. of loops in longitudinal mode $= \frac{6}{2} = 3$
16. (c) $v = \frac{\Delta\lambda}{\lambda} \times c = \frac{0.2}{100} \times 3 \times 10^8 = 6 \times 10^5$ m/s
17. (a)
18. (c) $n_1 = 256 = \frac{v}{4\ell_1} = \frac{v}{4 \times 25.4}$
$\therefore v = 256 \times 101.6$ cm/s
$$n_2 = \frac{v}{4\ell_2} = \frac{256 \times 101.6}{4 \times 25.6} = 254 \text{ Hz}$$
No. of beats/sec $= n_1 - n_2 = 256 - 254 = 2$
19. (b) $\frac{v_1}{v_2} = \sqrt{\frac{\rho_2}{\rho_1}}$
20. (c) Resultant amplitude is $\sqrt{a^2 + a^2}$ i.e. $\sqrt{2}\,a$
21. (b) $v = \frac{v}{2l} = \frac{60}{2 \times 1} = 30$ Hz

22. (b) $\omega = \frac{2\pi}{0.01}$ and $k = \frac{2\pi}{0.30}$

$v = \frac{\omega}{k} = \frac{2\pi}{0.01} \times \frac{0.30}{2\pi} = 30 \text{ m s}^{-1}$

23. (c) Intensity doubles, dB level increases by 3 dB.

24. (b) $y = A\sin^2(kx - \omega t)$

$\Rightarrow y = \frac{A}{2}[1 - \cos 2(kx - \omega t)]$

$\omega' = 2\omega,\ 2\pi v' = 2\omega,\ v' = \frac{\omega}{\pi}$

25. (c)

26. (N) The speed of sound in a gas is given by

$v = \frac{\sqrt{\gamma RT}}{M}$

$\therefore \frac{v_{O_2}}{v_{He}} = \sqrt{\frac{\gamma_{O_2}}{M_{O_2}} \times \frac{M_{He}}{\gamma_{He}}} = \sqrt{\frac{1.4}{32} \times \frac{4}{1.67}} = 0.3237$

$\therefore v_{He} = \frac{v_{O_2}}{0.3237} = \frac{460}{0.3237} = 1421 \text{ m/s}$

None of the option is correct.

27. (c) $10\log\frac{I}{I_0} = 10\log\frac{10^{-6}}{10^{-12}} = 10\log 10^6 = 60\text{dB}$

28. (a) Here, $m = \frac{5}{20}$ kg/m $= \frac{1}{4}$ kg/m

Tension in the middle of wire

T = weight of half the wire $= \frac{5}{2} \times g = \frac{5}{2} \times 10\text{ N} = 25\text{ N}$

As $v = \sqrt{T/m}$ $\quad \therefore\ v = \sqrt{\frac{25}{1/4}} = 10 \text{ m/s}$

29. (c)

30. (c) Velocity of wave $v = n\lambda$

where n = frequency of wave $\Rightarrow n = \frac{v}{\lambda}$

$n_2 = \frac{v_2}{\lambda_2} = \frac{396}{100 \times 10^{-2}} = 396\text{ Hz}$

no. of beats $= n_1 - n_2 = 4$

31. (a) $a\omega = 0.1 \times 2\pi \times 300 = 60\pi \text{ cm s}^{-1}$

32. (a) Doppler effect.

33. (c) Particle velocity

$v = \frac{d}{dt}\left[x_0 \sin 2\pi\left(nt - \frac{x}{\lambda}\right)\right]$

$= 2\pi n x_0 \cos 2\pi\left(nt - \frac{x}{\lambda}\right)$

$\therefore$ Maximum particle velocity $= 2\pi n x_0$

Wave velocity $= \frac{\lambda}{T} = n\lambda$

Given, $2\pi n x_0 = 4n\lambda \Rightarrow \lambda = \frac{2\pi n x_0}{4n} = \frac{\pi x_0}{2}$

34. (a) $\frac{v_A}{v_B} = \frac{D_B}{D_A} = \frac{1}{2}$

35. (a) Since Tension and mass per unit length remains unchanged, the frequency will be obtained in different mode.

36. (a)

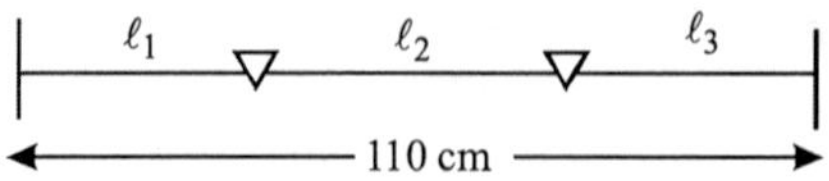

$n_1 : n_2 : n_3 = 3 : 2 : 1$

$n \propto \frac{1}{\ell}$

$\ell_1 : \ell_2 : \ell_3 = \frac{1}{3} : \frac{1}{2} : \frac{1}{1} = 2 : 3 : 6$

$\ell_1 + \ell_2 + \ell_3 = 110$

$\Rightarrow 2x + 3x + 6x = 110 \Rightarrow x = 10$

$\therefore$ The two bridges should be set at 2x i.e, 20 cm from one end and 6x i.e, 60 cm from the other end.

37. (b) $v_X = 258$ Hz or 242 Hz

$v_X = 258$ Hz or 282 Hz

$\Rightarrow$ frequency is 258 Hz

The total momentum will be zero and hence velocity will be zero just after collision. The pull of earth will make it fall down.

38. (b) Speed of pulse at a distance x from bottom, $v = \sqrt{gx}$.

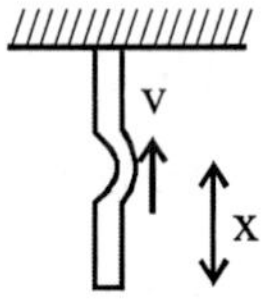

While traveling from mid point to the top, frequency remains unchanged.

$\frac{v_1}{\lambda_1} = \frac{v_2}{\lambda_2} \Rightarrow \frac{\sqrt{g(L/2)}}{\lambda_0} = \frac{\sqrt{gL}}{\lambda_2} \Rightarrow \lambda_2 = \sqrt{2}\lambda_0$

39. (b)

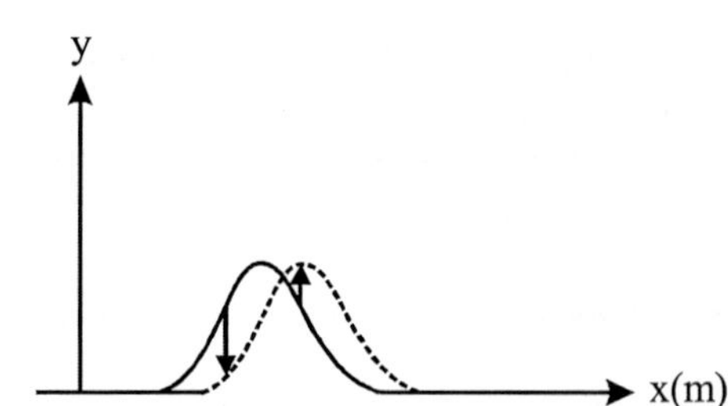

Dotted shape shows pulse position after a short time interval. Direction of the velocities are decided according to direction of displacements of the particles.

40. (c) Compare the given eqn. with the standard form

$y = a_0 \sin\left[\frac{2\pi x}{\lambda} - \frac{2\pi t}{T}\right]$

$\frac{2\pi}{\lambda} = 3,\ \lambda = 2\pi/3$ and $\frac{2\pi}{T} = 15$

$T = 2\pi/15$

Speed of propagation, $v = \frac{\lambda}{T} = \frac{2\pi/3}{2\pi/15} = 5$

41. (b) Equation of progressive wave is given by

$Y = A\sin 2\pi f t$

Given $Y_1 = 4\sin 500\pi t$ and $Y_2 = 2\sin 506\pi t$.

Comparing the given equations with equation of progressive wave, we get

$2f_1 = 500, \quad \Rightarrow f_1 = 250$

$2f_2 = 506 \quad \Rightarrow f_2 = 253$

Beats $= f_2 - f_1 = 253 - 250 = 3$ beats/sec

$= 3 \times 60 = 180$ beats/minute.

42. (c) $y = A\sin(\omega t - kx)$

Particle velocity,

$$v_p = \frac{dy}{dt} = A\omega\cos(\omega t - kx)$$

$\therefore \quad v_{p\,max} = A\omega$

wave velocity $= \frac{\omega}{k}$

$\therefore \quad A\omega = \frac{\omega}{k} \quad$ i.e., $A = \frac{1}{k}$ But $k = \frac{2\pi}{\lambda}$

$\therefore \quad \lambda = 2\pi A$

43. (c) We have, $v = n\lambda$

$\Rightarrow v \propto \lambda$ (as n remains constant)

Thus, as v increases 10 times, λ also increases 10 times.

44. (c) From $\Delta x = \frac{\lambda}{2\pi}\Delta\phi$, $\lambda = 2\pi\frac{\Delta x}{\Delta\phi} = \frac{2\pi(0.4)}{1.6\pi} = 0.5\,\text{m}$

$$\nu = \frac{v}{\lambda} = \frac{330}{0.5} = 660 \text{ Hz}$$

45. (d) $2\pi f_1 = 600\pi$

$f_1 = 300 \quad \ldots(1)$

$2\pi f_2 = 608\pi$

$f_2 = 304 \quad \ldots(2)$

$|f_1 - f_2| = 4$ beats

$$\frac{I_{max}}{I_{m.n}} = \frac{(A_1 + A_2)^2}{(A_1 + A_2)^2} = \frac{(5+4)^2}{(5-4)^2} = \frac{81}{1}$$

where A_1, A_2 are amplitudes of given two sound wave.

46. (b) At $t = 0, x = 0, y = 0$

$\phi = \pi$ rad

47. (a) Comparing the given equation

$y = 10^{-3}\sin(50t + 2x)$ with standard equation,

$y = a\sin(\omega t - kx)$

$\Rightarrow$ wave is moving along –ve x-axis with speed

$$v = \frac{\omega}{K} \Rightarrow v = \frac{50}{2} = 25 \text{ m/sec.}$$

48. (b) Given : Distance between one crest and one trough $= 1.5$ m

$$= (2n_1 + 1)\frac{\lambda}{2}$$

Distance between two crests $= 5$ m $= n_2\lambda$

$$\frac{1.5}{5} = \frac{(2n_1+1)}{2n_2} \Rightarrow 3n_2 = 10n_1 + 5$$

Here n_1 and n_2 are integer.

If $\quad n_1 = 1, n_2 = 5 \quad \therefore \lambda = 1$

$n_1 = 4, n_2 = 15 \quad \therefore \lambda = 1/3$

$n_1 = 7, n_2 = 25 \quad \therefore \lambda = 1/5$

Hence possible wavelengths $\frac{1}{1}, \frac{1}{3}, \frac{1}{5}$ metre.

49. (a) For first resonance, $\frac{\lambda}{4} = \ell_1 + e = 11$ cm

($\because$ end correction e = 1 cm given)

For second resonance, $\frac{3\lambda}{4} = \ell_2 + e$

$\Rightarrow \ell_2 = 3 \times 11 - 1 = 32$ cm

50. (a) In solids, Velocity of wave

$$V = \sqrt{\frac{Y}{\rho}} = \sqrt{\frac{9.27 \times 10^{10}}{2.7 \times 10^3}}$$

$v = 5.85 \times 10^3$ m/sec

Since rod is clamped at middle fundamental wave shape is as follow

$\frac{\lambda}{2} = L \Rightarrow \lambda = 2L$ [Figure: A — N — A, $\lambda/2$]

$\lambda = 1.2$m ($\because$ L = 60 cm = 0.6m (given)

Using $v = f\lambda$

$$\Rightarrow \quad f = \frac{v}{\lambda} = \frac{5.85 \times 10^3}{1.2}$$

$= 4.88 \times 10^3$ Hz $\simeq 5$ KHz

51. (d) Velocity of wave on string

$$V = \sqrt{\frac{T}{\mu}} = \sqrt{\frac{8}{5} \times 1000} = 40\text{m/s}$$

Here, T = tension and μ = mass/length

Wavelength of wave $\lambda = \frac{v}{n} = \frac{40}{100}$ m

Separation b/w successive nodes,

$$\frac{\lambda}{2} = \frac{40}{2 \times 100} = \frac{20}{100}\text{m} = 20 \text{ cm}$$

52. (a) If a closed pipe vibration in N[th] mode then frequency of vibration $n = \frac{(2N-1)v}{4l} = (2N-1)n_1$

(where n_1 = fundamental frequency of vibration)

Hence $20{,}000 = (2N - 1) \times 1500$

$\Rightarrow \quad N = 7.1 \approx 7$

$\therefore \quad$ Number of over tones = (No. of mode of vibration) – 1 $= 7 - 1 = 6$

53. (c) As there must be node at both ends and at the joint of the wire A and B so

$$\frac{V_A}{V_B} = \sqrt{\frac{u_B}{u_A}} = \frac{r_B}{r_A} = 2 = \frac{\lambda_A}{\lambda_B}$$

$$\Rightarrow \lambda_A = 2\lambda_B \quad \Rightarrow \quad \frac{P}{q} = \frac{1}{2}$$

54. (b) Given, $y = 0.3\sin(0.157x)\cos(200\pi t)$

So $k = 0.157$ and $w = 200\pi$

or f = 100 Hz, $v = \frac{w}{k} = \frac{200\pi}{0.157} = 4000$m/s

Now, using $f = \frac{nv}{2l} = \frac{4v}{2l} = \frac{2v}{l}$

$$\therefore l = \frac{2v}{f} = \frac{2 \times 4000}{100} = 80m$$

55. (b) $\frac{3\lambda}{2} = 2$ or $\lambda = \frac{4}{3}m$

Velocity, $v = f\lambda = 240 \times \frac{4}{3} = 320$ m/sec

Also $f_1 = \frac{240}{3} = 80$ Hz

56. (b) $V = f\lambda = f \times 2(\ell_2 - \ell_1)$
$= 480 \times 2(0.70 - 0.30)$
$= 384$ m/s

57. (a) Fundamental frequency, $f = 70$ Hz.
The fundamental frequency of wire vibrating under tension T is given by

$$f = \frac{1}{2L}\sqrt{\frac{T}{\mu}}$$

Here, μ = mass per unit length of the wire
L = length of wire

$$70 = \frac{1}{2L}\sqrt{\frac{540}{6 \times 10^{-3}}} \Rightarrow L \approx 2.14 \text{ m}$$

58. (c)

59. (d) $n_A = 425$ Hz, $n_B = ?$
Beat frequency x = 5 Hz which is decreasing ($5 \to 3$) after increasing the tension of the string B.
Also tension of string B increasing so

$n_B \uparrow$ ($\because n \propto \sqrt{T}$)

Hence $n_A - n_B\uparrow = x\downarrow \longrightarrow$ correct

$n_B\uparrow - n_A = x\downarrow \longrightarrow$ incorrect

$\therefore n_B = n_A - x = 425 - 5 = 420$ Hz

60. (a) Frequency of the sound produced by open flute.

$$f = 2\left(\frac{v}{2\ell}\right) = \frac{2 \times 330}{2 \times 0.5} = 660Hz$$

Velocity of observer, $v_0 = 10 \times \frac{5}{18} = \frac{25}{9} m/s$

As the source is moving towards the observer therefore, according to Doppler's effect.

$\therefore$ Frequency detected by observer,

$$f' = \left[\frac{v + v_0}{v}\right]f = \left[\frac{\frac{25}{9} + 330}{330}\right]660$$

$$= \frac{2995}{9 \times 330} \times 660 \text{ or, } f' = 665.55 \simeq 666 \text{ Hz}$$

Exercise 2 - Exemplar & Past Year Questions E&PYQs

Exemplar Questions

1. (b) As the water waves are produced by a motor boat on surfaces of water as well as inside the water are both longitudinal and transverse, because the waves, produce transverse as well as lateral vibrations in the particles of the medium.

2. (c) Let the frequency in the first medium is v and in the second medium is v'.

As we know that,
When waves passes from one medium to another its frequency does not change but its velocity and wavelength changes.

Hence, $v = v' \Rightarrow \frac{v}{\lambda} = \frac{v'}{\lambda'}$

(frequency are same for both medium)

$$\lambda' = \left(\frac{v'}{v}\right)\lambda$$

λ and λ', are wavelengths and v and v' speeds in first and second medium respectively.

So, $\lambda' = \left(\frac{2v}{v}\right)\lambda = 2\lambda$

3. (c) The speed of sound (longitudinal) wave in air is

$$v = \sqrt{\frac{\pi p}{\rho}}.$$

The density of water vapours is small (rises up) than the air, so on increasing humidity the density of medium increase the speed of sound in air.

For air λ and p are constants,

$v \propto \frac{1}{\sqrt{\rho}}$, where ρ is density of air.

$$\frac{v_2}{v_1} = \sqrt{\frac{\rho_2}{\rho_1}}$$

where ρ_1 is density of dry air and ρ_2 is density of moist air.

As $\rho_2 < \rho_1 = \frac{v_2}{v_1} > 1 \Rightarrow v_2 > v_1$

Hence, speed of sound wave in air increases with increase in humidity.

4. (c) As we know that,
$v_t = v_0(1 + 0.61t)$

Speed of sound wave in a medium $v \propto \sqrt{T}$

(where T is temperature of the medium)

Clearly, when temperature increase then the speed also increase as frequency does not change during propogation of wave by formula.

As, $v = \nu\lambda$

where ν is frequency and λ is wavelength.

Frequency (ν) remains fixed,

$v \propto \lambda$ or $\lambda \propto v$

So velocity v and wavelength (λ) both increases.

5. (b) Only energy is transmitted from one point to another and during propagation of any longitudinal waves in a medium transmission of energy through the medium without matter being transmitted.

6. (c) Mechanical transverse wave can propagates through a solid medium, the constituent of the medium oscillate perpendicular to wave motion causing change in shape. Thus each, element of the medium is subjected to shearing stress. Solids and strings have shear modulus, so sustain shearing stress.
Fluids have no shape of their own, they yield to shearing stress. Hence, transverse waves are possible in solids and strings but not in fluids.

7. (d)
(a) The density of medium changes due to compression and rarefraction. At compressed regions density is maximum and at rarefactions density is minimum.
(b) As density is changing very rapidly so temperature of medium increases. Hence Boyle's law is not obeyed.
(c) Bulk modulus of air remains same or constant.
(d) The time of compressions and rarefraction is very small i.e., we can assume adiabatic process, i.e. no transfer of heat from surroundings.

8. (b) As given that, Mass $M = 2.5$ kg
(Mass per unit length)

$$m = \frac{M}{l} = \frac{2.5\text{ kg}}{20} = \frac{125}{10} = 0.125\text{ kg/m}$$

Speed $v = \sqrt{\frac{T}{m}} = \sqrt{\frac{200}{0.125}}$

[speed of transverse waves in any string]

Distance $l = v \times t$

$$\Rightarrow 20 = \sqrt{\frac{200}{0.125}} \times t$$

$$t = 20 \times \sqrt{\frac{125}{2\times 10^5}} = 20 \times \sqrt{\frac{25\times 5}{2\times 10^5}}$$

$$= 20 \times \sqrt{25 \times \frac{1}{0.4\times 10^5}} = 20\times 5\sqrt{\frac{1}{4\times 10^4}} = \frac{20\times 5}{2\times 10^2}$$

$$t = \frac{1}{2} = 0.5\text{ sec.}$$

Past Years (2017-2020) NEET/AIPMT Questions

9. (c) Pressure change will be minimum at both ends. In fact, pressure variation is maximum at $\ell/2$ because the displacement node is pressure antinode.

10. (d) When sounded with a source of known frequency fundamental frequency
$= 250 \pm 4$ Hz $= 254$ Hz or 246 Hz
2nd harmonic if unknown frequency (suppose) 254 Hz $= 2 \times 254 = 508$ Hz
As it gives 5 beats
$\therefore 508 + 5 = 513$ Hz
Hence, unknown frequency is 254 Hz

11. (d) As $Y = A\sin(\omega t - kx + \phi)$

$$\omega = 2\pi f = \frac{2\pi}{\pi} = 2 \qquad [\because f = \frac{1}{\pi}]$$

$$k = \frac{2\pi}{\lambda} = \frac{2\pi}{2\pi} = 1 \qquad [\because \lambda = 2\pi]$$

$\therefore Y = 1\sin(2t - x + \phi) \qquad [\because A = 1\text{ m}]$

12. (b) $\frac{\Delta f}{f} = \frac{v}{C} \Rightarrow \frac{(\text{Beats})/2}{f} = \frac{v}{C}$

$$\Rightarrow \text{Beats} = \frac{2fv}{C} = 4.$$

13. (a) Total length of string $\ell = \ell_1 + \ell_2 + \ell_3$
(As string is divided into three segments)

But frequency $\propto \frac{1}{\text{length}} \quad \left(\because f = \frac{1}{2\ell}\sqrt{\frac{T}{m}}\right)$

so $\frac{1}{n} = \frac{1}{n_1} + \frac{1}{n_2} + \frac{1}{n_3}$

14. (d) In case of closed organ pipe frequency,

$$f_n = (2n+1)\frac{v}{4l}$$

for $n = 0, f_0 = 100$ Hz
$n = 1, f_1 = 300$ Hz
$n = 2, f_2 = 500$ Hz
$n = 3, f_3 = 700$ Hz
$n = 4, f_4 = 900$ Hz
$n = 5, f_5 = 1100$ Hz
$n = 6, f_6 = 1300$ Hz

Hence possible natural oscillation whose frequencies < 1250 Hz $= 6(n = 0, 1, 2, 3, 4, 5)$

15. (c) According to Doppler's effect
Apparent frequency

$$n' = n\left(\frac{v + v_0}{v + v_s}\right) = 1392\left(\frac{343 + 10}{343 + 5}\right).$$

$= 1412$ Hz

16. (b) Fundamental frequency of closed organ pipe

$$V_c = \frac{V}{4l_c}$$

Fundamental frequency of open organ pipe

$$V_0 = \frac{V}{2l_0}$$

Second overtone frequency of open organ pipe $= \frac{3V}{2l_0}$

From question,

$$\frac{V}{4l_c} = \frac{3V}{2l_0}$$

$\Rightarrow l_0 = 6l_c = 6 \times 20 = 120$ cm

17. (c) According to Doppler's effect in sound

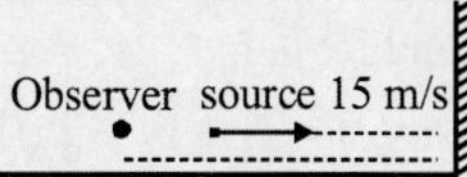

Apparent frequency,

$$n' = \frac{v}{v - v_s} n_0$$

$$= \frac{330}{330 - 15}(800) = \frac{330\times 800}{315} = 838\text{ Hz}$$

The frequency of sound observer hears in the echo reflected from the cliff is 838 Hz.

18. (c) For a closed organ pipe first minimum resonating length

$$L_1 = \frac{\lambda}{4} = 50\text{ cm}$$

$\therefore$ Next or second resonating length, L_2

$$= \frac{3\lambda}{4} = 150\text{ cm}$$

19. (a) Difference in two successive frequencies of closed pipe

$\frac{2v}{4l} = 260 - 220 = 40\text{ Hz}$

or $\frac{2v}{4l} = 40\text{ Hz} \Rightarrow \frac{v}{4\ell} = 20\text{Hz}$

Which is the fundamental frequency of system of closed organ pipe.

20. (b) Two successive resonance are produced at 20 cm and 73 cm of column length

$\therefore \quad \frac{\lambda}{2} = (73 - 20) \times 10^{-2}\text{ m}$

$\Rightarrow \quad \lambda = 2 \times (73 - 20) \times 10^{-2}$

Velocity of sound, $v = n\lambda$

$= 2 \times 320\,[73 - 20] \times 10^{-2}$

$= 339.2\text{ ms}^{-1}$

21. (a) For closed organ pipe, third harmonic

$$n = \frac{(2N-1)V}{4\ell} = \frac{3V}{4\ell} \quad (\because N = 2)$$

For open organ pipe, fundamental frequenty

$$n = \frac{NV}{2\ell} = \frac{V}{2\ell'} \quad (\because N = 1)$$

According to question, $\frac{3V}{4\ell} = \frac{V}{2\ell'}$

$$\Rightarrow \quad \ell' = \frac{4\ell}{3 \times 2} = \frac{2\ell}{3} = \frac{2 \times 20}{3} = 13.33\text{ cm}$$

22. (d)

23. (a) Frequency of string, $f = \frac{1}{2l}\sqrt{\frac{T}{m}}$

Frequency $\propto \sqrt{\text{Tension}}$

Difference of f_A and f_B is 6 Hz.

If tension decreases, f_B decreases and becomes f'_B.

Now, difference of f_A and $f'_B = 7$ Hz (increases)

So, $f_A > f_B$

$f_A - f_B = 6$ Hz

$\Rightarrow f_A = 530\text{ Hz} \Rightarrow f_B = 524\text{ Hz}$ (original)

Exercise 3 -Concept Application Problems 

1. (c) Let $I_1 = I_0$ and $I_2 = 4 I_0$

Resultant intensity, $I = I_1 + I_2 + 2\sqrt{I_1 I_2}\cos\phi$

$$= I_0 + 4 I_0 + 2\sqrt{I_0 4 I_0}\cos 0° = 9 I_0$$

When $\phi = \pi$, $I = I_0$

When $\phi = \pi/2$, $I = 5 I_0$

2. (a) For producing stationary waves, the two transverse waves must be travelling in opposite directions. Therefore, y_1 and y_2 is the only combination.

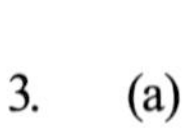

3. (a)

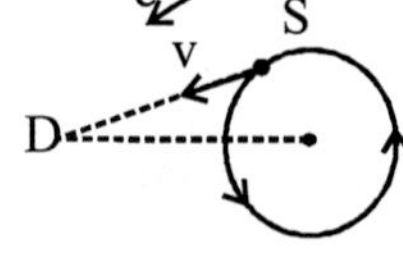

Largest frequency (f_1)

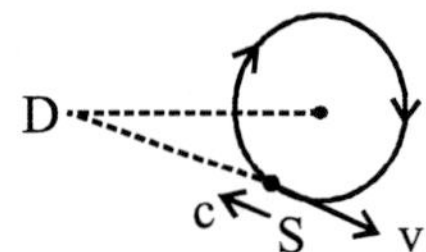

Lowest frequency (f_2)

Largest frequency will be detected when the source approaches detector along the line joining and the smallest frequency will be detected when the source recedes the detector along the line joining them

$$\frac{f_1}{f_2} = \frac{\left(\frac{c}{c-v}\right)f}{\left(\frac{c}{c+v}\right)f} = \frac{c+v}{c-v}$$

4. (d) In the spherical source, the amplitude A of wave is inversely proportional to the distance r i.e., $A \propto \frac{1}{r}$

Where r is distance of source from the point of consideration.

5. (a) Time taken for two syllables $t = \frac{2}{5}$ sec.

$x + x = v \times t = 330 \times \frac{2}{5} \qquad \therefore\ x = 66\text{ m}$

6. (c) At a given temperature, velocity of sound is not affected by pressure.

7. (b) $\Delta n = n \times \frac{v}{c} = \frac{4.5 \times 10^{14} \times 10^6}{3 \times 10^8} = 1.5 \times 10^{12}\text{ Hz}$

$\therefore\ n' = n - \Delta n = 4.5 \times 10^{14} - 1.5 \times 10^{12}$

$= 4.485 \times 10^{14}\text{ Hz}$

8. (c) Comparing it with $y(x, t) = A\cos(\omega t + \pi/2)\cos kx$.

If $kx = \pi/2$, a node occurs ; $\therefore\ 10\pi x = \pi/2 \Rightarrow x = 0.05$ m

If $kx = \pi$, an antinode occurs $\Rightarrow 10\pi x = \pi$

$\Rightarrow x = 0.1$ m

Also speed of wave $\omega/k = \frac{50\pi}{10\pi} = 5\text{m/s}$ and

$\lambda = 2\pi/k = 2\pi/10\pi = 0.2$ m

9. (c) $256 = n \times \frac{240}{60} = 4n \Rightarrow n = 64$

10. (d) $10\log\left(\frac{I}{I_0}\right) = 10 \times 12\log_{10}10 = 120$ dB

11. (c) Two possible frequencies of B are $256 \pm 4 = 260$ or 252. When A is loaded its frequency reduces from 256 to 248 say which would produce 4 beats/sec only if freq. of B is 252

12. (b) As passenger is a part of moving train, there is no relative motion between source and listener. Therefore, n' = n = 200 Hz

13. (b) Let the fundamental frequency of organ pipe be f

Case I : $f = 200 \pm 5 = 205$ Hz or 195 Hz

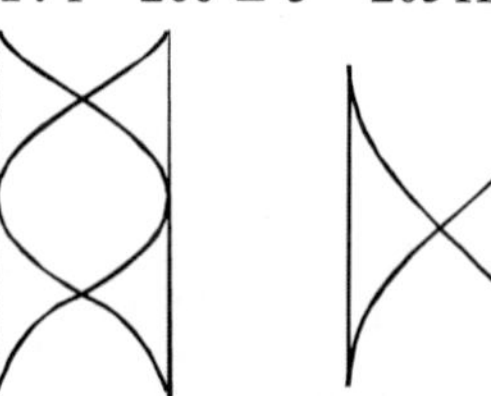

Case II : frequency of 2nd harmonic of organ pipe = 2f (as is clear from the second figure)

$2f = 420 \pm 10$ or $f = 210 \pm 5$ or $f = 205$ or 215

Hence fundamental frequency of organ pipe = 205 Hz

14. (d) $T = \frac{1}{500} s; \; t = \frac{T}{2} = \frac{1}{1000}$ s

15. (c) Velocity of source = 18 km h^{-1} = 5 m s^{-1}
(i) S moves towards listener (v_S)
(ii) listener moves towards source (v_L)
$\nu' = \frac{v + v_L}{v - v_S}\nu = 280$ Hz, Beats = $\nu' - \nu = 8$.

16. (a) $\sqrt{T/l}$ = constant; Tension decreases by a factor (8 – 1) / 8, length decreases by square root of this i.e. 0.77.

17. (a) $y(x, t) = 0.005 \cos(\alpha x - \beta t)$ (Given)
Comparing it with the standard equation of wave
$y(x, t) = a \cos(kx - \omega t)$ we get
$k = \alpha$ and $\omega = \beta$
But $k = \frac{2\pi}{\lambda}$ and $\omega = \frac{2\pi}{T} \Rightarrow \frac{2\pi}{\lambda} = \alpha$ and $\frac{2\pi}{T} = \beta$
Given that $\lambda = 0.08$ m and $T = 2.0$s
$\therefore \alpha = \frac{2\pi}{0.08} = 25\pi$ and $\beta = \frac{2\pi}{2} = \pi$

18. (c) Intensity at A, $I_A = \frac{P}{4\pi r^2}$;
intensity at B, $I_B = \frac{P}{4\pi (2r)^2}$
Sound level at A, $S_A = 10 \log \frac{I_A}{I_0}$;
Sound level at B, $S_B = 10 \log \frac{I_B}{I_0}$
Difference of sound level at A and B is
$S_A - S_B = 10 \log \frac{I_A}{I_0} - 10 \log \frac{I_B}{I_0} = 10 \log \left(\frac{I_A}{I_B}\right)$
$= 10 \log 4 = 20 \log 2 \approx 6$ dB

19. (b) $y_1 = 10^{-6} \sin(100t + x/50 + 0.5)$m
$= 10^{-6} \cos(100t + x/50 - \pi/2 + 0.5)$m
$y_2 = 10^{-6} \cos(100t + x/50)$m
$\therefore \quad \phi = \pi/2 - 0.5 = 1.07$ rad

20. (a) Here, $y_1 = a \sin(\omega t + kx + 0.57)$
and $y_2 = a \cos(\omega t + kx)$
$= a \sin\left[\frac{\pi}{2} + (\omega t + kx)\right]$
Phase difference, $\Delta\phi = \phi_2 - \phi_1$
$= \frac{\pi}{2} - 0.57 = 1$ radian

21. (a)

22. (a) As we know,
Pressure amplitude, $\Delta P_0 = aKB = S_0 KB = S_0 \times \frac{\omega}{V} \times \rho V^2$
$\left[\because K = \frac{\omega}{V}, V = \sqrt{\frac{B}{\rho}}\right]$
$\Rightarrow S_0 = \frac{\Delta P_0}{\rho V \omega} \approx \frac{10}{1 \times 300 \times 1000}$ m $= \frac{1}{30}$ mm $\approx \frac{3}{100}$ mm

23. (a) Using, $\beta = 10$
or $120 = 10 \log 10\left(\frac{I}{10^{-12}}\right)$ ...(i)
Also $I = \frac{P}{4\pi r^2} = \frac{2}{4\pi r^2}$ ...(ii)
On solving above equations, we get
$r = 40$ cm.

24. (a) On comparing with $P = P_0 \sin(wt - kx)$, we have $w = 1000$ rad/s, $K = 3$ m^{-1}
$\therefore v_0 = \frac{w}{k} = \frac{1000}{3} = 333.3$m/s
$\frac{v_1}{v_2} = \sqrt{\frac{T_1}{T_2}}$ or $\frac{333.3}{336} = \sqrt{\frac{273 + 0}{273 + t}}$
$\therefore$ t = 4°C

25. (a) Here, $l_1 = 17$ cm and $l_2 = 24.5$ cm, $V = 330$ m/s, $f = ?$
$\lambda = 2(l_2 - l_1) = 2 \times (24.5 - 17) = 15$ cm
Now, from $v = f\lambda \Rightarrow 330 = \lambda \times 15 \times 10^{-2}$
$\therefore \lambda = \frac{330}{15} \times 100 = \frac{1100 \times 100}{5} = 2200$ Hz

26. (c) Using, $V = f\lambda$
$\frac{V_1}{\lambda_1} = \frac{V_2}{\lambda_2} \Rightarrow \lambda_2 = \frac{V_2}{V_1}\lambda_1$
Again using,
$n = \frac{V}{\lambda} = \sqrt{\frac{T}{M}}\lambda_2 = \sqrt{\frac{T_2}{T_1}}\lambda_1$ $\quad T_2 = 8g$ (Top)
$= \sqrt{\frac{8g}{2g}}\lambda_1 = 2\lambda_1 = 12$ cm $\quad T_1 = 2g$ (Bottom)

T_2
12 m, 6 kg
$\lambda = 6$ cm T_1
2 kg

27. (a) Using $f = \frac{1}{2\ell}\sqrt{\frac{T}{\mu}}$,
where, T = tension and $\mu = \frac{\text{mass}}{\text{length}}$
$f_x = \frac{1}{2\ell}\sqrt{\frac{T_x}{\mu}}$ and $f_z = \frac{1}{2\ell}\sqrt{\frac{T_z}{\mu}}$
$\frac{f_x}{f_z} = \frac{450}{300} = \sqrt{\frac{T_x}{T_z}}$ $\quad \therefore \frac{T_x}{T_z} = \frac{9}{4} = 2.25$.

28. (b)

29. (a) Given, $l = 60$ cm, $m = 6$ g, $A = 1$ mm^2, $v = 90$ m/s and $Y = 16 \times 10^{11}$ Nm^{-2}
Using, $v = \sqrt{\frac{T}{m} \times l} \Rightarrow T = \frac{mv^2}{l}$
Again from, $Y = \frac{T}{A}\Delta L / L_0$
$\Delta L = \frac{Tl}{YA} = \frac{mv^2 \times l}{l(YA)}$
$= \frac{6 \times 10^{-3} \times 90^2}{16 \times 10^{11} \times 10^{-6}} = 3 \times 10^{-4} m = 0.03$ mm

30. (b) 31. (a)

32. (c) Beat frequency
= difference in frequencies of two waves
= 11 – 9 = 2 Hz

33. (d)

34. (d) According to question, tuning fork gives 1 beat/ second with (N) 3rd normal mode. Therefore, organ pipe will have frequency (256 ± 1) Hz. In open organ pipe,

frequency $n = \frac{NV}{2\ell}$

or, $255 = \frac{3 \times 340}{2 \times \ell} \Rightarrow \ell = 2\,m = 200$ cm

35. (a) Probable frequencies of tuning fork be $n \pm 5$

Frequency of sonometer wire, $n \propto \frac{1}{l}$

$\therefore \quad \frac{n+5}{n-5} = \frac{100}{95} \Rightarrow 95(n+5) = 100(n-5)$

or, $95\,n + 475 = 100\,n - 500$

or, $5\,n = 975$ or, $n = \frac{975}{5} = 195$ Hz

36. (b) Frequency heard by the observer

$$v_{observed} = \left(\frac{v_{sound}}{v_{sound} - v\cos\theta}\right) v_0$$

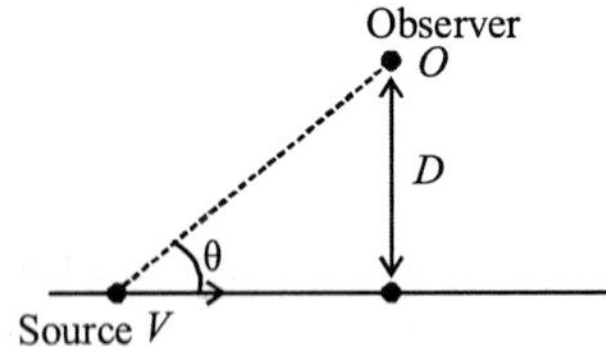

Initially θ will be less so cos θ more.

$\therefore v_{observed}$ more, then it will decrease.

37. (a) Let f_1 be the frequency heard by wall,

$$f_1 = \left(\frac{v}{v - v_c}\right) f_0$$

Here, v = Velocity of sound,

v_c = Velocity of Car,

f_0 = actual frequency of car horn

Let f_2 be the frequency heard by driver after reflection from wall.

$$f_2 = \left(\frac{v+v_c}{v}\right) f_1 = \left(\frac{v+v_c}{v-v_c}\right) f_0$$

$$\Rightarrow 480 = \left[\frac{345+v_c}{345-v_c}\right] 440 \Rightarrow \frac{12}{11} = \frac{345+v_c}{345-v_c}$$

$\Rightarrow v_c = 54$ km/hr

38. (a) From the Doppler's effect of sound, frequency appeared at wall

$$f_w = \frac{330}{330 - v} \cdot f \qquad ...(i)$$

Here, v = speed of bus,

f = actual frequency of source

Frequency heard after reflection from wall (f') is

$$f' = \frac{330+v}{330} \cdot f_w = \frac{330+v}{330-v} \cdot f \Rightarrow 490 = \frac{330+v}{330-v} \cdot 420$$

$$\Rightarrow v = \frac{330 \times 7}{91} \approx 25.38 \text{ m/s} = 91 \text{ km/s}$$

39. (d) Permanent magnets (P) are made of materials with large retentivity and large coercivity. Transformer cores (T) are made of materials with low retentivity and low coercivity.

40. (c)

41. (d) $f_1 = f\left(\frac{v - v_o}{v - v_s}\right) = f\left(\frac{1500-5}{1500-7.5}\right)$

No reflected signal,

$$f_2 = f_1\left(\frac{v + v_o}{v + v_s}\right) = f_1\left(\frac{1500+7.5}{1500+5}\right)$$

$$f_2 = 500\left(\frac{1500-5}{1500-7.5}\right)\left(\frac{1500+7.5}{1500+5}\right)$$

502 Hz

42. (c) $f_1 = f\frac{v - v_0}{v}$ and $f_2 = f\frac{v + v_0}{v}$

S_1 (L) $\xrightarrow{u}$ S_2

But frequency,

$$f_2 - f_1 = f \times \frac{2v_0}{v}$$

or $\quad 10 = 660 \times \frac{2u}{330} \quad \therefore u = 2.5$ m/s.

43. (b) Frequency of sound source (f_0) = 500 Hz

When observer is moving away from the source

Apparent frequency $f_1 = 480 = f_0\left(\frac{v - v'_0}{v}\right)$ ....(i)

And when observer is moving towards the source

$f_2 = 530 = f_0\left(\frac{v - v''_0}{v}\right)$ ....(ii)

From equation (i) $480 = 500\left(\frac{300 - v'_0}{300}\right)$

$v'_0 = 12$ m/s

From equation (ii) $530 = 500\left(1 + \frac{v''_0}{v}\right)$

$\therefore V''_0 = 18$ m/s

44. (a) When source is moving towards a stationary observer,

$$f_{app} = f_{source}\left(\frac{V-0}{V-50}\right)$$

$$1000 = f_{source}\left(\frac{350}{300}\right)$$

When source is moving away from observer

$$f' = f_{source}\left(\frac{350}{350+50}\right) = \frac{1000 \times 300}{350} \times \frac{350}{400} \approx 750 \text{ Hz}$$

45. (a) $f' = f\frac{v - v_0}{v + v_s}$

or $2000 = f\frac{340 - 20}{340 + 20} \quad \therefore f = 2250$ Hz.

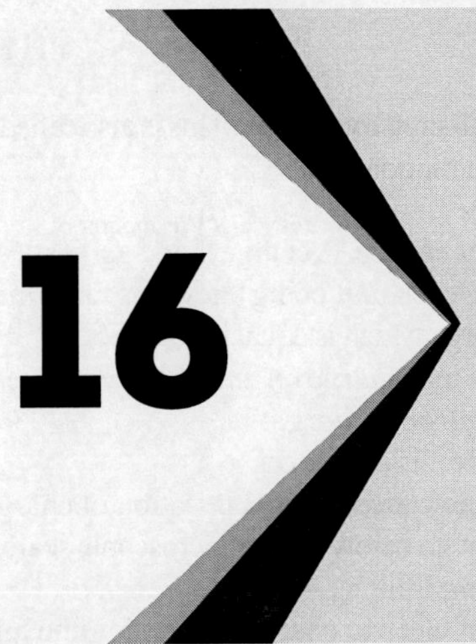

16 Electric Charges and Fields

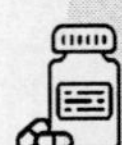

Topic 16.1 : Electric Charge, Conductors & Insulators, Coulomb's Law, Electric Field, Electric lines of Force, Electric Field for a Distribution of Direct & Continuous Charge and Motion of a Charged Particle in an Electric Field

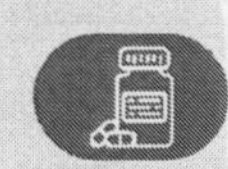

ELECTRIC CHARGE

Charge is something associated with matter due to which it produces and experiences electric and magnetic effects.

There are **two types of charges :**

(i) *Positive charge* and (ii) *Negative charge*

Positive and negative charges : Positive charge means the deficiency of electons while negative charge means excess of electrons. In any neutral body the net charge is equal to zero i.e., the sum of positive charges is equal to the sum of negative charges.

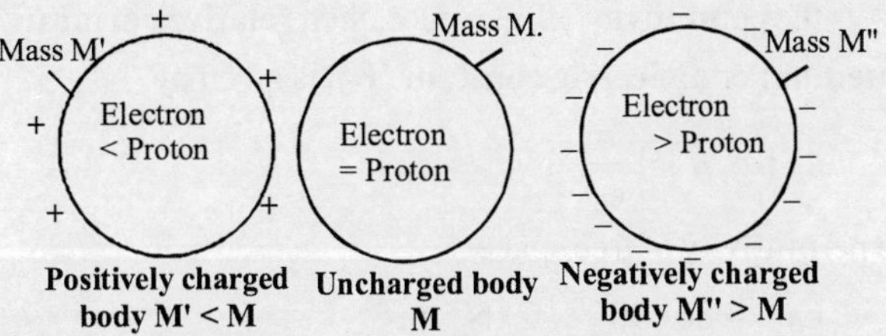

Charge is a scalar quantity and its **SI unit** is coulomb (C).

CONDUCTORS AND INSULATORS

The materials which allow electric charge (or electricity) to flow freely through them are called **conductors**. Metals are very good conductors of electricity. Silver, copper and aluminium are some of the best conductors of electricity. Our skin is also a conductor of electricity. Graphite is the only non-metal which is a conductor of electricity.

All metals, alloys and graphite have '*free electrons*', which can move freely throughout the conductor. These free electrons make metals, alloys and graphite good conductor of electricity.

Aqueous solutions of electrolytes are also conductors.

The materials which do not allow electric charge to flow through them are called **nonconductors** *or* **insulators**.

For example, most plastics, rubber, non-metals (except graphite), dry wood, wax, mica, porcelain, dry air etc., are insulators.

Insulators can be charged but do not conduct electric charge. Insulators do not have '*free electrons*' that is why insulators do not conduct electricity.

Induced charge can be lesser or equal to inducing charge (but never greater) and its max. value is given by

$Q' = -Q(1 - 1/k)$, where 'Q' is inducing charge and 'K' is the dielectric const. of the material of the uncharged body.

For metals $k = \infty \Rightarrow Q' = -Q$.

Methods of Charging

(i) **By friction** : By rubbing two suitable bodies, given in box one is charged by +ve and another by –ve charge in equal amount.

+ve	–ve
Glass rod	Silk
Fur	Ebonite rod
Dry hair	Comb
Wool	Amber

Note : Electric charges remain confined only to the rubbed portion of a non-conductor but in case of a conductor, they spread up throughout the conductor.

(ii) **By conduction :** Charging a neutral body by touching it with a charged body is called charging by conduction.

- It is important to note that when the bodies are charged by conduction, a charged and an uncharged bodies are brought into contact and then seperated, the two bodies may or may not have equal charges.
- If the two bodies are identical the charges on the two will be equal.
- If the two bodies are not identical, the charges will be different.
- The potential of the two bodies will always be the same.

(iii) **By induction :** Charging a body without bringing it in contact with a charged body is called charging by induction.

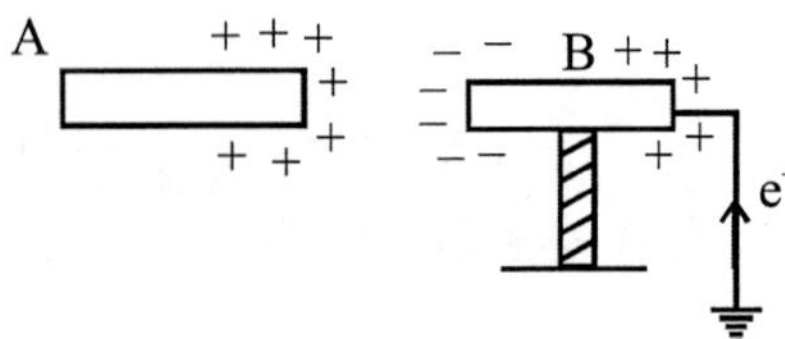

First rearrangement of charge takes place in metal rod B. When the rod B is connected to earth, electrons flow from earth to the rod B thus making it -vely charged

The magnitude of elementary positive or negative charge (electron) is same and is equal to 1.6×10^{-19} C.

Properties of Electric Charge

(i) **Similar charges repel and dissimilar charges attract each other.**

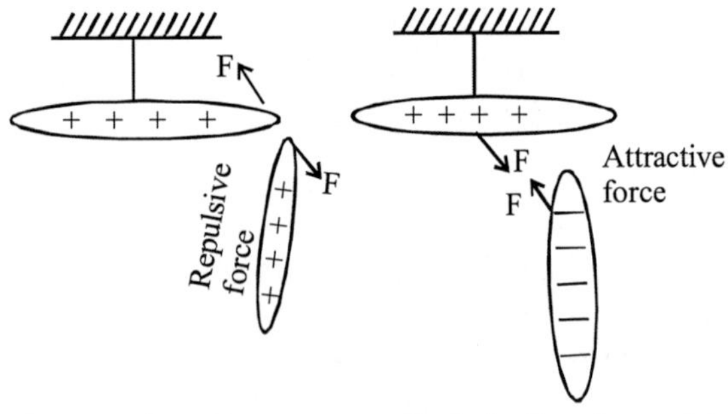

In rare situation you may find similar charged bodies attracting each other. Suppose a big positive charged body is placed near a small positively charged body then because of induction, opposite charge produced on the small body makes it to attract the other body.

(ii) **A charged body attracts light uncharged bodies, due to polarisation of uncharged body.**

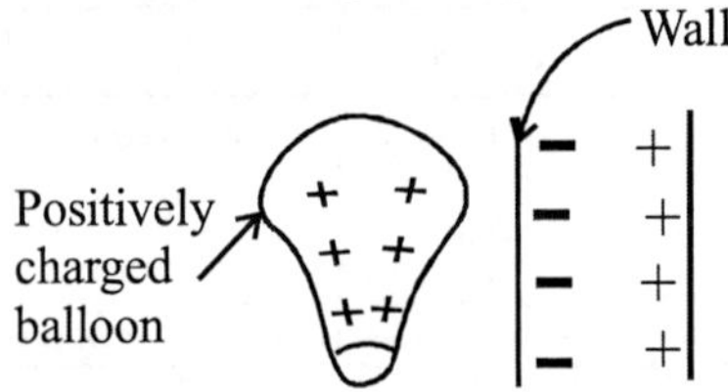

Fig : When a positively charged balloon is placed in contact with the wall, an opposite charge is induced with the wall, the balloon stick to the wall due to electrostatic attraction

(iii) **Charge is conserved** i.e., *the charge can neither be created nor be destroyed but it may simply be transferred from one body to the other.*

Thus we may say that the total charge in the universe is constant or we may say that charges can be created or destroyed in equal and opposite pair. *For example*

$$\gamma(\text{Energy} \geq 1.02\text{MeV}) \longrightarrow \underset{\text{Electron}}{e^-} + \underset{\text{Positron}}{e^+}$$

(Pair-production process)

- **Positron** is an antiparticle of electron. It has same mass as that of electron but equal negative charge.

$$e^- + e^+ \longrightarrow \gamma \text{ (Pair-annihilation process)}$$

(iv) **Charge is unaffected by motion**. This is also called charge invariance with motion

Mathematically, $(q)_{\text{at rest}} = (q)_{\text{in motion}}$

(v) ***Quantisation of charge.*** A charge is an aggregate of small unit of charges, each unit being known as fundamental or elementary charge which is equal to $e = 1.6 \times 10^{-19}$ C. This principle states that *charge on any body exists as integral mutliple of electronic charge.*

i.e. $\boldsymbol{q = ne}$ where n is an integer.

According to the concept of quantisation of charges, the charge q cannot go below e. On macroscopic scale, this is as good as taking limit $q_0 \to 0$.

Quantisation of electric charge is a basic (unexplained) law of nature. It is important to note that there is no analogous law of quantisation of mass.

Recent studies on high energy physics have indicated the presence of graphs with charge 2e/3, e/3. But since these cannot be isolated and are present in groups with total charge, therefore the concept of elementary charge is still valid.

COULOMB'S LAW

The force of attraction or repulsion between two point charges (q_1 and q_2) at finite separation (r) is directly proportional to the product of charges and inversely proportional to the square of distance between the charges and is directed along the line joining the two charges.

i.e., $F \propto \dfrac{q_1 q_2}{r^2}$ or $F = \dfrac{1}{4\pi\varepsilon} \cdot \dfrac{q_1 q_2}{r^2}$

q₁ ←— r —→ q₂

where ε is the permittivity of medium between the charges.

If ε_0 is the permittivity of free space, then **relative permittivity of medium** or **dielectric constant (K)**, is given by

$$\varepsilon_r \,(or\ K) = \frac{\varepsilon}{\varepsilon_0}$$

The permittivity of free space

$$\varepsilon_0 = 8.86 \times 10^{-12}\ \text{C}^2\text{N}^{-1}\text{m}^{-2}$$

and $\dfrac{1}{4\pi\varepsilon_0} = \dfrac{1}{4 \times 3.14 \times 8.86 \times 10^{-2}} = 9 \times 10^9\ \text{Nm}^2\text{C}^{-2}$.

Also $\dfrac{1}{4\pi\varepsilon_0} = 1$ in CGS system of unit.

Coulomb's law may also be expressed as

$$F = \frac{1}{4\pi\varepsilon_0\varepsilon_r} \cdot \frac{q_1 q_2}{r^2}$$

Let F_0 be the force between two charges placed in vacuum then

$$F_0 = \frac{1}{4\pi\varepsilon_0} \cdot \frac{q_1 q_2}{r^2}$$

r

$+q_1$ Medium with dielectric constant K $-q_2$

Hence $\frac{F_0}{F} = K$ $\left(\because F = \frac{1}{4\pi\varepsilon} \cdot \frac{q_1 q_2}{r^2} \text{ and } \frac{\varepsilon}{\varepsilon_0} = K \right)$

Therefore we can conclude that the force between two charges becomes 1/K times when placed in a medium of dielectric constant K.

The value of K for different media

Medium	Dielectric Constant (K)
Air	1.006
Vacuum	1.00
Water	1.00026
Mica	3 to 6
Metals	∞

Dielectric : A dielectric is an insulator. It is of two types -

(i) Polar dielectric and

(ii) Non-polar dielectric.

Significance of Permittivity Constant or Dielectric Constant : Permittivity constant is a measure of the inverse degree of permission of the medium for the charges to interact.

Dielectric strength : The maximum value of electric field that can be applied to the dielectric without its electric breakdown is called its dielectric strength.

Difference between electrostatic force and gravitational force :

Electrostatic force	*Gravitational force*
1. Much stronger	**1.** Much weaker as compared to electrostatic force
2. Can be attractive or repulsive	**2.** Only attractive
3. Depends on the nature of medium between charges	**3.** Does not depend on the nature of medium between masses

Note : Both electric and gravitational forces follow inverse square law.

Vector Form of Coulomb's Law :

$$\vec{F}_{12} = \frac{1}{4\pi\varepsilon_0 k} \frac{q_1 q_2}{r^3} \vec{r}_{12} = \frac{1}{4\pi\varepsilon_0 k} \frac{q_1 q_2}{r^2} \hat{r}_{12}$$

Superposition Principle For Discrete Charge Distribution : Force Between Multiple Charges

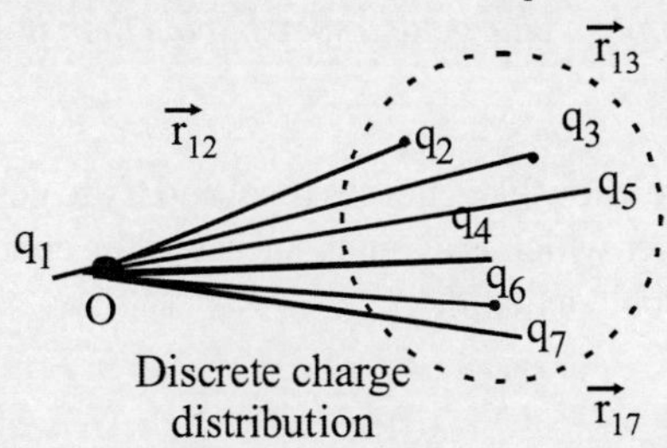

Discrete charge distribution

The electric force $\vec{F}_1$ on q_1 due to a number of charges placed in air or vacuum is given by

$$\vec{F}_1 = \frac{1}{4\pi\varepsilon_0} \sum_{i=1}^{n} \frac{q_1 q_i}{r_{1i}^2} \hat{r}_{1i} = \frac{1}{4\pi\varepsilon_0} \left[\frac{q_1 q_2}{r_{12}^2} \hat{r}_{12} + \frac{q_1 q_3}{r_{13}^2} \hat{r}_{13} + \ldots\ldots \right]$$

Note : Coulomb's law is valid if $r \geq 10^{-15}$ m and if charges are point charges

FORCE FOR CONTINUOUS CHARGE DISTRIBUTION

A small element having charge dq is considered on the body. The force on the charge q_1 is calculated as follows :

$$d\vec{F}_1 = \frac{1}{4\pi \in_0} \cdot \frac{q_1 dq}{r^2} \hat{r}$$

Now the total force $\vec{F}_1$ is calculated by integrating $d\vec{F}_1$ under proper limits.

i.e., $\vec{F}_1 = \int d\vec{F}_1 = \frac{1}{4\pi \in_0} \int \frac{q_1 dq}{r^2} \hat{r} = \frac{q_1}{4\pi \in_0} \int \frac{dq}{r} \hat{r}$

where $\hat{r}$ is a variable unit vector which points from each dq, towards the location of charge q_1 (where dq is a small charge element)

Types of Charge Distribution

(i) Volume charge distribution : If a charge, Q is uniformly distributed through a volume V, the charge per unit volume ρ (volume charge density) is defined by

$\rho = \frac{Q}{V}$; ρ has unit coulomb/m^3.

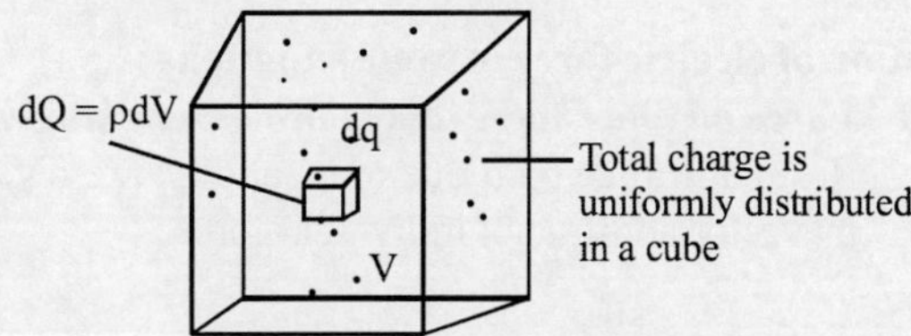

(ii) Surface charge distribution : If a charge Q is uniformly distributed on a surface of area A, the surface charge density σ, is defined by the following equation

$\sigma = \frac{Q}{A}$, σ has unit coulomb / m^2

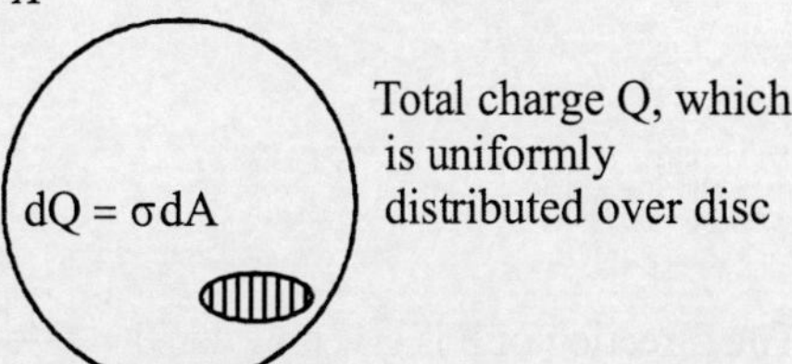

(iii) Linear charge distribution : If a charge q is uniformly distributed along a line of length λ, the linear charge density λ, is defined by

$\lambda = \frac{Q}{\ell}$, λ has unit coloumb/m.

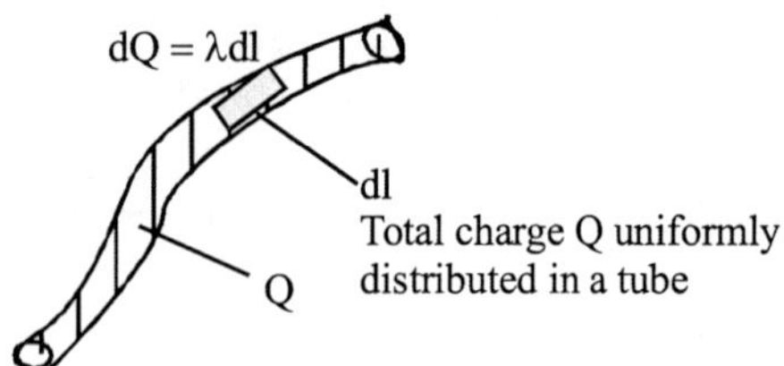

- If the charge is non uniformly distributed over a volume, surface, or line we would have to express the charge densities as

$$\rho = \frac{dQ}{dV}, \quad \sigma = \frac{dQ}{dA}, \quad \lambda = \frac{dQ}{dl},$$

where dQ is the amount of charge in a small volume, surface or length element.

- In general, when there is a distribution of direct and continuous charge bodies, we should follow the following steps to find force on a charge q due to all the charges :
  (1) Fix the origin of the coordinate system on charge q.
  (2) Draw the forces on q due to the surrounding charges considering one charge at a time.
  (3) Resolve the force in x and y-axis respectively and find ΣF_x and ΣF_y
  (4) The resultant force is $F = \sqrt{(\Sigma F_x)^2 + (\Sigma F_y)^2}$ and the direction is given by $\tan\theta = \frac{\Sigma F_x}{\Sigma F_y}$.

Calculation of electric force in some situations :

(a) Force on one charge due to two other charges :

Resultant force on q due to q_1 and q_2 are obtained by vector addition of individual forces

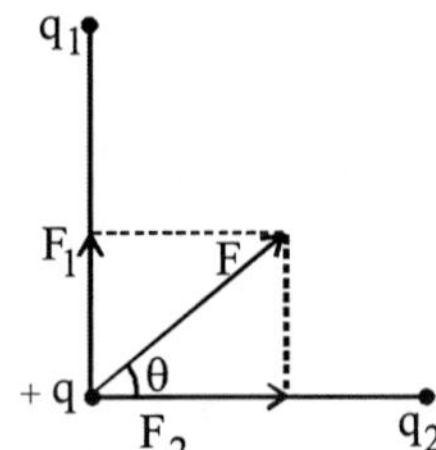

$$\vec{F} = \vec{F_1} + \vec{F_2}$$

$$|\vec{F}| = \sqrt{|\vec{F_1}|^2 + |\vec{F_2}|^2}$$

The direction of F is given by $\tan\theta = \frac{|\vec{F_1}|}{|\vec{F_2}|}$

(b) Force due to linear charge distribution :

Let AB is a long (length ℓ) thin rod with uniform distribution of total charge Q.

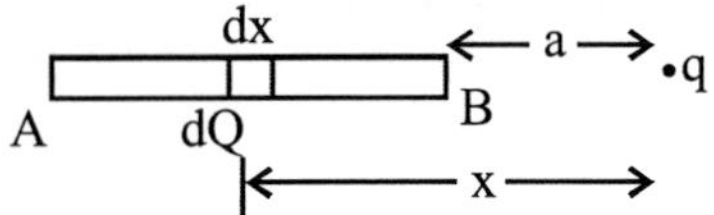

We calculate force of these charges i.e. Q on q which is situated at a distance a from the edge of rod AB.

Let, dQ is a small charge element in rod AB at a distance x from q.

The force on q due to this element will be

$$dF = \frac{q}{4\pi\varepsilon_o}\frac{dQ}{x^2} = \frac{q}{4\pi\varepsilon_o}\frac{\mu dx}{x^2}$$

where μ is linear charge density i.e., $\mu = Q/\ell$.

$$\text{so, } F = \int_a^{\ell+a} dF = \int_a^{\ell+a} \frac{q}{4\pi\epsilon_o}\cdot\frac{\mu}{x^2}dx$$

$$= \frac{q\mu}{4\pi\epsilon_0}\int_a^{\ell+a}\frac{1}{x^2}dx \text{ newton}$$

Problem Solving Tips

1. When the distance between the two charges placed in vacuum or a medium is increased K-times then the force between them decreases K^2-times. i.e., if F_0 and F be the initial and final forces between them, then

$$F = \frac{F_o}{K^2}$$

2. When the distance between the two charges placed in vacuum or a medium is decreased K-times then the force between them increases K^2-times. i.e., if F_o and F be the initial and final forces then

$$F = K^2F_o$$

3. When a medium of dielectric constant K is placed between the two charges then the force between them decreases by K-times. i.e., if F_o and F be the forces in vacuum and the medium respectively, then

$$F = \frac{F_o}{K}$$

4. When a medium of dielectric constant K between the charges is replaced by another medium of dielectric constant K' then the force decreases or increases by (K/K') times according as K' is greater than K or K' is less than K.

Example 1.

If we supply a charge to a soap bubble then it will expand. Why?

Solution :

Since we know like charges repel and try to get away from each other which is at outer surface of the conductor. So a soap bubble expand.

Example 2.

Calculate the net charge on a substance consisting of (a) 5 × 10^{14} electrons (b) a combination of 7 × 10^{13} protons and 4 × 10^{13} electrons.

Solution :

(a) The charge of one electron is -1.6×10^{-19}C. So net charge on a substance consisting of 5×10^{14} electrons is

$5\times10^{14}\times(-1.6\times10^{-19}\text{C}) = -8\times10^{-5}\text{C} = -80\mu\text{C}.$

(b) Similarly the net charge on a substance consisting of a combination of 7×10^{13} protons and 4×10^{13} electron is

$$[7\times10^{13}\times(1.6\times10^{-19}\text{C})]+[4\times10^{13}(-1.6\times10^{-19}-\text{C}]$$
$$=+4.8\,\mu\text{C}.$$

($\because$ the charge on one proton is $+1.6\times10^{19}$C)

Example 3.

Two protons in a molecule is separated by a distance 3×10^{-10} m. Find the electrostatic force exerted by one proton on the other.

Solution :

$\longmapsto 3\times10^{-10}\,\text{m} \longleftarrow$

1.6×10^{-19} C $\qquad$ 1.6×10^{-19} C

According to coulomb's law, the electrostatic force F between two charges q_1 and q_2, which are seperated by distance r is

$$F=\frac{1}{4\pi\varepsilon_o}\times\frac{q_1q_2}{r^2}$$

Here, $q_1 = q_2 = 1.6\times10^{-19}$C, $r = 3\times10^{-10}$ m

$$\text{so, } F=9\times10^{9}\,\frac{(1.6\times10^{-19})^2}{9\times10^{-20}}=2.56\times10^{-9}\,\text{C (Repulsive)}$$

Example 4.

When a piece of polythene is rubbed with wool, a charge of 2×10^{-7} C is developed on polythene. What is the amount of mass, which is transferred to polythene?

Solution :

No. of electrons transferred, $n=\frac{q}{e}$

$$\text{Mass transferred} = m_e\times n = m_e\times\left(\frac{q}{e}\right)$$

$$=9.1\times10^{-31}\times\left(\frac{2\times10^{-7}}{1.6\times10^{-19}}\right)$$

$$=11.38\times10^{-19}\ \text{kg}$$

Example 5.

Two negative charges of unit magnitude each and a positive charge q are placed along a straight line. At what position and for what value of q will the system be in equilibrium? Check whether it is stable, unstable or neutral equilibrium?

Solution :

Let the charge + q be held at a distance x_1 from unit negative charge at A, and at a distance x_2 from unit negative charge at B.

–1 $\qquad$ +q $\qquad$ –1

A $\qquad\qquad\qquad$ B

$\longleftarrow x_1 \longrightarrow\longleftarrow x_2 \longrightarrow$

$$\text{For equilibrium of q, } \frac{q(-1)}{4\pi\varepsilon_o x_1^2}=\frac{q(-1)}{4\pi\varepsilon_o x_2^2}$$

$\therefore x_1 = x_2$ i.e. q must be equidistant from A and B.

For equilibrium of unit negative charge at B.

Force on B due to charge at A + force on B due to q = 0

$$\frac{(-1)(-1)}{4\pi\varepsilon_o(x_1+x_2)^2}+\frac{q(-1)}{4\pi\varepsilon_o x_2^2}=0$$

$$\Rightarrow\ \frac{1}{4\pi\varepsilon_o(2x_2)^2}=\frac{-(-q)}{4\pi\varepsilon_o x_2^2}\quad(\because x_1 = x_2)$$

$q=\frac{1}{4}$ i.e. $\frac{1}{4}$th of the magnitude of either unit charge.

Stability : If q is displaced slightly towards A, force of attraction due to A exceeds the force of attraction due to B. Therefore, q will get displaced further towards A. Hence the equilibrium of q is unstable.

However, if q is displaced in a direction $\perp$ to A, net force would bring q back to its normal position. Therefore, the equilibrium will be stable.

Example 6.

Four identical point charges each of magnitude q are placed at the corners of a square of side a. Find the net electrostatic force on any of the charge.

Solution :

Let the concerned charge be at C then charge at C will experience the force due to charges at A, B and D. Let these forces respectively be $\vec{F}_A$, $\vec{F}_B$ and $\vec{F}_D$ thus forces are given as

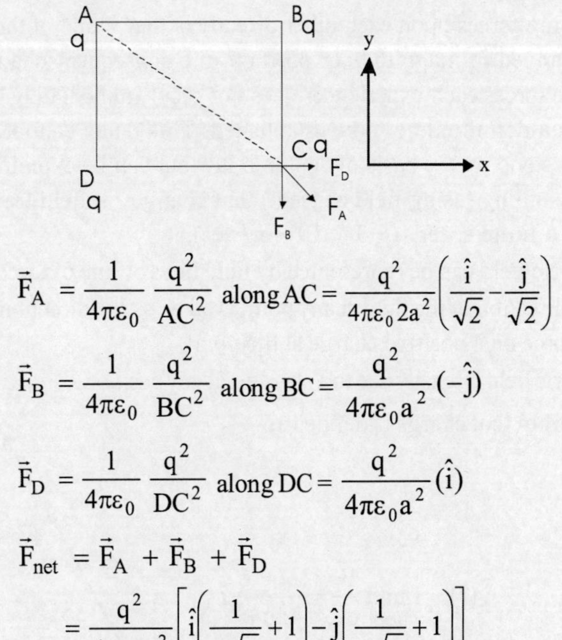

$$\vec{F}_A=\frac{1}{4\pi\varepsilon_0}\frac{q^2}{AC^2}\text{ along AC}=\frac{q^2}{4\pi\varepsilon_0 2a^2}\left(\frac{\hat{i}}{\sqrt{2}}-\frac{\hat{j}}{\sqrt{2}}\right)$$

$$\vec{F}_B=\frac{1}{4\pi\varepsilon_0}\frac{q^2}{BC^2}\text{ along BC}=\frac{q^2}{4\pi\varepsilon_0 a^2}(-\hat{j})$$

$$\vec{F}_D=\frac{1}{4\pi\varepsilon_0}\frac{q^2}{DC^2}\text{ along DC}=\frac{q^2}{4\pi\varepsilon_0 a^2}(\hat{i})$$

$$\vec{F}_{net}=\vec{F}_A+\vec{F}_B+\vec{F}_D$$

$$=\frac{q^2}{4\pi\varepsilon_0 a^2}\left[\hat{i}\left(\frac{1}{2\sqrt{2}}+1\right)-\hat{j}\left(\frac{1}{2\sqrt{2}}+1\right)\right]$$

$$\left|\vec{F}_{net}\right| = \sqrt{2}\left(\frac{1}{2\sqrt{2}}+1\right)\frac{q^2}{4\pi\varepsilon_0 a^2} = \left(\frac{1}{2}+\sqrt{2}\right)\frac{q^2}{4\pi\varepsilon_0 a^2}$$

Example 7.

Electric force between two point charges q and Q at rest is F. Now if a charge – q is placed next to q what will be the (a) force on Q due to q (b) total force on Q ?

Solution :

(a) As electric force between two body interaction, i.e., force between two particles, is independent of presence or absence of other particles, the force between Q and q will remain unchanged, i.e., F.

(b) An electric force is proportional to the magnitude of charges, total force on Q will be given by

$$\frac{F'}{F}=\frac{Qq'}{Qq}=\frac{q'}{q}=\frac{0}{q}=0 \quad [\text{as } q' = q + (-q) = 0]$$

i.e., the resultant or total force on Q will be zero.

ELECTRIC FIELD

The space around an electric charge, where it exerts a force on another charge is an **electric field.**

Electric force, like the gravitational force acts between the bodies that are not in contact with each other. To understand these forces, we involve the concept of force field. When a mass is present somewhere, the properties of space in vicinity can be considered to be so altered in such a way that another mass brought to this region will experience a force there. The space where alteration is caused by a mass is called its Gravitational field and any other mass is thought of as interacting with the field and not directly with the mass responsible for it.

Similarly an electric charge produces an electric field around it so that it interacts with any other charges present there. One reason it is preferable not to think of two charges as exerting forces upon each other directly is that if one of them is changed in magnitude or position, the consequent change in the forces each experiences does not occur immediately but takes a definite time to be established. This delay cannot be understood on the basis of coulomb law but can be explained by assuming (using field concept) that changes in field travel with a finite speed. ($\approx 3 \times 10^8$ m / sec).

Electric field can be represented by field lines or line of force.

The direction of the field at any point is taken as the direction of the force on a positive charge at the point.

Electric field intensity due to a charge q at any position ($\vec{r}$) from that charge is defined as

$$\vec{E} = \frac{\vec{F}}{q_0}$$

$$\vec{E}(r) = \underset{q_0 \to 0}{\text{Limit}}\frac{\vec{F}}{q_0} = \frac{1}{4\pi\varepsilon}\frac{q}{r^2}\hat{r}$$

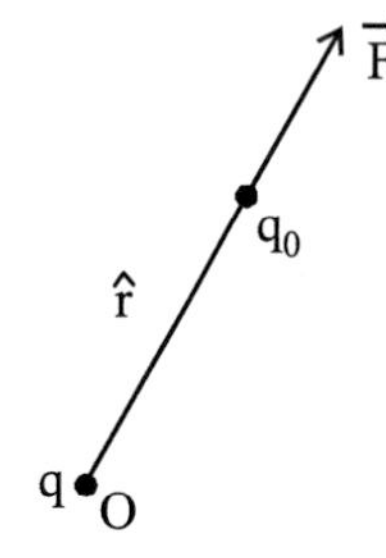

where $\vec{F}$ is the force experienced by a small positive test charge q_0 due to charge q. Its **SI unit** is NC^{-1}. It is a vector quantity. If there are more charges responsible for the field, then

$$\vec{E} = \vec{E_1} + \vec{E_2} + \vec{E_3} + ...$$

where $\vec{E_1}, \vec{E_2}, \vec{E_3}$,........ are the electric field intensities due to charges q_1, q_2, q_3 ......respectively.

ELECTRIC LINES OF FORCE

These are the imaginary lines of force and the tangent at any point on the lines of force gives the direction of the electric field at that point.

Properties of Electric Lines of Froce

(i) The lines of force diverge out from a positive charge and converge at a negative charge. i.e. the lines of force are always directed from higher to lower potential.

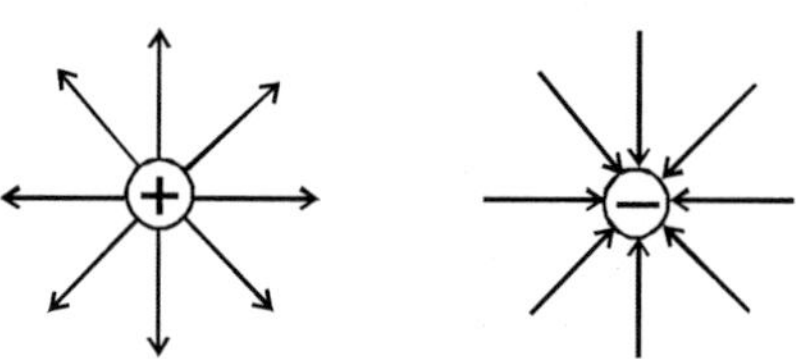

(ii) The electric lines of force contract length wise indicating unlike charges attract each other and expand laterally indicating like charges repel each other.

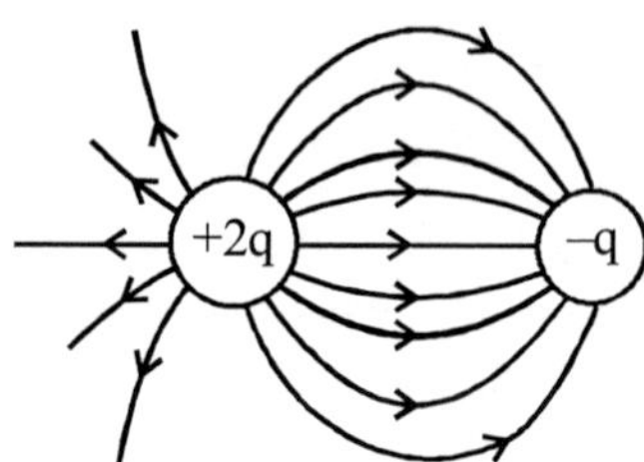

(iii) The number of lines that originate from or terminate on a charge is proportional to the magnitude of charge.

i.e., $\dfrac{|q_1|}{|q_2|} = \dfrac{N_1}{N_2}$

(iv) Two electric lines of force never intersect each other.

(v) They begin from positive charge and end on negative charge i.e., they do not make closed loop (while magnetic field lines form closed loop).

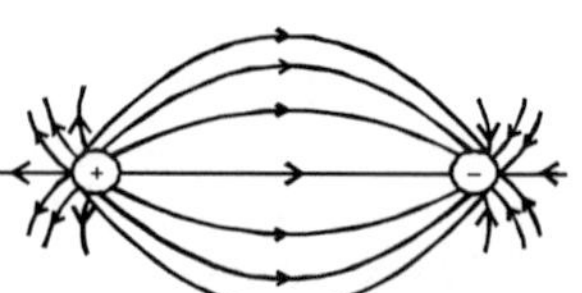

(vi) **Where the electric lines of force are**

(a) close together, the field is strong (see fig.1)

(b) far apart, the field is weak (see fig.2)

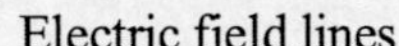

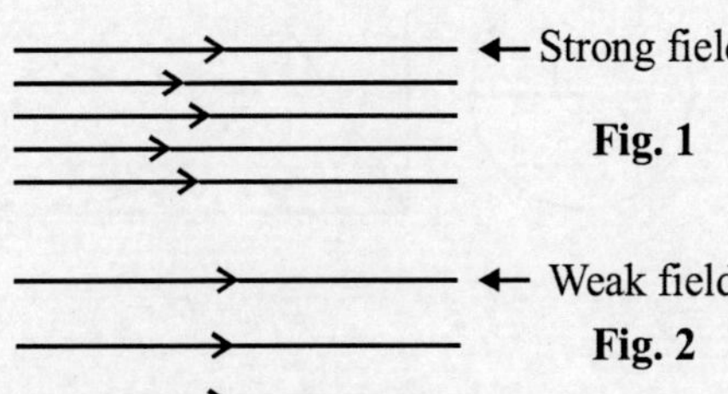

(vii) Electric lines of force generate or terminate at charges /surfaces at right angles.

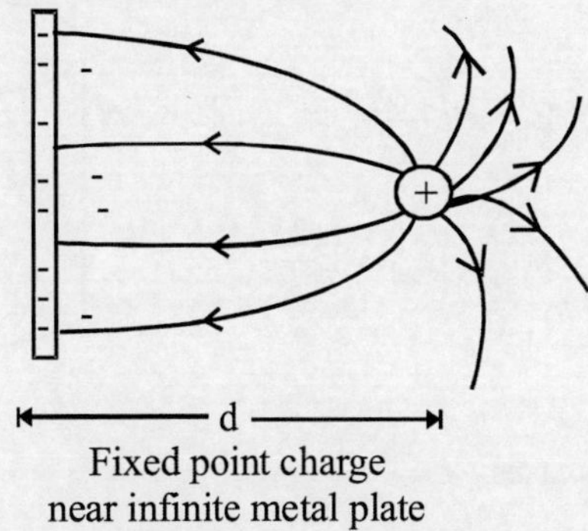

Fixed point charge near infinite metal plate

Electric Field for Continuous Charge Distribution :

If the charge distribution is continuous, then the electric field strength at any point may be calculated by dividing the charge into infinitesimal elements. If dq is the small element of charge within the charge distribution, then the electric field $d\vec{E}$ at point P at a distance r from charge element dq is

$$d\vec{E} = \frac{1}{4\pi\varepsilon}\frac{dq}{r^2}\hat{r};$$

Non conducting sphere (dq is small charge element)

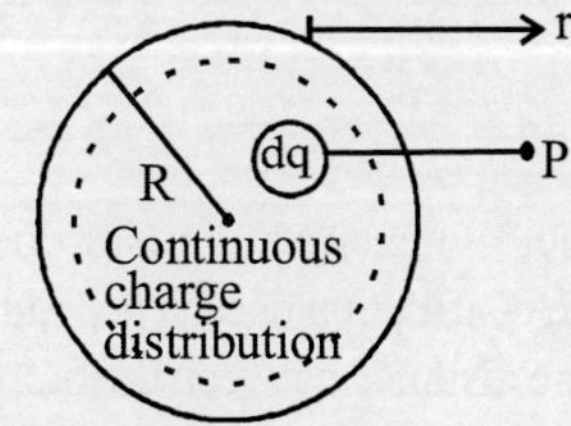

$dq = \lambda dl$ (line charge density)
$= \sigma\, ds$ (surface charge density)
$= \rho dv$ (volume charge density)

The net field strength due to entire charge distribution is given by

$$\vec{E} = \frac{1}{4\pi\varepsilon}\int \frac{dq}{r^2}\hat{r}$$

where the integration extends over the entire charge distribution.

Note : Electric field intensity due to a point charge q, at a distance $(r_1 + r_2)$ where r_1 is the thickness of medium of dielectric constant K_1 and r_2 is the thickness of medium of dielectric constant K_2 as shown in fig. is given by

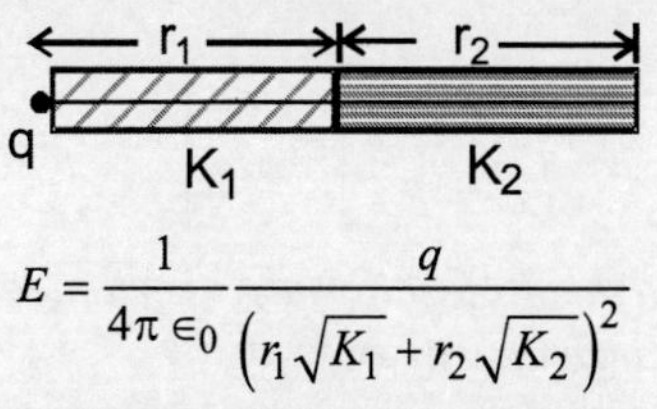

$$E = \frac{1}{4\pi\in_0}\frac{q}{\left(r_1\sqrt{K_1} + r_2\sqrt{K_2}\right)^2}$$

CALCULATION OF ELECTRIC FIELD INTENSITY FOR A DISTRIBUTION OF DIRECT AND CONTINOUS CHARGE

1. Fix origin of the coordinate system where electric field intenstiy is to be found.
2. Draw the direction of electric field intensity due to the surrounding charges considering one charge at a time.
3. Resolve the electric field intensity in x and y-axis respectively and find ΣE_x and ΣE_y
4. The resultant intensity is $E = \sqrt{(\Sigma E_x)^2 + (\Sigma E_y)^2}$ and $\tan\theta = \frac{\Sigma E_y}{\Sigma E_x}$ where θ is the angle between $\vec{E}$ and x-axis.
5. To find the force acting on the charge placed at the origin, the formula F = qE is used.

Energy density : Energy in unit volume of electric field is called energy density and is given by $u = \frac{1}{2}\varepsilon_o E^2$,

where E = electric field and ε_o = permitivity of vacuum

Electric Field due to Various Charge Distribution :

(i) *Electric Field due to an isolated point charge*

$$E = k\frac{q}{x^2}$$

(ii) *A circular ring of radius R with uniformly distributed charge*

$$E = k\frac{Qx}{(R^2 + x^2)^{3/2}}$$

When x >> R, $E = k\frac{Q}{x^2}$

[The charge on ring behaves as point charge]

E is max when $x = \pm\frac{R}{\sqrt{2}}$. Also $E_{max} = \frac{Q}{6\sqrt{3}\pi\varepsilon_0 R^2}$

(iii) *A circular disc of radius R with uniformly distributed charge with surface charge density σ*

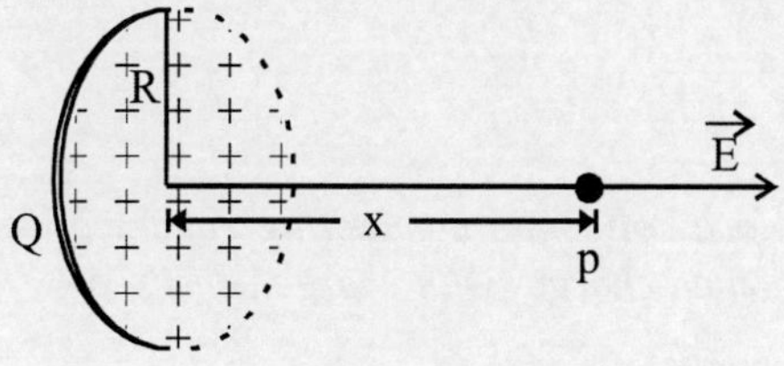

$$E = \frac{2kQ}{R^2}\left[1 - \frac{x}{\sqrt{x^2 + R^2}}\right] = \frac{\sigma}{2\varepsilon_0}\left[1 - \frac{x}{\sqrt{x^2 + R^2}}\right]$$

(iv) *An infinite sheet of uniformly distributed charges with surface charge density σ*

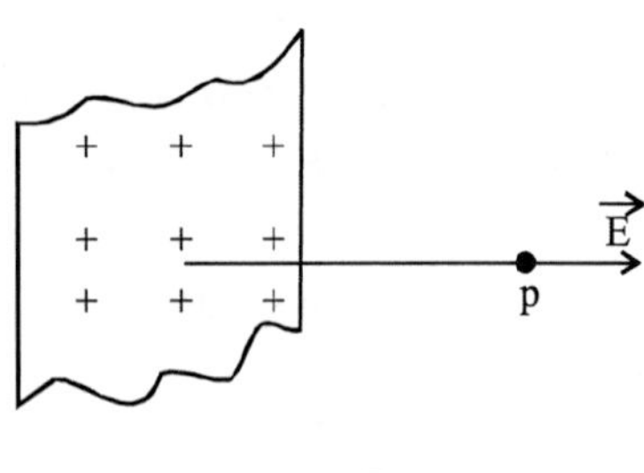

$$E = \frac{\sigma}{2\varepsilon_0}$$

(v) *A finite length of charge with linear charge density λ*

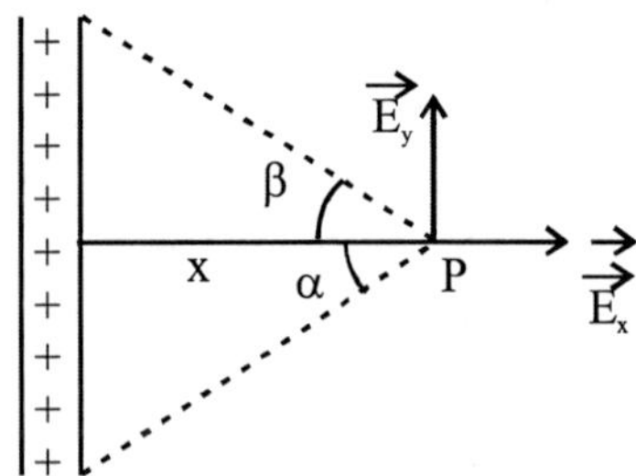

$$E_x = \frac{k\lambda}{x}[\sin\alpha + \sin\beta] \text{ and } E_y = \frac{k\lambda}{x}[\cos\alpha - \cos\beta]$$

Special case :

For Infinite length of charge, $\alpha = \beta = \frac{\pi}{2}$

$$\therefore \quad E_x = \frac{2k\lambda}{x} \text{ and } E_y = 0$$

(vi) *Due to a spherical shell of uniformly distributed charges with surface charge density σ*

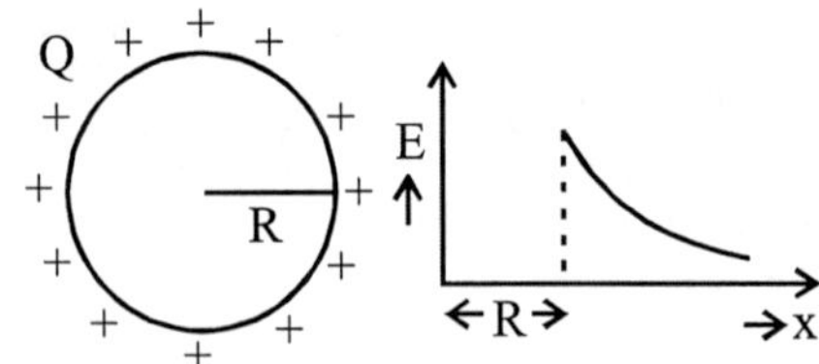

$E_{in} = 0\ (x < R)$

$$E_{surface} = k\frac{Q}{R^2} = \frac{\sigma}{\varepsilon_0}\ (x = R)$$

$$E_{out} = k\frac{Q}{x^2}$$

(vii) *Due to a solid non conducting sphere of uniformly distributed charges with charge density ρ*

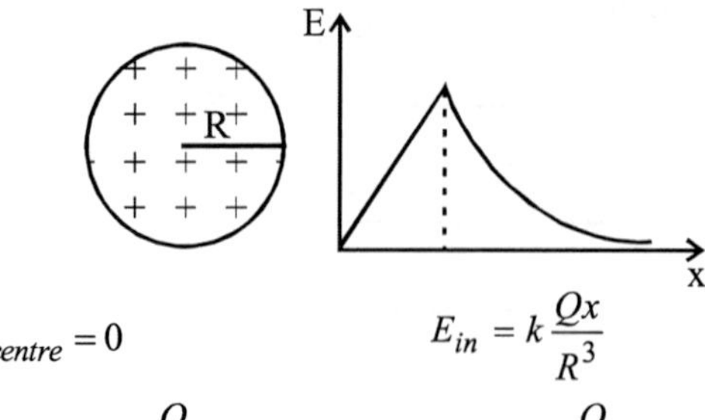

$E_{centre} = 0$ $\qquad E_{in} = k\frac{Qx}{R^3}$

$E_{surface} = k\frac{Q}{R^2}$ $\qquad E_{out} = k\frac{Q}{x^2}$

(viii) *Due to a solid non-conducting cylinder with linear charge denisty λ*

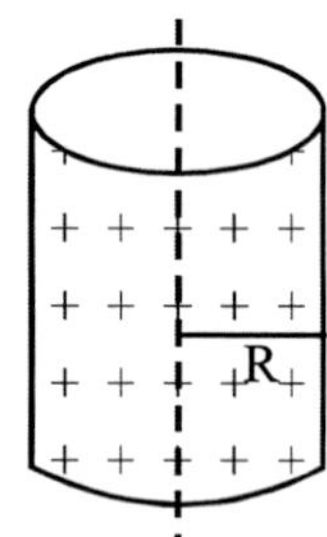

$$E_{axis} = 0,\ E_{in} = k\frac{2\lambda x}{R^2},$$

$$E_{surface} = k\frac{2\lambda}{R},\ E_{out} = k\frac{2\lambda}{x}$$

In above cases, $k = \frac{1}{4\pi \in_0}$

Problem Solving Tips

1. If the electric lines of force are parallel and equally spaced, the field is uniform.
2. If E_0 and E be the electric field intensity at a point due to a point charge or a charge distribution in vacuum and in a medium of dielectric constant K then
$$E = KE_0$$
3. If E and E' be the electric field intensity at a point in the two media having dielectric constant K and K' then
$$\frac{E'}{E} = \frac{K'}{K}$$
4. The electric field intensity at a point due to a ring with uniform charge distribution doesn't depend upon the radius of the ring if the distance between the point and the centre of the ring is much greater than the radius of the ring. The ring simply behaves as a point charge.
5. The electric field intensity inside a hollow sphere is zero but has a finite value at the surface $\left(= \frac{KQ}{R^2}\right)$ and outside it ($= \frac{KQ}{x^2}$; x being the distance of the point from the centre of the sphere).
6. The electric field intensity at a point outside a hollow sphere (or spherical shell) does not depend upon the radius of the sphere. It just behaves as a point charge.
7. The electric field intensity at the centre of a non-conducting solid sphere with uniform charge distribution is zero. At other points inside it, the electric field varies directly with the distance from the centre (i.e. $E \propto x$; x

being the distance of the point from the centre). On the surface, it is constant but varies inversely with the square of the distance from the centre (i.e. $E \propto \frac{1}{x^2}$). Note that the field doesn't depend on the radius of the sphere for a point outside it. It simply behaves as a point charge.

8. The electric field intensity at a point on the axis of non-conducting solid cylinder is zero. It varies directly with the distance from the axis inside it (i.e. $E \propto x$). On the surface, it is constant and varies inversely with the distance from the axis for a point outside it (i.e. $E \propto \frac{1}{x}$).

MOTION OF A CHARGED PARTICLE IN AN ELECTRIC FIELD

Let a charged particle of mass m and charge q be placed in an uniform electric field $\vec{E}$, then electric force on the charge particle is

$$\vec{F} = q\vec{E}$$

$\therefore$ *Acceleration,* $\vec{a} = \frac{q\vec{E}}{m}$ (constant)

(a) The velocity of the charged particle at time t is,

$v = u + at = at = \frac{qE}{m}t$ (Particle initially at rest)

or $v = \frac{qE}{m}t$

(b) Distance travelled by particle is $S = \frac{1}{2}at^2 = \frac{1}{2}\frac{qE}{m}t^2$

(c) Kinetic energy gained by particle, $K = \frac{1}{2}mv^2 = \frac{q^2E^2t^2}{2m}$

If a charged particle is entering the electric field in perpendicular direction.

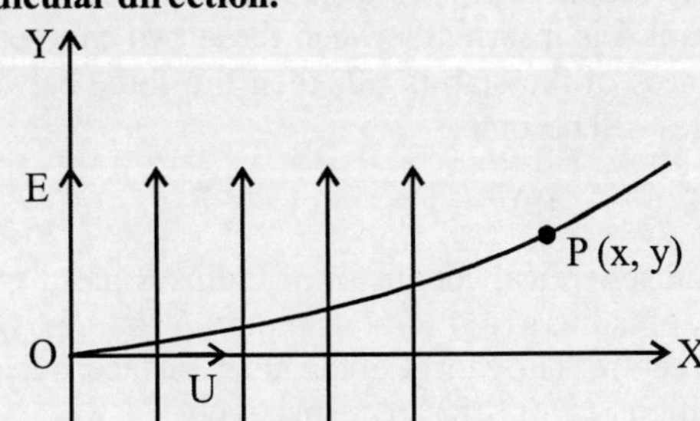

Let $\vec{E} = E\hat{j}$ and the particle enters the field with speed u along x-axis.

Acceleration along Y-axis, $a_y = \frac{qE}{m}$

The initial component of velocity along y-axis is zero. Hence the deflection of the particle along y-axis after time t is

$y = u_y t + \frac{1}{2}.\frac{qE}{m}t^2 = 0 + \frac{1}{2}a_y t^2;$

$\therefore y = \frac{1}{2}.\frac{qE}{m}t^2$ ......(i)

Distance covered by particle in x-axis,

$x = ut$ ...... (ii) ($\because$ acceleration $a_x = 0$)

Eliminating t from equation (i) & (ii),

$$y = \frac{qE}{2m}.\frac{x^2}{u^2} \text{ i.e. } y \propto x^2.$$

This shows that *the path of charged particle in perpendicular field is* ***parabola***.

If the width of the region in which the electric field exists be ℓ then

(i) the particle will leave the field at a distance from its original path in the direction of field, given by

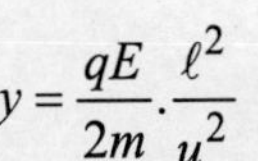

$$y = \frac{qE}{2m}.\frac{\ell^2}{u^2}$$

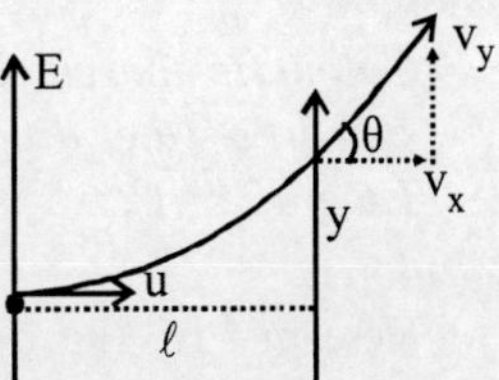

(ii) The particle will leave the region in the direction of the tangent drawn to the parabola at the point of escape.

(iii) The velocity of the particle at the point of escape is given by

$v = \sqrt{v_x^2 + v_y^2}$, where $v_x = u$ and

$v_y = u_y + a_y t = 0 + \frac{qE}{m}t$

$= \frac{qEt}{m} = \frac{qE\ell}{mu} \quad \left(\because t = \frac{\ell}{u}\right)$

$\therefore v = \sqrt{u^2 + \left(\frac{qE\ell}{mu}\right)^2}$

(iv) The direction of the particle in which it leaves the field is given by

$\tan\theta = \frac{v_y}{v_x} = \frac{qE\ell}{mu.u} = \frac{qE\ell}{mu^2} \Rightarrow \theta = \tan^{-1}\left(\frac{qE\ell}{mu^2}\right)$

Example 8.

Point charge q moves from point P to point S along the path PQRS (as shown in fig.) in a uniform electric field E pointing co-parallel to the positive direction of X-axis. The coordinates of the points P, Q, R and S are (a, b, 0), (2 a, 0, 0), (a, –b, 0) and (0, 0, 0) respectively.

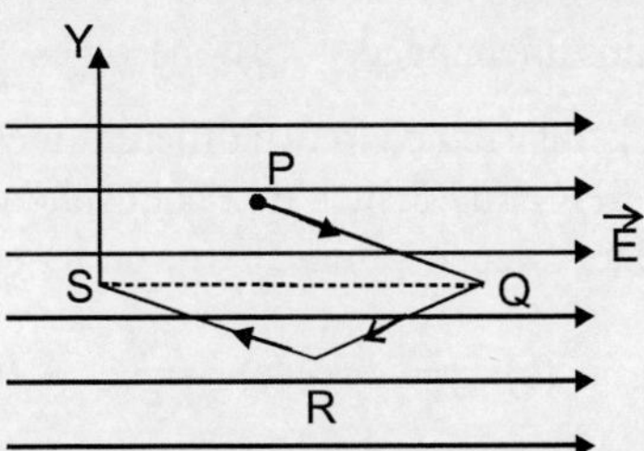

The workdone by the field in the above case is given by the expression

(a) q E A *(b) – q E A*

(c) q E A $\sqrt{2}$ *(d)* $qE\sqrt{[(2a)^2 + b^2]}$

Solution : **(b)**

$W = \vec{F}.\vec{S} = qE\vec{i}.\vec{S}$

Now $W_{P\to Q} = qE\vec{i}\cdot(a\vec{i} + b\vec{j}) = qEa$

$$W_{Q\to R} = qE\vec{i}\cdot(-a\vec{i}+b\vec{j}) = -qEa$$

(workdone against field is taken as negative)

$$W_{R\to S} = qE\vec{i}\cdot(-a\vec{i}+b\vec{j}) = -qEa$$

$$W = W_{P\to Q} + W_{Q+R} + W_{R\to S}$$

$$= qEa - qEa - qEa = -qEa$$

Example 9.

Calculate the electric field strength required to just support a water drop of mass 10^{-7} kg and having charge 1.6×10^{-19} C.

Solution :

Here, $m = 10^{-7}$ kg, $q = 1.6 \times 10^{-19}$ C

Step 1 : Let E be the electric field strength required to support the water drop.

Force acting on the water drop due to electric field E is

$$F = qE = 1.6 \times 10^{-19} E$$

Weight of drop acting downward,

$$W = mg = 10^{-7} \times 9.8 \text{ newton.}$$

Step 2 : Drop will be supported if F and W are equal and opposite.

i.e., $1.6 \times 10^{-19} E = 9.8 \times 10^{-7}$

or $$E = \frac{9.8\times10^{-7}}{1.6\times10^{-19}}$$

$$= 6.125 \times 10^{12} \text{ N C}^{-1}.$$

Example 10.

Can a metal sphere of radius 1cm hold a charge of 1 coulomb.

Solution :

Electric field at the surface of the sphere.

$$E = \frac{KQ}{R^2} = \frac{9\times10^9\times1}{(1\times10^{-2})^2} = 9\times10^{13}\frac{V}{m}$$

This field is much greater than the dielectric strength of air (3×10^6 v/m), the air near the sphere will get ionised and charge will leak out. Thus a sphere of radius 1 cm cannot hold a charge of 1 coulomb in air.

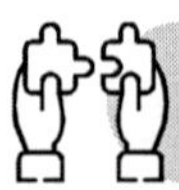

16.1 Concept Practice Problems

CPP

1. Identify the wrong statement in the following. Coulomb's law correctly describes the electric force that
   (a) binds the electrons of an atom to its nucleus
   (b) binds the protons and neutrons in the nucleus of an atom
   (c) binds atoms together to form molecules
   (d) binds atoms and molecules together to form solids
2. Two charges are at a distance d apart. If a copper plate of thickness $\frac{d}{2}$ is kept between them, the effective force will be
   (a) F/2 (b) zero (c) 2F (d) $\sqrt{2}$ F
3. When air is replaced by a dielectric medium of force constant K, the maximum force of attraction between two charges, separated by a distance
   (a) decreases K-times (b) increases K-times
   (c) remains unchanged (d) becomes $\frac{1}{K^2}$ times
4. Charge Q is distributed to two different metallic spheres having radii R and 2R such that both spheres have equal surface charge density, then charge on large sphere is
   (a) $\frac{4Q}{5}$ (b) $\frac{Q}{5}$ (c) $\frac{3Q}{5}$ (d) $\frac{5Q}{4}$
5. Among two discs A and B, first have radius 10 cm and charge 10^{-6} μC and second have radius 30 cm and charge 10^{-5}μC. When they are touched, charge on both q_A and q_B respectively will, be
   (a) $q_A = 2.75\mu C$, $q_B = 3.15\mu C$
   (b) $q_A = 1.09\mu C$, $q_B = 1.53\mu C$
   (c) $q_A = q_B = 5.5\mu C$
   (d) None of these
6. Two particle of equal mass m and charge q are placed at a distance of 16 cm. They do not experience any force. The value of $\frac{q}{m}$ is
   (a) 1 (b) $\sqrt{\frac{\pi\varepsilon_0}{G}}$
   (c) $\sqrt{\frac{G}{4\pi\varepsilon_0}}$ (d) $\sqrt{4\pi\varepsilon_0 G}$
7. Force between two identical charges placed at a distance of r in vacuum is F. Now a slab of dielectric of dielectric contrant 4 is inserted between these two charges. If the thickness of the slab is r/2, then the force between the charges will become
   (a) F (b) $\frac{3}{5}$F (c) $\frac{4}{9}$F (d) $\frac{F}{2}$
8. A solid sphereical conductor of radius R has a spherical cavity of radius a (a < R) at its centre. A charge +Q is kept at the centre. The cahrge at the inner surface, outer and at a position r (a < r < R) are respectively
   (a) +Q, –Q, 0 (b) –Q, +Q, 0
   (c) 0, –Q, 0 (d) +Q, 0, 0
9. A glass rod rubbed with silk is used to charge a gold leaf electroscope and the leaves are observed to diverge. The electroscope thus charged is exposed to X-rays for a short period. Then
   (a) the divergence of leaves will not be affected
   (b) the leaves will diverge further
   (c) the leaves will collapse
   (d) the leaves will melt
10. If a charge q is placed at the centre of the line joining two equal charges Q such that the system is in equilibrium then the value of q is
    (a) Q/2 (b) –Q/2 (c) Q/4 (d) –Q/4

ANSWER KEY																			
1	(b)	2	(b)	3	(a)	4	(a)	5	(c)	6	(d)	7	(c)	8	(b)	9	(b)	10	(d)

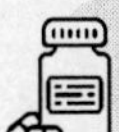

Topic 16.2 : Electric Dipole, Electric Flux and Gauss's Law

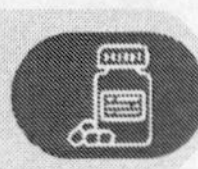

ELECTRIC DIPOLE

Two equal and opposite charges separated by a finite distance constitute an **electric dipole**. If –q and +q are charges at distance 2ℓ apart, then **dipole moment**,

$$p = q \times 2\ell$$

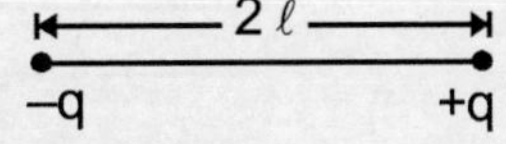

Its **SI unit** is coulomb metre.

Its direction is from –q to +q. It is a vector quantity.

The **torque** τ on a dipole in uniform electric field as shown in figure is given by, $\tau = qE \times 2\ell \sin\theta = \vec{p} \times \vec{E}$

So τ is maximum, when dipole is $\perp$ to field & minimum (=0) when dipole is parallel or antiparallel to field.

If $\vec{p} = p_x\hat{i} + p_y\hat{j} + p_z\hat{k}$ and $\vec{E} = E_x\hat{i} + E_y\hat{j} + E_z\hat{k}$

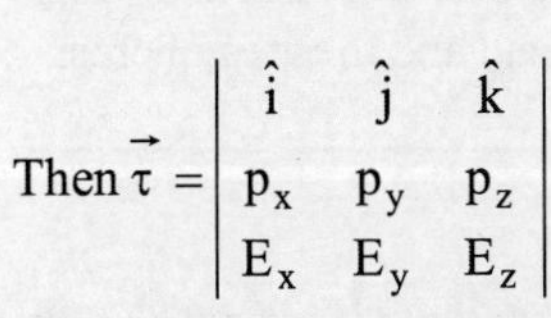

Then $\vec{\tau} = \begin{vmatrix} \hat{i} & \hat{j} & \hat{k} \\ p_x & p_y & p_z \\ E_x & E_y & E_z \end{vmatrix}$

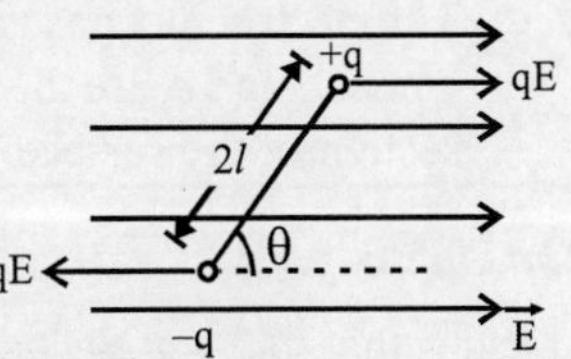

The work done in rotating the dipole from equilibrium through an angle $d\theta$ is given by

$$dW = \tau d\theta = pE\sin\theta\, d\theta$$

and from $\theta_1 \to \theta_2$,

$$W = \int_{\theta_1}^{\theta_2} dW = \int_{\theta_1}^{\theta_2} pE\sin\theta\, d\theta$$

If $\theta_1 = 0$ i.e., equilibrium position, then

$$W = \int_0^{\theta_2} pE\sin\theta d\theta = pE(1 - \cos\theta_2)$$

Workdone in rotating an electric dipole in uniform electric field from θ_1 to θ_2 is $W = pE\,(\cos\theta_1 - \cos\theta_2)$

Potential energy of an electric dipole in an electric field is,

$$U = -\vec{p}.\vec{E} \text{ i.e. } U = -pE\cos\theta$$

where θ is the angle between $\vec{E}$ and $\vec{p}$.

We can also write

$$U = p_xE_x + p_yE_y + p_zE_z$$

Electric Field due to an Electric Dipole

(a) *Along the axial line (or end-on position)*

2l; –q; +q; $\vec{p}$; x; P; $\vec{E}$

$\vec{p}$ and $\vec{E}$ are parallel

$$E_{ax} = \frac{1}{4\pi \epsilon_0} \cdot \frac{2px}{(x^2 - \ell^2)^2} \quad \textit{when } x >> l$$

(b) *Along equatorial line (or broad-side on position)*

$\vec{E}$; $\leftarrow p$; x; –q; ℓ; ℓ; +q

$$E_{eq} = \frac{1}{4\pi \epsilon_0} \cdot \frac{p}{(x^2 + \ell^2)^{3/2}} \quad \text{when } x >> l$$

When $\vec{p}$ and $\vec{E}$ are anti parallel then,

$$E_{ax} = 2E_{eq}$$

(c) *At any point (from the dipole)*

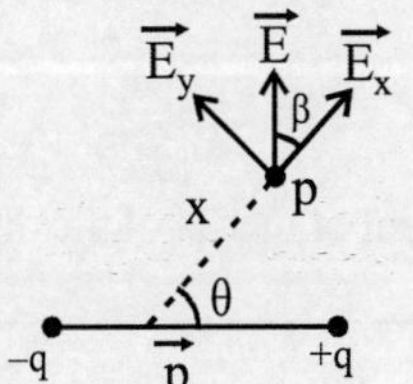

$$E = \frac{1}{4\pi \epsilon_0} \frac{p}{x^3}\sqrt{3\cos^2\theta + 1}\,;\ \tan\beta = \frac{1}{2}\tan\theta$$

Electric field intensity due to a point charge varies inversely as cube of the distance and in case of quadrupole it varies inversely as the fourth power of distance from the quadrupole.

Electric Force between Two Dipoles

The electrostatic force between two dipoles of dipole moments p_1 and p_2 lying at a seperation r is

$$F = \frac{1}{4\pi \epsilon_0} \frac{6p_1p_2}{r^4} \quad \textit{when dipoles are placed co-axially}$$

$$F = \frac{1}{4\pi \epsilon_0} \frac{3p_1p_2}{r^4} \quad \textit{when dipoles are placed perpendicular to each other.}$$

Problem Solving Tips

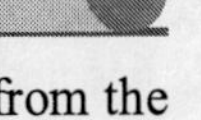

1. The dipole moment of a dipole has a direction from the negative charge to the positive charge.
2. If the separation between the charges of the dipole is increased (or decreased) K-times, the dipole moment increases (or decreases) by K-times.

3. The torque experienced by a dipole placed in a uniform electric field has value always lying between zero and pE, where p is the dipole moment and E, the uniform electric field. It varies directly with the separation between the charges of the dipole.
4. The work done in rotating a dipole in a uniform electric field varies from zero (minimum) to 2pE (maximum). Also, it varies directly with the separation between the charges of the dipole.
5. The potential energy of the dipole in a uniform electric field always lies between +pE and –pE.
6. The electric field intensity at a point due to an electric dipole varies inversely with the cube of the distance of the point from its centre if the distance is much greater than the length of the dipole.
7. The electric field at a point due to a small dipole in end-on position is double of its value in broad side-on position,

   i.e. $E_{\text{End-on}} = 2E_{\text{Broad side-on}}$
8. For a small dipole, the electric field tends from infinity at a point very close to the axis of the dipole to zero at a point at infinity.
9. The force between two dipoles increases (or decreases) by K^4-times as the distance between them decreases (or increases) by K-times.
10. **Time period of a dipole** in uniform electric field is

$$T = 2\pi\sqrt{\frac{I}{pE}}$$

where I = moment of inertia of the dipole about the axis of rotation.

Example 11.

Calculate the electric field intensity due to a dipole of length 10 cm and having a charge of 500 μ C at a point on the axis distant 20 cm from one of the charges in air.

Solution :

Given : $q = 500 \times 10^{-6}$C, a = 10 cm or $a/2 = 5 \times 10^{-2}$ m,

$r = (20 + 5)$ cm $= 25 \times 10^{-2}$ m,

$p = q \times a = (500 \times 10^{-6}) \times (10 \times 10^{-2}) = 5 \times 10^{-5}$ C-m

The electric intensity on the axial line of the dipole is given by

$$E_{\text{axial}} = \frac{1}{4\pi\varepsilon_0} \times \frac{2rp}{\left[r^2 - \left(\frac{a}{2}\right)^2\right]^2}$$

$$E_{\text{axial}} = (9 \times 10^9) \times \frac{2 \times (25 \times 10^{-2}) \times (5 \times 10^{-5})}{10^{-8}[(25)^2 - (5)^2]^2}$$

$$= 3.25 \times 10^7 \text{ NC}^{-1}$$

ELECTRIC FLUX

***Electric flux** is a measure of the number of electric field lines passing through the surface.* If surface is not open & encloses some net charge, then net number of lines that go through the surface is proportional to net charge within the surface.

For uniform electric field when the angle between area vector $\left(\vec{A}\right)$ and electric field $\left(\vec{E}\right)$ has the same value throughout the area, $\phi = \vec{E} \cdot \vec{A} \Rightarrow \phi = EA\cos\theta$

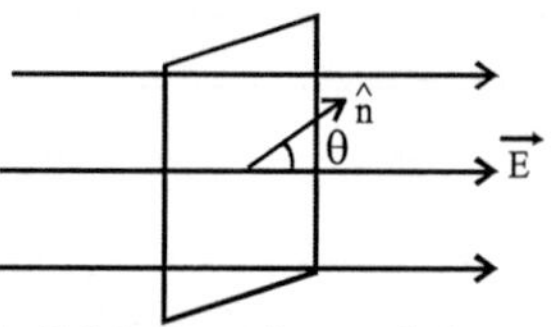

For uniform electric field when the angle between the area vector and electric field is not constant throughout the area

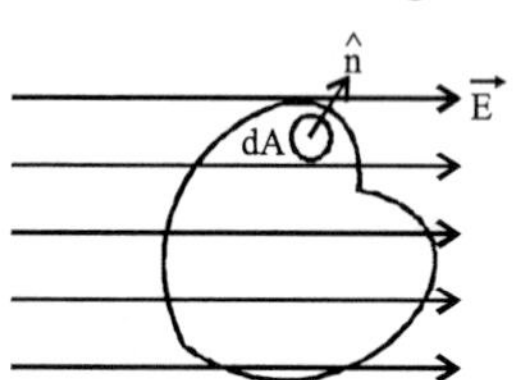

$$d\phi = \vec{E} \cdot \vec{dA} \Rightarrow \phi = \int \vec{E} \cdot \vec{dA} \Rightarrow \phi = \int EdA\cos\theta = E\int dA\cos\theta$$

Problem Solving Tips

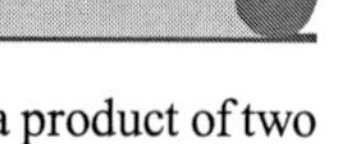

1. The electric flux is a scalar although it is a product of two vectors $\vec{E}$ and $\vec{A}$ (because it is a scalar product of the two).
2. The electric flux has values lying between –EA and +EA, where E and A are the electric field and the area of cross-section of the surface.

GAUSS'S LAW

It states that, *the net electric flux through a closed surface in vacuum is equal to $1/\varepsilon_o$ times the net charge enclosed within the surface.*

i.e., $\varphi = \oint_s \vec{E}.\vec{dA} = \oint \vec{E}.\vec{n}dA = \frac{Q_{in}}{\varepsilon_o}$

where Q_{in} represents the net charge inside the gaussian surface S.

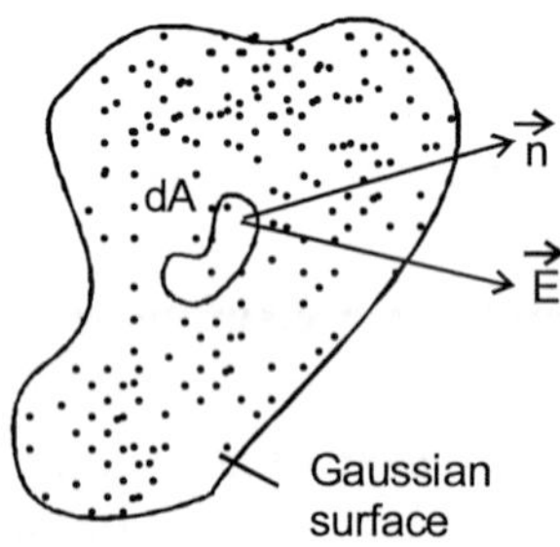

Closed surface of irregular shape which enclosed total charge Q_{in}

In principle, Gauss's law can always be used to calculate the electric field of a system of charges or a continuous distribution of charge. But in practice it is useful only in a limited number of situation, where there is a high degree of symmetry such as spherical, cylindrical etc.

(i) The net electric flux through any closed surface depends only on the charge inside that surface. In the figures, the net flux through S is q_1/ε_o, the net flux through S' is $(q_2 + q_3)/\varepsilon_o$ and the net flux, through S" is zero.

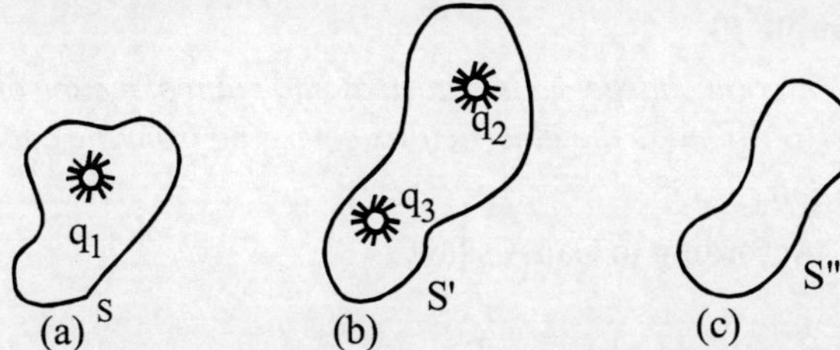

(ii) A point charge Q is located outside a closed surface S. In this case note that the number of lines entering the surface equals to the number of lines leaving the surface. In other words the net flux through a closed surface is zero, if there is no charge inside.

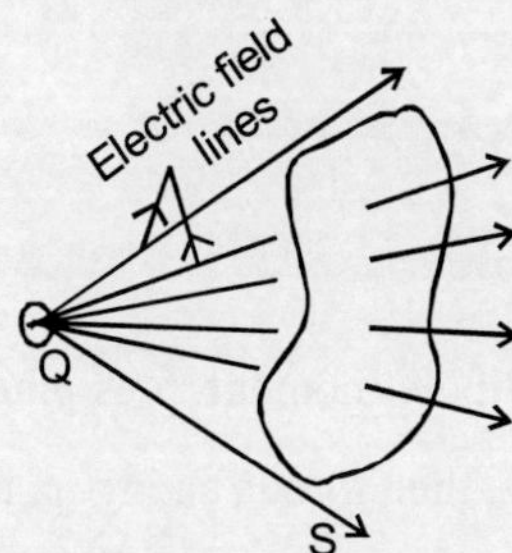

(iii) The net flux across surface A is zero

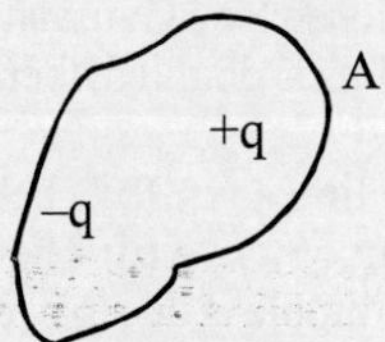

i.e., $\phi = \oint \vec{E}.d\vec{S} = \frac{Q_{in}}{\varepsilon_o} = 0$ because $Q_{in} = -q + q = 0$

Applications of Gauss's Law :

(i) **To determine electric field due to a point charge :**

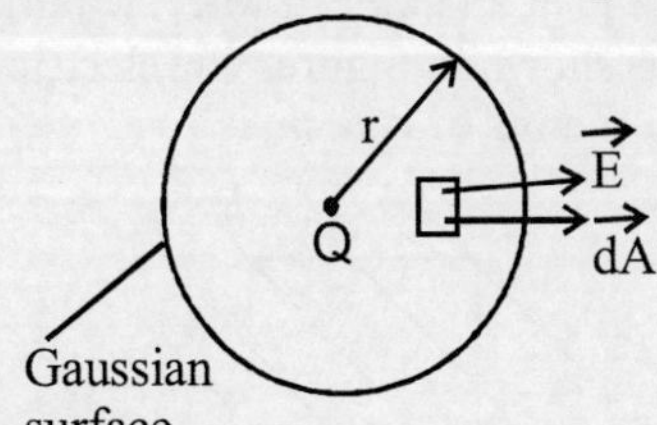

The point charge Q is at the centre of spherical surface shown in figure. Gaussian surface and $\vec{E}$ is parallel to $d\vec{A}$ (direction normal to Gaussian surface) at every point on the Gaussian surface.

so, $\phi_c = \oint \vec{E}.d\vec{A} = \oint EdA = \frac{Q}{\varepsilon_o}$

$$\Rightarrow E = \frac{Q}{4\pi\varepsilon_o r^2} \qquad \left(\because A = 4\pi r^2\right)$$

(ii) **To determine electric field due to a cylindrically symmetric charge distribution :**

We calculate the electric field at a distance r from a uniform positive line charge of infinite length whose charge per unit length is λ = constant. The flux through the plane surfaces of the Gaussian cylinder is zero, since $\vec{E}$ is parallel to the plane of end surface ($\vec{E}$ is perpendicular to $d\vec{A}$). The total charge inside the Gaussian suface is $\lambda\ \ell$, where λ is linear charge density and ℓ is the length of cylinder.

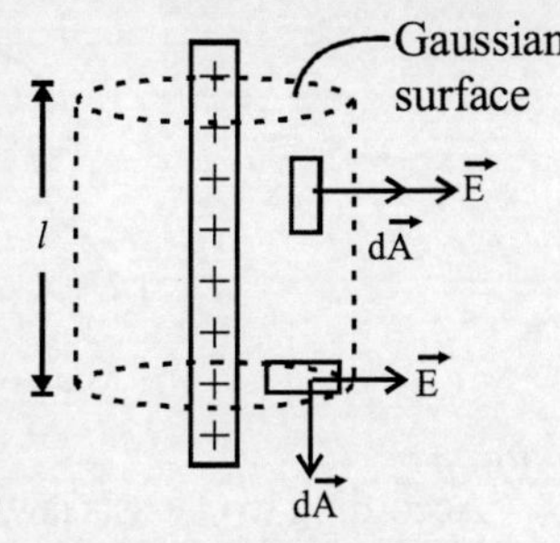

Now applying Gauss's law and noting $\vec{E}$ is parallel to $d\vec{A}$ everywhere on cylindrical surface, we find that

$$\phi_c = \oint_{\substack{\text{Gaussian}\\ \text{surface}}} \vec{E}.d\vec{A} = (\text{flux})_{\text{both ends}} + (\text{flux})_{\text{cylindrical surface}}$$

$$= 0 + E\,.\,2A$$

$$2E\,.\,\pi\, r\, \ell = \frac{Q_{in}}{\varepsilon_o} = \frac{\lambda\ell}{\varepsilon_o} \text{ or } E = \frac{\lambda}{2\pi\varepsilon_o r}$$

Problem Solving Tips

1. The closed imaginary surfaces drawn around a charge are called Gaussian surfaces.
2. If the flux emerging out of a Gaussian surface is zero then it is not necessary that the intensity of electric field is zero.
3. In the Gauss's law,

$$\oint \vec{E}.\,d\vec{A} = \frac{Q_{in}}{\epsilon_0}$$

$\vec{E}$ is the resultant electric field due to all charges lying inside or outside the Gaussian surface, but Q_{in} is the charge lying only inside the surface.

4. The net flux of the electric field through a closed surface due to all the charges lying inside or outside the surface is equal to the flux due to the charges only enclosed by the surface.
5. The electric flux through any closed surface does not depend on the dimensions of the surface but it depends only on the net charge enclosed by the surface.

Example 12.

The following figure shows a surface S which is enclosing –2q charge. The charge +q is kept outside the surface S. Calculate the net outward/ inward flux from the surface S.

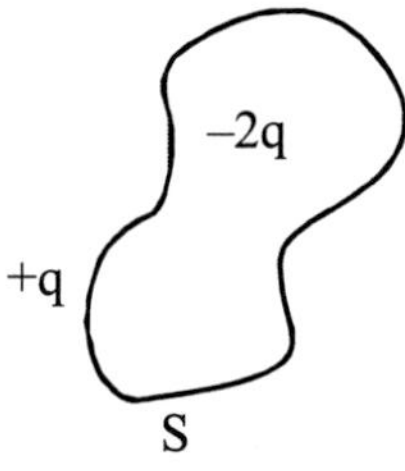

Solution :

According to Gauss's law, the net flux is

$$\phi = \frac{1}{\varepsilon_0} \times \text{net charge enclosed by closed surface} = \frac{-2q}{\varepsilon_0}$$

(Because +q is outside the surface S, so net flux due to +q is zero)

Example 13.

A point charge +q is placed at mid point of a cube of side 'L'. What is the electric flux emerging from the cube ?

Solution :

According to Gauss's law,

$$\phi_{\text{net closed surface}} = \frac{q}{\varepsilon_0}$$

$$= \frac{\text{Net charge enclosed by closed surface}}{\varepsilon_0}$$

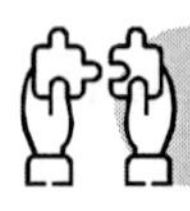

16.2 Concept Practice Problems

CPP

11. What is the angle between the electric dipole moment and the electric field due to it on the axial line?

(a) 0º (b) 90º
(c) 180º (d) None of these

12. In a region of space having a uniform electric field E, a hemispherical bowl of radius r is placed. The electric flux ϕ through the bowl is

(a) $2\pi RE$ (b) $4\pi R^2E$ (c) $2\pi R^2E$ (d) πR^2E

13. A cylinder of radius R and length ℓ is placed in a uniform electric field E parallel to the axis of the cylinder. The total flux over the curved surface of the cylinder is

(a) zero (b) πR^2E (c) $2\pi R^2E$ (d) $E/\pi R^2$

14. An electric dipole when placed in a uniform electric field **E** will have minimum potential energy if the dipole moment makes the following angle with **E**.

(a) π (b) $\pi/2$ (c) zero (d) $3\pi/2$

15. At the centre of a cubical box + Q charge is placed. The value of total flux that is coming out a wall is

(a) Q/ε_0 (b) $Q/3\varepsilon_0$ (c) $Q/4\varepsilon_0$ (d) $Q/6\varepsilon_0$

16. A charge q is placed at the centre of the open end of a cylindrical vessel. The flux of the electric field through the surface of the vessel is

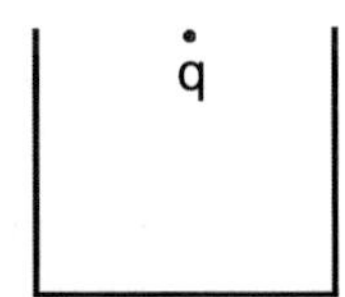

(a) zero (b) q/ε_0 (c) $q/2\varepsilon_0$ (d) $2q/\varepsilon_0$

17. If a dipole of dipole moment $\vec{p}$ is placed in a uniform electric field $\vec{E}$, then torque acting on it is given by

(a) $\vec{\tau} = \vec{p}.\vec{E}$ (b) $\vec{\tau} = \vec{p} \times \vec{E}$
(c) $\vec{\tau} = \vec{p} + \vec{E}$ (d) $\vec{\tau} = \vec{p} - \vec{E}$

18. A charge Q is enclosed by a Gaussian spherical surface of radius R. If the radius is doubled, then the outward electric flux will

(a) increase four times (b) be reduced to half
(c) remain the same (d) be doubled

19. The formation of a dipole is due to two equal and dissimilar point charges placed at a

(a) short distance (b) long distance
(c) above each other (d) none of these

20. A square surface of side *L* meter in the plane of the paper is placed in a uniform electric field *E* (volt/m) acting along the same plane at an angle θ with the horizontal side of the square as shown in Figure. The electric flux linked to the surface, in units of volt. *m*, is

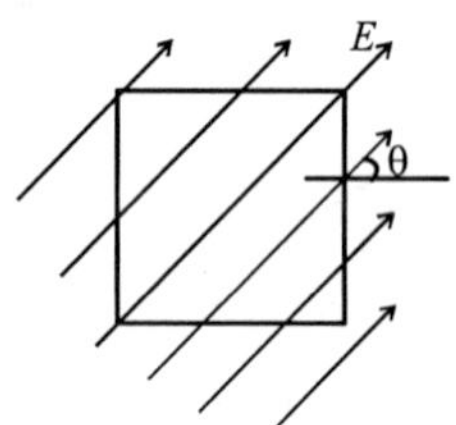

(a) EL^2 (b) $EL^2 \cos\theta$
(c) $EL^2 \sin\theta$ (d) zero

ANSWER KEY

11	(a)	12	(c)	13	(a)	14	(c)	15	(d)	16	(a)	17	(b)	18	(c)	19	(a)	20	(d)

CONCEPT MAP

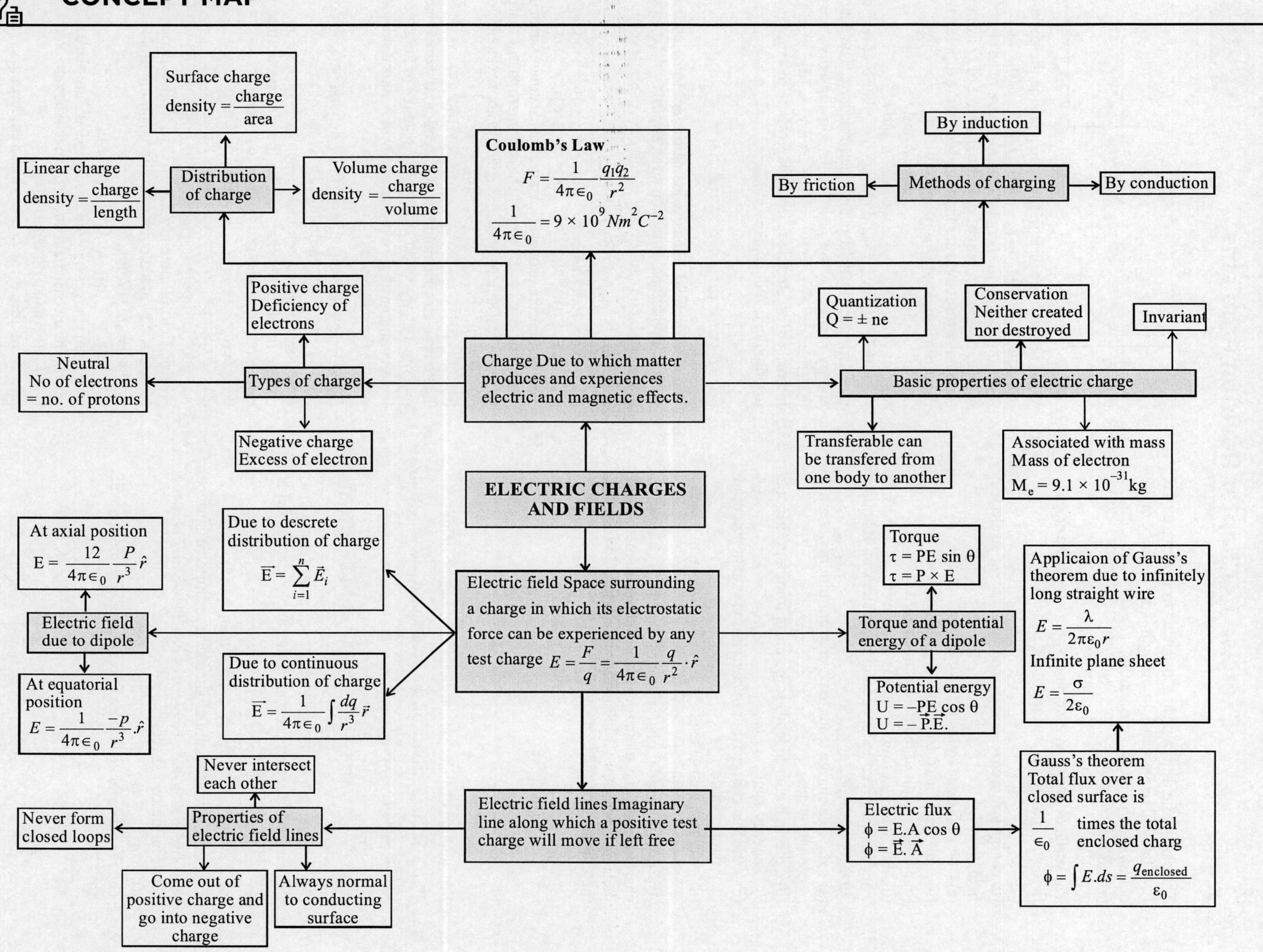
Surface charge density = $\frac{\text{charge}}{\text{area}}$
Linear charge density = $\frac{\text{charge}}{\text{length}}$
Distribution of charge
Volume charge density = $\frac{\text{charge}}{\text{volume}}$
Coulomb's Law
$F = \frac{1}{4\pi\epsilon_0}\frac{q_1q_2}{r^2}$
$\frac{1}{4\pi\epsilon_0} = 9 \times 10^9 Nm^2C^{-2}$
By induction
By friction
Methods of charging
By conduction
Positive charge Deficiency of electrons
Neutral No of electrons = no. of protons
Types of charge
Negative charge Excess of electron
Charge Due to which matter produces and experiences electric and magnetic effects.
Quantization $Q = \pm ne$
Conservation Neither created nor destroyed
Invariant
Basic properties of electric charge
Transferable can be transfered from one body to another
Associated with mass Mass of electron $M_e = 9.1 \times 10^{-31}$ kg
ELECTRIC CHARGES AND FIELDS
At axial position $E = \frac{12}{4\pi\epsilon_0}\frac{P}{r^3}\hat{r}$
Electric field due to dipole
At equatorial position $E = \frac{1}{4\pi\epsilon_0}\frac{-p}{r^3}.\hat{r}$
Due to descrete distribution of charge $\vec{E} = \sum_{i=1}^{n}\vec{E}_i$
Due to continuous distribution of charge $\vec{E} = \frac{1}{4\pi\epsilon_0}\int\frac{dq}{r^3}\vec{r}$
Electric field Space surrounding a charge in which its electrostatic force can be experienced by any test charge $E = \frac{F}{q} = \frac{1}{4\pi\epsilon_0}\frac{q}{r^2}\cdot\hat{r}$
Torque $\tau = PE \sin\theta$ $\tau = P \times E$
Torque and potential energy of a dipole
Potential energy $U = -PE \cos\theta$ $U = -\vec{P}.\vec{E}$.
Applicaion of Gauss's theorem due to infinitely long straight wire $E = \frac{\lambda}{2\pi\varepsilon_0 r}$
Infinite plane sheet $E = \frac{\sigma}{2\varepsilon_0}$
Never intersect each other
Never form closed loops
Properties of electric field lines
Come out of positive charge and go into negative charge
Always normal to conducting surface
Electric field lines Imaginary line along which a positive test charge will move if left free
Electric flux $\phi = E.A \cos\theta$ $\phi = \vec{E}.\vec{A}$
Gauss's theorem Total flux over a closed surface is $\frac{1}{\epsilon_0}$ times the total enclosed charg
$\phi = \int E.ds = \frac{q_{enclosed}}{\varepsilon_0}$

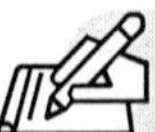

Exercise 1 - Chapter Revision Problems

CRP

1. The electric field strength at a distance r from a charge q is E. What will be electric field strength if the distance of the observation point is increased to 2 r?
(a) E/2 (b) E/4
(c) E/6 (d) None of these

2. The surface density on the copper sphere is σ. The electric field strength on the surface of the sphere is
(a) σ (b) $\sigma/2$ (c) $Q/2\varepsilon_0$ (d) Q/ε_0

3. If a charge is moved against the coulomb force of an electric field, then
(a) work is done by the electric field
(b) energy is used from some outside source
(c) the strength of the field is decreased
(d) the energy of the system is decreased

4. The charge given to any conductor resides on its outer surface, because
(a) the free charge tends to be in its minimum potential energy state
(b) the free charge tends to be in its minimum kinetic energy state
(c) the free charge tends to be in its maximum potential energy state.
(d) the free charge tends to be in its maximum kinetic energy state

5. An infinite parallel plane sheet of a metal is charged to charge density σ coulomb per square metre in a medium of dielectric constant K. Intensity of electric field near the metallic surface will be
(a) $E=\frac{\sigma}{\varepsilon_0 K}$ (b) $E=\frac{\sigma}{2\varepsilon_0}$
(c) $E=\frac{\sigma}{2\varepsilon_0 K}$ (d) $E=\frac{K\sigma}{2\varepsilon_0}$

6. In a medium of dielectric constant K, the electric field is $\vec{E}$. If ϵ_0 is permittivity of the free space, the electric displacement vector is
(a) $\frac{K\vec{E}}{\epsilon_0}$ (b) $\frac{\vec{E}}{K\epsilon_0}$ (c) $\frac{\epsilon_0 \vec{E}}{K}$ (d) $K\epsilon_0 \vec{E}$

7. Two conducting spheres of radii r_1 and r_2 are charged to the same surface charge density. The ratio of electric fields near their surface is
(a) r_1^2/r_2^2 (b) r_2^2/r_1^2 (c) r_1/r_2 (d) 1 : 1

8. Two thin infinite parallel sheets have uniform surface densities of charge $+\sigma$ and $-\sigma$. Electric field in the space between the two sheets is
(a) σ/ε_0 (b) $\sigma/2\varepsilon_0$ (c) $2\sigma/\varepsilon_0$ (d) zero

9. The E-r curve for an infinite linear charge distribution will be

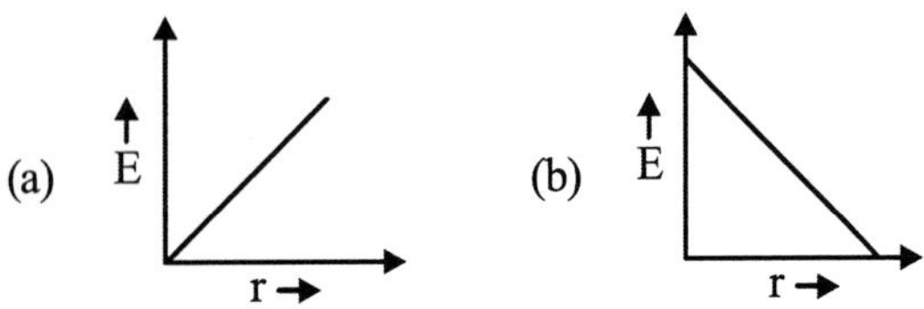

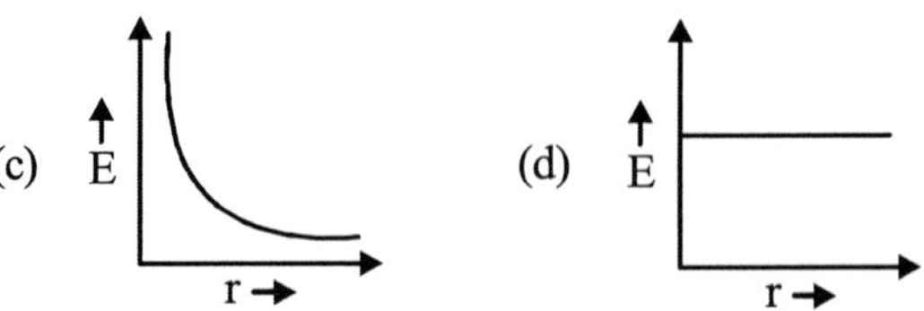

10. What is the value of E in the space outside the sheets?
(a) σ/ε_0 (b) $\sigma/2\varepsilon_0$ (c) $E \neq 0$ (d) $2\sigma/\varepsilon_0$

11. A point Q lies on the perpendicular bisector of an electrical dipole of dipole moment p. If the distance of Q from the dipole is r (much larger than the size of the dipole), then the electric field at Q is proportional to
(a) p^{-1} and r^{-2} (b) p and r^{-2}
(c) p^2 and r^{-3} (d) p and r^{-3}

12. A particle of mass m and charge q is placed at rest in a uniform electric field E and then released. The kinetic energy attained by the particle after moving a distance y is
(a) qEy^2 (b) qE^2y (c) qEy (d) q^2Ey

13. Intensity of an electric field (E) depends on distance r, due to a dipole, is related as
(a) $E \propto \frac{1}{r}$ (b) $E \propto \frac{1}{r^2}$ (c) $E \propto \frac{1}{r^3}$ (d) $E \propto \frac{1}{r^4}$

14. The electric field intensity just sufficient to balance the earth's gravitational attraction on an electron will be: (given mass and charge of an electron respectively are 9.1×10^{-31}kg and 1.6×10^{-19}C.)
(a) -5.6×10^{-11} N/C (b) -4.8×10^{-15} N/C
(c) -1.6×10^{-19} N/C (d) -3.2×10^{-19} N/C

15. The insulation property of air breaks down when the electric field is 3×10^6 Vm^{-1}. The maximum charge that can be given to a sphere of diameter 5 m is approximately
(a) 2×10^{-2} C (b) 2×10^{-3} C
(c) 2×10^{-4} C (d) 2×10^{-5} C

16. There is an electric field E in X-direction. If work done in moving a charge 0.2 C through a distance of 2m along a line making an angle of 60 degree with X-axis is 4.0 joule, what is the value of E?
(a) $\sqrt{3}$ newton per coulomb (b) 4 netwon per coulomb
(c) 5 newton per coulomb (d) None of these

17. A hollow insulated conduction sphere is given a positive charge of 10 μC. What will be the electric field at the centre of the sphere if its radius is 2 metres?
(a) Zero (b) 5 μCm^{-2}
(c) 20 μCm^{-2} (d) 8 μCm^{-2}

18. An electric dipole is placed at an angle of 30° with an electric field of intensity 2×10^5 NC^{-1}, It experiences a torque of 4 Nm. Calculate the charge on the dipole if the dipole length is 2 cm.
(a) 8mC (b) 4mC (c) 8μC (d) 2mC

19. Two point charges q_1 = 4μC and q_2 = 9 μC are placed 20 cm apart. The electric field due to them will be zero on the line joining them at a distance of
(a) 8 cm from q_1 (b) 8 cm form q_2
(c) $\frac{80}{13}$ cm from q_1 (d) $\frac{80}{13}$ cm from q_2

20. Three charge q, Q and 4q are placed in a straight line of length l at points distant 0, $\frac{1}{2}$ and l respectively from one end. In order to make the net froce on q zero, the charge Q must be equal to

(a) –q (b) – 2q (c) $\frac{-q}{2}$ (d) q

21. The spatial distribution of electric field due to charges (A, B) is shown in figure. Which one of the following statements is correct ?

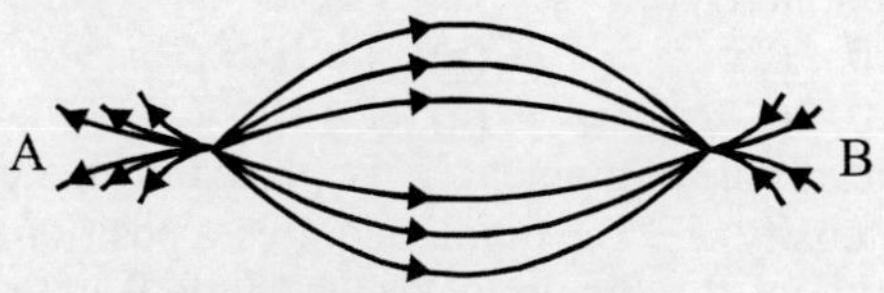

(a) A is +ve and B –ve, |A| > |B|
(b) A is –ve and B +ve, |A| = |B|
(c) Both are +ve but A > B
(d) Both are –ve but A > B

22. ABC is an equilateral triangle. Charges +q are placed at each corner as shown as fig. The electric intensity at centre O will be

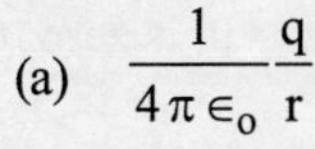

(a) $\frac{1}{4\pi\epsilon_0}\frac{q}{r}$

(b) $\frac{1}{4\pi\epsilon_0}\frac{q}{r^2}$

(c) $\frac{1}{4\pi\epsilon_0}\frac{3q}{r^2}$

(d) zero

23. A simple pendulum has a length ℓ, mass of bob m. The bob is given a charge q. The pendulum is suspended between the vertical plates of the charged parallel plate capacitor. If E is the field strength between the plates, then time period T equal to

(a) $2\pi\sqrt{\frac{\ell}{g}}$

(b) $2\pi\sqrt{\frac{\ell}{g+\frac{qE}{m}}}$

(c) $2\pi\sqrt{\frac{\ell}{g-\frac{qE}{m}}}$

(d) $2\pi\sqrt{\frac{\ell}{\sqrt{g^2+\left(\frac{qE}{m}\right)^2}}}$

24. A metallic sphere is placed in a uniform electric field. The line of force follow the path (s) shown in the figure as

(a) 1
(b) 2
(c) 3
(d) 4

25. A soap bubble is given negative charge, its radius will
(a) increase (b) decrease
(c) remain unchanged (d) fluctuate

26. A and B are two identically spherical charged bodies which repel each other with force F, kept at a finite distance. A third uncharged sphere of the same size is brought in contact with sphere B and removed. It is then kept at mid point of A and B. Find the magnitude of force on C.

(a) $\frac{F}{2}$ (b) $\frac{F}{8}$ (c) F (d) Zero

27. There exists a non-uniform electric field along x-axis as shown in the figure below. The field increases at a uniform rate along +ve x-axis. A dipole is placed inside the field as shown. Which one of the following is correct for the dipole?

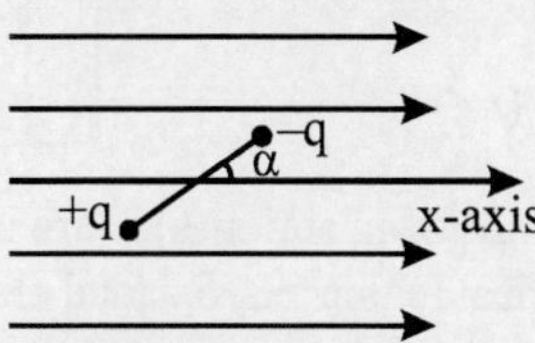

(a) Dipole moves along positive x-axis and undergoes a clockwise rotation
(b) Dipole moves along negative x-axis and undergoes a clockwise rotation
(c) Dipole moves along positive x-axis and undergoes a anticlockwise rotation
(d) Dipole moves along negative x-axis and undergoes a anticlockwise rotation

28. The electric dipole is situated is an electric field as shown in fig 1. The dipole and electric field are both in the plane of the paper. The dipole is rotated about an axis perpendicular to plane of paper passing through A in anticlockwise direction. If the angle of rotation (θ) is measured with respect to the direction of electric field, then the torque (τ) experienced by the dipole for different values of the angle of rotation θ will be represented in fig. 2, by

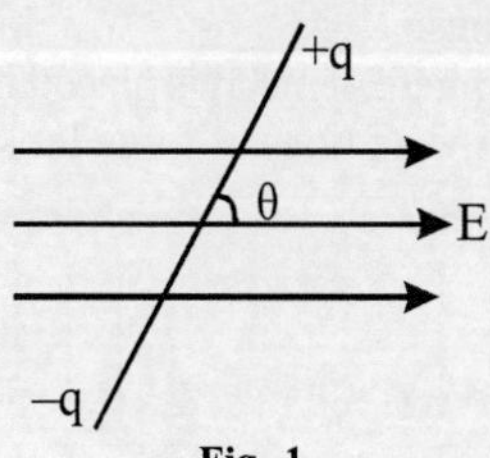

Fig. 1

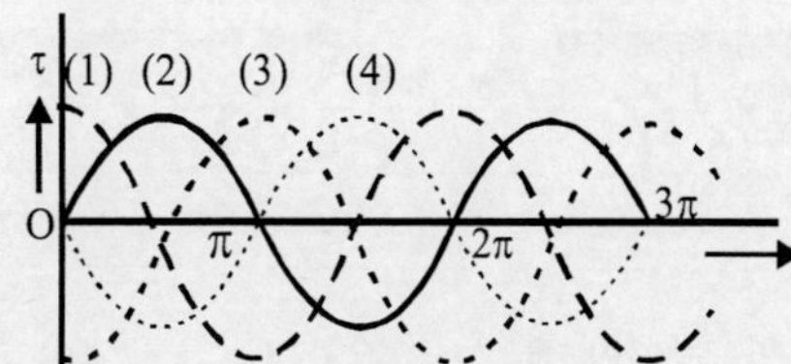

Fig. 2

(a) curve (1) (b) curve (2)
(c) curve (3) (d) curve (4)

29. A charge +q is at a distance L/2 above a square of side L. Then what is the flux linked with the surface?

(a) $\frac{q}{4\varepsilon_0}$ (b) $\frac{2q}{3\varepsilon_0}$ (c) $\frac{q}{6\varepsilon_0}$ (d) $\frac{6q}{\varepsilon_0}$

30. Positive and negative point charges of equal magnitude are kept at $\left(0, 0, \frac{a}{2}\right)$ and $\left(0, 0, \frac{-a}{2}\right)$ respectively. The work done by the electric field when another positive point charge is moved from (–a, 0, 0) to (0, a, 0) is
(a) positive (b) negative
(c) zero
(d) depends on the path connecting the initial and final positions

31. The electrostatic potential (ϕ_r) of a spherical symmetric system kept at origin, is shown in the figure, and given as

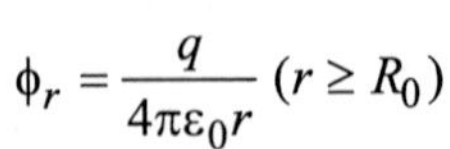

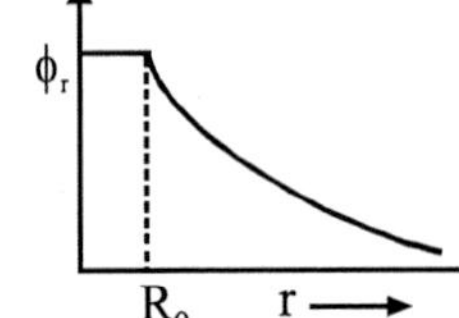

$$\phi_r = \frac{q}{4\pi\varepsilon_0 R_0} \; (r \le R_0)$$

Which of the following option(s) is/are incorrect
(a) For spherical region $r \le R_0$ total electrostatic energy stored is zero
(b) Within $r = 2R_0$ total charge is q.
(c) There will be no charge anywhere except at $r = R_0$
(d) None of these

32. A solid conducting sphere of radius a has a net positive charge 2Q. A conducting spherical shell of inner radius b and outer radius c is concentric with the solid sphere and has a net charge – Q. The surface charge density on the inner and outer surfaces of the spherical shell will be

(a) $-\frac{2Q}{4\pi b^2}, \frac{Q}{4\pi c^2}$

(b) 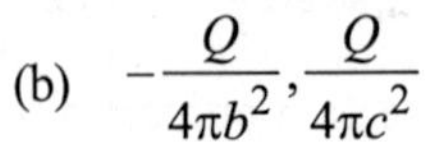

(c) 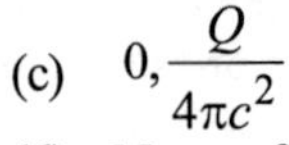

(d) None of these

33. An uncharged sphere of metal is placed in between charged plates as shown. The lines of force look like

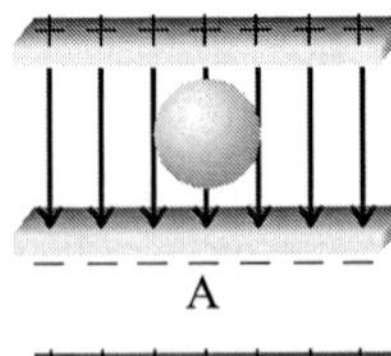

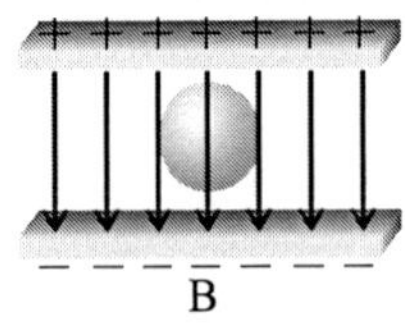

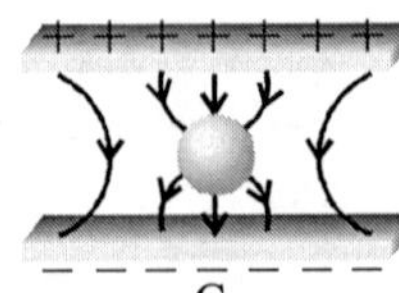

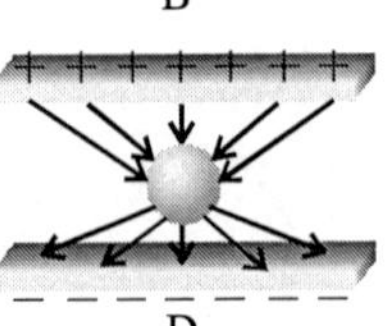

(a) A (b) B (c) C (d) D

34. The electric intensity due to a dipole of length 10 cm and having a charge of 500 μC, at a point on the axis at a distance 20 cm from one of the charges in air, is
(a) 6.25×10^7 N/C (b) 9.28×10^7 N/C
(c) 13.1×10^{11} N/C (d) 20.5×10^7 N/C

35. Two positive ions, each carrying a charge q, are separated by a distance d. If F is the force of repulsion between the ions, the number of electrons missing from each ion will be (e being the charge of an electron)

(a) $\frac{4\pi\varepsilon_0 Fd^2}{e^2}$ (b) $\sqrt{\frac{4\pi\varepsilon_0 Fe^2}{d^2}}$

(c) $\sqrt{\frac{4\pi\varepsilon_0 Fd^2}{e^2}}$ (d) $\frac{4\pi\varepsilon_0 Fd^2}{q^2}$

36. Two metallic spheres of radii 1 cm and 3 cm are given charges of -1×10^{-2} C and 5×10^{-2} C, respectively. If these are connected by a conducting wire, the final charge on the bigger sphere is
(a) 2×10^{-2} C (b) 3×10^{-2} C
(c) 4×10^{-2} C (d) 1×10^{-2} C

37. An electric dipole of moment $'p'$ is placed in an electric field of intensity $'E'$. The dipole acquires a position such that the axis of the dipole makes an angle θ with the direction of the field. Assuming that the potential energy of the dipole to be zero when = 90°, the torque and the potential energy of the dipole will respectively be
(a) $pE\sin\theta, -pE\cos\theta$ (b) $pE\sin\theta, -2pE\cos\theta$
(c) $pE\sin\theta, 2pE\cos\theta$ (d) $pE\cos\theta, -pE\cos\theta$

38. Three charges + Q, q, + Q are placed respectively, at distance, d/2 and d from the origin, on the x-axis. If the net force experienced by + Q, placed at $x = 0$, is zero, then value of q is:
(a) –Q/4 (b) +Q/2 (c) +Q/4 (d) –Q/2

39. Charges Q_1 and Q_2 are at points A and B of a right angle triangle OAB (see figure). The resultant electric field at point O is perpendicular to the hypotenuse, then Q_1/Q_2 is proportional to :

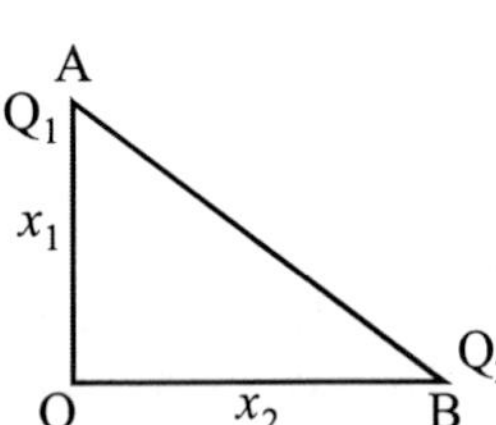

(a) $\frac{x_1^3}{x_2^3}$ (b) $\frac{x_2}{x_1}$ (c) $\frac{x_1}{x_2}$ (d) $\frac{x_2^2}{x_1^2}$

40. Consider the force F on a charge 'q' due to a uniformly charged spherical shell of radius R carrying charge Q distributed uniformly over it. Which one of the following statements is true for F, if 'q' is placed at distance r from the centre of the shell?

(a) $F = \frac{1}{4\pi\varepsilon_0}\frac{Qq}{R^2}$ for $r<R$ (b) $\frac{1}{4\pi\varepsilon_0}\frac{Qq}{R^2} > F > 0$ for $r<R$

(c) $F = \frac{1}{4\pi\varepsilon_0}\frac{Qq}{R^2}$ for $r>R$ (d) $F = \frac{1}{4\pi\varepsilon_0}\frac{Qq}{R^2}$ for all r

41. Two charged thin infinite plane sheets of uniform surface charge density σ_+ and σ_-, where $|\sigma_+| > |\sigma_-|$, intersect at right angle. Which of the following best represents the electric field lines for this system ?

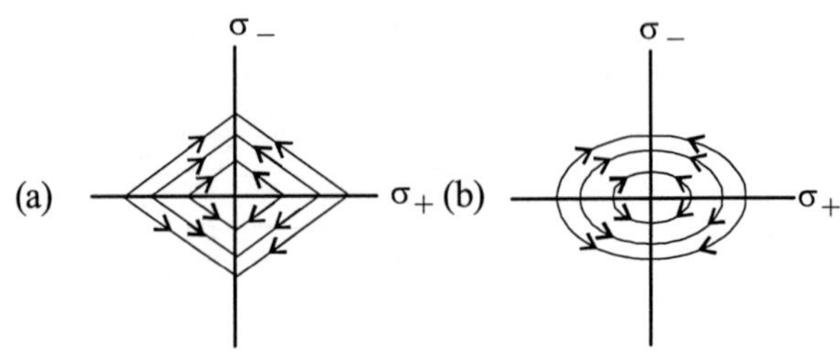

(c) (d)

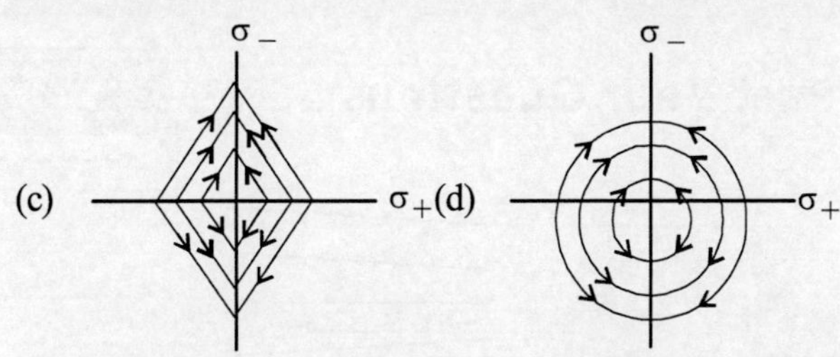

42. A particle of charge q and mass m is subjected to an electric field $E = E_0(1 - ax^2)$ in the x-direction, where a and E_0 are constants. Initially the particle was at rest at $x = 0$. Other than the initial position the kinetic energy of the particle becomes zero when the distance of the particle from the origin is :

(a) a (b) $\sqrt{\frac{2}{a}}$ (c) $\sqrt{\frac{3}{a}}$ (d) $\sqrt{\frac{1}{a}}$

43. A charged particle (mass m and charge q) moves along X axis with velocity V_0. When it passes through the origin it enters a region having uniform electric field $\vec{E} = -E\hat{j}$ which extends upto $x = d$. Equation of path of electron in the region $x > d$ is :

Y, $\vec{E}$, O, X, V_0, d

(a) $y = \frac{qEd}{mV_0^2}(x - d)$ (b) $y = \frac{qEd}{mV_0^2}\left(\frac{d}{2} - x\right)$

(c) $y = \frac{qEd}{mV_0^2}x$ (d) $y = \frac{qEd^2}{mV_0^2}x$

44. A small point mass carrying some positive charge on it, is released from the edge of a table. There is a uniform electric field in this region in the horizontal direction. Which of the following options then correctly describe the trajectory of the mass ? (Curves are drawn schematically and are not to scale).

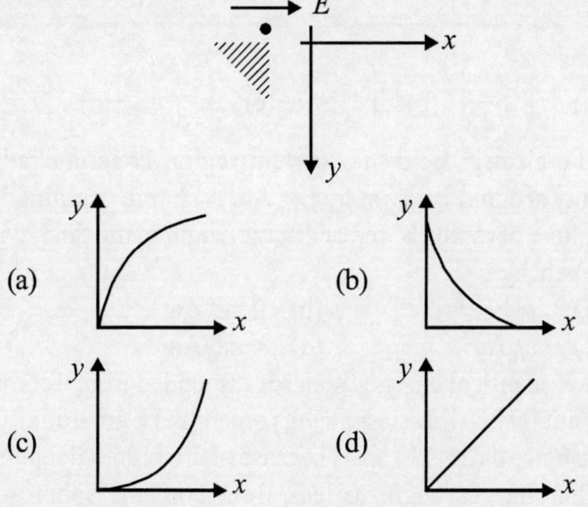

45. An electric dipole of moment $\vec{p} = (\hat{i} - 3\hat{j} + 2\hat{k}) \times 10^{-29}$ C.m is at the origin (0, 0, 0). The electric field due to this dipole at $\vec{r} = +\hat{i} + 3\hat{j} + 5\hat{k}$

(note that $\vec{r}.\vec{p} = 0$) is parallel to:

(a) $(+\hat{i} - 3\hat{j} - 2\hat{k})$ (b) $(-\hat{i} + 3\hat{j} - 2\hat{k})$

(c) $(+\hat{i} + 3\hat{j} - 2\hat{k})$ (d) $(-\hat{i} - 3\hat{j} + 2\hat{k})$

46. A particle of mass m and charge q is released from rest in a uniform electric field. If there is no other force on the particle, the dependence of its speed v on the distance x travelled by it is correctly given by (graphs are schematic and not drawn to scale)

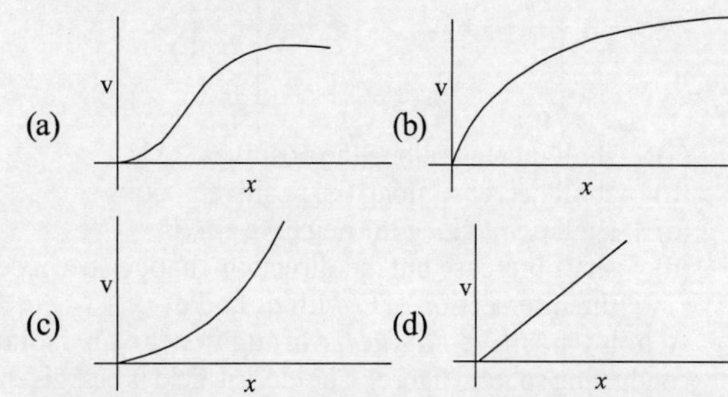

47. A particle of mass m and charge q has an initial velocity $\vec{v} = v_0\hat{j}$. If an electric field $\vec{E} = E_0\hat{i}$ and magnetic field $\vec{B} = B_0\hat{i}$ act on the particle, its speed will double after a time:

(a) $\frac{2mv_0}{qE_0}$ (b) $\frac{3mv_0}{qE_0}$ (c) $\frac{\sqrt{3}mv_0}{qE_0}$ (d) $\frac{\sqrt{2}mv_0}{qE_0}$

48. Four point charges $-q, +q, +q$ and $-q$ are placed on y-axis at $y = -2d$, $y = -d$, $y = +d$ and $y = +2d$, respectively. The magnitude of the electric field E at a point on the x-axis at $x = D$, with $D >> d$, will behave as:

(a) $E \propto \frac{1}{D^3}$ (b) $E \propto \frac{1}{D}$

(c) $E \propto \frac{1}{D^4}$ (d) $E \propto \frac{1}{D^2}$

49. The bob of a simple pendulum has mass 2 g and a charge of 5.0 ¼C. It is at rest in a uniform horizontal electric field of intensity 2000 V/m. At equilibrium, the angle that the pendulum makes with the vertical is :
(take $g = 10$ m/s²)

(a) $\tan^{-1}(2.0)$ (b) $\tan^{-1}(0.2)$

(c) $\tan^{-1}(5.0)$ (d) $\tan^{-1}(0.5)$

50. Two point charges q_1 ($\sqrt{10}$ μC) and q_2 (– 25 μC) are placed on the x-axis at $x = 1$ m and $x = 4$ m respectively. The electric field (in V/m) at a point $y = 3$ m on y-axis is,

$$\left[\text{take } \frac{1}{4\pi \epsilon_0} = 9 \times 10^9 \text{ Nm}^2\text{C}^{-2}\right]$$

(a) $(63\hat{i} - 27\hat{j}) \times 10^2$ (b) $(-63\hat{i} + 27\hat{j}) \times 10^2$

(c) $(81\hat{i} - 81\hat{j}) \times 10^2$ (d) $(-81\hat{i} + 81\hat{j}) \times 10^2$

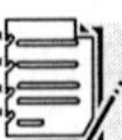

Exercise 2 - Exemplar & Past Year Questions

E&PYQs

Exemplar Questions

1. In figure two positive charges q_2 and q_3 fixed along the y-axis, exert a net electric force in the + x-direction on a charge q_1 fixed along the x-axis. If a positive charge Q is added at (x, 0), the force on q_1

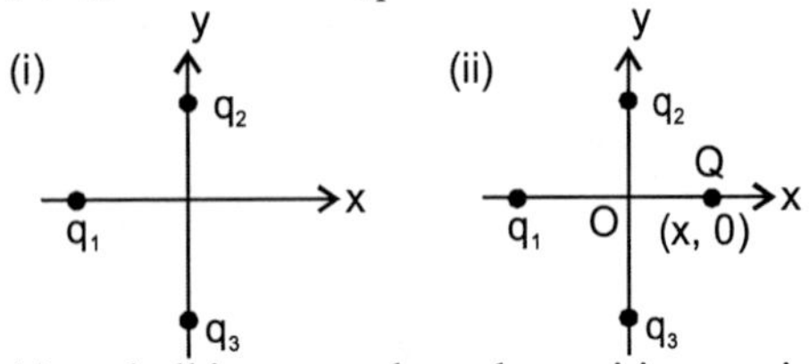

(a) shall increase along the positive x-axis
(b) shall decrease along the positive x-axis
(c) shall point along the negative x-axis
(d) shall increase but the direction changes because of the intersection of Q with q_2 and q_3

2. A point positive charge is brought near an isolated conducting sphere (figure). The electric field is best given by

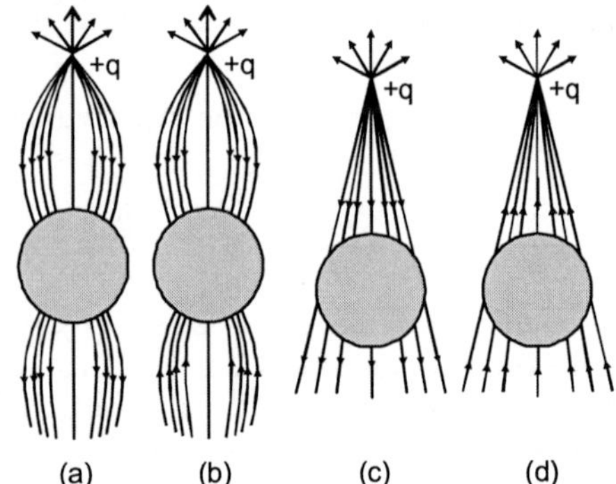

3. The electric flux through the surface

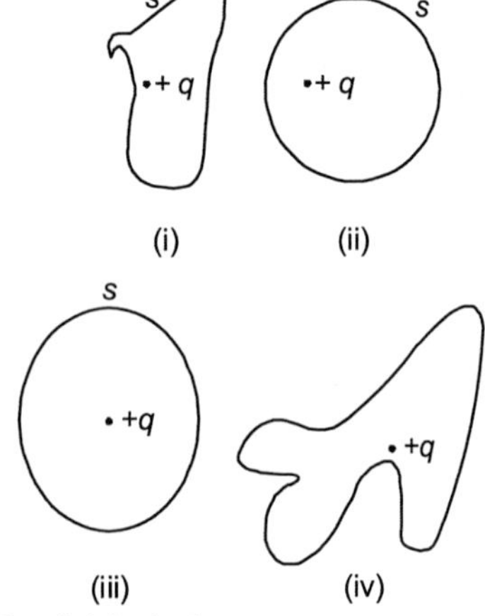

(a) in Fig. (iv) is the largest
(b) in Fig. (iii) is the least
(c) in Fig. (ii) is same as Fig. (iii) but is smaller than Fig. (iv)
(d) is the same for all the figures

4. Figure shows electric field lines in which an electric dipole P is placed as shown. Which of the following statements is correct?

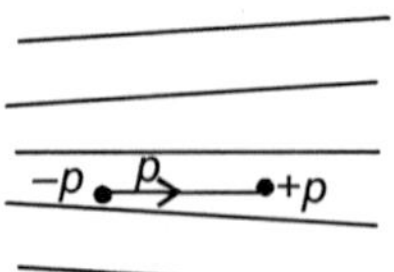

(a) The dipole will not experience any force
(b) The dipole will experience a force towards right
(c) The dipole will experience a force towards left
(d) The dipole will experience a force upwards

5. A point charge + q is placed at a distance d from an isolated conducting plane. The field at a point P on the other side of the plane is
(a) directed perpendicular to the plane and away from the plane
(b) directed perpendicular to the plane but towards the plane
(c) directed radially away from the point charge
(d) directed radially towards the point charge.

6. A hemisphere is uniformely charged positively. The electric field at a point on a diameter away from the centre is directed
(a) perpendicular to the diameter
(b) parallel to the diameter
(c) at an angle tilted towards the diameter
(d) at an angle tilted away from the diameter

NEET/AIPMT (2013-2020) Questions

7. Two pith balls carrying equal charges are suspended from a common point by strings of equal length. The equilibrium separation between them is r. Now the strings are rigidly clamped at half the height. The equilibrium separation between the balls now become **[2013]**

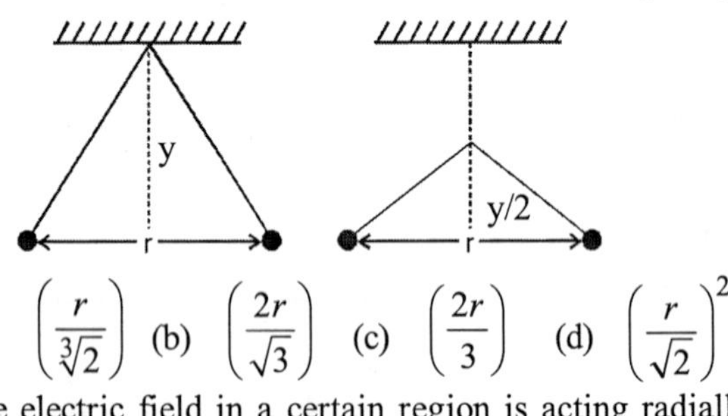

(a) $\left(\frac{r}{\sqrt[3]{2}}\right)$ (b) $\left(\frac{2r}{\sqrt{3}}\right)$ (c) $\left(\frac{2r}{3}\right)$ (d) $\left(\frac{r}{\sqrt{2}}\right)^2$

8. The electric field in a certain region is acting radially outward and is given by E = Aa. A charge contained in a sphere of radius 'a' centred at the origin of the field, will be given by **[2015]**
(a) $A\,\varepsilon_0\,a^2$ (b) $4\,\pi\varepsilon_0\,Aa^3$
(c) $\varepsilon_0\,Aa^3$ (d) $4\,\pi\varepsilon_0\,Aa^2$

9. Two identical charged spheres suspended from a common point by two massless strings of lengths l, are initially at a distance d (d << l) apart because of their mutual repulsion. The charges begin to leak from both the spheres at a constant rate. As a result, the spheres approach each other with a velocity v. Then v varies as a function of the distance x between the spheres, as : **[2016]**

(a) $v \propto x^{\frac{1}{2}}$ (b) $v \propto x$

(c) $v \propto x^{-\frac{1}{2}}$ (d) $v \propto x^{-1}$

10. Suppose the charge of a proton and an electron differ slightly. One of them is – e, the other is (e + Δe). If the net of electrostatic force and gravitational force between two hydrogen atoms placed at a distance d (much greater than atomic size) apart is zero, then Δe is of the order of [Given mass of hydrogen $m_h = 1.67 \times 10^{-27}$ kg] ***[2017]***

(a) 10^{-23}C (b) 10^{-37} C (c) 10^{-47} C (d) 10^{-20} C

11. An electron falls from rest through a vertical distance h in a uniform and vertically upward directed electric field E. The direction of electric field is now reversed, keeping its magnitude the same. A proton is allowed to fall from rest in it through the same vertical distance h. The time of fall of the electron, in comparison to the time of fall of the proton is ***[2018]***

(a) smaller (b) 5 times greater
(c) equal (d) 10 times greater

12. Two point charges A and B, having charges +Q and –Q respectively, are placed at certain distance apart and force acting between them is F. If 25% charge of A is transferred to B, then force between the charges becomes : ***[2019]***

(a) F (b) $\frac{9F}{16}$ (c) $\frac{16F}{9}$ (d) $\frac{4F}{3}$

13. Two parallel infinite line charges with linear charge densities +λ C/m and –λ C/m are placed at a distance of 2R in free space. What is the electric field mid-way between the two line charges? ***[2019]***

(a) zero (b) $\frac{2\lambda}{\pi \epsilon_0 R}$ N/C

(c) $\frac{\lambda}{\pi \epsilon_0 R}$ N/C (d) $\frac{\lambda}{2\pi\varepsilon_0 R}$ N/C

14. A hollow metal sphere of radius R is uniformly charged. The electric field due to the sphere at a distance r from the centre : ***[2019]***

(a) increases as r increases for r < R and for r > R
(b) zero as r increases for r < R, decreases as r increases for r > R
(c) zero as r increases for r < R, increases as r increases for r > R
(d) decreases as r increases for r < R and for r > R

15. A sphere encloses an electric dipole with charges $\pm 3 \times 10^{-6}$ C. What is the total electric flux across the sphere? ***[NEET Odisha 2019]***

(a) 6×10^{-6} Nm²/C (b) -3×10^{-6} Nm²/C
(c) Zero (d) 3×10^{-6} Nm²/C

16. A spherical conductor of radius 10 cm has a charge of 3.2×10^{-7} C distributed uniformly. What is the magnitude of electric field at a point 15 cm from the centre of the sphere? ***[2020]***

$\left(\frac{1}{4\pi \epsilon_0} = 9 \times 10^9 \text{ Nm}^2/\text{C}^2\right)$

(a) 1.28×10^5 N/C (b) 1.28×10^6 N/C
(c) 1.28×10^7 N/C (d) 1.28×10^4 N/C

Exercise 3 - Concept Application Problems CAP

1. If electric field in a region is radially outward with magnitude E = Ar, the charge contained in a sphere of radius r centred at the origin is

(a) $\frac{1}{4\pi\varepsilon_o} A r^3$ (b) $4\pi\varepsilon_o A r^3$

(c) $\frac{1}{4\pi\varepsilon_o}\frac{A}{r^3}$ (d) $\frac{4\pi\varepsilon_o A}{r^3}$

2. An electric dipole has the magnitude of its charge as q and its dipole moment is p. It is placed in uniform electric field E. If its dipole moment is along the direction of the field, the force on it and its potential energy are respectively.

(a) q.E and max. (b) 2 q.E and min.
(c) q.E and min (d) zero and min.

3. If the dipole of moment 2.57×10^{-17} cm is placed into an electric field of magnitude 3.0×10^4 N/C such that the fields lines are aligned at 30° with the line joining P to the dipole, what torque acts on the dipole?

(a) 7.7×10^{-13} Nm (b) 3.855×10^{-13} Nm
(c) 3.855×10^{-15} Nm (d) 7.7×10^{-15} Nm

4. A drop of oil of density ρ and radius r carries a charge q when placed in an electric field E, it moves upwards with a velocity v. If ρ_0 is the density of air, η be the viscosity of the air, then which of the following force is directed upwards?

(a) qE (b) 6πηrv

(c) $\frac{4}{3}\pi r^3(\rho - \rho_0)g$ (d) None of these

5. An electric dipole is placed along the x-axis at the origin O. A point P is at a distance of 20 cm from this origin such that OP makes an angle π/3 with the x-axis. If the electric field at P makes an angle θ with the x-axis, the value of θ would be

(a) $\frac{\pi}{3}$ (b) $\frac{\pi}{3} + \tan^{-1}\left(\frac{\sqrt{3}}{2}\right)$

(c) $\frac{2\pi}{3}$ (d) $\tan^{-1}\left(\frac{\sqrt{3}}{2}\right)$

6. Two identical thin rings, each of radius a meter, are coaxially placed at a distance R meter apart. If Q_1 coulomb and Q_2 coulomb are respectively the charges uniformly spread on the two rings, the work done in moving a charge q coulomb from the centre of one ring to that of the other is

(a) Zero (b) $\frac{q(Q_1 - Q_2)(\sqrt{2}-1)}{4\sqrt{2}\pi\varepsilon_0 a}$

(c) $\frac{q\sqrt{2}(Q_1+Q_2)}{4\pi\varepsilon_0 a}$ (d) $\frac{q(Q_1+Q_2)(\sqrt{2}+1)}{4\sqrt{2}\pi\varepsilon_0 a}$

7. An electric dipole of moment $\vec{P}$ is placed in a uniform electric field $\vec{E}$ such that $\vec{P}$ points along $\vec{E}$. If the dipole is slightly rotated about an axis perpendicular to the plane containing $\vec{E}$ and $\vec{P}$ and passing through the centre of the dipole, the dipole executes simple harmonic motion. Consider I to be the moment of inertia of the dipole about the axis of rotation. What is the time period of such oscillation?
(a) $\sqrt{(pE/I)}$ (b) $2\pi\sqrt{(I/pE)}$
(c) $2\pi\sqrt{(I/2pE)}$ (d) None of these

8. A short electric dipole of dipole moment $\vec{p}$ is placed at a distance r from the centre of a solid metallic sphere of radius a (<< r) as shown in the figure. The electric field intensity at the centre of sphere C due to induced charge on the sphere is

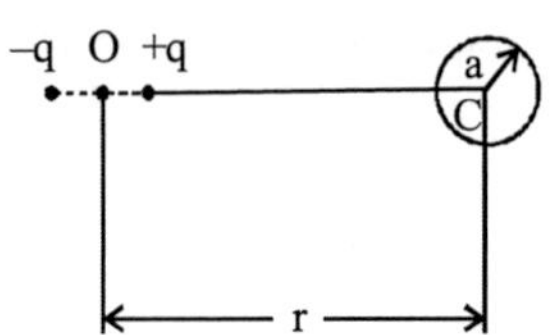

(a) zero (b) $\frac{1}{4\pi\varepsilon_0}\frac{2p}{r^3}$ along CO
(c) $\frac{1}{4\pi\varepsilon_0}\frac{2p}{r^3}$ along OC (d) $\frac{1}{4\pi\varepsilon_0}\frac{p}{r^3}$ along CO

9. Two pith balls carrying equal charges are suspended from a common point by strings of equal length. The equilibrium separation between them is r. Now the strings are rigidly clamped at half the height. The equilibrium separation between the balls now become

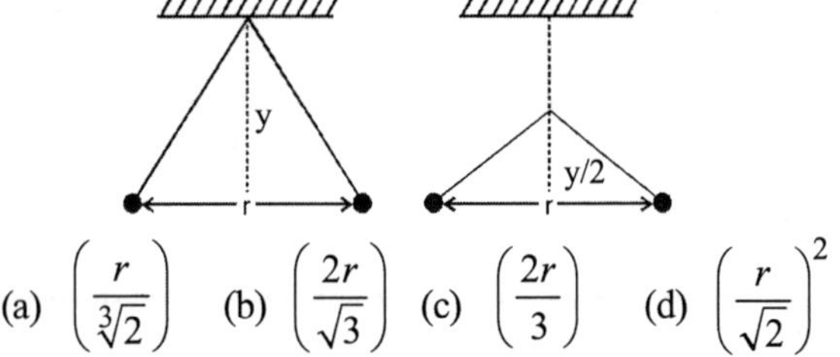

(a) $\left(\frac{r}{\sqrt[3]{2}}\right)$ (b) $\left(\frac{2r}{\sqrt{3}}\right)$ (c) $\left(\frac{2r}{3}\right)$ (d) $\left(\frac{r}{\sqrt{2}}\right)^2$

10. Charge is distributed within a sphere of radius R with a volume charge density $p(r) = \frac{A}{r^2}e^{-2r/a}$ where A and a are constants. If Q is the total charge of this charge distribution, the radius R is:

(a) $a\log\left(1-\frac{Q}{2\pi aA}\right)$ (b) $\frac{a}{2}\log\left(\frac{1}{1-\frac{Q}{2\pi aA}}\right)$

(c) $a\log\left(\frac{1}{1-\frac{Q}{2\pi aA}}\right)$ (d) $\frac{a}{2}\log\left(1-\frac{Q}{2\pi aA}\right)$

11. Two identical conducting spheres A and B, carry equal charge. They are separated by a distance much larger than their diameter, and the force between them is F. A third identical conducting sphere, C, is uncharged. Sphere C is first touched to A, then to B, and then removed. As a result, the force between A and B would be equal to
(a) $\frac{3F}{4}$ (b) $\frac{F}{2}$ (c) F (d) $\frac{3F}{8}$

12. Two balls of same mass and carrying equal charge are hung from a fixed support of length l. At electrostatic equilibrium, assuming that angles made by each thread is small, the separation, x between the balls is proportional to :
(a) l (b) l^2 (c) $l^{2/3}$ (d) $l^{1/3}$

13. Consider a sphere of radius R which carries a uniform charge density ρ. If a sphere of radius $\frac{R}{2}$ is carved out of it, as shown, the ratio $\frac{|\vec{E}_A|}{|\vec{E}_B|}$ of magnitude of electric field $\vec{E}_A$ and $\vec{E}_B$, respectively, at points A and B due to the remaining portion is:
(a) $\frac{21}{34}$
(b) $\frac{18}{34}$
(c) $\frac{17}{54}$
(d) $\frac{18}{54}$

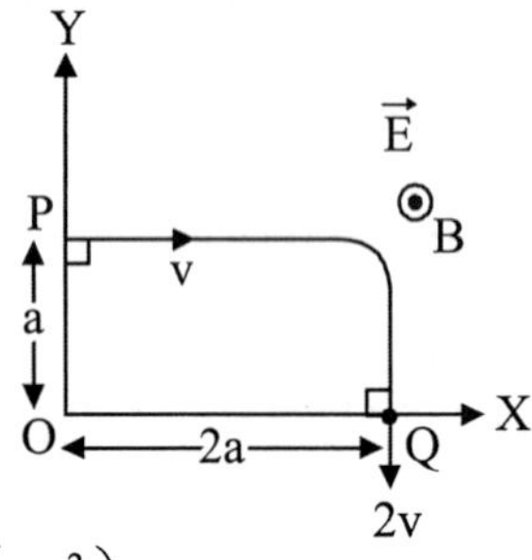

14. A charged particle of mass 'm' and charge 'q' moving under the influence of uniform electric field $E\hat{i}$ and a uniform magnetic field $B\hat{k}$ follows a trajectory from point P to Q as shown in figure. The velocities at P and Q are respectively, $v\hat{i}$ and $-2v\hat{j}$. Then which of the following statements (A, B, C, D) are the correct? (Trajectory shown is schematic and not to scale)

Y
$\vec{E}$
P
B
v
a
O
2a
Q
X
2v

(A) $E = \frac{3}{4}\left(\frac{mv^2}{qa}\right)$
(B) Rate of work done by the electric field at P is $\frac{3}{4}\left(\frac{mv^2}{a}\right)$
(C) Rate of work done by both the fields at Q is zero
(D) The difference between the magnitude of angular momentum of the particle at P and Q is 2 mav.
(a) (A), (C), (D) (b) (B), (C), (D)
(c) (A), (B), (C) (d) (A), (B), (C), (D)

15. Three charged particles A, B and C with charges $-4q$, $2q$ and $-2q$ are present on the circumference of a circle of radius d. The charged particles A, C and centre O of the circle formed an equilateral triangle as shown in figure. Electric field at O along x-direction is:

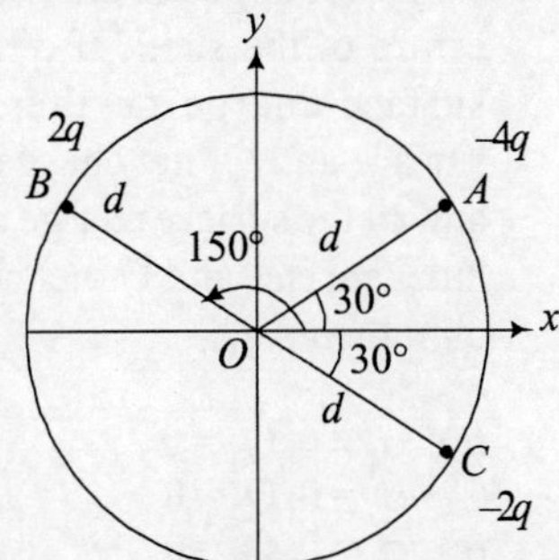

(a) $\frac{\sqrt{3}q}{\pi \epsilon_0 d^2}$ (b) $\frac{2\sqrt{3}q}{\pi \epsilon_0 d^2}$ (c) $\frac{\sqrt{3}q}{4\pi \epsilon_0 d^2}$ (d) $\frac{3\sqrt{3}q}{4\pi \epsilon_0 d^2}$

16. Two infinite planes each with uniform surface charge density $+\sigma$ are kept in such a way that the angle between them is 30°. The electric field in the region shown between them is given by:

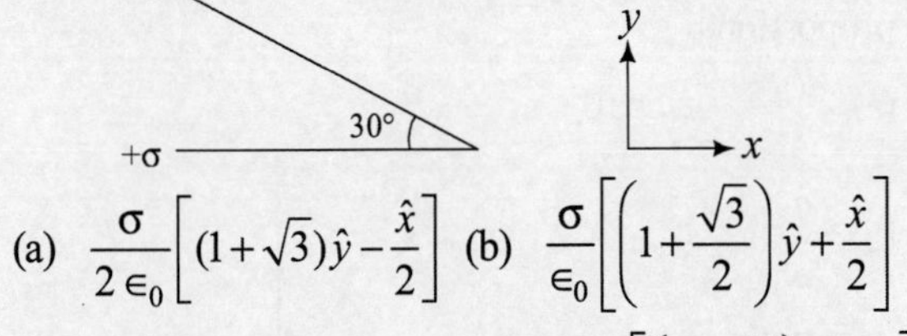

(a) $\frac{\sigma}{2\epsilon_0}\left[(1+\sqrt{3})\hat{y}-\frac{\hat{x}}{2}\right]$ (b) $\frac{\sigma}{\epsilon_0}\left[\left(1+\frac{\sqrt{3}}{2}\right)\hat{y}+\frac{\hat{x}}{2}\right]$

(c) $\frac{\sigma}{2\epsilon_0}\left[\left(1+\sqrt{3}\right)\hat{y}+\frac{\hat{x}}{2}\right]$ (d) $\frac{\sigma}{2\epsilon_0}\left[\left(1-\frac{\sqrt{3}}{2}\right)\hat{y}-\frac{\hat{x}}{2}\right]$

17. A simple pendulum of length L is placed between the plates of a parallel plate capacitor having electric field E, as shown in figure. Its bob has mass m and charge q. The time period of the pendulum is given by:

(a) $2\pi\sqrt{\frac{L}{\left(g+\frac{qE}{m}\right)}}$

(b) $2\pi\sqrt{\frac{L}{\sqrt{g^2-\frac{q^2E^2}{m^2}}}}$

(c) $2\pi\sqrt{\frac{L}{\left(g-\frac{qE}{m}\right)}}$

(d) $2\pi\sqrt{\frac{L}{\sqrt{g^2+\left(\frac{qE}{m}\right)^2}}}$

18. For a uniformly charged ring of radius R, the electric field on its axis has the largest magnitude at a distance h from its centre. Then value of h is:

(a) $\frac{R}{\sqrt{5}}$ (b) $\frac{R}{\sqrt{2}}$ (c) R (d) $R\sqrt{2}$

19. A body of mass M and charge q is connected to a spring of spring constant k. It is oscillating along x-direction about its equilibrium position, taken to be at $x = 0$, with an amplitude A. An electric field E is applied along the x-direction. Which of the following statements is correct?

(a) The total energy of the system is $\frac{1}{2}m\omega^2A^2+\frac{1}{2}\frac{q^2E^2}{k}$

(b) The new equilibrium position is at a distance: $\frac{2qE}{k}$ from $x=0$

(c) The new equilibrium position is at a distance: $\frac{qE}{2k}$ from $x=0$

(d) The total energy of the system is $\frac{1}{2}m\omega^2A^2-\frac{1}{2}\frac{q^2E^2}{k}$

20. A solid ball of radius R has a charge density ρ given by $\rho=\rho_0\left(1-\frac{r}{R}\right)$ for $0 \le r \le R$. The electric field outside the ball is:

(a) $\frac{\rho_0 R^3}{\varepsilon_0 r^2}$ (b) $\frac{4\rho_0 R^3}{3\varepsilon_0 r^2}$ (c) $\frac{3\rho_0 R^3}{4\varepsilon_0 r^2}$ (d) $\frac{\rho_0 R^3}{12\varepsilon_0 r^2}$

21. Two identical electric point dipoles have dipole moments $\vec{P_1}=P\hat{i}$ and $\vec{P_2}=-P\hat{i}$ and are held on the x axis at distance 'a' from each other. When released, they move along x-axis with the direction of their dipole moments remaining unchanged. If the mass of each dipole is 'm', their speed when they are infinitely far apart is:

(a) $\frac{P}{a}\sqrt{\frac{1}{\pi\varepsilon_0 ma}}$ (b) $\frac{P}{a}\sqrt{\frac{1}{2\pi\varepsilon_0 ma}}$

(c) $\frac{P}{a}\sqrt{\frac{2}{\pi\varepsilon_0 ma}}$ (d) $\frac{P}{a}\sqrt{\frac{2}{2\pi\varepsilon_0 ma}}$

22. In finding the electric field using Gauss law the formula $|\vec{E}|=\frac{q_{enc}}{\epsilon_0|A|}$ is applicable. In the formula ϵ_0 is permittivity of free space, A is the area of Gaussian surface and q_{enc} is charge enclosed by the Gaussian surface. This equation can be used in which of the following situation?

(a) Only when the Gaussian surface is an equipotential surface. Only when the Gaussian surface is an

(b) equipotential surface and $|\vec{E}|$ is constant on the surface.

(c) Only when $|\vec{E}|$ = constant on the surface.

(d) For any choice of Gaussian surface.

23. Shown in the figure is a shell made of a conductor. It has inner radius a and outer radius b, and carries charge Q. At its centre is a dipole $\vec{p}$ as shown. In this case:

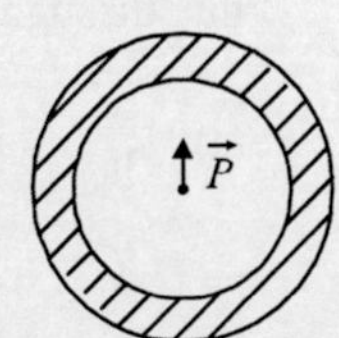

(a) surface change density on the inner surface is uniform and equal to $\frac{Q/2}{4\pi a^2}$

(b) electric field outside the shell is the same as that of a point charge at the centre of the shell.

(c) surface charge density on the outer surface depends on $|\vec{P}|$

(d) surface charge density on the inner surface of the shell is zero everywhere.

24. Let a total charge 2 Q be distributed in a sphere of radius R, with the charge density given by $\rho(r) = kr$, where r is the distance from the centre. Two charges A and B, of – Q each, are placed on diametrically opposite points, at equal distance, a, from the centre. If A and B do not experience any force, then.

(a) $a = 8^{-1/4}R$ (b) $a = \frac{3R}{2^{1/4}}$

(c) $a = 2^{-1/4}R$ (d) $a = R/\sqrt{3}$

25. An electric dipole is formed by two equal and opposite charges q with separation d. The charges have same mass m. It is kept in a uniform electric field E. If it is slightly rotated from its equilibrium orientation, then its angular frequency ω is :

(a) $\sqrt{\frac{qE}{md}}$ (b) $\sqrt{\frac{2qE}{md}}$ (c) $2\sqrt{\frac{qE}{md}}$ (d) $\sqrt{\frac{qE}{2md}}$

26. An electric field of 1000 V/m is applied to an electric dipole at angle of 45°. The value of electric dipole moment is 10^{-29} C.m. What is the potential energy of the electric dipole?

(a) -20×10^{-18} J (b) -7×10^{-27} J

(c) -10×10^{-29} J (d) -9×10^{-20} J

27. Charges – q and + q located at A and B, respectively, constitute an electric dipole. Distance AB = 2a, O is the mid point of the dipole and OP is perpendicular to AB. A charge Q is placed at P where OP = y and $y >> 2a$. The charge Q experiences an electrostatic force F. If Q is now moved along the equatorial line to P′ such that OP′ $= \left(\frac{y}{3}\right)$, the force on Q will be close to: $\left(\frac{y}{3} >> 2a\right)$

(a) 3 F

(b) $\frac{F}{3}$

(c) 9 F

(d) 27 F

28. A charge Q is placed at a distance a/2 above the centre of the square surface of edge a as shown in the figure. The electric flux through the square surface is:

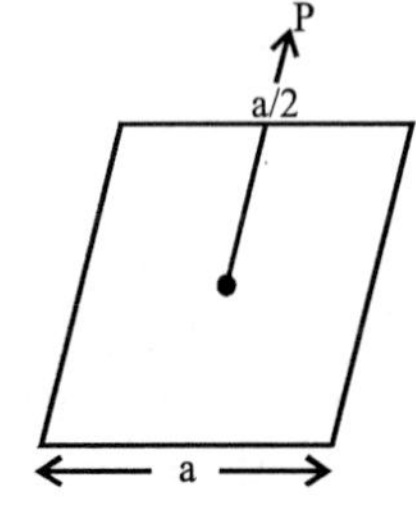

(a) $\frac{Q}{3\varepsilon_0}$

(b) $\frac{Q}{6\varepsilon_0}$

(c) $\frac{Q}{2\varepsilon_0}$

(d) $\frac{Q}{\varepsilon_0}$

29. Shown in the figure are two point charges +Q and –Q inside the cavity of a spherical shell. The charges are kept near the surface of the cavity on opposite sides of the centre of the shell. If σ_1 is the surface charge on the inner surface and Q_1 net charge on it and σ_2 the surface charge on the outer surface and Q_2 net charge on it then :

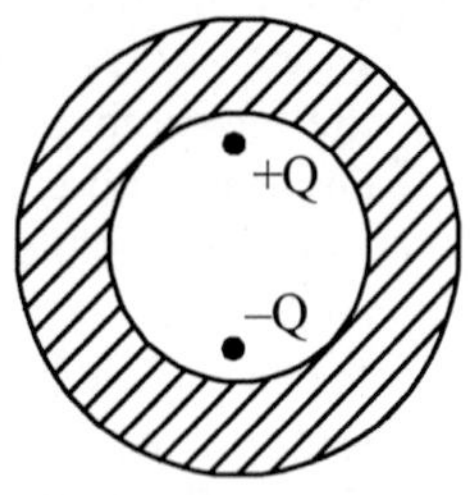

(a) $\sigma_1 \neq 0, Q_1 = 0$; $\sigma_2 = 0, Q_2 = 0$ (b) $\sigma_1 \neq 0, Q_1 = 0$; $\sigma_2 \neq 0, Q_2 = 0$

(c) $\sigma_1 = 0, Q_1 = 0$; $\sigma_2 = 0, Q_2 = 0$ (d) $\sigma_1 \neq 0, Q_1 \neq 0$; $\sigma_2 \neq 0, Q_2 \neq 0$

30. A charge Q is placed at each of the opposite corners of a square. A charge q is placed at each of the other two corners. If the net electrical force on Q is zero, then Q/q equals:

(a) –1 (b) 1 (c) $-\frac{1}{\sqrt{2}}$ (d) $-2\sqrt{2}$

31. Three charges $-q_1$, $+q_2$ and $-q_3$ are place as shown in the figure. The x - component of the force on $-q_1$ is proportional to

(a) $\frac{q_2}{b^2} - \frac{q_3}{a^2}\cos\theta$

(b) $\frac{q_2}{b^2} + \frac{q_3}{a^2}\sin\theta$

(c) $\frac{q_2}{b^2} + \frac{q_3}{a^2}\cos\theta$

(d) $\frac{q_2}{b^2} - \frac{q_3}{a^2}\sin\theta$

32. A long cylindrical shell carries positive surface charge σ in the upper half and negative surface charge - σ in the lower half. The electric field lines around the cylinder will look like figure given in : (*figures are schematic and not drawn to scale*)

(a) 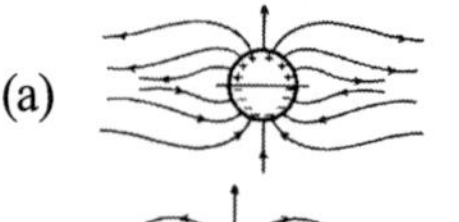 (b) 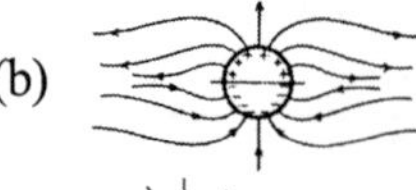

(c) 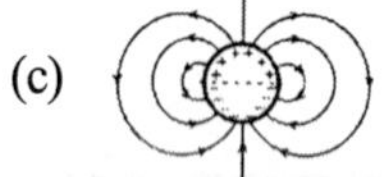 (d) 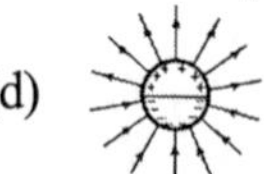

33. A wire of length L (=20 cm), is bent into a semicircular arc. If the two equal halves of the arc were each to be uniformly charged with charges $\pm$ Q, $[|Q| = 10^3\varepsilon_0$ Coulomb where ε_0 is the permittivity (in SI units) of free space] the net electric field at the centre O of the semicircular arc would be :

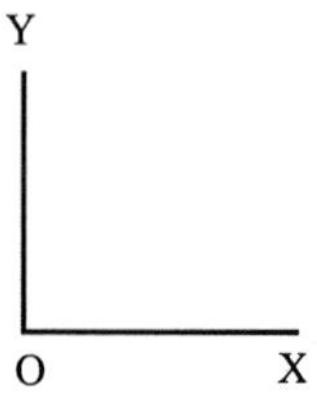

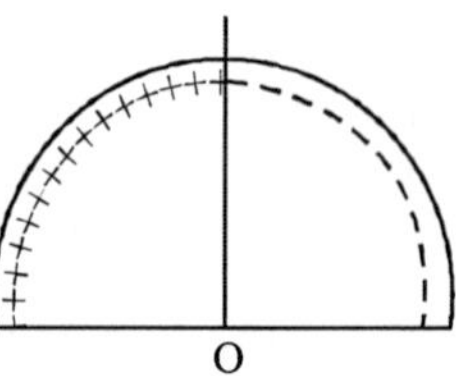

(a) $(50 \times 10^3 \text{N/C})\,\hat{j}$ (b) $(50 \times 10^3 \text{N/C})\,\hat{i}$

(c) $(25 \times 10^3 \text{N/C})\,\hat{j}$ (d) $(25 \times 10^3 \text{N/C})\,\hat{i}$

34. A thin disc of radius $b = 2a$ has a concentric hole of radius 'a' in it (see figure). It carries uniform surface charge 'σ' on it. If the electric field on its axis at height 'h' ($h << a$) from its centre is given as 'Ch' then value of 'C' is :

(a) $\frac{\sigma}{4a\epsilon_0}$ 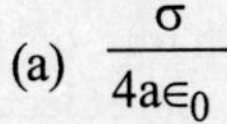

(b) $\frac{\sigma}{8a\epsilon_0}$

(c) $\frac{\sigma}{a\epsilon_0}$

(d) $\frac{\sigma}{2a\epsilon_0}$

35. A spherically symmetric charge distribution is characterised by a charge density having the following variations:

$\rho(r) = \rho_0\left(1 - \frac{r}{R}\right)$ for $r < R$

$\rho(r) = 0$ for $r \geq R$

Where r is the distance from the centre of the charge distribution ρ_o is a constant. The electric field at an internal point ($r < R$) is:

(a) $\frac{\rho_0}{4\varepsilon_o}\left(\frac{r}{3} - \frac{r^2}{4R}\right)$ (b) $\frac{\rho_0}{\varepsilon_o}\left(\frac{r}{3} - \frac{r^2}{4R}\right)$

(c) $\frac{\rho_0}{3\varepsilon_o}\left(\frac{r}{3} - \frac{r^2}{4R}\right)$ (d) $\frac{\rho_0}{12\varepsilon_o}\left(\frac{r}{3} - \frac{r^2}{4R}\right)$

36. The magnitude of the average electric field normally present in the atmosphere just above the surface of the Earth is about 150 N/C, directed inward towards the center of the Earth. This gives the total net surface charge carried by the Earth to be:

[Given $\varepsilon_o = 8.85 \times 10^{-12}$ C^2/N-m^2, $R_E = 6.37 \times 10^6$ m]

(a) +670 kC (b) −670 kC (c) −680 kC (d) +680 kC

37. The surface charge density of a thin charged disc of radius R is σ. The value of the electric field at the centre of the disc is $\frac{\sigma}{2\epsilon_0}$. With respect to the field at the centre, the electric field along the axis at a distance R from the centre of the disc :

(a) reduces by 70.7% (b) reduces by 29.3%

(c) reduces by 9.7% (d) reduces by 14.6%

38. A liquid drop having 6 excess electrons is kept stationary under a uniform electric field of 25.5 kVm^{-1}. The density of liquid is 1.26×10^3 kg m^{-3}. The radius of the drop is (neglect buoyancy).

(a) 4.3×10^{-7}m (b) 7.8×10^{-7}m

(c) 0.078×10^{-7}m (d) 3.4×10^{-7}m

39. In a uniformly charged sphere of total charge Q and radius R, the electric field E is plotted as function of distance from the centre, The graph which would correspond to the above will be:

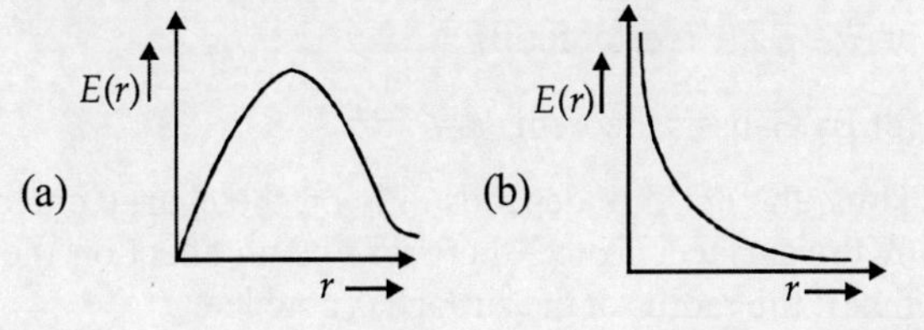

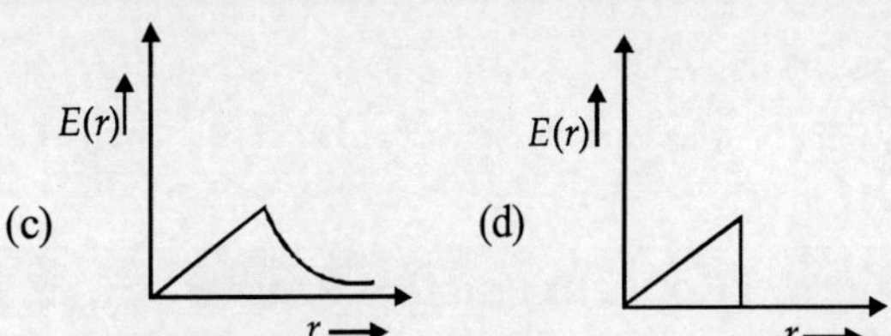

40. Three positive charges of equal value q are placed at vertices of an equilateral triangle. The resulting lines of force should be sketched as in

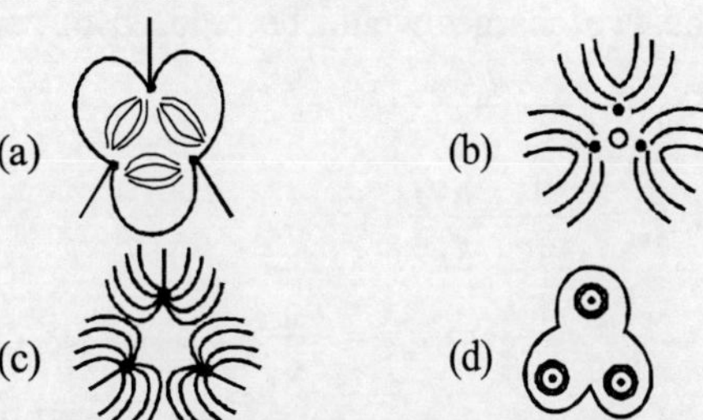

41. A charged ball B hangs from a silk thread S, which makes an angle θ with a large charged conducting sheet P, as shown in the figure. The surface charge density σ of the sheet is proportional to

(a) cot θ

(b) cos θ

(c) tan θ

(d) sin θ

42. Four charges equal to $-Q$ are placed at the four corners of a square and a charge q is at its centre. If the system is in equilibrium the value of q is

(a) $-\frac{Q}{2}(1+2\sqrt{2})$ (b) $\frac{Q}{4}(1+2\sqrt{2})$

(c) $-\frac{Q}{4}(1+2\sqrt{2})$ (d) $\frac{Q}{2}(1+2\sqrt{2})$

43. Two point charges $+ 8q$ and $- 2q$ are located at $x = 0$ and $x = L$ respectively. The location of a point on the x axis at which the net electric field due to these two point charges is zero is

(a) $\frac{L}{4}$ (b) $2L$ (c) $4L$ (d) $8L$

44. Four closed surfaces and corresponding charge distributions are shown below.

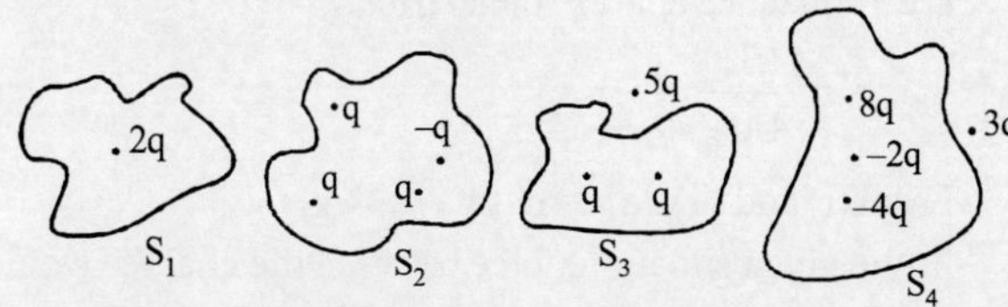

Let the respective electric fluxes through the surfaces be Φ_1, Φ_2, Φ_3, and Φ_4. Then :

(a) $\Phi_1 < \Phi_2 = \Phi_3 > \Phi_4$ (b) $\Phi_1 > \Phi_2 > \Phi_3 > \Phi_4$

(c) $\Phi_1 = \Phi_2 = \Phi_3 = \Phi_4$ (d) $\Phi_1 > \Phi_3 ; \Phi_2 < \Phi_4$

45. If the electric flux entering and leaving an enclosed surface respectively is ϕ_1 and ϕ_2, the electric charge inside the surface will be

(a) $(\phi_2 - \phi_1)\varepsilon_o$ (b) $(\phi_1 - \phi_2)/\varepsilon_o$

(c) $(\phi_2 - \phi_1)/\varepsilon_o$ (d) $(\phi_1 - \phi_2)\varepsilon_o$

Hints & Solutions

16.1 Concept Practice Problems

CPP

1. (b) Nuclear force binds the protons and neutrons in the nucleus of an atom.
2. (b) The dielectric constant for metal is infinity, the force between the two charges would be reduced to zero.
3. (a) In air, $F_{air} = \frac{1}{4\pi\varepsilon_0}\frac{q_1 q_2}{r^2}$

   In medium, $F_m = \frac{1}{4\pi\varepsilon_0}\frac{q_1 q_2}{Kr^2}$

   $\therefore \frac{F_m}{F_{air}} = \frac{1}{K} \Rightarrow F_m = \frac{F_{air}}{K}$ (decreases K-times)
4. (a) Let q and q' be the charges on spheres of radii R and 2R respectively.

   Given $q + q' = Q$ ...(i)

   Surface charge densities are

   $\sigma = \frac{q}{4\pi R^2}$ and $\sigma = \frac{q'}{4\pi(2R)^2}$

   Given $\sigma = \sigma'$ $\therefore \frac{q}{4\pi R^2} = \frac{q'}{4\pi(2R)^2}$ or, $q' = 4q$

   From eq. (i), $q' = Q - q$ or, $4q = Q - q$

   or, $Q = 5q$ ...(ii)

   $\therefore q' = Q - q = Q - \frac{Q}{5} = \frac{4Q}{5}$.
5. (c) The charge on disc A is 10^{-6} μC. The charge on disc B is 10×10^{-6} μC. The total charge on both = 11 μC. When touched, this charge will be distributed equally i.e. 5.5 μC on each disc.
6. (d) They will not experience any force if $|\vec{F}_G| = |\vec{F}_e|$

   $\Rightarrow G\frac{m^2}{(16\times10^{-2})^2} = \frac{1}{4\pi\varepsilon_0}\cdot\frac{q^2}{(16\times10^{-2})^2} \Rightarrow \frac{q}{m} = \sqrt{4\pi\varepsilon_0 G}$
7. (c) In vacuum, $F = \frac{1}{4\pi\varepsilon_0}\frac{q^2}{r^2}$ ...(i)

   Suppose, froce between the chrages is same when charges are r′ distance apart in dielectric.

   $\therefore F' = \frac{1}{4\pi\varepsilon_0}\frac{q^2}{kr'^2}$ ...(ii)

   From (i) and (ii), $kr'^2 = r^2$ or, $r = \sqrt{kr'}$

   In the given situation, force between the charges would be

   $$F' = \frac{1}{4\pi\varepsilon_0}\frac{q^2}{\left(\frac{r}{2} + \sqrt{4}\frac{r}{2}\right)^2} = \frac{4}{9}\frac{q^2}{4\pi\varepsilon_0 r^2} = \frac{4F}{9}$$
8. (b) The charge at the inner surface, outer surface and inside the conductor at P = (– Q, + Q, 0) as shown in the figure

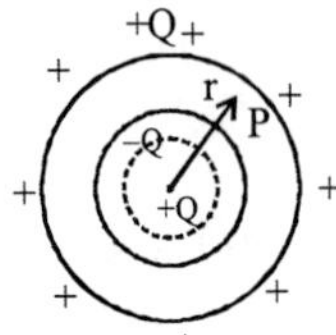

9. (b) Charge on glass rod is positive, so charge on gold leaves will also be positive. Due to X-rays, more electrons from leaves will be emitted, so leaves becomes more positive and diverge further.
10. (d) Let q charge is situated at the mid position of the line AB. The distance between AB is x. A and B be the positions of charges Q and Q respectively.

   Q A •- - - - - C • - - - - - B • Q ; ← x/2 → q ← x/2 → ; ← x →

   Let $AC = \frac{x}{2}$, $BC = \frac{x}{2}$

   The force on A due to charge q at C,

   $\vec{F}_{CA} = \frac{1}{4\pi\varepsilon_0}\cdot\frac{Q.q}{(x/2)^2}$ along $\overrightarrow{AC}$

   The force on A due to charge Q at B

   $\vec{F}_{AB} = \frac{1}{4\pi\varepsilon_0}\cdot\frac{Q^2}{x^2}$ along $\overrightarrow{BA}$

   The system is in equilibrium, then two oppositely directed force must be equal, i.e., total force on A is equal to zero.

   $\vec{F}_{CA} + \vec{F}_{AB} = 0 \Rightarrow \vec{F}_{CA} = -\vec{F}_{AB}$

   $\frac{1}{4\pi\varepsilon_0}\cdot\frac{4Q.q}{x^2} = \frac{-1}{4\pi\varepsilon_0}\cdot\frac{Q^2}{x^2} \Rightarrow q = -\frac{Q}{4}$

16.2 Concept Practice Problems

CPP

11. (a) Electric field $\vec{E}$ is along the dipole axis.

   $\therefore \theta = 0°$.
12. (c) $\phi = E(ds)\cos\theta = E(2\pi r^2)\cos 0° = 2\pi r^2 E$.
13. (a) For the curved surface, $\theta = 90°$

   $\therefore \phi = E\, ds\cos 90° = 0$.
14. (c) $U_p = -\mathbf{p}\cdot\mathbf{E} = -pE\cos\theta$

   $(U_p)_{minimum} = -pE$, when $\theta = 0°$
15. (d) According to Gauss' Law

   $\oint E.ds = \frac{Q_{\text{enclosed by closed surface}}}{\varepsilon_0} = \text{flux}$

   so total flux $= Q/\varepsilon_0$

   Since cube has six face, so flux coming out through one wall or one face is $Q/6\varepsilon_0$.
16. (a) The flux is zero according to Gauss' Law because it is a open surface which enclosed a charge q.
17. (b) **Given :** Dipole moment of the dipole = $\vec{p}$ and uniform electric field = $\vec{E}$. Torque (τ) = Either force × perpendicular distance between the two forces = qaEsinθ or $\tau = pE\sin\theta$ or $\vec{\tau} = \vec{p}\times\vec{E}$ (vector form)
18. (c) By Gauss's theorem, $\phi = \frac{Q_{in}}{\epsilon_0}$

   Thus, the net flux depends only on the charge enclosed by the surface. Hence, there will be no effect on the net flux if the radius of the surface is doubled.

19. (a) Dipole is formed when two equal and unlike charges are placed at a short distance.

20. (d) Electric flux, $\phi = EA\cos\theta$, where θ = angle between E and normal to the surface.

Here $\theta = \frac{\pi}{2} \Rightarrow \phi = 0$

Exercise 1 - Chapter Revision Problems CRP

1. (b) As new distance = 2 r and electric field due to single charge, $E \propto \frac{1}{r^2}$, therefore, new intensity = E/4.

2. (d) According to Gauss's theorem,

$\therefore E = \frac{q/4\pi R^2}{\epsilon_0}$ $[\because q/4\pi R^2 = \sigma]$

or $E = \sigma/\varepsilon_o$

3. (b) To overcome electrostatic repulsion forces, work will have to be done by external agency.

4. (a)

5. (c) Electric field intensity due to thin infinite plane sheet of charge,

$E = \frac{\sigma}{2\varepsilon} = \frac{\sigma}{2\varepsilon_0 K}$

[Where dielectric constant, $K = \frac{\varepsilon}{\varepsilon_0}$]

6. (d) Electric displacement vector, $\vec{D} = \varepsilon\vec{E}$

As, $\varepsilon = \varepsilon_0 K$ $\quad \therefore \vec{D} = \varepsilon_0 K\vec{E}$

7. (d) As $\sigma_1 = \sigma_2$

$\therefore \frac{Q_1}{4\pi r_1^2} = \frac{Q_2}{4\pi r_2^2}$ or $\frac{Q_1}{4\pi\varepsilon_o r_1^2} = \frac{Q_2}{4\pi\varepsilon_o r_2^2}$

$\therefore E_1 = E_2$ or $E_1/E_2 = 1 \Rightarrow E_1 : E_2 = 1:1$

8. (a) $E = E_1 - E_2 = \frac{\sigma}{2\varepsilon_o} - \left(\frac{-\sigma}{2\varepsilon_o}\right) = \sigma/\varepsilon_o$

The field intensity in between sheets having equal and opposite uniform surface densities of charge becomes constant. ie, an uniform electric field is produced and it is independent of the distance between the sheets.

9. (c) The field due to infinite linear charge distribution

$E = \frac{1}{4\pi\varepsilon_0}\int\frac{dq}{r} \Rightarrow E \propto \frac{1}{r}$ So hyperbola.

10. (c) Inside a charged conducting surface E = 0, but on or outside the surface $E \neq 0$.

$\therefore$ Electric intensity is discontinuous across a charged conducting surface.

11. (d) $E = \frac{p}{4\pi\varepsilon_0 . r^3}$

Apparently, $E \propto p$ and $E \propto \frac{1}{r^3} \propto r^{-3}$.

12. (c) K.E. acquired = work done = force × distance = q E × y = q E y

13. (c) Intensity of electric field due to a Dipole

$E = \frac{p}{4\pi\varepsilon_0 r^3}\sqrt{3\cos^2\theta + 1} \Rightarrow E \propto \frac{1}{r^3}$

14. (a) $-eE = mg$

$\vec{E} = -\frac{9.1\times10^{-31}\times10}{1.6\times10^{-19}} = -5.6\times10^{-11}\,N/C$

15. (b) $E = \frac{kQ}{r^2} \Rightarrow Q = \frac{E\times r^2}{k} = \frac{3\times10^6\times(2.5)^2}{9\times10^9} = 2\times10^{-3}\,C$

16. (d) Work done, W = F s cosθ = (q E) s cos θ

17. (a) Charge resides on the outer surface of a conducting hollow sphere of radius R. We consider a spherical surface of radius r < R.

By Gauss theorem

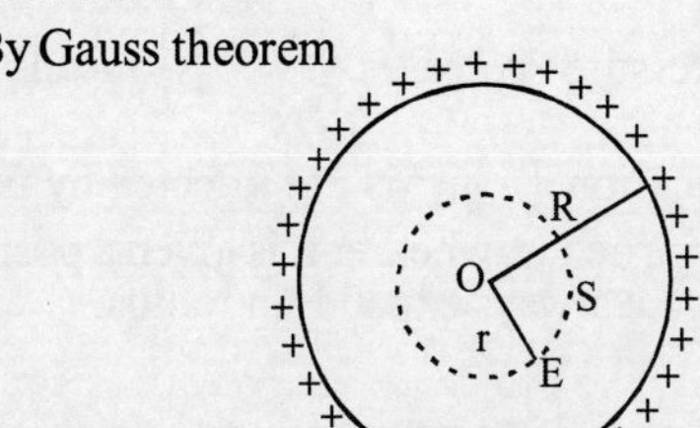

$\int_s \vec{E}.d\vec{s} = \frac{1}{\varepsilon_0} \times$ charge enclosed or $E \times 4\pi r^2 = \frac{1}{\varepsilon_0} \times 0$

$\Rightarrow E = 0$

i.e electric field inside a hollow sphere is zero.

18. (d) Torque, $\vec{\tau} = \vec{p}\times\vec{E} = pE\sin\theta$

$4 = p \times 2 \times 10^5 \times \sin 30°$

or, $p = \frac{4}{2\times10^5\times\sin 30°} = 4\times10^{-5}\,Cm$

Dipole moment, $p = q \times l$

$q = \frac{p}{l} = \frac{4\times10^{-5}}{0.02} = 2\times10^{-3}\,C = 2mC$

19. (a) $E_P = 0$

$\Rightarrow \frac{4}{x^2} = \frac{9}{(20-x)^2} \Rightarrow \frac{20-x}{x} = \frac{3}{2}$

$\Rightarrow 40 - 2x = 3x \Rightarrow x = 8\,cm$

20. (a) $(F_{net})_q = 0$

$\Rightarrow k\frac{Qq}{\left(\frac{\ell}{2}\right)^2} + k\frac{4q^2}{\ell^2} = 0$ (q —— $\ell/2$ —— Q —— $\ell/2$ —— 4q)

where $k = \frac{1}{4\pi\varepsilon_0} \Rightarrow 4Qq + 4q^2 = 0 \Rightarrow Q = -q$

21. (a) Since lines of force starts from A and ends at B, so A is +ve and B is –ve. Lines of forces are more crowded near A, so A > B.

22. (d) Unit positive charge at O will be repelled equally by three charges at the three corners of triangle.

By symmetry, resultant $\vec{E}$ at O would be zero.

23. (d) 24. (d)

25. (a) For a soap bubble (electrified)

excess pressure $= P = P_i - P_0 = \frac{4T}{r}$

T = surface tension, r = radius.

Force due to excess pressure balances surface tension. When bubble is charged

$$P_{excess} = P_{electrostatic} + \frac{4T}{r}$$

$$P_{electrostatic} = -\frac{\sigma^2}{2\varepsilon_0} = -\frac{1}{2\varepsilon_0}\frac{q^2}{16\pi^2 r^4}$$

$$P_{excess} = \frac{4}{r}\left[T - \frac{q^2}{128\pi^2\varepsilon_0 r^3}\right] \quad ....(A)$$

Surface tension decreases after electrification of bubble and therefore pressure decreases. $\left(P \propto \frac{1}{r}\right)$ means radius increases. In equation $(A), q^2$ is not affected by positive or negative charge hence, whether it is given a positive or a negative charge it always expands in radius.

26. (c)

27. (d) The dipole is placed in a non-uniform field, therefore a force as well as a couple acts on it. The force on the negative charge is more ($F \propto E$) and is directed along negative x-axis. Thus the dipole moves along negative x-axis and rotates in an anticlockwise direction.

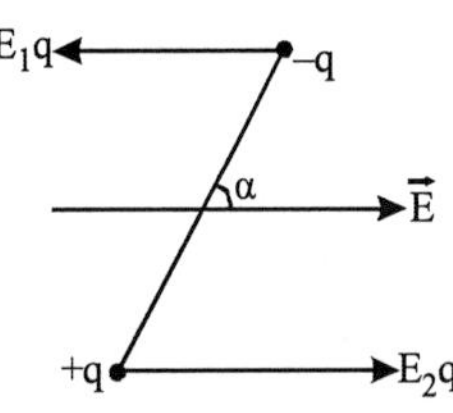

28. (b) $\tau = pE\sin\theta$, this is given by the second curve.

29. (c)

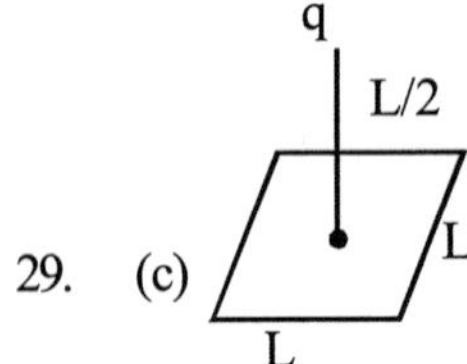

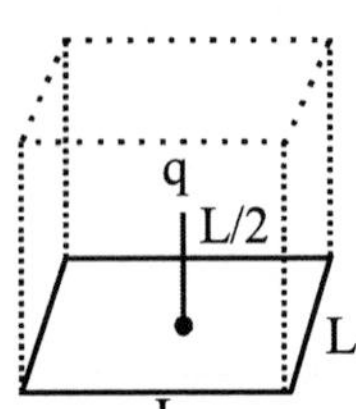

The given square of side L may be considered as one of the faces of a cube with edge L. Then given charge q will be considered to be placed at the centre of the cube. Then according to Gauss's theorem, the magnitude of the electric flux through the faces (six) of the cube is given by

$$\phi = q/\varepsilon_0$$

Hence, electric flux through one face of the cube for the given square will be

$$\phi' = \frac{1}{6}\phi = \frac{q}{6\varepsilon_0}$$

30. (c) The charges make an electric dipole. A and B points lie on the equitorial plane of the dipole. There fore potential at A = potential at B = 0

$W = Q(V_A - V_B) = q \times 0 = 0$

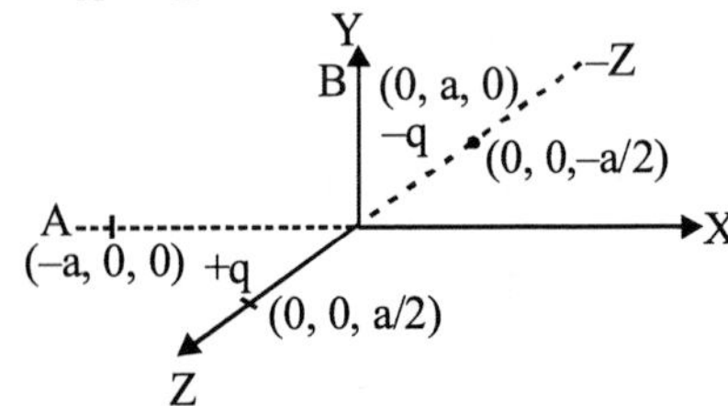

31. (a, b, c, d)

The potential shown is for charged spherical conductor.

32. (a) Surface charge density $(\sigma) = \frac{\text{Charge}}{\text{Surface area}}$

So $\sigma_{inner} = \frac{-2Q}{4\pi b^2}$

and $\sigma_{Outer} = \frac{Q}{4\pi c^2}$

– Q + 2Q = Q

–2Q

a b c

+2Q

33. (c) Electric lines of force never intersect the conductor. They are perpendicular and slightly curved near the surface of conductor.

34. (a) **Given :** Length of the dipole $(2l) = 10\text{cm} = 0.1\text{m}$ or $l = 0.05\text{ m}$

Charge on the dipole $(q) = 500\,\mu C = 500 \times 10^{-6}$ C and distance of the point on the axis from the mid-point of the dipole (r) $= 20 + 5 = 25\text{ cm} = 0.25\text{ m}$.

We know that the electric field intensity due to dipole on the given point (E)

$$= \frac{1}{4\pi\varepsilon_0} \times \frac{2(q.2l)r}{(r^2 - l^2)^2}$$

$$= 9\times10^9 \times \frac{2(500\times10^{-6}\times0.1)\times0.25}{[(0.25)^2 - (0.05)^2]^2}$$

$$= \frac{225\times10^3}{3.6\times10^{-3}} = 6.25\times10^7 \text{ N/C} \ (k = 1 \text{ for air})$$

35. (c) Let n be the number of electrons missing.

$$F = \frac{1}{4\pi\varepsilon_0}\cdot\frac{q^2}{d^2} \Rightarrow q = \sqrt{4\pi\varepsilon_0 d^2 F} = ne$$

$$\therefore \ n = \sqrt{\frac{4\pi\varepsilon_0 F d^2}{e^2}}$$

36. (b) At equilibrium potential of both sphere becomes same if charge of sp here one x and other sphere $Q - x$ then where $Q = 4 \times 10^{-2}\,C$

$v_1 = v_2$

$$\frac{kx}{1\text{cm}} = \frac{k(Q-x)}{3\text{cm}}$$

$3x = Q - x \Rightarrow 4x = Q$

$$x = \frac{Q}{4} = \frac{4\times10^{-2}}{4}C = 1\times10^{-2}$$

$Q' = Q - x = 3 \times 10^{-2}C$

37. (a) The torque on the dipole is given as

$\tau = PE\sin\theta$

The potential energy of the dipole in the electric field is given as

$U = -\,PE\cos\theta$

38. (a)

d

F_a F_b

+Q d/2 q d/2 +Q

Force due to charge + Q,

$$F_a = \frac{KQQ}{d^2}$$

Force due to charge q,

$$F_b = \frac{KQq}{\left(\frac{d}{2}\right)^2}$$

For equilibrium,

$$\vec{F}_a + \vec{F}_b = 0 \Rightarrow \frac{kQQ}{d^2} + \frac{kQq}{(d/2)^2} = 0 \qquad \therefore q = -\frac{Q}{4}$$

39. (c) Electric field due charge Q_2, $E_2 = \frac{kQ_2}{x_2^2}$

Electric field due charge Q_1, $E_1 = \frac{kQ_1}{x_1^2}$

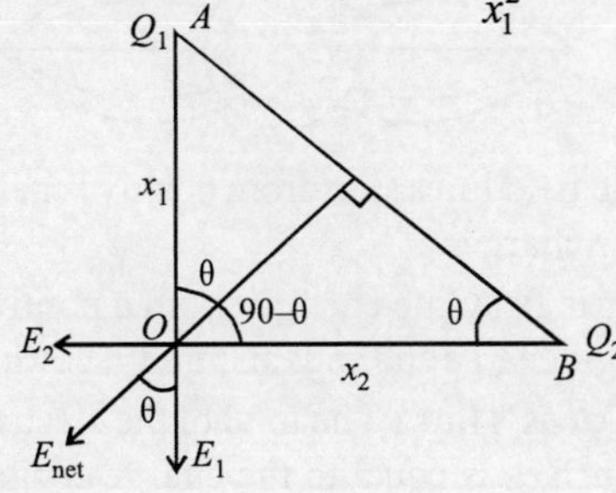

From figure,

$$\tan\theta = \frac{E_2}{E_1} = \frac{x_1}{x_2} \Rightarrow \frac{kQ_2}{x_2^2 \times \frac{kQ_1}{x_1^2}} = \frac{x_1}{x_2}$$

$$\Rightarrow \frac{Q_2 x_1^2}{Q_1 x_2^2} = \frac{x_1}{x_2} \Rightarrow \frac{Q_2}{Q_1} = \frac{x_2}{x_1} \text{ or, } \frac{Q_1}{Q_2} = \frac{x_1}{x_2}.$$

40. (c) For spherical shell

$E = \frac{1}{4\pi\varepsilon_0}\frac{Q}{r^2}$ (if $r \geq R$)

$= 0$ (if $r < R$)

Force on charge in electried field, $F = qE$

$\therefore F = 0$ (For $r < R$)

$F = \frac{1}{4\pi\varepsilon_0}\frac{Qq}{r^2}$ (For $r > R$)

41. (c) The electric field produced due to uniformly charged infinite plane is uniform. So option (b) and (d) are wrong. And +ve charge density σ_+ is bigger in magnitude so its field along Y direction will be bigger than field of –ve charge density $\sigma\_$ in X direction. Hence option (c) is correct.

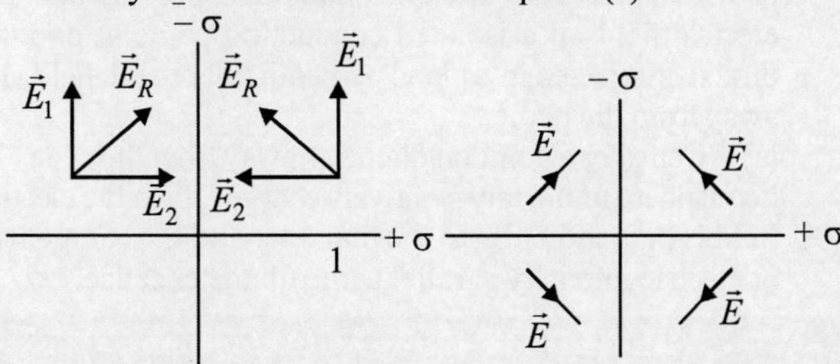

42. (c) Given,

Electric field, $E = E_0(1 - x^2)$

$\therefore$ Force, $F = qE = qE_0(1 - x^2)$

Also, $F = ma = mv\frac{dv}{dx}$ $\left(\because a = v\frac{dv}{dx}\right)$

$$\therefore mv\frac{dv}{dx} = qE_0(1 - x^2) \Rightarrow v\,dv = \frac{qE_0(1 - x^2)dx}{m}$$

Integrating both sides we get,

$$\Rightarrow \int_0^v v\,dv = \int_0^x \frac{qE_0(1 - x^2)dx}{m} \Rightarrow \frac{v^2}{2} = \frac{qE_0}{m}\left(x - \frac{9x^3}{3}\right) = 0$$

$$\Rightarrow x = \sqrt{\frac{3}{a}}$$

43. (b)

44. (d) Net force acting on the particle,

$\vec{F} = qE\hat{i} + mg\hat{j}$

Net acceleration of particle is constant, initial velocity is zero therefore path is straight line.

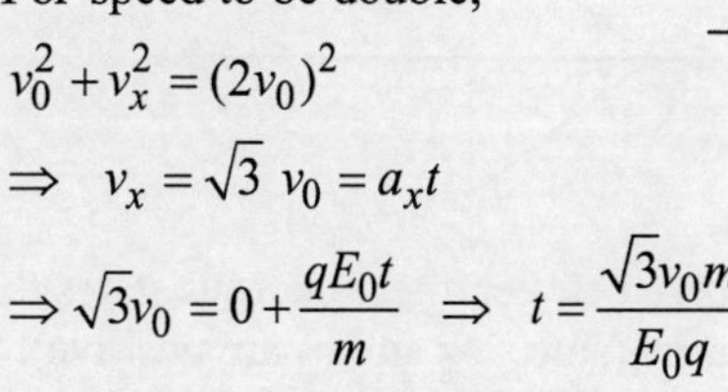

45. (c) Since $\vec{r} \cdot \vec{p} = 0$

$\vec{E}$ must be antiparallel to $\vec{p}$

$\therefore$ $\hat{E}$ is parallel to $\left(\hat{i} + 3\hat{j} - 2\hat{k}\right)$

46. (b) Using

$v^2 - u^2 = 2aS$ ...(i)

Here, $u = 0, s = x$

Also, $F_{electric} = ma$

$\Rightarrow qE = ma \Rightarrow a = \frac{qE}{m} \Rightarrow a = \frac{qE}{m}$

Substituting the values in (i) we get

$$v^2 = \frac{2qE}{m}.x$$

47. (c) In the x direction

$F_x = qE$

$\Rightarrow ma_x = qE$

$\Rightarrow \quad a_x = \frac{E_0 q}{m}$

For speed to be double,

$v_0^2 + v_x^2 = (2v_0)^2$

$\Rightarrow \quad v_x = \sqrt{3}\ v_0 = a_x t$

$\Rightarrow \sqrt{3}v_0 = 0 + \frac{qE_0 t}{m} \Rightarrow t = \frac{\sqrt{3}v_0 m}{E_0 q}$

48. (d) $\vec{E} = (\vec{E}_1 + \vec{E}_2) + (\vec{E}_3 + \vec{E}_4)$

or $E = 2E\cos\alpha - 2E\cos\beta$

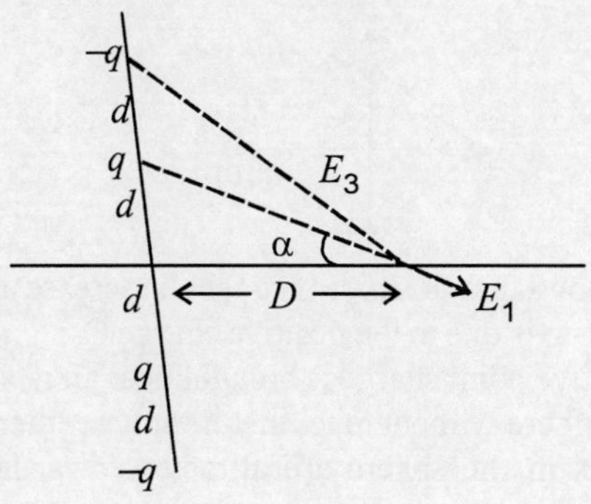

$$= \frac{2kq}{(D^2+d^2)} \times \frac{D}{\sqrt{D^2+d^2}} - \frac{2kq}{(D^2+(2d)^2} \times \frac{D}{\sqrt{D^2+(2d)^2}}$$

$$= \frac{2kqD}{(D^2+d^2)^{3/2}} - \frac{2kqD}{[D^2+(2d)^2]^{3/2}}$$

For d << D

$$E \propto \frac{D}{D^3} \propto \frac{1}{D^2}$$

49. (d) At equilibrium resultant force on bob must be zero, so
$T\cos\theta = mg$ ..... (i)
$T\sin\theta = qE$ ..... (ii)
Solving (i) and (ii) we get

$$\tan\theta = \frac{qE}{mg}$$

$$\tan\theta = \frac{5\times10^{-6}\times2000}{2\times10^{-3}\times10} = \frac{1}{2}$$

[Here, $q = 5\times10^{-6}$C, E = 2000 v/m, m = 2×10^{-3} kg]

$$\Rightarrow \tan^{-1}\left(\frac{1}{2}\right)$$

50. (a)

Exercise 2 - Exemplar & Past Year Questions E&PYQs

Exemplar Questions

1. (a) The force on q_1 depend on the force acting between q_1 and q_2 and q_1 and q_3 so that the net force acting on q_1 by q_2 and q_1 by q_3 is along the + x-direction, so the force acting between q_1, q_2 and q_1, q_3 is attractive force as shown in figure :

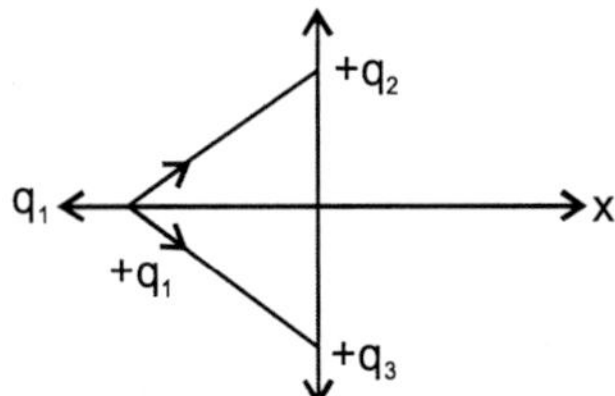

The attractive force between these charges states that q_1 is a negative charge (since, q_2 and q_3 are positive).
Then the force acting between q_1 and charge Q (positive) is also know as attractive force and then the net force on q_1 by q_2, q_3 and Q are along the same direction as shown in the figure.

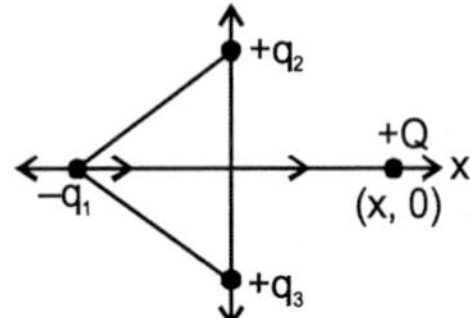

The figure shows that the force on q_1 shall increase along the positive x-axis due to the positive charge Q.

2. (a) If a positive point charge is brought near an isolated conducting sphere without touching the sphere, then the free electrons in the sphere are attracted towards the positive Charge and electric field passes through a charged body. This leaves an excess of positive charge on the (right) surface of sphere due to the induction process.
Both type of charges are bound in the (isolated conducting) sphere and cannot escape. They, therefore, reside on the surface.
Thus, the left surface of sphere has an excess of negative charge and the right surface of sphere has an excess of positive charge as shown in figure.

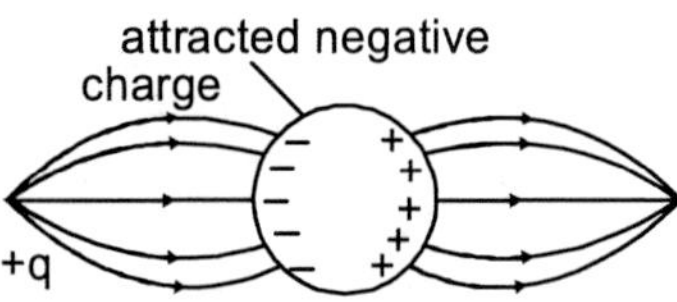

An electric field lines start from positive charge and ends at negative charge.
Also, electric field line emerges from a positive charge, in case of single charge and ends at infinity shown in figure (a).

3. (d) **By Gauss's law :** The total of the electric flux out of a closed surface is equal to the charge enclosed devided by the permittivity i.e., $\phi = \frac{Q}{\varepsilon_0}$.
Thus, electric flux through a surface doesn't depend on the shape, size or area of a surface but it depends on the number of charges enclosed by the surface. So all the given figures have same electric flux as all of them also has same single positive charge.

4. (c) The electric field lines, are directed away from positively charged source and directed toward negatively charged source. In electric field force are directly proportional to the electric field strength hence, higher the electric field strength greater the force and vice-versa. The space between the electric field lines is increasing, from left to right so strength of electric field decreases with the increase in the space between electric field lines. Then the force on charges also decreases from left to right. Thus, the force on charge –q is greater than force on charge +q in turn dipole will experience a force towards left.

5. (a) When a positive point charge +q is placed near an isolated conducting plane, some negative charge developes on the surface of the plane towards the charge and an equal positive charge developes on opposite side of the plane. This is called induction process and the electric field on a isolated conducting plane at point is directly projected in a plane perpendicular to the field and away from the plane.

6. (a) Consider a point on diameter away from the centre of hemisphere uniformly positively charged, then the electric field is perpendicular to the diameter and the component of electric intensity parallel to the diameter cancel out.

NEET/AIPMT (2013-2020) Questions

7. (a)

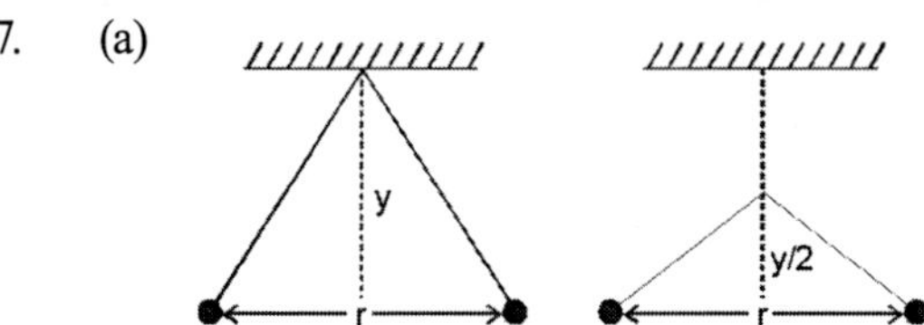

From figure, $\tan\theta = \frac{F_e}{mg} \Rightarrow \frac{r/2}{y} = \frac{\frac{kq^2}{r^2}}{mg}$

$\left[\because F = \frac{kq^2}{r^2} \text{ from coulomb's law}\right]$

$\Rightarrow r^3 \propto y \Rightarrow r'^3 \propto \frac{y}{2} \Rightarrow \frac{r'}{r} = \frac{1}{2^{1/3}} \Rightarrow r' = \frac{r}{\sqrt[3]{2}}$

8. (b) Net flux emmited from a spherical surface of radius a according to Gauss's theorem

$\phi_{net} = \frac{q_{in}}{\varepsilon_0}$

or, $(Aa)(4\pi a^2) = \frac{q_{in}}{\varepsilon_0}$

So, $q_{in} = 4\pi\varepsilon_0 A a^3$

9. (c) From figure $\tan\theta = \frac{F_e}{mg} \approx \theta$

$\frac{kq^2}{x^2 mg} = \frac{x}{2\ell}$

or $x^3 \propto q^2$ ...(1)

or $x^{3/2} \propto q$ ...(2)

Differentiating eq. (1) w.r.t. time

$3x^2\frac{dx}{dt} \propto 2q\frac{dq}{dt}$ but $\frac{dq}{dt}$ is constant

so $x^2(v) \propto q$ Replace q from eq. (2)

$x^2(v) \propto x^{3/2}$ or $v \propto x^{-1/2}$

10. (b) According to question, the net electrostatic force (F_E) = gravitational force (F_G)

$F_E = F_G$

or $\frac{1}{4\pi\varepsilon_0}\frac{\Delta e^2}{d^2} = \frac{Gm^2}{d^2}$

$\Rightarrow \Delta e = m\sqrt{\frac{G}{K}} \quad \left(\frac{1}{4\pi\varepsilon_0} = k = 9\times10^9\right)$

$= 1.67\times10^{-27}\sqrt{\frac{6.67\times10^{-11}}{9\times10^9}}$

$\Delta e \approx 1.436\times10^{-37}$ C

11. (a) As we know, $F = qE = ma$

$\Rightarrow a = \frac{qE}{m}$

$h = \frac{1}{2}\frac{qE}{m}t^2 \qquad \therefore t = \sqrt{\frac{2hm}{qE}}$

i.e., time $t \propto \sqrt{m}$ as 'q' is same for electron and proton. Since, electron has smaller mass so it will take smaller time.

12. (b) We know that,

$F = \frac{kQ^2}{r^2}$ +Q A ——— r ——— B −Q

If 25% of charges of A transfer to B then

$q_A = Q - \frac{Q}{4} = \frac{3Q}{4}$ and $q_B = -Q + \frac{Q}{4} = \frac{-3Q}{4}$

q_A ——— r ——— q_B

$F_1 = \frac{kq_Aq_B}{r^2} \Rightarrow F_1 = \frac{k\left(\frac{3Q}{4}\right)^2}{r^2} = \frac{9}{16}\frac{kQ}{r^2} = \frac{9F}{16}$

13. (c) Electric field due to line charge (1)

$\vec{E}_1 = \frac{\lambda}{2\pi\varepsilon_0 R}\hat{i}$ N/C

Electric field due to line charge (2)

$\vec{E}_2 = \frac{\lambda}{2\pi\varepsilon_0 R}\hat{i}$ N/C

$\vec{E}_{net} = \vec{E}_1 + \vec{E}_2$

$= \frac{\lambda}{2\pi\varepsilon_0 R}\hat{i} + \frac{\lambda}{2\pi\varepsilon_0 R}\hat{i}$

$= \frac{\lambda}{\pi\varepsilon_0 R}\hat{i}$ N/C

14. (b) Charge Q will be distributed over the surface of hollow metal sphere.

(i) For r < R (inside)

[At a point inside the hollow sphere]

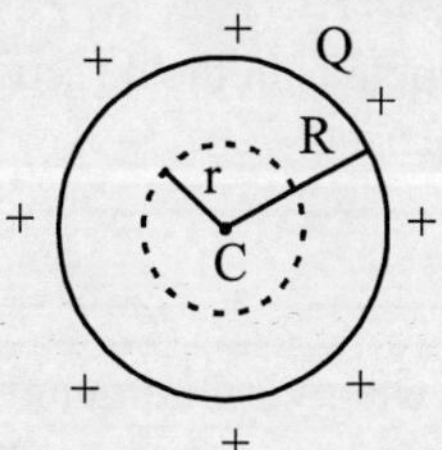

By Gauss's law, $\oint \vec{E}_{in}\cdot\vec{dS} = \frac{q_{en}}{\varepsilon_0} = 0$

As enclosed charge is = 0

So, $E_{in} = 0$ the electric field inside the hollow sphere is always zero.

(ii) For r > R (outside)

[At a point outside hollow sphere]

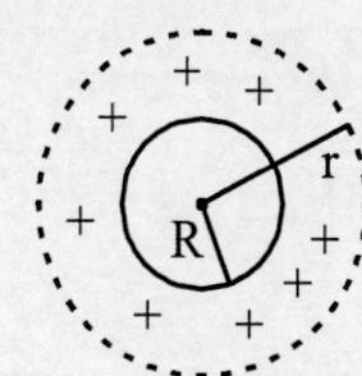

By Gauss's law, $\oint \vec{E}_0\cdot\vec{dS} = \frac{q_{en}}{\varepsilon_0} \quad (\because q_{en} = Q)$

$\therefore E_0 4\pi r^2 = \frac{Q}{\varepsilon_0}$

$\therefore E_0 \propto \frac{1}{r^2}$

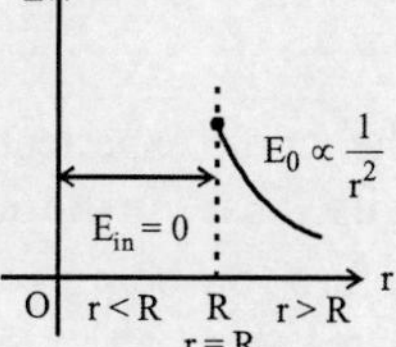

15. (c) $\phi_{Total} = \dfrac{q_{enclosed}}{\varepsilon_0}$

$\phi_{Total} = \dfrac{0}{\varepsilon_0} = 0$

16. (a) If the charge on a spherical conductor of radius *R* is *Q*, then electric field at distance *r* from centre is

$E = 0$ (if $r \angle R$)

$E = \dfrac{1}{4\pi \epsilon_0} \dfrac{Q}{r^2}$ (if $r \geq R$)

Electric field at a distance 15 cm from the centre of sphere will be

$$E = \frac{9 \times 10^9 \times 3.2 \times 10^{-7}}{225 \times 10^{-4}}$$

$= 0.128 \times 10^6 = 1.28 \times 10^5$ N/C

Exercise 3 - Concept Application Problems

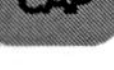

1. (b) $E = \dfrac{q}{4\pi\varepsilon_0 r^2} \Rightarrow Ar = \dfrac{q}{4\pi \epsilon_0 r^2} \Rightarrow q = 4\pi\varepsilon_0 Ar^3$

2. (d) When the dipole is in the direction of field then net force is $qE + (-qE) = 0$

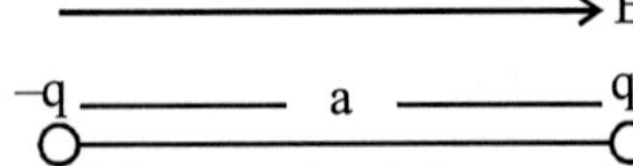

and its potential energy is minimum $= -p.E. = -qaE$

3. (b) $\tau = \left(2.57 \times 10^{-17} \text{Cm}\right)\left(3.0 \times 10^4 \dfrac{\text{N}}{\text{C}}\right)\left(\dfrac{1}{2}\right)$

$= 3.855 \times 10^{-13}$ Nm.

4. (a) Force due to electric field (F = q E) acts upwards.

5. (b) From figure, $\theta = \dfrac{\pi}{3} + \alpha$, where

$$\tan\alpha = \frac{E_2}{E_1} = \left(\frac{p\sin\theta}{4\pi \epsilon_0 r^3}\right)\left(\frac{4\pi \epsilon_0 r^3}{2p\cos\theta}\right) = \frac{1}{2}\tan\theta$$

$$\tan\left(\theta - \frac{\pi}{3}\right) = \frac{1}{2}\tan\frac{\pi}{3} = \frac{\sqrt{3}}{2}$$

or $\theta - \dfrac{\pi}{3} = \tan^{-1}\left(\dfrac{\sqrt{3}}{2}\right)$ or

$\alpha = \tan^{-1}\left(\dfrac{\sqrt{3}}{2}\right)$

or $\theta = \dfrac{\pi}{3} + \tan^{-1}\left(\dfrac{\sqrt{3}}{2}\right)$

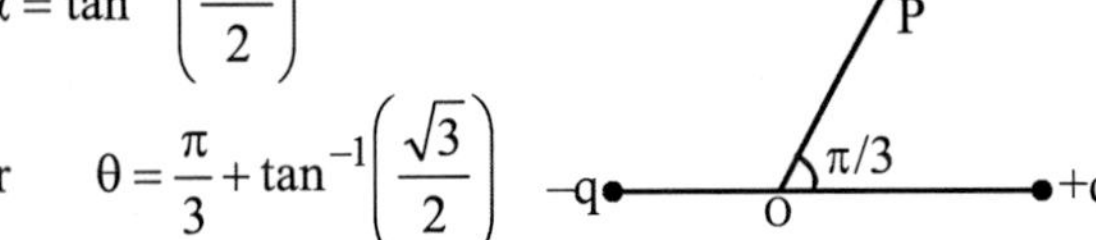

6. (b)

7. (b) The dipole experiences a torque pE sin θ tending to bring itself back in the direction of field.

Therefore, on being released (i.e. rotated) the dipole oscillates about an axis through its centre of mass and perpendicular to the field. If I is the moment of inertia of the dipole about the axis of rotation, then the equation of motion is $I.d^2\theta/dt^2 = -pE\sin\theta$

For small amplitude $\sin\theta \approx \theta$

Thus $d^2\theta/dt^2 = -(pE/I).\theta = -\omega^2\theta$

where $\omega = \sqrt{(pE/I)}$.

This is a S.H.M., whose period of oscillation is $T = 2\pi/\omega = 2\pi\sqrt{(I/pE)}$.

8. (b)

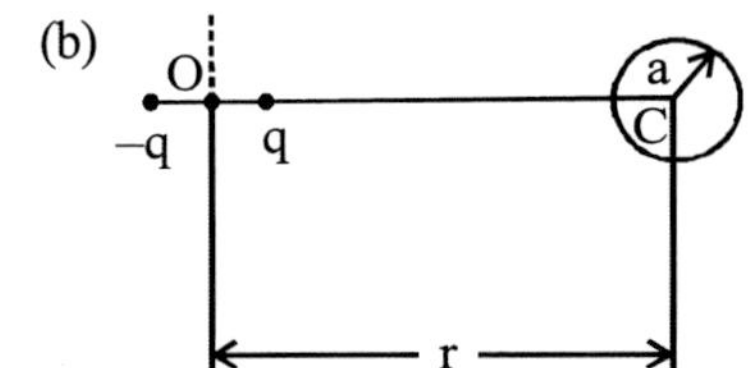

Electric field at C due to electric dipole

$= \dfrac{1}{4\pi\varepsilon_0}\dfrac{2p}{r^3}$ along OC

Electric field at C due to induced charge must be equal and opposite to electric field due to dipole as net field at C is zero.

9. (a)

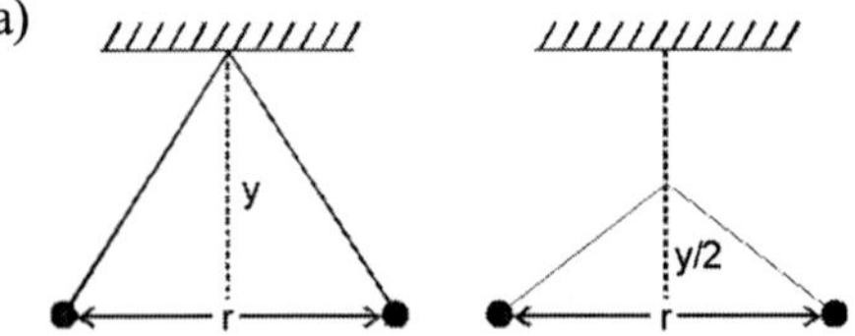

From figure, $\tan\theta = \dfrac{F_e}{mg} \Rightarrow \dfrac{r/2}{y} = \dfrac{\dfrac{kq^2}{r^2}}{mg}$

[$\because F = \dfrac{kq^2}{r^2}$ from Coulomb's law]

$\Rightarrow r^3 \propto y \Rightarrow r'^3 \propto \dfrac{y}{2} \Rightarrow \dfrac{r'}{r} = \dfrac{1}{2^{1/3}} \Rightarrow r' = \dfrac{r}{\sqrt[3]{2}}$

10. (b) $Q = \int \rho dv = \int_0^R \dfrac{A}{r^2} e^{-2r/a}\left(4\pi r^2 dr\right)$

$$= 4\pi A\int_0^R e^{-2r/a}dr = 4\pi A\left(\frac{e^{-2r/a}}{-\frac{2}{a}}\right)_0^R$$

$= 4\pi A\left(-\dfrac{a}{2}\right)\left(e^{-2R/a} - 1\right)$

$Q = 2\pi aA(1 - e^{-2R/a})$

$$R = \frac{a}{2}\log\left(\frac{1}{1 - \frac{Q}{2\pi aA}}\right)$$

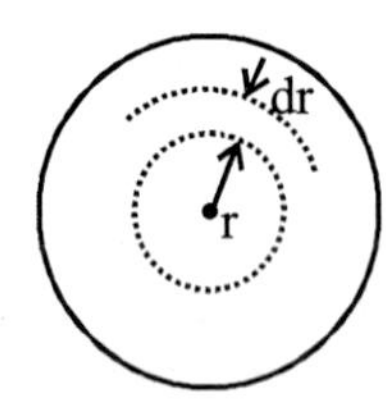

11. (d) Spheres A and B carry equal charge say 'q'

∴ Force between them, $F = \dfrac{kqq}{r^2}$

When A and C are touched, charge on both $q_A = q_C = \dfrac{q}{2}$

Then when B and C are touched, charge on B

$$q_B = \frac{\frac{q}{2}+q}{2} = \frac{3q}{4}$$

Now, the force between charge q_A and q_B

$$F' = \frac{kq_Aq_B}{r^2} = \frac{k\times\frac{q}{2}\times\frac{3q}{4}}{r^2} = \frac{3}{8}\frac{kq^2}{r^2} = \frac{3}{8}F$$

12. (d)

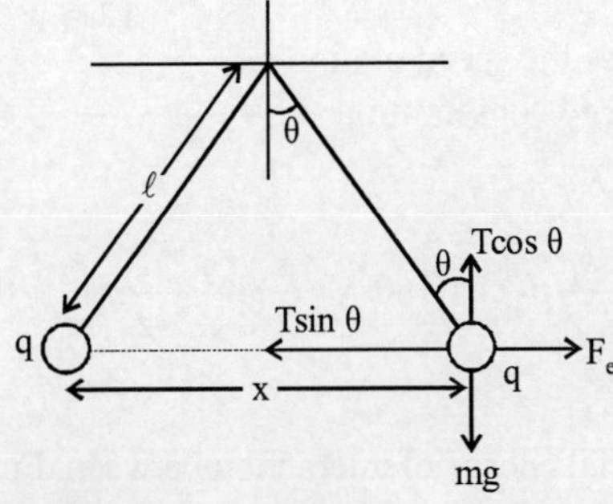

In equilibrium, $F_e = T\sin\theta$

$mg = T\cos\theta$

$$\tan\theta = \frac{F_e}{mg} = \frac{q^2}{4\pi\epsilon_0 x^2 \times mg}$$

also $\tan\theta \approx \sin = \dfrac{x/2}{\ell}$

Hence, $\dfrac{x}{2\ell} = \dfrac{q^2}{4\pi\epsilon_0 x^2\times mg} \Rightarrow x^3 = \dfrac{2q^2\ell}{4\pi\epsilon_0\, mg}$

$$\therefore x = \left(\frac{q^2\ell}{2\pi\epsilon_0\, mg}\right)^{1/3}$$

Therefore $x \propto \ell^{1/3}$

13. (b) Electric field at A $\left(R' = \dfrac{R}{2}\right)$

$$E_A.ds = \frac{q}{\varepsilon_0}$$

$$\Rightarrow \vec{E}_A = \frac{\rho\times\frac{4}{3}\pi\left(\frac{R}{2}\right)^3}{\varepsilon_0\cdot 4\pi\left(\frac{R}{2}\right)^2}$$

B A $\frac{3R}{2}$ R/2

$$\Rightarrow \vec{E}_A = \frac{\sigma(R/2)}{3\varepsilon_0} = \left(\frac{\sigma R}{6\varepsilon_0}\right)$$

Electric fields at 'B'

$$\vec{E}_B = \frac{k\times\rho\times\frac{4}{3}\pi R^3}{R^2} - \frac{k\times\rho\times\frac{4}{3}\pi\left(\frac{R}{2}\right)^3}{\left(\frac{3R}{2}\right)^2}$$

$$\Rightarrow \vec{E}_B = \frac{\sigma R}{3\varepsilon_0} - \left(\frac{1}{4\pi\varepsilon_0}\right)\frac{(\sigma)}{\left(\frac{3R}{2}\right)^2}\frac{4\pi}{3}\left(\frac{R}{2}\right)^3$$

$$\Rightarrow \vec{E}_B = \frac{\sigma R}{3\varepsilon_0} - \frac{\sigma R}{54\varepsilon_0} \Rightarrow E_B = \frac{17}{54}\left(\frac{\sigma R}{\varepsilon_0}\right)$$

$$\left|\frac{E_A}{E_B}\right| = \frac{1\times54}{6\times17} = \left(\frac{9}{17}\right) = \frac{9}{17}\times\frac{2}{2} = \frac{18}{34}$$

14. (c) (A) By work energy theorem

$$W_{mg} + W_{ele} = \frac{1}{2}m(2v)^2 - \frac{1}{2}m(v)^2$$

$$0 + qE_0 2a = \frac{3}{2}mv^2 \Rightarrow E_0 = \frac{3}{4}\frac{mv^2}{qa}$$

(B) Rate of work done at P = power of electric force

$$= qE_0V = \frac{3}{4}\frac{mv^3}{a}$$

(C) At, Q, $\dfrac{dw}{dt} = 0$ for both the fields

(D) The difference of magnitude of angular momentum of the particle at P and Q,

$$\Delta\vec{L} = \left(-m2v2a\hat{k}\right) - \left(-mva\hat{k}\right)$$

$$\left|\Delta\vec{L}\right| = 3mva$$

15. (a)

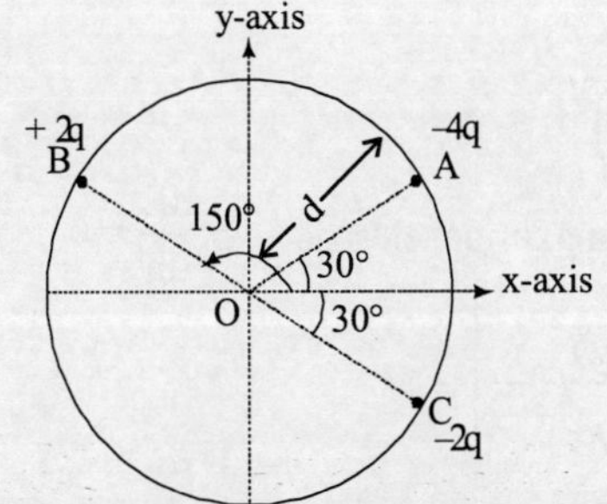

Electric field due to charge +2q at centre O

$$\vec{E}_1 = \frac{1}{4\pi\varepsilon_0}\times\frac{2q}{d^2}\left[\frac{\sqrt{3}\hat{i}-\hat{j}}{2}\right]$$

Electric field due to charge $-2q$ at centre O

$$\vec{E}_2 = \frac{1}{4\pi\varepsilon_0}\times\frac{2q}{d^2}\left[\frac{\sqrt{3}\hat{i}-\hat{j}}{2}\right]$$

Electric field due to charge $-4q$ at centre O

$$\vec{E}_3 = \frac{1}{4\pi\varepsilon_0}\times\frac{4q}{d^2}\left[\frac{\sqrt{3}\hat{i}+\hat{j}}{2}\right]$$

$\therefore$ Net electric field at point O

$$\vec{E}_0 = \vec{E}_1 + \vec{E}_2 + \vec{E}_3 = \frac{\sqrt{3}q}{\pi\varepsilon_0 d^2}\hat{i}$$

16. (d)

E₁ P +σ y 60° E₂ 30° x +σ

From figure,

$$\vec{E}_1 = \frac{\sigma}{2\varepsilon_0}\hat{y} \quad\text{and}\quad \vec{E}_2 = \frac{\sigma}{2\varepsilon_0}(-\cos 60°\hat{x} - \sin 60°\hat{y})$$

$$= \frac{\sigma}{2\varepsilon_0}\left(-\frac{1}{2}\hat{x} - \frac{\sqrt{3}}{2}\hat{y}\right)$$

Electric field in the region shown in figure (P)

$$\vec{E}_P = \vec{E}_1 + \vec{E}_2 = \frac{\sigma}{2\varepsilon_0}\left[-\frac{1}{2}\hat{x} + \left(1 - \frac{\sqrt{3}}{2}\right)\hat{y}\right]$$

$$\text{or, } \vec{E}_P = \frac{\sigma}{2\varepsilon_0}\left[\left(1 - \frac{\sqrt{3}}{2}\right)\hat{y} - \frac{\hat{x}}{2}\right]$$

17. (d) Time period of the pendulum (T) is given by

$$T = 2\pi\sqrt{\frac{L}{g_{\text{eff}}}}$$

$$g_{\text{eff}} = \frac{\sqrt{(mg)^2 + (qE)^2}}{m}$$

$$\Rightarrow g_{\text{eff}} = \sqrt{g^2 + \left(\frac{gE}{m}\right)^2} \Rightarrow T = 2\pi\sqrt{\frac{L}{\sqrt{g^2 + \left(\frac{qE}{m}\right)^2}}}$$

18. (b) Electric field on the axis of a ring of radius R at a distance h from the centre,

$$E = \frac{kQh}{\left(h^2 + R^2\right)^{3/2}}$$

Condition: for maximum electric field $\frac{dE}{dh} = 0$

$$\Rightarrow \frac{d}{dh}\left[\frac{kQh}{\left(R^2 + h^2\right)^{3/2}}\right] = 0$$

By using the concept of maxima and minima we get,

$$h = \frac{R}{\sqrt{2}}$$

19. (a) Equilibrium position will shift to point where resultant force = 0

$$kx_{eq} = qE \Rightarrow x_{eq} = \frac{qE}{k}$$

$$\text{Total energy} = \frac{1}{2}m\omega^2A^2 + \frac{1}{2}kx_{eq}^2$$

$$\text{Total energy} = \frac{1}{2}m\omega^2A^2 + \frac{1}{2}\frac{q^2E^2}{k}$$

20. (d) Charge density, $\rho = \rho_0\left(1 - \frac{r}{R}\right)$

$$dq = \rho dv$$

$$q_{in} = \int dq = \rho dv$$

$$= \rho_0\left(1 - \frac{r}{R}\right)4\pi r^2 dr \quad (\because dv = 4\pi r^2 dr)$$

$$= 4\pi\rho_0\int_0^R\left(1 - \frac{r}{R}\right)r^2 dr = 4\pi\rho_0\int_0^R r^2 dr - \frac{r^2}{R}dr$$

$$= 4\pi\rho_0\left[\left[\frac{r^3}{3}\right]_0^R - \left[\frac{r^4}{4R}\right]_0^R\right] = 4\pi\rho_0\left[\frac{R^3}{3} - \frac{R^4}{4R}\right]$$

$$= 4\pi\rho_0\left[\frac{R^3}{3} - \frac{R^3}{4}\right] = 4\pi\rho_0\left[\frac{R^3}{12}\right] = \frac{\pi\rho_0 R^3}{3}$$

$$E.4\pi r^2 = \left(\frac{\pi\rho_0 R^3}{3\epsilon_0}\right)$$

$\therefore$ Electric field outside the ball, $E = \frac{\rho_0 R^3}{12\epsilon_0 r^2}$

21. (b) Let v be the speed of dipole.
Using energy conservation

$$K_i + U_i = K_f + U_f$$

$$\Rightarrow 0 - \frac{2k \cdot p_1}{r^3}p_2\cos(180°) = \frac{1}{2}mv^2 + \frac{1}{2}mv^2 + 0$$

$\left(\because\right.$ Potential energy of interaction between dipole $\left. = \frac{-2p_1p_2\cos\theta}{4\pi\epsilon_0 r^3}\right)$

$$\Rightarrow mv^2 = \frac{2kp_1p_2}{r^3} \Rightarrow v = \sqrt{\frac{2kp_1p_2}{mr^3}}$$

When $p_1 = p_2 = p$ and $r = a$

$$v = \frac{p}{a}\sqrt{\frac{1}{2\pi\epsilon_0 ma}}$$

22. (a)
23. (b) Surface charge density depends only due to Q. Also

$$\oint\vec{E}.d\vec{A} = \frac{q_1\lambda}{\varepsilon_0}$$

or $\quad E \times 4\pi r^2 = \frac{Q}{\varepsilon_0} \Rightarrow E = \frac{1}{4\pi\varepsilon_0}\frac{Q}{r^2}, r \geq R$

24. (a)
25. (b) $\tau = -PE\sin\theta$
or $\quad I\alpha = -PE(\theta)$

$$\alpha = \frac{PE}{I}(-\theta)$$

On comparing with
$\alpha = -\omega^2\theta$

$$\omega = \sqrt{\frac{PE}{I}} = \sqrt{\frac{qdE}{2m\left(\frac{d}{2}\right)^2}} = \sqrt{\frac{2qE}{md}}$$

26. (b) Potential energy of a dipole is given by
$U = -\vec{P}.\vec{E}$
$= -PE\cos\theta$
[Where θ = angle between dipole and perpendicular to the field]
$= -(10^{-29})(10^3)\cos 45°$
$= -0.707 \times 10^{-26}\text{ J} = -7 \times 10^{-27}\text{J}$

27. (d) Electric field of equitorial plane of dipole

$$= -\frac{K\vec{P}}{r^3}$$

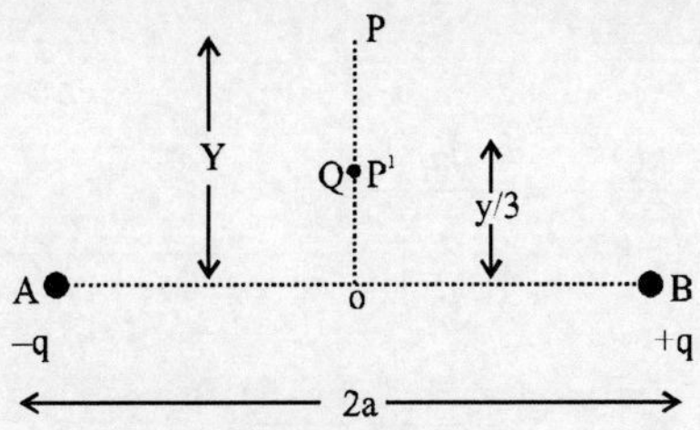

$\therefore$ At point P, $= +\frac{KP}{y^3}Q$

At Point P^1, $F^1 = +\frac{KPQ}{(y/3)^3} = 27F$.

28. (b) When cube is of side a and point charge Q is at the center of the cube then the total electric flux due to this charge will pass evenly through the six faces of the cube. So, the electric flux through one face will be equal to 1/6 of the total electric flux due to this charge.

Flux through 6 faces $= \frac{Q}{\epsilon_0}$

$\therefore$ Flux through 1 face, $= \frac{Q}{6\,\epsilon_0}$

29. (c) Inside the cavity net charge is zero.

$\therefore$ $Q_1 = 0$ and $\sigma_1 = 0$

There is no effect of point charges $+Q$, $-Q$ and induced charge on inner surface on the outer surface.

$\therefore$ $Q_2 = 0$ and $\sigma_2 = 0$

30. (d) Let F be the force between Q and Q. The force between q and Q should be attractive for net force on Q to be zero. Let F' be the force between Q and q. The resultant of F' and F' is R. For equilibrium

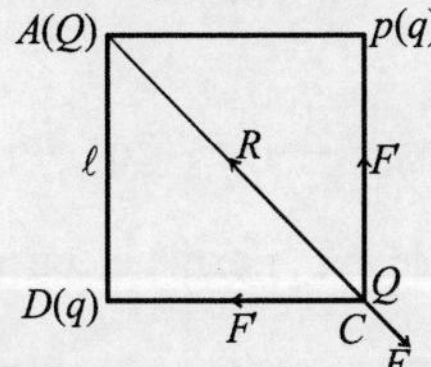

Net force on Q at C is zero.

$\therefore \vec{R} + \vec{F} = 0 \quad \Rightarrow \quad \sqrt{2}\,F' = -F$

$\Rightarrow \quad \sqrt{2} \times k\frac{Qq}{\ell^2} = -k\frac{Q^2}{(\sqrt{2}\,\ell)^2} \Rightarrow \frac{Q}{q} = -2\sqrt{2}$

31. (b)

32. (c) Field lines originate perpendicular from positive charge and terminate perpendicular at negative charge. Further this system can be treated as an electric dipole.

33. (d) Given: Length of wire $L = 20$ cm

charge $Q = 10^3 \varepsilon_0$

We know, electric field at the centre of the semicircular arc

$E = \frac{2K\lambda}{r}$

or, $E = \frac{2K\left(\frac{2Q}{\pi r}\right)}{r}\left[As\lambda = \frac{2Q}{\pi r}\right]$

$= \frac{4KQ}{\pi r^2} = \frac{4KQ\pi^2}{\pi L^2} = \frac{4\pi KQ}{L^2} = 25 \times 10^3\, N/C\hat{i}$

34. (a) Electric field due to complete disc ($R = 2a$) at a distance x and on its axis

$E_1 = \frac{\sigma}{2\varepsilon_0}\left[1 - \frac{x}{\sqrt{R^2 + x^2}}\right]$ $E_1 = \frac{\sigma}{2\varepsilon_0}\left[1 - \frac{h}{\sqrt{4a^2 + h^2}}\right]$

$= \frac{\sigma}{2\varepsilon_0}\left[1 - \frac{h}{2a}\right]$ $\left[\begin{matrix}\text{here } x = h \\ \text{and, } R = 2a\end{matrix}\right]$

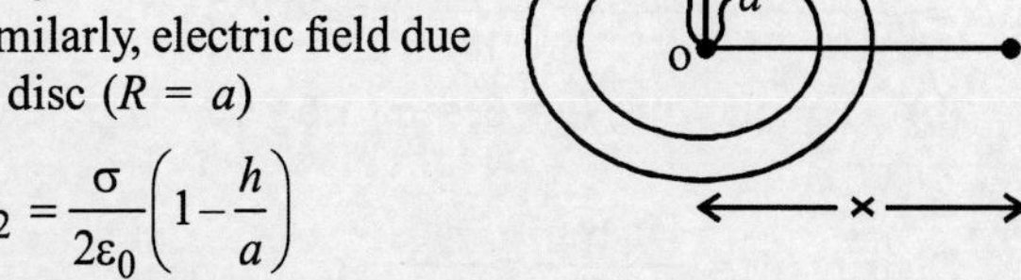

Similarly, electric field due to disc ($R = a$)

$E_2 = \frac{\sigma}{2\varepsilon_0}\left(1 - \frac{h}{a}\right)$

Electric field due to given disc

$E = E_1 - E_2$

$\frac{\sigma}{2\varepsilon_0}\left[1 - \frac{h}{2a}\right] - \frac{\sigma}{2\varepsilon_0}\left[1 - \frac{h}{a}\right] = \frac{\sigma h}{4\varepsilon_0 a}$

Hence, $c = \frac{\sigma}{4a\varepsilon_0}$

35. (b) Let us consider a spherical shell of radius x and thickness dx. Charge on this shell

$dq = \rho.4\pi x^2 dx = \rho_0\left(1 - \frac{x}{R}\right).4\pi x^2 dx$

$\therefore$ Total charge in the spherical region from centre to r (r < R) is

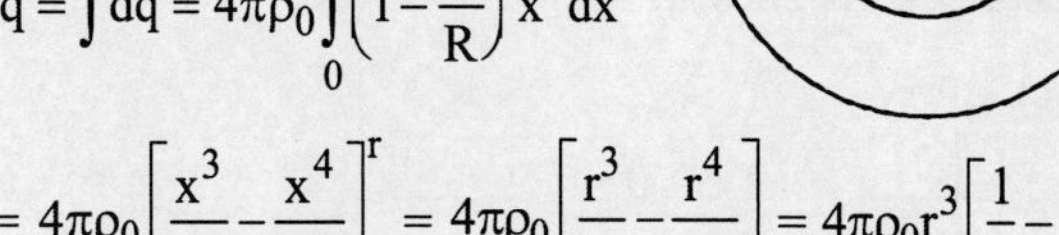

$q = \int dq = 4\pi\rho_0 \int_0^r \left(1 - \frac{x}{R}\right) x^2 dx$

$= 4\pi\rho_0\left[\frac{x^3}{3} - \frac{x^4}{4R}\right]_0^r = 4\pi\rho_0\left[\frac{r^3}{3} - \frac{r^4}{4R}\right] = 4\pi\rho_0 r^3\left[\frac{1}{3} - \frac{r}{4R}\right]$

$\therefore$ Electric field at r, $E = \frac{1}{4\pi\varepsilon_0}.\frac{q}{r^2}$

$= \frac{1}{4\pi\varepsilon_0}.\frac{4\pi\rho_0 r^3}{r^2}\left[\frac{1}{3} - \frac{r}{4R}\right] = \frac{\rho_0}{\varepsilon_0}\left[\frac{r}{3} - \frac{r^2}{4R}\right]$

36. (c) Given,

Electric field E = 150 N/C

Total surface charge carried by earth q = ?

or, $q = \epsilon_0 EA = \epsilon_0 E\pi r^2$.

$= 8.85 \times 10^{-12} \times 150 \times (6.37 \times 10^6)^2$.

$\simeq 680$ Kc

As electric field directed inward hence

$q = -680$ Kc

37. (a) Electric field intensity at the centre of the disc.

$E = \frac{\sigma}{2\,\epsilon_0}$ (given)

Electric field along the axis at any distance x from the centre of the disc

$$E' = \frac{\sigma}{2\epsilon_0}\left(1 - \frac{x}{\sqrt{x^2 + R^2}}\right)$$

From question, x = R (radius of disc)

$$\therefore E' = \frac{\sigma}{2\epsilon_0}\left(1 - \frac{R}{\sqrt{R^2 + R^2}}\right) = \frac{\sigma}{2\epsilon_0}\left(\frac{\sqrt{2}R - R}{\sqrt{2}R}\right) = \frac{4}{14}E$$

$\therefore$ % reduction in the value of electric field

$$= \frac{\left(E - \frac{4}{14}E\right) \times 100}{E} = \frac{1000}{14}\% \simeq 70.7\%$$

38. (b) $F = qE = mg \; (q = 6e = 6 \times 1.6 \times 10^{-19})$

$$\text{Density } (d) = \frac{\text{mass}}{\text{volume}} = \frac{m}{\frac{4}{3}\pi r^3} \text{ or } r^3 = \frac{m}{\frac{4}{3}\pi d}$$

Putting the value of d and m $\left(= \frac{qE}{g}\right)$ and solving we get r $= 7.8 \times 10^{-7}$ m

39. (a)

40. (c) Electric lines of force due to a positive charge is spherically symmetric.
All the charges are positive and equal in magnitude. So repulsion takes place. Due to which no lines of force are present inside the equilateral triangle and the resulting lines of force obtained as shown:

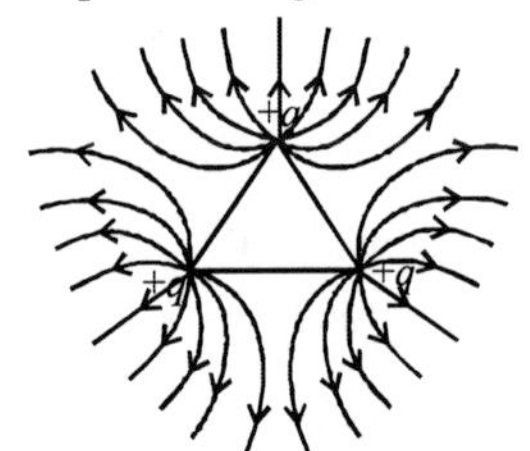

41. (c)

P, θ, T, $T\cos\theta$, $F = Eq = \frac{\sigma}{\varepsilon_0 K}q$, $T\sin\theta$, mg

$T\sin\theta = qE$ .... (i)

$T\cos\theta = mg$ .... (ii)

Dividing (i) by (ii),

$$\tan\theta = \frac{qE}{mg} = \frac{q}{mg}\left(\frac{\sigma}{\varepsilon_0 K}\right)\frac{\sigma q}{\varepsilon_0 K.mg}$$

$\therefore \sigma \propto \tan\theta$

42. (b) For the system to be equilibrium, net field at A should be zero

$$\sqrt{2}\,E_1 + E_2 = E_3$$

$$\therefore \frac{kQ \times \sqrt{2}}{a^2} + \frac{kQ}{(\sqrt{2}\,a)^2} = \frac{kq}{\left(\frac{a}{\sqrt{2}}\right)^2}$$

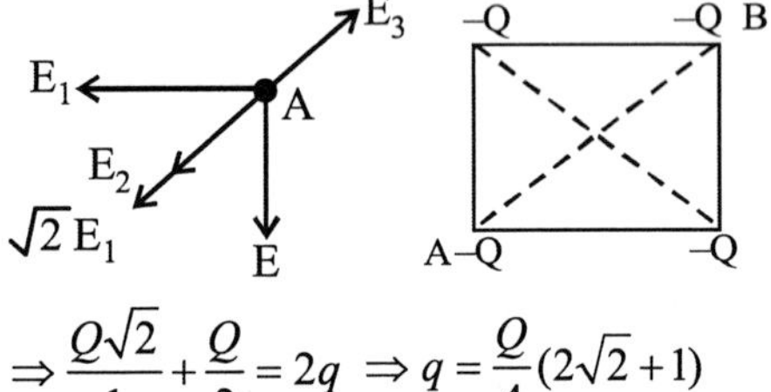

$$\Rightarrow \frac{Q\sqrt{2}}{1} + \frac{Q}{2} = 2q \Rightarrow q = \frac{Q}{4}(2\sqrt{2} + 1)$$

43. (b) At $P \frac{-K2q}{(x-L)^2} + \frac{K8q}{x^2} = 0$

$$\Rightarrow \frac{1}{(x-L)^2} = \frac{4}{x^2}$$

$$\text{or } \frac{1}{x-L} = \frac{2}{x}$$

$\Rightarrow x = 2x - 2L$ or $x = 2L$

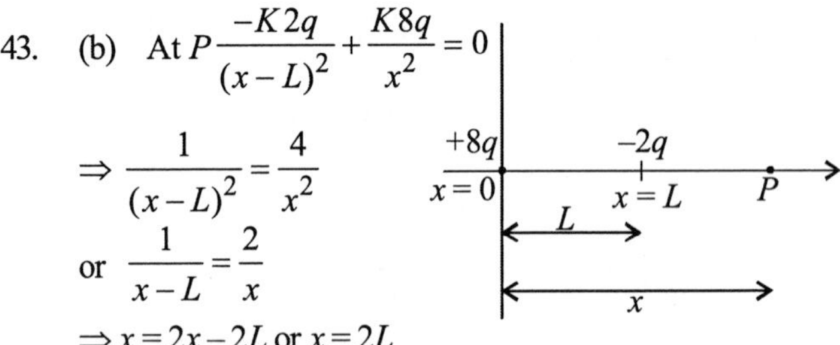

44. (c) The net flux linked with closed surfaces S_1, S_2, S_3 & S_4 are

For surface S_1, $\phi_1 = \frac{1}{\varepsilon_0}(2q)$

For surface S_2, $\phi_2 = \frac{1}{\varepsilon_0}(q + q + q - q) = \frac{1}{\varepsilon_0}2q$

For surface S_3, $\phi_3 = \frac{1}{\varepsilon_0}(q + q) = \frac{1}{\varepsilon_0}(2q)$

For surface S_4, $\phi_4 = \frac{1}{\varepsilon_0}(8q - 2q - 4q) = \frac{1}{\varepsilon_0}(2q)$

Hence, $\phi_1 = \phi_2 = \phi_3 = \phi_4$ i.e. net electric flux is same for all surfaces.

Keep in mind, the electric field due to a charge outside (S_3 and S_4), the Gaussian surface contributes zero net flux through the surface, because as many lines due to that charge enter the surface as leave it.

45. (a) The electric flux ϕ_1 entering an enclosed surface is taken as negative and the electric flux ϕ_2 leaving the surface is taken as positive, by convention. Therefore the net flux leaving the enclosed surface, $\phi = \phi_2 - \phi_1$

According to Gauss theorem

$$\phi = \frac{q}{\epsilon_0} \qquad \Rightarrow q = \epsilon_0\phi = \epsilon_0(\phi_2 - \phi_1)$$

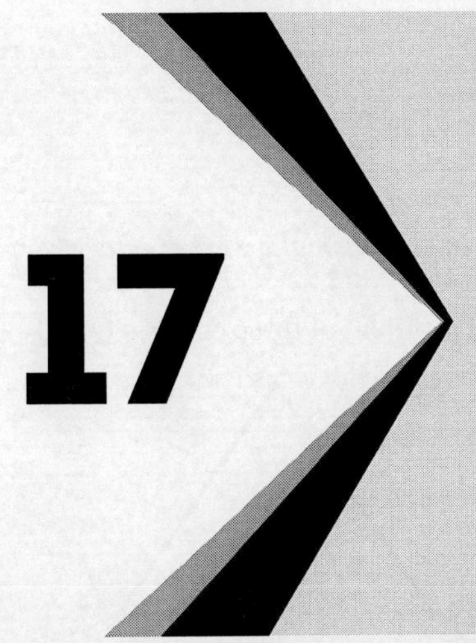

Electrostatic Potential and Capacitance

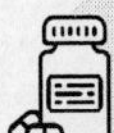

Topic 17.1 : Electrostatic Potential, Potential Energy of a System of Charges and Equipotential Surface

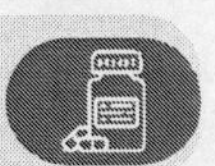

ELECTROSTATIC POTENTIAL

Electric potential *at a point in an electric field is defined as the amount of work done in bringing a unit positive test charge from infinity to that point along any arbitrary path.* (Infinity is taken as point of zero potential). It is denoted by V ;

$$V=\frac{W}{q_0}=\frac{\text{work done in bringing unit positive test charge from infinity to some point}}{\text{unit positive test charge}}$$

Its **SI unit** is JC^{-1} or volt. It is a scalar quantity.

Also, **electric potential at any point** in an electric field is defined as the negative line integral of the electric field vector $\vec{E}$ from a point infinitely away from all charges to that point

i.e. $V=-\int_{\infty}^{r}\vec{E}.\vec{dr}$

P ←———— ∞ +IC

Potential due to a Point Charge

The **electric potential due to a point charge** q at separation r is given by

$$V=\frac{1}{4\pi\varepsilon}\cdot\frac{q}{r}$$

(Please note that we have to write q with its sign in this formula)

Potential difference between two points is the work done in bringing unit positive charge from one point to another.

Q B A ; r_B ; r_A

$$V_{AB}=V_B-V_A=-\int_A^B E.dr=\frac{-Q}{4\pi\varepsilon_o}\cdot\left(\frac{l}{r_B}-\frac{l}{r_A}\right)\ J/C$$

Electric Potential due to Continuous Charge Distribution

The potential due to a continuous charge distribution is the sum of potentials of all the infinitesimal charge elements in which the distribution may be divided.

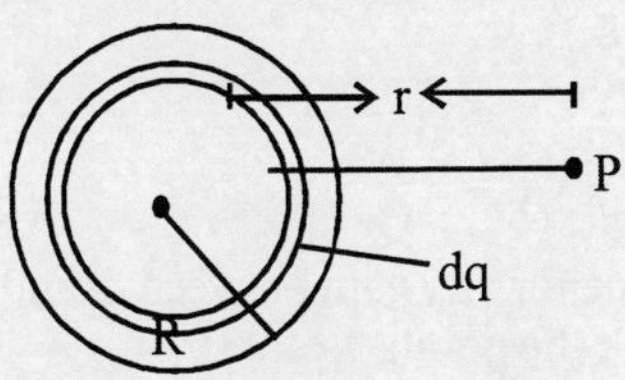

i.e. $V=\int dV=\int\frac{dq}{4\pi\varepsilon_o r}$ where $dV=\frac{dq}{4\pi\varepsilon_o r}$

Potential due to a System of Charges

The electric potential due to a system of charges $q_1, q_2, ...q_n$ is $V=V_1+V_2+...+V_n$

$$=\frac{1}{4\pi\varepsilon}\cdot\left(\frac{q_1}{r_1}+\frac{q_2}{r_2}+...+\frac{q_n}{r_n}\right)=\frac{1}{4\pi\varepsilon}\sum\frac{q_i}{r_i}$$

where r_i is the point from charge q_i and ε is the permitivity of medium in which the charges are situated.

Potential at any point P due to a point chage q at a distance (r_1+r_2) where r_1 is the thickness of medium of dielectric constant x_1 and r_2 is the thickness of the medium of dielectric constant k_2

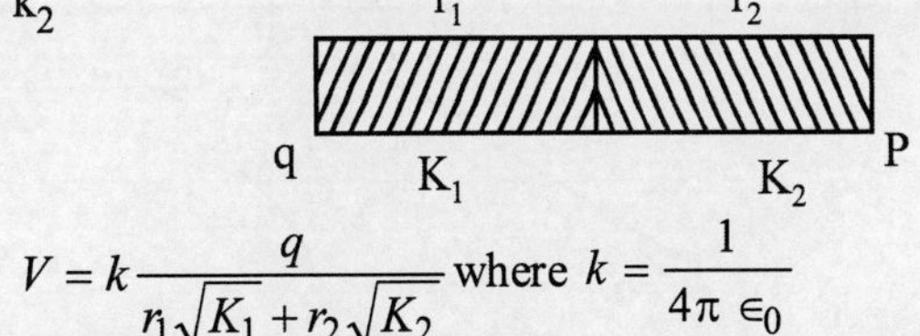

$$V=k\frac{q}{r_1\sqrt{K_1}+r_2\sqrt{K_2}}\text{ where }k=\frac{1}{4\pi\in_0}$$

Relation between electric field and potential

The relation between electric field (E) and potential (V) is

$$E=-\frac{dV}{dr}$$

For 3-D we can write

$$E_x=-\frac{\partial V}{\partial x},\ E_y=-\frac{\partial V}{\partial y}\text{ and }E_z=-\frac{\partial V}{\partial z}$$

So **electric field is equal to negative potential gradient.**

In this relation negative sign indicates that in the direction of electric field, potential decreases. Consider two points A and B situated in a uniform electric field at a distance d then,

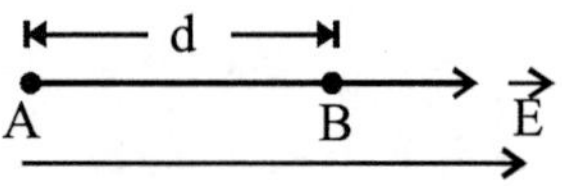

The potential difference between A and B is

$$V_{AB} = Ed$$

Conservative nature of electric field

The electric field is conservative in nature. In figure the work, W_{AB} has the same value whatever path is taken in moving the test charge.

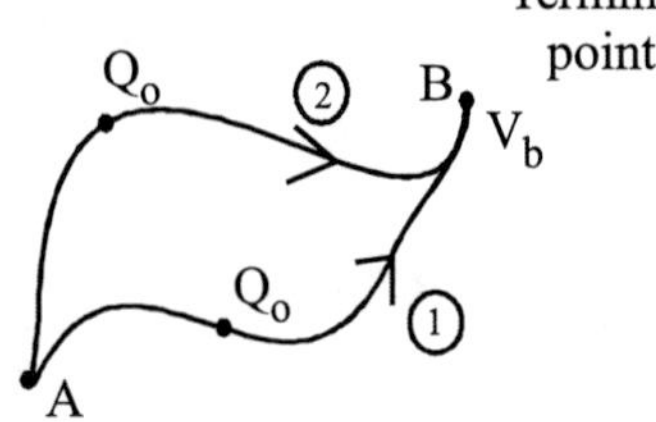

so, $V_{AB} = V_B - V_A = \frac{W_{AB}}{Q}$

has the same value for any path between A and B and V_B and V_A are unique for the points A and B.

Note : We cannot find the absolute value of potential therefore conventionally, we take infinity as the point of zero potential. If need arises, we can assume any point to be the point of zero potential and find the potential of other points on this basis.

POTENTIAL ENERGY OF A SYSTEM OF CHARGES

Potential energy can be defined only for those forces, which are conservative, such as gravitational and electrostatic forces. *The potential energy of a charge between two points is defined as the amount of work done in bringing the charge from one point to another.*

i.e. $V_B - V_A = \frac{W_{ext}}{q} = -\int_A^B \vec{E}.\vec{dr}$

Calculation of external work done against the field and a point charge Q in moving a test charge q from A to B. For a conservative field the work done by any path is same. The sectional force is – qE.

If A is at infinity then at infinity since potential is zero we assume infinity as reference point, $V_A = 0$

$$\Rightarrow V_B = -q\int_{\infty}^{B} E.dl$$

Potential energy of a system of two charges Q_1 and Q_2 is,

$$U = \frac{1}{4\pi\epsilon_0}\frac{Q_1 Q_2}{r^2}$$

[Please note that in this formula we have to write charges with sign]

Potential energy of a system of three charges Q_1, Q_2 and Q_3

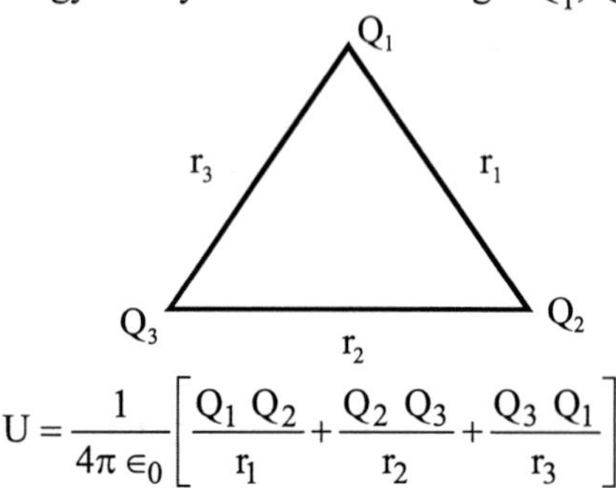

$$U = \frac{1}{4\pi\epsilon_0}\left[\frac{Q_1 Q_2}{r_1} + \frac{Q_2 Q_3}{r_2} + \frac{Q_3 Q_1}{r_3}\right]$$

Problem Solving Tips

1. For an assembly of n charges [Total number of intersection ${}^nC_2 = \frac{n(n-1)}{2}$] the potential energy is

$$U = \frac{1}{2}\left[k\sum_{\substack{i,j \\ i\neq j}}^{n} \frac{q_i q_j}{r_{ij}}\right]$$

2. For a system of two charges.

   If U_{system} = –ve, then there is net force of attraction between the charges of the system.

   If U_{system} = +ve, then there is net force of repulsion between the charges of the system

   U_{system} = max for unstable equilibrium

   U_{system} = min for stable equilibrium

   Also $F = -\frac{dU}{dx} = 0$

3. The energy required to take away the charges of a dipole at infinite distance $U = k\frac{q^2}{2l}$

4. The work done when a charge q is moved across a potential difference of V volt is given by W = qV

5. When one electronic charge (1.6×10^{-19} coulomb i.e., charge of electron) is moved across one volt the work done is called **one electron volt (eV).** Thus

   $1eV = (1 \text{ volt}) \times (1.6\times10^{-19} \text{ coulomb}) = 1.6\times10^{-19}$ joule.

EQUIPOTENTIAL SURFACE

It is that surface where the potential at any point of the surface has the same value. The electric lines of force and the equipotential surface are mutually perpendicular to each other. No work is done in moving a charge from one point to other on an equipotential surface. Work is done in moving a charge from one equipotential surface to another.

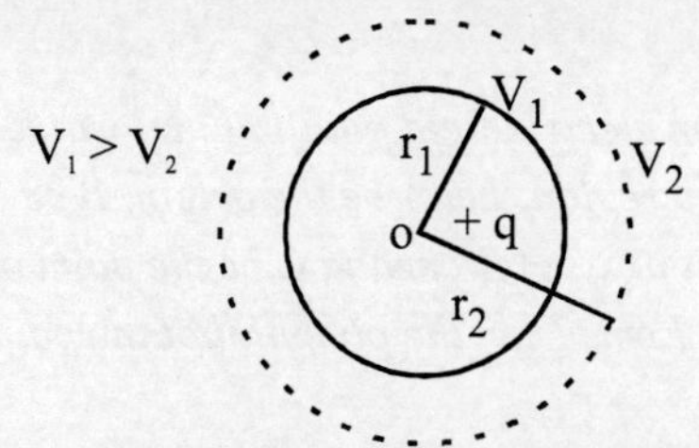

Spherical equipotential surface for point charge

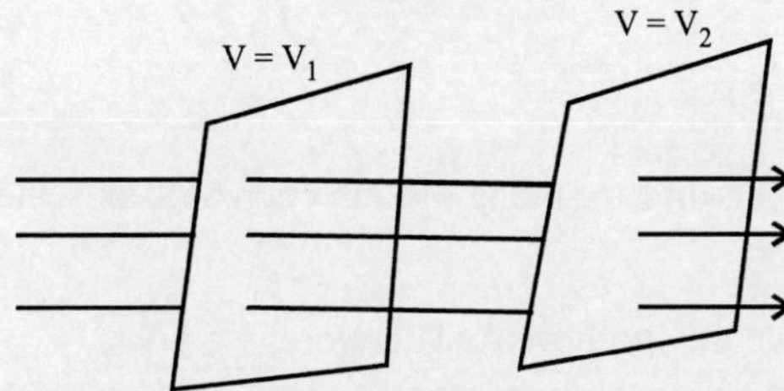

Plane equipotential surface for uniform field

- Equipotential surface do not cut each other.
- The density of the equipotential lines gives an idea of the strength of electric field at that point. Higher the density, larger is the field strength.

Potential Due to Various Charge Distribution

(i) **Electric potential due to isolated point charge**

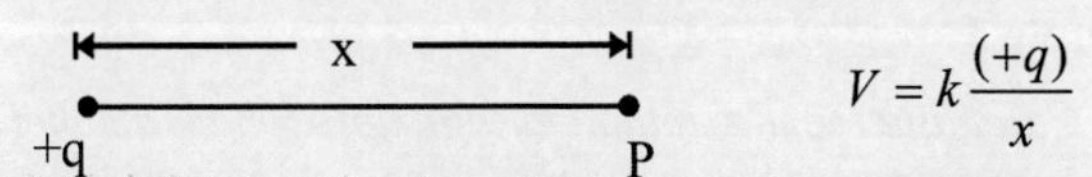

$$V = k\frac{(+q)}{x}$$

(ii) A **circular ring** of radius R with uniformly distributed charge Q

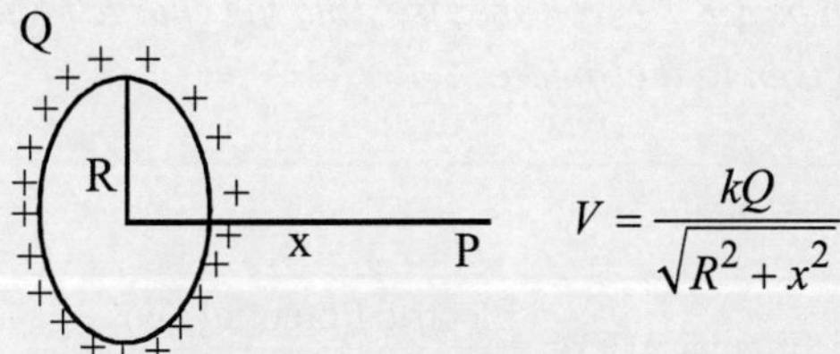

$$V = \frac{kQ}{\sqrt{R^2 + x^2}}$$

- Potential V does not depend on the way of charge distriubution on the ring (uniform / non-uniform).

(iii) **A circular disc** of radius R with uniformly distributed charge with surface charge density σ

$$V = \frac{\sigma}{2\varepsilon_0}\left[\sqrt{R^2 + x^2} - x\right]$$

(iv) A **finite length of charge** with linear charge density λ

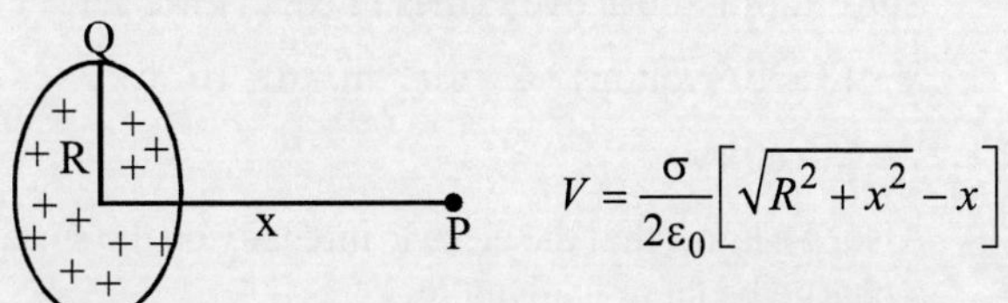

$$V = k\lambda \log_e\left(\frac{x + L}{x}\right)$$

(v) Due to a **spherical shell** of uniformly distributed charge with surface charge density σ

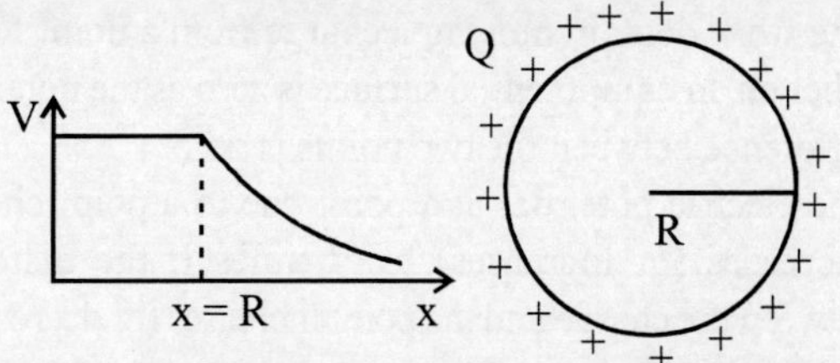

$$V_{in} = k\frac{Q}{R},\ V_{surface} = k\frac{Q}{R},\ V_{out} = k\frac{Q}{x}$$

(vi) Due to a **solid sphere** of uniformly distributed charge with volume charge density ρ.

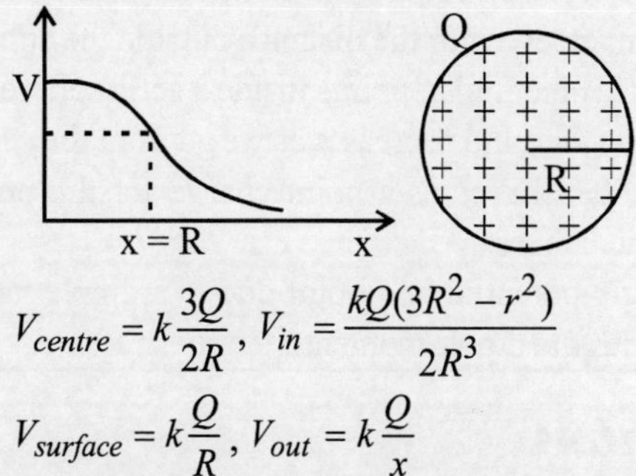

$$V_{centre} = k\frac{3Q}{2R},\ V_{in} = \frac{kQ(3R^2 - r^2)}{2R^3}$$

$$V_{surface} = k\frac{Q}{R},\ V_{out} = k\frac{Q}{x}$$

Potential due to Electric dipole

(a) Along axial line :

$$V_{axial} = k\frac{p}{x^2 - l^2}$$

when $x >> l$ $V_{axial} = \frac{kp}{x^2}$

(b) Along equatorial line :

$V_{eq} = zero$

(c) At any point from the dipole :

$$V = k\frac{p\cos\theta}{(x^2 - l^2\cos^2\theta)}$$

Problem Solving Tips

1. Electric field inside a charged conductor is zero

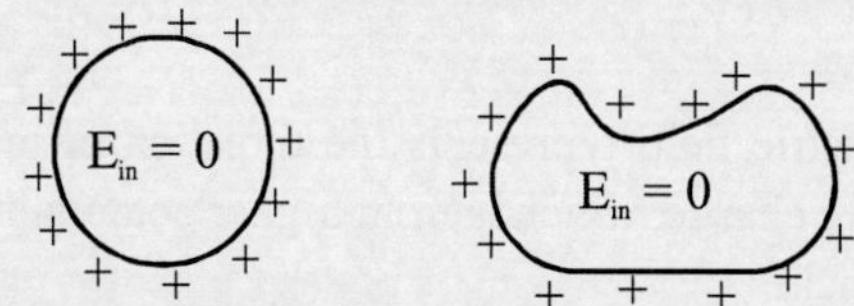

Spherical conductor Irregular shaped conductor

But in both the cases the potential at all the points of the surface will remain the same. But charges will have same distribution on spherical conductor and in case of irregularly shaped conductor the charge distribution will be non-uniform. At sharp points, charge density has greatest value.

2. Electronic lines of force are always perpendicular to the equipotential surfaces.

3. The work done in moving a charge from a point to the other on an equipotential surface is zero as the potential difference between the two points is zero.
4. The electric potential at a point due to a point charge decreases (or increases) by K-times if the distance between the charge and the point increases (or decreases) by K-times.
5. A ring with a charge distribution behaves as a point charge for the points very far from its centre.
6. The electric potential is constant inside a hollow charged sphere and it is also equal to its value on the surface but it varies inversely with the distance outside the sphere.
7. The electric potential at points inside a solid sphere has a non-zero value and decreases as we go from the centre outwards. It behaves as a point charge for the points outside the sphere.
8. The electric potential at a point due to a dipole varies directly with the dipole moment.

MISCONCEPTIONS

✘ ***Incorrect :*** Where electric field is zero, electric potential is also zero.

✔ ***Correct :*** It is not always correct, for example in a charged conducting shell, electric field inside the shell E = 0 but potential is not zero.

✘ ***Incorrect :*** Where electric potential is zero, electric field is also zero.

✔ ***Correct :*** It is not always correct. In the case of equitorial plane of an electric dipole the electric potential is zero but the electric field is non-zero.

Example 1

A uniform electric field pointing in positive y-direction exists in a region. Let A be the origin, B be the point on the x-axis at x = 2 cm and C be the point on the y-axis at y = 2 cm. Then the potential at the points A, B and C satisfy:

(a) $V_A < V_B$ (b) $V_A > V_B$
(c) $V_A < V_C$ (d) $V_A > V_C$

Solution : (d)

As electric field represents the direction of motion of positive charge, which is from higher potential to lower potential,
therefore, from fig, we find $V_A = V_B$ and $V_A > V_C$

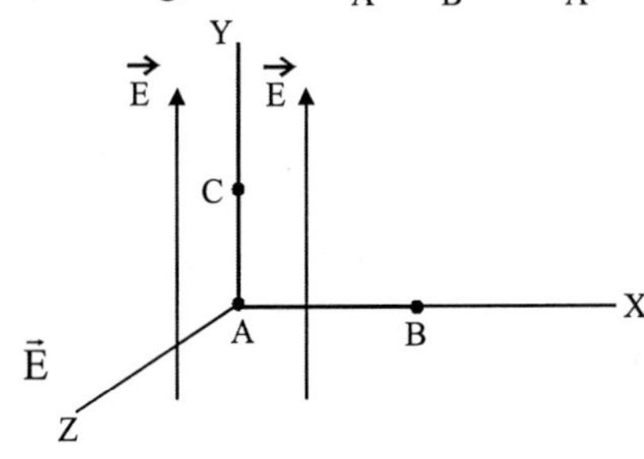

Example 2

A uniform electric field pointing in positive x-direction exists in a region. Let A be the origin, B be the point on the x-axis at x = + 1 cm and C be the point on the y-axis at y = + 1 cm. Then the potential at the points A, B and C satisfy

(a) $V_A < V_B$ (b) $V_A > V_B$
(c) $V_A < V_C$ (d) $V_A > V_C$

Solution : (b)

As $\vec{E}$ is directed along +ve direction of X-axis, therefore, $V_A > V_B$

C is vertically above A. Therefore, $V_A = V_C$.

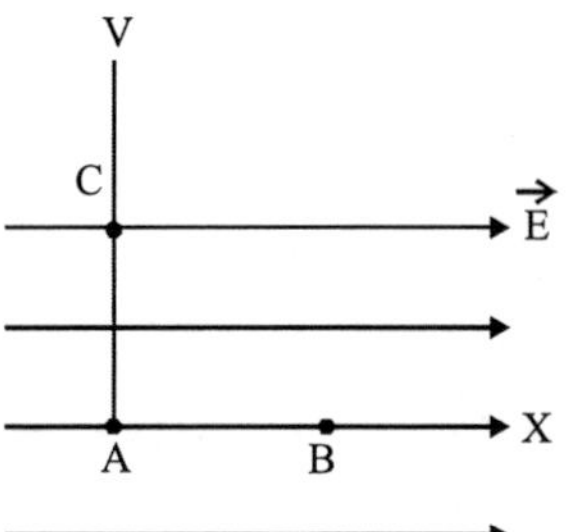

Example 3

Calculate the maximum voltage upto which a sphere of radius 2 cm can be charged in air under normal conditions, assuming that maximum electric intensity in air can be 3 × 10⁶ volt/m. Also, find the charge required to be given to the sphere.

Solution :

We know that

$$\text{Electric intensity (E)} = \frac{\text{Electric Potential (V)}}{\text{Distance (r)}}$$

$$\Rightarrow V = Er \qquad \text{......(1)}$$

Given, $E = 3 \times 10^6$ volt/m, $r = 2$ cm $= 2 \times 10^{-2}$ m.

Substituting the above values in eq. (1), we get

$V = (3 \times 10^6 \text{ volt/m}) \times 2 \times 10^{-2} \text{ m} = 6 \times 10^4$ volt.

$\Rightarrow V = 60$ kV

Also, we know that the electric intensity on the surface of a charged sphere is given by

$$E = \frac{1}{4\pi \epsilon_0} \cdot \frac{Q}{r^2}; \quad Q = \text{charge on the sphere}$$

$$\Rightarrow 3\times10^6 = (9\times10^9)\times\frac{Q}{(2\times10^{-2})^2}$$

$$\Rightarrow Q = 1.33\times10^{-7} \text{ coulomb.}$$

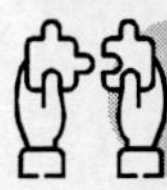

17.1 Concept Practice Problems

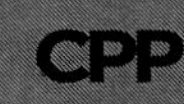

1. A sphere of radius R has uniform volume charge density. The electric potential at a points (r <R) is
(a) due to the charge inside a sphere of radius r only
(b) due to the entire charge of the sphere
(c) due to the charge in the spherical sheel of inner and outer radii r and R, only
(d) independent of r

2. Three charges 2 q, – q and – q are located at the vertices of an equilateral triangle. At the centre of the triangle
(a) the field is zero but potential is non-zero
(b) the field is non-zero, but potential is zero
(c) both field and potential are zero
(d) both field and potential are non-zero

3. Two conducting spheres of radii r_1 and r_2 are equally charged. The ratio of their potentials is
(a) r_1/r_2 (b) r_2/r_1 (c) r_1^2/r_2^2 (d) r_2^2/r_1^2

4. The electric potential due to a small electric dipole at a large distance r from the centre of the dipole is proportional to
(a) r (b) 1/r (c) $1/r^2$ (d) $1/r^3$

5. An electron of mass m and charge e is accelerated from rest through a potential difference V in vacuum. Its final speed will be
(a) $\sqrt{\frac{2eV}{m}}$ (b) $\sqrt{\frac{eV}{m}}$ (c) eV/2m (d) eV/m

6. A positive point charge q is carried from a point B to a point A in the electric field of a point charge + Q at O. If the permitivity of free space is ε_0, the work done in the process is given by
(a) $\frac{qQ}{4\pi\varepsilon_o}\left(\frac{1}{a}+\frac{1}{b}\right)$ (b) $\frac{qQ}{4\pi\varepsilon_o}\left(\frac{1}{a}-\frac{1}{b}\right)$
(c) $\frac{qQ}{4\pi\varepsilon_o}\left(\frac{1}{a^2}-\frac{1}{b^2}\right)$ (d) $\frac{qQ}{4\pi\varepsilon_o}\left(\frac{1}{a^2}+\frac{1}{b^2}\right)$

7. Two concentric, thin metallic spheres of radii R_1 and R_2 $(R_1 > R_2)$ bear charges Q_1 and Q_2 respectively. Then the potential at distance r between R_1 and R_2 will be $\left(k=\frac{1}{4\pi\varepsilon_0}\right)$
(a) $k\left(\frac{Q_1+Q_2}{r}\right)$ (b) $k\left(\frac{Q_1}{r}+\frac{Q_2}{R_2}\right)$
(c) $k\left(\frac{Q_2}{r}+\frac{Q_1}{R_1}\right)$ (d) $k\left(\frac{Q_1}{R_1}+\frac{Q_2}{R_2}\right)$

8. An alpha particle is accelerated through a potential difference of 10^6 volt. Its kinetic energy will be
(a) 1 MeV (b) 2 MeV (c) 4 MeV (d) 8 MeV

9. A hollow metal sphere of radius 5 cm is charged such that the potential on its surface is 10 V. The potential at a distance of 2 cm from the centre of the sphere is
(a) zero (b) 10 V (c) 4 V (d) 10/3 V

10. Find the dipole moment of a system where the potential 2.0×10^{-5} V at a point P, 0.1m from the dipole is 3.0×10^4. (Use $\theta = 30°$).
(a) 2.57×10^{-17} Cm (b) 1.285×10^{-15} Cm
(c) 1.285×10^{-17} Cm (d) 2.57×10^{-15} Cm

ANSWER KEY

1	(a)	2	(b)	3	(b)	4	(c)	5	(a)	6	(b)	7	(c)	8	(b)	9	(b)	10	(a)

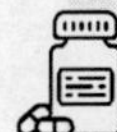

Topic 17.2 : Electrostatics of Conductors, Capacitors & Capacitance, Energy Stored in a Capacitor, Parallel Plate Capacitor, Combination of Capacitors and Charging & Discharging a Capacitor

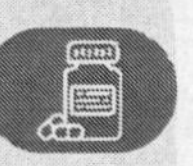

ELECTROSTATICS OF CONDUCTORS

Conductor is a substance that can be used to carry or conduct electric charges. Metals like silver. Copper, aluminium etc. are good conductors of electricity.

Regarding electrostatics of conductors following points are worth noting.

(i) Inside a conductor, electric field is zero.

(ii) The interior of a conductor can have no excess charge in static situation.

(iii) Electric field at the surface of a charged conductor is

$$\vec{E} = \frac{\sigma}{\epsilon_0}\hat{n}$$

where, s = surface charge density

$\hat{n}$ = unit vector normal to the surface in the outward direction.

(iv) Electric field just outside a charged conductor is perpendicular to the surface of the conductor at every point.

(v) Electrostatic potential is constant throughout the volume of the conductor and has the same value as on its surface.

(vi) Surface density of charge is different at different points.

CAPACITORS AND CAPACITANCE

A capacitor *or* ***condenser*** *is a device that stores electrical energy.* It generally consists of two conductors carrying equal but opposite charges.

The ability of a capacitor to hold a charge is measured by a quantity called the ***capacitance.*** Let us consider two uncharged identical conductors X and Y and create a P.D. (Potential Difference) V between them by connecting with battery B as shown in figure.

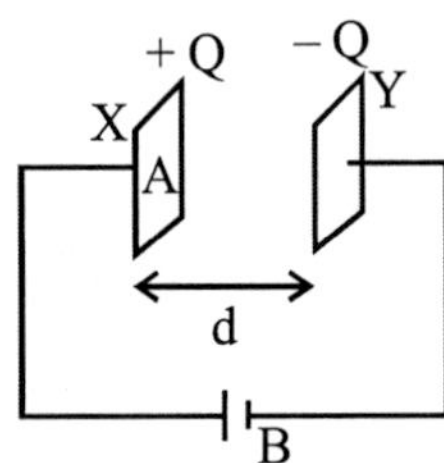

Fig- A capacitor consists of electrically insulated conductors carrying equal positive and negative charge

After connection with the battery, the two conductors X and Y have equal but opposite charges. Such a combination of charged conductors is a device called a capacitor. The P.D. between X and Y is found to be proportional to the charge Q on capacitor. *The capacitance C, of a capacitor is defined as the ratio of the magnitude of the charge on either conductor to the magnitude of P.D. between them.*

$$V \propto Q \Rightarrow \frac{Q}{V} = \text{constant} = (\text{Capacitance}).$$

Capacitance is always a positive quantity.

The **S.I. unit** of capacitance is coulomb per volt or farad (F).

Further more, the value of ***capacitance depends*** *on size, shape, relative positions of plate, and the medium between the plates. The value of C does not depend on the charge of the plate or p.d. between the plates.*

ENERGY STORED IN A CAPACITOR

If Q is charge, V is p.d, C is the capacitance of the capacitor then the energy stored is $U = \frac{1}{2}CV^2 = \frac{1}{2}QV = \frac{Q^2}{2C}$

Sharing of Charges

When the two charged conductors of capacitances C_1 and C_2 at potentials V_1 and V_2 respectively, are connected by a conducting wire, the charge flows from higher to lower potential, until the potentials of the two conductors are equal.

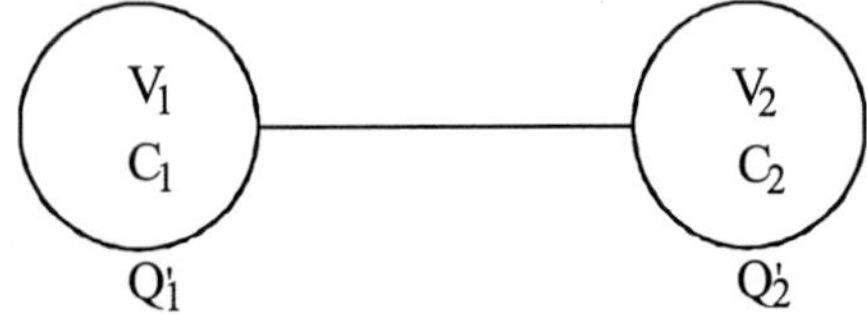

The common potential after sharing of charges,

$$V = \frac{\text{Net charge}}{\text{Net capacitance}} = \frac{Q_1 + Q_2}{C_1 + C_2} = \frac{C_1V_1 + C_2V_2}{C_1 + C_2}$$

The charges after sharing on two conductors will be

$$Q_1' = C_1V \text{ and } Q_2' = C_2V \text{ i.e., } \frac{Q_1}{Q_2} = \frac{C_1}{C_2} = \frac{Q_1'}{Q_2'}$$

There is a loss of energy during sharing, converted to heat given by

$$\Delta U = U_{\text{initial}} - U_{\text{final}} = \left[\frac{1}{2}C_1V_1^2 + \frac{1}{2}C_2V_2^2\right] - \frac{1}{2}(C_1 + C_2)V^2$$

$$\text{or, } \Delta u = \frac{C_1C_2(V_1 - V_2)^2}{2(C_1 + C_2)}$$

PARALLEL PLATE CAPACITOR

It consists of two parallel metallic plates of any shape, each of area A and at a distance d apart.

The capacitance of the capacitor is given by $C = \frac{\varepsilon_0 A}{d}$

Effect of Dielectric on Capacitance

When a dielectric slab is placed between the plates of a parallel plate capacitor, the charge induced on its plates due to polarisation of dielectric is $q_p = Q\left(1 - \frac{1}{K}\right)$

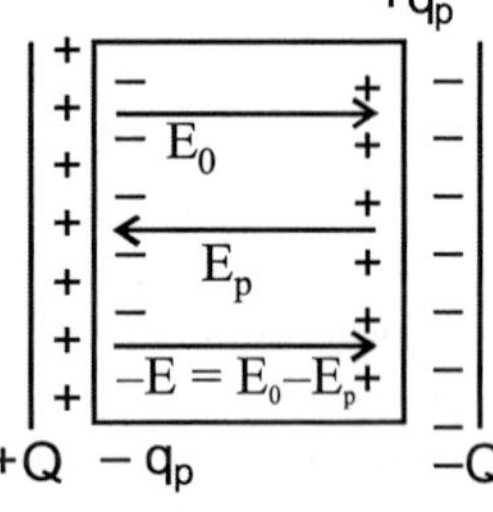

where K = dielectric constant.

When an electric field is applied across a dielectric, induced charges appear on the surface of dielectric which is shown in the above figure. These induced charges produce their own field which acts in the opposite direction of the applied field. Hence, total field is reduced, i.e., $E_0 - E_p = E$, where E_0 is the applied field, E_p is the induced field and E is the resultant field.

E is given by $\frac{E_0}{K}$, where K is the dielectric constant.

If medium between the plates is having a dielectric of dielectric constant K then the capacitance is given $C = \left(\frac{K\varepsilon_0 A}{d}\right)$

If the space between the plates is partly filled with dielectric then the capacitance of the capacitor will be given by,

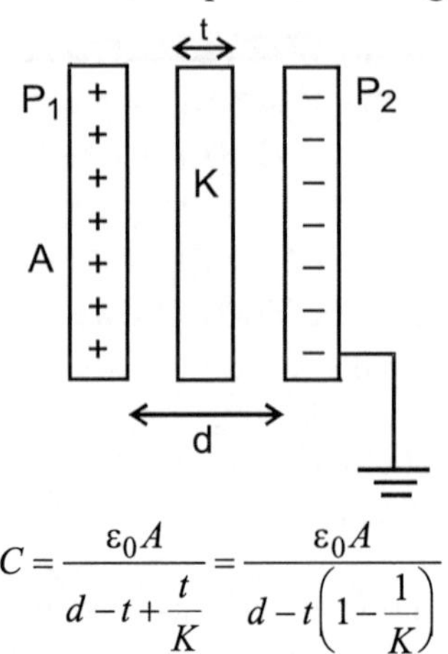

$$C = \frac{\varepsilon_0 A}{d - t + \frac{t}{K}} = \frac{\varepsilon_0 A}{d - t\left(1 - \frac{1}{K}\right)},$$

where t is the thickness of the dielectric with dielectric constant K.

Problem Solving Tips

1. The unit farad is quite a big unit for practical purposes. Even the capacitance of a huge body like earth is 711 μF.
2. A capacitor is a device which stores charges and produces electricity whenever required.
3. If the two plates of a capacitor is connected with a conducting wire, sparking takes place which shows that electrical energy is converted into heat and light energy.
4. A capacitor allows A.C. but doesn't allow D.C. to pass through it.
5. The capacitance of a capacitor increases with insertion of a dielectric between its plates and decreases with increase in the separation between the plates.
6. The capacitance of a capacitor increases K times if a medium of dielectric constant K is inserted between its plates.
7. The energy of a capacitor for a particular separation between the plates is the amount of work done in separating the two plates to that separation if they are made to touch to each other.
8. The loss of energy when the two charged conductors are connected by a wire doesn't depend on the length of the wire.

Example 4

A parallel plate capacitor is maintained at a certain potential difference. When a 3 mm slab is introduced between the plates, in order to maintain the same potential difference, the distance between the plates is increased by 2.4 mm. Find the dielectric constant of the slab.

Solution :

The capacity of a parallel plate capacitor in air is given by

$$C = \frac{\varepsilon_0 A}{d} \qquad ...(1)$$

By introducing a slab of thickness t, the new capacitance C′ becomes

$$C' = \frac{\varepsilon_0 A}{d' - t(1 - 1/K)} \qquad ...(2)$$

The charge (Q = CV) remains the same in both the cases. Hence

$$\frac{\varepsilon_0 A}{d} = \frac{\varepsilon_0 A}{d' - t(1-1/K)} \quad \text{or } d = d' - t\left(1 - \frac{1}{K}\right)$$

$d' = d + 2.4 \times 10^{-3}$ m, $t = 3$ mm $= 3 \times 10^{-3}$ m.

Substituting these values, we have

$$d = d + (2.4 \times 10^{-3}) - 3 \times 10^{-3}\left(1 - \frac{1}{K}\right)$$

or $\quad (2.4 \times 10^{-3}) = 3 \times 10^{-3}\left(1 - \frac{1}{K}\right)$

Solving it, we get K = 5.

SPHERICAL CAPACITOR

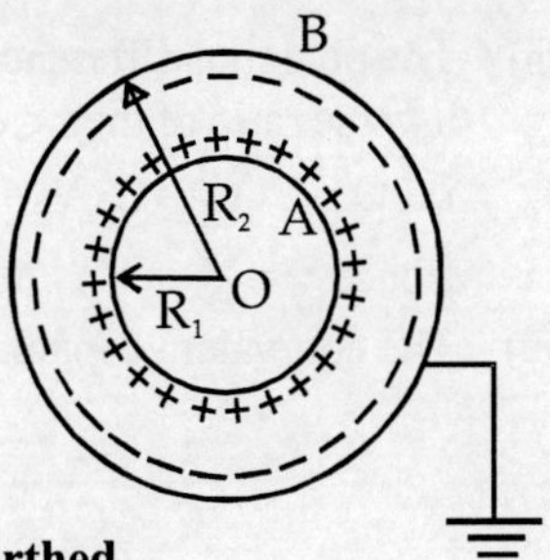

It consists of two concentric spherical conductors of radii R_1 and R_2. The space between two conductors is filled by a dielectric of dielectric constant K.

(a) **When outer conductor is earthed,**

Capacitance of spherical capacitor,

$$C = \frac{4\pi \epsilon_0 R_1 R_2}{R_2 - R_1} \qquad \text{(without dielectric)}$$

$$C = \frac{(4\pi\varepsilon_o K) R_1 R_2}{(R_2 - R_1)} \qquad \text{(with dielectric)}$$

(b) **When inner sphere is earthed,**

$$C = \frac{4\pi\varepsilon_o K\, R_1 R_2}{R_2 - R_1} + 4\pi\varepsilon_o R_2$$

This is because the combination behaves as two capacitors in parallel, one is a capacitor formed by two concentric spherical shells and the other is an isolated spherical shell of radius R_2.

CYLINDRICAL CAPACITOR

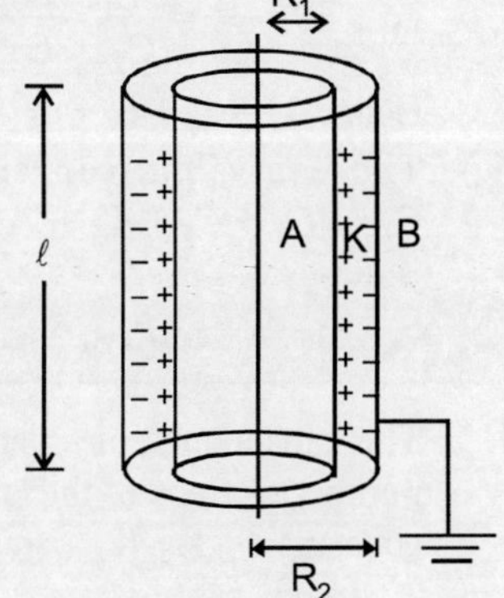

It consists of two-coaxial cylindrical conductors of radii R_1 and R_2, the outer surface of outer conductor being earthed. The space between the two is filled with a dielectric of dielectric constant K.

The capacitance of cylindrical condenser of length ℓ

$$C = \frac{2\pi \epsilon_0 \ell}{\log_e\left(\frac{R_2}{R_1}\right)} \qquad \text{(without dielectric)}$$

$$C = \frac{2\pi \epsilon_o K\ell}{\log_e\left(\frac{R_2}{R_1}\right)} \qquad \text{(with dielectric)}$$

COMBINATION OF CAPACITORS

Series Combination

(i) In this combination, the positive plate of one capacitor is connected to the negative plate of the other.

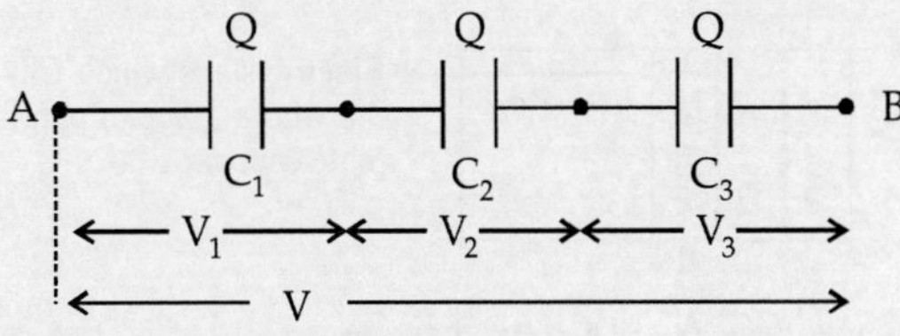

(ii) The charges of individual capacitor are equal.

(iii) The potential difference is shared by the capacitors in the inverse ratio of their capacities

i.e. $Q = C_1V_1 = C_2V_2 = C_3V_3$

Hence $V = V_1 + V_2 + V_3$

(iv) The equivalent capacitance (C) between A and B is

$$\frac{1}{C} = \frac{1}{C_1} + \frac{1}{C_2} + \frac{1}{C_3} + ... + \frac{1}{C_n}$$

Parallel Combination

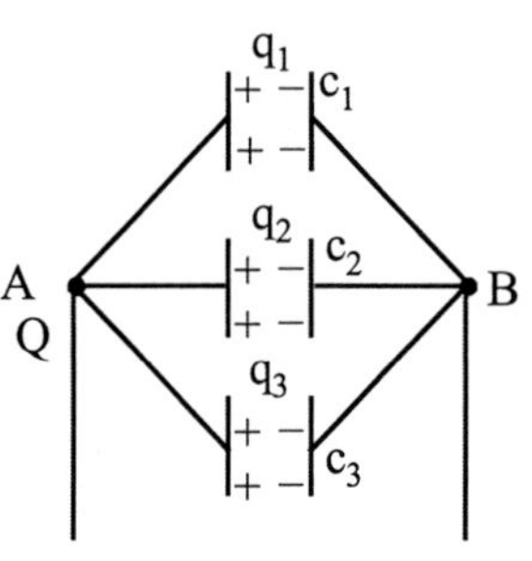

(i) In this arrangement, +ve plates of all the condensers are connected to one point and negative plates of all the condensers are connected to the other point.

(ii) The Potential difference across the individual capacitor is same.

(iii) The total charge shared by the individual capacitor is in direct ratio of their capacities

i.e. $V = \frac{q_1}{C_1} = \frac{q_2}{C_2} = \frac{q_3}{C_3}$

Hence, $Q = q_1 + q_2 + q_3$

(iv) The equivalent capacitance between A and B is $C_{eq} = C_1 + C_2 + C_3 + ... + C_n$

Problem Solving Tips

1. The capacitance of a parallel plate capacitor having a number of slabs of thickness t_1, t_2, t_3 .... and dielectric constant K_1, K_2, K_3 .... respectively between the plates is

$$C = \frac{\varepsilon_0 A}{\left(\frac{t_1}{K_1} + \frac{t_2}{K_2} + \frac{t_3}{K_3} + ...\right)}$$

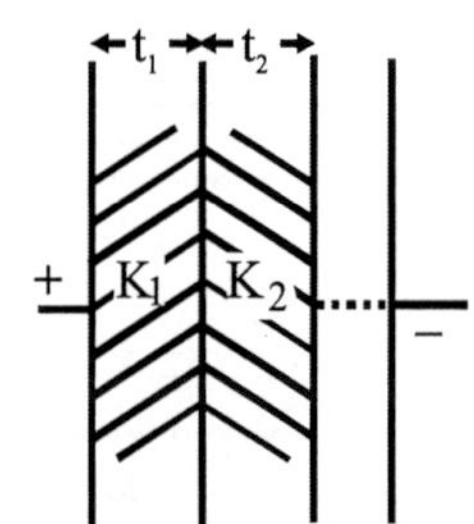

2. When a number of dielectric slabs of same thickness (d) and different areas of cross-section A_1, A_2, A_3 ... having dielectric constants K_1, K_2, K_3, ... respectively are placed between the plates of a parallel plate capacitor then the capacitance is given by

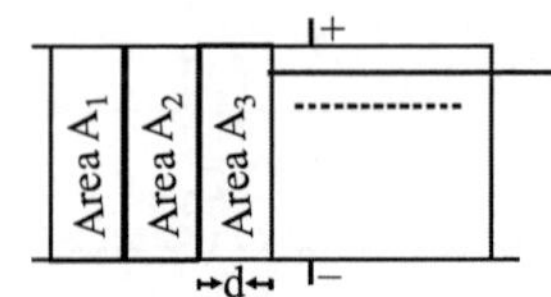

Electric slabs which fill the whole space of parallel plate capacitor

$$C = \frac{\varepsilon_0(K_1A_1 + K_2A_2 + K_3A_3 + ...)}{d}$$

3. When five capacitors are connected in wheatstone bridge arrangement as shown, such that $\frac{C_1}{C_2} = \frac{C_3}{C_4}$, the bridge is balanced and C_5 becomes ineffective. No charge is stored on C_5. Therefore C_1, C_2 and C_3, C_4 are in series. The two series combinations are in parallel between A and C. Hence equivalent capacitance can be calculated.

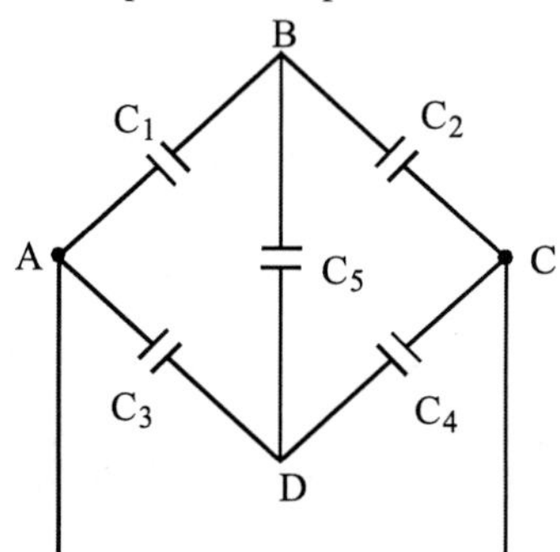

Relation between Three Electric Vectors $\vec{D}, \vec{P}$ and $\vec{E}$

If an electric field E is applied across a parallel plate capacitor filled with a dielectric of dielectric constant K (or permittivity ε), then

Polarisation P = induced charge per unit area (opposite to free charge) $= \frac{q'}{A}$

Electric displacement $D = \varepsilon E = \varepsilon_0 E + P$

i.e. Polarisation $P = (\varepsilon - \varepsilon_0)E = (K\varepsilon_0 - \varepsilon_0)E$

Electric susceptibility, $\chi_e = P/E$

Relation between dielectric constant K and electric susceptibility χ_e is

$$K = 1 + \frac{\chi_e}{\varepsilon_0}$$

Effect of filling dielectric With battery connected

When there is no dielectric

Capacitance $C_0 = \frac{A\varepsilon_0}{d}$

Potential difference between the plates V

Charge on a plate Q = CV

Energy $E_0 = \frac{1}{2}C_0V^2$

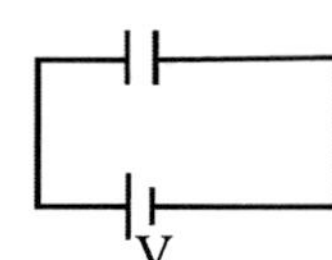

Electric field $E_0 = \frac{V}{d}$

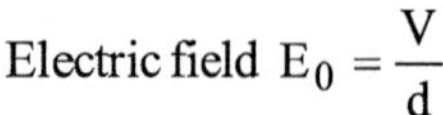

When dielectric is inserted

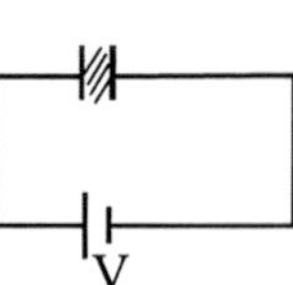

$C = \frac{KA\varepsilon_0}{d} = KC_0$

$Q = KC_0V = KQ_0$

$U = \frac{1}{2}KC_0V^2 = KE_0$

$E = \frac{V}{d} = E_0$

Effect of filling a dielectric in a capacitor after disconnection of battery

	+Q −Q, V	+Q −Q
Capacitance	C_0	$C = K\,C_0$
Charge	Q_0	$Q = Q_0$
P.D	$V_0 = \dfrac{Q_0}{C_0}$	$V = \dfrac{Q_0}{C} = \dfrac{V_0}{K}$
Potential energy	$U_0 = \dfrac{1}{2}C_0V_0^2$	$U = \dfrac{1}{2}KC_0\left(\dfrac{V_0}{K}\right)^2 = \dfrac{U_0}{K}$

CHARGING AND DISCHARGING A CAPACITOR

Charging a Capacitor

When an uncharged capacitor is connected across a source of constant potential difference such as a cell, it takes a finite time to get fully charged, although this time interval may be small. This time-interval depends on the capacity of the capacitor and the resistance in the circuit.

During the period of charging :

1. The charge on the capacitor increases from 'zero' to the final steady charge.
2. The potential difference developed across the capacitor opposes the constant potential difference of the source.
3. The charge on the capacitor 'grows' only as long as the potential difference of source is greater than the potential difference across the capacitor. This transport of the charge from the source to the capacitor constitutes a transient current in the circuit.
4. As the charge on the capacitor increases, more energy is stored in the capacitor.
5. When the capacitor is fully charged, potential difference across the capacitor is equal to the potential difference of the source and the transient current tends to zero.

If V_0 = constant potential difference of the source

R = pure resistance in the circuit

C = capacity of the capacitor

Q_0 = final charge on the capacitor, when fully charged

q = charge on the capacitor at time 't' from the starting of the charging

V = potential difference across the capacitor at time 't'

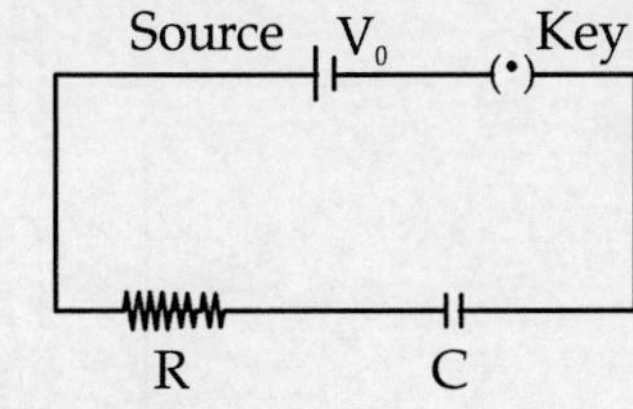

Then $\dfrac{Q_0}{V_0} = \dfrac{q}{V} = C$

and i = current in the circuit at time 't' = $\dfrac{dq}{dt}$

At time 't' by Kirchhoff's law

$$V_0 - R\frac{dq}{dt} - \frac{q}{C} = 0 \qquad \text{i.e.} \quad \frac{dq}{CV_0 - q} = \frac{1}{CR}dt$$

Integrating and putting in the initial condition q = 0 at t = 0, we get

$$q = CV_0\left[1 - e^{-\frac{1}{CR}t}\right]$$

Special cases :

(i) At t = 0, q = 0.

(ii) When t increases, q increases.

(iii) As $t \to \infty$, $q \to Q_0 = CV_0$ $\therefore q = Q_0\left[1 - e^{-\frac{1}{CR}t}\right]$

(iv) At t = CR ['CR' has dimensions of time]

$$q = Q_0\left[1 - \frac{1}{e}\right] = 0.631Q_0$$

This value of t = CR is called the '**time constant**' of the (CR) circuit.

Discharging of a Capacitor

If after charging the capacitor, the source of constant potential difference is disconnected and the charged capacitor is shorted through a resistance 'R', then by Kirchhoff's law, at time 't' from the instant of shorting,

$$\frac{q}{C} + R\frac{dq}{dt} = 0$$

Putting,

(i) the initial condition, $q = Q_0$ at t = 0 and

(ii) the final condition, q = 0 at $t \to \infty$,

the solution to the above equation is

$$q = Q_0 e^{-\frac{1}{CR}t}$$

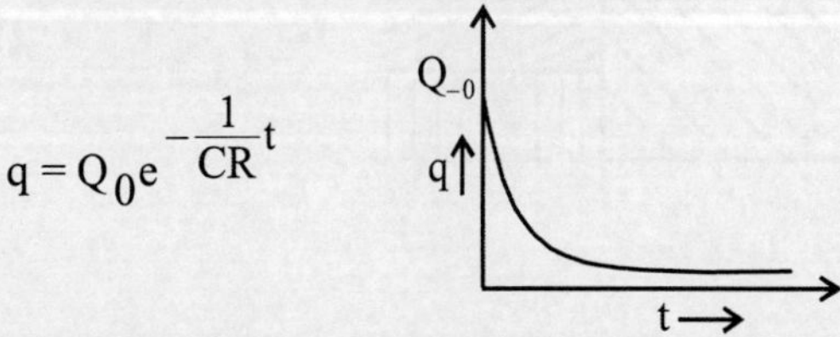

Problem Solving Tips

1. If *n* small drops each having a charge *q*, capacity '*C*' and potential *V* coalesc to form a big drop, then
   (i) the charge on the big drop = *nq*
   (ii) capacity of big drop = $n^{1/3}\,C$
   (iii) potential of big drop = $n^{2/3}\,V$
   (iv) potential energy of big drop = $n^{5/3}\,U$
   (v) surface density of charge on the big drop = $n^{1/3}$ × surface density of charge on one small drop.
2. **Charged soap bubble :** Four types of pressure act on a charged soap bubble.
   (i) Pressure due to air outside the bubble P_O, acting inwards.

(ii) Pressure due to surface tension of soap solution P_T, acting inwards.

(iii) Pressure due to air inside the bubble, P_i, acting outwards.

(iv) Electric pressure due to charging, $P_e = \frac{\sigma^2}{2\varepsilon_o}$, acting outwards.

In equilibrium, $P_i + P_e = P_O + P_T$

or, $P_i - P_O = P_T - P_e$

or, $P_{excess} = P_T - P_e$

$\therefore \quad P_{excess} = \frac{4T}{r} - \frac{\sigma^2}{2\varepsilon_o}$

Where T = surface tension of soap solution,

σ = surface charge density of bubble.

If $P_i = P_O$ then $P_i - P_O = P_T - P_e = 0$ or $P_T = P_e$

$$\frac{4T}{r} = \frac{\sigma^2}{2\varepsilon_o} = \frac{1}{2\varepsilon_o}\left(\frac{q}{4\pi r^2}\right)^2$$

Hence for maintaining the equilibrium of charged soap bubble, $\sigma = \sqrt{\frac{8\varepsilon_o T}{r}}$

$$q = 8\pi r\sqrt{2\varepsilon_o rT}$$

3. Force of attraction between the plates of a parallel plate capacitor $= \frac{q^2}{2\varepsilon_0 AK}$

where, A = area of the plates of capacitor and
K = dielectric constant of the medium filled between the plates.
In terms of electric field, the force of attraction
$F = \frac{1}{2}\varepsilon_0 KE^2$

4. **Uses of capacitor :**
- In LC oscillators
- As filter circuits
- Tuner circuit in radio etc.

5. The total energy stored in an array of capacitors (in series or in parallel) is the sum of the individual energies stored in each capacitor.

COMBINATION OF CAPACITOR : EQUIVALENT CAPACITANCE

(i) $\equiv C_1 = K_1\frac{A\varepsilon_0}{d/2}$, $C_2 = K_2\frac{A\varepsilon_0}{d/2}$ $\quad \frac{1}{C_{eq}} = \frac{1}{C_1} + \frac{1}{C_2}$ $\left[d = \frac{d}{2} + \frac{d}{2} \text{ and area of each plate} = A\right]$

(ii) 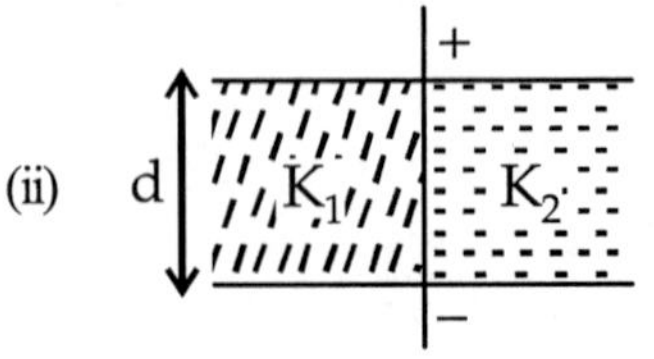

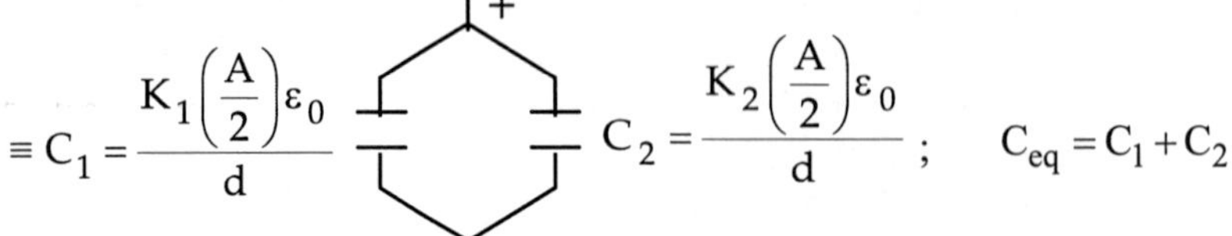

$\equiv C_1 = \frac{K_1\left(\frac{A}{2}\right)\varepsilon_0}{d}$ $\quad C_2 = \frac{K_2\left(\frac{A}{2}\right)\varepsilon_0}{d}$; $\quad C_{eq} = C_1 + C_2$

(iii) 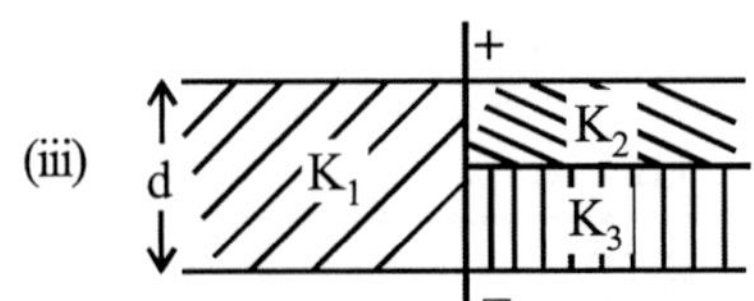

$\equiv C_1 = \frac{K_1(A/2)\varepsilon_0}{d}$ $\quad C_2 = \frac{K_2(A/2)\varepsilon_0}{d/2}$ $\quad C_3 = \frac{K_3(A/2)\varepsilon_0}{d/2}$ $\quad C_{eq} = C_1 + \frac{C_2C_3}{C_2C_3}$

(iv) 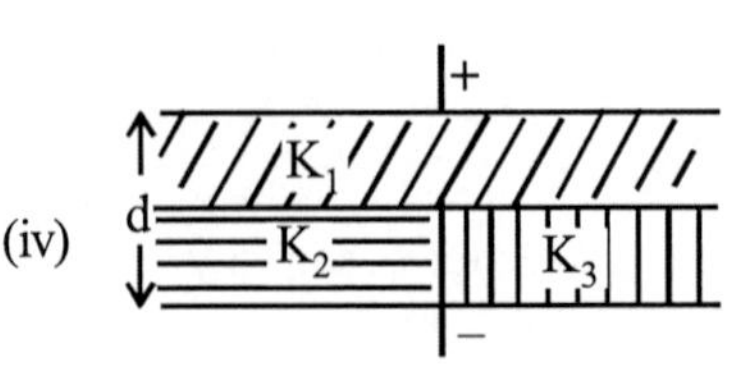

$C_1 = K_1\frac{A\varepsilon_0}{d/2}$

$\equiv C_2 = \frac{K_2\varepsilon_0(A/2)}{d/2}$ $\quad C_3 = \frac{K_3\varepsilon_0(A/2)}{d/2}$ $\quad \frac{1}{C_{eq}} = \frac{1}{C_1} + \frac{1}{C_2 + C_3}$

(v) 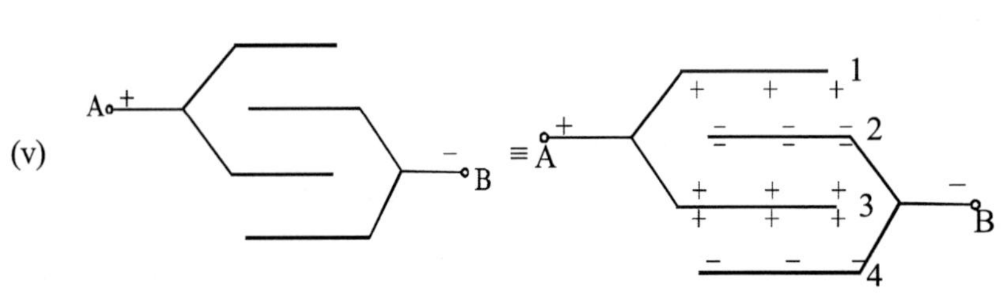

$\equiv$ 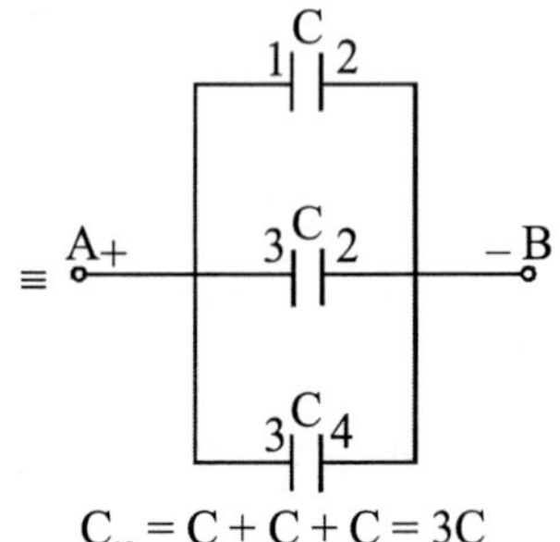

$C_{eq} = C + C + C = 3C$

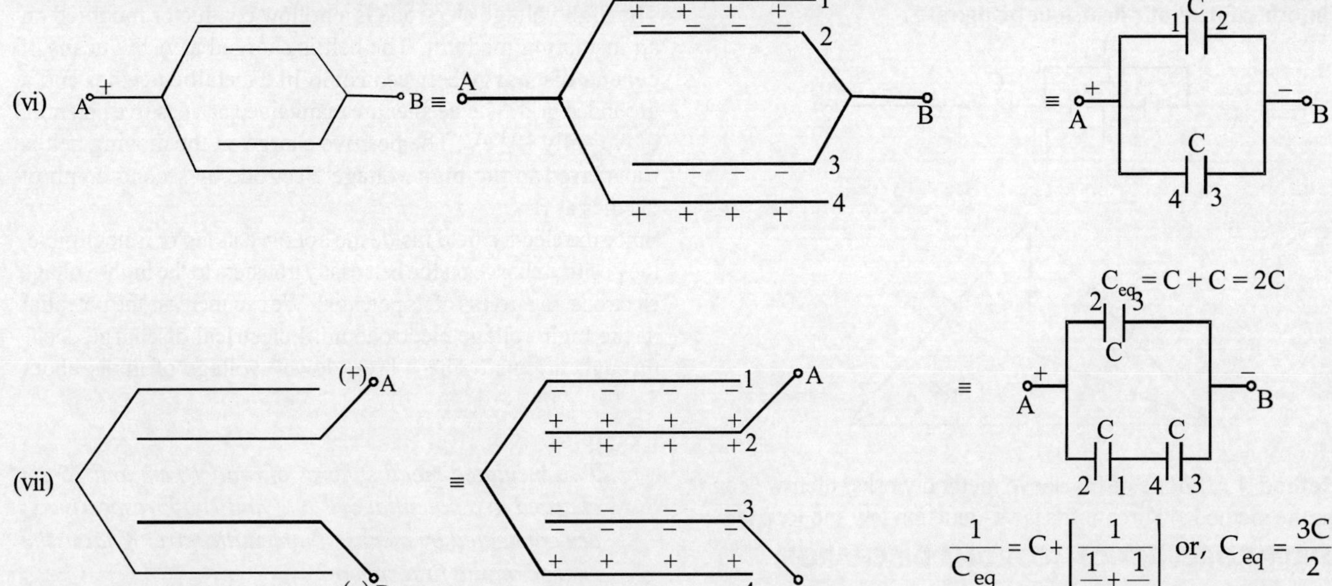

SOME METHODS OF FINDING EQUIVALENT CAPACITANCE

Method 1 : Successive Reduction

This method is applicable only when the capacitor can be clearly identified as in series or in parallel.

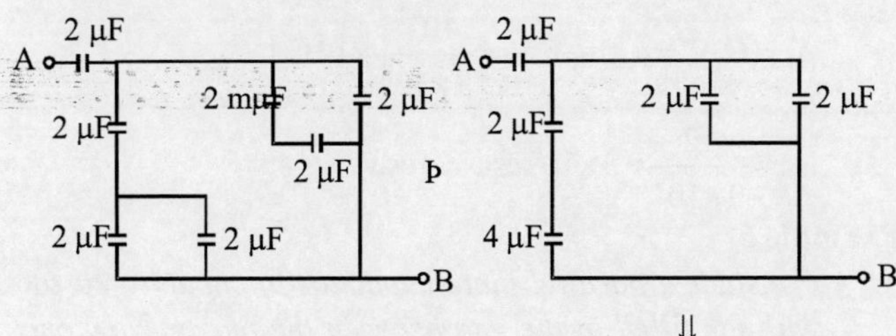

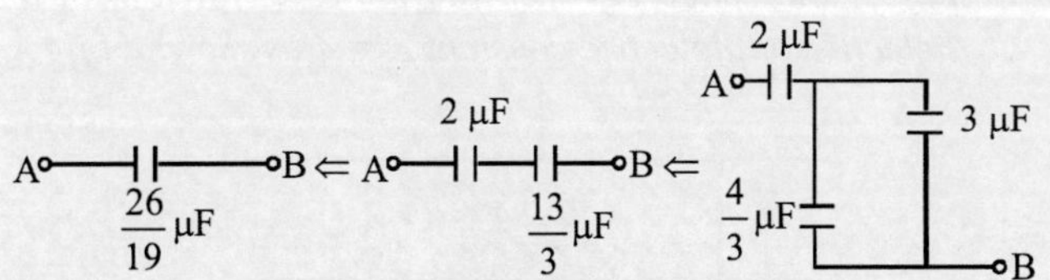

Method 2 : Using Symmetry

X A C E C B Y

C D

A

The above circuit is symmetrical about XAEBY axis. This is because the upper part of the circuit is mirror image of lower part.

Therefore $V_C = V_E = V_D$. The circuit can be redrawn as

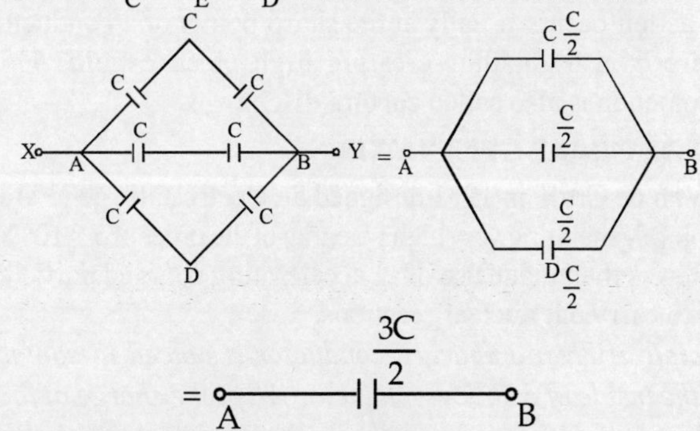

Method 3 : Wheatstone bridge

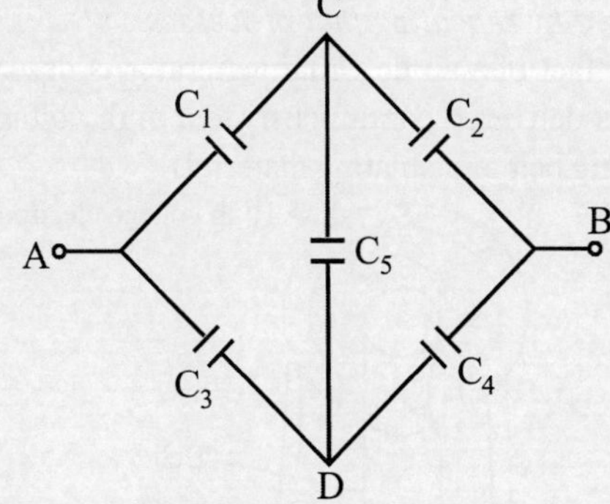

If $\frac{C_1}{C_3} = \frac{C_2}{C_4}$ then the wheatstone bridge is balanced. In this case there will be no charge accumulation in C_5 when battery is attached across A and B. Therefore the equivalent circuit is the capacitance C_1 and C_2 are in series. Similarly C_3 and C_4 is in series. Therefore the equivalent capacitance occurs between A and B is

$$\frac{1}{C_{eq}} = \frac{1}{C_1 + C_2} + \frac{1}{C_3 + C_4}$$

The other forms of wheatstone bridge are :

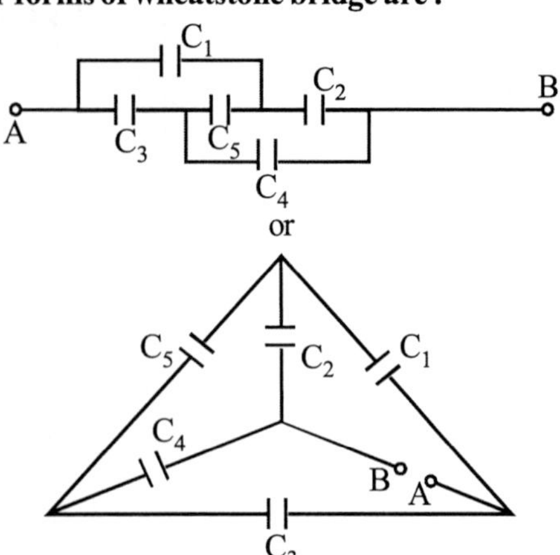

Method 4 : If none of the above method works, then we can use the method of Kirchhoff's laws - junction law and loop law.

SHARP POINT ACTION (CORONA DISCHARGE)

When the electric field (σ/ε_0) on a point on the surface of a conductor exceeds the electric strength of air, then the air becomes conducting and the surface of conductor loses charge. This action occurs usually at the sharp points of a conductor as here σ is high, thus creating high electric field. This phenomenon is also called **corona discharge**.

VAN DE GRAAF GENERATOR

R.J. Van de Graff in 1931 designed an electrostatic generator capable of generating very high potential of the order of 5×10^6 V, which was then made use of an accelerating charged particles so as to carry out nuclear reactions.

Principle : *When a charged conductor is placed in contact with the inside of a hollow conductor, all of the charge of first conductor is transferred to the hollow conductor. i.e., the charge on hollow conductor or its potential can be increased by any limit by repeating that processes.*

The basic fact of Van de Graaf generator is described in fig. (Charge is delivered continuously to a high voltage electrode on a moving belt of insulating material).

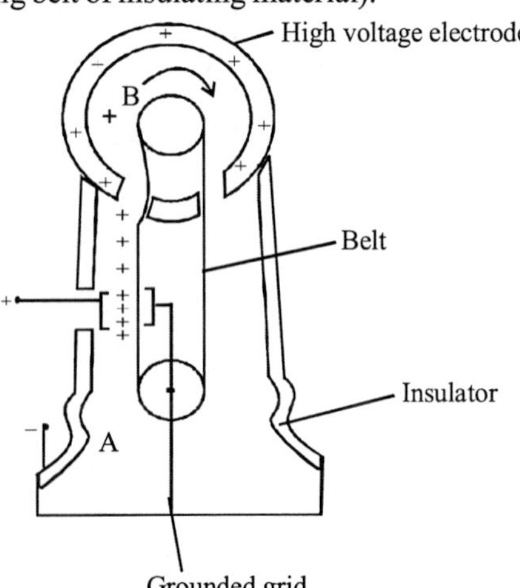

Schematic diagram of a Van de Graaf generator. Charge is transferred to hollow conductor at the top by means of a rotating belt. The charge is deposited on the belt at point A and is transferred to hollow conductor at point B.

The high voltage electrode is a hollow conductor mounted on an insulating medium. The belt is charged at A by means of **corona discharge** between comb-like metallic needles and a grounded grid. The needles are maintained at a positive potential of typically 10^4 eV. The positive charge on the moving belt is transferred to the high voltage electrode by second comb of needles at B.

Since the electric field inside the hollow conductor is negligible, the positive charge on the belt easily transfers to the high- voltage electrode, regardless of its potential. We can increase the potential of the high voltage electrode until electrical discharge occur through the air . The " breakdown" voltage of air is about 3×10^6 V/m.

Example 5

Two insulated metal spheres of radii 10 cm and 15 cm charged to a potential of 150 V and 100 V respectively, are connected by means of a metallic wire. What is the charge on the first sphere?

Solution :

Here, $r_1 = 10$ cm, $r_2 = 15$cm

$V_1 = 150$ V, $V_2 = 100$ V

Common potential

$$V = \frac{C_1V_1 + C_2V_2}{C_1 + C_2} = \frac{4\pi\epsilon_0 (r_1 V_1 + r_2 V_2)}{4\pi\epsilon_0 (r_1 + r_2)}$$

$= 120$ volt

$$q_1 = C_1V = 4\pi\epsilon_0 r_1 V = \frac{10^{-1}}{9\times10^9}\times 12C$$

$$= \frac{12}{9\times10^9}\times 3\times10^9 \text{ esu} = 4 \text{esu}$$

Example 6

Consider a parallel plate capacitor of capacity 10 μF with air filled in the gap between the plates. Now one half of the space between the plates is filled with a dielectric of dielectric constant K = 4 as shown in fig.

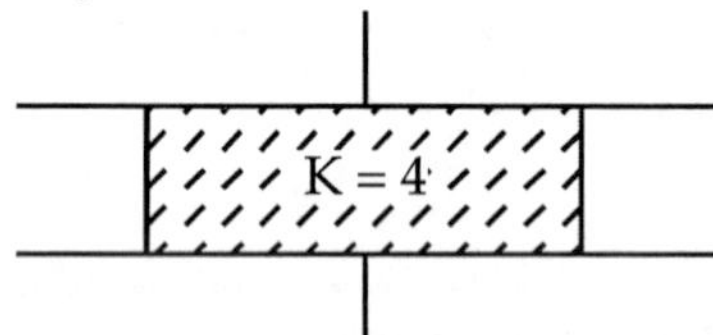

The capacity of the capacitor changes to

(a) 25 μF *(b) 20 μF*
(c) 40 μF *(d) 5 μF*

Solution : (a)

The arrangement is equivalent to three capacitors in parallel

$$C_1 = \frac{\varepsilon_0 A/4}{d} = \frac{10}{4} = 2.5\,\mu F;$$

$$C_2 = \frac{K\varepsilon_0 A/2}{d} = 4\times\frac{10}{2} = 20\,\mu F;$$

$$C_3 = \frac{\varepsilon_0 A/4}{d} = \frac{10}{2} = 2.5\,\mu F$$

$$\therefore\ C_{eq} = C_1 + C_2 + C_3 = 2.5 + 20 + 2.5 = 25\mu F$$

Example 7

A parallel plate capacitor is filled with dielectric as shown in fig. Its capacitance has ratio with that and without of dielectric as

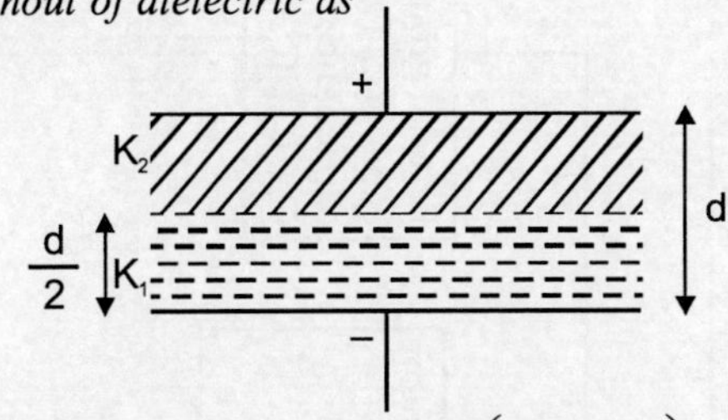

(a) $(K_1 + K_2)$ (b) $\left(\frac{K_1+K_2}{K_1-K_2}\right)$

(c) $\left(\frac{2K_1K_2}{K_1+K_2}\right)$ (d) $\left(\frac{K_1+K_2}{K_1K_2}\right)$

Solution : (c)

Without dielectric, $C_0 = \frac{\varepsilon_0 A}{d}$

With dielectric as shown,

$C_1 = \frac{K_1\varepsilon_0 A}{d/2} = 2K_1C_0$; $C_2 = \frac{K_2\varepsilon_0 A}{d/2} = 2K_2C_0$;

As C_1, C_2 are in series,

$\therefore \frac{1}{C_s} = \frac{1}{C_1} + \frac{1}{C_2} = \frac{C_2 + C_1}{C_1C_2}$;

$\therefore C_s = \frac{C_1C_2}{C_1+C_2} = \frac{2K_1C_0\,2K_0C_0}{2C_0(K_1+K_2)} = \frac{2K_1K_2C_0}{K_1+K_2}$

$\frac{C_s}{C_0} = \frac{2K_1K_2}{K_1+K_2}$

17.2 Concept Practice Problems

CPP

11. Force between two plates of a capacitor is

(a) $\frac{Q}{\varepsilon_0 A}$ (b) $\frac{Q^2}{2\varepsilon_0 A}$ (c) $\frac{Q^2}{\varepsilon_0 A}$ (d) $\frac{Q^2}{4\varepsilon_0 A}$

12. Eight drops of mercury of equal radius and possessing equal charge combine to form a big drop. The capacitance of bigger drop as compared to each small drop is

(a) 16 times (b) 8 times (c) 4 times (d) 2 times

13. The capacitance of a metallic sphere is 1 μF, then it's radius is nearly

(a) 1.11 m (b) 10 m (c) 9 km (d) 1.11 cm

14. A parallel plate capacitor is charged to a certain voltage. Now, if the dielectric material (with dielectric constant k) is removed then the

(a) capacitance increases by a factor of k
(b) electric field reduces by a factor k
(c) voltage across the capacitor decreases by a factor k
(d) None of these

15. Two capacitors of capacitances C_1 and C_2 are connected in parallel across a battery. If Q_1 and Q_2 respectively be the charges on the capacitors, then $\frac{Q_1}{Q_2}$ will be equal to

(a) $\frac{C_2}{C_1}$ (b) $\frac{C_1}{C_2}$ (c) $\frac{C_1^2}{C_2^2}$ (d) $\frac{C_2^2}{C_1^2}$

16. A conductor carries a certain charge. When it is connected to another uncharged conductor of finite capacity, then the energy of the combined system is

(a) more than that of the first conductor
(b) less than that of the first conductor
(c) equal to that of the first conductor
(d) uncertain

17. The magnitude of the electric field E in the annular region of a charged cylindrical capacitor

(a) is same throughout
(b) is higher near the outer cylinder than near the inner cylinder
(c) varies as $\frac{1}{r}$, where r is the distance from the axis
(d) varies as $\frac{1}{r^2}$, where r is the distance from the axis

18. A parallel plate condenser with oil between the plates (dielectric constant of oil K = 2) has a capacitance C. If the oil is removed, then capacitance of the capacitor becomes

(a) $\sqrt{2}C$ (b) 2C (c) $\frac{C}{\sqrt{2}}$ (d) $\frac{C}{2}$

19. An air capacitor C connected to a battery of e.m.f. V acquires a charge q and energy E. The capacitor is disconnected from the battery and a dielectric slab is placed between the plates. Which of the following statements is correct ?

(a) V and q decrease but C and E increase
(b) V remains unchange, but q, E and C increase
(c) q remains unchanged, C increases, V and E decrease
(d) q and C increase but V and E decrease.

20. A parallel plate condenser has a uniform electric field E(V/m) in the space between the plates. If the distance between the plates is d(m) and area of each plate is A(m²) the energy (joules) stored in the condenser is

(a) E^2Ad/ϵ_0 (b) $\frac{1}{2}\epsilon_0 E^2$

(c) $\epsilon_0 EAd$ (d) $\frac{1}{2}\epsilon_0 E^2Ad$

ANSWER KEY

11	(b)	12	(d)	13	(c)	14	(d)	15	(b)	16	(b)	17	(c)	18	(d)	19	(c)	20	(d)

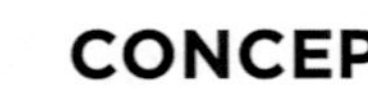

CONCEPT MAP

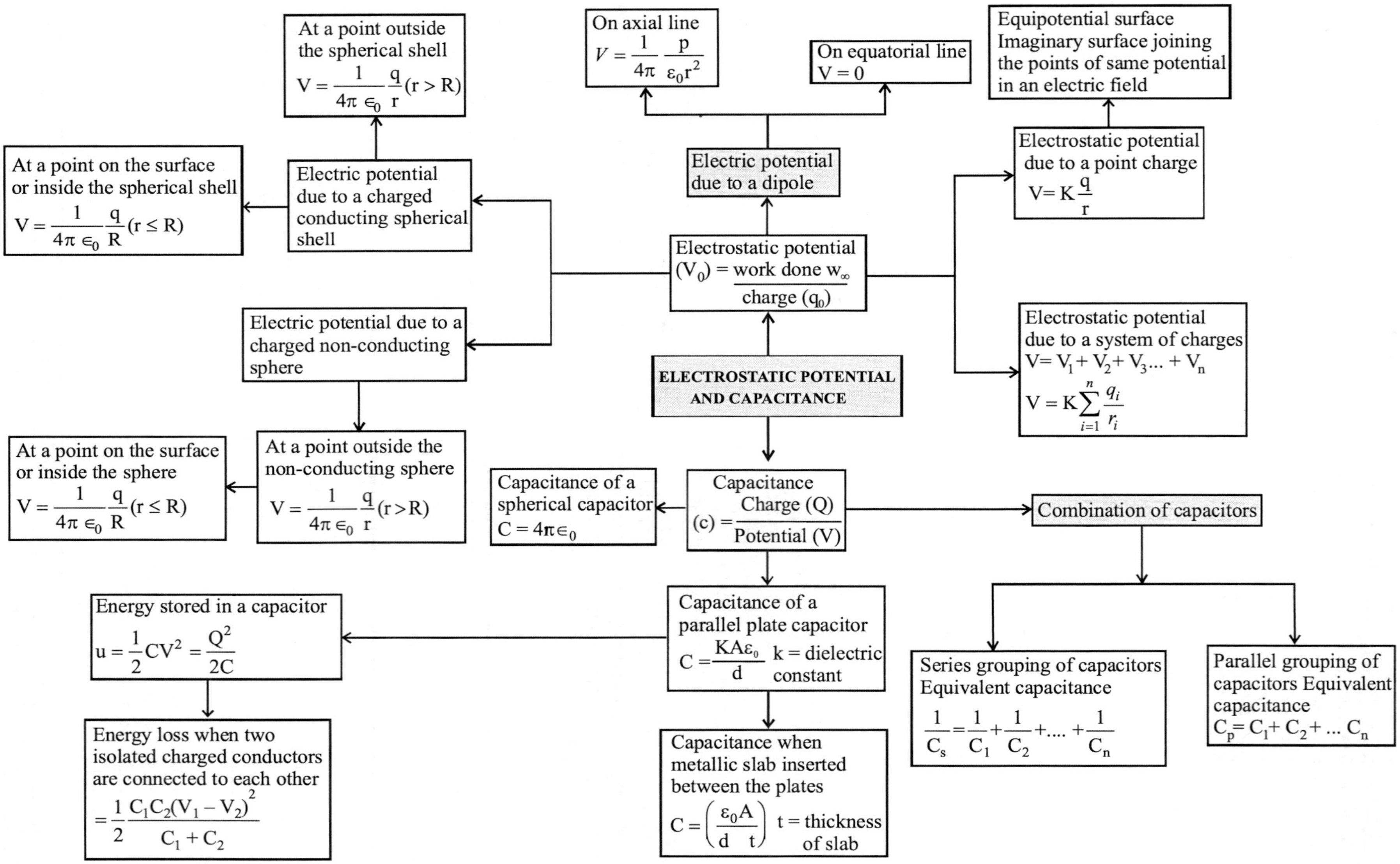

ELECTROSTATIC POTENTIAL AND CAPACITANCE

- Electrostatic potential $(V_0) = \frac{\text{work done } w_\infty}{\text{charge } (q_0)}$
  - Electric potential due to a dipole
    - On axial line $V = \frac{1}{4\pi}\frac{p}{\varepsilon_0 r^2}$
    - On equatorial line $V = 0$
  - Electrostatic potential due to a point charge $V = K\frac{q}{r}$
    - Equipotential surface: Imaginary surface joining the points of same potential in an electric field
  - Electrostatic potential due to a system of charges $V = V_1 + V_2 + V_3 ... + V_n$; $V = K\sum_{i=1}^{n}\frac{q_i}{r_i}$
  - Electric potential due to a charged conducting spherical shell
    - At a point outside the spherical shell $V = \frac{1}{4\pi \epsilon_0}\frac{q}{r}(r > R)$
    - At a point on the surface or inside the spherical shell $V = \frac{1}{4\pi \epsilon_0}\frac{q}{R}(r \le R)$
  - Electric potential due to a charged non-conducting sphere
    - At a point outside the non-conducting sphere $V = \frac{1}{4\pi \epsilon_0}\frac{q}{r}(r > R)$
    - At a point on the surface or inside the sphere $V = \frac{1}{4\pi \epsilon_0}\frac{q}{R}(r \le R)$
- Capacitance $(c) = \frac{\text{Charge (Q)}}{\text{Potential (V)}}$
  - Capacitance of a spherical capacitor $C = 4\pi\epsilon_0$
  - Combination of capacitors
    - Series grouping of capacitors Equivalent capacitance $\frac{1}{C_s} = \frac{1}{C_1} + \frac{1}{C_2} + ... + \frac{1}{C_n}$
    - Parallel grouping of capacitors Equivalent capacitance $C_p = C_1 + C_2 + ... C_n$
  - Capacitance of a parallel plate capacitor $C = \frac{KA\varepsilon_0}{d}$, k = dielectric constant
    - Capacitance when metallic slab inserted between the plates $C = \left(\frac{\varepsilon_0 A}{d \quad t}\right)$ t = thickness of slab
    - Energy stored in a capacitor $u = \frac{1}{2}CV^2 = \frac{Q^2}{2C}$
      - Energy loss when two isolated charged conductors are connected to each other $= \frac{1}{2}\frac{C_1C_2(V_1 - V_2)^2}{C_1 + C_2}$

Exercise 1 - Chapter Revision Problems

CRP

1. A system of two parallel plates, each of area A, are separated by distances d_1 and d_2. The space between them is filled with dielectrics of permittivities ε_1 and ε_2. The permittivity of free space is ε_0. The equivalent capacitance of the system is

(a) $\frac{\varepsilon_1\varepsilon_2 A}{\varepsilon_2 d_1+\varepsilon_1 d_2}$ (b) $\frac{\varepsilon_1\varepsilon_2\varepsilon_0 A}{\varepsilon_1 d_1+\varepsilon_2 d_2}$

(c) $\frac{\varepsilon_0 A}{\varepsilon_1 d_1+\varepsilon_2 d_2}$ (d) $\frac{\varepsilon_0 A}{\varepsilon_1 d_2+\varepsilon_2 d_1}$

2. Two identical conducting balls having positive charges q_1 and q_2 are separated by a distance r. If they are made to touch each other and then separated to the same distance, the force between them will be

(a) less than before (b) same as before
(c) more than before (d) zero

3. A large insulated sphere of radius r charged with Q units of electricity is placed in contact with a small insulated uncharged sphere of radius r′ and is then separated. The charge on smaller sphere will now be

(a) $Q(r'+r)$ (b) $Q(r+r')$ (c) $\frac{Q}{r'+r}$ (d) $\frac{Qr'}{r'+r}$

4. The capacitance of the capacitor of plate areas A_1 and A_2 $(A_1 < A_2)$ at a distance d, as shown in figure is

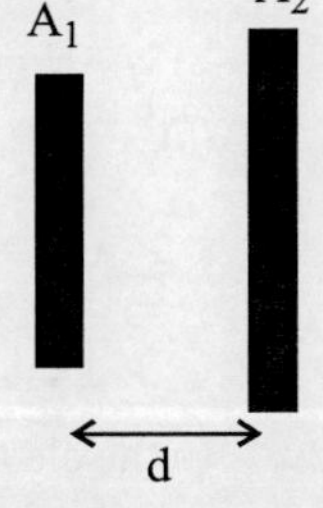

(a) $\frac{\epsilon_0 (A_1+A_2)}{2d}$

(b) $\frac{\epsilon_0 A_2}{d}$

(c) $\frac{\epsilon_0 \sqrt{A_1 A_2}}{d}$

(d) $\frac{\epsilon_0 A_1}{d}$

5. When air is replaced by a dielectric medium of force constant K, the maximum force of attraction between two charges, separated by a distance

(a) decreases K-times (b) increases K-times
(c) remains unchanged (d) becomes $\frac{1}{K^2}$ times

6. Two parallel metal plates having charges +Q and – Q face each other at a certain distance between them. If the plates are now dipped in kerosene oil tank, the electric field between the plates will

(a) remain same (b) become zero
(c) increases (d) decrease

7. A, B and C are three points in a uniform electric field. The electric potential is

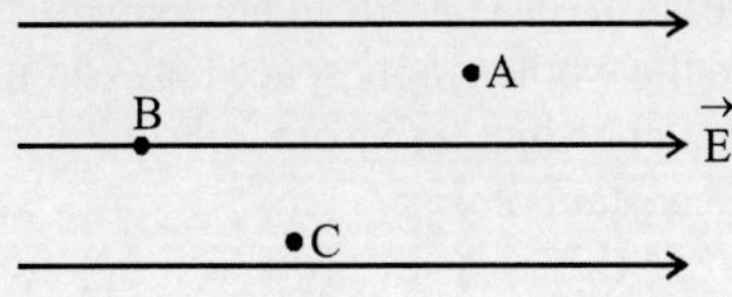

(a) maximum at B
(b) maximum at C
(c) same at all the three points A, B and C
(d) maximum at A

8. The positive terminal of 12 V battery is connected to the ground. Then the negative terminal will be at

(a) –6 V (b) +12 V (c) zero (d) –12 V

9. The electric potential at the surface of an atomic nucleus (Z = 50) of radius of 9×10^{-15} m is

(a) 80 V (b) 8×10^6 V (c) 9 V (d) 9×10^5 V

10. Three point charges +q, + 2q and – 4q where q = 0.1 μC, are placed at the vertices of an equilateral triangle of side 10 cm as shown in figure. The potential energy of the system is

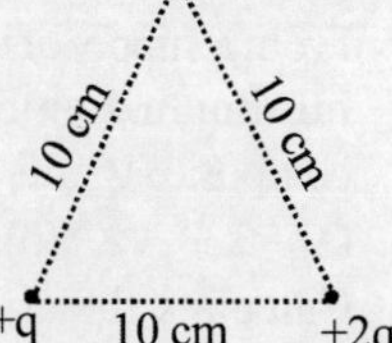

(a) 3×10^{-3} J

(b) -3×10^{-3} J

(c) 9×10^{-3} J

(d) -9×10^{-3} J

11. An air capacitor of capacity C = 10 μF is connected to a constant voltage battery of 12 volt. Now the space between the plates is filled with a liquid of dielectric constant 5. The (additional) charge that flows now from battery to the capacitor is

(a) 120 μC (b) 600 μC (c) 480 μC (d) 24 μC

12. A capacitor is charged to store an energy U. The charging battery is disconnected. An identical capacitor is now connected to the first capacitor in parallel. The energy in each of the capacitors is

(a) 3 U/2 (b) U (c) U/4 (d) U/2

13. Two capacitors when connected in series have a capacitance of 3 μF, and when connected in parallel have a capacitance of 16 μF. Their individual capacities are

(a) 1 μF, 2 μF (b) 6 μF, 2 μF
(c) 12 μF, 4 μF (d) 3 μF, 16 μF

14. The capacitor, whose capacitance is 6, 6 and 3μF respectively are connected in series with 20 volt line. Find the charge on 3μF.

6μF 6μF 3μF

20μF

(a) 30 μc

(b) 60 μF

(c) 15 μF

(d) 90 μF

15. A ball of mass 1 g carrying a charge 10^{-8} C moves from a point A at potential 600 V to a point B at zero potential. The change in its K.E. is

(a) -6×10^{-6} erg (b) -6×10^{-6} J
(c) 6×10^{-6} J (d) 6×10^{-6} erg

16. Two capacitors C_1 and C_2 in a circuit are joined as shown in figure. The potentials of points A and B are V_1 and V_2 respectively; then the potential of point D will be

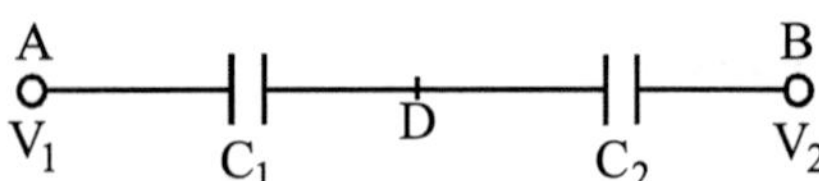

(a) $\frac{(V_1+V_2)}{2}$ (b) $\frac{C_2V_1+C_1V_2}{C_1+C_2}$

(c) $\frac{C_1V_1+C_2V_2}{C_1+C_2}$ (d) $\frac{C_2V_1+C_1V_2}{C_1+C_2}$

17. The plates of a parallel plate capacitor have an area of 90 cm^2 each and are separated by 2.5 mm. The capacitor is charged by a 400 volt supply. How much electrostatic energy is stored by the capacitor?

(a) 2.55×10^{-6} J (b) 1.55×10^{-6} J

(c) 8.15×10^{-6} J (d) 5.5×10^{-6} J

18. From a supply of identical capacitors rated 8 mF, 250V, the minimum number of capacitors required to form a composite 16 mF, 1000V is

(a) 2 (b) 4 (c) 16 (d) 32

19. Calculate the area of the plates of a one farad parallel plate capacitor if separation between plates is 1 mm and plates are in vacuum

(a) 18×10^8 m^2 (b) 0.3×10^8 m^2

(c) 1.3×10^8 m^2 (d) 1.13×10^8 m^2

20. A one microfarad capacitor of a TV is subjected to 4000 V potential difference. The energy stored in capacitor is

(a) 8 J (b) 16 J

(c) 4×10^{-3} J (d) 2×10^{-3} J

21. Two capacitors, $C_1 = 2\mu F$ and $C_2 = 8\ \mu F$ are connected in series across a 300 V source. Then

(a) the charge on each capacitor is 4.8×10^{-4} C

(b) the potential difference across C_1 is 60 V

(c) the potential difference across C_2 is 240 V

(d) the energy stroed in the system is 5.2×10^{-2} J

22. Two capacitors of capacitance C are connected in series. If one of them is filled with dielectric substance k, what is the effective capacitance ?

(a) $\frac{kC}{(1+k)}$ (b) $C(k+1)$

(c) $\frac{2kC}{1+k}$ (d) None of these

23. The potential at a point x (measured in μ m) due to some charges situated on the x-axis is given by $V(x) = 20/(x^2 - 4)$ volt

The electric field E at $x = 4\ \mu$ m is given by

(a) (10/9) volt/μ m and in the +ve x direction

(b) (5/3) volt/μ m and in the –ve x direction

(c) (5/3) volt/μ m and in the +ve x direction

(d) (10/9) volt/μ m and in the –ve x direction

24. Capacitance (in F) of a spherical conductor with radius 1 m is

(a) 1.1×10^{-10} (b) 10^6

(c) 9×10^{-9} (d) 10^{-3}

25. Two metal pieces having a potential difference of 800 V are 0.02 m apart horizontally. A particle of mass 1.96×10^{-15} kg is suspended in equilibrium between the plates. If e is the elementary charge, then charge on the particle is

(a) 8 (b) 6 (c) 0.1 (d) 3

26. Identical charges – q each are placed at 8 corners of a cube of each side b. Electrostatic potential energy of a charge + q which is placed at the centre of cube will be

(a) $\frac{-4\sqrt{2}\,q^2}{\pi\,\varepsilon_0 b}$ (b) $\frac{-8\sqrt{2}\,q^2}{\pi\,\varepsilon_0 b}$

(c) $\frac{-4q^2}{\sqrt{3}\,\pi\varepsilon_0 b}$ (d) $\frac{-8\sqrt{2}\,q^2}{\pi\varepsilon_0 b}$

27. Two equally charged spheres of radii a and b are connected together. What will be the ratio of electric field intensity on their surfaces?

(a) $\frac{a}{b}$ (b) $\frac{a^2}{b^2}$ (c) $\frac{b}{a}$ (d) $\frac{b^2}{a^2}$

28. In a hollow spherical shell, potential (V) changes with respect to distance (s) from centre as

(a)

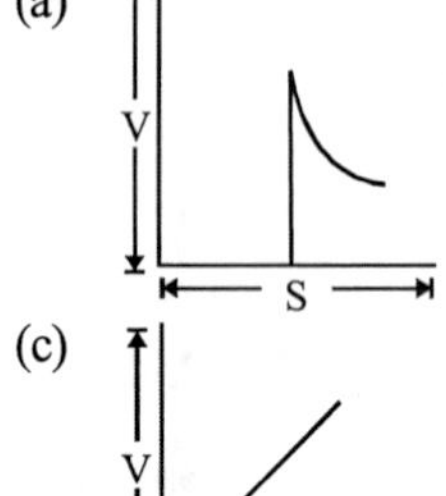

(b) (c)

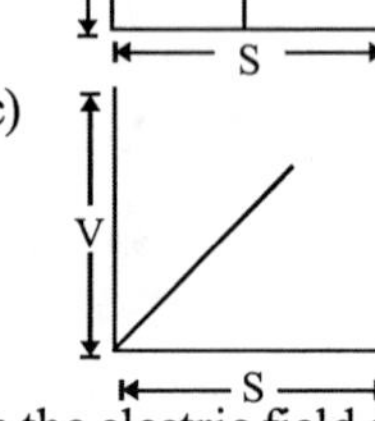

(d)

29. In the electric field of an point charge q, a certain charge is carried from point A to B, C, D and E. Then the work done is

(a) least along the path AB

(b) least along the path AD

(c) zero along any one of the path AB, AC, AD and AE

(d) least along AE

30. Three capacitors each of capacity 4μF are to be connected in such a way that the effective capacitance is 6 μF. This can be done by

(a) connecting two in parallel and one in series

(b) connecting all of them in series

(c) connecting them in parallel

(d) connecting two in series and one in parallel

31. If we increase 'd' of a parallel plate condenser to '2d' and fill wax to the whole empty space between its two plate, then capacitance increase from 1pF to 2pF. What is the dielectric constant of wax?

(a) 2 (b) 4 (c) 4 (d) 8

32. In the circuit shown, which of the following statements is true if V_1 (potential across C_1) is 30 V and V_2 (potential across C_2) is 20 V?

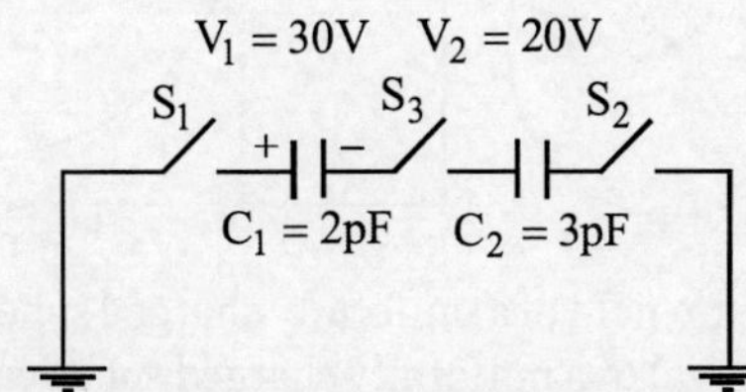

(a) With S_1 closed, $V_1 = 15$ V, $V_2 = 25$ V
(b) With S_3 closed, $V_1 = V_2 = 25$ V
(c) With S_1 and S_2 closed, $V_1 = V_2 = 0$
(d) With S_1 and S_3 closed, $V_1 = 30$ V, $V_2 = 20$ V

33. A parallel plate capacitor is located horizontally such that one of the plates is submerged in a liquid while the other is above the liquid surface. When plates are charged the level of liquid

Changed Liquid

(a) rises
(b) falls
(c) remains unchanged
(d) may rise or fall depending on the amount of charge

34. Three capacitors C_1, C_2 and C_3 are connected to a battery as shown. With symbols having their usual meanings, the correct conditions are

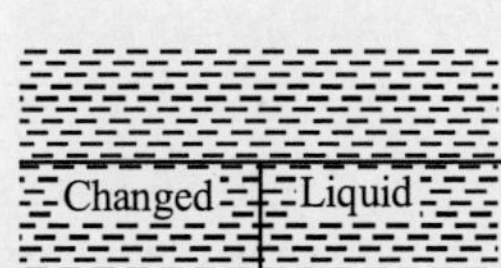

(a) $Q_1 = Q_2 = Q_3$ and $V_1 = V_2 = V$
(b) $V_1 = V_2 = V_3 = V$
(c) $Q_1 = Q_2 + Q_3$ and $V = V_1 = V_2$
(d) $Q_2 = Q_3$ and $V_2 = V_3$

35. Two parallel plate capacitors of capacitances C and 2C are connected in parallel and charged to a potential difference V. The battery is then disconnected and the region between the plates of the capacitor C is completely filled with a material fo dielectric constant K. The potential difference across the capacitors now becomes

(a) $\frac{3V}{K+2}$ (b) KV (c) $\frac{V}{K}$ (d) $\frac{3}{KV}$

36. The effective capacitance of combination of combination of equal capacitors between points A and B shown in figure is

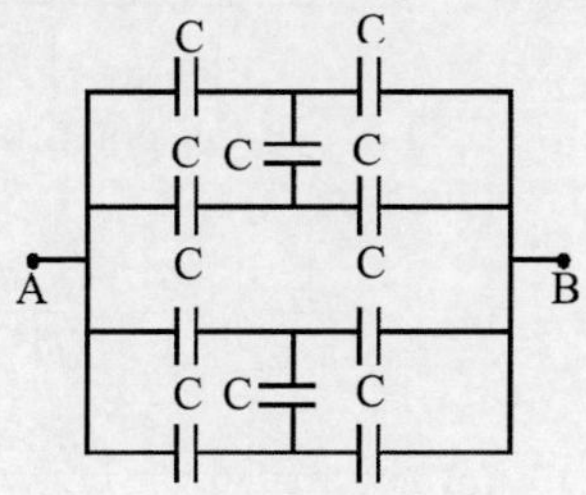

(a) C
(b) 2C
(c) 3C
(d) $\frac{C}{2}$

37. In the circuit given below, the charge in μC, on the capacitor having 5 μF is

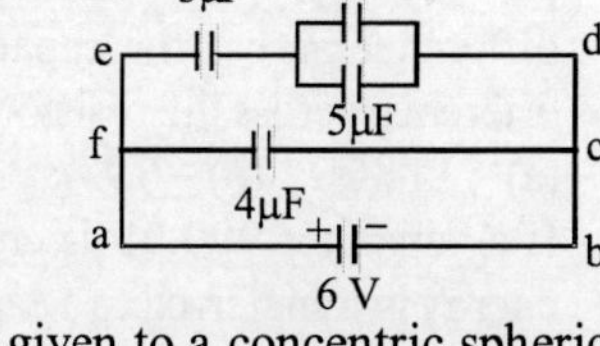

(a) 4.5
(b) 9
(c) 7
(d) 15

38. If a charge – 150 nC is given to a concentric spherical shell and a charge +50 nC is placed at its centre then the charge on inner and outer surface of the shell is

(a) –50 nC, –100 nC (b) +50 nC, –200 nC
(c) –50 nC, –200 nC (d) 50 nC, 100 nC

39. A battery is used to charge a parallel plate capacitor till the potential difference between the plates becomes equal to the electromotive force of the battery. The ratio of the energy stored in the capacitor and the work done by the battery will be

(a) 1/2 (b) 1 (c) 2 (d) 1/4

40. Four point charges q, q, q and – 3q are placed at the vertices of a regular tetrahedron of side L. The work done by electric force in taking all the charges to the centre of the tetrahedron is (where $k = \frac{1}{4\pi\varepsilon_0}$)

(a) $\frac{6kq^2}{L}$ (b) $\frac{-6kq^2}{L}$ (c) $\frac{12kq^2}{L}$ (d) zero

41. Two identical particles each of mass m and having charges –q and +q are revolving in a circle of radius r under the influence of electric attraction. Kinetic energy of each particle is $\left(k = \frac{1}{4\pi\varepsilon_0}\right)$

(a) $kq^2/4r$ (b) $kq^2/2r$ (c) $kq^2/8r$ (d) kq^2/r

42. If the potential of a capacitor having capacity 6 μF is increased from 10 V to 20 V, then increase in its energy will be

(a) 4×10^{-4} J (b) 4×10^{-4} J
(c) 9×10^{-4} J (d) 12×10^{-6} J

43. In the given circuit with steady current, the potential drop across the capacitor must be

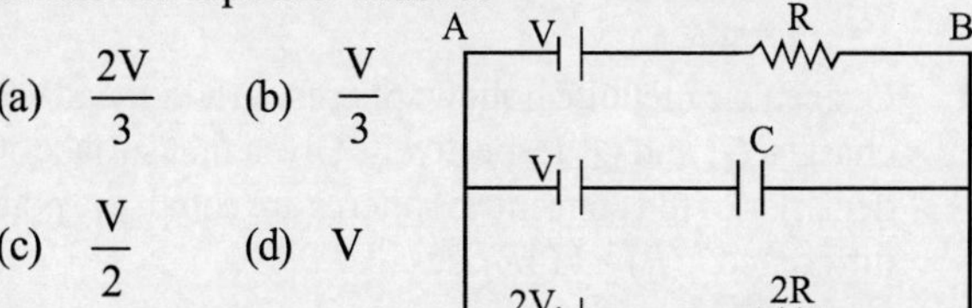

(a) $\frac{2V}{3}$ (b) $\frac{V}{3}$
(c) $\frac{V}{2}$ (d) V

44. A dielectric slab of thickness d is inserted in a parallel plate capacitor whose negative plate is at $x = 0$ and positive plate is at $x = 3d$. The slab is equidistant from the plates. the capacitor is given some charge. As one goes from 0 to $3d$

(a) the magnitude of the electric field remains the same
(b) the direction of the electric field remains the same
(c) the electric potential decreases continuously
(d) the electric potential increases at first, then decreases and again increases

45. A 4 μF capacitor, a resistance of 2.5 MΩ is in series with 12V battery. Find the time after which the potential difference across the capacitor is 3 times the potential diference across the resistor. [Given In (b) = 0.693]

(a) 13.86s (b) 6.93 *s* (c) 7*s* (d) 14 *s*

46. If a capacitor 900 μF is charged to 100 V and its total energy is transferred to a capacitor of capacitance 100 μF then its potential is

(a) 200 V (b) 30 V (c) 300 V (d) 400 V

47. What is the effective capacitance between points X and Y?

(a) 24 μF
(b) 18 μF
(c) 12 μF
(d) 6 μF

$C_1 = 6\mu F$, $C_3 = 6\mu F$, $C_5 = 20\mu F$, $C_2 = 6\mu F$, $C_4 = 6\mu F$; X, A, C, B, D, Y

48. In a parallel plate capacitor, the distance between the plates is d and potential difference across plates is V. Energy stored per unit volume between the plates of capacitor is

(a) $\frac{Q^2}{2V^2}$ (b) $\frac{1}{2}\varepsilon_0\frac{V^2}{d^2}$ (c) $\frac{1}{2}\frac{V^2}{\varepsilon_0 d^2}$ (d) $\frac{1}{2}\varepsilon_0\frac{V^2}{d}$

49. A capacitor C_1 is charged to a potential difference V. The charging battery is then removed and the capacitor is connected to an uncharged capacitor C_2. The potential difference across the combination is

(a) $\frac{VC_1}{(C_1+C_2)}$ (b) $V\left(1+\frac{C_2}{C_1}\right)$ (c) $V\left(1+\frac{C_1}{C_2}\right)$ (d) $\frac{VC_2}{(C_1+C_2)}$

50. As per this diagram a point charge +q is placed at the origin O. Work done in taking another point charge – Q from the point A [coordinates (0, a)] to another point B [coordinates (a, 0)] along the straight path AB is

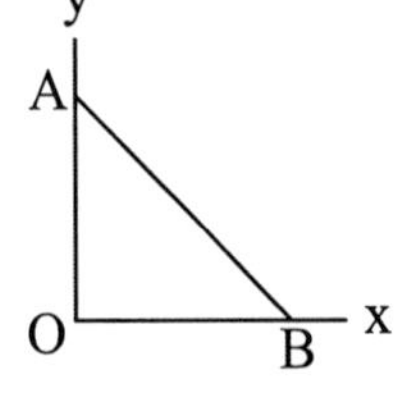

(a) zero

(b) $\left(\frac{-qQ}{4\pi\varepsilon_0}\frac{1}{a^2}\right)\sqrt{2}a$

(c) $\left(\frac{qQ}{4\pi\varepsilon_0}\frac{1}{a^2}\right)\cdot\frac{a}{\sqrt{2}}$

(d) $\left(\frac{qQ}{4\pi\varepsilon_0}\frac{1}{a^2}\right).\sqrt{2}a$

51. Concentric metallic hollow spheres of radii *R* and 4*R* hold charges Q_1 and Q_2 respectively. Given that surface charge densities of the concentric spheres are equal, the potential difference $V(R) - V(4R)$ is :

(a) $\frac{3Q_1}{16\pi\varepsilon_0 R}$ (b) $\frac{3Q_2}{4\pi\varepsilon_0 R}$ (c) $\frac{Q_2}{4\pi\varepsilon_0 R}$ (d) $\frac{3Q_1}{4\pi\varepsilon_0 R}$

52. A point dipole $= \vec{p} - p_o\hat{x}$ kept at the origin. The potential and electric field due to this dipole on the *y*-axis at a distance *d* are, respectively : (Take V = 0 at infinity)

(a) $\frac{|\vec{p}|}{4\pi\varepsilon_0 d^2}, \frac{\vec{p}}{4\pi\varepsilon_0 d^3}$ (b) $0, \frac{-\vec{p}}{4\pi\varepsilon_0 d^3}$

(c) $0, \frac{|\vec{p}|}{4\pi\varepsilon_0 d^3}$ (d) $\frac{|\vec{p}|}{4\pi\varepsilon_0 d^2}, \frac{-\vec{p}}{4\pi\varepsilon_0 d^3}$

53. The given graph shows variation (with distance r from centre) of:

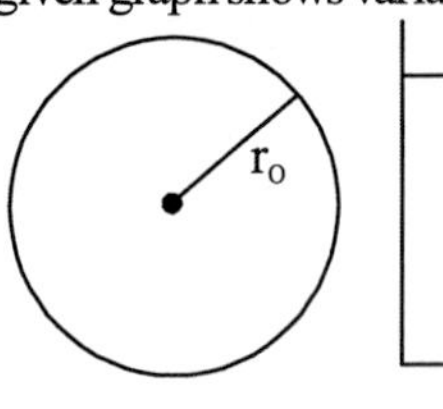

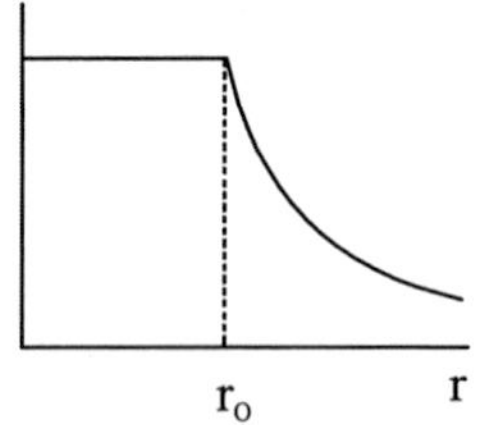

(a) Electric field of a uniformly charged sphere
(b) Potential of a uniformly charged spherical shell
(c) Potential of a uniformly charged sphere
(d) Electric field of a uniformly charged spherical shell

54. Consider two charged metallic spheres S_1 and S_2 of radii R_1 and R_2, respectively. The electric fields E_1 (on S_1) and E_2 (on S_2) on their surfaces are such that $E_1/E_2 = R_1/R_2$. Then the ratio V_1(on S_1)/V_2(on S_2) of the electrostatic potentials on each sphere is:

(a) R_1/R_2 (b) $(R_1/R_2)^2$ (c) (R_2/R_1) (d) $\left(\frac{R_1}{R_2}\right)^3$

55. A two point charges 4*q* and –*q* are fixed on the *x*-axis at $x = -\frac{d}{2}$ and $x = \frac{d}{2}$, respectively. If a third point charge '*q*' is taken from the origin to $x = d$ along the semicircle as shown in the figure, the energy of the charge will :

(a) increase by $\frac{3q^2}{4\pi\varepsilon_0 d}$

(b) increase by $\frac{2q^2}{3\pi\varepsilon_0 d}$

4*q* –*q*

(c) decrease by $\frac{q^2}{4\pi\varepsilon_0 d}$ (d) decrease by $\frac{4q^2}{3\pi\varepsilon_0 d}$

56. Hydrogen ion and singly ionized helium atom are accelerated, from rest, through the same potential difference. The ratio of final speeds of hydrogen and helium ions is close to :

(a) 1 : 2 (b) 10 : 7 (c) 2 : 1 (d) 5 : 7

57. In free space, a particle A of charge 1 μC is held fixed at a point P. Another particle B of the same charge and mass 4 μg is kept at a distance of 1 mm from P. If B is released, then its velocity at a distance of 9 mm from P is:

$\left[Take \frac{1}{4\pi\varepsilon_0} = 9\times10^9\, Nm^2C^{-2}\right]$

(a) 1.0m/s (b) 3.0×10^4 m/s
(c) 2.0×10^3 m/s (d) 1.5×10^2 m/s

58. A system of three charges are placed as shown in the figure:

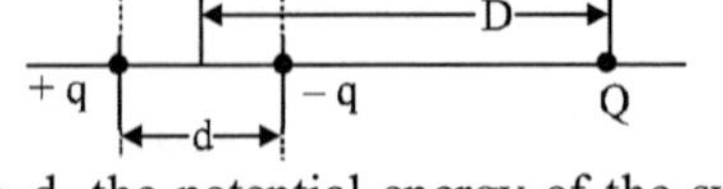

If D >> d, the potential energy of the system is best given by

(a) $\frac{1}{4\pi\epsilon_0}\left[\frac{-q^2}{d} - \frac{qQd}{2D^2}\right]$ (b) $\frac{1}{4\pi\epsilon_0}\left[\frac{-q^2}{d} + \frac{2qQd}{D^2}\right]$

(c) $\frac{1}{4\pi\epsilon_0}\left[+\frac{q^2}{d} + \frac{qQd}{D^2}\right]$ (d) $\frac{1}{4\pi\epsilon_0}\left[-\frac{q^2}{d} - \frac{qQd}{D^2}\right]$

59. Three charges Q, + q and + q are placed at the vertices of a right-angle isosceles triangle as shown below. The net electrostatic energy of the configuration is zero, if the value of Q is :

(a) +q

(b) $\frac{-\sqrt{2}q}{\sqrt{2}+1}$

(c) $\frac{-q}{1+\sqrt{2}}$

(d) –2q

60. A 10 μF capacitor is fully charged to a potential difference of 50 V. After removing the source voltage it is connected to an uncharged capacitor in parallel. Now the potential difference across them becomes 20 V. The capacitance of the second capacitor is :

(a) 15 μF (b) 30 μF (c) 20 μF (d) 10 μF

61. The parallel combination of two air filled parallel plate capacitors of capacitance C and *n*C is connected to a battery of voltage, V. When the capacitors are fully charged, the battery is removed and after that a dielectric material of dielectric constant K is placed between the two plates of the first capacitor. The new potential difference of the combined system is:

(a) $\frac{nV}{K+n}$ (b) V (c) $\frac{V}{K+n}$ (d) $\frac{(n+1)V}{(K+n)}$

62. In the given circuit, the charge on 4 μF capacitor will be :

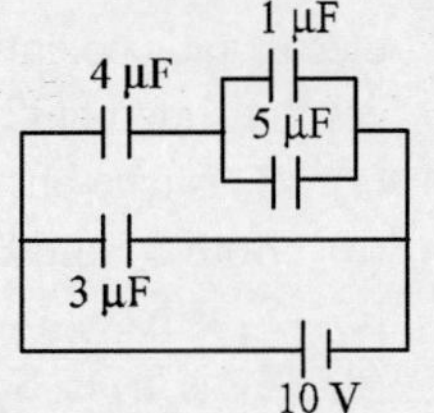

(a) 5.4 μC

(b) 9.6 μC

(c) 13.4 μC

(d) 24 μC

63. Figure shows charge (q) versus voltage (V) graph for series and parallel combination of two given capacitors. The capacitances are :

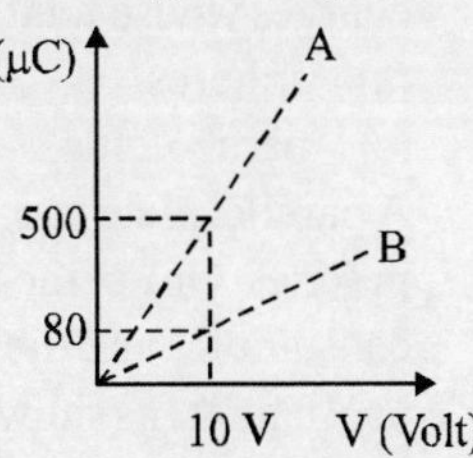

(a) 40 μF and 10 μF

(b) 60 μF and 40 μF

(c) 50 μF and 30 μF

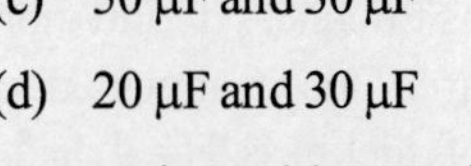

(d) 20 μF and 30 μF

64. A capacitor with capacitance 5μF is charged to 5 μC. If the plates are pulled apart to reduce the capacitance to 2 ¼F, how much work is done?

(a) 6.25×10^{-6} J (b) 3.75×10^{-6} J

(c) 2.16×10^{-6} J (d) 2.55×10^{-6} J

65. A parallel plate capacitor with plates of area 1 m^2 each, are at a separation of 0.1 m. If the electric field between the plates is 100 N/C, the magnitude of charge on each plate is :

(Take $\epsilon_0 = 8.85 \times 10^{-12} \frac{C^2}{N-M^2}$)

(a) 7.85×10^{-10} C (b) 6.85×10^{-10} C

(c) 8.85×10^{-10} C (d) 9.85×10^{-10} C

66. A parallel plate capacitor of capacitance 90 pF is connected to a battery of emf 20V. If a dielectric material of dielectric constant $k = \frac{5}{3}$ is inserted between the plates, the magnitude of the induced charge will be:

(a) 1.2 n C (b) 0.3 n C (c) 2.4 n C (d) 0.9 n C

67. The equivalent capacitance between *A* and *B* in the circuit given below is:

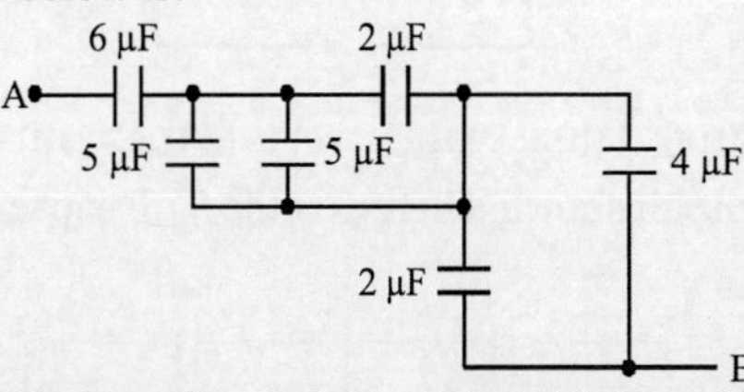

(a) 4.9 μF (b) 3.6 μF (c) 5.4 μF (d) 2.4 μF

68. A parallel plate capacitor with area 200cm^2 and separation between the plates 1.5cm, is connected across a battery of emf V. If the force of attraction between the plates is 25×10^{-6}N, the value of V is approximately:

$$\left(\varepsilon_0 = 8.85 \times 10^{-12} \frac{C^2}{N.m^2}\right)$$

(a) 150V (b) 100V (c) 250V (d) 300V

69. Three concentric metal shells A, B and C of respective radii *a*, *b* and *c* ($a < b < c$) have surface charge densities $+\sigma$, $-\sigma$ and $+\sigma$ respectively. The potential of shell B is:

(a) $\frac{\sigma}{\epsilon_0}\left[\frac{a^2-b^2}{a}+c\right]$ (b) $\frac{\sigma}{\epsilon_0}\left[\frac{a^2-b^2}{b}+c\right]$

(c) $\frac{\sigma}{\epsilon_0}\left[\frac{b^2-c^2}{b}+a\right]$ (d) $\frac{\sigma}{\epsilon_0}\left[\frac{b^2-c^2}{c}+a\right]$

70. The electric field in a region is given by $\vec{E} = (Ax + B)\hat{i}$, where E is in NC^{-1} and *x* is in metres. The values of constants are A = 20 SI unit and B = 10 SI unit. If the potential at $x = 1$ is V_1 and that at $x = -5$ is V_2, then $V_1 - V_2$ is :

(a) 320 V (b) –48V (c) 180 V (d) –520 V

71. A solid conducting sphere, having a charge Q, is surrounded by an uncharged conducting hollow spherical shell. Let the potential difference between the surface of the solid sphere and that of the outer surface of the hollow shell be V. If the shell is now given a charge of –4 Q, the new potential difference between the same two surfaces is :

(a) –2V (b) 2V (c) 4V (d) V

72. A capacitor *C* is fully charged with voltage V_0. After disconnecting the voltage source, it is connected in parallel with another uncharged capacitor of capacitance $\frac{C}{2}$. The energy loss in the process after the charge is distributed between the two capacitors is :

(a) $\frac{1}{2}CV_0^2$ (b) $\frac{1}{3}CV_0^2$ (c) $\frac{1}{4}CV_0^2$ (d) $\frac{1}{6}CV_0^2$

73. In the circuit shown in the figure, the total charge is 750 μC and the voltage across capacitor C_2 is 20 V. Then the charge on capacitor C_2 is :

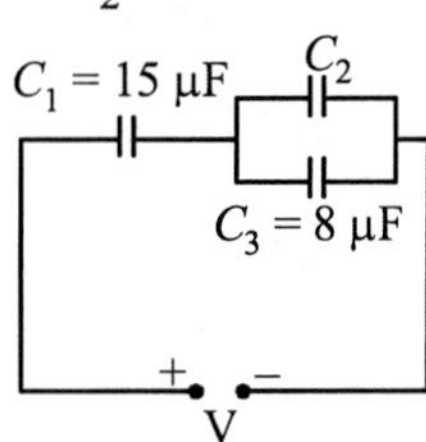

(a) 450 μC (b) 590 μC (c) 160 μC (d) 650 μC

74. In the circuit shown, charge on the 5 μF capacitor is :

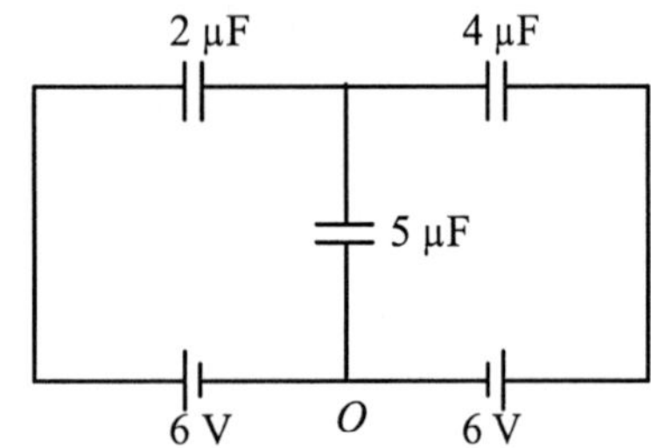

(a) 18.00 μC (b) 10.90 μC (c) 16.36 μC (d) 5.45 μC

75. There is a uniform spherically symmetric surface charge density at a distance R_o from the origin. The charge distribution is initially at rest and starts expanding because of mutual repulsion. The figure that represents best the speed V (R(t)) of the distribution as a function of its instantaneous radius R(t) is:

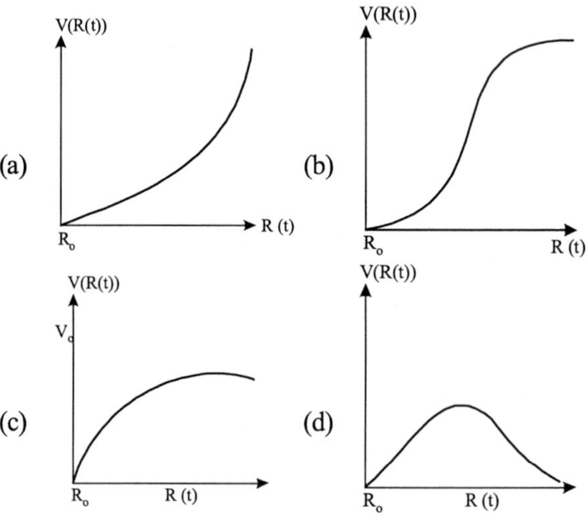

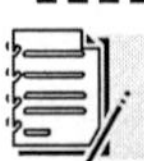

Exercise 2 - Exemplar & Past Year Questions

E&PYQs

Exemplar Questions

1. A capacitor of 4 μF is connected as shown in the circuit. The internal resistance of the battery is 0.5Ω. The amount of charge on the capacitor plates will be

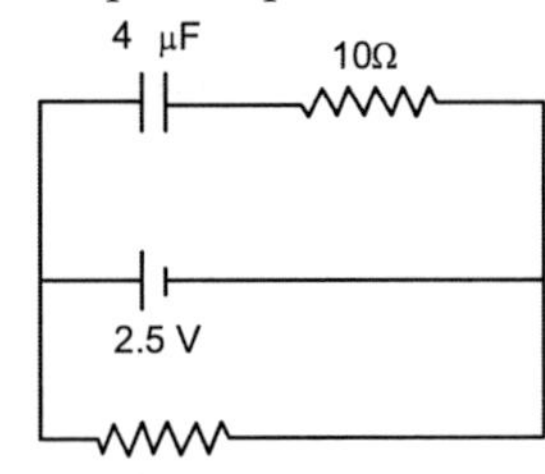

(a) 0 μC (b) 4 μC (c) 16 μC (d) 8 μC

2. A positively charged particle is released from rest in an uniform electric field. The electric potential energy of the charge
   (a) remains a constant because the electric field is uniform
   (b) increases because the charge moves along the electric field
   (c) decreases because the charge moves along the electric field
   (d) decreases because the charge moves opposite to the electric field

3. The electrostatic potential on the surface of a charged conducting sphere is 100V. Two statements are made in this regard S_1 at any point inside the sphere, electric intensity is zero. S_2 at any point inside the sphere, the electrostatic potential is 100V. Which of the following is a correct statement?
   (a) S_1 is true but S_2 is false
   (b) Both S_1 and S_2 are false
   (c) S_1 is true, S_2 is also true and S_1 is the cause of S_2
   (d) S_1 is true, S_2 is also true but the statements are independant

4. Equipotentials at a great distance from a collection of charges whose total sum is not zero are approximately
   (a) spheres (b) planes
   (c) paraboloids (d) ellipsoids

5. A parallel plate capacitor is made of two dielectric blocks in series. One of the blocks has thickness d_1 and dielectric constant K_1 and the other has thickness d_2 and dielectric constant K_2 as shown in figure. This arrangement can be thought as a dielectric slab of thickness d $(= d_1 + d_2)$ and effective dielectric constant K. The K is

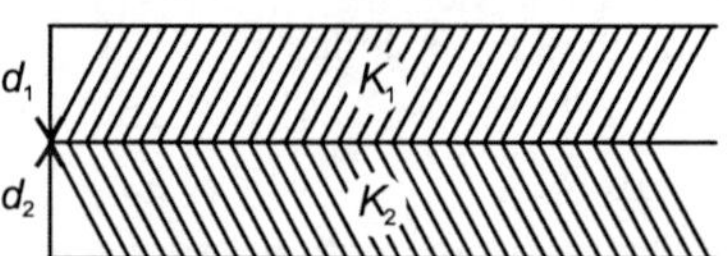

(a) $\dfrac{K_1d_1 + K_2d_2}{d_1 + d_2}$ (b) $\dfrac{K_1d_1 + K_2d_2}{K_1 + K_2}$

(c) $\dfrac{K_1K_2(d_1 + d_2)}{(K_1d_1 + K_2d_2)}$ (d) $\dfrac{2K_1K_2}{K_1 + K_2}$

NEET/AIPMT (2013-2020) Questions

6. A, B and C are three points in a uniform electric field. The electric potential is ***[2013]***

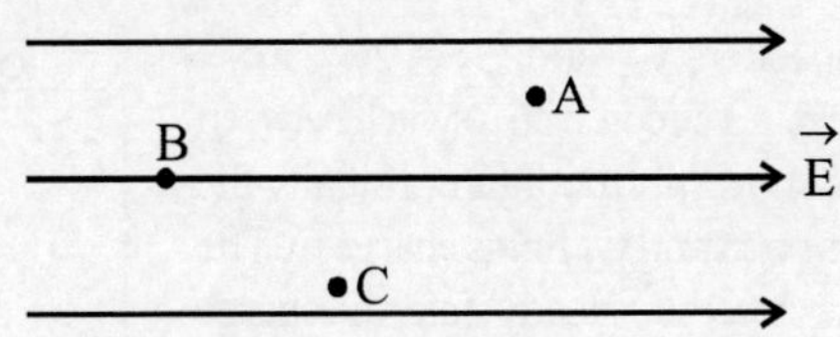

(a) maximum at B
(b) maximum at C
(c) same at all the three points A, B and C
(d) maximum at A

7. A conducting sphere of radius R is given a charge Q. The electric potential and the electric field at the centre of the sphere respectively are: ***[2014]***

(a) Zero and $\frac{Q}{4\pi\varepsilon_0 R^2}$ (b) $\frac{Q}{4\pi\varepsilon_0 R}$ and Zero

(c) $\frac{Q}{4\pi\varepsilon_0 R}$ and $\frac{Q}{4\pi\varepsilon_0 R^2}$ (d) Both are zero

8. In a region, the potential is represented by $V(x, y, z) = 6x - 8xy - 8y + 6yz$, where V is in volts and x, y, z are in metres. The electric force experienced by a charge of 2 coulomb situated at point (1, 1, 1) is : ***[2014]***

(a) $6\sqrt{5}$ N (b) 30 N (c) 24 N (d) $4\sqrt{35}$ N

9. A parallel plate air capacitor of capacitance C is connected to a cell of emf V and then disconnected from it. A dielectric slab of dielectric constant K, which can just fill the air gap of the capacitor, is now inserted in it. Which of the following is incorrect ? ***[2015]***

(a) The energy stored in the capacitor decreases K times.
(b) The chance in energy stored is $\frac{1}{2}CV^2\left(\frac{1}{K}-1\right)$
(c) The charge on the capacitor is not conserved.
(d) The potential difference between the plates decreases K times.

10. If potential (in volts) in a region is expressed as $V(x, y, z) = 6xy - y + 2yz$, the electric field (in N/C) at point (1, 1, 0) is : ***[2015 RS]***

(a) $-(6\hat{i}+5\hat{j}+2\hat{k})$ (b) $-(2\hat{i}+3\hat{j}+\hat{k})$
(c) $-(6\hat{i}+9\hat{j}+\hat{k})$ (d) $-(3\hat{i}+5\hat{j}+3\hat{k})$

11.

A capacitor of 2μF is charged as shown in the diagram. When the switch S is turned to position 2, the percentage of its stored energy dissipated is : ***[2016]***

(a) 0% (b) 20% (c) 75% (d) 80%

12. A capacitor is charged by a battery. The battery is removed and another identical uncharged capacitor is connected in parallel. The total electrostatic energy of resulting system:

(a) decreases by a factor of 2 ***[2017]***
(b) remains the same
(c) increases by a factor of 2
(d) increases by a factor of 4

13. The electrostatic force between the metal plates of an isolated parallel plate capacitor C having a charge Q and area A, is ***[2018]***

(a) independent of the distance between the plates
(b) linearly proportional to the distance between the plates
(c) inversely proportional to the distance between the plates
(d) proportional to the square root of the distance between the plates

14. Two identical capacitors C_1 and C_2 of equal capacitance are connected as shown in the circuit. Terminals a and b of the key k are connected to charge capacitor C_1 using battery of emf V volt. Now disconnecting *a* and *b* the terminals *b* and *c* are connected. Due to this, what will be the percentage loss of energy? ***[NEET Odisha 2019]***

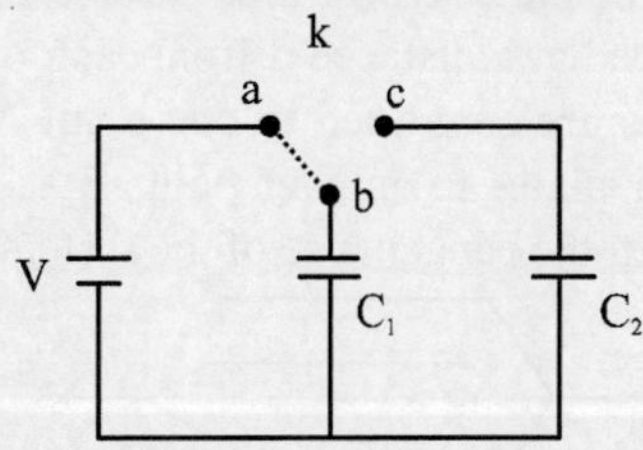

(a) 25% (b) 75% (c) 0% (d) 50%

15. In a certain region of space with volume 0.2 m^3, the electric potential is found to be 5 V throughout. The magnitude of electric field in this region is : ***[2020]***

(a) 0.5 N/C (b) 1 N/C (c) 5 N/C (d) zero

16. A short electric dipole has a dipole moment of 16×10^{-9} C m. The electric potential due to the dipole at a point at a distance of 0.6 m from the centre of the dipole, situated on a line making an angle of 60° with the dipole axis is : ***[2020]***

$$\left(\frac{1}{4\pi\epsilon_0} = 9\times10^9\,\text{N m}^2/\text{C}^2\right)$$

(a) 200 V (b) 400 V (c) zero (d) 50 V

17. The capacitance of a parallel plate capacitor with air as medium is 6 μF. With the introduction of a dielectric medium, the capacitance becomes 30 μF. The permittivity of the medium is: ($\epsilon_0 = 8.85 \times 10^{-12}\,C^2N^{-1}m^{-2}$) ***[2020]***

(a) $1.77 \times 10^{-12}\,C^2N^{-1}m^{-2}$ (b) $0.44 \times 10^{-10}\,C^2N^{-1}m^{-2}$
(c) $5.00\,C^2N^{-1}m^{-2}$ (d) $0.44 \times 10^{-13}\,C^2N^{-1}m^{-2}$

Exercise 3 - Concept Application Problems

CAP

1. A battery of e.m.f. V volt, resistors R_1 and R_2, a condenser C and switches S_1 and S_2 are connected in a circuit shown. The condenser will get fully charged to V volt when

(a) S_1 and S_2 are both closed
(b) S_1 and S_2 are both open
(c) S_1 is open and S_2 is closed
(d) S_1 is closed and S_2 is open

2. The four capacitors, each of 25 μ F are connected as shown in fig. The dc voltmeter reads 200 V. The charge on each plate of capacitor is

(a) $\pm 2\times10^{-3}$C
(b) $\pm 5\times10^{-3}$C
(c) $\pm 2\times10^{-2}$C
(d) $\pm 5\times10^{-2}$C

3. The capacity of a parallel plate condenser is 10 μF, when the distance between its plates is 8 cm. If the distance between the plates is reduced to 4 cm, then the capacity of this parallel plate condenser will be

(a) 5 μF (b) 10 μF (c) 20 μF (d) 40 μF

4. Four metallic plates each with a surface area of one side A, are placed at a distance d from each other. The two outer plates are connected to one point A and the two other inner plates to another point B as shown in the figure. Then the capacitance of the system is

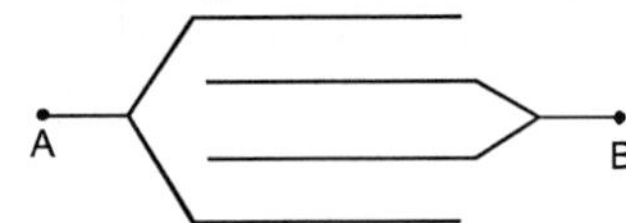

(a) $\frac{\varepsilon_0 A}{d}$ (b) $\frac{2\varepsilon_0 A}{d}$ (c) $\frac{3\varepsilon_0 A}{d}$ (d) $\frac{4\varepsilon_0 A}{d}$

5. Two spherical conductors A and B of radii a and b (b>a) are placed concentrically in air. The two are connected by a copper wire as shown in figure. Then the equivalent capacitance of the system is

(a) $4\pi\varepsilon_0 \frac{ab}{b-a}$
(b) $4\pi\varepsilon_0(a+b)$
(c) $4\pi\varepsilon_0 b$
(d) $4\pi\varepsilon_0 a$

6. A parallel plate capacitor with air between the plates is charged to a potential difference of 500V and then insulated. A plastic plate is inserted between the plates filling the whole gap. The potential difference between the plates now becomes 75V. The dielectric constant of plastic is

(a) 10/3 (b) 5 (c) 20/3 (d) 10

7. Two capacitors C_1 and $C_2 = 2C_1$ are connected in a circuit with a switch between them as shown in the figure. Initially the switch is open and C_1 holds charge Q. The switch is closed. At steady state, the charge on each capacitor will be

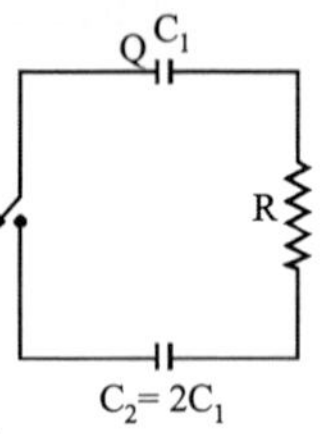

(a) Q, 2Q (b) $\frac{Q}{3}, \frac{2Q}{3}$

(c) $\frac{3Q}{2}, 3Q$ (d) $\frac{2Q}{3}, \frac{4Q}{3}$

8. A charge +q is fixed at each of the points $x = x_0$, $x = 3x_0$, $x = 5x_0$, ... upto ∞ on X-axis and charge –q is fixed on each of the points $x = 2x_0$, $x = 4x_0$, $x = 6x_0$, ... upto ∞ . Here x_0 is a positive constant. Take the potential at a point due to a charge Q at a distance r from it to be $\frac{Q}{4\pi\varepsilon_0 r}$. Then the potential at the origin due to above system of charges will be

(a) zero (b) $\frac{q}{8\pi\varepsilon_0 x_0 \log_e 2}$

(c) infinity (d) $\frac{q \log_e 2}{4\pi\varepsilon_0 x_0}$

9. A parallel plate capacitor of capacitance C is connected to a battery and is charged to a potential difference V. Another capacitor of capacitance 2C is similary charged to a potential difference 2V. The charging battery is now disconnected and the capacitors are connected in parallel to each other in such a way that the positive terminal of one is connected to the negative terminal of the other. The final energy of the configuration is

(a) zero (b) $\frac{3}{2}CV^2$ (c) $\frac{25}{6}CV^2$ (d) $\frac{9}{2}CV^2$

10. A solid conducting sphere having a charge Q is surrounding by an uncharged concentric conducting hollow spherical shell. Let the potential difference between the surface of the solid sphere and that of the outer surface of the hollow shell be V. If the shell is now given a charge of – 3Q, the new potential difference between the same two surfaces is

(a) V (b) 2V (c) 4V (d) –2 V

11. A circuit is connected as shown in the figure with the switch S open. When the switch is closed, the total amount of charge that flows from Y to X is

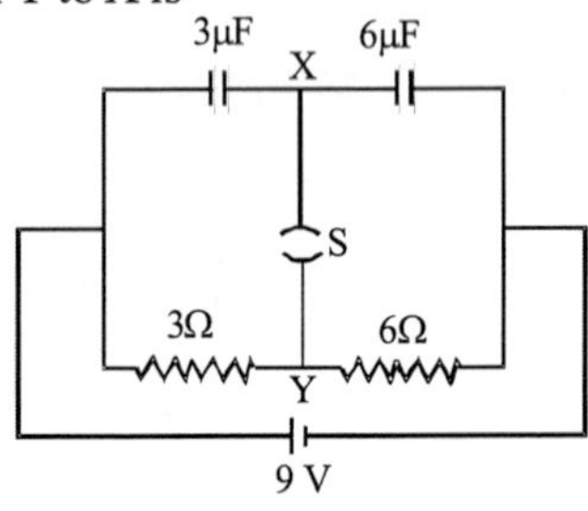

(a) 0
(b) 54 μC
(c) 27μC
(d) 81 μC

12. If a slab of insulating material 4×10^{-5} m thick is introduced between the plates of a parallel plate capacitor, the distance between the plates has to be increased by 3.5×10^{-5} m to restore the capacity to original value. Then the dielectric constant of the material of slab is
(a) 8 (b) 6 (c) 12 (d) 10

13. Two spherical conductors A and B of radii a and b (b > a) are placed concentrically in air. B is given charge +Q and A is earthed. The equivalent capacitance of the system is
(a) 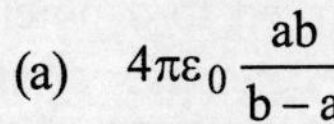 $4\pi\varepsilon_0 \dfrac{ab}{b-a}$
(b) $4\pi\varepsilon_0 (a+b)$
(c) $4\pi\varepsilon_0 b$
(d) $4\pi\varepsilon_0 \left(\dfrac{b^2}{b-a}\right)$

14. The capacitance of a parallel plate capacitor is C_a (Fig. a). A dielectric of dielectric constant K is inserted as shown in fig (b) and (c). If C_b and C_c denote the capacitances in fig (b) and (c), then

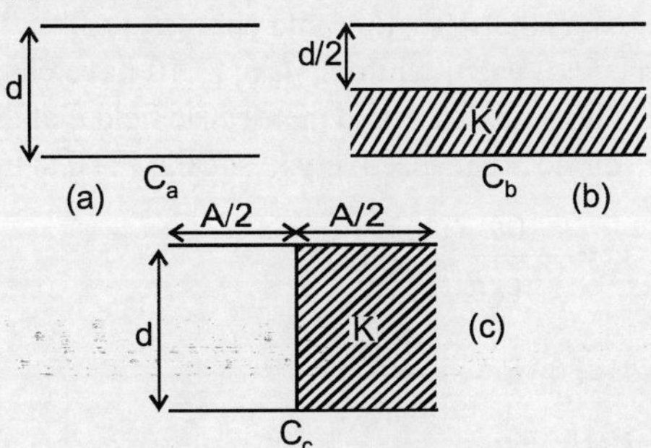

(a) both $C_b, C_c > C_a$ (b) $C_c > C_a$ while $C_b > C_a$
(c) both $C_b, C_c < C_a$ (d) $C_a = C_b = C_c$

15. Two small conductors A and B are given charges q_1 and q_2 respectively. Now they are placed inside a hollow metallic conductor C carrying a charge Q. If all the three conductors A, B and C are connected by a conducting wire as shown, the charges on A, B and C will be respectively
(a) $\dfrac{q_1+q_2}{2}, \dfrac{q_1+q_2}{2}, Q$
(b) $\dfrac{Q+q_1+q_3}{3}, \dfrac{Q+q_1+q_2}{3}, \dfrac{Q+q_1+q_2}{3}$
(c) 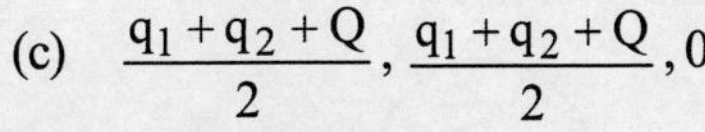 $\dfrac{q_1+q_2+Q}{2}, \dfrac{q_1+q_2+Q}{2}, 0$
(d) $0, 0, Q+q_1+q_2$

16. Between the plates of a parallel plate capacitor dielectric plate is introduced just to fill the space between the plates. The capacitor is charged and later disconnected from the battery. The dielectric plate is slowly drawn out of the capacitor parallel to plates. The plot of the potential difference V across the plates and the length of the dielectric plate drawn out is

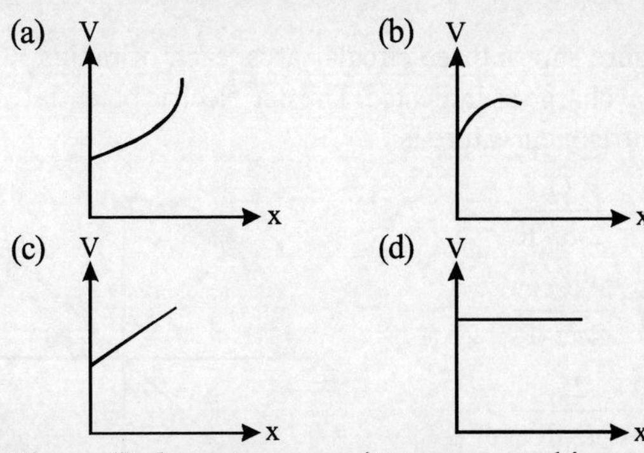

17. Figure (i) shows two capacitors connected in series and connected by a battery. The graph (ii) shows the variation of potential as one moves from left to right on the branch AB containing the capacitors. Then
(a) $C_1 = C_2$
(b) $C_1 < C_2$
(c) $C_1 > C_2$
(d) C_1 and C_2 cannot be compared

C_1 C_2 A B E (i)

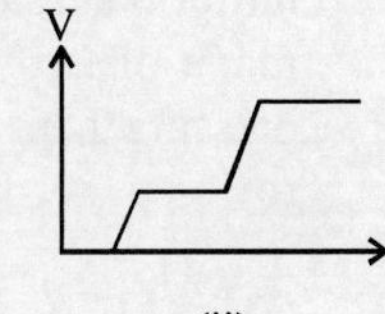

(ii)

18. Two vertical metallic plates carrying equal and opposite charges are kept parallel to each other like a parallel plate capacitor. A small spherical metallic ball is suspended by a long insulated thread such that it hangs freely in the centre of the two metallic plates. The ball, which is uncharged, is taken slowly towards the positively charged plate and is made to touch that plate. Then the ball will
(a) stick to the positively charged plate
(b) come back to its original position and will remain there
(c) oscillate between the two plates touching each plate in turn
(d) oscillate between the two plates without touch them

19. A parallel plate capacitor is connected to a battery. The quantities charge, voltage, electric field and energy associated with this capacitor are given by Q_0, V_0, E_0, and U_0 respectively. A dielectric slab is now introduced to fill the space between the plates with the battery still in connection. The corresponding quantities now given by Q, V, E and U are related to the previous ones as
(a) $Q > Q_0$ (b) $V > V_0$ (c) $E > E_0$ (d) $U < U_0$

20. A parallel plate capacitor of plate area A and plate separation d is charged to potential difference V and then the battery is disconnected. A slab of dielectric constant K is then inserted between the plates of capacitor so as to fill the space between the plates. If Q, E and W denote respectively, the magnitude of charge on each plate electric field between the plates (after the slab is inserted), and work done on the system, in question, in the process of inserting the slab, then which is wrong ?
(a) $Q = \dfrac{\varepsilon_0 AV}{d}$ (b) $Q = \dfrac{\varepsilon_0 KAV}{d}$
(c) $E = \dfrac{V}{Kd}$ (d) $W = \dfrac{\varepsilon_0 AV^2}{2d}\left(1 - \dfrac{1}{K}\right)$

21. Figure shows three circular arcs, each of radius R and total charge as indicated. The net electric potential at the centre of curvature is

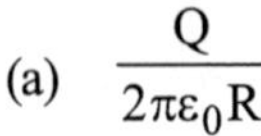

(a) $\frac{Q}{2\pi\varepsilon_0 R}$

(b) $\frac{Q}{4\pi\varepsilon_0 R}$

(c) $\frac{2Q}{\pi\varepsilon_0 R}$

(d) $\frac{Q}{\pi\varepsilon_0 R}$

22. A uniformly charged thin spherical shell of radius R carries uniform surface charge density of σ per unit area. It is made of two hemispherical shells, held together by pressing them with force F (see figure). F is proportional to

(a) $\frac{1}{\varepsilon_0}\sigma^2 R^2$ (b) $\frac{1}{\varepsilon_0}\sigma^2 R$

(c) $\frac{1}{\varepsilon_0}\frac{\sigma^2}{R}$ (d) $\frac{1}{\varepsilon_0}\frac{\sigma^2}{R^2}$

23. In the given circuit if point C is connected to the earth and a potential of +2000V is given to the point A, the potential at B is

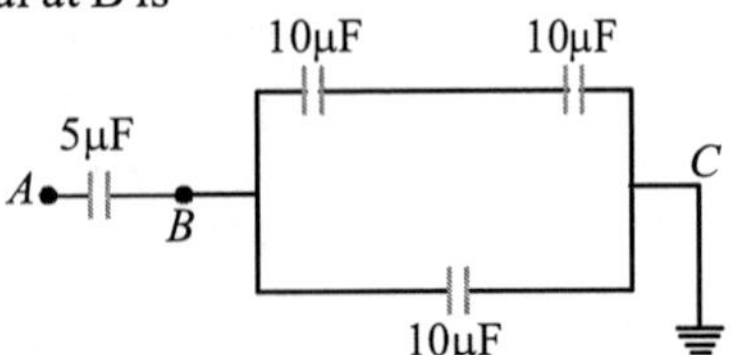

(a) 1500V (b) 1000V (c) 500V (d) 400V

24. Two charges q_1 and q_2 are placed 30 cm apart, as shown in the figure. A third charge q_3 is moved along the arc of a circle of radius 40 cm from C to D. The change in the potential energy of the system is $\frac{q_3}{4\pi\in_0}$k, , where k is

(a) $8q_1$

(b) $6q_1$

(c) $8q_2$

(d) $6q_2$

25. A network of four capacitors of capacity equal to $C_1 = C$, $C_2 = 2C$, $C_3 = 3C$ and $C_4 = 4C$ are conducted to a battery as shown in the figure. The ratio of the charges on C_2 and C_4 is

(a) 4/7

(b) 3/22

(c) 7/4

(d) 22/3

26. A series combination of n_1 capacitors, each of value C_1, is charged by a source of potential difference 4 V. When another parallel combination of n_2 capacitors, each of value C_2, is charged by a source of potential difference V, it has the same (total) energy stored in it, as the first combination has. The value of C_2, in terms of C_1, is then

(a) $\frac{2C_1}{n_1 n_2}$ (b) $16\frac{n_2}{n_1}C_1$ (c) $2\frac{n_2}{n_1}C_1$ (d) $\frac{16C_1}{n_1 n_2}$

27. A condenser of capacity C is charged to a potential difference of V_1. The plates of the condenser are then connected to an ideal inductor of inductance L. The current through the inductor when the potential difference across the condenser reduces to V_2 is

(a) $\left(\frac{C(V_1^2 - V_2^2)}{L}\right)^{1/2}$ (b) $\left(\frac{C(V_1 - V_2)^2}{L}\right)^{1/2}$

(c) $\frac{C(V_1^2 - V_2^2)}{L}$ (d) $\frac{C(V_1 - V_2)}{L}$

28. Ten charges are placed on the circumference of a circle of radius R with constant angular separation between successive charges. Alternate charges 1, 3, 5, 7, 9 have charge $(+q)$ each, while 2, 4, 6, 8, 10 have charge $(-q)$ each. The potential V and the electric field E at the centre of the circle are respectively : (Take $V = 0$ at infinity)

(a) $V = \frac{10q}{4\pi\varepsilon_0 R}; E = 0$

(b) $V = 0; E = \frac{10q}{4\pi\varepsilon_0 R^2}$

(c) $V = 0; E = 0$

(d) $V = \frac{10q}{4\pi\varepsilon_0 R}; E = \frac{10q}{4\pi\varepsilon_0 R^2}$

29. Two isolated conducting spheres S_1 and S_2 of radius $\frac{2}{3}R$ and $\frac{1}{3}R$ have 12 μC and –3 μC charges, respectively, and are at a large distance from each other. They are now connected by a conducting wire. A long time after this is done the charges on S_1 and S_2 are respectively :

(a) 4.5 μC on both (b) +4.5 μC and –4.5 μC

(c) 3 μC and 6 μC (d) 6 μC and 3 μC

30. A charge Q is distributed over two concentric conducting thin spherical shells radii r and R $(R > r)$. If the surface charge densities on the two shells are equal, the electric potential at the common centre is :

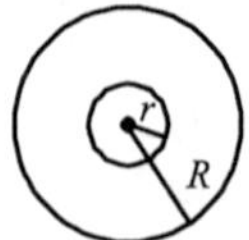

(a) $\frac{1}{4\pi\varepsilon_0}\frac{(R+r)}{2(R^2+r^2)}Q$ (b) $\frac{1}{4\pi\varepsilon_0}\frac{(2R+r)}{(R^2+r^2)}Q$

(c) $\frac{1}{4\pi\varepsilon_0}\frac{(R+2r)Q}{2(R^2+r^2)}$ (d) $\frac{1}{4\pi\varepsilon_0}\frac{(R+r)}{(R^2+r^2)}Q$

31. A uniformly charged ring of radius 3a and total charge q is placed in xy-plane centred at origin. A point charge q is moving towards the ring along the z-axis and has speed v at z = 4a. The minimum value of v such that it crosses the origin is :

(a) $\sqrt{\frac{2}{m}}\left(\frac{4}{15}\frac{q^2}{4\pi\varepsilon_0 a}\right)^{1/2}$ (b) $\sqrt{\frac{2}{m}}\left(\frac{1}{5}\frac{q^2}{4\pi\varepsilon_0 a}\right)^{1/2}$

(c) $\sqrt{\frac{2}{m}}\left(\frac{2}{15}\frac{q^2}{4\pi\varepsilon_0 a}\right)^{1/2}$ (d) $\sqrt{\frac{2}{m}}\left(\frac{1}{15}\frac{q^2}{4\pi\varepsilon_0 a}\right)^{1/2}$

32. A charge Q is distributed over three concentric spherical shells of radii a, b, c (a < b < c) such that their surface charge densities are equal to one another. The total potential at a point at distance r from their common centre, where r < a, would be:

(a) $\frac{Q}{12\pi\epsilon_0}\frac{ab+bc+ca}{abc}$ (b) $\frac{Q(a^2+b^2+c^2)}{4\pi\epsilon_0(a^3+b^3+c^3)}$

(c) $\frac{Q}{4\pi\epsilon_0(a+b+c)}$ (d) $\frac{Q(a+b+c)}{4\pi\epsilon_0(a^2+b^2+c^2)}$

33. Two electric dipoles, A, B with respective dipole moments $\vec{d}_A = -4\,qa\,\hat{i}$ and $\vec{d}_B = -2\,qa\,\hat{i}$ are placed on the *x*-axis with a separation R, as shown in the figure

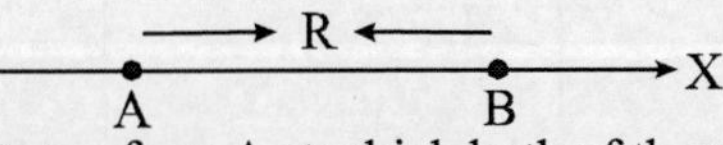

The distance from A at which both of them produce the same potential is:

(a) $\frac{R}{\sqrt{2}+1}$ (b) $\frac{\sqrt{2}R}{\sqrt{2}+1}$ (c) $\frac{R}{\sqrt{2}-1}$ (d) $\frac{\sqrt{2}R}{\sqrt{2}-1}$

34. A solid sphere of radius *R* carries a charge $Q+q$ distributed uniformaly over its volume. A very small point like piece of it of mass *m* gets detached from the bottom of the sphere and falls down vertically under gravity. This piece carries charge *q*. If it acquires a speed *v* when it has fallen through a vertical height *y* (see figure), then : (assume the remaining portion to be spherical).

(a) $v^2 = y\left[\frac{qQ}{4\pi\varepsilon_0 R^2 ym}+g\right]$

(b) $v^2 = y\left[\frac{qQ}{4\pi\varepsilon_0 R(R+y)m}+g\right]$

(c) $v^2 = 2y\left[\frac{Qq\,R}{4\pi\varepsilon_0 (R+y)^3 m}+g\right]$

(d) $v^2 = 2y\left[\frac{qQ}{4\pi\varepsilon_0 R(R+y)m}+g\right]$

35. A positive point charge is released from rest at a distance r_0 from a positive line charge with uniform density. The speed (v) of the point charge, as a function of instantaneous distance *r* from line charge, is proportional to :

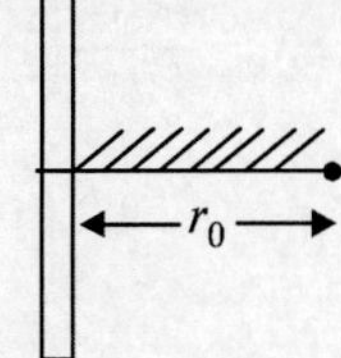

(a) $v \propto e^{+r/r_0}$

(b) $v \propto \sqrt{ln\left(\frac{r}{r_0}\right)}$

(c) $v \propto ln\left(\frac{r}{r_0}\right)$

(d) $v \propto \left(\frac{r}{r_0}\right)$

36. Four equal point charges Q each are placed in the xy plane at (0, 2), (4, 2), (4, – 2) and (0, – 2). The work required to put a fifth charge Q at the origin of the coordinate system will be:

(a) $\frac{Q^2}{4\pi\varepsilon_0}\left(1+\frac{1}{\sqrt{3}}\right)$ (b) $\frac{Q^2}{4\pi\varepsilon_0}\left(1+\frac{1}{\sqrt{5}}\right)$

(c) $\frac{Q^2}{2\sqrt{2}\,\pi\varepsilon_0}$ (d) $\frac{Q^2}{4\pi\varepsilon_0}$

37. Two capacitors of capacitances C and 2C are charged to potential differences V and 2V, respectively. These are then connected in parallel in such a manner that the positive terminal of one is connected to the negative terminal of the other. The final energy of this configuration is :

(a) $\frac{25}{6}CV^2$ (b) $\frac{3}{2}CV^2$ (c) zero (d) $\frac{9}{2}CV^2$

38. Effective capacitance of parallel combination of two capacitors C_1 and C_2 is 10 μF. When these capacitors are individually connected to a voltage source of 1 V, the energy stored in the capacitor C_2 is 4 times that of C_1. If these capacitors are connected in series, their effective capacitance will be:

(a) 4.2 μF (b) 3.2 μF (c) 1.6 μF (d) 8.4 μF

39. A capacitor is made of two square plates each of side '*a*' making a very small angle a between them, as shown in figure. The capacitance will be close to:

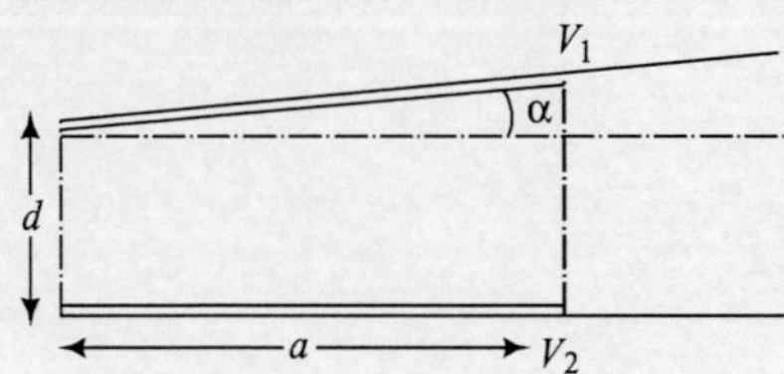

(a) $\frac{\epsilon_0 a^2}{d}\left(1-\frac{\alpha a}{2d}\right)$ (b) $\frac{\epsilon_0 a^2}{d}\left(1-\frac{\alpha a}{4d}\right)$

(c) $\frac{\epsilon_0 a^2}{d}\left(1+\frac{\alpha a}{d}\right)$ (d) $\frac{\epsilon_0 a^2}{d}\left(1-\frac{3\alpha a}{2d}\right)$

40. A parallel plate capacitor has plates of area A separated by distance '*d*' between them. It is filled with a dielectric which has a dielectric constant that varies as $k(x) = K(1 + \alpha x)$ where '*x*' is the distance measured from one of the plates. If $(\alpha d) << 1$, the total capacitance of the system is best given by the expression:

(a) $\frac{AK\epsilon_0}{d}\left(1+\frac{\alpha d}{2}\right)$

(b) $\frac{A\epsilon_0 K}{d}\left(1+\left(\frac{\alpha d}{2}\right)^2\right)$

(c) $\frac{A\epsilon_0 K}{d}\left(1+\frac{\alpha^2 d^2}{2}\right)$

(d) $\frac{AK\epsilon_0}{d}(1+\alpha d)$

41. Find the capacitance between P and Q (Fig). Each Capacitor has cpacitance C.

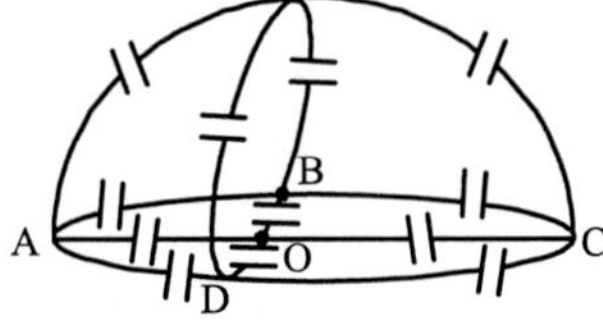

(a) 2C
(b) 3C
(c) 8C
(d) 6C

42. Voltage rating of a parallel plate capacitor is 500 V. Its dielectric can withstand a maximum electric field of 10^6 V/m. The plate area is 10^{-4} m^2. What is the dielectric constant if the capacitance is 15 pF ?
(given $\varepsilon_0 = 8.86 \times 10^{-12}$ C^2/Nm^2)

(a) 3.8 (b) 8.5 (c) 4.5 (d) 6.2

43. A parallel plate capacitor has 1μF capacitance. One of its two plates is given + 2μC charge and the other plate, +4μC charge. The potential difference developed across the capacitor is :

(a) 3V (b) 1V (c) 5V (d) 2V

44. In the figure shown, after the switch 'S' is turned from position 'A' to position 'B', the energy dissipated in the circuit in terms of capacitance 'C' and total charge 'Q' is:

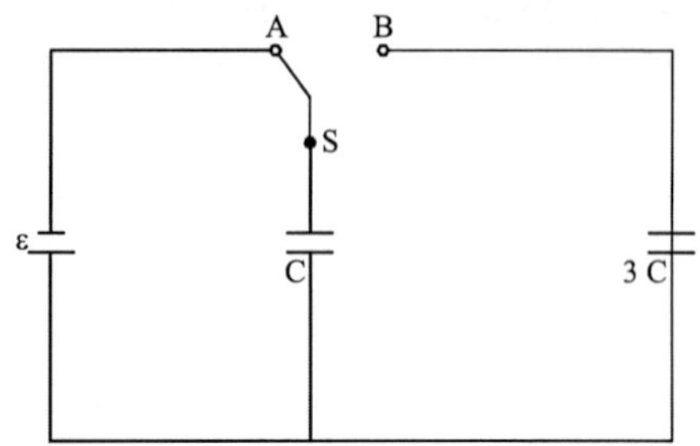

(a) $\frac{1}{8}\frac{Q^2}{C}$ (b) $\frac{3}{8}\frac{Q^2}{C}$ (c) $\frac{5}{8}\frac{Q^2}{C}$ (d) $\frac{3}{4}\frac{Q^2}{C}$

45. In the circuit shown, find C if the effective capacitance of the whole circuit is to be 0.5 μF. All values in the circuit are in μF.

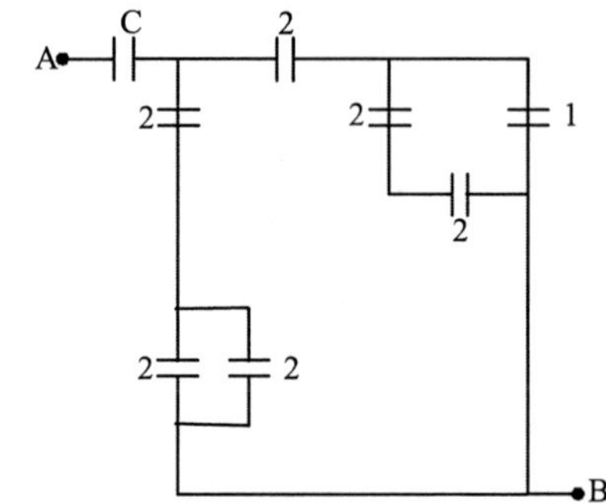

(a) $\frac{7}{11}$ μF (b) $\frac{6}{5}$ μF (c) 4 μF (d) $\frac{7}{10}$ μF

Hints & Solutions

17.1 Concept Practice Problems

CPP

1. (a) Inside the sphere, electric potential is due to the charge inside the sphere.
2. (b) Potential at the centre of the triangle,

$$V = \frac{\Sigma q}{4\pi\varepsilon_0 r} = \frac{2q - q - q}{4\pi\varepsilon_0 r} = 0$$

Obviously, $E \neq 0$

3. (b) As $V = \frac{Q}{4\pi\varepsilon_0 r}$ i.e. $V \propto \frac{1}{r}$

$\therefore \frac{V_1}{V_2} = \frac{r_2}{r_1}$

4. (c) Due to small dipole, $V \propto \frac{1}{r^2}$.
5. (a) K.E. = Work done = eV

$\frac{1}{2}mv^2 = eV \quad \therefore \; v = \sqrt{\frac{2eV}{m}}$

6. (b) $W_{BA} = q(V_A - V_B)$

$$= q\left[\frac{Q}{4\pi\varepsilon_0 a} - \frac{Q}{4\pi\varepsilon_0 b}\right] = \frac{qQ}{4\pi\varepsilon_0}\left[\frac{1}{a} - \frac{1}{b}\right]$$

7. (c) $V_r = \frac{Q_2}{4\pi\varepsilon_0 r} + \frac{Q_1}{4\pi\varepsilon_0 R_1}$

$$V_r = \frac{1}{4\pi\varepsilon_0}\left(\frac{Q_2}{r} + \frac{Q_1}{R_1}\right)$$

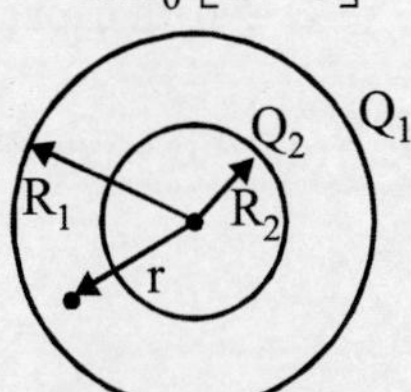

8. (b) Charge on α particle, q = 2 e.
K.E. = work done = $q \times V = 2e \times 10^6 V = 2$ MeV.
9. (b) Potential at any point inside the sphere = potential at the surface of the sphere = 10V.
10. (a) $\frac{Vr^2}{k\cos\theta} = qd = \frac{(2.0\times10^{-5}\,V)(0.1m)^2}{\left\{9.0\times10^9\,\frac{m}{\left(\frac{C}{V}\right)}\right\}\left(\frac{\sqrt{3}}{2}\right)} = 2.57\times10^{-17}$ Cm.

Note that the units cancel to leave units appropriate for a dipole moment.

17.2 Concept Practice Problems

CPP

11. (b) The magnitude of electric field by any one plate is

$\frac{\sigma}{2\varepsilon_0}$ or $\frac{Q}{2A\varepsilon_0}$

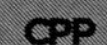

Now force magnitude is $|Q||E|$ i.e. $|F| = \frac{Q^2}{2A\varepsilon_0}$

12. (d)
13. (c)
14. (d)
15. (b) In parallel, potential is same, say V

$$\frac{Q_1}{Q_2} = \frac{C_1 V}{C_2 V} = \frac{C_1}{C_2}$$

16. (b) Energy will be lost during transfer of charge (heating effect).
17. (c) $E \propto \frac{\lambda}{2\pi\varepsilon_0 r}$ hence $E \propto \frac{1}{r}$
18. (d) When oil is placed between space of plates

$C = \frac{2A\varepsilon_0}{d}$ ... (1) $\quad \left[\because C = \frac{KA\varepsilon_0}{d}, \text{ where } K = 2\right]$

When oil is removed $C' = \frac{A\varepsilon_0}{d}$ .... (2)

on comparing both equation, weget $C' = C/2$

19. (c) When a battery across the plates of capacitor is disconnected and dielectric slab is placed in between the plates, then
(i) capacity C increases
(ii) charge q remains unchanged
(iii) potential V decreases
(iv) energy E decreases
20. (d) $U = \frac{1}{2}CV^2$

$$U = \frac{1}{2}\left(\frac{A\epsilon_0}{d}\right)(Ed)^2 = \frac{1}{2}A\epsilon_0 E^2 d$$

Exercise 1 - Chapter Revision Problems

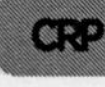

1. (a)

A — ε_1 | ε_2 — A; d_1, d_2

$$\frac{1}{C_S} = \frac{1}{C_1} + \frac{1}{C_2} \Rightarrow \frac{1}{C_S} = \frac{1}{\frac{\varepsilon_1 A}{d_1} + \frac{\varepsilon_2 A}{d_2}}$$

$$\Rightarrow \frac{1}{C_S} = \frac{1}{A}\left(\frac{d_1}{\varepsilon_1} + \frac{d_2}{\varepsilon_2}\right) \Rightarrow C_S = \frac{A\varepsilon_1\varepsilon_2}{\varepsilon_2 d_1 + \varepsilon_1 d_2}$$

2. (c)
3. (d) Common potential, $V = \frac{Q}{4\pi\varepsilon_0 r} + \frac{0}{4\pi\varepsilon_0 r}$

$$= \frac{Q + 0}{4\pi\varepsilon_0 (r + r')}$$

$\therefore$ charge on smaller sphere of radius r' is

$$4\pi\varepsilon_0 r' \times V = \frac{Qr'}{r + r'}$$

4. (d) $C = \frac{\epsilon_0 A}{d}$

$A \rightarrow$ common area, Here $A = A_1$

5. (a) In air $F_{air} = \frac{1}{4\pi\varepsilon_0}\frac{q_1 q_2}{r^2}$

In medium $F_m = \frac{1}{4\pi\varepsilon_0}\frac{q_1 q_2}{Kr^2}$

$\therefore \frac{F_m}{F_{air}} = \frac{1}{K} \Rightarrow F_m = \frac{F_{air}}{K}$ (decreases K-times)

6. (d) Electric field $E = \frac{\sigma}{\varepsilon} = \frac{Q}{A\varepsilon}$

ε of kerosine oil is more than that of air.

As ε increases, E decreases.

7. (a) Potential at B, V_B is maximum

$$V_B > V_C > V_A$$

8. (d) When negative terminal is grounded, positive terminal of battery is at +12 V. When positive terminal is grounded, the negative terminal will be at –12 V.

9. (b) $V = \frac{q}{4\pi\varepsilon_o r} = \frac{(Ze)}{4\pi \epsilon_0 r}$

$$9\times10^9 \frac{(50\times1.6\times10^{-19})}{9\times10^{-15}} = 8\times10^6 V$$

10. (d) $U = \frac{1}{4\pi\varepsilon_0}\left(\frac{2q^2}{a} - \frac{8q^2}{a} - \frac{4q^2}{a}\right)$

$$\Rightarrow U = \frac{1}{4\pi\varepsilon_0}\left(-\frac{10q^2}{a}\right)$$

$$\Rightarrow U = -\frac{9\times10^9\times10\times(0.1\times10^{-6})^2}{\left(\frac{10}{100}\right)}$$

$\Rightarrow U = -9\times10^{-3}$ J

11. (c) $q_1 = C_1 V = 10\times12 = 120\mu C$

$q_2 = C_2 V = KC_1 \times V = 5\times10\times12 = 600\mu C$

Additional charge that flows

$= q_2 - q_1 = 600 - 120 = 480\,\mu C.$

12. (c) As battery is disconnected, total charge Q is shared equally by two capacitors.

Energy of each capacitor $= \frac{(Q/2)^2}{2C} = \frac{1}{4}\frac{Q^2}{2C} = \frac{1}{4}U.$

13. (c)

14. (a) In series $\frac{1}{C} = \frac{1}{C_1} + \frac{1}{C_2} + \frac{1}{C_3}$ and charge on each capacitor is same.

15. (c) As work is done by the field, K.E. of the body increases by

$$K.E. = W = q(V_A - V_B)$$

$$= 10^{-8}(600 - 0) = 6\times10^{-6} J$$

16. (c) Consider the potential at D be 'V'.

Potential drop across C_1 is $(V - V_1)$ and C_2 is $(V_2 - V)$

$\therefore q_1 = C_1(V - V_1),\ q_2 = C_2(V_2 - V)$

As $q_1 = q_2$ [capacitors are in series]

$\therefore C_1(V - V_1) = C_2(V_2 - V)$

$$v = \frac{C_1V_1 + C_2V_2}{C_1 + C_2}$$

17. (a) Here, A = 90 cm² = 90×10^{-4} m²;
d = 2.5 mm = 2.5×10^{-3} m; V = 400 volt

$$C = \frac{\varepsilon_0 A}{d} = \frac{8.854\times10^{-12}\times90\times10^{-4}}{2.5\times10^{-3}}$$

$= 3.187\times10^{-11}$ F

$$W = \frac{1}{2}CV^2 = \frac{1}{2}\times3.187\times10^{-11}\times(400)^2$$

$= 2.55\times10^{-6}$ J

18. (d) Let 'n' such capacitors are in series and such 'm' such branch are in parallel.

$\therefore\ 250\times n = 1000\quad \therefore\ n = 4\quad$ ...(i)

Also $\frac{8}{n}\times m = 16$

$m = \frac{16\times n}{8} = 8\quad$ ...(ii)

$\therefore$ No. of capacitor $= 8\times4 = 32$

19. (d) For a parallel plate capacitor $C = \frac{\varepsilon_0 A}{d}$

$$\therefore\ A = \frac{Cd}{\varepsilon_0} = \frac{1\times10^{-3}}{8.85\times10^{-12}} = 1.13\times10^8 m^2$$

This corresponds to area of square of side 10.6 km which shows that one farad is very large unit of capacitance.

20. (a) $E = \frac{1}{2}CV^2 = \frac{1}{2}\times1\times10^{-6}\times(4000)^2 = 8J.$

21. (a) $C_s = \frac{2\times8}{2+8} = 1.6\mu F$

Since, $Q = C_s V = 1.6\times10^{-6}\times300$

$Q = 4.8\times10^{-4}$ C

$$V_1 = \frac{4.8\times10^{-4}}{2\times10^{-6}} = 240V$$

$$V_2 = \frac{4.8\times10^{-4}}{8\times10^{-6}} = 60V$$

$$U = \frac{Q^2}{2C_1} + \frac{Q^2}{2C_2}$$

$$\Rightarrow U = \frac{\left(4.8\times10^{-4}\right)^2}{2}\left(\frac{1}{1.6\times10^{-6}}\right)$$

$\Rightarrow U = 3\times2.4\times10^{-2}$ J

$\Rightarrow U = 7.2\times10^{-2}$ J

22. (a)

23. (a) Here, $V(x)=\frac{20}{x^2-4}$ volt

We know that $E=-\frac{dV}{dx}=-\frac{d}{dx}\left(\frac{20}{x^2-4}\right)$

or, $E=+\frac{40x}{(x^2-4)^2}$

At $x=4\,\mu m$,

$$E=+\frac{40\times 4}{(4^2-4)^2}=+\frac{160}{144}=+\frac{10}{9}\text{ volt}/\mu m.$$

Positive sign indicates that $\vec{E}$ is in +ve x-direction.

24. (a) Capacitance of spherical conductor = $4\pi\varepsilon_0 a$ where a is radius of conductor.

Therefore, $C=\frac{1}{9\times10^9}\times 1=\frac{1}{9}\times10^{-9}$

$=0.11\times10^{-9}\text{ F}=1.1\times10^{-10}\text{ F}$

25. (d) In equilibrium, $F=qE=(ne)\frac{V}{d}=mg$

$$n=\frac{mgd}{eV}=\frac{1.96\times10^{-15}\times9.8\times0.02}{1.6\times10^{-19}\times800}=3$$

26. (c) Length of body diagonal = $\sqrt{3}\,b$

$\therefore$ Distance of centre of cube from each corner, $r=\frac{\sqrt{3}}{2}b$

Total P.E. of charge + q at the centre

$$=\frac{8q(-q)}{4\pi\varepsilon_0 r}=\frac{-8q^2}{4\pi\varepsilon_0(\sqrt{3}\,b/2)}=\frac{-4q^2}{\pi\varepsilon_0\sqrt{3}\,b}$$

27. (c)

28. (b) In shell, q charge is uniformly distributed over its surface, it behaves as a conductor.

V= potential at surface = $\frac{q}{4\pi\varepsilon_0 R}$ and

inside $V=\frac{q}{4\pi\varepsilon_0 R}$

Because of this it behaves as an equipotential surface.

29. (c) Since, all A, B, C, D and E lie on an equipotential surface so,

$$W=0$$

30. (d) For series $C'=\frac{C_1\times C_2}{C_1+C_2}=\frac{4\times4}{4+4}=2\mu F$

For parallel $C_{eq}=C'+C_2=2+4=6\mu F$

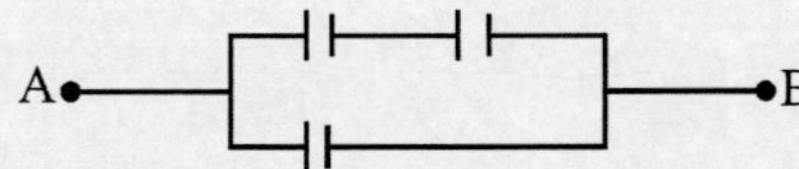

31. (b) $C=\frac{K\varepsilon_0 A}{d}$

$1\times10^{-12}=\frac{1\times\epsilon_0 A}{d}$ .... (1)

$2\times10^{-12}=\frac{K\times\epsilon_0 A}{2d}$ .... (2)

$\frac{(2)}{(1)}\Rightarrow\frac{K}{2}=2$ or $K=4$

32. (d) When S_1 and S_3 is closed $V_1=30$ V and potential drop across C_2 becomes 20 V.

33. (a) The molecules of liquid will convert into induced dipole, get oriented along the electric field produced between the plates and rise due to force of attraction.

34. (c) C_2 and C_3 are parallel so $V_2=V_3$
C_1 and combination of C_2 & C_3 is in series.
So, $V=V_2+V_1$ or $V=V_3+V_1$
and also $Q_1=Q_2+Q_3$

35. (a) Initial charge on first capacitor is $CV=Q_1$.
Initial charge on second capacitor is $2CV=Q_2$.
Final capacitance of first capacitor is KC
If V' is the common potential then

$$V'=\frac{Q_1+Q_2}{C_1'+C_2}\Rightarrow V'=\frac{CV+2CV}{KC+2C}=\frac{3V}{2+K}$$

36. (b)

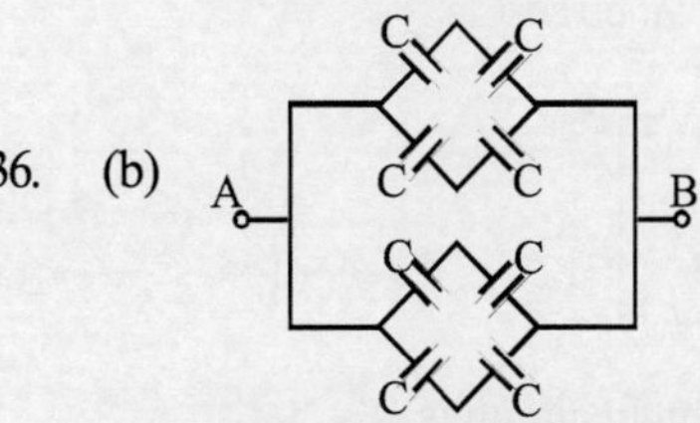

The figure shows two independent balanced wheatstone Brides connected in parallel each having a capacitance C.
So, $C_{net}=C_{AB}=2C$

37. (b) Potential difference across the branch de is 6 V. Net capacitance of de branch is 2.1 μF
So, $q=CV$
$\Rightarrow q=2.1\times6\,\mu C$
$\Rightarrow q=12.6\,\mu C$
Potential across 3 μF capacitance is

$$V=\frac{12.6}{3}=4.2\text{ volt}$$

Potential across 2 and 5 combination in parallel is
$6-4.2=1.8$ V
So, $q'=(1.8)(5)=9\,\mu C$

38. (a) Whenever a charge (+50 nC) is kept inside a hollow metallic spherical shell, it induces an equal and opposite charge on the inner surface and an equal and same type of charges on the outer surface.
$\therefore$ Inside, induced charge is – 50 nC and outside, +50 nC – 150 nC already present.

39. (a)

40. (b) $U_i=k\left[\frac{(-3q)\,q}{L}\times3+\frac{(q)\times(q)}{L}\times3\right]=\frac{-6kq^2}{L}$

$U_f=0$

Work done by electric field = – Change in potential energy

$$=U_i-U_f=\frac{-6kq^2}{L}$$

41. (c)

$$\frac{mv^2}{r}=\frac{kq^2}{(2r)^2}\ ;\ mv^2=\frac{kq^2}{4r}$$

Kinetic energy of each particle

$$=\frac{1}{2}mv^2=\frac{kq^2}{8r}$$

42. (c) Capacitance of capacitor (C) = 6 μF = 6 × 10^{-6} F; Initial potential (V_1) = 10 V and final potential (V_2) = 20 V. The increase in energy (ΔU)

$$=\frac{1}{2}C(V_2^2-V_1^2)=\frac{1}{2}\times(6\times10^{-6})\times[(20)^2-(10)^2]$$

$$=(3\times10^{-6})\times300=9\times10^{-4}\,J.$$

43. (b) As the capacitors offer infinite resistance to steady current so, the equivalent circuit is

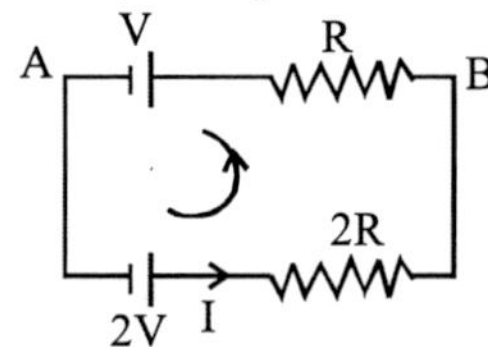

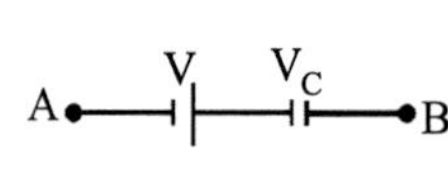

Using ohm's law, current in circuit is

$$2V-V=I(2R+R)\Rightarrow I=\frac{V}{3R}$$

The voltage drop across

$$V_{AB}=2V-\frac{V}{3R}\times2R=\frac{4}{3}V$$

$$V_{AB}=\frac{4}{3}V=V+V_C$$

$\Rightarrow$ Voltage drop across C = $\frac{1}{3}$V.

44. (c) Even after introduction of dielectric slab, direction of electric field will be perpendicular to the plates and directed from positive plate to negative plate.

Further, magnitude of electric field in air $=\frac{\sigma}{\varepsilon_0}$

Magnitude of electric field in dielectric $=\frac{\sigma}{K\varepsilon_0}$

Similarly electric lines always flows from higher to lower potential, therefore, electric potential inceases continuously as we move from x = 0 to x = 3d.

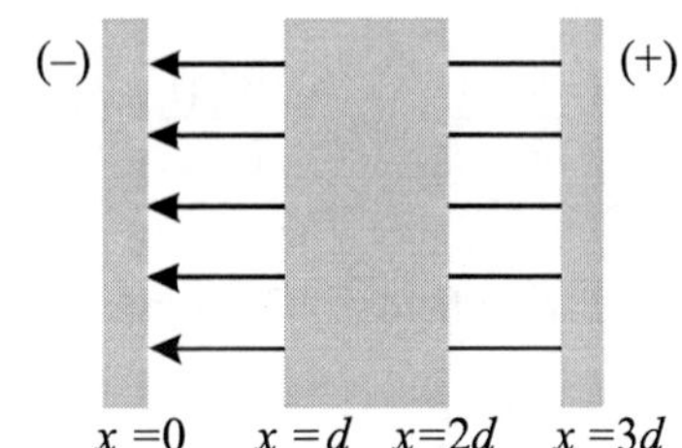

45. (a) $V_R=\frac{V_0}{4}=V_0e^{-\frac{t}{RC}}\Rightarrow\frac{1}{4}=e^{\frac{t}{10}}$

$$\Rightarrow4=e^{\frac{t}{10}}\Rightarrow\log_e4=\frac{t}{10}\Rightarrow t=10\log4=13.86s$$

(RC = 2.5 × 10^6 × 4 × 10^{-6} = 10)

46. (c) $\frac{1}{2}C_1V_1^2=\frac{1}{2}C_2V_2^2$

because total energy is transferred (given).

$$\therefore\ \frac{1}{2}\times900\times10^{-6}\times100^2=\frac{1}{2}\times100\times10^{-6}\times V^2$$

$\therefore V^2=90000\Rightarrow V=300$ V.

47. (d)

48. (c) Energy stored per unit volume

$$=\frac{1}{2}\varepsilon_0E^2=\frac{1}{2}\varepsilon_0\left(\frac{V}{d}\right)^2=\frac{1}{2}\varepsilon_0\frac{V^2}{d^2}\quad\left(\because E=\frac{V}{d}\right)$$

49. (a) Charge Q = C_1V

Total capacity of combination (parallel) C = C_1+C_2

$$P.D.=\frac{Q}{C}=\frac{C_1V}{C_1+C_2}$$

50. (a) We know that potential energy of two charge system is given by $U=\frac{1}{4\pi\epsilon_0}\frac{q_1q_2}{r}$

According to question,

$$U_A=\frac{1}{4\pi\epsilon_0}\frac{(+q)(-Q)}{a}=-\frac{1}{4\pi\varepsilon_0}\frac{Qq}{a}$$

and $U_B=\frac{1}{4\pi\epsilon_0}\frac{(+q)(-Q)}{a}=-\frac{1}{4\pi\varepsilon_0}\frac{Qq}{a}$

$$\Delta U=U_B-U_A=0$$

When known that for conservative force,

$$W=-\Delta U=0$$

51. (a) We have given two metallic hollow spheres of radii R and $4R$ having charges Q_1 and Q_2 respectively.

Potential on the surface of inner sphere (at A)

$$V_A=\frac{kQ_1}{R}+\frac{kQ_2}{4R}$$

Potential on the surface of outer sphere (at B)

$$V_B=\frac{kQ_1}{4R}+\frac{kQ_2}{4R}\qquad\left(\text{Here, }k=\frac{1}{4\pi\varepsilon_0}\right)$$

Potential difference,

$$\Delta V=V_A-V_B=\frac{3}{4}\cdot\frac{kQ_1}{R}=\frac{3}{16\pi\epsilon_0}\cdot\frac{Q_1}{R}$$

52. (b) The electric potential at the bisector is zero and electric field is antiparallel to the dipole moment.

$$\therefore\quad V=0\text{ and }\vec{E}=\frac{1}{4\pi\varepsilon_0}\left(\frac{-\vec{P}}{d^3}\right)$$

53. (b) Electric potential is constant inside a charged spherical shell.

54. (b)

55. (d) Change in potential energy, $\Delta u = q(V_f - V_i)$

Potential of $-q$ is same as initial and final point of the path.

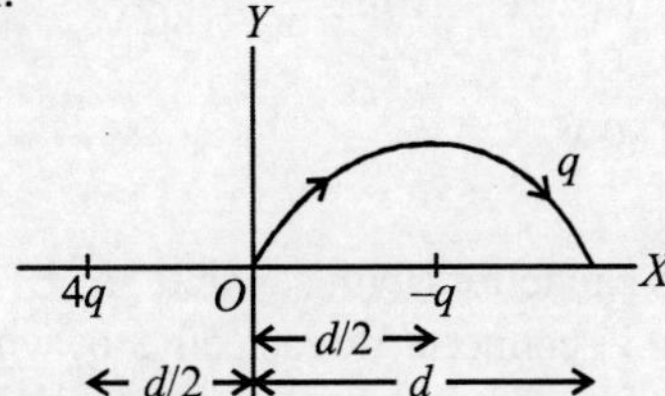

$$\Delta u = q\left(\frac{k4q}{3d/2} - \frac{k4q}{d/2}\right) = -\frac{4q^2}{3\pi\varepsilon_0 d}$$

–ve sign shows the energy of the charge is decreasing.

56. (c) According to work energy theorem, gain in kinetic energy is equal to work done in displacement of charge.

$$\therefore \quad \frac{1}{2}mv^2 = q\Delta V$$

Here, ΔV = potential difference between two positions of charge q.

For same q and ΔV.

$$v \propto \frac{1}{\sqrt{m}}$$

Mass of hydrogen ion $m_H = 1$

Mass of helium ion $m_{He} = 4$

$$\therefore \quad \frac{v_H}{v_{He}} = \sqrt{\frac{4}{1}} = 2:1.$$

57. (c) Using conservation of energy

$$U_i = U_F + \frac{1}{2}mv^2$$

$$\frac{kq_1q_2}{r_1} = \frac{kq_1q_2}{r_2} + \frac{1}{2}mv^2$$

$$\Rightarrow \frac{1}{2}mv^2 = kq_1q_2\left[\frac{1}{r_1} - \frac{1}{r_2}\right]$$

$$v^2 = \frac{2kq_1q_2}{m}\left[\frac{1}{r_1} - \frac{1}{r_2}\right]$$

$$= \frac{2\times 9\times 10^9 \times 10^{-12}}{4\times 10^{-6}\times 10^{-3}}\left[1 - \frac{1}{9}\right] = 4\times 10^{+6}$$

$v = 2\times 10^3$ m/s

58. (d) $$U = \frac{1}{4\pi\epsilon_0}\left[\frac{q(-q)}{d} + \frac{qQ}{\left(D + \frac{d}{2}\right)} + \frac{(-q)Q}{\left(D - \frac{d}{2}\right)}\right]$$

$$= \frac{1}{4\pi\epsilon_0}\left[-\frac{q^2}{d} - \frac{qQd}{D^2}\right], \text{ Ignoring } \frac{d^2}{4}$$

59. (b) Net electrostatic energy for the system

$$U = K\left[\frac{q^2}{a} + \frac{Qq}{a} + \frac{Qq}{a\sqrt{2}}\right] = 0$$

$$\Rightarrow q = -Q\left[1 + \frac{1}{\sqrt{2}}\right]$$

$$\Rightarrow Q = \frac{-q\sqrt{2}}{\sqrt{2}+1}$$

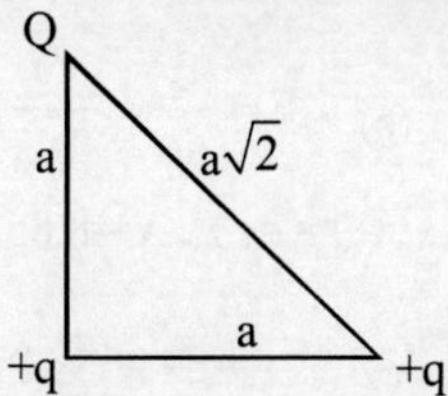

60. (a) Given,

Capacitance of capacitor, $C_1 = 10\ \mu F$

Potential difference before removing the source voltage, $V_1 = 50$ V

If C_2 be the capacitance of uncharged capacitor, then common potential is

$$V = \frac{C_1V_1 + C_2V_2}{C_1 + C_2} \Rightarrow 20 = \frac{10\times 50 + 0}{20 + C} \Rightarrow C = 15\ \mu F$$

61. (d) $$V' = \frac{CV + (nC)V}{kC + nC}$$

$$\frac{(n+1)V}{k+n}$$

62. (d) $V_1 + V_2 = 10$

and $4V_1 = 6V_2$

On solving above equations, we get

$V_1 = 6$ V

Charge on 4 μf,

$q = CV_1 = 4\times 6 = 24\ \mu C$.

4μF 6μF

10V

63. (a) Equivalent capacitance in series combination (C') is given by

$$\frac{1}{C'} = \frac{1}{C_1} + \frac{1}{C_2} \Rightarrow C' = \frac{C_1C_2}{C_1 + C_2}$$

For parallel combination equivalent capacitance

$C'' = C_1 + C_2$

For parallel combination

$q = 10(C_1 + C_2)$

$q_1 = 500\ \mu C$

$500 = 10(C_1 + C_2)$

$C_1 + C_2 = 50\mu F$ ....(i)

For Series Combination–

$$q_2 = 10\frac{C_1C_2}{(C_1 + C_2)}$$

$80 = 10\frac{C_1C_2}{50}$ From equation ....(ii)

$C_1C_2 = 400$ ....(iii)

From equation (i) and (ii)

$C_1 = 10\mu F \quad C_2 = 40\mu F$

64. (b) $$\omega = \omega_f - v_i = \frac{q}{2}\left(\frac{1}{C_f} - \frac{1}{C_i}\right)$$

$$= \frac{(5\times 10)^2}{2}\left(\frac{1}{2} - \frac{1}{5}\right)\times 10^6$$

$= 3.75\times 10^{-6}$ J

65. (c) $E = \frac{\sigma}{\varepsilon_0} = \frac{Q}{A\varepsilon_0}$

$\therefore Q = \varepsilon_0 . E. A = 8.85 \times 10^{-12} \times 100 \times 1$
$= 8.85 \times 10^{-10} C$

66. (a) Charge on Capacitor, $Q_i = CV$
After inserting dielectric of dielectric constant
$= K\ Q_f = (kC)V$
Induced charges on dielectric
$Q_{ind} = Q_f - Q_i = KCV - CV$

$$(K-1)CV = \left(\frac{5}{3}-1\right) \times 90\,\text{pF} \times 2\text{V} = 1.2\text{nc}$$

67. (d) The simplified circuit of the circuit given in question as follows:

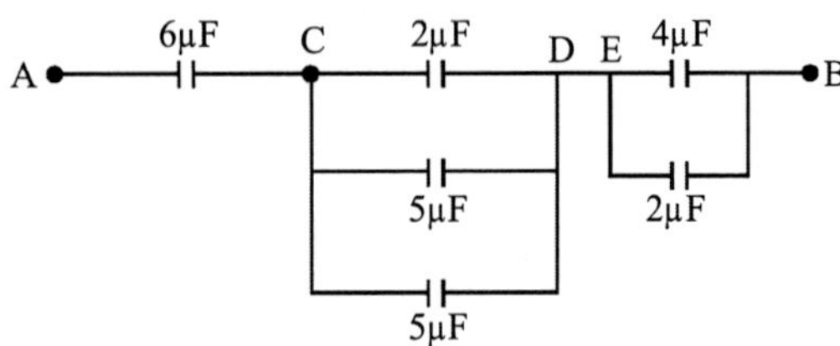

The equivalent capacitance between C & D capacitors of 2μF, 5μF and 5 μF are in parallel.

$\therefore$ $C_{CD} = 2 + 5 + 5 = 12\ \mu F$ ($\because$ In parallel grouping $C_{eq} = C_1 + C_2 + ... + C_n$)

Similarly equivalent capacitance between E & B $C_{EB} = 4 + 2 = 6\mu F$

Now equivalent capacitance between A & B

$$\frac{1}{C_{eq}} = \frac{1}{6} + \frac{1}{12} + \frac{1}{6} = \frac{5}{12}$$

$\Rightarrow C_{eq} = \frac{12}{5} = 2.4\ \mu F$ ($\because$ In series grouping, $\frac{1}{C_{eq}} = \frac{1}{C_1} + \frac{1}{C_2} + ... + \frac{1}{C_n}$)

68. (c)

69. (b) Potential outside the shell, $V_{outside} = \frac{KQ}{r}$

where r is distance of point from the centre of shell

Potential inside the shell, $V_{inside} = \frac{KQ}{R}$

where 'R" is radius of the shell

$$V_B = \frac{Kq_A}{r_b} + \frac{Kq_B}{r_b} + \frac{Kq_C}{r_c}$$

$$V_B = \frac{1}{4\pi\epsilon_0}\left[\frac{\sigma 4\pi a^2}{b} - \frac{\sigma 4\pi b^2}{b} + \frac{\sigma 4\pi c^2}{c}\right]$$

$$V_B = \frac{\sigma}{\epsilon_0}\left[\frac{a^2 - b^2}{b} + c\right]$$

70. (c) Given, $\vec{E} = (Ax + B)\hat{i}$

or $E = 20x + 10$

Using $V = \int E dx$, we have

$$V_2 - V_1 = \int_{-5}^{1} (20x + 10)dx = -180\ \text{V}$$

or $V_1 - V_2 = 180$ V

71. (d)

72. (d) When two capacitors with capacitance C_1 and C_2 at potential V_1 and V_2 connected to each other by wire, charge begins to flow from higher to lower potential till they acquire common potential. Here, some loss of energy takes place which is given by.

Heat loss, $H = \frac{C_1 C_2}{2(C_1 + C_2)}(V_1 - V_2)^2$

In the equation, put $V_2 = 0$, $V_1 = V_0$

$$C_1 = C,\ C_2 = \frac{C}{2}$$

Loss of heat $= \frac{C \times \frac{C}{2}}{2\left(C + \frac{C}{2}\right)}(V_0 - 0)^2 = \frac{C}{6}V_0^2$

$$H = \frac{1}{6}CV_0^2$$

73. (b) According to question,

$Q = 750\mu C = q_2 + q_3$

Capacitors C_2 and C_3 are in parallel hence,
Voltage across C_2 = voltage across C_3 = 20 V
Change on capacitor C_3,

$q_3 = C_3 \times V_3 = 8 \times 20 = 160\mu C$

$\therefore q_2 = 750\mu C - 160\mu C = 590\mu C$

74. (a)

Let q_1 and q_2 be the charge on the capacitors of 2μF and 4μF. Then charge on capacitor of 5μF

$Q = q_1 + q_2$

$\Rightarrow 5V_0 = 2(6 - V_0) + 4(6 - V_0)$

$\Rightarrow 5V_0 = 12 - 2V_0 + 24 - 4V_0$

$\Rightarrow 11V_0 = 36 \Rightarrow V_0 = \frac{36}{11}V$

$\Rightarrow Q = 5V_0 = \frac{180}{11}\mu C$

75. (c) Total energy of charge distribution is constant at any instant t.

$$U_f + K_f = U_i + K_i$$

i.e., $\frac{1}{2}mV^2 + \frac{KQ^2}{2R} = 0 + \frac{KQ^2}{2R_0}$

$\therefore \frac{1}{2}mV^2 = \frac{KQ^2}{2R_0} - \frac{KQ^2}{2R}$

$\therefore V = \sqrt{\frac{2}{m}\frac{KQ^2}{2}\left(\frac{1}{R_0} - \frac{1}{R}\right)}$

$\therefore V = \sqrt{\frac{KQ^2}{m}\left(\frac{1}{R_0} - \frac{1}{R}\right)} = C\sqrt{\frac{1}{R_0} - \frac{1}{R}}$

Also the slope of V – R curve will go on decreasing.

Exercise 2 - Exemplar & Past Year Questions E&PYQs

Exemplar Questions

1. (d) As capacitor offers infinite resistance in dc-circuit. So, current flows through 2Ω resistance from left to right, given by

$$I = \frac{V}{R+r} = \frac{2.5V}{2+0.5} = \frac{2.5}{2.5} = 1\text{ A}$$

So, the potential difference across 2Ω resistance

$V = IR = 1 \times 2 = 2$ volt.

Since, capacitor is in parallel with 2Ω resistance, so it also has 2V potential difference across it.

As current does not flow through capacitor branch so no potential drop will be accross 10Ω resistance. The charge on capacitor

$q = CV = (4\ \mu F) \times 2V = 8\ \mu C$

2. (c) The direction of electric field is always perpendicular to the direction of electric field and equipotential surface maintained at high electrostatic potential to other equipotential surface maintained at low electrostatic potential.

The positively charged particle experiences the electrostatic force in the direction of electric field i.e., from high electrostatic potential to low electrostatic potential. Thus, the work done by the electric field on the positive charge, so electrostatic potential energy of the positive charge decreases because speed of charged particle moves in the direction of field due to force $q\vec{E}$.

3. (c) As we know that the relation between electric field intensity E and electric potential V is

$$E = -\frac{dV}{dr}$$

Electric field intensity E = 0 then $\frac{dV}{dr} = 0$

This imply that V = constant

Thus, E = 0 inside the charged conducting sphere then the constant electrostatic potential 100V at every where inside the sphere and it verifies the shielding effect also.

4. (a) Here we have to findout the shape of equipotential surface, these surface are perpendicular to the field lines, so there must be electric field which can not be without charge.

So, the collection of charges, whose total sum is not zero, with regard to great distance can be considered as a point charge. The equipotentials due to point charge are spherical in shape as electric potential due to point charge q is given by

$$V = K_e\frac{q}{r}$$

This suggest that electric potentials due to point charge is same for all equidistant points. The locus of these equidistant points which are at same potential, form spherical surface.

The lines of field from point charge are radial. So the equipotential surface perpendicular to field lines from a sphere.

5. (c)

NEET/AIPMT (2013-2020) Questions

6. (a) Potential at B, V_B is maximum

$$V_B > V_C > V_A$$

As in the direction of electric field potential decreases.

7. (b) Due to conducting sphere

At centre, electric field E = 0

And electric potential $V = \frac{Q}{4\pi\epsilon_0 R}$

8. (d) $\vec{E} = -\frac{\partial V}{\partial x}\hat{i} - \frac{\partial V}{\partial y}\hat{j} - \frac{\partial V}{\partial z}\hat{k}$

$= -[(6-8y)\hat{i} + (-8x-8+6z)\hat{j} + (6y)\hat{k}]$

At (1, 1, 1), $\vec{E} = 2\hat{i} + 10\hat{j} - 6\hat{k}$

$\Rightarrow (\vec{E}) = \sqrt{2^2 + 10^2 + 6^2} = \sqrt{140} = 2\sqrt{35}$

$\therefore\ F = q\vec{E} = 2 \times 2\sqrt{35} = 4\sqrt{35}$

9. (c) Capacitance of the capacitor, $C = \frac{Q}{V}$

After inserting the dielectric, new capacitance

$C^1 = K.C$

New potential difference

$V^1 = \frac{V}{K}$

$u_i = \frac{1}{2}cv^2 = \frac{Q^2}{2C}\quad (\because Q = cv)$

$u_f = \frac{Q^2}{2f} = \frac{Q^2}{2kc} = \frac{C^2V^2}{2KC} = \left(\frac{u_i}{k}\right)$

$\Delta u = u_f - u_i = \frac{1}{2}cv^2\left\{\frac{1}{k} - 1\right\}$

As the capacitor is isolated, so change will remain conserved p.d. between two plates of the capacitor

$L = \frac{Q}{KC} = \frac{V}{K}$

10. (a) Potential in a region

$V = 6xy - y + 2yz$

As we know the relation between electric potential and electric field is $\vec{E} = \frac{-dV}{dx}$

$$\vec{E} = \left(\frac{\partial V}{\partial x}\hat{i} + \frac{\partial V}{\partial y}\hat{j} + \frac{\partial V}{\partial z}\hat{k}\right)$$

$$\vec{E} = \left[(6y\hat{i} + (6x - 1 + 2z)\hat{j} + (2y)\hat{k}\right]$$

$$\vec{E}_{(1,1,0)} = -(6\hat{i} + 5\hat{j} + 2\hat{k})$$

11. (d) **When S and 1 are connected**

The 2μF capacitor gets charged. The potential difference across its plates will be V.

The potential energy stored in 2 μF capacitor

$$U_i = \frac{1}{2}CV^2 = \frac{1}{2} \times 2 \times V^2 = V^2$$

When S and 2 are connected

The 8μF capacitor also gets charged. During this charging process current flows in the wire and some amount of energy is dissipated as heat. The energy loss is

$$\Delta U = \frac{1}{2}\frac{C_1 C_2}{C_1 + C_2}(V_1 - V_2)^2$$

Here, $C_1 = 2\mu F, C_2\ 8\ \mu F, V_1 = V, V_2 = 0$

$$\therefore \ \Delta U = \frac{1}{2} \times \frac{2 \times 8}{2 + 8}(V - 0)^2 = \frac{4}{5}V^2$$

The percentage of the energy dissipated

$$= \frac{\Delta U}{Ui} \times 100 = \frac{\frac{4}{5}V^2}{V^2} \times 100 = 80\%$$

12. (a) When battery is replaced by another uncharged capacitor

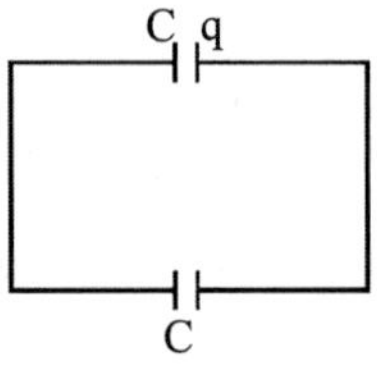

As uncharged capacitor is connected parallel

So, C' = 2C

and $V_c = \dfrac{q_1 + q_2}{C_1 + C_2}$

$$V_c = \frac{q + 0}{C + C} \Rightarrow V_c = \frac{V}{2}$$

Initial Energy of system, $U_i = \frac{1}{2}CV^2$ ...(i)

Final energy of system, $U_f = \frac{1}{2}(2C)\left(\frac{V}{2}\right)^2$

$$= \frac{1}{2}CV^2\left(\frac{1}{2}\right) \quad ...(ii)$$

From equation (i) and (ii)

$$U_f = \frac{1}{2}U_i$$

i.e., Total electrostatic energy of resulting system decreases by a factor of 2

13. (a) Electrostatic force between the metal plates

$$F_{plate} = \frac{Q^2}{2A_{\varepsilon_0}}$$

For isolated capacitor Q = constant

Clearly, F is independent of the distance between plates.

14. (d) $U_i = \frac{1}{2}CV^2$

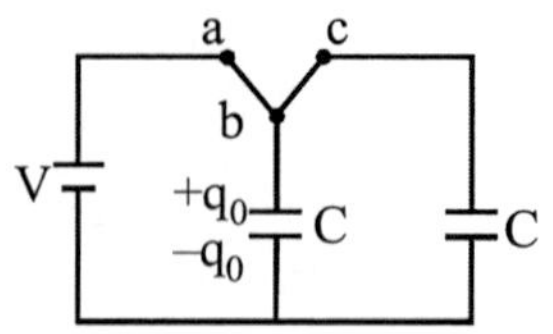

On switching key at point c

$$\frac{q_0 - q}{C} = \frac{q}{C}$$

$$2q = q_0$$

$$q = \left(\frac{q_0}{2}\right)$$

$$U_f = \frac{1}{2}\left(\frac{q_0}{2}\right)^2 \times \frac{1}{C} + \frac{1}{2}\left(\frac{q_0}{2}\right)^2 \times \frac{1}{C}$$

$$U_f = \frac{1}{4}CV^2$$

loss = 50%

15. (d) Since, electric potential is constant throughout the volume, hence electric field, $E = -\frac{dV}{dr} = 0$.

16. (a) Given,

Dipole moment of short electric dipole,

$p = 16 \times 10^{-9}$ C m.

Distance from centre of dipole, $r = 0.6$ m

Electric potential, $V = \dfrac{kp\cos\theta}{r^2}$

$$\Rightarrow V = \frac{9 \times 10^9 \times 16 \times 10^{-9} \times \cos 60}{0.36} = 200 \text{ V}$$

17. (b) Capacitance of a parallel plate capacitor with air is

$$C = \frac{\varepsilon_0 A}{d} \quad ...(i)$$

Here, A = area of plates of capacitor,

d = distance between the plates

Capacitance of a same parallel plate capacitor with introduction of dielectric medium of dielectric constant K is

$$C' = \frac{K\varepsilon_0 A}{d} \quad ...(ii)$$

Dividing (ii) by (i)

$$\Rightarrow \frac{C'}{C} = K \Rightarrow \frac{30}{6} = K \Rightarrow K = 5 \Rightarrow K = \frac{\varepsilon}{\varepsilon_0}$$

$$\Rightarrow \varepsilon = K\varepsilon_0 = 5 \times 8.85 \times 10^{-12} = 0.44 \times 10^{-10}\ C^2N^{-1}m^{-2}$$

Exercise 3 - Concept Application Problems CAP

1. (d) When S_1 is closed and S_2 is opened, the capacitor will get charged to a potential difference of V volts.
2. (b) Charge on each plate of each capacitor

$$Q = \pm CV = \pm 25 \times 10^6 \times 200 = \pm 5 \times 10^{-3} C$$

3. (c) C = 10 μF ; d = 8 cm

C' = ? ; d' = 4 cm

$$C = \frac{A \in_0}{d} \Rightarrow C \alpha \frac{1}{d}$$

If d is halved then C will be doubled.

Hence C' = 2C = 2 × 10 μF = 20 μF

4. (b) It consists of two capacitors in parallel, therefore, the total capacitance is = $\dfrac{2 \in_0 A}{d}$

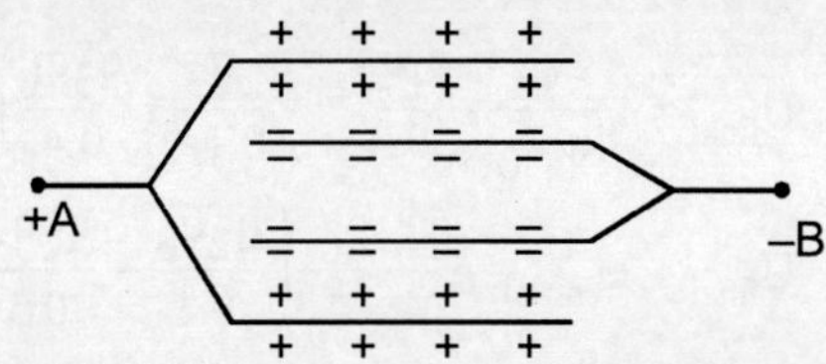

(The plates of B, having negative charge do not constitute a capacitor).

5. (c) All the charge given to inner sphere will pass on to the outer one. So capacitance that of outer one is $4\pi \in_0 b$.

6. (c) $V_0 = \frac{q}{C_0}$

$V = \frac{q}{C} \Rightarrow \frac{V}{V_0} = \frac{C_0}{C} \Rightarrow \frac{C_0}{C} = \frac{500}{75} = \frac{20}{3}$

By definition, $C = kC_0 \Rightarrow k = \frac{20}{3}$

7. (b) In steady state, both the capacitors are at the same potential,

i.e., $\frac{Q_1}{C_1} = \frac{Q_2}{C_2}$ or $\frac{Q_1}{C} = \frac{Q_2}{2C}$ or $Q_2 = 2Q_1$

Also $Q_1 + Q_2 = Q$

$\therefore Q_1 = \frac{Q}{3}, Q_2 = \frac{2Q}{3}$

8. (d) Potential at origin

$= (V_1 + V_3 + V_5 + ...) - (V_2 + V_4 + V_6 + ...)$

$\Rightarrow \frac{q}{4\pi\varepsilon_0}\left[\frac{1}{x_0} - \frac{1}{2x_0} + \frac{1}{3x_0} ..... \infty\right]$

$\Rightarrow \frac{q}{4\pi\varepsilon_0 x_0}\left[1 - \frac{1}{2} + \frac{1}{3} - \frac{1}{4} ..... \infty\right]$

$\Rightarrow \frac{q}{4\pi\varepsilon_0 x_0}\log_e(1+1) \Rightarrow \frac{q}{4\pi\varepsilon_0 x_0}\log_e 2$

9. (b) Energy stored,

$U = \frac{1}{2}C_{aq}V^2_{net} = \frac{1}{2}(3C)V^2 = \frac{3}{2}CV^2$

10. (a)

Situation 1 :

$V_1 - V_2 = V = K\frac{Q}{r_1} - K\frac{Q}{r_2} = KQ\left[\frac{1}{r_1} - \frac{1}{r_2}\right]$

Situation 2 :

$V'_1 - V'_2 = V' = \left[\frac{KQ}{r_1} - \frac{3KQ}{r_2}\right] - \left[\frac{KQ}{r_2} - \frac{3KQ}{r_2}\right]$

$= KQ\left[\frac{1}{r_1} - \frac{1}{r_2}\right] = V$

11. (c) When steady state is reached, the current I coming from the battery is given by

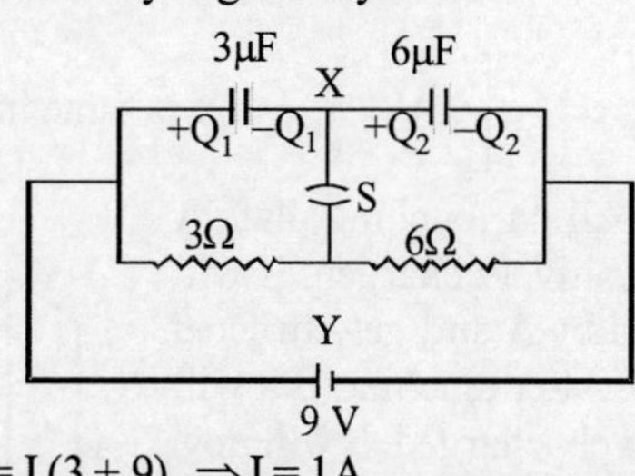

$9 = I(3+9) \Rightarrow I = 1A$

$\Rightarrow$ potential difference across 3 Ω resistance = 3V and potential difference across 6 Ω resistance = 6V

$\Rightarrow$ p.d. across 3 μF capacitor = 3V and p.d. across 6μF capacitor = 6V

$\therefore$ Charge on 3 μF capacitor, $Q_1 = 3 \times 3 = 9\ \mu C$

Charge on 6μF capacitor, $Q_2 = 6 \times 6 = 36\ \mu C$

$\Rightarrow$ Charge $(-Q_1)$ is shifted from the positive plate of 6μF capacitor. The remaining charge on the positive plate of 6 μF capacitor is shifted through the switch.

$\therefore$ Charge passing through the switch

$= 36 - 9 = 27\ \mu C$

12. (a) As $x = t\left(1 - \frac{1}{K}\right)$, where x is the addition distance of plate, to restore the capacity of original value.

$\therefore\ 3.5 \times 10^{-5} = 4 \times 10^{-5}\left(1 - \frac{1}{K}\right)$.

Solving, we get, K = 8.

13. (d)

14. (a) $C_a = \frac{\in_0 A}{d}$ and $C_b = \frac{\in_0 A}{\frac{d}{2} + \frac{d}{2K}} = \frac{2\in_0 A(1+K)}{d}$

and $C_c = \frac{\in_0 \frac{A}{2}}{d} + \frac{\in_0 \frac{A}{2}K}{d} = \frac{\in_0 A}{2d}(1+K)$

or $C_b = \frac{\in_0 A}{d}2(1+K) > C_a$

or $C_c = \frac{\in_0 A}{d}\frac{1+K}{2} > C_a$ $\quad \therefore C_b$ and $C_c > C_a$.

15. (d) Charge given to a hollow conductor resides only on the outer surface.

16. (b) $C = C_1 + KC_2 = \frac{(\ell - x)b \in_0}{d} + \frac{Kxb \in_0}{d}$

$= \frac{b \in_0}{d}[\ell - x + Kx]$

$C = \frac{b \in_0}{d}[\ell + x(K-1)]$

$V = \frac{q}{C} = \frac{qd}{b \in_0 [\ell + x(K-1)]}$

as x decreases, V increases.

17. (c) Since, potential difference across C_2 is greater than C_1.

$$\Rightarrow C_1 > C_2 \left[\because V = \frac{q}{C} \text{ and q is same in series}\right]$$

18. (c) The ball on touching plate A will get positively charged. It will be repelled by A and get attracted towards B. After touching B it will get negatively charged. It will now be repelled by B and get attracted towards A. Thus it will remain oscillating and at the extreme position touch the plates.

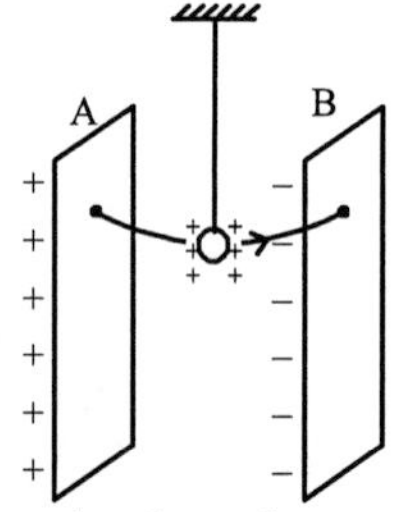

19. (a) Since battery is still in connection, so, $V = V_0$

$\Rightarrow Q_0 = C_0V_0$ and $Q = kC_0V_0$

$\Rightarrow Q = kQ_0$

Since, $k > 1$

$\Rightarrow Q > Q_0$

Also, $U_0 = \frac{1}{2}Q_0V_0$ and

$U = \frac{1}{2}QV = kU_0 \quad \{\therefore Q = kQ_0 \text{ and } V = V_0\}$

Hence, $U > U_0$

20. (b)

21. (a) $V = V_1 + V_2 + V_3 = \frac{1}{4\pi \epsilon_0}.\frac{Q}{R} + \frac{1}{4\pi \epsilon_0}\left(\frac{-2Q}{R}\right)$

$$+\frac{1}{4\pi \epsilon_0}\left(\frac{3Q}{R}\right) = \frac{1}{4\pi \epsilon_0}\left(\frac{2Q}{R}\right)$$

22. (a) The electrostatic pressure at a point on the surface of a uniformly charged sphere $= \frac{\sigma^2}{2\epsilon_0}$

$\therefore$ The force on a hemispherical shell $= \frac{\sigma^2}{2\epsilon_0} \times \pi R^2$

23. (c) The given circuit can be redrawn as follows

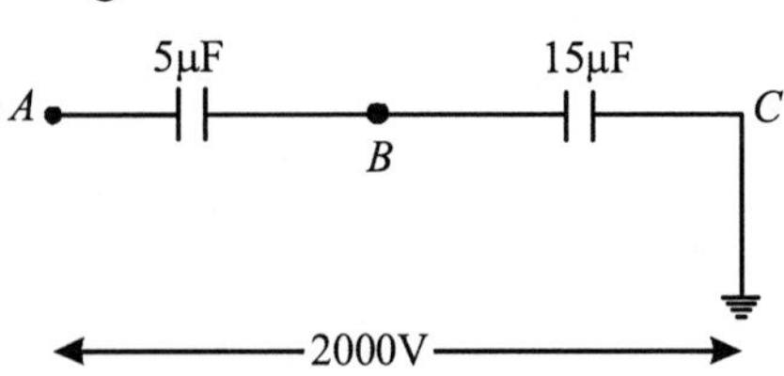

$$(V_A - V_B) = \left(\frac{15}{5+15}\right) \times 2000 \Rightarrow V_A - V_B = 1500V$$

$\Rightarrow 2000 - V_B = 1500V \Rightarrow V_B = 500V$

24. (c) We know that potential energy of discrete system of charges is given by

$$U = \frac{1}{4\pi \epsilon_0}\left(\frac{q_1q_2}{r_{12}} + \frac{q_2q_3}{r_{23}} + \frac{q_3q_1}{r_{31}}\right)$$

According to question,

$$U_{initial} = \frac{1}{4\pi \epsilon_0}\left(\frac{q_1q_2}{0.3} + \frac{q_2q_3}{0.5} + \frac{q_3q_1}{0.4}\right)$$

$$U_{final} = \frac{1}{4\pi \epsilon_0}\left(\frac{q_1q_2}{0.3} + \frac{q_2q_3}{0.1} + \frac{q_3q_1}{0.4}\right)$$

$$U_{final} - U_{initial} = \frac{1}{4\pi \epsilon_0}\left(\frac{q_2q_3}{0.1} - \frac{q_2q_3}{0.5}\right)$$

$$= \frac{1}{4\pi \epsilon_0}\left[10q_2q_3 - 2q_2q_3\right] = \frac{q_3}{4\pi \epsilon_0}(8q_2)$$

25. (b)

26. (d) In series, $C_{eff} = \frac{C_1}{n_1}$

$\therefore$ Energy stored,

$$E_S = \frac{1}{2}C_{eff}V_S^2 = \frac{1}{2}\frac{C_1}{n_1}16V^2 = 8V^2\frac{C_1}{n_1}$$

In parallel, $C_{eff} = n_2C_2$

$\therefore$ Energy stored, $E_p = \frac{1}{2}n_2C_2V^2$

$$\therefore \frac{8V^2C_1}{n_1} = \frac{1}{2}n_2C_2V^2 \Rightarrow C_2 = \frac{16C_1}{n_1n_2}$$

27. (a) $q = CV_1 \cos wt$

$\Rightarrow i = \frac{dq}{dt} = -\omega C v_1 \sin \omega t$

Also, $\omega^2 = \frac{1}{LC}$ and $V = V_1 \cos \omega t$

At $t = t_1$, $V = V_2$ and $i = -\omega CV_1 \sin \omega t_1$

$\therefore \cos \omega t_1 = \frac{V_2}{V_1}$ (–ve sign gives direction)

Hence, $i = V_1\sqrt{\frac{C}{L}}\left(1 - \frac{V_2^2}{V_1^2}\right)^{1/2} = \left(\frac{C(V_1^2 - V_2^2)}{L}\right)^{1/2}$

28. (c) Potential at the centre, $V_C = \frac{KQ_{net}}{R}$

$\because Q_{net} = 0$

$\therefore V_C = 0$

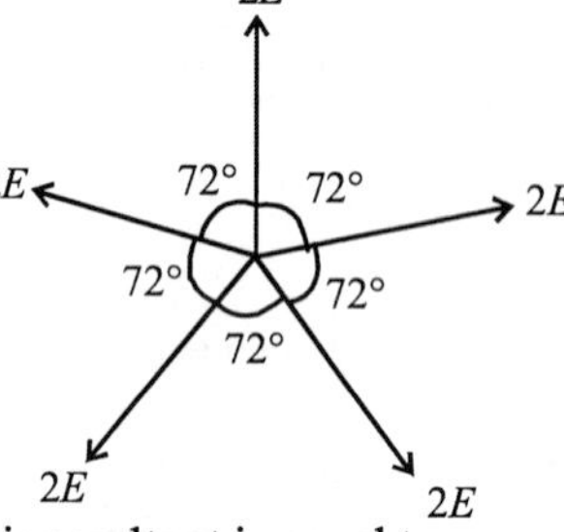

Let E be electric field produced by each charge at the centre, then resultant electric field will be $E_C = 0$, since equal electric field vectors are acting at equal angle so their resultant is equal to zero.

29. (d) Total charge $Q_1 + Q_2 = Q'_1 + Q'_2$

$$= 12\mu C - 3\mu C = 9\mu C$$

Two isolated conducting sphres S_1 and S_2 are now connected by a conducting wire.

$$\therefore V_1 = V_2 = \frac{KQ'_1}{\frac{2}{3}R} = \frac{KQ'_2}{\frac{R}{3}} = 12 - 3 = 9\,\mu C$$

$Q'_1 = 2Q'_2 \Rightarrow 2Q'_2 + Q'_2 = 9\mu C$

$\therefore Q'_1 = 6\mu C$ and $Q'_2 = 3\mu C$

30. (d) Let σ be the surface charge density of the shells.

Charge on the inner shell,

$Q_1 = \sigma 4\pi r^2$

Charge on the outer shell,

$Q_2 = \sigma 4\pi R^2$

∴ Total charge, $Q = \sigma 4\pi (r^2 + R^2)$

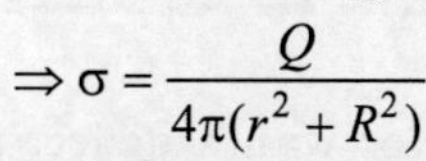

$\Rightarrow \sigma = \dfrac{Q}{4\pi(r^2 + R^2)}$

Potential at the common centre,

$$V_C = \frac{KQ_1}{r} + \frac{KQ_2}{R} \quad \left(\text{where } K = \frac{1}{4\pi\varepsilon_0}\right)$$

$$= \frac{K\sigma 4\pi r^2}{r} + \frac{K\sigma 4\pi R^2}{R} = K\sigma 4\pi (r + R)$$

$$= \frac{KQ 4\pi (r+R)}{4\pi (r^2 + R^2)} = \frac{1}{4\pi\varepsilon_0} \frac{(r+R)Q}{(r^2 + R^2)}$$

31. (c) Potential at any point of the charged ring

$$V_P = \frac{Kq}{\sqrt{R^2 + Z^2}}$$

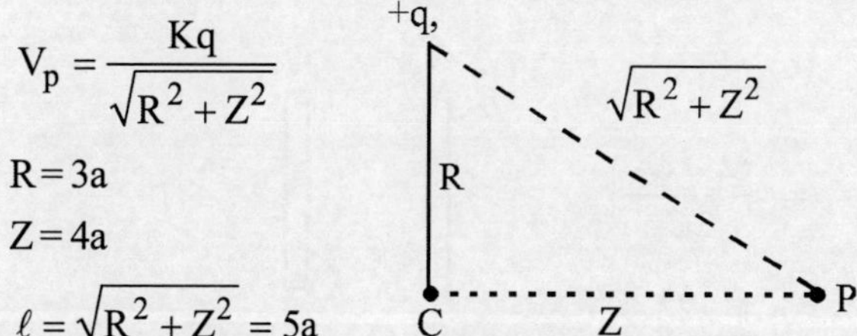

R = 3a

Z = 4a

$\ell = \sqrt{R^2 + Z^2} = 5a$

The minimum velocity (v_0) should just sufficient to reach the point charge at the center, therefore

$$\frac{1}{2} m v_0^2 = q[V_C - V_P] = q\left[\frac{Kq}{3a} - \frac{Kq}{5a}\right]$$

$$v_0^2 = \frac{4Kq^2}{15ma} = \frac{4}{15} \frac{1}{4\pi\varepsilon_0} \frac{q^2}{ma}$$

$$\Rightarrow v_0 = \sqrt{\frac{2}{m}} \left(\frac{2q^2}{15 \times 4\pi\varepsilon_0 a}\right)^{\frac{1}{2}}$$

32. (d) Potential at point P, $V = \dfrac{kQ_a}{a} + \dfrac{kQ_b}{b} + \dfrac{kQ_c}{c}$

Since surface charge densities are equal to one another

i.e., $\sigma_a = \sigma_b = \sigma_c$

$\therefore Q_a : Q_b : Q_c :: a^2 : b^2 : c^2$

$$\therefore Q_a = \left[\frac{a^2}{a^2 + b^2 + c^2}\right] Q$$

$$Q_b = \left[\frac{b^2}{a^2 + b^2 + c^2}\right] Q$$

$$Q_c = \left[\frac{c^2}{a^2 + b^2 + c^2}\right] Q$$

$$\therefore V = \frac{Q}{4\pi \in_0} \left[\frac{(a+b+c)}{a^2 + b^2 + c^2}\right]$$

33. (d) Let at a distance 'x' from point B, both the dipoles produce same potential

$$\therefore \frac{4qa}{(R+x)} = \frac{2qa}{(x^2)}$$

$$\Rightarrow \sqrt{2}x = R + x \Rightarrow x = \frac{R}{\sqrt{2} - 1}$$

Therefore distance from A at which both of them produce the same potential

$$= \frac{R}{\sqrt{2} - 1} + R = \frac{\sqrt{2}R}{\sqrt{2} - 1}$$

34. (d) By using energy conservation,

$$\Delta KE + (\Delta PE)_{\text{Electro}} + (\Delta PE)_{\text{gravitational}} = 0$$

$$\frac{1}{2} m V^2 + \left(k\frac{Qq}{R+y} - k\frac{Qq}{R}\right) + (-mgy) = 0$$

$$\Rightarrow \frac{1}{2} m V^2 = mgy + kQq\left(\frac{1}{R} - \frac{1}{R+y}\right)$$

$$\Rightarrow V^2 = 2gy + \frac{2kQq}{m} \frac{y}{R(R+y)}$$

$$\text{or, } V^2 = 2y\left[\frac{qQ}{4\pi\varepsilon_0 R(R+y)m} + g\right]$$

35. (b) Using, $[K + U]_i = [K + U]_f$

or $0 + Vq = mv^2 + v'q$

or $mv^2 = (V - V')q$

$$= -q\int_{r_0}^{r} E dr = q\int_{r_0}^{r} \frac{\lambda}{2\pi \in_0 r} dr = \frac{\lambda q}{2\pi \in_0}\left(\frac{\ln^3}{r_0}\right)$$

$$\Rightarrow v \propto \sqrt{ln\frac{r}{r_0}}$$

36. (b)

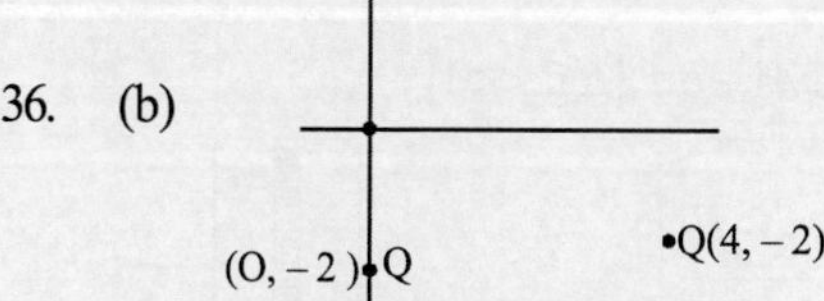

Potential at origin

$$v = \frac{KQ}{2} + \frac{KQ}{2} + \frac{KQ}{\sqrt{20}} + \frac{KQ}{\sqrt{20}}$$

and potential at $\infty = 0 = KQ\left(1 + \dfrac{1}{\sqrt{5}}\right)$

∴ Work required to put a fifth charge Q at origin W = VQ

$$= \frac{Q^2}{4\pi\varepsilon_0}\left(1 + \frac{1}{\sqrt{5}}\right)$$

37. (b) When capacitors *C* and 2*C* capacitance are charged to V and 2V respectively.

$Q_1 = CV \quad Q_2 = 2C \times 2V = 4CV$

When connected in parallel
By conservation of charge

$$4CV - CV = (C + 2C)V_{common}$$

$$V_{common} = \frac{3CV}{3C} = V$$

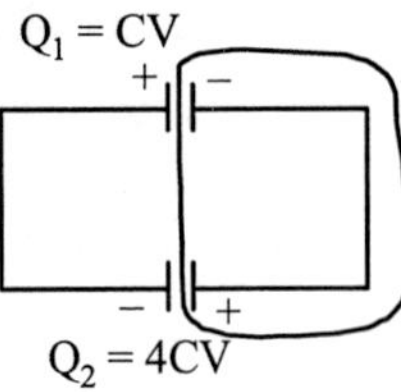

Therefore final energy of this configuration,

$$U_f = \left(\frac{1}{2}CV^2 + \frac{1}{2} \times 2CV^2\right) = \frac{3}{2}CV^2$$

38. (c) In parallel combination, $C_{eq} = C_1 + C_2 = 10\ \mu F$
When connected across $1\ V$ battery, then

$$\frac{U_1}{U_2} = \frac{\left(\frac{1}{2}C_1V^2\right)}{\left(\frac{1}{2}C_2V^2\right)} = \frac{1}{4} \Rightarrow \frac{C_1}{C_2} = \frac{1}{4}$$

$\therefore C_2 = 8\ \mu F$ and $C_1 = 2\ \mu F$
Now C_1 and C_2 are connected in series combination,

$$\therefore C_{equivalent} = \frac{C_1C_2}{C_1 + C_2} = \frac{2 \times 8}{2 + 8} = \frac{16}{10} = 1.6\mu F$$

39. (a)

40. (a) Given, $K(x) = K(1 + \alpha x)$

Capacitance of element, $C_{el} = \frac{K\varepsilon_0 A}{dx}$

$$\Rightarrow C_{el} = \frac{\varepsilon_0 K(1 + \alpha x)A}{dx}$$

$$\therefore \int d\left(\frac{1}{C}\right) = \frac{1}{C_{el}} = \int_0^d \left(\frac{dx}{\varepsilon_0 KA(1 + \alpha x)}\right)$$

$$\Rightarrow \frac{1}{C} = \frac{1}{\varepsilon_0 KA\alpha}[ln(1 + \alpha x)]_0^d$$

$$\Rightarrow \frac{1}{C} = \frac{1}{\varepsilon_0 KA\alpha} ln(1 + \alpha d)[\alpha d << 1]$$

$$= \frac{1}{\varepsilon_0 KA\alpha}\left[\alpha d - \frac{\alpha^2 d^2}{2}\right]$$

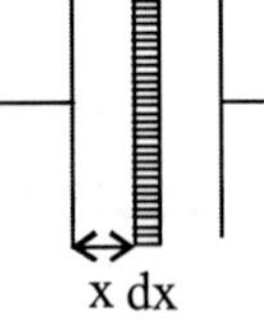

$$= \frac{1}{\varepsilon_0 KA}\left[1 - \frac{\alpha d}{2}\right]$$

$$\therefore C = \frac{\varepsilon_0 KA}{d\left(1 - \frac{\alpha d}{2}\right)} \Rightarrow C = \frac{\varepsilon_0 KA}{d}\left(1 + \frac{\alpha d}{2}\right)$$

41. (a) A, B, C and D are equipotential points (see fig.)

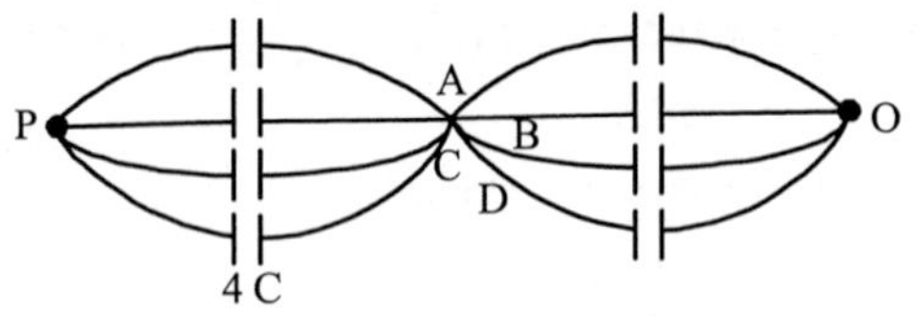

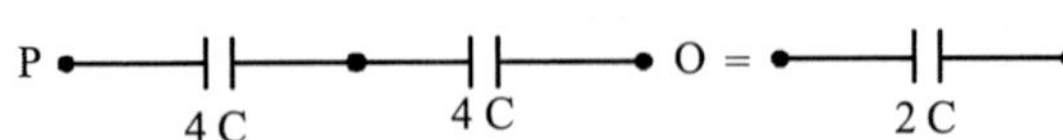

42. (b) Capacitance of a capacitor with a dielectric of dielectric constant k is given by

$$C = \frac{k \in_0 A}{d}$$

$$\because E = \frac{V}{d} \qquad \therefore C = \frac{k \in_0 AE}{V}$$

$$15 \times 10^{-12} = \frac{k \times 8.86 \times 10^{-12} \times 10^{-4} \times 10^6}{500}$$

$k = 8.5$

43. (b) $V = \frac{Q}{C}$

$$= \left(\frac{Q_1 - Q_2}{2C}\right)$$

$$= \left(\frac{4 - 2}{2 \times 1}\right) = 1\ V$$

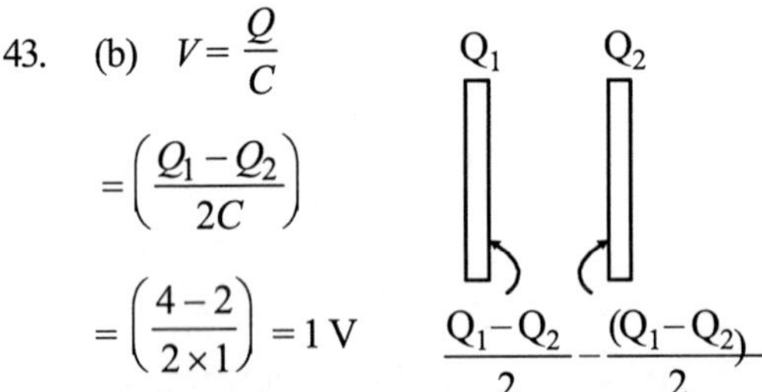

44. (b) Energy stored in the system initially

$$U_i = \frac{1}{2}CE^2$$

$$U_f = \frac{1}{2}\frac{Q^2}{C_{eq}} = \frac{(CE)^2}{2 \times 4C} = \frac{1}{2}\frac{CE^2}{4}$$

[As $Q = CE$, and $C_{eq} = 4C$]

$$\Delta U = \frac{1}{2}CE^2 \times \frac{3}{4} = \frac{3}{8}CE^2 = \frac{3}{8}\frac{Q^2}{C}$$

45. (a) For series combination

$$\frac{1}{C_{eq}} = \frac{1}{C_1} + \frac{1}{C_2}$$

$$\Rightarrow \frac{\frac{7C}{3}}{\frac{7}{3} + C} = \frac{1}{2}$$

$\Rightarrow 14C = 7 + 3C$

$\Rightarrow C = \frac{7}{11}\mu F$

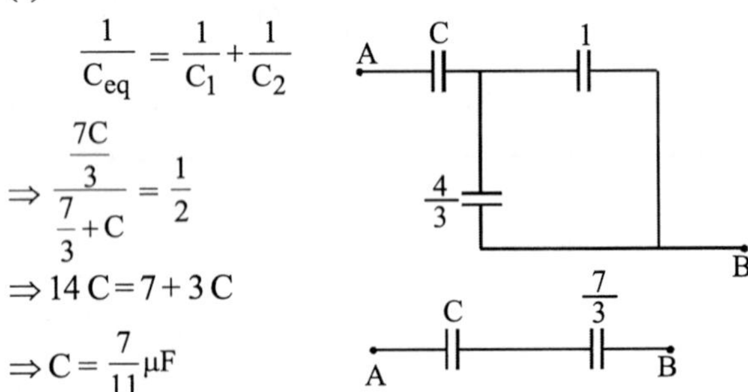

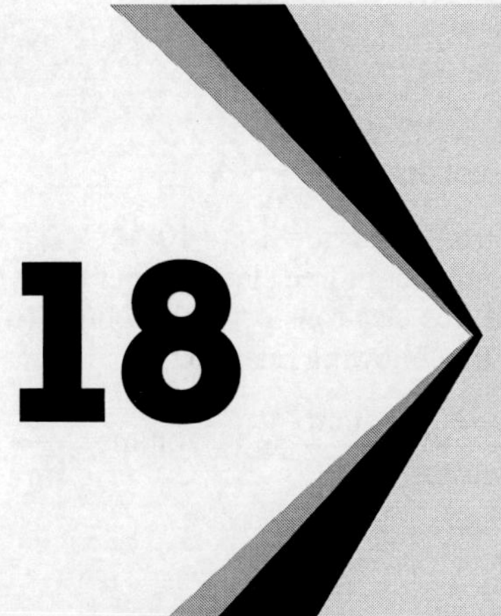

18 Current Electricity

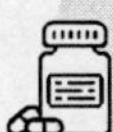

Topic 18.1 : Electric Current, Current Density, Drift Velocity, Ohm's Law & Electrical Resistance, Series & Parallel Combination of Resistors and Colour Coding for Carbon Resistor

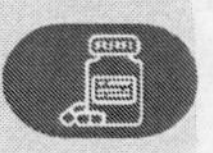

ELECTRIC CURRENT

It is the rate of flow of charge through any cross section.

i.e. $I = \frac{dq}{dt}$

Conventionally, the direction of flow of positive charge is taken as the direction of electric current. It is a scalar quantity and its **S.I. unit** is ampere (A).

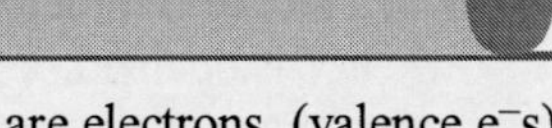

Problem Solving Tips

(i) Current carriers in conductor are electrons, (valence e^-s) ions in electrolytes, electrons & holes in semiconductor and positive ions /electrons in gases.

(ii) Charge of electron = 1.6×10^{-19}c

(iii) 1 ampere = 6.25×10^{18} electrons/sec

(iv) Though direction is associated with current (opposite to the motion of electrons), but it is not a vector quantity as it does not follow rules of vector addition.

(v) For a current to flow through a cross-section, there must be a net flow of charge through that cross-section.
In a metal like copper there are around 10^{28} free electrons per m^3 moving randomly in all direction with speeds of the order of 10^6 m/s even in the absence of electric field. But since the number of electrons passing through a cross-section from left to right is equal to the number of electrons passing from right to left in a given time, therefore the net charge flow is zero and hence the electric current is zero.

(vi) A conductor remains uncharged when current flows in it. i.e. Net charge in a current carrying conductor is zero.

CURRENT DENSITY

Current density at a point inside a conductor is defined as the amount of current flowing per unit cross sectional area around that point of the conductor, provided the area is held in a direction normal to the direction of current.

i.e. *Current density*, $J = \frac{I}{A}$

If area is not normal to current, then area normal to current is A' = A cos θ (see the figure)

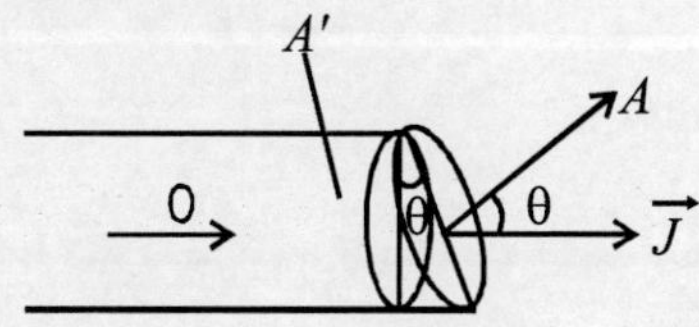

$$J = \frac{I}{A\cos\theta} \text{ or } I = JA\cos\theta \text{ or } I = \vec{J}.\vec{A} = \int \vec{J}.\vec{A}$$

Its **SI unit** is Am^{-2}

Current density can also be related to electric field as

$$\vec{j} = \sigma\vec{E} = \frac{\vec{E}}{\rho}$$

where σ is conductivity of the substance & ρ is specific resistance of the substance.

J is a vector quantity and its direction is same as that of $\vec{E}$. **Dimensions** of J are $[M^{\circ}L^{-2}T^{\circ}A]$

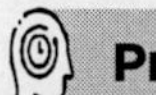

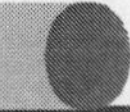

Problem Solving Tips

(i) Electric current is a macroscopic physical quantity where as current density is a microscopic physical quantity.

(ii) For a given conductor current does not change with change in cross-sectional area.

DRIFT VELOCITY $(\vec{V_d})$

When the ends of a conductor are connected to the two terminals of a battery, an electric field is set up in the conductor from the positive terminal to the negative terminal. The free electrons in the conductor experiences a force opposite to the direction of the electric field and hence get accelerated. However this process of acceleration is soon interrupted by collision with ions of solid. The average time for which each electron is accelerated before suffering a collision is called the **mean free time** or **mean relaxation time.**

Thus, the free electrons within the metal, in addition to its random motion acquire a small velocity towards the positive end of conductor. This velocity is called **drift velocity.** It is given by

$$\vec{v}_d = -\frac{e\vec{E}\tau}{m},$$

where e is the charge and m is the mass of electron.

$\vec{E}$ is the electric field established in conductor and τ is the average relaxation time.

Negative sign is because the directions of $\vec{E}$ and $\vec{v}_d$ (for electron) are opposite.

$$E = \frac{V}{l}$$

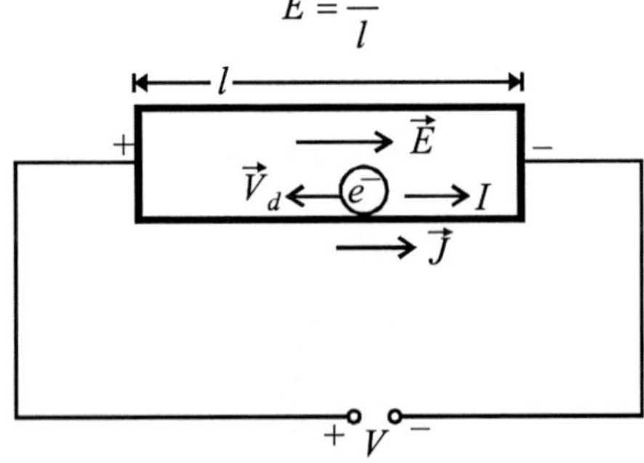

where V is the potential difference across ends of the conductor of length ℓ. The uniform current I, flowing through the conductor is given by

$$I = neAv_d$$

where n = number of free electrons per unit volume, A = area of cross-section, v_d = drift velocity

In vector form, $\Rightarrow \vec{J} = -ne\vec{v}_d$

The negative sign is because the direction of drift velocity of electron is opposite to $\vec{J}$.

Mobility - *Drift velocity per unit electric field is called mobility.* It is denoted by μ.

$$\mu = \frac{\vec{V}_d}{E}$$

Its **S.I. unit** is m^2/volt-sec.

Problem Solving Tips

1. Drift velocity is very small, it is of the order of 10^{-4}m/s which is negligible as compared to thermal speed of e^-s at room temperature ($\simeq 10^5$ m/s)
2. The drift velocity is given by

$$v_d = \frac{J}{ne},$$

where, J = current density $= \frac{I}{A}$

e = electronic charge = 1.6×10^{-19} C

n = the number of free electrons per unit volume

3. The number of free electrons per unit volume (n) can be determined by the following relation :

$$n = \frac{\text{No. of free } e^- \text{ per atom}}{\text{Volume}} \quad \text{and} \quad \text{volume} = \frac{M}{N_0 d}.$$

$$n = \frac{N_0 d}{M} \times x,$$

where N_0 = Avogadro number

d = density of the metal

M = molecular weight

and x = number of free electrons per atom

3. For steady current :

$$J = \frac{I}{A};\ E = \frac{I}{\sigma A};\ V_d = \frac{I}{neA}$$

This means that for a given material and steady current in case of non-uniform cross-section of material

$$J \propto \frac{1}{A};\ E \propto \frac{1}{A};\ V_d \propto \frac{1}{A}$$

4. Variation of drift velocity :

$$V_d = \frac{E}{ne} = \frac{1}{ne}\frac{V}{l};\ V_d \propto E$$

when length is doubled, v_d becomes half and when V is doubled, v_d becomes twice.

Example 1.

The current in a wire varies with time according to the relation $i = 4 + 2t^2$

How many coulomb of charge pass a cross-section of wire in time interval t = 5s to t = 10s?

Solution :

$$i = \frac{dq}{dt} \Rightarrow dq = i\,dt \Rightarrow dq = (4 + 2t^2)\,dt$$

$$\text{On integrating } q = \int_5^{10} (14 + 2t^2)dt = \left[14t + 2\frac{t^3}{3}\right]_5^{10}$$

$$= 603.33 \text{ C}$$

Example 2.

The current density at a point is $\vec{J} = \left(2 \times 10^4 \frac{A}{m^2}\right)\hat{j}$. *Find the rate of charge flow through a cross-sectional area* $\vec{S}$ *such that*

(i) $\vec{S} = (2cm^2)\hat{j}$,

(ii) $\vec{S} = (4cm^2)\hat{i}$ and (iii) $\vec{S} = (2\hat{i} + 3\hat{j}\,cm^2)$

Solution :

The rate of charge flow = current

$$i = \vec{J}d\vec{S}$$

(i) Current $i = (2 \times 10^4 A/m^2)\hat{j}.(2 \times 10^{-4} m^2)\hat{j} = 2A$

[using $\hat{j}.\hat{j} = 1$]

(ii) Current $i = (2 \times 10^4 A/m^2)\hat{j}.(4 cm^2)\hat{i} = 0$

[using $\hat{j}.\hat{i} = 0$]

(iii) Current $i = (2 \times 10^4 A/m^2)\hat{j}.(2\hat{i} + 3\hat{j}) \times 10^{-4} m^2 = 6A$

OHM'S LAW AND ELECTRICAL RESISTANCE

When a potential difference is applied across the ends of a conductor, a current I is set up in the conductor.

According to ***Ohm's law*** *"Keeping the given physical conditions such as temperature, mechanical strain etc. constant, the current (I) produced in the conductor is directly proportional to the potential difference (V) applied across the conductor".*

i.e., $I \propto V$ or $I = KV$ ... (1)

where K is a constant of proportionality called the **conductance** of the given conductor.

Alternatively, $V \propto I$ or $V = RI$ ... (2)

where the constant **R is called the electrical resistance** or **simply resistance** of the given conductor.

From above two eqs. it is clear that $R = 1/K$.

If a substance follows Ohm's law, then a linear relationship exists between V & I as shown by figure 1. These substance are called **Ohmic substance.** Some substances do not follow Ohm's law, these are called **non-ohmic substance** (shown by figure 2)

Diode valve, triode valve and electrolytes, thermistors are some examples of non-ohmic conductors.

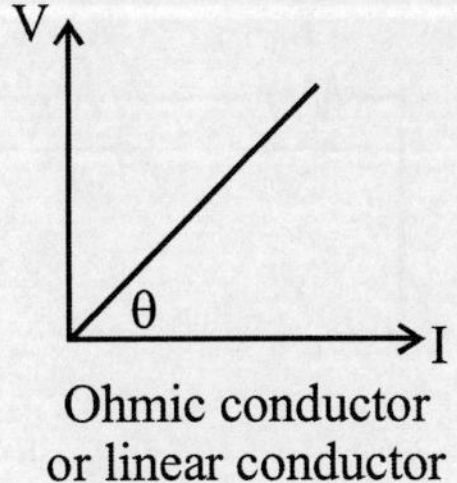

Ohmic conductor or linear conductor
Fig. 1

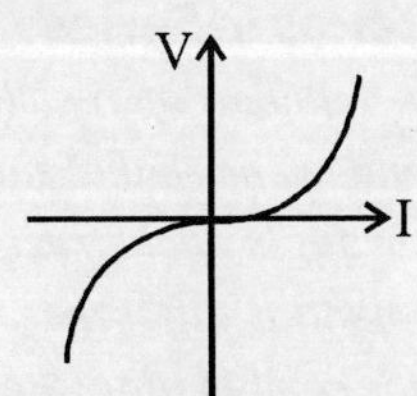

Non-linear conductor or non-ohmic conductor
Fig. 2

Slope of V-I Curve of a conductor provides the resistance of the conductor

$$\text{slope} = \tan\theta = \frac{V}{I}$$

The **SI unit** of resistance R is volt/ampere = ohm (Ω)

Electrical Resistance

On application of potential difference across the ends of a conductor, the free e^-s of the conductor starts drifting towards the positive end of the conductor. While drifting they make collisions with the ions/atoms of the conductor & hence their motion is obstructed. *The net hindrance offered by a conductor to the flow of free e^-s or simply current is called electrical resistance.*

It depends upon the **size, geometry, temperature** and **nature** of the conductor.

Resistivity : For a given conductor of uniform cross-section A and length ℓ, the electrical resistance R is directly proportional to length ℓ and inversely proportional to cross-sectional area A

i.e., $R \propto \frac{\ell}{A}$ or $R = \frac{\rho\ell}{A}$ or $\rho = \frac{RA}{\ell}$

ρ is called **specific resistance** or **electrical resistivity.**

Also, $\rho = \frac{m}{ne^2\tau}$

The **SI unit** of resistivity is ohm - m.

Conductivity(σ) : It is the reciprocal of resistivity i.e. $\sigma = \frac{1}{\rho}$.

The **SI unit** of conductivity is $Ohm^{-1}m^{-1}$ or mho/m.

Ohm's law may also be expressed as, $J = \sigma E$

where J = current density and E = electric field strength

Conductivity, $\sigma = \frac{ne^2\tau}{m}$ where n is free electron density, τ is relaxation time and m is mass of electron.

(i) The value of ρ is very low for conductor, very high for insulators & alloys, and in between those of conductors & insulators for semiconductors.

(ii) Resistance is the property of object while resistivity is the property of material.

Materials and their resistivity

	Material	Resistivity (ρ) (at 0°c) (in Ω m)
(i)	Silver	1.6×10^{-8}
(ii)	Copper	1.7×10^{-8}
(iii)	Aluminium	2.8×10^{-8}
(iv)	Tungsten	5.2×10^{-8}
(v)	Platinum	10.6×10^{-8}
(vi)	Manganin	42×10^{-8}
(vii)	Carbon	35×10^{-6}
(viii)	Germanium	.46
(ix)	Silicon	2300
(x)	Glass	$\sim 10^{13}$
(xi)	Mica	$\sim 2 \times 10^{15}$

MISCONCEPTION

Since $R = \rho\frac{l}{A}$ ⇒ $R \propto l$

It is incorrect to think that if the length of a resistor is doubled its resistance will become twice.

If you look by an eye of physicist you will find that when l change, A will also change. This is discussed in the following article.

Case of Reshaping a Resistor

On reshaping, volume of a material is constant.
i.e., Initial volume = final volume

or, $A_i \ell_i = A_f \ell_f$ ... (i)

where ℓ_i, A_i are initial length and area of cross-section of resistor and ℓ_f, A_f are final length and area of cross-section of resistor. If initial resistance before reshaping is R_i and final resistance after reshaping is R_f then

$$\frac{R_i}{R_f} = \frac{\rho \frac{\ell_i}{A_i}}{\rho \frac{\ell_f}{A_f}} = \frac{\ell_i}{\ell_f} \times \frac{A_f}{A_i} \quad ...(ii)$$

From eqs. (i) and (ii), $\frac{R_i}{R_f} = \left(\frac{l_i}{l_f}\right)^2 \Rightarrow R \propto l^2$

This means that resistance is proportional to the square of the length during reshaping of a resistor wire.

Also from eqs. (i) and (ii), $\frac{R_i}{R_f} = \left(\frac{A_f}{A_i}\right)^2 \Rightarrow R \propto \frac{1}{A^2}$

This means that resistance is inversely proportional to the square of the area of cross-section during reshaping of resistor.
Since $A = \pi r^2$ (for circular cross-section)

$$\therefore R \propto \frac{1}{r^4}$$

where r is radius of cross section.

Effect of Temperature on Resistance and Resistivity

Resistance of a conductor is given by $R_t = R_0 (1 + \alpha \Delta t)$
Where α = temperature coefficient of resistance and Δt = change in temperature

For metallic conductors : If ρ_1 and ρ_2 be resistivity of a conductor at temperature t_1 and t_2, then

$$\rho_2 = \rho_1 (1 + \alpha \Delta T)$$

where α = temperature coefficient of resistivity and

$\Delta T = t_2 - t_1$ = change in temperature

The value of α is positive for all metallic conductors.

$\therefore \quad \rho_2 > \rho_1$

In other words, with rise in temperature, the positive ions of the metal vibrate with higher amplitude and these obstruct the path of electrons more frequently. Due to this the mean path decreases and the relaxation time also decreases. This leads to increase in resistivity.

Please note that the value of α for most of the metals is $\frac{1}{273} K^{-1}$

For alloys : In case of alloys, the rate at which the resistance changes with temperature is less as compared to pure metals. For example, an alloy manganin has a resistance which is 30-40 times that of copper for the same dimensions.
Also the value of α for manganin is very small $\approx 0.00001°C^{-1}$. Due to the above properties manganin is used in preparing wires for standard resistance (heaters), resistance boxes etc.
Please note that eureka and constantan are other alloys for which ρ is high. These are used to detect small temperature, protect picture tube/ windings of generators, transformers etc.

For semiconductors : The resistivity of semi-conductors decreases with rise in temperature. For semi conductor the value of α is negative.

$$\rho = \frac{m}{ne^2 \tau}$$

With rise in temperature, the value of n increases. Please note that τ decreases with rise in temperature. But the value of increase in n is dominating for the value of ρ in this case.

For electrolytes : The resistivity decreases with rise in temperature. This is because the viscosity of electrolyte decreases with increase in temperature so that ions get more freedom to move.

For insulators : The resistivity increases nearly exponentially with decrease in temperature. Conductivity of insulators is almost zero at 0 K.

Superconductors : There are certain materials for which the resistance becomes zero below a certain temperature. This temperature is called the **critical temperature**. Below critical temperature the material offers no resistance to the flow of e^-s. The material in this case is called a **superconductor**. The reason for super conductivity is that the electrons in superconductors are not mutually independent but are mutually coherent. This coherent cloud of e^-s makes no collision with the ions of superconductor and hence no resistance is offered to the flow of e^-s For example, R = 0 for Hg at 4.2 K and R = 0 for Pb at 7.2 K. These substances are called superconductors at that critical temperature.

Superconductors are used *(a) in making very strong electromagnets, (b) to produce very high speed computers (c) in transmission of electric power (d) in the study of high energy particle physics and material science.*

SERIES AND PARALLEL COMBINATION OF RESISTORS

Resistances in Series

When a number of resistances are joined end to end so that same current flows through each, resistor when some potential difference is applied across the combination, the conductor are said to be connected in series.

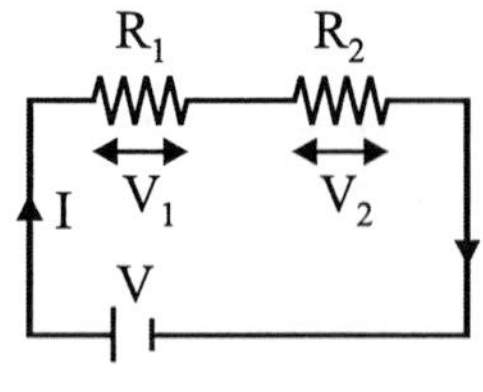

The equivalent resistance in series is given by

$$(R_{eq})_s = R_1 + R_2 + ... + R_n$$

Equivalent resistance of same resistances connected in series is always greater than the greatest of individual resistance.

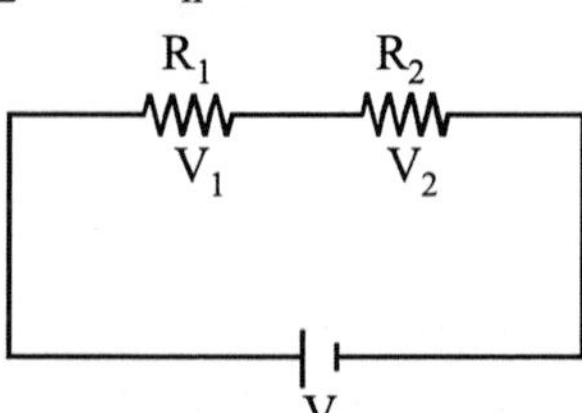

Potential division rule in series combination :

$$V_1 = \frac{VR_1}{R_1 + R_2}; \quad V_2 = \frac{VR_2}{R_1 + R_2}$$

Resistances in Parallel

Two or more resistors are said to be connected in parallel if the same potential difference exits across all resistors.

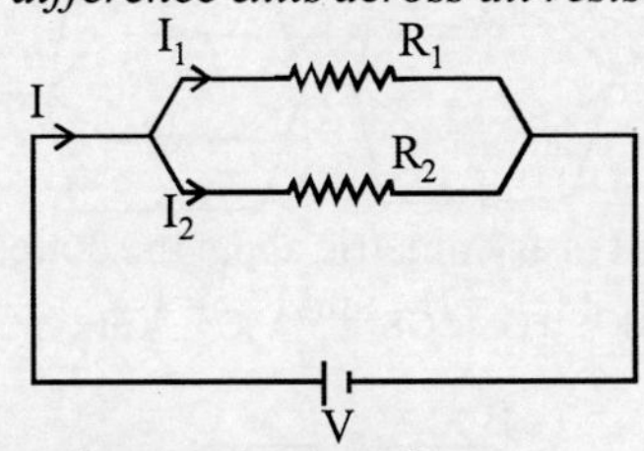

The equivalent resistance is given by

$$\frac{1}{(R_{eq})_p} = \frac{1}{R_1} + \frac{1}{R_2} + ... + \frac{1}{R_n}$$

The equivalent resistance in a parallel combination is always less than the value of the least individual resistance in the circuits.

Current division rule in parallel combination

$$I_1 = \frac{IR_2}{R_1 + R_2} \; ; \; I_2 = \frac{IR_1}{R_1 + R_2}$$

In a given combination of resistors, when you want to detect whether the resistances are in series or in parallel then see that if the same current flows through two resistors then these are in series and if same potential difference is there across two resistors then these are in parallel potential diff across each resistor is the same & is equal to the applied potential difference.

HOW TO FIND EQUIVALENT RESISTANCE ?

Successive Reduction

This method is applicable only when the resistors can be clearly identified as in series or parallel. Let us take some example to find resistance between ends A and B

Ex. (i)

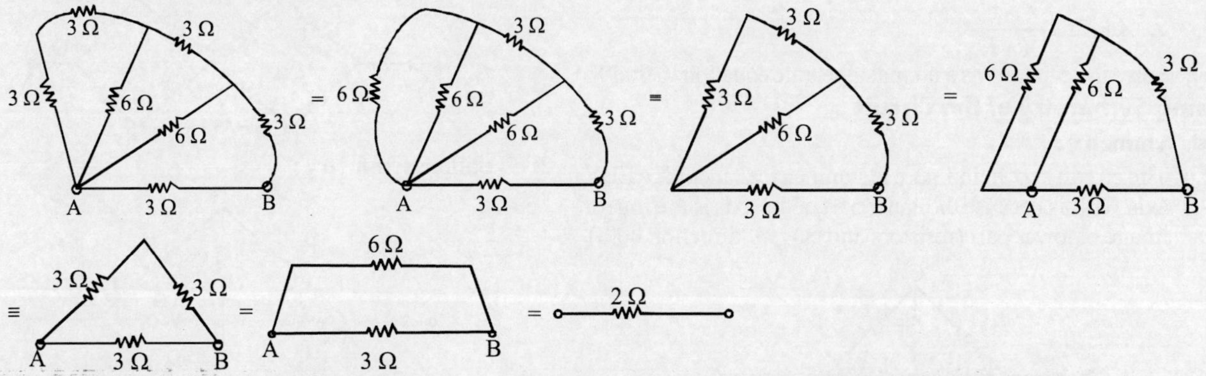

Ex. (ii)

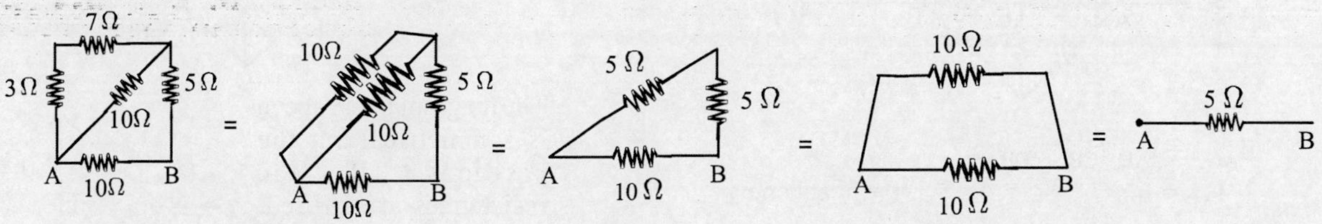

Ex. (iii)

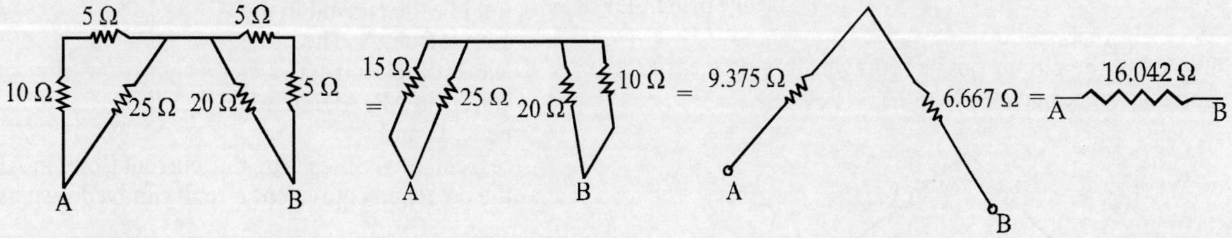

Ex. (iv)

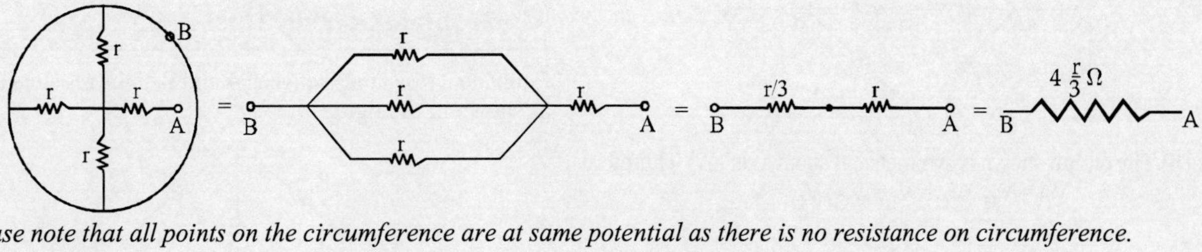

Please note that all points on the circumference are at same potential as there is no resistance on circumference.

Ex. (vi) Infinite series :

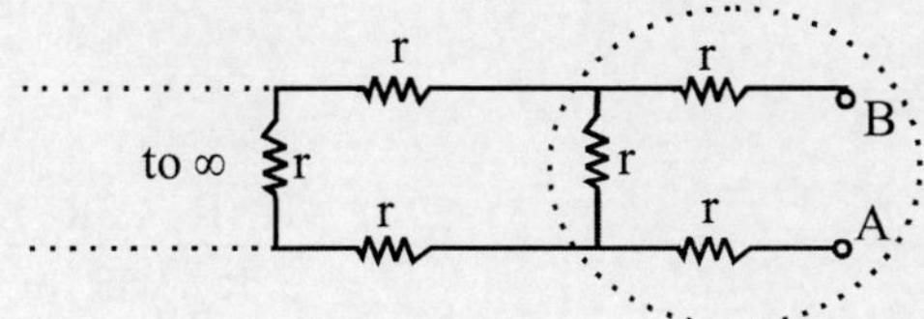

We observe that there is a repetitive unit extending to infinity on left hand side. We assume that the equivalent resistance of all the unit except one (shown dotted) is equal to X ohm. The equivalent circuit will be as shown below.

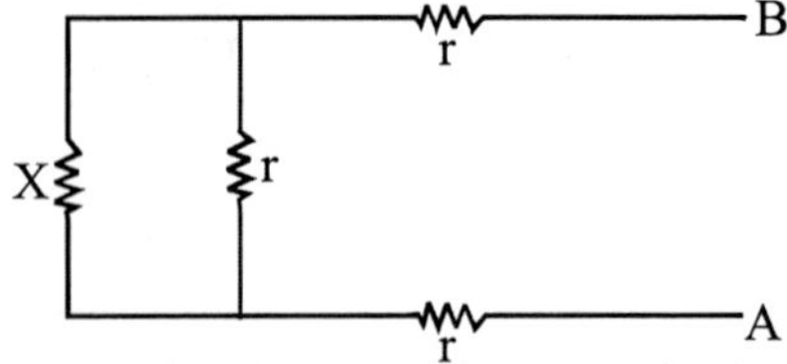

The equivalent resistance across A and B is

$$R_{AB} = r + \frac{X \times r}{X + r} + r$$

Please note that R_{AB} can be taken as X because if you add one unit to the sum of infinite units, then it will be approximately the same.

$$\therefore\ X = 2r + \frac{X \times r}{X + r}$$

Solve the equation as a normal algebraic equation to find X.

Using Symmetry of the Circuit

Axis symmetry :

Ex.(i) The circuit shown in figure is symmetrical about XAEBY axis. This is because the upper part of the axis is the mirror image of lower part (resistors and current direction both)

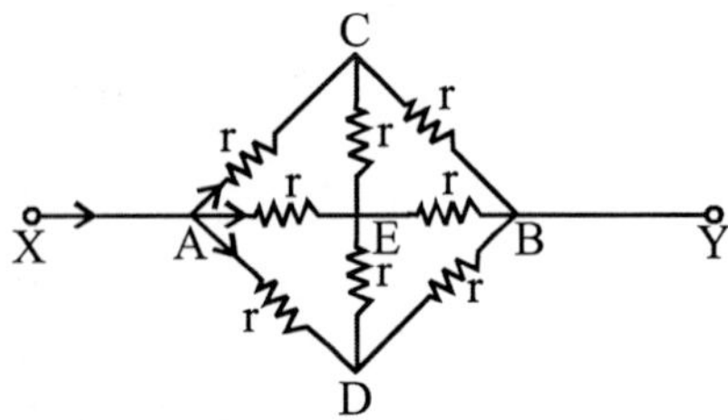

$\therefore\ I_{AC} = I_{AD}; I_{CB} = I_{DB};$

$I_{AE} = I_{EB}$ ($\because$ $V_C = V_E = V_D$ wheatstone bridge principle)

$\Rightarrow\ I_{CE} = I_{ED} = 0$

Therefore the circuit can be redrawn. It is now easier to find resistance between X and Y.

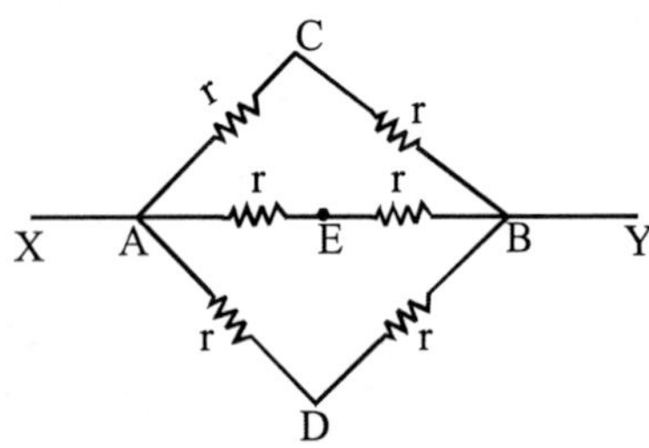

Ex.(ii) The circuit shown is symmetrical about axis XY. Therefore

$$V_B = V_H;\ V_C = V_I = V_G;\ V_D = V_F$$

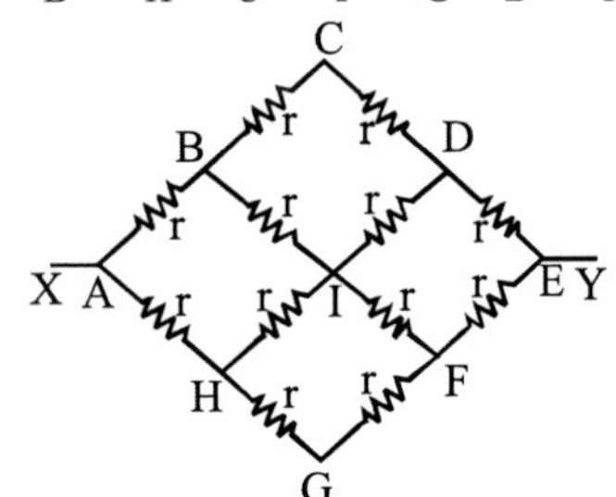

Therefore the circuit can be redrawn as

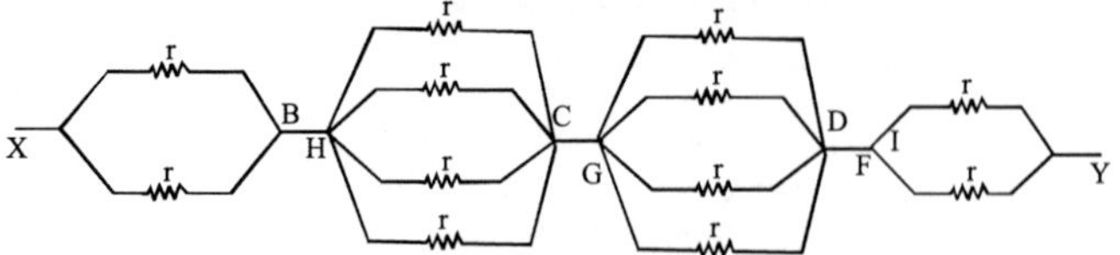

Ex.(iii) The circuit is asymmetric about the dotted line

$\therefore\ I_{BG} = I_{GC};\ I_{FG} = I_{GE}$ and $I_{AG} = I_{GB}$

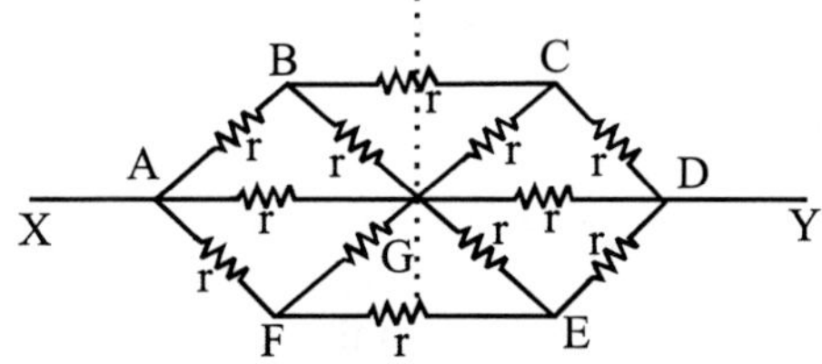

Therefore the equivalent circuit is

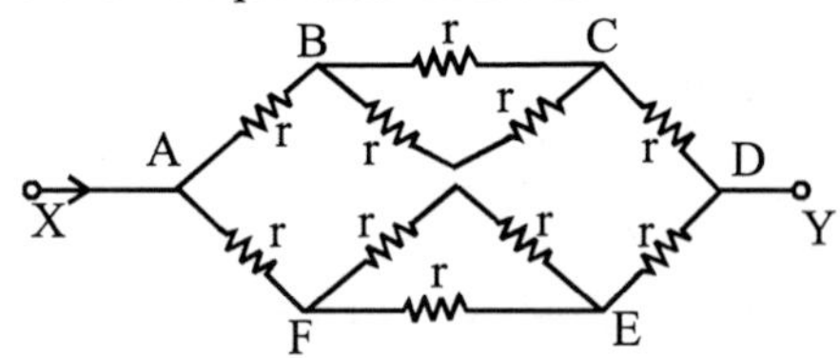

2. Shifted symmetry :

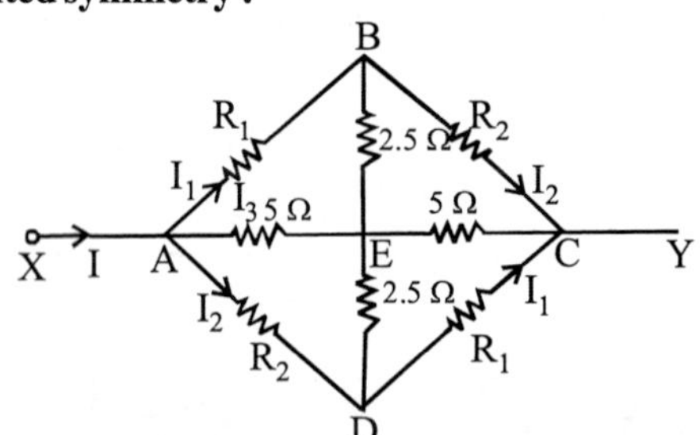

The diagram given above is symmetrical but the positions of the resistances are shifted. Let I be the current in the circuit from A. The same leaves the circuit at C. Let current in AB, AD and AE be I_1, I_2 and I_3 respectively. Since the same current flows in AE and EC, the detached equivalent circuit can be drawn as

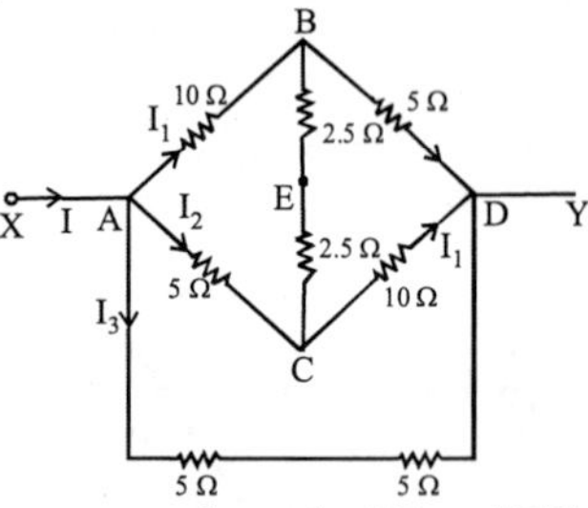

Problem Solving Tips

Equivalent resistance between A and B of the resistors connected as shown in the figure

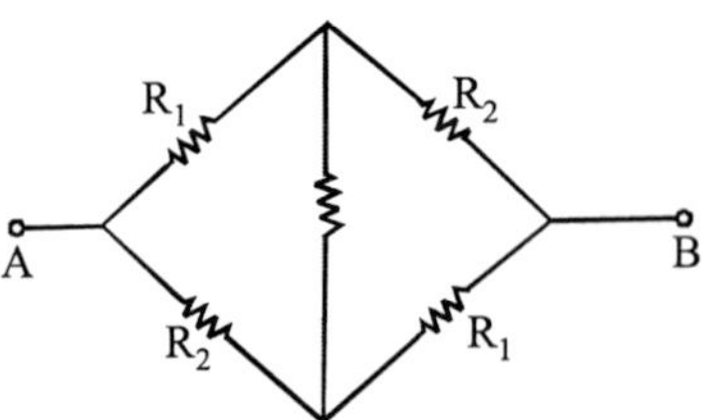

Wheatstone bridge

$$R_{AB} = \frac{R_1(R_1 + 3R_2)}{R_2 + 3R_1}$$

3. Path symmetry :
All paths from one point to another which have the same setting of resistances have the same amount of currents.

Example :

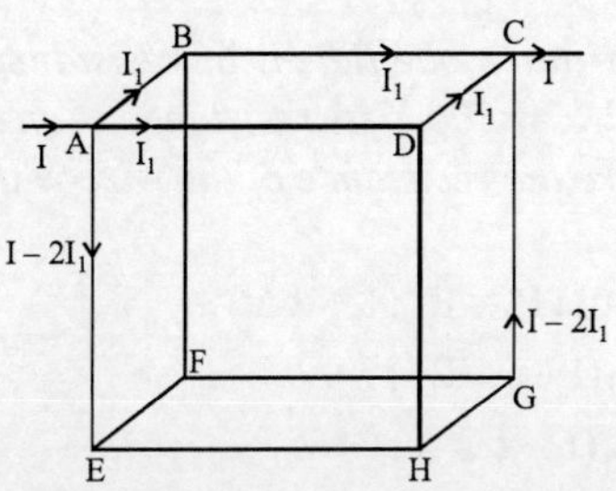

Twelve wires each having resistance r are joined to form a cube. We have to find the equivalent resistance across A and B.

By path symmetry, $I_{AB} = I_{BC} = I_{AD} = I_{DC} = I$

$\therefore \quad I_{AE} = I - 2I_1 \Rightarrow I_{GC} = I - 2I_1,$

Since current in AB = current in BC

$\Rightarrow \quad I_{BF} = 0$

Also $\quad I_{AD} = I_{DC} \Rightarrow I_{DH} = 0$

The equivalent circuit will be as shown. The resistance now clearly visible as in series and in parallel.

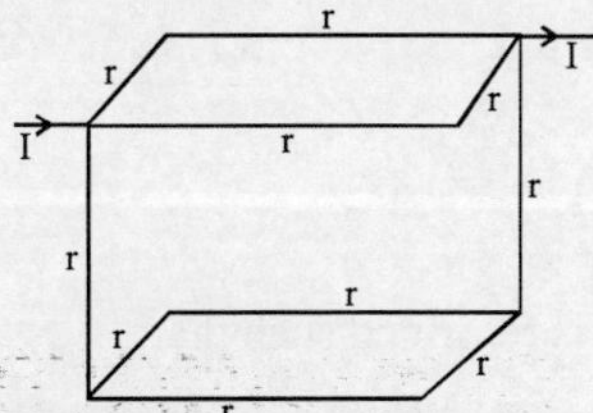

4. Star -delta connection :

$$R_a = \frac{r_1 r_3}{r_1 + r_2 + r_3}; \quad R_b = \frac{r_1 r_2}{r_1 + r_2 + r_3};$$

$$R_c = \frac{r_2 r_3}{r_1 + r_2 + r_3};$$

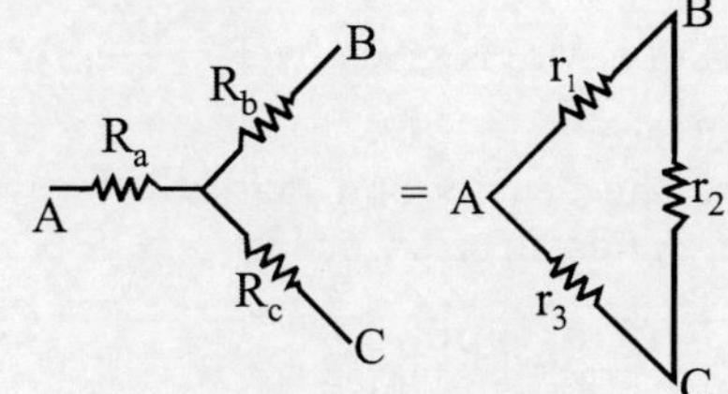

$$r_1 = \frac{R_a R_b + R_b R_c + R_c R_a}{R_c};$$

$$r_2 = \frac{R_a R_b + R_b R_c + R_c R_a}{R_a};$$

$$r_3 = \frac{R_a R_b + R_b R_c + R_c R_a}{R_b};$$

Using delta to star conversion

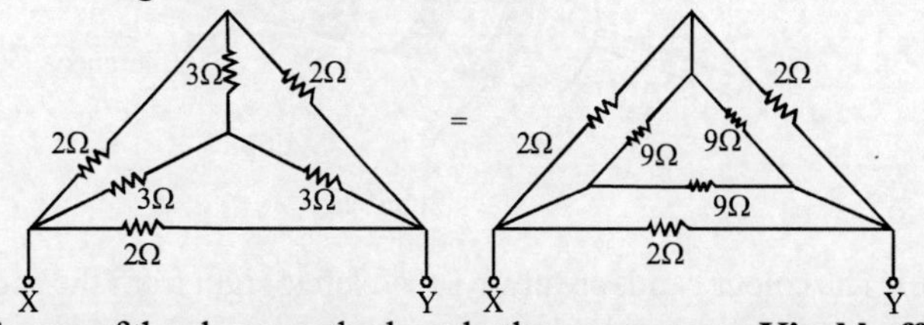

If none of the above method works then we may use **Kirchhoff's method** which will be discussed later

MISCONCEPTIONS

1. Resistors are not just in series or in parallel if they look so geometrically, e.g. the resistors in the diagram are not in parallel but in series.

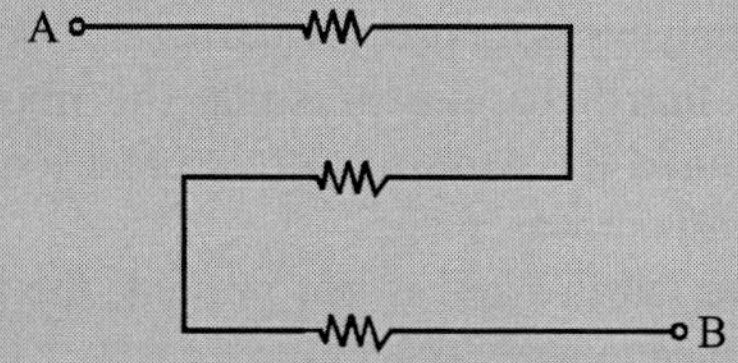

These resistors across A and B are in series, as same current passes through them.

2. This is a common thinking that current which comes out from the positive terminal of a battery is used up till it reaches the negative terminal. But infact the current remains the same in a branch. In fact a potential drop takes place across a resistor.

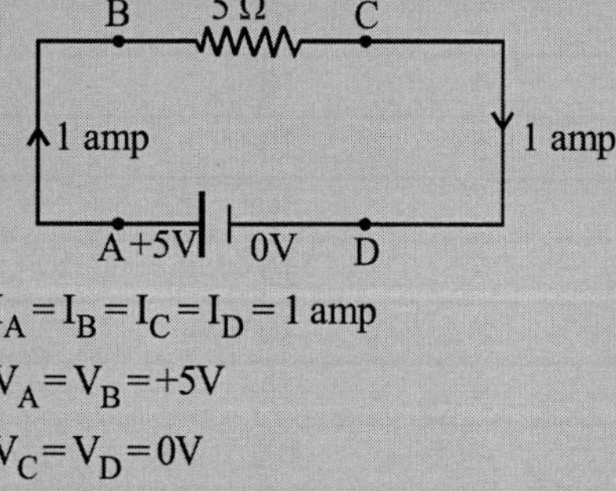

$I_A = I_B = I_C = I_D = 1$ amp

$V_A = V_B = +5V$

$V_C = V_D = 0V$

This means that a potential drop of 5V takes place across the resistor

3. ✗ ***Incorrect :*** If two resistances are not in series then it is in parallel and vice-versa.

✓ ***Correct :*** The above thinking is incorrect. We may have resistances which are neither in series nor in parallel.

COLOUR CODING FOR CARBON RESISTOR AND THEIR STANDARD VALUES

(i) It is a system of colour coding used to indicate the values of resistors.

(ii) For the fixed, moulded composition resistor, four colour bands are printed on one end of the outer casing as shown below.

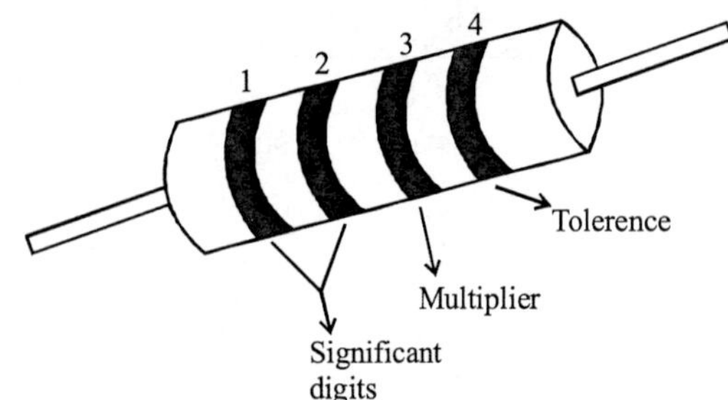

(iii) The colour bands are always read left to right from the end that has the bands closest to it.

(iv) (a) The first and second colour bands, represent the first and second significant digits respectively, of the resistance value.

(b) The third colour band is for the number of zeros that follow the second digit.

(c) In case the third band is gold or silver, it represents a multiplying factor of 0.1 or 0.01.

(d) The fourth band represents the manufacture's tolerance. It is a measure of the precision with which the resistor was made.

(e) If the fourth band is not present, the tolerance is assumed to be ± 20%.

(v) **Standard value of colour codes for carbon resistors**

Colour	Digit	Multiplier	Tolerance
Black	0	$10^0 = 1$	
Brown	1	$10^1 = 10$	
Red	2	10^2	
Orange	3	10^3	
Yellow	4	10^4	
Green	5	10^5	
Blue	6	10^6	
Violet	7	10^7	
Grey	8	10^8	
White	9	10^9	
Gold	–	0.1	± 5%
Silver	–	0.01	± 10%
No colour	–	–	± 20%

To learn the above table of colour codes of resistors let us learn this interesting sentence :

BB ROY of Great Britain has a Very Good Wife.

In the above sentence the capital letters have the following meaning :

B ⇒ Black B ⇒ Brown
R ⇒ Red O ⇒ Orange
Y ⇒ Yellow G ⇒ Green
V ⇒ Violet G ⇒ Grey
W ⇒ White

Remember the colour in the above order and the corresponding digits from 0 to 9 and also the multiplier with the power to 10 from 0 to 9.

Commercial resistors are of two types

(a) **Wire round resistor** made by winding of wires of an alloy manganins, constantan and nichrome.

(b) **Carbon resistors** have low cost and are compact.

Example 3.

The temperature coefficient of resistance of a wire is $0.00125°C^{-1}$. At 300 K its resistance is one ohm. At what temperature the resistance of the wire will be 2 ohm?

Solution :

From formula $R_t = R_0(1 + \propto \Delta t)$

$R_{300} = R_0(1 + \alpha \times 27) = 1$

$R_t = R_0(1 + \propto \Delta \times t) = 2$

$\therefore \quad \dfrac{1+27\alpha}{1+\alpha t} = \dfrac{1}{2}$

or $2 + 54\alpha = 1 + \alpha t$

$\Rightarrow 2 + 54(0.00125) = 1 + (0.00125)t$

$\therefore t = 854°C = 1127\,K$

Example 4.

A cylindrical copper rod is reformed to twice its original length with no change in volume. The resistance between its ends before the change was R. Now its resistance will be

(a) 8 R (b) 6 R (c) 4 R (d) 2 R

Solution : (c)

$$R = \frac{\rho \ell_1}{\pi r_1^2} \quad ...(1)$$

Now the rod is reformed such that

$l_2 = 2l_1$ and $\pi r_1^2 \ell_1 = \pi r_2^2 \ell_2$ (no change in volume)

or $(r_1^2 / r_2^2) = (\ell_2 / \ell_1)$

$$\therefore \quad R_2 = \frac{\rho \ell_2}{\pi r_2^2} \quad ...(2)$$

From eqns. (1) and (2), we get

$$\frac{R}{R_2} = \frac{\ell_1}{\ell_2} \cdot \frac{r_2^2}{r_1^2} = \frac{\ell_1}{\ell_2} \cdot \frac{\ell_1}{\ell_2} = \frac{1}{2} \cdot \frac{1}{2}$$

$\therefore \quad R_2 = 4\,R$

Example 5.

A copper wire is stretched to make 0.1% longer. What is the percentage change in its resistance?

Solution :

The resistance R of a wire is given by $R = \dfrac{\rho \ell}{A}$, where

ρ = specific resistance

Let d and m be the density and mass of the wire, respectively then $A\ell d = m$ or $A = m/\ell d$

$$\therefore R = \frac{\rho \ell \times \ell d}{m} = \frac{\rho \ell^2 d}{m} = \left(\frac{\rho d}{m}\right) \times \ell^2$$

Taking log, of both sides, we get

$$\log_e R = \log_e \left(\frac{\rho d}{m}\right) + 2_e \log_e \ell$$

Differentiating $\dfrac{dR}{R} = \dfrac{2d\ell}{\ell}$ $\left(\because \dfrac{\rho d}{m} = \text{constant}\right)$

$$\frac{dR}{R}\times 100 = 2\left(\frac{d\ell}{\ell}\times 100\right)\% = 2\times(0.1)$$

$\therefore$ Percentage change in resistance $= 2\times(0.1)\,\% = 0.2\%$

So the resistance increases by 0.2%.

Example 6.

Determine the equivalent resistance of the arrangement of resistances shown in fig between the points A and B.

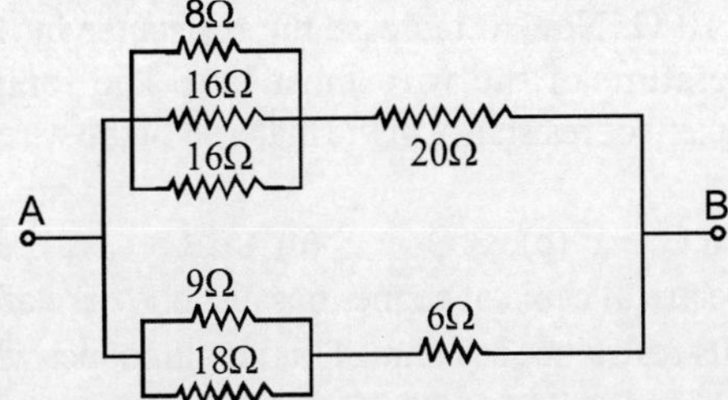

Solution :

8Ω, 16Ω, and 16Ω resistances are connected in parallel. Their equivalent resistance is given by R'

$$\frac{1}{R'} = \frac{1}{8} + \frac{1}{16} + \frac{1}{16} = \frac{2+1+1}{16} = \frac{4}{16}$$

$\therefore$ R' = 4Ω.

This is in series with 20Ω. So upper part of AB has a resistance

$4 + 20 = 24\,\Omega$ ...(1)

For lower part, 9Ω and 18Ω resistances are connected in parallel. Their equivalent resistance R" is given by

$$\frac{1}{R''} = \frac{1}{9} + \frac{1}{18} = \frac{2+1}{18} = \frac{3}{18} \Rightarrow R'' = 18/3 = 6\Omega$$

This is in series with 6Ω. So the resistance of lower part of AB is $6 + 6 = 12\Omega$ ...(2)

The upper and lower parts of AB are in parallel. Hence the equivalent resistance between A and B is given by

$$\frac{1}{R} = \frac{1}{24} + \frac{1}{12} = \frac{1+2}{24} = \frac{3}{24} \Rightarrow R = 24/3 = 8\Omega$$

Example 7.

What will be the equivalent resistance between the two points A and D of fig?

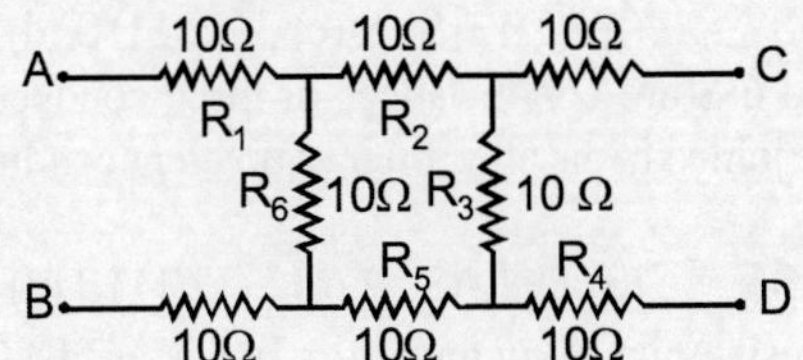

Solution :

Resistances R_2 and R_3 are in series.

$\therefore R' = R_2 + R_3 = 10 + 10 = 20\,\Omega$

Similarly, R_5 and R_6 are in series.

$\therefore R'' = R_5 + R_6 = 10 + 10 = 20\,\Omega$

Further, R' and R" are in parallel

$$\therefore R''' = \frac{R'R''}{R'+R''} = \frac{20\times 20}{20+20} = 10\Omega$$

Resistance between A and D $= R_1 + R''' + R_4 = 10 + 10 + 10 = 30\Omega$

Example 8.

A wire has a resistance of 16.0 ohm. It is melted and drawn to a wire half its initial length. What will be the new resistance of the wire ?

Solution :

The factor by which the length is changed is $n = \frac{\ell'}{\ell} = \frac{1}{2}$

The new resistance R' is given by

$$R' = R\,(n^2) = 16\,\Omega\left(\frac{1}{2}\right)^2 = 4\Omega$$

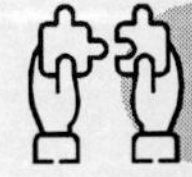

18.1 Concept Practice Problems CPP

1. When a current I is set up in a wire of radius r, the drift velocity is v_d. If the same current is set up through a wire of radius 2 r, the drift velocity will be
   (a) $4\,v_d$ (b) $2\,v_d$ (c) $v_d/2$ (d) $v_d/4$
2. The electric resistance of a certain wire of iron is R. If its length and radius are both doubled, then
   (a) the resistance and the specific resistance, will both remain unchanged
   (b) the resistance will be doubled and the specific resistance will be halved
   (c) the resistance will be halved and the specific resistance will remain unchanged
   (d) the resistance will be halved and the specific resistance will be doubled
3. A given resistor has the following colour scheme of the various strips on it : Brown, black, green and silver. Its value in ohm is
   (a) $1.0\times 10^4 \pm 10\%$ (b) $1.0\times 10^5 \pm 10\%$
   (c) $1.0\times 10^6 \pm 10\%$ (d) $1.0\times 10^7 \pm 10\%$
4. A conductor carries a current of 50 μ A. If the area of cross-section of the conductor is 50 mm^2, then value of the current density in Am^{-2} is
   (a) 0.5 (b) 1 (c) 10^{-3} (d) 10^{-6}
5. Two wires A and B of the same material, having radii in the ratio 1 : 2 and carry currents in the ratio 4 : 1. The ratio of drift speed of electrons in A and B is
   (a) 16 : 1 (b) 1 : 16 (c) 1 : 4 (d) 4 : 1
6. A flow of 10^7 electrons per second in a conducting wire constitutes a current of
   (a) 1.6×10^{-26} A (b) 1.6×10^{26} A
   (c) 1.6×10^{-12} A (d) 1.6×10^{12} A
7. A wire X is half the diameter and half the length of a wire Y of similar material. The ratio of resistance of X to that of Y is
   (a) 8 : 1 (b) 4 : 1 (c) 2 : 1 (d) 1 : 1

8. 2, 4 and 6 S are the conductances of three conductors. When they are joined in series, their equivalent conductance will be
(a) 12 S (b) (1/12) S (c) (12/11) S (d) (11/12) S

9. 2, 4 and 6 S are conductances of three conductors. When they are joined in parallel, their equivalent conductance will be
(a) 12 S (b) (1/12) S (c) (12/11) S (d) (11/12) S

10. If the resistance of a conductor is 5Ω at 50° C & 7Ω at 100° C, then mean temperature coefficient of resistance (of material) is
(a) 0.013/°C (b) 0.004/°C (c) 0.006/°C (d) 0.008/°C

11. If negligibly small current is passed though a wire of length 15 m & resistance of 5Ω, having uniform cross section of 6×10^{-7} m², then coefficient of resistivity of material is
(a) 1×10^{-7}Ω–m (b) 2×10^{-7}Ω–m
(c) 3×10^{-7}Ω–m (d) 4×10^{-7}Ω–m

12. What is the equivalent resistance between the points A and D in given figure?

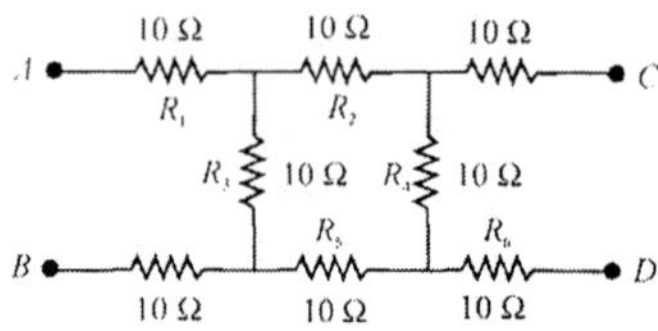

(a) 10 Ω (b) 20 Ω (c) 30 Ω (d) 40 Ω

13. Two wires of same metal have the same length but their cross-sections are in the ratio 3 : 1. They are joined in series. The resistance of the thicker wire is 10 Ω. The total resistance of the combination is
(a) 5/2 Ω (b) 40/3 Ω (c) 40 Ω (d) 100 Ω

14. The resistance of a wire at room temperature 30°C is found to be 10 Ω. Now to increase the resistance by 10%, the temperature of the wire must be [The temperature coefficient of resistance of the material of the wire is 0.002 per °C]
(a) 36°C (b) 83°C (c) 63°C (d) 33°C

15. An electrical cable of copper has just one wire of radius 9 mm. Its resistance is 5 ohm. This single copper wire of the cable is replaced by 6 different well insulated copper wires each of radius 3 mm. The total resistance of the cable will now be equal to
(a) 7.5 ohm (b) 45 ohm (c) 90 ohm (d) 270 ohm

ANSWER KEY

1	(d)	2	(c)	3	(c)	4	(b)	5	(a)	6	(c)	7	(c)	8	(c)	9	(a)	10	(a)
11	(b)	12	(c)	13	(c)	14	(b)	15	(a)										

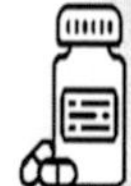

Topic 18.2 : Joule's Law of Heating, Electric Power, Electromotive Force & Internal Resistance of a Cell, Combination of Cells Kirchhoff's Law & Electrical Circuit

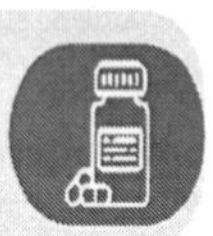

JOULE'S LAW OF HEATING

It states that the amount of heat produced in a conductor is directly proportional to the

(i) square of the current flowing through the conductor, (q, T – constt) i.e. $H \propto i^2$

(ii) resistance of the conductor (i, T – constt.)
i.e. $H \propto R$

(iii) time for which the current is passed (i, R, – constt)
i.e., $H \propto t$

$$\text{Thus } H = i^2 RT \, joule = \frac{i^2RT}{4.2} \, cal$$

ELECTRIC POWER

It is defined as the rate at which work is done in maintaining the current in electric circuit.

Electric power, $P = VI = I^2 R = V^2 / R$ watt or joule/second.

Electric energy : The electric energy consumed in a circuit is defined as *the total work done in maintaining the current in an electric circuit for a given time.*

Electric energy = $VIt = Pt = I^2 Rt = V^2 t / R$

The **S.I. unit** of electric energy is joule (denoted by J) where 1 joule = 1 watt × 1 second = 1 volt × 1 ampere × 1 sec.

In **household circuits** the electrical appliances are connected in parallel and the electrical energy consumed is measured in kWh (kilo watt hour).

$$1\, kWh\, (1\, B.O.T.\, unit) = 1000\, Wh = 3.6 \times 10^6 J$$

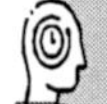

Problem Solving Tips

For Series Combination :

1. If resistances (or electrical appliances) are connected in series, the current through each resistance is same. Then power of an electrical appliance

$$P \propto R \text{ and } V \propto R \qquad (\because P = i^2Rt)$$

It means *in series combination of resistances, the potential difference and power consumed will be more in larger resistance.*

2. (i) When the appliances of power P_1, P_2, P_3... are connected in series, the effective power consumed (P) is

$$\frac{1}{P}=\frac{1}{P_1}+\frac{1}{P_2}+\frac{1}{P_3}...+\frac{1}{P_n}$$ i.e., the effective power is less than the power of individual appliance.

(ii) If n appliances, each of equal resistance R, are connected in series with a voltage source V, the power dissipated P_s will be

$$P_s=\frac{V^2}{nR} \quad ...(i)$$

3. When two lamps of different wattage are connected in series in a house the lamp of lower wattage glows more brightly.

For Parallel Combination :

1. If resistances (i.e. electrical appliances) are connected in parallel, the potential difference across each resistance is same. Then $P \propto 1/R$ and $I \propto 1/R$.
It means *in parallel combination of resistances the current and power consumed will be more in smaller resistance.*
2. When the appliances of power P_1, P_2, P_3.... are in parallel, the effective power consumed (P) is
$$P=P_1+P_2+P_3 \ ... +P_n$$
i.e. the effective power of various electrical appliances is more than the power of individual appliance.
3. If n appliances, each of resistance R, are connected in parallel with a voltage source V, the power dissipated P_p will be
$$P_P=\frac{V^2}{(R/n)}=\frac{nV^2}{R} \quad ...(ii)$$
From eq^{ns}. (i) and (ii),
$$\frac{P_P}{P_S}=n^2 \text{ or } P_P=n^2 P_S$$
This shows that power consumed by n equal resistances in parallel is n^2 times that of power consumed in series if voltage remains same.
4. In parallel grouping of bulbs across a given source of voltage, the bulb of greater wattage will give more brightness and will allow more current through it, but will have lesser resistance and same potential difference across it.
5. For a given voltage V, if resistance is changed from R to R/n, power consumed changes from P to nP.
$P=V^2/R$; when $R'=R/n$,
then $P'=V^2/(R/n)=n V^2/R=nP$.
6. Filament of lower wattage bulb is thinner than that of higher wattage bulb i.e. filament of 60 watt bulb is thinner than that of 100 watt bulb.
7. If I is the current through the fuse wire of length ℓ, radius r, specific resistance ρ and Q is the rate of loss of heat per unit area of a fuse wire, then at steady state,
$$I^2R=QA \text{ or } \frac{I^2\rho\ell}{\pi r^2}=Q\times 2\pi r\ell$$
or $$I^2=\frac{2\pi^2 Q}{\rho}r^3 \Rightarrow I \,\alpha\, r^{3/2}$$
Hence current capacity of a fuse is independent of its length and varies with its radius as $r^{3/2}$.
8. If t_1 and t_2 are the time taken by two different coils for producing same heat with same supply, then
(i) If they are connected in series to produce same heat, time taken, $t=t_1+t_2$
(ii) If they are connected in parallel to produce same heat, time taken is, $t=\frac{t_1 t_2}{t_1+t_2}$
9. When a bulb glows the temperature of the filament is of the order of 3000K.
10. To avoid lengthy calculations *use* $P=I^2R$ *in series combination and* $P=\frac{V^2}{R}$ *in parallel combination* and P = VI when we want to find power of a device and V and I are known.
11. The resistance of an appliance, can be formed by rated voltage and power is $R=\frac{V_{rated}^2}{P_{rated}}$
Now this resistance does not change (remember resistance depends only on the parameters of resistors and not on the voltage across it or the current flowing through it, if we neglect the changes occurring due to change in temperature).
12. The maximum current that can be safely passed through an appliance (a resistor) is $I=\frac{P_{rated}}{V_{rated}}$.
13. Bulbs get fused sometimes when switched on. This is because with the rise in temperature the resistance increases and power decreases ($P=V^2/R$). Therefore the bulb glows brighter in the beginning and get fused.
14. A lead-acid secondary cell is discharged if the relative density of electrolyte drop to 1.18 and e.m.f. of 1.8V.
15. Hot wire galvanometer is based on heating effect of current. Its deflection θ is directly proportional to the heating effect (i.e. I^2). It works on A.C. as well as D.C.
16. Two wires of same material and same length but having different diameters connected in parallel produce more heat than when connected in series. i.e., $H_{parallel}>H_{series}$.
17. If t_1 and t_2 be the time taken by two heaters to boil a given mass of a liquid, then the time taken to boil the same amount of the liquid, when both heaters are connected in parallel is given by
$$t_p=\frac{t_1t_2}{t_1+t_2}.$$
18. If t_1 and t_2 be the time taken by two heaters to boil a given amount of a liquid, then the time taken to boil the same amount of the liquid, when both heaters are connected in series is given by
$$t_s=t_1+t_2.$$
19. If I be the current at which a fuse wire of radius R blows, then $\frac{I^2}{R^3}$ constant. i.e., for two fuse wires of radii R_1 and R_2 and maximum bearing current I_1, and I_2, we have
$$\frac{I_1^2}{R_1^3}=\frac{I_2^2}{R_2^3}.$$

20. If the two resistors R_1 and R_2 are first connected in series and then parallel then the ratio of heat produced in the two cases (series to parallel) is given by

$$\frac{H_s}{H_p}=\frac{(R_1+R_2)^2}{R_1R_2}$$

21. If two resistances R_1 and R_2 are connected in parallel and a current is passed in them such that heat produced in them is H_1 and H_2 respectively, then

$$\frac{H_1}{H_2}=\frac{R_2}{R_1}.$$

Example 9.

A bulb has voltage rating of 220 V and power rating of 40 W. How can this bulb be made to glow with normal brightness if a voltage source of e.m.f. 330 V is available?

Solution :

Here V = 220 V; P = 40 W

Resistance of the bulb, $R=\frac{V^2}{P}=\frac{(220)^2}{40}=1210\Omega$

Current in the circuit, $I=\frac{330}{1210+S}$

Potential difference across the bulb,

$$IR=\left(\frac{330}{1210+S}\right)1210$$

As per question, $220=\frac{330\times1210}{1210+S}$

On solving, we get $S=605\ \Omega$

Hence to glow bulb, a resistance of 605Ω should be connected in series.

Example 10.

If two bulbs of wattage 25 and 30 W, each rated at 220 volts are connected in series with a 440 volt supply, which bulb will fuse?

Solution :

Resistance of 25 W bulb, $R_1=\frac{(220)^2}{25}\Omega$;

Current $I_1=\frac{25}{220}A$

Resistance of 30 W bulb, $R_2=\frac{(220)^2}{30}\Omega$,

Current $I_2=\frac{30}{220}A$

When bulbs are connected in series, effective resistance is

$$R=R_1+R_2=(220)^2\left[\frac{1}{25}+\frac{1}{30}\right]=220\times220\times\frac{11}{150}\Omega$$

When supply voltage is 440 V, then current is

$$I'=\frac{440}{R}=\frac{440\times150}{220\times220\times11}=\frac{27.27}{220}A$$

As $I'>I_1$ but less than I_2, hence the bulb of 25 watt will fuse.

Example 11.

What will happen when 40 W, 220 V lamp and 100 W, 220 V lamp are connected in series across 440V lamp?

Solution :

Resistance of first lamp,

$R_1=220\times220/40=1210\ \Omega$.

Resistance of second lamp,

$R_2=220\times220/100=484\ \Omega$.

Total resistance in series = 1210 + 484 = 1694 Ω.

Current in the circuit when supply voltage is 440 V will be,

$$I=\frac{440}{1694}=0.26\,A$$

Voltage drop across $R_1=0.26\times1210=314.6$ V

Voltage drop across $R_2=0.26\times484=112.84$V

Therefore 40 W bulb will fuse because lamp can tolerate only 220 V.

Example 12.

A fuse wire with a circular cross section and having diameter of 0.4 mm blows with a current of 3 amp. The value of the current for which another fuse wire made of the same material but having circular cross-section with diameter of 0.06 mm will blow is

(a) 3 amp. (b) $3\times\sqrt{(3/2)}$ amp.
(c) $3\times(3/2)$ amp. (d) $3\times(3/2)^{3/2}$ amp.

***Solution :* (d)**

For a fuse wire $I^2\propto r^3$

$$\therefore\quad \frac{I_1^2}{I_2^2}=\frac{r_1^3}{r_2^3}$$

where $r_1=\frac{0.04}{2}=0.02$ cm and $r_2=\frac{0.06}{2}=0.03$ cm.

$$\therefore\quad \frac{(3)^2}{I_2^2}=\left(\frac{0.02}{0.03}\right)^3=\left(\frac{2}{3}\right)^3$$

or $I_2^2=(3)^2\left(\frac{3}{2}\right)^3$ or $I_2=3\times\left(\frac{3}{2}\right)^{3/2}$

ELECTROMOTIVE FORCE AND INTERNAL RESISTANCE OF A CELL

An emf (electromotive force) device has a positive terminal (at high potential) and a negative terminal (at low potential). This device is responsible for moving positive charge within itself from negative terminal to positive terminal.

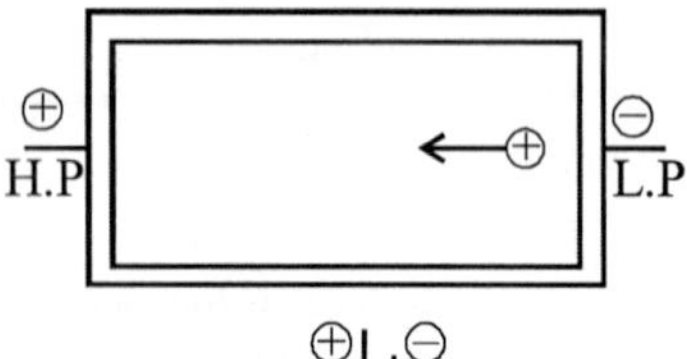

For this to happen, work is done by some agency in the emf device. The energy required to do this work is chemical energy (as in a battery), mechanical energy (as in electric generator), temperature difference (as in a thermopile).

The emf is thus given by the formula

$$E=\frac{dW}{dq}$$

The **S.I unit** of emf is $\frac{J}{C}$ = volt(V)

Problem Solving Tips

1. Electromotive force is not a force but a potential difference.
2. E.m.f. can be defined as the work done in moving a charge once around a closed circuit.

Internal Resistance (r)

The potential difference across a real source of emf is not equal to its emf. The reason is that the charge which is moving inside the emf device also suffers resistance. This resistance is called **internal resistance** of the emf device.

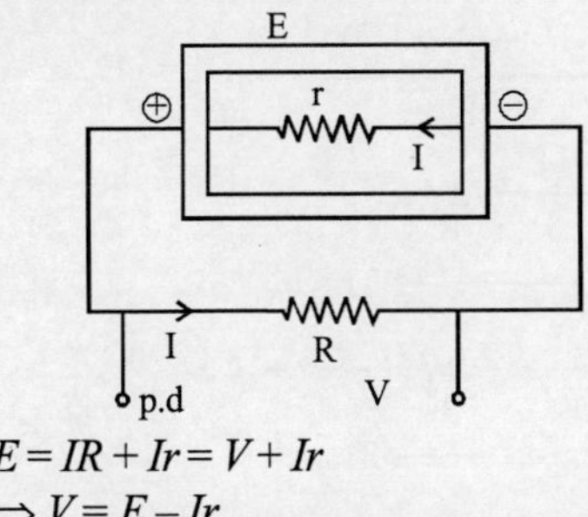

$E = IR + Ir = V + Ir$

$\Rightarrow V = E - Ir$

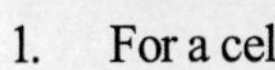

Problem Solving Tips

1. For a cell

Circuit	Mode	Expression
(i) 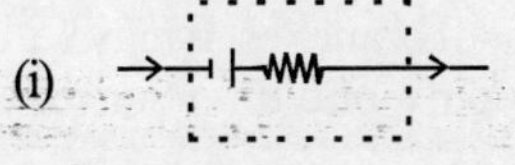	Discharging	$V = E - Ir \quad \therefore V < E$
(ii) 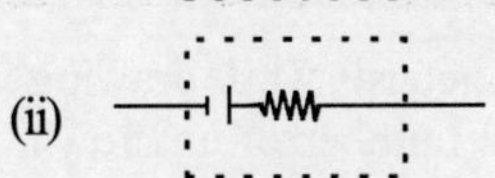	No current	$V = E$
(iii) 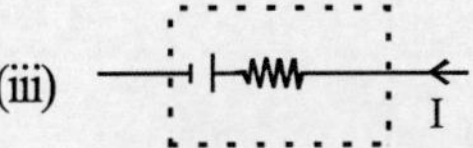	Charging	$V = E + Ir \quad \therefore V > E$

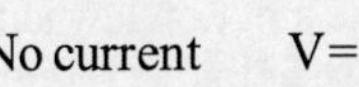

2. Emf is the property of a cell but terminal potential difference depends on the current drawn from the cell.

Short Circuiting

When the terminals of an emf device are connected with a conducting path without any external resistance then

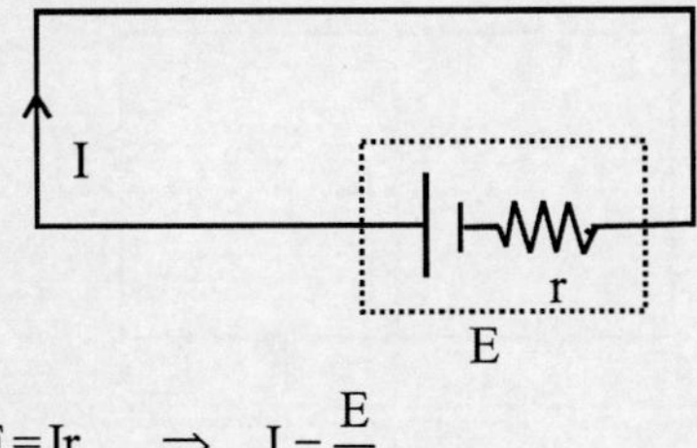

$E = Ir \quad \Rightarrow \quad I = \frac{E}{r}$

Since internal resistance has a very small value, therefore a very high current flows in the circuit producing a large amount of heat. This condition is called **short circuiting**.

Note : During short circuiting, the terminal potential difference is zero.

COMBINATION OF CELLS

Series Combination of Cells

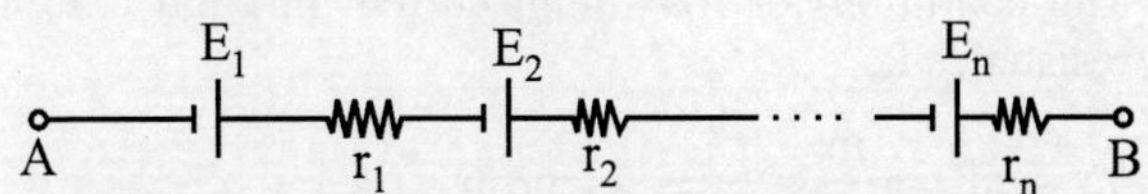

Equivalent Emf $E_{AB} = E_1 + E_2 + ... + E_n$

Equivalent internal resistance, $R_{AB} = r_1 + r_2 + ... + r_n$

Parallel Combination of Cells

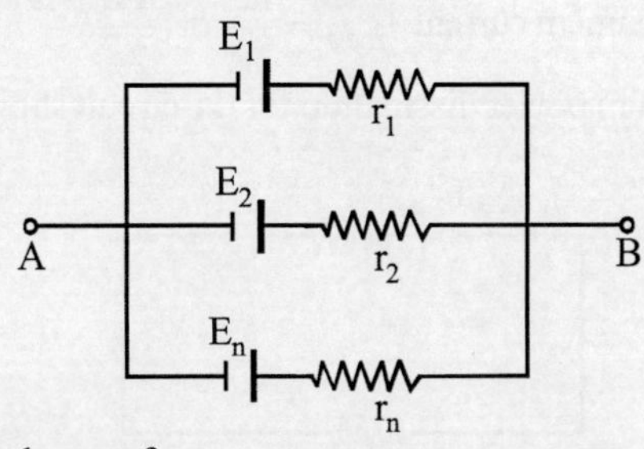

Equivalent emf

$$E_{AB} = \frac{\frac{E_1}{r_1} + \frac{E_2}{r_2} + ... + \frac{E_n}{r_n}}{\frac{1}{r_1} + \frac{1}{r_2} + ... \frac{1}{r_n}}$$

Equivalent internal resistance

$$\frac{1}{R_{AB}} = \frac{1}{r_1} + \frac{1}{r_2} + ... + \frac{1}{r_n}$$

Mixed Grouping of Cells :

If the cells are connected as shown below then they are said to be in mixed grouping.

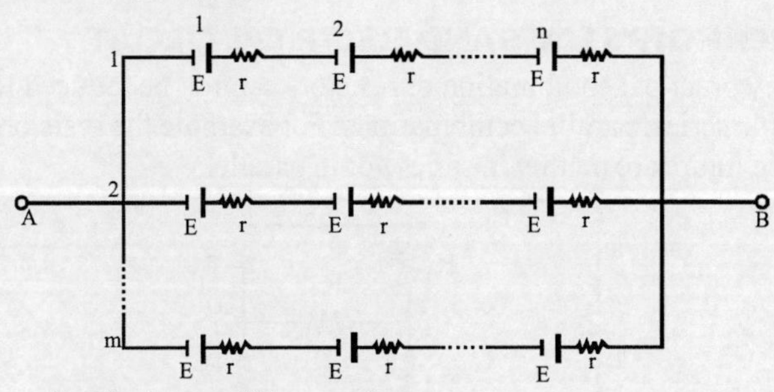

Equivalent emf $E_{AB} = nE$

Equivalent resistance $= \frac{nr}{m}$

Where n = no. of cells in a row. and

M = no. of rows

If this equivalent cell is attached to an external resistance R then

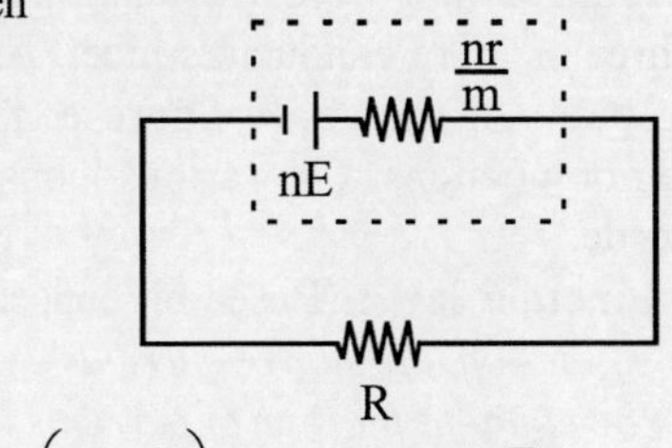

$$nE = I\left(R + \frac{nr}{m}\right) \Rightarrow I = \frac{nmE}{mR + nr}$$

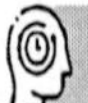

Problem Solving Tips

(i) The condition for maximum current through external resistance R

$nr = mR \Rightarrow \frac{m}{n} = \frac{r}{R} \Rightarrow R = nr/m$

In other words, when external resistance is equal to total internal resistances of all the cells.

The maximum current $I_{max} = \frac{nE}{2R}$ or $\frac{mE}{2r}$

(ii) Maximum power dissipation for the circuit shown in fig.

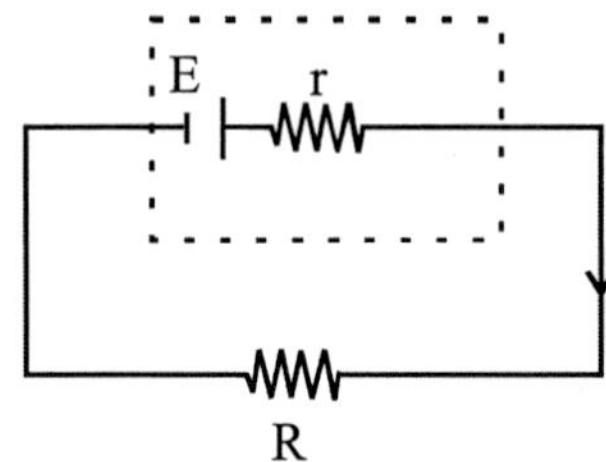

Power $P = I^2R = \left(\frac{E}{R+r}\right)^2 R = \frac{E^2R}{(R+r)^2}$

For maximum power across the resistor, $\frac{dP}{dR} = 0$

On solving, we get $R = r$

This is the condition for maximum power dissipation.

(iii) If identical cells are connected in a loop in order, then emf between any two points in the loop is zero.

(iv) If n identical cells are connected in series and m are wrongly connected then $E_{net} = nE - 2mE$

KIRCHHOFF'S LAWS AND ELECTRICAL CIRCUIT

Many practical combination of resistors cannot be reduced to simple series, parallel combinations. For example the resistors in the figure are neither in series nor in parallel.

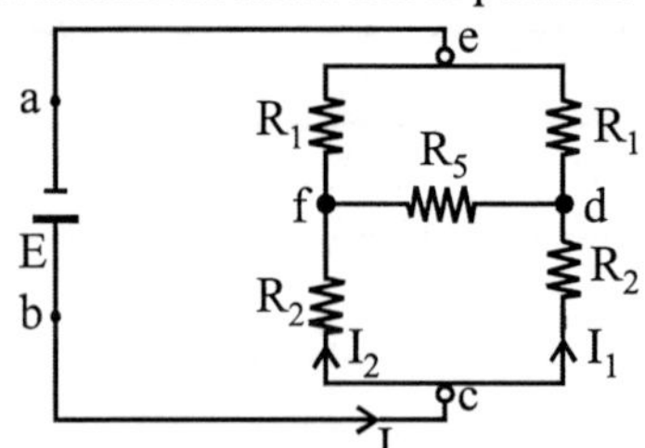

The use of Ohm's law is not sufficient to solve such problems. Kirchoff's laws are used in such cases.

We will often use the term junction and loop, so let us first understand the meaning of these words. A junction in a circuit is a point where three or more conductors meet. A loop is a closed conducting path. In the above figure e, f, d, c are junctions. a, b, are not junctions. The various loops are efde, cdfc, eabcf and eabcde.

(i) Kirchhoff's junction law : (Based on conservation of charge) *At any junction, the sum of currents entering the junction must be equal to the sum of currents leaving it.* If this is not so, charges will accumulate at the junction. This cannot happen as this would mean high/low potential maintained at a point in a wire without external influence. When we apply this rule at junction c, we get $I = I_1 + I_2$

(ii) Kirchhoff's loop law : (Based on energy conservation) *The algebraic sum of changes in potential around any closed loop of a circuit must be zero.*

Sign convention for using loop law. If we move a loop element (resistor, emf device, capacitor, inductor etc.) in the direction of increasing potential, we take the potential difference positive and vice-versa.

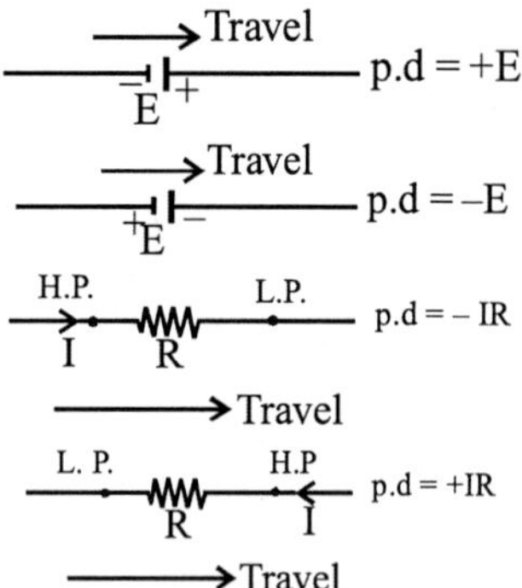

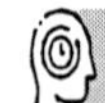

Problem Solving Tips

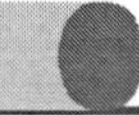

(i) Draw a circuit diagram large enough to show all resistors, emf device, capacitors, currents clearly.

(ii) Take into account the resistance of voltmeter/ammeter/ internal resistance of a cell (if given).

(iii) **Assume** the direction of current in all branches. It may be noted here that one branch has only one direction of current.

It is best to use junction law simultaneously while drawing currents. This helps to reduce the number of unknown quantities.

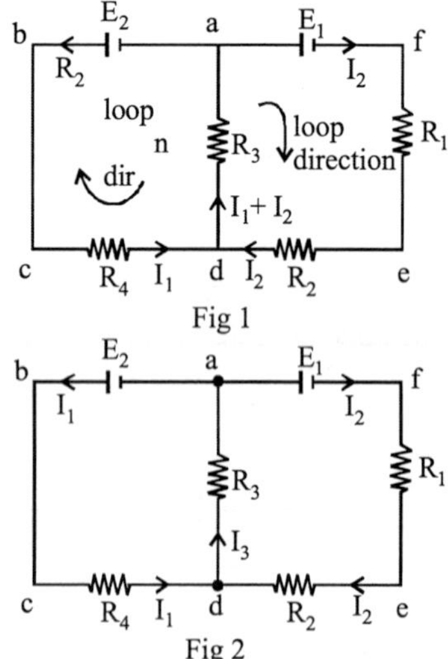

In the above circuits we arbitrarily assumed the direction of current I_1 in branch abcd as anti-clockwiswe and the direction of current I_2 in branch afed as clockwise.

In figure 1 we have two unknown currents (I_1, I_2) whereas figure 2 we have three unknown currents (I_1, I_2 and I_3). The first figure is a better option for solving problems. In figure 1 we used junction rule at d simultaneously while labelling currents.

(iv) In a branch containing a capacitor, the current is zero when d.c is applied and steady state conditions are achieved.

(v) Now we need as many independent equations as there are conditions unknowns. If we have to find a particular unknown, we should ensure that, the unknown appears in one of the equations made by us.

(vi) For making equations choose the loop and travel the loop completely. We may travel the loop in clockwise or anti-clockwise direction. While using second law use sign conventions properly.

(vii) Solve the equations formed to find the unknown quantities. If any value of current comes out to be negative then that particular current is in the opposite direction to that assumed.

Applications

Let us use second law in the loop abcda of figure 1 taking the loop in anti-clockwise direction starting from a.

$$+E_2 - I_1R_4 - (I_1 + I_2)R_3 = 0$$

For loop afeda, moving the loop in clockwise direction we get –

$$E_1 - I_2R_1 - I_2R_2 - (I_1 + I_2)R_3 = 0$$

Node method to apply Kirchoff's law (Open loop method)

Step 1 : We select a reference node and assume its potential to be (zero/x)V

Step 2 : We calculate the voltage of other selected points w.r.t. the reference node

Step 3: We find some independent node (whose voltage is not known). We apply Kirchoff's law to find the relevant values.

Example 13.

Find current through branch BD

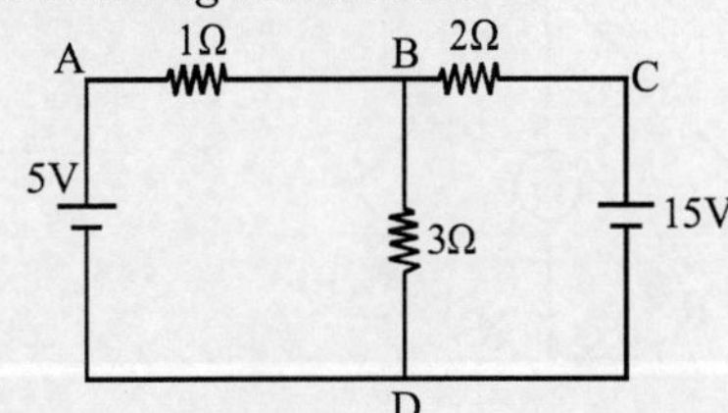

Solution :

Let $V_D = 0V$

$\therefore V_A = +5V$ and $V_C = +15\,V$

Let the voltage of B = V_B

Applying Kirchhoff's junction law at B

$$\frac{5 - V_B}{1} + \frac{15 - V_B}{2} + \frac{0 - V_B}{3} = 0 \Rightarrow V_B = 6.82 \text{ Volt}$$

$$\text{Current through BD} = \frac{6.82 - 0}{3} = 2.27\text{A}$$

Example 14.

Calculate the currents I_1, I_2 and I_3 in the circuit shown in figure.

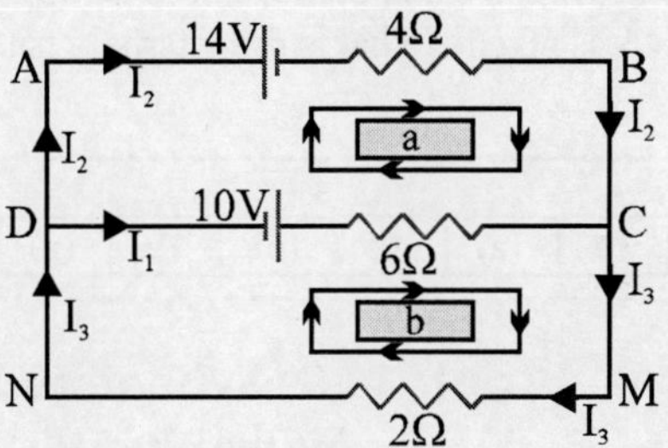

Solution :

Junction rule at C yields

$I_1 + I_2 - I_3 = 0$ i.e., $I_1 + I_2 = I_3$ .... (1)

while loop for meshes a and b yields respectively :

$-14 - 4I_2 + 6I_1 - 10 = 0$

i.e., $3I_1 - 2I_2 = 12$ .... (2)

and, $10 - 6I_1 - 2I_3 = 0$

i.e., $3I_1 + I_3 = 5$ .... (3)

Substituting I_3 from equation (1) in (3)

$4I_1 + I_2 = 5$

Solving equations (2) and (4) for I_1 and I_2, we find

$I_1 = 2A$ and $I_2 = -3A$

And hence equation (1) yields, $I_3 = -1A$

The fact that I_2 and I_3 are negative implies that actual direction of I_2 and I_3 are opposite to that shown in the circuit.

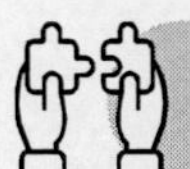

18.2 Concept Practice Problems

CPP

16. A cell of internal resistance r is connected across an external resistance nr. Then the ratio of the terminal voltage to the emf of the cell is

(a) $\frac{1}{n}$ (b) $\frac{1}{n+1}$ (c) $\frac{n}{n+1}$ (d) $\frac{n-1}{n}$

17. A battery of e.m.f. 10 V and internal resistance 0.5 Ω is connected across a variable resistance R. The value of R for which the power delivered in it is maximum is given by

(a) 0.5 Ω (b) 1.0 Ω (c) 2.0 Ω (d) 0.25 Ω

18. Two electric bulbs whose resistance are in the ratio 1 : 2 are arranged in parallel to a constant voltage source. The powers dissipated in them have the ratio

(a) 1 : 2 (b) 1 : 1 (c) 2 : 1 (d) 1 : 4

19. A cell when balanced with potentiometer gave a balance length of 50 cm. 4.5 Ω external resistance is introduced in the circuit, now it is balanced on 45 cm. The internal resistance of cell is

(a) 0.25 Ω (b) 0.5 Ω (c) 1.0 Ω (d) 1.5 Ω

20. An electric fan and a heater are marked as 100 W, 220 V and 1000 W, 220 V respectively. The resistance of heater is

(a) equal to that of fan (b) lesser than that of fan
(c) greater than that of fan (d) zero

21. Two identical cells connected in series send 1.0A current through a 5 Ω resistor. When they are connected in parallel, they send 0.8 A current through the same resistor. What is the internal resistance of the cell?

(a) 0.5 Ω (b) 1.0 Ω (c) 1.5 Ω (d) 2.5 Ω

22. Water boils in the electric kettle in 15 minutes after switching on. If the length of heating wire is decreased to 2/3 of its initial value, then the same amount of water will boil with the same supply voltage in

(a) 8 minutes (b) 10 minutes
(c) 12 minutes (d) 15 minutes

23. Three equal resistors, connected across a source of e.m.f. together dissipate 10 watt of power. What will be the power dissipated in watts if the same resistors are connected in parallel across the same source of e.m.f.

(a) 10 (b) 10/3 (c) 30 (d) 90

24. Null point with 1V cell comes out to be 55 cm and with $R = 10\Omega$ it is 50 cm. What is the internal resistance of the cell ?

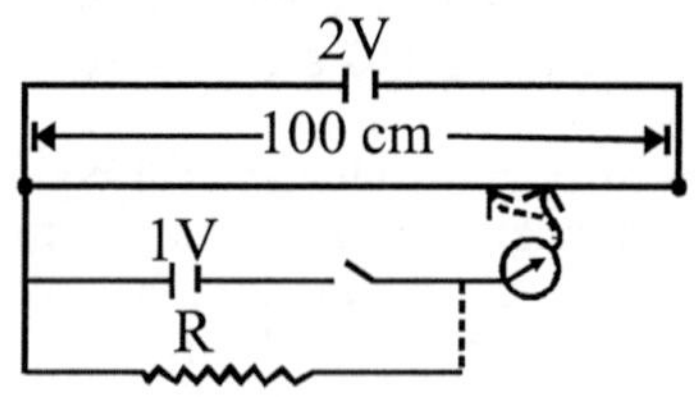

(a) 0.5Ω (b) 0.4Ω (c) 1Ω (d) 0.2Ω

25. A fuse wire with a radius of 1 mm blows at 1.5 A. If the fuse wire of the same material should blow at 3.0 A, the radius of the wire must be

(a) $4^{1/3}$ mm (b) $\sqrt{2}$ mm (c) 0.5 mm (d) 8.0 mm

ANSWER KEY																			
16	(c)	17	(a)	18	(c)	19	(a)	20	(b)	21	(d)	22	(b)	23	(d)	24	(c)	25	(a)

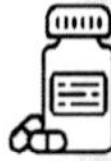

Topic 18.3 : Wheatstone Bridge, Meter Bridges, Potentiometer, Measuring Instrument-Voltmeter and Ammeter

WHEATSTONE BRIDGE

The condition for balanced wheatstone bridge

$$E_{AB} = (\pi_{AB})_T - (\pi_{AB})_{T_0} + \sigma_A(T - T_o) - \sigma_B(T - T_o)$$

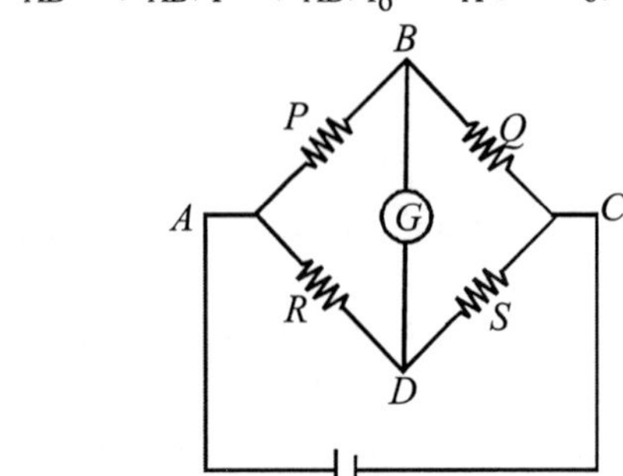

$$\frac{P}{Q} = \frac{R}{S} \text{ also } \frac{P}{R} = \frac{Q}{S}$$

Note that when battery and galvanometer of a Wheatstone bridge is interchanged, the balance position remains undisturbed, while sensitivity of the bridge changes.

In the balanced condition, the resistance in the branch BD may be neglected

Example : *Resistance connected to BC may be neglected.*

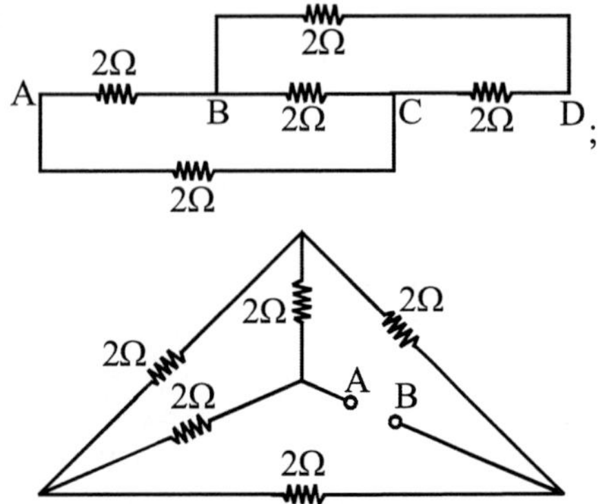

Note : In a Wheatstone bridge, the deflection in a galvanometer does not change, if the battery and the galvanometer are interchanged

Measuring temperature with the help of Wheatstone bridge

$$\text{At balancing } \frac{P}{R + \Delta R} = \frac{Q}{S(1 + \alpha\Delta T)}$$

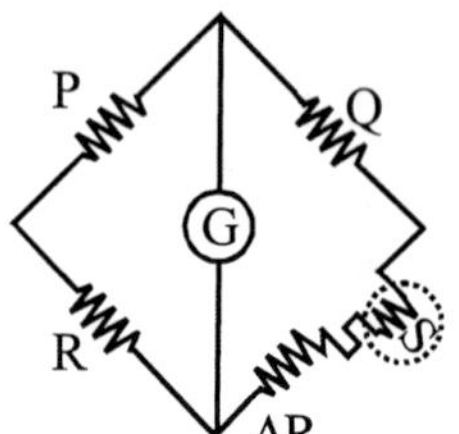

When $P = Q$ then $\Delta R = S\,\alpha\,\Delta T$ $[\because R \approx S]$

$$\therefore \Delta T = \frac{\Delta R}{S\alpha}$$

MISCONCEPTIONS

× **Incorrect** If the current flows in a wire, there has to be a potential difference. The potential drop takes place only when current passes through a resistor.

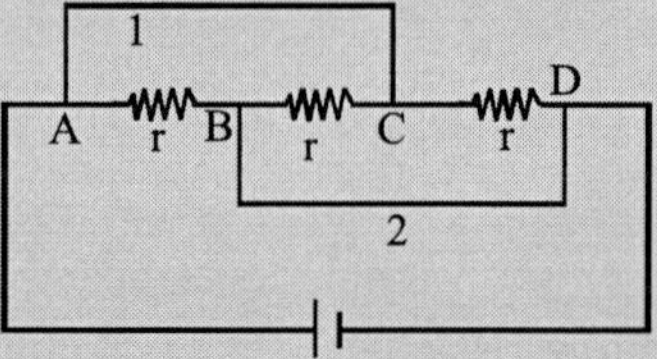

✓ **Correct** In the diagram, the three resistors are in parallel. The potential at A is equal to the potential at C. Current flows in wire 1 but there is no potnetial drop across A and C.

× **Incorrect** If potential difference between the points is zero, there is zero current between the two points.

✓ **Coorect** There is no p.d. between A and C still current flows in segment 1.

Example 15.

Find the potential difference between the points A and B in fig.

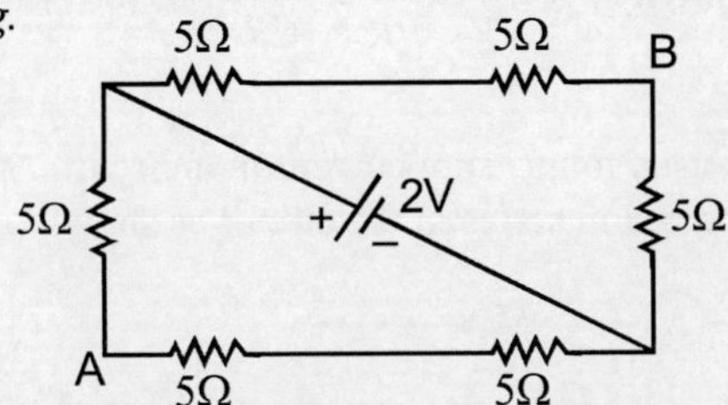

Solution :

The upper three resistances of the cell are in series. Their equivalent resistance is 15Ω. Similarly lower three resistances are in series. Their equivalent resistance is also 15Ω. The upper and lower equivalent resistances are connected in parallel. So, resultant resistance of the circuit is given by

$$\frac{1}{R}=\frac{1}{15}+\frac{1}{15}=\frac{2}{15} \text{ or } R=\frac{15}{2}\Omega$$

Current from the cell, $i=\frac{2}{(15/2)}=\frac{4}{15}$ amp.

In order to calculate potential difference between points A and B, see fig.

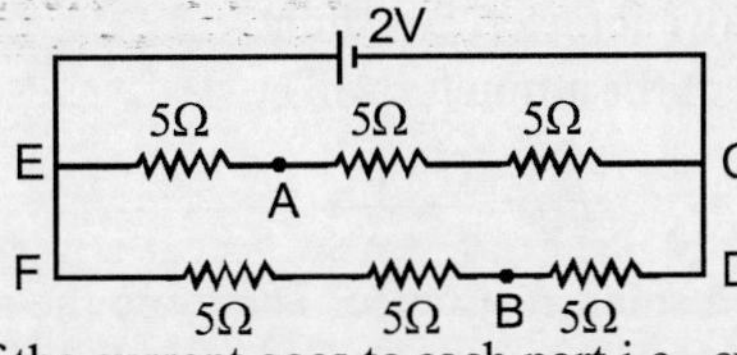

Half of the current goes to each part i.e., current in each part is (2/15) amp. Consider the loop AEFDCA, we have

$$V_{AB}=-\frac{2}{15}\times 5+\frac{2}{15}\times 5+\frac{2}{15}\times 5=V_A-V_B$$

$$=\frac{2}{15}\times 5=\frac{2}{3} \text{ volt} \quad \text{or} \quad V_A=2-\frac{2}{15}\times 5=\frac{4}{3} \text{ volt},$$

$$V_B=2-\frac{2}{15}\times 10=\frac{2}{3} \text{ volt so } V_{AB}=V_A-V_B=\frac{2}{3} \text{ volt}$$

METER BRIDGE OR SLIDE WIRE BRIDGE

Principle: Based on balanced Wheatstone bridge principle.

Use : To find unknown resistance

Working : Let P be the unknown resistance.

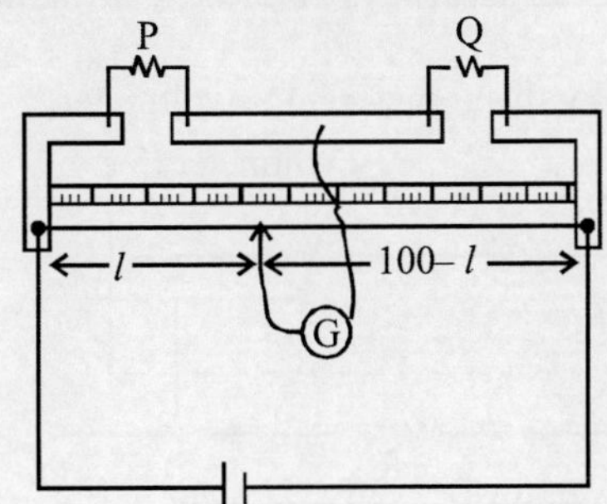

At balance point

$$\frac{P}{l}=\frac{Q}{100-l}$$

Q is known and l can be calculated.

POTENTIOMETER

Principle : The p.d. across a resistance wire is directly proportional to its length provided I, r and A are constant.

$$V=IR=I\rho\frac{l}{A}$$

$\Rightarrow V \propto l$ [I, ρ and A are constant]

Working : PQ is the resistance wire of potentiometer generally made up of constantan or nichrome. One end P is connected to the positive terminal of the battery B while negative terminal is connected to Q through a Rheostat (Rh) and key (K). This is the main circuit.

A cell whose emf has to be measured is also connected to the potential wire in such a way that the positive terminal is connected with P and negative terminal is connected to a galvanometer and then to a jockey (J) which is free to slide along the wire

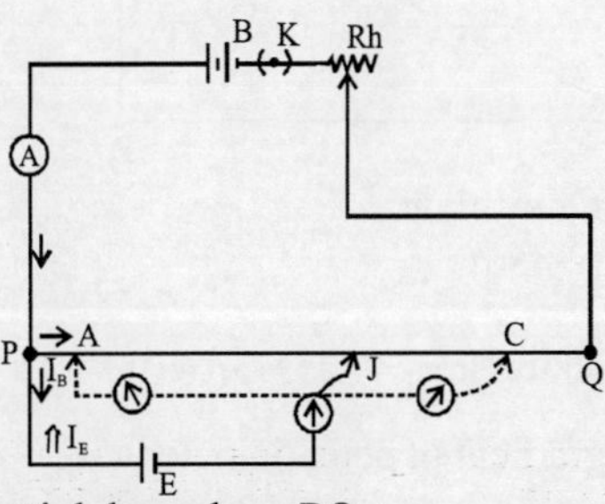

There is a potential drop along PQ.

The potential drop per unit length along PQ is called ***potential gradient.***

When the jockey is pressed on some point, current flows from E to P (⇒). Also current that comes from B after reaching P divides into two parts. One part moves towards A and the other towards E (→). Three cases may arise.

(a) $I_B > I_E$. This happens when $V_{PC} > E$. One side deflection in galvanometer

(b) $I_B = I_E$. This happens when $V_{PC} = E$, Zero deflection in galvanometer

(c) $I_B < I_E$. This happens when $V_{PA} < E$. Other side defection in galvanometer

Note :

- At null point since no current flows through E therefore it is said to be in the condition of open circuit.
- More is the length of potentiometer, higher is the sensitivity of potentiometer and smaller is the potential gradient.
- Potentiometer will work only when B > E. Also the positive terminal of the batteries is connected at P. If any of the above conditions is not followed, we do not get a null point.

Uses : (i) Comparison of emfs of cells $\frac{E_1}{E_2}=\frac{l_1}{l_2}$

(ii) To find internal resistance of a cell $r=\left(\frac{l}{l'}\right)R$

emf can be measured by potentiometer and not voltmeter.

Example 16.

A 10 m long wire AB of uniform area of cross-section and 20Ω resistance is used as a potentiometer wire. This wire is connected in series with a battery of 5V and a resistor of 480Ω. An unknown emf is balanced at 600 cm of the wire as shown in the figure.

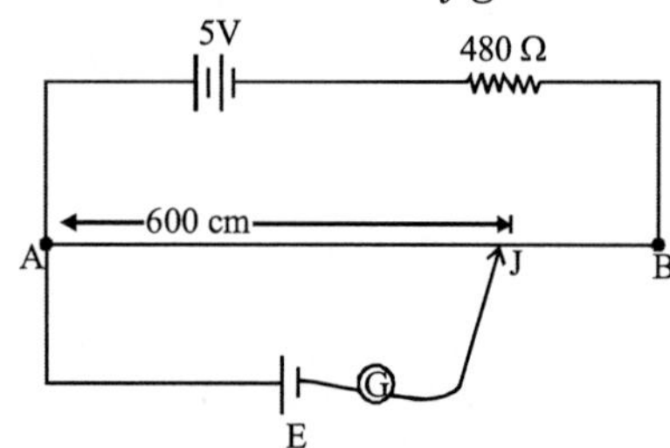

Calculate :

(i) *The potential gradient for the potentiometer wire*

(ii) *The value of unknown emf E*

Solution :

(i)

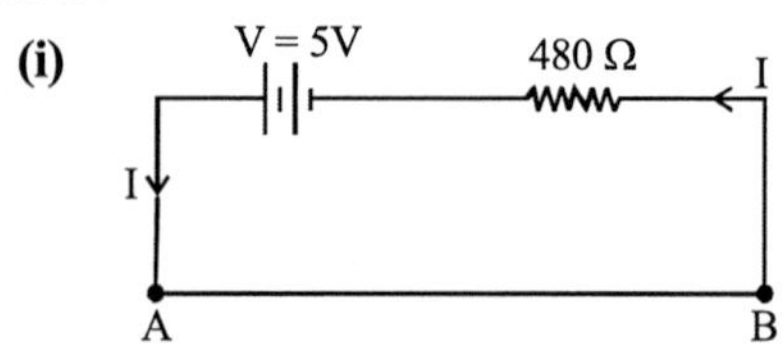

Applying Ohm's law

$V = I(R_{AB} + 480)$

$5 = I(20 + 480)$ $[R_{AB} = 20\,\Omega \text{ (given)}] \Rightarrow I = \frac{5}{500} = 0.01A$

Potential gradient of potentiometer wire

$$= \frac{V_{AB}}{\ell_{AB}} = \frac{0.2}{10} = 0.02 Vm^{-1}$$

(ii) With reference to the current given in question, the emf E and the potential drop across AJ should be equal for the balancing : E = (potential gradient of potentiometer wire) × balancing length = 0.02 × 6 = 0.12 V

Example 17.

A uniform potential gradient is established across a potentiometer wire. Two cells of emf E_1 and E_2 connected to support and oppose each other are balanced over ℓ_1 = 6m and ℓ_2 = 2m. Find E_1/E_2.

Solution :

$E_1 + E_2 = x\ell_1 = 6x$ and $E_1 - E_2 = 2x$

$$\frac{E_1 + E_2}{E_1 - E_2} = \frac{6}{2} \quad \text{or} \quad \frac{E_1}{E_2} = \frac{2}{1}$$

MEASURING INSTRUMENTS

Galvanometer

It is an instrument used to detect small currents in a circuit. The current required for full scale deflection in the galvanometer is called full scale deflection current and is denoted by I_g.

Current sensitivity of a galvanometer.

It is defined as the deflection produced in the galvanometer, when unit current flows through it.

Current sensitivity, $I_s = \frac{\theta}{I} = \frac{NBA}{C}$ and its **unit** is rad A^{-1}

Current sensitivity can be increased either by decreasing C i.e. restoring torque per unit twist or increasing B.

Voltage sensitivity of a galvanometer

It is defined as the deflection produced in the galvanometer when a unit voltage is applied across the two terminals of the galvanometer.

Voltage sensitivity $V_S = \frac{\theta}{V} = \frac{\theta}{IR} = \frac{NBA}{CR}$, its **unit** is rad V^{-1}

Ammeter

Ammeter is used to measure current in a circuit. Ammeter is always connected in series in the circuit as shown.

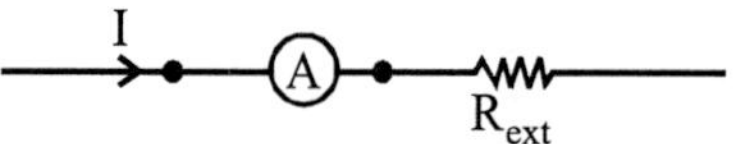

Conversion of a galvanometer into an ammeter

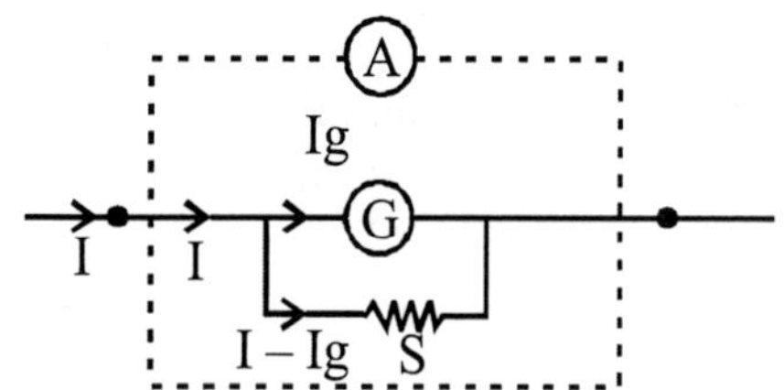

For this, we connect ***a small resistance S (called shunt)*** *in parallel with the galvanometer.*

Mathematically, $I_g \times G = (I - I_g)S$

where I is the maximum current which ammeter can measure. G is the resistance of galvanometer and Ig is the current of full scale deflection in galvanometer. S is shunt.

The **resistance of the ammeter** will be

$$\frac{1}{R_A} = \frac{1}{G} + \frac{1}{S} \quad R_A = \frac{G \times S}{G + S}$$

Since shunt is a small resistance. Therefore the resistance of ammeter is very small.

The above arrangement is made so that when we connect ammeter in series to measure current, it does not change the original current to a large extent. The change is infact very small. Also since galvanometer is a sensitive device and cannot take large currents, this arrangement serves the purpose. Most of the current entering the ammeter passes through the shunt as current always prefer low resistance path.

An **ideal ammeter** is one which has zero resistance.

The range of ammeter can be increased but cannot be decreased below Ig.

Voltmeter

Voltmeter is used to measure potential difference across a resistor. Voltmeter is always connected in parallel across a resistor.

Conversion of a galvanometer into a voltmeter

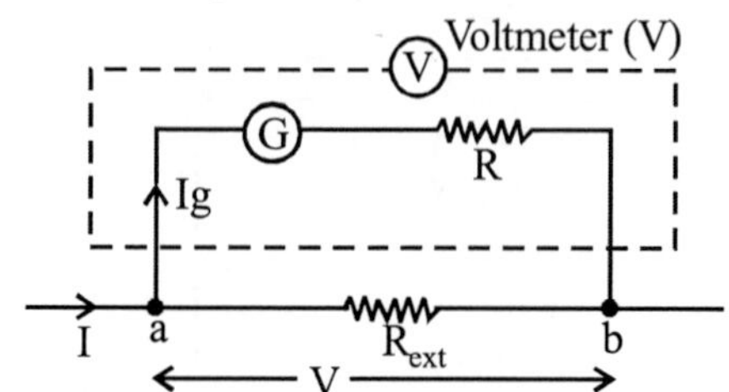

For this, we connect a large resistance R in series with the galvanometer.

The potential difference which has to be measured is across the external resistance i.e. across points a and b.

Let it be V. Then

$$V = I_g (G + R)$$

where V is the maximum potential difference that the voltmeter can measure and R is the large resistance connected in series with the galvanometer

The resistance of the voltmeter will be $R_V = G + R$

Since R is a large resistance. Therefore resistance of voltmeter is very large.

An **ideal voltmeter** is one which has infinite resistance.

The range of voltmeter can be increased and decreased.

Note : When ammeter/voltmeter is connected in the circuit, the current or voltage indicated by these is less than the actual values in their absence.

Example 18.

A galvanometer of coil resistance 20 ohm, gives a full scale deflection with a current of 5 mA. What arrangements should be made in order to measure currents upto 1.0 A ?

Solution :

The upper limiting value of current to be measured is to be increased by a factor

$$n = \frac{1.0A}{5A} = 200$$

∴ Resistance of the shunt required will be

$$S = \frac{G}{n-1} = \frac{20\Omega}{200-1} \approx 0.1\,\Omega$$

Hence, a shunt of resistance $0.1\ \Omega$ should be connected in parallel across the galvanometer coil.

Example 19.

A voltmeter having 100Ω resistance can measure a potential difference of 25V. What resistance R is required to be connected in series, to make it read voltage upto 250 V ?

Solution :

The upper limiting value of voltage is to be increased by a factor

$$n = \frac{250V}{25V} = 10$$

∴ Resistance, $R = (n-1)\,G = (10-1)\,100 = 900\,\Omega$

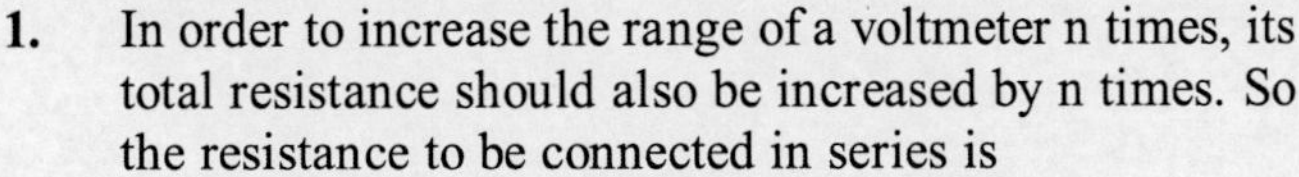

1. In order to increase the range of a voltmeter n times, its total resistance should also be increased by n times. So the resistance to be connected in series is
$R = (n-1)\,G$
2. In order to increase the range of an ammeter n times, the value of shunt resistance to be connected in parallel is
$S = G/(n-1)$
3. For galvanometers with their coil in uniform magnetic field B
$$I = \frac{C\theta}{NAB\sin\alpha}$$
C = torsional rigidity of suspension wire.
For galvanometer with concave pole-pieces – radial magnetic field is produced, $\alpha = 90°$
$I = (C/NAB)\theta$ or $I = K\theta$

Note : All galvanometers used in practice have concave pole-pieces, for making the radial magnetic field.

Example 20.

A galvanometer has a resistance of 30 Ω and current of 2 mA is needed to give full scale deflection. What is the resistance needed and how is it to be connected to convert the galvanometer

(a) *into an ammeter of 0.3 ampere range*

(b) *into voltmeter of 0.2 volt range*

Solution :

(a) We know that $i_g = \left(\frac{S}{S+G}\right) i$

Substituting the given values, we get

$$2\times10^{-3} = \left(\frac{S}{S+30}\right)\times0.3$$

Solving it, we get S = (30/149) Ω

So, a resistance of (30/149) Ω must be connected in parallel with the galvanometer.

(b) In this case, $i_g = \left(\frac{V}{R+G}\right)$ or $R = \frac{V}{i_g} - G$

$$\therefore\ R = \frac{0.2}{2\times10^{-3}} - 30 = 100 - 30 = 70\Omega$$

So, a resistance of 70 Ω must be connected in series with the galvanometer.

Example 21.

A voltmeter has a resistance of G ohm and range V volt. What will be the value of resistance used in series to convert it into voltmeter of range nV volt?

Solution :

We know that, $R = \frac{V}{I_g} - G$

The voltmeter gives full scale deflection for potential difference V. Its resistance is G

Hence $I_g = (V/G)$

$$\therefore\ R = \frac{nV}{(V/G)} - G = nG - G = (n-1)G$$

Example 22.

In the circuit shown in fig., Find the reading of voltmeter.

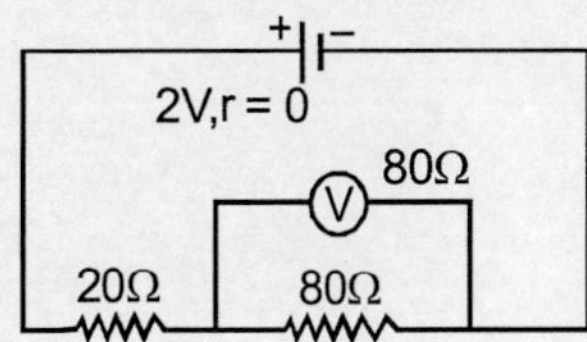

Solution :

The equivalent resistance of the circuit is given by

$$R_{eq.} = 20 + \frac{80 \times 80}{80 \times 80} = 20 + 40 = 60\Omega$$

Current through the circuit $I = \frac{V}{R} = (2/60) = (1/30)$ amp

Reading of voltmeter

$= \text{current} \times R_T$

$$= \frac{1}{30} \times \left(\frac{80 \times 80}{80 + 80}\right) = \frac{40}{30} = 1.33\,\text{V}$$

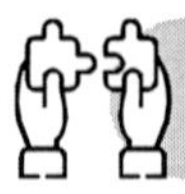

18.3 Concept Practice Problems

CPP

26. In a metre bridge, the balancing length from the left end (standard resistance of one ohm is in the right gap) is found to be 20 cm. The value of the unknown resistance is

(a) 0.8 Ω (b) 0.5 Ω (c) 0.4 Ω (d) 0.25 Ω

27. An ammeter has a resistance of G ohm and a range of I amp. The value of resistance used in parallel to convert it into an ammeter of range nI amp is

(a) nG (b) (n – 1)G (c) G/n (d) G/(n – 1)

28. Potentiometer measures potential more accurately because

(a) it measures potential in open circuit
(b) it uses sensitive galvanometer for null deflection
(c) it uses high resistance potentiometer wire
(d) it measures potential in closed circuit

29. A potentiometer consists of a wire of length 4m and resistance 10Ω. It is connected to a cell of e.m.f. 3V. The potential gradient of wire is

(a) 5V/m (b) 2V/m (c) 5V/m (d) 10V/m

30. Potentiometer wire of length 1 m is connected in series with 490Ω resistance and 2 V battery. If 0.2 mV/cm is the potential gradient, then resistance of the potentiometer wire is

(a) 4.9 Ω (b) 7.9 Ω (c) 5.9 Ω (d) 6.9 Ω

31. A galvanometer of 50 ohm resistance has 25 divisions. A current of 4×10^{-4} ampere gives a deflection of one division. To convert this galvanometer into a voltmeter having a range of 25 volts, it should be connected with a resistance of

(a) 2450 Ω in series. (b) 2500 Ω in series.
(c) 245 Ω in series. (d) 2550 Ω in series.

32. In an experiment to measure the internal resistance of a cell, by a potentiometer, it is found that the balance point is at a length of 2 m, when the cell is shunted by a 5 Ω resistance and is at a length of 3 m when the cell is shunted by a 10 Ω resistance. The internal resistance of the cell is then

(a) 1.5 Ω (b) 10 Ω (c) 15 Ω (d) 1 Ω

33. In the circuit shown below, if the resistance of voltmeter is 4 kΩ, then the error in the reading of voltmeter will be

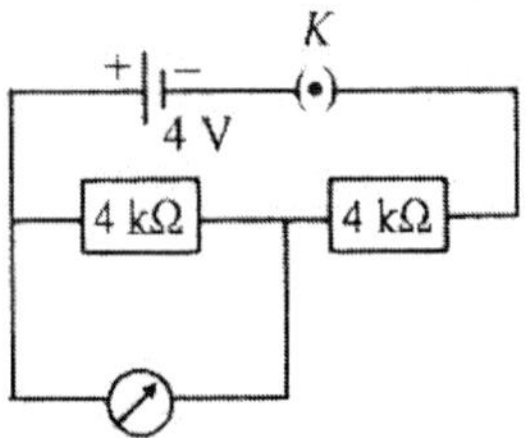

(a) 50% (b) 68% (c) 17% (d) 33.3%

34. A milli voltmeter of 25 milli volt range is to be converted into an ammeter of 25 ampere range. The value (in ohm) of necessary shunt will be

(a) 0.001 (b) 0.01 (c) 1 (d) 0.05

35. The resistance of the four arms P, Q, R and S in a Wheatstone's bridge are 10 ohm, 30 ohm, 30 ohm and 90 ohm, respectively. The e.m.f. and internal resistance of the cell are 7 volt and 5 ohm respectively. If the galvanometer resistance is 50 ohm, the current drawn from the cell will be

(a) 0.2 A (b) 0.1 A (c) 2.0 A (d) 1.0 A

ANSWER KEY

26	(d)	27	(d)	28	(a)	29	(a)	30	(a)	31	(a)	32	(b)	33	(d)	34	(a)	35	(a)

CONCEPT MAP

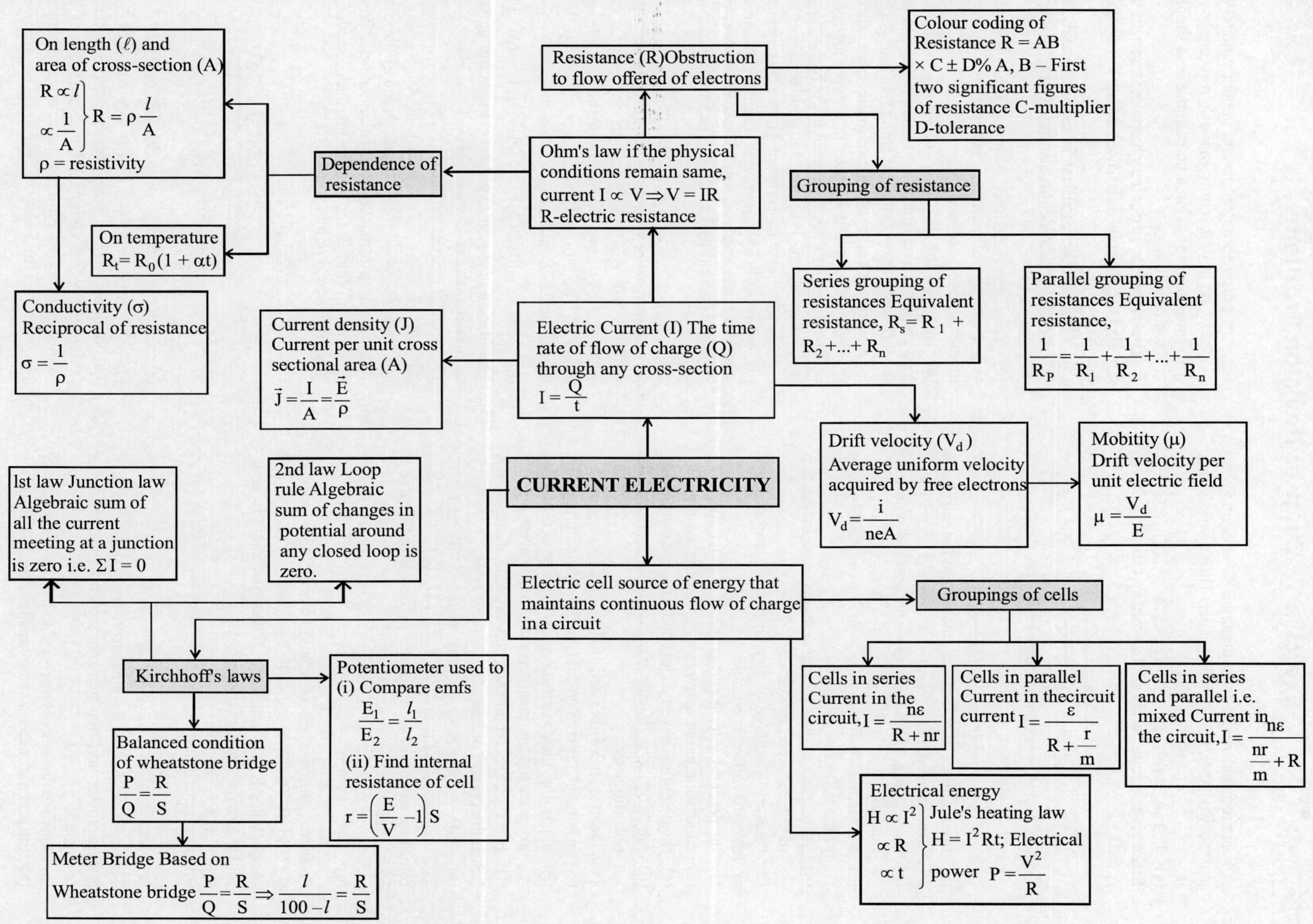

CURRENT ELECTRICITY

Electric Current (I) The time rate of flow of charge (Q) through any cross-section $I = \frac{Q}{t}$

Ohm's law if the physical conditions remain same, current $I \propto V \Rightarrow V = IR$ R-electric resistance

Resistance (R)Obstruction to flow offered of electrons

Colour coding of Resistance $R = AB \times C \pm D\%$ A, B – First two significant figures of resistance C-multiplier D-tolerance

Grouping of resistance

Series grouping of resistances Equivalent resistance, $R_s = R_1 + R_2 + ... + R_n$

Parallel grouping of resistances Equivalent resistance, $\frac{1}{R_P} = \frac{1}{R_1} + \frac{1}{R_2} + ... + \frac{1}{R_n}$

Dependence of resistance

On length (ℓ) and area of cross-section (A) $R \propto l$, $\propto \frac{1}{A}$ $\Big\} R = \rho \frac{l}{A}$ ρ = resistivity

On temperature $R_t = R_0(1 + \alpha t)$

Conductivity (σ) Reciprocal of resistance $\sigma = \frac{1}{\rho}$

Current density (J) Current per unit cross sectional area (A) $\vec{J} = \frac{I}{A} = \frac{\vec{E}}{\rho}$

Drift velocity (V_d) Average uniform velocity acquired by free electrons $V_d = \frac{i}{neA}$

Mobility (μ) Drift velocity per unit electric field $\mu = \frac{V_d}{E}$

Electric cell source of energy that maintains continuous flow of charge in a circuit

Groupings of cells

Cells in series Current in the circuit, $I = \frac{n\varepsilon}{R + nr}$

Cells in parallel Current in thecircuit current $I = \frac{\varepsilon}{R + \frac{r}{m}}$

Cells in series and parallel i.e. mixed Current in the circuit, $I = \frac{n\varepsilon}{\frac{nr}{m} + R}$

Electrical energy $H \propto I^2$, $\propto R$, $\propto t$ $\Big\}$ Jule's heating law $H = I^2Rt$; Electrical power $P = \frac{V^2}{R}$

Kirchhoff's laws

Ist law Junction law Algebraic sum of all the current meeting at a junction is zero i.e. $\Sigma I = 0$

2nd law Loop rule Algebraic sum of changes in potential around any closed loop is zero.

Potentiometer used to (i) Compare emfs $\frac{E_1}{E_2} = \frac{l_1}{l_2}$ (ii) Find internal resistance of cell $r = \left(\frac{E}{V} - 1\right)S$

Balanced condition of wheatstone bridge $\frac{P}{Q} = \frac{R}{S}$

Meter Bridge Based on Wheatstone bridge $\frac{P}{Q} = \frac{R}{S} \Rightarrow \frac{l}{100 - l} = \frac{R}{S}$

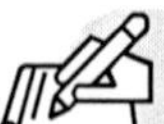

Exercise 1 - Chapter Revision Problems

CRP

1. A 4 ohm resistance wire is bent through 180° at its mid point and the two halves are twisted together. Then the resistance is
   (a) 1 Ω (b) 2 Ω (c) 5 Ω (d) 8 Ω
2. In the given circuit, as the sliding contact C is moved from A to B

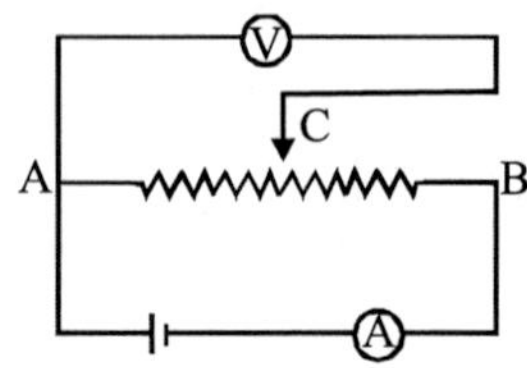

   (a) the readings of both the ammeter and the voltmeter remain constant
   (b) the reading of both the ammeter and the voltmeter increase
   (c) the reading of the ammeter remains constant but that of the voltmeter increases
   (d) the reading of the ammeter remains constant but that of the voltmeter decreases
3. For measuring voltage of any circuit, potentiometer is preferred to voltmeter because
   (a) the potentiometer is cheap and easy to handle.
   (b) calibration in the voltmeter is sometimes wrong.
   (c) the potential draws no current during measurement.
   (d) range of the voltmeter is not as wide as that of the potentiometer.
4. Two identical fuses are rated at 10 A. If they are joined
   (A) in parallel, the combination acts as a fuse of rating 20 A
   (B) in parallel, the combination acts as a fuse of rating 5 A
   (C) in series, the combination acts as a fuse of rating 10 A
   (D) in series, the combination acts as a fuse of rating 20 A
   Select the correct options.
   (a) A, B (b) A, C (c) B, D (d) B, C, D
5. The resistance of the coil of an ammeter is R. The shunt required to increase its range n-fold should have a resistance
   (a) $\frac{R}{n}$ (b) $\frac{R}{n-1}$ (c) $\frac{R}{n+1}$ (d) nR
6. A current source drives a current in a coil of resistance R_1 for a time t. The same source drives current in another coil of resistance R_2 for same time. If heat generated is same, find internal resistance of source.
   (a) $\frac{R_1R_2}{R_1+R_2}$ (b) R_1+R_2
   (c) zero (d) $\sqrt{R_1R_2}$
7. The emf developed is measured with the help of a potentiometer and not by a moving coil millivoltmeter because
   (a) the potentiometer is more accurate than the voltmeter
   (b) the potentiometer is more sensitive than voltmeter
   (c) the potentiometer makes measurement without drawing any current from the thermocouple
   (d) measurement using a potentiometer is simpler than with a voltmeter
8. Is it possible that any battery has some constant value of e.m.f but the potential difference between the plates is zero?
   (a) No
   (b) Yes, if another identical battery is joined in series.
   (c) Yes, if another identical battery is joined in opposition in series.
   (d) Yes, if another similar battery is joined in parallel.
9. Which of the following in electricity is analogous to momentum mv in dynamics ?
   (a) IV (b) IL (c) QL (d) IQ
10. You are given a resistance coil and a battery. In which of the following cases is largest amount of heat generated ?
   (a) When the coil is connected to the battery directly
   (b) When the coil is divided into two equal parts and both the parts are connected to the battery in parallel
   (c) When the coil is divided into four equal parts and all the four parts are connected to the battery in parallel
   (d) When only half the coil is connected to the battery
11. A primary cell has an e.m.f. of 1.5 volt. When short-circuited it gives a current of 3 ampere. The internal resistance of the cell is
   (a) 4.5 ohm (b) 2 ohm
   (c) 0.5 ohm (d) (1/4.5) ohm
12. A 100-W bulb and a 25-W bulb are designed for the same voltage. They have filaments of the same length and material. The ratio of the diameter of the 100-W bulb to that of the 25-W bulb is
   (a) 4 : 1 (b) 2 : 1 (c) $\sqrt{2}:1$ (d) 1 : 2
13. The amount of charge Q passed in time t through a cross-section of a wire is $Q = 5t^2 + 3t + 1$.
   The value of current at time t = 5 s is
   (a) 9 A (b) 49 A
   (c) 53 A (d) None of these
14. The four wires from a larger circuit intersect at junction A as shown. What is the magnitude and direction of the current between points A and B ?

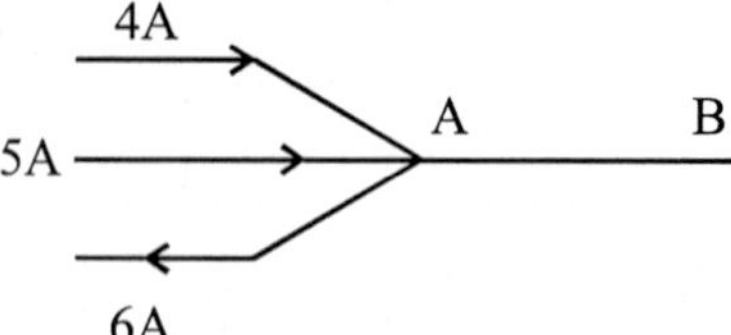

   (a) 2 A from A to B (b) 2A from B to A
   (c) 3A from A to B (d) 2A from B to A
15. The deflection in a galvanometer decreases from 25 divisions to 5 divisions when a resistor of 20Ω is connected in series. Find resistance of galvanometer.
   (a) 4 Ω (b) 5 Ω (c) 6 Ω (d) 7 Ω

16. In the equation AB = C, A is the current density, C is the electric field, Then B is
(a) resistivity (b) conductivity
(c) potential difference (d) resistance

17. A dynamo develops 0.5 A at 6 V. The energy which is generated in one second is
(a) 0.083 J (b) 3 J
(c) 12 J (d) None of these

18. A potentiometer wire, 10 m long, has a resistance of 40Ω. It is connected in series with a resistance box and a 2 V storage cell. If the potential gradient along the wire is 0.1 m V/cm, the resistance unplugged in the box is
(a) 260 Ω (b) 760 Ω (c) 960 Ω (d) 1060 Ω

19. If R_1 and R_2 are the filament resistances of 200 W and a 100 W bulb respectively both designed to run at the same voltage, then
(a) R_2 is four times of R_1 (b) R_1 is four times of R_2
(c) R_2 is two times of R_1 (d) R_1 is two times of R_2

20. Two identical batteries each of e.m.f. 2 V and internal resistance 1 Ω are available to produce heat in an external resistance by passing a current through it. The maximum power that can be developed across R using these batteries is
(a) 3.2 W (b) 2.0 W (c) 1.28 W (d) 8/9 W

21. A heater of 220 V heat a volume of water in 5 minutes time. A heater of 110 V heats the same volume of water in
(a) 5 minutes (b) 8 minutes
(c) 10 minutes (d) 20 minutes

22. The internal resistance of a primary cell is 4Ω. It generates a current of 0.2 A in an external reistance of 21 Ω. The rate of chemical energy consumed in providing the current is
(a) 0.42 J s^{-1} (b) 0.84 J s^{-1} (c) 1 J s^{-1} (d) 5 J s^{-1}

23. An electric lamp is marked 60 W, 220 V. The cost of kilo watt hour of electricity is ₹ 1.25. The cost of using this lamp on 220 V for 8 hours is
(a) ₹0.25 (b) ₹0.60 (c) ₹1.20 (d) ₹4.00

24. If current flowing in a conductor changes by 1% then power consumed will change by
(a) 10% (b) 2% (c) 1% (d) 100%

25. Each of the resistance in the network shown in fig. is equal to R. The resistance between the terminals A and B is

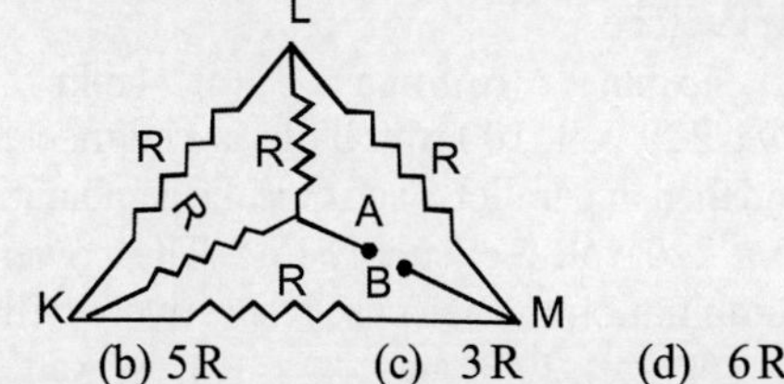

(a) R (b) 5 R (c) 3 R (d) 6 R

26. Four resistors are connected as shown in fig. A 6 V battery of negligible resistance is connected across terminal AC. The potential difference across terminals B, D will be

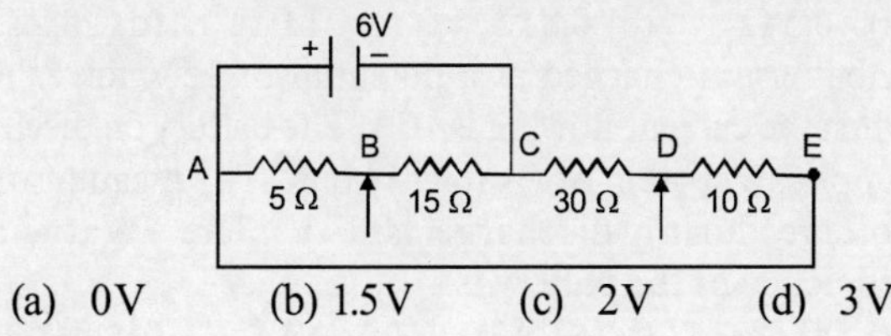

(a) 0V (b) 1.5 V (c) 2V (d) 3 V

27. A non-conducting ring of radius R has charge Q distributed unevenly over it. If it rotates with an angular velocity ω, the equivalent current will be
(a) zero (b) Qω (c) $Q\frac{\omega}{2\pi}$ (d) $Q\frac{\omega}{2\pi R}$

28. All the edges of a block with parallel faces are unequal. Its longest edge is twice its shortest edge. The ratio of the maximum to minimum resistance between parallel faces is
(a) 2 (b) 4
(c) 8
(d) indeterminate unless the length of the third edge is specified

29. In the network shown below, the ring has zero resistance. The equivalent resistance between the point A and B is
(a) 2R
(b) 4R
(c) 7R
(d) 10R

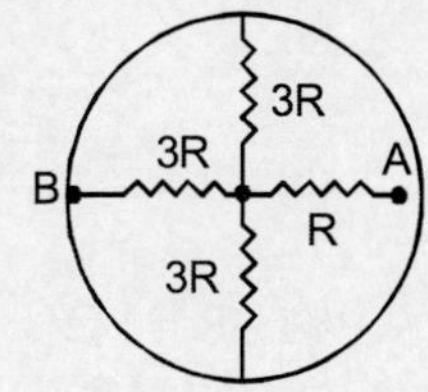

30. The belt of an electrostatic generator is 50 cm wide and travels at 30 cm/sec. The belt carries charge into the sphere at a rate corresponding to 10^{-4} ampere. What is the surface density of charge on the belt.
(a) 6.7×10^{-5} Cm^{-2}/s (b) 6.7×10^{-4} Cm^{-2}/s
(c) 6.7×10^{-7} Cm^{-2}/s (d) 6.7×10^{-8} Cm^{-2}/s

31. A wire has a resistance 12 Ω. It is bent in the form of a circle. The effective resistance between two points on any diameter is
(a) 6 Ω (b) 3 Ω (c) 12 Ω (d) 24 Ω

32. Current I_1 in the following circuit is

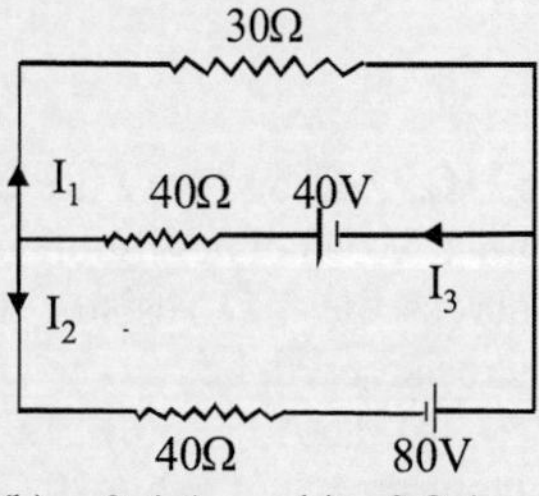

(a) 0.4A (b) – 0.4 A (c) 0.8 A (d) – 0.8 A

33. Three resistances are connected to form a T-shape as shown in the figure. Then the current in the 4K resistor is:

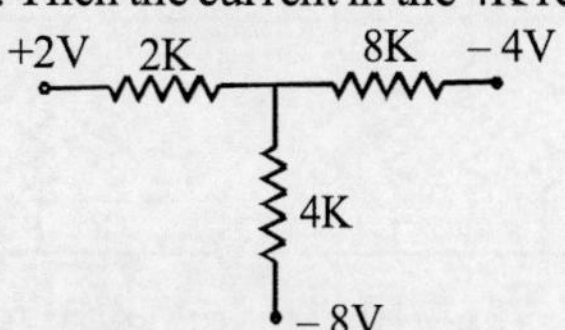

(a) 0.93mA (b) 1.42mA (c) 2.5mA (d) 1.57mA

34. Determine the current in 2Ω resistor.

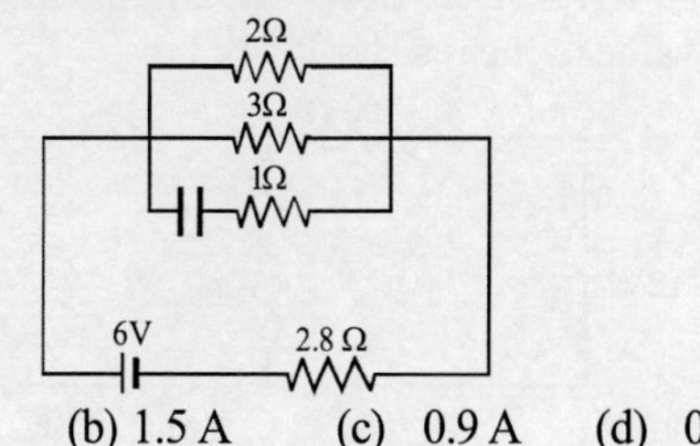

(a) 1 A (b) 1.5 A (c) 0.9 A (d) 0.6 A

35. There is an infinite wire grid with cells in the form of equilateral triangles. The resistance of each wire between neighbouring joint connections is R_0. The net resistance of the whole grid between the points A and B as shown is

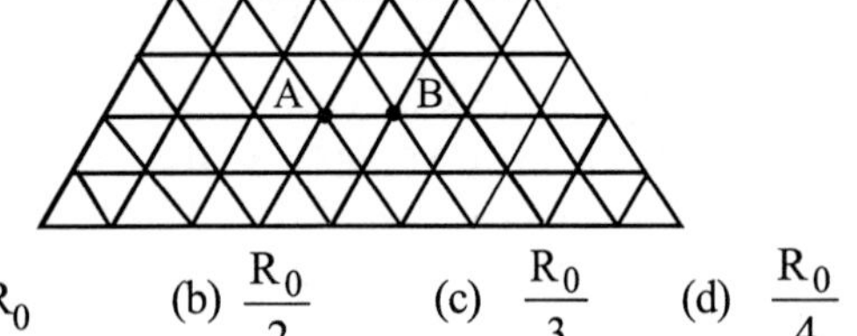

(a) R_0 (b) $\frac{R_0}{2}$ (c) $\frac{R_0}{3}$ (d) $\frac{R_0}{4}$

36. Twelve indentical resistors each of value 1Ω are connected as shown. Net resistance between C and D (R) is

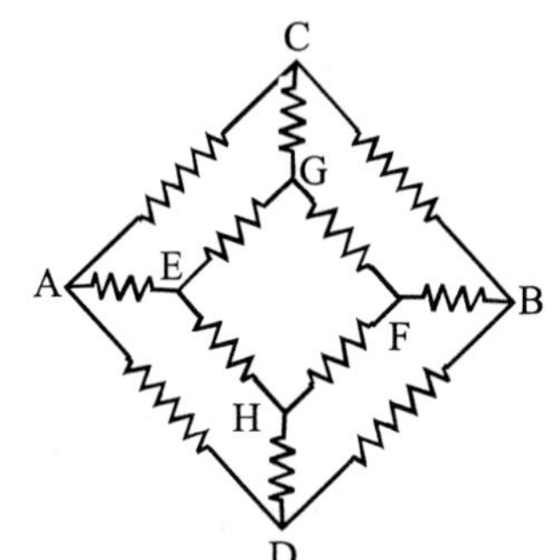

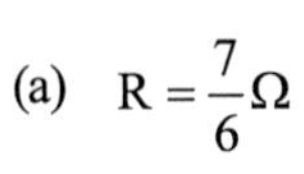
(a) $R = \frac{7}{6}\Omega$

(b) $R = \frac{4}{3}\Omega$

(c) $R = 1\Omega$

(d) $R = \frac{3}{4}\Omega$

37. In the network shown, each resistance is equal to R. The equivalent resistance between adjacent corners A and D is

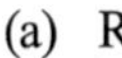
(a) R

(b) $\frac{2}{3}R$

(c) $\frac{3}{7}R$

(d) $\frac{8}{15}R$

38. Resistances 1 Ω, 2 Ω and 3 Ω are connected to form a triangle. If a 1.5 V cell of negligible internal resistance is connected across the 3 Ω resistor, the current flowing through this resistor will be

(a) 0.25 A (b) 0.5 A (c) 1.0 A (d) 1.5 A

39. Seven resistances, each of value 20 Ω, are connected to a 2 V battery as shown in the figure. The ammeter reading will be

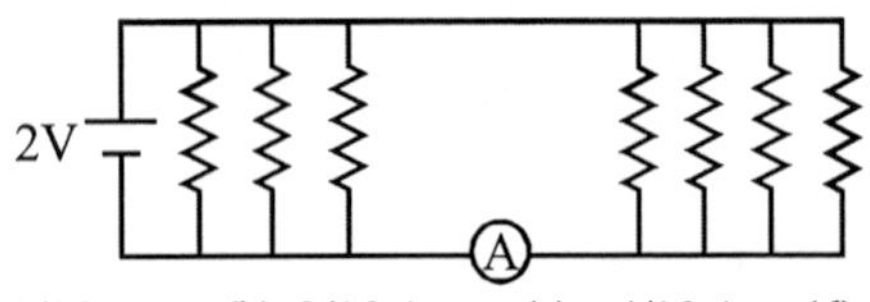

(a) 1/10 A (b) 3/10 A (c) 4/10 A (d) 7/10 A

40. In the circuit, the galvanometer G shows zero deflection. If the batteries A and B have negligible internal resistance, the value of the resistor R will be

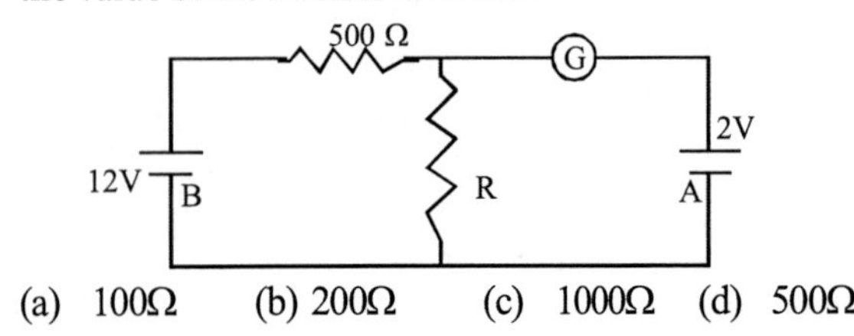

(a) 100Ω (b) 200Ω (c) 1000Ω (d) 500Ω

41. A 4 μ F conductor is charged 50 volts and then its plates are joined through a resistance of 1 k Ω. The heat produced in the resistance is

(a) 0.16 J (b) 1.28 J (c) 0.64 J (d) 0.32 J

42. A wire of resistance 20 Ω is covered with ice and a voltage of 210 V is applied across the wire, then rate of melting the ice is

(a) 0.85 g/s (b) 1.92 g/s
(c) 6.56 g/s (d) All of these

43. A 5–ampere fuse wire can withstand a maximum power of 1 watt in the circuit. The resistance of the fuse wire is

(a) 0.04 Ω (b) 0.2 Ω (c) 5 Ω (d) 0.4 Ω

44. Three equal resistors connected across a source of e.m.f. together dissipate 10 watt of power. What will be the power dissipated in watt if the same resistors are connected in parallel across the same source of e.m.f.?

(a) 10/3 (b) 10 (c) 30 (d) 90

45. Two 1000 W heaters when connected in parallel across 220 V supply produced heat Q_P in time t. If they are connected in series across the same power supply the heat produced in the same time is Q_S. What is Q_P/Q_S?

(a) 4 (b) 2 (c) 0.5 (d) 0.25.

46. A heating coil is labelled 100 W, 220 V. The coil is cut in half and the two pieces are joined in parallel to the same source. The energy now liberated per second is

(a) 25 J (b) 50 J (c) 200 J (d) 400 J

47. Five resistances have been connected as shown in the figure. The effective resistance between A & B is

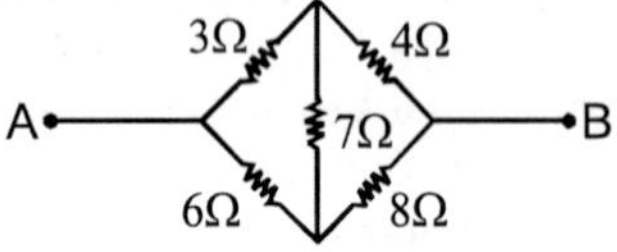

(a) 14/3Ω (b) 20/3Ω (c) 14Ω (d) 21Ω

48. An electric kettle has two heating coils. When one of the coils is connected to an a.c. source, the water in the kettle boils in 10 minutes. When the other coil is used the water boils in 40 minutes. If both the coils are connected in parallel, the time taken by the same quantity of water to boil will be

(a) 15 min (b) 8 min (c) 4 min (d) 25 min

49. Two 220 volt, 100 watt bulbs are connected first in series and then in parallel. Each time the combination is connected to a 220 volt a.c. supply line. The power drawn by the combination in each case respectively will be

(a) 50 watt, 200 watt (b) 50 watt, 100 watt
(c) 100 watt, 50 watt (d) 200 watt, 150 watt

50. The internal resistance of a 2.1 V cell which gives a current of 0.2 A through a resistance of 10 Ω is

(a) 0.5 Ω (b) 0.8 Ω (c) 1.0 Ω (d) 0.2 Ω

51. A battery is charged at a potential of 15V for 8 hours when the current flowing is 10A. The battery on discharge supplies a current of 5A for 15 hour. The mean terminal voltage during discharge is 14V. The "Watt-hour" efficiency of the battery is

(a) 87.5% (b) 82.5% (c) 80% (d) 90%

52. When three identical bulbs of 60 watt, 200 volt rating are connected in series to a 200 volt supply, the power drawn by them will be
(a) 20 watt (b) 60 watt (c) 180 watt (d) 10 watt

53. In India electricity is supplied for domestic use at 220 V. It is supplied at 110 V in USA. If the resistance of a 60 W bulb for use in India is R, the resistance of a 60 W bulb for use in USA will be
(a) R/2 (b) R (c) 2R (d) R/4

54. For the network shown in the figure the value of the current i is

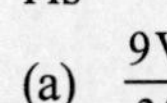

(a) $\frac{9V}{35}$
(b) $\frac{18V}{5}$
(c) $\frac{5V}{9}$
(d) $\frac{5V}{18}$

55. In the circuit shown in the figure, if potential at point A is taken to be zero, the potential at point B is

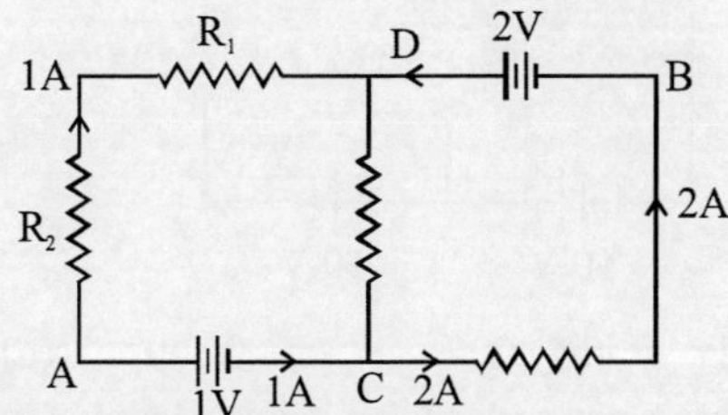

(a) –1V (b) +2V (c) –2V (d) +1V

56. The power dissipated in the circuit shown in the figure is 30 Watts. The value of R is
(a) 20 Ω
(b) 15 Ω
(c) 10 Ω
(d) 30 Ω

57. Cell having an emf ε and internal resistance r is connected across a variable external resistance R. As the resistance R is increased, the plot of potential difference V across R is given by

(a)
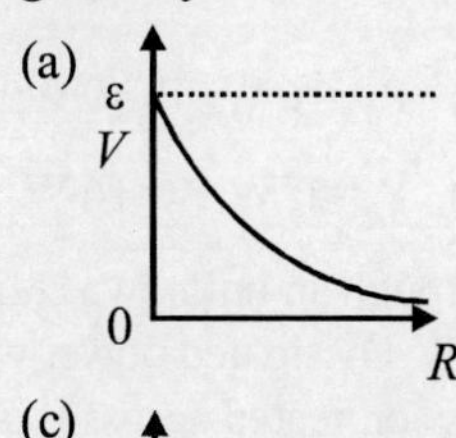

(b)

(c)
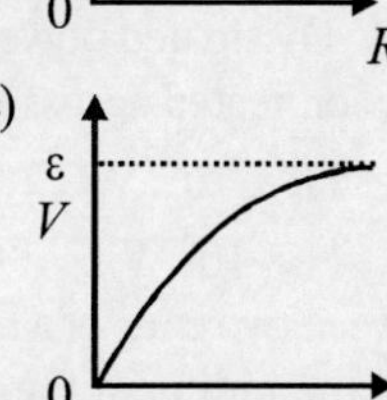

(d)
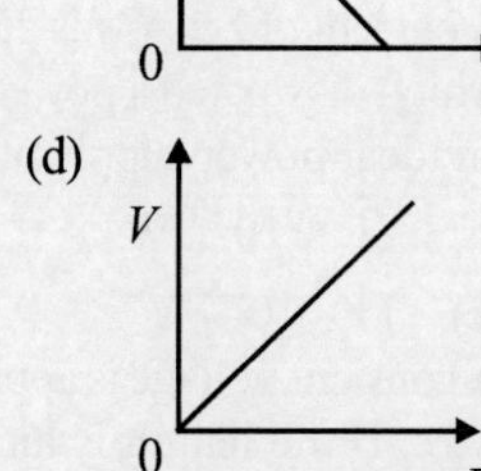

58. In the circuit shown the cells A and B have negligible resistances. For $V_A = 12V$, $R_1 = 500\Omega$ and $R = 100\Omega$ the galvanometer (G) shows no deflection. The value of V_B is

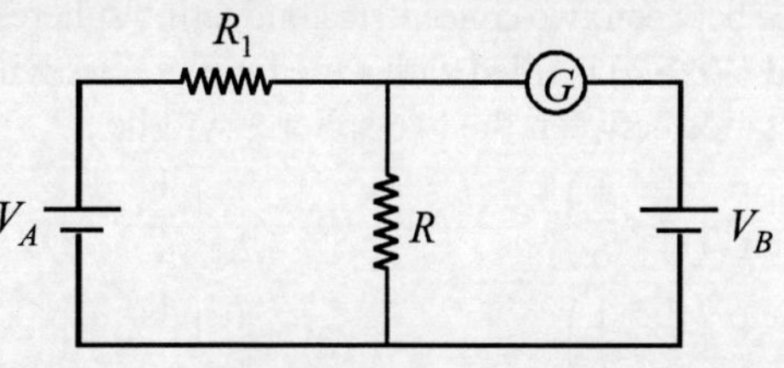

(a) 4 V (b) 2 V (c) 12 V (d) 6 V

59. If voltage across a bulb rated 220 Volt-100 Watt drops by 2.5% of its rated value, the percentage of the rated value by which the power would decrease is
(a) 20% (b) 2.5% (c) 5% (d) 10%

60. A wire of resistance 4 Ω is stretched to twice its original length. The resistance of stretched wire would be
(a) 4 Ω (b) 8 Ω (c) 16 Ω (d) 2 Ω

61. To verify Ohm's law, a student connects the voltmeter across the battery as, shown in the figure. The measured voltage is plotted as a function of the current, and the following graph is obtained :

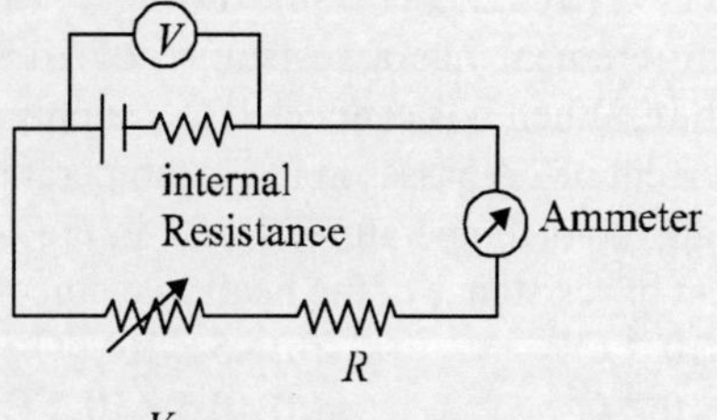

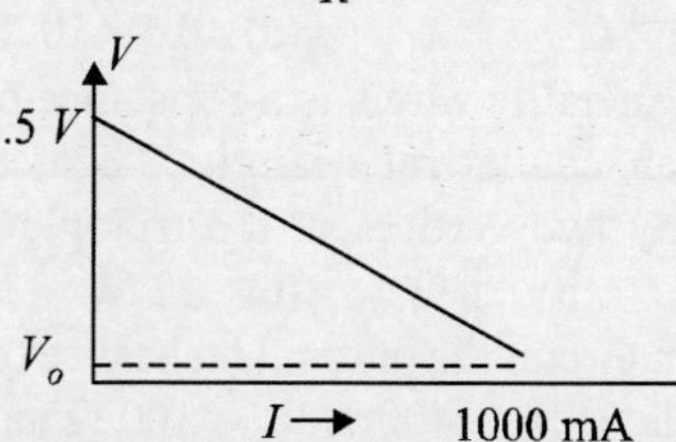

If V_0 is almost zero, identify the correct statement:
(a) The emf of the battery is 1.5 V and its internal resistance is 1.5 Ω
(b) The value of the resistance R is 1.5 Ω
(c) The potential difference across the battery is 1.5 V when it sends a current of 1000 mA
(d) The emf of the battery is 1.5 V and the value of R is 1.5 Ω

62. In an experiment, the resistance of a material is plotted as a function of temperature (in some range). As shown in the figure, it is a straight line.

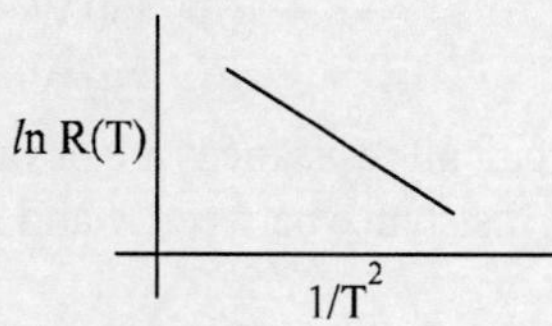

One may canclude that:

(a) $R(T) = \frac{R_0}{T^2}$ (b) $R(T) = R_0 e^{-T_0^2/T^2}$

(c) $R(T) = R_0 e^{-T^2/T_0^2}$ (d) $R(T) = R_0 e^{T^2/T_0^2}$

63. Space between two concentric conducting spheres of radii a and b ($b > a$) is filled with a medium of resistivity ρ. The resistance between the two spheres will be :

(a) $\frac{\rho}{4\pi}\left(\frac{1}{a}-\frac{1}{b}\right)$ (b) $\frac{\rho}{2\pi}\left(\frac{1}{a}-\frac{1}{b}\right)$

(c) $\frac{\rho}{2\pi}\left(\frac{1}{a}+\frac{1}{b}\right)$ (d) $\frac{\rho}{4\pi}\left(\frac{1}{a}+\frac{1}{b}\right)$

64. A resistance is shown in the figure. Its value and tolerance are given respectively by:

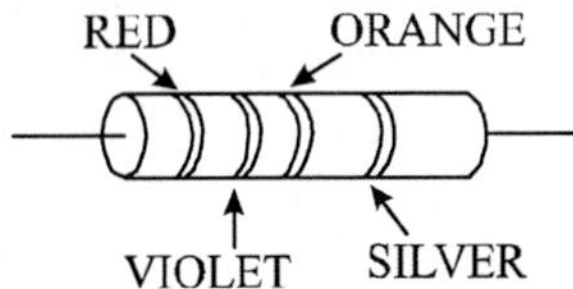

(a) 270 Ω, 10% (b) 27 kΩ, 10%
(c) 27 kΩ, 20% (d) 270 Ω, 5%

65. A copper wire is stretched to make it 0.5% longer. The percentage change in its electrical resistance if its volume remains unchanged is:

(a) 2.0% (b) 2.5% (c) 1.0% (d) 0.5%

66. A heating element has a resistance of 100Ω at room temperature. When it is connected to a supply of 220 V, a steady current of 2 A passes in it and temperature is 500°C more than room temperature. What is the temperature coefficient of resistance of the heating element?

(a) $1 \times 10^{-4}\,°C^{-1}$ (b) $5 \times 10^{-4}\,°C^{-1}$
(c) $2 \times 10^{-4}\,°C^{-1}$ (d) $0.5 \times 10^{-4}\,°C^{-1}$

67. A uniform metallic wire has a resistance of 18 Ω and is bent into an equilateral triangle. Then, the resistance between any two vertices of the triangle is:

(a) 4 Ω (b) 8 Ω (c) 12 W (d) 2 W

68. In the given circuit the internal resistance of the 18 V cell is negligible. If R_1 = 400Ω, R_3 = 100 Ω and R_4 = 500 Ω and the reading of an ideal voltmeter across R_4 is 5 V, then the value of R_2 will be:

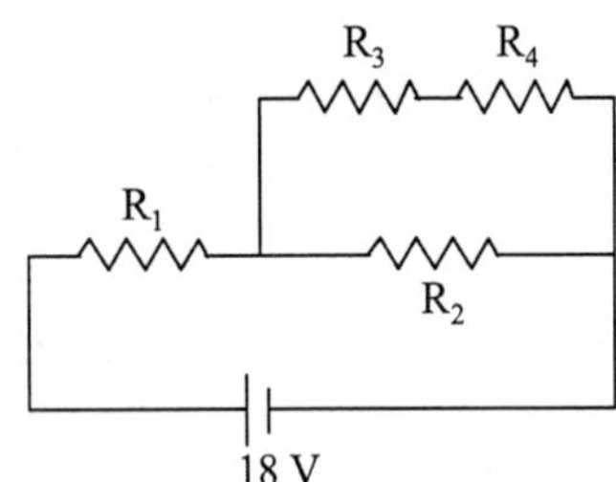

(a) 300 W (b) 450 W
(c) 550 W (d) 230 W

69. In the given circuit all resistances are of value R ohm each. The equivalent resistance between A and B is :

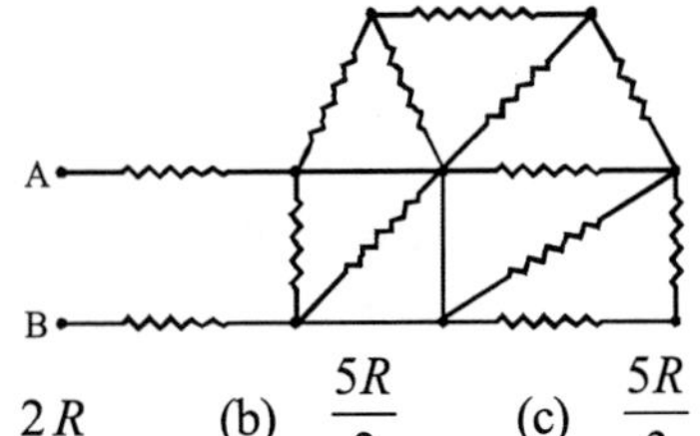

(a) $2R$ (b) $\frac{5R}{2}$ (c) $\frac{5R}{3}$ (d) $3R$

70. The value of current i_1 flowing from A to C in the circuit diagram is :

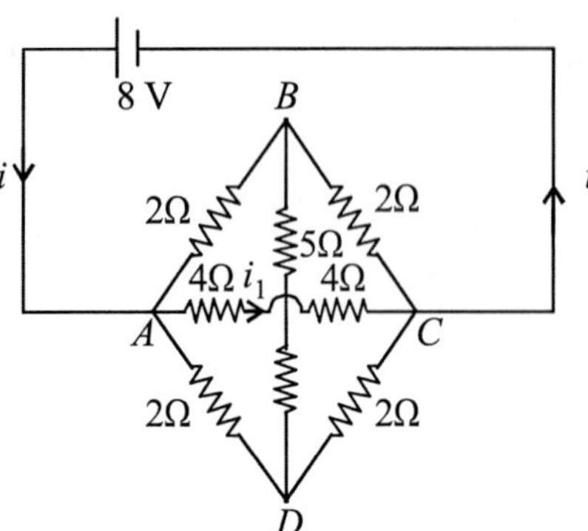

(a) 2 A (b) 4 A (c) 1 A (d) 5 A

71. In the given circuit the cells have zero internal resistance. The currents (in Amperes) passing through resistance R_1 and R_2 respectively, are:

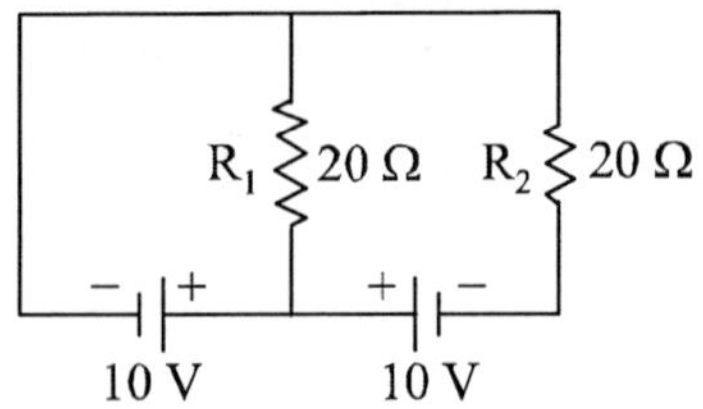

(a) 1, 2 (b) 2, 2 (c) 0.5, 0 (d) 0, 1

72. The resistive network shown below is connected to a D.C. source of 16 V. The power consumed by the network is 4 Watt. The value of R is :

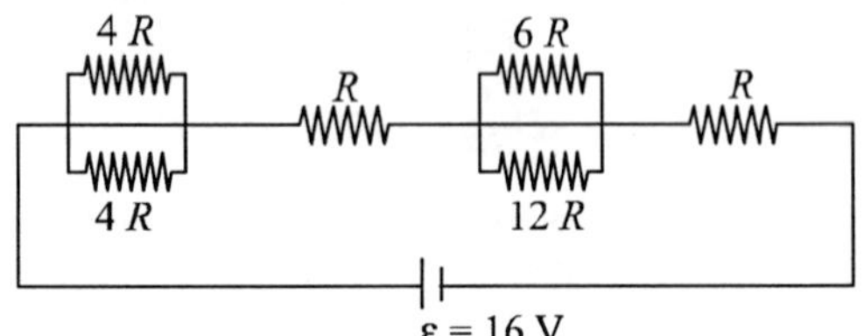

(a) 6Ω (b) 8Ω (c) 1Ω (d) 16Ω

73. Two electric bulbs, rated at (25 W, 220 V) and (100 W, 220 V), are connected in series across a 220 V voltage source. If the 25 W and 100 W bulbs draw powers P_1 and P_2 respectively, then:

(a) P_1=16 W, P_2=4 W (b) P_1=16 W, P_2=9 W
(c) P_1=9 W, P_2=16 W (d) P_1=4 W, P_2=16 W

74. A current of 2 mA was passed through an unknown resistor which dissipated a power of 4.4 W. Dissipated power when an ideal power supply of 11 V is connected across it is:

(a) 11×10^{-5} W (b) 11×10^{-3} W
(c) 11×10^{-4} W (d) 11×10^{5} W

75. A constant voltage is applied between two ends of a metallic wire. If the length is halved and the radius of the wire is doubled, the rate of heat developed in the wire will be:

(a) Increased 8 times (b) Doubled
(c) Halved (d) Unchanged

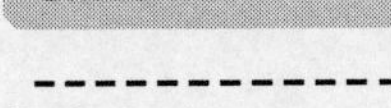

Exercise 2 - Exemplar & Past Year Questions

E&PYQs

Exemplar Questions

1. Consider a current carrying wire (current I) in the shape of a circle.
   (a) source of emf
   (b) electric field produced by charges accumulated on the surface of wire
   (c) the charges just behind a given segment of wire which push them just the right way by repulsion
   (d) the charges ahead
2. Two batteries of emf ε_1 and $\varepsilon_2(\varepsilon_2 > \varepsilon_1)$ and internal resistances r_1 and r_2 respectively are connected in parallel as shown in figure.
   (a) Two equivalent emf ε_{eq} of the two cells is between ε_1 and ε_2, i.e., $\varepsilon_1 < \varepsilon_{eq} < \varepsilon_2$
   (b) The equivalent emf ε_{eq} is smaller than ε_1
   (c) The ε_{eq} is given by $\varepsilon_{eq} = \varepsilon_1 + \varepsilon_2$ always
   (d) ε_{eq} is independent of internal resistances r_1 and r_2

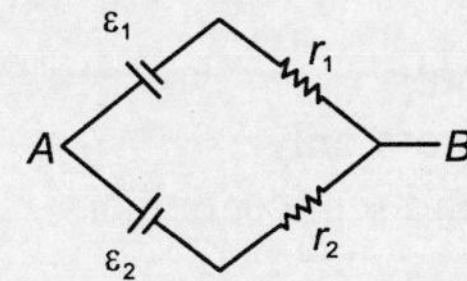

3. A resistance R is to be measured using a meter bridge, student chooses the standard resistance S to be 100Ω. He finds the null point at $l_1 = 2.9$ cm. He is told to attempt to improve the accuracy.
   Which of the following is a useful way?
   (a) He should measure I_1 more accurately
   (b) He should change 5 to 1000Ω and repeat the experiment
   (c) He should change S to 3Ω and repeat the experiment
   (d) He should given up hope of a more accurate measurement with a meter bridge
4. Two cells of emfs approximately 5 V and 10 V are to be accurately compared using a potentiometer of length 400 cm.
   (a) The battery that runs the potentiometer should have voltage of 8V
   (b) The battery of potentiometer can have a voltage of 15 V and R adjusted so that the potential drop across the wire slightly exceeds 10 V
   (c) The first portion of 50 cm of wire itself should have a potential drop of 10 V
   (d) Potentiometer is usually used for comparing resistances and not voltages
5. A metal rod of length 10 cm and a rectangular cross-section of $1\text{cm} \times \frac{1}{2}$ cm is connected to a battery across opposite faces. The resistance will be
   (a) maximum when the battery is connected across $1 \text{ cm} \times \frac{1}{2}$ cm faces
   (b) maximum when the battery is connected across 10 cm × 1 cm faces
   (c) maximum when the battery is connected across 10 cm $\times \frac{1}{2}$ cm faces
   (d) same irrespective of the three faces
6. Which of the following characteristics of electrons determines the current in a conductor?
   (a) Drift velocity alone
   (b) Thermal velocity alone
   (c) Both drift velocity and thermal velocity
   (d) Neither drift nor thermal velocity

NEET/AIPMT (2013-2020) Questions

7. The internal resistance of a 2.1 V cell which gives a current of 0.2 A through a resistance of 10 Ω is **[2013]**
   (a) 0.5 Ω (b) 0.8 Ω (c) 1.0 Ω (d) 0.2 Ω
8. The resistance of the four arms P, Q, R and S in a Wheatstone's bridge are 10 ohm, 30 ohm, 30 ohm and 90 ohm, respectively. The e.m.f. and internal resistance of the cell are 7 volt and 5 ohm respectively. If the galvanometer resistance is 50 ohm, the current drawn from the cell will be **[2013]**
   (a) 0.2 A (b) 0.1 A (c) 2.0 A (d) 1.0 A
9. Ten identical cells connected in series are needed to heat a wire of length one meter and radius '*r*' by 10°C in time '*t*'. How many cells will be required to heat the wire of length two meter of the same radius by the same temperature in time '*t*'? **[NEET Kar. 2013]**
   (a) 10 (b) 20 (c) 30 (d) 40
10. A potentiometer circuit has been set up for finding the internal resistance of a given cell. The main battery used across the potentiometer wire, has an emf of 2.0 V and a negligible internal resistance. The potentiometer wire itself is 4m long, When the resistace R, connected across the given cell, has values of
    (i) infinity (ii) 9.5Ω
    The balancing lengths', on the potentiometer wire are found to be 3 m and 2.85 m, respectively. The value of internal resistance of the cell is **[2014]**
    (a) 0.25Ω (b) 0.95Ω (c) 0.5Ω (d) 0.75Ω
11. In an ammeter 0.2% of main current passes through the galvanometer. If resistance of galvanometer is G, the resistance of ammeter will be : **[2014]**
    (a) $\frac{1}{499}G$ (b) $\frac{499}{500}G$ (c) $\frac{1}{500}G$ (d) $\frac{500}{499}G$
12. Two cities are 150 km apart. Electric power is sent from one city to another city through copper wires. The fall of potential per km is 8 volt and the average resistance per km is 0.5 Ω. The power loss in the wires is : **[2014]**
    (a) 19.2 W (b) 19.2 kW (c) 19.2 J (d) 12.2 kW
13. Across a metallic conductor of non-uniform cross section a constant potential difference is applied. The quantity which remains constant along the conductor is : **[2015]**
    (a) current (b) drift velocity
    (c) electric field (d) current density

14. A potentiometer wire has length 4 m and resistance 8Ω. The resistance that must be connected in series with the wire and an accumulator of e.m.f. 2V, so as to get a potential gradient 1 mV per cm on the wire is *[2015]*
(a) 40 Ω (b) 44 Ω (c) 48 Ω (d) 32 Ω

15. A, B and C are voltmeters of resistance R, 1.5 R and 3R respectively as shown in the figure. When some potential difference is applied between X and Y, the voltmeter readings are V_A, V_B and V_C respectively. Then *[2015]*

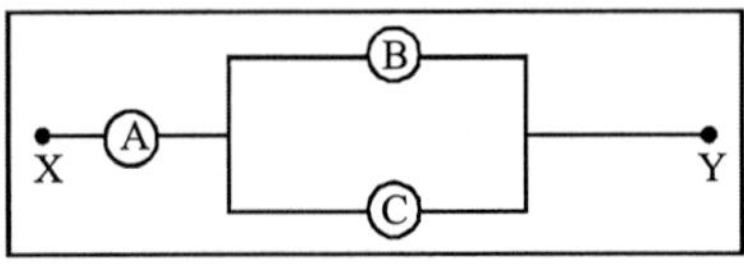

(a) $V_A \neq V_B = V_C$ (b) $V_A = V_B \neq V_C$
(c) $V_A \neq V_B \neq V_C$ (d) $V_A = V_B = V_C$

16. A circuit contains an ammeter, a battery of 30V and a resistance 40.8Ω all connected in series. If the ammeter has a coil of resistance 480Ω and a shunt of 20Ω, the reading in the ammeter will be: *[2015 RS]*
(a) 0.25 A (b) 2A (c) 1 A (d) 0.5 A

17. The charge flowing through a resistance R varies with time t as $Q = at - bt^2$, where a and b are positive constants. The total heat produced in R is: *[2016]*
(a) $\frac{a^3R}{6b}$ (b) $\frac{a^3R}{3b}$ (c) $\frac{a^3R}{2b}$ (d) $\frac{a^3R}{b}$

18. A potentiometer wire is 100 cm long and a constant potential difference is maintained across it. Two cells are connected in series first to support one another and then in opposite direction. The balance points are obtained at 50 cm and 10 cm from the positive end of the wire in the two cases. The ratio of emf's is : *[2016]*
(a) 5 : 1 (b) 5 : 4 (c) 3 : 4 (d) 3 : 2

19. A potentiometer is an accurate and versatile device to make electrical measurements of E.M.F. because the method involves *[2017]*
(a) Potential gradients
(b) A condition of no current flow through the galvanometer
(c) A combination of cells, galvanometer and resistances
(d) Cells

20. The resistance of a wire is 'R' ohm. If it is melted and stretched to 'n' times its original length, its new resistance will be :- *[2017]*
(a) $\frac{R}{n}$ (b) n^2R (c) $\frac{R}{n^2}$ (d) nR

21. A carbon resistor of (47 ± 4.7) kΩ is to be marked with rings of different colours for its identification. The colour code sequence will be *[2018]*
(a) Violet – Yellow – Orange – Silver
(b) Yellow – Violet – Orange – Silver
(c) Green – Orange – Violet – Gold
(d) Yellow – Green – Violet – Gold

22. A set of 'n' equal resistors, of value 'R' each, are connected in series to a battery of emf 'E' and internal resistance 'R'. The current drawn is I. Now, the 'n' resistors are connected in parallel to the same battery. Then the current drawn from battery becomes 10 I. The value of 'n' is *[2018]*
(a) 10 (b) 11 (c) 9 (d) 20

23. Which of the following acts as a circuit protection device? *[2019]*
(a) fuse (b) conductor
(c) inductor (d) switch

24. The solids which have the negative temperature coefficient of resistance are: *[2020]*
(a) insulators only
(b) semiconductors only
(c) insulators and semiconductors
(d) metals

25. The color code of a resistance is given below

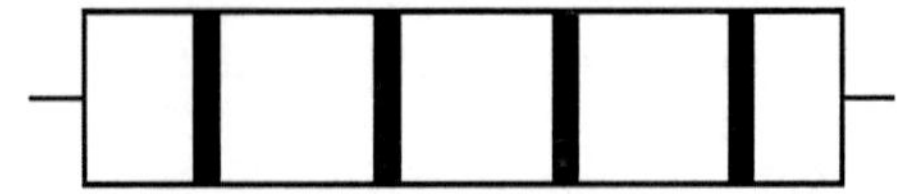

Yellow Violet Brown Gold

The values of resistance and tolerance, respectively, are *[2020]*
(a) 47 kΩ, 10% (b) 4.7 kΩ, 5%
(c) 470 Ω, 5% (d) 470 kΩ, 5%

26. A charged particle having drift velocity of 7.5×10^{-4} m s^{-1} in an electric field of 3×10^{-10} Vm^{-1}, has a mobility in $m^2 V^{-1} s^{-1}$ of: *[2020]*
(a) 2.5×10^6 (b) 2.5×10^{-6}
(c) 2.25×10^{-15} (d) 2.25×10^{15}

Exercise 3 - Concept Application Problems CAP

1. Three copper wires of lengths and cross sectional areas are (ℓ, A), (2 ℓ, A/2) and (ℓ/2, 2A). Resistance is minimum in
(a) wire of cross-sectional area A/2
(b) wire of cross-sectional area A
(c) wire of cross-sectional area 2A
(d) same in all the three cases

2. In an household electric circuit, which of the following is/are correct?
(A) All electric appliances drawing power are joined in parallel
(B) A switch may be either in series or in parallel with the appliance which it controls
(C) If a switch is in parallel with an appliance, it will draw power when the switch is in the 'off' position (open)
(D) If a switch is in parallel with an appliance, the fuse will blow (burn out) when the switch is put 'on' closed.
(a) A, D (b) A, C, D (c) B, C, D (d) A, B, D

3. If R_1 and R_2 are respectively the filament resistances of a 200 watt bulb and a 100 watt bulb designed to operate on the same voltage
   (a) R_1 is two times R_2 (b) R_2 is two times R_1
   (c) R_2 is four times R_1 (d) R_1 is four times R_2
4. A torch bulb rated as 4.5 W, 1.5 V is connected as shown in fig. The e.m.f. of the cell, needed to make the bulb glow at full intensity is

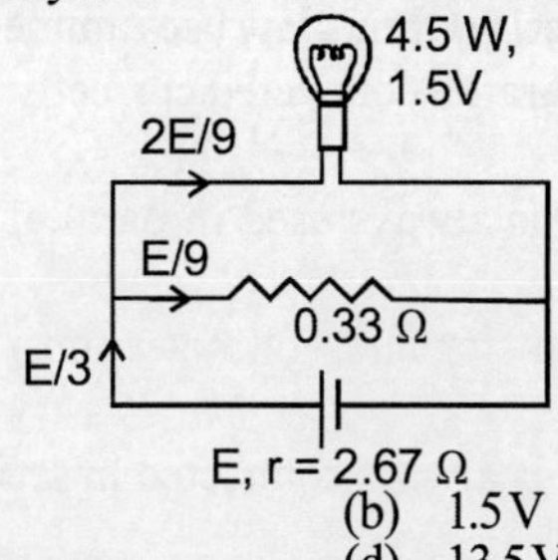

   (a) 4.5 V (b) 1.5 V
   (c) 2.67 V (d) 13.5 V
5. A capacitor of 10μ F has a pot. difference of 40 volts across it. If it is discharged in 0.2 second, the average current during discharge is
   (a) 2 mA (b) 4 mA (c) 1 mA (d) 0.5 mA
6. Two heating wires of equal length are first connected in series and then in parallel to a constant voltage source. The rate of heat produced in two cases is (parallel to series)
   (a) 1 : 4 (b) 4 : 1 (c) 1 : 2 (d) 2 : 1
7. A wire of radius r and another wire of radius 2r, both of same material and length are connected in series to each other. The combination is connected across a battery. The ratio of the heats produced in the two wires will be
   (a) 4.00 (b) 2.00 (c) 0.50 (d) 0.25
8. To get maximum current in a resistance of 3 ohms, one can use n rows of m cells (connected in series) connected in parallel. If the total number of cells is 24 and the internal resistance of a cell is 0.5 ohms then
   (a) m = 12, n = 2 (b) m = 8, n = 3
   (c) m = 2, n = 12 (d) m = 6, n = 4
9. A 4 m long wire of resistance 8 Ω is connected in series with a battery of e.m.f. 2 V and a resistor of 7 Ω. The internal resistance of the battery is 1 Ω. What is the potential gradient along the wire?
   (a) $1.00\ \text{V m}^{-1}$ (b) $0.75\ \text{V m}^{-1}$
   (c) $0.50\ \text{V m}^{-1}$ (d) $0.25\ \text{V m}^{-1}$
10. The length of a given cylindrical wire is increased by 100%. Due to the consequent decrease in diameter the change in the resistance of the wire will be
    (a) 100% (b) 50% (c) 300% (d) 200%
11. Two resistances R_1 and R_2 are made of different materials. The temperature coefficient of the material of R_1 is α and that of material of R_2 is – β. The resistance of the series combination of R_1 and R_2 will not change with temperature if $\frac{R_1}{R_2}$ equal to
    (a) $\frac{\alpha}{\beta}$ (b) $\frac{\alpha+\beta}{\alpha-\beta}$ (c) $\frac{\alpha^2+\beta^2}{2\alpha\beta}$ (d) $\frac{\beta}{\alpha}$
12. The equivalent resistance between A and B is

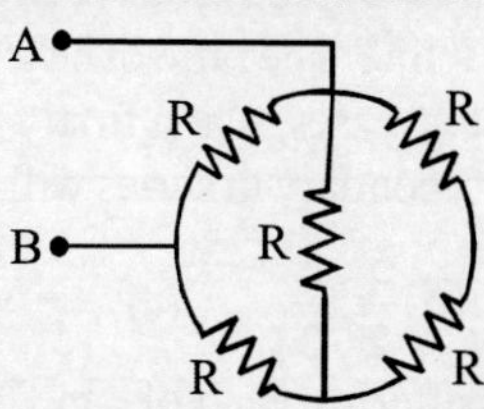

    (a) $\frac{8R}{5}$ (b) $\frac{5R}{8}$ (c) $\frac{3R}{8}$ (d) $\frac{7R}{8}$
13. Twelve resistors each of resistance 16Ω are connected in the circuit as shown. The net resistance between AB is

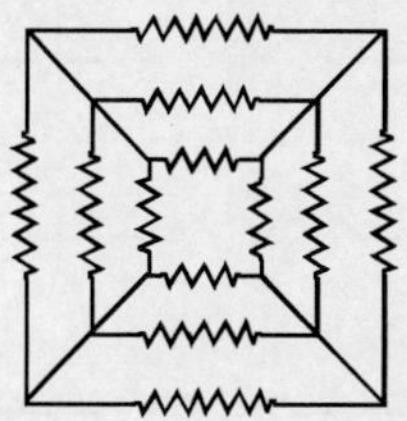

    (a) 1Ω (b) 2Ω(c) 3Ω (d) 4Ω
14. A battery of e.m.f E and internal resistance r is connected to a variable resistor R as shown. Which one of the following is true ?

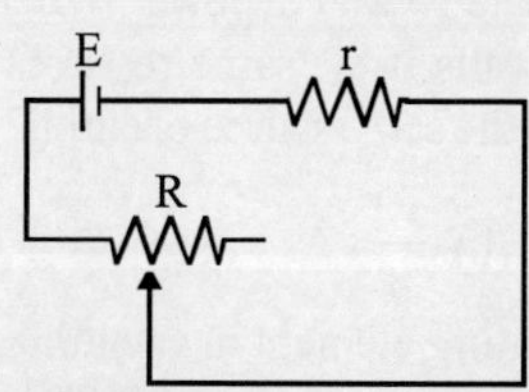

    (a) Potential difference across the terminals of the battery is maximum where R = r
    (b) Power delivered to resistor is maximum when R = r
    (c) Current in the circuit is maximum when R = r
    (d) Current in the circuit is maximum when R >> r
15. The numerical value of charge on either plate of capacitor C shown in figure is

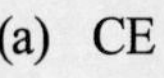

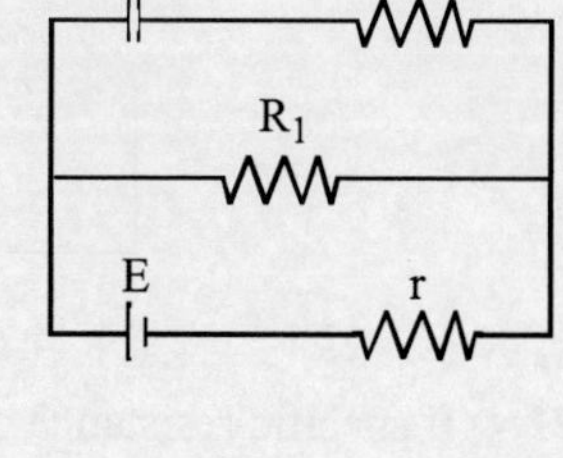

    (a) CE
    (b) $\frac{CER_1}{R_1+r}$
    (c) $\frac{CER_2}{R_2+r}$
    (d) $\frac{CER_1}{R_2+r}$
16. In the circuit shown, the internal resistance of the cell is negligible. The steady state current in the 2Ω resistor is

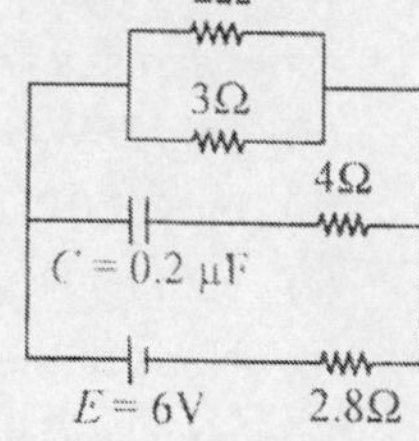

    (a) 0.6 A
    (b) 0.9 A
    (c) 1.2 A
    (d) 1.5 A

17. Two bulbs of 500 W and 200 W are manufactured to operate on 220 V line. The ratio of heat produced in 500 W and 200 W, in two cases, when firstly they are connected in parallel and secondary in series will be

(a) $\frac{5}{2}:\frac{2}{5}$ (b) $\frac{5}{2}:\frac{5}{2}$ (c) $\frac{2}{5}:\frac{5}{2}$ (d) $\frac{2}{5}:\frac{2}{5}$

18. Two identical batteries, each of e.m.f. 2 volt and internal resistance 1.0 ohm are available to produce heat in a resistance R = 0.5 Ω, by passing a current through it. The maximum power that can be developed across R using these batteries is

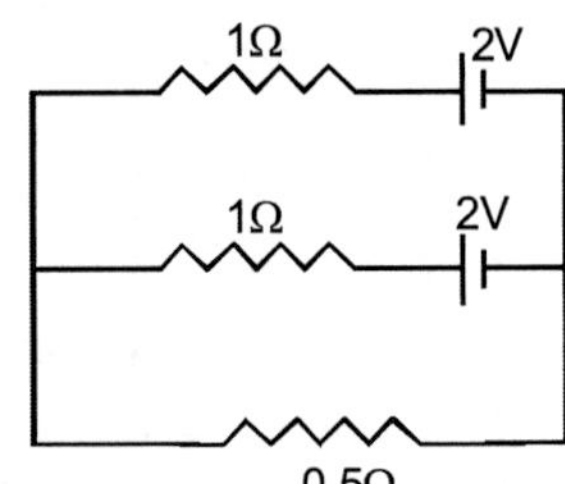

(a) 1.28 W (b) 2.0 W (c) 8/9 W (d) 3.2 W

19. Three equal resistors connected across a source of e.m.f. together dissipate 10 watt of power. What will be the power dissipated in watts if the same resistors are connected in parallel across the same source of e.m.f.?

(a) 10 (b) $\frac{10}{3}$ (c) 30 (d) 90

20. An electric heating element in vacuum is surrounded by a cavity at constant temperature of 227°C; it consumes 60W of power to maintain a temperature of 727°C. What is the power consumed by the element to maintain a temperature of 1227° C?

(a) 101 W (b) 304 W (c) 90 W (d) 320 W

21. In the circuit shown in figure, the 5Ω resistance develops 20.00 cal/s due to the current flowing through it. The heat developed in 2 Ω resistance (in cal/s) is

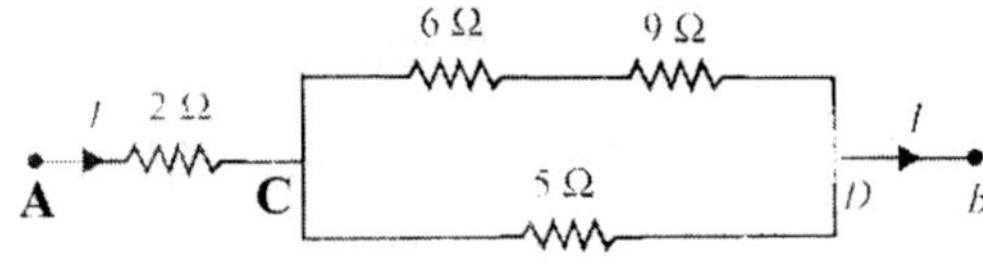

(a) 23.8 (b) 14.2 (c) 11.9 (d) 7.1

22. If specific resistance of a potentiometer wire is 10^{-7}Ωm current flowing through it, is 0.1 amp and cross sectional area of wire is 10^{-6} m^2, then potential gradient will be

(a) 10^{-2} volt/m (b) 10^{-4} volt/m
(c) 10^{-6} volt/m (d) 10^{-8} volt/m

23. If 25W, 220 V and 100 W, 220 V bulbs are connected in series across a 440 V line, then

(a) only 25W bulb will fuse
(b) only 100W bulb will fuse
(c) both bulbs will fuse
(d) None of these

24. Five equal resistances each of resistance R are connected as shown in the figure. A battery of V volts is connected between A and B. The current flowing in AFCEB will be

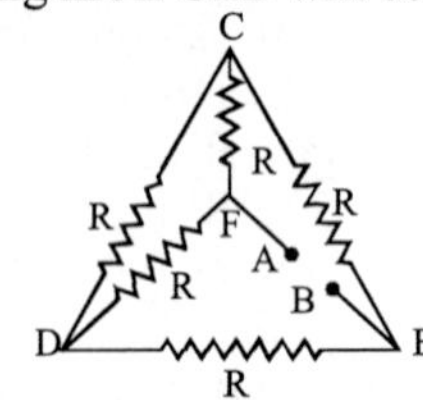

(a) $\frac{2V}{R}$ (b) $\frac{3V}{R}$
(c) $\frac{V}{R}$ (d) $\frac{V}{2R}$

25. A circuit to verify Ohm's law uses ammeter and voltmeter in series or parallel connected correctly to the resistor. In the circuit :

(a) ammeter is always used in parallel and voltmeter is series
(b) Both ammeter and voltmeter must be connected in parallel
(c) ammeter is always connected in series and voltmeter in parallel
(d) Both, ammeter and voltmeter must be connected in series

26. Consider four conducting materials copper, tungsten, mercury and aluminium with resistivity ρ_C, ρ_T, ρ_M and ρ_A respectively. Then :

(a) $\rho_C > \rho_A > \rho_T$ (b) $\rho_M > \rho_A > \rho_C$
(c) $\rho_A > \rho_T > \rho_C$ (d) $\rho_A > \rho_M > \rho_C$

27. A current of 5 A passes through a copper conductor (resistivity) = 1.7×10^{-8}Wm) of radius of cross-section 5 mm. Find the mobility of the charges if their drift velocity is 1.1×10^{-3} m/s.

(a) 1.8m^2/Vs (b) 1.5m^2/Vs
(c) 1.3 m^2/Vs (d) 1.0m^2/Vs

28. In a conductor, if the number of conduction electrons per unit volume is 8.5×10^{28} m^{-3} and mean free time is 25 *fs* (femto second), it's approximate resistivity is: (m_e = 9.1×10^{-31} kg)

(a) 10^{-6}Ω m (b) 10^{-7} Ωm
(c) 10^{-8} Ωm (d) 10^{-5} Ωm

29. A 200 Ω resistor has a certain color code. If one replaces the red color by green in the code, the new resistance will be :

(a) 100 Ω (b) 400 Ω (c) 300 Ω (d) 500 Ω

30. The charge on a capacitor plate in a circuit, as a function of time, is shown in the figure:

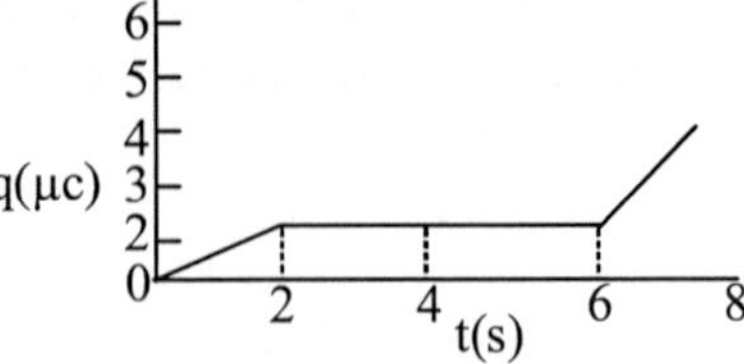

What is the value of current at t = 4 s ?

(a) Zero (b) 3 μA (c) 2 μA (d) 1.5 μA

31. Drift speed of electrons, when 1.5 A of current flows in a copper wire of cross section 5 mm^2, is v. If the electron density in copper is 9×10^{28}/m^3 the value of v in mm/s close to (Take charge of electron to be = 1.6×10^{-19}C)

(a) 0.02 (b) 3 (c) 2 (d) 0.2

32. A carbon resistance has following colour code. What is the value of the resistance?

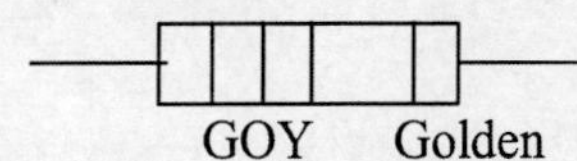

(a) 530 kΩ ± 5% (b) 5.3 kΩ ± 5%
(c) 6.4 MΩ ± 5% (d) 64 MΩ ± 10%

33. A copper rod of cross-sectional area A carries a uniform current I through it. At temperature T, if the volume charge density of the rod is ρ, how long will the charges take to travel a distance d ?

(a) $\frac{2\rho dA}{IT}$ (b) $\frac{2\rho dA}{I}$ (c) $\frac{\rho dA}{I}$ (d) $\frac{\rho dA}{IT}$

34. In the given circuit diagram, a wire is joining points B and D. The current in this wire is:

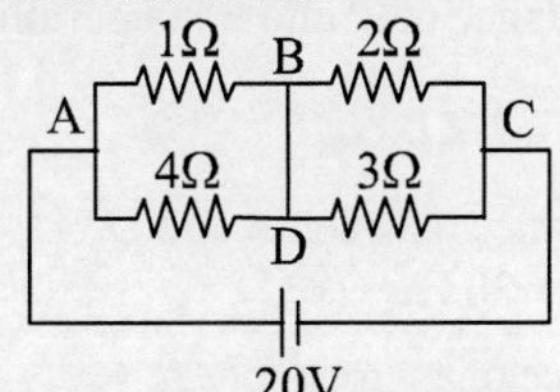

(a) 0.4A (b) 2A (c) 4A (d) zero

35. The current I_1 (in A) flowing through 1 Ω resistor in the following circuit is:

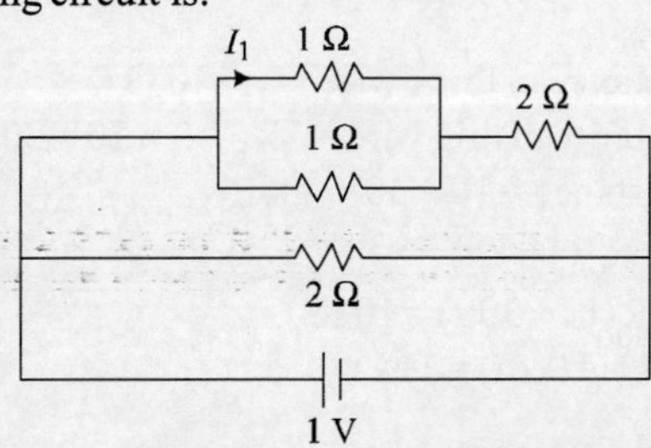

(a) 0.4 (b) 0.5 (c) 0.2 (d) 0.25

36. A metal wire of resistance 3 Ω is elongated to make a uniform wire of double its previous length. This new wire is now bent and the ends joined to make a circle. If two points on the circle make an angle 60° at the centre, the equivalent resistance between these two points will be

(a) $\frac{12}{5}\Omega$ (b) $\frac{5}{2}\Omega$ (c) $\frac{5}{3}\Omega$ (d) $\frac{7}{2}\Omega$

37.

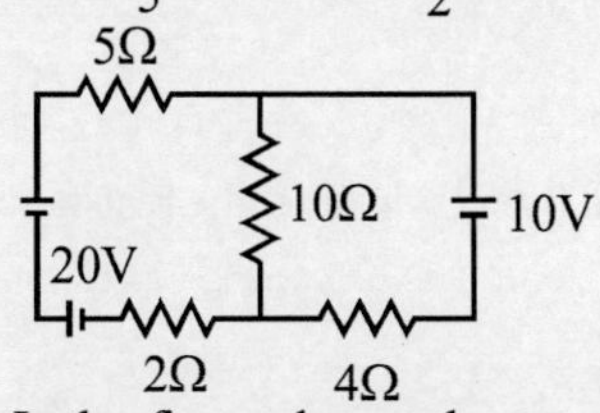

In the figure shown, the current in the 10 V battery is close to :

(a) 0.71 A from positive to negative terminal
(b) 0.42 A from positive to negative terminal
(c) 0.21 A from positive to negative terminal
(d) 0.36 A from negative to positive terminal

38. In the circuit, given in the figure currents in different branches and value of one resistor are shown. Then potential at point B with respect to the point A is :

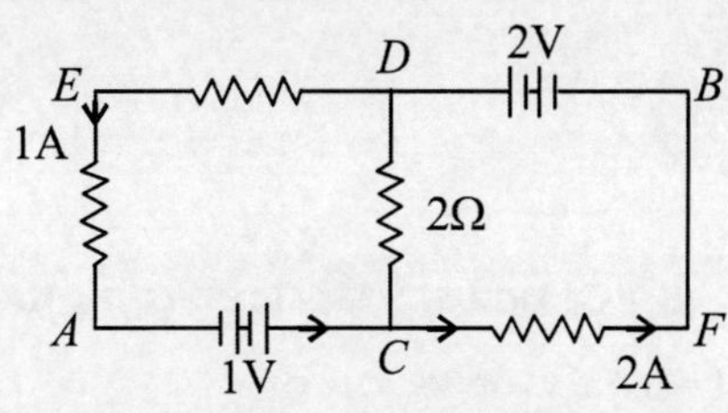

(a) +2 V (b) −2 V (c) −1 V (d) +1 V

39. For the circuit shown, with $R_1 = 1.0\,\Omega$, $R_2 = 2.0\,\Omega$, $E_1 = 2$ V and $E_2 = E_3 = 4$ V, the potential difference between the points '*a*' and '*b*' is approximately (in V) :

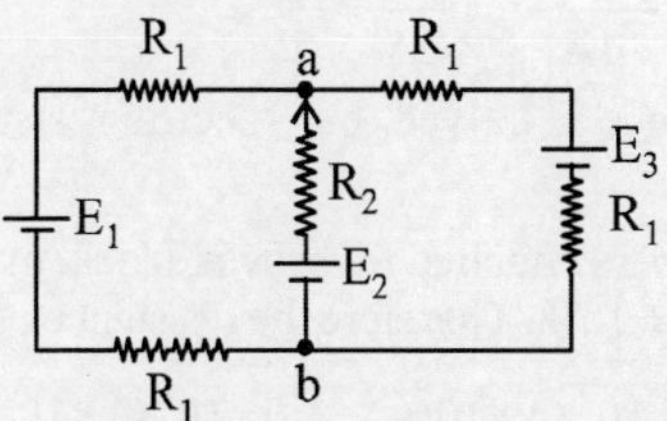

(a) 2.7 (b) 2.3 (c) 3.7 (d) 3.3

40. A cell of internal resistance r drives current through an external resistance R. The power delivered by the cell to the external resistance will be maximum when :

(a) $R = 0.001\,r$ (b) $R = 1000\,r$
(c) $R = 2r$ (d) $R = r$

41. Two batteries with e.m.f. 12 V and 13 V are connected in parallel across a load resistor of 10Ω. The internal resistances of the two batteries are 1Ω and 2Ω respectively. The voltage across the load lies between:

(a) 11.6 V and 11.7 V (b) 11.5 V and 11.6 V
(c) 11.4 V and 11.5 V (d) 11.7 V and 11.8 V

42. An electrical power line, having a total resistance of 2 Ω, delivers 1 kW at 220 V. The efficiency of the transmission line is approximately :

(a) 72% (b) 91% (c) 85% (d) 96%

43. In a building there are 15 bulbs of 45 W, 15 bulbs of 100 W, 15 small fans of 10 W and 2 heaters of 1 kW. The voltage of electric main is 220 V. The minimum fuse capacity (rated value) of the building will be:

(a) 10 A (b) 25 A (c) 15 A (d) 20 A

44. One kg of water, at 20°C, is heated in an electric kettle whose heating element has a mean (temperature averaged) resistance of 20 Ω. The rms voltage in the mains is 200 V. Ignoring heat loss from the kettle, time taken for water to evaporate fully, is close to :

[Specific heat of water = 4200 J/(kg°C), Latent heat of water = 2260 kJ/kg]

(a) 16 minutes (b) 22 minutes
(c) 3 minutes (d) 3 minutes

45. Two equal resistances when connected in series to a battery, consume electric power of 60 W. If these resistance are now connected in parallel combination to the same battery, the electric power consumed will be :

(a) 60 W (b) 240 W (c) 120 W (d) 30 W

Hints & Solutions

18.1 Concept Practice Problems

1. (d) $I = n A e v_d$ or $v_d \propto 1/\pi r^2$

2. (c) $R = \frac{\rho \ell_1}{A_1}$, now $\ell_2 = 2\ell_1$
$A_2 = \pi(r_2)^2 = \pi(2r_1)^2 = 4\pi r_1^2 = 4A_1$
$\therefore \quad R_2 = \frac{\rho(2\ell_1)}{4A_1} = \frac{\rho \ell}{2A} = \frac{R}{2}$
$\therefore$ Resistance is halved, but specific resistance remains the same.

3. (c) Numbers attached for brown, black, green and silver are 1, 0, 5, ± 10%. Therefore the resistance of given resistor
$= 10 \times 10^5 \Omega \pm 10\% \; = 1.0 \times 10^6 \Omega \pm 10\%$.

4. (b) Current density J = I/A
$= 50 \times 16^{-6} / 50 \times 10^{-6} = 1 \text{ Am}^{-2}$

5. (a) Current flowing through the conductor, I = n e v A. Hence
$$\frac{4}{1} = \frac{nev_{d_1}\pi(1)^2}{nev_{d_2}\pi(2)^2} \text{ or } \frac{v_{d_1}}{v_{d_2}} = \frac{4 \times 1}{1} = \frac{16}{1}.$$

6. (c) $I = q/t = 10^7 \times 1.6 \times 10^{-19}/1 \; = 1.6 \times 10^{-12} A$

7. (c) $R = \frac{\rho \ell}{(\pi D^2/4)}$ or $R \propto \frac{\ell}{D^2}$.
$$\frac{R_x}{R_y} = \frac{\ell_x}{D_x^2} \times \frac{D_y^2}{\ell_y} = \frac{\ell_y/2}{(D_y/2)^2} \times \frac{D_y^2}{\ell_y} = \frac{2}{1}$$

8. (c) $R_1 = \frac{1}{2}\Omega;\ R_2 = \frac{1}{4}\Omega;\ R_3 = \frac{1}{6}\Omega$
In series; $R_s = R_1 + R_2 + R_3 \; = \frac{1}{2} + \frac{1}{4} + \frac{1}{6} = \frac{11}{12}$
$\therefore \sigma_s = \frac{1}{R_s} = \left(\frac{12}{11}\right)$

9. (a) $R_1 = 1/2\Omega, R_2 = 1/4\Omega; R_3 = 1/6\Omega$
In parallel; $\frac{1}{R_p} = \frac{1}{R_1} + \frac{1}{R_2} + \frac{1}{R_3} = 2 + 4 + 6 = 12$
$\therefore \sigma_p = \frac{1}{R_p} = 12 \text{ S}$

10. (a) [Hint ⇒ $R_t = R_o(1 + \alpha t)$]
$5\Omega = R_0(1 + \alpha \times 50)$ and $7\Omega = R_0(1 + \alpha \times 100)$
or $\frac{5}{7} = \frac{1 + 50\alpha}{1 + 100\alpha}$ or $\alpha = \frac{2}{150} = 0.0133/°C$

11. (b) (Hint ⇒ $\rho = \frac{R.A}{\ell}$ = Coefficient of resistivity)

12. (c) The effective circuit will be as shown in the figure.

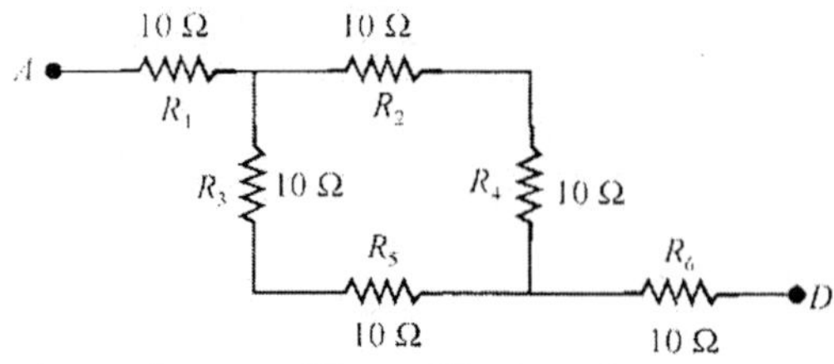

Effective resistance of R_2 and R_4 in series,
$R' = 10 + 10 = 20\,\Omega$.
Effective resistance of R_3 and R_5 in series,
$R'' = 10 + 10 = 20\,\Omega$
Net total resistance of R' and R'' in parallel is
$$R_1 = \frac{20 \times 20}{20 + 20} = 10\Omega.$$
$\therefore$ Total resistance between A and D
$= 10 + 10 + 10 = 30\,\Omega$.

13. (c) Resistance of a wire = $\rho l / A$.
For the same length and same material,
$\frac{R_2}{R_1} = \frac{A_1}{A_2} = \frac{3}{1}$ or, $R_2 = 3R_1$
The resistance of thick wire, $R_1 = 10\,\Omega$
The resistance of thin wire = $3R_1 = 3 \times 10 = 30\,\Omega$.
Total resistance = $10 + 30 = 40\Omega$.

14. (b) $R_t = R_0(1 + \alpha t)$
Initially, $R_0(1 + 30\alpha) = 10\,\Omega$
Finally, $R_0(1 + \alpha t) = 11\,\Omega$
$\therefore \frac{11}{10} = \frac{1 + \alpha t}{1 + 30\alpha}$
or, $10 + (10 \times 0.002 \times t) = 11 + 330 \times 0.002$
or, $0.02t = 1 + 0.66 = 1.066$ or $t = \frac{1.66}{0.02} = 86°C$.

15. (a) Let the resistance of single copper wire be R_1. If ρ is the specific resistance of copper wire, then
$$R_1 = \frac{\rho \times \ell}{A_1} = \frac{\rho \times \ell}{\pi r_1^2} \quad ...(1)$$
When the wire is replaced by six wires, let the resistance of each wire be R_2. Then
$$R_2 = \frac{\rho \times \ell}{A_2} = \frac{\rho \times \ell}{\pi r_2^2} \quad ...(2)$$
From eqs. (1) and (2), we get
$$\frac{R_1}{R_2} = \frac{r_2^2}{r_1^2} \text{ or } \frac{5}{R_2} = \frac{(3 \times 10^3)^2}{(9 \times 10^{-3})^2};\ R_2 = 45\Omega$$
These six wires are in parallel. Hence the resistance of the combination would be $R_2 = 7.5\,\Omega$

18.2 Concept Practice Problems

16. (c) Internal resistance = r, External resistance = nr.
Let terminal voltage = V

then $V = E - Ir \Rightarrow V = E - \frac{Er}{(n+1)r}$

$V = \frac{nE}{n+1} \Rightarrow \frac{V}{E} = \frac{n}{n+1}$

17. (a) According to maximum power theorem, the power in the circuit is maximum if the value of external resistance is equal to the internal resistance of battery.

18. (c) $P = V^2/R$ or $P \propto 1/R \therefore \frac{P_1}{P_2} = \frac{R_2}{R_1} = \frac{2}{1}$.

19. (a)

20. (b) As $R \propto V^2/P$ or $R \propto 1/P$, so resistance of heater is less than that of fan.

21. (d) Case (I): $E + E = (r + r + 5)\,1$ or $2E = 2r + 5$ ...(i)

Case (II): $E = \left(\frac{r \times r}{r + r} + 5\right) \times 0.8$ or $E = \left(\frac{r}{2} + 5\right) 0.8$

or $E = 0.4r + 4.0$ ...(ii)

Multiplying (ii) by 2 and equating with (i), we get

$2r + 5 = 0.8r + 8$ or $1.2r = 3$ or $r = \frac{3}{1.2} = 2.5$

22. (b) $H = \frac{V^2}{R} \times 15 \times 60 = \frac{V^2}{(2/3)R} \times t$

or $t = \frac{2}{3} \times 15 \times 60 = 600\,s = 10$ minutes.

23. (d) (Hint: $P = V^2/R$)

24. (c) Length of wire $= 100$cm.

$2V$ = voltage of battery, $1V$ = voltage of a cell

When current flows along wire electric potential falls continuously along wire.

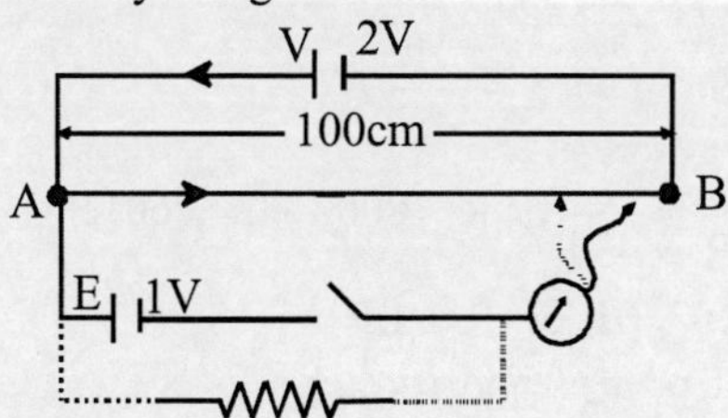

Potential gradient = fall in potential length, $K = \frac{E}{l}$

because in null point position, $E = V$

$\therefore \frac{E_1}{E_2} = \frac{l_1}{l_2} = \frac{R_1}{R_2}$ ....(1)

For internal resistance, $E = E_1, r = E_2$

$E = iR + ir$

$E - V = ir \qquad (\because i = V/R) \; r = \left(\frac{E}{V} - 1\right)R$

$\Rightarrow r = \left(\frac{l_1}{l_2} - 1\right)R. = 10\left(\frac{55}{50} - 1\right) = 10\left(\frac{5}{50}\right) = 1\Omega$

25. (a) The temperature of the wire increases to such a value at which, the heat produced per second equals heat lost per second due to radiation i.e.

$I^2\left(\frac{\rho \ell}{\pi r^2}\right) = H \times 2\pi r \ell$, where H is heat lost per second per unit area due to radiation. Hence, $I^2 \propto r^3$

so $\frac{I_1^2}{I_2^2} = \frac{r_1^3}{r_2^3}$ or $r_2 = r_1\,(I_2/I_1)^{2/3}$

$= 1 \times (3.0/1.5)^{2/3} = 4^{1/3}$ mm.

18.3 Concept Practice Problems

26. (d) $\frac{P}{Q} = \frac{l}{(100 - l)}$ or $P = \frac{l}{100 - l} \times Q = \frac{20}{80} \times 1 = 0.25\Omega$.

27. (d) $S = \frac{I_g}{I - I_g} \times G = \frac{I}{(nI - I)} \times G = \frac{G}{(n-1)}$

28. (a)

29. (a) **Hint:** Potential gradient $= \frac{\text{Pot. Difference}}{\text{length of wire}} = \frac{V_A - V_B}{\ell}$

30. (a) Pot. gradient = 0.2mV/cm

$= \frac{0.2 \times 10^{-3}}{10^{-2}} = 2 \times 10^{-2}\,V/m$

Emf of cell $= 2 \times 10^{-2} \times 1m = 2 \times 10^{-2}\,V = 0.02\,V$

As per the condition of potentiometer

$0.02\,(R + 490) = 2\,(R)$ or $1.98\,R = 9.8$

$\Rightarrow R = \frac{9.8}{1.98} = 4.9\,\Omega$

31. (a) $R_g = 50\Omega, I_g = 25 \times 4 \times 10^{-4}\Omega = 10^{-2}\,A$

Range of V = 25 volts

$V = I_g(HR + R_g)$

$\therefore HR = \frac{V}{I_g} - R_g = 2450\Omega$

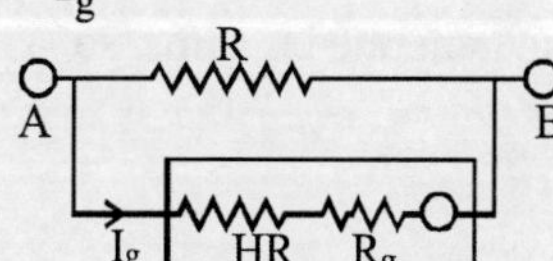

32. (b) In case of internal resistance measurement by potentiometer,

$\frac{V_1}{V_2} = \frac{\ell_1}{\ell_2} = \frac{\{ER_1/(R_1 + r)\}}{\{ER_2/(R_2 + r)\}} = \frac{R_1(R_2 + r)}{R_2(R_1 + r)}$

Here $\ell_1 = 2m$, $\ell_2 = 3m$, $R_1 = 5\Omega$ and $R_2 = 10\Omega$

$\therefore \frac{2}{3} = \frac{5(10 + r)}{10(5 + r)}$ or $20 + 4r = 30 + 3r$ or $r = 10\,\Omega$

33. (d)

34. (a) Galvanometer is converted into ammeter, by connected a shunt, in parallel with it.

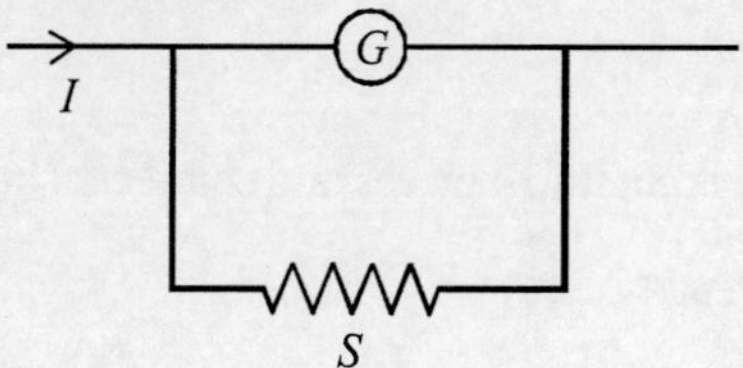

$$\frac{GS}{G+S}=\frac{V_G}{I}=\frac{25\times10^{-3}}{25}$$

$$\frac{GS}{G+S}=0.001\Omega$$

Here $S << G$ so $S=0.001\ \Omega$

35. (a) Given : V = 7 V

r = 5Ω

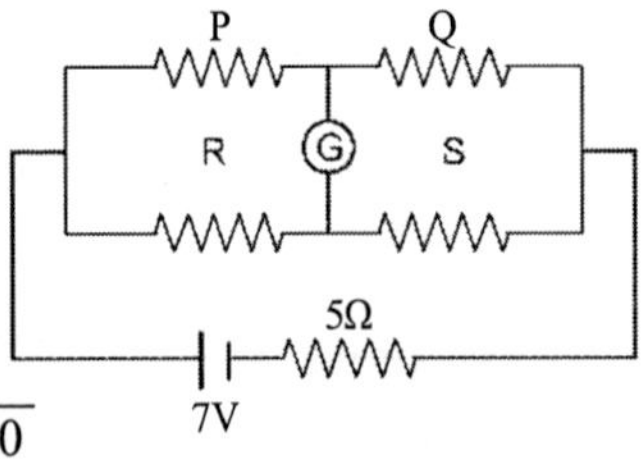

$$R_{eq}=\frac{40\times120}{40+120}\Omega$$

$$I=\frac{V}{R}=\frac{7}{5+\frac{40\times120}{40+120}}$$

$$=\frac{7}{5+30}=\frac{1}{5}=0.2\text{ A}.$$

Exercise 1 - Chapter Revision Problems CRP

1. (a) $R=\rho\ell/A;\ R'=\frac{\rho\ell'}{A'}=\frac{\rho(\ell/2)}{2A}=\frac{1}{4}R.$
2. (c) As we more from A to B the potential difference across AC increases and hence the reading of voltmeter also increases. But currnet flowing through ammeter remains almost constant.
3. (c) 4. (b)
5. (b) $S=\frac{I_gR}{nI_g-I_g}\Rightarrow S=\frac{I_g}{(n-1)I_g}R$
6. (d) Let internal resistance of source = R

Current in coil of resistance $R_1=I_1=\frac{V}{R+R_1}$

Current in coil of resistance $R_2=I_2=\frac{V}{R+R_2}$

Further, as heat generated is same, so

$$I_1^2R_1t=I_2^2R_2t$$

or $$\left(\frac{V}{R+R_1}\right)^2R_1=\left(\frac{V}{R+R_2}\right)^2R_2$$

$$\Rightarrow R_1(R+R_2)^2=R_2(R+R_1)^2$$

$$\Rightarrow R^2R_1+R_1R_2^2+2RR_1R_2$$

$$=R^2R_2+R_1^2R_2+2RR_1R_2\ ?$$

$$\Rightarrow R^2(R_1-R_2)=R_1R_2(R_1-R_2)$$

$$\Rightarrow R=\sqrt{R_1R_2}$$

7. (c) 8. (c)
9. (b) $m\cong L,\ v\cong I$
10. (c) $R=\frac{\rho\ell}{A}$

When wire is cut into 4 pieces and connected in parallel.

$$R_{eff.}=\frac{R}{16}\Rightarrow P_C=16P$$

$$P_A:P_B:P_C:P_D::\frac{V^2}{R}:\frac{V^2}{R/4}:\frac{V^2}{R/16}:\frac{V^2}{R/2}$$

11. (c) $r=E/I=1.5/3=0.5$ ohm.
12. (b) $\frac{R_1}{R_2}=\frac{V^2/P_1}{V^2/P_2}=\frac{P_2}{P_1}$

$$=\frac{\rho\ell/\pi(d_1/2)^2}{\rho\ell/\pi(d_2/2)^2}=\frac{d_2^2}{d_1^2}=\frac{100W}{25W}$$

$$\Rightarrow\frac{d_2}{d_1}=\frac{10}{5}=\frac{2}{1}$$

13. (c) $I=\frac{dQ}{dt}=10t+3$

At t = 5s, I = 10 × 5 + 3 = 53 A

14. (c) Kirchhoff's junction rule states that the algebraic sum of all currents into and out of any branch point is zero : ΣI = 0. By convention, the sign of current entering a junction is positive and current leaving a junction is negative. $4A+5A-6A+I_{AB}=0$, therefore $I_{AB}=-3A$. The wire between points A and B carries a current of 3A away from the junction.
15. (b) **Case (I) :** When resistor is not connected

Using $V=IR\Rightarrow V=25(R_G)$ .... (i)

Case (II) : When resistor is connected

$V=5(20+R_G)=100+5R_G$ .... (ii)

From (i) and (ii), $20R_G=100\Rightarrow R_G=5\Omega$

16. (a) $J=\sigma E\Rightarrow J\rho=E$

J is current density, E is electric field

so B = ρ = resistivity.

17. (b) Energy produced = V I t = 6 × 0.5 × 1 = 3.0 J.
18. (b) Potential gradient along wire

$$=\frac{\text{potential difference along wire}}{\text{length of wire}}$$

or, $0.1\times10^{-3}=\frac{I\times40}{1000}$ V/cm

or, Current in wire, $I=\frac{1}{400}$ A

or, $\frac{2}{40+R}=\frac{1}{400}$ or $R=800-40=760\Omega$

19. (c) As $R=V^2/P$ or $R\propto 1/P$

so $R_2/R_1=P_1/P_2=200/100=2$

or $R_2=2R_1$.

20. (b) For maximum current, the two batteries should be connected in series. The current will be maximum when external resistance is equal to the total internal resistance of cells i.e. 2 Ω. Hence power developed across the resistance R will be

$$=I^2R=\left(\frac{2E}{R+2r}\right)^2R=\left(\frac{2\times2}{2+2}\right)\times2=2\text{ W}.$$

21. (d) Heat produced, $H=\frac{V^2t}{R}$. When voltage is halved, the heat produced becomes one fourth. Hence time taken to heat the water becomes four time.

22. (c) Chemical energy consumed per sec = heat energy produced per sec.
$= I^2 (R + r) = (0.2)^2 (21 + 4) = 1 Js^{-1}$.

23. (b) Energy consumed per day = P × t = 60 × 8 = 480 watt hour = 480/1000 = 0.48 kWh or unit of electricity.
Hence the cost = 0.48 × 1.25 = Re 0.60.

24. (b) As $P = I^2 R$, so $P_1 = (1.01\, I)^2 R$
$= 1.02 I^2 R = 1.02 P.$

It means % increase in power $= \left(\frac{P_1}{P} - 1\right) \times 100 = 2\%.$

25. (a)

26. (a) The given figure is a circuit of balanced Wheatstone's bridge. Point B and D would be at the same potential i.e., potential difference between these points is zero.

27. (c) With each rotation, charge Q crosses any fixed point P near the ring. Number of rotations per second = ω/2π.

$\therefore$ charge crossing P per second = current = $\frac{Q\omega}{2\pi}$

28. (b) Let the edges be 2ℓ, a, and ℓ, in decreasing order.

$R_{max} = \rho \frac{2\ell}{a\ell} = \frac{2\rho}{a}, \quad R_{min} = \rho \frac{\ell}{2\ell a} = \frac{\rho}{2a}; \quad \frac{R_{max}}{R_{min}} = 4.$

29. (a) As the ring has no resistance, the three resistances of 3R each are in parallel.

$\Rightarrow \frac{1}{R'} = \frac{1}{3R} + \frac{1}{3R} + \frac{1}{3R} = \frac{1}{R} \Rightarrow R' = R$

$\therefore$ between point A and B equivalent resistance = R+R = 2R

30. (b) $J = I/A = 10^{-4}/(0.30 \times 0.50).$

$= 6.7 \times 10^{-4} Cm^{-2}/s = 6.7 \times 10^{-4} Am^{-2}$

31. (b) Resistance of the wire of a semicircle = 12/2 = 6Ω
For equivalent resistance between two points on any diameter, 6Ω and 6Ω are in parallel.

or

If a wire of resistance R is bent in the form of a circle, the effective resistance between the ends of a diameter = R/4.

32. (b)

33. (d) Let potential of X be x.
Now current from AX and BX will pass through XC.

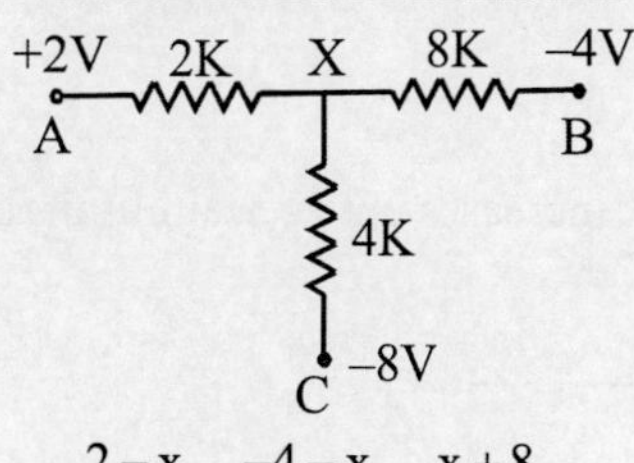

so $\frac{2-x}{2} + \frac{-4-x}{8} = \frac{x+8}{4}$

$2 - x + \frac{-4-x}{4} = \frac{x}{2} + 4 \quad -x - 1 - \frac{x}{4} = \frac{x}{2} + 2$

$-\frac{5x}{4} - \frac{x}{2} = 3 \quad -\frac{7x}{4} = 3 \Rightarrow \text{or } x = -\frac{12}{7}$

So current in 4K will be $\frac{-\frac{12}{7}+8}{4} = \frac{44}{28} = \frac{11}{7} = 1.57\,A$

34. (c) At steady state the capacitor will be fully charged and thus there will be no current in the 1Ω resistance. So the effective circuit becomes

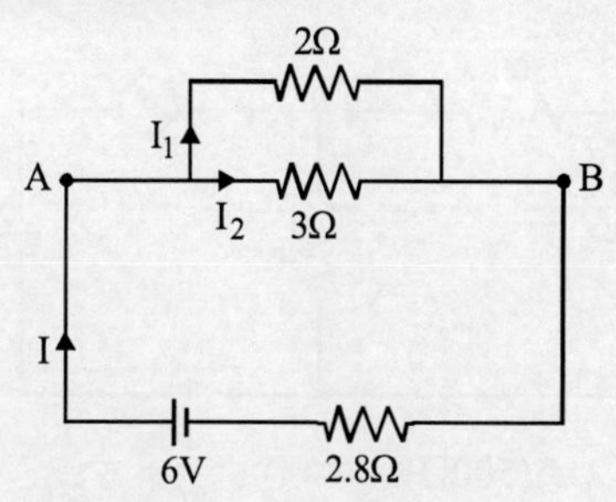

Net current from the 6V battery,

$I = \frac{6}{\left(\frac{2\times3}{2+3}\right) + \frac{2.8}{1}} = \frac{6}{1.2+2.8} = \frac{3}{2} = 1.5A$

Between A and B, voltage is same in both resistances, $2I_1 = 3I_2$ where $I_1 + I_2 = I = 1.5$

$\Rightarrow \quad 2I_1 = 3(1.5 - I_1) \Rightarrow I_1 = 0.9A$

35. (c) By principle of symmetry and superposition,

$2 \times \frac{I}{6} \times R_0 = I\, R_{eq.} \Rightarrow R_{eq.} = \frac{R_0}{3}$

(Current $\frac{I}{6}$ in AB is due to division in current entering at A and current $\frac{I}{6}$ is due to current returning from infinity of grid).

36. (d) Current in arm AE and FB is zero.
So,

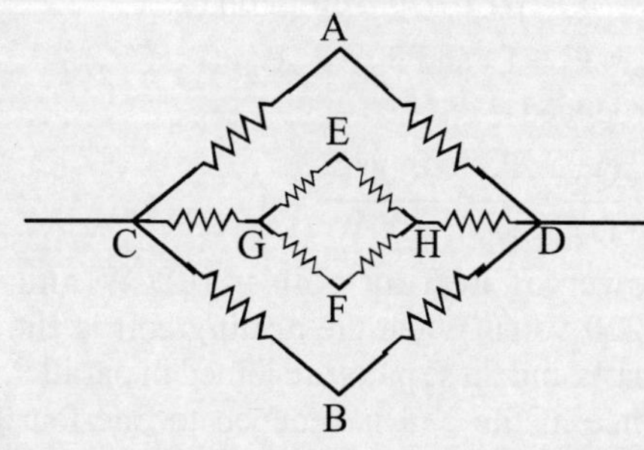

37. (d)

38. (b) Equivalent resistance between A and B = series combination of 1 Ω and 2 Ω in parallel with 3 Ω resistor..

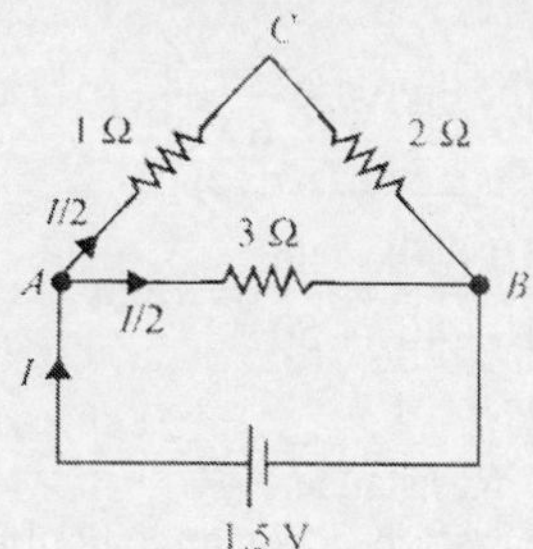

$\frac{1}{R}=\frac{1}{3}+\frac{1}{3}=\frac{2}{3}$ or $R = 1.5\,\Omega$.

$\therefore$ Current in the circuit is $I = V/R = 1.5/1.5 = 1A$.

Since the resistance in arm ACB = resistance in arm AB = $3\,\Omega$, the current divides equally in the two arms. Hence the current through the $3\,\Omega$ resistor = $I/2 = 0.5$ A.

39. (c)

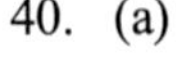

40. (a)

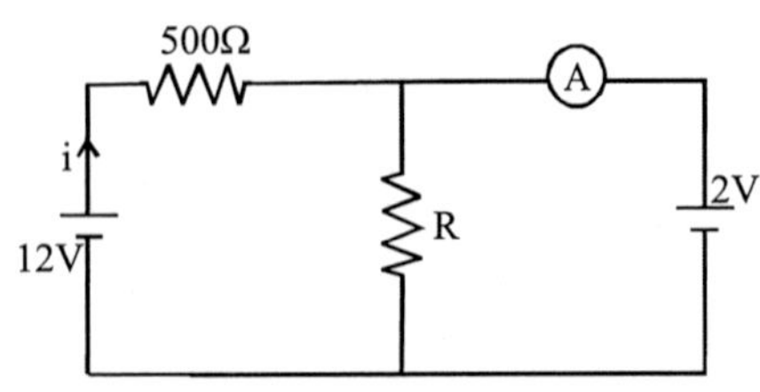

$12-2=(500\Omega)i \Rightarrow i=\frac{10}{500}=\frac{1}{50}$

Again, $i=\frac{12}{500+R}=\frac{1}{50}$

$\Rightarrow 500+R=600 \Rightarrow R=100\,\Omega$

41. (d) The energy stored in the capacitor = $\frac{1}{2}CV^2$. This energy will be converted into heat in the resistor.

42. (c) $H = mL = V^2t/RJ$ or $m=\frac{V^2t}{JRL}$

$=\frac{(210)^2\times 1}{4.2\times 20\times 80}=6.56\,g/s.$

43. (a) $R=\frac{P}{I^2}=\frac{1}{25}=0.04\Omega$

44. (d) $R_s = 3R$ and $R_P=\frac{R}{3}$

$P_S=\frac{V^2}{3R}=10W$ and

$P_P = V^2/(R/3) = 3V^2/R = 9P_S = 90$ W.

45. (a) $P_P = P_1 + P_2$ and $P_S = P_1P_2/(P_1+P_2)$

Heat produced = Pt.

Hence, $\frac{Q_P}{Q_S}=\frac{P_P}{P_S}=\frac{2000\,W}{500\,W}=4.$

46. (d) Power of heating coil = 100 W and voltage (V) = 220 volts. When the heating coil is cut into two equal parts and these parts are joined in parallel, then the resistance of the coil is reduced to one-fourth of the previous value. Therefore energy liberated per second becomes 4 times i.e., $4 \times 100 = 400$ J.

47. (a) **Hint :** The wheatstone bridge is balanced, when P/Q = R/S, In the this case $\frac{3}{6}=\frac{4}{8}$, so bridge is balanced & 7Ω resistance is not effective)

48. (b) Time $=\frac{10\times 40}{10+40}=\frac{400}{50}=8\,\text{min}$

49. (a) Power $\propto \frac{1}{\text{Resistance}}$

In series combination, Resistance doubles

Hence, Power will be halved.

In parallel combination, resistance halved

Hence, power will be double.

50. (a)

51. (a) Efficiency is given by

$\eta=\frac{\text{output Power}}{\text{input Power}}=\frac{5\times 15\times 14}{10\times 8\times 15}=8.75$ or $87.5\,\%$

52. (a) $\frac{1}{P_{eq}}=\frac{1}{P_1}+\frac{1}{P_2}+\frac{1}{P_3}$ or $\frac{1}{P_{eq}}=\frac{3}{60}\Rightarrow P_{eq}=20$ watt.

53. (d) $P=\frac{V^2}{R}\Rightarrow R=\frac{V^2}{P}=\frac{(220)^2}{60}=\frac{4(110)^2}{60}$;

$R'=\frac{(110)^2}{60}=\frac{R}{4}$

54. (d) It is balanced Wheatstone bridge. Hence bridge 4Ω can be eliminated.

$\therefore\ R_{eq}=\frac{6\times 9}{6+9}=\frac{18}{5}$ $\quad\therefore\ I=\frac{V}{R_{eq}}=\frac{5V}{18}$

55. (d) Current from D to C = 1A

$\therefore V_D - V_C = 2\times 1 = 2V$

$V_A = 0 \quad \therefore V_C = 1V, \ \therefore V_D - V_C = 2$

$\Rightarrow V_D - 1 = 2 \quad \therefore V_D = 3V$

$\therefore V_D - V_B = 2 \quad \therefore 3 - V_B = 2 \ \therefore V_B = 1V$

56. (c)

57. (c) The current through the resistance *R*

$I=\left(\frac{\varepsilon}{R+r}\right)$

The potential difference across *R*

$V=IR=\left(\frac{\varepsilon}{R+r}\right)R$

$V=\frac{\varepsilon}{\left(1+\frac{r}{R}\right)}$

when $R = 0$, $V = 0$,

$R = \infty$, $v = \varepsilon$

Thus *V* increases as *R* increases upto certain limit, but it does not increase further.

58. (b)

Since deflection in galvanometer is zero so current will flow as shown in the above diagram.

current $I=\frac{V_A}{R_1+R}=\frac{12}{500+100}=\frac{12}{600}$

So $\quad V_B = IR = \dfrac{12}{600} \times 100 = 2V$

59. (c) Resistance of bulb is constant

$$P = \frac{V^2}{R} \Rightarrow \frac{Dp}{p} = \frac{2DV}{V} + \frac{DR}{R}$$

$$\frac{Dp}{p} = 2 \times 2.5 + 0 = 5\%$$

60. (c) Resistance $R = \dfrac{\rho\ell}{A}$

$\because \ell' = 2\ell \quad \therefore A' = \dfrac{A}{2}$

$$\therefore R' \rho\frac{2\ell}{\frac{A}{2}} = 4R = 4 \times 4\,\Omega = 16\,\Omega$$

Therefore the resistance of new wire becomes 16 Ω

61. (a) When $i = 0$, $V = e = 1.5$ volt

62. (b) Equation of straight line from graph

$y = -mx + c$

$$\Rightarrow l\text{n}R = -m\left(\frac{1}{T^2}\right) + c$$

here, m & c are constants

$$R = e^{\left[-m\left(\frac{1}{T^2}\right)+c\right]} = e^{-m\left(\frac{1}{T^2}\right)} \times e^c$$

$$R(T) = R_0 e^{\frac{-T_0^2}{T^2}}$$

63. (a) $dR = \dfrac{(\rho)(dx)}{4\pi x^2}$

$$R = \int dR$$

$$\int dR = \rho\int_a^b \frac{dx}{4\pi x^2}$$

$$\Rightarrow R = \frac{\rho}{4\pi}\left[\frac{-1}{x}\right]_a^b$$

$$R = \left(\frac{\rho}{4\pi}\right)\cdot\left(\frac{1}{a} - \frac{1}{b}\right)$$

64. (b) Color code : Bl, Br, R, O, Y, G, B, V, Gr, W
0, 1, 2, 3, 4, 5, 6, 7, 8 9

$R = AB \times C \pm D\%$ where D = tolerance

$D_{gold} = \pm 5\%$, $D_{silver} = \pm 10\%$; $D_{no\ colour} = \pm 20\%$

Red voilet orange silver

$R = 27 \times 10^3\ \Omega \pm 10\% = 27\,k\Omega \pm 10\%$

65. (c) Resistance, $R = \dfrac{\rho\ell}{A}$

$$R = \rho\frac{\ell}{A} \times \frac{\ell}{\ell} = \frac{\rho\ell^2}{V}\ [\gg \text{Volume}(V) = A\gg.]$$

Since resistivity and volume remains constant therefore % change in resistance

$$\frac{\Delta R}{R} = \frac{2\Delta\ell}{\ell} = 2 \times (0.5) = 1\%$$

66. (c) Resistance after temperature increases by 500°C i.e.,

$$R_t = \frac{V}{I} = \frac{220}{2} = 110\Omega$$

$R_0 = 100$ (given) temperature coefficient of resistance, $\alpha = ?$

using $R_t = R_0(1 + \alpha t)$

$110 = 100(1 + \alpha 500)$

$$\alpha = \frac{10}{100 \times 500}$$

or, $\quad \alpha = 2 \times 10^{-4}\,{}^\circ C^{-1}$

67. (a)

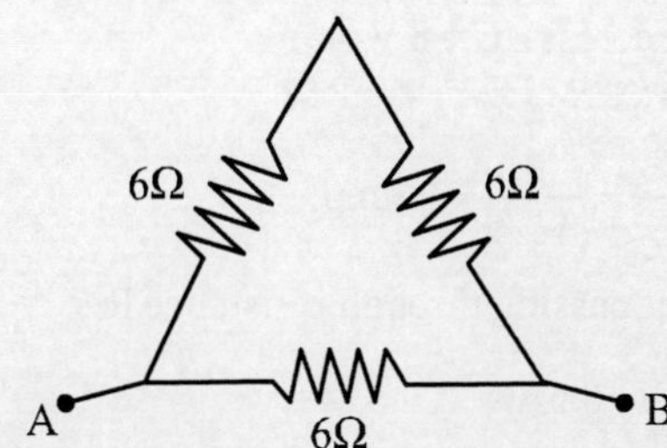

Resistance, $R \propto l$ so resistance of each side of the equilateral triangle = 6 Ω

Resistance R_{eq} between any two vertices

$$\frac{1}{R_{eq}} = \frac{1}{12} + \frac{1}{6} \Rightarrow R_{eq.} = 4\Omega$$

68. (a) Across R_4 reading of voltmeter, $V_4 = 5V$

$$\text{Current, } i_4 = \frac{V_4}{R_4} = 0.01\,A$$

$V_3 = i_1 R_3 = 1V$

$V_3 + V_4 = 6V = V_2$

$V_1 + V_3 + V_4 = 18V$

$\Rightarrow V_1 = 12\,V$

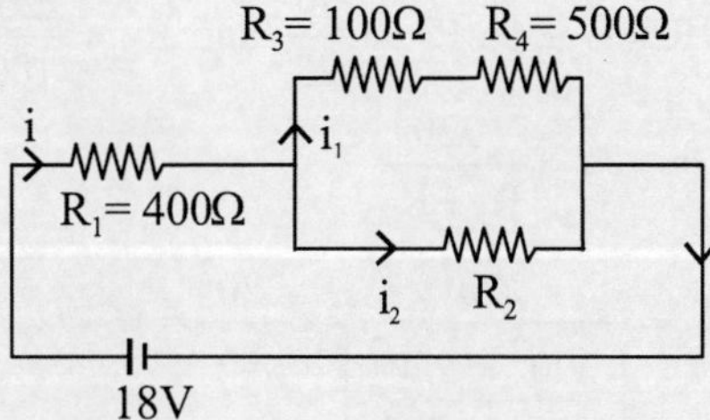

$$i = \frac{V_1}{R_1} = 0.03A$$

$$i = i_1 + i_2 \Rightarrow i_2 = i - i_1 = 0.03 - 0.01A = 0.02\,A$$

$$\therefore R_2 = \frac{V_2}{i_2} = \frac{6}{0.02} = 300\Omega$$

69. (a) $R_{series} = R_1 + R_2 + ... + R_n$

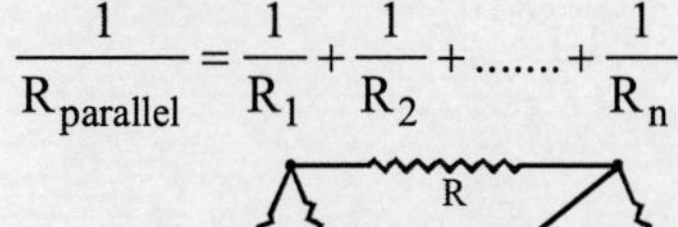

$$\frac{1}{R_{parallel}} = \frac{1}{R_1} + \frac{1}{R_2} + ... + \frac{1}{R_n}$$

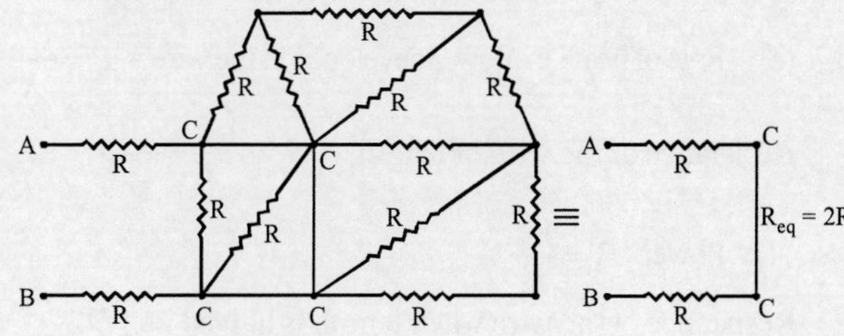

70. (c) The equivalent circuit can be drawn as

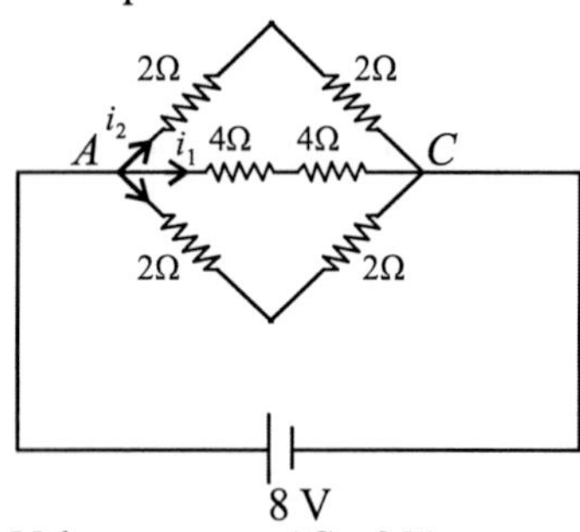

Voltage across $AC = 8$ V

Resistance $R_{AC} = 4 + 4 = 8\ \Omega$

$$i_1 = \frac{V}{R_{AC}} = \frac{8}{4+4} = 1 \text{ Amp}$$

71. (c) Current passing through resistance R_1,

$$i_1 = \frac{v}{R_1} = \frac{10}{20} = 0.5\text{A}$$

and, $i_2 = 0$

72. (b) Equivalent resistance,

$$R_{eq} = \frac{4R \times 4R}{4R + 4R} + R + \frac{6R \times 12R}{6R + 12R} + R$$

$= 2R + R + 4R + R$

$= 8R.$

Using, $P = \dfrac{V^2}{R_{eq}} \Rightarrow 4 = \dfrac{16^2}{8R}$

$\therefore \quad R = \dfrac{16^2}{4 \times 8} = 8$ W

73. (a) As $R = \dfrac{V^2}{P}$, so $R_1 = \dfrac{220^2}{25}$ and $R_2 = \dfrac{220^2}{100}$

Current flown $i = \dfrac{220}{R_1 + R_2}$

$$P_1 = i^2 R_1 = \frac{220^2}{\left(\frac{220^2}{25} + \frac{220^2}{100}\right)} \times \frac{220^2}{25} = 16 \text{ W}$$

Similarly, $P_2 = i^2 R_2 = 4$ W

74. (a) Power, $P = I^2 R$

$4.4 = 4 \times 10^{-6} \times R$

$\Rightarrow R = 1.1 \times 10^6 \Omega$

When supply of 11 v is connected

Power, $P' = \dfrac{v^2}{R} = \dfrac{11^2}{1.1} \times \dfrac{11^2}{1.1} \times 10^{-6}$

$= 11 \times 10^{-5}$ W

75. (a) Rate of heat i.e., Power developed in the wire $= P = \dfrac{V^2}{R}$

Resistance of the wire of length, L $R_1 = \dfrac{\rho L}{A} = \dfrac{\rho L}{\pi r^2}$

$\therefore \quad$ Power, $P_1 = \dfrac{V^2}{R_1}$

Resistance of the wire when length is halved i.e., $L/2$

$$R_2 = \frac{\rho \frac{L}{2}}{\pi (2r)^2} = \frac{\rho L}{\pi 8 r^2} = \frac{R_1}{8}$$

$\therefore \quad$ Power, $P_2 = \dfrac{V}{\frac{R_1}{8}} = \dfrac{8V}{R_1}$

or, $P_2 = 8P_1$ i.e., power increased 8 times of previous or original wire.

Exercise 2 - Exemplar & Past Year Questions E&PYQs

Exemplar Questions

1. (b) As we know, electric current per unit area I/A, is called current density j i.e., $j = \dfrac{I}{A}$

The SI units of the current density are A/m^2.

The current density is also directed along E and is also a vector and the relationship is

$$j = \sigma E$$

Current density changes due to electric field produced by charges accumulated on the surface of wire.

2. (a) As we know the equivalent emf (ε_{eq}) in the parallel combination

$$\varepsilon_{eq} = \frac{\varepsilon_2 r_1 + \varepsilon_1 r_2}{r_1 + r_2}$$

So according to formula the equivalent emf ε_{eq} of the two cells in parallel combination is between ε_1 and ε_2. Thus ($\varepsilon_1 < \varepsilon_{eq} < \varepsilon_2$).

3. (c) Adjusting the blance point near the middle of the bridge, i.e.. when l_1 is close to 50 cm. requires a suitable choice of S, R is unknown resistance :

Since, $\dfrac{R}{S} = \dfrac{Rl_1}{R(100 - l_1)}$

$\dfrac{R}{S} = \dfrac{l_1}{100 - l_1}$ or $R = S\left[\dfrac{l_1}{100 - l_1}\right]$

$R = S\left[\dfrac{2.9}{97.1}\right]$

So, here, R : S = 2.9 : 97.1 implies that the S is nearly 33 times to that of R. In orded to make this ratio 1 : 1 it is necessary to reduce the value of S nearly $\dfrac{1}{33}$ times i.e., nearly 3 Ω.

4. (b) The potential drop across wires of potentiometer should be more than emfs of primary cells. Here, values of emfs of two cells are given as 5V and 10V, so the potential drop along the potentiometer wire must be more than 10V. So battery should be of 15V and about 4V potential is droped by using variable resistance.

5. (a) As we known that the resistance of wire is $R = \rho \dfrac{l}{A}$

For maximum value of R, l must be higher and A should be lower and it is possible only when the battery is connected across area of cross section $= 1\text{cm} \times \left(\dfrac{1}{2}\right)$cm.

6. (a) We know that the relationship between current and drift speed is

$$I = neAv_d$$

Where, I is the current and V_d is the drift velocity.

So, $I \propto V_d$

Hence, only drift velocity determines the current in a conductor.

NEET/AIPMT (2013-2020) Questions

7. (a) Given : emf $\varepsilon = 2.1$ V

$I = 0.2$ A, $R = 10\Omega$

Internal resistance r = ?

From formula.

$\varepsilon - Ir = V = IR$

$2.1 - 0.2r = 0.2 \times 10$

$2.1 - 0.2r = 2$ or $0.2r = 0.1$

$\Rightarrow r = \frac{0.1}{0.2} = 0.5\,\Omega$

8. (a) Given : V = 7 V

$r = 5\Omega$

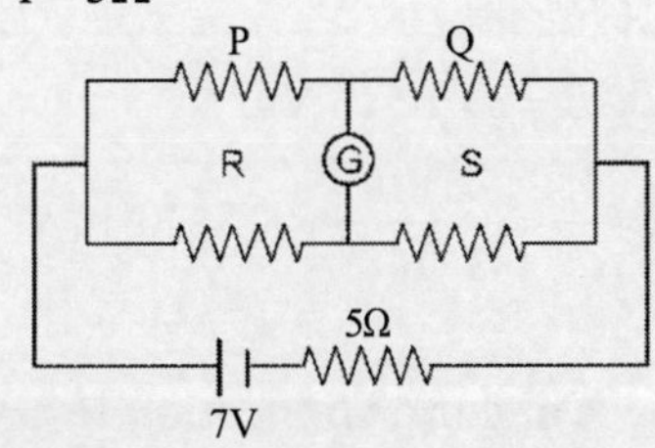

$R_{eq} = \frac{40\times120}{40+120}\Omega$

$I = \frac{V}{R} = \frac{7}{5+\frac{40\times120}{40+120}}$

$= \frac{7}{5+30} = \frac{1}{5} = 0.2$ A.

9. (b) Resistance is directly proportionl to length of the wire. As length is doubled so mass is doubled and resistance is doubled.

We have

$\frac{(10E)^2}{R}t = mS\Delta T$, Now $\frac{(nE)^2 t}{2R} = (2m)S\Delta T$

$\Rightarrow \frac{n^2E^2t}{2R} = 2\frac{10^2E^2t}{R}$

$\Rightarrow n = 20$

10. (c) Internal resistance of the cell,

$r = \left(\frac{E-V}{V}\right)R = \left(\frac{\ell_1-\ell_2}{\ell_2}\right)R$

$= \left(\frac{3-2.85}{2.85}\right)\times(9.5)\,\Omega = 0.5\,\Omega$

11. (c) As 0.2% of main current passes through the galvanometer hence $\frac{998}{1000}$I current through the shunt.

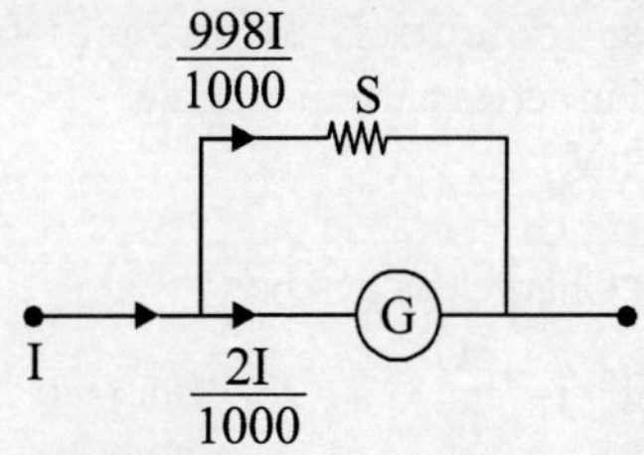

$\left(\frac{2I}{1000}\right)G = \left(\frac{998I}{1000}\right)S \Rightarrow S = \frac{G}{499}$

Total resistance of Ammeter

$R = \frac{SG}{S+G} = \frac{\left(\frac{G}{499}\right)G}{\left(\frac{G}{499}\right)+G} = \frac{G}{500}$

12. (b) Total resistance $R = (0.5\,\Omega/\text{km}) \times (150\text{ km}) = 75\,\Omega$

Total voltage drop = (8 V/km) × (150 km)

= 1200 V

Power loss $= \frac{(\Delta V)^2}{R} = \frac{(1200)^2}{75}$ W

= 19200 W = 19.2 kW

13. (a) Here, metallic conductor can be considered as the combination of various conductors connected in series. And in series combination current remains same.

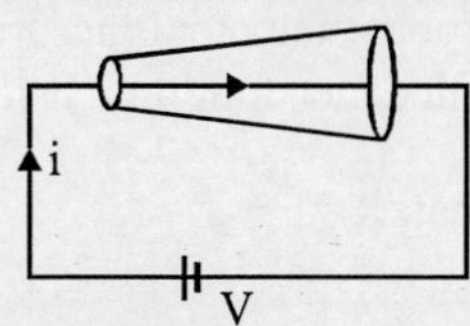

14. (d) Total potential difference across potentiometer wire $= 10^{-3} \times 400$ volt = 0.4 volt

potential gradient $= \frac{1\text{mv}}{\text{cm}}$

$= 10^{-3}$ v/cm $= 10^{-1}\frac{\text{v}}{\text{m}}$

Let resistance of RΩ connected in series.

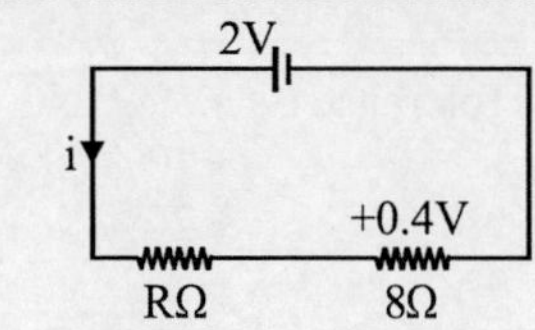

So, $\frac{2}{R+8} = \frac{10^{-1}\times4}{8} = \frac{1}{20}$

$\Rightarrow R + 8 = 40$ or, $R = 32\,\Omega$

15. (d) Effective resistance of B and

$= \frac{R_B \cdot R_C}{R_B + R_C} = \frac{1.5R\times3R}{1.5R+3R} = \frac{4.5R^2}{4.5R} = R$

i.e., equal to resistance of voltmeter A.

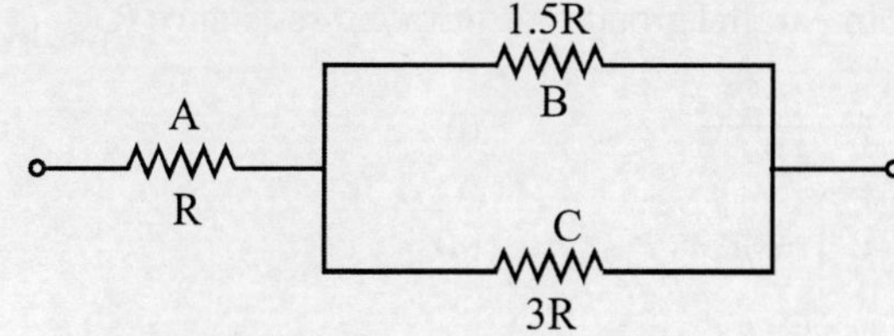

In parallel potential difference is same so, $V_B = V_C$ and in series current is same

So, $V_A = V_B = V_C$

16. (d)

17. (a) **Given:** Charge $Q = at - bt^2$

$\therefore$ Current $i = \frac{\partial Q}{\partial t} = a - 2bt$ {for $i = 0 \Rightarrow t = \frac{a}{2b}$}

From joule's law of heating, heat produced

$dH = i^2 Rdt$

$$H = \int_0^{a/2b} (a - 2bt)^2 \, Rdt$$

$$H = \left.\frac{(a-2bt)^3 R}{-3 \times 2b}\right|_0^{\frac{a}{2b}} = \frac{a^3 R}{6b}$$

18. (d) When two cells are connected in series i.e., $E_1 + E_2$ the balance point is at 50 cm. And when two cells are connected in opposite direction i.e., $E_1 - E_2$ the balance point is at 10 cm. According to principle of potential

$$\frac{E_1 + E_2}{E_1 - E_2} = \frac{50}{10}$$

$$\Rightarrow \frac{2E_1}{2E_2} = \frac{50+10}{50-10} \Rightarrow \frac{E_1}{E_2} = \frac{3}{2}$$

19. (b) Reading of potentiometer is accurate because during taking reading it does not draw any current from the circuit.

20. (b) We know that, $R = \frac{\rho \ell}{A}$

or $R = \frac{\rho \ell^2}{\text{Volume}} \Rightarrow R \propto \ell^2$

According to question $\ell_2 = n\ell_1$

$$\frac{R_2}{R_1} = \frac{n^2 l_1^2}{l_1^2} \quad \text{or,} \quad \frac{R_2}{R_1} = n^2$$

$\Rightarrow R_2 = n^2 R_1$

21. (b) Colour code for carbon resistor

0	Black		
1	Brown	Tolerance :	± 5% Gold
2	Red		± 10% Silver
3	Orange		± 20% No colour
4	Yellow		
5	Green		
6	Blue		
7	Violet		
8	Grey		
9	White		

$(47 \pm 4.7)\,k\Omega = 47 \times 10^3 \pm 10\%$

$\therefore$ Yellow - Violet - Orange - Silver

22. (a) In series grouping equivalent resistance $R_{series} = nR$

In parallel grouping equivalent resistance $R_{parallel} = \frac{R}{n}$

$$I = \frac{E}{nR + R} \quad ...(i)$$

$$10\,I = \frac{E}{\frac{R}{n} + R} \quad ...(ii)$$

Dividing eq. (ii) by (i),

$$10 = \frac{(n+1)R}{\left(\frac{1}{n} + 1\right)R}$$

Solving we get, n = 10

23. (a)

24. (c) For metals temperature coefficient of resistance is positive while for insulators and semiconductors, temperature coefficient of resistance is negative.

25. (c) According to colour coding -

Yellow	Violet	Brown	Gold
4	7	1	5%

First colour gives first digit, second colour gives the second digit and third colour gives the multiplier and fourth colour gives tolerance.

$\therefore$ Resistance,

$R = 47 \times 10^1 \pm 5\% = 470 \pm 5\%\Omega$

26. (a) Given,

Drift velocity of charged particle,

$V_d = 7.5 \times 10^{-4}$ m/s

Electric field, $E = 3 \times 10^{-10}$ Vm^{-1}

Mobility, $\mu = \frac{V_d}{E} = \frac{7.5 \times 10^{-4}}{3 \times 10^{-10}} = 2.5 \times 10^6 \, m^2 V^{-1} s^{-1}$

Exercise 3 - Concept Application Problems 

1. (c) $R \propto \frac{\ell}{A}$;

So, the resistance of the wire will be minimum when the area of cross-section is maximum and length is minimum.

2. (b)

3. (b) $R_1 = \frac{V^2}{P_1}$ and $R_2 = \frac{V^2}{P_2}$

$\therefore \frac{R_2}{R_1} = \frac{P_1}{P_2} = \frac{200}{100} = 2$ ($\because$ V = constant)

$R_2 = 2R_1$

4. (d) Resistance of bulb $R_b = \frac{(1.5)^2}{4.5} = 0.5\Omega$

Current drawn from battery $= \frac{E}{2.67 + 0.33} = \frac{E}{3}$

Share of bulb $= \frac{2}{3} \times \frac{E}{3} = \frac{2E}{9}$

$\therefore \left(\frac{2E}{9}\right)^2 \times 0.5 = 4.5$ or E = 13.5 V.

5. (a) Current $I = \frac{q}{t} = \frac{CV}{t} = \frac{(10 \times 10^6) \times 40}{0.2} = 2 \times 10^{-3} A$

6. (b) If R is the resistance of each wire, total resistance in series = R + R = 2 R; and total resistance in parallel $= \frac{R \times R}{R + R} = \frac{R}{2}$.

Heat produced per second (= V^2/R) will be four times in parallel than in series.

7. (a) $H = I^2 Rt$. Here $R_1 = \rho\frac{l}{\pi r^2}$ and

$R_2 = \rho\frac{l}{\pi(2r)^2}$ That is, $R_1 = 4R_2$. Hence, $\frac{H_1}{H_2} = 4$

8. (a) Let, we connect 24 cells in n rows of m cells, then if I is the current in external circuit then

$$I = \frac{mE}{mr/n + R} \quad ...(1)$$

For I to be maximum, (mr + nR) should be minimum.

It is minimum for $R = \frac{mr}{n}$ ...(2)

So maximum current in external circuit is

$$I = \frac{mE}{2R} \quad ...(3)$$

here R = 3, r = 0.5 so equation (2) become $\frac{m}{n} = 6$

so n = 2, m = 12

9. (d) Current in the potentiometer, $I = \frac{2}{8+7+1} = \frac{1}{8}A.$

Voltage drop across potentiometer wire $= \frac{1}{8} \times 8 = 1V$

$\therefore$ Potential gradient of potentiometer wire $= \frac{1}{4} = 0.25\ V/m$

10. (c) $\frac{R_1}{R_2} = \left(\frac{\ell_1}{\ell_2}\right)^2 \Rightarrow \frac{R}{R'} = \left(\frac{1}{2}\right)^2$

$\Rightarrow R' = 4R$ or $\Delta R = 3R$

$\therefore$ % change in resistance of wire

$= \frac{3R}{R} \times 100 = 300\%$

11. (d) $R_1 + R_2$ = Constant, R_1 will increase, R_2 will decrease.

$R_1\alpha\Delta T - R\beta\Delta T = 0 \Rightarrow R_1\alpha\Delta T = R_2\beta\Delta T$

$\therefore \frac{R_1}{R_2} = \frac{\beta}{\alpha}$

12. (b) The equivalent circuit can be redrawn as

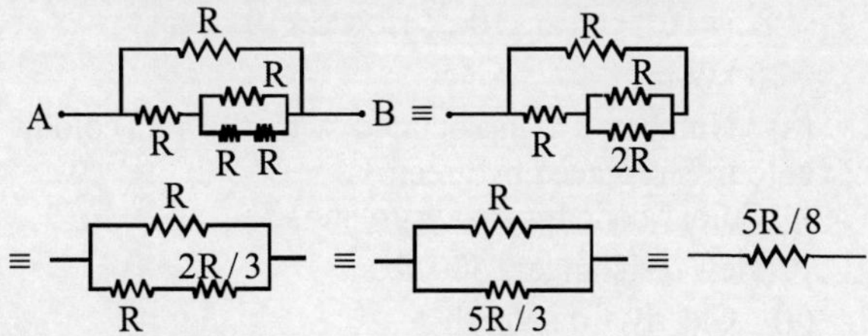

13. (d)

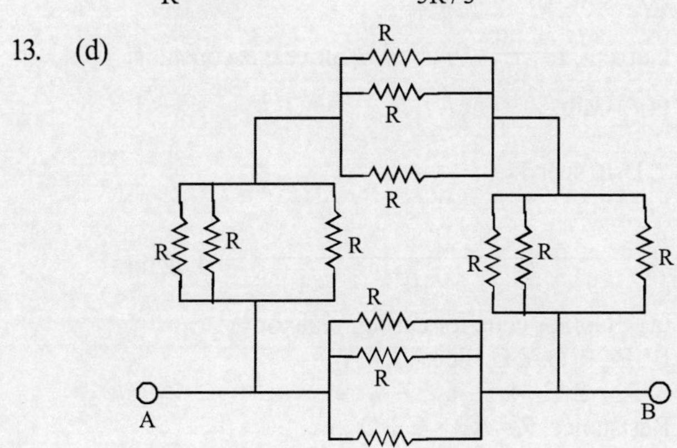

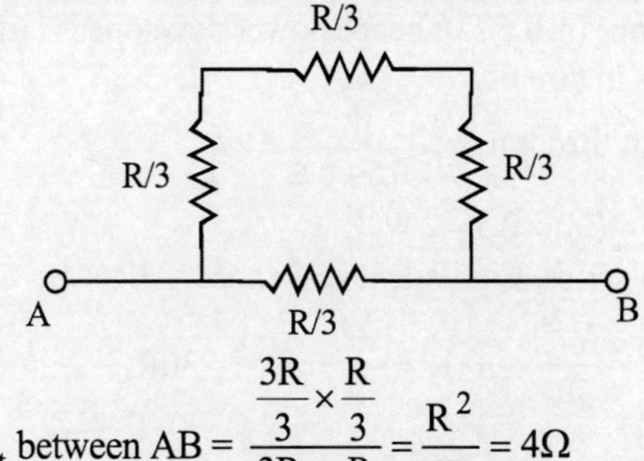

$$R_{net} \text{ between AB} = \frac{\frac{3R}{3} \times \frac{R}{3}}{\frac{3R}{3} + \frac{R}{3}} = \frac{R^2}{4R} = 4\Omega$$

14. (b,c) $I = \frac{E}{R+r} = \frac{E}{(\sqrt{R} - \sqrt{r})^2 + 2\sqrt{R}\sqrt{r}}$

I is maximum when R = r

$P = I^2R$, when I is max, P is also max.

$P_{max} = I^2_{max}R$.

15. (b) Current in branch of capacitor is zero.

$R_{net} = R + r$

$I = \frac{E}{R+r}$ potential across capacitor is equal to potential across resistance R_1.

$V_1 = \frac{E}{R_1 + r}R_1$ So charge $= CV_1 = \frac{ECR_1}{R+r}$

16. (b) Given Capacitance of the capacitor, C = 0.2 μF and e.m.f. of cell, E = 6V.

Reactance of a capacitor for a cell, which is a DC source, is infinity. Therefore, no current flows in 4Ω resistance. Resistances 2 Ω and 3 Ω (both in upper arm) are connected in parallel. Therefore, their equivalent resistance

$(R') = \frac{2\times 3}{2+3} = 1.2\Omega$

Now, R′ and 2.8 Ω are in series combination. Therefore, equivalent resistance of the circuit,

R = R′ + 2.8 = 1.2 + 2.8 = 4 Ω

Current drawn in the circuit, $I = \frac{E}{R} = \frac{6}{4} = 1.5A$

Therefore, potential difference across 2 Ω resistance, V = IR = 1.5 × 1.2 = 1.8 V

Thus, current in 2 Ω resistance $(I_1) = \frac{V}{2} = \frac{1.8}{2} = 0.9A$

17. (a) In parallel, $\frac{H_1}{H_2} = \frac{P_1 t}{P_2 t} = \frac{P_1}{P_2} = \frac{500}{200} = \frac{5}{2}$

In series, $\frac{H_1}{H_2} = \frac{I^2 R_1 t}{I^2 R_2 t} = \frac{R_1}{R_2} = \frac{V^2/P_1}{V^2/P_2}$

$= \frac{P_2}{P_1} = \frac{200}{500} = \frac{2}{5}$.

18. (b) Total internal resistance of two cells $= \frac{1\times 1}{1+1} = 0.5\Omega$.

Since internal resistance of coil is equal to external resistance (= 0.5 Ω), hence power developed is maximum by cells in circuit.

Current through $R = \frac{2}{0.5+0.5} = 2\,A$

Power $= (2)^2 \times 0.5 = 2\,W$.

19. (d) In series, Equivalent resistance = 3R

Power $= \frac{V^2}{3R} \Rightarrow 10 = \frac{V^2}{3R} \Rightarrow V^2 = 30R$

In parallel, $\frac{1}{R'} = \frac{1}{R} + \frac{1}{R} + \frac{1}{R} = \frac{3}{R}$

∴ Equivalent resistance $R' = \frac{R}{3}$

∴ Power $= \frac{V^2}{R'} = \frac{30R}{R/3} = 90\,W$

20. (d) $P = \frac{H}{t} = \sigma(T_1^4 - T_2^4)$

$T_1 = 727 + 273 = 1000\,K$, $T_2 = 227 + 273 = 500\,K$, $P = 60$ watt
In the second case, $T_1' = 1227 + 273 = 1500\,K$,

$T_2' = 500\,K$, $P' = ?$

$$\frac{P'}{P} = \frac{(1500)^4 - (500)^4}{(1000)^4 - (500)^4} = \frac{(500)^4[3^4 - 1]}{(500)^4[2^4 - 1]} \Rightarrow \frac{80}{15}$$

$\Rightarrow P' = 60 \times \frac{80}{15} = 320$ watt.

21. (b) Let I_1 be the current throug 5 Ω resistance, I_2 through (6 + 9) Ω resistance. Then as per question,

$I_1^2 \times 5 = 20$ or, $I_1 = 2A$.

Potential difference across C and D = 2 × 5 = 10V

Current $I_2 = \frac{10}{6+9} = \frac{2}{3}A$.

Heat produced per second in 2 Ω

$= I^2R\left(\frac{8}{3}\right)^2 \times 2 = 14.2\,cal/s$.

22. (a) Potential gradient $= \frac{V_A - V_B}{\ell} = \frac{i \times \rho}{A} = \frac{0.1 \times 10^{-7}}{10^{-6}}$

$= 10^{-2}\,V/m$

23. (a) As for an electric appliance $R = (V_s^2 / P)$, so for same specified voltage V_s,

$\frac{R_{25}}{R_{100}} = \frac{100}{25} = 4$ i.e, $R_{25} = 4R$ with $R_{100} = R$

Now, in series potential divides in proportion to resistance.

So, $V_1 = \frac{R_1}{(R_1 + R_2)} V$ i.e., $V_{25} = \frac{4}{5} \times 440 = 352V$

and, $V_2 = \frac{R_2}{(R_1 + R_2)} V$ i.e., $V_{100} = \frac{1}{5} \times 440 = 88V$

From this it is clear that voltage across 100 W bulb (= 88 V) is lesser than specified (220 V) while across 25 W bulb (=352 V) is greater than specified (220 V), so 25 W bulb will fuse.

24. (d) A balanced Wheatstone's bridge exists between A & B. $R_{eq} = R$
current through circuit is V/R
current through AFCEB = V/2R

25. (c) **Ammeter :** In series connection, the same current flows through all the components. It aims at measuring the current flowing through the circuit and hence, it is connected in series.

Voltmeter : A voltmeter measures voltage change between two points in a circuit. So we have to place the voltmeter in parallel with the cicuit component.

26. (b) $\rho_M = 98 \times 10^{-8}$

$\rho_A = 2.65 \times 10^{-8}$

$\rho_C = 1.724 \times 10^{-8}$

$\rho_T = 5.65 \times 10^{-8}$

$\therefore \rho_M > \rho_T > \rho_A > \rho_C$

27. (d) Charge mobility

$(\mu) = \frac{V_d}{E}$ [Where V_d = drift velocity]

and resistivity $(\rho) = \frac{E}{j} = \frac{EA}{I} \Rightarrow E = \frac{I(\rho)}{A}$

$\Rightarrow \mu = \frac{V_d}{E} = \frac{V_d A}{I_\rho}$

$$= \frac{1.1 \times 10^{-3} \times \pi \times \left(5 \times 10^{-3}\right)^2}{5 \times 1.7 \times 10^{-8}}$$

$\mu = 1.0 \frac{m^2}{V_s}$

28. (c) $\rho = \frac{m}{ne^2\tau}$

$$= \frac{9.1 \times 10^{-31}}{8.5 \times 10^{28} \times (1.6 \times 10^{-19})^2 \times 25 \times 10^{-15}}$$

$= 10^{-8}$ W-m

29. (d) Number 2 is associated with the red colour. This colour is replaced by green.

∵ Colour code figure for green is 5

∴ New resistance = 500 Ω

30. (a) Clearly, from graph

Current, $I = \frac{dq}{dt} = 0$ at $t = 4s$ [Since q is constant]

31. (a) Using, $I = neAv_d$

∴ Drift speed $v_d = \frac{1}{neA}$

$$\frac{1.5}{9 \times 10^{28} \times 1.6 \times 10^{-19} \times 5 \times 10^{-6}} = 0.02\ mms^{-1}$$

32. (a) Colour code for carbon resistor
Bl, Br, R, O, Y, G, Blue, V, Gr, W
0 1 2 3 4 5 6 7 8 9
Resistance, R = AB × C ± D

Bands A and B are the first two significant figures of resistance
B and C indicates the decimal multiplier or the number of zeros that follow A and B
B and D is tolerance: Gold = ± 5%,
Silver = ± 10 % No colour = ± 20%

$R = 53\times10^4 \pm 5\% = 530 k\Omega \pm 5\%$

33. (c) Charge density $\rho = \frac{\text{charge}}{\text{volume}} = \frac{q}{Ad} \Rightarrow q = \rho Ad$

Also, $q = IT \Rightarrow T = \frac{q}{I} = \frac{\rho Ad}{I}$

34. (b) 35. (c)

36. (c) When length becomes double its resistance becomes $(R \mu l^2)$

$R = 4\times 3 = 12$ W

$R_{eq} = \frac{2\times10}{12} = \frac{5}{3}\Omega$

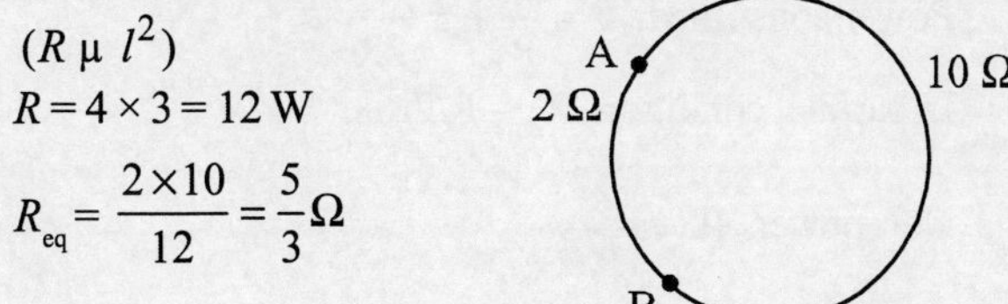

37. (c)

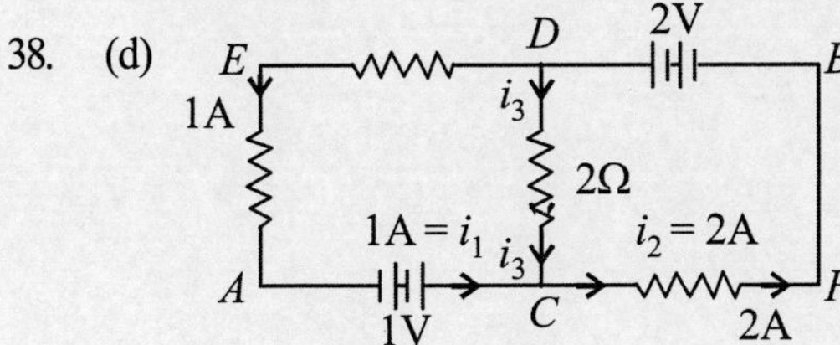

Using Kirchoff's loop law in loop *ABCD*

$-5i_2 - 10(i_1 + i_2) - 2i_2 + 20 = 0$

$\Rightarrow -10i_1 - 17i_2 + 20 = 0$ ...(i)

Using Kirchoff's loop law in loop *BEFC*

$\Rightarrow -10 + 4i_1 + 10(i_1 + i_2) = 0$

$\Rightarrow 14i_1 + 10i_2 + 10 = 0$ ...(ii)

Multiplying equation (i) by 10, we have

$(10i_1 + 17i_2 = 20)\times 10$

$\Rightarrow 100i_1 - 170i_2 = 200$ ...(iii)

Multiplying equation (ii) by 17, we have

$(14i_1 + 10i_2 = 10)\times 17$

$\Rightarrow 238i_1 - 170i_2 = 170$ ...(iv)

On solving equations (iii) and (iv), we get

$-138i_1 = 30 \Rightarrow i_1 = -\frac{30}{138} = -0.217$

i_1 is negative it means current flows from positive to negative terminal.

38. (d)

Let us assume the potential at $A = V_A = 0$
Using Kirchoff's junction rule at *C*, we get

$i_1 + i_3 = i_2$

$1A + i_3 = 2A \Rightarrow i_3 = 2A$

Now using Kirchoff's loop law along *ACDB*

$V_A + 1 + i_3(2) - 2 = V_B$

$\Rightarrow V_A + 1 + i_3(1) - 2 = V_B$

$\Rightarrow V_B - V_A = 3 - 2 = 1$ volt

39. (d) Applying parallel combination of batteries

$$\frac{\frac{E_1}{1+1}+\frac{E_2}{2}+\frac{E_3}{1+1}}{\frac{1}{1+1}+\frac{1}{2}+\frac{1}{1+1}}$$

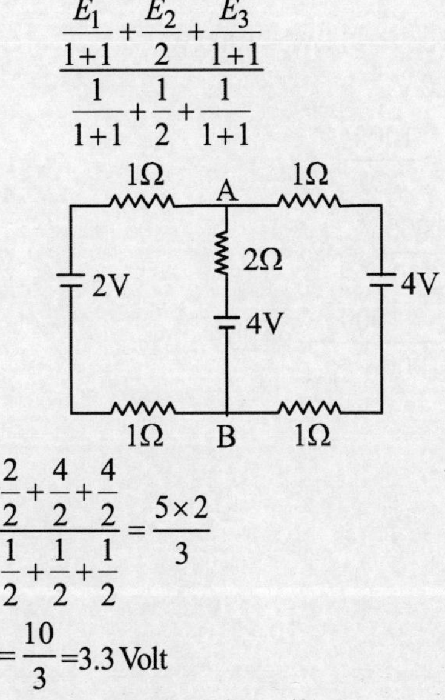

$$\frac{\frac{2}{2}+\frac{4}{2}+\frac{4}{2}}{\frac{1}{2}+\frac{1}{2}+\frac{1}{2}} = \frac{5\times2}{3}$$

$= \frac{10}{3} = 3.3$ Volt

40. (d) $i = \left(\frac{\varepsilon}{R+r}\right)$

Power delivered to R.

$P = i^2R = \left(\frac{\varepsilon}{R+r}\right)^2 R$

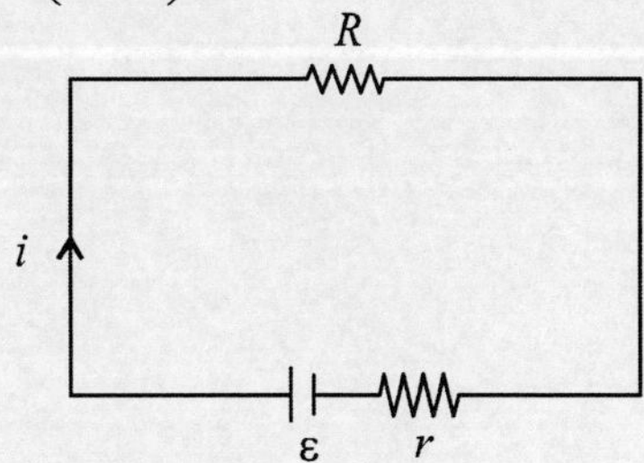

P to be maximum, $\frac{dP}{dR} = 0$

or $\frac{d}{dR}\left[\left(\frac{\varepsilon}{R+r}\right)^2 R\right] = 0$

or $R = r$

41. (b)

Using Kirchhoff's law at *P* we get

$$\frac{V-12}{1}+\frac{V-13}{2}+\frac{V-0}{10}=0$$

[Let potential at P, Q, U = 0 and at R = V

$$\Rightarrow \frac{V}{1}+\frac{V}{2}+\frac{V}{10}=\frac{12}{1}+\frac{13}{2}+\frac{0}{10}$$

$$\Rightarrow \frac{10+5+1}{10}V=\frac{24+13}{2} \Rightarrow V\left(\frac{16}{10}\right)=\frac{37}{2}$$

$$\Rightarrow V=\frac{37\times 10}{16\times 2}=\frac{370}{32}=11.56 \text{ volt}$$

42. (b) Given : Power, $P = 1$ kW = 1000 W
$R = 2\Omega$, $V = 220$ V

$$\text{Current, } I=\frac{P}{V}=\frac{1000}{220}$$

$$P_{\text{loss}}=I^2R=\left(\frac{1000}{220}\right)^2\times 2$$

$$\therefore \text{Efficiency}=\frac{1000}{1000+P_{\text{loss}}}\times 100=96\%.$$

43. (d) Net Power, P
$= 15\times 45+15\times 100+15\times 10+2\times 1000$
$= 15\times 155+2000$ W
Power, $P = VI$

$$\Rightarrow I=\frac{P}{V}$$

$$\therefore I_{\text{main}}=\frac{15\times 155+2000}{220}=19.66\ A\approx 20A$$

44. (b)

45. (b) When two resistances are connected in series, $R_{eq}=2R$

$$\text{Power consumed, } P=\frac{\varepsilon^2}{R_{eq}}=\frac{\varepsilon^2}{2R}$$

In parallel condition, $R_{eq} = R/2$.

$$\text{New power, } P'=\frac{\varepsilon^2}{(R/2)}$$

or $P' = 4P = 240$ W ($\because P = 60$ W)

19 Moving Charges and Magnetism

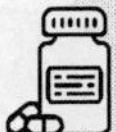

Topic 19.1 : Oersted Experiment, Magnetic Field, Magnetic Field Due to Current Carrying Conductor, Biot-Savart's Law and Ampere's Circuital Law

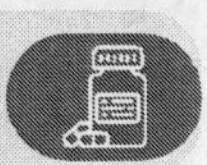

OERSTED EXPERIMENT

In 1802 Gian Domenico Romagnosi, an Italian lawyer and judge, found that a steady electric current flowing in wire affected a magnetic needle placed near it. He published his observation in a local newspaper (called Gazetta di Trentino). But nobody noticed this phenomenon.

In 1820 Hans Christian **Oersted** (a Danish Physicist) rediscovered this phenomenon. He noted that a magnetic compass needle, brought close to a straight wire carrying a steady electric current, aligned itself perpendicular to the wire i.e., the direction of magnetic field B is tangential to a circle which has the wire as centre, and which has its plane perpendicular to the wire (Fig 1-a). Oersted also noticed that on reversing the direction of current; the direction of magnetic field is reversed.

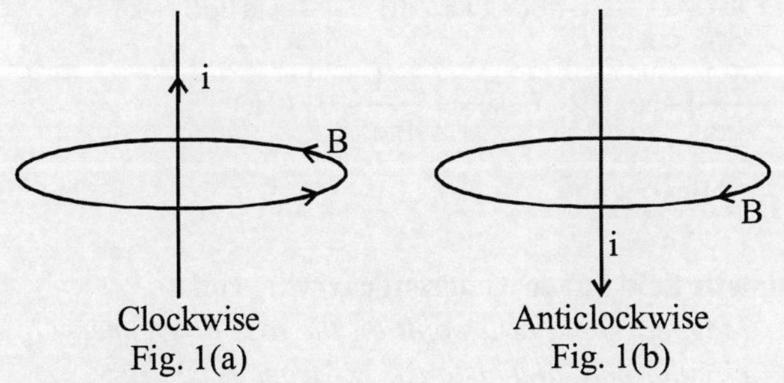

Clockwise
Fig. 1(a)

Anticlockwise
Fig. 1(b)

In first case when current is in upward direction, magnetic field is clockwise (Fig 1-a) and when the current is downward, magnetic field is anticlockwise (Fig. 1-b).

MAGNETIC FIELD

It is a region of space around a magnet or current carrying conductor or a moving charge in which its magnetic effect can be felt.

The conductor carrying current is electrically neutral but a magnetic field is associated with it.

The **SI unit** of magnetic field induction is tesla (T) or weber/m^2 and **cgs unit** is gauss. 1 gauss = 10^{-4} T

Comparison between electric field and magnetic field

Electric field	*Magnetic field*
1. Source is an electric charge (q).	1. Source is a current element $(I\vec{d\ell})$.
2. Isolated charge exists	2. Isolated poles do not exist.
3. Electric field at a point due to a point charge is in the plane containing the point and the charge.	3. Magnetic field at a point due to a current element is perpendicular to the plane containing the point and the current element.
4. It obeys inverse square law (a long range force).	4. It also obeys inverse square law (a long range force).
5. It obeys principle of superposition as the field is linear related to charge.	5. It also obeys principle of superposition.
6. Angle dependence is not present.	6. Angle dependence is present.
7. Line of electric lines of force do not form closed loops.	7. Lines of magnetic lines of force form closed loops.
8. Electric field changes kinetic energy of a charged particle.	8. Magnetic field does not change kinetic energy of a charged particle.
9. A charged particle whether at rest or in motion in an electric field experiences a force due to electric field.	9. A charged particle at rest do not experience force due to magnetic field.

MAGNETIC FIELD DUE TO CURRENT CARRYING CONDUCTOR, BIOT-SAVART'S LAW

The magnetic induction $\vec{dB}$ at any point outside the current path due to a small current element of length $\vec{d\ell}$ (in the direction of the current) is given by Biot-Savart's law

$$\vec{dB} = \frac{\mu_0}{4\pi}\frac{I(\vec{d\ell}\times\vec{r})}{r^3}$$

or, $$|\vec{dB}| = \frac{\mu_0}{4\pi}\frac{I\,d\ell\sin\theta}{r^2}$$

A, P, i, θ, dl, $\vec{r}$, B

Also, $\vec{dB} = \frac{\mu_0}{4\pi}\frac{q(\vec{v}\times\vec{r})}{r^3}$ where $\vec{v}$ is the drift velocity of charge where $\mu_0 = 4\pi\times10^{-7}$ TmA^{-1}.

Direction of $\overrightarrow{dB}$

The direction of $\overrightarrow{dB}$ is perpendicular to both $\vec{d\ell}$ and $\vec{r}$, governed by the right hand thumb rule of the cross-product of $\vec{d\ell}$ and $\vec{r}$.

The magnetic fields going into the page and coming out of the page are represented as follows :

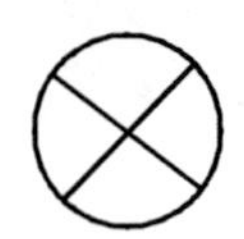

Magnetic field going into the page

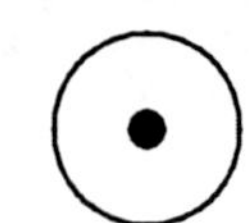

Magnetic field coming out of the page.

Magnetic Field due to Various Current Carrying Conductors

Magnetic field due to finite sized conductor :

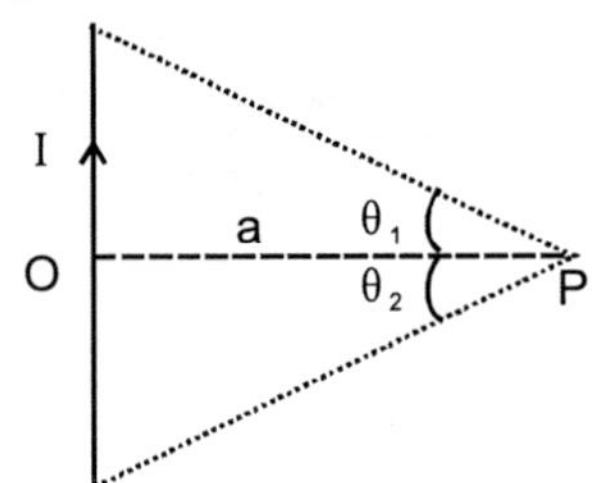

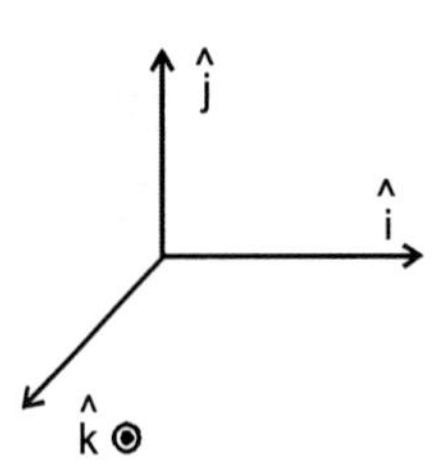

$$\vec{B}_{(at\ P)} = \frac{\mu_0 I}{2\pi a}(\sin\theta_1 + \sin\theta_2)(-\hat{k})$$

$$\Rightarrow B = \frac{\mu_0}{4\pi}\frac{2I}{a}(\sin\theta_1 + \sin\theta_2)$$

Elucidation

$$d\vec{B} = \frac{\mu_0 I}{4\pi r^3}\left(d\vec{\ell}\times\vec{r}\right) \quad r = a\sec\theta,\ \ \ell = a\tan\theta$$

$$\Rightarrow d\ell = a\sec^2\theta\, d\theta \Rightarrow d\vec{\ell} = a\sec^2\theta d\theta\hat{j}$$

$$\vec{r} = -a\tan\theta\hat{j} + a\hat{i}$$

$$\Rightarrow d\vec{B} = \frac{\mu_0 I a\sec^2\theta d\theta}{4\pi a^3\sec^3\theta}\hat{j}\times(-a\tan\theta\hat{j} + a\hat{i})$$

$$= \frac{\mu_0 I\sec^2\theta d\theta}{4\pi a\sec^3\theta}(-\hat{k}) = \frac{\mu_0 I\cos\theta d\theta}{4\pi a}(-\hat{k})$$

$$\therefore B = \int_{-\theta_1}^{\theta_2}\frac{\mu_0 I}{4\pi a}\cos\theta d\theta = \frac{\mu_0 I}{4\pi a}\int_{(-\theta_1)}^{\theta_2}\cos\theta d\theta$$

$$\Rightarrow B = \frac{\mu_0 I}{4\pi a}[\sin\theta_2 + \sin\theta_1] \text{ (Pointing into the plane of paper)}$$

Magnetic field near the end of a finite sized conductor :

$$\underset{(at\ P)}{\vec{B}} = \frac{\mu_0 I}{4\pi a}\sin\theta$$

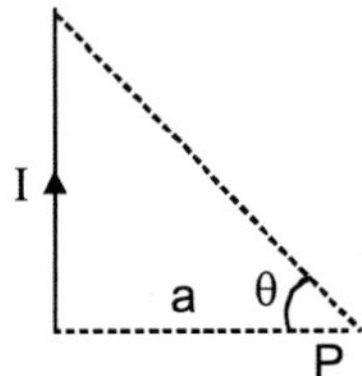

Magnetic field due to an infinitely long conductor :

$$\underset{(at\ P)}{\vec{B}} = \frac{\mu_0 I}{2\pi a}(-\hat{k}) \Rightarrow B = \frac{\mu_0}{4\pi}\frac{2I}{a}$$

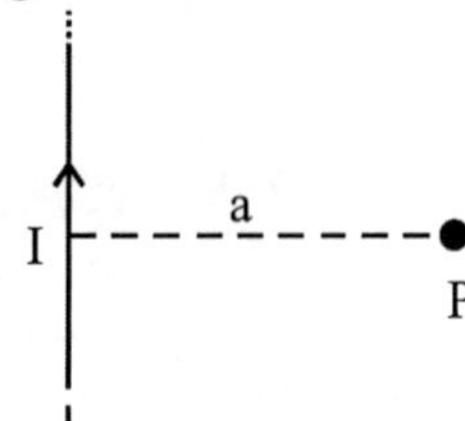

Elucidation

Magnetic field in the case of infinitely long wire

$$dB = \int_{-\pi/2}^{\pi/2}\frac{\mu_0 I}{4\pi a}\cos\theta d\theta$$

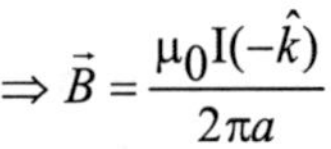

$$\Rightarrow \vec{B} = \frac{\mu_0 I(-\hat{k})}{2\pi a}$$

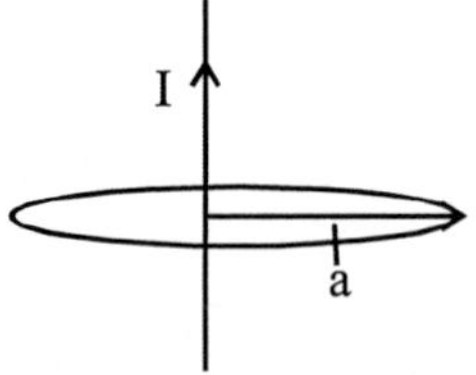

Magnetic field near the end of a long conductor :

$$\underset{(at\ P)}{B} = \frac{\mu_0 I}{4\pi a}$$

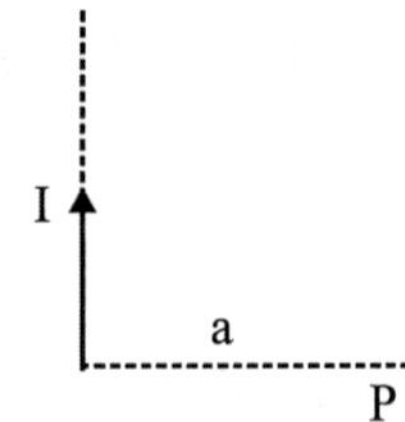

Elucidation

$r = a\ \text{cosec}\ \theta$, $\ell = a\cot\theta$,

$d\ell = a\ \text{cosec}^2\theta\ d\theta$

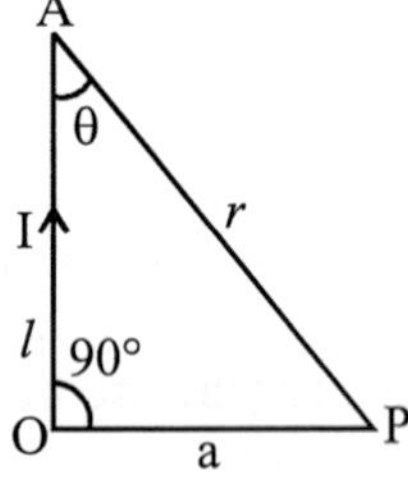

$$d\vec{B} = \frac{\mu_0\vec{dl}\times r}{4\pi r^3}$$

$$= \frac{\mu_0 I a\ \text{cosec}^2\theta d\theta\hat{j}}{4\pi a^3\text{cosec}^2\theta}\times(a\hat{j} - a\cot\theta\hat{j})$$

$$= \frac{\mu_0 I}{4\pi a}\frac{\text{cosec}\ \theta}{\text{cosec}^3\theta}d\theta(-\hat{k}) \Rightarrow \overrightarrow{dB} = \frac{\mu_0 I}{4\pi a}\sin\theta d\theta\ (-\hat{k})$$

$$\vec{B} = \frac{\mu_0 I}{4\pi a}[-\cos\theta]_{\pi/2}^{\pi}(-\hat{k}) = \left(\frac{\mu_0 I}{4\pi a} - 0\right)(-\hat{k})$$

$$\Rightarrow \vec{B} = \frac{\mu_0 I}{4\pi a}(-\hat{k})$$

Magnetic field due to a current carrying coil :

(i) *Magnetic field at a point on the axis of symmetry of a circular coil, at a distance "x" from its centre :*

$B = \mu_0 NI\ a^2/2(a^2 + x^2)^{3/2}$

or, $B = \dfrac{\mu_o}{4\pi}\dfrac{2\pi NIa^2}{(a^2 + x^2)^{3/2}}$

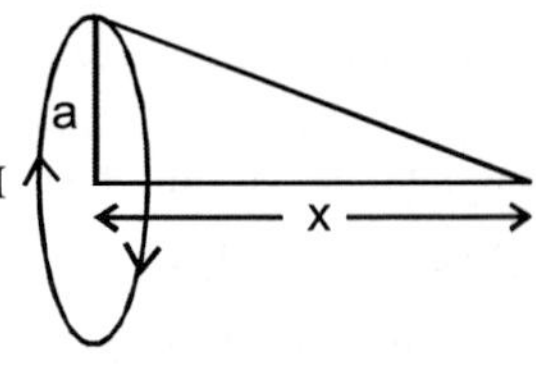

N = total number of turns

a = coil radius

The direction of $\vec{B}$ is given by Right hand screw rule.

Right hand screw rule : *If direction of rotation of right handed screw-head is the directon of current in a circular conductor then the direction of its advance is the direction of magnetic field.* This is applicable even if the current, magnetic field are interchanged, as in case of current flowing through a straight conductor.

Elucidation

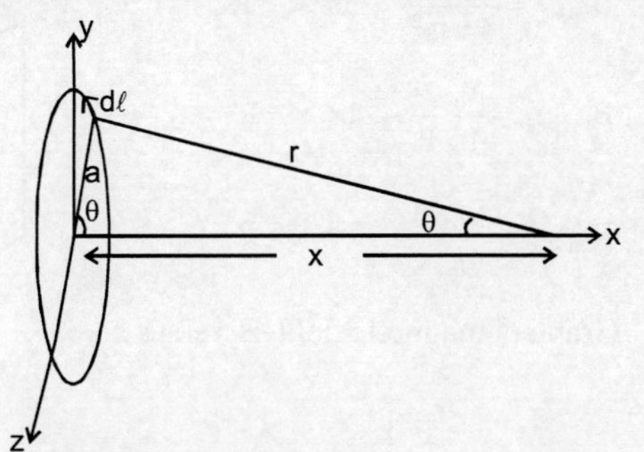

Let for a particular angle, position of small length element dl is given by its coordinates as

$z = -a\cos\theta,\ y = a\sin\theta$.

Now, $\vec{a} = -a\cos\theta\hat{k} + a\sin\theta\hat{j}$,

$\vec{r} = -\vec{a} + x\hat{i} = x\hat{i} - a\sin\theta\hat{j} + a\cos\theta\hat{k}$

Also we have $\ell = r\theta \Rightarrow d\ell = rd\theta$.

Now $\vec{d\ell} \perp \vec{a}$ at any instant

$\therefore \vec{d\ell} = d\ell(\sin\theta\hat{k} + \cos\theta\hat{j})$, $\vec{dB} = \dfrac{\mu_0 I}{4\pi r^3}\left(\vec{d\ell} \times \vec{r}\right)$

$$\Rightarrow \vec{dB} = \frac{\mu_0 Ird\theta}{4\pi r^3}(\sin\theta\hat{k} + \cos\theta\hat{j}) \times (x\hat{i} - a\sin\theta\hat{j} + a\cos\theta\hat{k})$$

$$= \frac{\mu_0 Ird\theta}{4\pi(x^2+a^2)^{3/2}}(x\sin\theta\hat{j} + a\sin^2\theta\hat{i} + x\cos\theta\hat{k} + a\cos^2\theta\hat{i})$$

$$= \frac{\mu_0 Ird\theta}{4\pi(x^2+a^2)^{3/2}}[x(\sin\theta\hat{j} + \cos\theta\hat{k}) + a\hat{i}]$$

$$\Rightarrow \vec{B} = \int \vec{dB}$$

$$= \frac{\mu_0 Ia}{4\pi(x^2+a^2)^{3/2}}[x\,|-\cos\theta\hat{j} + \sin\theta\hat{k}\,|_0^{2\pi} + a(2\pi - 0)\hat{i}]$$

$$\vec{B} = \frac{\mu_0 I 2\pi a(\hat{i})}{4\pi(x^2+a^2)^{3/2}}$$

If number of turns of coil are N, then

$$|\vec{B}| = \frac{\mu_0 I 2\pi Na(\hat{i})}{4\pi(x^2+a^2)^{3/2}} = \frac{\mu_0 INa(\hat{i})}{2(x^2+a^2)^{3/2}}$$

$$\Rightarrow \quad B = \frac{\mu_0}{4\pi}\frac{2\pi NIa}{(x^2+a^2)^{3/2}}$$

(ii) *At the centre of a circular coil,* $B = \mu_0 NI/2a = \dfrac{\mu_0}{4\pi}\dfrac{2\pi NI}{a}$

(iii) *Magnetic field at the centre of a circular arc carrying current*

$$\underset{(at\ P)}{\vec{B}} = \frac{\mu_0 I}{2a} \times \frac{\theta}{360}(-\hat{k}) \Rightarrow B = \frac{\mu_0}{4\pi}\frac{I\theta}{a}$$

where θ is in radian.
In this case the direction of magnetic field $\vec{B}$ is into the page.

Magnetic field inside a current carrying solenoid

(i) *Finite size solenoid*

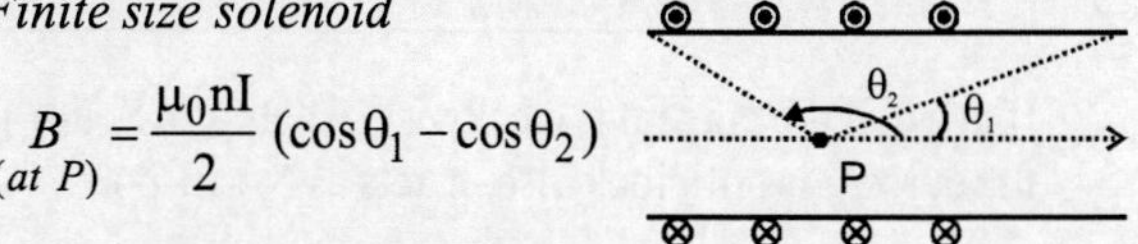

$$\underset{(at\ P)}{B} = \frac{\mu_0 nI}{2}(\cos\theta_1 - \cos\theta_2)$$

(ii) *Near the end of a finite solenoid*

$$B = \frac{\mu_0 nI}{2}\cos\theta;\ (\theta_1 = \theta\ \&\ \theta_2 = \pi/2)$$

(iii) *In the middle of a very long solenoid,* $B = \mu_0 nI$

(iv) *Near the end of a very long solenoid*

$$B = \frac{\mu_0 nI}{2}$$

n is the number of turns per unit length of solenoid.

(v) *Magnetic field in the endless solenoid (toroid) is same throughout and is* $\mu_0 nI$.

(vi) *Magnetic field outside a solenoid or toroid is zero.*

AMPERE'S CIRCUITAL LAW

The line integral of magnetic field across a closed loop is equal to 40 times the net correct inside the loop

i.e., $\oint \vec{B}.\vec{dl} = \mu_0 I$

where I is the net current inside the loop.

(1) The direction of the magnetic field at a point on one side of a conductor of any shape is equal in magnitude but opposite in direction of the field at an equidistant point on the other side of the conductor.

(2) If the magnetic field at a point due to a conductor of any shape is B_o if it is placed in vacuum then the magnetic field at the same point in a medium of relative permeability μ_r is given by $B = \mu_r B_o$.

(3) If the distance between the point and an infinitely long conductor is decreased (or increased) by K-times then the magnetic field at the point increases (or decreases) by K-times.

(4) The magnetic field at the centre of a circular coil of radius smaller than other similar coil with greater radius is more than that of the latter.

(5) For two circular coils of radii R_1 and R_2 having same current and same number of turns, we have

$\dfrac{B_1}{B_2} = \dfrac{R_2}{R_1}$, where B_1 and B_2 are the magnetic fields at their centres.

(6) The magnetic field at a point outside a thick straight wire carrying current is inversely proportional to the distance but magnetic field at a point inside the wire is directly proportional to the distance.

Problem Solving Tips

1. If in a coil the current is clockwise, it acts as a South-pole. If the current is anticlockwise, it acts as North-pole.

2. No magnetic field occurs at point P, Q and R due to a thin current element $I\vec{dl}$.

3. Magnetic field intensity in a thick current carrying conductor at any point x is

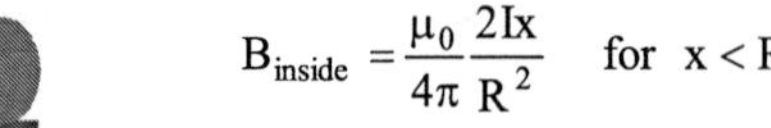

$$B_{inside} = \frac{\mu_0}{4\pi}\frac{2Ix}{R^2} \quad \text{for } x < R$$

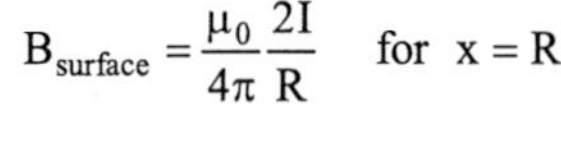

$$B_{surface} = \frac{\mu_0}{4\pi}\frac{2I}{R} \quad \text{for } x = R$$

$$B_{outside} = \frac{\mu_0}{4\pi}\frac{2I}{x} \quad \text{for } x > R$$

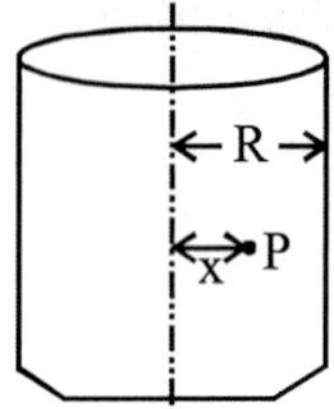

4. Graph of magnetic field $\vec{B}$ versus x

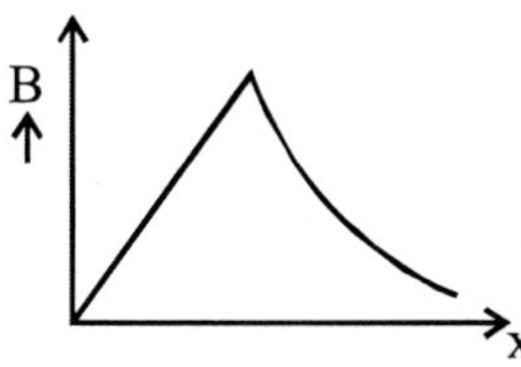

5. Magnetic field is zero at all points inside a current carrying hollow conductor.

Magnitude and direction of magnetic field due to different configuration of current carrying conductor.

S.No.	Configuration of current carrying conductor	Point of observation	Magnetic field	
			Magnitude	Direction
1.	Two long linear and parallel current carrying conductors Wire 1 Wire 2	At P, the mid point between the two wires. The distance of P from each wire is r/2. At P', distant x from wire 2 as shown. At P'', distant x' from wire 1 as shown.	$B = 0$ $B = \frac{\mu_0}{4\pi}2I\left[\frac{1}{x}+\frac{1}{r+x}\right]$ $B = \frac{\mu_0}{4\pi}2I\left[\frac{1}{r-x'}-\frac{1}{x'}\right]$	Normal to the plane of paper, inwards. Normal to the plane of paper, outwards.
2.	Square loop	At the centre.	$B = 4\left[\frac{\mu_0}{4\pi}\frac{I}{a/2}\left(\sin 45° + \sin 45°\right)\right]$	Normal to the plane of paper, inwards.
3.	Two concentric circular coils having turns n_1 and n_2	At the centre.	$B = \frac{\mu_0}{4\pi}2\pi I\left[\frac{n_1}{a}-\frac{n_2}{b}\right]$	If $\frac{n_1}{a} > \frac{n_2}{b}$ Perpendicular to the plane of paper inwards.
4.	Straight wire and loop	At the centre.	$B = 0$	

5.	Straight wire & semi-circular loop	At the centre.	$B = \frac{\mu_0}{4\pi}\frac{\pi I}{a}$	Normal to the plane of paper, inwards.
6.	Circular loop	At the centre of loop.	$B = \frac{\mu_0}{4\pi}\left[\frac{2\pi I}{a} - \frac{2I}{a}\right]$	Normal to the plane of paper, inwards.
7.	Two concentric circular arcs	At the common centre.	$B = \frac{\mu_0}{4\pi} I\theta \left[\frac{1}{a} - \frac{1}{b}\right]$	Normal to the plane of paper, outwards.
8.	Semi-circular area and straight conductors	At the centre of the semi-circle.	$B = \frac{\mu_0}{4\pi}\frac{\pi I}{r} + \frac{\mu_0}{4\pi}\frac{I}{r}$	Normal to the plane of paper, outwards.
9.	Two concentric coils mutually normal to each other.	At the common centre.	$B = \sqrt{B_1^2 + B_2^2}$ where $B_1 = \frac{\mu_0}{4\pi}\frac{2\pi n_1 I}{a}$, $B_2 = \frac{\mu_0}{4\pi}\frac{2\pi n_2 I}{b}$	According to law of vectors addition.

Example 1.

In fig., there are two semi-circles of radii r_1 and r_2 in which a current i is flowing. Find the magnetic induction at centre O.

Solution :

$$B = B_1 + B_2 = \frac{\mu_0}{4\pi}\times\frac{\pi i}{r_1} + \frac{\mu_0}{4\pi}\times\frac{\pi i}{r_2}$$

$$= \frac{\mu_0 i}{4}\left[\frac{1}{r_1} + \frac{1}{r_2}\right] = \frac{\mu_0 i}{4}\left[\frac{r_1 + r_2}{r_1 r_2}\right]$$

Example 2.

Two circular coils X and Y having equal number of turns and carry equal currents in the same sense and subtend same solid angle at point O. If the smaller coil X is midway between O and Y, then if we represent the magnetic induction due to bigger coil Y at O as B_Y and due to smaller coil X at O as B_X then find $\frac{B_Y}{B_X}$.

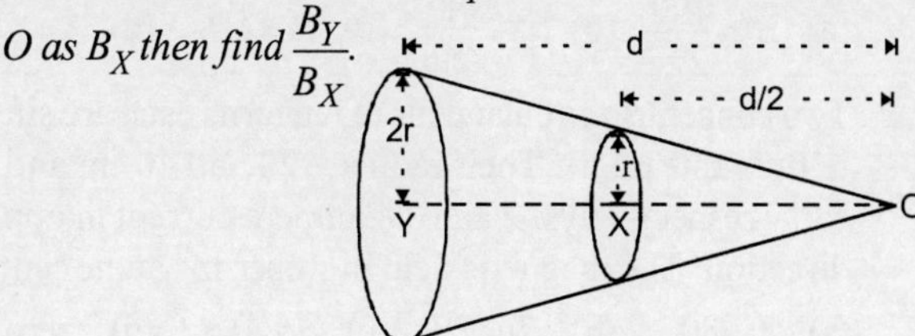

Solution :

Magnetic induction at O due to coil Y is given by

$$B_Y = \frac{\mu_0}{4\pi} \times \frac{2\pi I(2r)^2}{[(2r)^2 + (d)^2]^{3/2}} \quad ...(1)$$

Similarly, the magnetic induction at O due to coil X is given by

$$B_X = \frac{\mu_0}{4\pi} \times \frac{2\pi I(r)^2}{[(r)^2 + (d/2)^2]^{3/2}} \quad ...(2)$$

From eqs. (1) and (2), $\frac{B_Y}{B_X} = \frac{1}{2}$

Example 3.

A cell is connected between two points of a uniformly thick circular conductor. i_1 and i_2 are the currents flowing in two parts of the circular conductor of radius a. What will be the magnetic field at the centre of the loop?

Solution :

Let ℓ_1, ℓ_2 be the lengths of the two parts PRQ and PSQ of the conductor and ρ be the resistance per unit length of the conductor. The resistance of the portion PRQ will be $R_1 = \ell_1\rho$

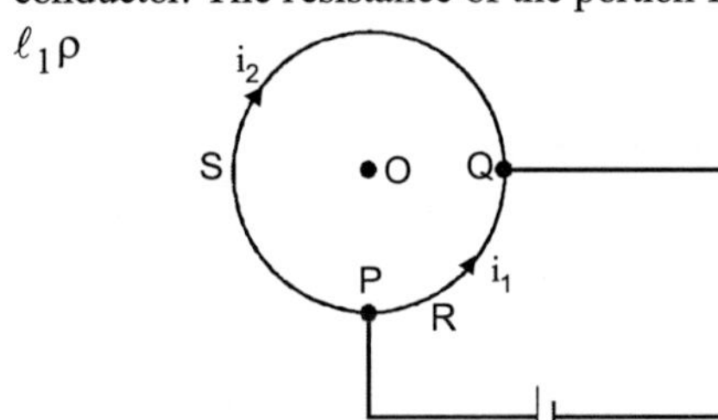

The resistance of the portion PSQ will be $R_2 = \ell_2\rho$

Pot. diff. across P and Q $= i_1R_1 = i_2R_2$

or $i_1\ell_1\rho = i_2\ell_2\rho$ or $i_1\ell_1 = i_2\ell_2$ ......(i)

Magnetic field induction at the centre O due to currents through circular conductors PRQ and PSQ will be

$$B_1 - B_2 = \frac{\mu_0}{4\pi}\frac{i_1\ell_1 \sin 90°}{r^2} - \frac{\mu_0}{4\pi}\frac{i_2\ell_2 \sin 90°}{r^2} = 0$$

Example 4.

A current passing through a circular coil of two turns produces magnetic field B at its centre. The coil is then rewound so as to have four turns and the same current is passed through it. The magnetic field at its centre now is

(a) 2 B *(b)* $\frac{B}{2}$ *(c)* $\frac{B}{4}$ *(d)* 4 B

Solution : (d)

$$B = \frac{\mu_0}{4\pi}\frac{2\pi nI}{r} \text{ i.e. } B \propto \frac{n}{r};$$

Given, $L = 2\pi r_1 \times 2 = 2\pi r_2 \times 4$; $r_1/r_2 = 4/2 = 2$

$$\frac{B_2}{B_1} = \frac{n_2}{n_1} \times \frac{r_1}{r_2} = \frac{4}{2} \times 2 = 4 \quad \text{or } B_2 = 4B_1 = 4B.$$

Example 5.

Compute the flux density in air at a point of 9 cm from the long straight wire carrying a current of 6A.

Solution :

Given : $a = 9 \text{ cm} = 9 \times 10^{-2}\text{ m}, I = 6A$

$$B = \frac{\mu_o I}{2\pi a} = \frac{4\pi \times 10^{-7} \times 6}{2\pi \times 9 \times 10^{-2}} = 1.33 \times 10^{-5}\text{ T}$$

Example 6.

Calculate the flux density at a distance of 1 cm from a very long straight wire carrying a current of 5A. At what distance from the wire will the field flux density neutralize that due to the earth's horizontal component flux density 2×10^{-5} T? ($\mu_0 = 4\pi \times 10^{-7}$ Hm^{-1})

Solution :

$$B = \frac{\mu_o I}{2\pi a} = \frac{4\pi \times 10^{-7} \times 5}{2\pi \times 1 \times 10^{-2}} = 10^{-4}\text{T}$$

For the second part,

$$a = \frac{\mu_o I}{2\pi B} = \frac{4\pi \times 10^{-7} \times 5}{2\pi \times 2 \times 10^{-5}} = 5 \times 10^{-2} = 5 \text{ cm}$$

Example 7.

A wire 28m long is bent into N turns of circular coil of diameter 14 cm forming a solenoid of length 60 cm. Calculate the flux density inside it when a current of 5 amp passed through it. ($\mu_0 = 12.57 \times 10^{-7}$ m^{-1})

Solution :

Given : $d = 14\text{cm} = 0.14\text{m}$ $\ell = 60\text{cm} = 0.6\text{ m}$

By the question, $N \times \pi d = 28$ m.

$$N \times \pi \times 0.14 = 28$$

$$\therefore N = \frac{28}{0.14 \times \pi} = 63.66 \text{ turns.}$$

$$B = \mu_0 nI = \mu_0 \frac{N}{\ell} I = 12.57 \times 10^{-7} \times \frac{63.66}{0.6} \times 5$$

$$= 6.67 \times 10^{-4}\text{T}$$

19.1 Concept Practice Problems

CPP

1. The magnetic field near the end of a long conductor at a distance *r* is

(a) $B = \frac{\mu_0 I}{2\pi d}$ (b) $B = \frac{\mu_0 I}{4\pi d}$ (c) $B = \frac{\mu_0 I}{\pi d}$ (d) $B = \frac{2\mu_0 I}{d}$

2. Two concentric circular coils of ten turns each are situated in the same plane. Their radii are 20 and 40 cm and they carry respectively 0.2 and 0.4 ampere current in opposite direction. The magnetic field in weber/m^2 at the centre is

(a) $\mu_0/80$ (b) $7\mu_0/80$ (c) $(5/4)\mu_0$ (d) zero

3. If we double the radius of a coil keeping the current through it unchanged, then the magnetic field at any point at a large distance from the centre becomes approximately

(a) double (b) three times
(c) four times (d) one-fourth

4. A long solenoid carrying a current produces a magnetic field B along its axis. If the current is double and the number of turns per cm is halved, the new value of the magnetic field is

(a) 4B (b) B/2 (c) B (d) 2B

5. Tesla is the unit of
(a) magnetic flux (b) magnetic field
(c) magnetic induction (d) magnetic moment

6. A portion of a conductive wire is bent in the form of a semicircle of radius r as shown below in fig. At the centre of semicircle, the magnetic induction will be

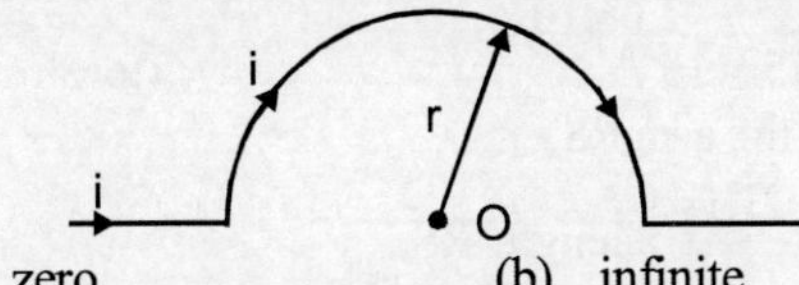

(a) zero (b) infinite
(c) $\frac{\mu_0}{4\pi}.\frac{\pi i}{r}$ gauss (d) $\frac{\mu_0}{4\pi}.\frac{\pi i}{r}$ tesla

7. A helium nucleus makes a full rotation in a circle of radius 0.8 meter in 2 sec. The value of the magnetic field induction B in tesla at the centre of circle will be
(a) $2\times10^{-19}\,\mu_0$ (b) $10^{-19}/\mu_0$
(c) $10^{-19}\,\mu_0$ (d) $2\times10^{-20}/\mu_0$

8. A solenoid of length 1.5 m and 4 cm diameter possesses 10 turns per cm. A current of 5A is flowing through it, the magnetic induction at axis inside the solenoid is
($\mu_0 = 4\pi\times10^{-7}$ weber amp^{-1} m^{-1})
(a) $4\pi\times10^{-5}$ gauss (b) $2\pi\times10^{-5}$ gauss
(c) $4\pi\times10^{-5}$ tesla (d) $2\pi\times10^{-5}$ tesla

9. The magnetic flux density B at a distance r from a long straight wire carrying a steady current varies with r as

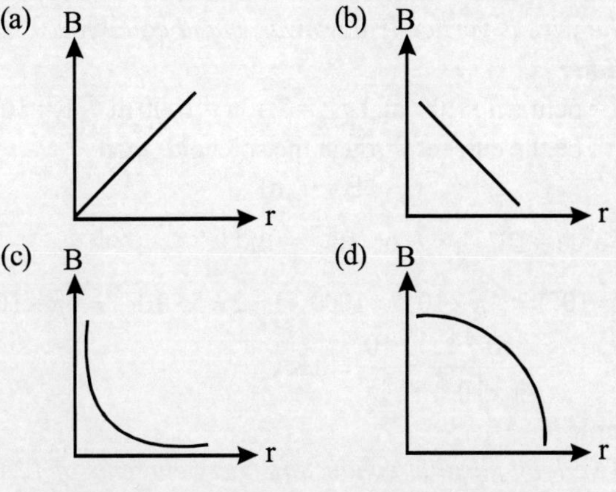

10. A current of I ampere flows along an infinitely long straight thin walled hollow metallic cylinder of radius r. The magnetic field at any point inside the cylinder at a distance x from the axis of the cylinder is
(a) ∞ (b) $\frac{\mu_0 I}{2\pi r}$ (c) $\frac{\mu_0 I}{2\pi x}$ (d) zero

ANSWER KEY

1	(b)	2	(d)	3	(c)	4	(c)	5	(b)	6	(d)	7	(c)	8	(d)	9	(c)	10	(d)

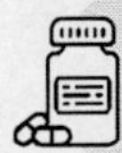

Topic 19.2 : Force on a Conductor, Torque on a Coil and Force Between two Parallel Current Carrying Conductors

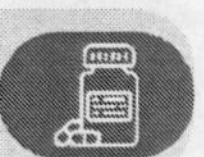

FORCE ON A CONDUCTOR

The force on a conductor is given by

$$F = BI\ell \sin\alpha$$

where ℓ is the length of the conductor in meter; B is the flux density of field in tesla (Wb/m^2); I is the current in ampere and α is the angle which the conductor makes with the direction of the field.

Special case :

If $\alpha = 90°$, then $F = BI\ell$

The direction of the force is given by Fleming's left hand rule.

TORQUE ON A COIL

The torque acting on a rectangular coil placed with its plane parallel to a uniform magnetic field of flux density B is given by

$$\tau = BINA$$

where N is the number of turns in the coil, A is the area and I is the current.

If the plane of the coil makes an angle α with the direction of the field, then

$$\tau = BINA\cos\alpha.$$

FORCE BETWEEN TWO PARALLEL CURRENT CARRYING CONDUCTORS

When a current flows in a conductor, the free charges (electrons in case of a metal wire) move. Each free charge movement generates a force which adds up to give the force on the conductor.

Force between infinitely long conductors placed parallel to each other at distance d.

$$\textit{Force per unit length} = \frac{F}{\ell} = \frac{\mu_0}{4\pi}\frac{2I_1 I_2}{d}$$

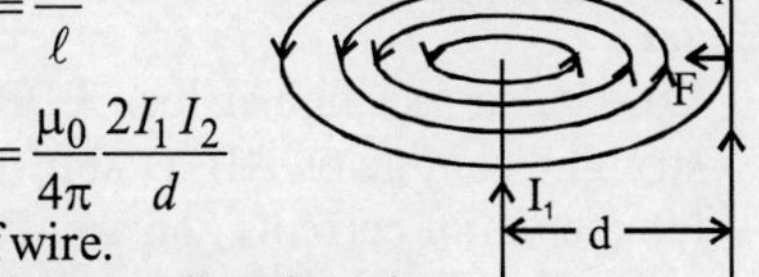

where ℓ is the length of wire.

If currents are pointing in same direction, the force is of attractive nature and if currents are oppositely directed the force is of repulsive nature.

Torque on a current loop in uniform magnetic field $\vec{B}$ is given by $\vec{\tau} = (\vec{M}\times\vec{B})$ where $\vec{M}$ is the magnetic moment of coil.

$\vec{M} = N\,I\,A\hat{n}$ where $\hat{n}$ is the unit vector normal to the plane of the loop.

Example 8.

A horizontal wire, of lenth 5 cm and carrying a current of 2A placed in the middle of a long solenoid and right angles to its axis. The solenoid has 1000 turns per metre and carries a steady current I. Calculate I if the force on the wire is vertically downwards and equal to 10^{-4} N.

Solution :

$l = 5cm = 5 \times 10^{-2} m, I_{wire} = 2A, n = 1000 m^{-1}, F = 10^{-4} N$

If I be the current through the solenoid, then

$$B = \mu_0 nI$$

$$\text{Force} = BI_{wire} \times \ell \text{ or } 10^{-4} = \mu_0 NI \times I_{wire} \times 1$$

$$\text{or } 10^{-4} = 4\pi \times 10^{-7} \times 1000 \times I \times 2 \times 5 \times 10^{-2} = 4\pi \times 10^{-5} I$$

$$\therefore I = \frac{10^{-4}}{4\pi \times 10^{-5}} = \frac{10}{4\pi} = 0.8A$$

Example 9.

Two long parallel conductors carry currents of 12A and 8A respectively in the same direction. If the wires are 10cm apart, find where the third parallel wire also carrying a current must be placed so that the force experienced by it shall be zero.

Solution :

For the force on the third conductor to be zero, the direction of the flux density due to the current flowing in the two wires must be opposite in the position of the wire.

$\therefore$ Third wire must be placed between the wire. Let the third wire placed at a distance x m from the wire carrying 12A,

then, $B_1 = B_2$

$$\frac{\mu_o I_1}{2\pi x} = \frac{\mu_o I_2}{2\pi(0.1 - x)}.$$

$$\text{or} \quad \frac{12}{x} = \frac{8}{0.1 - x} \text{ or } \frac{3}{x} = \frac{2}{0.1 - x}$$

$$\text{or} \quad 0.3 = 5x = \frac{0.3}{5} = 0.06 \text{ m}$$

Example 10.

A rectangular loop of sides 25 cm and 10 cm carrying a current of 15 A is placed with its longer side parallel to a long straight conductor 2.0 cm apart carrying a current of 25 A. What is the net force on the loop?

Solution :

Consider a rectangular loop PQRS placed near a long straight conductor AB as shown in Fig. Due to the interaction of currents, the arm PQ of the loop will get attracted while arm RS will get repelled. Forces on the arms QR and SP will be equal and opposite and hence cancel out.

Here, $PQ = 25 \text{ cm} = 25 \times 10^{-2}$ m,

$PS = 10 \text{ cm} = 10 \times 10^{-2}$ m

Distance of PQ from AB,

$r_1 = 2.0 \text{ cm} = 2.0 \times 10^{-2}$ m

Distance of RS from AB,

$r_2 = 2.0 + 10 = 12.0$ cm

$= 12.0 \times 10^{-2}$ m

Current through long wire AB, $I_1 = 25$ A

Current through rectangular loop, $I_2 = 15$ A

$$\therefore \text{Force on the arm PQ, } F_1 = \frac{\mu_0}{4\pi} \frac{2I_1 I_2}{r_1} \times \text{length PQ}$$

$$F_1 = \frac{10^{-1} \times 2 \times 25 \times 15 \times 25 \times 10^{-2}}{2.0 \times 10^{-2}}$$

$= 9.375 \times 10^{-4}$ (towards AB)

Force on the arm RS,

$$F_2 = \frac{\mu_0}{4\pi} \frac{2I_1 I_2}{r_2} \times \text{length RS}$$

$$= \frac{10^{-7} \times 2 \times 25 \times 15 \times 25 \times 10^{-2}}{12 \times 10^{-2}}$$

$= 1.563 \times 10^{-4}$ (away from AB)

$\therefore$ Effective force on the loop,

$F = F_1 - F_2 = 9.375 \times 10^{-4} - 1.563 \times 10^{-4} = 7.812 \times 10^{4}$ N (towards AB)

Example 11.

A narrow vertical rectangular coil is suspended from the middle of its upper side with its plane parallel to a uniform horizontal magnetic field of 0.02 T. The coil has 10 turns and the lengths of its vertical and horizontal sides are 0.1 m and 0.05 m respectively. Calculate the torque on the coil when a current of 5A is passed into it. What would be the new value of the torque if the plane of the vertical coil was initially at 60° to the magnetic field and a current of 5A was passed into the coil.

Solution :

$B = 0.02$ T, $N = 10$ turns

$A = l \times b = 0.1 \times 0.05 = 0.005 \text{ m}^2$

$I = 5A$

$\text{Torque} = BINA = 0.02 \times 5 \times 10 \times 0.005$

$= 0.005 \text{ Nm} = 5 \times 10^{-3}$ Nm

New value of the torque when the plane of the vertical coil was at 60° to the magnetic field.

$= BINA \cos\theta = 5 \times 10^{-3} \cos 60°$

$= 5 \times 10^{-3} \times \frac{1}{2} = 2.5 \times 10^{-3}$ Nm.

Example 12.

A rectangular coil of 50 turns hungs vertically in a uniform magnetic field of magnitude 10^{-2} T, so that the plane of the coil is parallel to the field, the mean height of the coil is 5cm and its mean width is 2cm. Calculate the strength of the current the must pass through the coil in order to deflect it 30° if the torsional constant of the suspension is 10^{-9} Nm per degree.

Solution :

$N = 50$ turns, $B = 10^{-2}$T, $q = 30°$

$C = 10^{-9}$ Nm per degree,

$A = 5 \times 2 \text{ cm}^2 = 10 \times 10^{-4} \text{ m}^2 = 10^{-3} \text{ m}^2$

$\text{Torque} = BINA \cos\theta = C\theta$

$$\therefore I = \frac{C\theta}{BNA\cos\theta} = \frac{10^{-9} \times 30}{10^{-2} \times 50 \times 10^{-3} \cos 30^o} = 6.9 \times 10^{-5}$$

$A = 69\mu A$

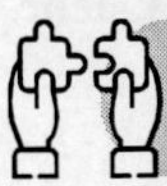

19.2 Concept Practice Problems

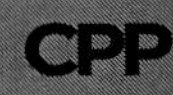

11. A current carrying coil is subjected to a uniform magnetic field. The coil will orient so that its plane becomes
(a) inclined at 45° to the magnetic field
(b) inclined at any arbitrary angle to the magnetic field
(c) parallel to the magnetic field
(d) perpendicular to the magnetic field

12. A current carrying conductor placed in a magnetic field experiences maximum force when angle between current and magnetic field is
(a) $3\pi/4$ (b) $\pi/2$ (c) $\pi/4$ (d) zero

13. A current of 3 A is flowing in a linear conductor having a length of 40 cm. The conductor is placed in a magnetic field of strength 500 gauss and makes an angle of 30° with the direction of the field. It experiences a force of magnitude
(a) 3×10^{-4} N (b) 3×10^{-2} N
(c) 3×10^{2} N (d) 3×10^{4} N

14. A circular loop of area 0.02 m^2 carrying a current of 10A, is held with its plane perpendicular to a magnetic field induction 0.2 T. The torque acting on the loop is
(a) 0.01 Nm (b) 0.001 Nm (c) zero (d) 0.8Nm

15. Through two parallel wires A and B, 10A and 2A of currents are passed respectively in opposite directions. If the wire A is infinitely long and the length of the wire B is 2m, then force on the conductor B, which is situated at 10 cm distance from A, will be
(a) 8×10^{-7} N (b) 8×10^{-5} N
(c) 4×10^{-7} N (d) 4×10^{-5} N

16. A circular loop of area 0.02 m^2 carrying a current of 10A, is held with its plane perpendicular to a magnetic field induction 0.2 T. The torque acting on the loop is
(a) 0.01 Nm (b) 0.001 Nm (c) zero (d) 0.8Nm

17. Two thin, long, parallel wires, separated by a distance 'd' carry a current of 'i' A in the same direction. They will
(a) repel each other with a force of $\mu_0 i^2/(2\pi d)$
(b) attract each other with a force of $\mu_0 i^2/(2\pi d)$
(c) repel each other with a force of $\mu_0 i^2/(2\pi d^2)$
(d) attract each other with a force of $\mu_0 i^2/(2\pi d^2)$

18. Four wires, each of length 2.0 m, are bent into four loops P, Q, R and S and then suspended in a uniform magnetic field. If the same current is passed in each, then the torque will be maximum on the loop

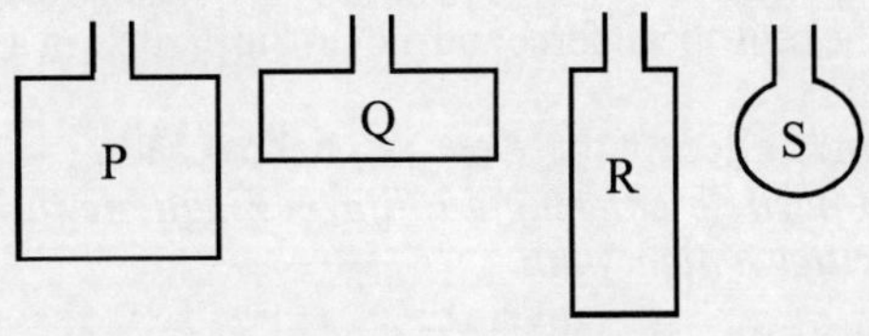

(a) P (b) Q (c) R (d) S

19. A current loop in a magnetic field
(a) can be in equilibrium in one orientation
(b) can be in equilibrium in two orientations, both the equilibrium states are unstable
(c) can be in equilibrium in two orientations, one stable while the other is unstable
(d) experiences a torque whether the field is uniform or non-uniform in all orientations

20. A straight wire of length 0.5 metre and carrying a current of 1.2 ampere is placed in uniform magnetic field of induction 2 tesla. The magnetic field is perpendicular to the length of the wire. The force on the wire is
(a) 2.4 N (b) 1.2 N (c) 3.0 N (d) 2.0 N

ANSWER KEY

11	(d)	12	(b)	13	(b)	14	(c)	15	(b)	16	(c)	17	(b)	18	(d)	19	(c)	20	(b)

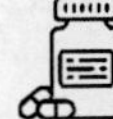

Topic 19.3 : Force Acting on a Charged Particle Moving in a Uniform Magnetic Field and Moving Coil Galvanometer

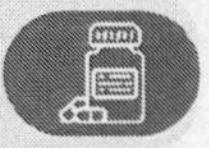

FORCE ACTING ON A CHARGED PARTICLE MOVING IN A UNIFORM MAGNETIC FIELD

The force acting on a particle having a charge q and moving with velocity $\vec{v}$ in a uniform magnetic field $\vec{B}$ is given by

$\vec{F} = q(\vec{v} \times \vec{B}) \Rightarrow F = qvB\sin\theta$,

where θ is the angle between $\vec{v}$ and $\vec{B}$

Case (i) If $\theta = 0, F = 0$. Also if $\theta = 180°, F = 0$

If a charged particle enters a uniform magnetic field in the direction of magnetic field or in the opposite direction of magnetic field, the force acting on the charged particle is zero.

Case (ii) If $\theta = 90°, F = qvB$

In this case the force acting on the particle is maximum and this force acts as centripetal force which makes the charged particle move in a circular path.

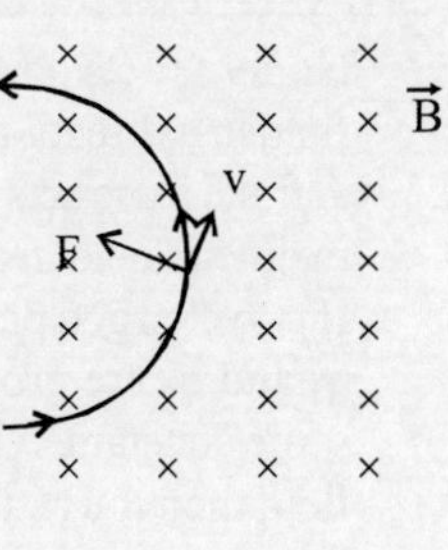

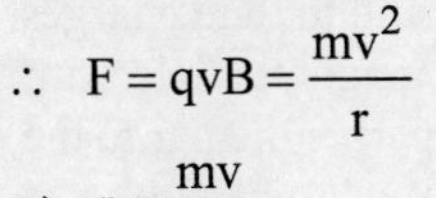

$$\therefore \ F = qvB = \frac{mv^2}{r}$$

$$\Rightarrow r = \frac{mv}{qB}$$

where r is the radius of the circular path.

It is important to note that this force cannot change the speed of the charged particle and hence its kinetic energy. But it changes the velocity of charged particle (due to change in direction) and hence also causes a change in momentum.
Also the work done by the force is zero as the force is acting perpendicular to the direction of motion.

Case (iii) If $\theta = \alpha$ is any other angle then the path taken is helical. The velocity of the charged particle can be split into two parts for better understnading.

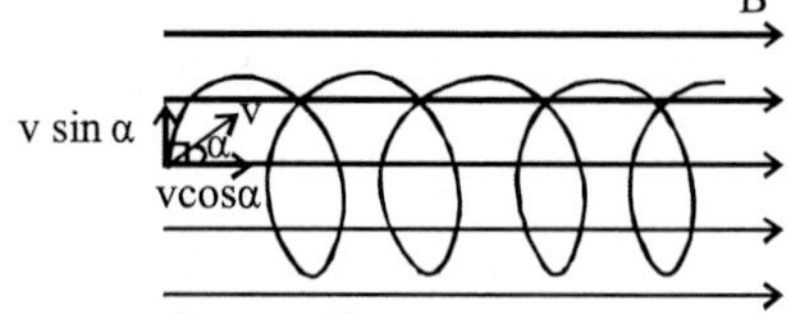

(a) $v \cos \alpha$: The force on charged particle due to this component is zero. This component is responsible in moving the charged particle uniformly in the direction of $\vec{B}$.

(b) $v \sin \alpha$: The force acting on charged particle due to this component is $q(v \sin \alpha) B \sin 90° = qvB \sin \alpha$. This acts as the centripetal force and moves the particle in a circular path.

The combined effect of these two is a helical path.

A charged particle entering a uniform magnetic field at an angle executes helical path.

Radius of the helix, $R = \dfrac{mv \sin \alpha}{qB}$

Angular frequency of rotation, $\omega = (2\pi / T) = qB / m$

Pitch of the helix $= (v \cos \alpha) T = \dfrac{2\pi mv \cos \alpha}{qB}$.

Direction of force $\vec{F}$: We can use the rule of cross product. The direction of $\vec{F}$ is perpendicular to the plane containing $\vec{v}$ and $\vec{B}$ and can be found by right hand thumb rule. It is important to note that if q is positive, we will get the correct direction of $\vec{F}$ by right hand thumb rule. But if q is negative, we have to reverse the direction of force.

Flemings left hand rule : *It states that if the fore finger, the central finger and the thumb of the left hand are stretched at right angles to each other then if the central finger represents the direction of current and fore finger represents field, the thumb will represent the direction of motion or force experienced by the current carrying conductor.*

Lorentz Force Equation

For a charged particle q moving in a region of simultaneously applied electric field $\vec{E}$ and magnetic field $\vec{B}$, the force experienced by it is given by

$$\vec{F} = q[\vec{E} + (\vec{v} \times \vec{B})]$$

Problem Solving Tips

1. No force acts on a charged particle if it enters a magnetic field in a direction parallel or antiparallel to the field.
2. A finite force acts on a charged particle if it enters a uniform magnetic field in a direction with finite angle with the field.
3. If two charged particles of masses m_1 and m_2 and charges q_1 and q_2 are projected in a uniform magnetic field with same constant velocity in a direction perpendicular to the field then the ratio of their radii ($R_1 : R_2$) is given by
$$\frac{R_1}{R_2} = \frac{m_1}{m_2} \times \frac{q_2}{q_1}$$
4. The force on a conductor carrying current in a magnetic field is directly proportional to the current, the length of conductor and the magnetic field.
5. If the distance between the two parallel conductors is decreased (or increased) by k-times then the force between them increases (or decreases) k-times.
6. The momentum of the charged particle moving along the direction of magnetic field does not change, since the force acting on it due to magnetic field is zero.
7. Lorentz force between two charges q_1 and q_2 moving with velocity v_1, v_2 separated by distance r is given by:
$$F_m = \frac{\mu_0}{4\pi} \cdot \frac{(q_1 v_1)(q_2 v_2)}{r^2}$$
8. If the charges move, the electric as well as magnetic fields are produced. In case the charges move with speeds comparable to the speed of light, magnetic and electric force between them would become comparable.
9. A current carrying coil is in stable equilibrium if the magnetic dipole moment $\vec{M}$, is parallel to $\vec{B}$ and is in unstable equilibrium when $\vec{M}$ is antiparallel to $\vec{B}$.
10. Magnetic moment is independent of the shape of the loop. It depends on the area of the loop.
11. A straight conductor and a conductor of any shape in the same plane and between the same two end points carrying equal current in the same direction, when placed in the same magnetic field experience the same force.
12. There is net repulsion between two similar charges moving parallel to each other inspite of attractive magnetic force between them. This is because of electric force of repulsion which is much more stronger than the magnetic force.
13. The speed of the charged particle can only be changed by an electric force.

MOVING COIL GALVANOMETER

The moving coil galvanometer was first devised by Kelvin and later on modified by D'Arsonaval. This is used for detection and measurement of small electric current.

The **principle of a moving coil galvanometer** is based on the fact that when a current carrying coil is placed in a magnetic field, it experiences a torque.

Construction: A moving coil ballistic galvanometer is shown in figure.

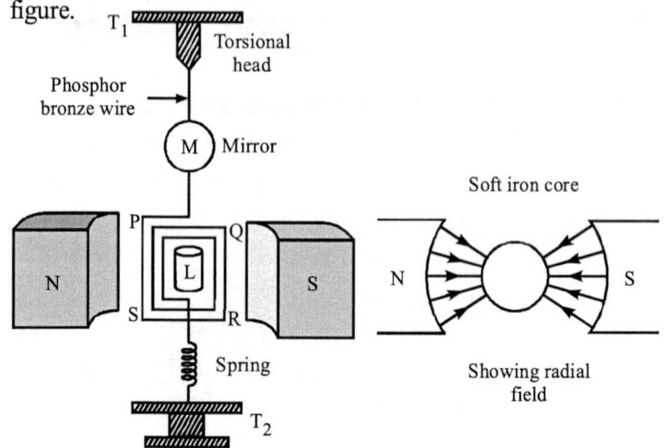

It essentially consists of a rectangular coil PQRS or a cylindrical coil of large number of turns of fine insulated wire wound over a non-conducting frame of ivory or bamboo. This coil is suspended by means of phosphor bronze wire between the pole pieces of a powerful horse shoe magnet NS. The poles of the magnet are curved to make the field radial. The lower end of the coil, is attached to a spring of phosphor-bronze wire. The spring and the free ends of phosphor bronze wire are joined to two terminals T_2 and T_1 respectively on the top of the case of the instrument. L is a soft iron core. A small mirror M is attached on the suspension wire. Using lamp and scale arrangement, the deflection of the coil can be recorded. The whole arrangement is enclosed in a non-metallic case.

Theory : Let the coil be suspended freely in the magnetic field.
Suppose, n = number of turns in the coil
A = area of the coil
B = magnetic field induction of radial magnetic field in which the coil is suspended.
Here, the magnetic field is radial, i.e., the plane of the coil always remains parallel to the direction of magnetic field, and hence the torque acting on the coil

$$\tau = niAB \quad \ldots(1)$$

Due to this torque, the coil rotates. As a result, the suspension wire gets twisted. Now a restoring torque is developed in the suspension wire. The coil will rotate till the deflecting torque acting on the coil due to flow of current through it is balanced by the restoring torque developed in the suspension wire due to twisting. Let C be the restoring couple for unit twist in the suspension wire and θ be the angle through which the coil has turned. The couple for this twist θ is Cθ.
In equilibrium, deflecting couple = restoring couple

$\therefore$ ni AB = Cθ or i = Cθ/ (nAB)

or i = Kθ (where C/nAB = K) ...(2)

K is a constant for galvanometer and is known as galvanometer constant. Hence $i \propto \theta$

Therefore, the deflection produced in the galvanometer is directly proportional to the current flowing through it.

Current sensitivity of the galvanometer : *The current sensitivity of a galvanometer is defined as the deflection produced in the galvanometer when a unit current is passed through it.*

We know that, niAB = Cθ

$$\therefore \quad \text{Current sensitivity, } i_s = \frac{\theta}{i} = \frac{nAB}{C}$$

where C = restoring couple per unit twist

The **SI unit** of current sensitivity is radian per ampere or deflection per ampere.

Voltage sensitivity of the galvanometer : *The voltage sensitivity of the galvanometer is defined as the deflection produced in the galvanometer when a unit voltage is applied across the terminals of the galvanometer.*

$$\therefore \quad \text{Voltage sensitivity, } V_s = \frac{\theta}{V}$$

If R be the resistance of the galvanometer and a current is passed through it, then

$$V = iR$$

$$\therefore \quad \text{Voltage sensitivity, } V_s = \frac{\theta}{iR} = \frac{nAB}{CR}$$

The **SI. unit** of voltage sensitivity is radian per ampere or deflection per ampere.

Conditions for sensitivity : A galvanometer is said to be more sensitive if it shows a large deflection even for a small value of current.

We know that, $\theta = \frac{nAB}{C} i$

For a given value of *i*, θ will be large if (i) n is large, (ii) A is large, (iii) B is large, and (iv) C is small.

Regarding above factors, n and A cannot be increased beyond a certain limit. By increasing n, the resistance of the galvanometer will increase and by increasing A, the size of the galvanometer will increase. So, the sensitivity will decrease. Therefore, B is increased. The value of B can be increased by using strong horse shoe magnet. Further, the value of C can be decreased. The value of C for quartz and phosphor-bronze is very small. So, the suspension wire of quartz or phosphor-bronze is used. The value of C is further decreased if the wire is hammered into a flat strip.

Example 13.

Two particles X and Y having equal charges, after being accelerated throught the same potential difference, enter a region of uniform magnetic field and describe circular paths of radii R_1 and R_2 respectively. Find the ratio of mass of X to that of Y.

Solution :

$$\frac{1}{2}mv^2 = qV \quad \therefore v = (2qV/m)^{1/2}$$

(where V is the potential difference)

$$\text{Centripetal force } \frac{mv^2}{R} = qvB \quad \therefore v = \left(\frac{qB}{m}\right)R$$

$$\text{Hence } \left(\frac{2qV}{m}\right)^{1/2} = \left(\frac{qB}{m}\right)R \text{ or } R = \left(\frac{2mV}{q}\right)^{1/2} \times \frac{1}{B}$$

Here V, q and B are constant. Hence $R \propto \sqrt{m}$

$$\therefore \quad \frac{m_1}{m_2} = \left(\frac{R_1}{R_2}\right)^2$$

Example 14.

An electron beam moving with a velocity of 10^6 ms^{-1} through a uniform magnetic field of 0.1T, which is perpendicular to the direction of the beam. Calculate the force on an electron if the electron charge is 1.6×10^{-19}C.

Solution :

$v = 10^{-6} ms^{-1}$, B = 0.IT, $q = 1.6 \times 10^{-19}$C

$F = Bqv = 0.1 \times 10^6 \times 10^{19} = 1.6 \times 10^{-14}$ N

Example 15.

A copper wire has 1.0×10^{29} free electrons per cubic metre, a cross sectional area of $2.0\ mm^2$ and carries a current of 5.0A. Calculate the force acting on each electron if the wire is now placed in a magnetic field of flux density 0.15 T which is perpendicular to the wire ($e = 1.6 \times 10^{19}$C)

Solution :

$n = 10 \times 10^{29}\, m^{-3}, A = 2.0\, mm^2 = 2 \times 10^{-6}\, m^2$

$I = 5.0A, B = 0.15\, T, F = ?.$

$I = nevA \text{ or } v = \frac{I}{nev}$

$F = Bev = \frac{Be \times I}{neA} = \frac{BI}{nA} = \frac{0.15 \times 5}{1.0 \times 10^{29} \times 2 \times 10^{-6}}$

$= 3.75 \times 10^{-24}\, N$

Example 16.

If the coil of a moving coil galvanometer having 10 turns and of resistance 4Ω is removed and is replaced by a second coil having 100 turns and of resistance 160Ω. Calculate

(a) the factor by which the current sensitivity changes and

(b) the factor by which the voltage sensitivity changes.

Solution :

Given : $N_1 = 10$ turns, $R = 4\Omega$

$N_2 = 100$ turns, $R_2 = 160\Omega$

(a) Current sensitivity with the Ist coil, $\left(\frac{\theta}{I}\right)_1 = \frac{N_1 AB}{C}$

Current sensitivity with the 2nd coil $\left(\frac{\theta}{I}\right)_2 = \frac{N_2 AB}{C}$

$\therefore \frac{\left(\frac{\theta}{I}\right)_2}{\left(\frac{\theta}{I}\right)_1} = \frac{N_2}{N_1} = \frac{100}{10} = 10$

(b) Voltage sensitivity with the Ist coil $\left(\frac{\theta}{V}\right)_1 = \frac{N_1 AB}{CR_1}$

Voltage sensitivity with the 2nd coil $\left(\frac{\theta}{V}\right)_2 = \frac{N_2 AB}{CR_2}$

$\therefore \frac{\left(\frac{\theta}{V}\right)_2}{\left(\frac{\theta}{V}\right)_1} = \frac{N_2}{N_1}\frac{R_1}{R_2} = \frac{100}{10} \times \frac{4}{160} = \frac{1}{4}$

19.3 Concept Practice Problems

CPP

21. An electron enters a region where magnetic field (B) and electric field (E) are mutually perpendicular, then
(a) it will always move in the direction of B
(b) it will always move in the direction of E
(c) it always possesses circular motion
(d) it can go undeflected also

22. A proton, deutron and an α-particle enter a magnetic field perpendicular to field with same velocity. What is the ratio of the radii of circular paths?
(a) 1 : 2 : 2 (b) 2 : 1 : 1 (c) 1 : 1 : 2 (d) 1 : 2 : 1

23. If an electron and a proton having same momenta enter perpendicular to a magnetic field, then
(a) curved path of electron and proton will be same (ignoring the sense of revolution)
(b) they will move undeflected
(c) curved path of electron is more curved than that of the proton
(d) path of proton is more curved

24. In cyclotron the gyro radius is
(a) proportional to momentum
(b) proportional to energy
(c) inversely proportional to momentum
(d) inversely proportional to energy

25. The current sensitivity of a moving coil galvanometer depends on
(a) the number of turns in the coil
(b) moment of inertia of the coil
(c) current sent through galvanometer
(d) eddy current in Al frame

26. The radius of motion of a charged particle oscillating in a magnetic field is
(a) $\frac{mB}{qv}$ (b) $\frac{mv}{qB}$ (c) $\frac{mq}{vB}$ (d) $\frac{qv}{mB}$

27. In cyclotron the charged particle may be accelerated upto energies
(a) Several eV (b) MeV
(c) BeV (d) Kev

28. In cyclotron the resonance condition is
(a) the frequency of revolution of charged particle is equal to the frequency of A.C. voltage sources
(b) the frequency of revolution of charged particle is equal to the frequency of applied magnetic field
(c) the frequency of revolution of charged particle is equal to the frequency of rotation of earth
(d) the frequency of revolution of charged particle, frequency of A.C. source and frequency of magnetic field are equal

29. Two parallel wires carrying currents in the same direction attract each other because of
(a) mutual inductance between them
(b) potential difference between them
(c) electric forces between them
(d) magnetic forces between them

30. If a current is passed through a spring then the spring will
(a) expand (b) compress
(c) remains same (d) None of these.

ANSWER KEY

21	(d)	22	(a)	23	(a)	24	(a)	25	(a)	26	(b)	27	(b)	28	(a)	29	(d)	30	(b)

CONCEPT MAP

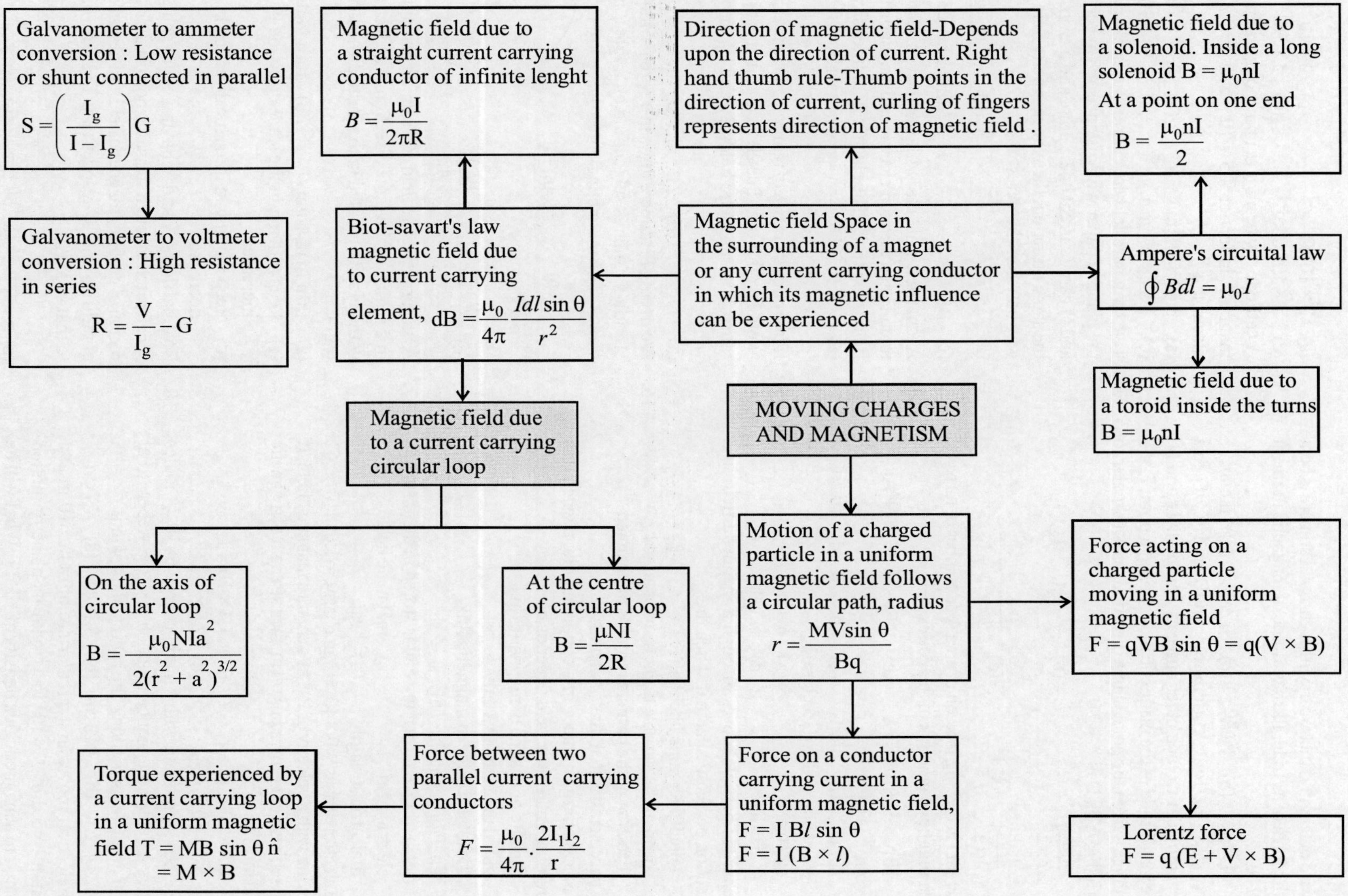

MOVING CHARGES AND MAGNETISM

Magnetic field Space in the surrounding of a magnet or any current carrying conductor in which its magnetic influence can be experienced

Direction of magnetic field-Depends upon the direction of current. Right hand thumb rule-Thumb points in the direction of current, curling of fingers represents direction of magnetic field .

Biot-savart's law magnetic field due to current carrying element, $dB = \frac{\mu_0}{4\pi}\frac{Idl\sin\theta}{r^2}$

Magnetic field due to a straight current carrying conductor of infinite lenght $B = \frac{\mu_0 I}{2\pi R}$

Magnetic field due to a current carrying circular loop

- On the axis of circular loop $B = \frac{\mu_0 NIa^2}{2(r^2 + a^2)^{3/2}}$
- At the centre of circular loop $B = \frac{\mu NI}{2R}$

Ampere's circuital law $\oint Bdl = \mu_0 I$

Magnetic field due to a solenoid. Inside a long solenoid $B = \mu_0 nI$

At a point on one end $B = \frac{\mu_0 nI}{2}$

Magnetic field due to a toroid inside the turns $B = \mu_0 nI$

Galvanometer to ammeter conversion : Low resistance or shunt connected in parallel $S = \left(\frac{I_g}{I - I_g}\right)G$

Galvanometer to voltmeter conversion : High resistance in series $R = \frac{V}{I_g} - G$

Motion of a charged particle in a uniform magnetic field follows a circular path, radius $r = \frac{MV\sin\theta}{Bq}$

Force acting on a charged particle moving in a uniform magnetic field $F = qVB\sin\theta = q(V \times B)$

Lorentz force $F = q(E + V \times B)$

Force on a conductor carrying current in a uniform magnetic field, $F = IBl\sin\theta$, $F = I(B \times l)$

Force between two parallel current carrying conductors $F = \frac{\mu_0}{4\pi}.\frac{2I_1I_2}{r}$

Torque experienced by a current carrying loop in a uniform magnetic field $T = MB\sin\theta\,\hat{n} = M \times B$

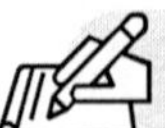

Exercise 1 - Chapter Revision Problems

CRP

1. A wire of length L metre carrying a current I ampere is bent in the form of a circle. Its magnitude of magnetic moment will be
   (a) $IL/4\pi$ (b) $I^2L^2/4\pi$ (c) $IL^2/4\pi$ (d) $IL^2/8\pi$
2. Two straight long conductors AOB and COD are perpendicular to each other and carry currents I_1 and I_2. The magnitude of the magnetic induction at a point P at a distance a from the point O in a direction perpendicular to the plane ABCD is
   (a) $\frac{\mu_0}{2\pi a}(I_1+I_2)$ (b) $\frac{\mu_0}{2\pi a}(I_1-I_2)$
   (c) $\frac{\mu_0}{2\pi a}(I_1^2+I_2^2)^{\frac{1}{2}}$ (d) $\frac{\mu_0}{2\pi a}\frac{I_1 I_2}{I_1+I_2}$
3. Current i is flowing in a coil of area A & number of turns N, then magnetic moment of the coil is M is equal to
   (a) NiA (b) Ni/A (c) $Ni/\sqrt{A}$ (d) N^2Ai
4. 1 Wbm^{-2} is equal to
   (a) 10^4 G (b) 10^2 G (c) 10^{-2} G (d) 10^{-4} G
5. Cyclotron is used to accelerate
   (a) electrons (b) neutrons
   (c) α particles (d) negative ions
6. A charged particle moves through a magnetic field in a direction perpendicular to it. Then the
   (a) velocity remains unchanged
   (b) speed of the particle remains unchanged
   (c) direction of the particle remains unchanged
   (d) acceleration remains unchanged
7. The total charge induced in a conducting loop when it is moved in a magnetic field depends on
   (a) the rate of change of magnetic flux
   (b) initial magnetic flux only
   (c) the total change in magnetic flux
   (d) final magnetic flux only
8. Energy in a current carrying coil is stored in the form of
   (a) electric field (b) magnetic field
   (c) dielectric strength (d) heat
9. An electron (mass = 9×10^{-31} kg, charge = 1.6×10^{-19} C) moving with a velocity of 10^6 m/s enters a magnetic field. If it describes a circle of radius 0.1m, then strength of magnetic field must be
   (a) 4.5×10^{-5} T (b) 1.4×10^{-5} T
   (c) 5.5×10^{-5} T (d) 2.6×10^{-5} T
10. An electron moving with kinetic energy 6×10^{-16} joules enters a field of magnetic induction 6×10^{-3} weber/m^2 at right angle to its motion. The radius of its path is
    (a) 3.42 cm (b) 4.23 cm (c) 5.17 cm (d) 7.7 cm
11. An electron moves in a circular arc of radius 10 m at a contant speed of 2×10^7 ms^{-1} with its plane of motion normal to a magnetic flux density of 10^{-5} T. What will be the value of specific charge of the electron?
    (a) 2×10^4 C kg^{-1} (b) 2×10^5 C kg^{-1}
    (c) 5×10^6 C kg^{-1} (d) 2×10^{11} C kg^{-1}
12. A cathode ray beam is bent in a circle of radius 2 cm by a magnetic induction 4.5×10^{-3} weber/m^2. The velocity of electron is
    (a) 3.43×10^7 m/s (b) 5.37×10^7 m/s
    (c) 1.23×10^7 m/s (d) 1.58×10^7 m/s
13. Two long parallel wires P and Q are held perpendicular to the plane of paper with distance of 5 m between them. If P and Q carry current of 2.5 amp. and 5 amp. respectively in the same direction, then the magnetic field at a point half-way between the wires is
    (a) $\mu_0/17$ (b) $\sqrt{3}\mu_0/2\pi$
    (c) $\mu_0/2\pi$ (d) $3\mu_0/2\pi$
14. A charged particle with velocity 2×10^3 m/s passes undeflected through electric and magnetic field. Magnetic field is 1.5 tesla. The electric field intensity would be
    (a) 2×10^3 N/C (b) 1.5×10^3 N/C
    (c) 3×10^3 N/C (d) $4/3\times10^{-3}$ N/C
15. If in a circular coil A of radius R, current I is flowing and in another coil B of radius 2R a current 2I is flowing, then the ratio of the magnetic fields B_A and B_B, produced by them will be
    (a) 1 (b) 2 (c) 1/2 (d) 4
16. A current of I ampere flows in a wire forming a circular arc of radius r metres subtending an angle θ at the centre as shown. The magnetic field at the centre O in tesla is
    (a) $\frac{\mu_0 I\theta}{4\pi r}$ (b) $\frac{\mu_0 I\theta}{2\pi r}$
    (c) $\frac{\mu_0 I\theta}{2r}$ (d) $\frac{\mu_0 I\theta}{4r}$

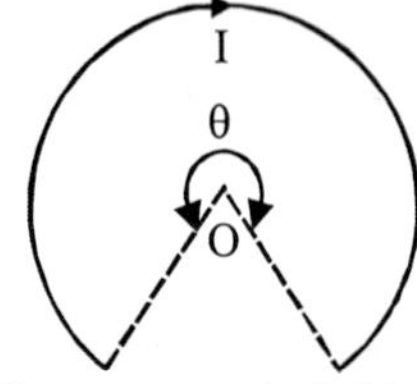

17. A uniform electric field and a uniform magnetic field exist in a region in the same direction. An electron is projected with velocity pointed in the same direction. The electron will
    (a) turn to its right (b) turn to its left
    (c) keep moving in the same direction but its speed will increase
    (d) keep moving in the same direction but its speed will decrease
18. Two particles X and Y having equal charge, after being accelerated through the same potential difference enter a region of uniform magnetic field and describe circular paths of radii R_1 and R_2 respectively. The ratio of the mass of X to that of Y is
    (a) $\sqrt{\frac{R_1}{R_2}}$ (b) $\left(\frac{R_2}{R_1}\right)^2$ (c) $\left(\frac{R_1}{R_2}\right)^2$ (d) $\sqrt{\frac{R_2}{R_1}}$

19. A square coil of side a carries a current I. The magnetic field at the centre of the coil is

(a) $\frac{\mu_0 I}{a\pi}$ (b) $\frac{\sqrt{2}\mu_0 I}{a\pi}$

(c) $\frac{\mu_0 I}{\sqrt{2}\,a\pi}$ (d) $\frac{2\sqrt{2}\,\mu_0 I}{a\pi}$

20. Protons and α-particles of equal momenta enter a uniform magnetic field normally. The radii of their orbits will have the ratio.

(a) 1 (b) 2 (c) 0.5 (d) 4

21. What is cyclotron frequency of an electron with an energy of 100 e V in the earth's magnetic field of 1×10^{-4} weber / m^2 if its velocity is perpendicular to magnetic field?

(a) 0.7 MHz (b) 2.8 MHz (c) 1.4 MHz (d) 2.1 MHz

22. A horizontal overhead powerline is at height of 4m from the ground and carries a current of 100A from east to west. The magnetic field directly below it on the ground is ($\mu_0 = 4\pi \times 10^{-7}$ TmA^{-1})

(a) 2.5×10^{-7} T southward (b) 5×10^{-6} T northward

(c) 5×10^{-6} T southward (d) 2.5×10^{-7} T northward

23. If an electron describes half a revolution in a circle of radius r in a magnetic field B, the energy acquired by it is

(a) zero (b) $\frac{1}{2}mv^2$ (c) $\frac{1}{4}mv^2$ (d) $\pi r \times Bev$

24. The orbital speed of electron orbiting around a nucleus in a circular orbit of radius 50 pm is 2.2×10^6 ms^{-1}. Then the magnetic dipole moment of an electron is

(a) 1.6×10^{-19} Am^2 (b) 5.3×10^{-21} Am^2

(c) 8.8×10^{-24} Am^2 (d) 8.8×10^{-26} Am^2

25. A proton and an α-particle enter a uniform magnetic field perpendicularly with the same speed. If proton takes 25 μ second to make 5 revolutions, then the time period for the α-particle would be

(a) 50 μ sec (b) 25 μ sec (c) 10 μ sec (d) 5 μ sec

26. In fig, what is the magnetic field induction at point O

(a) $\frac{\mu_0 i}{4\pi r}$

(b) $\frac{\mu_0 i}{4r} + \frac{\mu_0 i}{2\pi r}$

(c) $\frac{\mu_0 i}{4r} + \frac{\mu_0 i}{4\pi r}$

(d) $\frac{\mu_0 i}{4r} - \frac{\mu_0 i}{4\pi r}$

27. Three wires are situated at the same distance. A current of 1A, 2A, 3A flows through these wires in the same direction. What is ratio of F_1/F_2, where F_1 is force on 1 and F_2 on 2?

(a) 7/8

(b) 1

(c) 9/8

(d) None of these

28. A charged particle (charge q) is moving in a circle of radius R with uniform speed v. The associated magnetic moment μ is given by

(a) qvR^2 (b) $qvR^2/2$ (c) qvR (d) qvR/2

29. A straight wire of diameter 0.5 mm, carrying a current of 1A is replaced by another wire of 1mm diameter carrying the same current. The strength of magnetic field far away is

(a) unchanged

(b) quarter of its earlier value

(c) half of the earlier value

(d) twice the earlier value

30. The magnetic field (dB) due to small element (dl) at a distance ($\vec{r}$) from element carrying current i, is

(a) $dB = \frac{\mu_0}{4\pi} i \left(\frac{\vec{dl} \times \vec{r}}{r}\right)$ (b) $dB = \frac{\mu_0}{4\pi} i^2 \left(\frac{\vec{dl} \times \vec{r}}{r^2}\right)$

(c) $dB = \frac{\mu_0}{4\pi} i^2 \left(\frac{\vec{dl} \times \vec{r}}{r^2}\right)$ (d) $dB = \frac{\mu_0}{4\pi} i \left(\frac{\vec{dl} \times \vec{r}}{r^3}\right)$

31. A 10eV electron is circulating in a plane at right angles to a uniform field at a magnetic induction 10^{-4} Wb/m^2 (= 1.0 gauss). The orbital radius of the electron is

(a) 12 cm (b) 16 cm (c) 11 cm (d) 18 cm

32. A current carrying loop in the form of a right angle isosceles triangle ABC is placed in a uniform magnetic field acting along AB. If the magnetic force on the arm BC is F, what is the force on the arm AC?

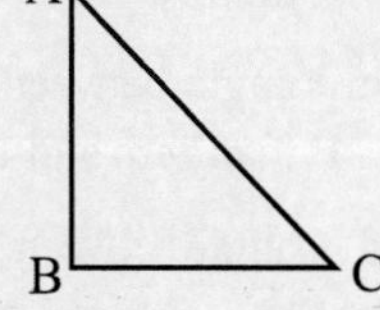

(a) $-\sqrt{2}\,\vec{F}$

(b) $-\vec{F}$

(c) $\vec{F}$

(d) $\sqrt{2}\,\vec{F}$

33. Two similar coils of radius *R* are lying concentrically with their planes at right angles to each other. The currents flowing in them are *I* and 2 *I*, respectively. The resultant magnetic field induction at the centre will be

(a) $\frac{\sqrt{5}\mu_0 I}{2R}$ (b) $\frac{3\mu_0 I}{2R}$ (c) $\frac{\mu_0 I}{2R}$ (d) $\frac{\mu_0 I}{R}$

34. An alternating electric field, of frequency *v*, is applied across the dees (radius = *R*) of a cyclotron that is being used to accelerate protons (mass = *m*). The operating magnetic field (*B*) used in the cyclotron and the kinetic energy (*K*) of the proton beam, produced by it, are given by

(a) $B = \frac{mv}{e}$ and $K = 2m\pi^2 v^2 R^2$

(b) $B = \frac{2\pi mv}{e}$ and $K = m^2 \pi v R^2$

(c) $B = \frac{2\pi mv}{e}$ and $K = 2m\pi^2 v^2 R^2$

(d) $B = \frac{mv}{e}$ and $K = m^2 \pi v R^2$

35. A proton carrying 1 MeV kinetic energy is moving in a circular path of radius *R* in uniform magnetic field. What should be the energy of an α-particle to describe a circle of same radius in the same field?

(a) 2 MeV (b) 1 MeV (c) 0.5 MeV (d) 4 MeV

36. A charged particle moves through a magnetic field in a direction perpendicular to it. Then the

(a) velocity remains unchanged
(b) speed of the particle remains unchanged
(c) direction of the particle remains unchanged
(d) acceleration remains unchanged

37. A conducting circular loop of radius r carries a constant current i. It is placed in a uniform magnetic field B such that B is perpendicular to the plane of the loop. The magnetic force acting on the loop is :

(a) irB (b) $2\pi riB$ (c) zero (d) πriB

38. A proton moving vertically downward enters a magnetic field pointing towards north. In which direction proton will deflect?

(a) East (b) West (c) North (d) South

39. When a charged particle moving with velocity $\vec{v}$ is subjected to a magnetic field of induction $\vec{B}$, the force on it is non-zero. This implies that

(a) angle between $\vec{v}$ and $\vec{B}$ is necessarily 90°
(b) angle between $\vec{v}$ and $\vec{B}$ can have any value other than 90°
(c) angle between $\vec{v}$ and $\vec{B}$ can have any value other than zero and 180°
(d) angle between $\vec{v}$ and $\vec{B}$ is either zero or 180°

40. A coil carrying electric current is placed in uniform magnetic field, then

(a) torque is formed
(b) e.m.f is induced
(c) both (a) and (b) are correct
(d) none of the above

41. A charge moving with velocity v in X-direction is subjected to a field of magnetic induction in negative X-direction. As a result, the charge will

(a) remain unaffected
(b) start moving in a circular path Y–Z plane
(c) retard along X-axis
(d) move along a helical path around X-axis

42. The magnetic field at a distance r from a long wire carrying current i is 0.4 tesla. The magnetic field at a distance 2r is

(a) 0.2 tesla (b) 0.8 tesla (c) 0.1 tesla (d) 1.6 tesla

43. A uniform magnetic field acts at right angles to the direction of motion of electron. As a result, the electron moves in a circular path of radius 2cm. If the speed of electron is doubled, then the radius of the circular path will be

(a) 2.0 cm (b) 0.5 cm (c) 4.0 cm (d) 1.0 cm

44. A beam of protons with speed $4 \times 10^5\ \text{ms}^{-1}$ enters a uniform magnetic field of 0.3 T at an angle of 60° to the magnetic field. The pitch of the resulting helical path of protons is close to : (Mass of the proton = 1.67×10^{-27} kg, charge of the proton = 1.69×10^{-19} C)

(a) 2 cm (b) 5 cm (c) 12 cm (d) 4 cm

45. Proton with kinetic energy of 1 MeV moves from south to north. It gets an acceleration of $10^{12}\ \text{m/s}^2$ by an applied magnetic field (west to east). The value of magnetic field: (Rest mass of proton is 1.6×10^{-27} kg)

(a) 0.71 mT (b) 7.1 mT (c) 0.071 mT (d) 71 mT

46. A proton, an electron, and a Helium nucleus, have the same energy. They are in circular orbits in a plane due to magnetic field perpendicular to the plane. Let r_p, r_e and r_{He} be their respective radii, then,

(a) $r_e > r_p = r_{He}$ (b) $r_e < r_p = r_{He}$
(c) $r_e < r_p < r_{He}$ (d) $r_e > r_p > r_{He}$

47. In an experiment, electrons are accelerated, from rest, by applying a voltage of 500 V. Calculate the radius of the path if a magnetic field 100 mT is then applied.
[Charge of the electron = 1.6×10^{-19} C
Mass of the electron = 9.1×10^{-31} kg]

(a) 7.5×10^{-3} m (b) 7.5×10^{-2} m
(c) 7.5 m (d) 7.5×10^{-4} m

48. Magnitude of magnetic field (in SI units) at the centre of a hexagonal shape coil of side 10 cm, 50 turns and carrying current I (Ampere) in units of $\frac{\mu_0 I}{\pi}$ is :

(a) $250\sqrt{3}$ (b) $50\sqrt{3}$ (c) $500\sqrt{3}$ (d) $5\sqrt{3}$

49. The magnitude of the magnetic field at the center of an equilateral triangular loop of side 1 m which is carrying a current of 10 A is : [Take $\mu_0 = 4\pi \times 10^{-7}\ \text{NA}^{-2}$]

(a) 18 μT (b) 9 μT (c) 3 μT (d) 1 μT

50. The dipole moment of a circular loop carrying a current I, is m and the magnetic field at the centre of the loop is B_1. When the dipole moment is doubled by keeping the current constant, the magnetic field at the centre of the loop is B_2. The ratio $\frac{B_1}{B_2}$ is:

(a) 2 (b) $\sqrt{3}$ (c) $\sqrt{2}$ (d) $\frac{1}{\sqrt{2}}$

51. Find the magnetic field at point P due to a straight line segment AB of length 6 cm carrying a current of 5 A. (See figure) ($\mu_0 = 4\pi \times 10^{-7}$ N-A^{-2})

(a) 2.0×10^{-5}T
(b) 1.5×10^{-5}T
(c) 3.0×10^{-5}T
(d) 2.5×10^{-5}T

52. Choose the correct sketch of the magnetic field lines of a circular current loop shown by the dot ⊙ and the cross ⊗.

(a) 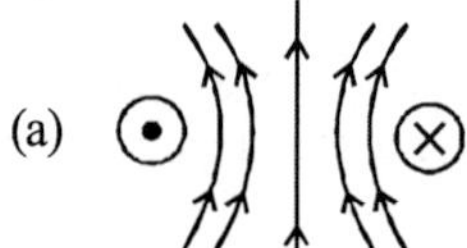 (b) 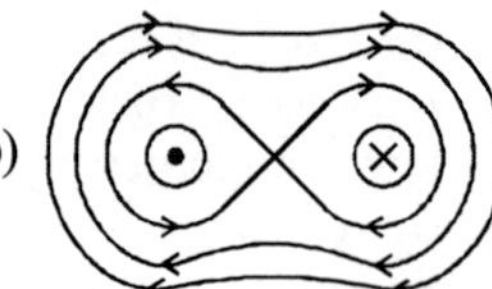

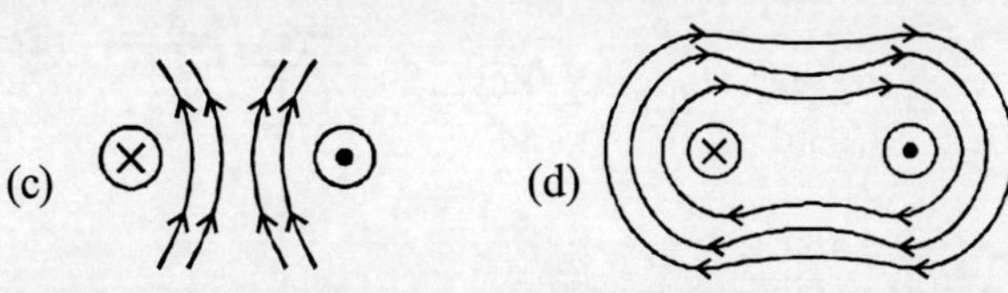

53. A current i is flowing in a straight conductor of length L. The magnetic induction at a point on its axis at a distance $\frac{L}{4}$ from its centre will be :

(a) Zero (b) $\frac{\mu_0 i}{2\pi L}$ (c) $\frac{\mu_0 i}{\sqrt{2}L}$ (d) $\frac{4\mu_0 i}{\sqrt{5}\pi L}$

54. An electric current is flowing through a circular coil of radius R. The ratio of the magnetic field at the centre of the coil and that at a distance $2\sqrt{2}R$ from the centre of the coil and on its axis is :

(a) $2\sqrt{2}$ (b) 27 (c) 36 (d) 8

55. A long straight wire of radius a carries a steady current i. The current is uniformly distributed across its cross section. The ratio of the magnetic field at $a/2$ and $2a$ is

(a) 1/2 (b) 1/4 (c) 4 (d) 1

56. A current I flows along the length of an infinitely long, straight, thin walled pipe. Then

(a) the magnetic field at all points inside the pipe is the same, but not zero
(b) the magnetic field is zero only on the axis of the pipe
(c) the magnetic field is different at different points inside the pipe
(d) the magnetic field at any point inside the pipe is zero

57. If in a circular coil A of radius R, current I is flowing and in another coil B of radius $2R$ a current $2I$ is flowing, then the ratio of the magnetic fields B_A and B_B, produced by them will be

(a) 1 (b) 2 (c) 1/2 (d) 4

58. A circular coil having N turns and radius r carries a current I. It is held in the XZ plane in a magnetic field B. The torque on the coil due to the magnetic field is :

(a) $\frac{Br^2 I}{\pi N}$ (b) $B\pi r^2 IN$ (c) $\frac{B\pi r^2 I}{N}$ (d) Zero

59. A charge q is spread uniformly over an insulated loop of radius r . If it is rotated with an angular velocity ω with respect to normal axis then the magnetic moment of the loop is

(a) $\frac{1}{2}q\omega r^2$ (b) $\frac{4}{3}q\omega r^2$ (c) $\frac{3}{2}q\omega r^2$ (d) $q\omega r^2$

60. The time period of a charged particle undergoing a circular motion in a uniform magnetic field is independent of its

(a) speed (b) mass
(c) charge (d) magnetic induction

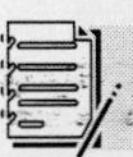

Exercise 2 - Exemplar & Past Year Questions

E&PYQs

Exemplar Questions

1. Two charged particles traverse identical helical paths in a completely opposite sense in a uniform magnetic field $\mathbf{B} = B_0\hat{\mathbf{k}}$.

(a) They have equal z-components of momenta
(b) They must have equal charges
(c) They necessarily represent a particle, anti-particle pair
(d) The charge to mass ratio satisfy

$$\left(\frac{e}{m}\right)_1 + \left(\frac{e}{m}\right)_2 = 0$$

2. Biot-Savart law indicates that the moving electrons (velocity v) produce a magnetic field **B** such that

(a) B is perpendicular of
(b) B is parallel to v
(c) it obeys inverse cube law
(d) it is along the line joining the electron and point of observation.

3. A current carrying circular loop of radius R is placed in the x-y plane with centre at the origin. Half of the loop with $x > 0$ is now bent so that it now lies in the y-z plane.

(a) The magnitude of magnetic moment now diminishes
(b) The magnetic moment does not change
(c) The magnitude of B at (0, 0, z), $z > R$ increases
(d) The magnitude of B at (0, 0, z), $z >> R$ is unchanged

4. An electron is projected with uniform velocity along the axis of a current carrying long solenoid. Which of the following is true?

(a) The electron will be accelerated along the axis
(b) The electron path will be circular about the axis
(c) The electron will experience a force at 45° to the axis and hence execute a helical path
(d) The electron will continue to move with uniform velocity along the axis of the solenoid

5. In a cyclotron, a charged particle

(a) undergoes acceleration all the time
(b) speeds up between the dees because of the magnetic field
(c) speeds up in a dees
(d) slows down within a dee and speeds up between dees

NEET/AIPMT (2013-2020) Questions

6. A current loop in a magnetic field ***[2013]***

(a) can be in equilibrium in one orientation
(b) can be in equilibrium in two orientations, both the equilibrium states are unstable
(c) can be in equilibrium in two orientations, one stable while the other is unstable
(d) experiences a torque whether the field is uniform or non-uniform in all orientations

7. A circular coil *ABCD* carrying a current *i* is placed in a uniform magnetic field. If the magnetic force on the segment *AB* is $\vec{F}$, the force on the remaining segment *BCDA* is ***[NEET Kar. 2013]***

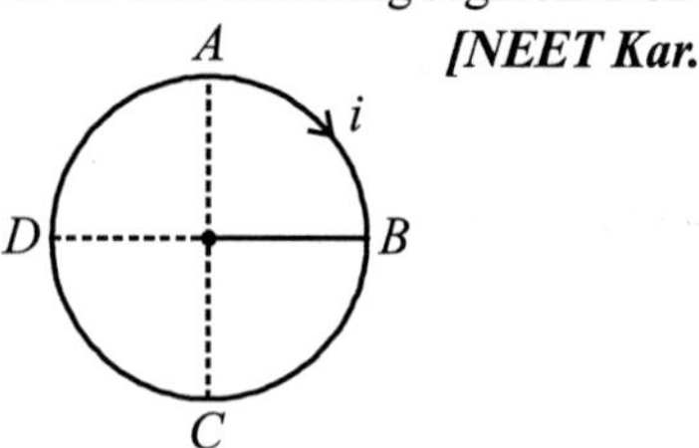

(a) $\vec{F}$ (b) $-\vec{F}$ (c) $3\vec{F}$ (d) $-3\vec{F}$

8. Two identical long conducting wires AOB and COD are placed at right angle to each other, with one above other such that 'O' is their common point for the two. The wires carry I_1 and I_2 currents respectively. Point 'P' is lying at distance 'd' from 'O' along a direction perpendicular to the plane containing the wires. The magnetic field at the point 'P' will be : ***[2014]***

(a) $\frac{\mu_0}{2\pi d}\left(\frac{I_1}{I_2}\right)$ (b) $\frac{\mu_0}{2\pi d}(I_1 + I_2)$

(c) $\frac{\mu_0}{2\pi d}(I_1^2 - I_2^2)$ (d) $\frac{\mu_0}{2\pi d}(I_1^2 \times I_2^2)^{1/2}$

9. An electron moving in a circular orbit of radius r makes n rotations per second. The magnetic field produced at the centre has magnitude: ***[2015]***

(a) Zero (b) $\frac{\mu_0 n^2 e}{r}$ (c) $\frac{\mu_0 ne}{2r}$ (d) $\frac{\mu_0 ne}{2\pi r}$

10. A proton and an alpha particle both enter a region of uniform magnetic field B, moving at right angles to field B. If the radius of circular orbits for both the particles is equal and the kinetic energy acquired by proton is 1 MeV the energy acquired by the alpha particle will be: ***[2015 RS]***

(a) 0.5 MeV (b) 1.5 MeV (c) 1 MeV (d) 4 MeV

11. A rectangular coil of length 0.12 m and width 0.1 m having 50 turns of wire is suspended vertically in a uniform magnetic field of strength 0.2 weber/m^2. The coil carries a current of 2A. If the plane of the coil is inclined at an angle of 30° with the direction of the field, the torque required to keep the coil in stable equilibrium will be : ***[2015 RS]***

(a) 0.20 Nm (b) 0.24 Nm (c) 0.12 Nm (d) 0.15 Nm

12. A long straight wire of radius a carries a steady current I. The current is uniformly distributed over its cross-section. The ratio of the magnetic fields B and B', at radial distances $\frac{a}{2}$ and 2a respectively, from the axis of the wire is : ***[2016]***

(a) $\frac{1}{4}$ (b) $\frac{1}{2}$ (c) 1 (d) 4

13. A 250-turn rectangular coil of length 2.1 cm and width 1.25 cm carries a current of 85 μA and subjected to magnetic field of strength 0.85 T. Work done for rotating the coil by 180° against the torque is ***[2017]***

(a) 4.55 μJ (b) 2.3 μJ (c) 1.15 μJ (d) 9.1 μJ

14. An arrangement of three parallel straight wires placed perpendicular to plane of paper carrying same current 'I along the same direction is shown in fig. Magnitude of force per unit length on the middle wire 'B' is given by ***[2017]***

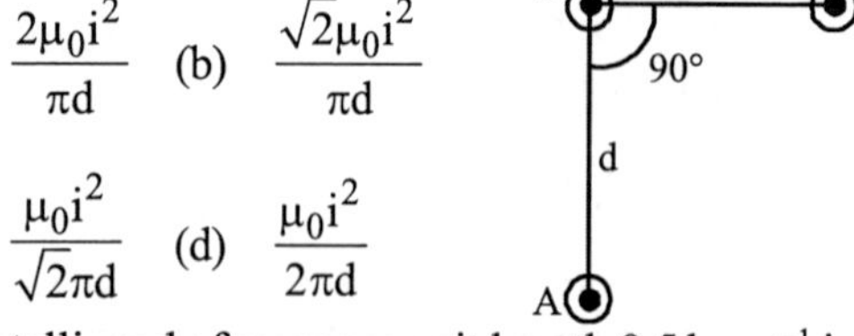

(a) $\frac{2\mu_0 i^2}{\pi d}$ (b) $\frac{\sqrt{2}\mu_0 i^2}{\pi d}$

(c) $\frac{\mu_0 i^2}{\sqrt{2}\pi d}$ (d) $\frac{\mu_0 i^2}{2\pi d}$

15. A metallic rod of mass per unit length 0.5 kg m^{-1} is lying horizontally on a smooth inclined plane which makes an angle of 30° with the horizontal. The rod is not allowed to slide down by flowing a current through it when a magnetic field of induction 0.25 T is acting on it in the vertical direction. The current flowing in the rod to keep it stationary is ***[2018]***

(a) 7.14A (b) 5.98A (c) 11.32A (d) 14.76A

16. Current sensitivity of a moving coil galvanometer is 5 div/mA and its voltage sensitivity (angular deflection per unit voltage applied) is 20 div/V. The resistance of the galvanometer is ***[2018]***

(a) 40 Ω (b) 25 Ω (c) 500 Ω (d) 250 Ω

17. Ionized hydrogen atoms and α-particles with same momenta enters perpendicular to a constant magnetic field, B. The ratio of their radii of their paths $r_H : r_\alpha$ will be : ***[2019]***

(a) 2 : 1 (b) 1 : 2 (c) 4 : 1 (d) 1 : 4

18. A cylindrical conductor of radius R is carrying a constant current. The plot of the magnitude of the magnetic field, B with the distance, *d*, from the centre of the conductor, is **correctly** represented by the figure : ***[2019]***

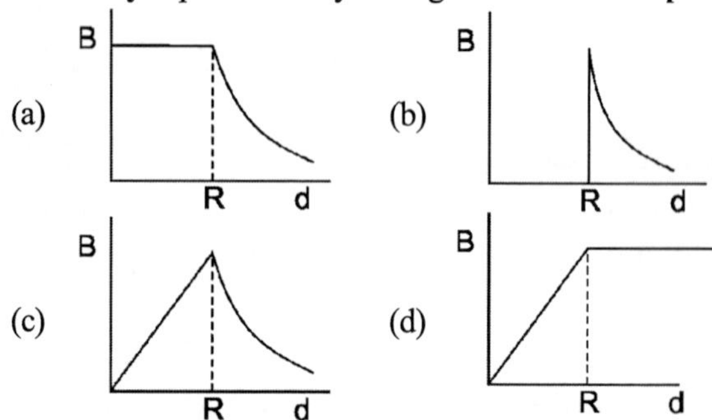

19. Two toroids 1 and 2 have total no. of turns 200 and 100 respectively with average radii 40 cm and 20 cm respectively. If they carry same current *i*, the ratio of the magnetic fields along the two loops is, ***[NEET Odisha 2019]***

(a) 1 : 2 (b) 1 : 1 (c) 4 : 1 (d) 2 : 1

20. A straight conductor carrying current *i* splits into two parts as shown in the figure. The radius of the circular loop is *R*. The total magnetic field at the centre *P* of the loop is, ***[NEET Odisha 2019]***

(a) $\frac{\mu_0 i}{2R}$, inward (b) Zero

(c) $3\mu_0 i/32R$, outward (d) $3\mu_0 i/32R$, inward

21. A long solenoid of 50 cm length having 100 turns carries a current of 2.5 A. The magnetic field at the centre of the solenoid is : ($\mu_0 = 4\pi \times 10^{-7}$ T m A^{-1}) ***[2020]***

(a) 3.14×10^{-4} T (b) 6.28×10^{-5} T

(c) 3.14×10^{-5} T (d) 6.28×10^{-4} T

Exercise 3 - Concept Application Problems

CAP

1. An infinite straight conductor carrying current 2 I is split into a loop of radius r as shown in fig. The magnetic field at the centre of the coil is

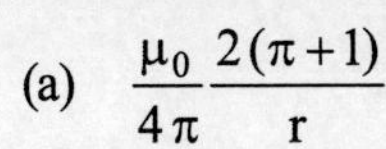

(a) $\frac{\mu_0}{4\pi}\frac{2(\pi+1)}{r}$

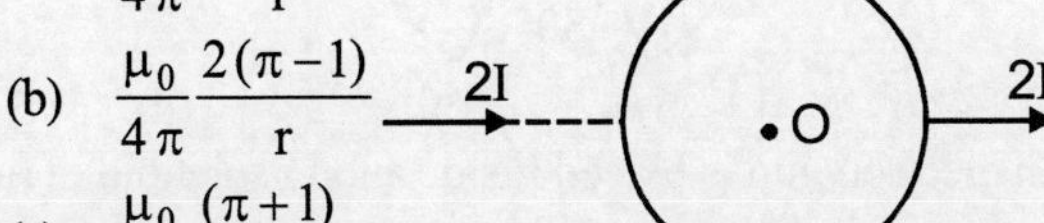

(b) $\frac{\mu_0}{4\pi}\frac{2(\pi-1)}{r}$

(c) $\frac{\mu_0}{4\pi}\frac{(\pi+1)}{r}$

(d) zero

2. A long wire is bent into shape ABCDE as shown in fig., with BCD being a semicircle with centre O and radius r metre. A current of I amp. flows through it in the direction A→B→C→D→E. Then the magnetic induction at the point O of the figure in vacuum is

(a) $\mu_0\left[\frac{I}{2\pi r}+\frac{I}{4r}\right]$

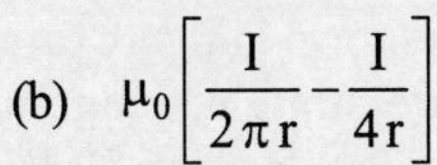

(b) $\mu_0\left[\frac{I}{2\pi r}-\frac{I}{4r}\right]$

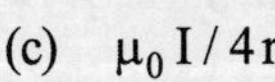

(c) $\mu_0 I/4r$

(d) $\mu_0 I/\pi r$

3. A conducting circular loop of radius r carries a constant current i. It is placed in a uniform magnetic field $\vec{B}_0$ such that $\vec{B}_0$ is perpendicular to the plane of the loop. The magnetic force acting on the loop is

(a) irB_0 (b) $2\pi irB_0$ (c) zero (d) πirB_0

4. An electron traveling with a speed u along the positive x-axis enters into a region of magnetic field where $B = -B_0\hat{k}$ $(x > 0)$. It comes out of the region with speed v then

(a) $v = u$ at $y > 0$

(b) $v = u$ at $y < 0$

(c) $v > u$ at $y > 0$

(d) $v > u$ at $y < 0$

5. A square current carrying loop is suspended in a uniform magnetic field acting in the plane of the loop. If the force on one arm of the loop is $\vec{F}$, the net force on the remaining three arms of the loop is

(a) $3\vec{F}$ (b) $-\vec{F}$ (c) $-3\vec{F}$ (d) $\vec{F}$

6. A current loop consists of two identical semicircular parts each of radius R, one lying in the x-y plane and the other in x-z plane. If the current in the loop is i., the resultant magnetic field due to the two semicircular parts at their common centre is

(a) $\frac{\mu_0 i}{\sqrt{2}R}$ (b) $\frac{\mu_0 i}{2\sqrt{2}R}$ (c) $\frac{\mu_0 i}{2R}$ (d) $\frac{\mu_0 i}{4R}$

7. A uniform electric field and uniform magnetic field are acting along the same direction in a certain region. If an electron is projected in the region such that its velocity is pointed along the direction of fields, then the electron

(a) will turn towards right of direction of motion

(b) speed will decrease

(c) speed will increase

(d) will turn towards left direction of motion

8. Charge q is uniformly spread on a thin ring of radius R. The ring rotates about its axis with a uniform frequency f Hz. The magnitude of magnetic induction at the centre of the ring is

(a) $\frac{\mu_0 qf}{2R}$ (b) $\frac{\mu_0 q}{2fR}$ (c) $\frac{\mu_0 q}{2\pi fR}$ (d) $\frac{\mu_0 qf}{2\pi R}$

9. A magnetic needle suspended parallel to a magnetic field requires $\sqrt{3}$ J of work to turn it through 60°. The torque needed to maintain the needle in this position will be

(a) $2\sqrt{3}$J (b) 3J (c) $\sqrt{3}$J (d) $\frac{3}{2}$J

10. An electron moves in a circular orbit with a uniform speed v. It produces a magnetic field B at the centre of the circle. The radius of the circle is proportional to

(a) $\sqrt{\frac{B}{v}}$ (b) $\frac{B}{v}$ (c) $\sqrt{\frac{v}{B}}$ (d) $\frac{v}{B}$

11. The magnetic induction at a point P which is at a distance of 4 cm from a long current carrying wire is 10^{-3} T. The field of induction at a distance 12 cm from the current will be

(a) 3.33×10^{-4} T (b) 1.11×10^{-4} T

(c) 3×10^{-3} T (d) 9×10^{-3} T

12. An electron is moving along $+x$ direction with a velocity of 6×10^6 ms^{-1}. It enters a region of uniform electric field of 300 V/cm pointing along $+y$ direction. The magnitude and direction of the magnetic field set up in this region such that the electron keeps moving along the x direction will be :

(a) 3×10^{-4} T, along $+z$ direction

(b) 5×10^{-3} T, along $-z$ direction

(c) 5×10^{-3} T, along $+z$ direction

(d) 3×10^{-4} T, along $-z$ direction

13. A particle of charge q and mass m is moving with a velocity $-v\hat{i}(v\neq0)$ towards a large screen placed in the Y-Z plane at a distance d. If there is a magnetic field $\vec{B}=B_0\hat{k}$, the minimum value of v for which the particle will not hit the screen is:

(a) $\frac{qdB_0}{3m}$ (b) $\frac{2qdB_0}{m}$ (c) $\frac{qdB_0}{m}$ (d) $\frac{qdB_0}{2m}$

14. A charged particle carrying charge 1 μC is moving with velocity $(2\hat{i}+3\hat{j}+4\hat{k})$ ms^{-1}. If an external magnetic field of $(5\hat{i}+3\hat{j}-6\hat{k})\times10^{-3}$ T exists in the region where the particle is moving then the force on the particle is $\vec{F}\times10^{-9}$ N. The vector $\vec{F}$ is :

(a) $-0.30\hat{i}+0.32\hat{j}-0.09\hat{k}$ (b) $-30\hat{i}+32\hat{j}-9\hat{k}$

(c) $-300\hat{i}+320\hat{j}-90\hat{k}$ (d) $-3.0\hat{i}+3.2\hat{j}-0.9\hat{k}$

15. A proton and an α-particle (with their masses in the ratio of 1 : 4 and charges in the ratio 1 : 2) are accelerated from rest through a potential difference V. If a uniform magnetic field (B) is set up perpendicular to their velocities, the ratio of the radii $r_p : r_\alpha$ of the circular paths descrfibed by them will be:

(a) $1:\sqrt{2}$ (b) $1:2$ (c) $1:3$ (d) $1:\sqrt{3}$

16. The region between $y = 0$ and $y = d$ contains a magnetic field $\vec{B} = B\hat{z}$. A particle of mass m and charge q enters the region with a velocity $\vec{v} = v\hat{i}$. if $d = \frac{mv}{2qB}$, the acceleration of the charged particle at the point of its emergence at the other side is :

(a) $\frac{qvB}{m}\left(\frac{1}{2}\hat{i}-\frac{\sqrt{3}}{2}\hat{j}\right)$ (b) $\frac{qvB}{m}\left(\frac{\sqrt{3}}{2}\hat{i}+\frac{1}{2}\hat{j}\right)$

(c) $\frac{qvB}{m}\left(\frac{-\hat{j}+\hat{i}}{\sqrt{2}}\right)$ (d) $\frac{qvB}{m}\left(\frac{\hat{i}+\hat{j}}{\sqrt{2}}\right)$

17. An electron, a proton and an alpha particle having the same kinetic energy are moving in circular orbits of radii r_e, r_p, r_α respectively in a uniform magnetic field B. The relation between r_e, r_p, r_α is:

(a) $r_e > r_p = r_\alpha$ (b) $r_e < r_p = r_\alpha$

(c) $r_e < r_p < r_\alpha$ (d) $r_e < r_\alpha < r_p$

18. The velocity of certain ions that pass undeflected through crossed electric field $E = 7.7$ k V/m and magnetic field $B = 0.14$ T is

(a) 18 km/s (b) 77 km/s (c) 55 km/s (d) 1078 km/s

19. In a region, steady and uniform electric and magnetic fields are present. These two fields are parallel to each other. A charged particle is released from rest in this region. The path of the particle will be a

(a) helix (b) straight line

(c) ellipse (d) circle

20. If an electron and a proton having same momenta enter perpendicular to a magnetic field, then

(a) curved path of electron and proton will be same (ignoring the sense of revolution)

(b) they will move undeflected

(c) curved path of electron is more curved than that of the proton

(d) path of proton is more curved.

21. A wire *A*, bent in the shape of an arc of a circle, carrying a current of 2 A and having radius 2 cm and another wire *B*, also bent in the shape of arc of a circle, carrying a current of 3 A and having radius of 4 cm, are placed as shown in the figure. The ratio of the magnetic fields due to the wires *A* and *B* at the common centre *O* is :

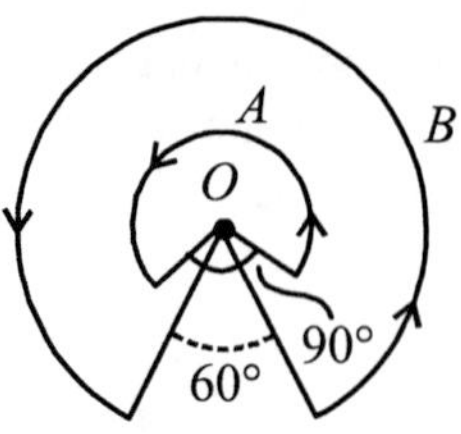

(a) 4 : 6 (b) 6 : 4 (c) 2 : 5 (d) 6 : 5

22. An electron gun is placed inside a long solenoid of radius R on its axis. The solenoid has n turns/length and carries a current I. The electron gun shoots an electron along the radius of the solenoid with speed *v*. If the electron does not hit the surface of the solenoid, maximum possible value of *v* is (all symbols have their standard meaning):

(a) $\frac{e\mu_0 nIR}{m}$ (b) $\frac{e\mu_0 nIR}{2m}$

(c) $\frac{e\mu_0 nIR}{4m}$ (d) $\frac{2e\mu_0 nIR}{m}$

23. A very long wire *ABDMNDC* is shown in figure carrying current *I*. *AB* and *BC* parts are straight, long and at right angle. At *D* wire forms a circular turn *DMND* of radius *R*.

AB, *BC* parts are tangential to circular turn at *N* and *D*. Magnetic field at the centre of circle is:

(a) $\frac{\mu_0 I}{2\pi R}\left(\pi+\frac{1}{\sqrt{2}}\right)$

(b) $\frac{\mu_0 I}{2\pi R}\left(\pi-\frac{1}{\sqrt{2}}\right)$

(c) $\frac{\mu_0 I}{2\pi R}(\pi+1)$

(d) $\frac{\mu_0 I}{2R}$

24. Two very long, straight, and insulated wires are kept at 90° angle from each other in *xy*-plane as shown in the figure.

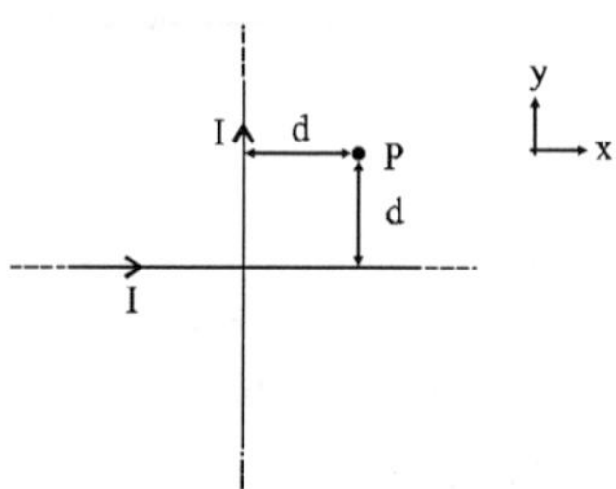

These wires carry currents of equal magnitude I, whose directions are shown in the figure. The net magnetic field at point P will be :

(a) Zero (b) $-\frac{\mu_0 I}{2\pi d}(\hat{x}+\hat{y})$

(c) $\frac{+\mu_0 I}{\pi d}(\hat{z})$ (d) $\frac{\mu_0 I}{2\pi d}(\hat{x}+\hat{y})$

25. One of the two identical conducting wires of length L is bent in the form of a circular loop and the other one into a circular coil of N identical turns. If the same current is passed in both, the ratio of the magnetic field at the central of the loop (B_1) to that at the centre of the coil (B_C), *i.e.*, $\frac{B_L}{B_C}$ will be:

(a) N (b) $\frac{1}{N}$ (c) N^2 (d) $\frac{1}{N^2}$

26. A current of 1A is flowing on the sides of an equilateral triangle of side 4.5×10^{-2}m . The magnetic field at the centre of the triangle will be:

(a) 4×10^{-5}Wb/m^2 (b) Zero
(c) 2×10^{-5}Wb/m^2 (d) 8×10^{-5}Wb/m^2

27. A square loop of side $2a$ and carrying current I is kept is xz plane with its centre at origin. A long wire carrying the same current I is placed parallel to z-axis and passing through point (0, b, 0), ($b >> a$). The magnitude of torque on the loop about z-axis will be :

(a) $\frac{2\mu_0 I^2 a^2}{\pi b}$ (b) $\frac{2\mu_0 I^2 a^2 b}{\pi(a^2+b^2)}$

(c) $\frac{\mu_0 I^2 a^2 b}{2\pi(a^2+b^2)}$ (d) $\frac{\mu_0 I^2 a^2}{2\pi b}$

28. A square loop of side $2a$, and carrying current I, is kept in XZ plane with its centre at origin. A long wire carrying the same current I is placed parallel to the z-axis and passing through the point (0, b, 0), ($b >> a$). The magnitude of the torque on the loop about z-axis is given by :

(a) $\frac{\mu_0 I^2 a^2}{2\pi b}$ (b) $\frac{\mu_0 I^2 a^3}{2\pi b^2}$ (c) $\frac{2\mu_0 I^2 a^2}{\pi b}$ (d) $\frac{2\mu_0 I^2 a^3}{\pi b^2}$

29. A small circular loop of conducting wire has radius a and carries current I. It is placed in a uniform magnetic field B perpendicular to its plane such that when rotated slightly about its diameter and released, it starts performing simple harmonic motion of time period T. If the mass of the loop is m then :

(a) $T=\sqrt{\frac{2m}{IB}}$ (b) $T=\sqrt{\frac{\pi m}{2IB}}$

(c) $T=\sqrt{\frac{2\pi m}{IB}}$ (c) $T=\sqrt{\frac{\pi m}{IB}}$

30. Three straight parallel current carrying conductors are shown in the figure. The force experienced by the middle conductor of length 25 cm is:

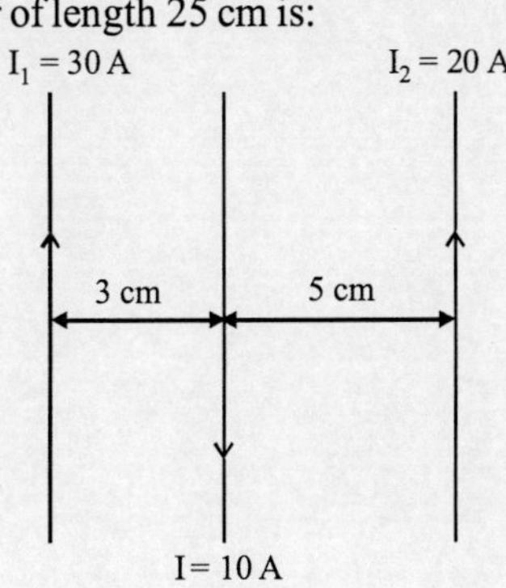

(a) 3×10^{-4} N toward right
(b) 6×10^{-4} N toward right
(c) 9×10^{-4} N toward right
(d) Zero

31. A coil of one turn is made of a wire of certain length and then from the same length a coil of two turns is made. If the same current is passed in both the cases, then the ratio of the magnetic inductions at their centres will be

(a) 2 : 1 (b) 1 : 4 (c) 4 : 1 (d) 1 : 2

32. A particle having the same charge as of electron moves in a circular path of radius 0.5 cm under the influence of a magnetic field of 0.5T. If an electric field of 100V/m makes it to move in a straight path then the mass of the particle is (Given charge of electron = 1.6×10^{-19}C)

(a) 9.1×10^{-31} kg (b) 1.6×10^{-27} kg
(c) 1.6×10^{-19} kg (d) 2.0×10^{-24} kg

33. A charged particle going around in a circle can be considered to be a current loop. A particle of mass m carrying charge q is moving in a plane wit speed v under the influence of magnetic field $\vec{B}$. The magnetic moment of this moving particle :

(a) $\frac{mv^2 \vec{B}}{2B^2}$ (b) $-\frac{mv^2 \vec{B}}{2\pi B^2}$ (c) $-\frac{mv^2 \vec{B}}{B^2}$ (d) $-\frac{mv^2 \vec{B}}{2B^2}$

34. An infinitely long straight wire contains a uniformly continuous current of 10A. The radius of the wire is 4×10^{-2} m. The magnetic field at 2×10^{-2} m from the centre of the wire will be:

(a) 0 (b) 2.5×10^{-5}T
(c) 5.0×10^{-5}T (d) none of these.

35. A moving coil galvanometer has a resistance of 900 Ω. In order to send only 10% of the main current through this galvanometer, the resistance of the required shunt is

(a) 0.9 Ω (b) 100 Ω (c) 405 Ω (d) 90 Ω

36. A square loop is carrying a steady current I and the magnitude of its magnetic dipole moment is m. If this square loop is changed to a circular loop and it carries the same current, the magnitude of the magnetic dipole moment of circular loop will be :

(a) $\frac{m}{\pi}$ (b) $\frac{3m}{\pi}$ (c) $\frac{2m}{\pi}$ (d) $\frac{4m}{\pi}$

37. A thin ring of 10 cm radius carries a uniformly distributed charge. The ring rotates at a constant angular speed of 40 À rad s^{-1} about its axis, perpendicular to its plane. If the magnetic field at its centre is 3.8×10^{-9} T, then the charge carried by the ring is close to ($\mu_0 = 4\pi \times 10^{-7}$ N/A^2).

(a) 2×10^{-6}C (b) 3×10^{-5}C (c) 4×10^{-5}C (d) 7×10^{-6}C

38. Electron move at right angle to a magnetic field of 1.5×10^{-2} tesla with speed of 6×10^7 m/s. If the specific charge of the electron is 1.7×10^{11} C/kg. The radius of circular path will be

(a) 3.31 cm (b) 4.31cm (c) 1.31 cm (d) 2.35 cm

39. The magnetic field due to a current carrying circular loop of radius 3 cm at a point on the axis at a distance of 4 cm from the centre is 54 μT. What will be its value at the centre of loop?

(a) 125 μT (b) 150 μT (c) 250 μT (d) 75 μT

40. A rectangular coil (Dimension 5 cm × 2.5 cm) with 100 turns, carrying a current of 3 A in the clock-wise direction, is kept centered at the origin and in the X-Z plane. A magnetic field of 1 T is applied along X-axis. If the coil is tilted through 45° about Z-axis, then the torque on the coil is:

(a) 0.38 Nm (b) 0.55 Nm
(c) 0.42 Nm (d) 0.27 Nm

41. A deutron of kinetic energy 50 keV is describing a circular orbit of radius 0.5m, in a plane perpendicular to magnetic field $\vec{B}$. The kinetic energy of a proton that discribes a circular orbit of radius 0.5m in the same plane with the same magnetic field $\vec{B}$ is

(a) 200 keV (b) 50 keV (c) 100 keV (d) 25 keV

42. Two equal electric currents are flowing perpendicular to each other as shown in figure. AB and CD are perpendicular to each other and symmetrically placed with respect to the currents. Where do we expect the resultant magnetic field to be zero?

(a) on AB
(b) on CD
(c) on both AB & CD
(d) on both OD & BO

43. A cell is connected between two points of a uniformly thick circular conductor and i_1 and i_2 are the currents flowing in two parts of the circular conductor of radius a. The magnetic field at the centre of the loop will be

(a) zero (b) $\frac{\mu_0}{4\pi}(I_1 - I_2)$

(c) $\frac{\mu_0}{2a}(I_1 + I_2)$ (d) $\frac{\mu_0}{a}(I_1 + I_2)$

44. Under the influence of a uniform magnetic field a charged particle is moving in a circle of radius R with constant speed v. The time period of the motion

(a) depends on both R and v
(b) is independent of both R and v
(c) depends on R and not v
(d) depends on v and not on R

45. A long, straight wire of radius a carries a current distributed uniformly over its cross-section. The ratio of the magnetic fields due to the wire at distance $\frac{a}{3}$ and $2a$, respectively from the axis of the wire is:

(a) $\frac{2}{3}$ (b) 2 (c) $\frac{1}{2}$ (d) $\frac{3}{2}$

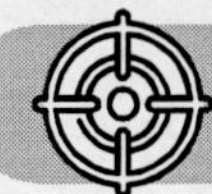

Hints & Solutions

19.1 Concept Practice Problems

1. (b) Magnetic field $B = \frac{\mu_0 I}{4\pi d}$ at a distance *d* near the end of a long conductor.

2. (d) $B = \frac{\mu_0}{4\pi} \cdot \frac{2\pi n i_1}{r_1} - \frac{\mu_0}{4\pi} \cdot \frac{2\pi n i_2}{r_2} = \frac{\mu_0}{2}\left[\frac{n i_1}{r_1} - \frac{n i_2}{r_2}\right]$

3. (c) $B_{axis} = \left(\frac{\mu_0 NI}{2x^3}\right)R^2$

$B \propto R^2$

So, when radius is doubled, magnetic field becomes four times.

4. (c) $B = \mu_0 N_0 i$; $B_1 = (\mu_0)\left(\frac{N_0}{2}\right)(2\,i) = \mu_0 N_0 i = B$

$\Rightarrow B_1 = B$

5. (b) Tesla is the unit of magnetic field.
6. (d) The straight part will not contribute magnetic field at the centre of the semicircle because every element of the straight part will be 0° or 180° with the line joining the centre and the element

Due to circular portion, the field is $\frac{1}{2}\frac{\mu_0 i}{2r} = \frac{\mu_0 i}{4r}$

Hence total field at O $= \frac{\mu_0 i}{4r}$ tesla

7. (c) $B = \frac{\mu_0}{4\pi}\frac{2\pi i}{r}$ where

$i = \frac{2e}{t} = \frac{2 \times 1.6 \times 10^{-19}}{2} = 1.6 \times 10^{-19}$ A

$\therefore\ B = \frac{\mu_0 i}{2r} = \frac{\mu_0 \times 1.6 \times 10^{-19}}{2 \times 0.8} = \mu_0 \times 10^{-19}$ T

8. (d) $B = \mu_0 nI = 4\pi \times 10^{-7} \times 10 \times 5 = 2\pi \times 10^{-5}$ T.
9. (c)
10. (d) Since no current is enclosed inside the hollow conductor. Hence $B_{inside} = 0$.

19.2 Concept Practice Problems

11. (d) The plane $\perp \vec{B}$.
12. (b) $F = iBl \sin\theta$. This is maximum when $\sin\theta = 1$ or $\theta = \pi/2$.
13. (b) $F = I\ell B \sin\theta = 3 \times 0.40 \times (500 \times 10^{-4}) \times \sin 30° = 3 \times 10^{-2}$ N.
14. (c) Torque on loop $\tau = nIAB\cos\theta$; Here $\theta = 90°$

$\therefore\ \tau = 0$.

15. (b) $F = \frac{\mu_0}{4\pi}\frac{2I_1I_2}{r} \times \ell$

$= \frac{10^{-7} \times 2 \times 10 \times 2}{0.1} \times 2 = 8 \times 10^{-5}$ N

16. (c)
17. (b) $\frac{F}{\ell} = \frac{\mu_0 i_1 i_2}{2\pi d} = \frac{\mu_0 i^2}{2\pi d}$

(attractive as current is in the same direction)

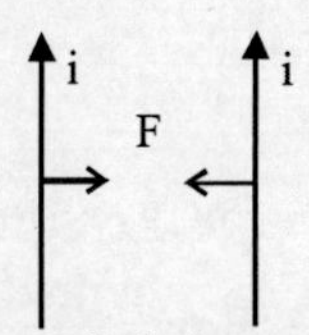

18. (d) For a given perimeter the area of circle is maximum. So magnetic moment of (S) is greatest.
19. (c) A current loop in a magnetic field is in equilibrium in two orientations one is stable and another unstable.

$\because\ \vec{\tau} = \vec{M} \times \vec{B} = MB\sin\theta$

If $\theta = 0° \Rightarrow \tau = 0$ (stable)

If $\theta = \pi \Rightarrow \tau = 0$ (unstable)

Do not experience a torque in some orientations

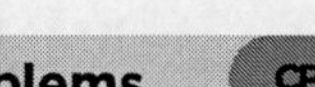

Hence option (c) is correct.

20. (b) $F = Bi\ell = 2 \times 1.2 \times 0.5 = 1.2$ N

19.3 Concept Practice Problems

21. (d) When $\vec{E}$ and $\vec{B}$ are mutually $\perp$ then electron can go undeflected also.
22. (a) $r = \frac{mv}{Bq}$ or, $r \propto \frac{m}{q}$ for the same value of v and B.
23. (a) $r = mv/Bq$ is same for both.
24. (a) $Bqv = \frac{mv^2}{r} \Rightarrow r = \frac{mv}{Bq}$
25. (a) Current sensitivity $= \frac{nBA}{K}$

where K is constant of torsional rigidity.

26. (b)
27. (b) In cyclotron, energy with which aceleration takes place is in term of MeV.
28. (a)
29. (d)
30. (b) It will compress due to the force of attraction between two adjacent coils carrying current in the same direction.

Exercise 1 - Chapter Revision Problems

1. (c) If r is the radius of the circle,

then $L = 2\pi r$ or, $r = \frac{L}{2\pi}$

Area $= \pi r^2 = \pi L^2/4\pi^2 = L^2/4\pi$

2. (c) The point P is lying symmetrically w.r.t. the two long straight current carrying conductors. The magnetic fields at P due to these current carrying conductors are mutually perpendicular.
3. (a) 4. (a) 5. (c)
6. (b) Magnetic force acts perpendicular to the velocity. Hence speed remains constant.

7. (c) $e = \frac{d\phi}{dt}; i = \frac{e}{R} = \frac{1}{R}\frac{d\phi}{dt}$

Total charge induced $= \int i\, dt = \int \frac{1}{R}\frac{d\phi}{dt}.dt$

$$= \frac{1}{R}\int_{\phi_1}^{\phi_2} d\phi = \frac{1}{R}(\phi_2 - \phi_1)$$

8. (b) Energy is stored in magnetic field.

9. (c) $Bqv = \frac{m v^2}{r}$ or $B = \frac{m v}{rq} = \frac{(9 \times 10^{-31}) \times 10^6}{0.1 \times (1.6 \times 10^{-19})}$

$= 5.5 \times 10^{-5}$ T

10. (a) $E_k = \frac{1}{2}mv^2$ or $mv = \sqrt{2E_k m}$ and

$r = \frac{mv}{Bq} = \frac{\sqrt{2E_k m}}{Bq}$

11. (d) $Bqv = mv^2/r$ or $q/m = v/rB$.

12. (d) $v = \frac{Bqr}{m} = \frac{4.5 \times 10^{-3} \times 1.6 \times 10^{-19} \times 2 \times 10^{-2}}{9.1 \times 10^{-31}}$

$= 1.58 \times 10^7$ m/s

13. (c) $B = \frac{\mu_0}{4\pi}\frac{2i_2}{(r/2)} - \frac{\mu_0}{4\mu}\frac{2i_1}{(r/2)} = \frac{\mu_0}{4\pi}\frac{4}{r}(i_2 - i_1)$

$= \frac{\mu_0}{4\pi}\frac{4}{5}(5 - 2.5) = \frac{\mu_0}{2\pi}$.

14. (c) $E = vB = 2 \times 10^3 \times 1.5 = 3 \times 10^3$ V/m.

15. (a) In coil A, $B = \frac{\mu_0}{4\pi}\frac{2\pi I}{R}$. $\quad \therefore B \propto \frac{I}{R}$;

Hence, $\frac{B_1}{B_2} = \frac{I_1}{R_1} \cdot \frac{R_2}{I_2} = \frac{2}{2} = 1$

16. (a) $B = \frac{\mu_0 I}{2r} \times \frac{\theta}{2\pi} = \frac{\mu_0 I\theta}{4\pi r}$

17. (d) No magnetic force acts on the electron and force due to electric field will act opposite to its initial direction of motion. Hence its velocity decreases in magnitude.

18. (c) $r = \frac{1}{B}\sqrt{\frac{2mV}{q}}$

$\frac{R_1}{R_2} = \sqrt{\frac{m_x}{m_y}} \Rightarrow \frac{m_x}{m_y} = \left(\frac{R_1}{R_2}\right)^2$

19. (d) $B_{total} = 4B_{side}$

$B_{total} = 4\frac{\mu_0 I}{2\pi\left(\frac{a}{2}\right)}\left[\sin\frac{\pi}{4} + \sin\frac{\pi}{4}\right]$

$B_{total} = \frac{2\sqrt{2}\mu_0 I}{a\pi}$

20. (b) $r = \frac{mv}{qB} = \frac{p}{qB} \Rightarrow \frac{r_p}{r_\alpha} = \frac{q_\alpha}{q_p} = \frac{2e}{e} = \frac{2}{1}$

21. (b)

22. (c) The magnetic field is

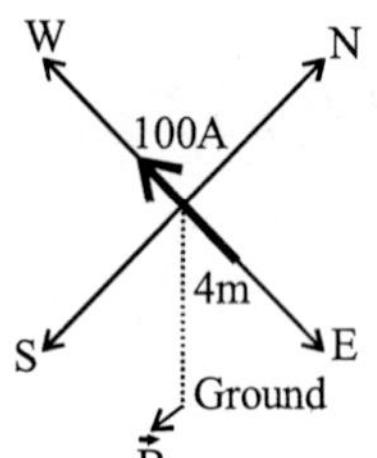

$B = \frac{\mu_0}{4\pi}\frac{2I}{r}$

$= 10^{-7} \times \frac{2 \times 100}{4}$

$= 5 \times 10^{-6}$ T

According to right hand palm rule, the magnetic field is directed towards south.

23. (a) Since magnetic force is always perpendicular to the velocity of electron, so it can only change the direction of velocity of electron, but it (the magnetic force) cannot accelerate or deaccelerate the electron.

24. (c) Magnetic dipole moment

$m = iA = \frac{e}{T} \times \pi r^2 = \frac{e}{(2\pi r/v)} \times \pi r^2 = \frac{erv}{2}$.

$= \frac{1.6 \times 10^{-19} \times 50 \times 10^{-12} \times 2.2 \times 10^6}{2}$

$= 8.8 \times 10^{-24}$ Am^2.

25. (c) Time taken by proton to make one revolution

$= \frac{25}{5} = 5\mu$ sec.

As $T = \frac{2\pi m}{qB}$; so $\frac{T_2}{T_1} = \frac{m_2}{m_1} \times \frac{q_1}{q_2}$

or $T_2 = T_1\frac{m_2 q_1}{m_1 q_2} = \frac{5 \times 4m_1}{m_1} \times \frac{q}{2q} = 10\ \mu$ sec.

26. (c) B at O will be due to the following portions

(i) Vertical straight portion. This is zero.

(ii) Circular portion. This is given by

$B_{circular} = \frac{1}{2}\frac{\mu_0 i}{2r} = \frac{\mu_0 i}{4r}$

(iii) Straight horizontal portion. This is given by

$B_{straight} = \frac{\mu_0 i}{4\pi r}$ $\quad \therefore B_{Total} = \frac{\mu_0 i}{4r} + \frac{\mu_0 i}{4\pi r}$

27. (a) Due to flow of current in same direction at adjacent side, an attractive magnetic force will be produced.

28. (d) Magnetic moment $\mu = IA$

Since $T = \frac{2\pi R}{v}$

Also, $I = \frac{q}{T} = \frac{qv}{2\pi R}$

$\therefore \mu = \left(\frac{qv}{2\pi R}\right)\left(\pi R^2\right) = \frac{qvR}{2}$.

29. (a) [Hint $\Rightarrow B = \frac{\mu_0 i}{2\pi r}$, where r is distance of point from the wire, where we want to calculate the magnetic field. It is clear from expression that B is independent of thickness of wire.]

30. (d)

31. (b) [Hint $\Rightarrow \frac{mv^2}{r} = qvB$].

32. (b)

33. (a) The magnetic field, due the coil, carrying current I Ampere

$$B_1 = \frac{m_0 I}{2R}$$

The magnetic field due to the coil, carrying current $2I$ Ampere

$$B_2 = \frac{m_0(2I)}{2R}$$

The resultant B

$$B_{net} = \sqrt{B_1^2 + B_2^2 + 2B_1B_2\cos q},\ \theta = 90°$$

$$B_{net} = \sqrt{B_1^2 + B_2^2} = \frac{m_0(2I)}{2R}\sqrt{1+4} = \frac{\sqrt{5}\,m_0 I}{2R}$$

34. (c) Time period of cyclotron is

$$T = \frac{1}{\upsilon} = \frac{2\pi m}{eB};\ B = \frac{2\pi m}{e}\upsilon;\ R = \frac{m\upsilon}{eB} = \frac{p}{eB}$$

$$\Rightarrow P = eBR = e \times \frac{2\pi m\upsilon}{e}R = 2\pi m\upsilon R$$

$$\text{K.E.} = \frac{p^2}{2m} = \frac{(2\pi m\upsilon R)^2}{2m} = 2\pi^2 m\upsilon^2 R^2$$

35. (b) According to the principal of circular motion in a magnetic field

$$F_c = F_m \Rightarrow \frac{mv^2}{R} = qVB$$

$$\Rightarrow R = \frac{mv}{qB} = \frac{P}{qB} = \frac{\sqrt{2m.k}}{qB}$$

$$R_\alpha = \frac{\sqrt{2(4m)K'}}{2qB}$$

$$\frac{R}{R_\alpha} = \sqrt{\frac{K}{K'}}$$

but $R = R_\alpha$ (given)

Thus $K = K' = 1$ MeV

36. (b) Magnetic force acts perpendicular to the velocity. Hence speed remains constant.

37. (c) The force on each point on loop is radially outward and so net force = 0

38. (a) Proton will represent the direction of current, so the direction of current is vertically downward. By Fleming's left hand rule, force acting on the proton in east direction.

39. (c) As $\vec{F} = q\vec{V}\vec{B}\sin\theta$

F is zero for sin 0° or sin 180° and is non-zero for angle between $\vec{V}$ and $\vec{B}$ any value other than zero and 180°.

40. (a) A current carrying coil has magnetic dipole moment. Hence, a torque $\vec{p}_m \times \vec{B}$ acts on it in magnetic field.

41. (a) The force acting on a charged particle in magnetic field is given by

$\vec{F} = q(\vec{v} \times \vec{B})$ or $F = qvB\sin\theta$,

When angle between v and B is 180°,

$F = 0$

42. (a) $B = \frac{\mu_0 i}{2\pi r}$ or $B \propto \frac{1}{r}$

When r is doubled, the magnetic field becomes half, i.e., now the magnetic field will be 0.2 T.

43. (c) $r = \frac{mv}{qB}$ or $r \propto v$

As v is doubled, the radius also becomes double. Hence, radius = 2 × 2 = 4 cm

44. (d) Pitch = $(v\cos\theta)T$ and $T = \frac{2\pi m}{qB}$

$$\therefore \text{Pitch} = (V\cos\theta)\frac{2\pi m}{qB}$$

$$= (4\times10^5\cos 60°)\frac{2\pi}{0.3}\left(\frac{1.67\times10^{-27}}{1.69\times10^{-19}}\right) = 4\text{ cm}$$

45. (a)

$\vec{B}$ (to the right); $\vec{v}$, $a = 10^{12}$ m/s²; q, E = 1Mev, Proton; North, South, West, East

As we know, magnetic force $F = qvB = ma$

$$\therefore \vec{a} = \left(\frac{qvB}{m}\right) \text{ perpendicular to velocity.}$$

$$\therefore \text{Also } v = \sqrt{\frac{2KE}{m}} = \sqrt{\frac{2\times e\times10^6}{m}}$$

$$\therefore a = \frac{qvB}{m} = \frac{eB}{m}\sqrt{\frac{2\times e\times10^6}{m}}$$

$$\therefore 10^{12} = \left(\frac{1.6\times10^{-19}}{1.67\times10^{-27}}\right)^{\frac{3}{2}}.\sqrt{2}\times10^3 B$$

$$\therefore B \simeq \frac{1}{\sqrt{2}}\times10^{-3}T = 0.71\text{ mT (approx)}$$

46. (b) As mvr = qvB ⇒ $r = \frac{mv}{qB} = \frac{\sqrt{2mK.E.}}{qB}$

[As: $\frac{1}{2}mv^2 = K.E.$

$\Rightarrow m^2v^2 = 2mK.E.$

$\Rightarrow mv = \sqrt{2mK.E.}$]

For proton, electron and α-particle,

$m_{He} = 4m_p$ and $m_p >> m_e$

Also $a_{He} = 2q_p$ and $q_p = q_e$

∴ As KE of all the particles is same then,

$r\ \alpha\ \frac{\sqrt{m}}{q}$ $\therefore r_{He} = r_p > r_e$

47. (d) Radius of the path (r) is given by $r = \frac{mv}{qB}$

$$r = \frac{\sqrt{2mk}}{eB}\quad (\because p = mv = \sqrt{2mk})$$

$$= \frac{\sqrt{2meV}}{eB}\quad (\because k = eV)$$

$$r = \frac{\sqrt{\frac{2m}{e}V}}{B} = \frac{\sqrt{\frac{2\times9.1\times10^{-31}}{1.6\times10^{-19}}(500)}}{100\times10^{-3}}$$

$$r = \frac{\sqrt{\frac{9.1}{0.16} \times 10^{-10}}}{10^{-1}} = \frac{3}{.4} \times 10^{-4}$$

$$= 7.5 \times 10^{-4}$$

48. (c)

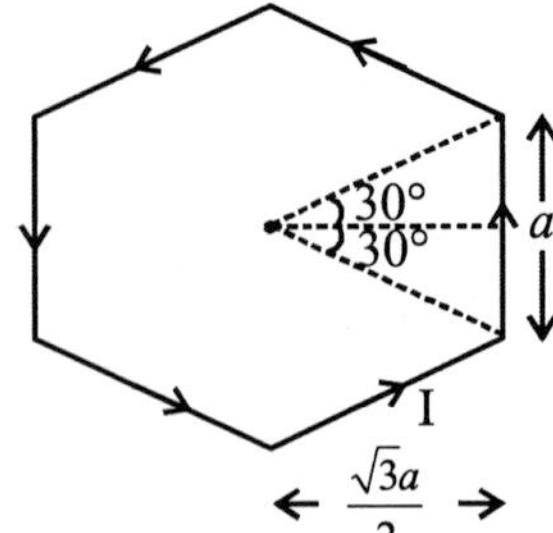

Magnetic field due to one side of hexagon

$$B = \frac{\mu_0 I}{4\pi \frac{\sqrt{3}a}{2}} (\sin 30° + \sin 30°)$$

$$\Rightarrow B = \frac{\mu_0 I}{2\sqrt{3}a}\left(\frac{1}{2} + \frac{1}{2}\right) = \frac{\mu_0 I}{2\sqrt{3}a\pi}$$

Now, magnetic field due to one hexagon coil

$$B = 6 \times \frac{\mu_0 I}{2\sqrt{3}a\pi}$$

Again magnetic field at the centre of hexagonal shape coil of 50 turns,

$$B = 50 \times 6 \times \frac{\mu_0 I}{2\sqrt{3}a\pi} \qquad \left[\because a = \frac{10}{100} = 0.1 \text{ m}\right]$$

$$\text{or, } B = \frac{150\mu_0 I}{\sqrt{3} \times 0.1 \times \pi} = 500\sqrt{3}\frac{\mu_0 I}{\pi}$$

49. (a) $r = \left(\frac{1}{3}\right)(a \sin 60)$

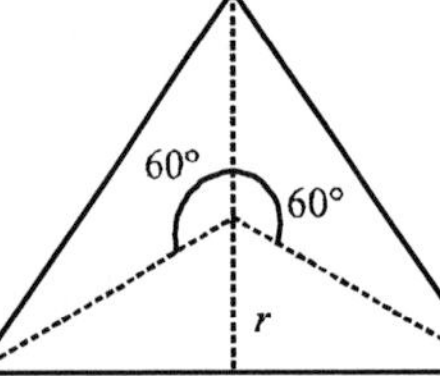

$$r = \frac{a}{3} \times \frac{\sqrt{3}}{2} = \left(\frac{a}{2\sqrt{3}}\right)$$

$$B_0 = 3\left[\frac{\mu_0 I}{4\pi r}(\sin 60° + \sin 60°)\right]$$

$$= \frac{3\mu_0 I}{4\pi\left(\frac{a}{2\sqrt{3}}\right)} \times (2)\left(\frac{\sqrt{3}}{2}\right) = \frac{9}{2}\left(\frac{\mu_0 I}{\pi a}\right)$$

$$= \frac{9 \times 2 \times 10^{-7} \times 10}{1} = 18\,\mu\text{T}$$

50. (c) Magnetic field at the centre of loop, $B_1 = \frac{\mu_0 I}{2R}$

Dipole moment of circular loop is m = IA

$m_1 = I.A = I.\pi R^2$ {R = Radius of the loop}

If moment is doubled (keeping current constant) R becomes $\sqrt{2}R$

$$m_2 = I.\pi\left(\sqrt{2}R\right)^2 = 2.I\pi R^2 = 2m_1$$

$$B_2 = \frac{\mu_0 I}{2\left(\sqrt{2}R\right)} \qquad \therefore \frac{B_1}{B_2} = \frac{\frac{\mu_0 I}{2R}}{\frac{\mu_0 I}{2\left(\sqrt{2}R\right)}} = \sqrt{2}$$

51. (b) $B = \frac{\mu_0}{4\pi}, \frac{i}{r}(\sin\alpha + \sin\beta)$

Here $r = \sqrt{5^2 - 3^2} = 4$ cm

$\alpha = \beta = 37°$

$\therefore \quad B = 10^{-7} \times \frac{5}{4} 2\sin 37° = 1.5 \times 10^{-5}$ T

52. (a) If magnetic field is perpendicular and into the plane of the paper, it is represented by cross ⊗ and if the direction of the magnetic field is perpendicular out of the plane of the paper it is represented by dot ⊙.

53. (a) Magnetic field at any point lies on axial position of current carrying conductor B = 0

54. (b) Given : Radius = R

Distance $x = 2\sqrt{2}R$

$$\frac{B_{centre}}{B_{axis}} = \left(1 + \frac{x^2}{R^2}\right)^{3/2} = \left(1 + \frac{(2\sqrt{2}R)^2}{R^2}\right)^{3/2}$$

$$= (9)^{3/2} = 27$$

55. (d) Since uniform current is flowing through a straight wire, current enclosed in the amperean path formed at a distance $r_1\left(= \frac{a}{2}\right)$ is

a/2 P₁ P₂

$$i = \left(\frac{\pi r_1^2}{\pi a^2}\right) \times I,$$

where I is total current

Using Ampere circuital law,

$$\oint B \cdot \vec{dl} = \mu_0 i$$

$$\Rightarrow B_1 = \frac{\mu_0 \times \text{current enclosed}}{\text{Path}}$$

$$\Rightarrow B_1 = \frac{\mu_0 \times \left(\frac{\pi r_1^2}{\pi a^2}\right) \times I}{2\pi r_1} = \frac{\mu_0 \times I r_1}{2\pi a^2}$$

Now, magnetic field induction at point P_2,

$$B_2 = \frac{\mu_0}{2\pi} \cdot \frac{I}{(2a)} = \frac{\mu_0 I}{4\pi a}.$$

$$\therefore \frac{B_1}{B_2} = \frac{\mu_0 I r_1}{2\pi a^2} \times \frac{4\pi a}{\mu_0 I}$$

$$\Rightarrow \frac{B_1}{B_2} = \frac{2r_1}{a} = \frac{2 \times \frac{a}{2}}{a} = 1.$$

56. (d) There is no current inside the pipe. From Ampere's circuital law $\oint \vec{B} \cdot \vec{dl} = \mu_0 I$

$\because I = 0$

$\therefore B = 0$

57. (a) Magnetic field induction at the centre of current carrying circular coil of radius r is

$$B = \frac{\mu_0}{4\pi}\frac{I}{R} \times 2\pi$$

Here $B_A = \frac{\mu_0}{4\pi}\frac{I}{R} \times 2\pi$

and $B_B = \frac{\mu_0}{4\pi}\frac{2I}{2R} \times 2\pi \Rightarrow \frac{B_A}{B_B} = \frac{I/R}{2I/2R} = 1$

58. (b) $|\vec{\tau}| = |\vec{\mu} \times \vec{B}|$ $[\mu = NIA]$

$= NIA \times B \sin 90° [A = \pi r^2]$

$\Rightarrow \tau = NI\pi r^2 B$

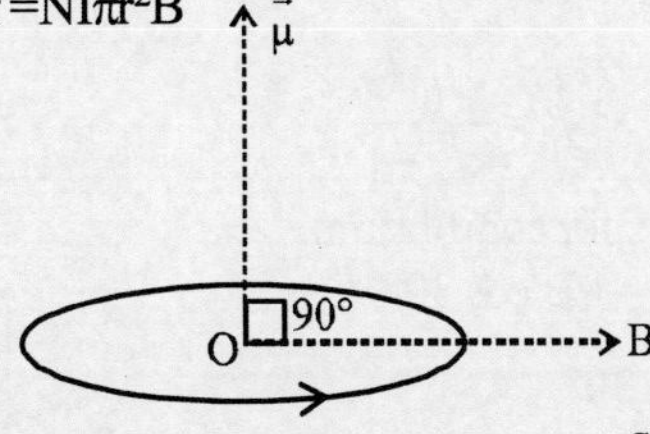

59. (a) Magnetic moment, $\mu = IA = \frac{qv}{2\pi r}(\pi r^2)$

or, $\mu = \frac{qr\omega}{2\pi r}(\pi r^2) = \frac{1}{2}qr^2\omega$

60. (a) The time period of a charged particle of charge q and mass m moving in a magnetic field (B) is $T = \frac{2\pi m}{qB}$

Clearly time period is independent of speed of the particle.

Exercise 2 - Exemplar & Past Year Questions 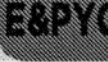

Exemplar Questions

1. (d) As we know that the uniqueness of helical path is determined by its pitch

$$P(\text{Pitch}) = \frac{2\pi m v \cos\theta}{Bq}$$

Where θ is angle of velocity of charge particle with x-axis

For the given pitch d correspond to charge particle, we have

$$\frac{q}{m} = \frac{2\pi v \cos\theta}{BP} = \text{constant}$$

If motion is not helical, $(\theta = 0)$

As charged particles traverse identical helical paths in a completely opposite direction in a same magnetic field **B**, LHS for two particles should be same and of opposite sign.

$$\therefore \quad \left(\frac{e}{m}\right)_1 + \left(\frac{e}{m}\right)_2 = 0$$

2. (a) By Biot-Savart law

$$dB = \frac{Idl \sin\theta}{r^2} = \left(\frac{I \times dl}{r}\right)$$

In Biot-Savat's law, magnetic field **B**||idl × **r** and *idl* due to flow of electron is in opposite direction of v and by direction of cross product of two vectors

$$B \perp V$$

So, the magnetic field is ⊥ to the direction of flow of charge.

3. (a) As the direction of magnetic moment of circular loop of radius R placed in the x-y plane is along z-direction and given by $M = I(\pi r^2)$, when half of the loop with $x > 0$ is now bent so that it now lies in the y-z plane, the magnitudes of magnetic field moment of each semicircular loop of radius R lie in the x-y plane and the y-z plane is $M' = I(\pi r^2)/4$ and the direction of magnetic field moments are along z-directlon and x-direction respectively.

Then resultant is :

$$M_{net} = \sqrt{M'^2 + M'^2} = \sqrt{2}\,M' = \sqrt{2}\,I(\pi r^2)/4$$

So, $M_{net} < M$ or M diminishes.

Hence, the magnitude of magnetic moment is now diminishes.

4. (d) Magnetic Lorentz force : $F = qVB \sin\theta$

Magnetic Lorentz force electron is projected with uniform velocity along the axis of a current carrying long solenoid $F = -qvB \sin 180° = 0 (\theta = 0°)$ as magnetic field and velocity are parallel and electric field is zero (E = 0) due to this magnetic field (B) perpendicular to the direction of motion (V). So it will not affect the velocity of moving charge particle. So the electron will continue to move with uniform velocity along the axis of the solenoid

5. (a) There is crossed electric and magnetic field between dees so the charged particle accelerates by electric field between dees towards other dees.

So, the charged particle undergoes acceleration as

(i) speeds up between the dees because of the oscillating electric field.

(ii) speed remain the same inside the dees because of the magnetic field but direction undergoes change continuously.

Hence, the charge particle accelerates inside and between Dees always.

NEET/AIPMT (2013-2020) Questions

6. (c) A current loop in a magnetic field is in equilibrium in two orientations one is stable and another unstable.

$\because \quad \vec{\tau} = \vec{M} \times \vec{B} = MB \sin\theta$

If $\theta = 0° \Rightarrow \tau = 0$ (stable)

If $\theta = \pi \Rightarrow \tau = 0$ (unstable)

Do not experience a torque in some orientations

Hence option (c) is correct.

7. (b) Here, $\vec{F}_{AB} + \vec{F}_{BCDA} = \vec{0}$

$\Rightarrow \vec{F}_{BCDA} = -\vec{F}_{AB} = -\vec{F} \quad (\because F_{AB} = \vec{F})$

8. (d) Net magnetic field, $B = \sqrt{B_1^2 + B_2^2}$

$$= \sqrt{\left(\frac{\mu_0 I_1}{2\pi d}\right)^2 + \left(\frac{\mu_0 I_2}{2\pi d}\right)^2} \left(\because B_1 = \frac{\mu_0 I_1}{2\pi d} \text{ and } B_2 = \frac{\mu_0 I_2}{2\pi d}\right)$$

$$= \frac{\mu_0}{2\pi d}\sqrt{I_1^2 + I_2^2}$$

9. (c) Radius of circular orbit = r
No. of rotations per second = n

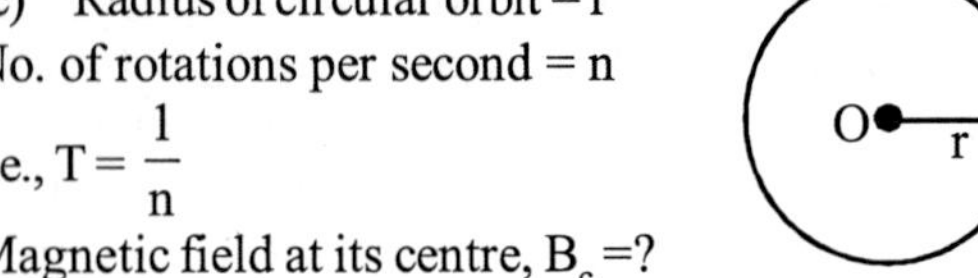

i.e., $T = \frac{1}{n}$
Magnetic field at its centre, B_c =?
As we know, current

$$i = \frac{e}{T} = \frac{e}{(1/n)} = en = \text{equivalent current}$$

Magnetic field at the centre of circular orbit,

$$B_c = \frac{\mu_0 i}{2r} = \frac{\mu_0 ne}{2r}$$

10. (c) As we know, $F = qvB = \frac{mv^2}{R}$

$$\therefore \quad R = \frac{mv}{qB} = \frac{\sqrt{2m(kE)}}{qB}$$

Since R is same so, $KE \propto \frac{q^2}{m}$
Therefore KE of α particle

$$= \frac{q^2}{m} = \frac{(2)^2}{4} = 1 \text{ MeV}$$

11. (a) Here, number of turns of coil, N = 50
Current through the coil I = 2A
Area $A = l \times b = 0.12 \times 0.1 m^2$
Magnetic field $\vec{B} = 0.2\ \omega/m^2$

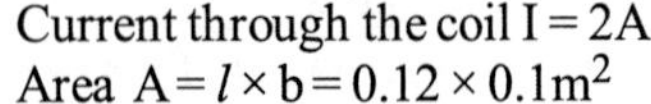

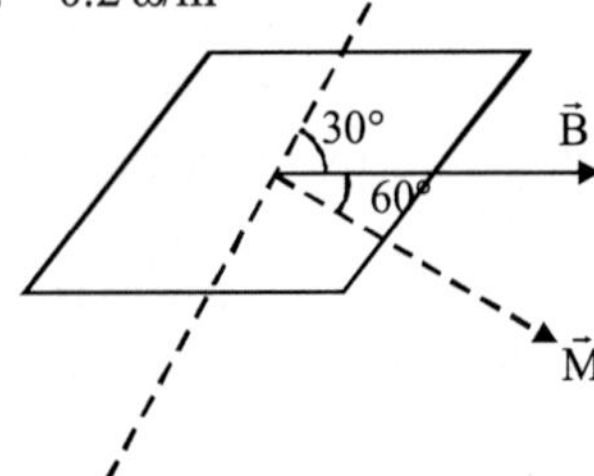

Torque required to keep the coil in stable equilibrium.

$$\tau = \vec{M} \times \vec{B} = MB \sin 60° = NiAB \sin 60°$$

$$= 50 \times 2 \times 0.12 \times 0.1 \times 0.2 \times \frac{\sqrt{3}}{2}$$

$$= 12\sqrt{3} \times 10^{-2} = 0.20784 \text{ Nm}$$

12. (c) For points inside the wire i.e., $(r \le R)$
Magnetic field $B = \frac{\mu_0 Ir}{2\pi R^2}$
For points outside the wire $(r \ge R)$
Magnetic field, $B' = \frac{\mu_0 I}{2\pi R}$

$$\therefore \quad \frac{B}{B'} = \frac{\frac{\mu_0 I(a/2)}{2\pi a^2}}{\frac{\mu_0 I}{2\pi(2a)}} = 1:1$$

13. (d) Work done, $W = MB(\cos\theta_1 - \cos\theta_2)$
When it is rotated by angle 180° then
W = MB (cos0° – cos 180°) = MB (1 + 1)
W = 2MB
W = 2 (NIA) B
$= 2 \times 250 \times 85 \times 10^{-6}[1.25 \times 2.1 \times 10^{-4}] \times 85 \times 10^{-2}$
= 9.1 μJ

14. (c) Force per unit length between two parallel current carrying conductors,

$$F = \frac{\mu_0 i_1 i_2}{2\pi d}$$

Since same current flowing through both the wires
$i_i = i_2 = i$ — F_1[due to wire A]

so $F_1 = \frac{\mu_0 i^2}{2\pi d} = F_2$

F_2[due to wire C]

∴ Magnitude of force per unit length on the middle wire 'B'

$$F_{net} = \sqrt{F_1^2 + F_2^2} = \frac{\mu_0 i^2}{\sqrt{2}\pi d}$$

15. (c) From figure, for equilibrium,
$mg \sin 30° = I\ell B \cos 30°$

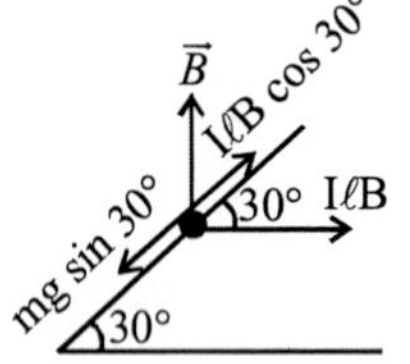

$$\Rightarrow \quad I = \frac{mg}{\ell B} \tan 30°$$

$$= \frac{0.5 \times 9.8}{0.25 \times \sqrt{3}} = 11.32 \text{ A}$$

16. (d) Current sensitivity of moving coil galvanometer

$$I_s = \frac{NBA}{C} \quad \text{...(i)}$$

Voltage sensitivity of moving coil galvanometer,

$$V_s = \frac{NBA}{CR_G} \quad \text{...(ii)}$$

Dividing eqn. (i) by (ii)
Resistance of galvanometer

$$R_G = \frac{I_s}{V_s} = \frac{5 \times 1}{20 \times 10^{-3}} = \frac{5000}{20} = 250\,\Omega$$

17. (a) Radius of the path $= r = \frac{mv}{qB} = \frac{P}{qB}$

For H^+ion, $r_H = \frac{p_H}{eB}$

For α particle

$$r_\alpha = \frac{p_\alpha}{2eB} \text{ and } \frac{r_H}{r_\alpha} = \frac{\frac{p}{eB}}{\frac{p}{2eB}} \quad [\text{as given } p_H = p_\alpha = p]$$

$$\Rightarrow \frac{r_H}{r_\alpha} = \frac{2}{1}$$

18. (c) Inside $(d < R)$
Magnetic field inside conductor

$$B = Kd \quad \text{..... (i)}$$

This is straight line passing through origin
At surface $(d = R)$

$$B = \frac{\mu_0}{2\pi} \frac{1}{d}$$

Maximum at surface
Outside $(d > R)$

$$B = \frac{\mu_0}{2\pi} \frac{1}{d}$$

or $B \propto \frac{1}{d}$ ∴ Hyperbolic

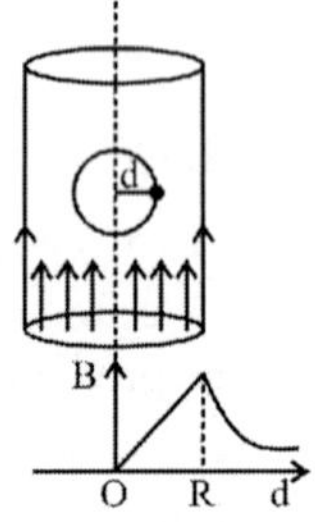

19. (b) $B = \dfrac{\mu_0 N \cdot I}{2\pi R}$

$\therefore \dfrac{B_1}{B_2} = \dfrac{N_1 R_2}{N_2 R_1} = \dfrac{200}{100}\dfrac{20}{40} = 1$

So, $\dfrac{B_1}{B_2} = 1$

20. (b) Net magnetic field at point '

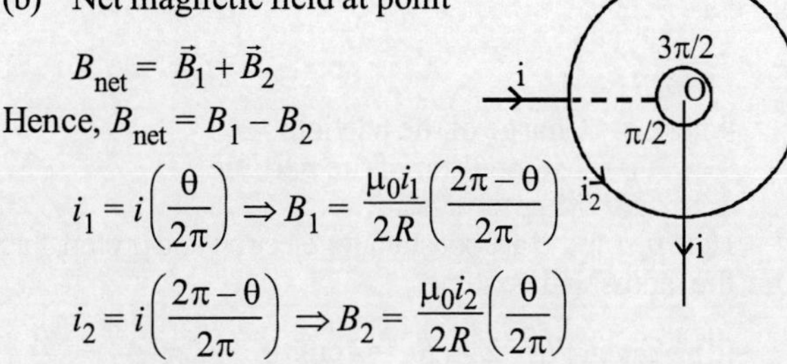

$B_{net} = \vec{B}_1 + \vec{B}_2$

Hence, $B_{net} = B_1 - B_2$

$i_1 = i\left(\dfrac{\theta}{2\pi}\right) \Rightarrow B_1 = \dfrac{\mu_0 i_1}{2R}\left(\dfrac{2\pi - \theta}{2\pi}\right)$

$i_2 = i\left(\dfrac{2\pi - \theta}{2\pi}\right) \Rightarrow B_2 = \dfrac{\mu_0 i_2}{2R}\left(\dfrac{\theta}{2\pi}\right)$

Here $\theta = \dfrac{\pi}{2}$

$B_{net} = B_1 - B_2 = 0$

21. (d) Magnetic field at the centre of solenoid,

$B_{solenoid} = \mu_0 nl$

Given : No. of turns / length,

$n = \dfrac{N}{L} = \dfrac{100}{50 \times 10^{-2}} = 200$ turns/ m

Current, $I = 2.5$ A

$\therefore B_{solenoid} = \mu_0 nI = 4\pi \times 10^{-7} \times 200 \times 2.5$

$= 6.28 \times 10^{-4}$ T

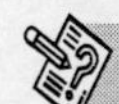

Exercise 3 - Concept Application Problems CAP

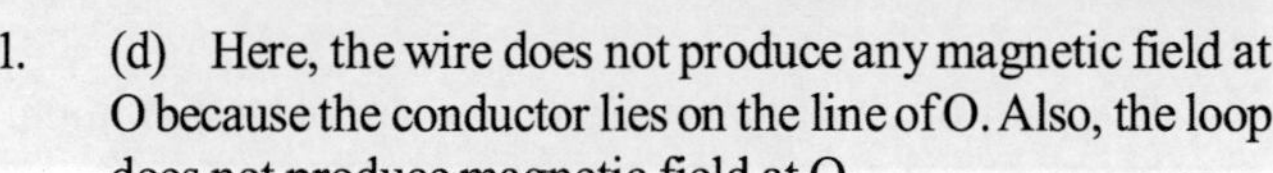

1. (d) Here, the wire does not produce any magnetic field at O because the conductor lies on the line of O. Also, the loop does not produce magnetic field at O.

2. (a) $B = \dfrac{\mu_0}{4\pi}\left[\dfrac{I}{r} + \dfrac{\pi I}{r} + \dfrac{I}{r}\right] \dfrac{\mu_0}{4\pi}\left[\dfrac{2I}{r} + \dfrac{\pi I}{r}\right]$

$= \mu_0\left[\dfrac{I}{2\pi r} + \dfrac{I}{4r}\right]$

(The direction of $\vec{B}$ is into the page.)

3. (c) The magnetic field is perpendicular to the plane of the paper. Let us consider two diametrically opposite elements. By Fleming's Left hand rule on element AB the direction of force will be Leftwards and the magnitude will be

dF = Idl B sin 90° = IdlB

On element CD, the direction of force will be towards right on the plane of the papper and the magnitude will be dF = IdlB.

4. (b) From Lorentz equation

$F = -eu\,\hat{i} \times B_0(-\hat{k}) = -euB_0\hat{j}$

hence it will complete a semicircular arc and comes out of the region at a position y, such that $y < 0$

5. (b) The force on the two arms parallel to the field is zero.

$\therefore$ Force on remaining arms $= -F$

6. (b) Magnetic fields due to the two parts at their common centre are respectively,

$B_y = \dfrac{\mu_0 i}{4R}$ and $B_z = \dfrac{\mu_0 i}{4R}$

Resultant field $= \sqrt{B_y^2 + B_z^2}$

$= \sqrt{\left(\dfrac{\mu_0 i}{4R}\right)^2 + \left(\dfrac{\mu_0 i}{4R}\right)^2} = \sqrt{2}.\dfrac{\mu_0 i}{4R} = \dfrac{\mu_0 i}{2\sqrt{2}R}$

7 (b) $\vec{v}$ and $\vec{B}$ are in same direction so that magnetic force on electron becomes zero, only electric force acts. But force on electron due to electric field is opposite to the direction of velocity.

8. (a) Magnetic field at the centre of the ring is $\dfrac{\mu_0 qf}{2R}$

9. (b) According to work energy theorem

$W = U_{final} - U_{initial} = MB\,(\cos 0 - \cos 60°)$

$W = \dfrac{MB}{2} = \sqrt{3}$J ...(i)

$\tau = \vec{M} \times \vec{B} = MB\sin 60° = \left(\dfrac{MB\sqrt{3}}{2}\right)$ ...(ii)

From equation (i) and (ii)

$\tau = \dfrac{2\sqrt{3} \times \sqrt{3}}{2} = 3$J

10. (d) $r = \dfrac{mv}{qB} \Rightarrow r \propto \dfrac{v}{B}$

11. (a) $B = \dfrac{\mu_0 I}{2\pi r} \Rightarrow B \propto \dfrac{1}{r}$

As the distance is increased to three times, the magnetic induction reduces to one third. Hence,

$B = \dfrac{1}{3} \times 10^{-3}$ tesla $= 3.33 \times 10^{-4}$ tesla

12. (c)

13. (c) In uniform magnetic field particle moves in a circular path, if the radius of the circular path is 'r', particle will not hit the screen.

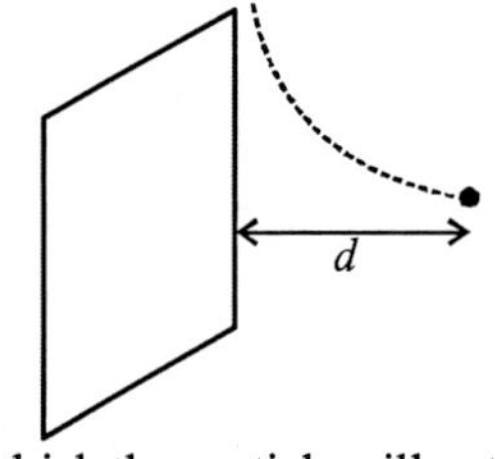

$r = \frac{mv}{qB_0}$ $\left[\because \frac{mv^2}{r} = qvB_0\right]$

Hence, minimum value of v for which the particle will not hit the screen.

$v = \frac{qB_0 d}{m}$

14. (a) [Given: $q = 1\mu C = 1\times10^{-6} C$;

$\vec{V} = (2\hat{i} + 3\hat{j} + 4\hat{k})$ m/s and

$\vec{B} = (5\hat{i} + 3\hat{j} - 6\hat{k}) \times 10^{-3}$ T]

$$\vec{F} = q(\vec{V} \times \vec{B}) = 10^{-6} \times 10^{-3} \begin{vmatrix} \hat{i} & \hat{j} & \hat{k} \\ 2 & 3 & 4 \\ 5 & 3 & -6 \end{vmatrix}$$

$= (-30\hat{i} + 32\hat{j} - 9\hat{k}) \times 10^{-9}$ N

$\therefore \vec{F} = (-30\hat{i} + 32\hat{j} - 9\hat{k})$

15. (a) Radius of the circular path will be $r = \frac{mv}{qB}$

$\Rightarrow r = \frac{\sqrt{2mKE}}{qB}$ $(\because p = mv = \sqrt{2mKE})$

$\because KE = q\Delta V$

$\therefore r = \frac{\sqrt{2mq\Delta V}}{qB} \Rightarrow r \propto \sqrt{\frac{m}{q}}$ $\therefore \frac{r_p}{r_\alpha} = \frac{1}{\sqrt{2}}$

16. (BONUS)

Assuming particle enters from (0, d)

$r = \frac{mv}{qB}$, $d = \frac{r}{2}$

$a = \frac{qVB}{m}\left[\frac{-\sqrt{3}i - j}{2}\right]$

this option is not given in the all above four choices.

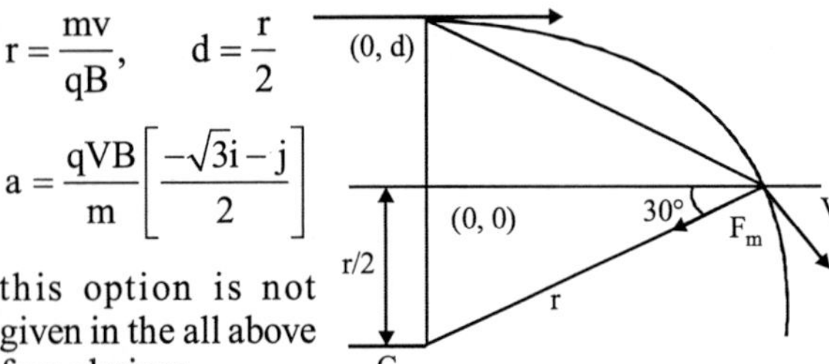

17. (b) As we know, radius of circular path in magnetic field

$r = \frac{\sqrt{2Km}}{qB}$

For electron, $r_e = \frac{\sqrt{2Km_e}}{eB}$ ....(i)

For proton, $r_p = \frac{\sqrt{2Km_p}}{eB}$ ....(ii)

For α particle, $r_\alpha = \frac{\sqrt{2Km_a}}{q_\alpha B} = \frac{\sqrt{2K4m_p}}{2eB} = \frac{\sqrt{2Km_p}}{eB}$ ...(iii)

$\therefore$ $r_e < r_p = r_\alpha$ $(\because m_e < m_p)$

18. (c) As velocity $v = \frac{E}{B} = \frac{7.7 \times 10^3}{0.14} = 55$ km/s

19. (b) The charged particle will move along the lines of electric field (and magnetic field). Magnetic field will exert no force. The force by electric field will be along the lines of uniform electric field. Hence the particle will move in a straight line.

20. (a) When a moving charged particle is subjected to a perpendicular magnetic field, then it describes a circular path of radius.

$r = \frac{p}{qB}$

where q = Charge of the particle

p = Momentum of the particle

B = Magnetic field

Here p, q and B are constant for electron and proton, therefore the radius will be same.

21. (d) Given : $I_A = 2$ A, $R_A = 2$ cm, $\theta_A = 2\pi - \frac{\pi}{2} = \frac{3\pi}{2}$

$I_B = 3$ A, $R_B = 4$ cm, $\theta_B = 2\pi - \frac{\pi}{3} = \frac{5\pi}{3}$

Using, magnetic field, $B = \frac{\mu_0 I\theta}{4\pi R}$

$$\frac{B_A}{B_B} = \frac{I_A}{I_B} \times \frac{\theta_A R_B}{\theta_B R_A} = \frac{2 \times \frac{3\pi}{2} \times 4}{3 \times \frac{5\pi}{3} \times 2} = \frac{6}{5}$$

22. (b) Magnetic field inside the solenoid is given by

$B = \mu_0 nI$ .... (i)

Here, n = number of turns per unit length

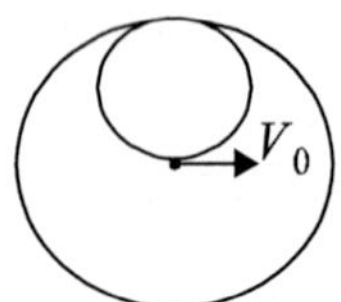

The path of charge particle is circular. The maximum possible radius of electron $= \frac{R}{2}$

$\therefore \frac{mV_{max}}{qB} = \frac{R}{2}$

$\Rightarrow V_{max} = \frac{qBR}{2m} = \frac{eR\mu_0 nI}{2m}$ (using (i))

23. (a)

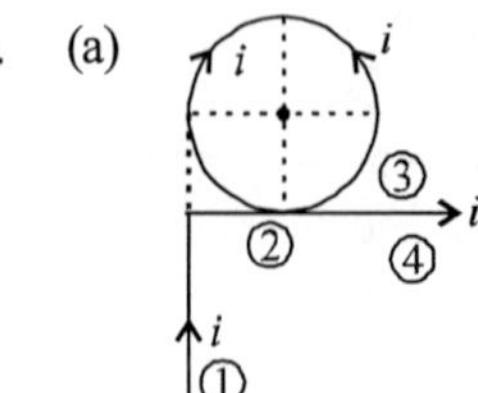

$B_0 = B_1 + B_2 + B_3 + B_4$

$= \frac{\mu_0 I}{4\pi R}[\sin 90° - \sin 45°] + \frac{\mu_0 I}{2R} + \frac{\mu_0 I}{4\pi R}$ $[\sin 45° + \sin 90°]$

$$= -\frac{\mu_0 I}{4\pi R}\left(1 - \frac{1}{\sqrt{2}}\right) + \frac{\mu_0 I}{2R} + \frac{\mu_0 I}{4\pi R}\left(1 + \frac{1}{\sqrt{2}}\right)$$

$$\overrightarrow{B_0^{\odot}} = \frac{\mu_0 I}{2\pi R}\left(\pi + \frac{1}{\sqrt{2}}\right)^{\odot}$$

24. (a) $\vec{B} = \vec{B_1} + \vec{B_2}$

$$= \frac{\mu_0}{2\pi}\cdot\left(\frac{i^o}{d}.\hat{k} + \frac{i^o}{d}\left(-\hat{k}\right)\right) = 0$$

25. (d) L = 2πR L = N × 2πr

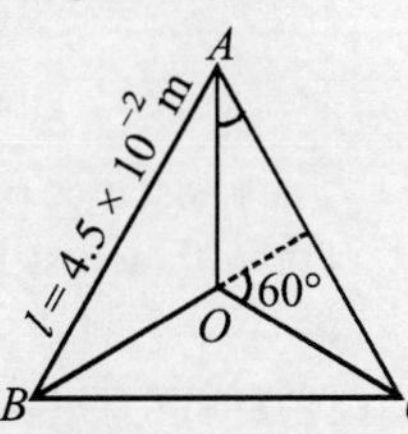

$R = Nr \Rightarrow r = \frac{R}{N}$

$$B_{Loop} = \frac{\mu_0 i}{2R} \quad B_{coil} = \frac{\mu_0 Ni}{2r} = \frac{\mu_0 Ni}{2\left(\frac{R}{N}\right)} = \frac{\mu_0 N^2 i}{2R}$$

$$\therefore \frac{B_L}{B_C} = \frac{1}{N^2}$$

26. (a) Here, side of the triangle, $l = 4.5 \times 10^{-2}$ m, current, I = 1A magnetic field at the centre of the triangle 'O' $B = ?$

From figure, $\tan 60° = \sqrt{3} = \frac{1}{2d}$

$$\Rightarrow \quad d = \frac{l}{2\sqrt{3}} = \left(\frac{4.5 \times 10^{-2}}{2\sqrt{3}}\right)\text{m}$$

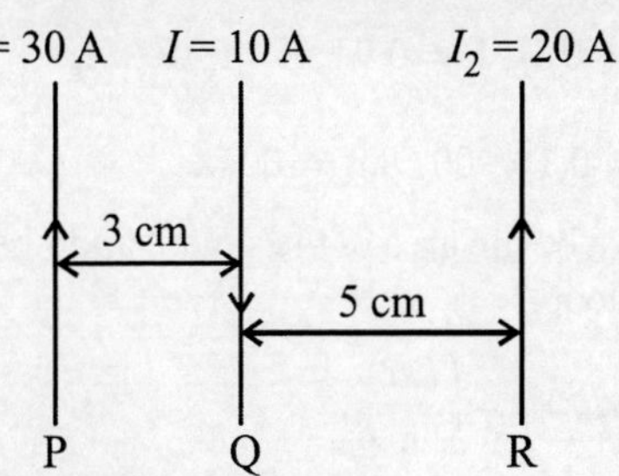

Magnetic field, $B = \frac{\mu_0 i}{4\pi d}(\cos\theta_1 + \cos\theta_2)$

Putting value of $\mu = 4\pi \times 10^{-7}$ and θ_1 and θ_2 we will get $B = 4 \times 10^{-5}$ Wb/m²

27. (b)

28. (c) Torque on the loop,

$$\overline{\tau} = \overline{M} \times \overline{B} = MB\sin\theta = MB\sin 90°$$

Magnetic field, $B = \frac{\mu_0 I}{2\pi d}$

$$\therefore \tau = I_1(2a)^2\left(\frac{\mu_0 I_2}{2\pi d}\right)\sin 90° = \frac{2\mu_0 I_1 I_2}{\pi d} \times a^2 = \frac{2\mu_0 I^2 a^2}{\pi d}$$

29. (c) Torque on circular loop, $\tau = MB\sin\theta$

where, M = magnetic moment

B = magnetic field

Now, using $\tau = I\alpha$

$$\therefore \quad \tau = MB\sin\theta = I\alpha \Rightarrow \quad \pi R^2 IB\theta = \frac{mR^2\alpha}{2}$$

($\because m = IA$ and moment of inertia of circular loop, $I = \frac{mR^2}{2}$)

$$\Rightarrow \quad \pi R^2 IB\,\theta = \frac{mR^2}{2}\omega\theta$$

$$\Rightarrow \omega = \sqrt{\frac{2\pi IB}{m}} \quad \Rightarrow \quad \frac{2\pi}{T} = \sqrt{\frac{2\pi IB}{m}}$$

$$\Rightarrow T = \sqrt{\frac{2\pi m}{IB}}$$

30. (a) $I_1 = 30$ A $\quad I = 10$ A $\quad I_2 = 20$ A

Also given; length of wire Q = 25 cm = 0.25 m

Force on wire Q due to wire R

$$F_{QR} = 10^{-7} \times \frac{2 \times 20 \times 10}{0.05} \times 0.25$$

$= 20 \times 10^{-5}$ N (Towards left)

Force on wire Q due to wire P

$$F_{QP} = 10^{-7} \times \frac{2 \times 30 \times 10}{0.03} \times 0.25$$

$= 50 \times 10^{-5}$ N (Towards right)

Hence, $F_{net} = F_{QP} - F_{QR}$

$= 50 \times 10^{-5}$ N $- 20 \times 10^{-5}$ N

$= 3 \times 10^{-4}$ N towards right

31. (b) Let ℓ be length of wire

Ist case : $\ell = 2\pi r \Rightarrow r = \frac{\ell}{2\pi}$

$$B = \frac{\mu_0 I}{2\pi r} = \frac{\mu_0 I}{\ell}$$

2nd Case : $\ell = 2(2\pi r') \Rightarrow r' = \frac{\ell}{4\pi}$

$$B' = \frac{\mu_0 In}{2\pi\frac{\ell}{4\pi}} = \frac{2\mu_0 I}{\frac{\ell}{2}} \quad \text{(where n = 2)}$$

on putting the value of B $\Rightarrow B' = 4\left(\frac{\mu_0 I}{l}\right) = 4B$

32. (d) As particle is moving along a circular path

$$\therefore R = \frac{mv}{qB} \qquad \text{...(i)}$$

Path is straight line, then

qE = qvB

$$E = vB \Rightarrow v = \frac{E}{B} \qquad \text{....(ii)}$$

From equation (i) and (ii)

$$m = \frac{qB^2R}{E} = \frac{1.6 \times 10^{-19} \times (0.5)^2 \times 0.5 \times 10^{-2}}{100}$$

$\therefore m = 2.0 \times 10^{-24}$ kg

33. (d)

34. (b) $B = \frac{\mu_0}{2\pi}.\frac{ir}{R^2} = 2 \times 10^{-7} \times 10 \times \frac{2 \times 10^{-2}}{(4 \times 10 - 2)^2}$

$= 2.5 \times 10^{-5}$ T

35. (b) $I_g = 0.1I, I_s = 0.9I; S = I_g R_g / I_s$

$= 0.1 \times 900 / 0.9 = 100\,\Omega.$

36. (d) Let a be the area of the square and r be the radius of circular loop.

$2\pi r = 4a \Rightarrow r = \left(\frac{2a}{\pi}\right)$

For square
$M = (I)\,a^2$
For circular loop
$M_1 = (I)\pi r^2$

$M_1 = (I)(\pi)\left(\frac{4a^2}{\pi^2}\right) = \frac{4Ia^2}{\pi} = \frac{4M}{\pi} \quad (\because M = Ia^2)$

37. (b) If q is the charge on the ring, then

$i = \frac{q}{T} = \frac{q\omega}{2\pi}$

Magnetic field,

$B = \frac{\mu_0 i}{2R}$

$= \frac{\mu_0\left(\frac{q\omega}{2\pi}\right)}{2R}$

or $\quad 3.8 \times 10^{-9} = \left(\frac{\mu_0}{4\pi}\right)\frac{q\omega}{R} = \left(10^{-7}\right)\frac{q \times 40\pi}{0.10}$

$\therefore \; q = 3 \times 10^{-5}\,C.$

38. (d) $B = 1.5 \times 10^{-2}$ T, $\theta = 90°$, $\sin\theta = 1$

$v = 6 \times 10^7$ m/s, $\frac{e}{m} = 1.7 \times 10^{11}$ C/kg

$r = \frac{mv}{Be} = \frac{6\times10^7}{1.5\times10^{-2}\times1.7\times10^{11}}$

$= 2.35 \times 10^{-2}$m $= 2.35$ cm

39. (c) The magnetic field at a point on the axis of a circular loop at a distance x from centre is,

$B = \frac{\mu_0 i\, a^2}{2(x^2 + a^2)^{3/2}}$

Magnetic field at the centre of loop is

$B' = \frac{\mu_0 i}{2a} \qquad \therefore B' = \frac{B\cdot(x^2+a^2)^{3/2}}{a^3}$

Put $x = 4$ & $a = 3$

$\Rightarrow B' = \frac{54(5^3)}{3\times3\times3} = 250\,\mu T$

40. (d) $\tau = MB\sin45° = N\,(iA)\,B\sin 45°$

$= 100 \times 3(5\times2.5)\times10^{-4}\times1\times\frac{1}{\sqrt{2}}$

$= 0.27$ N-m

41. (c) So $r_{deutron} = \frac{\sqrt{2m_d E_d}}{Bq}$; $r_{proton} = \frac{\sqrt{2m_p E_p}}{Bq}$

For same radius, B and q

$m_p E_p = m_d E_d \Rightarrow E_p = \frac{m_d}{m_p} E_d = \frac{2}{1} \times 50 = 100\text{keV}$

42. (a) The direction of the magnetic field due to a current is given by right hand curled fingers rule. Therefore at AB axis, the components of magnetic field will cancel each other and the resultant magnetic field will be zero on AB.

43. (a) Let ℓ_1, ℓ_2 be the lengths of the two parts PRQ and PSQ of the conductor and ρ be the resistance per unit length of the conductor. The resistance of the portion PRQ will be $R_1 = \ell_1\,\rho$

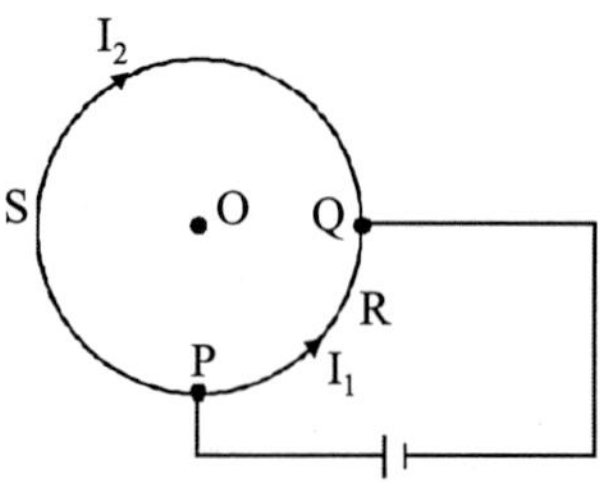

The resistance of the portion PSQ will be $R_2 = \ell_2\,\rho$
Pot. diff. across P and Q $= I_1 R_1 = I_2 R_2$
or $I_1 \ell_1 \rho = I_2 \ell_2 \rho$ or $I_1 \ell_1 = I_2 \ell_2$ ...(1)
Magnetic field induction at the centre O due to currents through circular conductors PRQ and PSQ will be

$= B_1 - B_2 = \frac{\mu_0}{4\pi}\frac{I_1\ell_1 \sin 90°}{r^2} - \frac{\mu_0}{4\pi}\frac{I_2\ell_2 \sin 90°}{r^2} = 0.$

44. (b) In a uniform magnetic field, a charged particle is moving in a circle of radius R with constant speed v.

$\therefore \; \frac{mv^2}{R} = Bqv \quad$ or, $R = \frac{mv}{Bq}$ .....(1)

Time period, $T = \frac{2\pi R}{v} = \frac{2\pi mv}{Bqv} = \frac{2\pi m}{Bq}$ .....(2)

Time period T does not depend on both R and v because when v is changed, R is also changed proportionately and for period, it is R/v that is taken.

45. (a) Let a be the radius of the wire
Magnetic field at point A (inside)

$B_A = \frac{\mu_0 ir}{2\pi a^2} = \frac{\mu_0 i\frac{a}{3}}{2\pi a^2} = \frac{\mu_0 i}{\pi a^2}\frac{a}{6} = \frac{\mu_0 i}{6\pi a}$

Magnetic field at point B (outside)

$B_B = \frac{\mu_0 i}{2\pi(2a)}$

$\therefore \; \frac{B_A}{B_B} = \frac{\frac{\mu_0 i}{6\pi a}}{\frac{\mu_0 i}{2\pi(2a)}} = \frac{4}{6} = \frac{2}{3}$

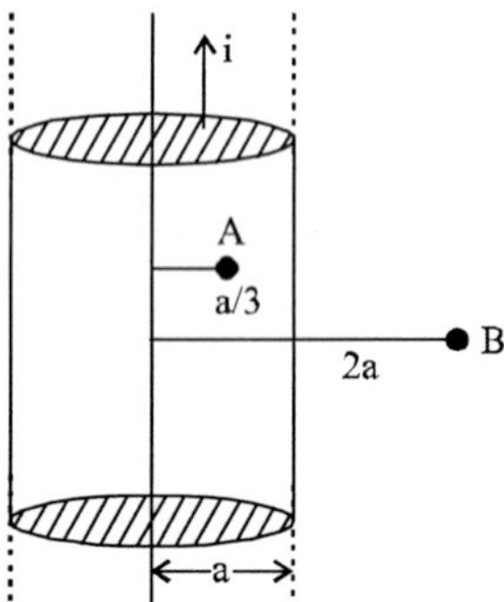

20 Magnetism and Matter

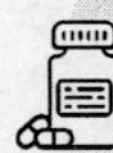

Topic 20.1 : Natural Magnet, Bar Magnet, Magnetic Field, Magnetic Lines of Force, Magnetic Moment, Coulomb's Law, Torque on a Magnet, Gauss's Law in Magnetism, Magnetic Field and Potential

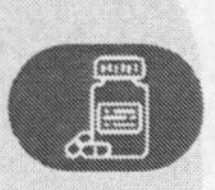

NATURAL MAGNET

A natural magnet is an ore of iron (Fe_3O_4) which

(i) attracts small pieces of iron, cobalt and nickel towards it.

(ii) when suspendeded freely, comes to rest along north-south direction.

The magnets which are obtained artificially are called artificial magnets, e.g. a bar magnet, a magnetic needle, horse shoe magnet etc.

BAR MAGNET

A bar magnet consists of two equal and opposite magnetic poles separated by a small distance. Poles are not exactly at the ends. The shortest distance between two poles is called effective length (L_e) and is less than its geometric length (L_g).

For bar magnet $L_e = 2l$ and $L_e = (5/6)\, L_g$.

For semicircular magnet $L_g = \pi R$ and $L_e = 2R$.

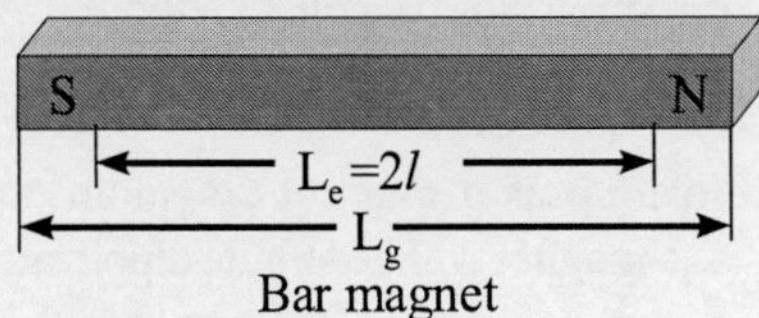

Bar magnet

Properties of Magnets

(i) **Attractive property :** A magnet attracts small pieces of iron, cobalt, nickel, etc. and other magnetic subsances.

(ii) **Directive property :** A freely suspended magnet aligns itself nearly in the geographical north-south direction.

(iii) **Law of magnetic poles :** Like magnetic poles repel, and unlike magnetic poles attract each other.

According to **Gauss's theorem in magnetism**, surface integral of magnetic field intensity over a surface (closed or open) is always zero i.e. $\oint \vec{B}.d\vec{s}$ (or $\int \vec{B}.d\vec{s}$) = 0.

This theorem establishes that the poles always exist in equal and unlike pairs.

(iv) **Magnetic poles exist in pairs :** Isolated magnetic poles do not exist. If we break a magnet into two pieces, we get two smaller dipole magnets.

(v) Repulsion is a sure test of magnetism.

MAGNETIC FIELD

The space around a magnet within which its influence can be experienced is called its magnetic field.

Uniform magnetic field : A uniform magnetic field is one where the strength of the magnetic field is the same at all points of the field. In a uniform field, all the magnetic lines of force are parallel to one another. But in **non-uniform magnetic field** the strength of magnetic field is not same at all points of the field and also the magnetic lines of force are not parallel.

Atom as a Magnetic Dipole

Every atom of a magnetic material behaves as a magnetic dipole, because electrons in the atom revolve round the nucleus. The magnetic moment M associated with an atomic dipole as

$$M = \frac{neh}{4\pi m} = n\mu_B$$

where n = 1, 2, 3 ..... denotes the no. of orbits and $\mu_B = \frac{eh}{4\pi m}$.

Least value of dipole moment of atom = 9.27×10^{-24} Am^2.

μ_B is called **Bohr magneton.**

Most of the magnetic moment is produced due to electron spin, the contribution of the orbital revolution is very small.

MAGNETIC LINES OF FORCE

Magnetic line of force is an imaginary curve the tangent to which at a point gives the direction of magnetic field at that point or the magnetic field line is the imaginary path along which an isolated north pole will tend to move if it is free to do so.

Properties of Magnetic Lines of Force

(i) Magnetic lines of force are hypothetical lines use to depict magnetic field in a region and understand certain phenomenon in magnetism.

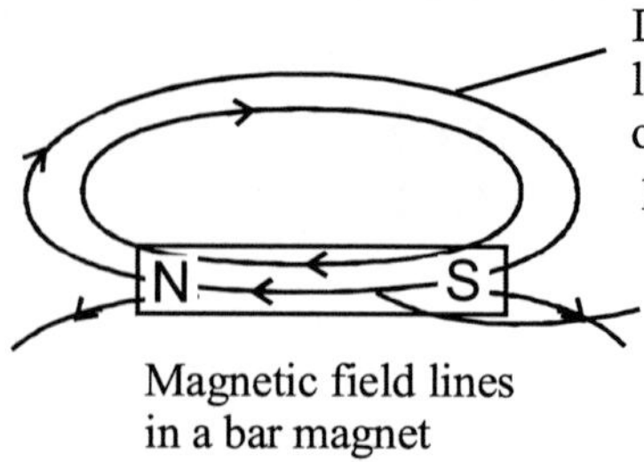

Magnetic field lines in a bar magnet

(ii) Tangent to field line at a point gives us the direction of magnetic field intensity $\vec{B}$ at that point. *No two magnetic lines of force can intersect each other* because magnetic field will have two directions at the point of intersection.

(iii) Magnetic lines of force are continuous curve from north to south, outside the body of the magnet and from south to north inside the body of the magnet.

(iv) The number of lines originating or terminating on a pole is proportional to its pole strength.
Magnetic flux = number of magnetic lines of force
$= \mu_0 \times m$
Where μ_0 is number of lines associated with unit pole.

(v) The number of lines of force per unit area at a point gives magnitude of field at that point. The crowded lines show a strong field while distant lines represent a weak field.

(vi) The magnetic lines of force have a tendency to contract longitudinally like a stretched elastic string producing attraction between opposite pole.

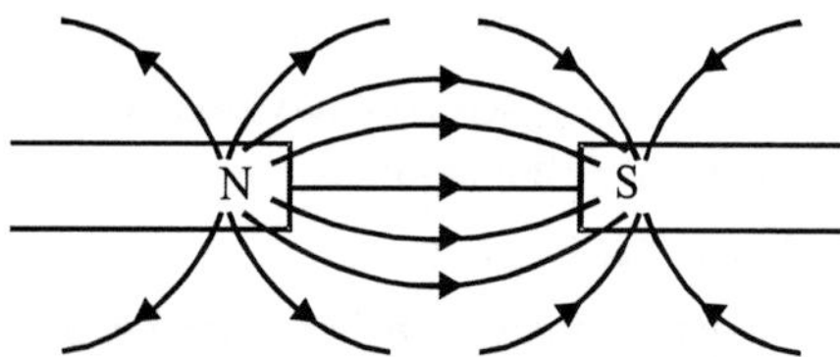

Longitudnal contraction (attraction)

(vii) The magnetic lines of force have a tendency to repel each other laterally resulting in repulsion between similar poles.

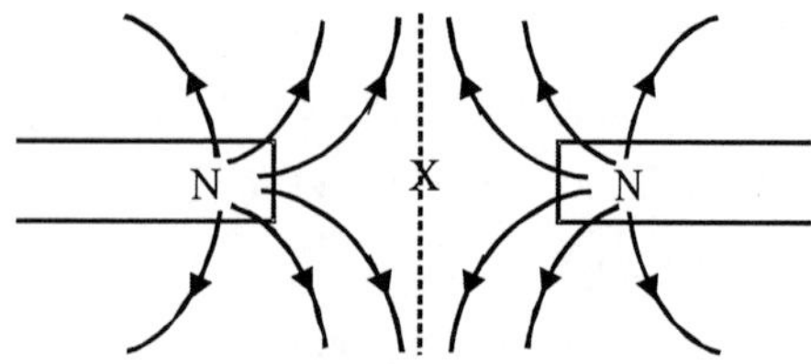

Lateral expansion (repulsion)

(viii) The region of space with no magnetic field has no lines of force. At neutral point where resultant field is zero there cannot be any line of force.

SOME TERMS RELATED TO MAGNETISM

Magnetic poles : These are the regions of apparently concentrated magnetic strength where the magnetic attraction is maximum.

It means that pole of a magnet is located not at a point but over a region. Magnetic poles exist in pairs. An isolated magnetic pole (north or south) does not exist. If a magnet is cut into two pieces, then instead of obtaining separate N-pole and S-pole, each of the two parts are found to behave as complete magnets.

Magnetic axis : The line passing through the poles of a magnet is called its magnetic axis.

Magnetic equator : The line passing through the centre of the magnet and at right angles ot the magnetic axis is called the magnetic equator of the magnet.

Magnetic length : The shortest distance between the two poles of a magnet is called its magnetic length. It is less than the geometrical length of the magnet. This magnetic length is also called an effective length.

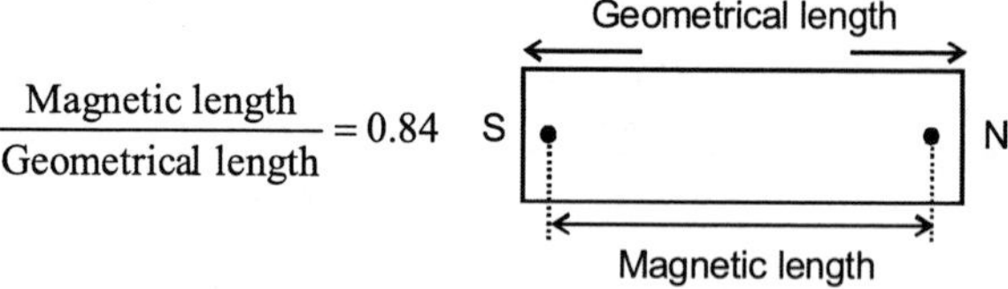

MAGNETIC MOMENT

The magnetic moment of a magnet in magnitude is equal to the product of pole strength with effective length (i.e. magnetic length). Its direction is along the axis of magnet from south pole to north pole.

$$\vec{M} = m \times 2\ell \times (\vec{n}) \Rightarrow |\vec{M}| = 2m\ell$$

If the same bar magnet is bent in a semicircle then

$$\pi r = 2l \Rightarrow r = \frac{2l}{\pi}$$

m r m

Net magnetic moment

$$M' = m \times 2r = m \times 2 \times \frac{2l}{\pi} = m \times \frac{4l}{\pi} = \frac{2M}{\pi}$$

Where m is pole strength, 2ℓ is effective length and $\vec{n}$ is unit vector having a direction from S-pole to N-pole.

The **SI unit** of $\vec{M}$ is A m^2, which is equivalent to J/T.

Circular current loop as a magnet : A small plane loop of current behaves as a magnet with a definite dipole moment given by

$$\vec{M} = I A\hat{n}$$

where A is the area of the loop, I the current in the loop and $\hat{n}$ is a unit vector perpendicular to the plane of the loop, and its direction is decided by the sense of flow of current I using the Fleming's right hand rule.

Relation between magnetic moment and angular momentum

$$\vec{M} = \frac{q}{2m}\vec{L}$$

Where q is the total charge on a body of mass m rotating about a fixed axis.

Magnetic moment, pole strength and effective length when a magnet is cut

Magnet placed after cutting	Pole strength	Effective length	Magnetic moment after cutting
N S Breadth, Length	m	2ℓ	$M = 2m\ell$
N S X X′	m/2	2ℓ	$M_1 = \frac{m}{2}.2\ell = \frac{M}{2}$
Y S N Y′	m	ℓ	$M_2 = m\ell = \frac{M}{2}$
Y N S X X′ Y′	m/2	ℓ	$M_3 = \frac{m\ell}{2} = \frac{M}{4}$
2*l* m m	m	2*l*	$M = m \times 2l$

COULOMB'S LAW OF MAGNETIC FORCE

It states that :

(i) *The force of attraction or repulsion between two magnetic poles is directly proportional to the product of their pole strengths.*

(ii) *The force of attraction or repulsion between two magnetic poles is inversely proportional to the square of the distance between them*. This law is also known as **inverse square law**.

i.e., $F \propto m_1 m_2$ and $F \propto \frac{1}{r}$ or, $F = \frac{\mu_0}{4\pi}.\frac{m_1\, m_2}{r^2}$

where m_1 and m_2 are the pole strengths of the two magnetic poles, r is the distance between them and μ_0 is the permeability of free space.

Unit magnetic pole : A unit magnetic pole may be defined as the pole which when placed in vacuum at a distance of one metre from an identical pole, repels it with a force of 10^{-7} newton.

TORQUE ON A MAGNET IN A MAGNETIC FIELD

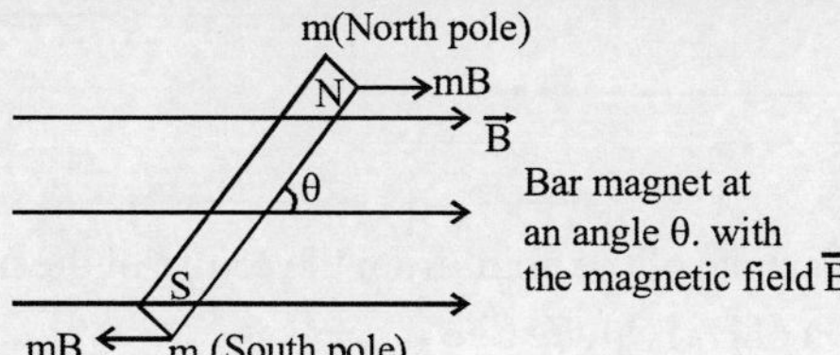

A magnet of dipole moment M suspended freely in a magnetic field B experiences a torque $\vec{\tau}$ given by

$\vec{\tau} = \vec{M} \times \vec{B}$; $\tau = MB \sin\theta$

where θ is the angle between $\vec{M}$ and $\vec{B}$

It is clear from the expression that $|\vec{\tau}_{max}| = MB$

i.e., *when dipole is perpendicular to field the torque is maximum and when they are parallel, the torque is minimum*

(for $\theta = 0$ or $180° \rightarrow |\vec{\tau}| = 0$).

The net force acting on a bar magnet placed

→ in a uniform magnetic field is zero

→ in a non-uniform magnetic field is non-zero

Let the length of a bar magnet be 2ℓ and pole strength be m, the magnetic field is B, and the angle between B and bar magnet is θ. Force on north pole is mB along the field and that on south pole is mB opposite to the field.

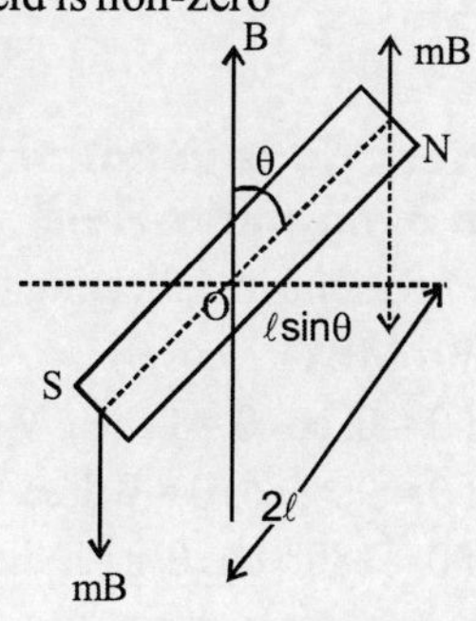

The torque of these two forces about O is
$\tau = 2mB\ell\sin\theta = MB\sin\theta$

$\vec{\tau} = \vec{M} \times \vec{B}$
where M is the magnetic moment of the magnet. ($\because M = 2m\ell$)
This torque tries to align the magnet with the field.

Work Done by External Agent in Rotating the Magnet

If an external agent rotates the magnet slowly, the agent has to exert a torque MBsinθ opposite to that exerted by the field.
Work done by the agent in changing the angle from θ to θ + dθ is $dW = (MB\sin\theta)\,d\theta$

$$W_{ext} = \int_{\theta_0}^{\theta} (MB\sin\theta)d\theta$$

$$W_{ext} = MB(\cos\theta_0 - \cos\theta)$$

W_{ext} is stored as potential energy of the field-magnet system. Thus

$U(\theta) - U(\theta_0) = MB(\cos\theta_0 - \cos\theta)$

If we take $U(\theta_0) = 0$ for $\theta_0 = 90°$, then

Potential energy

$U(\theta) = U(\theta) - U(90°) = -MB\cos\theta = -\vec{M}\cdot\vec{B}$

(i) When $\theta = 0$, $U = -MB$ (minimum PE)
(ii) When $\theta = 90°$, $U = 0$
(iii) When $\theta = 180°$, $U = MB$ (maximum PE)

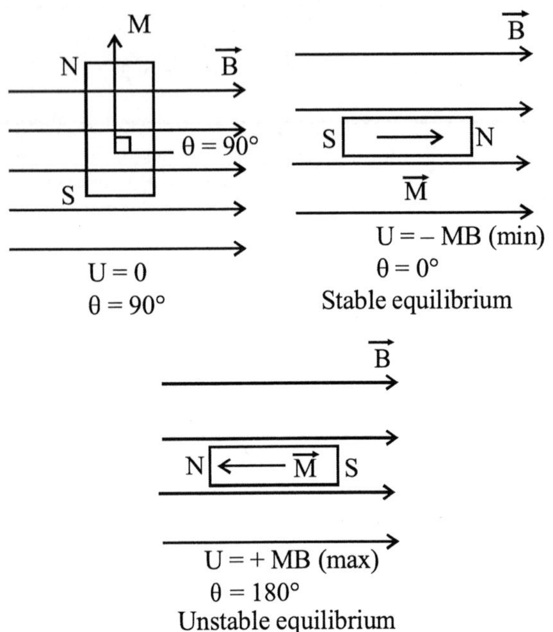

Work done in Rotating a Uniform Magnetic Dipole in a Magnetic Field

Work done in deflecting the dipole through an angle θ is,
$W = MB(1 - \cos\theta)$
If $\theta = 0$, $\cos\theta = 1$ then $W = MB(1-1) = 0$
If $\theta = 90°$, $\cos\theta = 0$ then $W = MB$
If $\theta = 180°$, $\cos\theta = -1$, then $W = 2MB$

GAUSS'S LAW IN MAGNETISM

The surface integral of magnetic field $\vec{B}$ over a closed surface S is always zero.

Mathematically $\oint_S \vec{B}\cdot\vec{da} = 0$

(1) Isolated magnetic poles do not exist is a direct consequence of gauss's law in magnetism.
(2) The total magnetic flux linked with a closed surface is always zero.
(3) If a number of magnetic field lines are leaving a closed surface, an equal number of field lines must also be entering the surface.

Magnetic Flux

The magnetic flux through a given area may be defined as the total number of magnetic lines of force passing through this area. It is equal to the product of the normal components of the magnetic field B and the area over which it is uniform. In general,
Magnetic flux, $\phi = \int_A \vec{B}.\vec{dA} = \int_A BdA\cos\theta$, where θ is angle between normal to the area dA with magnetic field B.

Magnetic flux linked with a closed surface is zero i.e., $\oint_S \vec{B}.\vec{dA} = 0$

The **S.I. Unit** of magnetic flux is weber (Wb) : If a magnetic field of 1 tesla passes normally through a surface of area 1 square metre, then the magnetic flux linked with this surface is said to be 1 weber.

Oscillations of a Bar Magnet in a Magnetic Field

A freely suspended magnet of magnetic moment M and of moment of inertia I oscillates simple harmonically in a magnetic field B with frequency

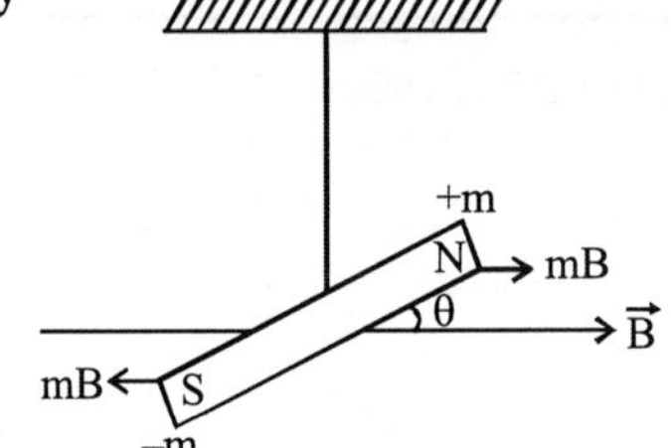

Freely suspended bar magnet, at an angle θ with the magnetic field $\vec{B}$

$$\nu = \frac{1}{2\pi}\sqrt{\frac{MB}{I}}, \therefore \text{ Time period, } T = 2\pi\sqrt{\frac{I}{MB}}$$

MAGNETIC FIELD DUE TO A BAR MAGNET

(i) **Magnetic field intensity B_1 due to a bar magnet at any point on the axial line of the magnet is** $B_1 = \frac{\mu_0}{4\pi}\frac{2Md}{(d^2 - \ell^2)^2}$

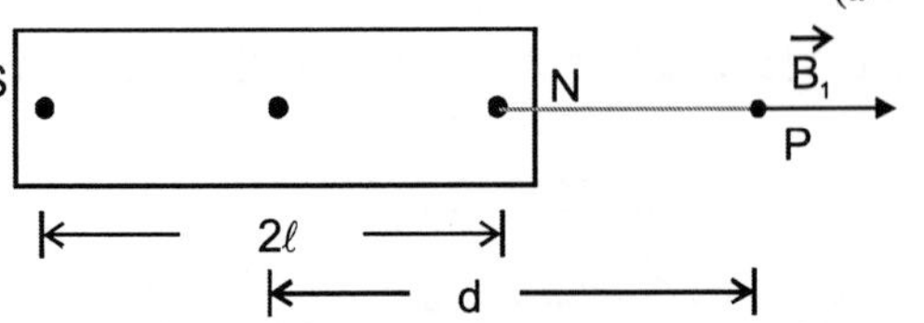

where d = distance of the point from the centre of the magnet. The direction of B_1 is along SN.

$B_N = \frac{\mu_0}{4\pi} \frac{m}{(d-\ell)^2}$ where, m is pole strength.

B_N is magnetic field due to north pole, it is directed away from the magnet.

$B_S = \frac{\mu_0}{4\pi} \frac{m}{(d+\ell)^2}$ it is directed towards the magnet.

$$\therefore B = B_N - B_S \Rightarrow B = \frac{\mu_0 m}{4\pi}\left[\frac{1}{(d-\ell)^2} - \frac{1}{(d+\ell)^2}\right]$$

$$= \frac{\mu_0 m(4\ell d)}{4\pi (d^2-\ell^2)^2} = \frac{\mu_0}{4\pi}\frac{2Md}{(d^2-\ell^2)^2} \qquad [\because M = m(2L)]$$

If $d >> \ell$, $B = \frac{\mu_0}{4\pi}\frac{2M}{d^3}$

(ii) Magnetic field intensity (B_2) due to A bar magnet at any point on the equatorial line of the bar magnet is

$$B_2 = \frac{\mu_0}{4\pi}\frac{M}{(d^2+\ell^2)^{3/2}}$$

The direction of B_2 is along a line parallel to NS.

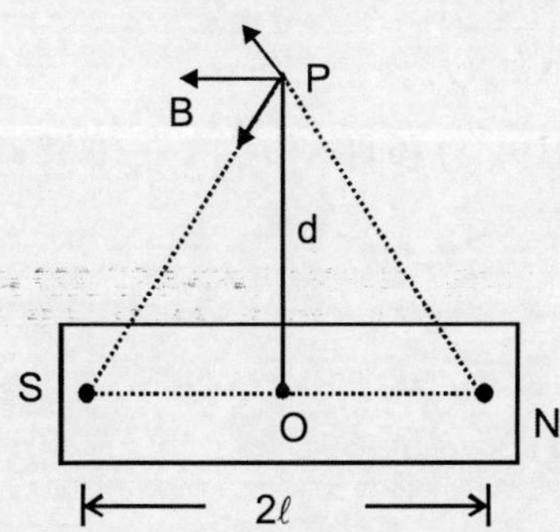

$B_N = \frac{\mu_0}{4\pi}\frac{m\overrightarrow{NP}}{NP^3}$, $B_S = \frac{\mu_0}{4\pi}\frac{m\overrightarrow{PS}}{PS^3}$

Now, $NP = PS = (d^2+\ell^2)^{3/2}$

Resultant field at P is, $\vec{B} = \overrightarrow{B_N} + \overrightarrow{B_S}$

$$\Rightarrow \vec{B} = \frac{\mu_0}{4\pi}.\frac{m}{(d^2+\ell^2)^{3/2}}(\overrightarrow{NP}+\overrightarrow{PS}) = \frac{\mu_0}{4\pi}.\frac{m}{(d^2+\ell^2)^{3/2}}(\overrightarrow{NS})$$

$$|\vec{B}| = \frac{\mu_0}{4\pi}\frac{2ml}{(d^2+\ell^2)^{3/2}} = \frac{\mu_0}{4\pi}\frac{M}{(d^2+\ell^2)^{3/2}}$$

If $d >> \ell$, $|\vec{B}| = \frac{\mu_0}{4\pi}\frac{M}{d^3}$

The magnetic field at any point having polar coordinates (r, θ) relative to centre of magnet or loop

$B = \frac{\mu_0}{4\pi}\frac{M}{r^3}\sqrt{(1+3\cos^2\theta)}$ and direction is given by

$\tan\alpha = \frac{1}{2}\tan\theta$

MAGNETIC POTENTIAL

The magnetic potential at a point is defined as the work done in carrying a unit N-pole from infinity to that point against the field. It may also be defined as the quantity whose space rate of variation in any direction gives the intensity of the magnetic field

i.e., $$B = -\frac{dV_B}{dx}$$

(i) **Magnetic potential due to a point dipole, at a distance r from the pole of strength m** is given by

$$V_B = \frac{\mu_0}{4\pi}.\frac{m}{r} \text{ (joule/Wb)}$$

B due to a pole of Pole strength m at a distance r is given by $B = \frac{\mu_0}{4\pi}\frac{m}{r^2}$

Now V_0 at A is the work done is bringing a unit pole from infinity to A.

$$\therefore V_A - V_\infty = \int_\infty^r a\frac{\mu_0 m}{4\pi r^2}dr \Rightarrow V_A = \frac{\mu_0 m}{4\pi r}$$

(ii) **Potential due to a magnetic dipole at a point in end-side on position** is $V_B = \frac{\mu_0}{4\pi}.\left(\frac{m}{r^2-\ell^2}\right)$, where $M = 2ml$.

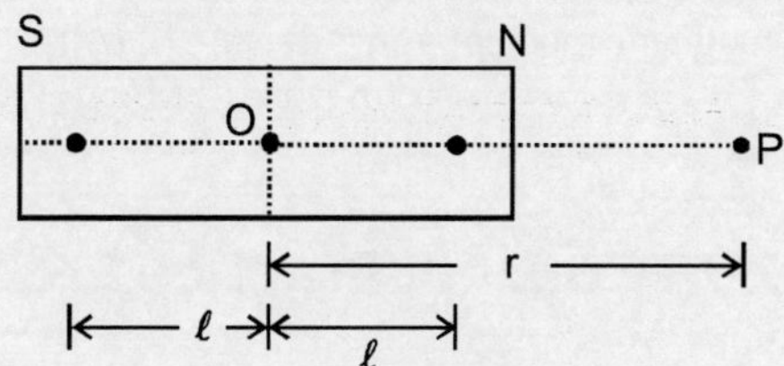

If $\ell^2 << r^2$ then $V_B = \frac{\mu_0}{4\pi}\frac{m}{r^2}$

(iii) **Potential due to a magnetic pole at a point in the broad side-on position**. Net potential at P = 0. The potential at any point lying on the magnetic equator of a magnet is zero in CGS and MKS system.

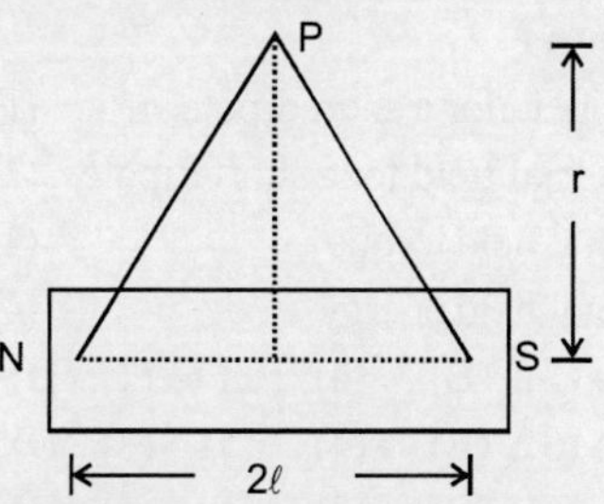

(iv) **The magnetic potential at a point lying on a line passing through the centre and making angle θ with the axis**

$V_B = \frac{\mu_0}{4\pi}\frac{M\cos\theta}{(r^2-\ell^2)}$ and for small dipole, $r >> \ell$

$$V_B = \frac{\mu_0}{4\pi}\frac{M\cos\theta}{r^2}$$

Example 1.

Two identical thin bar magnets each of length ℓ and pole strength m are placed at right angles to each other, with north pole of one touching south pole of the other, then find the magnetic moment of the system.

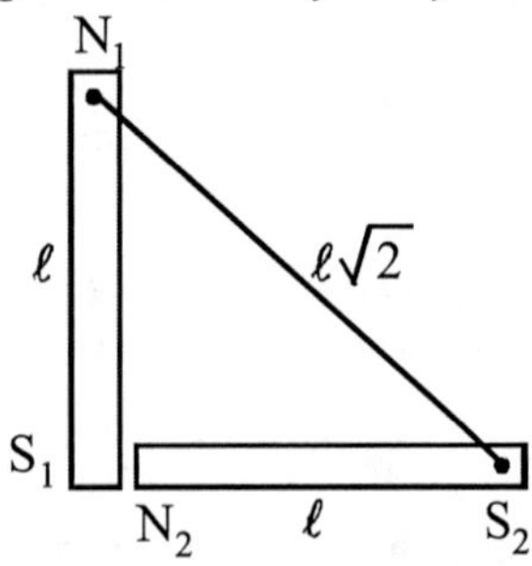

Solution :

Initial magnetic moment of each magnet = m × ℓ.
As is clear from fig., S_1 and N_2 neutralize each other.
Effective distance between

N_1 and $S_2 = \sqrt{\ell^2 + \ell^2} = \ell\sqrt{2}$ $\quad \therefore \; M' = m\ell\sqrt{2}$.

Example 2.

A steel wire of length ℓ has a magnetic moment M. It is then bent into a semi-circular arc. Find the new magnetic moment.

Solution :

Let d be the diameter of semi-circle.

$\therefore \; \ell = (\pi d/2)$ or $d = (2\ell/\pi)$

New magnetic moment = $m \times d = m \times (2\ell/\pi)$
$= 2m\ell/\pi = (2M/\pi)$

Example 3.

Work done in turning a magnet of magnetic moment M by an angle 90° from the magnetic meridian is n times the corresponding work done to turn through an angle of 60°, where n is

(a) 1/2 (b) 2
(c) 1/4 (d) 1

***Solution :* (b)**

$W_1 = -MB(\cos 90° - \cos 0°) = MB$
$W_2 = -MB(\cos 60° - \cos 0°)$

$$= -MB\left(\frac{1}{2} - 1\right) = \frac{1}{2}MB = \frac{1}{2}W_1$$

As $W_1 = n\,W_2$; $\quad \therefore \; n = 2$

Example 4.

In a hydrogen atom, an electron revolves with a frequency of 6.8×10^9 megahertz in an orbit of diameter 1.06 Å. What will be the equivalent magnetic moment?

Solution :

$\nu = 6.8 \times 10^9$ MHz $= 6.8 \times 10^{15}$ Hz,

$$r = \frac{1.06}{2} = 0.53\text{ Å} = 0.53 \times 10^{-10}\text{ m}$$

$$M = IA = \left(\frac{e}{1/\nu}\right)\pi r^2 = e\nu\pi r^2$$

$$= (1.6 \times 10^{-19})\,(6.80 \times 10^{15}) \times \frac{22}{7}(0.53 \times 10^{-10})^2$$

$$= 9.7 \times 10^{-24}\text{ A m}^2$$

20.1 Concept Practice Problems

CPP

1. For bar magnet effective length (L_e) related with geometrical length (L_g) as

(a) $Le = \frac{6}{5}L_g$ (b) $Le = \frac{5}{6}L_g$
(c) $Le = L_g$ (d) $Le = 2L_g$

2. Match the columns I and II.

	Column I		Column II
(A)	Axial field for a short dipole	(1)	$-M.B$
(B)	Equatorial field for a short dipole	(2)	$M \times B$
(C)	External field torque	(3)	$\mu_0 2M/4\pi r^3$
(D)	External field energy	(4)	$-\mu_0 M/4\pi r^3$

(a) (A)→(3); (B)→(4); (C)→(2); (D)→(1)
(b) (A)→(3); (B)→(4); (C)→(3); (D)→(1)
(c) (A)→(4); (B)→(3); (C)→(2); (D)→(1)
(d) (A)→(2); (B)→(1); (C)→(4); (D)→(3)

3. The magnetic lines of force inside a bar magnet

(a) are from N-pole to S-pole of magnet
(b) do not exist
(c) depend upon the area of cross section of bar magnet
(d) are from S-pole of magnet

4. A circular loop carrying a current is replaced by an equivalent magnetic dipole. A point on the axis of the loop is in

(a) end-on position (b) broadside-on position
(c) both (d) None of these

5. A magnet of magnetic moment 20 C.G.S. units is freely suspended in a uniform magnetic field of intensity 0.3 C.G.S. units. The amount of work done in deflecting it by an angle of 30° in C.G.S. units is

(a) 6 (b) $3\sqrt{3}$ (c) $3(2-\sqrt{3})$ (d) 3

6. A magnet of length 0.1 m and pole strength 10^{-4} *A.m.* is kept in a magnetic field of 30 Wb/m^2 at an angle 30°. The couple acting on it is .... $\times 10^{-4}$ *Nm.*

(a) 7.5 (b) 3.0 (c) 1.5 (d) 6.0

7. A bar magnet having centre O has a length of 4 cm. Point P_1 is in the broad side-on and P_2 is in the end side-on position with $OP_1 = OP_2 = 10$ metres. The ratio of magnetic intensities H at P_1 and P_2 is

(a) $H_1 : H_2 = 16 : 100$ (b) $H_1 : H_2 = 1 : 2$
(c) $H_1 : H_2 = 2 : 1$ (d) $H_1 : H_2 = 100 : 16$

8. The force between magnetic poles when their pole strength and the distance between them both doubled is
(a) twice the previous value
(b) half the previous value
(c) four times the previous value
(d) not change

9. A permanent magnet in the shape of a thin cylinder of length 10 cm has magnetisation (M) = 10^6 A m^{-1}. Its magnetization current I_M is
(a) 10^5 A (b) 10^6 A
(c) 10^7 A (d) 10^8 A

10. Assume that each iron atom has a permanent magnetic moment equal to 2 Bohr magnetons (1 Bohr magneton = 9.27×10^{-24} A-m^2). The density of atoms in iron is 8.52×10^{28} atoms/m^3. Find the maximum magnetic moment per unit volume.
(a) 1.5×10^2 A|m (b) 1.58×10^6 A|m
(c) 1.2×10^5 A|m (d) 1.3×10^6 A|m

ANSWER KEY

1	(b)	2	(a)	3	(d)	4	(a)	5	(c)	6	(c)	7	(b)	8	(d)	9	(a)	10	(b)

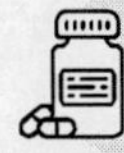

Topic 20.2 : Earth's Magnetism, Classification of Magnetic Materials and Magnetic Equipments

EARTH'S MAGNETISM

Magnetic field of earth extends nearly upto five times the radius of earth i.e., 3.2×10^4 km.

The magnetic field of earth is fairly uniform and can be represented by equidistant parallel lines.

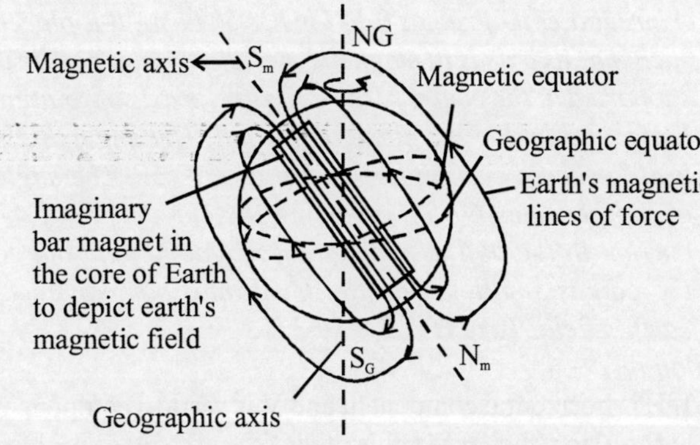

Geographic meridian : The geographic meridian at a place is the vertical plane passing through the geographic north & south at that place.

Magnetic meridian : The magnetic meridian at a place is the vertical plane passing through the magnetic axis of a freely suspended small magnet. The earth's magnetic field acts in the plane of magnetic meridian.

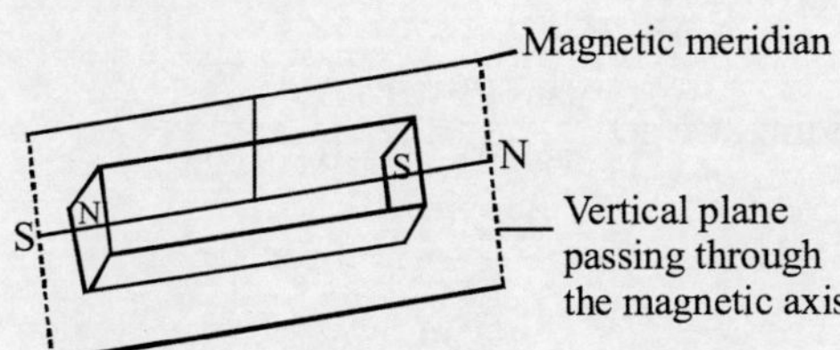

Elements of Earth's Magnetic Field

The earth's magnetic field at a place can be completely described by three independent parameters called elements of earth's magnetic field. These are :

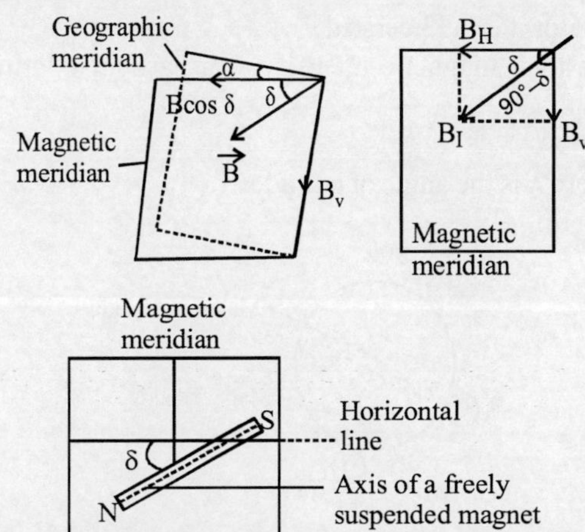

(i) **Magnetic declination (θ) :** *The angle between the geographic meridian and the magnetic meridian at a place is called the magnetic declination at that place.*

(ii) **Angle of dip (δ) :** *The angle made by the earth's total magnetic field $\vec{B}$ with the horizontal is called angle of dip at any place.*

$$\tan\delta = \frac{B_H}{B_V}$$

True and apparent dip

When the plane of the dip circle is in the magnetic meridian, then the needle stops in the actual direction of the Earth's magnetic field. The angle made by the needle with the horizontal in this condition is called **true dip**.

In case, the plane of the dip circle is not in the magnetic meridian then the angle made by the needle with the horizontal is called **apparent dip**. In this case the vertical component of earth's magnetic field remains the same but the effective horizontal component $B'_H = B_H \cos\theta$

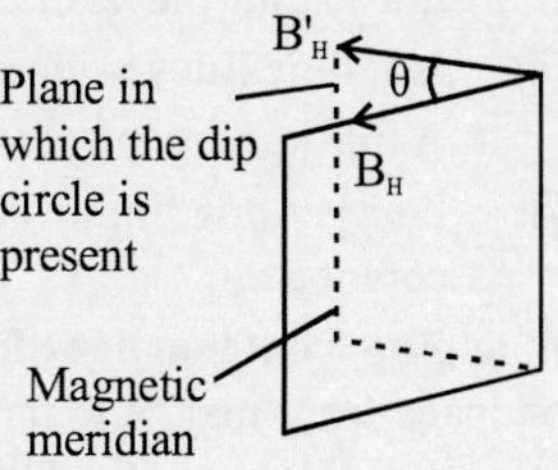

$$\tan\delta' = \frac{B'_V}{B'_H} = \frac{B_V}{B_H\cos\theta}$$

where δ' = apparent dip

δ = true dip

If the dip circle is rotated by 90°, the new apparent dip δ'' and δ' and δ are related as $\cot^2\delta = \cot^2\delta' + \cot^2\delta''$

(iii) Horizontal component of earth's magnetic field (B_H) : It is the *component of the earth's total magnetic field $\vec{B}$ in the horizontal diection and is given by, $B_H = B\cos\delta$*

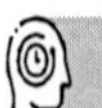

Problem Solving Tips

1. Dip circle is an instrument used to measure angle of dip at a place.
2. At poles total magnetic intensity is 0.66 oersted and at equator it is 0.33 oersted
   The total magnetic intensity at a particular latitude is
   $I = I_0\sqrt{1+3\sin^2\lambda}$
   where λ is the angle of latitude

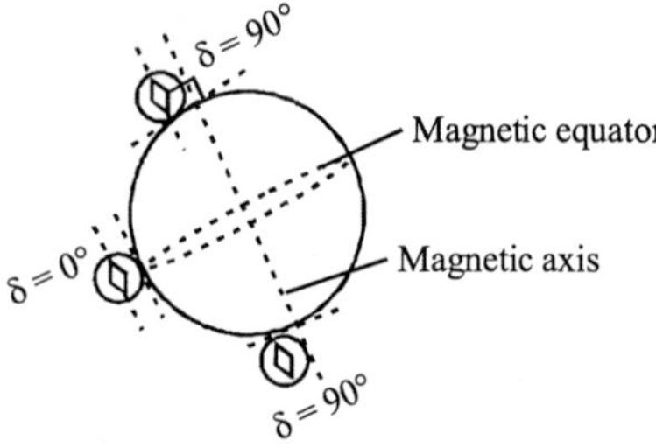

   The angle of dip $\delta = 0°$ at magnetic equator and $\delta = 90°$ at magnetic poles.
3. A spectacular effect due to earth's magnetism is observed near the magnetic poles of earth. This effect is called **aurora-borealis in the north** and **aurora - austorlis in south**. It is shown by patterns of coloured lights.

Magnetic Maps

Magnetic surveys all over the earth have been carried out and magnetic maps have been prepared which show the values of magnetic element throughout the world. Lines can be drawn to join places having the same value of a particular magnetic element.

(i) **Isogonic lines :** These join places of equal declination. A line joining places of zero declination is called **agonic line.**

(ii) **Isoclinic lines :** These join places of equal dip.
A line joining the places of zero-dip is called **aclinic line.**

(iii) **Isodynamic lines :** These join places of equal horizontal component.

Shielding from magnetic fields : For shielding a certain region of space from magnetic field, we surround the region by soft iron rings. Magnetic field lines will be drawn into the rings and the space enclosed will be free of magnetic field.

Neutral Points

Neutral points are the points where the net field intensity due to the field of the bar magnet and field of earth is zero. When magnet is placed with its north pole towards geographic north, neutral points lie **on equatorial line of the magnet**. At each neutral point,

$$B_2 = \frac{\mu_0}{4\pi}\frac{M}{(d^2+\ell^2)^{3/2}} = H$$

where H = horizontal component of earth's magnetic field.

When the bar magnet is placed with its north pole towards geographic south, the neutral points lie **on the axial line of the magnet**. At each neutral point,

$$B_1 = \frac{\mu_0}{4\pi}\frac{M}{(d^2-\ell^2)^2} = H$$

Relation between the units of quantities associated with magnetic field :

$1A = 1JT^{-1}m^{-2} = 1J\,Wb^{-1}$

$1T = 1JA^{-1}m^{-2} = 1Wb\,m^{-2}$

$1Wb = 1JA^{-1} = 1Tm^2$

$[B] = NA^{-1}m^{-1} = T = Wb\,m^{-2}$

$[M] = A\,m^2 = JT^{-1} = J\,m^2\,Wb^{-1}$

$[\mu_0] = NA^{-2} = T^2\,m^2\,N^{-1} = Wb^2\,J^{-1}\,m^{-1}$

Example 5.

A circular coil of radius 0.157 m has 50 turns. It is placed such that its axis is in magnetic meridian. A dip needle is supported at the centre of the coil with its axis of rotation horizontal and in the plane of the coil. The angle of dip is 30°, when a current flows through the coil. The angle of dip becomes 60° on reversing the current. Find the current in the coil assuming that magnetic field due to the coil is smaller than the horizontal component of earth's field. Take $H = 3\times10^{-5}$ T.

Solution :

If H is horizontal component and V is vertical component at the place, then true value of dip (δ) at the place is given by, $\tan\delta = \frac{V}{H}$

If B is magnetic field intensity at the centre of coil due to current I in circular coil and B is along H, then $\tan 30° = \frac{V}{H+B}$.

On reversing the direction of current, the direction of B is reversed.

$$\therefore \tan 60° = \frac{V}{H-B}$$

Dividing, we get $\frac{\tan 60°}{\tan 30°} = \frac{H+B}{H-B} = \frac{\sqrt{3}}{1/\sqrt{3}} = 3$

$$\therefore B = H/2 \Rightarrow B = \frac{3\times10^{-5}}{2} = 1.5\times10^{-5}\,T$$

For a circular coil, $B = \frac{\mu_0 nI}{2r}$

$$\therefore 1.5\times10^{-5} = \frac{(4\pi\times10^{-7})\times50\times I}{2\times0.157}$$

$$\therefore I = \frac{1.5\times10^{-5}\times2\times0.157}{4\pi\times10^{-7}\times50} = 0.75\,A.$$

Example 6.

If θ_1 and θ_2 are angles of dip in two vertical planes at right angle to each other and θ is true dip then prove $\cot^2\theta = \cot^2\theta_1 + \cot^2\theta_2$.

Solution :

If the vertical plane in which dip is θ_1 subtends an angle α with meridian than other vertical plane in which dip is θ_2 and is perpendicular to first will make an angle of $90° - \alpha$ with magnetic meridian. If θ_1 and θ_2 are apparent dips then

$$\tan\theta_1 = \frac{B_V}{B_H \cos\alpha};$$

$$\tan\theta_2 = \frac{B_V}{B_H \cos(90-\alpha)} = \frac{B_V}{B_H \sin\alpha}$$

$$\cot^2\theta_1 + \cot^2\theta_2 = \frac{1}{(\tan\theta_1)^2} + \frac{1}{(\tan\theta_2)^2}$$

$$= \frac{B_H^2\cos^2\alpha + B_H^2\sin^2\alpha}{B_V^2} = \frac{B_H^2}{B_V^2} = \left(\frac{B\cos\theta}{B\sin\theta}\right)^2 = \cot^2\theta$$

so $\cot^2\theta_1 + \cot^2\theta_2 = \cot^2\theta$

TERMS RELATED TO MAGNETISM

Magnetic intensity $(\vec{H})$: When a magnetic material is placed in a magnetic field, it becomes magnetised. *The capability of the magnetic field to magnetise a material is expressed by means of a magnetic vector $\vec{H}$, called the 'magnetic intensity' of the field.* The relation between magnetic induction B and magnetising field $\vec{H}$ $H = \frac{B}{\mu}$, μ being permeability of medium.

Intensity of magnetisation (I) : When a material is placed in a magnetising field, it acquires magnetic moment M. *The intensity of magnetisation is defined as the magnetic moment per unit volume* i.e., $I_m = \frac{M}{V}$

V being volume of mateiral. If the material is in the form of a bar of cross-sectional area A, length 2ℓ and pole strength m, then

$$M = m \times 2\ell; V = A \times 2\ell \qquad \therefore I_m = \frac{M}{V} = \frac{m.2\ell}{A.2\ell} = \frac{m}{A}$$

Magnetic susceptibility (χ) : *The magnetic susceptibility is defined as the intensity of magnetisation per unit magentising field.*

i.e., $\chi = \frac{I_m}{H}$

Magnetic permeability (μ) : The magnetic permeability of a material is the measure of degree to which the material can be permited by a magnetic field and is defined as *the ratio of magnetic induction (B) in the material to the magnetising field*

i.e. $\mu = \frac{B}{H}$

Relation between Magnetic Susceptibility and Permeability

We have magnetic induction in mateiral, $B = \mu H$

Also $B = B_0 + B_m$

where B_0 = magnetic induction in vacuum produced by magnetising field

B_m = magnetic induction due to magnetisation of material.

But $B_0 = \mu_0 H$ and $B_m = \mu_0 I_m \Rightarrow B = \mu_0[H + I_m]$

$$\therefore B = \mu_0 H\left[1 + \frac{I_m}{H}\right] = B_0[1+\chi]; \quad \therefore B/B_0 = [1+\chi]$$

$$\therefore B/B_0 = \frac{\mu H}{\mu_0 H} = \mu/\mu_0 = \mu_r, \text{ the relative magnetic permeability}$$

$$\boxed{\therefore \mu_r = 1+\chi}$$

This is required relation.

CLASSIFICATION OF MAGNETIC MATERIALS

According to the behaviour of substances in magnetic field, they are classified into three categories:

1. **Diamagnetic Substances :** *These are the substances which when placed in a strong magnetic field acquire a feeble magnetism opposite to the direction of magnetising field.* The **examples** are copper, gold, antimony, bismuth, alcohol, water, quartz, hydrogen, etc.

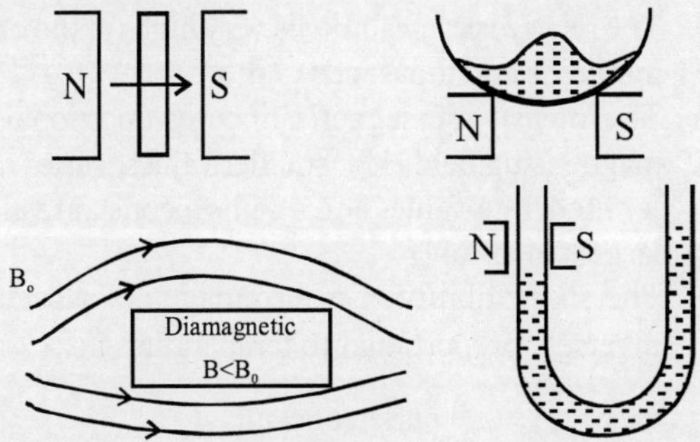

Behaviour of diamagnetic substance in an external magnetic field $\vec{B}$

The characteristics of diamagnetic substances are

(a) They are feebly repelled by a strong magnet
(b) Their susceptibility is negative (i.e. $\chi < 0$)
(c) Their relative permeability is less than 1. (i.e. $\mu_r < 1$)
(d) Their susceptibility is independent of magnetising field and temperature (except for Bismuth at low temperature)

2. **Paramagnetic Substances :** *These are the materials which when placed in a strong magnetic field acquire a feeble magnetism in the same sense as the applied magnetic field.* The **examples** are platinum, aluminium, chromium, manganese, $CuSO_4$, O_2, air, etc.

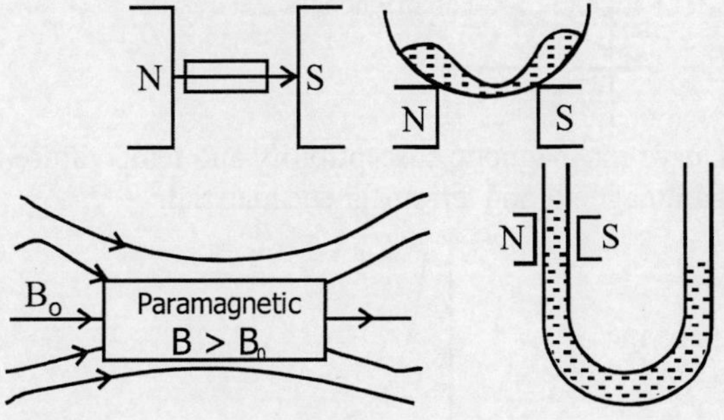

Behaviour of paramagnetic substance in an external field $\vec{B}_0$

The characteristics of paramagnetic substances are

(a) They are attracted by a strong magnet

(b) Their susceptibility is positive but very small ($\chi > 0$)

(c) Their relative permeability is slightly greater than unity. ($\mu > 1$)

(d) Their susceptibility and permeability do not change with the variation of magnetising field.

(e) Their susceptibility is inversely proportional to temperature, $\left(\text{i.e. } \chi \alpha \frac{1}{T}\right)$.

(f) They are found in those material which have atoms containing odd number of electrons

3. **Ferromagnetic Substances :** *These are the substances which are strongly magnetised by relatively weak magnetising field in the same sense as the magnetising field.* The **examples** are Ni, Co, iron and their alloys.

The characteristics of ferromagnetic substances are

(a) They are attracted even by a weak magnet.

(b) The susceptibility is very large and positive. ($\chi >> 0$)

(c) The relative permeability is very high (of the order of hundreds and thousands). ($\mu >> 1$)

(d) The intensity of magnetisation is proportional to the magnetising field H for smaller values, varies rapidly for moderate values and attains a constant value for larger values of H.

(e) The susceptibility of a ferromagnetic substance is inversely proportional to temperature i.e., $\chi \propto 1/T$

$\Rightarrow \chi = \frac{C}{T}$; C = curie constant .

This is called **Curie law**. *At a temperature called* **curie temperature**, *ferromagnetic substance becomes paramagnetic*. The curie temperatures for Ni, Fe and Co are 360°C, 740°C and 1100°C respectively.

(f) They are found in those material which have domains and can be converted into strong magnets

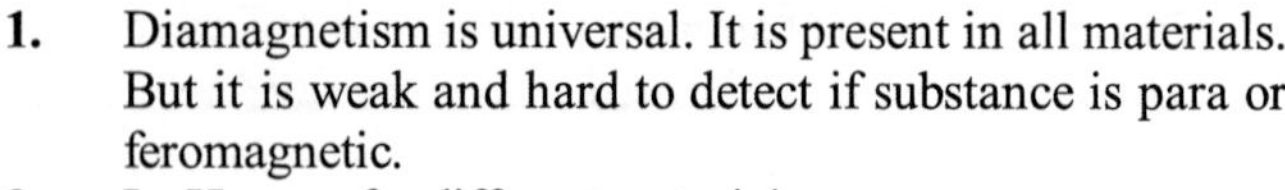

Problem Solving Tips

1. Diamagnetism is universal. It is present in all materials. But it is weak and hard to detect if substance is para or feromagnetic.

2. I – H curve for different materials

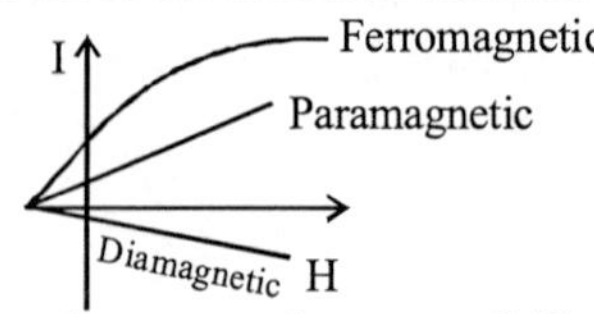

3. Curve for magnetic susceptibility and temperature for a paramagnetic and ferromagnetic material.

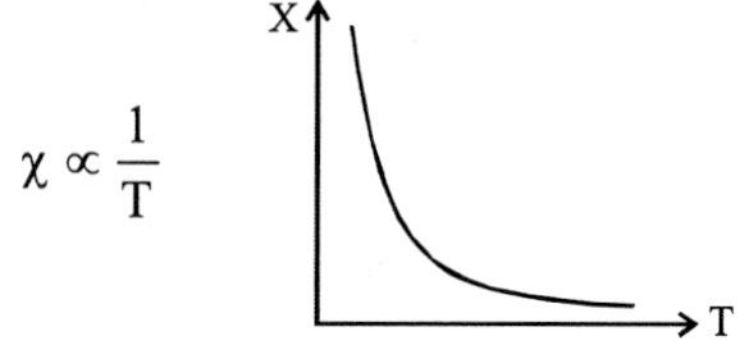

HYSTERESIS

When a bar of ferromagnetic material is magnetised by a varying magnetic field and the intensity of magnetisation I_m induced is measured for different values of magnetising field H, the graph of I versus H is as shown in fig

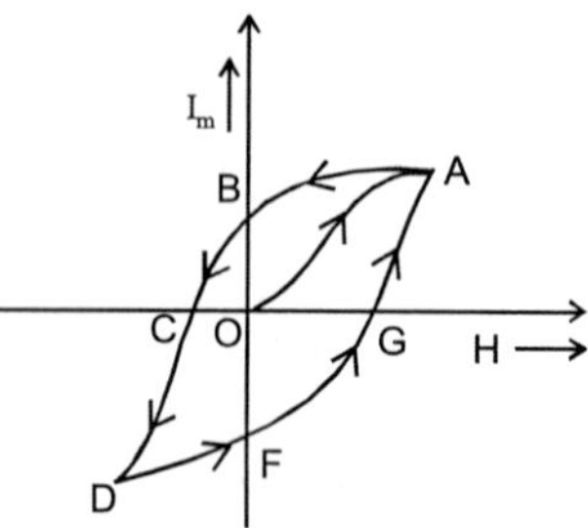

The graph shows :

(i) When magnetising field is increased from O the intensity of magnetisation I_m increases and becomes maximum (i.e. point A). This maximum value is called the **saturation value**.

(ii) When H is reduced, I_m reduces but is not zero when H = 0. The remainder value OB of magnetisation when H = 0 is called the residual magnetism or **retentivity**. OB is retentivity.

(iii) When magnetic field H is reversed, the magnetisaiton decreases and for a particular value of H, it becomes zero i.e., for H = OC, I = 0. This value of H is called the **coercivity**.

(iv) When field H is further increased in reverse direction, the intensity of magnetisation attains saturation value in reverse direction (i.e., point D).

(v) When H is decreased to zero and changed direction in steps, we get the part DFGA.

Properties of Soft Iron and Steel

For soft iron, the susceptibility, permeability and retentivity are greater while coercivity and hysteresis loss per cycle are smaller than those of steel.

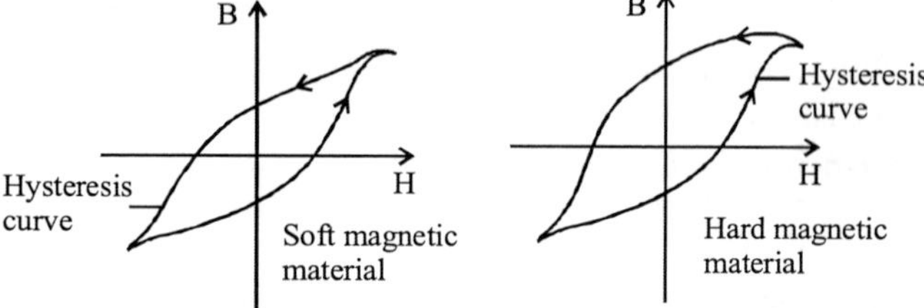

PERMANENT MAGNETS AND ELECTROMAGNETS

Permanent magnets are made of steel and cobalt while electromagnets are made of soft iron.

An electromagnet is made by inserting a soft iron core into the interior of a solenoid. Soft iron does not retain a significant permanent magnetization when the solenoid's field is turned off–soft iron does not make a good permanent magnet. When current flows in the solenoid, magnetic dipoles in the iron tend to line up with the field due to the solenoid. The net effect is that the field inside the iron is intensified by a factor known as the relative permeability. The relative permeability is analogous in magnetism to the dielectric constant in electricity. However, the dielectric constant is the factor by which the electric field is weakened, while the relative permeability is the factor by which the magnetic field is strengthened. The reactive permeability of a ferromagnet can be in the hundreds or even thousands– the intensification of the magnetic field is significant. Not only that, but in an electromagnet the strength and even direction of the magnetic field can be changed by changing the current in the solenoid.

Problem Solving Tips

1. By alloying soft-iron with 4% silicon 'transformer steel' is produced. It has a higher relative permeability and is an ideal material for cores of transformers. Alloys of iron and nickel called 'permalloys', also have very large permeabilities.
2. Energy spent per unit volume of specimen is complete cycle of magnetisation is numerically equal to area of I – H loop

	Perme-ability	Suscep-tibility	Intensity of magnetisation	Reten-tivity	Coerc-ivity	Hysteresis loss
Soft iron	high	high	high	high	low	low
Steel	low	low	low	low	high	high

⇒ Steel is most suitable for making parmanent magnet

⇒ Soft iron is most suitable for making core of an electromagnet.

Example 7.

A magnetising field of 1600 Am^{-1} produces a magnetic flux of 2.4×10^{-5} weber in a bar of iron of cross section 0.2 cm^2. Calculate permeability and susceptibility of the bar.

Solution :

Here, $H = 1600\ Am^{-1}$, $\phi = 2.4 \times 10^{-5}$ Wb.

$A = 0.2\ cm^2 = 0.2 \times 10^{-4}\ m^2$, $\mu = ?\ \chi_m = ?$

$$B = \frac{\phi}{A} = \frac{2.4\times10^{-5}}{0.2\times10^{-4}} = 1.2\ \text{weber}/m^2\ ;$$

$$\mu = \frac{B}{H} = \frac{1.2}{1600} = 7.5\times10^{-4}\,TA^{-1}m\ ;$$

$$[\because \text{As } \mu = \mu_0(1+\chi_m)]$$

$$\therefore \chi_m = \frac{\mu}{\mu_0} - 1 = \frac{7.5\times10^{-4}}{4\pi\times10^{-7}} - 1\ ;$$

$$\chi_m = \frac{7.5\times10^{3}}{4\pi} - 1 = 597.1 - 1 = 596.1$$

Example 8.

A solenoid of 500 turns/m is carrying a current of 3A. Its core is made of iron which has a relative permeability of 5000. Determine the magnitude of magnetic intensity, magnetisation and magnetic field inside the core.

Solution :

Magnetic intensity

$H = ni = 500 \times 3 = 1500$ A/m

$\mu_r = 1 + \chi_m$ so $\chi_m = \mu_r - 1 = 4999 \approx 5000$

Intensity of magnetisation

$I = \chi H = 5000 \times 1500 = 7.5 \times 10^6$ A/m

Magnetic field $B = \mu_r \mu_0 H = 5000 \times 4\pi \times 10^{-7} \times 1500$

$= 9.4$ tesla.

TANGENT GALVANOMETER

It is an instrument used for measuring small current. It is based on tangent law. It is a moving magnet and fixed coil type galvanometer.

Tangent Law : *If a small magnetic needle is under the influence of two crossed magnetic fields (B) and (H) and suffers a deflection θ from field H, then by tangent law, $B = H \tan \theta$.*

Formula for current : If a current passing through the coil of n turns and mean radius r of a tangent galvanometer placed in magnetic meridian causes a deflection θ in the magnetic needle kept at the centre of the coil, then

$$I = \left(\frac{2rH}{\mu_0 n}\right)\tan\theta\ ;\ I = K\tan\theta \text{ where } K = \frac{2rH}{\mu_0 n}$$ and is called the **reduction factor.**

DEFLECTION MAGNETOMETER

It's working is based on the principle of tangent law.

(a) **Tan A Position :** In this position the magneto- meter is set perpendicular to magnetic meridian so that, magnetic field due to magnet is in axial position and perpendicular to earth's field and hence

$$\frac{\mu_0}{4\pi}\frac{2Md}{(d^2 - l^2)^2} = H\tan\theta$$

where d = distance of needle from centre of magnet and $2l$ = length of magnet.

(b) **TanB position :** The arms of magnetometer are set in magnetic meridian, so that the field is at equatorial position

and hence, $H\tan\theta = \dfrac{\mu_0}{4\pi}\dfrac{M}{(d^2 - l^2)^{3/2}}$

Magnetic field of earth extends nearly upto five times the radius of earth i.e., 3.2×10^4 km.

The magnetic field of earth is fairly uniform and can be represented by equidistant parallel lines.

VIBRATION MAGNETOMETER

It is an instrument for comparing the magnetic moments of two magnets and for comparing their magnetic fields.

The time period of a bar magnet vibrating in the vibration magnetometer kept in magnetic meridian is given by

$$T = 2\pi\sqrt{\frac{I}{MH}} \qquad \therefore \quad M = \frac{4\pi^2 I}{T^2 H}$$

where $I = \left(\dfrac{m(l^2 + b^2)}{12}\right)$ is the moment of inertia of the vibrating magnet, m = mass of magnet, $2l$ = length of magnet, b = breadth of magnet.

Example 9.

A vibration magnetometer consists of two identical bar magnets, placed one over the other, such that they are mutually perpendicular and bisect each other. The time period of oscillation in a horizontal magnetic field is 4 second. If one of the magnets is taken away, find the period of oscillation of the other in the same field.

Sol. For a vibration magnetometer, we know that

$T = 2\pi\sqrt{I/MH}$

Let M be the magnetic moment and M.I, moment of inertia of each magnet,

$\therefore M' = \sqrt{M^2 + M^2} = M\sqrt{2}$

and net $M.I' = M.I + M.I = 2M.I$

$$\therefore\ T' = 2\pi\sqrt{\frac{2\ M.I.}{M\sqrt{2}H}} = 2\times\sqrt{\frac{\sqrt{2}M.I.}{MH}} \quad ....(1)$$

When one of the magnets is taken away,

$M'' = M,\ MI'' = MI,$

$$\therefore\ T'' = 2\pi\sqrt{\frac{M.I}{MH}} \quad ...(2)$$

Divide eqn. (2) by (1),

$$\frac{T''}{T'} = \frac{1}{(2)^{1/4}} \text{ or } T'' = \frac{T'}{(2)^{1/4}} = \frac{4}{2^{1/4}} = 3.34 \text{ s}$$

Example 10.

The period of oscillation of a magnet in a vibration magnetometer is 2 sec. What will be the period of oscillation of a magnet whose magnetic moment is four times that of the first magnet?

Sol. $T = 2\pi\sqrt{\left(\frac{I}{MB_H}\right)}$

$$T' = 2\pi\sqrt{\left(\frac{I}{4MB_H}\right)} = \frac{1}{2}\left[2\pi\sqrt{\frac{I}{(MB_H)}}\right] = \frac{1}{2}\times 2 = 1.5$$

20.2 Concept Practice Problems

CPP

11. The magnetic compass is not useful for navigation near the magnetic poles, since

(a) R = 0 (b) V = 0 (c) H = 0 (d) $\theta = 0°$

12. The most appropriate magnetization M versus magnetising field H curve for a paramagnetic substance is

(a) A

(b) B

(c) C

(d) D

M, +, 0, –, H, C, A, B, D

13. Identify the correctly matched pair

(a) Diamagnetic - Gadolinium
(b) Soft ferromagnetic - Alnico
(c) Hard ferromagnetic - Copper
(d) Paramagnetic - Sodium

14. Materials suitable for permanent magnet, must have which of the following properties?

(a) High retentivity, low coercivity and high permeability.
(b) Low retentivity, low coercivity and low permeability.
(c) Low retentivity, high coercivity and low permeability.
(d) High retentivity, high coercivity and high permeability.

15. Match the column I & II.

Column I	Column II
(A) Horizontal component	(1) $B_E \sin\theta$
(B) Vertical component	(2) $\frac{B_V}{B_H}$
(C) $\tan\theta$	(3) $B_E \cos\theta$
(D) Tangent law	(4) $B = B_H \tan\theta$

(a) A→(3); B→(2); C→(1); D→(4)
(b) A→(3); B→(1); C→(2); D→(4)
(c) A→(2); B→(3); C→(1); D→(4)
(d) A→(1); B→(3); C→(2); D→(4)

16. A material is placed in a magnetic field and it is thrown out of it. The material is

(a) diamagnetic (b) paramagnetic
(c) ferromagnetic (d) non-magnetic

17. A current carrying coil is placed with its axis perpendicular to *N-S* direction. Let horizontal component of earth's magnetic field be H_0 and magnetic field inside the loop be H. If a magnet is suspended inside the loop, it makes angle θ with H. Then θ =

(a) $\tan^{-1}\left(\frac{H_0}{H}\right)$ (b) $\tan^{-1}\left(\frac{H}{H_0}\right)$

(c) $\operatorname{cosec}^{-1}\left(\frac{H}{H_0}\right)$ (d) $\cot^{-1}\left(\frac{H_0}{H}\right)$

18. A domain in a ferromagnetic substance is in the form of a cube of side length 1 μm. If it contains 8×10^{10} atoms and each atomic dipole has a dipole moment of 9×10^{-24} A m^2, then the magnetization of the domain is

(a) 7.2×10^5 A m^{-1} (b) 7.2×10^3 A m^{-1}
(c) 7.2×10^9 A m^{-1} (d) 7.2×10^{12} A m^{-1}

19. The magnetic needle of a tangent galvanometer is deflected at an angle 30° due to a magnet. The horizontal component of earth's magnetic field 0.34×10^{-4} *T* is along the plane of the coil. The magnetic intensity is

(a) 1.96×10^{-4} *T* (b) 1.96×10^{-5} *T*
(c) 1.96×10^{4} *T* (d) 1.96×10^{5} *T*

20. A compass needle made of pure iron (with density 7900 kg/m^3) has a length *L* of 3.0 cm, a width of 1.00 mm, and a thickness of 0.50 mm. The magnitude of the magnetic dipole moment of an iron atom is $M_{Fe} = 2.1\times10^{-23}$ *J/T*. If the magnetisation of the needle is equivalent to the alignment of 10% of the atoms in the needle, what is the magnitude of the needle's magnetic dipole moment $\vec{M}$?

(a) 2.7×10^{-1} J/T (b) 2.7×10^{-2} J/T
(c) 2.7×10^{-3} J/T (d) 2.7×10^{-4} J/T

ANSWER KEY

11	(c)	12	(a)	13	(d)	14	(d)	15	(b)	16	(a)	17	(a)	18	(a)	19	(b)	20	(c)

CONCEPT MAP

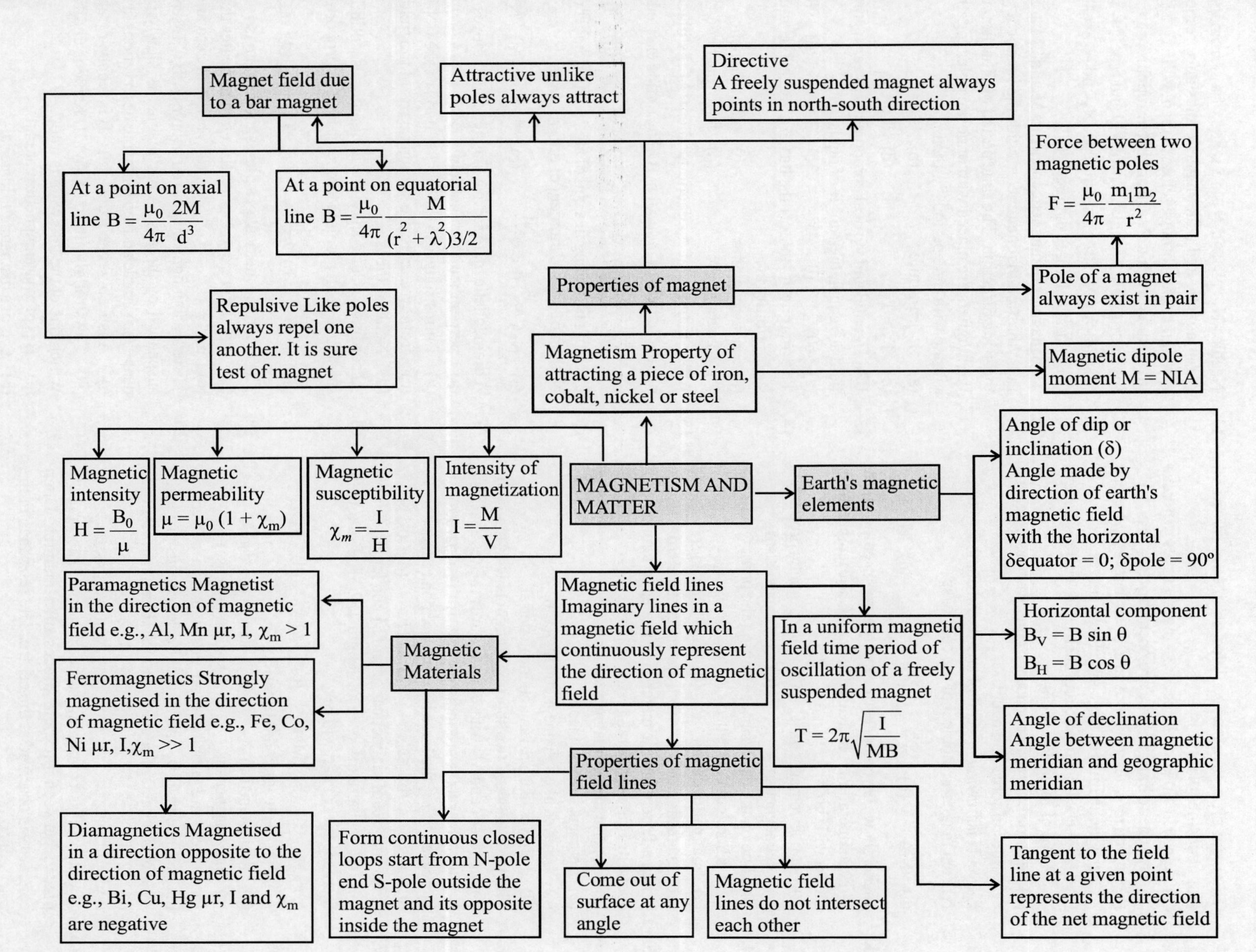
Magnet field due to a bar magnet
Attractive unlike poles always attract
Directive A freely suspended magnet always points in north-south direction
At a point on axial line $B = \frac{\mu_0}{4\pi}\frac{2M}{d^3}$
At a point on equatorial line $B = \frac{\mu_0}{4\pi}\frac{M}{(r^2 + \lambda^2)3/2}$
Force between two magnetic poles $F = \frac{\mu_0}{4\pi}\frac{m_1 m_2}{r^2}$
Properties of magnet
Pole of a magnet always exist in pair
Repulsive Like poles always repel one another. It is sure test of magnet
Magnetism Property of attracting a piece of iron, cobalt, nickel or steel
Magnetic dipole moment M = NIA
Angle of dip or inclination (δ) Angle made by direction of earth's magnetic field with the horizontal δequator = 0; δpole = 90º
Magnetic intensity $H = \frac{B_0}{\mu}$
Magnetic permeability $\mu = \mu_0 (1 + \chi_m)$
Magnetic susceptibility $\chi_m = \frac{I}{H}$
Intensity of magnetization $I = \frac{M}{V}$
MAGNETISM AND MATTER
Earth's magnetic elements
Paramagnetics Magnetist in the direction of magnetic field e.g., Al, Mn μr, I, $\chi_m > 1$
Magnetic field lines Imaginary lines in a magnetic field which continuously represent the direction of magnetic field
In a uniform magnetic field time period of oscillation of a freely suspended magnet $T = 2\pi\sqrt{\frac{I}{MB}}$
Horizontal component $B_V = B \sin\theta$ $B_H = B \cos\theta$
Magnetic Materials
Ferromagnetics Strongly magnetised in the direction of magnetic field e.g., Fe, Co, Ni μr, I,$\chi_m >> 1$
Angle of declination Angle between magnetic meridian and geographic meridian
Properties of magnetic field lines
Diamagnetics Magnetised in a direction opposite to the direction of magnetic field e.g., Bi, Cu, Hg μr, I and χ_m are negative
Form continuous closed loops start from N-pole end S-pole outside the magnet and its opposite inside the magnet
Come out of surface at any angle
Magnetic field lines do not intersect each other
Tangent to the field line at a given point represents the direction of the net magnetic field

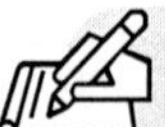

Exercise 1 - Chapter Revision Problems

CRP

1. The main difference between electric lines of force and magnetic lines of force is
   (a) electric lines of force are closed curves whereas magnetic lines of force are open curves
   (b) electric lines of force are open curves whereas magnetic lines of force are closed curves
   (c) magnetic lines of force cut each other whereas electric lines of force do not cut
   (d) electric lines of force cut each other whereas magnetic lines of force do not cut
2. Current i is flowing in a coil of area A and number of turns N, then magnetic moment of the coil, M is
   (a) NiA (b) $\frac{Ni}{A}$ (c) $\frac{Ni}{\sqrt{A}}$ (d) N^2Ai
3. Nickel shows ferromagnetic property at room temperature. If the temperature is increased beyond Curie temperature, then it will show
   (a) anti ferromagnetism (b) no magnetic property
   (c) diamagnetism (d) paramagnetism
4. The line on the earth surface joining the point where the field is horizontal, is called
   (a) magnetic equator (b) magnetic line
   (c) magnetic axis (d) magnetic inertia
5. When a ferromagnetic material is heated to temperature above its Curie temperature, the material
   (a) is permanently magnetized
   (b) remains ferromagnetic
   (c) behaves like a diamagnetic material
   (d) behaves like a paramagnetic material
6. The force between two short bar magnets with magnetic moments M_1 and M_2 whose centres are r metres apart is 8 N when their axes are in same line. if the separation is increased to 2 r, the force between them in reduced to
   (a) 4 N (b) 2 N (c) 1 N (d) 0.5 N
7. A bar magnet of magnetic moment M and length L is cut into two equal parts each of length L/2. The magnetic moment of each part will be
   (a) M (b) M/4 (c) $\sqrt{2}$M (d) M/2
8. A superconductor exhibits perfect :
   (a) ferrimagnetism (b) ferromagnetism
   (c) paramagnetism (d) diamagnetism
9. In end on and broadside on position of a deflection magnetometer, if θ_1 and θ_2 are the deflections produced by short magnets at equal distances, then $\tan\theta_1/\tan\theta_2$ is
   (a) 2 : 1 (b) 1 : 2
   (c) 1 : 1 (d) None of these
10. A watch glass containing some powdered substance is placed between the pole pieces of a magnet. Deep concavity is observed at the centre. The substance in the watch glass is
    (a) iron (b) chromium
    (c) carbon (d) wood
11. Needles N_1, N_2 and N_3 are made of a ferromagnetic, a paramagnetic and a diamagnetic substance respectively. A magnet when brought close to them will
    (a) attract N_1 and N_2 strongly but repel N_3
    (b) attract N_1 strongly, N_2 weakly and repel N_3 weakly
    (c) attract N_1 strongly, but repel N_2 and N_3 weakly
    (d) attract all three of them
12. Two magnets of magnetic moments M and 2M are placed in a vibration magnetometer, with the identical poles in the same direction. The time period of vibration is T_1. If the magnets are placed with opposite poles together and vibrate with time period T_2, then
    (a) T_2 is infinite (b) $T_2 = T_1$
    (c) $T_2 > T_1$ (d) $T_2 < T_1$
13. If horizontal and vertical components of earths magnetic field are equal, then angle of dip is
    (a) 60° (b) 45° (c) 30° (d) 90°
14. The magnetic materials having negative magnetic susceptibility are
    (a) non-magnetic (b) para magnetic
    (c) dia magnetic (d) ferro magnetic
15. A bar magnet, of magnetic moment $\vec{M}$, is placed in a magnetic field of induction $\vec{B}$. The torque exerted on it is
    (a) $\vec{M}\cdot\vec{B}$ (b) $-\vec{M}\cdot\vec{B}$ (c) $\vec{M}\times\vec{B}$ (d) $\vec{B}\times\vec{M}$
16. Current i is flowing in a coil of area A and number of turns N, then magnetic moment of the coil M is
    (a) NiA (b) $\frac{Ni}{A}$ (c) $\frac{Ni}{\sqrt{A}}$ (d) N^2Ai
17. A diamagnetic material in a magnetic field moves
    (a) perpendicular to the field
    (b) from stronger to the weaker parts of the field
    (c) from weaker to the stronger parts of the field
    (d) None of these
18. According to Curie's law, the magnetic susceptibility of a substance at an absolute temperature T is proportional to
    (a) T^2 (b) $\frac{1}{T}$ (c) T (d) $\frac{1}{T^2}$
19. The magnetic moment of a diamagnetic atom is
    (a) equal to zero (b) much greater than one
    (c) unity (d) between zero and one
20. There are four light-weight-rod samples A,B,C,D separately suspended by threads. A bar magnet is slowly brought near each sample and the following observations are noted
    (i) A is feebly repelled (ii) B is feebly attracted
    (iii) C is strongly attracted (iv) D remains unaffected
    Which one of the following is true ?
    (a) B is of a paramagnetic material
    (b) C is of a diamagnetic material
    (c) D is of a ferromagnetic material
    (d) A is of a non-magnetic material

21. A bar magnet 8 cms long is placed in the magnetic merdian with the N-pole pointing towards geographical north. Two netural points separated by a distance of 6 cms are obtained on the equatorial axis of the magnet. If horizontal component of earth's field = 3.2×10^{-5} T, then pole strength of magnet is
(a) 5 ab-amp × c (b) 10 ab-amp × cm
(c) 2.5 ab-amp × cm (d) 20 ab-amp × cm

22. Two isolated point poles of strength 30 A-m and 60 A-m are placed at a distance of 0.3m. The force of repulsion is
(a) 2×10^{-3} N (b) 2×10^{-4} N
(c) 2×10^{5} N (d) 2×10^{-5} N

23. The magnetic moment of a magnet is 0.1 amp × m^2. It is suspended in a magnetic field of intensity 3×10^{-4} weber/m^2. The couple acting upon it when deflected by 30° from the magnetic field is
(a) 1×10^{-5} N m (b) 1.5×10^{-5} N m
(c) 2×10^{-5} N m (d) 2.5×10^{-5} N m

24. When 2 ampere current is passed through a tangent galvanometer, it gives a deflection of 30°. For 60° deflection, the current must be
(a) 1 amp. (b) $2\sqrt{3}$ amp.
(c) 4 amp. (d) 6 amp.

25. The variation of magnetic susceptibility (x) with temperature for a diamagnetic substance is best represented by

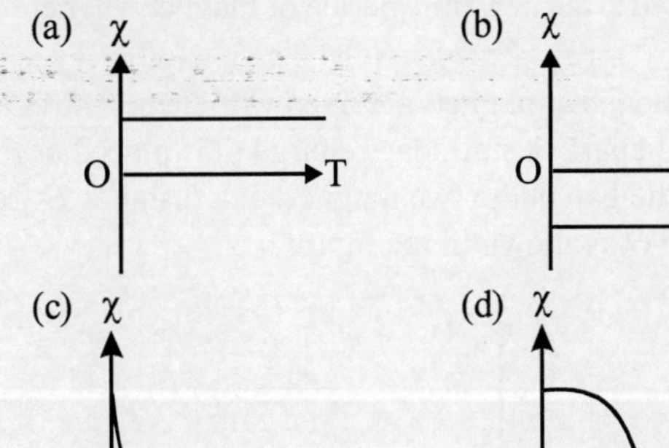

26. At a temperatur of 30°C, the susceptibility of a ferromagnetic material is found to be χ. Its susceptibility at 333°C is
(a) χ (b) 0.5χ (c) 2χ (d) 11.1χ

27. Of the following fig., the lines of magnetic induction due to a magnet SN, are given by

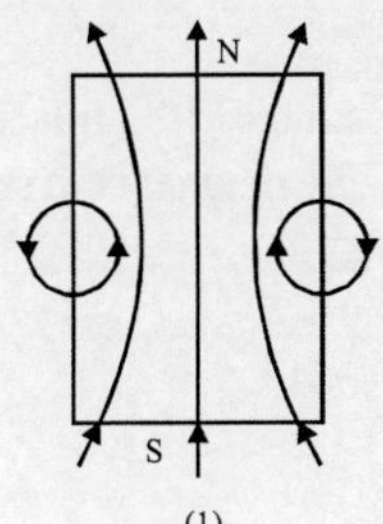

(1)

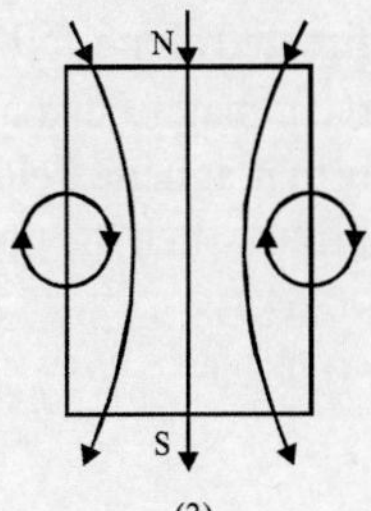

(2)

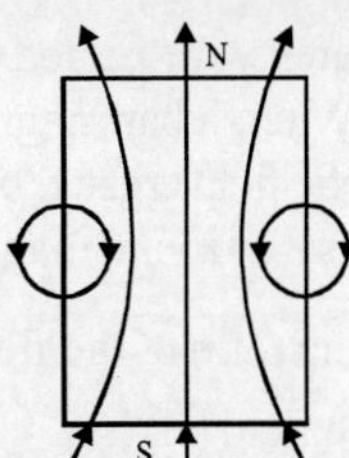

(3)

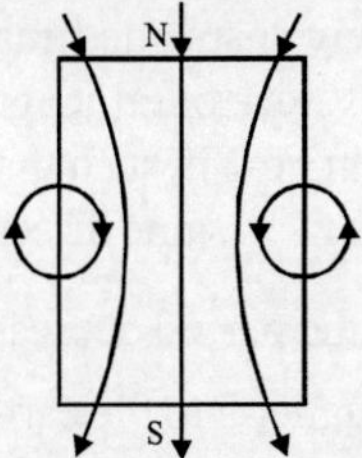

(4)

(a) 1 (b) 2 (c) 3 (d) 4

28. The B – H curve (i) and (ii) shown in fig. associated with

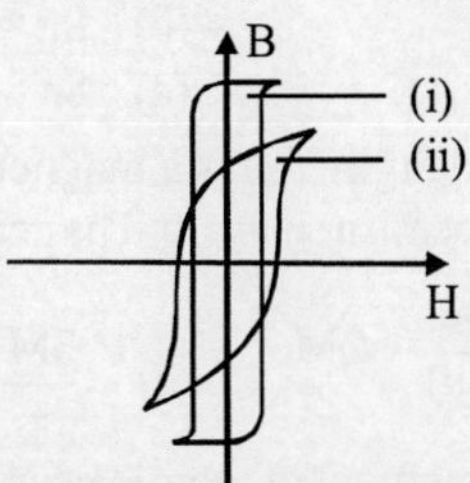

(a) (i) diamagnetic and (ii) paramagnetic substance
(b) (i) paramagnetic and (ii) ferromagnetic substance
(c) (i) soft iron and (ii) steel respectively
(d) (i) steel and (ii) soft iron respectively

29. A thin bar magnet of length 2 ℓ and breadth 2 b pole strength m and magnetic moment M is divided into four equal parts with length and breadth of each part being half of original magnet. Then the pole strength of each part is
(a) m (b) m/2 (c) 2m (d) m/4

30. In the above question, magnetic moment of each part is
(a) M/4 (b) M (c) M/2 (d) 2 M

31. Two points A and B are situated at a distance x and 2x respectively from the nearer pole of a magnet 2 cm long. The ratio of magnetic field at A and B is
(a) 4 : 1 exactly (b) 4 : 1 approximately
(c) 8 : 1 approximately (d) 1 : 1 approximately

32. Two bar magnets of the same mass, same length and breadth but having magnetic moments M and 2M are joined together pole for pole and suspended by a string. The time period of assembly in a magnetic field of strength H is 3 seconds. If now the polarity of one of the magnets is reversed and combination is again made to oscillate in the same field, the time of oscillation is
(a) $\sqrt{3}$ sec (b) $3\sqrt{3}$ sec
(c) 3 sec (d) 6 sec

33. Two short magnets have equal pole strengths but one is twice as long as the other. The shorter magnet is placed 20 cms in tan A position from the compass needle. The longer magnet must be placed on the other side of the magnetometer for no deflection at a distance equal to
(a) 20 cms (b) $20(2)^{1/3}$ cms
(c) $20(2)^{2/3}$ cms (d) $20(2)^{3/3}$ cms

34. Two magnets are held together in a vibration magnetometer and are allowed to oscillate in the earth's magnetic field with like poles together. 12 oscillations per minute are made but for unlike poles together only 4 oscillations per minute are executed. The ratio of their magnetic moments is
(a) 3 : 1 (b) 1 : 3 (c) 3 : 5 (d) 5 : 4

35. A freely suspended magnet oscillates with period T in earth's horizontal magnetic field. When a bar magnet is brought near it, such that the magnetic field created by bar magnet is in same direction as earth's horizontal magnetic field, the period decreases to $\frac{T}{2}$. The ratio of the field of the magnet F to the earth's magnetic field (H) is
(a) 1 : 3 (b) 1 : 1 (c) 3 : 1 (d) 9 : 1

36. If relative permeability of iron is 2000. Its absolute permeability in S.I. units is
(a) $8\pi \times 10^{-4}$ (b) $8\pi \times 10^{-3}$
(c) $800/\pi$ (d) $8\pi \times 10^{9}/\pi$

37. A steel wire of length ℓ has a magnetic moment M. It is then bent into a semicircular arc. The new magnetic moment is
(a) $\frac{M}{\pi}$ (b) $\frac{2M}{\pi}$ (c) $\frac{3M}{\pi}$ (d) $\frac{4M}{\pi}$

38. The magnetic moment of atomic neon is equal to
(a) zero (b) $\frac{1}{2}\mu_B$ (c) μ_B (d) $\frac{3}{2}\mu_B$

39. The net magnetic moment of two identical magnets each of magnetic moment M_0, inclined at 60° with each other is
(a) M_0
(b) $\sqrt{2}\, M_0$
(c) $\sqrt{3}\, M_0$
(d) $2M_0$

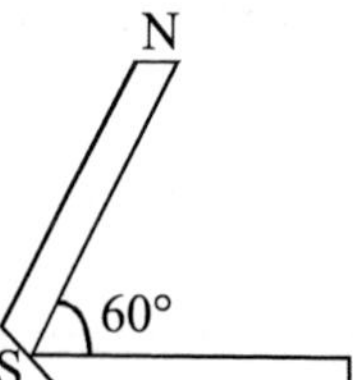

40. A magnetic needle vibrates in a vertical plane parallel to the magnetic meridian about a horizontal axis passing through its centre. Its frequency is n. If the plane of oscillation is turned about a vertical axis by 90°C, the frequency of its oscillation in vertical plane will be
(a) n (b) zero
(c) less than n (d) more than n

41. A thin rectangular magnet suspended freely has a period of oscillation of 4 s. If it is broken into two halves (each having half the original length) and one of the pieces is suspended similarly. The period of its oscillation will be
(a) 4 s (b) 2 s (c) 0.5 s (d) 0.25 s

42. A steel wire of length ℓ has a magnetic moment M. It is bent in L-shape (Figure). The new magnetic moment is
(a) M
(b) $\frac{M}{\sqrt{2}}$
(c) $\frac{M}{2}$
(d) 2M

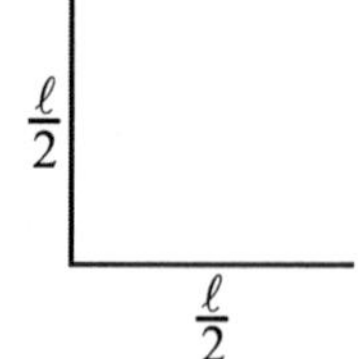

43. The time period of oscillation of a magnet in a vibration magnetometer is 1.5 sec. The time period of oscillation of another magnet similar in size, shape and mass but having 1/4 magnetic moment than that of the 1st magnet oscillating at the same place will be
(a) 0.75 sec (b) 1.5 sec
(c) 3.0 sec (d) 6.0 sec

44. If a toroid uses bismuth for its core, the field in the core compared to that in empty core will be slightly
(a) greater (b) smaller
(c) equal (d) None of these

45. Relative permittivity and permeability of a material ε_r and μ_r, respectively. Which of the following values of these quantities are allowed for a diamagnetic material?
(a) $\varepsilon_r = 0.5, \mu_r = 1.5$ (b) $\varepsilon_r = 1.5, \mu_r = 0.5$
(c) $\varepsilon_r = 0.5, \mu_r = 0.5$ (d) $\varepsilon_r = 1.5, \mu_r = 1.5$

46. The work done in turning a magnet of magnetic moment M by an angle of 90° from the meridian, is n times the corresponding work done to turn it through an angle of 60°. The value of n is given by
(a) 2 (b) 1 (c) 0.5 (d) 0.25

47. Iron is ferromagnetic
(a) above 770°C (b) below 770°C
(c) at all temperature (d) above 1100°C

48. A vibration magnetometer placed in magnetic meridian has a small bar magnet. The magnet executes oscillations with a time period of 2 sec in earth's horizontal magnetic field of 24 microtesla. When a horizontal field of 18 microtesla is produced opposite to the earth's field by placing a current carrying wire, the new time period of magnet will be
(a) 1 *s* (b) 2 *s* (c) 3 *s* (d) 4 *s*

49. Two identical bar magnets are fixed with their centres at a distance d apart. A stationary charge *Q* is placed at *P* in between the gap of the two magnets at a distance *D* from the centre *O* as shown in the figure.

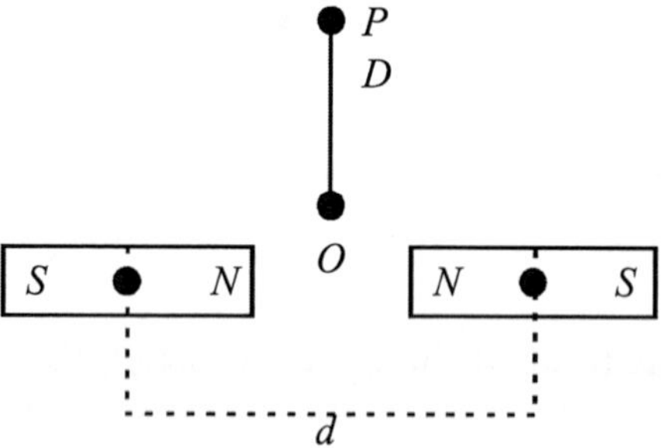

The force on the charge *Q* is
(a) directed perpendicular to the plane of paper
(b) zero
(c) directed along *OP*
(d) directed along *PO*

50. A short bar magnet of magnetic moment $0.4\,J\,T^{-1}$ is placed in a uniform magnetic field of 0.16 T. The magnet is in stable equilibrium when the potential energy is
(a) −0.64 J (b) zero
(c) −0.082 J (d) 0.064 J

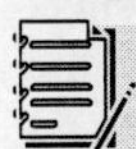

Exercise 2 - Exemplar & Past Year Questions

E&PYQs

Exemplar Questions

1. A toroid of n turns, mean radius R and cross-sectional radius a carries current I. It is placed on a horizontal table taken as xy-plane. Its magnetic moment m
(a) is non-zero and points in the z-direction by symmetry
(b) points along the axis of the toroid ($m = m\phi$)
(c) is zero, otherwise there would be a field falling as $\frac{1}{r^3}$ at large distances outside the toroid
(d) is pointing radially outwards

2. The magnetic field of the earth can be modelled by that of a point dipole placed at the centre of the earth. The dipole axis makes an angle of 11.3° with the axis of the earth. At Mumbai, declination is nearly zero. Then,
(a) the declination varies between 11.3° W to 11.3° E
(b) the least declination is 0°
(c) the plane defined by dipole axis and the earth axis passes through Greenwich
(d) declination averaged over the earth must be always negative

3. In a permanent magnet at room temperature.
(a) magnetic moment of each molecule is zero
(b) the individual molecules have non-zero magnetic moment which are all perfectly aligned
(c) domains are partially aligned
(d) domains are all perfectly aligned

4. A paramagnetic sample shows a net magnetisation of 8 Am^{-1} when placed in an external magnetic field of 0.6 T at a temperature of 4 K. When the same sample is placed in an external magnetic field of 0.2 T at a temperature of 16 K, the magnetisation will be
(a) $\frac{32}{3}Am^{-1}$ (b) $\frac{2}{3}Am^{-1}$ (c) $6Am^{-1}$ (d) $2.4Am^{-1}$

NEET/AIPMT (2013-2020) Questions

5. A bar magnet of length 'ℓ' and magnetic dipole moment 'M' is bent in the form of an arc as shown in figure. The new magnetic dipole moment will be **[2013]**
(a) $\frac{3}{\pi}M$
(b) $\frac{2}{\pi}M$
(c) $\frac{M}{2}$
(d) M

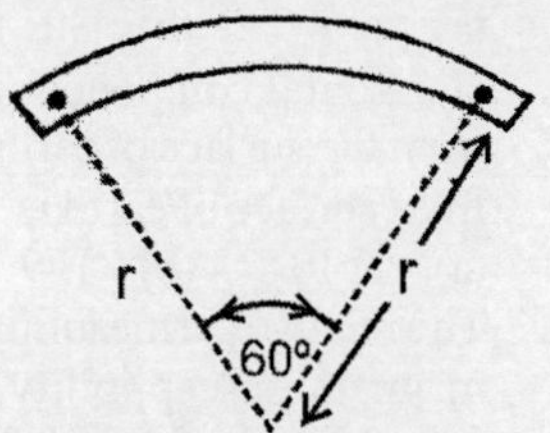

6. A bar magnet of magnetic moment *M* is placed at right angles to a magnetic induction *B*. If a force *F* is experienced by each pole of the magnet, the length of the magnet will be **[NEET Kar. 2013]**
(a) F/MB (b) MB/F (c) BF/M (d) MF/B

7. The magnetic susceptibility is negative for : **[2016]**
(a) diamagnetic material only
(b) paramagnetic material only
(c) ferromagnetic material only
(d) paramagnetic and ferromagnetic materials

8. If θ_1 and θ_2 be the apparent angles of dip observed in two vertical planes at right angles to each other, then the true angle of dip θ is given by :- **[2017]**
(a) $\tan^2\theta = \tan^2\theta_1 + \tan^2\theta_2$
(b) $\cot^2\theta = \cot^2\theta_1 - \cot^2\theta_2$
(c) $\tan^2\theta = \tan^2\theta_1 - \tan^2\theta_2$
(d) $\cot^2\theta = \cot^2\theta_1 + \cot^2\theta_2$

9. A thin diamagnetic rod is placed vertically between the poles of an electromagnet. When the current in the electromagnet is switched on, then the diamagnetic rod is pushed up, out of the horizontal magnetic field. Hence the rod gains gravitational potential energy. The work required to do this comes from **[2018]**
(a) the current source
(b) the magnetic field
(c) the induced electric field due to the changing magnetic field
(d) the lattice structure of the material of the rod

10. At a point A on the earth's surface the angle of dip, $\delta = +25°$. At a point B on the earth's surface the angle of dip, $\delta = -25°$. We can interpret that: **[2019]**
(a) A and B are both located in the northern hemisphere.
(b) A is located in the southern hemisphere and B is located in the northern hemisphere.
(c) A is located in the northern hemisphere and B is located in the southern hemisphere.
(d) A and B are both located in the southern hemisphere.

11. An iron rod of susceptibility 599 is subjected to a magnetising field of 1200 $A\,m^{-1}$. The permeability of the material of the rod is : ($\mu_0 = 4\pi \times 10^{-7}\,T\,m\,A^{-1}$) **[2020]**
(a) $8.0 \times 10^{-5}\,T\,m\,A^{-1}$ (b) $2.4\pi \times 10^{-5}\,T\,m\,A^{-1}$
(c) $2.4\pi \times 10^{-7}\,T\,m\,A^{-1}$ (d) $2.4\pi \times 10^{-4}\,T\,m\,A^{-1}$

Exercise 3 - Concept Application Problems

CAP

1. The magnet of pole strength m and magnetic moment M is cut into two pieces along its axis. Its pole strength and magnetic moment now becomes
(a) $\frac{m}{2}, \frac{M}{2}$ (b) $m, \frac{M}{2}$ (c) $\frac{m}{2}, M$ (d) m, M

2. A bar magnet is oscillating in the Earth's magnetic field with a period T. What happens to its period and motion if its mass is quadrupled?
(a) Motion remains S.H. and period remains nearly constant

(b) Motion remains S.H. with time period $= \frac{T}{2}$
(c) Motion remains S.H. with time period = 2T
(d) Motion remains S.H. with time period = 4T

3. For protecting a sensitive equipment from the external electric arc, it should be
(a) wrapped with insulation around it when passing current through it
(b) placed inside an iron can
(c) surrounded with fine copper sheet
(d) placed inside an aluminium can

4. If a diamagnetic substance is brought near north or south pole of a bar magnet, it is
(a) attracted by the poles
(b) repelled by the poles
(c) repelled by north pole and attracted by the south pole
(d) attracted by the north pole and repelled by the south pole

5. If the magnetic dipole moment of an atom of diamagnetic material, paramagnetic material and ferromagnetic material are denoted by μ_d, μ_p and μ_f respectively, then
(a) $\mu_d = 0$ and $\mu_p \neq 0$ (b) $\mu_d \neq 0$ and $\mu_p = 0$
(c) $\mu_p = 0$ and $\mu_f \neq 0$ (d) $\mu_d \neq 0$ and $\mu_f \neq 0$

6. Two tangent galvanometers having coils of the same radius are connected in series. A current flowing in them produces deflections of 60° and 45° respectively. The ratio of the number of turns in the coils is
(a) 4/3 (b) $\frac{\sqrt{3}+1}{1}$ (c) $\frac{\sqrt{3}+1}{\sqrt{3}-1}$ (d) $\frac{\sqrt{3}}{1}$

7. Two identical magnetic dipoles of magnetic moments 1.0 A-m^2 each, placed at a separation of 2 m with their axis perpendicular to each other. The resultant magnetic field at point midway between the dipole is
(a) 5×10^{-7} T (b) $\sqrt{5} \times 10^{-7}$ T
(c) 10^{-7} T (d) 2×10^{-7} T

8. A curve between magnetic moment and temperature of magnet is

(a)
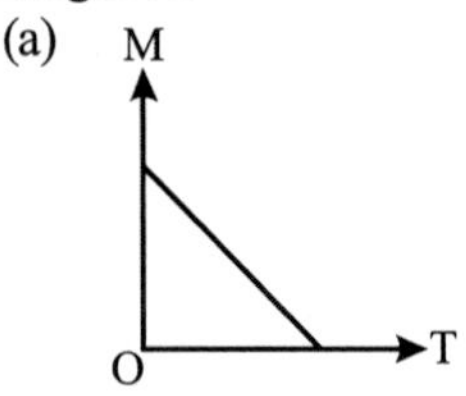

(b)
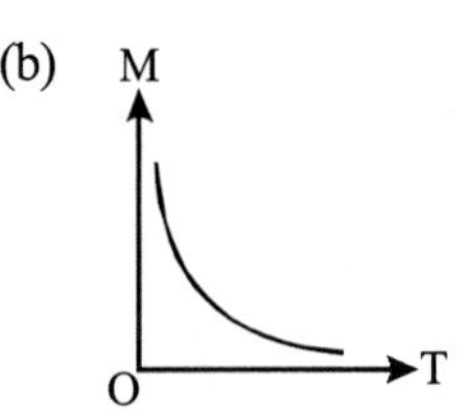

(c)
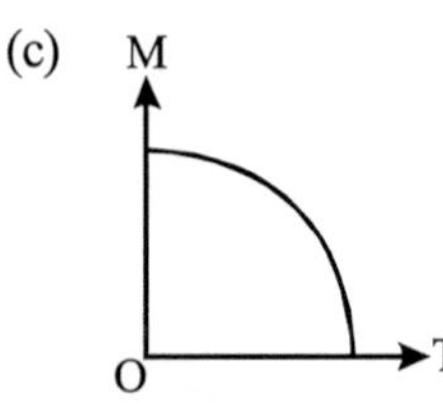

(d)
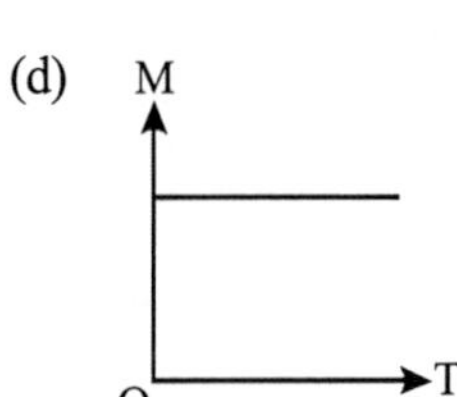

9. If a magnet is suspended at angle 30° to the magnetic meridian, the dip needle makes an angle of 45° with the horizontal. The real dip is
(a) $\tan^{-1}(\sqrt{3/2})$ (b) $\tan^{-1}(\sqrt{3})$
(c) $\tan^{-1}(\sqrt{3}/2)$ (d) $\tan^{-1}(2/\sqrt{3})$

10. A compass needle placed at a distance r from a short magnet in Tan A position shows a deflection of 60°. If the distance is increased to r $(3)^{1/3}$, then deflection of compass needle is
(a) 30° (b) $60 \times 3^{\frac{1}{3}}$ (c) $60 \times 3^{\frac{2}{3}}$ (d) $60 \times 3^{\frac{3}{3}}$

11. A dip needle lies initially in the magnetic meridian when it shows an angle of dip θ at a place. The dip circle is rotated through an angle x in the horizontal plane and then it shows an angle of dip θ′.
Then $\frac{\tan\theta'}{\tan\theta}$ is
(a) $\frac{1}{\cos x}$ (b) $\frac{1}{\sin x}$ (c) $\frac{1}{\tan x}$ (d) cos x

12. A dip circle is so set that its needle moves freely in the magnetic meridian. In this position, the angle of dip is 40°. Now the dip circle is rotated so that the plane in which the needle moves makes an angle of 30° with the magnetic meridian. In this position, the needle will dip by an angle
(a) 40° (b) 30°
(c) more than 40° (d) less than 40°

13. Work done in turning a magnet of magnetic moment M by an angle of 90° from the mgnetic meridian is n times the corresponding work done to turn through an angle of 60°, where n is
(a) 1/2 (b) 2 (c) 1/4 (d) 1

14. At a certain place, horizontal component is $\sqrt{3}$ times the vertical component. The angle of dip at this place is
(a) 0 (b) π/3
(c) π/6 (d) None of these

15. Torques τ_1 and τ_2 are required for a magnetic needle to remain perpendicular to the magnetic fields at two different places. The magnetic fields at those places are B_1 and B_2 respectively; then ratio $\frac{B_1}{B_2}$ is
(a) $\frac{\tau_2}{\tau_1}$ (b) $\frac{\tau_1}{\tau_2}$ (c) $\frac{\tau_1+\tau_2}{\tau_1-\tau_2}$ (d) $\frac{\tau_1-\tau_2}{\tau_1+\tau_2}$

16. Time periods of vibation of two bar magnets in sum and difference positions are 4 sec and 6 sec respectively. The ratio of their magnetic moments M_1 / M_2 is
(a) 6 : 4 (b) 30 : 16 (c) 2.6 : 1 (d) 1.5 : 1

17. Horizontal component of earth's field at a height of 1 m from the surface of earth is H. Its value at a height of 10 m from surface of earth is
(a) H/10 (b) H/9 (c) H/100 (d) H

18. The relative permeability of a medium is 0.075. What is its magnetic susceptibility?
(a) 0.925 (b) –0.925 (c) 1.075 (d) –1.075

19. The moment of a magnet (15 cm × 2 cm × 1 cm) is 1.2 A-m^2. What is its intensity of magnetisation?
(a) 4×10^4 A m^{-1} (b) 2×10^4 A m^{-1}
(c) 10^4 A m^{-1} (d) None of these

20. At a certain place, the angle of dip is 30° and the horizontal component of earth's magnetic field is 0.50 oerested. The earth's total magnetic field (in oerested) is
(a) $\sqrt{3}$ (b) 1 (c) $\frac{1}{\sqrt{3}}$ (d) $\frac{1}{2}$

21. A coil in the shape of an equilateral triangle of side l is suspended between the pole pieces of a permanent magnet such that $\vec{B}$ is in plane of the coil. If due to a current i in the triangle a torque τ acts on it, the side l of the triangle is

(a) $\frac{2}{\sqrt{3}}\left(\frac{\tau}{B.i}\right)^{\frac{1}{2}}$ (b) $2\left(\frac{\tau}{\sqrt{3}B.i}\right)^{\frac{1}{2}}$

(c) $\frac{2}{\sqrt{3}}\left(\frac{\tau}{B.i}\right)$ (d) $\frac{1}{\sqrt{3}}\frac{\tau}{B.i}$

22. A small bar magnet placed with its axis at 30° with an external field of 0.06 T experiences a torque of 0.018 Nm. The minimum work required to rotate it from its stable to unstable equilibrium position is :

(a) 6.4×10^{-2} J (b) 9.2×10^{-3} J

(c) 7.2×10^{-2} J (d) 11.7×10^{-3} J

23. A circular coil has moment of inertia 0.8 kg m^2 around any diameter and is carrying current to produce a magnetic moment of 20 Am^2. The coil is kept initially in a vertical position and it can rotate freely around a horizontal diameter. When a uniform magnetic field of 4 T is applied along the vertical, it starts rotating around its horizontal diameter. The angular speed the coil acquires after rotating by 60° will be :

(a) 10 rad s^{-1} (b) 10π rad s^{-1}

(c) 20π rad s^{-1} (d) 20 rad s^{-1}

24. Two magnetic dipoles X and Y are placed at a separation d, with their axes perpendicular to each other. The dipole moment of Y is twice that of X. A particle of charge q is passing through their midpoint P, at angle $\theta = 45°$ with the horizontal line, as shown in figure. What would be the magnitude of force on the particle at that instant? (d is much larger than the dimensions of the dipole)

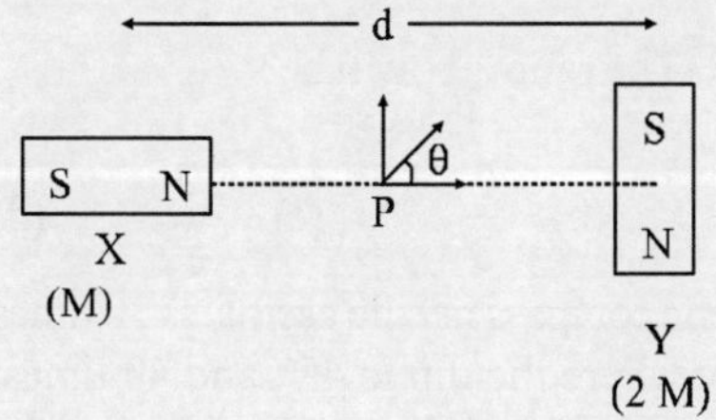

(a) $\left(\frac{\mu_0}{4\pi}\right)\frac{M}{\left(\frac{d}{2}\right)^3} \times qv$ (b) 0

(c) $\sqrt{2}\left(\frac{\mu_0}{4\pi}\right)\frac{M}{\left(\frac{d}{2}\right)^3} \times qv$ (d) $\left(\frac{\mu_0}{4\pi}\right)\frac{2M}{\left(\frac{d}{2}\right)^3} \times qv$

25. A magnet of total magnetic moment $10^{-2}\hat{i}$ A-m^2 is placed in a time varying magnetic field, B$\hat{i}$ (cosωt)where B = 1 Tesla and ω = 0.125 rad/s. The work done for reversing the direction of the magnetic moment at t = 1 second, is:

(a) 0.01 J (b) 0.007 J (c) 0.028 J (d) 0.014 J

26. A magnetic dipole in a constant magnetic field has :

(a) maximum potential energy when the torque is maximum

(b) zero potential energy when the torque is minimum.

(c) zero potential energy when the torque is maximum.

(d) minimum potential energy when the torque is maximum.

27. A magnetic dipole is acted upon by two magnetic fields which are inclined to each other at an angle of 75°. One of the fields has a magnitude of 15 mT. The dipole attains stable equilibrium at an angle of 30° with this field. The magntidue of the other field (in mT) is close to :

(a) 1 (b) 11 (c) 36 (d) 1060

28. A 25 cm long solenoid has radius 2 cm and 500 total number of turns. It carries a current of 15 A. If it is equivalent to a magnet of the same size and magnetization $\vec{M}$ (magnetic moment/volume), then $|\vec{M}|$ is :

(a) 30000π Am^{-1} (b) 3π Am^{-1}

(c) 30000 Am^{-1} (d) 300 Am^{-1}

29. An iron rod of volume 10^{-3} m^3 and relative permeability 1000 is placed as core in a solenoid with 10 turns/cm. If a current of 0.5 A is passed through the solenoid, then the magnetic moment of the rod will be :

(a) 50×10^2 Am^2 (b) 5×10^2 Am^2

(c) 500×10^2 Am^2 (d) 0.5×10^2 Am^2

30. A paramagnetic sample shows a net magnetisation of 6 A/m when it is placed in an external magnetic field of 0.4 T at a temperature of 4 K. When the sample is placed in an external magnetic field of 0.3 T at a temperature of 24 K, then the magnetisation will be :

(a) 1 A/m (b) 4 A/m (c) 2.25 A/m (d) 0.75 A/m

31. A perfectly diamagnetic sphere has a small spherical cavity at its centre, which is filled with a paramagnetic substance. The whole system is placed in a uniform magnetic field $\vec{B}$. Then the field inside the paramagnetic substance is :

(a) $\vec{B}$

(b) zero

(c) much large than $|\vec{B}|$ and parallel to $\vec{B}$

(d) much large than $|\vec{B}|$ but opposite to $\vec{B}$

32. Magnetic materials used for making permanent magnets (P) and magnets in a transformer (T) have different properties of the following, which property best matches for the type of magnet required?

(a) T : Large retentivity, small coercivity

(b) P : Small retentivity, large coercivity

(c) T : Large retentivity, large coercivity

(d) P : Large retentivity, large coercivity

33.

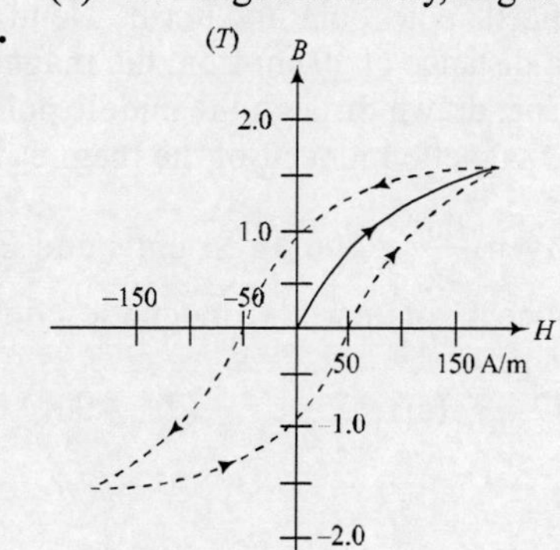

The figure gives experimentally measured B vs. H variation in a ferromagnetic material. The retentivity, co-ercivity and saturation, respectively, of the material are:
(a) 1.5 T, 50 A/m and 1.0 T
(b) 1.5 T, 50 A/m and 1.0 T
(c) 150 A/m, 1.0 T and 1.5 T
(d) 1.0 T, 50 A/m and 1.5 T

34. A paramagnetic material has 10^{28} atoms/m^3. Its magnetic susceptibility at temperature 350 K is 2.8×10^{-4}. Its susceptibility at 300 K is:
(a) 3.267×10^{-4} (b) 3.672×10^{-4}
(c) 3.726×10^{-4} (d) 2.672×10^{-4}

35. A paramagnetic substance in the form of a cube with sides 1 cm has a magnetic dipole moment of 20×10^{-6} J/T when a magnetic intensity of 60×10^3 A/m is applied. Its magnetic susceptibility is:
(a) 3.3×10^{-2} (b) 4.3×10^{-2}
(c) 2.3×10^{-2} (d) 3.3×10^{-4}

36. At some location on earth the horizontal component of earth's magnetic field is 18×10^{-6} T. At this location, magnetic needle of length 0.12 m and pole strength 1.8 Am is suspended from its mid-point using a thread, it makes 45° angle with horizontal in equilibrium. To keep this needle horizontal, the vertical force that should be applied at one of its ends is:
(a) 3.6×10^{-5} N (b) 1.8×10^{-5} N
(c) 1.3×10^{-5} N (d) 6.5×10^{-5} N

37. A bar magnet is demagnetized by inserthing it inside a solenoid of length 0.2 m, 100 turns, and carrying a current of 5.2 A. The coercivity of the bar magnet is:
(a) 285 A/m (b) 2600 A/m
(c) 520 A/m (d) 1200 A/m

38. The B-H curve for a ferromagnet is shown in the figure. The ferromagnet is placed inside a long solenoid with 1000 turns/cm.. The current that should be passed in the solenoid to demagnetise the ferromagnet completely is:
(a) 2 mA
(b) 1 mA
(c) 40 μA
(d) 20 μA

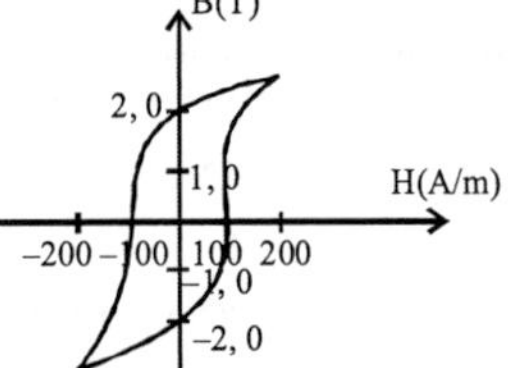

39. A short bar magnet is placed in the magnetic meridian of the earth with north pole pointing north. Neutral points are found at a distance of 30 cm from the magnet on the East – West line, drawn through the middle point of the magnet. The magnetic moment of the magnet in Am^2 is close to: (Given $\frac{\mu_0}{4\pi} = 10^{-7}$ in SI units and B_H =Horizontal component of earth's magnetic field = 3.6×10^{-5} tesla)
(a) 14.6 (b) 19.4 (c) 9.7 (d) 4.9

40. An example of a perfect diamagnet is a superconductor. This implies that when a superconductor is put in a magnetic field of intensity B, the magnetic field B_s inside the superconductor will be such that:
(a) $B_s = -B$ (b) $B_s = 0$
(c) $B_s = B$ (d) $B_s < B$ but $Bs \neq 0$

41. Three identical bars A, B and C are made of different magnetic materials. When kept in a uniform magnetic field, the field lines around them look as follows:

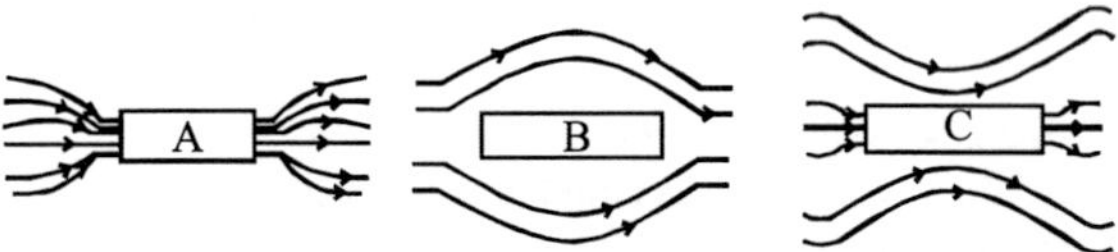

Make the correspondence of these bars with their material being diamagnetic (D), ferromagnetic (F) and paramagnetic (P):
(a) $A \leftrightarrow D, B \leftrightarrow P, C \leftrightarrow F$
(b) $A \leftrightarrow F, B \leftrightarrow D, C \leftrightarrow P$
(c) $A \leftrightarrow P, B \leftrightarrow F, C \leftrightarrow D$
(d) $A \leftrightarrow F, B \leftrightarrow P, C \leftrightarrow D$

42. The mid points of two small magnetic dipoles of length d in end-on positions, are separated by a distance x, (x >> d). The force between them is proportional to x^{-n} where n is:

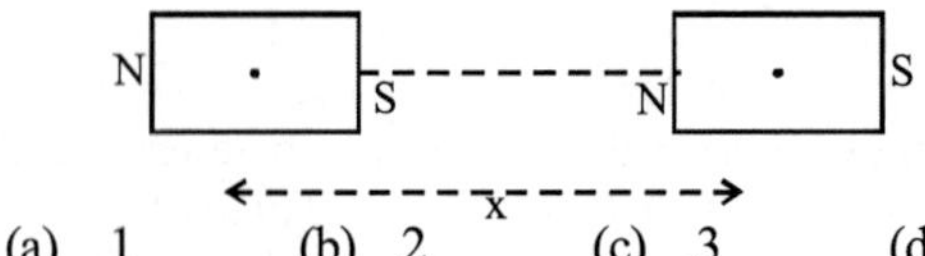

(a) 1 (b) 2 (c) 3 (d) 4

43. A ring is hung on a nail. It can oscillate, without slipping or sliding (i) in its plane with a time period T_1 and, (ii) back and forth in a direction perpendicular to its plane, with a period T_2. The ratio $\frac{T_1}{T_2}$ will be :
(a) $\frac{2}{\sqrt{3}}$ (b) $\frac{2}{3}$ (c) $\frac{3}{\sqrt{2}}$ (d) $\frac{\sqrt{2}}{3}$

44. A magnetic compass needle oscillates 30 times per minute at a place where the dip is 45°, and 40 times per minute where the dip is 30°. If B_1 and B_2 are respectively the total magnetic field due to the earth and the two places, then the ratio B_1/B_2 is best given by :
(a) 1.8 (b) 0.7 (c) 3.6 (d) 2.2

45. A hoop and a solid cylinder of same mass and radius are made of a permanent magnetic material with their magnetic moment parallel to their respective axes. But the magnetic moment of hoop is twice of solid cylinder. They are placed in a uniform magnetic field in such a manner that their magnetic moments make a small angle with the field. If the oscillation periods of hoop and cylinder are T_h and T_c respectively, then:
(a) $T_h = T_c$ (b) $T_h = 2\,T_c$
(c) $T_h = 1.5\,T_c$ (d) $T_h = 0.5\,T_c$

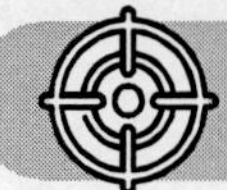

Hints & Solutions

20.1 Concept Practice Problems

1. (b) $L_e = \frac{5}{6} L_g$
2. (a) (A)→3; (B)→4; (C)→2; (D)→1
3. (d) 4. (a)
5. (c) Work done $W = MB_H (1 - \cos\theta)$
$= 20 \times 0.3(1 - \cos 30°) = 6\left(1 - \frac{\sqrt{3}}{2}\right) = 3(2 - \sqrt{3})$
6. (c) $\tau = MB \sin\theta = m \times (2\ell) \times B \sin\theta$
$= 10^{-4} \times 0.1 \times 30 \sin 30° = 1.5 \times 10^{-4}\ Nm$
7. (b) Magnetic intensity on end side -on position is twice than broad side on position.
8. (d) $F = k\frac{m_1 m_2}{r^2}$
9. (a) As $BI = \mu_0 MI_M = \mu_0(I + I_M)$
Here, $I = 0$
Then $\mu_0 MI = \mu_0(I_M)$
$\Rightarrow\ I_M = MI = 10^6 \times 0.1^3\ 10^{-5}$ A
10. (b) The total magnetic moment per unit volume.
$= \frac{(8.52\times10^{28})\times(2\times9.27\times10^{-24})}{1} = 1.58 \times 10^6$ A/m

20.2 Concept Practice Problems

11. (c) Near the magnetic poles H = 0
12. (a) For paramagnetic substance magnetization M is proportional to magnetising field H, and M is positive.
13. (d)
14. (d) Materials suitable for permanent magnets should have high retentivity, high coercivity and high permeability.
15. (b) 16. (a)
17. (a) $\tan\theta = \frac{H_0}{H} \Rightarrow \theta = \tan^{-1}\left(\frac{H_0}{H}\right)$
18. (a) The volume of the cube is
$V = (10^{-6}\ m)^3 = 10^{-18}\ m^3$
Net dipole moment $m_{net} = 8 \times 10^{10} \times 9 \times 10^{-24}\ Am^2$
$= 72 \times 10^{-14}\ Am^2$
Intensity of magnetization is magnetic moment developed per unit volume.
$\therefore$ magnetization, $M = \frac{m_{net}}{volume}$
$= \frac{72\times10^{-14}\ A\ m^2}{10^{-18}\ m^3} = 72\times10^4\ A\ m^{-1} = 7.2 \times 10^5\ Am^{-1}$
19. (b) We know that
$\frac{B}{B_H} = \tan q$ or $B = B_H \tan\theta = 0.34 \times 10^{-4} \tan 30°$
$= 1.96 \times 10^{-5}$ T
20. (c) The volume of the needle,
$V = (3 \times 10^{-2}) \times (1 \times 10^{-3}) \times (0.5 \times 10^{-3}) = 1.5 \times 10^{-8}\ m^3$
The mass of the needle = ρV
$= 7900 \times 1.5 \times 10^{-8}$
$= 1.183 \times 10^{-4}$ kg
The number of atoms in the needle
$= \left[\frac{1.185\times10^{-4}}{56\times10^{-3}}\right]\times6.02\times10^{23}$
$= 1.27 \times 10^{21}$
The needle's dipole moment
$M = \frac{1}{10}(1.27\times10^{21})\times(2.1\times10^{-23})$
$= 2.7 \times 10^{-3}$ J/T

Exercise 1 - Chapter Revision Problems

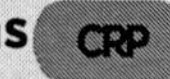

1. (b) 2. (a) 3. (d) 4. (a) 5. (d)
6. (d) As $F \propto \frac{1}{r^4}$ and r becomes twice, therefore, F becomes $\frac{1}{2^4} = \frac{1}{16}$ times
$\therefore\ \frac{1}{16}\times 8 = 0.5$ N.
7. (d) As magnetic moment = pole strength x length and length is halved without affecting pole strength, therefore, magnetic moment becomes half.
8. (d) A superconductor exhibits perfect diamagnetism.
9. (a) $\frac{\tan\theta_1}{\tan\theta_2} = \frac{2}{1}$
10. (a) Iron is ferromagnetic.
11. (b) Ferromagnetic substance has magnetic domains whereas paramagnetic substances have magnetic dipoles which get attracted to a magnetic field.
Diamagnetic substances do not have magnetic dipole but in the presence of external magnetic field due to their orbital motion these substance are repelled.
12. (c) $T_1 = 2\pi\sqrt{\frac{K_1 + K_2}{(M + 2M)H}} = 2\pi\sqrt{\frac{K}{3MH}}$
$T_2 = 2\pi\sqrt{\frac{K}{(2M - M)H}} = 2\pi\sqrt{\frac{K}{MH}}$
Obviously $T_2 > T_1$
13. (b) $\tan\theta = \frac{B_V}{B_H} = 1, B_V = B_H$
$\theta = \tan^{-1}(1) = 45°$
14. (c) χ_m is negative for diamagnetic materials.
15. (c) We know that when a bar magnet is placed in the magnetic field at an angle θ, then torque acting on the bar magnet

$(\tau) = MB\sin\theta = \vec{M}\times\vec{B}$

Note : This torque τ has a tendency to make the axis of the magnet parallel to the direction of the magnetic field.

16. (a) Magnetic moment linked with one turn = iA
Magnetic moment linked with N turn
= iNA amp-m^2.
Here A = Area of current loop.

17. (b) A diamagnetic material in a magnetic field moves, from stronger to the weaker parts of the field.

18. (b) According to Curie's law, $\chi_m \propto \frac{1}{T}$

19. (a) The magnetic moment of a diamagnetic atom is equal to zero.

20. (a) A → diamagnetic B → paramagnetic
C → Ferromagnetic D → Non-magnetic

21. (a) Here, $2\ell = 8\,\text{cm},\ \ell = 4\,\text{cm},\ d = \frac{6}{2} = 3\,\text{cm}.$

At neutral point,

$$H = B = \frac{\mu_0}{4\pi}\frac{M}{(d^2+\ell^2)^{3/2}}$$

$$= 10^{-7}\frac{M}{(5\times10^{-2})^3} = \frac{M}{1250}$$

$$\therefore\ M = 1250\,H = 1250\times3.2\times10^{-5}\ \text{Am}^2$$

$$m = \frac{M}{2\ell} = \frac{1250\times3.2\times10^{-5}}{8\times10^{-2}}\text{A m.}$$

$$= 0.5\ \text{Am} = 0.5\times\frac{1}{10}\text{ab amp}\times100\ \text{cm}$$

$$= 5\ \text{ab-amp cm.}$$

22. (a) $F = \frac{\mu_0}{4\pi}\frac{m_1 m_2}{r^2} = 10^{-7}\times\frac{30\times60}{(0.3)^2} = 2\times10^{-3}\,\text{N}.$

23. (b) $\tau = MB\sin\theta = 0.1\times3\times10^{-4}\sin30°$
or $\tau = 1.5\times10^{-5}$ N–m.

24. (d) As $\frac{i_2}{i_1} = \frac{\tan\theta_2}{\tan\theta_1}$

25. (b)

26. (b) According to Curie's law, $\chi_m = \frac{\mu_0 C}{T}$
where C is Curie constant, T = temperature

$$\therefore \chi_m \alpha \frac{1}{T}$$

$$\frac{\chi_{m_1}}{\chi_{m_2}} = \frac{T_2}{T_1} = \frac{273+333}{273+30} = \frac{606}{303} = 2$$

$$\therefore \chi_{m_2} = \chi_{m_1}/2 = 0.5\chi_{m_1} = 0.5\chi.\left(\because \chi_{m_1} = \chi\right)$$

27. (a) As lines of magnetic induction B are continuous curves, they run continuously through the bar and outside, as shown in Fig. (1).

28. (c) The loop (i) is for soft iron and the loop (ii) is for steel in Fig.

29. (b) As breadth of each part is half the original breadth, therefore, pole strength becomes half (i.e. m/2).

30. (a) As length of each part also becomes half, therefore magnetic moment M = pole strength × length

$$\Rightarrow \frac{1}{2}\times\frac{1}{2} = \frac{1}{4}\text{th i.e. M/4.}$$

31. (c) Taking distances from the centre of the magnet,

$$\frac{B_1}{B_2} = \left(\frac{x_2}{x_1}\right)^3 = \left(\frac{2x+1}{x+1}\right)^3 = 8:1,\ \text{approximately.}$$

32. (b) $\frac{T_2^2}{T_1^2} = \frac{2M+M}{2M-M} = 3 \quad \therefore\ T_2 = T_1\sqrt{3} = 3\sqrt{3}\,\text{s.}$

33. (b) Here, $d_1 = 20$ cm, $M_2 = 2M_1$, $d_2 = ?$

$$\frac{M_2}{M_1} = \frac{d_2^3}{d_1^3} = 2 \Rightarrow d_2 = 2^{1/3}d_1 = 20(2)^{1/3}\ \text{cm}$$

34. (d) Here, $T_1 = \frac{60}{12} = 5\,\text{s},\ T_2 = \frac{60}{4} = 15\,\text{s}$

$$\frac{M_1}{M_2} = \frac{T_2^2+T_1^2}{T_2^2-T_1^2} = \frac{15^2+5^2}{15^2-5^2} = \frac{250}{200} = \frac{5}{4}$$

35. (c) $T_1 = 2\pi\sqrt{\frac{I}{HM}}$,

$$T_2 = 2\pi\sqrt{\frac{I}{(H+F)M}}$$

$$\frac{T_1^2}{T_2^2} = \frac{H+F}{H} = \frac{T^2}{T^2/4} = \frac{4}{1} \Rightarrow H+F = 4H \Rightarrow 3H = F$$

36. (a) $\mu = \mu_0\mu_r = (4\pi\times10^{-7})\times2000 = 8\pi\times10^{-4}$ S.I. units

37. (b) Let pole strength = m
So, $M = m\ell$
When wire is in form of arc, then the distance between poles $= \frac{2\ell}{\pi}$

So, $M' = \frac{m2\ell}{\pi} = \frac{2M}{\pi}$

38. (a) Magnetic moment is cancelled and $\mu_{net} = 0$.

39. (c) $M_{net} = \sqrt{M_0^2+M_0^2+2M_0^2\cos60°}$

$$= \sqrt{3M_0^2} = \sqrt{3}M_0$$

40. (c) $n = \frac{1}{2\pi}\sqrt{\frac{MB}{I}}$
When it is turned by an angle 90° the effective field is vertical = V and B > V
So, new frequency < n.

41. (b) $T = 2\pi\sqrt{\frac{I}{MB}}$

$$I = \frac{m}{2}\left(\frac{\ell}{2}\right)^2 \Rightarrow I' = \frac{I}{8}$$

$$M' = \frac{M}{2}$$

So, $T' = 2\pi\sqrt{\frac{I}{4MB}} \Rightarrow T' = \frac{T}{2} = 2\ \text{sec}.$

42. (b) Magnetic moment, $M = m\ell$

$\frac{M}{\ell} = m$, where m is the polestrength.

Therefore distance between poles

$= \sqrt{(\ell/2)^2 + (\ell/2)^2} = \frac{\ell}{\sqrt{2}}$

So, $M' = \frac{m\ell}{\sqrt{2}} = \frac{M}{\sqrt{2}}$

43. (c) $\frac{T_2}{T_1} = \sqrt{\frac{M_1}{M_2}} = \sqrt{\frac{M_1}{\frac{1}{4}M_1}} = 2$

$\therefore T_2 = 2T_1 = 3\text{ s}$

44. (b) Field in the core with Bismuth will be smaller because bismuth is diamagnetic.

45. (b) For a diamagnetic material, the value of μ_r is less than one.

For any material, the value of ϵ_r is always greater than 1.

46. (a) Magnetic moment = M; Initial angle through which magnet is turned $(\theta_1) = 90°$ and final angle which magnet is turned $(\theta_2) = 60°$. Work done in turning the magnet through

$90°(W_1) = MB(\cos 0° - \cos 90°) = MB(1-0) = MB.$

Similarly, $W_2 = MB(\cos 0° - \cos 60°)$

$= MB\left(1 - \frac{1}{2}\right) = \frac{MB}{2}.$

$\therefore W_1 = 2W_2$ or $n = 2$.

47. (b)

48. (d) Time period of a vibration magnetometer,

$T \propto \frac{1}{\sqrt{B}} \Rightarrow \frac{T_1}{T_2} = \sqrt{\frac{B_2}{B_1}}$

$\Rightarrow T_2 = T_1\sqrt{\frac{B_1}{B_2}}$

$= 2\sqrt{\frac{24\times10^{-6}}{6\times10^{-6}}} = 4\,s$

49. (b) Force on a charged particle is given by $F = qvB$. Here $v = 0$ and also resultant B is zero.

$\therefore$ Force = 0

50. (a) For stable equilibrium

$U = -MB = -(0.4)(0.16) = -0.064\text{ J}$

Exercise 2 - Exemplar & Past Year Questions E&PYQs

Exemplar Questions

1. (c) Toroid is a hollow circular ring on which a large number of turns of a wire are closely wound. Thus, in this case magnetic field is only confined inside the body of toroid. So no magnetic field outside the toroid and magnetic field only inside the toroid.

In case of toroid, the magnetic field is in the form of concentric magnetic lines of force and there is no magnetic field outside the body of toroid. This is because the loop encloses no current. Thus, the magnetic moment of toroid is zero.

In other case, if we take r as a large distance outside the toroid, then $m \propto \frac{1}{r^3}$. Which is not possible.

2. (a)

3. (d) We know that a permanent magnet is a substance which at room temperature retain ferromagnetic property for a long period of time. The individual atoms in a ferromagnetic material possess a dipole moment as in a paramagnetic material. However, they interact with one another in such a way that they spontaneously align themselves in a common direction over a macroscopic volume i.e., domain.

Hence, in a permanent magnet at room temperature, domains are all perfectly aligned.

4. (b) According to the Curie law, the intensity of magnetisation (I) is directly proportional to the magnetic field induction and inversely proportional to the temperature (t) in kelvin.

So, I magnetisation $\propto \frac{\text{B (magnetic field induction)}}{\text{t(temperature in kelvin)}}$

$\Rightarrow \frac{I_2}{I_1} = \frac{B_2}{B_1} \times \frac{t_1}{t_2}$ ... (i)

As given that : $I_1 = 8\text{ Am}^{-1}, I_2 = ?$

$B_1 = 0.6\text{ T}, t_1 = 4\text{K}$

$B_2 = 0.2\text{ T}, t_2 = 16\text{K}$

by putting the value of $B_1, B_2, t_1, t_2 I_1$ in equation (i)

So, $\frac{0.2}{0.6} \times \frac{4}{16} = \frac{I_2}{8}$

We get, $I_2 = 8 \times \frac{1}{12}$

$I_2 = \frac{2}{3}\text{ A/m}$

NEET/AIPMT (2013-2020) Questions

5. (a) Magnetic dipole moment

$M = m \times \ell \quad M' = m \times r$

From figure

$\ell = \frac{\pi r}{3}$ or $r = \frac{3\ell}{\pi}$

so, $M' = m \times r = \frac{m \times 3\ell}{\pi} = \frac{3}{\pi}M$

ℓ
r sin 30°
r sin 30°
r
30°
30°
60°

6. (b) $FL = MB\,(= \text{Torque}) \Rightarrow L = \frac{MB}{F}$

7. (a) Magnetic susceptibility χ for dia-magnetic materials only is negative and low $|\chi| = -1$; for paramagnetic substances low but positive $|\chi| = 1$ and for ferromagnetic substances positive and high $|\chi| = 10^2$.

8. (d) If θ_1 and θ_2 are opparent angles of dip

Let α be the angle which one of the plane make with the magnetic meridian.

$\tan\theta_1 = \frac{v}{H\cos\alpha}$

i.e., $\cos\alpha = \frac{v}{H\tan\theta_1}$ ...(i)

$\tan\theta_2 = \frac{v}{H\sin\alpha}$,

i.e., $\sin\alpha = \frac{v}{H\tan\theta_2}$ ...(ii)

Squaring and adding (i) and (ii), we get

$$\cos^2\alpha + \sin^2\alpha = \left(\frac{V}{H}\right)^2\left(\frac{1}{\tan^2\theta_1} + \frac{1}{\tan^2\theta_2}\right)$$

i.e., $1 = \frac{V^2}{H^2}\left[\cot^2\theta_1 + \cot^2\theta_2\right]$

or $\frac{H^2}{V^2} = \cot^2\theta_1 + \cot^2\theta_2$

i.e., $\cot^2\theta = \cot^2\theta_1 + \cot^2\theta_2$

9. (a) Rod gains gravitational potential energy which comes from energy of current source.
10. (c) As we know that the angle of dip is the angle between earth's resultant magnetic field from horizontal.

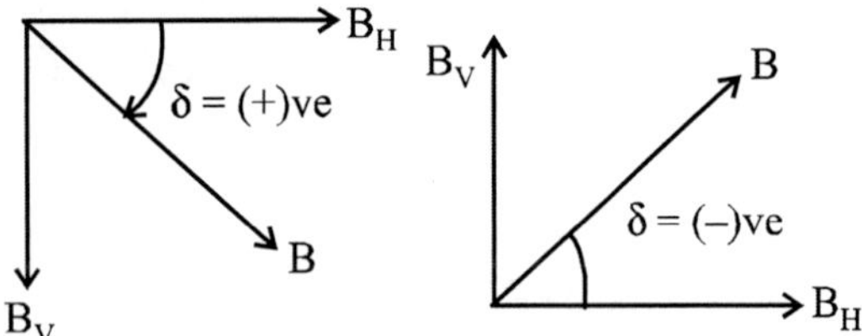

At equator, dip is zero. At Northern hemisphere, dip is positive. At southern hemisphere, dip is negative.

11. (d) Given : Magnetic susceptibility of iron, $\chi_m = 599$
Using, $\mu_r = 1 + \chi_m = 600$
$\mu = \mu_r\mu_0 = 600 \times 4\pi \times 10^{-7} = 2400\pi \times 10^{-7}$
Hence, permeability of the material of the rod,
$\mu = 2.4\pi \times 10^{-4}$ T m A^{-1}

Exercise 3 - Concept Application Problems CAP

1. (a) When cut along the axis, area of cross-section becomes half. Therefore, pole strength is halved and M = m (2 ℓ), is also halved.
2. (c) $T \propto \sqrt{I}$; $I \alpha M \Rightarrow T \alpha \sqrt{M}$

$$\frac{T_1}{T_2} = \sqrt{\frac{M_1}{M_2}} \Rightarrow T_2 = 2T_1 = 2T$$

3. (b) The iron can produces a magnetic screening for the equipment as lines of magnetic force can not enter iron enclosure.
4. (b) Diamagnetic substances do not have any unpaired electron. and they magnetised in direction opposite to that of magnetic field. Hence when they are brought to North or South pole of Bar magnet, they are repelled by poles.
5. (a) The magnetic dipole moment of diamagnetic material is zero as each of its pair of electrons have opposite spins, i.e., $\mu_d = 0$.

Paramagnetic substances have dipole moment > 0, i.e. $\mu_p \neq 0$, because of excess of electrons in its molecules spinning in the same direction.
Ferro-magnetic substances are very strong magnets and they also have permanent magnetic moment, i.e. $\mu_f \neq 0$.

6. (d) In series, same current flows through two tangent galvanometers.
7. (b) As the axes are perpendicular, mid point lies on axial line of one magnet and on equatorial line of other magnet.

$$\therefore B_1 = \frac{\mu_0}{4\pi}\frac{2M}{d^3} = \frac{10^{-7} \times 2 \times 1}{1^3} = 2 \times 10^{-7}$$

and $B_2 = \frac{\mu_0}{4\pi}\frac{M}{d^3} = 10^{-7}$

$\therefore$ Resultant field $= \sqrt{B_1^2 + B_2^2} = \sqrt{5} \times 10^{-7}$ T

8. (c)
9. (d) Angle of dip, $\delta = 45°$

$$\therefore \tan\delta' = \frac{\tan\delta}{\cos\theta} = \frac{\tan 45}{\cos 30°} = \frac{1}{\sqrt{3}/2} = \frac{2}{\sqrt{3}}$$

$\therefore$ Real dip $\delta' = \tan^{-1}(2/\sqrt{3})$

10. (a) $\frac{\tan\theta_2}{\tan\theta_1} = \frac{d_1^3}{d_2^3} = \frac{r^3}{[r(3)^{1/3}]^3} = \frac{1}{3}$

$\tan\theta_2 = \frac{1}{3}\tan\theta_1 = \frac{\tan 60}{3} = \frac{\sqrt{3}}{3} = \frac{1}{\sqrt{3}}$ $\therefore \theta_2 = 30°$

11. (a) $\tan\theta = \frac{V}{H}, \tan\theta' = \frac{V}{H\cos x}$; $\frac{\tan\theta'}{\tan\theta} = \frac{1}{\cos x}$
12. (d) $\delta_1 = 40°, \delta_2 = 30°, \delta = ?$

$$\cot\delta = \sqrt{\cot^2\delta_1 + \cot^2\delta_2}$$
$$= \sqrt{\cot^2 40° + \cot^2 30°}$$
$$\cot\delta = \sqrt{1.19^2 + 3} = 2.1$$

$\therefore \delta = 25°$ i.e. $\delta < 40°$.

13. (b) $W_1 = -MB(\cos 90° - \cos 0°) = MB$
$W_2 = -MB(\cos 60° - \cos 0°)$

$$= -MB\left(\frac{1}{2} - 1\right) = \frac{1}{2}MB = \frac{1}{2}W_1$$

As $W_1 = n W_2$ $\therefore n = 2$

14. (c) $\tan\delta = \frac{V}{H} = \frac{V}{\sqrt{3}V} = \frac{1}{\sqrt{3}}$

$\therefore \delta = 30° = \pi/6$ radian

15. (c) $\tau = MB\sin\theta$ $(\theta = 90°)$

$\tau = MB \Rightarrow \frac{B_1}{B_2} = \frac{\tau_1}{\tau_2}$ (since magnetic moment is same)

16. (c) $\frac{M_1}{M_2} = \frac{T_2^2 + T_1^2}{T_2^2 - T_1^2} = \frac{6^2 + 4^2}{6^2 - 4^2} = \frac{52}{20} = (2.6):1$
17. (d) The value of H is fairly uniform.

18. (b) From $\mu_r = 1 + \chi_m$;

Magnetic suscaptibility, $\chi_m = \mu_r - 1$

$\chi_m = 0.075 - 1 = -0.925.$

19. (a) Intensity of magnetisation

$$I_m = \frac{M}{V} = \frac{1.2}{(15 \times 2 \times 1)10^{-6}} = 4 \times 10^4 \text{ A m}^{-1}$$

20. (c) $B = \frac{H}{\cos\theta} = \frac{0.50}{\cos 30^\circ} = \frac{0.50 \times 2}{\sqrt{3}} = 1/\sqrt{3}$

21. (b)

22. (c) Here, $\theta = 30^\circ$, $\tau = 0.018$ N-m, $B = 0.06$ T

Torque on a bar magnet :

$\tau = MB\sin\theta$

$0.018 = M \times 0.06 \times \sin 30^\circ$

$\Rightarrow 0.018 = M \times 0.06 \times \frac{1}{2} \Rightarrow M = 0.6 \text{ A-m}^2$

Position of stable equilibrium ($\theta = 0^\circ$)

Position of unstable equilibrium ($\theta = 180^\circ$)

Minimum work required to rotate bar magnet from stable to unstable equilibrium

$\Delta U = U_f - U_i = -MB\cos 180^\circ - (-MB\cos 0^\circ)$

$W = 2MB = 2 \times 0.6 \times 0.06$

$\therefore W = 7.2 \times 10^{-2}$ J

23. (a) Given,

Moment of inertia of circular coil, $I = 0.8$ kg m^2

Magnetic moment of circular coil, $M = 20$ Am^2

Rotational kinetic energy of circular coil,

$\text{KE} = \frac{1}{2} I\omega^2$

Here, ω = angular speed of coil

Potential energy of bar magnet = – $MB\cos\phi$

From energy conservation

$\frac{1}{2} I\omega^2 = U_{in} - U_f = -MB\cos 60^\circ - (-MB)$

$\Rightarrow \frac{MB}{2} = \frac{1}{2} I\omega^2$

$\Rightarrow \frac{20 \times 4}{2} = \frac{1}{2}(0.8)\omega^2$

$\Rightarrow 100 = \omega^2 \Rightarrow \omega = 10$ rad

24. (b)

25. (c) Work done, W = 2 m·B

= 2 × 10^{-2} × 1 cos (0.125)

= 0.02 J

26. (c) Potential energy of dipole,

U = – pE cos θ

Torque experienced by dipole

τ = pE sin θ

Torque will be maximum (τ_{max}) when θ = 90° then potential energy U = 0

27. (b) We know that, magnetic dipole moment

$M = NiA\cos\theta$ i.e., $M \propto \cos\theta$

When two magnetic fields are inclined at an angle of 75° the equilibrium will be at 30°, so

$\cos\theta = \cos(75° - 30°) = \cos 45° = \frac{1}{\sqrt{2}}$

$\frac{x}{\sqrt{2}} = \frac{15}{2} \backslash\ x » 11$

28. (c) $\vec{M}$ (mag. moment/volume) = $\frac{NiA}{A\ell}$

$= \frac{Ni}{\ell} = \frac{(500)15}{25 \times 10^{-2}} = 30000 \text{ Am}^{-1}$

29. (b) Given,

Volume of iron rod, $V = 10^{-3}$ m^3

Relative permeability, $\mu_r = 1000$

Number of turns per unit length, $n = 10$

Magnetic moment of an iron core solenoid,

$M = (\mu_r - 1) \times NiA$

$\Rightarrow M = (\mu_r - 1) \times Ni\frac{V}{l} \Rightarrow M = (\mu_r - 1) \times \frac{N}{l} iV$

$\Rightarrow M = 999 \times \frac{10}{10^{-2}} \times 0.5 \times 10^{-3} = 499.5 \approx 500.$

30. (d)

31. (b) When magnetic field is applied to a diamagnetic substance, it produces magnetic field in opposite direction so net magnetic field inside the cavity of sphere will be zero. So, field inside the paramagnetic substance kept inside the cavity is zero.

32. (d) Permanent magnets (P) are made of materials with large retentivity and large coercivity. Transformer cores (T) are made of materials with low retentivity and low coercivity.

33. (d)

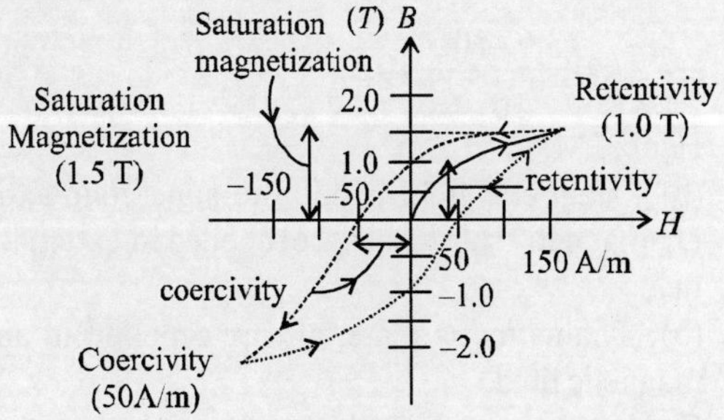

Saturation (T) B
magnetization
Saturation Magnetization (1.5 T)
2.0
1.0
–150
–50
50
150 A/m
H
–1.0
–2.0
Retentivity (1.0 T)
retentivity
coercivity
Coercivity (50A/m)

34. (a) According to Curie law for paramagnetic substance,

$\chi \propto \frac{1}{T_C} \Rightarrow \frac{\chi_1}{\chi_2} = \frac{T_{C_2}}{T_{C_1}}$

$\frac{2.8 \times 10^{-4}}{\chi_2} = \frac{300}{350}$

$\chi_2 = \frac{2.8 \times 350 \times 10^{-4}}{300} = 3.266 \times 10^{-4}$

35. (d) Magnetic susceptibility,

$\chi = \frac{I}{H}$

where, $I = \frac{\text{Magnetic moment}}{\text{Volume}} = \frac{20\times10^{-6}}{10^{-6}} = 20\ N/m^2$

Now, $\chi = \frac{20}{60\times10^3} = \frac{1}{3}\times10^{-3} = 3.3\times10^{-4}$

36. (d) using, MB sinθ = F ℓ Sinθ (τ)

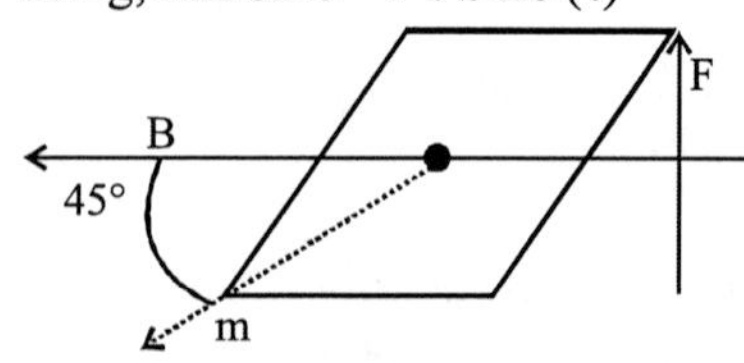

$MB\sin 45° = F\frac{\ell}{2}\sin 45°$

$F = 2MB = 2\times1.8\times18\times10^{-6} = 6.5\times10^{-5} N$

37. (b) Corecivity, $H = \frac{B}{\mu_0}$ and $B = \mu_0 ni\left(n = \frac{N}{\ell}\right)$

or, $H = \frac{N}{\ell}i = \frac{100}{0.2}\times5.2 = 2600\ A/m$

38. (b) Given Number of turns,
$n = 1000$ turns/cm $= 1000\times100$ turns/m
Coercivity of ferromagnet, H = 100 A/m
Current to demagnetise the ferromagnet, I = ?
Using, H = nI
or, $100 = 10^5\times I$

$\therefore\ I = \frac{100}{10^5} = 1\ mA$

39. (c) Here, r = 30cm = 0.3cm

we know $\frac{\mu_0 M}{4\pi r^3} = B_H = 3.6\times10^{-5}$

$\Rightarrow M = \frac{3.6\times10^{-5}}{10^{-7}}(0.3)^3$

Hence, $M = 9.7\ Am^2$

40. (b) Magnetic field inside the superconductor is zero. Diamagnetic substances are repelled in external magnetic field.

41. (b) Diamagnetic materials are repelled in an external magnetic field.
Bar *B* represents diamagnetic materials.

42. (d) In magnetic dipole

Force $\propto \frac{1}{r^4}$

In the given question,
Force $\propto x^{-n}$
Hence, n = 4

43. (a) Let I_1 and I_2 be the moment of inertia in first and second case respectively.

$I_1 = 2MR^2$

$I_2 = MR^2 + \frac{MR^2}{2} = \frac{3}{2}MR^2$

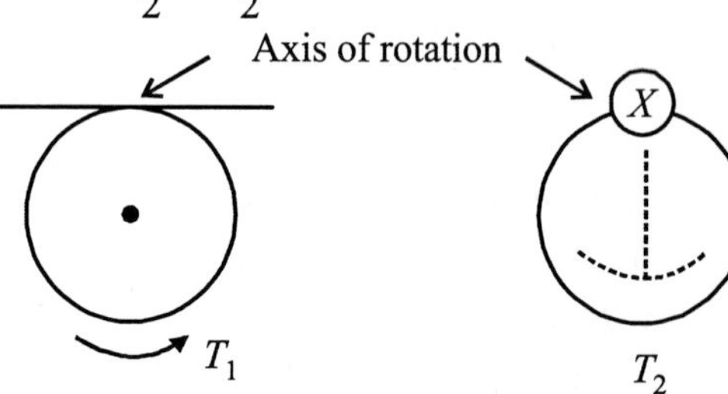

Time period, $T = 2\pi\sqrt{\frac{I}{mgd}}$

$T \propto I$

$\therefore \frac{T_1}{T_2} = \sqrt{\frac{I_1}{I_2}} = \sqrt{\frac{2MR^2}{\frac{3}{2}MR^2}} = \frac{2}{\sqrt{3}}$

44. (Bonus) We have, $T = 2\pi\sqrt{\frac{I}{MB_x}}$ $\therefore \frac{T_1^2}{T_2^2} = \frac{Bx_2}{Bx_1}$

or $\left(\frac{2}{1.5}\right)^2 = \frac{B_2\cos 45°}{B_1\cos 30°} = \frac{B_2\times2}{\sqrt{2}\times B_1\times\sqrt{3}}$

$\left(\frac{4}{3}\right)^2 = \frac{B_2}{B_1}\times\frac{2}{\sqrt{6}}$ $\therefore \frac{B_1}{B_2} = \frac{9}{8\sqrt{6}} = 0.46$

45. (a) Using, time /oscillation period,

$T = 2\pi\sqrt{\frac{I}{MB}}$

Where, M = magnetic moment, I moment of inertia and B = magnetic field

$T_h = 2\pi\sqrt{\frac{mR^2}{(2MB)}}$ and $T_c = 2\pi\sqrt{\frac{1/2mR^2}{MB}}$

Clearly, $T_h = T_c$

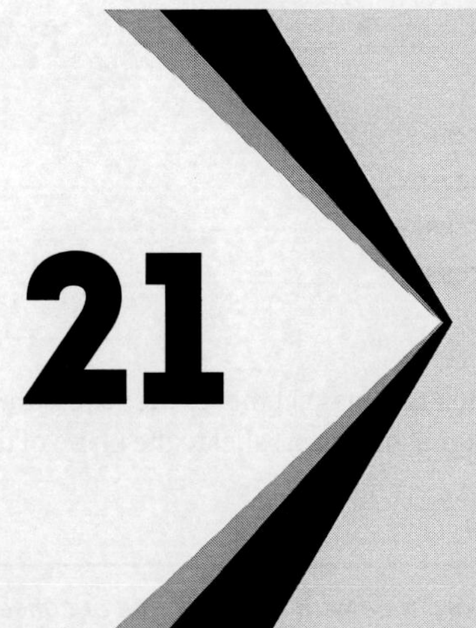

21 Electromagnetic Induction

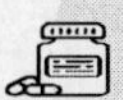

Topic 21.1 : The Experiments of Faraday & Henry, Magnetic Flux, Faraday's Law, Lenz's Law, Methods of Inducing EMF and Eddy Currents

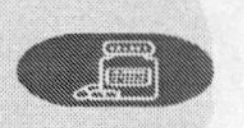

THE EXPERIMENTS OF FARADAY AND HENRY

The discovery and understanding of electromagnetic induction are based on a long series of experiments carried out by Faraday and Henry. These experiments are illustrated by the following figures.

When the bar magnet is pushed towards the coil, the pointer in the galvanometer G deflects.

Current is induced in coil C_1 due to motion of the current carrying coil C_2

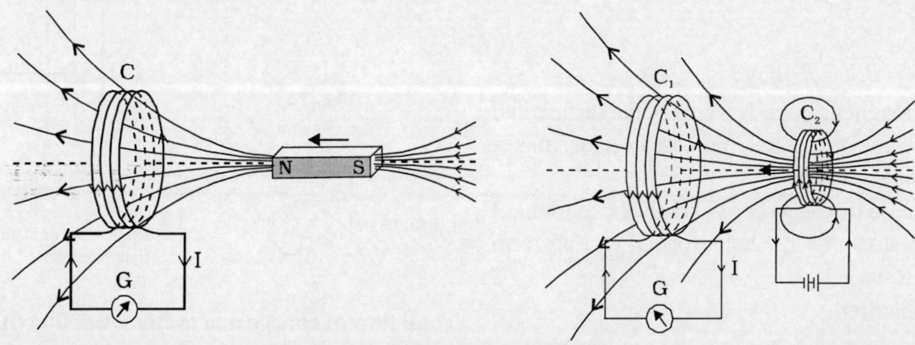

S. No.	Experiment	Observation	
1.	Place a magnet near a conducting loop with a galvanometer in the circuit.	No current flows through the galvanometer.	N S
2.	Move the magnet towards the loop.	The galvanometer register a current.	N S
3.	Reverse the direction of motion of the magnet.	The galvanometer deflection reverses.	N S
4.	Reverse the polarity of the magnet and move the magnet towards the loop.	The galvanometer deflection reverses.	S N
5.	Keep magnet fixed and move the coil towards the magnet.	The galvanometer register a current.	N S

6.	Increases the speed of the magnet.	The deflection in the galvanometer increases.
7.	Increase the strength of the magnet.	The deflection in the galvanometer increases.
8.	Increase the diameter of the coil.	The deflection in the galvanometer increases.
9.	Fix the speed of the magnet but repeat the experiment with the magnet closer to the coil.	The deflection in the galvanometer increases.
10.	Move the magnet at an angle to the plane of the coil.	Deflection decreases, it is maximum when the magnet moves perpendicular to the plane of the coil and is zero when the magnet moves parallel to the plane of the coil.
11.	Increase the number of turns of the coil.	Magnitude of current increases.

MAGNETIC FLUX

The number of magnetic lines of force crossing a surface is called magnetic flux linked with the surface.

It is represented by ϕ.

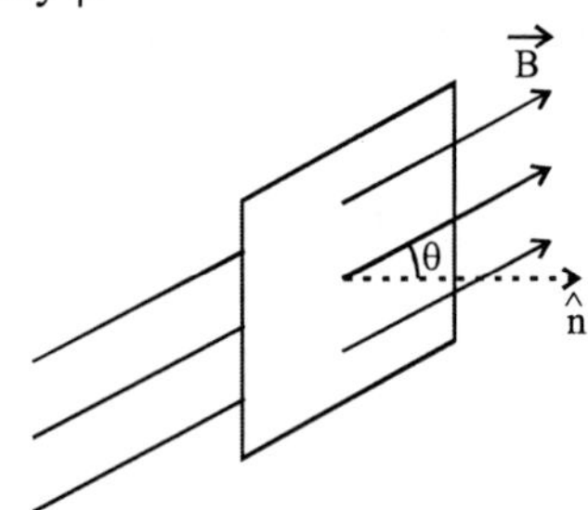

Magnetic flux $\phi = \vec{B}.\vec{A} = BA\cos\theta$

where B is strength of magnetic field, A is area of the surface and θ is the angle which normal to the area (unit area vector) makes with the direction of magnetic field.

The **S.I. unit** of magnetic flux is weber which is the amount of magnetic flux over an area of 1 m^2 held normal to a uniform magnetic field of one tesla.

The **c.g.s. unit** of ϕ is maxwell.

1 weber = 10^8 maxwell.

FARADAY'S LAW OF ELECTROMAGNETIC INDUCTION

Whenever the number of magnetic lines of force (flux) linked with any closed circuit change, an induced current flows through the circuit which lasts only so long as the change lasts. An increase in the number of lines of force produces an inverse current, while a decrease of such lines produces a direct current.

The induced emf is equal to the negative rate of change of magnetic flux.

i.e. $$e = \frac{-d\phi}{dt}$$

The -ve sign shows that the induced emf opposes the change in magnetic flux (Lenz's law).

LENZ'S LAW

The direction of induced e.m.f. is given by Lenz's law. According to this law, *the direction of induced e.m.f. in a circuit is always such that it opposes the every cause which produces it.*

Thus, $$e = \frac{-d\phi}{dt}$$

Lenz's law is in accordance with the principle of conservation of energy. Infact, work done in moving the magnet w.r.t. the coil changes into electric energy producing induced current.

There is also another law for finding the direction of induced current. This is **Fleming's right hand rule**. According to this rule, if *we stretch the right-hand thumb and two nearby fingers perpendicular to one another such that the first finger points in the direction of magnetic field and the thumb in the direction of motion of the conductor, then the middle finger will point in the direction of the induced current.*

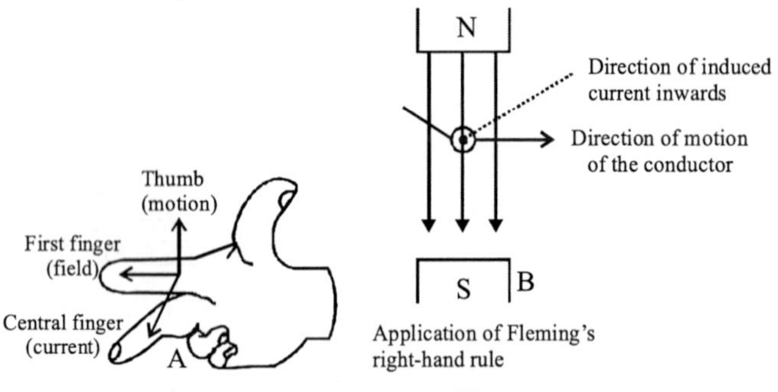

Total flow of charge due to change of flux ($\Delta\phi$):

$$Q = N\Delta\phi / R = \frac{(\text{No. of turns} \times \text{change in magnetic flux})}{\text{Resistance}}$$

METHODS OF INDUCING E.M.F.

As is known, e.m.f. is induced in a circuit only when amount of magnetic flux linked with the circuit changes. As $\phi = BA\cos\theta$, therefore **three methods of producing induced e.m.f. :**

(i) By changing B, (ii) By changing A and, (iii) By changing θ (orientation of the coil). When a conductor of length ℓ moves with a velocity v in a magnetic field of strength B so that magnetic flux linked with the circuit changes, the e.m.f. induced (ε) is given by

$$\varepsilon = B\ell v.$$

Induced e.m.f. and its direction

Case (i) **In conducting rod:** The induced e.m.f. is generated because of rotation of a conducting rod in a perpendicular magnetic field

$$e = -\frac{B\ell^2\omega}{2} \quad \text{also, } e = -BAf$$

where f = frequency of rotation and

$A = \pi r^2$, where r is the radius of circle in which this rod moves, hence $r = \ell$. ω = angular velocity, ℓ = length of conducting rod.

Case (ii) **In disc:** Induced e.m.f generated in a disc rotating with a constant angular velocity in a perpendicular magnetic field

$$e = -BAf = -B\pi r^2 f = -\frac{Br^2\omega}{2}$$

where A = area of disc = πr^2, r = radius of disc, ω = angular velocity of disc.

Case (iii) **In two coils:** When two coils are arranged as shown in the figure

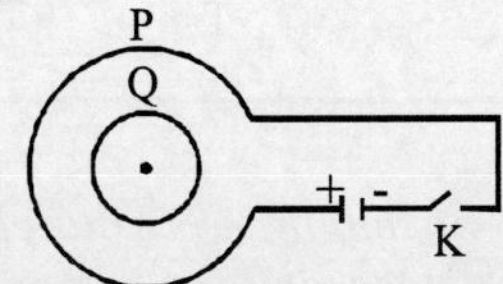

(a) if key K is closed then current in P will flow in clockwise direction and consequently induced current in Q will flow in anticlockwise direction. (see fig. a)

(b) when key K is opened then current in P falls from maximum to zero and consequently induced current in Q will flow in clockwise direction. (see fig. b)

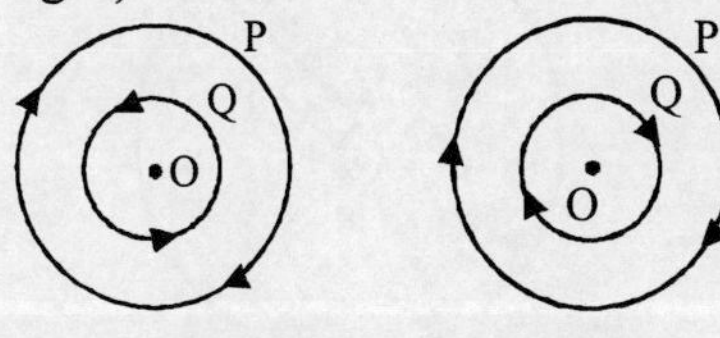

(a) (b)

Case (iv) **In three coils arranged coaxially :** Three coils P, Q and R are arranged coaxially as shown in figure. Equal currents are flowing in coils P and R . Coils Q and R are fixed. Coil P is moved towards Q. The induced current in Q will be in anti-clockwise direction so that it may oppose the approach of P according to Lenz's law. As the face of P towards Q is a south pole hence plane of Q towards P will also be a south pole.

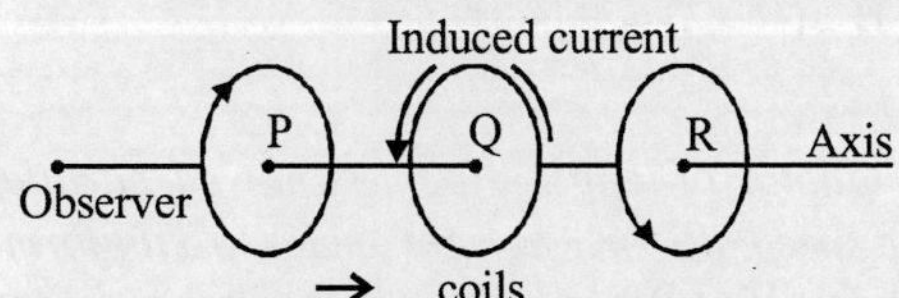

As there is no relative motion between Q and R, hence no current is induced in Q due to R.

Case (v) **Current increases in straight conductor :** When current in the straight conductor is increased then

(a) the direction of induced current in the loop will be clockwise so that it may oppose the increase of magnetic flux in the loop in downward direction.

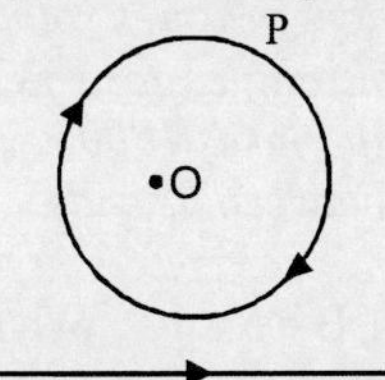

(b) the direction of induced current in the loop will be anti-clockwise so that it may oppose the increase of magnetic flux in the loop in upward direction.

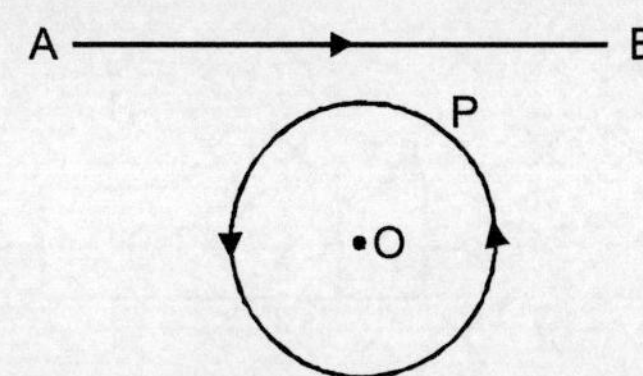

Case (vi) **Magnet dropped freely in long vertical copper tube:** The resistance of copper tube is quite negligible and hence maximum induced current are generated in it due to the motion of the magnet. Due to these induced current the motion of magnet is opposed to maximum. Consequently the acceleration of the magnet will be zero ($a = g - g = 0$).

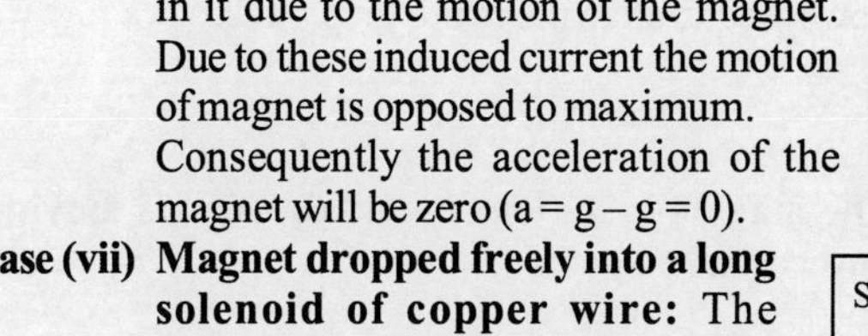

Case (vii) **Magnet dropped freely into a long solenoid of copper wire:** The resistance of copper solenoid is much higher than that of copper tube. Hence the induced current in it, due to motion of magnet, will be much less than that in the tube. Consequently the opposition to the motion of magnet will be less and the magnet will fall with an acceleration (a) less than g. (i.e. $a < g$).

Case (viii) **Motional EMF:** Induced emf in a conducting rod moving perpendicular through a uniform magnetic field as shown

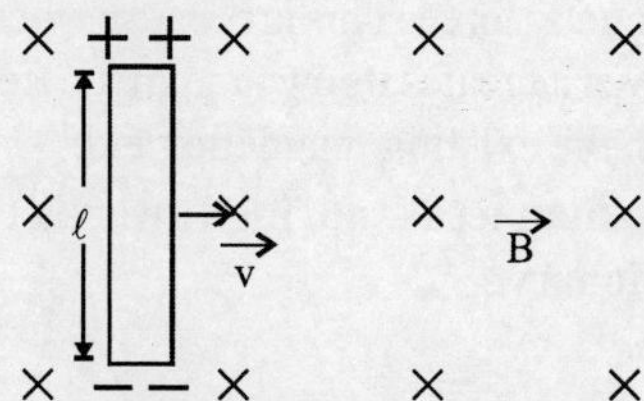

The induced emf produced across the rod

$$e = B\ell v = \int_0^{\ell} (\vec{v} \times \vec{B}).d\ell$$

This is also called motional emf and *it develops when a metal rod cuts magnetic lines of force.*

Special case : If the rod moves in the magnetic field making an angle θ with it, then induced emf $e = B_n v\ell = Bv\ell \sin\theta$.

MISCONCEPTION

✗ ***Incorrect.*** When there is no change in magnetic flux no induced current is produced.

✓ ***Correct.*** Consider the case (viii) discussed above. There is no change in the magnetic flux throgh the rod, still induced emf is produced.

Case (ix) A straight conductor (slider) moving with velocity v on a U shaped wire placed in a uniform magnetic field.

The induced current produced is $I = \frac{B\ell v}{R}$

Case (x) When a rectangular loop perpendicular to the magnetic field is pulled out, then forces $\overrightarrow{F_1}$ and $\overrightarrow{F_3}$ being equal and opposite cancel out.

$$F_2 = BI\ell = B\left(\frac{B\ell v}{R}\right)\ell = \frac{B^2\ell^2 v}{R}$$

Power required to move the loop out

$$P = F_2 \times v = \frac{B^2\ell^2 v^2}{R}$$

Case (xi) The magnet is stationary and the loop is moving towards the magnet.

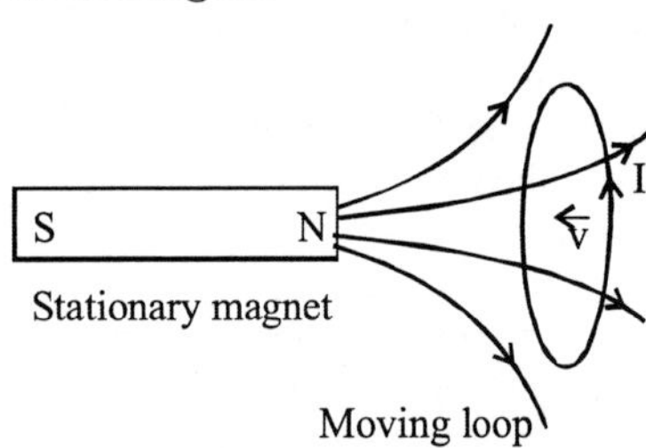

The induced emf or current I is shown which is in accordance to Lenz's law. In this case the magnetic force causes the charge to move. We know that if a charged particle is in motion in a field it experiences a magnetic force. This is because when charged particle moves it creates its own magnetic field which interacts with the existing magnetic field.

Case (xii) The magnet is moving towards the loop which is stationary.

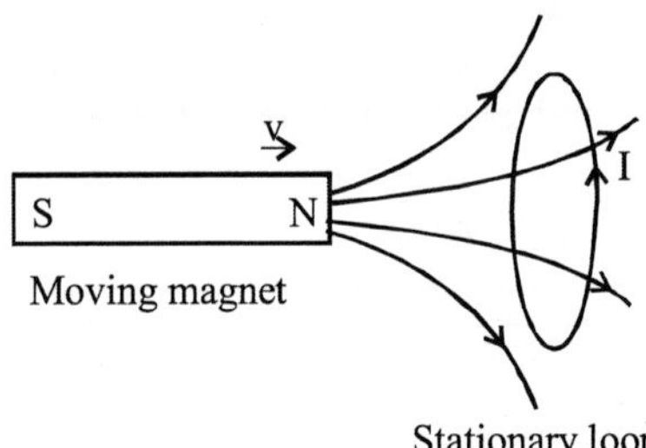

The induced emf or current I is shown which is in accordance to Lenz's law. Here the varying magnetic field at the location of loop (due to the movement of magnet) creates an electric field.

We should remember certain points regarding the induced electric field produced due to changing magnetic field.

- Induced electric field lines form closed loops (different from the electric field lines used to depict electric field produced due to charges)
- Induced electric field is non-conservative in nature (again a difference from the electric field produced by electric charges)

Mathematically, $e = \oint \vec{E}.\vec{dl} = -\frac{d\phi}{dt} \neq 0$

Note :

1. An emf is induced in a circuit where the magnetic flux is changing even if the circuit is open. But obviously no current will flow. If we close the circuit, the current will start flowing.
2. In a loop moving in a uniform magnetic field, when the loop remains in the field, the net emf induced is zero.

Example 1.

A copper rod of length ℓ is rotated about one end perpendicular to the uniform magnietic field B with constant angular velocity ω. What will be the induced e.m.f. between two ends ?

Solution :

Consider a small element of the rod of length dx at a distance x from the centre O.

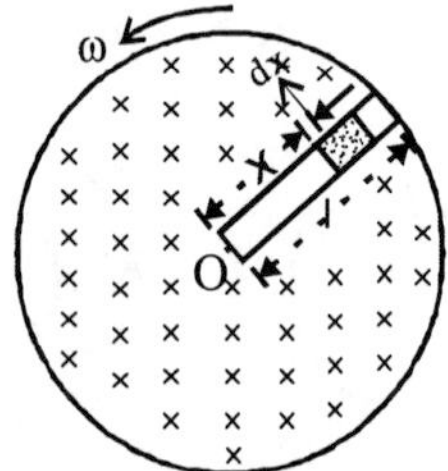

Let v be the linear velocity of the element at right angles to the magnetic field B. The e.m.f. developed across the element is $de = B\,v\,dx = B(\omega x)\,dx$ $(\because v = \omega x)$

The e.m.f. across the entire rod of length ℓ is given by

$$e = \int de = B\omega\int_0^{\ell} x\,dx = B\omega\left[\frac{x^2}{2}\right]_0^{\ell}$$

$$= B\omega(\ell^2/2) = \frac{1}{2}B\omega\ell^2$$

Example 2.

A conductor of length 10 cm is moved parallel to itself with a speed of 10 m/s at right angles to a uniform magnetic induction 10^{-4} Wb/m². *What is the induced e.m.f. in it?*

Solution :

Given : $\ell = 10\text{ cm} = 0.1\text{ m}, v = 10\text{ m/s}$

$B = 10^{-4}\text{ Wb/m}^2$

e.m.f. induced in conductor

$$e = B\ell V = 10^{-4} \times 0.1 \times 10 = 10^{-4}\text{ V}$$

Example 3.

A metal rod of length 1 m is rotated about one of its ends in a plane right angles to a field of inductance 2.5 × 10^{-3} Wb/m². If it makes 1800 revolutions/min. Calculate induced e.m.f. between its ends.

Solution :

Given : $\ell = 1\text{m}, B = 5 \times 10^{-3}\text{ Wb/m}^2$

$$f = \frac{1800}{60} = 30\text{ rotations/sec}$$

In one rotation, the moving rod of the metal traces a circle of radius $r = \ell$

$\therefore$ Area swept in one rotation $= \pi r^2$

$$\frac{d\phi}{dt} = \frac{d}{dt}(BA) = B.\frac{dA}{dt} = \frac{B\pi r^2}{T} = B f \pi r^2$$

$$= (5 \times 10^{-3}) \times 3.14 \times 30 \times 1 = 0.471 \text{ V}$$

$\therefore$ e.m.f. induced in a metal rod = 0.471 V

Example 4.

A coil having 100 turns and area 0.001 metre^2 is free to rotate about an axis. The coil is placed perpendicular to a magnetic field of 1.0 weber/metre^2. If the coil is rotate rapidly through an angle of 180°, how much charge will flow through the coil? The resistance of the coil is 10 ohm.

Solution :

The flux linked with the coil when the plane of the coil is perpendicular to the magnetic field is

$$\phi = nAB\cos\theta = nAB.$$

Change in flux on rotating the coil by 180° is

$$d\phi = nAB - (-nAB) = 2nAB$$

$$\therefore \text{ induced charge} = \frac{d\phi}{R}$$

$$= \frac{2nAB}{dt} = \frac{2 \times 100 \times 0.001 \times 1}{10}$$

$$= 0.01 \text{ coulomb}$$

Example 5.

Predict the direction of induced current in the situations described by the following fig. (1) to (5).

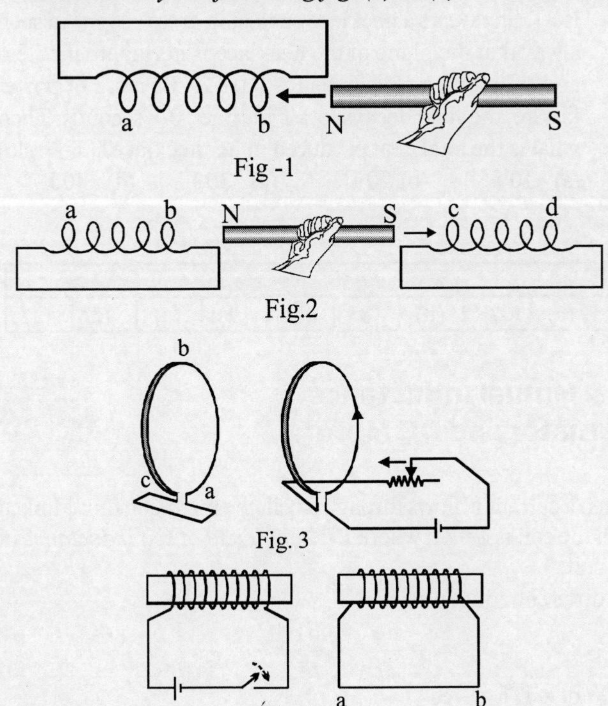

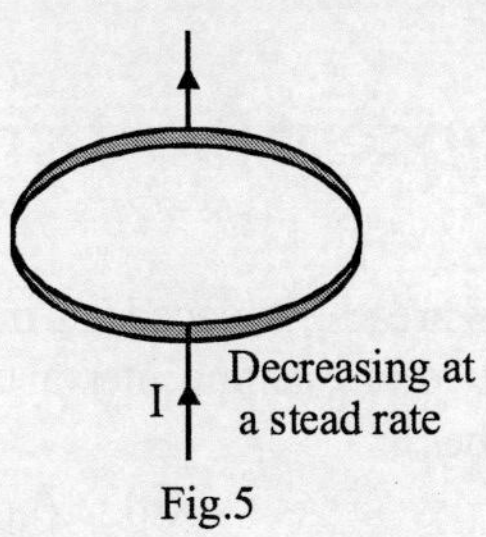

Fig.5

Solution :

Applying Lenz's law

Fig. (1) along $a \rightarrow b$

Fig. (2) along $b \rightarrow a$

Fig. (3) along $c \rightarrow a$

Fig. (4) along $a \rightarrow b$

Fig. (5) no induced current since field lines lie in the plane of the loop.

EDDY CURRENTS

The induced circulating currents produced in a metal itself due to change in magnetic flux linked with the metal are called eddy currents. These currents were discovered by Foucault, so they are also known as Foucault Currents.

The direction of eddy currents is given by Lenz's law.

Eddy currents produced in a metallic block moving in a non-uniform magnetic field is shown in fig.

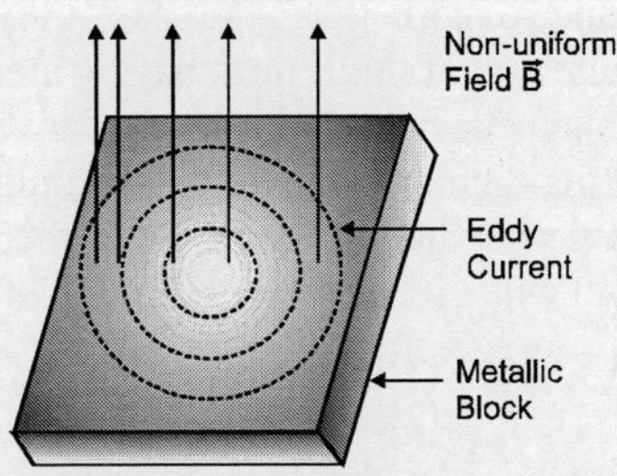

Applications of Eddy Current

Like friction, eddy currents are helpful in some fields and have to be increased, while in some other fields they are undesirable and have to be minimised.

(1) Dead beat galvanometer.
(2) Energy meter.
(3) Speedometer.
(4) Electric brakes.
(5) Single phase AC motor.
(6) Induction furnace.
(7) Diathermy

Note : In a moving coil galvanometer, damping is necessary to avoid oscillation of display needle. This is brought into practice with the help of eddy currents. The winding of the coil of galvanometer is done on a metallic frame. When the coil rotates the magnetic flux linked with the metallic frame changes due to which eddy currents are developed which oppose the rotation of the coil. This is called **dead beat galvanometer.**

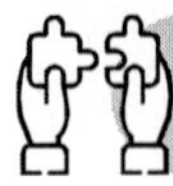

21.1 Concept Practice Problems

CPP

1. A coil having an area A_0 is placed in a magnetic field which changes from B_0 to 4 B_0 in time interval t. The e.m.f. induced in the coil will be
   (a) $3A_0 B_0/t$ (b) $4A_0 B_0/t$
   (c) $3B_0/A_0t$ (d) $4A_0/B_0t$
2. Eddy currents are produced when
   (a) a metal is kept in varying magnetic field
   (b) a metal is kept in steady magnetic field
   (c) a circular coil is placed in a magnetic field
   (d) through a circular coil, current is passed
3. An electron moves along the line PQ which lies in the same plane as a circular loop of conducting wire as shown in figure. What will be the direction of the induced current in the loop ?
   (a) Anticlockwise
   (b) Clockwise
   (c) Alternating
   (d) No current will be induced

   loop
   P Q
4. Induced emf in the coil depends upon
   (a) conductivity of coil
   (b) amount of flux
   (c) rate of change of linked flux
   (d) resistance of coil
5. A rectangular coil of single turn, having area A, rotates in a uniform magnetic field B with an angular velocity ω about an axis perpendicular to the field. If initially the plane of the coil is perpendicular to the field, then the average induced emf when it has rotated through 90° is
   (a) $\frac{\omega BA}{\pi}$ (b) $\frac{\omega BA}{2\pi}$ (c) $\frac{\omega BA}{4\pi}$ (d) $\frac{2\omega BA}{\pi}$
6. According to Faraday's law of electromagnetic induction
   (a) electric field is produced by time varying magnetic flux.
   (b) magnetic field is produced by time varying electric flux.
   (c) magnetic field is associated with a moving charge.
   (d) None of these
7. The magnetic flux across a loop of resistance 10Ω is given by $\phi = 5t^2 - 4t + 1$ weber. How much current is induced in the loop after 0.2 sec.
   (a) 0.4 A (b) 0.2 A (c) 0.04 A (d) 0.02 A
8. A metal rod moves at a constant velocity in a direction perpendicular to its length. A constant uniform magnetic field exists in space in a direction perpendicular to the rod as well its velocity. Select correct statements (s) from the following.
   (a) The entire rod is at the same potential
   (b) There is an electric field in the rod
   (c) The electric potential is highest at the centre
   (d) The electric potential is lowest at its centre and increases towards its ends
9. As a result of change in the magnetic flux linked to the closed loop shown in the figure, an e.m.f. V volt is induced in the loop. The work done (in joule) in taking a charge Q coulomb once along the loop is

   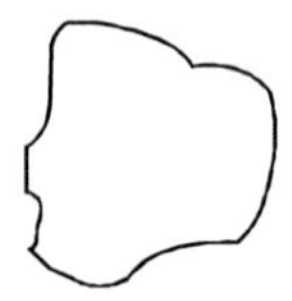

   (a) QV (b) 2QV (c) QV/2 (d) zero
10. A physicist works in a laboratory where the magnetic field is 2T. She wears a necklace enclosing area 0.01 m^2 in such a way that the plane of the necklace is normal to the field and is having a resistance R= 0.01 Ω. Because of power failure, the field decays to 1 T in time 10^{-3} seconds. Then what is the total heat produced in her necklace? (T= tesla)
    (a) 10 J (b) 20 J (c) 30 J (d) 40 J

ANSWER KEY

1	(a)	2	(a)	3	(a)	4	(c)	5	(d)	6	(a)	7	(b)	8	(b)	9	(a)	10	(a)

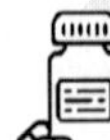

Topic 21.2 : Self Inductance & Mutual Inductance AC Generator/Dynamo/Alternator and DC Motor

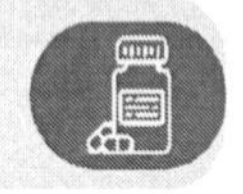

SELF INDUCTANCE AND MUTUAL INDUCTANCE

Self Inductance

The property of a coil by virtue of which the coil opposes any change in the strength of the current flowing through it, by inducing an e.m.f. in itself is called self inductance.

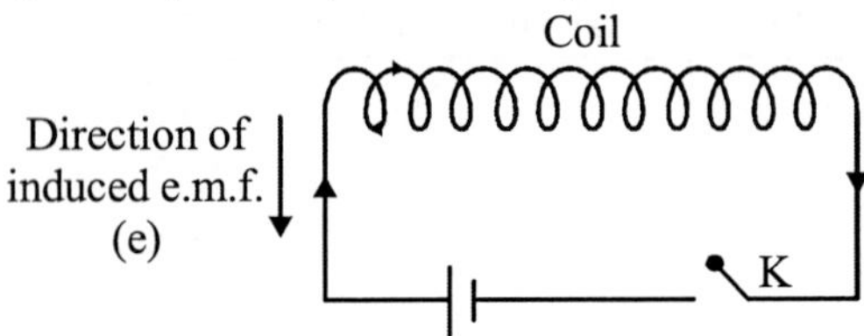

When a current I flows through a coil, the magnetic flux ϕ linked with the coil is $\phi = LI$, where *L is coefficient of self inductance* of the coil.

On differentiating, we get

$$\frac{d\phi}{dt} = L\frac{dI}{dt} = -e$$

If $dI/dt = 1$; $L = -e$.

Hence coefficient of *self inductance of a coil is equal to e.m.f. induced in the coil when rate of change of current through the same coil is unity.* Coefficient of self induction of a coil is also defined as the magnetic flux linked with a coil when 1 ampere current flows through the same coil.

The value of L depends on geometry of the coil and is given by $L = \frac{\mu_0 N^2 A}{\ell}$.

where ℓ is length of the coil (solenoid), N is total number of turns of solenoid and A is area of cross section of the solenoid.

The **S.I. unit** of L is henry. Coefficient of self induction of a coil is said to be one henry when a current change at the rate of 1 ampere/sec. in the coil induces an e.m.f. of one volt in the coil.

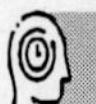

Problem Solving Tips

1. Energy stored in a coil (inductor) $= \frac{1}{2}Li^2$

   where L is the self-inductance and i current flowing through the inductor.

   The energy stored in the magnetic field of the coil.

   $$E = \frac{1}{2}Li^2 = \frac{1}{2}(\mu_0 n^2 A\ell)\left(\frac{B}{\mu_0 n}\right)^2$$

   $$= \left(\frac{B^2}{2\mu_0}\right)A\ell = \left(\frac{B^2}{2\mu_0}\right) \times \text{volume}$$

2. The self inductance is a measure of the coil to oppose the flow of current through it. The role of self-inductance in an electrical circuit is the same as that of the inertia in mechanics. Therefore it is called **electrical inertia**.
3. The magnetic energy density (energy stored per unit volume) in a solenoid $= \frac{B^2}{2\mu_0}$

Mutual Inductance

Mutual induction is the property of two coils by virtue of which each opposes any change in the strength of current flowing through the other by developing an induced e.m.f.

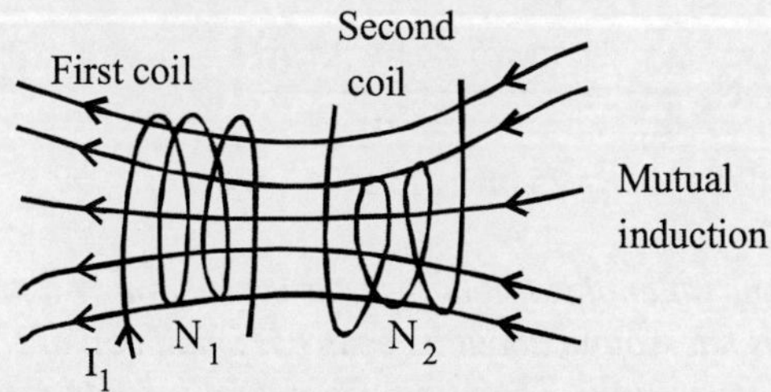

Coefficient of mutual inductance (M) of two coils is said to be one henry, when a current change at the rate of 1 ampere/sec. in one coil induces an e.m.f. of one volt in the other coil. The value of M depends on geometry of two coils, distance between two coils, relative placement of two coils etc.

The coefficient of mutual inductance of two long co-axial solenoids, each of length ℓ, area of across section A, wound on an air core is $M = \frac{\mu_0 N_1 N_2 A}{\ell}$] ...(1)

where N_1 and N_2 are total number of turns of the two solenoids. The mutual inductance M is defined by the equation

$$N_2\phi_2 = MI_1$$

where I_1 is the current in coil 1, due to which flux ϕ_2 is linked with each turn of secondary coil.

Now we can calculate, e.m.f. e_2 induced in secondary by a changing current in first coil. From Faraday's law

$$e_2 = -\frac{d}{dt}(N_2\phi_2) = -M\frac{dI_1}{dt}$$

If $\frac{dI_1}{dt} = 1 \Rightarrow e_2 = -M$ ...(2)

The two definitions for M defined by equations (1) and (2) are equivalent. We can express these two equations in words as :

(i) M is numerically equal to the flux-linkage in one circuit, when unit current flows through the other. (we use this definition to calculate M)

(ii) M is numerically equal to the e.m.f. induced in one circuit, when the current changes in the other at the rate of one ampere in each second. (it is used to describe the mutual behavior of two circuits).

For a pair of coils, $M_{12} = M_{21} = \mu_0 N_1 N_2 A/\ell$, when wound on one another.

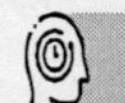

Problem Solving Tips

1. **Coefficient of self inductance of two coils in series** :

   L_1 L_2 $L_s = L_1 + L_2$

   The effective self inductance is $L_s = L_1 + L_2$

   If M is the coefficient of mutual inductance between the two coils when they have flux linkage in the same sense, then $L = L_1 + L_2 + 2M$

   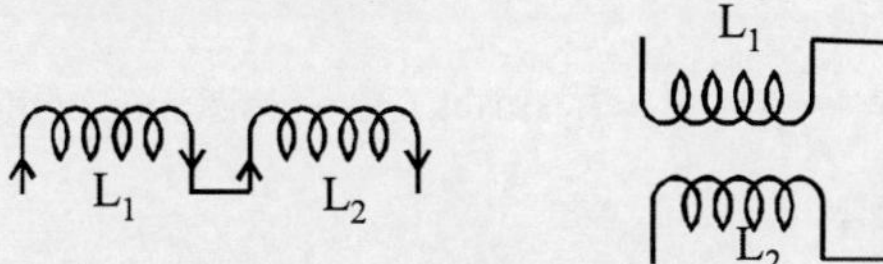

   And for flux linkage in opposite direction

   $$L = L_1 + L_2 - 2M$$

2. **Coefficient of self inductance of two coils in parallel :**

   L_1 L_2 $\equiv$ L_p

   $$\frac{1}{L_p} = \frac{1}{L_1} + \frac{1}{L_2}$$

(i) The coefficient of coupling between two coils having self inductance L_1 & L_2 and coefficient of mutual inductance M is

$$K = \frac{\pm M}{\sqrt{L_1 L_2}}$$

(ii) Generally the value of K is less than 1.

(iii) If K is 1, then the coupling of two coils is tight while if K < 1, then coupling is loose.

- Inductance is pure geometrical factor, and is independent of current or applied e.m.f.
- If the angle between the axis of two closely placed coil is θ then M ∝ cos θ.

AC GENERATOR/DYNAMO/ALTERNATOR

An electrical machine used to convert mechanical energy into electrical energy is known as AC generator/alternator or dynamo.

Principle : It works on the principle of electromagnetic induction, i.e., when a coil is rotated in uniform magnetic field, an induced emf is produced in it.

Working :

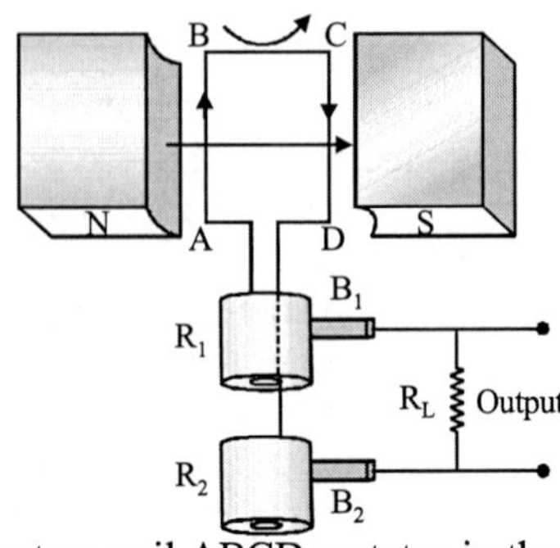

When the armature coil ABCD rotates in the magnetic field provided by the strong field magnet, it cuts the magnetic lines of force. Thus the magnetic flux linked with the coil changes and hence induced emf is set up in the coil. The direction of the induced emf or the current in the coil is determined by the Fleming's right hand rule.

The current flows out through the brush B_1 in one direction of half of the revolution and through the brush B_2 in the next half revolution in the reverse direction. This process is repeated. Therefore, emf produced is of alternating nature.

$$e = -\frac{Nd\phi}{dt} = NBA\omega \sin\omega t = e_0 \sin\omega t\text{ , where } e_0 = NBA\omega$$

$$I = \frac{e}{R} = \frac{e_0}{R}\sin\omega t = I_0 \sin\omega t\text{ , } R \to \text{resistance of the circuit}$$

DC MOTOR

A D.C. motor converts direct current energy from a battery into mechanical energy of rotation.

Principle : It is based on the fact that when a coil carrying current is held in a magnetic field, it experiences a torque, which rotates the coil.

Working :

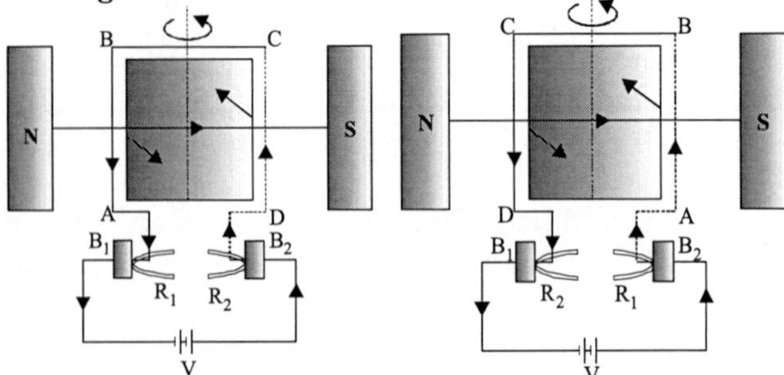

The battery sends current through the armature coil in the direction shown in fig. Applying Fleming's left hand rule, CD experiences a force directed inwards and perpendicular to the plane of the coil. Similarly, AB experiences a force directed outwards and perpendicular to the plane of the coil. These two forces being equal, unlike and parallel form a couple. The couple rotates the armature coil in the anticlockwise direction. After the coil has rotated through 180°, the direction of the current in AB and CD is reversed, fig. Now CD experiences an outward force and AB experiences an inward force. The armature coil thus continues rotating in the same i.e., anticlockwise direction.

Efficiency of the d.c. motor : Since the current I is being supplied to the armature coil by the external source of e.m.f. V, therefore,
Input electric power = VI
According to Joule's law of heating,
Power lost in the form of heat in the coil = $I^2 R$
If we assume that there is no other loss of power, then
Power converted into external work
i.e., Output mechanical power = $VI - I^2 R = (V - IR) I = EI$
$\therefore$ Efficiency of the d.c. motor

$$\eta = \frac{\text{Output mechanical power}}{\text{Input electric power}}$$

or $$\eta = \frac{EI}{VI} = \frac{E}{V} = \frac{\textit{Back e.m.f.}}{\textit{Applied e.m.f.}}$$

Uses of D.C Motor

1. The D.C. motors are used in D.C. fans (exhaust, ceiling or table) for cooling and ventilation.
2. They are used for pumping water.
3. Big D.C. motors are used for running tram-cars and even trains.

Example 6.

Two coils are wound on the same iron rod so that the flux generated by one also passes through the other. The primary has 100 loops and secondary has 200 loops. When a current of 2 A flows through the primary the flux in it is 25 x 10^{-4} Wb. Determine value of M between the coils.

Solution :

$$|e_s| = N_s \frac{d\phi_s}{dt} \text{ and } |e_s| = M\frac{di_p}{dt};$$

$$\therefore N_s \frac{d\phi_s}{dt} = M\frac{di_p}{dt} \quad \text{or}$$

$$M = N_s \frac{d\phi_s}{di_p} = \frac{200(2.5\times10^{-4} - 0)}{(2-0)}$$

$$= 2.5\times10^{-2} = 25\text{ mH}$$

Example 7.

A long solenoid of length L, cross section A having N_1 turns has wound about its centre is small coil of N_2 turns as shown in fig. Then find the mutual inductance of two circuits.

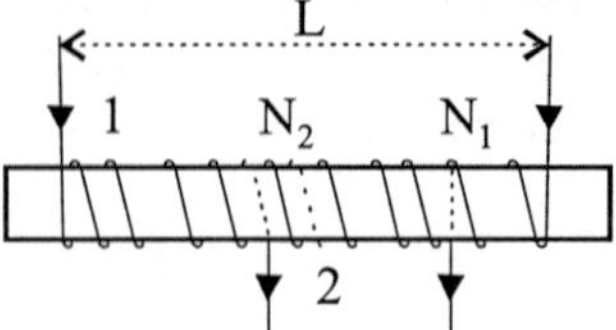

Solution :

Magnetic flux at the centre of solenoid $B_1 = \mu_0(N_1/L)i_1$

Magnetic flux through each turn of the coil of area A,

$$\phi_1 = B_1 A = \frac{\mu_0 N_1 i_1}{L} \times A$$

Magnetic flux linked with the coil of turns N_2,

$$\phi_2 = \phi_1 \times N_2 = \frac{\mu_0 N_1 N_2 i_1 A}{L}$$

According to the definition of mutual inductance $\phi_2 = Mi_1$

$$\therefore\ Mi_1 = \frac{\mu_0 N_1 N_2 i_1}{L} A \text{ or } M = \frac{\mu_0 N_1 N_2 A}{L}$$

Example 8.

A small coil of radius r is placed at the centre of a large coil of radius R, where R >>r. The two coils are coplanar. The mutual induction between the coils is proportional to

(a) r/R (b) r^2/R
(c) r^2/R^2 (d) r/R^2

Solution : (b)

Let I be the current flows in the large coil.

$\therefore$ Mag. field at the centre of coil $B = \frac{\mu_0 I}{2R}$

Mag. flux linked with smaller coil

$$\phi = \pi r^2 B = \pi r^2 \left(\frac{\mu_0 I}{2R}\right)$$

But $\phi = MI$ $\quad \therefore\ M = \frac{\phi}{I} = \frac{\pi r^2 \mu_0}{2R}$ or $M \propto r^2/R$

Example 9.

The mutual inductance of a pair of coils is 0.75 H. If current in the primary coil changes from 0.5 A to zero in 0.01 s find average induced e.m.f. in secondary coil.

Solution :

Given : $M = 0.75\text{ H}$ and $\frac{dI}{dt} = \frac{0.5-0}{0.01} = 50\text{ A/s}$

$\therefore$ Average induced e.m.f. in secondary coil,

$$e = M\frac{dI}{dt} = 0.75 \times 50 = 37.5\text{ V}$$

Example 10.

Find the self inductance of a coil in which an e.m.f. of 10 V is induced when the current in the circuit changes uniformly from 1 A to 0.5 A in 0.2 sec.

Solution :

Given : $e = 10\text{ V}$ and $\frac{dI}{dt} = \frac{1-0.5}{0.2} = \frac{0.5}{0.2} = 2.5\text{ A/s}$

Self inductance of coil $L = \frac{e}{dI/dt} = \frac{10}{2.5} = 4\text{ H}$

$\left[\because\ e = L\frac{dI}{dt} \text{ (Considering Magnitude only)}\right]$

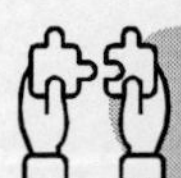

21.2 Concept Practice Problems CPP

11. If N is the number of turns in a coil, the value of self inductance varies as
(a) N^0 (b) N (c) N^2 (d) N^{-2}

12. An inductor may store energy in
(a) its electric field
(b) its coils
(c) its magnetic field
(d) both in electric and magnetic fields

13. The mutual inductance of a pair of coils, each of N turns, is M henry. If a current of I ampere in one of the coils is brought to zero in t second, the emf induced per turn in the other coil, in volt, will be
(a) $\frac{MI}{t}$ (b) $\frac{NMI}{t}$ (c) $\frac{MN}{It}$ (d) $\frac{MI}{Nt}$

14. Two solenoids of same cross-sectional area have their lengths and number of turns in ratio of 1 : 2. The ratio of self-inductance of two solenoids is
(a) 1 : 1 (b) 1 : 2 (c) 2 : 1 (d) 1 : 4

15. The back e.m.f. in a d.c. motor is maximum, when
(a) the motor has picked up max speed
(b) the motor has just started moving
(c) the speed of motor is still on the increase
(d) the motor has just been switched off

16. The mutual inductance between two coils depends on
(a) medium between the coils
(b) separation between the two coils
(c) orientation of the two coils
(d) All of the above

17. If coefficient of self induction of a coil is 1 H, an e.m.f. of 1V is induced, if
(a) current flowing is 1A
(b) current variation rate is 1 As^{-1}
(c) current of 1A flows for one sec.
(d) None of these

18. A small square loop of wire of side ℓ is placed inside a large square loop of side L (L >> ℓ). The loop are coplanar and their centres coincide. The mutual inductance of the system is proportional is
(a) $\frac{\ell}{L}$ (b) $\frac{\ell^2}{L}$ (c) $\frac{L}{\ell}$ (d) $\frac{L^2}{\ell}$

19. A wire loop is rotated in a uniform magnetic field about an axis perpendicular to the field. The direction of the current induced in the loop reverses once each
(a) quarter revolution (b) half revolution
(c) full revolution (d) two revolutions

20. If the number of turns per unit length of a coil of solenoid is doubled, the self-inductance of the solenoid will
(a) remain unchanged (b) be halved
(c) be doubled (d) become four times

ANSWER KEY

11	(c)	12	(c)	13	(a)	14	(b)	15	(a)	16	(d)	17	(b)	18	(b)	19	(b)	20	(d)

CONCEPT MAP

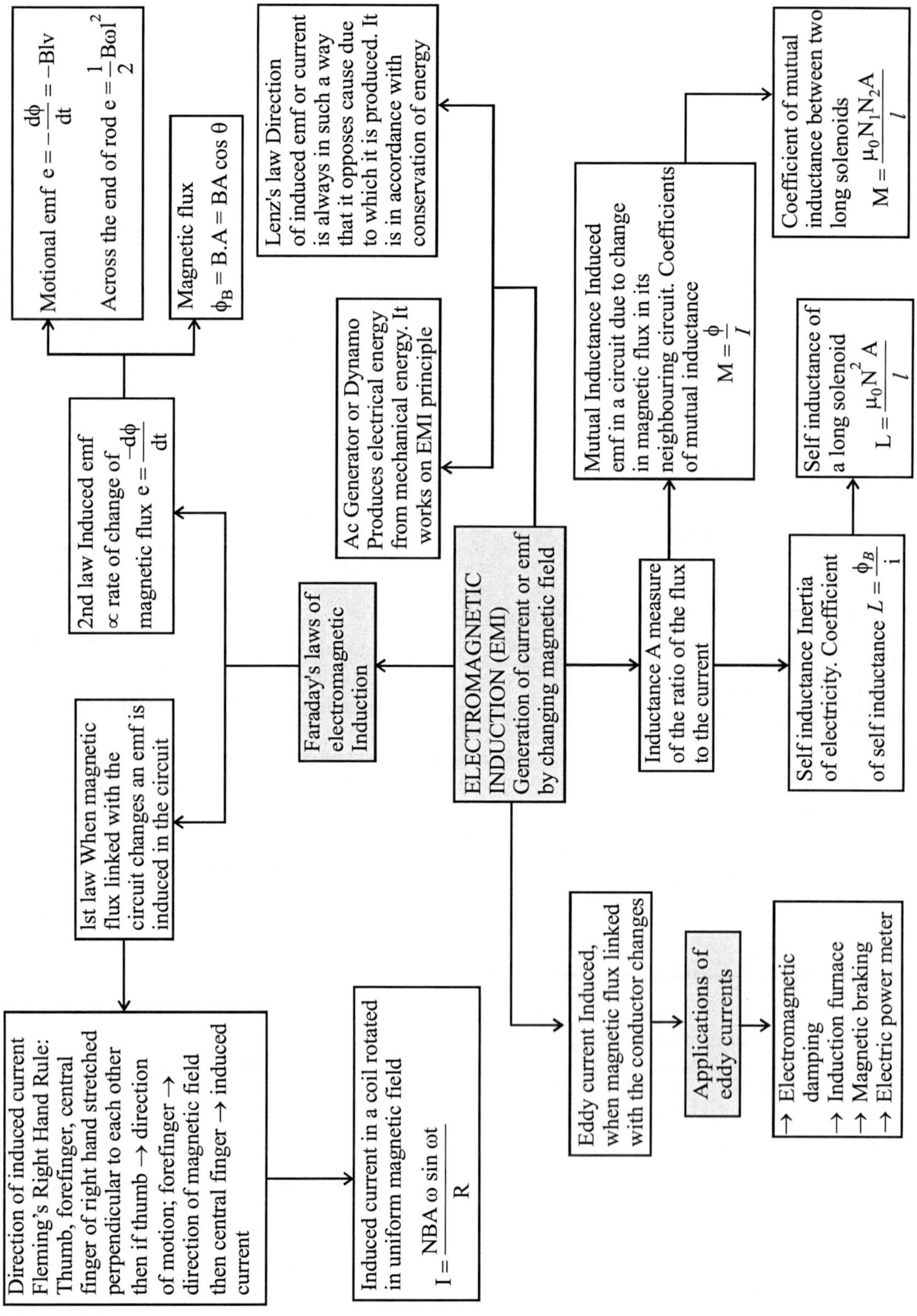

ELECTROMAGNETIC INDUCTION (EMI) Generation of current or emf by changing magnetic field

Faraday's laws of electromagnetic Induction

- Ist law When magnetic flux linked with the circuit changes an emf is induced in the circuit
  - Direction of induced current Fleming's Right Hand Rule: Thumb, forefinger, central finger of right hand stretched perpendicular to each other then if thumb → direction of motion; forefinger → direction of magnetic field then central finger → induced current
    - Induced current in a coil rotated in uniform magnetic field $I = \frac{NBA\,\omega \sin \omega t}{R}$
- 2nd law Induced emf ∝ rate of change of magnetic flux $e = \frac{-d\phi}{dt}$
  - Motional emf $e = -\frac{d\phi}{dt} = -Blv$
    Across the end of rod $e = \frac{1}{2}B\omega l^2$
  - Magnetic flux $\phi_B = B.A = BA\cos\theta$

Ac Generator or Dynamo Produces electrical energy from mechanical energy. It works on EMI principle

Lenz's law Direction of induced emf or current is always in such a way that it opposes cause due to which it is produced. It is in accordance with conservation of energy

Eddy current Induced, when magnetic flux linked with the conductor changes

Applications of eddy currents

→ Electromagnetic damping
→ Induction furnace
→ Magnetic braking
→ Electric power meter

Inductance A measure of the ratio of the flux to the current

- Mutual Inductance Induced emf in a circuit due to change in magnetic flux in its neighbouring circuit. Coefficients of mutual inductance $M = \frac{\phi}{I}$
  - Coefficient of mutual inductance between two long solenoids $M = \frac{\mu_0 N_1 N_2 A}{l}$
- Self inductance Inertia of electricity. Coefficient of self inductance $L = \frac{\phi_B}{i}$
  - Self inductance of a long solenoid $L = \frac{\mu_0 N^2 A}{l}$

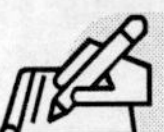

Exercise 1 - Chapter Revision Problems

CRP

1. If mutual inductance (M) of a system, M = 0 then self inductance L
(a) must be zero
(b) may or may not be zero
(c) must be non-zero
(d) no relation between L and M

2. Two identical coaxial circular loops carry current i each circulating in the clockwise direction. If the loops are approaching each other, then
(a) current in each loop increases
(b) current in each loop remains the same
(c) current in each loop decreases
(d) current in one-loop increases and in the other it decreases

3. The total charge induced in a conducting loop when it is moved in a magnetic field depend on
(a) the rate of change of magnetic flux
(b) initial magnetic flux only
(c) the total change in magnetic flux
(d) final magnetic flux only

4. If rotational velocity of a dynamo armature is doubled, then induced e.m.f. will become
(a) half (b) two times
(c) four times (d) unchanged

5. Choke coil works on the principle of
(a) transient current (b) self induction
(c) mutual induction (d) wattless current

6. A current $i = 2\sin(\pi t/3)$ amp is flowing in an inductor of 2 henry. The amount of work done in increasing the current from 1.0 amp to 2.0 amp is
(a) 1 J (b) 2 J (c) 3 J (d) 4 J

7. Fig shown below represents an area $A = 0.5\ m^2$ situated in a uniform magnetic field $B = 2.0$ weber/m^2 and making an angle of 60° with respect to magnetic field.

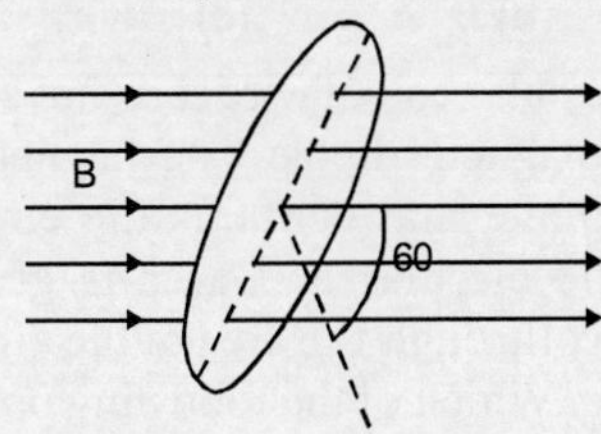

The value of the magnetic flux through the area would be equal to
(a) 2.0 weber (b) $\sqrt{3}$ weber
(c) $\sqrt{3}/2$ weber (d) 0.5 weber

8. In a coil of area 10 cm^2 and 10 turns with magnetic field directed perpendicular to the plane and is changing at the rate of 10^8 Gauss/second. The resistance of the coil is 20Ω. The current in the coil will be
(a) 0.5 A (b) 5 A (c) 50 A (d) 5×10^8 A

9. A generator has an e.m.f. of 440 Volt and internal resistance of 4000 hm. Its terminals are connected to a load of 4000 ohm. The voltage across the load is
(a) 220 volt (b) 440 volt (c) 200 volt (d) 400 volt

10. When the current in a coil changes from 2 amp. to 4 amp. in 0.05 sec., an e.m.f. of 8 volt is induced in the coil. The coefficient of self inductance of the coil is
(a) 0.1 henry (b) 0.2 henry
(c) 0.4 henry (d) 0.8 henry

11. A coil has 200 turns and area of 70 cm^2. The magnetic field perpendicular to the plane of the coil is 0.3 Wb/m^2 and take 0.1 sec to rotate through 180°. The value of the induced e.m.f. will be
(a) 8.4 V (b) 84 V (c) 42 V (d) 4.2 V

12. If a current increases from zero to one ampere in 0.1 second in a coil of 5 mH, then the magnitude of the induced e.m.f. will be
(a) 0.005 volt (b) 0.5 volt (c) 0.05 volt (d) 5 volt

13. A 100 millihenry coil carries a current of 1 ampere. Energy stored in its magnetic field is
(a) 0.5 J (b) 1 J (c) 0.05 J (d) 0.1 J

14. The armature of a dc motor has 20W resistance. It draws a current of 1.5 A when run by a 220 V dc supply. The value of the back emf induced in it is
(a) 150 V (b) 170 V (c) 180 V (d) 190 V

15. A coil having 500 square loops each of side 10 cm is placed normal to a magnetic field which increases at the rate of 1 Wb/m^2. The induced e.m.f. is
(a) 0.1 V (b) 5.0 V (c) 0.5 V (d) 1.0 V

16. Magnetic flux ϕ in weber in a closed circuit of resistance 10Ω varies with time ϕ (sec) as $f = 6t^2 - 5t + 1$. The magnitude of induced current at t = 0.25s is
(a) 0.2 A (b) 0.6 A (c) 1.2 A (d) 0.8 A

17. The current in a coil of L = 40 mH is to be increased uniformly from 1A to 11A in 4 milli sec. The induced e.m.f. will be
(a) 100 V (b) 0.4 V (c) 440 V (d) 40 V

18. Consider the situation shown. The wire AB is sliding on fixed rails with a constant velocity. If the wire AB is replaced by semi-circular wire, the magnitude of induced e.m.f. will

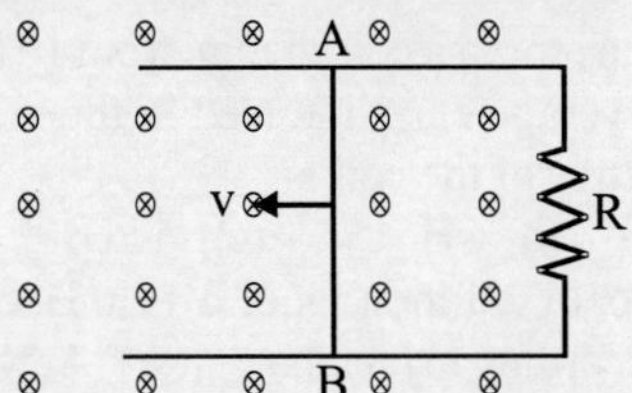

(a) increase (b) decrease
(c) remain the same
(d) increase or decrease depending on whether the semi-circle buldges towards the resistance or away from it.

19. A coil is wound on a frame of rectangular cross-section. If all the linear dimensions of the frame are increased by a factor 2 and the number of turns per unit length of the coil remains the same, self-inductance of the coil increases by a factor of
(a) 4 (b) 8 (c) 12 (d) 16

20. A conductor of length 0.4 m is moving with a speed of 7 m/s perpendicular to a magnetic field of intensity 0.9 Wb/m^2. The induced e.m.f. across the conductor is
(a) 1.26V (b) 2.52V (c) 5.04V (d) 25.2V

21. The inductance between A and D is
(a) 3.66 H
(b) 9 H
(c) 0.66 H
(d) 1 H

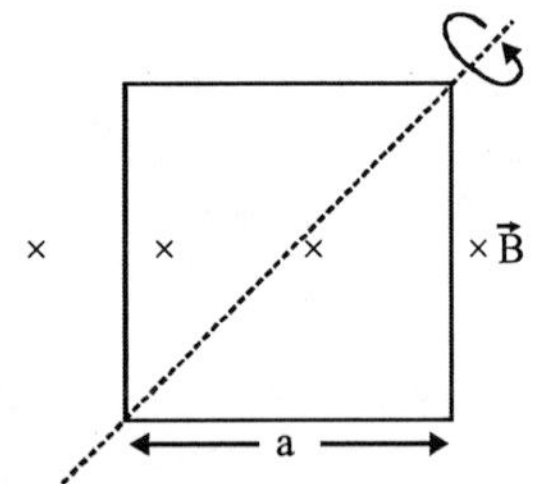

22. Two identical circular loops of metal wire are lying on a table without touching each other. Loop A carries a current which increases with time. In response the loop B
(a) remains stationary
(b) is attracted by loop A
(c) is repelled by loop A
(d) rotates about is CM with CM fixed

23. A square loop of side a is rotating about its diagonal with angular velocity ω in a perpendicular magnetic field $\vec{B}$. It has 10 turns. The emf induced is

(a) $B a^2 \sin \omega t$ (b) $B a^2 \cos \omega t$
(c) $5\sqrt{2}\, B a^2$ (d) $10 B a^2 \sin \omega t$

24. In fig., final value of current in 10Ω resistor, when plug of key K is inserted is

(a) $\frac{3}{10}$A

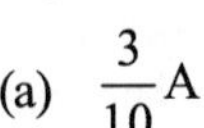

(b) $\frac{3}{20}$A
(c) $\frac{3}{11}$A
(d) zero

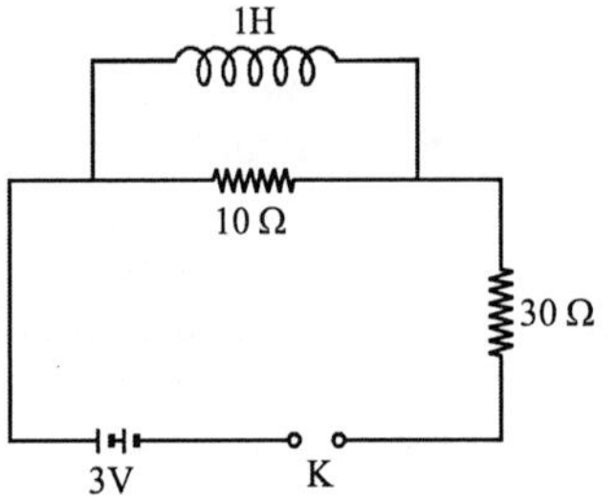

25. A varying current in a coil change from 10A to zero in 0.5 sec. If the average e.m.f induced in the coil is 220V, the self-inductance of the coil is
(a) 5H (b) 6H (c) 11H (d) 12H

26. In an inductor of self-inductance L = 2 mH, current changes with time according to relation $i = t^2 e^{-t}$. At what time emf is zero?
(a) 4s (b) 3s (c) 2s (d) 1s

27. The magnetic flux through a circuit of resistance R changes by an amount Δϕ in a time Δt. Then the total quantity of electric charge Q that passes any point in the circuit during the time Δt is represented by
(a) $Q = R.\frac{\Delta\phi}{\Delta t}$ (b) $Q = \frac{1}{R}.\frac{\Delta\phi}{\Delta t}$
(c) $Q = \frac{\Delta\phi}{R}$ (d) $Q = \frac{\Delta\phi}{\Delta t}$

28. A rod *PQ* of length *L* moves with a uniform velocity *v* parallel to a long straight wire carrying a current *i*, the end *P* remaining at a distance *r* from the wire. The emf induced across the rod is
(a) $\frac{\mu_0 i v^2}{2\pi}\ln\left(\frac{r+L}{r}\right)$ (b) $\frac{\mu_0 i^2 v^2}{2\pi}\ln\left(\frac{r^2+L}{r}\right)$
(c) $\frac{\mu_0 i v}{2\pi}\ln\left(\frac{r+L}{r}\right)$ (d) $\frac{\mu_0 i v}{2\pi}\ln\left(\frac{r^2+L^2}{L^2}\right)$

29. A coil of self-inductance L is connected in series with a bulb B and an AC source. Brightness of the bulb decreases when
(a) number of turns in the coil is reduced
(b) a capacitance of reactance $X_C = X_L$ is included in the same circuit
(c) an iron rod is inserted in the coil
(d) frequency of the AC source is decreased

30. A magnetic field of 2×10^{-2} T acts at right angles to a coil of area 100 cm^2, with 50 turns. The average e.m.f. induced in the coil is 0.1 V, when it is removed from the field in t sec. The value of t is
(a) 10 s (b) 0.1 s (c) 0.01 s (d) 1 s

31. A rectangular coil of 20 turns and area of cross-section 25 sq. cm has a resistance of 100Ω. If a magnetic field which is perpendicular to the plane of coil changes at a rate of 1000 tesla per second, the current in the coil is
(a) 1 A (b) 50 A (c) 0.5 A (d) 5 A

32. If the magnetic flux linked with a coil through which a current of x A is set up is y Wb, then the coefficient of self inductance of the coil is
(a) (x – y) henry (b) $\frac{x}{y}$henry
(c) $\frac{y}{x}$henry (d) x y henry

33. The plane in which eddy currents are produced in a conductor is inclined to the plane of the magnetic field at an angle equal to
(a) 45° (b) 0° (c) 180° (d) 90°

34. Consider a circular coil of wire carrying constant current *I*, forming a magnetic dipole. The magnetic flux through an infinite plane that contains the circular coil and excluding the circular coil area is given by ϕ_i. The magnetic flux through the area of the circular coil area is given by ϕ_0. Which of the following option is correct?
(a) $\phi_i = \phi_0$ (b) $\phi_i > \phi_0$ (c) $\phi_i < \phi_0$ (d) $\phi_i = -\phi_0$

35. At time $t = 0$ magnetic field of 1000 Gauss is passing perpendicularly through the area defined by the closed loop shown in the figure. If the magnetic field reduces linearly to 500 Gauss, in the next 5 s, then induced EMF in the loop is:

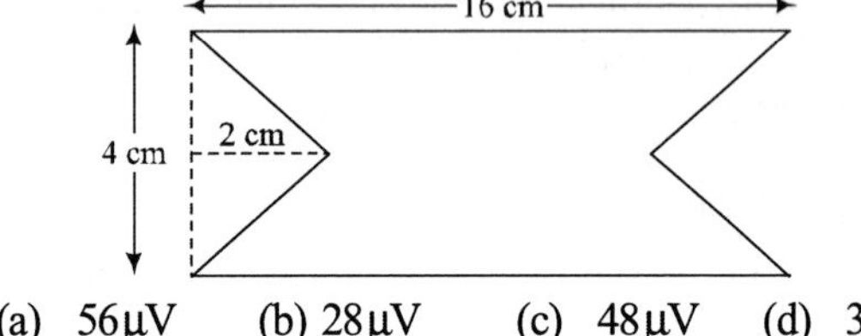

(a) 56μV (b) 28μV (c) 48μV (d) 36μV

36. Two coils 'P' and 'Q' are separated by some distance. When a current of 3A flows through coil 'P', a magnetic flux of 10^{-3} Wb passes through 'Q'. No current is passed through 'Q'. When no current passes through 'P' and a current of 2A passes through 'Q', the flux through 'P' is:
(a) 6.67×10^{-4} Wb (b) 3.67×10^{-3} Wb
(c) 6.67×10^{-3} Wb (d) 3.67×10^{-4} Wb

37. The self induced emf of a coil is 25 volts. When the current in it is changed at uniiform rate from 10 A to 25 A in 1s, the change in the energy of the inductance is:
(a) 740 J (b) 437.5 J
(c) 540 J (d) 637.5 J

38. A conducting circular loop made of a thin wire, has area 3.5×10^{-3}m^2 and resistance 10Ω. It is placed perpendicular to a time dependent magnetic field B (t) = (0.4T) sin (50πt). The the net charge flowing through the loop during t = 0 s and t = 10 ms is close to:
(a) 14 mC (b) 7 mC (c) 21 mC (d) 6 mC

39. A 10 m long horizontal wire extends from North East to South West. It is falling with a speed of 5.0 ms^{-1}, at right angles to the horizontal component of the earth's magnetic field, of 0.3×10^{-4} Wb/m^2. The value of the induced emf in wire is :
(a) 1.5×10^{-3} V (b) 1.1×10^{-3} V
(c) 2.5×10^{-3}V (d) 0.3×10^{-3} V

40. There are two long co-axial solenoids of same length *l*. The inner and outer coils have radii r_1 and r_2 and number of turns per unit length n_1 and n_2, respectively. The ratio of mutual inductance to the self-inductance of the inner-coil is :

(a) $\frac{n_1}{n_2}$ (b) $\frac{n_2}{n_1} \cdot \frac{r_1}{r_2}$ (c) $\frac{n_2}{n_1} \cdot \frac{r_2^2}{r_1^2}$ (d) $\frac{n_2}{n_1}$

41. A copper wire is wound on a wooden frame, whose shape is that of an equilateral triangle. If the linear dimension of each side of the frame is increased by a factor of 3, keeping the number of turns of the coil per unit length of the frame the same, then the self inductance of the coil:
(a) decreases by a factor of 9
(b) increases by a factor of 27
(c) increases by a factor of 3
(d) decreases by a factor of $9\sqrt{3}$

42. A solid metal cube of edge length 2 cm is moving in a positive *y*-direction at a constant speed of 6 m/s. There is a uniform magnetic field of 0.1 T in the positive *z*-direction. The potential difference between the two faces of the cube perpendicular to the *x*-axis, is:
(a) 12 mV (b) 6 mV (c) 1 mV (d) 2 mV

43. A coil of cross-sectional area A having n turns is placed in a uniform magnetic field B. When it is rotated with an angular velocity ω, the maximum e.m.f. induced in the coil will be

(a) nBAω (b) $\frac{3}{2}$nBAω (c) 3nBAω (d) $\frac{1}{2}$nBAω

44. An ideal capacitor of capacitance 0.2 μF is charged to a potential difference of 10V. The charging battery is then disconnected. The capacitor is then connected to an ideal inductor of self inductance 0.5mH. The current at a time when the potential difference across the capacitor is 5V, is:
(a) 0.17A (b) 0.15A (c) 0.34A (d) 0.25A

45. At the centre of a fixed large circular coil of radius R, a much smaller circular coil of radius r is placed. The two coils are concentric and are in the same plane. The larger coil carries a current I. The smaller coil is set to rotate with a constant angular velocity ω about an axis along their common diameter. Calculate the emf induced in the smaller coil after a time t of its start of rotation

(a) $\frac{\mu_0 I}{2R}\omega r^2 \sin\omega t$ (b) $\frac{\mu_0 I}{4R}\omega\pi r^2 \sin\omega t$

(c) $\frac{\mu_0 I}{2R}\omega\pi r^2 \sin\omega t$ (d) $\frac{\mu_0 I}{4R}\omega r^2 \sin\omega t$

46. A boat is moving due east in a region where the earth's magnetic field is 5.0×10^{-5} NA^{-1} m^{-1} due north and horizontal. The boat carries a vertical aerial 2 m long. If the speed of the boat is 1.50 ms^{-1}, the magnitude of the induced emf in the wire of aerial is:
(a) 0.75 mV (b) 0.50 mV (c) 0.15 mV (d) 1 mV

47. A coil having n turns and resistance *R*Ω is connected with a galvanometer of resistance 4*R*Ω. This combination is moved in time *t* seconds from a magnetic field W_1 weber to W_2 weber. The induced current in the circuit is

(a) $-\frac{(W_2 - W_1)}{Rnt}$ (b) $-\frac{n(W_2 - W_1)}{5\ Rt}$

(c) $-\frac{(W_2 - W_1)}{5\ Rnt}$ (d) $-\frac{n(W_2 - W_1)}{Rt}$

48. A circular wire of radius r rotates about its own axis with angular speed ω in a magnetic field B perpendicular to its plane, then the induced e.m.f. is

(a) $\frac{1}{2}$Brω^2 (b) Brω^2 (c) 2Brω^2 (d) zero

49. Charge Q is uniformly distributed on a thin insulating ring of mass m which is initially at rest. To what angular velocity will the ring be accelerated when a magnetic field B, perpendicular to the plane of the ring, is switched on?

(a) $\frac{QB}{2m}$ (b) $\frac{3QB}{2m}$ (c) $\frac{QB}{m}$ (d) $\frac{QB}{4m}$

50. A circular loop of radius 0.3 cm lies parallel to amuch bigger circular loop of radius 20 cm. The centre of the small loop is on the axis of the bigger loop. The distance between their centres is 15 cm. If a current of 2.0 A flows through the smaller loop, then the flux linked with bigger loop is
(a) 9.1×10^{-11} weber (b) 6×10^{-11} weber
(c) 3.3×10^{-11} weber (d) 6.6×10^{-9} weber

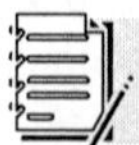

Exercise 2 - Exemplar & Past Year Questions

E&PYQs

Exemplar Questions

1. A square of side L metres lies in the xy-plane in a region, where the magnetic field is given by $B = B_0(2\hat{i} + 3\hat{j} + 4\hat{k})$ T, where B_0 is constant. The magnitude of flux passing through the square is
(a) $2B_0L^2$Wb (b) $3B_0L^2$Wb
(c) $4B_0L^2$Wb (d) $\sqrt{29}B_0L^2$Wb

2. A loop, made of straight edges has six corners at A(0, 0, 0), B(L, 0, 0), C(L, L, 0), D(0, L, 0), E(0, L, L) and F(0, 0, L). A magnetic field $B = B_0(\hat{i} + \hat{k})$ T is present in the region. The flux passing through the loop ABCDEFA (in that order) is
(a) B_0L^2 Wb (b) $2B_0L^2$Wb
(c) $\sqrt{2}B_0L^2$ Wb (d) $4B_0L^2$Wb

3. A cylindrical bar magnet is rotated about its axis. A wire is connected from the axis and is made to touch the cylindrical surface through a contact. Then,
(a) a direct current flows in the ammeter A
(b) no current flows through the ammeter A
(c) an alternating sinusoidal current flows through the ammeter A with a time period $T = \frac{2\pi}{\omega}$
(d) a time varying non-sinusoidal current flows through the ammeter A.

4. There are two coils A and B as shown in figure a current starts flowing in B as shown, when A is moved towards B and stops when A stops moving. The current in A is counter clockwise. B is kept stationary when A moves. We can infer that
(a) there is a constant current in the clockwise direction in A
(b) there is a varying current in A
(c) there is no current in A
(d) there is a constant current in the counter clockwise direction in A

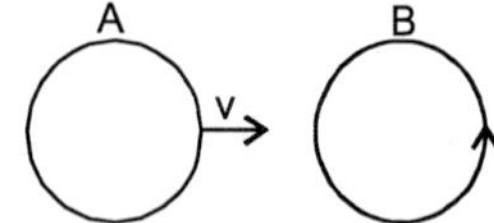

5. Same as problem 4 except the coil A is made to rotate about a vertical axis (figure). No current flows in B if A is at rest. The current in coil A, when the current in B (at t = 0) is counter-clockwise and the coil A is as shown at this instant, t = 0, is
(a) constant current clockwise
(b) varying current clockwise
(c) varying current counter clockwise
(d) constant current counter clockwise

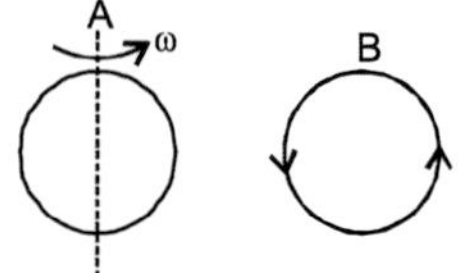

6. The self inductance L of a solenoid of length *l* and area of cross-section A, with a fixed number of turns N increases as
(a) *l* and A increase
(b) *l* decreases and A increases
(c) *l* increases and A decreases
(d) both *l* and A decrease

NEET/AIPMT (2013-2020) Questions

7. A wire loop is rotated in a magnetic field. The frequency of change of direction of the induced e.m.f. is ***[2013]***
(a) twice per revolution
(b) four times per revolution
(c) six times per revolution
(d) once per revolution

8. A current of 2.5 A flows through a coil of inductance 5 H. The magnetic flux linked with the coil is ***[NEET Kar. 2013]***
(a) 2 Wb (b) 0.5 Wb (c) 12.5 Wb (d) Zero

9. A thin semicircular conducting ring (PQR) of radius 'r' is falling with its plane vertical in a horizontal magnetic field B, as shown in figure. The potential difference developed across the ring when its speed is v, is : ***[2014]***

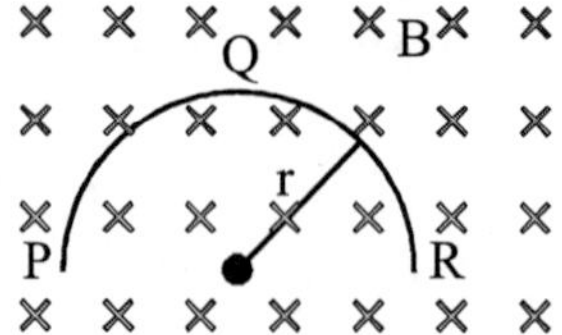

(a) Zero
(b) $Bv\pi r^2/2$ and P is at higher potnetial
(c) πrBv and R is at higher potnetial
(d) $2rBv$ and R is at higher potential

10. A conducting square frame of side 'a' and a long staight wire carrying current I are located in the same plane as shown in the figure. The frame moves to the right with a constant velocity 'V'. The emf induced in the frame will be proportional to ***[2015]***

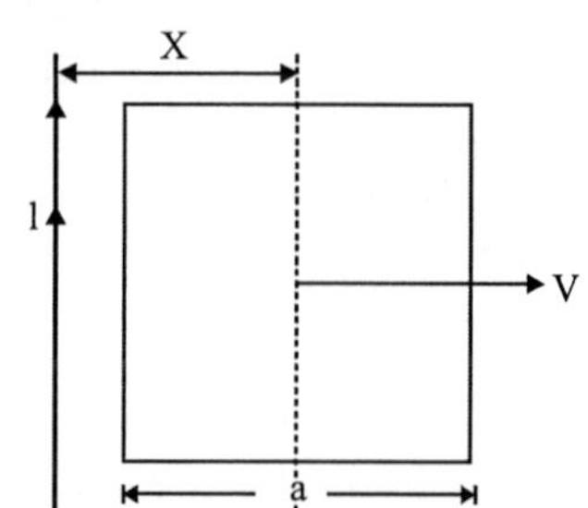

(a) $\frac{1}{(2x-a)^2}$ (b) $\frac{1}{(2x+a)^2}$
(c) $\frac{1}{(2x-a)(2x+a)}$ (d) $\frac{1}{x^2}$

11. A long solenoid of diameter 0.1 m has 2×10^4 turns per meter. At the centre of the solenoid, a coil of 100 turns and radius 0.01 m is placed with its axis coinciding with the solenoid axis. The current in the solenoid reduces at a constant rate to 0A from 4 A in 0.05 s. If the resistance of the coil is $10\pi^2\Omega$. the total charge flowing through the coil during this time is : ***[2017]***

(a) 16 μC (b) 32 μC (c) 16 π μC (d) 32 π μC

12. The magnetic potential energy stored in a certain inductor is 25 mJ, when the current in the inductor is 60 mA. This inductor is of inductance ***[2018]***

(a) 0.138 H (b) 138.88 H (c) 13.89 H (d) 1.389 H

13. A 800 turn coil of effective area $0.05\ m^2$ is kept perpendicular to a magnetic field $5\ 10^{-5}$ T. When the plane of the coil is rotated by 90° around any of its coplanar axis in 0.1 s, the emf induced in the coil will be : ***[2019]***

(a) 2 V (b) 0.2 V
(c) 2×10^{-3} V (d) 0.02 V

14. In which of the following devices, the eddy current effect is not used ? ***[2019]***

(a) induction furnace
(b) magnetic braking in train
(c) electromagnet
(d) electric heater

15. A cycle wheel of radius 0.5 m is rotated with constant angular velocity of 10 rad/s in a region of magnetic field of 0.1 *T* which is perpendicular to the plane of the wheel. The EMF generated between its centre and the rim is ***[NEET Odisha 2019]***

(a) zero (b) 0.25 V
(c) 0.125 V (d) 0.5 V

Exercise 3 - Concept Application Problems

CAP

1. A copper disc of radius 0.1 m rotated about its centre with 10 revolutions per second in a uniform magnetic field of 0.1 tesla with its plane perpendicular to the field. The e.m.f. induced across the radius of disc is

(a) $\frac{\pi}{10}$ volt (b) $\frac{2\pi}{10}$ volt
(c) $\pi \times 10^{-2}$ volt (d) $2\pi \times 10^{-2}$ volt

2. In the figure the flux through the loop perpendicular to the plane of the coil and directed into the paper is varying according to the relation $\phi = 6t^2 + 7t + 1$ where ϕ is in milliweber and t is in second. The magnitude of the emf induced in the loop at t = 2 s and the direction of induce current through R are

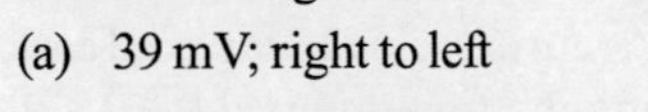

(a) 39 mV; right to left
(b) 39 mV; left to right
(c) 31 mV; right to left
(d) 31 mV; left to right

3. A circular coil and a bar magnet placed nearby are made to move in the same direction. If the coil covers a distance of 1 m in 0.5. sec and the magnet a distance of 2 m in 1 sec, the induced e.m.f. produced in the coil is

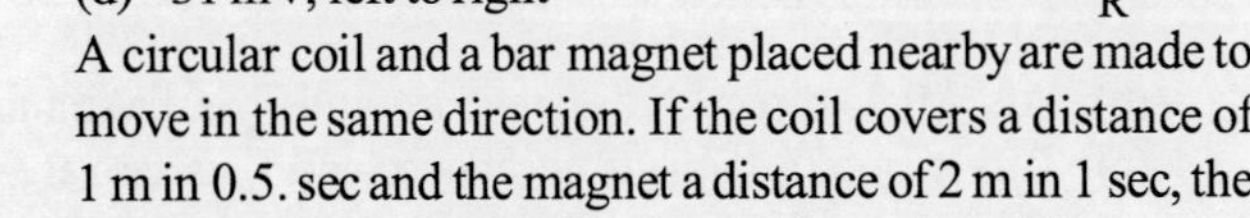

(a) zero (b) 0.5 V (c) 1 V (d) 2 V

4. The self inductance of the motor of an electric fan is 10 H. In order to impart maximum power at 50 Hz, it should be connected to a capacitance of

(a) 8μF (b) 4μF (c) 2μF (d) 1μF

5. The flux linked with a coil at any instant 't' is given by $\phi = 10t^2 - 50t + 250$. The induced emf at t = 3s is

(a) –190 V (b) –10 V (c) 10 V (d) 190 V

6. A conducting square loop of side L and resistance R moves in its plane with a uniform velocity v perpendicular to one of its side. A magnetic induction B constant in time and space, pointing perpendicular and into the plane of the loop exists everywhere.

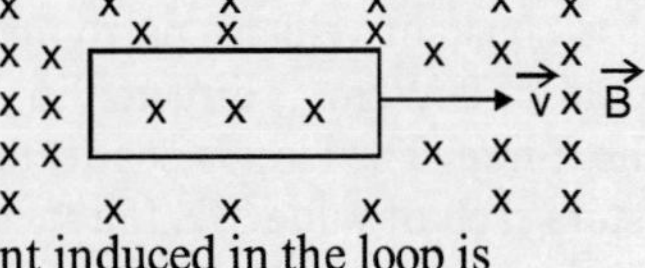

The current induced in the loop is

(a) $\frac{B\ell v}{R}$ clockwise

(b) $\frac{B\ell v}{R}$ anticlockwise

(c) $\frac{2B\ell v}{R}$ anticlockwise

(d) zero

7. The two rails of a railway track, insulated from each other and the ground, are connected to millivoltmeter. What is the reading of the millivoltmeter when a train passes at a speed of 180 km/hr along the track, given that the vertical component of earth's magnetic field is 0.2×10^{-4} wb/m^2 and rails are separated by 1 metre

(a) 10^{-2} volt (b) 10mV (c) 1 volt (d) 1mV

8. A long solenoid having 200 turns per cm carries a current of 1.5 amp. At the centre of it is placed a coil of 100 turns of cross-sectional area 3.14×10^{-4} m^2 having its axis parallel to the field produced by the solenoid. When the direction of current in the solenoid is reversed within 0.05 sec, the induced e.m.f. in the coil is

(a) 0.48 V (b) 0.048 V (c) 0.0048 V (d) 48 V

9. Two coils have a mutual inductance 0.005H. The current changes in first coil according to equation $I = I_0 \sin \omega t$ where $I_0 = 10$A and $\omega = 100\pi$ radian/sec. The max. value of e.m.f. in second coil is

(a) 2π (b) 5π (c) π (d) 4π

10. A metal conductor of length 1 m rotates vertically about one of its ends at angular velocity 5 radians per second. If the horizontal component of earth's magnetic field is 0.2×10^{-4}T, then the e.m.f. developed between the two ends of the conductor is

(a) 5mV (b) 50μV (c) 5μV (d) 50mV

11. Two identical induction coils each of inductance L are jointed in series are placed very close to each other such that the winding direction of one is exactly opposite to that of the other, what is the net inductance?

(a) L^2 (b) 2L (c) L/2 (d) zero

12. A thin circular ring of area A is held perpendicular to a uniform magnetic field of induction B. A small cut is made in the ring and a galvanometer is connected across the ends such that the total resistance of the circuit is R. When the ring is suddenly squeezed to zero area, the charge flowing through the galvanometer is

(a) $\frac{BR}{A}$ (b) $\frac{AB}{R}$ (c) ABR (d) $\frac{B^2A}{R^2}$

13. A horizontal telegraph wire 0.5 km long running east and west in a part of a circuit whose resistance is 2.5 Ω. The wire falls to $g = 10.0\ m/s^2$ and $B = 2 \times 10^{-5}$ weber/m^2, then the current induced in the circuit is

(a) 0.7 amp (b) 0.04 amp
(c) 0.02 amp (d) 0.01 amp

14. A square metal loop of side 10 cm and resistance 1 Ω is moved with a constant velocity partly inside a uniform magnetic field of 2 Wbm^{-2}, directed into the paper, as shown in the figure. The loop is connected to a network of five resistors each of value 3Ω. If a steady current of 1 mA flows in the loop, then the speed of the loop is

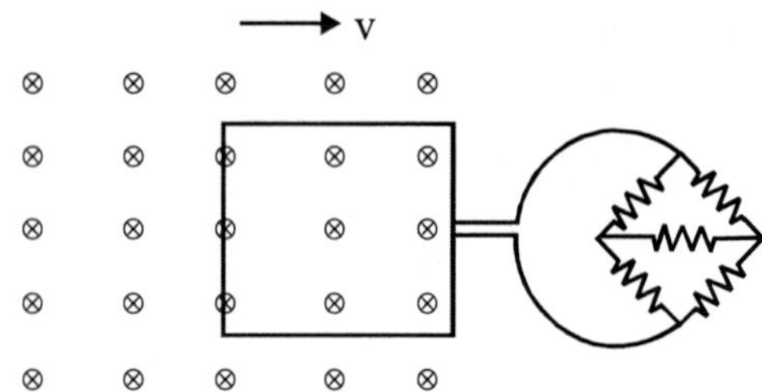

(a) 0.5 cms^{-1} (b) 1 cms^{-1} (c) 2 cms^{-1} (d) 4 cms^{-1}

15. In a circuit given in figure 1 and 2 are ammeters. Just after key K is pressed to complete the circuit, the reading is

(a) zero in both 1 and 2
(b) maximum in both 1 and 2
(c) zero in 1 and maximum in 2
(d) maximum in 1 and zero in 2

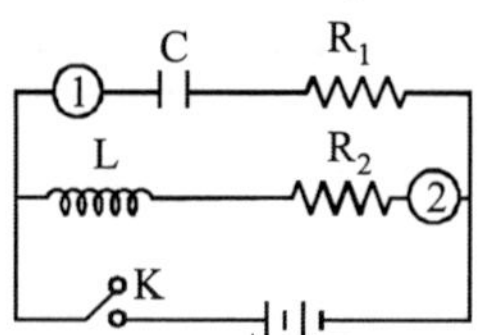

16. A solenoid has 2000 turns wound over a length of 0.3 m. Its cross-sectional area is $1.2 \times 10^{-3}\ m^2$. Around its central section a coil of 300 turns is wound. If an initial current of 2 A flowing in the solenoid is reversed in 0.25 s, the emf induced in the coil will be

(a) 2.4×10^{-4} V (b) 2.4×10^{-2} V
(c) 4.8×10^{-4} V (d) 4.8×10^{-2} V

17. Two coaxial solenoids are made by winding thin insulated wire over a pipe of cross-sectional area A = 10 cm^2 and length = 20 cm. If one of the solenoid has 300 turns and the other 400 turns, their mutual inductance is
($\mu_0 = 4\pi \times 10^{-7}$ TmA^{-1})

(a) $2.4\pi \times 10^{-5}$ H (b) $4.8\pi \times 10^{-4}$ H
(c) $4.8\pi \times 10^{-5}$ H (d) $2.4\pi \times 10^{-4}$ H

18. A conducting circular loop is placed in a uniform magnetic field, $B = 0.025\ T$ with its plane perpendicular to the loop. The radius of the loop is made to shrink at a constant rate of 1 mm s^{-1}. The induced e.m.f. when the radius is 2 cm, is

(a) $2\pi\mu V$ (b) $\pi\mu V$ (c) $\frac{\pi}{2}\mu V$ (d) $2\mu V$

19. In a coil of resistance 10 Ω, the induced current developed by changing magnetic flux through it, is shown in figure as a function of time. The magnitude of change in flux through the coil in weber is

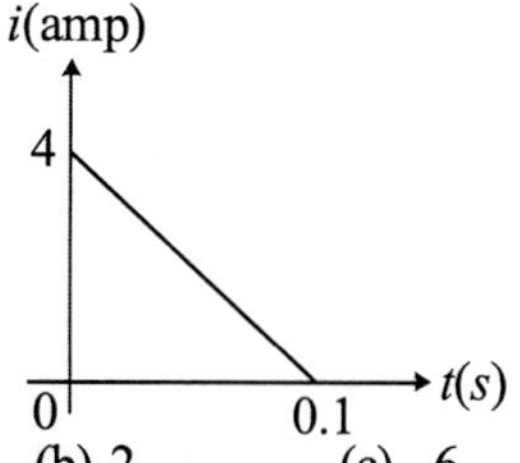

(a) 8 (b) 2 (c) 6 (d) 4

20. A coil of resistance 400Ω is placed in a magnetic field. If the magnetic flux ϕ (wb) linked with the coil varies with time t (sec) as $\phi = 50t^2 + 4$. The current in the coil at $t = 2$ sec is

(a) 0.5 A (b) 0.1 A (c) 2 A (d) 1 A

21. A uniform magnetic field B exists in a direction perpendicular to the plane of a square loop made of a metal wire. The wire has a diameter of 4 mm and a total length of 30 cm. The magnetic field changes with time at a steady rate $dB/dt = 0.032$ Ts^{-1}. The induced current in the loop is close to (Resistivity of the metal wire is 1.23×10^{-8} Ω m)

(a) 0.43 A (b) 0.61 A (c) 0.34 A (d) 0.53 A

22. A long solenoid of radius R carries a time (t) - dependent current $I(t) = I_0 t(1 - t)$. A ring of radius $2R$ is placed coaxially near its middle. During the time interval $0 \le t \le 1$, the induced current (I_R) and the induced $EMF(V_R)$ in the ring change as:

(a) Direction of I_R remains unchanged and V_R is maximum at $t = 0.5$
(b) At $t = 0.25$ direction of I_R reverses and V_R is maximum
(c) Direction of I_R remains unchanged and V_R is zero at $t = 0.25$
(d) At $t = 0.5$ direction of I_R reverses and V_R is zero

23. A planar loop of wire rotates in a uniform magnetic field. Initially, at $t = 0$, the plane of the loop is perpendicular to the magnetic field. If it rotates with a period of 10 s about an axis in its plane then the magnitude of induced emf will be maximum and minimum, respectively at:

(a) 2.5 s and 7.5 s (b) 2.5 s and 5.0 s
(c) 5.0 s and 7.5 s (d) 5.0 s and 10.0 s

24. The mutual inductance of a pair of coils, each of N turns, is M henry. If a current of I ampere in one of the coils is brought to zero in t second, the emf induced per turn in the other coil, in volt, will be

(a) $\frac{MI}{t}$ (b) $\frac{NMI}{t}$ (c) $\frac{MN}{It}$ (d) $\frac{MI}{Nt}$

25. A generator of 220 V having internal resistance r = 10Ω and external resistance R = 100Ω. What is the power developed in the external circuit?
(a) 484 W (b) 400 W (c) 441 W (d) 369 W

26. The figure shows a square loop L of side 5 cm which is connected to a network of resistances. The whole setup is moving towards right with a constant speed of 1 cm s^{-1}. At some instant, a part of L is in a uniform magnetic field of 1 T, perpendicular to the plane of the loop. If the resistance of L is 1.7 Ω, the current in the loop at that instant will be close to :

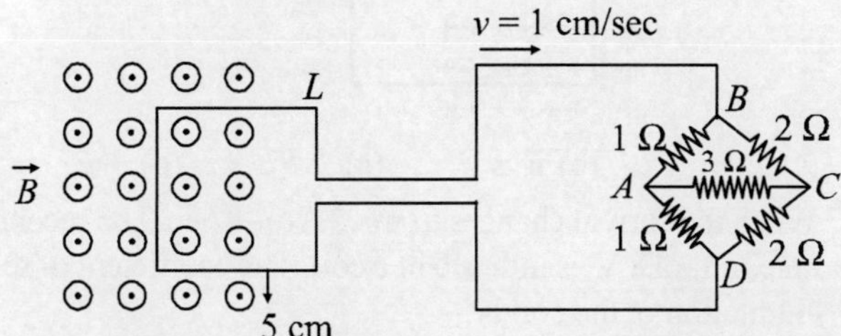

(a) 60μA (b) 170 μA (c) 150 μA (d) 115 μA

27. The total number of turns and cross-section area in a solenoid is fixed. However, its length L is varied by adjusting the separation between windings. The inductance of solenoid will be proportional to:
(a) L (b) L^2 (c) $1/L^2$ (d) 1/L

28. A thin strip 10 cm long is on a U shaped wire of negligible resistance and it is connected to a spring of spring constant 0.5 Nm^{-1} (see figure).

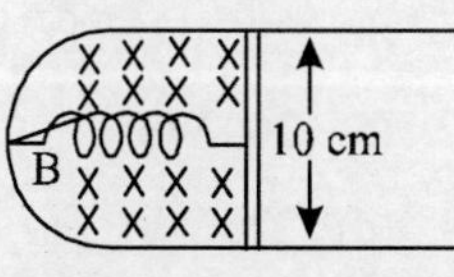

The assembly is kept in a uniform magnetic field of 0.1 T. If the strip is pulled from its equilibrium position and released, the number of oscillations it performs before its amplitude decreases by a factor of *e* is N. If the mass of strip is 50 grams, its resistance 10Ω and air drag negligible, N will be close to :
(a) 1000 (b) 50000 (c) 5000 (d) 10000

29. An insulating thin rod of length l has a linear charge density $\rho(x) = \rho_0 \frac{x}{l}$ on it. The rod is rotated about an axis passing through the origin ($x = 0$) and perpendicular to the rod. If the rod makes n rotations per second, then the time averaged magnetic moment of the rod is:
(a) $\pi n \rho l^3$ (b) $\frac{\pi}{3} n \rho l^3$ (c) $\frac{\pi}{4} n \rho l^3$ (d) $n \rho l^3$

30. A copper rod of mass m slides under gravity on two smooth parallel rails, with separation 1 and set at an angle of θ with the horizontal. At the bottom, rails are joined by a resistance R. There is a uniform magnetic field B normal to the plane of the rails, as shown in the figure. The terminal speed of the copper rod is:

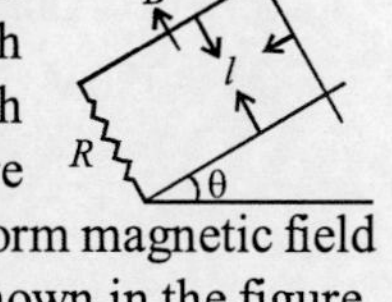

(a) $\frac{mgR\cos\theta}{B^2l^2}$ (b) $\frac{mgR\sin\theta}{B^2l^2}$

(c) $\frac{mgR\tan\theta}{B^2l^2}$ (d) $\frac{mgR\cot\theta}{B^2l^2}$

31. A square frame of side 10 cm and a long straight wire carrying current 1 A are in the plate of the paper. Starting from close to the wire, the frame moves towards the right with a constant speed of 10 ms^{-1} (see figure).

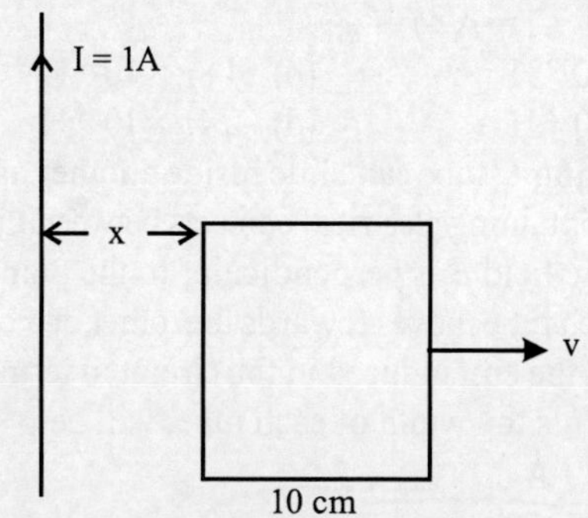

The e.m.f induced at the time the left arm of the frame is at x = 10 cm from the wire is:
(a) 2 μV (b) 1 μV (c) 0.75 μV (d) 0.5 μV

32. A metallic rod of length 'ℓ' is tied to a string of length 2ℓ and made to rotate with angular speed ω on a horizontal table with one end of the string fixed. If there is a vertical magnetic field 'B' in the region, the e.m.f. induced across the ends of the rod is

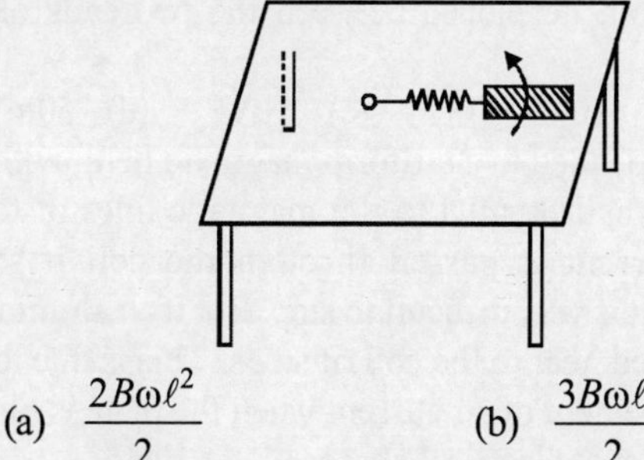

(a) $\frac{2B\omega\ell^2}{2}$ (b) $\frac{3B\omega\ell^2}{2}$

(c) $\frac{4B\omega\ell^2}{2}$ (d) $\frac{5B\omega\ell^2}{2}$

33. A rectangular loop has a sliding connector PQ of length l and resistance R Ω and it is moving with a speed v as shown. The set-up is placed in a uniform magnetic field going into the plane of the paper. The three currents I_1, I_2 and I are

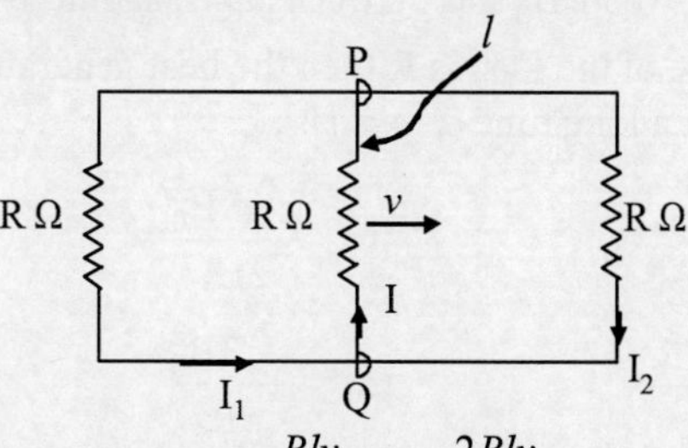

(a) $I_1 = -I_2 = \frac{Blv}{6R}$, $I = \frac{2Blv}{6R}$

(b) $I_1 = I_2 = \frac{Blv}{3R}$, $I = \frac{2Blv}{3R}$

(c) $I_1 = I_2 = I = \frac{Blv}{R}$

(d) $I_1 = I_2 = \frac{Blv}{6R}$, $I = \frac{Blv}{3R}$

34. Two coaxial solenoids are made by winding thin insulated wire over a pipe of cross-sectional area $A = 10\ cm^2$ and length = 20 cm. If one of the solenoid has 300 turns and the other 400 turns, their mutual inductance is
$(\mu_0 = 4\pi \times 10^{-7}\ Tm A^{-1})$
(a) $2.4\pi \times 10^{-5}$ H (b) $4.8\pi \times 10^{-4}$ H
(c) $4.8\pi \times 10^{-5}$ H (d) $2.4\pi \times 10^{-4}$ H

35. One conducting *U* tube can slide inside another as shown in figure, maintaining electrical contacts between the tubes. The magnetic field *B* is perpendicular to the plane of the figure. If each tube moves towards the other at a constant speed v, then the emf induced in the circuit in terms of *B*, *l* and v where *l* is the width of each tube, will be

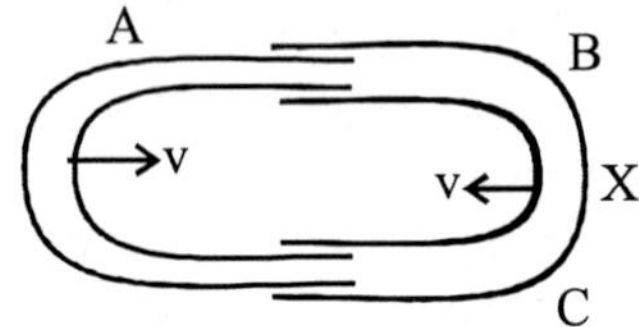

(a) $-Blv$ (b) Blv (c) $2\ Blv$ (d) zero

36. A metal conductor of length 1 m rotates vertically about one of its ends at angular velocity 5 radians per second. If the horizontal component of earth's magnetic field is 0.2×10^{-4}T, then the e.m.f. developed between the two ends of the conductor is
(a) 5mV (b) 50μV (c) 5μV (d) 50mV

37. A coil is suspended in a uniform magnetic field, with the plane of the coil parallel to the magnetic lines of force. When a current is passed through the coil it starts oscillating; It is very difficult to stop. But if an aluminium plate is placed near to the coil, it stops. This is due to :
(a) developement of air current when the plate is placed
(b) induction of electrical charge on the plate
(c) shielding of magnetic lines of force as aluminium is a paramagnetic material.
(d) electromagnetic induction in the aluminium plate giving rise to electromagnetic damping.

38. A conducting metal circular–wire–loop of radius r is placed perpendicular to a magnetic field which varies with time as $B = B_0 e^{-t/\tau}$, where B_0 and τ are constants, at time t = 0. If the resistance of the loop is R then the heat generated in the loop after a long time ($t \to \infty$) is ;

(a) $\dfrac{\pi^2 r^4 B_0^4}{2\tau R}$ (b) $\dfrac{\pi^2 r^4 B_0^2}{2\tau R}$

(c) $\dfrac{\pi^2 r^4 B_0^2 R}{\tau}$ (d) $\dfrac{\pi^2 r^4 B_0^2}{\tau R}$

39. A conducting square loop of side *L* and resistance *R* moves in its plane with a uniform velocity v perpendicular to one of its sides. A magnetic induction *B* constant in time and space, pointing perpendicular and into the plane at the loop exists everywhere with half the loop outside the field, as shown in figure. The induced emf is

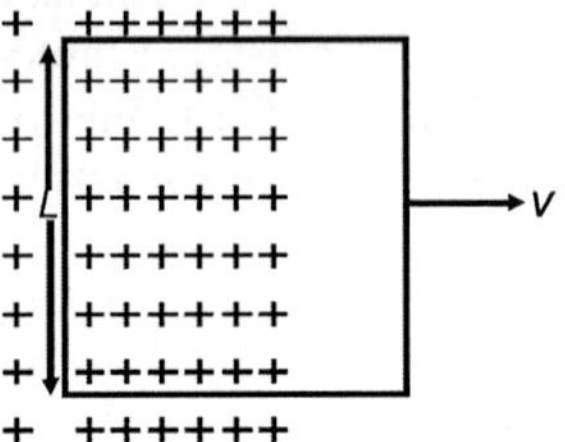

(a) zero (b) RvB (c) vBL/R (d) vBL

40. When the current changes from +2 A to –2A in 0.05 second, an e.m.f. of 8 V is induced in a coil. The coefficient of self -induction of the coil is
(a) 0.2H (b) 0.4H (c) 0.8H (d) 0.1H

41. In a coil of resistance 100Ω, a current is induced by changing the magnetic flux through it as shown in the figure. The magnitude of change in flux through the coil is

(a) 250 Wb
(b) 275 Wb
(c) 200 Wb
(d) 225 Wb

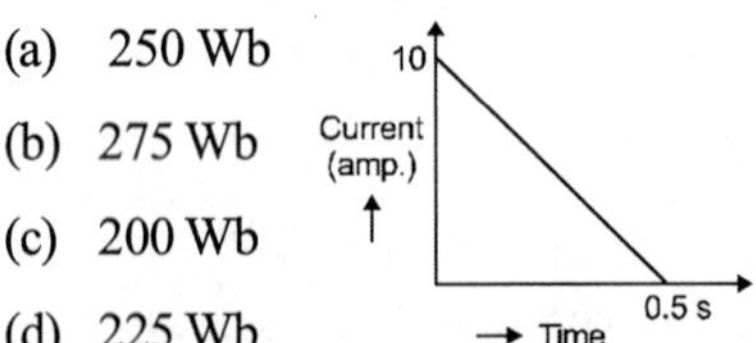

42. When current in a coil changes from 5 A to 2 A in 0.1 s, average voltage of 50 V is produced. The self - inductance of the coil is :
(a) 6H (b) 0.67H (c) 3H (d) 1.67H

43. A coil of circular cross-section having 1000 turns and 4 cm^2 face area is placed with its axis parallel to a magnetic field which decreases by 10^{-2} Wb m^{-2} in 0.01 s. The e.m.f. induced in the coil is:
(a) 400mV (b) 200mV (c) 4mV (d) 0.4mV

44. Two coils of self inductances 2 mH and 8 mH are placed so close together that the effective flux in one coil is completely linked with the other. The mutual inductance between these coils is
(a) 6mH (b) 4mH (c) 16mH (d) 10mH

45. The flux linked with a coil at any instant '*t*' is given by $\phi = 10t^2 - 50t + 250$. The induced emf at $t = 3s$ is
(a) –190V (b) –10V (c) 10V (d) 190V

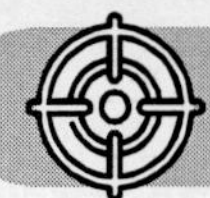

Hints & Solutions

21.1 Concept Practice Problems

1. (a) Induced e.m.f. $\varepsilon = \frac{d\phi}{dt} = \frac{dBA}{dt} = A_0 \frac{dB}{dt}$

$$= A_0\left(\frac{4B_0 - B_0}{t}\right) = 3A_0 B_0 / t$$

2. (a)
3. (a) 4. (c)
5. (d) Initially flux, $\phi = BA\cos 0 = BA$

After rotating through an angle 90°.
Flux through the coil is zero.
So, $\Delta\phi = BA$

Angular speed = w, so, time period $= \frac{2\pi}{\omega} = T$

$\frac{T}{4}$ is time taken to rotate 90°.

So, $\frac{\Delta\phi}{\Delta t} = \frac{BA}{T/4} = \frac{2BA\omega}{\pi}$

6. (a) Farady's law states that time varying magnetic flux can induce an e.m.f.
7. (b)
8. (b) Due to shifting of electrons, one end of the rod becomes positive and the other end negative. This developes a electric field in the rod.
9. (a) $V = \frac{W}{Q} \Rightarrow W = QV$
10. (a)

21.2 Concept Practice Problems

11. (c) 12. (c)
13. (a) $E = \frac{d}{dt}(NMI) \Rightarrow E = NM\frac{dI}{dt} \Rightarrow E = \frac{NMI}{t}$

emf induced per unit turn $= \frac{E}{N} = \frac{MI}{t}$

14. (b) From $L = \frac{\mu_0 N^2 A}{l} \alpha \frac{N^2}{l}$

we get, $\frac{L_1}{L_2} = \frac{(1/2)^2}{1/2} = \frac{1}{2}$

15. (a) The back e.m.f. in a motor is induced e.m.f., which is maximum, when speed of rotation of the coil is maximum.
16. (d) Mutual inductance between two coils depends on all the three factors given here.
17. (b) From $e = LdI/dt$, $dI/dt = \frac{e}{L} = \frac{1}{1} = 1As^{-1}$
18. (b)
19. (b) It is because after every 1/2 revolution the current becomes zero and mode of change in flux changes thereafter (If before the current becomes zero, the mode of flux change was from left to right then after the current becomes zero the mode of flux change becomes right to left).
20. (d) Self inductance of a solenoid $= \frac{\mu n^2 A}{\ell}$

So, self induction $\propto n^2$
So, inductance becomes 4 times when n is doubled.

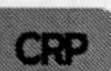

Exercise 1 - Chapter Revision Problems

1. (b) Mutual inductance $M = k\sqrt{L_1 L_2}$
2. (c)
3. (c) $q = \int idt = \frac{1}{R}\int edt = \frac{1}{R}\int\left(\frac{-d\phi}{dt}\right)dt = \frac{1}{R}\int d\phi$

(taking only magnitude of e)

Hence, total charge induced in the conducting loop depends upon the total change in magnetic flux.

4. (b) $e \propto \omega$
5. (b) 6. (c)
7. (d) $\phi = BA\cos\theta = 2.0 \times 0.5 \times \cos 60° = \frac{2.0 \times 0.5}{2}$

$= 0.5$ weber.

8. (b) $\varepsilon = \frac{d\phi}{dt} = nA\frac{dB}{dt}$

$\therefore \varepsilon = 10 \times (10 \times 10^{-4})(10^4)$ (10^8 Gauss/sec $= 10^4$ T/s)
$= 100$ V.
$I = (\varepsilon/R) = (100/20) = 5$ amp.

9. (d) Total resistance of the circuit $= 4000 + 400 = 4400$ W

Current flowing $i = \frac{V}{R} = \frac{440}{4400} = 0.1$ amp.

Voltage across load $= Ri = 4000 \times 0.1 = 400$ volt.

10. (b) $\varepsilon = M\frac{di}{dt}$ or $8 = M\left[\frac{(4-2)}{0.05}\right]$

$\therefore M = \frac{8 \times 0.05}{2} = 0.2$ henry

11. (a) Change in flux $= 2BAN$

$\therefore$ Induced e.m.f. $= \frac{2 \times 0.3 \times 200 \times 70 \times 10^{-4}}{0.1}$

12. (c) $\varepsilon = (5 \times 10^{-3})(1/0.1) = 0.05$ V.

13. (c) Energy stored U is given by

$$U=\frac{1}{2}Li^2=\frac{1}{2}\times(100\times10^{-3})\ (1)^2=0.05\,J.$$

14. (d)

15. (b) $e=\frac{d\phi}{dt}=\frac{d}{dt}(NBA)=NA\frac{dB}{dt}=500\times10^{-2}\times1=5.0\,V$

16. (a) $e=\frac{-d\phi}{dt}=\frac{-d}{dt}\left(6t^2-5t+1\right)=-12t+5$

$e=-12\,(0.25)+5=2$ volt

$$i=\frac{e}{R}=\frac{2}{10}=0.2A.$$

17. (a) $e=\frac{LdI}{dt}=\frac{40\times10^{-3}(11-1)}{4\times10^{-3}}=100V$

18. (c) E.m.f. will remain same because change in area per unit time will be same in both cases.

19. (b) Self inductance $=\mu_0 n^2 AL=\mu_0 n^2(\ell\times b)\times L$

n = Total number of turns/length

L = Length of inductor

l = Length of rectangular cross section

b = breadth of rectangular cross-section

So, when all linear dimensions are increased by a factor of 2. The new self inductance becomes L' = 8L.

20. (b) Length of conductor (l) = 0.4 m; Speed (v) = 7 m/s and magnetic field (B) = 0.9 Wb/ m^2. Induced e.m.f. (ε) = Blv cos q = 0.9 × 0.4 × 7 × cos 0° = 2.52 V.

21. (d) The given circuit clearly shows that the inductors are in parallel we have, $\frac{1}{L}=\frac{1}{3}+\frac{1}{3}+\frac{1}{3}$ or L= 1H

22. (c) An opposite current induced in B in accordance to Lenz's law. So the two loops repel each other.

23. (d) $\phi=n\,BA\cos\theta=10\,B\,a^2\cos\omega t$

$$e=-\frac{d\phi}{dt}=-\frac{d}{dt}\left(10\,B\,a^2\cos\omega t\right)=10\,B\,a^2\sin\omega t\,(\omega).$$

24. (d) As resistance of 1 H coil is zero, the entire current flows through the coil. Current through 10Ω resistance is zero.

25. (c) Initial current (I_1) = 10 A; Final current (I_2)= 0; Time (t) = 0.5 sec and induced e.m.f. (e) = 220 V.

$$-L\frac{dI}{dt}=-L\frac{(I_2-I_1)}{t}=-L\frac{(0-10)}{0.5}=20L$$

or $L=\frac{220}{20}=11$ H

(where L = Self inductance of coil)

26. (c) L = 2mH, $i=t^2e^{-t}$

$$E=-L\frac{di}{dt}=-L[-t^2e^{-t}+2te^{-t}]$$

when E = 0

$-e^{-t}t^2+2te^{-t}=0$

$2t\,e^{-t}=e^{-t}t^2$

t = 2 sec.

27. (c) $\frac{\Delta\phi}{\Delta t}=\varepsilon=iR\Rightarrow\Delta\phi=(i\Delta t)R=QR\Rightarrow Q=\frac{\Delta\phi}{R}$

28. (c)

29. (c) By inserting iron rod in the coil,

L ↑ z ↑ I ↓ so brightness ↓

30. (b) $e=\frac{-(\phi_2-\phi_1)}{t}=\frac{-(0-NBA)}{t}=\frac{NBA}{t}$

$$t=\frac{NBA}{e}=\frac{50\times2\times10^{-2}\times10^{-2}}{0.1}=0.1\,s$$

31. (c) $i=\frac{e}{R}=\frac{nAdB/dt}{R}$

$$=\frac{20\times(25\times10^{-4})\times1000}{100}=0.5A$$

32. (c)

33. (d)

34. (d) As magnetic field lines form close loop, hence every magnetic field line creating magnetic flux through the inner region (ϕ_i) must be passing through the outer region. Since flux in two regions are in opposite region.

$\therefore\ \phi_i=-\phi_0$

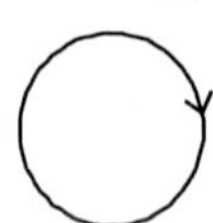

35. (a)

36. (a) $Q_{coil}=(NQ)\propto i$

So, $\frac{Q_1}{Q_2}=\frac{i_1}{i_2}=\frac{3}{2}$

or $Q_2=\frac{2}{3}Q_1=\frac{2}{3}\times10^{-3}=6.67\times10^{-4}$ Wb

37. (b) According to faraday's law of electromagnetic induction, $e=\frac{-d\phi}{dt}$

$L\times\frac{di}{dt}=25\Rightarrow L\times\frac{15}{1}=25$ or $L=\frac{5}{3}H$

Change in the energy of the inductance,

$$\Delta E=\frac{1}{2}L\left(i_1^2-i_2^2\right)=\frac{1}{2}\times\frac{5}{3}\times(25^2-10^2)$$

$$=\frac{5}{6}\times525=437.5\,J$$

38. [Bonus]

Net charge $Q=\frac{\Delta\phi}{R}=\frac{1}{10}A(B_f-B_i)=\frac{1}{10}\times3.5\times10^{-3}$

$$\left(0.4\sin\frac{\pi}{2}-0\right)$$

$$=\frac{1}{10}(3.5\times10^{-3})(0.4-0)=1.4\times10^{-4}$$

39. (a) Induced emf, $\varepsilon=Bv\ell$

$=0.3\times10^{-4}\times5\times10$

$=1.5\times10^{-3}$ V

40. (d) The rate of mutual inductance is given by
$M=\mu_0 n_1 n_2 \pi r_1^2$ ...(i)
The rate of self inductance is given by
$L=\mu_0 n_1^2 \pi r_1^2$ ...(ii)
Dividing (i) by (ii) $\Rightarrow \frac{M}{L}=\frac{n_2}{n_1}$

41. (c)

42. (a) Potential difference between two faces perpendicular to x-axis
$=lV.B=2\times10^{-2}(6\times0.1)=12mV$

43. (a) Induced emf in a coil, $e=-\frac{d\phi}{dt}=NBA\sin\omega t$
Also, $e=e_0\sin\omega t$
$\therefore$ Maximum emf induced, $e_0=nBA\omega$

44. (a) Given: Capacitance, $C=0.2\,\mu F=0.2\times10^{-6}F$
Inductance $L=0.5\,mH=0.5\times10^{-3}H$
Current I = ?
Using energy conservation
$$\frac{1}{2}CV^2=\frac{1}{2}CV_1^2+\frac{1}{2}LI^2$$
$$\frac{1}{2}\times0.2\times10^{-6}\times10^2+0$$
$$=\frac{1}{2}\times0.2\times10^{-6}\times5^2+\frac{1}{2}\times0.5\times10^{-3}I^2$$
$\therefore\ I=\sqrt{3}\times10^{-1}A=0.17A$

45. (c) According to Faraday's law of electromagnetic induction,
$$e=-\frac{d\phi}{dt}\text{ and }\phi=BA\cos\omega t=B\pi r^2\cos\omega t$$
$$\Rightarrow\ e=-\frac{d}{dt}(\pi r^2B\cos\omega t)=\pi r^2B\sin\omega t(\omega)$$
$$\therefore\ e=\frac{\mu_0 I}{2R}\pi\omega r^2\sin\omega t\ \left(\because B=\frac{\mu_0 I}{2R}\right)$$

46. (d) As magnetic field lines form close loop, hence every magnetic field line creating magnetic flux through the inner region (ϕ_i) must be passing through the outer region. Since flux in two regions are in opposite region.

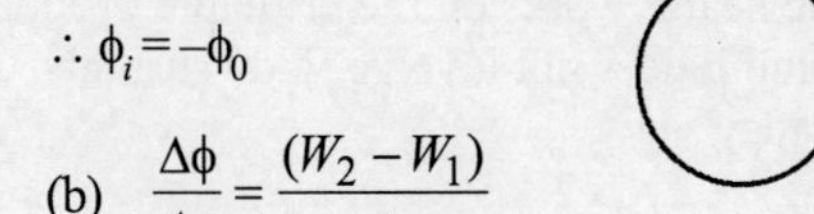

$\therefore \phi_i=-\phi_0$

47. (b) $\frac{\Delta\phi}{\Delta t}=\frac{(W_2-W_1)}{t}$
$R_{tot}=(R+4R)\Omega=5R\Omega$
$$i=\frac{nd\phi}{R_{tot}dt}=\frac{-n(W_2-W_1)}{5Rt}$$
($\because W_2$ & W_1 are magnetic flux)

48. (d) The e.m.f. is induced when there is change of flux. As in this case there is no change of flux, hence no e.m.f. will be induced in the wire.

49. (a)

50. (a) As we know, Magnetic flux, $\phi=B.A$
$$\frac{\mu_0(2)(20\times10^{-2})^2}{2[(0.2)^2+(0.15)^2]}\times\pi(0.3\times10^{-2})^2$$
On solving
$=9.216\times10^{-11}=9.2\times10^{-11}$ weber

Exercise 2 - Exemplar & Past Year Questions 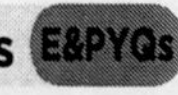

Exemplar Questions

1. (c) As we know that, the magnetic flux linked with uniform surface of area A in uniform magnetic field is $\phi=B.A$
The direction of A is perpendicular to the plane of square and square line in x-y plane in a region.
$A=L^2k$
As given that, $B=B_0(2\hat{i}+3\hat{j}+4\hat{k})$
So, $\phi=B.A=B_0(2\hat{i}+3\hat{j}+4\hat{k}).L^2\hat{k}$
$=4B_0L^2$ Wb

2. (b) The loop can be considered in two planes, Plane of ABCDA lies x-y plane whose area vector $A_1=|A|\hat{k}$, $A_1=L^2\hat{k}$
whereas plane of ADEFA lies in y-z plane whose area vector $A_2=|A|\hat{i}$, $A_2=L^2\hat{i}$.
Then the magnetic flux linked with uniform surface of area A in uniform magnetic field is

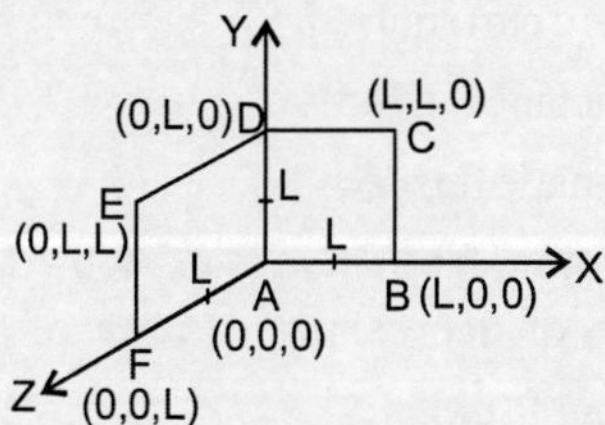

$\phi=B.A$
$A=A_1+A_2=(L^2\hat{k}+L^2\hat{i})$
and $B=B_0(\hat{i}+\hat{k})$
Now, $\phi=B.A=B_0(\hat{i}+\hat{k})\cdot(L^2\hat{k}+L^2\hat{i})$
$=2B_0L^2$ Wb

3. (b)

4. (d) When the coil A stops moving the current in B b ecome ze ro, it possible only if the current in A is constant. If the current in A would be variable, there must be an induced emf (current) in B even if the A stops moving. So there is a constant current in same direction or counter clockwise direction in A as in B by lenz's law.

5. (a) By Lenz's law, at (t = 0) the current in B is counter-clockwise and the coil A is considered above to it. The

counterclockwise flow of the current in B is equivalent to north pole of magnet and magnetic field lines are emanating upward to coil A.

When coil A start rotating at t = 0, the current in A is constant along clockwise direction by Lenz's rule. As flux changes across coil A by rotating it near the N-pole formed by flowing current in B, in anticlockwise.

6. (b) The self-inductance of a long solenoid of cross-sectional area A and length l, having n turns per unit length, filled the inside of the solenoid with a material of relative permeability is given by

$L = \mu_r\mu_0 n^2 Al$

$\therefore \quad n = N/l$

$$L = \mu_r\mu_0\left[\frac{N^2.A}{l.l}\right].l$$

$$L = \mu_r\mu_0 [N^2A/l] \quad \left(L \propto A, L \propto \frac{1}{l}\right)$$

As μ_r and N are constant here so, to increase L for a coil, area A must be increased and l must be decreased.

NEET/AIPMT (2013-2020) Questions

7. (a) This is the case of periodic EMI

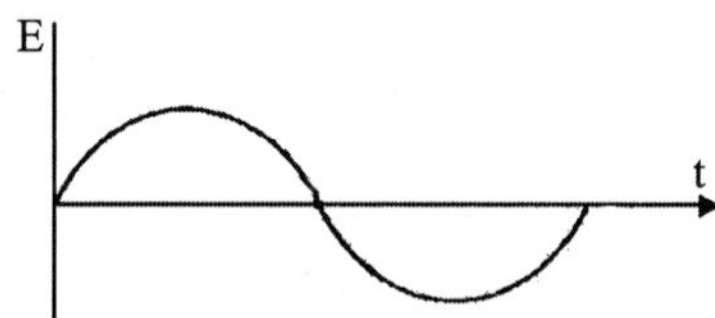

From graph, it is clear that direction is changing once in $\frac{1}{2}$ cycle.

8. (c) Given: current I = 2.5 A

Inductance, L = 5H

Magnatic flux, ϕ = ?

We know, $\phi = LI \Rightarrow 5 \times 2.5$ Wb = 12.5 Wb

9. (d) Rate of decreasing of area of semicircular ring

$$= \frac{dA}{dt} = (2r)V$$

From Faraday's law of electromagnetic induction

$$e = -\frac{d\theta}{dt} = -B\frac{dA}{dt} = -B(2rV)$$

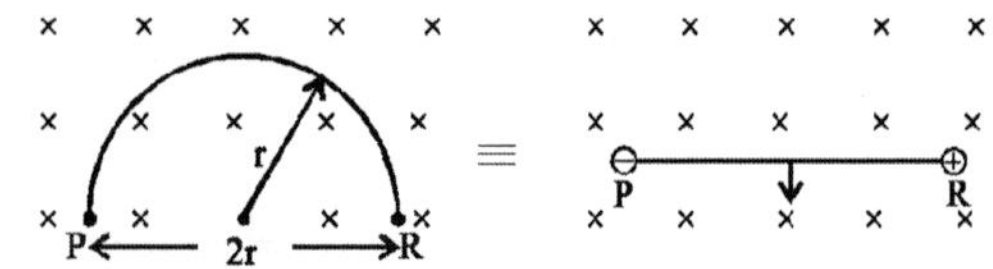

As induced current in ring produces magnetic field in upward direction hence R is at higher potential.

10. (c) Emf induced in side 1 of frame $e_1 = B_1 V\ell$

$$B_1 = \frac{\mu_0 I}{2\pi(x - a/2)}$$

Emf induced in side 2 of frame $e_2 = B_2 V\ell$

$$B_2 = \frac{\mu_0 I}{2\pi(x + a/2)}$$

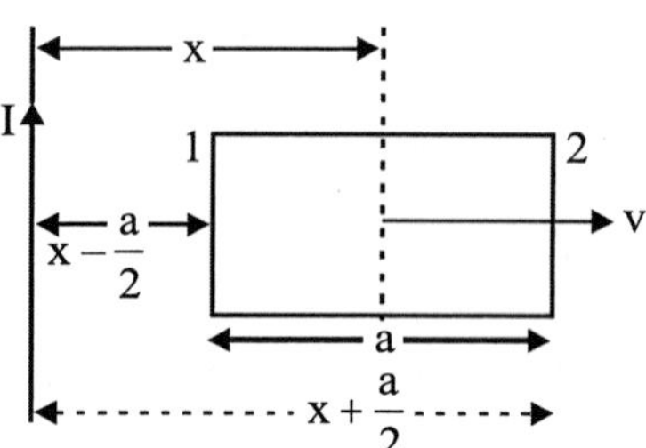

Emf induced in square frame

$e = B_1 V\ell - B_2 V\ell$

$$= \frac{\mu_0 I}{2\pi(x - a/2)}\ell v - \frac{\mu_0 I}{2\pi(x + a/2)}\ell v$$

$$\text{or, } e \propto \frac{1}{(2x - a)(2x + a)}$$

11. (b)

12. (c) From question energy stored in inductor, $U = 25 \times 10^{-3}$ J

Current, I = 60 mA

Energy stored in inductor $U = \frac{1}{2}LI^2$

$$25 \times 10^{-3} = \frac{1}{2} \times L \times (60 \times 10^{-3})^2$$

$$L = \frac{25 \times 2 \times 10^6 \times 10^{-3}}{3600} = 13.89 \text{ Hm}$$

13. (d) Magnetic field $B = 5 \times 10^{-5}$ T

Number of turns in coil N = 800

Area of coil $A = 0.05 \text{ m}^2$

Time taken to rotate = Δt = 0.1 s

Initial angle $\theta_1 = 0°$

Final angle $\theta_2 = 90°$

Change in magnetic flux $\Delta\phi$

$= NBA\cos 90° - BA\cos 0°$

$= -NBA$

$= -800 \times 5 \times 10^{-5} \times 0.05$

$= -2 \times 10^{-2}$ weber

$$\theta = -\frac{\Delta\phi}{\Delta t} = \frac{-(-)2 \times 10^{-3}\text{ Wb}}{0.1\text{ s}} = 0.02 \text{ V}$$

14. (d) An electric heater works on the principle of Joule's heating effect and it does not involve Eddy currents.

15. (c) Using Faraday's law,

$$e = \frac{Bl^2\omega}{2} = \frac{1}{2} \times 0.1 \times \left(\frac{1}{2}\right)^2 \times 10 = \frac{1}{8} = 0.125 \text{ V}$$

Exercise 3 - Concept Application Problems CAP

1. (c) e.m.f. induced $= \frac{1}{2}BR^2\omega = \frac{1}{2}BR^2(2\pi n)$

$$= \frac{1}{2} \times (0.1) \times (0.1)^2 \times 2\pi \times 10 = (0.1)^2 \pi \text{ volts}$$

2. (d) $\phi = 6t^2 + 7t + 1 \Rightarrow \frac{d\phi}{dt} = 12t + 7$

At time, t = 2 sec.

$\frac{d\phi}{dt} = 24 + 7 = 31$ volt

Direction of current is from left to right according to Flemmings right hand rule.

3. (a) Vel. of coil $= \frac{1}{0.5} = 2\text{m/s}$

velocity of magnet $= \frac{2}{1} = 2\text{m/s}$.

As they are made to move in the same direction, their relative velocity is zero. Therefore, induced e.m.f. = 0.

4. (d) For maximum power, $X_L = X_C$, which yields

$C = \frac{1}{(2\pi n)^2 L} = \frac{1}{4\pi^2 \times 50 \times 50 \times 10}$

$\therefore\ C = 0.1 \times 10^{-5} F = 1\mu F$

5. (b) $\phi = 10t^2 - 50t + 250$

$e = -\frac{d\phi}{dt} = -(20t - 50)$

$e_{t=3} = -10$ V

6. (d) Since the magnetic field is uniform the flux f through the square loop at any time t is constant, because

$f = B \times A = B \times L^2 =$ constant

$\therefore\ \varepsilon = -\frac{d\phi}{dt} =$ zero

7. (d) $\varepsilon = Blv$

$= (0.2 \times 10^{-4})(1)(180 \times 5/18) = 10^{-3}\text{ V} = 1\text{ mV}$

8. (b) $B = \mu_0 ni = (4\pi \times 10^{-7})(200 \times 10^{-2}) \times 1.5$

$= 3.8 \times 10^{-2}\text{ Wb/m}^2$

Magnetic flux through each turn of the coil

$\phi = BA = (3.8 \times 10^{-2})(3.14 \times 10^{-4}) = 1.2 \times 10^{-5}$ weber

When the current in the solenoid is reversed, the change in magnetic flux

$= 2 \times (1.2 \times 10^{-5}) = 2.4 \times 10^{-5}$ weber

Induced e.m.f. $= N\frac{d\phi}{dt} = 100 \times \frac{2.4 \times 10^{-5}}{0.05} = 0.048$ V.

9. (b) $\varepsilon = \frac{M}{dt} dI = 0.005 \times I_0 \cos\omega t \times \omega$

and $\varepsilon_{max} = 0.005 \times I_0 \times \omega = 5\pi$

10. (b) l = 1m, w = 5 rad/s, $B = 0.2 \times 10^{-4}$ T

$\varepsilon = \frac{B\omega\ell}{2} = \frac{0.2 \times 10^{-4} \times 5 \times 1}{2} = 50\mu V$

11. (d) When two inductance coil are joined in series, such that the winding of one is exactly opposite to each other the emf produced in the two coils are out of phase such that they cancel out.

12. (b) The individual emf produced in the coil $e = \frac{-d\phi}{dt}$

$\therefore$ The current induced will be $i = \frac{|e|}{R} \Rightarrow i = \frac{1}{R}\frac{d\phi}{dt}$

But $i = \frac{dq}{dt} \Rightarrow \frac{dq}{dt} = \frac{1}{R}\frac{d\phi}{dt} \Rightarrow \int dq = \frac{1}{R}\int d\phi \Rightarrow q = \frac{BA}{R}$

13. (c) $i = \frac{\varepsilon}{R} = \frac{1}{R}\frac{d\phi}{dt}$

Here $df = B \times A = (2 \times 10^{-5}) \times (0.5 \times 10^{+3} \times 5)$

dt = time taken by the wire to fall at ground

$= (2h/g)^{1/2} = (10/10)^{1/2} = 1\text{sec}.$

$\therefore\ i = \frac{1}{2.5}\left[\frac{(2 \times 10^{-5}) \times (0.5 \times 10^3 \times 5)}{1}\right] = 0.02$ amp.

14. (c) $\varepsilon = B\ell v = 2 \times 10^{-1} \times v = 0.2$ v

$I = \frac{\varepsilon}{R} = 10^{-3} \Rightarrow \frac{0.2v}{4} = 10^{-3}$

[Since effective resistance R of bridge is $R = \frac{6 \times 6}{6 + 6} = 3\Omega$

so total resistance $= 1 + 3 = 4\Omega$]

$\Rightarrow v = 2\text{ cm s}^{-1}$

15. (c) Capacitor is a dc blocking element and hence no current flow in (1).

An inductor offers a zero resistance path to flow of dc and hence maximum current flows through (2).

16. (b) $n = \frac{N}{\ell} = \frac{2000}{0.3} = \frac{20000}{3}$

$\xi = \frac{d}{dt}(NBA) = NA\frac{dB}{dt}$

Since $B = \mu_0 nI$

$\Rightarrow\ \xi = (\mu NAn)\frac{dt}{dt}\ \Rightarrow\ \xi = 0.024$ V

17. (d) $M = \frac{\mu_0 N_1 N_2 A}{\ell} = \frac{4\pi \times 10^{-7} \times 300 \times 400 \times 100 \times 10^{-4}}{0.2}$

$= 2.4\pi \times 10^{-4}$ H

18. (b) Magnetic flux linked with the loop is $\phi = B\pi r^2$

$|e| = \frac{d\phi}{dt} = B\pi \cdot 2r\frac{dr}{dt}$

When $r = 2$ cm, $\frac{dr}{dt} = 1\text{ mm } s^{-1}$

$e = 0.025 \times \pi \times 2 \times 2 \times 10^{-2} \times 10^{-3}$

$= 0.100 \times \pi \times 10^{-5} = \pi \times 10^{-6} V = \pi\mu V$

19. (b) The charge through the coil = area of current-time $(i - t)$ graph

$q = \frac{1}{2} \times 0.1 \times 4 = 0.2$ C

$q = \frac{\Delta\phi}{R}$ $\because$ Change in flux $(\Delta\phi) = q \times R$

$q = 0.2 = \frac{\Delta\phi}{10}$

$\Delta\phi = 2$ weber

20. (a) According, to Faraday's law of induction

Induced e.m.f. $\varepsilon = -\dfrac{d\phi}{dt} = -(100t)$

Induced current i at $t = 2$ sec.

$= \left|\dfrac{\varepsilon}{R}\right| = +\dfrac{100 \times 2}{400} = +0.5\,\text{Amp}$

21. (b) Given,

Length of wire, $l = 30$ cm

Radius of wire, $r = 2$ mm $= 2 \times 10^{-3}$ m

Resistivity of metal wire, $\rho = 1.23 \times 10^{-8}\,\Omega\text{m}$

Emf generated, $|e| = \dfrac{d\phi}{dt} = \dfrac{dB}{dt}(A)$ $(\because \phi = \text{B.A.})$

Current, $i = \dfrac{e}{R}$

But, resistance of wire, $R = \rho\dfrac{l}{A}$

$\therefore i = \left|\dfrac{dB}{dt}\right|\dfrac{(A)^2}{\rho l} = \dfrac{0.032 \times \{\pi \times 2 \times 10^{-3}\}^2}{1.23 \times 10^{-8} \times 0.3} = 0.61\,\text{A}.$

22. (d) According to question,

$I(t) = I_0 t(1-t)$

$\therefore I = I_0 t - I_0 t^2$

$\phi = B.A$

$\phi = (\mu_0 nI) \times (\pi R^2)$

$(\because B = \mu_0 nI \text{ and } A = \pi R^2)$

$V_R = \dfrac{-d\phi}{dt}$

$V_R = \mu_0 n\pi R^2 (I_0 - 2I_0 t)$

$\Rightarrow V_R = 0$ at $t = \dfrac{1}{2}s$

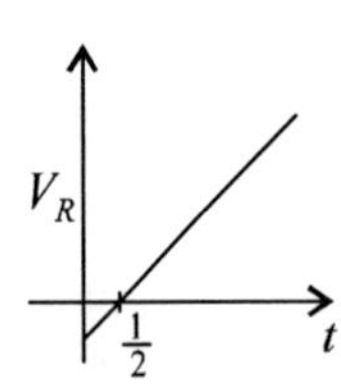

V_R, $\frac{1}{2}$, t

23. (b) We have given, time period, $T = 10$s

$\therefore$ Angular velocity, $\omega = \dfrac{2\pi}{10} = \dfrac{\pi}{5}$

Magnetic flux, $\phi(t) = BA\cos\omega t$

Emf induced, $E = \dfrac{-d\phi}{dt} = BA\omega\sin\omega t = BA\omega\sin(\omega t)$

Induced emf, $|\varepsilon|$ is maximum when $\omega t = \dfrac{\pi}{2}$

$\Rightarrow t = \dfrac{\frac{\pi}{2}}{\frac{\pi}{5}} = 2.5$ s

For induced emf to be minimum i.e zero

$\omega t = \pi \Rightarrow t = \dfrac{\pi}{\frac{\pi}{5}} = 5\,s$

$\therefore$ Induced emf is zero at t = 5 s

24. (a) $\text{E} = \dfrac{d}{dt}(\text{NMI}) \Rightarrow \text{E} = \text{NM}\dfrac{dI}{dt} \Rightarrow \text{E} = \dfrac{\text{NMI}}{t}$

emf induced per unit turn $= \dfrac{\text{E}}{\text{N}} = \dfrac{\text{MI}}{t}$

25. (b) $V = 200$V; $r = 10\Omega$

$R' = 10 + 100\Omega = 110\Omega$

$I = \dfrac{V}{R'} = \dfrac{220}{100} = 2A$

$P = I^2R = 4 \times 100 = 400\,W$

26. (b) Induced emf,

$e = Bv\ell = 1 \times 10^{-2} \times 0.05 = 5 \times 10^{-4}$ V

Equivalent resistance,

$R = \dfrac{4 \times 2}{4+2} + 1.7 = \dfrac{4}{3} + 1.7 \simeq 3\,\Omega$

Current, $i = \dfrac{e}{R} = \dfrac{5 \times 10^{-4}}{3} \simeq 170\,\mu\text{A}$

27. (d) Inductance $= \dfrac{\mu_0 N^2 A}{L}$

28. (c)

29. (c)

$\text{X} = l$

1⟵x⟶dx

Magnetic moment, M = NIA

$dQ = \rho\, dx$

$dI = \dfrac{dQ}{2\pi}.\omega$ and $dM = dI \times A$

$= \dfrac{\omega}{2\pi}.\dfrac{\rho_0}{\ell}.x\pi x^2\, dx \Rightarrow M = \dfrac{\rho_0}{\ell}n\pi\int_0^{\ell} x^3\, dx$

$= \dfrac{\pi}{4}.n\rho\ell^3$

30. (b) From Faraday's law of electomagnetic induction,

$e = \dfrac{d\phi}{dt} = \dfrac{d(BA)}{lt} = \dfrac{d(Bll)}{dt}$

$= \dfrac{Bdl \times l}{dt} = BVl$

Also, $F = ilB = \left(\dfrac{BV}{R}\right)(l^2B) = \dfrac{B^2l^2V}{R}$

At equilibrium

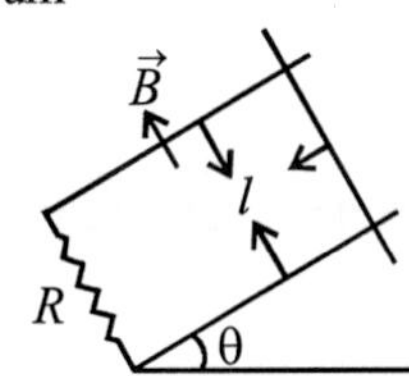

$mg\sin\theta = \dfrac{B^2lV}{R} \Rightarrow V = \dfrac{mgR\sin\theta}{B^2l^2}$

31. (b)

32. (d) Here, induced e.m.f.

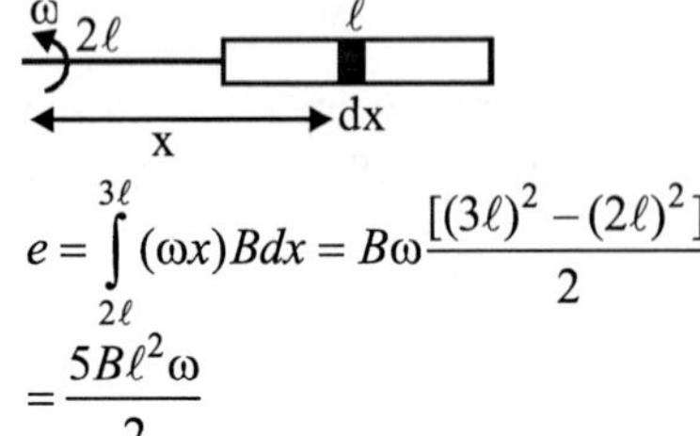

$e = \int_{2\ell}^{3\ell}(\omega x)Bdx = B\omega\dfrac{[(3\ell)^2 - (2\ell)^2]}{2}$

$= \dfrac{5B\ell^2\omega}{2}$

33. (b) Due to the movement of resistor R, an emf equal to Blv will be induced in it as shown in figure clearly,

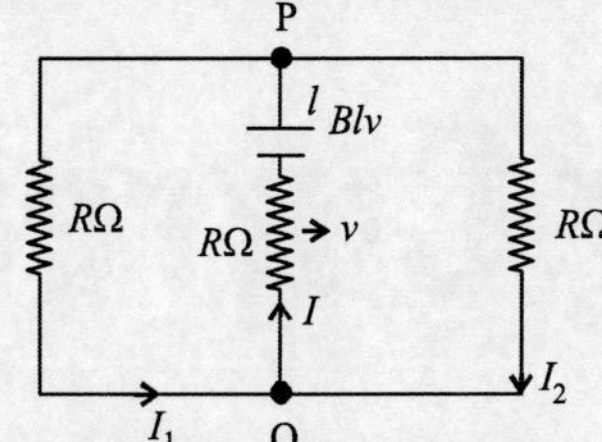

$I = I_1 + I_2$ Also, $I_1 = I_2$
Solving the circuit,

we get $I_1 = I_2 = \frac{Blv}{3R}$

and $I = 2I_1 = \frac{2Blv}{3R}$

34. (d) Given, Area of cross-section of pipe,
$A = 10\text{ cm}^2$
Length of pipe, $\ell = 20$ cm

$M = \frac{\mu_0 N_1 N_2 A}{\ell}$

$= \frac{4\pi \times 10^{-7} \times 300 \times 400 \times 100 \times 10^{-4}}{0.2}$

$M = \frac{\mu_0 N_1 N_2 A}{\ell}$

$= 2.4\pi \times 10^{-4}$ H

35. (c) Relative velocity of the tube of width l,
$= v - (-v)\ v = 2v$
∴ Induced emf. $= B.l\,(2v)$

36. (b) Given, length of conductor $\ell = 1$m,
Angular speed, $\omega = 5$ rad/s,
Magnetic field, $B = 0.2 \times 10^{-4}\ T$
EmF generated between two ends of conductor

$\varepsilon = \frac{B\omega l^2}{2} = \frac{0.2 \times 10^{-4} \times 5 \times 1}{2} = 50\mu V$

37. (d) Because of the Lenz's law of conservation of energy. Length of straight wire, $\ell = 20$m Earth's Magneti field, $B = 0.30 \times 10^{-4}$ Wb/m^2.

38. (b) Electric flux is given by
$\phi = B.A$

$\phi = B_0 \pi r^2 e^{-t/\tau} \qquad \left(\because B = B_0 e^{-t/t}\right)$

Induced E.m.f. $\varepsilon = \frac{d\phi}{dt} = \frac{B_0 \pi r^2}{\tau^2} e^{-t/\tau}$

Heat $= \int_0^\infty \frac{\varepsilon^2}{R} = \frac{\pi^2 r^4 B_0^2}{2\tau R}$

39. (d) As the side BC is outside the field, no emf is induced across BC. Further, sides AB and CD are not cutting any flux. So, they will not centribute in flux.
Only side AD is cutting the flux 50 emf will be induced due to AD only.
The induced emf is

$e = \frac{-d\phi}{dt} = -\frac{d(\vec{B}\cdot\vec{A})}{dt} = \frac{-d\,(BA\cos 0^\circ)}{dt}$

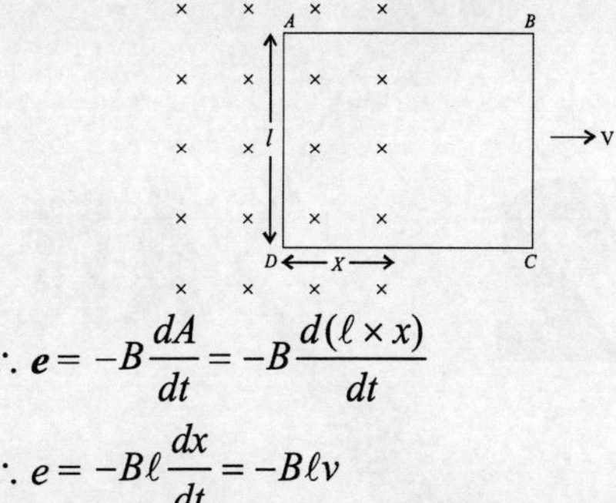

$\therefore e = -B\frac{dA}{dt} = -B\frac{d(\ell \times x)}{dt}$

$\therefore e = -B\ell\frac{dx}{dt} = -B\ell v$

40. (d) Induced emf,

$e = -\frac{\Delta\phi}{\Delta t} = \frac{-\Delta(LI)}{\Delta t} = -L\frac{\Delta I}{\Delta t}$

$\therefore |e| = L\frac{\Delta I}{\Delta t}$

$\Rightarrow 8 = L \times \frac{[2-(-2)]}{0.05}$

$\Rightarrow L = \frac{8 \times 0.05}{4} = 0.1\text{H}$

41. (a) According to Faraday's law of electromagnetic induction, $\varepsilon = \frac{d\phi}{dt}$
Also, $\varepsilon = iR$

$\therefore \quad iR = \frac{d\phi}{dt} \quad \Rightarrow \quad \int d\phi = R\int i dt$

Magnitude of change in flux $(d\phi) = R \times$ area under current vs time graph

or, $d\phi = 100 \times \frac{1}{2} \times \frac{1}{2} \times 10 = 250$ Wb

42. (d) According to Faraday's law of electromagnetic induction,

Induced emf, $e = \frac{Ldi}{dt}$

$50 = L\left(\frac{5-2}{0.1\text{sec}}\right)$

$\Rightarrow \quad L = \frac{50 \times 0.1}{3} = \frac{5}{3} = 1.67$ H

43. (a) Given: No. of turns $N = 1000$
Face area, $A = 4\text{ cm}^2 = 4 \times 10^{-4}\text{ m}^2$
Change in magnetic field,
$\Delta B = 10^{-2}$ wbm^{-2}
Time taken, $t = 0.01\text{s} = 10^{-2}$ sec
Emf induced in the coil $e = ?$
Applying formula,

Induced emf, $e = \frac{-d\phi}{dt} = N\left(\frac{\Delta B}{\Delta t}\right)A\cos\theta$

$= \frac{1000 \times 10^{-2} \times 4 \times 10^{-4}}{10^{-2}} = 400$ mV

44. (b) Mutual Inductance of two coils
$M = \sqrt{M_1 M_2} = \sqrt{2\text{mH} \times 8\text{mH}} = 4\text{mH}$

45. (b) Electric flux, $\phi = 10t^2 - 50t + 250$

Induced emf, $e = -\frac{d\phi}{dt} = -(20t - 50)$

$e_{t=3} = -10\ V$

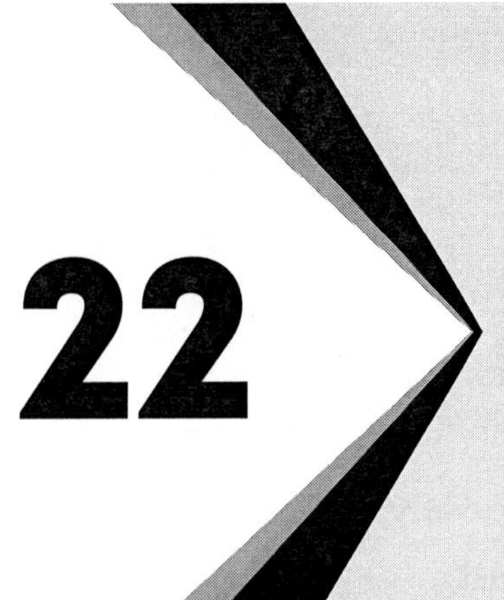

22 Alternating Current

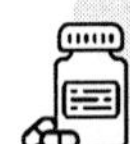

Topic 22.1: Alternating & Direct Current, Average & RMS Value of Current, Resistance Offered by Various Elements to AC, Impedances and Phases of AC Circuit Containing Different Elements, Q-factor and Power in an AC Circuit

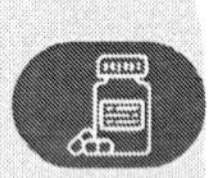

ALTERNATING AND DIRECT CURRENT

*An **alternating current** (A.C.) is one which periodically changes in magnitude and direction.* It increases from zero to a maximum value, then decreases to zero and reverses in direction, increases to a maximum in this direction and then decreases to zero.

The source of alternating emf may be a dynamo or an electronic oscillator.

The alternating emf E at any instant may be expressed as

$$E = E_0 \sin\omega t$$

where ω is the angular frequency of alternating emf and E_0 is the peak value of emf.

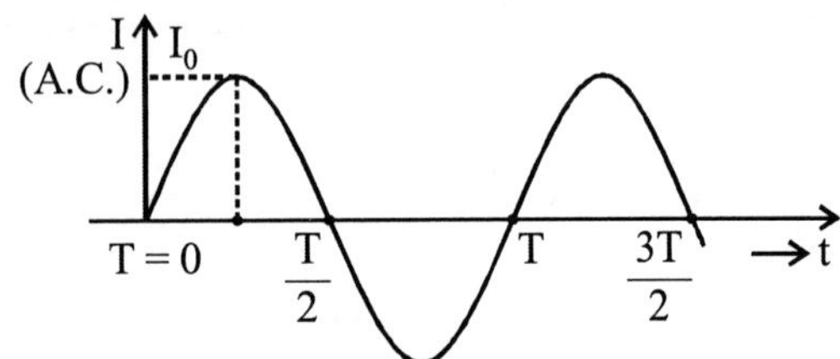

***Direct current** (D.C.) is that current which may or may not change in magnitude but it does not change its direction.*

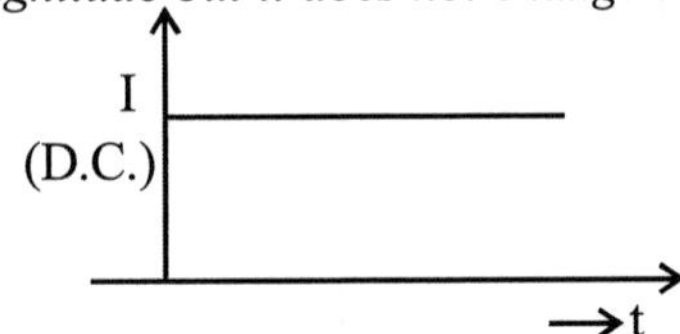

Advantages of A.C. over D.C.

(i) The generation of A.C. is cheaper than that of D.C.

(ii) Alternating voltage can be easily stepped up or stepped down by using a transformer.

(iii) A.C. can be easily converted into D.C. by rectifier. D.C. is converted to A.C. by an inverter.

(iv) A.C. can be transmitted to a long distance without appreciable loss.

AVERAGE AND RMS VALUE OF ALTERNATING CURRENT

The average value of AC over one full cycle is zero since there are equal positive and negative half cycles.

The average current for half cycle is $2I_0/\pi$ where I_0 is the peak value of current.

The root mean square (rms) value of AC is

$$I_{rms} = \frac{I_0}{\sqrt{2}}$$

where I_0 is the peak or maximum value of alternating current.

*The **rms value** of alternating current can also be defined as the direct current which produces the same heating effect in a given resistor in a given time as is produced by the given A.C. flowing through same resistor for the same time.* Due to this reason the rms value of current is also known as **effective** or **virtual value of current**.

$$\therefore \quad I_{effective} = I_{virtual} = I_{rms} = \frac{I_0}{\sqrt{2}}$$

Similarly the rms value of alternating voltgae is called the effective or virtual value of alternating voltage (or emf).

$$\therefore \quad E_{effective} = E_{virtual} = E_{rms} = \frac{E_0}{\sqrt{2}}$$

Problem Solving Tips

(1) **Time period :** The time taken by A.C. to go through one cycle of changes is called its period. It is given as $T = \frac{2\pi}{\omega}$

(2) **Phase :** It is that property of wave motion which tells us the position of the particle at any instant as well as its direction of motion. It is measured either by the angle which the particle makes with the mean position or by fraction of time period.

(3) **Phase angle :** Angle associated with the wave motion (sine or cosine) is called phase angle.

(4) **Lead :** Out of the current and emf the one having greater phase angle will lead the other e.g., in equation

$$i = i_0 \sin\left(\omega t + \frac{\pi}{2}\right) \text{ and } e = e_0 \sin \omega t,$$

the current leads the emf by an angle $\frac{\pi}{2}$.

(5) **Lag :** Out of current and emf the one having smaller phase angle will lag the other. In the above equations, the emf lags the current by $\frac{\pi}{2}$.

RESISTANCE OFFERED BY VARIOUS ELEMENTS (INDUCTOR, RESISTOR AND CAPACITOR) TO A.C.

Alternating current in a circuit may be controlled by resistance, inductance and capacitance, while the direct current is controlled only by resistance.

(i) **Impedance (Z) :** *In alternating current circuit, the ratio of emf applied and consequent current produced is called the impedance* and is denoted by Z,

i.e., $Z = \frac{E}{I} = \frac{E_0}{I_0} = \frac{E_{rms}}{I_{rms}}$

Physically impedance of ac circuit is the hindrance offered by resistance along with either inductance or capacitance or both in the circuit to the flow of ac through it. Its unit is ohm.

(ii) **Reactance (X) :** *The hindrance offered by inductance or capacitance or both to the flow of ac in an ac circuit is called reactance* and is denoted by X. Thus when there is no ohmic resitance in the cirucit, the reactance is equal to impedance. The reactance due to inductance alone is called inductive reactance and is denoted by X_L, while the reactance due to capacitance alone is called the capacitive reactance and is denoted by X_C. Its unit is also ohm.

(iii) **Admittance (Y) :** *The inverse of impedance is called the admittance* and is denoted by Y, i.e., $Y = \frac{1}{Z}$

Its SI unit is ohm^{-1}.

IMPEDANCES AND PHASES OF AC CIRCUIT CONTAINING DIFFERENT ELEMENTS

As already pointed out that in an ac circuit the current and applied emfs are not necessarily in same phase. The applied emf (E) and current produced (I) may be expresed as

$E = E_0 \sin \omega t$ and $I = I_0 \sin(\omega t + \phi)$ with $I_0 = E_0 / Z$

where E_0 and I_0 are peak values of alternating emf and current.

Circuit Containing only Resistor (R)

Consider a pure ohmic resistor (zero inductance) of resistance R connected to an alternating source of emf $E = E_0 \sin\omega t$.

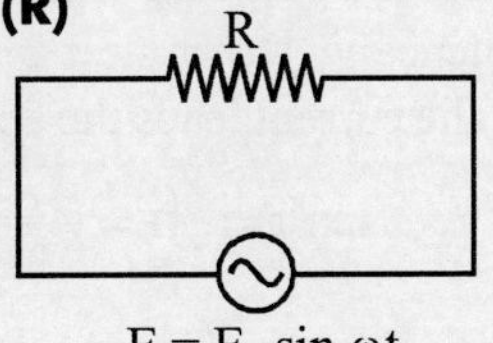

Then current I in the circuit is

$$I = \frac{E}{R} = \frac{E_0 \sin \omega t}{R} = I_0 \sin \omega t, \text{ where } I_0 = E_0 / R$$

Comparing this with standard equation, we get that **impedance of circuit, Z = R** and **phase difference between current & emf = 0.**

Hence we conclude that *in a purely resistive ac circuit the current and voltage are in same phase and impedance of circuit is equal to the ohmic resistance.*

Phasor diagram : •——→——→—— X (I, E)

Graph of emf or current versus ωt :

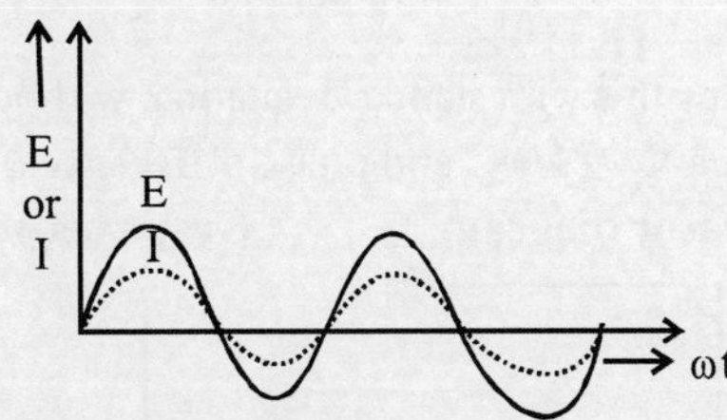

Circuit Contianing only Inductor (L)

Consider a pure inductor (zero ohmic resistance) of inductance L connected to an alternating source of emf $E = E_0 \sin \omega t$.

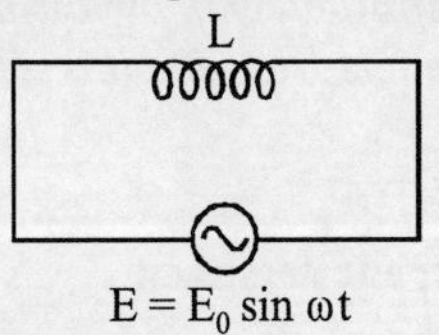

Then current I in the circuit is

$$I = I_0 \sin\left(\omega t - \frac{\pi}{2}\right) \quad \text{where } I_0 = \frac{E_0}{\omega L}$$

Comparing this with standard equation, we get

$Z = \omega L$ and phase difference $\phi = \pi/2$.

Hence we conclude that *in a purely inductive circuit the current lags behind the applied voltage by an angle π/2 and the impedance to the circuit is ωL and this is called as* ***inductive reactance.***

Graph of emf or current versus ωt

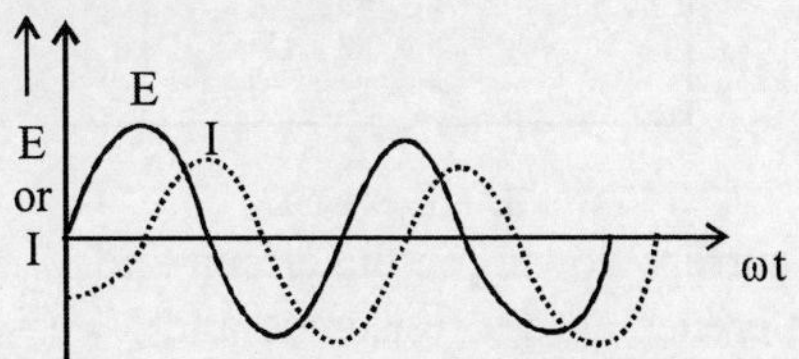

Phasor diagram **Graph between X_L and f**

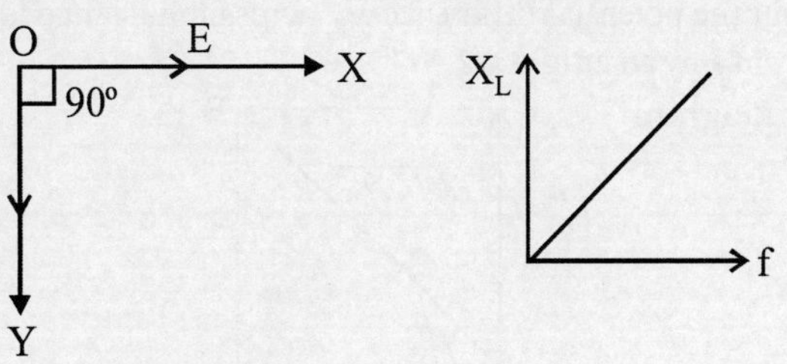

Circuit Containing only Capacitor

Consider a capacitor of capacitance C connected to an alternating source of emf, $E = E_0 \sin \omega t$.

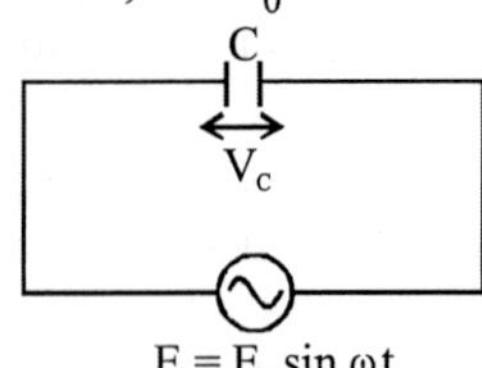

Then the current through capacitor is given by,

$$I = I_0 \sin\left(\omega t + \frac{\pi}{2}\right)$$

Comparing this with standard equation, we find that **capacitive reactance $X_C = 1/\omega C$** and **phase difference $\phi = +\pi/2$**

Phasor diagram **Graph between X_C and f**

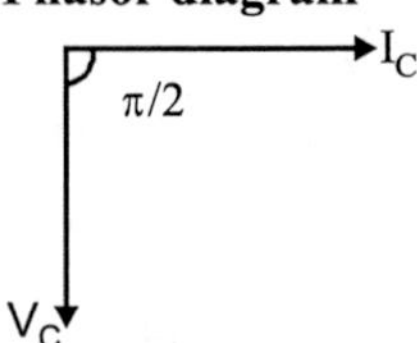

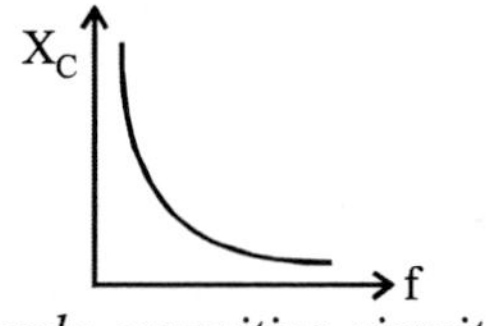

Hence we conclude that *in a purely capacitive circuit the current leads the applied emf by an angle π/2 and the impedance of the circuit is 1/ωC and this is known as capacitive reactance* $Z = X_C = \frac{1}{\omega C}$.

Graph of emf or current versus ωt

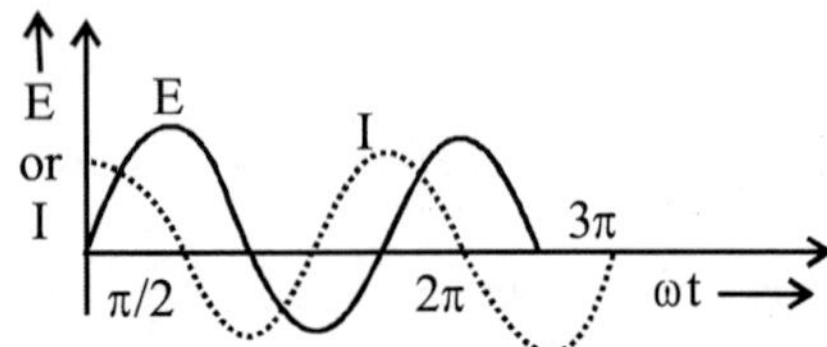

Circuit Containing Resistance and Inductance in Series (LR Series Circuit)

Consider a circuit containing resistance R and inductance L in series having an alternating emf $E = E_0 \sin \omega t$.

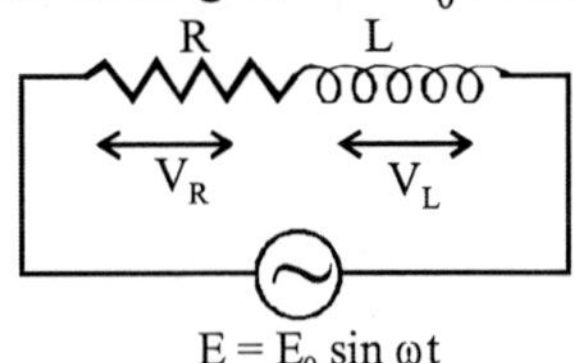

Let I be the current flowing in the circuit and V_R (= **IR**) the potential difference across resistance and V_L (= ωL.**I**) the potential difference across inductance.

The current **I** and the potential difference V_R are always in phase but the potential difference V_L across inductance leads the current **I** by an anlgle π/2.

Phasor diagram

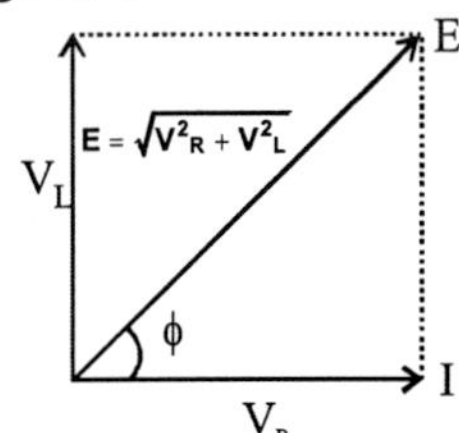

From phasor diagrom, resultant voltage is given by,

$$E = \sqrt{(V_R^2 + V_L^2)} = \sqrt{(RI)^2 + (\omega L.I)^2}$$

Graph of emf or current versus ωt

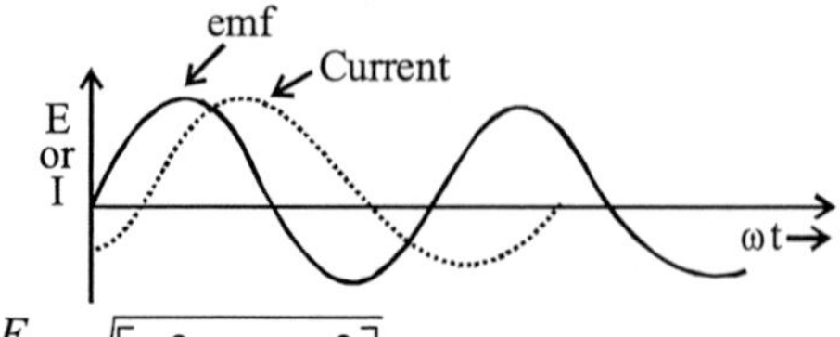

$\therefore \quad \frac{E}{I} = \sqrt{\left[R^2 + (\omega L)^2\right]}$

$\therefore$ Impedance of R – L circuit,

$$Z = \frac{E}{I} = \sqrt{(R^2 + X_L^2)} \quad \text{where } X_L = \omega L$$

It is obvious that *the current lags behind the emf by angle ϕ given by,*

$$\phi = \tan^{-1}\left(\frac{V_L}{V_R}\right) = \tan^{-1}\left(\frac{X_L}{R}\right) = \tan^{-1}\left(\frac{\omega L}{R}\right)$$

Circuit Containing Resistance and Capacitance in Series (C–R Series Circuit)

Consider a circuit containing resistance R and capacitance C in series having an alternating emf $E = E_0 \sin \omega t$.

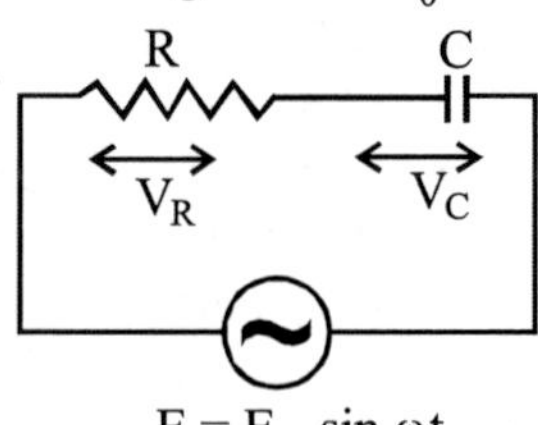

Let I be the current flowing in the circuit, V_R the potential difference across resistance and V_C the potential difference across capacitance.

Phasor diagram

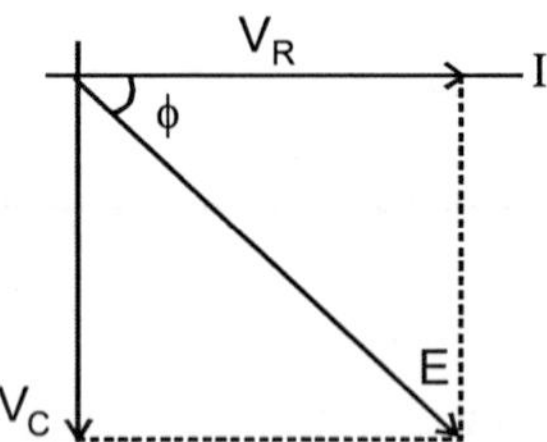

From phasor diagram the resultant emf is given by

$$E = \sqrt{(V_R^2 + V_C^2)} = \sqrt{(R\mathbf{I})^2 + (X_C\mathbf{I})^2]}$$

$\therefore$ Impedance, $Z = E/\mathbf{I} = \sqrt{(R^2 + X_C^2)}$, where

$$X_C = \left(\frac{1}{\omega C}\right)$$

The potential difference V_R and current **I** are in same phase and the potential difference V_C lags behind the current **I** (and hence V_R) by angle π/2

The current leads the applied emf by an angle ϕ given by

$$\tan\varphi = \frac{V_C}{V_R} = \frac{X_C\mathbf{I}}{R\mathbf{I}} = \frac{X_C}{R}$$

or $\tan\phi = \left(\frac{X_C}{R}\right) \Rightarrow \phi = \tan^{-1}\left(\frac{1/\omega C}{R}\right) = \tan^{-1}\left(\frac{1}{\omega CR}\right)$

Graph of emf or current versus ωt

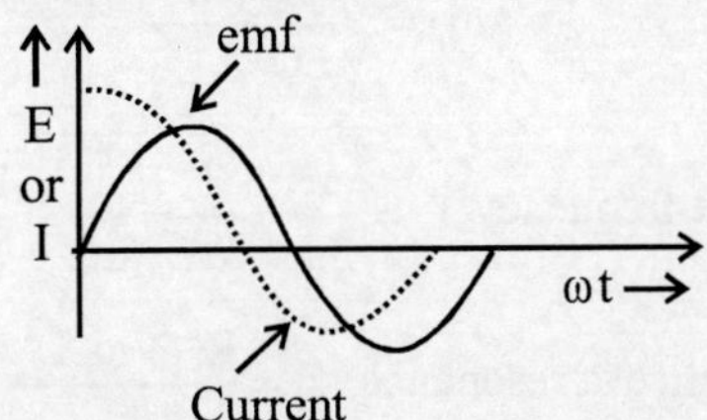

Circuit Containing Inductance and Capacitance in Series (Series LC Circuit)

Consider a circuit containing inductance L and capacitance C in series having an alternating emf

$$E = E_0 \sin \omega t.$$

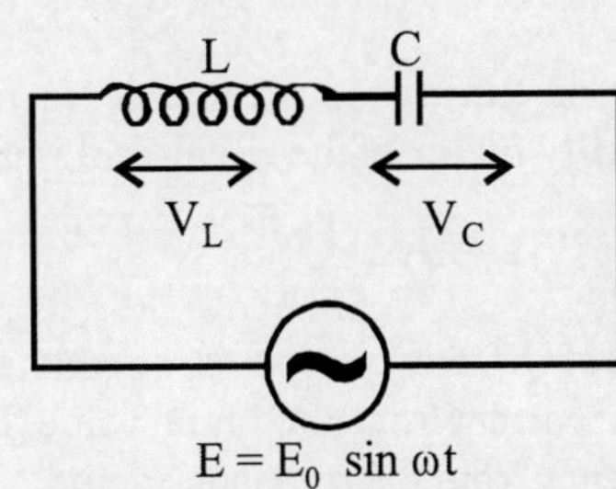

$E = E_0 \sin \omega t$

Let I be the current flowing in circuit, V_L the potential difference across inductance L and V_C the p.d. across capacitance C.

Phasor diagram :

The p.d. V_C lags behind the current by angle π/2 and the p.d. V_L leads the current by angle π/2.

∴ Resultant applied emf, $E = V_C - V_L = X_C\mathbf{I} - X_L\mathbf{I}$

∴ Reactance of circuit,

$$X = E/\mathbf{I} = X_C - X_L = \left(\frac{1}{\omega C} - \omega L\right)$$

The current leads applied emf by $\phi = \pi/2$.

In case of $X_C = X_L$, $Z = 0$, then $\frac{1}{\omega C} = \omega L$ or $\omega = \frac{1}{\sqrt{(LC)}}$

∴ Frequency $f = \omega/2\pi = \frac{1}{2\pi\sqrt{(LC)}}$

At certain frequency the impedance of the circuit is minimum and the current is maximum.

This frequency is called the **resonant frequency**.

Circuit Containing Resistance, Inductance and Capacitance in Series (Series LCR Circuit)

Consider a circuit containing a resistance R, inductance L and capacitance C in series having an alternating emf

$$E = E_0 \sin \omega t.$$

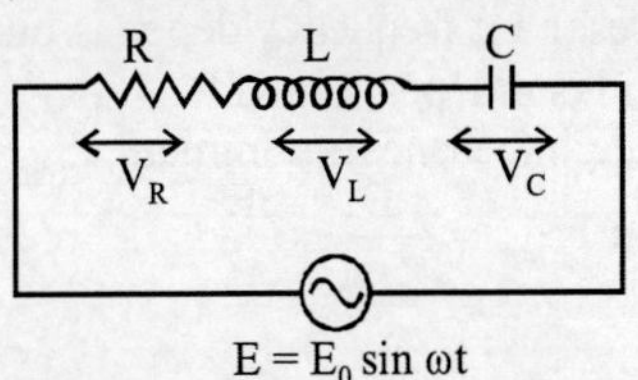

$E = E_0 \sin \omega t$

Let **I** be the current flowing in circuit. V_R, V_L and V_C are respective potential differences across resistance R, inductance L and capacitance C.

Phasor diagram :

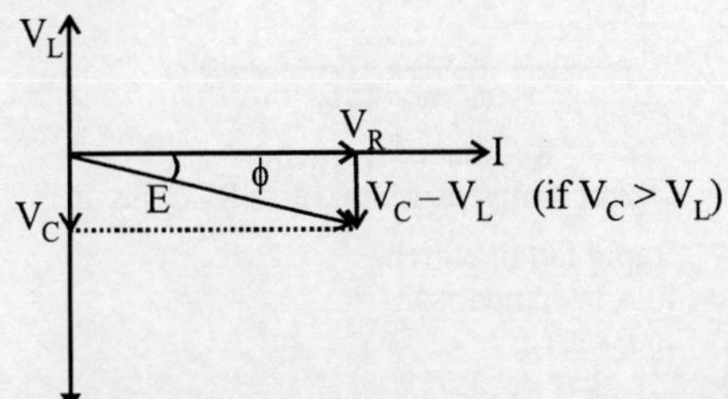

The p.d. V_R is in phase with current **I**. The p.d. V_C lags behind the current by angle π/2. The p.d. V_L leads the current by angle π/2.

∴ Resultant applied emf, $E = \sqrt{[V_R^2 + (V_C - V_L)^2]}$

i.e., $E = \sqrt{\{(R\mathbf{I})^2 + (\mathbf{I}X_C - \mathbf{I}X_L)^2\}}$

∴ Impedance, $Z = \frac{E}{\mathbf{I}} = \sqrt{\{R^2 + (X_C - X_L)^2\}}$

The phase leads of current over applied emf is given by

$$\tan\varphi = \frac{V_C - V_L}{V_R} = \frac{IX_C - IX_L}{RI} = \frac{X_C - X_L}{R}$$

i.e., $\varphi = \tan^{-1}\left(\frac{X_C - X_L}{R}\right)$

It is concluded that :

(a) If $X_C > X_L$, the value of ϕ is positive, i.e., current leads the applied emf.

(b) If $X_C < X_L$, the value of ϕ is negative, i.e., current lags behind the applied emf.

(c) If $X_C = X_L$, the value of ϕ is zero, i.e., current and emf are in same phase. This is called the case of **resonance** and resonant frequency for condition $X_C = X_L$, is given by :

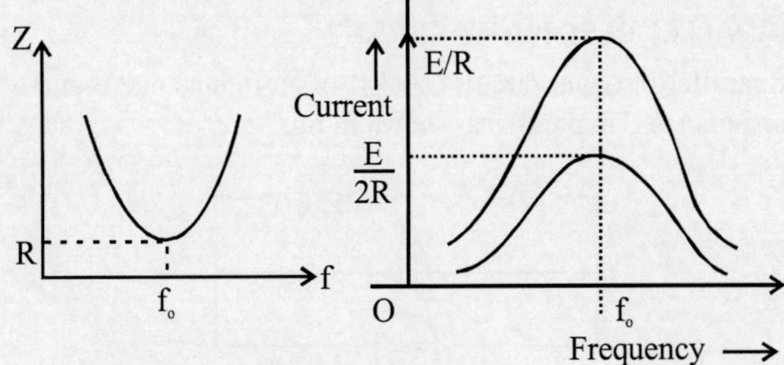

$$\frac{1}{\omega C} = \omega L \text{ i.e., } \omega = \frac{1}{\sqrt{LC}}$$

$$\therefore \quad f_o = \omega/2\pi = \frac{1}{2\pi\sqrt{(LC)}}.$$

Thus the resonant frequency depends on the product of L and C and is independent of R.

At resonance, impedance is minimum, $Z_{min} = R$ and current is maximum $\mathbf{I}_{max} = \frac{E}{Z_{min}} = \frac{E}{R}$

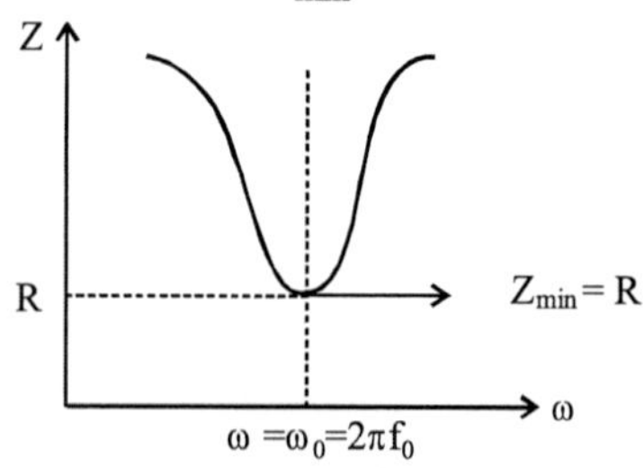

Resonance frequency

Circuit impedence in series RLC circuit

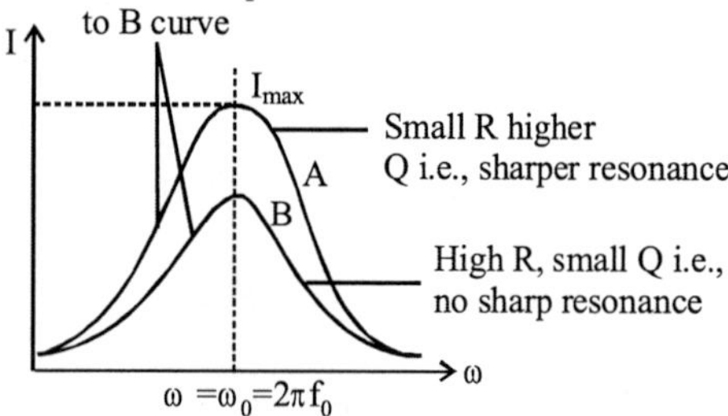

Resonance frequency

Current amplitude in series RLC circuit

It is interesting to note that before resonance the current leads the applied emf, at resonance it is in phase, and after resonance it lags behind the emf. LCR series circuit is also called as **acceptor circuit** and parallel LCR circuit is called **rejector circuit**.

MISCONCEPTIONS

✗ ***Incorrect.*** Adding impedances / reactances /resistors algebrically.

✓ ***Correct.*** For these physical quantities, vector additon must be done

✗ ***Incorrect.*** Kirchoff's laws are applicable in D.C. circuit only

✓ ***Correct.*** Kirchoff's laws are applicable in A.C. circuit also (which may include inductor and capacitor).

PARALLEL RESONANT CIRCUIT

A parallel resonant circuit consists of an inductance L and a capacitance C in parallel as shown in fig.

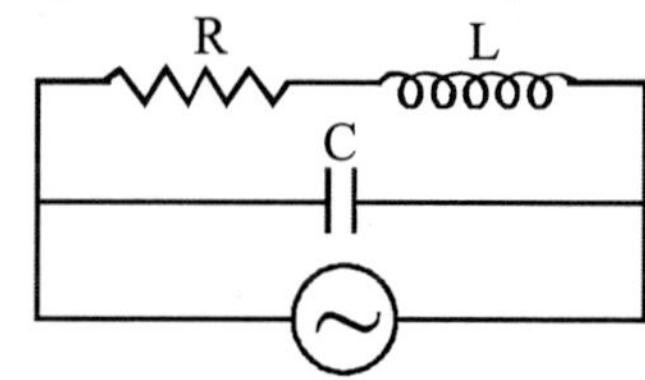

$E = E_0 \sin \omega t$

The condition of resonance is again that the current and applied emf must be in same phase. The condition gives angular resonant frequency.

$$\omega_r = \sqrt{\frac{1}{LC} - \frac{R^2}{L^2}}$$

$\therefore$ Resonant frequency $f_r = \frac{\omega_r}{2\pi} = \frac{1}{2\pi}\sqrt{\frac{1}{LC} - \frac{R^2}{L^2}}$

The impedance at resonance, $Z = \frac{R^2 + \omega^2 L^2}{R} = \frac{L}{RC}$

In parallel resonant circuit the impedance is maximum and the current is minimum.

If $R \to 0$, then $f_r = \frac{1}{2\pi\sqrt{(LC)}}$ and $Z \to \infty$.

Q - FACTOR

The sharpness of tuning at resonance is measured by **Q-factor** or **quality factor** of the circuit and is given by

$$Q = \frac{1}{R}\sqrt{\frac{L}{C}}$$

Higher the value of Q-factor, sharper is the resonance i.e. more rapid is the fall of current from maximum value ($\mathbf{I}_0$) with slight change in frequency from the resonance value.

It is clear from the figure that at low value of θ, the resonance is poor. However the bandwidth increases

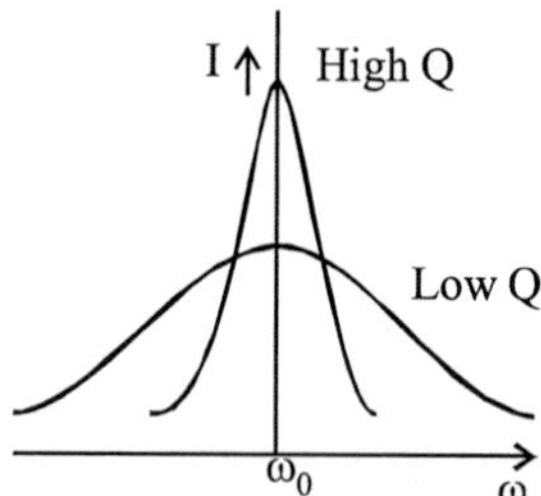

The figure given below explains the concept of bandwidth and cut-off frequency.

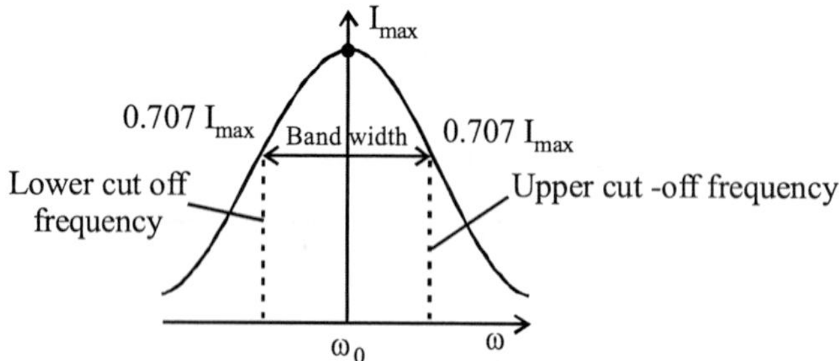

when $\omega < \omega_0$	$X_C < X_L$
when $\omega > \omega_0$	$X_L > X_C$
when $\omega = \omega_0$	$X_C = X_L$

Bandwidth : *It is the band of allowed frequencies and is defined as the difference between upper and lower cut-off frequencies, the frequency at which power becomes half of maximum value and current becomes* $I_{max}/\sqrt{2}$.

POWER IN AN A.C. CIRCUIT

The power is defined as the rate at which work is being done in the circuit. In ac circuit, the current and emf are not necessarily in the same phase, therefore we write

$E = E_0 \sin \omega t$ & $I = I_0 \sin(\omega t + \phi)$.

The instaneous power, $P = EI$

$= E_0 \sin \omega t \, I_0 \sin(\omega t + \phi)$,

The *average power* $P_{av} = E_{rms} I_{rms} \cos \phi$

$$\therefore \quad P_{av} = \frac{E_0}{\sqrt{2}} \frac{I_0}{\sqrt{2}} \cos \phi$$

In this expression $\cos \phi$ is known as **power factor.** The value of $\cos \phi$ depends on the nature of the circuit. For L, C and L-C circuit, the power factor is zero ($\because \phi = 90^\circ$); for R-circuit $\cos \phi = 1$ ($\because \phi = 0$) and for all other circuit $\cos \phi = R/Z$, where Z = impedance.

If $R = 0$, $\cos \phi = 0$ and $P_{av} = 0$ i.e., in a circuit with no resistance, the power loss is zero. Such a circuit is called the **wattless circuit** and the current flowing is called the **wattless current.**

Power is of two types

(i) Reactive power	$P_{reactive} = V_{rms} I_{rms} \sin \phi$ This is also called wattless power. It is not read by energy meter
(ii) Active power	$P_{active} = V_{rms} I_{rms} \cos \phi$ It is read by energy meter

Half Power Points

The values of ω at which the average power is half of its maximum value (at resonant frequency) are called half power points.

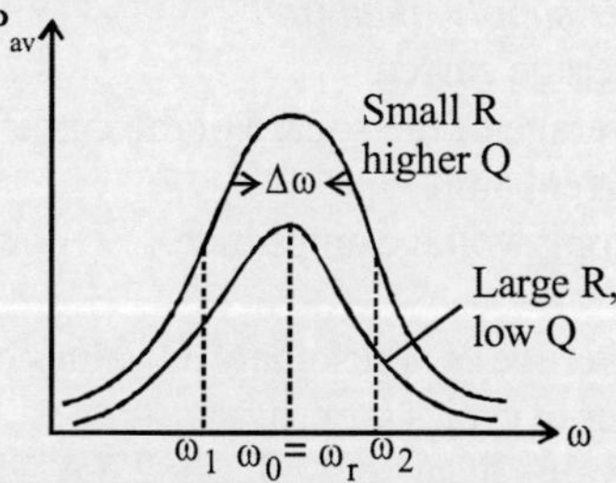

Plot of average power versus frequency for a series RLC circuit. The upper curve is for a small R & lower broad curve is for large value of R.

It is clear from the figure that for smaller R, value of Q_0 is high (Q_0 is Quality factor of circuit) & hence sharper resonance i.e. greater rate of fall of average power maximum average power P_{av} changes with slight change in frequency from resonant frequency.

The Quality factor, Q_0 is defined as, $Q_0 = \dfrac{\omega_0}{\Delta\omega}$

Where $\Delta\omega = \omega_2 - \omega_1$ and ω_2 & ω_1 are **half power points.**

Now, since $\Delta\omega \approx \dfrac{R}{L}$; so $Q_0 \approx \dfrac{\omega_0 L}{R}$

Whereas $\omega_1 = \omega_0 - \dfrac{\omega_0}{Q_0}$; $\omega_2 = \omega_0 + \dfrac{\omega_0}{Q_0}$

In concise term, we can write as, $\omega = \omega_r\left(1 \pm \dfrac{1}{Q_0}\right)$

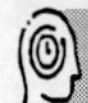

Problem Solving Tips

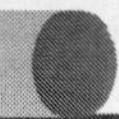

1. Unless mentioned otherwise, all a.c. currents and voltages are r.m.s. values.
2. For resonance to occur, the presence of both L and C elements in the circuit is a must.
3. In series resonant circuit, current is maximum at resonance. In a parallel resonant circuit, current is minimum (or zero) at resonance but p.d across the combination is maximum.
4. To depict oscillatory motion mathematically we may use sines, cosines or their linear combination. This is because changing the zero position transforms one into another.
5. While adding voltage across different elements in an a.c. circuit we should take care of their phases.
6. The average current over a complete cycle in an a.c circuit is zero but the average power is not zero.
7. An inductor offers negligibly low resistance path to d.c. and a resistive path for a.c.
8. A capacitor acts as a block for d.c and a low resistance path to a.c.
9.

Inductive reactance	Capacitive reactance
$X_L = \omega L = 2\pi f L$ $\Rightarrow X_L \propto f$	$X_C = \dfrac{1}{\omega C} = \dfrac{1}{2\pi f C}$ $\Rightarrow X_C \propto \dfrac{1}{f}$
Current through pure inductor lags behind emf by 90°	Current through pure capacitor leads emf by 90°
For d.c $f = 0 \therefore X_L = 0$	For d.c $f = 0 \Rightarrow X_C = \infty$
For a.c as f increases X_L increases	For a.c as f increases X_C decreases

10.

Series Resonant circuit	Parallel resosant circuit
$X_L = X_C$	$\dfrac{1}{X_L} = \dfrac{1}{X_C}$
$\nu_r = \dfrac{1}{2\pi\sqrt{LC}}$	$\nu_r = \dfrac{1}{2\pi}\sqrt{\dfrac{1}{LC} - \dfrac{R^2}{L^2}}$
$Z = \sqrt{R^2 + (X_L - X_C)^2}$	$\dfrac{1}{Z} = \sqrt{\dfrac{1}{R^2} + \left(C\omega - \dfrac{1}{L\omega}\right)^2}$

11. The principle of electric meter is heating effect of current. These meters give the reading of I_{rms}. It is important to note that these meters can measure D.C. as well as A.C.
12. D.C. flows through the cross-section of the conductor whereas A.C. flows mainly along the surface of the conductor. This is also known as **Skin Effect**. The skin effect is directly proportional to the frequency.

Example 1.

Calculate the r.m.s. value of e.m.f. given by
$E = 8 \sin \omega t + 6 \sin 2 \omega t$ volts.

Solution :

The mean square value is given by $E = \overline{E^2}$

$$\therefore \quad \overline{E^2} = \overline{(8\sin \omega t + 6\sin 2\omega t)^2}$$

$$= 64\overline{\sin^2 \omega t} + 96\overline{\sin \omega t . \sin 2\omega t} + 36\overline{\sin^2 2\omega t}$$

We know that $\overline{\sin^2 \omega t} = \frac{1}{2}$, $\overline{\sin^2 2\omega t} = \frac{1}{2}$, and

$\overline{\sin \omega t}.\overline{\sin 2\omega t} = 0$

$$\therefore \quad \overline{E^2} = 64 \times \frac{1}{2} + 96 \times 0 + 36 \times \frac{1}{2} = 32 + 18 = 50$$

or $\quad E_{r.m.s.} = \sqrt{(\overline{E^2})} = \sqrt{50} = 7.07$ volt

Example 2.

When 100 volt D.C. is applied across a solenoid a current of 1.0 amp flows in it. When 100 volt A.C. is applied across the same coil, the current drops to 0.5 amp. If the frequency of the A.C. source is 50 Hz, then determine the impedance and inductance of the solenoid.

Solution :

In case of D.C., $\omega = 0$ and hence $Z = R$

$$\therefore \quad Z = R = \frac{E}{I} = \frac{100}{1} = \mathbf{100\Omega}$$

For A.C., $Z = \left[R^2 + (2\pi n L)^2\right]^{1/2}$

$$= [(100)^2 + (100\pi L)^2]^{1/2}$$

(where $\omega = 2\pi n$ & n is frequency of AC source)

$$\therefore \quad 200 = [(100)^2 + (100\pi L)^2]^{1/2}$$

$\left\{\because Z = \frac{100}{0.5} = 200\Omega\right\}$ Solving we get $L =$ **0.55 henry**

Example 3.

A coil has an inductance of 0.7 henry and is joined in series with a resistance of 220 Ω. When an alternating e.m.f. of 220 V at 50 cycles per second, is applied to it, then what will be the wattless component of current in the circuit?

Solution :

Here, $X_L = \omega L = 2\pi n L = 2\pi \times 50 \times 0.7 \times = 220\,\Omega$
$R = 220\,\Omega$

$$Z = \sqrt{R^2 + X_L^2} = \sqrt{220^2 + 220^2} = 220\sqrt{2} \text{ ohm.}$$

$\therefore$ wattless component of current is

$$\mathbf{I} = \frac{E_O}{Z} = \frac{220}{220\sqrt{2}} = \frac{1}{\sqrt{2}} = 0.707\text{A}$$

Example 4.

A 60 volt-10 watt bulb is operated at 100 volt-60 Hz a.c. The inductance required is

(a) 2.56 H (b) 0.32 H
(c) 0.64 H (d) 1.28 H

Solution : (d)

$$\mathbf{I} = \frac{P}{V} = \frac{10}{60} = \frac{1}{6}\text{A};$$

$$R = \frac{V^2}{P} = \frac{60 \times 60}{10} = 360\Omega; \quad Z = \frac{V}{I} = \frac{100}{1/6} = 600\Omega$$

$$X_L^2 = Z^2 - R^2 = 600^2 - 360^2 = (600 + 360)(600 - 360)$$

$$X_L = \sqrt{960 \times 240} = 240 \times 2 = 480\Omega$$

$$\omega L = 2\pi n L = X_L = 480$$

$$L = \frac{X_L}{2\pi n} = \frac{480}{120\pi} = 1.28\text{H}$$

Example 5.

An a.c. circuit consists of only an inductor of inductance 2H. If the current is represented by a sine wave of amplitude 0.25 amp. and frequency 60 Hz, calculate the effective potential difference across the inductor.

Solution :

The effective potential difference across the inductor is given by

$$V_{eff} = I_{eff}\, X_L = \frac{I_0}{\sqrt{2}} .2\pi f L; \; V_{eff} = V_{rms}$$

Given that $I_0 = 0.25$ amp, f = 60 Hz, L = 2H

$$\therefore \quad V_{eff} = \frac{0.25}{\sqrt{2}} \times 2 \times 3.14 \times 60 \times 2 = 133.2 \text{ Volt}$$

Example 6.

If a domestic appliance draws 2.5 A from a 220-V, 60- Hz A.C. power supply, then find

(a) the average current
(b) the average of the square of the current
(c) the current amplitude
(d) the supply voltage amplitude.

Solution :

(a) The average of sinusoidal AC values over any whole number of cycles is zero.
(b) RMS value of current = I_{rms} = 2.5 A

$$\therefore \quad (I^2)_{av} = (I_{rms})^2 = 6.25\text{ A}^2$$

(c) $I_{rms} = \frac{I_m}{\sqrt{2}}$

$\therefore$ Current amplitude $= \sqrt{2} I_{rms} = \sqrt{2}(2.5\text{A}) = 3.5\text{ A}$

(d) $V_{rms} = 220\text{V} = \frac{V_m}{\sqrt{2}}$

$\therefore$ Supply voltage amplitude

$$V_m = \sqrt{2}(V_{rms}) = \sqrt{2}(220V) = 311\text{ V.}$$

Example 7.

A 100 μF capacitor in series with a 40 Ω resistance is connected to a 110 V, 60 Hz supply.

(a) What is the maximum current in the circuit?
(b) What is the time lag between current maximum and voltage maximum?

Solution :

(a) Here, $C = 100\ \mu F = 100 \times 10^{-6}\ F, R = 40\ \Omega$,

$V_{rms} = 110\ V, f = 60\ Hz$

Peak voltage, $V_0 = \sqrt{2}\ .\ V_{rms} = 100\sqrt{2} = 155.54\ V$

Circuit impedance, $Z = \sqrt{R^2 + \dfrac{1}{\omega^2 C^2}}$

$$= \sqrt{40^2 + \frac{1}{(2 \times \pi \times 60 \times 100 \times 10^{-6})^2}}$$

$$= \sqrt{1600 + 703.60} = \sqrt{2303.60} = 48\ \Omega$$

Hence, maximum current in coil,

$$I_0 = \frac{V_0}{Z} = \frac{155.54}{48} = 3.24\ A$$

(b) Phase lead angle (for current),

$$\theta = \tan^{-1}\frac{1}{\omega C R} = \tan^{-1}\frac{1}{2 \times 3.14 \times 60 \times 100 \times 10^{-6} \times 40}$$

$= \tan^{-1} 0.66315 = 33° 33'$ (taken 33.5°)

Time lead, $t = \dfrac{\theta}{\omega} = \dfrac{\theta}{2\pi\nu} = \dfrac{33.5}{360 \times 60} = 0.001551$ sec

$= 1.551 \times 10^{-3}$ sec

Voltage will lag current by = 1.551 ms.

Example 8.

30.0 μF capacitor is connected to a 220 V, 50 Hz source. Find the capacitive reactance and the current (rms and peak) in the circuit. If the frequency is doubled, what happens to the capacitive reactance and the current?

Solution :

The capacitive reactance is $X_C = \dfrac{1}{2\pi fC} = 106\Omega$

The rms current is $I_{rms} = \dfrac{V_{rms}}{X_C} = 2.08A$

The peak current is $I_m = \sqrt{2} I_{rms} = 2.96A$

This current oscillates between 2.96A and – 2.96A and is ahead of the voltage by 90°.

If the frequency is doubled, the capacitive reactance is halved and consequently, the current is doubled.

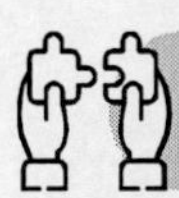

22.1 Concept Practice Problems

CPP

1. The maximum value of a.c. voltage in a circuit is 707 V. Its r.m.s. value is
   (a) 70.7 V (b) 100 V (c) 500 V (d) 707 V
2. In an a.c. circuit, the r.m.s. value of current, I_{rms} is related to the peak current, I_0 by the relation
   (a) $I_{rms} = \sqrt{2}\, I_0$ (b) $I_{rms} = \pi I_0$
   (c) $I_{rms} = \dfrac{1}{\pi} I_0$ (d) $I_{rms} = \dfrac{1}{\sqrt{2}} I_0$
3. A bulb and a capacitor are connected in series to a source of alternating current. If its frequency is increased, while keeping the voltage of the source constant, then bulb will
   (a) give more intense light
   (b) give less intense light
   (c) give light of same intensity before
   (d) stop radiating light
4. In a pure capacitive A.C. circuit current and voltage differ in phase by
   (a) 0° (b) 45° (c) 90° (d) 180°
5. A capacitor has capacitance C and reactance X, if capacitance and frequency become double, then reactance will be
   (a) 4X (b) X/2 (c) X/4 (d) 2X
6. In the circuit of Fig, the bulb will become suddenly bright if
   (a) contact is made or broken
   (b) contact is made
   (c) contact is broken
   (d) won't become bright at all
7. In a circuit L, C and R are connected in series with an alternating voltage source of frequency f. The current leads the voltage by 45°. The value of C is
   (a) $\dfrac{1}{\pi f(2\pi fL - R)}$ (b) $\dfrac{1}{2\pi f(2\pi fL - R)}$
   (c) $\dfrac{1}{\pi f(2\pi fL + R)}$ (d) $\dfrac{1}{2\pi f(2\pi fL + R)}$
8. In LCR circuit if resistance increases quality factor
   (a) increases finitely (b) decreases finitely
   (c) remains constant (d) None of these
9. In an A.C. circuit with phase voltage V and current I, the power dissipated is
   (a) VI (b) V^2I (c) VI^2 (d) V^2I^2
10. The power factor of an AC circuit having resistance (R) and inductance (L) connected in series and an angular velocity ω is
    (a) R/ωL (b) $R/(R^2 + \omega^2L^2)^{1/2}$
    (c) ωL/R (d) $R/(R^2 - \omega^2L^2)^{1/2}$

ANSWER KEY

1	(c)	2	(d)	3	(a)	4	(c)	5	(c)	6	(c)	7	(d)	8	(b)	9	(a)	10	(b)

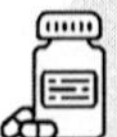

Topic 22.2 : Varying Current, Decay of Current, LC Oscillations and Transformer

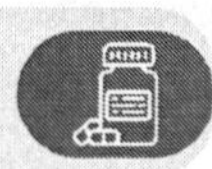

VARYING CURRENT

When the key in a D.C. circuit (containing a D.C. source of emf, inductance coil, resistance and capacitor) is closed or opened, the current in the circuit varies. This is known as varying current as it varies w.r.t. time and takes a final value after a short while.

Growth of Current

If K is closed at $t = 0$ so at $t = 0$, current in the circuit $I = 0$

After closing the key K at time t let current in the circuit = I and for small time in the circuit, current varies with time, so if rate of change of current with time $= \frac{dI}{dt}$ then due to phenomenon of self induction, induced emf across inductance $= -L\frac{dI}{dt}$

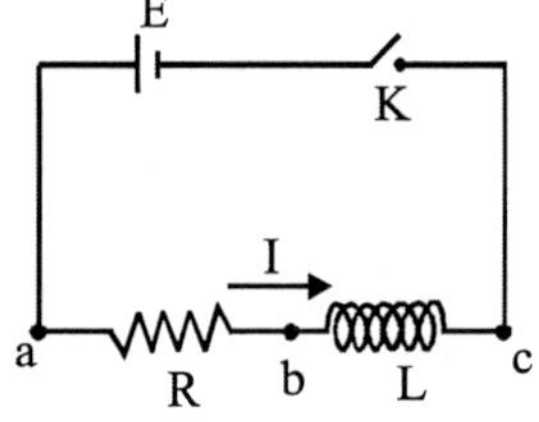

Potential difference across the resistance = IR

During growth of current in L-R circuit, if we applying Kirchhoff's loop rule then

$$E + \left(-L\frac{dI}{dt}\right) = IR$$

On solving it we get the value of current at any time t during growth of current in LR-circuit. $I = I_0\left(1 - e^{-\frac{R}{L}t}\right)$

Graph showing how current varies with time

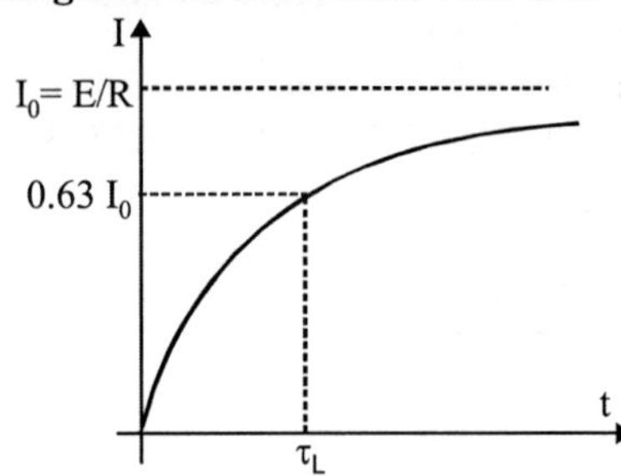

Time Constant

$\frac{L}{R}$ has dimensions of time. It is called **inductive time constant** of LR-circuit.

$$\text{At } t = \frac{L}{R}; \quad I = I_0(1 - e^{-\frac{R}{L}\cdot\frac{L}{R}}) = I_0(1 - e^{-1}) = I_0\left(\frac{e-1}{e}\right)$$

$$= I_0\left(\frac{2.71-1}{2.71}\right) = 0.632\, I_0$$

The ***inductive time constant*** *of an LR-circuit is the time in which the current grows from zero to 0.632 (or 63.2%) of its maximum value.* When $t \to \infty$.

$$I = I_0\left(1 - e^{-\frac{R}{L}\cdot\infty}\right) = I_0\left(1 - e^{-\infty}\right) = I_0(1 - 0)$$

Potential difference across resistance :

$$V_R = E\left(1 - e^{-\frac{R}{L}t}\right) \quad ; V_L = L\frac{dI}{dt}$$

$$I = I_0 - I_0 e^{-\frac{R}{L}t} \quad ;$$

$$\frac{dI}{dt} = 0 - I_0\, e^{-\frac{R}{L}t}\left(-\frac{R}{L}\right)$$

$$V_L = E\, e^{-\frac{R}{L}t}$$

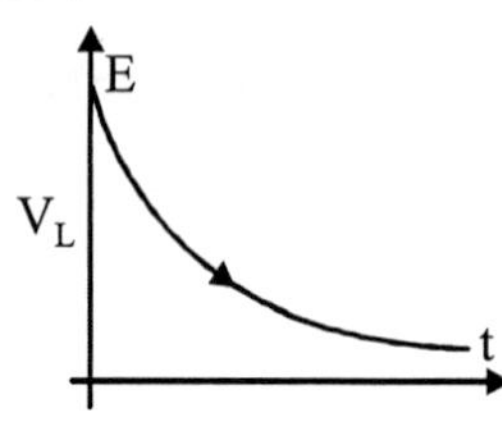

Initially, an inductor acts to oppose changes in the current through it. A long time later, it acts like ordinary connecting wire.

DECAY OF CURRENT

Let the current has reached its steady state value I_0 through inductor. Now switch K in the circuit shown in fig. has been closed.

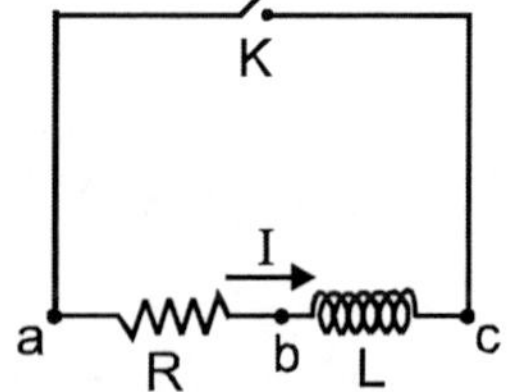

Let this time is $t = 0$.

Let at $t = 0$ current in the circuit (which is maximum) $= I_0$

After time t current in the circuit = I

Applying Kirchhoff's loop rule to this circuit

$$0 + \left(-L\frac{dI}{dt}\right) = IR \quad \text{(since there is no source of e.m.f.)}$$

$$\text{or} \quad L\frac{dI}{dt} = -IR \quad \text{or} \quad \frac{dI}{I} = -\frac{R}{L}dt$$

The eq^n. gives the value of current at any time t during decay of current in LR-circuit.

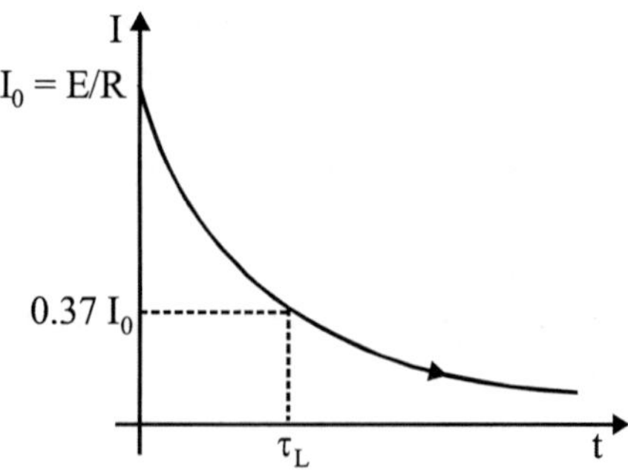

Again, dimensions of $\frac{L}{R}$ are same as that of time

The inductive time constant of the LR-circuit can also be defined by using equation

Setting $t = \frac{L}{R}$ in equation., we get

$$I = I_0\, e^{-\frac{R}{L}\cdot\frac{L}{R}} = I_0\, e^{-1} = \frac{1}{e}I_0 \qquad \text{or } I \cong 0.37\, I_0.$$

As $t \to \infty$, $\quad I \to 0$

$V_R = IR$

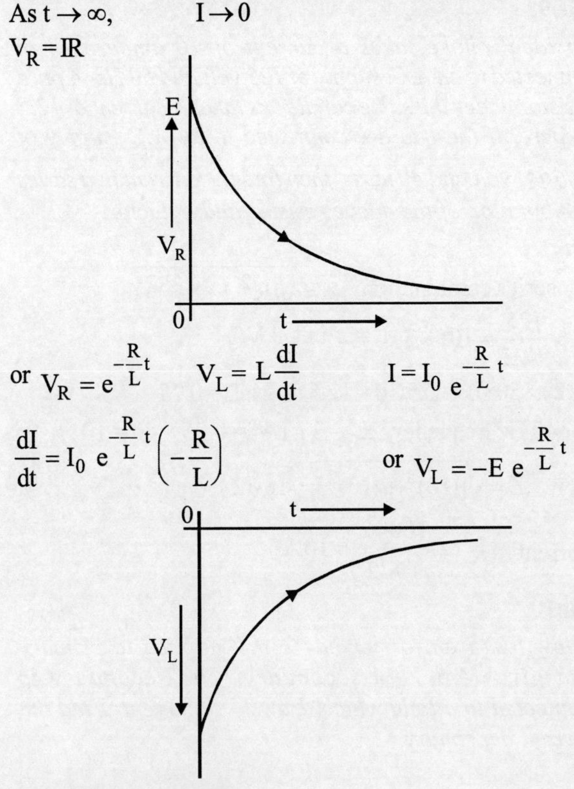

or $V_R = e^{-\frac{R}{L}t}$ $\quad V_L = L\frac{dI}{dt}$ $\quad I = I_0\, e^{-\frac{R}{L}t}$

$\frac{dI}{dt} = I_0\, e^{-\frac{R}{L}t}\left(-\frac{R}{L}\right)$ $\quad$ or $V_L = -E\, e^{-\frac{R}{L}t}$

LC OSCILLATIONS

If a charged capacitor C is short-circuited though an inductor L, the charge and current in the circuit start oscillating simple harmonically. If the resistance of the circuit is zero, no energy is dissipated as heat. Assume an idealized situation in which energy is not radiated away from the circuit. With these idealizations-zero resistance and no radiation, the oscillations in the circuit persist indefinitely and the energy is transferred from the capacitor's electric field to the inductor's magnetic field back and forth. The total energy associated with the circuit is constant. This is analogous to the transfer of energy in an oscillating mechanical system from potential energy to kinetic energy and back, with constant total energy.

Let us now derive an equation for the oscillations in an L-C circuit.

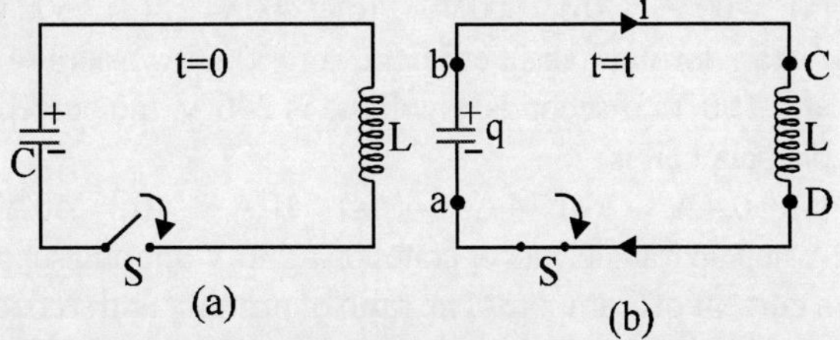

Refer figure (a) : The capacitor is charged to a potential difference V such that charge on capacitor $q_0 = CV$

Here q_0 is the maximum charge on the capacitor. At time $t = 0$, it is connected to an inductor through a switch S. At time $t = 0$, switch S is closed.

Refer figure (b) : When the switch is closed, the capacitor starts discharging. Let at time t charge on the capacitor is $q\ (< q_0)$ and since, it is further decreasing there is a current i in the circuit in the direction shown in figure.

The potential difference across capacitor = potential difference across inductor,

or $V_b - V_a = V_c - V_d \quad \therefore \quad \frac{q}{C} = L\left(\frac{di}{dt}\right)$ ...(i)

Now, as the charge is decreasing,

$i = \left(\frac{-dq}{dt}\right)$ $\quad$ or $\quad \frac{di}{dt} = -\frac{d^2q}{dt^2}$

Substituting this value of $\frac{di}{dt}$ in equation (i), we get

$\frac{q}{C} = -L\left(\frac{d^2q}{dt^2}\right)$ $\quad$ or $\quad \frac{d^2q}{dt^2} = -\left(\frac{1}{LC}\right)q$ ...(ii)

This is the standard equation of simple harmonic motion $\left(\frac{d^2x}{dt^2} = -\omega^2 x\right)$

Here $\omega = \frac{1}{\sqrt{LC}}$ or $f = \frac{1}{2\pi\sqrt{LC}}$ ...(iii)

The general solution of equation (ii),

is $q = q_0 \cos(\omega t \pm \phi)$

In case $\phi = 0$ as $q = q_0$ at $t = 0$.

Thus, we can say that charge in the circuit oscillates with angular frequency given by equation (iii). Thus,

In L-C oscillations, q, i and $\frac{di}{dt}$ all oscillate harmonically with same angular frequency ω. But the phase difference between q and i or between i and $\frac{di}{dt}$ is $\pi/2$. Their amplitudes are q_0, $q_0\omega$ and $\omega_2 q_0$ respectively. So

$q = q_0 \cos\omega t$, then

$i = \frac{dq}{dt} = -q_0\omega \sin\omega t$; $\quad \frac{di}{dt} = -q_0\omega^2 \cos\omega t$

Similarly potential energy across capacitor (U_C) and across inductor (U_L) also oscillate with double the frequency 2ω.

TRANSFORMER

A ***transformer*** *is a device for converting high voltage into low voltage and vice versa, without change in power.*

There are two types of transformers.

(a) **Step up transformer :** *It converts low voltage into high voltage.*

(b) **Step down transformer :** *It converts high voltage into low voltage.*

The **principle of a transformer** is based on mutual induction and a transformer always works on AC. The input is appleid across primary terminals and output is obtained across secondary terminals.

The ratio of number of turns in secondary and primary is called the turn ratio

i.e., $\frac{n_S}{n_P}$ = *turn ratio* K.

If E_P and E_S are alternating voltages, I_P and I_S the alternating currents across primary and secondary terminals respectively then, $\frac{E_S}{E_P} = \frac{n_S}{n_P} = K = \frac{I_P}{I_S}$.

Efficiency of transformer,

$$\eta = \frac{Output\ power}{Input\ power} = \frac{P_{out}}{P_{in}} = \frac{E_S I_S}{E_P I_P}$$

Comparative study of step-up transformer and step-down transformer.

Step - up transformer	Step - down transformer
1. $E_s > E_P$	1. $E_s < E_p$
2. $N_s > N_p$	2. $N_s < N_p$
3. $I_S < I_p$	3. $I_s > I_p$
4. $Z_s < Z_p$	4. $Z_s < Z_p$
5. $k > 1$	5. $k < 1$

Power losses in a transformer :

(a) **Copper loss.** This is due to resistance of the winding of primary and secondary coil ($I^2 R$)

(b) **Iron loss or Eddy current loss.**

(c) **Loss due to leakage of magnetic flux.**

(d) **Hysteresis :** Due to repeated magnetisation and demagnetisation of iron core.

(e) **Humming loss :** Due to vibration.

Inspite of all these losses, we have transformers with efficiency of 70% – 90%.

Example 9.

An ideal choke takes a current of 10 ampere when connected to an A.C. supply of 125 volt and 50 Hz. A pure resistor under the same conditions takes a current of 12.5 ampere. If the two are connected to an A.C. supply of $100\sqrt{2}$ volt and 40 hertz, then find the current in a series combination of the above resistor and inductor.

Solution :

For series combination, $Z = \sqrt{[R^2 + (X_L)^2]}$

$R = \frac{125}{12.5} = 10\,\Omega$, $\omega L = 2\pi f L = V/I$

$\therefore\ 2\pi \times 50 \times L = 125/10 = 12.5$ or $2\pi L = 0.25$

For 40 Hz frequency, $X_L = 2\pi L \times f = 0.25 \times 40 = 10\,\Omega$

Now $Z = \sqrt{[(10)^2 + (10)^2]} = 10\sqrt{2}$;

Current $= \frac{I_0}{Z} = \frac{100\sqrt{2}}{10\sqrt{2}} = 10\,A$

Example10.

A low loss transformer has 230 V applied to primary and gives 4.6 V in secondary. The secondary is connected to a load which draws 5 A current. Find the current in primary.

Solution :

Assuming no loss of power $E_p I_p = E_s I_s$

$\therefore\ I_p = \frac{E_s I_s}{E_p} = 4.6 \times \frac{5}{230} = 0.1\,A$

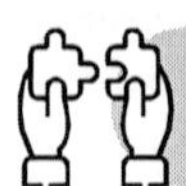

22.2 Concept Practice Problems

CPP

11. In step-up transformer, relation between number of turns in primary (Np) and number of turns in secondary (Ns) coils is
(a) Ns > Np (b) Np > Ns (c) Ns = Np (d) Np = 2Ns

12. The time taken by the current to rise to 0.63 of its maximum value in a d.c. circuit containing inductance (L) and resistance (R) depends on
(a) L only (b) R only (c) $\frac{L}{R}$ (d) LR

13. In an oscillating LC circuit the max. charge on the capacitor is Q. The charge on capacitor when the energy is stored equally between electric and magnetic field is
(a) Q/2 (b) $Q/\sqrt{3}$ (c) $Q/\sqrt{2}$ (d) Q

14. The core of any transformer is laminated so as to
(a) reduce the energy loss due to eddy currents
(b) make it light weight
(c) make it robust and sturdy
(d) increase secondary voltage

15. The time constant of C–R circuit is
(a) 1/CR (b) C/R (c) CR (d) R/C

16. A step down transformer reduces 220 V to 110 V. The primary draws 5 ampere of current and secondary supplies 9 ampere. The efficiency of transformer is
(a) 20% (b) 44% (c) 90% (d) 100%

17. The primary of a transformer has 400 turns while the secondary has 2000 turns. If the power output from the secondary at 1000 V is 12 kW, what is the primary voltage?
(a) 200 V (b) 300 V (c) 400 V (d) 500 V

18. A transformer has an efficiency of 80%. It works at 4 kW and 100 V. If secondary voltage is 240 V, the current in primary coil is
(a) 0.4 A (b) 4 A (c) 10 A (d) 40 A

19. A step up transformer operates on a 230 V line and supplies a current of 2 ampere. The ratio of primary and secondary winding is 1:25. The current in primary is
(a) 25 A (b) 50 A (c) 15 A (d) 12.5 A

20. A step-up transformer has transformation ratio of 3 : 2. What is the voltage in secondary, if voltage in primary is 30 V?
(a) 45 V (b) 15 V (c) 90 V (d) 300 V

ANSWER KEY

11	(a)	12	(c)	13	(c)	14	(a)	15	(c)	16	(c)	17	(a)	18	(d)	19	(b)	20	(a)

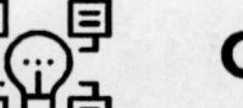

CONCEPT MAP

ALTERNATING CURRENT
Direction of current Changes alternatively and its magnitude changes continuously

Alternating current(I) and alternating voltage (V)
$I = I_0 \sin \omega t$; $V = V_0 \sin \omega t$

RMS value of alternating current and voltage
$I_{rms} = \frac{I_0}{\sqrt{2}}$ $V_{rms} = \frac{V_0}{\sqrt{2}}$

Mean or average value of alternating current and voltage
$I_{mean} = \frac{2I_0}{\pi}$ $V_{mean} = \frac{2V_0}{\pi}$

Peak current (I_0) and voltage V_0 : The maximum value of current and voltage
$I_0 = \sqrt{2}\, I_{rms}$ $V_0 = \sqrt{2}\, V_{rms}$

Transformer Device Changes a low voltage of high current into a high voltage of low current and vice-versa

Step-up transformer
$K > 1$ $K = \frac{N_s}{N_p} = \frac{E_s}{E_p} = \frac{I_p}{I_s}$

Step-down transformer
$K < 1$ $K = \frac{N_p}{N_s} = \frac{E_p}{E_s} = \frac{I_s}{I_p}$

AC Circuit

RC Circuit
Current: $I = I_0 \sin(\omega t + \phi)$
Voltage: $V = \sqrt{V_R^2 + V_C^2}$
Impedance: $Z = \sqrt{R^2 + X_C^2}$
Phase difference: $\tan^{-1} \frac{1}{\omega CR}$
Power factor: $\cos\phi = \frac{R^2}{\sqrt{R^2 + X_C^2}}$
Leading quantity: Current

LC Circuit
Current: $I = I_0 \sin\left(\omega t \pm \frac{\pi}{2}\right)$
Voltage: $V = V_L - V_C$
Impedance : $Z = X_L - X_C$
Phase difference: $\phi = 90^\circ$
Power factor : $\cos\phi = 0$
Leading quantity:
Either voltage or current

LR Circuit
Current: $I = I_0 \sin(\omega t + \phi)$
Voltage : $V = \sqrt{V_R^2 + V_L^2}$
Impedance: $Z = \sqrt{R^2 + X_L^2}$
Phase difference: $\phi = \tan^{-1} \frac{\omega L}{R}$
Power factor : $\cos\phi = \frac{R}{\sqrt{R^2 + X_L^2}}$
Leading quantity : voltage

Power in an Ac. Circuit
$P_{av} = V_{rms} I_{rms} \cos\theta$

LCR series Circuit
Current : $I = I_0 \sin(\omega t \pm \phi)$: Voltage:
$V = \sqrt{R^2 + (V_L - V_C)^2}$
Impedance $Z = \sqrt{R^2 + (X_L - X_C)^2}$;
Phase difference $\frac{X_L - X_C}{R}$
At resonance $X_L = X_C \Rightarrow Z_{min} = R$
Band-width: $\Delta\omega = \frac{R}{L}$; Quality factor
$Q = \frac{1}{R}\sqrt{\frac{L}{C}}$

Inductive (L) Circuit
Current : $I = I_0 \sin\left(\omega t - \frac{\pi}{2}\right)$
Phase difference between V and I : $\phi = 90^\circ$ or $\pi/2$
Power factor : $\cos\phi = 0$
Power : $P = 0$
Phasor : Voltage leads the current by $\pi/2$

Capacitive (C) Circuit
Current : $I = I_0 \sin(\omega t + \pi/2)$
Phase difference between V and I : $\phi = 90^\circ$ or $-\pi/2$ Power factor : $\cos\phi = 0$ Power : $P = 0$
Phasor : Current leads the voltage by $\pi/2$

Resistive (R) Circuit
Current : $I = I_0 \sin \omega t$
Phase difference between V and I : $\phi = 0^\circ$ Power factor: $\cos\phi = 1$
Power : $P = \frac{V_0 I_0}{2}$
Phasor : Current and voltage both in same phase

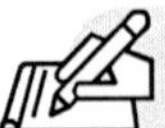

Exercise 1 - Chapter Revision Problems

CRP

1. In a RLC circuit capacitance is changed from C to 2 C. For the resonant frequency to remain unchanged, the inductance should be changed from L to
(a) 4L (b) 2L (c) L/2 (d) L/4

2. An LCR series circuit, connected to a source E, is at resonance. Then the voltage across
(a) R is zero
(b) R equals applied voltage
(c) C is zero
(d) L equals applied voltage

3. In a LCR circuit at resonance which of these will effect the current in circuit
(a) R only (b) L and R only
(c) R and C only (d) all L, C and R

4. Which of the following will have the dimensions of time
(a) LC (b) R/L (c) L/R (d) C/L

5. A.C. power is transmitted from a power house at a high voltage as
(a) the rate of transmission is faster at high voltages
(b) it is more economical due to less power loss
(c) power cannot be transmitted at low voltages
(d) a precaution against theft of transmission lines

6. Which of the following statement is incorrect ?
(a) In LCR series ac circuit, as the frequency of the source increases, the impedence of the circuit first decreases and then increases.
(b) If the net reactance of an LCR series ac circuit is same as its resistance, then the current lags behind the voltage by 45°.
(c) At resonance, the impedence of an ac circuit becomes purely resistive.
(d) Below resonance, voltage leads the current while above it, current leads the voltage.

7. Resonance frequency of LCR series a.c. circuit is f_0. Now the capacitance is made 4 times, then the new resonance frequency will become
(a) $f_0/4$ (b) $2f_0$ (c) f_0 (d) $f_0/2$.

8. In a series resonant circuit, having L,C and R as its elements, the resonant current is i. The power dissipated in circuit at resonance is
(a) $\dfrac{i^2R}{(\omega L - 1/\omega C)}$ (b) zero
(c) $i^2\omega L$ (d) i^2R.
Whereas ω is angular resonant frequency

9. An inductance L having a resistance R is connected to an alternating source of angular frequency ω. The Quality factor Q of inductance is
(a) $R/\omega L$ (b) $(\omega L/R)^2$ (c) $(R/\omega L)^{1/2}$ (d) $\omega L/R$

10. Energy in a current carrying coil is stored in the form of
(a) electric field (b) magnetic field
(c) dielectric strength (d) heat

11. In an A.C. circuit, the current flowing in inductance is $I = 5 \sin(100t - \pi/2)$ amperes and the potential difference is $V = 200 \sin(100t)$ volts. The power consumption is equal to
(a) 1000 watt (b) 40 watt
(c) 20 watt (d) Zero

12. If resistance of 100Ω, and inductance of 0.5 henry and capacitance of 10×10^6 farad are connected in series through 50 Hz A.C. supply, then impedance is
(a) 1.8765 Ω (b) 18.76 Ω
(c) 187.6 Ω (d) 101.3 Ω

13. Using an A.C. voltmeter the potential difference in the electrical line in a house is read to be 234 volt. If the line frequency is known to be 50 cycles/second, the equation for the line voltage is
(a) $V = 165 \sin(100\pi t)$ (b) $V = 331 \sin(100\pi t)$
(c) $V = 220 \sin(100\pi t)$ (d) $V = 440 \sin(100\pi t)$

14. An inductance of negligible resistance whose reactance is 22 Ω at 200 Hz is connected to 200 volts, 50 Hz power line. The value of inductance is
(a) 0.0175 henry (b) 0.175 henry
(c) 1.75 henry (d) 17.5 henry

15. An inductive circuit contains resistance of 10 ohms and an inductance of 2 henry. If an A.C. voltage of 120 Volts and frequency 60 Hz is applied to this circuit, the current would be nearly
(a) 0.32 Amp (b) 0.16 Amp
(c) 0.48 Amp (d) 0.80 Amp

16. In an a.c. circuit V and **I** are given by
$V = 100 \sin(100t)$ volts
$\mathbf{I} = 100 \sin(100t + \pi/3)$ mA
the power dissipated in the circuit is
(a) 10^4 watt (b) 10 watt (c) 2.5 watt (d) 5.0 watt

17. The primary winding of a transformer has 100 turns and its secondary winding has 200 turns. The primary is connected to an A.C. supply of 120 V and the current flowing in it is 10 A. The voltage and the current in the secondary are
(a) 240 V, 5 A (b) 240 V, 10 A
(c) 60 V, 20 A (d) 120 V, 20 A

18. In the circuit shown in fig, the resonant frequency is
(a) 75 kc/s
(b) 750 kc/s
(c) 7.5 kc/s
(d) 75 mc/s

19. An alternating voltage E (in volts) = $200\sqrt{2} \sin 100t$ is connected to one micro farad capacitor through an a.c. ammeter. The reading of the ammeter shall be
(a) 100 mA (b) 20 mA (c) 40 mA (d) 80 mA

20. The r.m.s value of an a.c. of 50 Hz is 10 amp. The time taken by the alternating current in reaching from zero to maximum value and the peak value of current will be
(a) 2×10^{-2} sec and 14.14 amp
(b) 1×10^{-2} sec and 7.07 amp
(c) 5×10^{-3} sec and 7.07 amp
(d) 5×10^{-3} sec and 14.14 amp

21. The frequency of A.C. mains in India is
(a) 30 c/s (b) 50 c/s (c) 60 c/s (d) 120 c/s

22. A 12 Ω resistor and a 0.21 henry inductor are connected in series to an a.c. source operating at 20 volt, 50 cycle. The phase angle between the current and source voltage is
(a) 30º (b) 40º (c) 80º (d) 90º

23. An alternating current is given by
$i = i_1 \cos\omega t + i_2 \sin\omega t$
The rms current is given by
(a) $\frac{i_1 + i_2}{\sqrt{2}}$ (b) $\frac{|i_1 + i_2|}{\sqrt{2}}$ (c) $\sqrt{\frac{i_1^2 + i_2^2}{2}}$ (d) $\sqrt{\frac{i_1^2 + i_2^2}{\sqrt{2}}}$

24. The impedance in a circuit containing a resistance of 1 Ω and an inductance of 0.1 H in series, for AC of 50 Hz, is
(a) $100\sqrt{10}\Omega$ (b) $10\sqrt{10}\Omega$
(c) 100Ω (d) $\sqrt{10}\Omega$

25. Determine the rms value of the emf given by
E (in volt) = 8 sin (ω t) + 6sin (2 ω t)
(a) $5\sqrt{2}$V (b) $7\sqrt{2}$V (c) 10V (d) $10\sqrt{2}$V

26. A transformer is used to light a 140 W, 24 V bulb from a 240 V a.c. mains. The current in the main cable is 0.7 A. The efficiency of the transformer is
(a) 63.8% (b) 83.3% (c) 16.7% (d) 36.2%

27. An AC voltage source has an output of $V = 200\sin 2\pi ft$. This source is connected to a 100 Ω resistor. RMS current in the resistance is
(a) 1.41 A (b) 2.41 A (c) 3.41 A (d) 0.71 A

28. In an A.C. circuit, a resistance of R ohm is connected in series with an inductance L. If phase angle between voltage and current be 45°, the value of inductive reactance will be
(a) R/4 (b) R/2 (c) R
(d) cannot be found with given data

29. The ratio of mean value over half cycle to r.m.s. value of A.C. is
(a) $2:\pi$ (b) $2\sqrt{2}:\pi$ (c) $\sqrt{2}:\pi$ (d) $\sqrt{2}:1$

30. In series combination of R, L and C with an A.C. source at resonance, if R = 20 ohm, then impedence Z of the combination is
(a) 20 ohm (b) zero (c) 10 ohm (d) 400 ohm

31. In an LR circuit f = 50 Hz, L=2H, E=5 volts, R=1 Ω then energy stored in inductor is
(a) 50 J (b) 25 J
(c) 100 J (d) None of these

32. A capacitor in an ideal LC circuit is fully charged by a DC source, then it is disconnected from DC source, the current in the circuit
(a) becomes zero instantaneously
(b) grows , monotonically
(c) decays monotonically
(d) oscillate infinitely

33. Which one of the following curves represents the variation of impedance (Z) with frequency f in series LCR circuit?

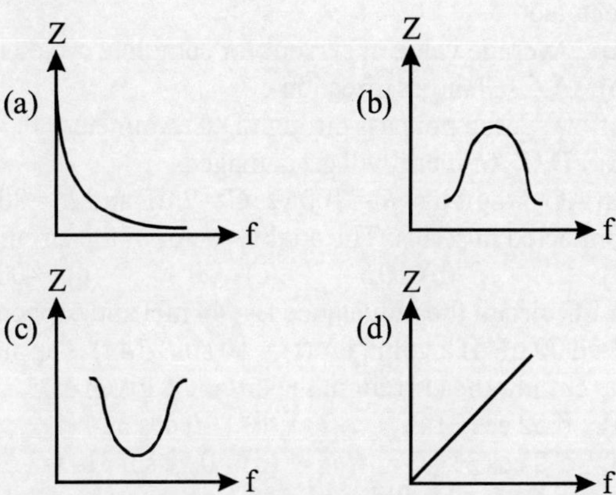

34. A steady potential difference of 10 V produces heat at a rate x in a resistor. The peak value of the alternating voltage which will produce heat at a rate $\frac{x}{2}$ in the same resistor is
(a) 5V (b) $5\sqrt{2}$ V (c) 10V (d) $10\sqrt{2}$ V

35. In the circuit shown, when the switch is closed, the capacitor charges with a time constant
(a) RC
(b) 2RC
(c) $\frac{1}{2}$RC
(d) RC ln 2

C R + – B

36. In the question 86, if the switch is opened after the capacitor has been charged, it will discharges with a time constant
(a) RC (b) 2RC (c) $\frac{1}{2}$RC (d) RC ln 2

37. An alternating voltage of 220 V, 50 Hz frequency is applied across a capacitor of capacitance 2 μF. The impedence of the circuit is
(a) $\frac{\pi}{5000}$ (b) $\frac{1000}{\pi}$ (c) 500π (d) $\frac{5000}{\pi}$

38. The instantaneous voltage through a device of impedance 20 Ω is e = 80 sin 100 πt. The effective value of the current is
(a) 3 A (b) 2.828 A (c) 1.732 A (d) 4 A

39. An alternating voltage $v(t) = 220 \sin 100\pi t$ volt is applied to a purely resistive load of 50Ω. The time taken for the current to rise from half of the peak value to the peak value is :
(a) 5 ms (b) 2.2 ms (c) 7.2 ms (d) 3.3 ms

40. A sinusoidal voltage V(t) = 100 sin (500t) is applied across a pure inductance of L = 0.02 H. The current through the coil is:
(a) 10 cos (500 t) (b) – 10 cos (500t)
(c) 10 sin (500t) (d) – 10 sin (500t)

41. Alternating current can not be measured by D.C. ammeter because
(a) Average value of current for complete cycle is zero
(b) A.C. Changes direction
(c) A.C. can not pass through D.C. Ammeter
(d) D.C. Ammeter will get damaged.

42. An AC circuit has $R = 100\ \Omega$, $C = 2\ \mu F$ and $L = 80$ mH, connected in series. The quality factor of the circuit is :
(a) 2 (b) 0.5 (c) 20 (d) 400

43. In LC circuit the inductance L = 40 mH and capacitance C = 100 μF. If a voltage $V(t) = 10 \sin(314\,t)$ is applied to the circuit, the current in the circuit is given as:
(a) 0.52 cos 314 t (b) 10 cos 314 t
(c) 5.2 cos 314 t (d) 0.52 sin 314 t

44. For an RLC circuit driven with voltage of amplitude v_m and frequency $\omega_0 = \frac{1}{\sqrt{LC}}$ the current exhibits resonance. The quality factor, Q is given by:
(a) $\frac{\omega_0 L}{R}$ (b) $\frac{\omega_0 R}{L}$ (c) $\frac{R}{(\omega_0 C)}$ (d) $\frac{CR}{\omega_0}$

45. When resonance is produced in a series LCR circuit, then which of the following is not correct ?
(a) Current in the circuit is in phase with the applied voltage.
(b) Inductive and capacitive reactances are equal.
(c) If R is reduced, the voltage across capacitor will increase.
(d) Impedance of the circuit is maximum.

46. The plot given below is of the average power delivered to an LRC circuit versus frequency. The quality factor of the circuit is :

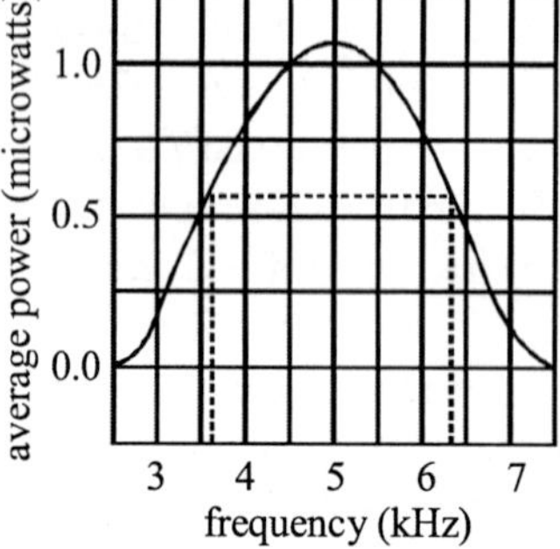

(a) 5.0
(b) 2.0
(c) 2.5
(d) 0.4

47. A series LR circuit is connected to an ac source of frequency ω and the inductive reactance is equal to 2R. A capacitance of capacitive reactance equal to R is added in series with L and R. The ratio of the new power factor to the old one is :
(a) $\sqrt{\frac{2}{3}}$ (b) $\sqrt{\frac{2}{5}}$ (c) $\sqrt{\frac{3}{2}}$ (d) $\sqrt{\frac{5}{2}}$

48. The core of any transformer is laminated so as to
(a) reduce the energy loss due to eddy currents
(b) make it light weight
(c) make it robust and strong
(d) increase the secondary voltage

49. A power transmission line feeds input power at 2300 V to a step down transformer with its primary windings having 4000 turns. The output power is delivered at 230 V by the transformer. If the current in the primary of the transformer is 5A and its efficiency is 90%, the output current would be:
(a) 50 A (b) 45 A (c) 35 A (d) 25 A

50. A transformer consisting of 300 turns in the primary and 150 turns in the secondary gives output power of 2.2kW. If the current in the secondary coil is 10 A, then the input voltage and current in the primary coil are :
(a) 220 V and 20 A (b) 440 V and 20 A
(c) 440 V and 5 A (d) 220 V and 10 A

Exercise 2 - Exemplar & Past Year Questions E&PYQs

Exemplar Questions

1. If the rms current in a 50 Hz AC circuit is 5 A, the value of the current 1/300 s after its value becomes zero is
(a) $5\sqrt{2}$A (b) $5\sqrt{3/2}$ A (c) 5/6 A (d) $5/\sqrt{2}$A

2. An alternating current generator has an internal reactance R_g and an internal reactance X_g. It is used to supply power to a passive load consisting of a resistance R_g and a reactance X_L. For maximum power to be delivered from the generator to the load, the value of X_L is equal to
(a) zero (b) X_g (c) $-X_g$ (d) R_g

3. When a voltage measuring device is connected to AC mains, the meter shows the steady input voltage of 220 V. This means
(a) input voltage cannot be AC voltage, but a DC voltage
(b) maximum input voltage is 220 V
(c) the meter reads not v but $<v^2>$ and is calibrated to read $\sqrt{<v^2>}$
(d) The pointer of the meter is stuck by some mechanical defect

4. To reduce the resonant frequency in an L-C-R series circuit with a generator
(a) the generator frequency should be reduced
(b) another capacitor should be added in parallel to the first
(c) the iron core of the inductor should be removed
(d) dielectric in the capacitor should be removed

5. Which of the following combinations should be selected for better tuning of an L-C-R circuit used for communication?
(a) $R = 20\,\Omega, L = 1.5\,H, C = 35\,\mu F$
(b) $R = 25\Omega, L = 2.5\,H, C = 45\,\mu F$
(c) $R = 15\Omega, L = 3.5\,H, C = 30\,\mu F$
(d) $R = 25\Omega, L = 1.5\,H, C = 45\,\mu F$

6. An inductor of reactance 1Ω and a resistor of 2Ω are connected in series to the terminals of a 6V (rms) AC source. The power dissipated in the circuit is
(a) 8 W (b) 12 W (c) 14.4 W (d) 18 W

7. The output of a step-down transformer is measured to be 24 V when connected to a 12 W light bulb. The value of the peak current is
(a) $1/\sqrt{2}$ A (b) $\sqrt{2}$ A (c) 2 A (d) $2\sqrt{2}$ A

NEET/AIPMT (2013-2020) Questions

8. A coil of self-inductance L is connected in series with a bulb B and an AC source. Brightness of the bulb decreases when *[2013]*
(a) number of turns in the coil is reduced
(b) a capacitance of reactance $X_C = X_L$ is included in the same circuit
(c) an iron rod is inserted in the coil
(d) frequency of the AC source is decreased

9. A transformer having efficiency of 90% is working on 200V and 3kW power supply. If the current in the secondary coil is 6A, the voltage across the secondary coil and the current in the primary coil respectively are :
(a) 300 V, 15A (b) 450 V, 15A *[2014]*
(c) 450V, 13.5A (d) 600V, 15A

10. A resistance 'R' draws power 'P' when connected to an AC source. If an inductance is now placed in series with the resistance, such that the impedance of the circuit becomes 'Z', the power drawn will be *[2015]*
(a) $P\sqrt{\frac{R}{Z}}$ (b) $P\left(\frac{R}{Z}\right)$ (c) P (d) $P\left(\frac{R}{Z}\right)^2$

11. An inductor 20 mH, a capacitor 50 μF and a resistor 40Ω are connected in series across a source of emf V = 10 sin 340 t. The power loss in A.C. circuit is : *[2016]*
(a) 0.51 W (b) 0.67 W (c) 0.76 W (d) 0.89 W

12. A small signal voltage $V(t) = V_0 \sin \omega t$ is applied across an ideal capacitor C : *[2016]*
(a) Current I (t), lags voltage V(t) by 90°.
(b) Over a full cycle the capacitor C does not consume any energy from the voltage source.
(c) Current I (t) is in phase with voltage V(t).
(d) Current I (t) leads voltage V(t) by 180°.

13. Figure shows a circuit that contains three identical resistors with resistance R = 9.0 Ω each, two identical inductors with inductance L = 2.0 mH each, and an ideal battery with emf ε = 18 V. The current 'i' through the battery just after the switch closed is *[2017]*

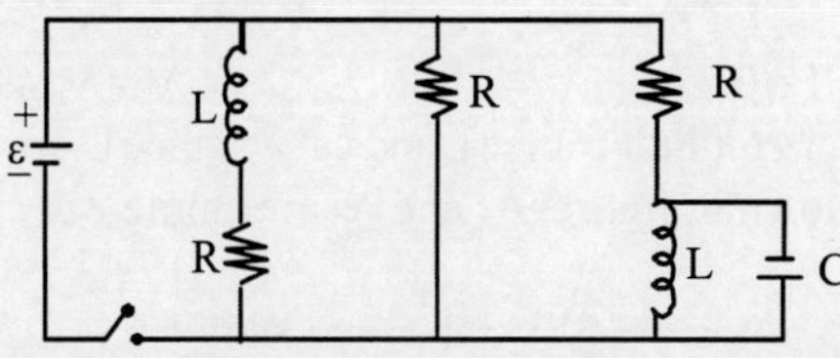

(a) 0.2 A (b) 2 A (c) 0 (d) 2 mA

14. An inductor 20 mH, a capacitor 100 μF and a resistor 50Ω are connected in series across a source of emf, V = 10 sin 314 t. The power loss in the circuit is *[2018]*
(a) 0.79 W (b) 0.43 W (c) 1.13 W (d) 2.74 W

15. A circuit when connected to an AC source of 12 V gives a current of 0.2 A. The same circuit when connected to a DC source of 12 V, gives a current of 0.4 A. The circuit is *[NEET Odisha 2019]*
(a) Series LCR (b) Series LR
(c) Series RC (d) Series LC

16. A 40 μF capacitor is connected to a 200 V, 50 Hz ac supply. The rms value of the current in the circuit is, nearly : *[2020]*
(a) 2.05 A (b) 2.5 A (c) 25.1 A (d) 1.7 A

17. A series LCR circuit is connected to an ac voltage source. When L is removed from the circuit, the phase difference between current and voltage is $\frac{\pi}{3}$. If instead C is removed from the circuit, the phase difference is again $\frac{\pi}{3}$ between current and voltage. The power factor of the circuit is : *[2020]*
(a) 0.5 (b) 1.0 (c) –1.0 (d) zero

Exercise 3 - Concept Application Problems CAP

1. A step down transformer is connected to 2400 volts line and 80 amperes of current is found to flow in output load. The ratio of the turns in primary and secondary coil is 20 : 1. If transformer efficiency is 100%, then the current flowing in the primary coil will be
(a) 1600 amp (b) 20 amp
(c) 4 amp (d) 1.5 amp

2. The primary winding of transformer has 500 turns whereas its secondary has 5000 turns. The primary is connected to an A.C. supply of 20 V, 50 Hz. The secondary will have an output of
(a) 2 V, 5 Hz (b) 200 V, 500 Hz
(c) 2V, 50 Hz (d) 200 V, 50 Hz

3. In the given circuit, the current drawn from the source is

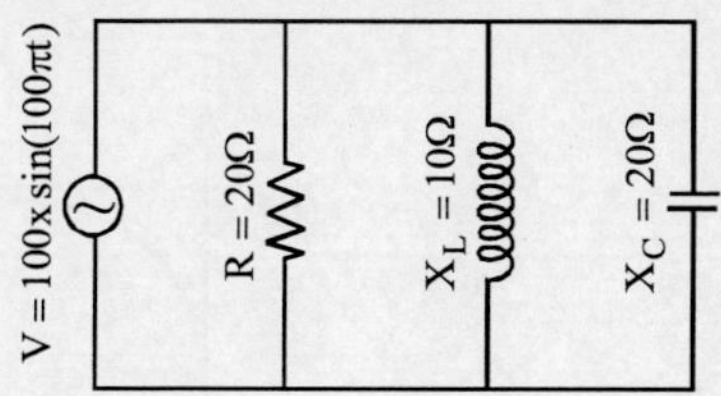

(a) 20 A (b) 10 A (c) 5 A (d) $5\sqrt{2}$ A

4. An alternating voltage $V = V_0 \sin \omega t$ is applied across a circuit. As a result, a current $I = I_0 \sin(\omega t - \pi/2)$ flows in it. The power consumed per cycle is
   (a) zero (b) $0.5\, V_0 I_0$
   (c) $0.707\, V_0 I_0$ (d) $1.414\, V_0 I_0$

5. For the circuit shown in the fig., the current through the inductor is 0.9 A while the current through the condenser is 0.4 A. Then
   (a) current drawn from generator $I = 1.13$ A
   (b) $\omega = 1/(1.5\, LC)$
   (c) $I = 0.5$ A
   (d) $I = 0.6$ A

C L $V = V_0 \sin \omega t$

6. In a circuit inductance L and capacitance C are connected as shown in figure. A_1 and A_2 are ammeters.

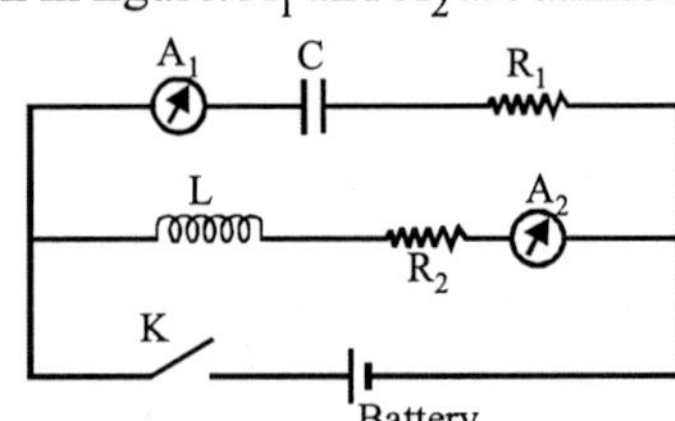

When key K is pressed to complete the circuit, then just after closing key (K), the readings of A_1 and A_2 will be
   (a) zero in both A_1 and A_2
   (b) maximum in both A_1 and A_2
   (c) zero in A_1 and maximum in A_2
   (d) maximum in A_1 and zero in A_2

7. The tuning circuit of a radio receiver has a resistance of $50\,\Omega$, an inductor of 10 mH and a variable capacitor. A 1 MHz radio wave produces a potential difference of 0.1 mV. The values of the capacitor to produce resonance is (Take $\pi^2 = 10$)
   (a) 2.5 pF (b) 5.0 pF (c) 25 pF (d) 50 pF

8. Two coils A and B are connected in series across a 240 V, 50 Hz supply. The resistance of A is $5\,\Omega$ and the inductance of B is 0.02 H. The power consumed is 3 kW and the power factor is 0.75. The impedance of the circuit is
   (a) $0.144\,\Omega$ (b) $1.44\,\Omega$ (c) $14.4\,\Omega$ (d) $144\,\Omega$

9. In LCR series circuit fed by a DC source, how does the amplitude of charge oscillations vary with time during discharge ?

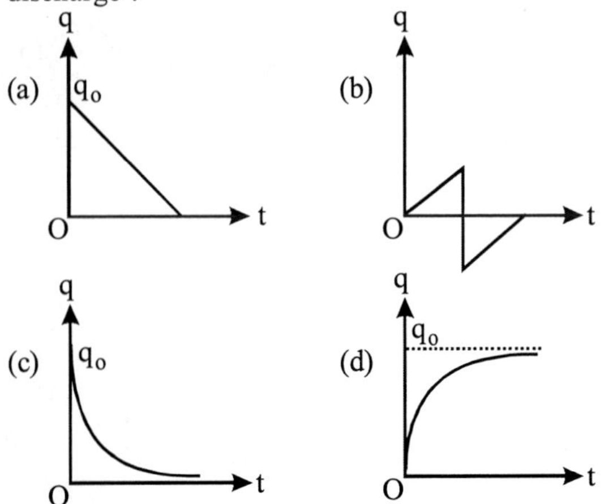

10. An inductive coil has a resistance of $100\,\Omega$. When an a.c. signal of frequency 1000 Hz is fed to the coil, the applied voltage leads the current by 45°. What is the inductance of the coil ?
   (a) 10mH (b) 12mH (c) 16mH (d) 20mH.

11. An inductor of self inductance 100 mH and a resistor of resistance 50Ω, are connected to a 2 V battery. The time required for the current to half its steady value is
   (a) 2 milli second (b) $2\, ln\,(0.5)$ milli second
   (c) $2\, ln\,(3)$ milli second (d) $2\, ln\,(2)$ milli second

12. The primary winding of transformers has 500 turns whereas its secondary has 5000 turns. The primary is connected to an A.C. supply of 20 V, 50 Hz. The secondary will have an output of
   (a) 2V, 5Hz (b) 200 V, 500 Hz
   (c) 2V, 50 Hz (d) 200 V, 50Hz

13. In an experiment, 200 V A.C. is applied at the ends of an LCR circuit. The circuit consists of an inductive reactance $(X_L) = 50\,\Omega$, capacitive reactance $(X_C) = 50\,\Omega$ and ohmic resistance $(R) = 10\,\Omega$. The impedance of the circuit is
   (a) 10Ω (b) 20Ω (c) 30Ω (d) 40Ω

14. In a region of uniform magnetic induction $B = 10^{-2}$ tesla, a circular coil of radius 30 cm and resistance π^2 ohm is rotated about an axis which is perpendicular to the direction of B and which forms a diameter of the coil. If the coil rotates at 200 rpm the amplitude of the alternating current induced in the coil is
   (a) $4\pi^2$ mA (b) 30 mA (c) 6 mA (d) 200 mA

15. In the given circuit the reading of voltmeter V_1 and V_2 are 300 volt each. The reading of the voltmeter V_3 and ammeter A are respectively
   (a) 150 V and 2.2 A
   (b) 220 V and 2.0 A
   (c) 220 V and 2.0 A
   (d) 100 V and 2.0 A

L C $R = 100\Omega$ V_1 V_2 V_3 A 220 V, 50 Hz

16. A small circular loop of wire of radius a is located at the centre of a much larger circular wire loop of radius b. The two loops are in the same plane. The outer loop of radius b carries an alternating current $I = I_o \cos(\omega t)$. The emf induced in the smaller inner loop is nearly :
   (a) $\dfrac{\pi\mu_0 I_o}{2} \cdot \dfrac{a^2}{b} \omega \sin(\omega t)$ (b) $\dfrac{\pi\mu_0 I_o}{2} \cdot \dfrac{a^2}{b} \omega \cos(\omega t)$
   (c) $\pi\mu_0 I_o \dfrac{a^2}{b} \omega \sin(\omega t)$ (d) $\dfrac{\pi\mu_0 I_o b^2}{a} \omega \cos(\omega t)$

17. A series L-R circuit is connected to a battery of emf V. If the circuit is switched on at $t = 0$, then the time at which the energy stored in the inductor reaches $\left(\dfrac{1}{n}\right)$ times of its maximum value, is :
   (a) $\dfrac{L}{R} \ln\left(\dfrac{\sqrt{n}}{\sqrt{n}-1}\right)$ (b) $\dfrac{L}{R} \ln\left(\dfrac{\sqrt{n}+1}{\sqrt{n}-1}\right)$
   (c) $\dfrac{L}{R} \ln\left(\dfrac{\sqrt{n}}{\sqrt{n}+1}\right)$ (d) $\dfrac{L}{R} \ln\left(\dfrac{\sqrt{n}-1}{\sqrt{n}}\right)$

18. A 750 Hz, 20 V (rms) source is connected to a resistance of 100 Ω, an inductance of 0.1803 H and a capacitance of 10 μF all in series. The time in which the resistance (heat capacity 2 J/°C) will get heated by 10°C. (assume no loss of heat to the surroundings) is close to :

(a) 418 s (b) 245 s (c) 365 s (d) 348 s

19. An inductance coil has a reactance of 100 Ω. When an AC signal of frequency 1000 Hz is applied to the coil, the applied voltage leads the current by 45°. The self-inductance of the coil is :

(a) 1.1×10^{-2} H (b) 1.1×10^{-1} H

(c) 5.5×10^{-5} H (d) 6.7×10^{-7} H

20. Consider the LR circuit shown in the figure. If the switch S is closed at t = 0 then the amount of charge that passes through the battery between t = 0 and $t = \frac{L}{R}$ is :

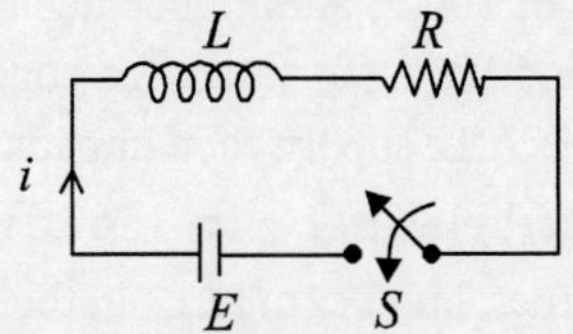

(a) $\frac{2.7EL}{R^2}$ (b) $\frac{EL}{2.7R^2}$ (c) $\frac{7.3EL}{R^2}$ (d) $\frac{EL}{7.3R^2}$

21. A coil of self inductance 10 mH and resistance 0.1 Ω is connected through a switch to a battery of internal resistance 0.9 Ω. After the switch is closed, the time taken for the current to attain 80% of the saturation value is [take *ln* 5 = 1.6]

(a) 0.324 s (b) 0.103 s (c) 0.002 s (d) 0.016 s

22. A 20 Henry inductor coil is connected to a 10 ohm resistance in series as shown in figure. The time at which rate of dissipation of energy (Joule's heat) across resistance is equal to the rate at which magnetic energy is stored in the inductor, is :

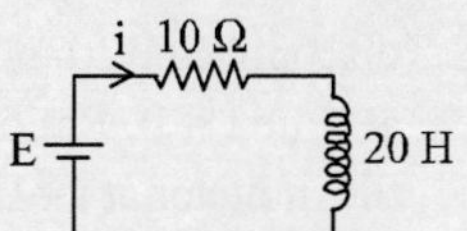

(a) $\frac{2}{ln\,2}$ (b) $\frac{1}{2} ln\,2$

(c) $2\,ln\,2$ (d) $ln\,2$

23. A circuit connected to an *ac* source of *emf* $e = e_0 \sin(100t)$ with *t* in seconds, gives a phase difference of $\frac{\pi}{4}$ between the *emf e* and current *i*. Which of the following circuits will exhibit this ?

(a) RL circuit with R = 1 kΩ and L = 10 mH

(b) RL circuit with R = 1 kΩ and L = 1 mH

(d) RC circuit with R = 1 kΩ and C = 1 μF

(d) RC circuit with R = 1 kΩ and C = 10 μF.

24. In the figure shown, a circuit contains two identical resistors with resistance R = 5 Ω and an inductance with L = 2 mH. An ideal battery of 15 V is connected in the circuit. What will be the current through the battery long after the switch is closed?

(a) 5.5 A

(b) 7.5 A

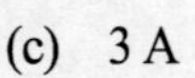

(c) 3 A

(d) 6 A

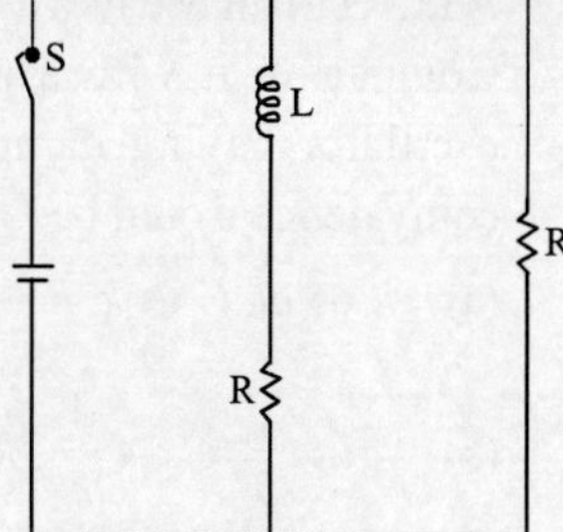

25.

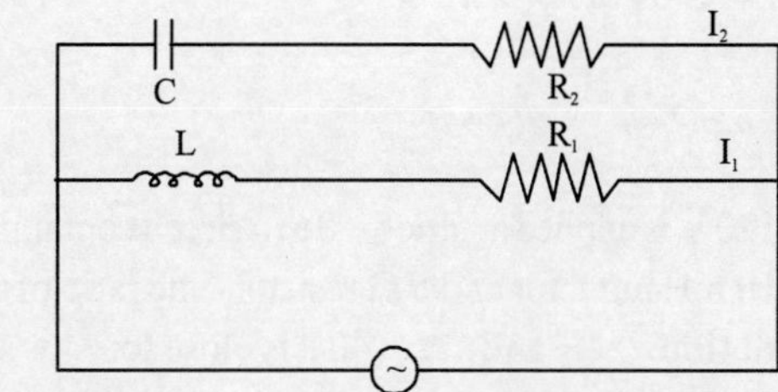

In the above circuit, $C = \frac{\sqrt{3}}{2}\mu F$, $R_2 = 20\ \Omega$, $L = \frac{\sqrt{3}}{10}$ H and $R_1 = 10\ \Omega$. Current in L-R_1 path is I_1 and in C-R_2 path it is I_2. The voltage of A.C source is given by, $V = 200\sqrt{2} \sin(100\,t)$ volts. The phase difference between I_1 and I_2 is :

(a) 60° (b) 30° (c) 90° (d) 0

26. A capacitor of 10 μF and an inductor of 1 H are joined in series. An ac of 50 Hz is applied to this combination. What is the impedance of the combination?

(a) $\frac{5(\pi^2 - 5)}{\pi}\Omega$ (b) $\frac{10^2(\pi^2 - 10)}{\pi}$

(c) $\frac{10(\pi^2 - 5)}{\pi}\Omega$ (d) $\frac{5(10 - \pi^2)}{\pi}\Omega$

27. A series AC circuit containing an inductor (20 mH), a capacitor (120 μF) and a resistor (60 Ω) is driven by an AC source of 24 V/50 Hz. The energy dissipated in the circuit in 60 s is:

(a) 5.65×10^2 J (b) 2.26×10^3 J

(c) 5.17×10^2 J (d) 3.39×10^3 J

28.

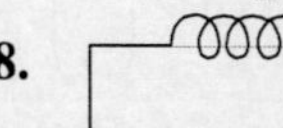

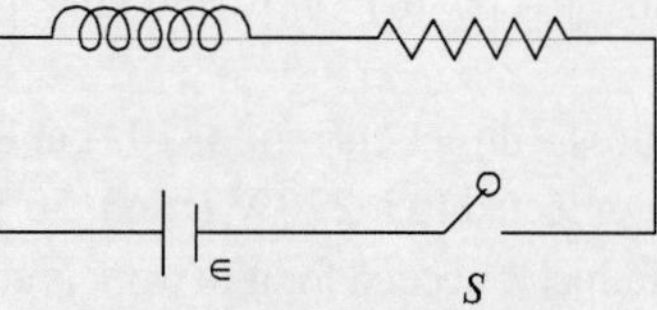

As shown in the figure, a battery of emf ∈ is connected to an inductor *L* and resistance *R* in series. The switch is closed at *t* = 0. The total charge that flows from the battery, between *t* = 0 and $t = t_c$ (t_c is the time constant of the circuit) is:

(a) $\frac{\in R}{eL^2}$ (b) $\frac{\in L}{R^2}\left(1 - \frac{1}{e}\right)$ (c) $\frac{\in L}{R^2}$ (d) $\frac{\in R}{eL^2}$

29. A LCR circuit behaves like a damped harmonic oscillator. Comparing it with a physical spring-mass damped oscillator having damping constant 'b', the correct equivalence would be:

(a) $L \leftrightarrow m, C \leftrightarrow k, R \leftrightarrow b$

(b) $L \leftrightarrow \frac{1}{b}, C \leftrightarrow \frac{1}{m}, R \leftrightarrow \frac{1}{k}$

(c) $L \leftrightarrow k, C \leftrightarrow b, R \leftrightarrow m$

(d) $L \leftrightarrow m, C \leftrightarrow \frac{1}{k}, R \leftrightarrow b$

30. An emf of 20 V is applied at time $t = 0$ to a circuit containing in series 10 mH inductor and 5 Ω resistor. The ratio of the currents at time $t = \infty$ and at $t = 40$ s is close to: (Take $e^2 = 7.389$)

(a) 1.06 (b) 1.15 (c) 1.46 (d) 0.84

31. In an a.c. circuit, the instantaneous e.m.f. and current are given by

$e = 100 \sin 30t$ and $i = 20 \sin\left(30t - \frac{\pi}{4}\right)$

In one cycle of a.c., the average power consumed by the circuit and the wattless current are, respectively:

(a) 50W, 10A (b) $\frac{1000}{\sqrt{2}}$ W, 10A

(c) $\frac{50}{\sqrt{2}}$ W, 0 (d) 50W, 0

32. A sinusoidal voltage of peak value 283 V and angular frequency 320/s is applied to a series LCR circuit. Given that R = 5 Ω, L = 25 mH and C = 1000 μF. The total impedance, and phase difference between the voltage across the source and the current will respectively be :

(a) 10 Ω and $\tan^{-1}\left(\frac{5}{3}\right)$ (b) 7 Ω and 45°

(c) 10 Ω and $\tan^{-1}\left(\frac{8}{3}\right)$ (d) 7 Ω and $\tan^{-1}\left(\frac{5}{3}\right)$

33. An arc lamp requires a direct current of 10 A at 80 V to function. If it is connected to a 220 V (rms), 50 Hz AC supply, the series inductor needed for it to work is close to :

(a) 0.044 H (b) 0.065 H (c) 80 H (d) 0.08 H

34. The equation of alternating current is :

$I = 50\sqrt{2} \sin 400\pi t$ amp. Then the frequency and root mean square of current are respectively

(a) 200 Hz, 50 amp (b) 400π Hz, $50\sqrt{2}$ amp

(c) 200 Hz, $50\sqrt{2}$ amp (d) 50 Hz, 200 amp

35. An inductor (L = 0.03 H) and a resistor (R = 0.15 kΩ) are connected in series to a battery of 15V emf in a circuit shown below. The key K_1 has been kept closed for a long time. Then at t = 0, K_1 is opened and key K_2 is closed simultaneously. At t = 1 ms, the current in the circuit will be : $(e^5 \cong 150)$

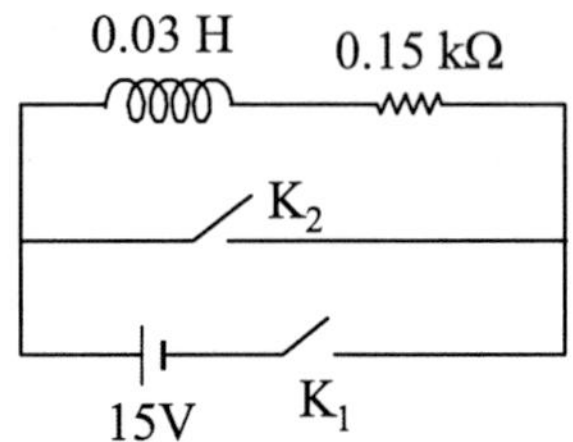

(a) 6.7 mA (b) 0.67 mA (c) 100 mA (d) 67 mA

36. If resistance of 100Ω, and inductance of 0.5 henry and capacitance of 10×10^6 farad are connected in series through 50 Hz A.C. supply, then impedance is

(a) 1.8765 Ω (b) 18.76 Ω (c) 187.6 Ω (d) 101.3 Ω

37. In a transformer, number of turns in the primary coil are 140 and that in the secondary coil are 280. If current in primary coil is 4 A, then that in the secondary coil is

(a) 4 A (b) 2 A (c) 6 A (d) 10 A.

38. In an LCR series a.c. circuit, the voltage across each of the components, L, C and R is 50V. The voltage across the LC combination will be

(a) 100 V (b) $50\sqrt{2}$ V

(c) 50 V (d) 0 V

39. In the circuit shown here, the point 'C' is kept connected to point 'A' till the current flowing through the circuit becomes constant. Afterward, suddenly, point 'C' is disconnected from point 'A' and connected to point 'B' at time t = 0. Ratio of the voltage across resistance and the inductor at t = L/R will be equal to:

(a) $\frac{e}{1-e}$

(b) 1

(c) –1

(d) $\frac{1-e}{e}$

40. When the rms voltages V_L, V_C and V_R are measured respectively across the inductor L, the capacitor C and the resistor R in a series LCR circuit connected to an AC source, it is found that the ratio $V_L : V_C : V_R = 1 : 2 : 3$. If the rms voltage of the AC sources is 100 V, the V_R is close to:

(a) 50 V (b) 70 V (c) 90 V (d) 100 V

41. In an LCR circuit as shown below both switches are open initially. Now switch S_1 is closed, S_2 kept open. (q is charge on the capacitor and τ = RC is Capacitive time constant). Which of the following statement is correct ?

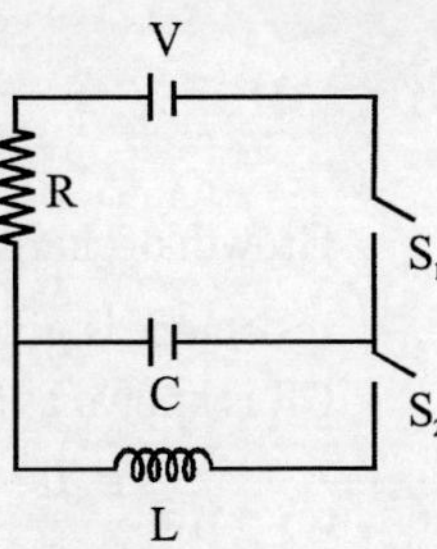

(a) Work done by the battery is half of the energy dissipated in the resistor
(b) At, $t = \tau$, $q = CV/2$
(c) At, $t = 2\tau$, $q = CV(1 - e^{-2})$
(d) At, $t = 2\tau$, $q = CV(1 - e^{-1})$

42. In a series L-C-R circuit, $C = 10^{-11}$ Farad, $L = 10^{-5}$ Henry and R = 100 Ohm, when a constant D.C. voltage E is applied to the circuit, the capacitor acquires a charge 10^{-9} C. The D.C. source is replaced by a sinusoidal voltage source in which the peak voltage E_0 is equal to the constant D.C. voltage E. At resonance the peak value of the charge acquired by the capacitor will be :

(a) 10^{-15} C (b) 10^{-6} C (c) 10^{-10} C (d) 10^{-8} C

43. An LCR circuit as shown in the figure is connected to a voltage source V_{ac} whose frequency can be varied.

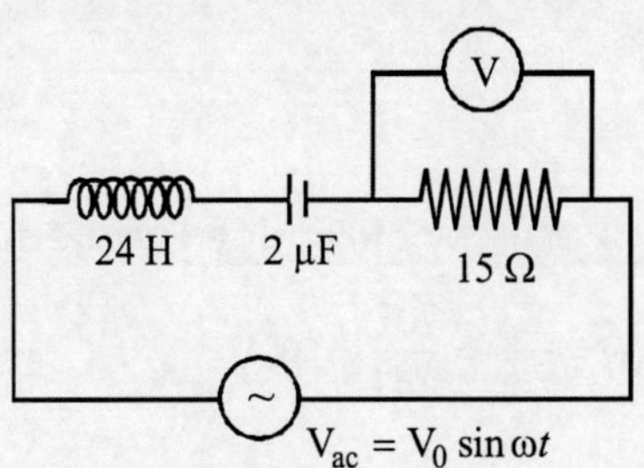

The frequency, at which the voltage across the resistor is maximum, is :

(a) 902 Hz (b) 143 Hz (c) 23 Hz (d) 345 Hz

44. The phase difference between the alternating current and emf is $\frac{\pi}{2}$. Which of the following cannot be the constituent of the circuit?

(a) *R, L* (b) *C* alone(c) *L* alone (d) *L, C*

45. A power transmission line feeds input power at 2300 V to a step down transformer with its primary windings having 4000 turns, giving the output power at 230 V. If the current in the primary of the transformer is 5 A, and its efficiency is 90%, the output current would be:

(a) 20 A (b) 40 A (c) 45 A (d) 25 A

Hints & Solutions

22.1 Concept Practice Problems CPP

1. (c) $E_{rms} = \frac{E_0}{\sqrt{2}} = \frac{707}{1.41} = 500V$
2. (d)
3. (a) When frequency of alternating current is increased, the effective resistance of capacitor $\left(X_L = \frac{1}{\omega L}\right)$ is decreased. As capacitive resistance decreases current in the circuit increases
4. (c)
5. (c) The reactance of capacitor $X = \frac{1}{\omega C}$ where w is frequency and C is the capacitance of capacitor.
6. (c) When a circuit is broken, the induced e.m.f. is largest. So the answer is (c).
7. (d) From figure,

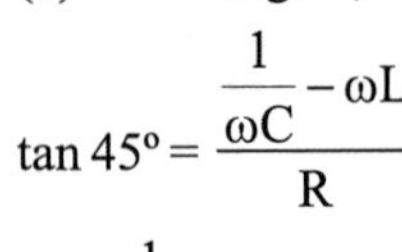

$$\tan 45° = \frac{\frac{1}{\omega C} - \omega L}{R}$$

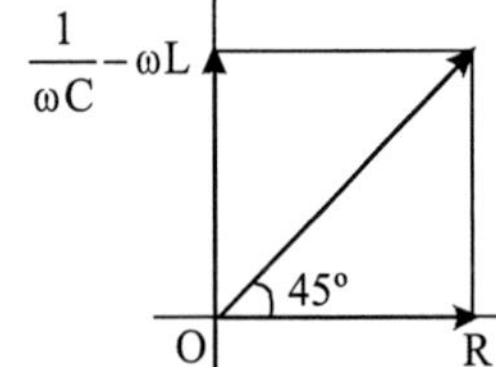

$$\Rightarrow \frac{1}{\omega C} - \omega L = R$$

$$\Rightarrow \frac{1}{\omega C} = R + \omega L$$

$$\Rightarrow C = \frac{1}{\omega(R + \omega L)} = \frac{1}{2\pi f(R + 2\pi fL)}$$

8. (b)
9. (a) Power, $P = VI$
10. (b) Power factor $= \frac{R}{Z} = \frac{R}{(R^2 + \omega^2 L^2)^{1/2}}$

22.2 Concept Practice Problems 

11. (a) In step-up transformer, Ns > Np
12. (c)
13. (c) In the case of maximum charge on capacitor, the whole energy is, stored in capacitor in the form of electric field which is

$$U = \frac{1}{2}\frac{Q^2}{C}$$

When energy in distributed equally between electric and magnetic field, then energy stored in electric field i.e. in capacitor is $U_1 = \frac{U}{2} = \left(\frac{1}{2}\frac{Q^2}{C}\right)\frac{1}{2}$

At that time if charge on capacitor is Q_1, then

$$U_1 = \frac{1}{2}\frac{Q_1^2}{C} = \frac{U}{2} = \frac{1}{4}\frac{Q^2}{C} \Rightarrow Q_1 = Q/\sqrt{2}$$

14. (a)
15. (c) The time constant for resonance circuit, $= CR$

Growth of charge in a circuit containing capacitance and resistance is given by the formula, $q = q_0(1 - e^{-t/CR})$ CR is known as time constant in this formula.

16. (c) $\eta = \frac{E_S I_S}{E_P I_P}$ $\therefore \eta = \frac{110 \times 9}{220 \times 5} = 0.9 \times 100\% = 90\%$
17. (a) $N_P = 400, N_S = 2000$ and $V_S = 1000$ V.

$\frac{V_P}{V_S} = \frac{N_P}{N_S}$ of, $V_P = \frac{V_S \times N_P}{N_S} = \frac{1000 \times 400}{2000} = 200V.$

18. (d) As $E_p I_p = P_i$ $\therefore I_p = \frac{P_i}{E_p} = \frac{4000}{100} = 40\,A.$
19. (b) $\frac{n_p}{n_s} = \frac{E_p}{E_s} = \frac{1}{25}$

$\therefore E_s = 25E_p$

But $E_S I_S = E_P I_P \Rightarrow I_P = \frac{E_S \times I_S}{E_p} \Rightarrow I_p = 50A$

20. (a) Transformation ratio $k = \frac{N_S}{N_P}$

Since $\frac{V_S}{V_P} = \frac{N_S}{N_P}$ $\therefore V_S = \frac{N_S}{N_P} \times V_P$

$V_S = \frac{3}{2} \times 30 = 45V$

Exercise 1 - Chapter Revision Problems 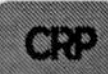

1. (c) We know that $f = \frac{1}{2\pi\sqrt{(LC)}}$,

when C is doubled, L should be halved so that resonant frequency remains unchanged.

2. (b)
3. (a) At resonance, $\omega L = \frac{1}{\omega C}$

Hence the impedance of the circuit would be just equal to R (minimum). In other words, the LCR-series circuit will behave as a purely resistive circuit. Due to this the current is maximum. This condition is known as resonance

$$\therefore \quad Z = R, \quad \text{Current} = \frac{V}{R}$$

4. (c) 5. (b)
6. (d) Option (d) is false because the reason why the voltage leads the current is because $\frac{1}{C\omega} > L\omega$ and if the voltage lags, the inductive reactance is greater than the capacitive reactance.
7. (d) In LCR series circuit, resonance frequency f_0 is given by

$$L\omega = \frac{1}{C\omega} \Rightarrow \omega^2 = \frac{1}{LC} \quad \therefore \omega = \sqrt{\frac{1}{LC}} = 2\pi f_0$$

$$\therefore f_0 = \frac{1}{2\pi\sqrt{LC}} \quad \text{or} \quad f_0 \alpha \frac{1}{\sqrt{C}}$$

When the capacitance of the circuit is made 4 times, its resonant frequency become f_0'

$$\therefore \frac{f_0'}{f_0} = \frac{\sqrt{C}}{\sqrt{4C}} \quad \text{or} \quad f_0' = \frac{f_0}{2}$$

8. (d) At resonance wL= 1/wC
and i = E/R, So power dissipated in circuit is P = i^2R.

9. (d) $Q = \dfrac{\text{Potential drop across capacitor or inductor}}{\text{Potential drop across R.}}$

$$= \frac{\omega L}{R}$$

10. (b) Energy stored in a coil = $\frac{1}{2}Li^2$
where, L is the self-inductance and *i* the current flowing through the inductor. Thus, energy is stored in the magnetic field of the coil.

11. (d) Power, $P = I_{r.m.s} \times V_{r.m.s} \times \cos\varphi$
In the given problem, the phase difference between voltage and current is p/2. Hence

$$P = I_{r.m.s} \times V_{r.m.s} \times \cos(\pi/2) = 0.$$

12. (c) $Z = \sqrt{R^2 + \left(\omega L - \dfrac{1}{\omega C}\right)^2}$
Here R = 100 W, L = 0.5 henry, C = 10 × 10^6 farad
$\omega = 2 p \pi = 100 \pi.$

13. (b) $V = V_0 \sin \omega t$
Voltage in r.m.s. value

$$V_0 = \sqrt{2} \times 234\text{ V} = 331 \text{ volt}$$

and $\omega t = 2\pi n t = 2\pi \times 50 \times t = 100\pi t$
Thus, the equation of line voltage is given by
V = 331 sin (100 π t)

14. (a) $X_L = \omega L = 2\pi n L$

$$\therefore L = \frac{X_L}{2\pi n} = \frac{22 \times 7}{2 \times 22 \times 200} H = 0.0175H$$

15. (b)

16. (c) $P = V_{r.m.s} \times I_{r.m.s} \times \cos\phi = \frac{1}{2} V_0 I_0 \cos\phi$

$$= \frac{1}{2} \times 100 \times (100 \times 10^{-3}) \cos\pi/3 = 2.5 \text{ W}$$

17. (a) $\dfrac{E_s}{E_p} = \dfrac{n_s}{n_p}$ or $E_s = E_p \times \left(\dfrac{n_s}{n_p}\right)$

$$\therefore E_s = 120 \times \left(\frac{200}{100}\right) = 240\text{V}$$

$$\frac{I_p}{I_s} = \frac{n_s}{n_p} \text{ or } I_s = I_p\left(\frac{n_p}{n_s}\right) \quad \therefore I_s = 10\left(\frac{100}{200}\right) = 5 \text{ amp}$$

18. (a)

19. (b) $I = \dfrac{E}{X_C} = E\omega C = \left(\dfrac{E_0}{\sqrt{2}} \times \omega C\right)$

$$\therefore I = 120 \times \left(\frac{200}{100}\right) = 240\text{V} = 20 \times 10^{-3} \text{ amp.}$$

20. (d) 21. (b)

22. (c) The phase angle is given by

$$\tan\phi = \frac{\omega L}{R} = \frac{2\pi \times 50 \times 0.21}{12} = 5.5$$

$$\phi = \tan^{-1} 5.5 = 80°$$

23. (c) 24. (b)

25. (a) $E = 8\sin\omega t + 6\sin 2\omega t$

$$\Rightarrow E_{peak} = \sqrt{8^2 + 6^2} = 10\text{ V}$$

$$E_{rms} = \frac{10}{\sqrt{2}} = 5\sqrt{2}\text{ V}$$

26. (b) Power of source = EI = 240 × 0.7 = 166

$$\Rightarrow \text{Efficiency} = \frac{140}{166} \Rightarrow \eta = 83.3\%$$

27. (a)

28. (c) $\tan\phi = \dfrac{\omega L}{R} = \dfrac{X_L}{R}$
Given $\phi = 45°$. Hence $X_L = R$.

29. (b) We know that $I_{rms} = I_0/\sqrt{2}$ and $I_m = 2I_0/\pi$

$$\therefore \frac{I_m}{I_{rms}} = \frac{2\sqrt{2}}{\pi}$$

30. (a)

31. (d) L = 2H, E = 5 volts, R = 1Ω

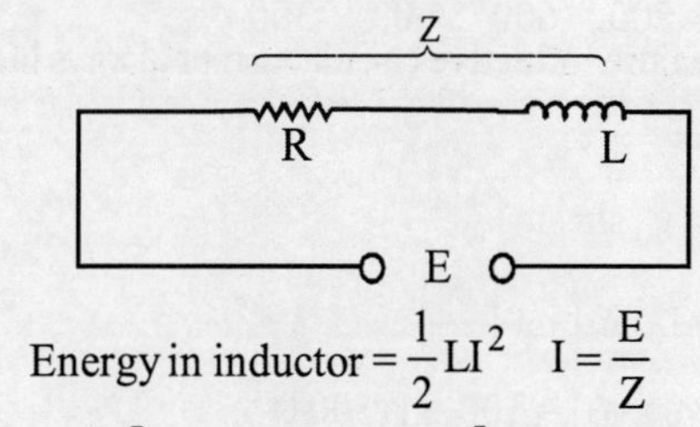

Energy in inductor = $\frac{1}{2}LI^2$ $\quad I = \frac{E}{Z}$

$$I = \frac{5}{\sqrt{R^2 + (\omega L)^2}} = \frac{5}{\sqrt{1 + 4\pi^2 \times 50^2 \times 4}}$$

$$= \frac{5}{\sqrt{1 + (200\pi)^2}} = \frac{5}{200\pi}$$

$$\text{Energy} = \frac{1}{2} \times 2 \times \frac{5 \times 5}{200 \times 200\pi^2} = 6.33 \times 10^{-5} \text{ joules}$$

32. (a)

33. (c) Impedance at resonant frequency is minimum in series LCR circuit.

$$\text{So, } Z = \sqrt{R^2 + \left(2\pi fL - \frac{1}{2\pi fC}\right)^2}$$

When frequency is increased or decreased, Z increases.

34. (c)

35. (a) The resistance in the middle plays no part in the charging process of C, as it does not alter either the potential difference across the RC combination or the current through it.

36. (b) C discharges through both resistance in series.

37. (d) Impedence of a capacitor is $X_C = 1/\omega C$

$$X_C = \frac{1}{2\pi fC} = \frac{1}{2\pi \times 50 \times 2 \times 10^{-6}} = \frac{5000}{\pi}.$$

38. (b) Given equation, $e = 80 \sin 100\pi t$ ...(i)
Standard equation of instantaneous voltage is given by
$e = e_m \sin\omega t$ ...(ii)
Compare (i) and (ii), we get $e_m = 80$ V
where e_m is the voltage amplitude.

Current amplitude $I_m = \frac{e_m}{Z}$ where Z = impendence
$= 80/20 = 4$ A.

$$I_{r.m.s} = \frac{4}{\sqrt{2}} = \frac{4\sqrt{2}}{2} = 2\sqrt{2} = 2.828 \text{ A}.$$

39. (d) As $V(t) = 220 \sin 100\pi t$

so, $I(t) = \frac{220}{50} \sin 100\pi t$

i.e., $I = I_m = \sin(100\pi t)$
For $I = I_m$

$$t_1 = \frac{\pi}{2} \times \frac{1}{100\pi} = \frac{1}{200} \text{ sec. and for } I = \frac{I_m}{2}$$

$$\Rightarrow \frac{I_m}{2} = I_m \sin(100\pi t_2) \Rightarrow \frac{\pi}{6} = 100\pi t_2$$

$$\Rightarrow t_2 = \frac{1}{600} s$$

$$\therefore t_{req} = \frac{1}{200} - \frac{1}{600} = \frac{2}{600} = \frac{1}{300} s = 3.3 \text{ ms}$$

40. (b) In a pure inductive circuit current always lags behind the emf by $\frac{\pi}{2}$.
If $v(t) = v_0 \sin\omega t$
then $I = I_0 \sin\left(\omega t - \frac{\pi}{2}\right)$
Now, given $v(t) = 100 \sin(500t)$

and $I_0 = \frac{E_0}{\omega L} = \frac{100}{500 \times 0.02}$ $[\because L = 0.02H]$

$$I_0 = 10\sin\left(500t - \frac{\pi}{2}\right) \Rightarrow I_0 = -10\cos(500t)$$

41. (a) D.C. ammeter measure average value of current. In AC current, average value of current in complete cycle is zero. Hence reading will be zero.

42. (a) Quality factor,

$$Q = \frac{1}{R}\sqrt{\frac{L}{C}} = \frac{1}{100}\sqrt{\frac{80 \times 10^{-3}}{2 \times 10^{-6}}}$$

$$= \frac{1}{100}\sqrt{40 \times 10^3} = \frac{200}{100} = 2$$

43. (a) Given, Inductance, $L = 40$ mH
Capacitance, $C = 100\ \mu F$
Impedance, $Z = X_C - X_L$

$$\Rightarrow Z = \frac{1}{\omega C} - \omega L \quad \left(\because X_c = \frac{1}{\omega C} \text{ and } X_L = \omega L\right)$$

$$= \frac{1}{314 \times 100 \times 10^{-6}} - 314 \times 40 \times 10^{-3} = 19.28\Omega$$

Current, $i = \frac{V_0}{Z}\sin(\omega t + \pi/2)$

$$\Rightarrow i = \frac{10}{19.28}\cos\omega t = 0.52\cos(314t)$$

44. (a) Quality factor $Q = \frac{\omega_0}{2\Delta\omega} = \frac{\omega_0 L}{R}$

45. (d) Impedance (Z) of the series LCR circuit is
$Z = \sqrt{R^2 + (X_L - X_C)^2}$
At resonance, $X_L = X_C$
Therefore, $Z_{minimum} = R$

46. (b)

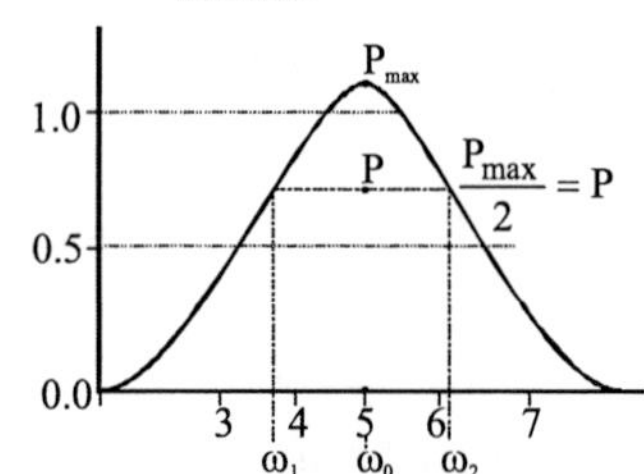

Quality factor of the circuit

$$= \frac{\omega_0}{\omega_2 - \omega_1} = \frac{5}{2.5} = 2.0$$

47. (d) Power factor $_{(old)}$

$$= \frac{R}{\sqrt{R^2 + X_L^2}} = \frac{R}{\sqrt{R^2 + (2R)^2}} = \frac{R}{\sqrt{5}R}$$

Power factor$_{(new)}$

$$= \frac{R}{\sqrt{R^2 + (X_L - X_C)^2}} = \frac{R}{\sqrt{R^2 + (2R - R)^2}} = \frac{R}{\sqrt{2}R}$$

$$\therefore \frac{\text{New power factor}}{\text{Old power factor}} = \frac{\frac{R}{\sqrt{2}R}}{\frac{R}{\sqrt{5}R}} = \sqrt{\frac{5}{2}}$$

48. (a) Laminated core provide less area of cross-section for the current to flow. Because of this, resistance of the core increases and current decreases there by decreasing the energy loss due to eddy current.

49. (b) Efficiency, $\eta = \frac{P_{out}}{P_{in}} = \frac{V_s I_s}{V_p I_p}$

$$\Rightarrow 0.9 = \frac{230 \times I_s}{2300 \times 5} \Rightarrow I_s = 0.9 \times 50 = 45\text{A}$$

Output current = 45A

50. (c) Power output $(V_2 I_2) = 2.2$ kW

$$\therefore V_2 = \frac{2.2\text{kW}}{(10\text{A})} = 220 \text{ volts}$$

$\therefore$ Input voltage for step-down transformer

$$\frac{V_1}{V_2} = \frac{N_1}{N_2} = 2$$

$V_{input} = 2 \times V_{output} = 2 \times 220 = 440$ V

Also $\frac{I_1}{I_2} = \frac{N_2}{N_1}$ $\therefore$ $I_1 = \frac{1}{2} \times 10 = 5\text{A}$

Exercise 2 - Exemplar & Past Year Questions E&PYQs

Exemplar Questions

1. (b) As given that, $\nu = 50$ Hz, $I_{rms} = 5A$, $t = \frac{1}{300}s$

As we know that $I_{rms} = \frac{I_0}{\sqrt{2}}$

$I_0 = \text{Peak value} = \sqrt{2}.I_{rms} = \sqrt{2}\times 5 = 5\sqrt{2}A$

at, $t = \frac{1}{300}\text{sec}$, $I = I_0 \sin\omega t = 5\sqrt{2}\sin 2\pi\nu t$

$= 5\sqrt{2}\sin 2\pi\times 50\times\frac{1}{300}$

$I = 5\sqrt{2}\sin\frac{\pi}{3} = 5\sqrt{2}\times\frac{\sqrt{3}}{2} = 5\sqrt{3/2}$ Amp

2. (c) To deliver maximum power from the generator to the load, total internal reactance must be equal to conjugate of total external reactance.

So, $X_{int} = X_{ext}$

$X_g = (X_L) = -X_L$

Hence, $X_L = -X_g$ (Reactance in external circuit)

3. (c) As we know that,

The voltmeter in AC reads rms values of voltage

$I_{rms} = \sqrt{2}I_0$ and $V_{rms} = \sqrt{2}v_0$

The voltmeter in AC circuit connected to AC mains reads mean value ($<v^2>$) and is calibrated in such a way that it gives rms value of $<v^2>$, which is multiplied by form factor $\sqrt{2}$ to give rms value V_{rms}.

4. (b) As we know that,

The resonant frequency in an L-C-R series circuit is

$$\nu_0 = \frac{1}{2\pi\sqrt{LC}}$$

So, to reduce ν_0 either increase L or increase C.

To increase capacitance, another capacitor must be connect in parallel with the first capacitor.

5. (c) As we know that, Quality factor (Q) of an L-C-R circuit must be higher so Q is

$$Q = \frac{1}{R}\sqrt{\frac{L}{C}}$$

where R is resistance, L is inductance and C is capacitance of the circuit.

So, for higher Q, L must be large, and C and R should be low.

Hence, option (c) is verify.

6. (c) As given that,

$X_L = 1\Omega, R = 2\Omega, E_{rms} = 6V, P_{av} = ?$

The average power dissipated in the L, R, series circuit with AC source

Then $P_{av} = E_{rms} I_{rms}\cos\phi$ ... (i)

$I_{rms} = \frac{I_0}{\sqrt{2}} = \frac{E_{rms}}{Z}$

$Z = \sqrt{R^2 + X_L^2} = \sqrt{4+1} = \sqrt{5}$

$I_{rms} = \frac{6}{\sqrt{5}}A$ and $\cos\phi = \frac{R}{Z} = \frac{2}{\sqrt{5}}$

By putting the value of I_{rms}, E_{rms}, $\cos\phi$ in equation (i), then,

$P_{av} = 6\times\frac{6}{\sqrt{5}}\times\frac{2}{\sqrt{5}} = \frac{72}{\sqrt{5}\sqrt{5}} = \frac{72}{5} = 14.4$ watt

7. (a) As given that,

Secondary voltage (V_S) is :

$V_S = 24$ Volt

Power associated with secondary is :

$P_S = 12$ Watt

As we know that $P_S = V_S I_S$

$I_S = \frac{P_S}{V_S} = \frac{12}{24} = \frac{1}{2}A = 0.5$ Amp

Peak value of the current in the secondary

$I_0 = I_S\sqrt{2} = 0.5\sqrt{2} = \frac{5}{10}\sqrt{2}\left[I_0 = \frac{1}{\sqrt{2}}\text{Amp}\right]$

NEET/AIPMT (2013-2020) Questions

8. (c) By inserting iron rod in the coil,

$L\uparrow z\uparrow I\downarrow$ so brightness $\downarrow$

9. (b) Efficiency $\eta = \frac{V_s I_s}{V_p I_p} \Rightarrow 0.9 = \frac{V_s(6)}{3\times 10^3}$

$\Rightarrow V_s = 450$ V

As $V_p I_p = 3000$ so

$I_p = \frac{3000}{V_p} = \frac{3000}{200}A = 15A$

10. (d)

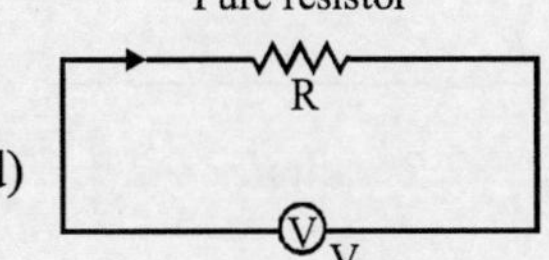

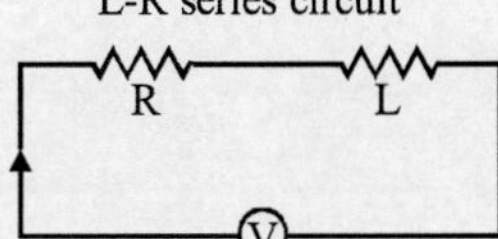

Phasor diagram

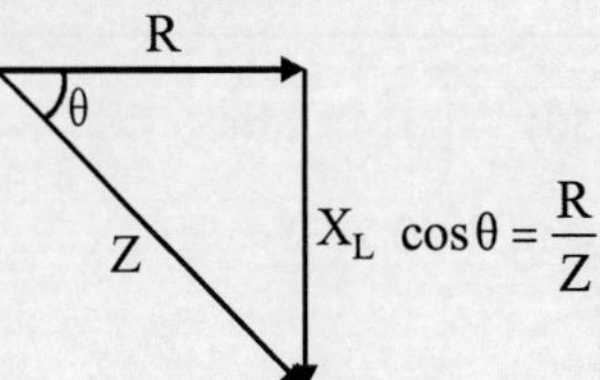

$\cos\theta = \frac{R}{Z}$

Z = impedance

For pure resistor circuit, power

$P = \frac{V^2}{R} \Rightarrow V^2 = PR$

For L-R series circuit, power

$P^1 = \frac{V^2}{Z}\cos\theta = \frac{V^2}{Z}.\frac{R}{Z} = \frac{PR}{Z^2}.R = P\left(\frac{R}{Z}\right)^2$

11. (a) Given: L = 20 mH; C = 50 μF; R = 40 Ω

$V = 10\sin 340t \quad \therefore V_{runs} = \frac{10}{\sqrt{2}}$

$X_C = \frac{1}{\omega C} = \frac{1}{340\times 50\times 10^{-6}} = 58.8\,\Omega$

$X_L = \omega L = 340 \times 20 \times 10^{-3} = 6.8\,\Omega$

Impedance, $Z = \sqrt{R^2 + (X_C - X_L)^2}$

$= \sqrt{40^2 + (58.8 - 6.8)^2} = \sqrt{4304}\,\Omega$

Power loss in A.C. circuit,

$$P = i_{rms}^2 R = \left(\frac{V_{rms}}{Z}\right)^2 R$$

$$= \left(\frac{10/\sqrt{2}}{\sqrt{4304}}\right)^2 \times 40 = \frac{50 \times 40}{4304} \simeq 0.51 \text{ W}$$

12. (b) As we know, power $P = V_{rms} \cdot I_{rms} \cos\phi$
as $\cos\phi = 0$ $(\because \phi = 90°)$
$\therefore$ Power consumed = 0 (in one complete cycle)

13. (b) 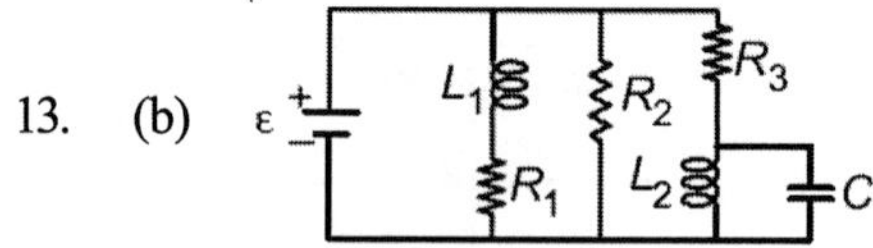

At t = 0, no current flows through R_1 and R_3

$\therefore$ 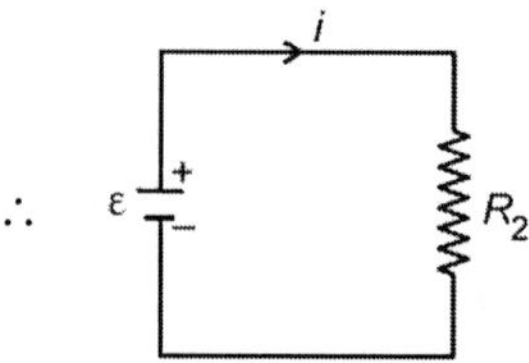

Current through battery just after the switch closed is

$$i = \frac{\varepsilon}{R_2} = \frac{18}{9} = 2\text{A}$$

14. (a) Power dissipated in an LCR series circuit connected to an a.c. source of emf E

$$P = E_{rms} i_{rms} \cos\phi = \frac{E_{rms}^2 R}{Z^2} = \frac{E_{rms}^2 R}{R^2 + \left(\omega L - \frac{1}{C\omega}\right)^2}$$

$$= \frac{\left(\frac{10}{\sqrt{2}}\right)^2 \times 50}{(50)^2 + \left(314 \times 20 \times 10^{-3} - \frac{1}{314 \times 100 \times 10^{-6}}\right)^2}$$

Solving we get, P = 0.79 W

15. (b) $I_1 = \dfrac{V}{Z}$

$$I_1 = \frac{12}{\sqrt{R^2 + (X_L - X_C)^2}} = 0.2\text{A}$$

In second case, the capacitor would provide infinite resistance but current is present in circuit, it means resistor and inductor can be present in the circuit.
Since current with AC source and DC source are different, inductor must be present with resistance.

16. (b) Given:
Capacitance, $C = 40\,\mu\text{F} = 40 \times 10^{-6}$ F
Frequency, $f = 50$ Hz

$\therefore \omega = 2\pi f = 100\pi$

$\varepsilon_{rms} = 200$ V

$$\therefore I_{rms} = \frac{\varepsilon_{rms}}{X_C} = \frac{\varepsilon_{rms}}{\frac{1}{C\omega}}$$

$= 200 \times 40 \times 10^{-6} \times 2\pi \times 50 = 2.5$ A.

17. (b) When L is removed,
Phase difference

$$\tan\phi = \frac{|X_C|}{R} = \tan\frac{\pi}{3} = \frac{X_C}{R} \quad ...(1)$$

When C is removed,
Phase difference

$$\tan\phi = \frac{|X_L|}{R} = \tan\frac{\pi}{3} = \frac{X_L}{R} \quad ...(2)$$

From eqs. (1) and (2), $X_L = X_C$

Since, $X_L = X_C$, the circuit is in resonance.
In this case, $Z = R$

$\therefore$ Power factor, $\cos\phi = \dfrac{R}{Z} = 1$.

Exercise 3 - Concept Application Problems CAP

1. (c) $\dfrac{I_s}{I_p} = \dfrac{n_p}{n_s}$; $\dfrac{80}{I_p} = \dfrac{20}{1}$ or $I_p = 4$ amp.

2. (d) The transformer converts A.C. high voltage into A.C. low voltage, but it does not cause any change in frequency.

$$\frac{E_s}{E_p} = \frac{N_s}{N_p} \Rightarrow E_s = \frac{N_s}{N_p} E_p = \frac{5000}{500} \times 20 = 200\text{V}$$

Thus output has voltage 200 V and frequency 50 Hz.

3. (d)

4. (a) The phase angle between voltage V and current I is $\pi/2$. Therefore, power factor $\cos\phi = \cos(\pi/2) = 0$. Hence the power consumed is zero.

5. (c) The current drawn by inductor and capacitor will be in opposite phase. Hence net current drawn from generator $= I_L - I_C = 0.9 - 0.4 = 0.5$ amp.

6. (d) Initially there is no D.C. current in inductive circuit and maximum D.C.current is in capacitive current. Hence, the current is zero in A_2 and maximum in A_1.

7. (a) $L = 10\text{ mHz} = 10^{-2}$ Hz
$f = 1\text{MHz} = 10^6$ Hz

$$f = \frac{1}{2\pi\sqrt{LC}}; \quad f^2 = \frac{1}{4\pi^2 LC}$$

$$\Rightarrow C = \frac{1}{4\pi^2 f^2 L} = \frac{1}{4 \times 10 \times 10^{-2} \times 10^{12}} = \frac{10^{-12}}{4} = 2.5 \text{ pF}$$

8. (c) $P = \dfrac{E_v^2 \cos\phi}{Z}$

$$P = 3000 = \frac{(240)^2 (0.75)}{Z} \text{d} \quad \Rightarrow Z = 14.4\Omega$$

9. (c) 10. (c)

11. (d) The time constant of the circuit is

$$\tau = \frac{L}{R} = \frac{100 \times 10^{-3}}{50} = 2 \times 10^{-3} \text{ s} = 2 \text{ milli second.}$$

Current at time t is given by $I = I_0 e^{-t/\tau}$ where I_0 is the steady current. Therefore, time for I to fall to $I_0/2$ is

$e^{-t/\tau} = \frac{1}{2}$ or, $e^{t/\tau} = 2$, $t = \tau \ell n(2) = 2\ell n(2)$ milli second.

12. (d)
13. (a) Given : Supply voltage $(V_{ac}) = 200$ V
Inductive reactance $(X_L) = 50$ W
Capacitive reactance $(X_C) = 50$ W
Ohmic resistance (R) = 10 W.
We know that impedance of the LCR circuit

$$(Z) = \sqrt{\{(X_L - X_C)^2 + R^2\}} = \sqrt{\{(50-50)^2 + (10)^2\}} = 10\Omega$$

14. (c) $I_0 = \frac{E_0}{R} = \frac{nBA\omega}{R}$
Given, $n = 1, B = 10^{-2}$ T,
$A = \pi(0.3)^2 m^2, R = \pi^2$
$f = (200/60)$ and $\omega = 2\pi(200/60)$
Substituting these values and solving, we get
$I_0 = 6 \times 10^{-3}$ A = 6mA
15. (b) As $V_L = V_C = 300\ V$, resonance will take place
$\therefore V_R = 220\ V$

Current, $I = \frac{220}{100} = 2.2 A$

$\therefore$ reading of $V_3 = 220\ V$
and reading of $A = 2.2\ A$
16. (a)
17. (a) Potential energy stored in the inductor

$$U = \frac{1}{2}LI^2$$

During growth of current,

$$i = I_{max}\left(1 - e^{-Rt/L}\right)$$

For U to be $\frac{U_{max}}{n}$; i has to be $\frac{I_{max}}{\sqrt{n}}$

$$\therefore \frac{I_{max}}{\sqrt{n}} = I_{max}(1 - e^{-Rt/L})$$

$$\Rightarrow e^{-Rt/L} = 1 - \frac{1}{\sqrt{n}} = \frac{\sqrt{n}-1}{\sqrt{n}}$$

$$\Rightarrow -\frac{Rt}{L} = \ln\left(\frac{\sqrt{n}-1}{\sqrt{n}}\right) \Rightarrow t = \frac{L}{R}\ln\left(\frac{\sqrt{n}}{\sqrt{n}-1}\right)$$

18. (d)
19. (a) Given,
Reactance of inductance coil, $Z = 100\Omega$
Frequency of AC signal, $v = 1000$ Hz
Phase angle, $\phi = 45°$

$$\tan\phi = \frac{X_L}{R} = \tan 45° = 1 \Rightarrow X_L = R$$

Reactance, $Z = 100 = \sqrt{X_L^2 + R^2}$

$$\Rightarrow 100 = \sqrt{R^2 + R^2}$$

$$\Rightarrow \sqrt{2}R = 100 \Rightarrow R = 50\sqrt{2}$$

$$\therefore X_L = 50\sqrt{2}$$

$$\Rightarrow L\omega = 50\sqrt{2} \quad (\because X_L = \omega L)$$

$$\Rightarrow L = \frac{50\sqrt{2}}{2\pi \times 1000} \quad (\because \omega = 2\pi v)$$

$$= \frac{25\sqrt{2}}{\pi}\text{ mH} = 1.1 \times 10^{-2}\text{ H}$$

20. (b) We have, $i = i_0(1 - e^{-t/c}) = \frac{\varepsilon}{R}(1 - e^{-t/c})$

Charge, $q = \int_0^\tau i dt$

$$= \frac{\varepsilon}{R}\int_0^\tau (1 - e^{-t/\tau})dt = \frac{E}{R}\frac{\tau}{e} = \frac{E}{R} \times \frac{(L/R)}{e} = \frac{EL}{2.7R^2}$$

21. (d) $I = I_0\left(1 - e^{-\frac{Rt}{L}}\right)$ Here $R = R_L + r = 1\Omega$

$$0.8I_0 = I_0\left(1 - e^{-\frac{t}{.01}}\right) \Rightarrow 0.8 = 1 - e^{-100t}$$

$$\Rightarrow e^{-100t} = 0.2 = \left(\frac{1}{5}\right)$$

$$\Rightarrow 100t = \ln 5 \Rightarrow t = \frac{1}{100}\ln 5 = 0.016\text{ s}$$

22. (c) $i^2 R = \left(\tau\frac{di}{dt}\right)i \Rightarrow \frac{di}{dt} = \frac{i}{\tau}$

$$\Rightarrow t = \tau\, ln2 = 2ln2 \left[\text{as } \tau = \frac{L}{R} = \frac{20}{10} = 2\right]$$

23. (d) $\omega = 100$ rad/s
We know that

$$\tan\phi = \frac{X_C}{R} = \frac{1}{\omega CR} \text{ or } \tan 45° = \frac{1}{\omega CR}$$

or $\omega CR = 1$
LHS: $\omega CR = 10 \times 10 \times 10^{-6} \times 10^3 = 1$
24. (d) Long time after switch is closed, the inductor will be idle so, the equivalent diagram will be as below

ε R R

$$I = \frac{\varepsilon}{\left(\frac{R \times R}{R + R}\right)} = \frac{2\varepsilon}{R} = \frac{2 \times 15}{5} = 6\text{ A}$$

25. (Bonus)
Capacitive reactance,

$$X_c = \frac{1}{\omega C} = \frac{4}{10^{-6} \times \sqrt{3} \times 100} = \frac{2 \times 10^4}{\sqrt{3}}$$

$$\tan\theta_1 = \frac{X_C}{R_2} = \frac{10^3}{\sqrt{3}}$$

θ_1 is close to 90°
For L-R circuit

$$X_L = \omega L = 100 \times \frac{\sqrt{3}}{10} = 10\sqrt{3}$$

i θ₁ V

$R_1 = 10$

$\tan\theta_2 = \frac{X_L}{R_1}$

$\tan\theta_2 = \sqrt{3} \Rightarrow \theta_2 = \tan^{-1}(\sqrt{3})$

$\theta_2 = 60°$

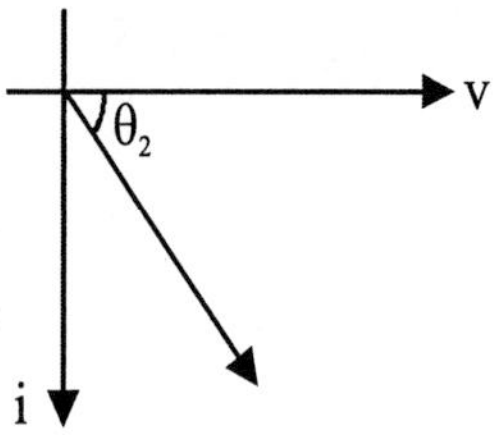

So, phase difference comes out 90° + 60° = 150°

If R_2 is 20 KΩ

then phase difference comes out to be 60 + 30 = 90°.

Therefore Ans. is **Bonus**

26. (b) Here, $X_L = \omega_L = 2\pi fL = 2\pi \times 50 \times 1 = 100\,\pi\,\Omega$

$$X_c = \frac{1}{\omega C} = \frac{1}{2\pi fC} = \frac{1}{2\pi \times 50 \times 10 \times 10^{-6}} = \frac{10^3}{\pi}\Omega$$

$$\text{So,}\quad X = |X_L - X_C| = \left|100\pi - \frac{10^3}{\pi}\right| = \left|10^2\left[\frac{\pi^2 - 10}{\pi}\right]\right|\Omega$$

27. (c)

28. (a) For series connection of a resistor and inductor, time variation of current is $I = I_0(1 - e^{-t/T_c})$

Here, $T_C = \frac{L}{R}$

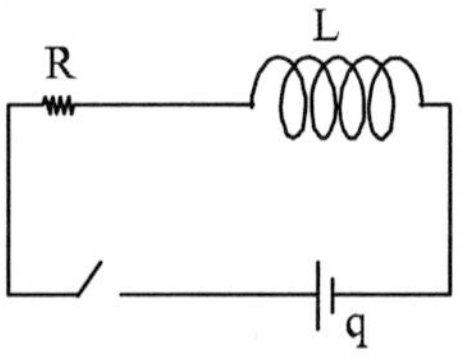

$$q = \int_0^{T_c} i\,dt$$

$$\Rightarrow \int dq = \int \frac{E}{R}\left(1 - e^{-t/t_c}\right)dt$$

$$\Rightarrow q = \frac{\in}{R}\left[t + t_C e^{-t/t_c}\right]_0^{t_c} \Rightarrow q = \frac{\in}{R}\left[t_C + \frac{t_C}{e} - t_C\right]$$

$$\Rightarrow q = \frac{\in}{R}\frac{L}{\text{Re}} \quad \therefore q = \frac{\in L}{R^2 e}$$

29. (d) In damped harmonic oscillation,

$$\frac{md^2x}{dt^2} = -kx - bv$$

$$\Rightarrow \frac{md^2x}{dt^2} + b\frac{dx}{dt} + kx = 0 \quad ....(i)$$

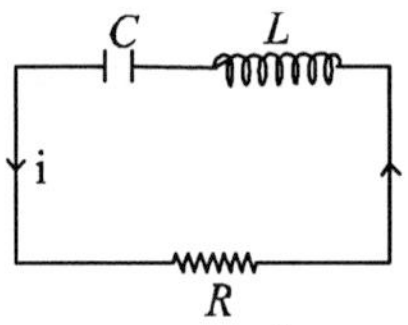

In LCR circuit, $\frac{-q}{C} - iR - \frac{Ldi}{dt} = 0$

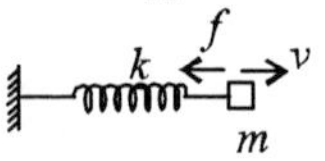

$$L\frac{d^2}{dt^2} + R\frac{dq}{dt} + \frac{q}{C} = 0 \quad ...(ii)$$

Comparing equations (i) & (ii)

$$L \leftrightarrow m,\ C \leftrightarrow \frac{1}{k},\ R \leftrightarrow b$$

30. (a) The current (I) in LR series circuit is given by

$$I = \frac{V}{R}\left(1 - e^{-\frac{tR}{L}}\right)$$

At $t = \infty$,

$$I_\infty = \frac{20}{5}\left(I - e^{\frac{-\infty}{L/R}}\right) = 4 \quad ...(i)$$

At $t = 40$s,

$$\left(1 - e^{\frac{-40 \times 5}{10 \times 10^{-3}}}\right) = 4(1 - e^{-20,000}) \quad ...(ii)$$

Dividing (i) by (ii) we get

$$\Rightarrow \frac{I_\infty}{I_{40}} = \frac{1}{1 - e^{-20,000}}$$

31. (b) As we know, average power $P_{avg} = V_{rms} I_{rms} \cos\theta$

$$= \left(\frac{V_0}{\sqrt{2}}\right)\left(\frac{I_0}{\sqrt{2}}\right)\cos\theta = \left(\frac{100}{\sqrt{2}}\right)\left(\frac{20}{\sqrt{2}}\right)\cos 45° \quad (\because \theta = 45°)$$

$$P_{avg} = \frac{1000}{\sqrt{2}}\text{ watt}$$

Wattless current $I = I_{rms}\sin\theta$

$$= \frac{I_0}{\sqrt{2}}\sin\theta = \frac{20}{\sqrt{2}}\sin 45° = 10\text{A}$$

32. (b) Given,

$V_0 = 283$ volt, $\omega = 320$, $R = 5\,\Omega$, $L = 25$ mH, $C = 1000\,\mu$F

$x_L = \omega L = 320 \times 25 \times 10^{-3} = 8\,\Omega$

$$x_C = \frac{1}{\omega C} = \frac{1}{320 \times 1000 \times 10^{-6}} = 3.1\,\Omega$$

Total impedance of the circuit :

$$Z = \sqrt{R^2 + (X_L - X_C)^2} = \sqrt{25 + (4.9)^2} = 7\,\Omega$$

Phase difference between the voltage and current

$$\tan\phi = \frac{X_L - X_C}{R}$$

$$\tan\phi = \frac{4.9}{5} \approx 1 \Rightarrow \phi = 45°$$

33. (b) Here $i = \frac{e}{\sqrt{R^2 + X_L^2}} = \frac{e}{\sqrt{R^2 + \omega^2 L^2}} = \frac{e}{\sqrt{R^2 + 4\pi^2 v^2 L^2}}$

$$10 = \frac{220}{\sqrt{64 + 4\pi^2(50)^2 L}} \quad [\because R = \frac{V}{I} = \frac{80}{10} = 8]$$

On solving we get L = 0.065 H

34. (a)

35. (b) $I(0) = \frac{15 \times 100}{0.15 \times 10^3} = 0.1A$

$I(\infty) = 0$

$$I(t) = [I(0) - I(\infty)]\, e^{\frac{-t}{L/R}} + i(\infty)$$

$$I(t) = 0.1\, e^{\frac{-t}{L/R}} = 0.1\, e^{\frac{R}{L}}$$

$$I(t) = 0.1\, e^{\frac{0.15 \times 1000}{0.03}} = 0.67\text{ mA}$$

36. (c) $Z = \sqrt{R^2 + \left(\omega L - \frac{1}{\omega C}\right)^2}$

Here R = 100 Ω, L = 0.5 henry, C = 10 × 10^6 farad

ω = 2(50) π = 100 π.

37. (b) Number of turns in primary

$N_p = 140$

Number of turns in secondary $N_s = 280, I_p = 4A, I_s = ?$

Using transformation ratio for a transformer $\frac{I_s}{I_p} = \frac{N_p}{N_s}$

$\Rightarrow \frac{I_s}{4} = \frac{140}{280}$

$\Rightarrow I_s = 2A$

38. (d) In a series LCR circuit voltage across the inductor and capacitor are in opposite phase

$\therefore$ Net voltage difference across

$LC = 50 - 50 = 0$

39. (c) Applying Kirchhoff's law of voltage in closed loop

$-V_R - V_C = 0 \Rightarrow \frac{V_R}{V_C} = -1$

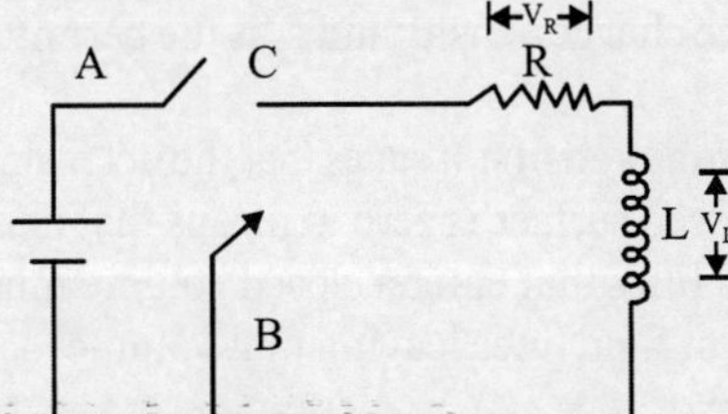

40. (c) Given, $V_L : V_C : V_R = 1:2:3$

$V = 100\,V$

$V_R = ?$

As we know,

$V = \sqrt{V_R^2 + (V_L - V_C)^2}$

Solving we get, $V_R \simeq 90V$

41. (c) Charge on he capacitor at any time t is given by $q = CV(1 - e^{t/\tau})$

at $t = 2\tau$

$q = CV(1 - e^{-2})$

42. (d)

43. (c) Frequency $f = \frac{1}{2\pi\sqrt{LC}} = \frac{1}{2 \times 3.4\sqrt{24 \times 2 \times 10^{-6}}}$

$\simeq 23\text{Hz}$

44. (a) Phase difference for *R–L* circuit lies between $\left(0, \frac{\pi}{2}\right)$

45. (c) Given : $V_P = 2300\,V, V_s = 230\,V, I_P = 5\,A, n = 90\% = 0.9$

Efficiency $n = 0.9 = \frac{P_s}{P_P} \Rightarrow P_s = 0.9\,P_p$

$V_s I_s = 0.9 \times V_P I_P \quad (\because P = VI)$

$I_s = \frac{0.9 \times 2300 \times 5}{230} = 45\,A$

23 Electromagnetic Waves

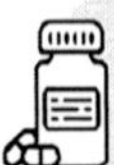

Topic 23.1 : Displacement Current, Maxwell's Modification of Ampere's Circuital Law and Electromagnetic Waves

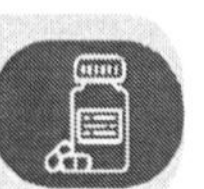

DISPLACEMENT CURRENT

It is that current which comes into play in a region, where electric field (and hence the electric flux) is changing with time.

The displacement current is given by, $I_D = \varepsilon_o \dfrac{d\phi_E}{dt}$

where ε_0 = absolute permittivity (or permitivity of free space)

and $\dfrac{d\phi_E}{dt}$ = rate of change of electric flux.

In case of a steady electric flux linked with a region, the displacement current is maximum.

The current in the electric circuit which arises due to flow of electrons in the connecting wires of the circuit, in a defined closed path is called ***conduction current****.*

MAXWELL'S MODIFICATION OF AMPERE'S CIRCUITAL LAW

In 1864, Maxwell showed that Ampere's circuital law is logically inconsistent for non-steady currents. He modified Ampere's law as $\oint \vec{B}.\overrightarrow{d\ell} = \mu_0\left(I + \varepsilon_0 \dfrac{d\phi_E}{dt}\right)$ (Sum of conduction current and displacement current)

The term $I_d = \varepsilon_0(d\phi_E/dt)$ is displacement current. It is that current which comes into existence, in addition to the conduction current, whenever the electric field and hence the electric flux changes with time.

Maxwell's Equation

Maxwell found that all the basic principles of electromagnetism can be formulated in terms of four fundamental equations, called Maxwell's equation. These are :

(i) Gauss's law for electrostatics : According to Gauss's law the total electric flux through any closed surface is equal to the net charge inside that surface divided by ε_0

i.e., $\oint \vec{E}.\overrightarrow{dA} = \dfrac{Q}{\varepsilon_o}$

This law relates the electric field to charge distribution, whereas electric field lines orignate from positive (+ive) charge and terminate on negative (–ive) charge. The differential form of this law is $\vec{\nabla}.\vec{E} = \dfrac{\rho}{\varepsilon_0}$

where ρ is volume charge density and ε_0 is the permittivity of free space.

(ii) Gauss's law for magnetism : It states that the net magnetic flux through a closed surface is zero. It means that number of magnetic field lines that enter a closed volume must be equal to number of field lines leaving that volume

i.e., $\oint \vec{B}.d\vec{A} = 0$

It means that magnetic mono pole cannot exists in nature. The differential form of this law is $\vec{\nabla}.\vec{B} = 0$

(iii) Faraday's law : This law states that the line integral of the electric field around any closed path (which equals the e.m.f.) equals the rate of change of magnetic flux through any surface area bounded by that path.

i.e., $\oint \vec{E}.\vec{d}\ell = \dfrac{d\phi_m}{dt}$

The **consequence of this law** is that, if we keep any conducting loop in a time varying magnetic field, then an induced current, flows in that conducting loop. The differential form of this law is $\vec{\nabla} \times \vec{E} = -\dfrac{dB}{dt}$

This law decribes a relationship between an electric field and a changing magnetic flux.

(iv) Modified Ampere-Maxwell law : It states that " the line integral of magnetic field around any closed path is determined by the sum of the net conduction current through that path and the rate of change of electric flux through any surface bounded by that path

i.e., $\oint \vec{B}.d\vec{S} = \mu_0 I + \varepsilon_o\mu_0 \dfrac{d\phi_e}{dt}$

It describes the relationship between magnetic and electric fields and electric current. The differential form of this law is

$$\vec{\nabla} \times \vec{B} = \mu_0 J + \mu_0 E_0 \frac{dE}{dt}$$

ELECTROMAGNETIC WAVES

Maxwell-on the basis of four basic equations of electromagnetism theoretically predicted the existence of electromagnetic waves. *An electromagentic wave is the one constituted by oscillating electric and magnetic fields which oscillate in two mutually perpendicular planes.* The wave itself propagates in a direction perpendicular to both of the directions of oscillations of electric and magnetic fields.

Properties of Electromagnetic Waves

(i) The direction of oscillations of E and B fields are perpendicular to each other as well as to the direction of propagation. Electromagnetic waves are transverse in nature.

(ii) The electric and magnetic field oscillate in same phase.

(iii) The electromagnetic waves travel through vacuum with the same speed of light

$$c = \frac{1}{\sqrt{\mu_0 \varepsilon_0}} = 3 \times 10^8 \text{ ms}^{-1}$$

(iv) *The energy density of electric field is* $\frac{1}{2}\varepsilon_o E^2$ *and that of magnetic field is* $\frac{1}{2}\frac{B^2}{\mu_0}$, so the *energy density of the electromagnetic wave is* $u = \frac{1}{2}\left[\varepsilon_o E^2 + \frac{B^2}{\mu_0}\right]$

where E and B are the instantaneous values of the electric and magnetic field vectors.

(v) The ratio $\frac{E}{B} = c = \frac{1}{\sqrt{\mu_0 \varepsilon_o}}$.

Production of Electromagnetic Waves

An accelerated charge emits electromagnetic waves. An oscillating charge, as in an LC-circuit has non-zero acceleration, it continues to emit electromagnetic waves. The frequency of electromagnetic waves is the same as that of the oscillating charge.

Hertz's experiment : In 1888, Hertz succeeded in experimentally confirming the existence of electromagnetic waves. By using oscillator LC-circuits, he not only produced and detected electromagnetic waves, but also demonstrated their properties of reflection, refraction and interference and established beyond doubt that light radiation has wave nature.

Problem Solving Tips

1. The amplitudes of electric and magnetic fields in free space, in electromagnetic waves are related by $E_0 = cB_0$ or $C = \frac{E_0}{B_0}$
2. The velocity of electromagnetic wave does not depend on amplitude of field vectors.
3. The electric vector of an electromagnetic wave is responsible for the optical effects & is called a light vector.
4. In a plane electromagnetic wave, the average energy densities of electric and magnetic fields are equal.

In vacuum, the average electric energy density is given by, $u_E = \frac{1}{2}\varepsilon_o E^2 = \frac{1}{2}\varepsilon_o (E_0/\sqrt{2})^2 = \frac{1}{4}\varepsilon_o E_0^2$

The average magnetic energy density is given by

$$u_B = \frac{B^2}{2\mu_0} = \frac{(B_0/\sqrt{2})^2}{2\mu_0} = \frac{B_0^2}{4\mu_0}$$

Also, $u_E = \frac{1}{4}\varepsilon_o E_0^2 = \frac{1}{4}\varepsilon_o (cB_0)^2 = \frac{1}{4}\varepsilon_o c^2 B_0^2$

$$= \frac{1}{4}\frac{\varepsilon_o B_0^2}{\varepsilon_o \mu_0} = \frac{B_0^2}{4\mu_0} = u_B$$

∴ Total average energy density

$$= u_E + u_B = 2u_E = 2u_B = \frac{1}{2}\varepsilon_o E_0^2 = \frac{B_0^2}{2\mu_0}$$

5. **Poynting vector:** When an electromagnetic wave advances, the electromagnetic energy flows in the direction $\vec{E} \times \vec{B}$. The total energy flowing perpendicularly per second per unit area into the space in free space is called a **poynting vector** $\vec{S}$ where

$$\vec{S} = c\varepsilon_0(\vec{E} \times \vec{B}) = (\vec{E} \times \vec{B})/\mu_0.$$

$$S = |\vec{S}| = \frac{1}{\mu_0} EB\sin 90° = \frac{EB}{\mu_0}$$

The **SI unit** of S is watt/m^2

6. The intensity of a sinusoidal plane electromagnetic wave is defined as average value of poynting vector taken over one cycle. Thus,

$$I = S_{av} = \frac{1}{\mu_0}\left(\frac{E_0}{\sqrt{2}}\right)\left(\frac{B_0}{\sqrt{2}}\right) = \frac{E_0 B_0}{2\mu_0} = \frac{E_0^2}{2\mu_0 c} = \frac{cB_0^2}{2\mu_0}$$

7. **Radiation pressure :** The pressure exerted by electromagnetic waves is called as **radiation pressure (P).** When an electromagnetic wave with Poynting vector $\vec{S}$ is incident on a perfectly absorbing surface, then radiation pressure on surface is $P = \frac{\vec{S}}{c}$.

Example 1.

In a plane electromagnetic wave the electric field varies with time having an amplitude 1 Vm^{-1}. The frequency of wave is 0.5 × 10^{15} Hz. The wave is propagating along Z-axis. What is the average energy density of (i) electric field (ii) magnetic field (iii) total field. (iv) What is amplitude of magnetic field?

Solution :

(i) Average energy density of electric field

$$U_E = \frac{1}{2}\varepsilon_0 E^2 = \frac{1}{2}\varepsilon_0\left(\frac{E_0}{\sqrt{2}}\right)^2 \quad \left[\because E = \frac{E_0}{\sqrt{2}}\right]$$

$$= \frac{1}{4}\varepsilon_0 E_0^2 = \frac{1}{4} \times (8.854 \times 10^{-12}) \times 1^2 = 2.21 \times 10^{-12} \text{ Jm}^{-3}.$$

(ii) Average energy density of magnetic field,
U_B = Average energy density of electric field
$= 2.21 \times 10^{-12}\ Jm^{-3}$

(iii) Total average energy density $U = U_E + U_B = 2\,U_E$
$= 2 \times 2.21 \times 10^{-12} = 4.42 \times 10^{-12}\ Jm^{-3}$

(iv) Amplitude of magnetic field, $B_0 = E_0/c$
$= 1/(3 \times 10^8) = 3.33 \times 10^{-9}\ T$

Example 2.

If ε_o and μ_0 represent the permittivity and permeability of vacuum and ε and μ represent the permittivity and permeability of medium, then refractive index of the medium is given by

(a) $\sqrt{\frac{\mu_0\varepsilon_o}{\mu\varepsilon}}$ (b) $\sqrt{\frac{\mu\varepsilon}{\mu_0\varepsilon_o}}$ (c) $\sqrt{\frac{\varepsilon}{\mu_0\varepsilon_o}}$ (d) $\sqrt{\frac{\mu_0\varepsilon_o}{\mu}}$

***Solution :* (b)**

$\because$ Velocity of light in medium $c = \frac{1}{\sqrt{\mu\varepsilon}}$

$\therefore$ Refractive index $= \frac{c_0}{c} = \frac{1/\sqrt{\mu_0\varepsilon_o}}{1/\sqrt{\mu\varepsilon}} = \sqrt{\frac{\mu\varepsilon}{\mu_0\varepsilon_o}}$

Example 3.

The magnetic field in a plane electromagnetic wave is given by $B = 2 \times 10^{-7} \sin(0.5\times 10^3 x + 1.5 \times 10^{11} t)$ T.
(a) What is the wavelength and frequency of the wave?
(b) Write an expression for the electric field.

Solution :

(a) Comparing the given equation with

$$B = B_0 \sin\left[2\pi\left(\frac{x}{\lambda} + \frac{t}{T}\right)\right]$$

we get, $\lambda = \frac{2\pi}{0.5\times 10^3}\ m = 1.26\ cm$

and $\frac{1}{T} = \nu = (1.5\times 10^{11})/2\pi = 23.9\ GHz$

(b) $E_0 = B_0 c = 2 \times 10^{-7}\ T \times 3 \times 10^8\ m/s = 6 \times 10^1\ V/m$

The electric field component is perpendicular to the direction of propagation and the direction of magnetic field. Therefore, the electric field component along the z-axis is obtained as

$E_z = 60 \sin(0.5 \times 10^3 x + 1.5 \times 10^{11} t)$ V/m

Example 4.

A plane electromagnetic wave of frequency 25 MHz travels in free space along the x-direction. At a particular point in space and time, $\vec{E} = 6.3\,\hat{j}$ V/m. What is $\vec{B}$ at this point?

Solution :

The magnitude of $\vec{B}$ is

$B = \frac{E}{c} = \frac{6.3\ V/m}{3\times 10^8\ m/s} = 2.1\times 10^{-8} T$

To find the direction, we note that $\vec{E}$ is along y-direction and the wave propagates along x-axis. Therefore, B should be in a direction perpendicular to both x- and y-axes. Using vector algebra, $\vec{E}\times\vec{B}$ should be along x-direction.

Since, $(+\hat{j})\times(+\hat{k}) = \hat{i}.\vec{B}$, $\vec{B}$ is along the z-direction.

Thus, $\vec{B} = 2.1\times 10^{-8}\hat{k} T$

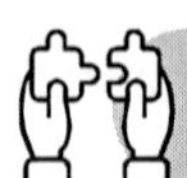

23.1 Concept Practice Problems

CPP

1. Displacement current goes through the gap between the plates of a capacitor when the charge on the capacitor
(a) is changing with time (b) decreases
(c) does not change (d) decreases to zero

2. If the frequency of EM radiations is halved then the energy of EM radiation will become
(a) double (b) remains unchanged
(c) becomes half (d) becomes one fourth

3. According to Maxwell's hypothesis, a changing electric field gives rise to
(a) an e.m.f
(b) electric displacement current
(c) magnetic field
(d) pressure gradient

4. A plane electromagnetic wave is incident on a material surface. If the wave delivers momentum p and energy E, then
(a) $p = 0, E = 0$ (b) $p \neq 0, E \neq 0$
(c) $p \neq 0, E = 0$ (d) $p = 0, E \neq 0$

5. In a plane electromagnetic wave propagating in space has an electric field of amplitude 9×10^3 V/m, then the amplitude of the magnetic field is
(a) 2.7×10^{12} T (b) 9.0×10^{-3} T
(c) 3.0×10^{-4} T (d) 3.0×10^{-5} T

6. A beam has intensity $2.5 \times 10^{14}\ Wm^{-2}$. The ratio of electric and magnetic fields in the beam is
(a) $2.98\times 10^8\ NC^{-1}T^{-1}$ (b) $8.32\times 10^5\ NCT^{-1}$
(c) $6.22\times 10^7\ NC^{-1}T^{-1}$ (d) $2.88\times 10^6\ NCT^{-1}$

7. An electromagnetic wave with frequency ω and wavelength λ travels in the $+y$ direction. Its magnetic field is along $+x$-axis. The vector equation for the associated electric field (of amplitude E_0) is

(a) $\vec{E} = -E_0\cos\left(\omega t + \frac{2\pi}{\lambda}y\right)\hat{x}$

(b) $\vec{E} = E_0\cos\left(\omega t - \frac{2\pi}{\lambda}y\right)\hat{x}$

(c) $\vec{E} = E_0\cos\left(\omega t - \frac{2\pi}{\lambda}y\right)\hat{z}$

(d) $\vec{E} = -E_0\cos\left(\omega t + \frac{2\pi}{\lambda}y\right)\hat{z}$

8. If a source is transmitting electromagnetic wave of frequency 8.2×10^6 Hz, then wavelength of the electromagnetic waves transmitted from the source will be
(a) 36.6m (b) 40.5m (c) 42.3m (d) 50.9m

9. For plane electromagnetic waves propagating in the z-direction, which one of the following combination gives the correct possible direction for $\vec{E}$ and $\vec{B}$ field respectively?
(a) $(2\hat{i}+3\hat{j})$ and $(\hat{i}+2\hat{j})$
(b) $(-2\hat{i}-3\hat{j})$ and $(3\hat{i}-2\hat{j})$
(c) $(3\hat{i}+4\hat{j})$ and $(4\hat{i}-3\hat{j})$
(d) $(\hat{i}+2\hat{j})$ and $(2\hat{i}-\hat{j})$

10. The amplitude of the electric field if the intensity of a plane electromagnetic wave is given as $2.0\ \text{Wm}^{-2}$ is
(a) $38.8\ \text{NC}^{-1}$ (b) $48.3\ \text{NC}^{-1}$
(c) $50.2\ \text{NC}^{-1}$ (d) $68.8\ \text{NC}^{-1}$

ANSWER KEY

1	(a)	2	(c)	3	(c)	4	(b)	5	(d)	6	(a)	7	(c)	8	(a)	9	(b)	10	(a)

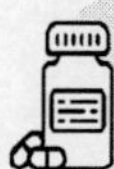

Topic 23.2 : Electromagnetic Spectrum and Uses of Electromagnetic Waves

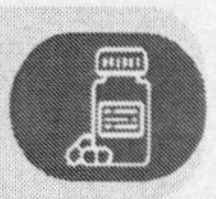

ELECTROMAGNETIC SPECTRUM

All the known radiations form a big family of electromagnetic waves according to frequency or wavelength. We call this family as the complete electromagnetic spectrum. It includes: *Gamma rays, X-rays, ultraviolet light, visible light, infrared light, microwaves and radio waves.*

S.No.	Name	Wavelength range (in m)	Frequency range (in Hz)	Source	Detection
1	Gamma rays	6×10^{-14} to 1×10^{-11}	5×10^{22} to 3×10^{19}	Nuclear origin	Photographic film, Geiger tubes, ionisation chamber
2	X-rays	1×10^{-11} to 3×10^{-8}	3×10^{19} to 1×10^{16}	Sudden deceleration of high energy electron (collision of electrons with target)	Photographic film, Geiger tubes, ionisation chamber
3	Ultra-violet	6×10^{-8} to 4×10^{-7}	5×10^{17} to 8×10^{14}	Excitation of atom, spark and arc lamp	Photocells, photographic film
4	Visible light	4×10^{-7} to 7×10^{-7}	8×10^{14} to 4×10^{14}	Excitation of valency electron	The eye, photocells, photographic film
5	Infrared	7×10^{-7} to 3×10^{-5}	4×10^{14} to 1×10^{13}	Excitation of atoms and molecules	Thermopiles, bolometer
6	Heat radiations	10^{-5} to 10^{-1}	3×10^{13} to 3×10^{9}	Hot bodies	
7	Micro-waves	10^{-3} to 0.3	3×10^{11} to 1×10^{9}	Oscillating current in special vacuum tube	Point contact diodes
8	Ultra high frequency	1×10^{-1} to 1	3×10^{9} to 3×10^{8}	Oscillating circuit	
9	Very high radio frequency	1 to 10	3×10^{8} to 3×10^{7}	Oscillating circuit	
10	Radio frequency	10 to 10^{4}	3×10^{7} to 3×10^{4}	Oscillating circuit	Receiver's aerial
11	Power frequency	5 × 106 to 6 × 106	60 to 50	Weak radiations from a.c. circuit	

USES OF ELECTROMAGNETIC WAVES

The following are some of the uses of electromagnetic waves

1. **Radio waves** are used in radio and T.V. communication systems.
2. **Microwaves** are used in microwave oven.
3. **Infrared radiations** are used (a) in revealing the secret writings on the ancient walls (b) in green houses to keep the plants warm (c) in warfare, for looking through haze, fog or mist as these radiations can pass through them.
4. **Ultraviolet radiations** are used in the detection of invisible writing, forged documents, finger prints in forensic laboratory and to preserve the food stuffs.
5. The **study of infrared, visible and ultraviolet radiations** help us to know through spectra, the structure of the molecules and arrangement of electrons in the external shells.
6. **X-rays** can pass through flesh and blood but not through bones. This property of X-rays is used in medical diagnosis, after X-rays photographs are made.

The study of X-rays has revealed the atomic structure and crystal structure.

7. The study of **γ-rays** provides us valueable information about the structure of the atomic nuclei
8. **Super high frequency electromagnetic waves** (3000 to 30,000 MHz) are used in radar and satellite communication.
9. **Electromagnetic waves (frequency 50 to 60 Hz)** are ued for lighting. These are weak waves having wavelength 5×10^6 to 6×10^6 m and can be produced from A.C. circuits.

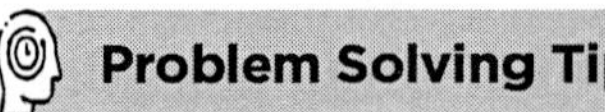

1. Green house effect : It is the phenomenon which keeps the earth's surface warm at night. The earth absorbs solar radiation and reflects back only infrared rays due to its low temperature. These rays are reflected back by the clouds and the gas molecules of the lower atmosphere. This keeps the earth's surface warm at night.

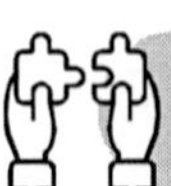

23.2 Concept Practice Problems

CPP

11. The range of wavelength of the UV rays is
(a) 10 Å to 100 Å (b) 10^9 Å to 10^{10} Å
(c) 8,000 Å to 10,000Å (d) 10,000 Å to 15,000 Å

12. The range of wavelength of visible light is
(a) 50 Å to 500 Å (b) 4000 Å to 8000 Å
(c) 9000 Å to 25,000 Å (d) 15,000 Å to 25,000 Å

13. Which of the following is the infrared wavelength?
(a) 10^{-4} cm (b) 10^{-5} cm
(c) 10^{-6} cm (d) 10^{-7} cm

14. What is the cause of "Green house effect"?
(a) Infrared rays (b) Ultraviolet rays
(c) X-rays (d) Radio waves

15. Which one of the following has the maximum energy?
(a) Radio waves (b) Infrared rays
(c) Ultraviolet rays (d) Micro waves

16. The velocity of all radio waves in free space is 3×10^8 m/s. The frequency of a radio wave of wavelength 150m is
(a) 20kHz (b) 2kHz (c) 2MHz (d) 1MHz

17. If $\lambda = 10$ Å then it corresponds to
(a) infrared (b) microwaves
(c) ultraviolet (d) X-rays

18. The waves used in telecommunication are
(a) IR (b) UV
(c) Microwave (d) Cosmic rays

19. The electromagnetic radiation used in food processing sterilizing agent is
(a) microwaves (b) UV rays
(c) gamma rays (d) radio waves

20. In electromagnetic spectrum, the frequencies γ-rays, X-rays and ultraviolet rays are denoted by n_1, n_2 and n_3 respectively then
(a) $n_1 > n_2 > n_3$ (b) $n_1 < n_2 < n_3$
(c) $n_1 > n_2 < n_3$ (d) $n_1 < n_2 > n_3$

ANSWER KEY

11	(b)	12	(b)	13	(a)	14	(a)	15	(c)	16	(c)	17	(d)	18	(c)	19	(b)	20	(a)

CONCEPT MAP

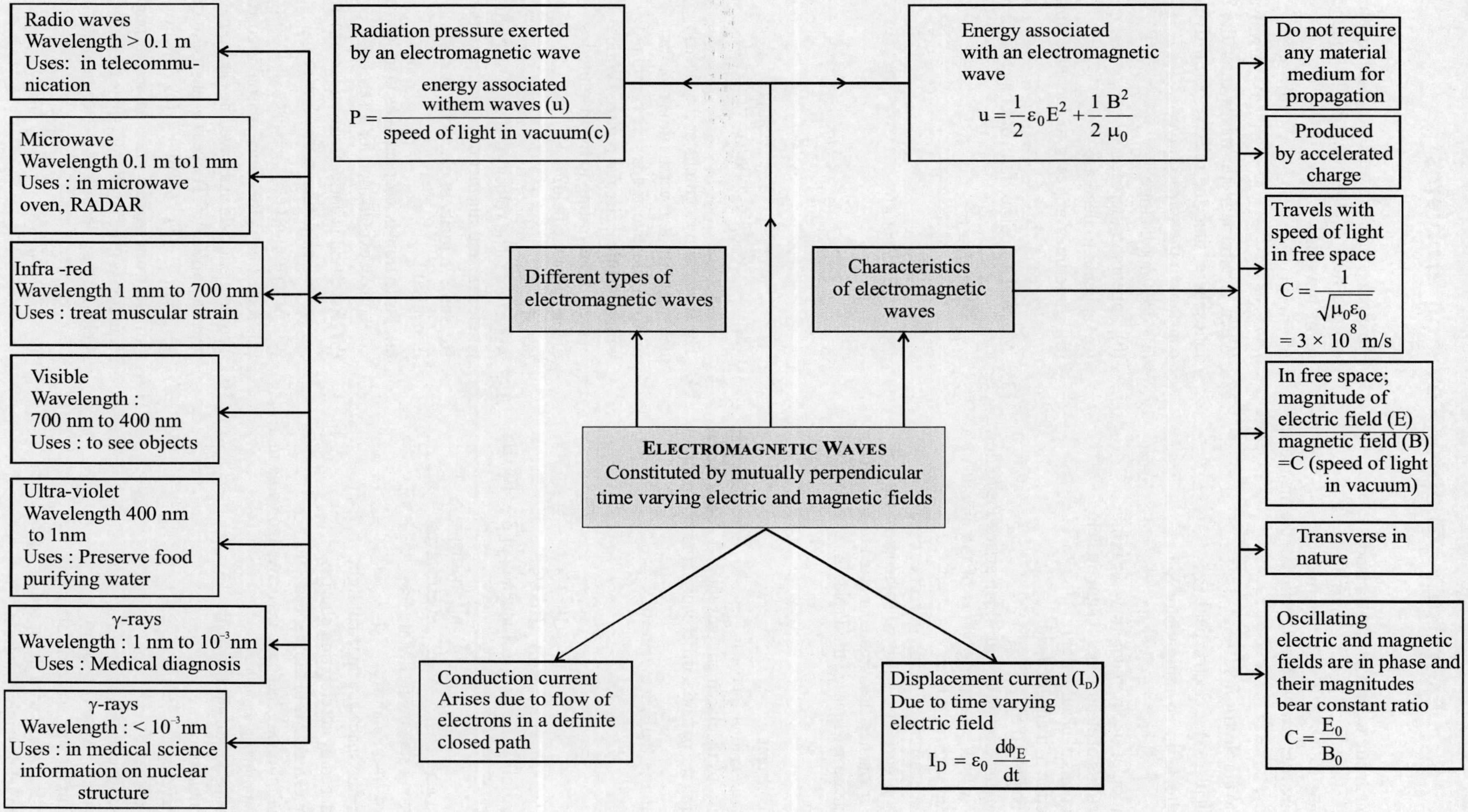

ELECTROMAGNETIC WAVES
Constituted by mutually perpendicular time varying electric and magnetic fields

Different types of electromagnetic waves

- Radio waves
  Wavelength > 0.1 m
  Uses: in telecommunication
- Microwave
  Wavelength 0.1 m to1 mm
  Uses : in microwave oven, RADAR
- Infra -red
  Wavelength 1 mm to 700 mm
  Uses : treat muscular strain
- Visible
  Wavelength :
  700 nm to 400 nm
  Uses : to see objects
- Ultra-violet
  Wavelength 400 nm to 1nm
  Uses : Preserve food purifying water
- γ-rays
  Wavelength : 1 nm to 10^{-3}nm
  Uses : Medical diagnosis
- γ-rays
  Wavelength : < 10^{-3}nm
  Uses : in medical science information on nuclear structure

Radiation pressure exerted by an electromagnetic wave

$$P = \frac{\text{energy associated withem waves (u)}}{\text{speed of light in vacuum(c)}}$$

Energy associated with an electromagnetic wave

$$u = \frac{1}{2}\varepsilon_0 E^2 + \frac{1}{2}\frac{B^2}{\mu_0}$$

Characteristics of electromagnetic waves

- Do not require any material medium for propagation
- Produced by accelerated charge
- Travels with speed of light in free space
  $C = \frac{1}{\sqrt{\mu_0 \varepsilon_0}}$
  $= 3 \times 10^8$ m/s
- In free space; $\frac{\text{magnitude of electric field (E)}}{\text{magnetic field (B)}}$ =C (speed of light in vacuum)
- Transverse in nature
- Oscillating electric and magnetic fields are in phase and their magnitudes bear constant ratio
  $C = \frac{E_0}{B_0}$

Conduction current
Arises due to flow of electrons in a definite closed path

Displacement current (I_D)
Due to time varying electric field

$$I_D = \varepsilon_0 \frac{d\phi_E}{dt}$$

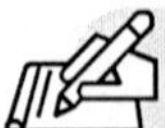

Exercise 1 - Chapter Revision Problems

CRP

1. The electromagnetic wave does not transport
(a) energy (b) charge
(c) momentum (d) information

2. In an electromagnetic wave, the direction of the magnetic induction $\vec{B}$ is
(a) parallel to the electric field $\vec{E}$
(b) perpendicular to the electric field $\vec{E}$
(c) antiparallel to the Poynting vector $\vec{S}$
(d) random

3. The polarisation of electromagnetic wave is in
(a) the directions of electric and magnetic field
(b) the directions of electric field
(c) the direction of magnetic field
(d) can not be polarized

4. The current in the electric circuit which arises due to flow of electrons in the connecting wires of the circuit in a defined closed path is called
(a) alternating current (b) direct current
(c) conduction current (d) displacement current

5. If a variable frequency ac source connected to a capacitor then with decrease in frequency, the displacement current will
(a) increase
(b) decrease
(c) remain constant
(d) first decrease then increase

6. An instantaneous displacement current of 1 A can be set up by changing the potential difference across the parallel plates capacitor (1.0 μF) at the rate of $\frac{dV}{dt}$.
here $\frac{dV}{dt}$ is
(a) $10^6\ Vs^{-1}$ (b) $10^3\ Vs^{-1}$
(c) $10^2\ Vs^{-1}$ (d) $10^1\ Vs^{-1}$

7. An electron oscillating with a frequency of 3×10^6 Hz, would generate
(a) X-rays (b) ultraviolet rays
(c) radio waves (d) microwaves

8. Select the wrong statement. EM waves
(a) are transverse in nature.
(b) travel in free space at a speed of light.
(c) are produced by accelerating charges.
(d) travel in all media with same speed.

9. Which of the following has/have zero average value in a plane electromagnetic wave?
(a) Both magnetic and electric field
(b) Electric field only
(c) Magnetic energy
(d) Electric energy

10. The electromagnetic waves
(a) travel with the speed of sound
(b) travel with the same speed in all media
(c) travel in free space with the speed of light
(d) do not travel through a medium

11. An electromagnetic wave propagating along north has its electric field vector upwards. Its magnetic field vector point towards
(a) north (b) east
(c) west (d) downwards

12. When electromagnetic waves enter the ionised layer of ionosphere, then the relative permittivity *i.e.*, dielectric constant of the ionised layer
(a) does not change
(b) appears to increase
(c) appears to decrease
(d) sometimes appears to increase and sometimes to decrease

13. Maxwell's modified form of Ampere's circuital law is
(a) $\oint_s \vec{B}\cdot\vec{ds} = 0$
(b) $\oint_s \vec{B}\cdot\vec{dl} = \mu_0 I$
(c) $\oint_s \vec{B}\cdot\vec{dl} = \mu_0 I + \frac{1}{\varepsilon_o}\frac{dq}{dt}$
(d) $\oint_s \vec{B}\cdot\vec{dl} = \mu_0 I + \mu_0 \varepsilon_o \frac{d\phi_E}{dt}$

14. The figure shows graphs of the electric field magnitude E versus time t for four uniform electric fields, all contained within identical circular regions. Which of them is according to the magnitudes of the magnetic field?

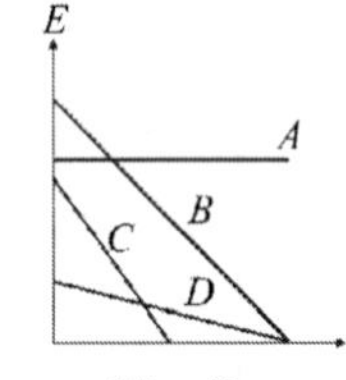

(a) A (b) B (c) C (d) D

15. **Assertion :** The velocity of electromagnetic waves depends on electric and magnetic properties of the medium.
Reason : Velocity of electromagnetic waves in free space is constant.
(a) Assertion is correct, reason is correct; reason is a correct explanation for assertion.
(b) Assertion is correct, reason is correct; reason is not a correct explanation for assertion
(c) Assertion is correct, reason is incorrect
(d) Assertion is incorrect, reason is correct.

16. The magnetic field in a travelling electromagnetic wave has a peak value of 20 nT. The peak value of electric field strength is
(a) 3 V/m (b) 6 V/m (c) 9 V/m (d) 12 V/m

17. An electromagnetic wave passes through space and its equation is given by $E = E_0 \sin(\omega t - kx)$ where E is electric field. Energy density of electromagnetic wave in space is
(a) $\frac{1}{2}\varepsilon_0 E_0^2$ (b) $\frac{1}{4}\varepsilon_0 E_0^2$ (c) $\varepsilon_0 E_0^2$ (d) $2\varepsilon_0 E_0^2$

18. A plane electromagnetic wave is incident on a plane surface of area A, normally and is perfectly reflected. If energy flux I strikes the surface in time t then average force exerted on the surface is (c = speed of light)
(a) zero (b) I/Atc (c) $\frac{2IA}{C}$ (d) I/c

19. The pressure exerted by an electromagnetic wave of intensity I (watts/m^2) on a nonreflecting surface is [c is the velocity of light]
(a) Ic (b) Ic^2 (c) I/c (d) I/c^2

20. An electromagnetic wave going through vacuum is described by $E = E_0\sin(kx - \omega t)$; $B = B_0 \sin(kx - \omega t)$. Which of the following equations is true?
(a) $E_0k = B_0\omega$ (b) $E_0\omega = B_0k$
(c) $E_0B_0 = \omega k$ (d) None of these

21. In an apparatus, the electric field was found to oscillate with an amplitude of 18 V/m. The magnitude of the oscillating magnetic field will be
(a) 4×10^{-6} T (b) 6×10^{-8} T
(c) 9×10^{-9} T (d) 11×10^{-11} T

22. A wave is propagating in a medium of electric dielectric constant 2 and relative magnetic permeability 50. The wave impedance of such a medium is
(a) 5Ω (b) 376.6Ω
(c) 1883Ω (d) 3776Ω

23. In a plane em wave, the electric field oscillates sinusoidally at a frequency 2×10^{10} Hz and amplitude 48 Vm^{-1}, then the amplitude of oscillating magnetic field is
(a) 16×10^{-8} T (b) 12×10^{-6} T
(c) 11×10^{-5} T (d) 6.6×10^{-3} T

24. When an electromagnetic wave enters an ionised layer of earth's atmosphere present in ionosphere
(a) the electron cloud will not oscillate in the electric field of the wave
(b) the electron cloud will oscillate in the electric field of wave in the phase of sinusoidal electromagnetic wave
(c) the electron cloud will oscillate in the electric field of wave in the opposite phase of sinusoidal electromagnetic wave
(d) the electron cloud will oscillate in the electric field of wave with a phase retardation of 90° for a sinusoidal electromagnetic wave.

25. An electromagnetic wave of intensity I falls on a surface kept in vacuum and exerts radiation pressure P on it. Which of the following statements are true?
I. Radiation pressure is I/c if the wave is totally absorbed.
II. Radiation pressure is I/c if the wave is totally reflected.
III. Radiation pressure is $2I/c$ if the wave is totally reflected.
(a) I and II (b) I and III
(c) III only (d) I, II and III

26. The amplitude of an electromagnetic wave in vacuum is doubled with no other changes made to the wave. As a result of this doubling of the amplitude, which of the following statements are incorrect?
I. The speed of wave propagation chages only
II. The frequency of the wave changes only
III. The wavelength of the wave changes only
(a) I and II (b) II and III
(c) I and III (d) I, II and III

27. Figure shows a parallel plate capacitor and the current in the connecting wires that is discharging the capacitor.

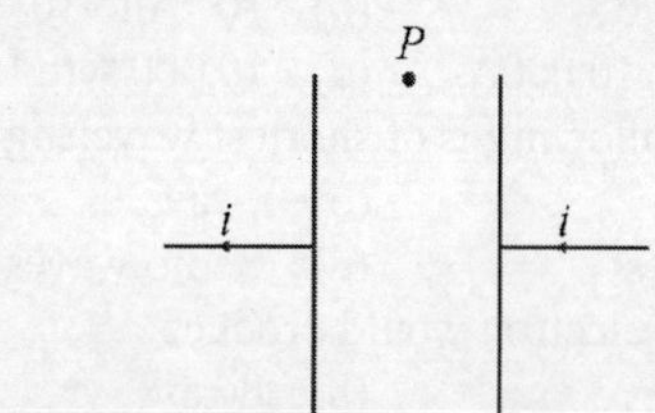

(a) The displacement current is leftward.
(b) The displacement current is rightward
(c) The electric field $\vec{E}$ is rightward
(d) The magnetic field at point P is out the page.

28. The transmitting antenna of a radiostation is mounted vertically. At a point 10 km due north of the transmitter the peak electric field is 10^{-3} Vm^{-1}. The magnitude of the radiated magnetic field is.
(a) 3.33×10^{-10} T (b) 3.33×10^{-12} T
(c) 10^{-3} T (d) 3×10^{5} T

29. A plane electromagnetic wave propagating in the X-direction has wavelength of 6.0 mm. The electric field is in the Y-direction and its maximum magnitude is 33 Vm^{-1}. The equation for the electric field as a function of x and t is
(a) $11\sin\pi\left(t-\frac{x}{c}\right)$ (b) $33\sin\left[\pi\times10^{11}\left(t-\frac{x}{c}\right)\right]$
(c) $33\sin\pi\left(t-\frac{x}{c}\right)$ (d) $11\sin\left[\pi\times10^{11}\left(t-\frac{x}{c}\right)\right]$

30. A circular ring of radius r is placed in a homogeneous magnetic field perpendicular to the plane of the ring. The field B changes with time according to equation $B = kt$, where, k is a constant and t is the time). The electric field in the ring is:
(a) $\frac{kr}{4}$ (b) $\frac{kr}{3}$ (c) $\frac{kr}{2}$ (d) $\frac{k}{2r}$

31. An electric charge oscillating with a frequency of 1 kilo cycles/sec can radiate electromagnetic waves of wavelength
(a) 800 km (b) 400 km (c) 300 km (d) 100 km

32. The charge on a parallel plate capacitor varies as $q = q_0 \cos 2\pi\nu t$. The plates are very large and close together (area = A, separation = d). Neglecting the edge effects, the displacement current through the capacitor is
(a) $2\pi\nu q_0 \sin 2\pi\nu t$ (b) $3/5\pi\nu q_0 \sin \pi\nu t$
(c) $4\pi\nu q_0 \sin 2\pi\nu t$ (d) None of these

33. A parallel plate capacitor with a and seperation d, is charged by a constant current I. Consider a plane surface of area $\frac{a}{2}$ parallel to the plates and drawn symmetrically between the plates. What is the displacement current through this area?
(a) $I/2$ (b) $I/3$ (c) $I/5$ (d) $I/7$

34. The amplitude of the electric field if the intensity of a plane electromagnetic wave is given as 2.0 Wm^{-2} is
(a) 38.8 NC^{-1} (b) 48.3 NC^{-1}
(c) 50.2 NC^{-1} (d) 68.8 NC^{-1}

35. The range of wavelength of the UV rays is
(a) 10 Å to 100 Å (b) 10^9 Å to 10^{10} Å
(c) 8,000 Å to 10,000Å (d) 10,000 Å to 15,000 Å

36. Which of the following is of shortest wavelength?
(a) X-rays (b) γ-rays
(c) Microwaves (d) Radio waves

37. An accelerated electron would produce
(a) γ-rays (b) β-rays
(c) α-rays (d) e.m. waves

38. Radio waves do not penetrate in the band of
(a) ionosphere (b) mesosphere
(c) troposphere (d) stratosphere

39. The ozone layer in the atmosphere absorbs
(a) only the radiowaves
(b) only the visible light
(c) only the γ-rays
(d) X-rays and ultraviolet rays

40. Which one of the following has the shortest wavelength?
(a) Infrared rays (b) Ultraviolet rays
(c) Microwaves (d) Gamma rays

41. Microwaves are electromagnetic waves with frequency in the range of
(a) Micro hertz (b) Giga hertz
(c) Mega hertz (d) Hertz

42. Ozone layer above earth's atmosphere will not
(a) prevent infrared radiations from sun reaching earth.
(b) prevent infra red radiations originated from earth from escaping earth's atmosphere.
(c) prevent ultraviolet rays from sun.
(d) reflect back radio waves.

43. The frequency of electromagnetic wave, which best suited to observe a particle of radii 3×10^{-4} cm is of the order of
(a) 10^{15} (b) 10^{14} (c) 10^{13} (d) 10^{12}

44. Various electromagnetic waves are given in column I and various frequency ranges in column II. Match the two columns.

Column I	Column II
(A) Radio waves	(1) 1×10^{16} to 3×10^{21} Hz
(B) γ–rays	(2) 1×10^{9} to 3×10^{11} HZ
(C) Microwaves	(3) 3×10^{18} to 5×10^{22} Hz
(D) X-rays	(4) 5×10^{5} to 10^{9} Hz.

(a) (A)$\to$(2); (B)$\to$(5); (C)$\to$(3); (D)$\to$(4)
(b) (A)$\to$(2); (B)$\to$(2); (C)$\to$(4); (D)$\to$(3)
(c) (A)$\to$(4); (B)$\to$(3); (C)$\to$(2); (D)$\to$(1)
(d) (A)$\to$(2); (B)$\to$(1); (C)$\to$(4); (D)$\to$(3)

45. Photons of an electromagnetic radiation has an energy 11 keV each. To which region of electromagnetic spectrum does it belong?
(a) X-ray region (b) Ultra violet region
(c) Infrared region (d) Visible region

46. Radio waves diffract around building, although light waves do not. The reason is that radio waves
(a) travel with speed larger than *c*
(b) have much larger wavelength than light
(c) are not electromagnetic waves
(d) None of these

47. **Assertion :** Infrared radiation plays an important role in maintaining the average temperature of earth.
Reason : Infrared radiations are sometimes referred to as heat waves.
(a) Assertion is correct, reason is correct; reason is a correct explanation for assertion.
(b) Assertion is correct, reason is correct; reason is not a correct explanation for assertion
(c) Assertion is correct, reason is incorrect
(d) Assertion is incorrect, reason is correct.

48. Which of the following wave can not be produced by charges accelerating in AC circuits having an inductor and capacitor?
(a) Radio wave (b) Microwave
(c) Infrared (d) None of these

49. The ozone layer converts the ultraviolet radiation to [which is used to heat the atmosphere and the earth's surface.]
(a) Infrared (b) Visible ray
(c) γ-ray (d) None of these

50. Which of the following statement is false for the properties of electromagnetic waves?
(a) Both electric and magnetic field vectors attain the maxima and minima at the same place and same time.
(b) The energy in electromagnetic wave is divided equally between electric and magnetic vectors
(c) Both electric and magnetic field vectors are parallel to each other and perpendicular to the direction of propagation of wave
(d) These waves do not require any material medium for propagation.

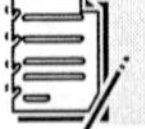

Exercise 2 - Exemplar & Past Year Questions

E&PYQs

Exemplar Questions

1. One requires 11 eV of energy to dissociate a carbon monoxide molecule into carbon and oxygen atoms. The minimum frequency of the appropriate electromagnetic radiation to achieve the dissociation lies in
(a) visible region (b) infrared region
(c) ultraviolet region (d) microwave region

2. A linearly polarised electromagnetic wave given as $E = E_0 \hat{i} \cos(kz - \omega t)$ is incident normally on a perfectly reflecting infinite wall at z = a. Assuming that the material of the wall is optically inactive, the reflected wave will be given as
(a) $E_r = E_0 \hat{i}(kz - \omega t)$ (b) $E_r = E_0 \hat{i} \cos(kz + \omega t)$
(c) $E_r = -E_0 \hat{i} \cos(kz + \omega t)$ (d) $E_r = E_0 \hat{i} \sin(kz - \omega t)$

3. Light with an energy flux of 20 W/cm^2 falls on a non-reflecting surface at normal incidence. If the surface has an area of 30 cm^2, the total momentum delivered (for complete absorption) during 30 min is
(a) 36×10^{-5} kg-m/s (b) 36×10^{-4} kg-m/s
(c) 108×10^{4} kg-m/s (d) 1.08×10^{7} kg-m/s

4. The electric field intensity produced by the radiations coming from 100 W bulb at a 3 m distance is E. The electric field intensity produced by the radiations coming from 50 W bulb at the same distance is
(a) $\frac{E}{2}$ (b) 2E (c) $\frac{E}{\sqrt{2}}$ (d) $\sqrt{2}E$

5. If E and B represent electric and magnetic field vectors of the electromagnetic wave, the direction of propagation of electromagnetic wave is along
(a) E (b) B (c) B×E (d) E×B

6. An EM wave radiates outwards from a dipole antenna, with E_0 as the amplitude of its electric field vector. The electric field E_0 which transports significant energy from the source falls off as
(a) $\frac{1}{r^3}$ (b) $\frac{1}{r^2}$ (c) $\frac{1}{r}$
(d) remains constant

NEET/AIPMT (2013-2020) Questions

7. An electromagnetic wave of frequency ν = 3.0 MHz passes from vacuum into a dielectric medium with relative permittivity ε = 4.0. Then *[NEET Kar. 2013]*
(a) wavelength is doubled and frequency is unchanged
(b) wavelength is doubled and frequency becomes half
(c) wavelength is halved and frequency remains unchanged
(d) wavelength and frequency both remain unchanged

8. Light with an energy flux of 25 × 10^4 Wm^{-2} falls on a perfectly reflecting surface at normal incidence. If the surface area is 15 cm^2, the average force exerted on the surface is : *[2014]*
(a) 1.25×10^{-6} N (b) 2.50×10^{-6} N
(c) 1.20×10^{-6} N (d) 3.0×10^{-6} N

9. The energy of the em waves is of the oder of 15 keV. To which part of the spectrum does it belong? *[2015 RS]*
(a) Infra-red rays (b) Ultraviolet rays
(c) γ-rays (d) X-rays

10. A radiation of energy 'E' falls normally on a perfectly reflecting surface. The momentum transferred to the surface is (C = Velocity of light) *[2015]*
(a) $\frac{2E}{C}$ (b) $\frac{2E}{C^2}$ (c) $\frac{E}{C^2}$ (d) $\frac{E}{C}$

11. Out of the following options which one can be used to produce a propagating electromagnetic wave ? *[2016]*
(a) A charge moving at constant velocity
(b) A stationary charge
(c) A chargeless particle
(d) An accelerating charge

12. In an electromagnetic wave in free space the root mean square value of the electric field is E_{rms} = 6V/m. The peak value of the magnetic field is :- *[2017]*
(a) 2.83×10^{-8} T (b) 0.70×10^{-8} T
(c) 4.23×10^{-8} T (d) 1.41×10^{-8} T

13. An em wave is propagating in a medium with a velocity $\vec{V} = V\hat{i}$. The instantaneous oscillating electric field of this em wave is along +y axis. Then the direction of oscillating magnetic field of the em wave will be along *[2018]*
(a) –z direction (b) +z direction
(c) –x direction (d) –y direction

14. Which colour of the light has the longest wavelength ? *[2019]*
(a) red (b) blue (c) green (d) violet

15. The ratio of contributions made by the electric field and magnetic field components to the intensity of an electromagnetic wave is :
(c = speed of electromagnetic waves) *[2020]*
(a) 1 : 1 (b) 1 : c (c) 1 : c^2 (d) c : 1

Exercise 3 - Concept Application Problems CAP

1. The oscillating electric and magnetic vectors of an electromagnetic wave are oriented along
(a) the same direction but differ in phase by 90°
(b) the same direction and are in phase
(c) mutually perpendicular directions and are in phase
(d) mutually perpendicular directions and differ in phase by 90°

2. Displacement current is
(a) continuous when electric field is changing in the circuit
(b) continuous when magnetic field is changing in the circuit
(c) continuous in both types of fields
(d) continuous through wires and resistance only

3. In an electromagnetic wave
(a) power is transmitted along the magnetic field
(b) power is transmitted along the electric field
(c) power is equally transferred along the electric and magnetic fields
(d) power is transmitted in a direction perpendicular to both the fields

4. The electric field of an electromagnetic wave travelling through vaccum is given by the equation $E = E_0 \sin(kx - \omega t)$. The quantity that is independent of wavelength is
(a) $k\omega$ (b) $\frac{k}{\omega}$ (c) $k^2\omega$ (d) ω

5. When an electromagnetic waves enter the ionised layer of ionosphere, the motion of electron cloud produces a space current and the electric field has its own capacitative displacement current, then
(a) the space current is in phase of displacement current
(b) the space current lags behind the displacement current by a phase 180°.
(c) the space current lags behind the displacement current by a phase 90°.
(d) the space current leads the displacement current by a phase 90°.

6. A plane electromagnetic wave travels in free space along x-axis. At a particular point in space, the electric field along y-axis is 9.3V m^{-1}. The magnetic induction (B) along z-axis is
(a) 3.1×10^{-8} T (b) 3×10^{-5} T
(c) 3×10^{-6} T (d) 9.3×10^{-6} T

7. The electric and the magnetic field associated with an E.M. wave, propagating along the +z-axis, can be represented by
(a) $\left[\vec{E} = E_0\hat{i}, \vec{B} = B_0\hat{j}\right]$ (b) $\left[\vec{E} = E_0\hat{k}, \vec{B} = B_0\hat{i}\right]$
(c) $\left[\vec{E} = E_0\hat{j}, \vec{B} = B_0\hat{i}\right]$ (d) $\left[\vec{E} = E_0\hat{j}, \vec{B} = B_0\hat{k}\right]$

8. In an electromagnetic wave, the electric and magnetic fields are 100 V m^{-1} and 0.265 A m^{-1}. The maximum energy flow is
(a) 26.5 W/m^2 (b) 36.5 W/m^2
(c) 46.7 W/m^2 (d) 765 W/m^2

9. A new system of unit is evolved in which the values of μ_0 and ϵ_0 are 2 and 8 respectively. Then the speed of light in this system will be
(a) 0.25 (b) 0.5 (c) 0.75 (d) 1

10. The figure here gives the electric field of an electromagnetic wave at a certain point and a certain instant. The wave is transporting energy in the negative z-direction. The direction of the magnetic field of the wave at that point and instant is

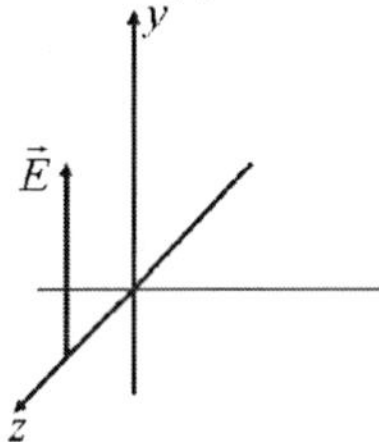

(a) + ve x-direction (b) –ve x-direction
(c) +ve z-direction (d) –ve y-direction

11. In order to establish an instantaneous displacemet current of 5 mA in the space between the plates of 5μF parallel plate capacitor, the potential difference need to apply is
(a) 100 Vs^{-1} (b) 200 Vs^{-1} (c) 300 Vs^{-1} (d) 1000Vs^{-1}

12. An electromagnetic wave of frequency $\upsilon = 3$ MHz passes from vacuum into a dielectric medium with permittivity $\varepsilon = 4$. Then
(a) wavelength and frequency both become half.
(b) wavelength is doubled and frequency remains unchanged.
(c) wavelength and frequncy both remain unchanged.
(d) wavelength is halved and frequency remains unchanged.

13. The electric field component of a monochromatic radiation is given by

$$\vec{E} = 2E_0\hat{i} \cos kz \cos \omega t$$

Its magnetic field $\vec{B}$ is then given by:
(a) $\frac{2E_o}{c}\hat{j} \sin kz \cos \omega t$ (b) $-\frac{2E_o}{c}\hat{j} \sin kz \sin \omega t$
(c) $\frac{2E_o}{c}\hat{j} \sin kz \sin \omega t$ (d) $\frac{2E_o}{c}\hat{j} \cos kz \cos \omega t$

14. The magnetic field in the plane electromagnetic field is given by: $B_y = 2 \times 10^{-7} \sin (0.5 \times 10^3 z + 1.5 \times 10^{11} t)$ T
The expression for the electric field may be given by
(a) $E_y = 2 \times 10^{-7} \sin(0.5 \times 10^3 z + 1.5 \times 10^{11} t)$ V/m
(b) $E_x = 2 \times 10^{-7} \sin(0.5 \times 10^3 z + 1.5 \times 10^{11} t)$ V/m
(c) $E_y = 60 \sin(0.5 \times 10^3 z + 1.5 \times 10^{11} t)$ V/m
(d) $E_x = 60 \sin(0.5 \times 10^3 z + 1.5 \times 10^{11} t)$ V/m

15. The magnetic field between the plates of radius 12 cm separated by distance of 4 mm of a parallel plate capacitor of capacitance 100 pF along the axis of plates having conduction current of 0.15 A is
(a) zero (b) 1.5 T (c) 15 T (d) 0.15 T

16. The energy contained in a cylinder of cross-section 10cm^2 and length 50cm along the x-axis if electric field in an electromagnetic wave is given by

$$E = 50 \sin \omega(t - x/c) \text{ is}$$

(a) 1.2×10^{-10} J (b) 5.5×10^{-12} J
(c) 2.3×10^{-10} J (d) 3.6×10^{-12} J

17. The magnetic field of a beam emerging from a filter facing a floodlight is given by
$B_0 = 12 \times 10^{-8} \sin(1.20 \times 10^7 z - 3.60 \times 10^{15} t)$ T.
What is the average intensity of the beam?
(a) $1.72 \times 10^2 \text{ W/m}^2$ (b) 1.72 W/m^2
(c) 2.31 W/m^2 (d) $2.31 \times 10^2 \text{ W/m}^2$

18. Suppose that the electric field amplitude of an em wave is $E_o = 120$ N/C and that its frequency is $\upsilon = 50$ Hz, then
(a) $B_o = 200$ T (b) $\omega = r \times 10^8$ rad/s
(c) $k = \left(\pi/4\right)$ rad/m (d) $\lambda = 92$m

19. Find the average energy density corresponding to maximum electric field, if magnetic field in a plane electromagnetic wave is given by
$B = 200 \times 10^{-6} \sin[(4 \times 10^{15})(t - x/c)]$
(a) 1.6 J m^{-3} (b) 0.16 J m^{-3}
(c) 0.016 J m^{-3} (d) 0.0016 J m^{-3}

20. Which of the following electromagnetic waves has the longest wavelength?
(a) uv-rays (b) Visible light
(c) Radio waves (d) Microwaves

21. The wavelength of X-ray is of the order of
(a) 1 metre (b) 1 cm
(c) 1 micron (d) 1 angstrom

22. If v_s, v_x and v_m are the speed of soft gamma rays, X-rays and microwaves respectively in vacuum, then
(a) $v_s > v_x > v_m$ (b) $v_s < v_x < v_m$
(c) $v_s > v_x < v_m$ (d) $v_s = v_x = v_m$

23. The waves which are electromagnetic in nature are
(a) sound waves and light waves
(b) water waves and radio waves
(c) light waves and X-rays
(d) sound waves and water waves

24. 10 cm is a wavelength corresponding to the spectrum of
(a) infrared rays (b) ultra-violet rays
(c) microwaves (d) γ-rays

25. The speed of electromagnetic wave in vacuum depends upon the source of radiation. It
(a) increases as we move from γ-rays to radio waves
(b) decreases as we move from γ-rays to radio waves
(c) is same for all of them
(d) None of these

26. It is possible to take pictures of those objects which are not fully visible to the eye using camera films sensitive to
(a) ultraviolet rays (b) infrared rays
(c) microwaves (d) radiowaves

27. X-rays, gamma rays and microwaves travelling in vaccum have
(a) same wavelength but different velocities
(b) same frequency but different velocities
(c) same velocity but different wavelength
(d) same velocity and same frequency

28. A radar sends the waves towards a distant object and receives the signal reflected by object. These waves are
(a) sound waves (b) light waves
(c) radio waves (d) microwaves

29. Radio waves and visible light in vacuum have
(a) same velocity but different wavelength
(b) same frequency
(c) different velocity
(d) same wavelength

30. We consider the radiation emitted by the human body. Which one of the following statements is true?
(a) The radiation emitted is in the infrared region.
(b) The radiation is emitted only during the day.
(c) The radiation is emitted during the summers and absorbed during winters.
(d) The radiation is emitted lies in the ultraviolet region and hence is not visible.

31. An electromagnetic wave of frequency 1×10^{14} hertz is propagating along z-axis. The amplitude of electric field is 4 V/m. If $\varepsilon_0 = 8.8 \times 10^{-12}$ $C^2/N\text{-}m^2$, then average energy density of electric field will be:
(a) 35.2×10^{-10} J/m³ (b) 35.2×10^{-11} J/m³
(c) 35.2×10^{-12} J/m³ (d) 35.2×10^{-13} J/m³

32. A point source of electromagnetic radiation has an average power output of 800 W. The maximum value of electric field at a distance 4.0 m from the source is
(a) 64.7 V/m (b) 57.8 V/m
(c) 56.72 V/m (d) 54.77 V/m

33. A plane electromagnetic wave in a non-magnetic dielectric medium is given by $\vec{E} = \vec{E}_0(4\times10^{-7}x - 50t)$ with distance being in meter and time in seconds. The dielectric constant of the medium is :
(a) 2.4 (b) 5.8 (c) 8.2 (d) 4.8

34. A plane electromagnetic wave travels in free space along X-direction. If the value of $\vec{B}$ (in tesla) at a particular point in space and time is $1.2 \times 10^{-8}\ \hat{k}$. The value of $\vec{E}$ (in Vm^{-1}) at that point is
(a) $1.2\,\hat{j}$ (b) $3.6\,\hat{k}$ (c) $1.2\,\hat{k}$ (d) $3.6\,\hat{j}$

35. The electric field associated with an e.m. wave in vacuum is given by $\vec{E} = \hat{i}\ 40\cos(kz - 6\times10^8 t)$, where E, z and t are in volt/m, meter and seconds respectively. The value of wave vector k is
(a) $2\ m^{-1}$ (b) $0.5\ m^{-1}$ (c) $6\ m^{-1}$ (d) $3\ m^{-1}$

36. A lamp emits monochromatic green light uniformly in all directions. The lamp is 3% efficient in converting electrical power to electromagnetic waves and consumes 100 W of power. The amplitude of the electric field associated with the electromagnetic radiation at a distance of 5 m from the lamp will be nearly:
(a) 1.34 V/m (b) 2.68 V/m (c) 4.02 V/m (d) 5.36 V/m

37. An electromagnetic wave in vacuum has the electric and magnetic field $\vec{E}$ and $\vec{B}$, which are always perpendicular to each other. The direction of polarization is given by $\vec{X}$ and that of wave propagation by $\vec{k}$. Then
(a) $\vec{X} \parallel \vec{B}$ and $\vec{k} \parallel \vec{B}\times\vec{E}$ (b) $\vec{X} \parallel \vec{E}$ and $\vec{k} \parallel \vec{E}\times\vec{B}$
(c) $\vec{X} \parallel \vec{B}$ and $\vec{k} \parallel \vec{E}\times\vec{B}$ (d) $\vec{X} \parallel \vec{E}$ and $\vec{k} \parallel \vec{B}\times\vec{E}$

38. The charge on a parallel plate capacitor varies as $q = q_0 \cos 2\pi\upsilon t$. The plates are very large and close together (area $= A$, separation $= d$). The displacement current through the capacitor is
(a) $q_0\ 2\pi\upsilon\ \sin\pi\upsilon t$ (b) $-\ q_0\ 2\pi\upsilon\ \sin 2\pi\upsilon t$
(c) $q_0\ 2\pi\ \sin\pi\upsilon t$ (d) $q_0\ \pi\upsilon\ \sin 2\pi\upsilon t$

39. Find the energy contained in a cylinder of cross-section 10 cm² and length 50 cm along x-axis, if $E = 50 \sin\omega(t - x/C)$ be the electric field in an electromagnetic wave
(a) 5.5×10^{-12} J (b) 1.5×10^{-11} J
(c) 6.2×10^{-10} J (d) 1.1×10^{-15} J

40. The rms value of the electric field of the light coming from the Sun is 720 N/C. The average total energy density of the electromagnetic wave is
(a) 4.58×10^{-6} J/m³ (b) 6.37×10^{-9} J/m³
(c) 81.35×10^{-12} J/m³ (d) 3.3×10^{-3} J/m³

41. A point source of electromagnetic radiation has an average power output of 1500 W. The maximum value of electric field at a distance of 3m from this sources in Vm^{-1} is
(a) 500 (b) 100 (c) $\frac{500}{3}$ (d) $\frac{250}{3}$

42. The electric field part of an electromagnetic wave in a medium is represented by $E_x = 0$;

$$E_y = 2.5\frac{N}{C}\cos\left[\left(2\pi\times10^6\frac{rad}{m}\right)t - \left(\pi\times10^{-2}\frac{rad}{s}\right)x\right];$$

$E_z = 0$. The wave is :
(a) moving along x direction with frequency 10^6 Hz and wave length 100 m.
(b) moving along x direction with frequency 10^6 Hz and wave length 200 m.
(c) moving along – x direction with frequency 10^6 Hz and wave length 200 m.
(d) moving along y direction with frequency $2\pi \times 10^6$ Hz and wave length 200 m.

43. In order to establish an instantaneous displacemet current of 1 mA in the space between the plates of 2μF parallel plate capacitor, the potential difference need to apply is
(a) $100\ Vs^{-1}$ (b) $200\ Vs^{-1}$
(c) $300\ Vs^{-1}$ (d) $500\ Vs^{-1}$

44. The magnetic component of a polarised wave of light is $B_x = (4.0 \times 10^{-6} T)\sin[(1.57 \times 10^7\ m^{-1})y + \omega t]$. The intensity of light is
(a) 1.9 kW/m² (b) 3.8 kW/m²
(c) 5.7 kW/m² (d) 7.6 kW/m²

45. The average electric field of electromagnetic waves in certain region of free space is $9 \times 10^{-4}\ NC^{-1}$. Then the average magnetic field in the same region is of the order of
(a) 27×10^{-4} T (b) 3×10^{-12} T
(c) $\left(\frac{1}{3}\right) \times 10^{-12}$ T (d) 3×10^{12} T

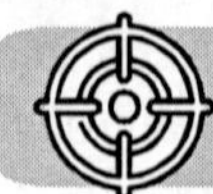

Hints & Solutions

23.1 Concept Practice Problems CPP

1. (a) Displacement current arises when electric field in a region is changing with time. It will be so if the charge on a capacitor is changing with time.
2. (c)
3. (c) According to Maxwell, a changing electric field is a source of magnetic field.
4. (b) An electromagnetic wave has both energy and momentum.
5. (d) $B_0 = \frac{E_0}{c} = \frac{9\times10^3}{3\times10^8} = 3\times10^{-5}T.$
6. (a)
7. (c) In an electromagnetic wave electric field and magnetic field are perpendicular to the direction of propagation of wave. The vector equation for the electric field is
$$\vec{E} = E_0 \cos\left(\omega t - \frac{2\pi}{\lambda}y\right)\hat{z}$$
8. (a) Here, $\lambda = \frac{c}{\nu} = \frac{3\times10^8}{8.2\times10^6} = 36.6\text{m}.$
9. (b) As we know, $\vec{E}\cdot\vec{B} = 0 \quad \because [\vec{E}\perp\vec{B}]$
and $\vec{E}\times\vec{B}$ should be along Z direction
As $(-2\hat{i}-3\hat{j})\times(3\hat{i}-2\hat{j}) = 5\hat{k}$
Hence option (b) is the correct answer.
10. (a) Intersity of a plane electromagnetic wave $= \frac{1}{2}\varepsilon_0 E_0^2 c$
$E = \sqrt{\frac{2I}{\varepsilon_0 c}} = 38.8\ \text{NC}^{-1}$

23.2 Concept Practice Problems CPP

11. (b) UV rays 10^9Å to 10^{10}Å
12. (b) The range of visible radiations is 4000Å to 8000 Å
13. (a) The wavelength of infrared region is 8×10^{-5} cm to 3×10^{-3} cm. So maximum wavelength of infrared region $= 8\times10^{-5}$ cm $\approx 10^{-4}$ cm.
14. (a) 15. (c)
16. (c) Here : Velocity of electromagnetic waves in free space and wavelength
$v = 3\times10^8$ m/s and $\lambda = 150\ m$
The frequency of radio waves is given by
$= \frac{v}{\lambda} = \frac{3\times10^8}{150} = 2\times10^6\text{Hz} = 2\text{ MHz}.$
17. (d) 18. (c) 19. (b)
20. (a) From electromagnetic spectrum, frequencies of γ-rays is greater than frequency of X-rays. Frequency of X-rays is greater than frequency of ultraviolet rays.

Exercise 1 - Chapter Revision Problems CRP

1. (b) The electromagnetic waves do not transport charge.
2. (b) In an electromagnetic wave the directions of magnetic induction is perpendicular to electric field.
3. (b) 4. (c)
5. (b) Current through capacitor,
$$I = \frac{E}{X_C} = \frac{E}{\frac{1}{\omega C}} = \omega CE = 2\pi\upsilon\ CE \text{ or } I \propto \upsilon.$$
∴ decrease in frequency υ of ac source decreases the conduction current. As displacement current is equal to conduction current, decrease in υ decreases displacement current in circuit.
6. (a) $i_d = c\times\frac{dv}{dt} \Rightarrow \frac{dv}{dt} = \frac{i_d}{c} = 10^6\text{Vs}^{-1}$
7. (c) 8. (d)
9. (a) Both magnetic and electric fields have zero average value in a plane e.m. wave.
10. (c) The electromagnetic waves of all wavelengths travel with the same speed in space which is equal to velocity of light.
11. (b) 12. (c) 13. (d)
14. (c) $\oint \vec{B}\cdot d\vec{\ell}\sqrt{b^2-4ac} = \mu_0 \epsilon_0 \frac{d\phi}{dt}$
or $B\times 2\pi r = \mu_0 \epsilon_0 A\left(\frac{dE}{dt}\right) \quad \therefore B \propto \left(\frac{dE}{dt}\right)$
15. (b) $v = \frac{1}{\sqrt{\mu\varepsilon}} = \frac{c}{\sqrt{\mu_r\varepsilon_r}}$
16. (b) From question, $B_0 = 20$ nT $= 20\times10^{-9}$T
$\vec{E}_0 = \vec{B}_0\times\vec{C}$
$|\vec{E}_0| = |\vec{B}_0|\cdot|\vec{C}| = 20\times10^{-9}\times3\times10^8 = 6$ V/m.
(∵ velocity of light in vacuum $C = 3\times10^8\ \text{ms}^{-1}$)
17. (a) Energy density (EM waves)
$$= \varepsilon_0 E_{rms}^2 = \varepsilon_0\left(\frac{E_0}{\sqrt{2}}\right)^2 = \frac{1}{2}\varepsilon_0 E_0^2$$
18. (c) Average force,
$$F = \frac{\Delta P}{t} = \frac{2IA}{C}$$
19. (c)
20. (a) $\frac{E_0}{B_0} = c\cdot$ also $k = \frac{2\pi}{\lambda}$ and $\omega = 2\pi v$
These relation gives $E_0 k = B_0\omega$
21. (b) Here, $E_0 = 18$ V/m; $B_0 = ?$
$$B_0 = \frac{E_0}{c} = \frac{18}{3\times10^8} = 6\times10^{-8}\,T$$
22. (c) 23. (a) 24. (d) 25. (b)
26. (d) Velocity of electromagnetic wave
$$c = \frac{1}{\sqrt{\mu_0\varepsilon_0}} = 3\times10^8\ m\ \text{s}^{-1}$$
It is independent of amplitude, frequency and wavelength of electromagnetic wave.
27. (a) According to conservation of charge, the displacement current must be leftward.

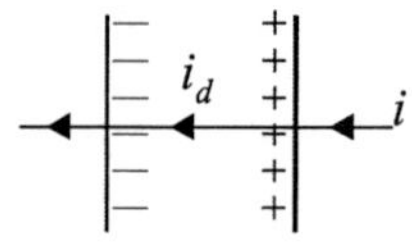

28. (b) $B_0 = \frac{E_0}{c}$

E_0 - Electric field, c - speed of light, B_0 - Magnetic Field.

$B_0 = \frac{10^{-3}}{3\times10^8} = 3.33\times10^{-12}\ T$

29. (b) $\omega = 2\pi\nu = \frac{2\pi c}{\lambda} = \frac{2\pi\times3\times10^8}{6\times10^{-3}} = \pi\times10^{11}$ rad/sec

The equation for the electric field, along *y*-axis in the electromagnetic wave is

$Ey = E_0 \sin\omega\left(t-\frac{x}{c}\right) = 33\sin\left[\pi\times10^{11}\left(t-\frac{x}{c}\right)\right]$

30. (c) $\oint \vec{E}\cdot d\vec{\ell} = -\frac{d\phi_B}{dt}$ or $E(2\pi r) = \frac{d}{dt}(kt\times\pi r^2)$ $\therefore E = \frac{kr}{2}$

31. (c)

32. (a) As we know that,

As the displacement current through the capacitor is,

$I_d = I_c = \frac{dq}{dt}$ ... (i)

As given that, $q = q_0\cos2\pi\nu t$

Putting this value of *q* in Eq (i), we get

So, $I_d = I_c = \frac{d}{dt}(q_0\cos^2\pi\nu t)$

$I_d = I_c = -q_0\sin2\pi\nu t\times2\pi\nu$

$I_d = I_c = 2\pi\nu q_0\sin2\pi\nu t$

33. (a)

34. (a) Intersity of a plane electromagnetic wave $= \frac{1}{2}\varepsilon_0E_0^2c$

$E = \sqrt{\frac{2I}{\varepsilon_0c}} = 38.8\ NC^{-1}$

35. (b) 36. (b) 37. (d)

38. (a) Radiowaves are reflected by ionosphere.

39. (d) 40. (d) 41. (b)

42. (d) Ozone layer will absorb ultraviolet rays; reflect the infrared radiation and does not reflect back radiowaves.

43. (a)

44. (c) (A)→(4); (B)→(3); (C)→(2); (D)→(1)

The frequency ranges of various waves are as under : Radiowaves ; 5×10^5 to 10^9 Hz; γ-rays ; 3×10^{18} to 5×10^{22} Hz Microwaves; 1×10^9 to 3×10^{11} Hz; X-rays; 1×10^{16} to 3×10^{21} Hz.

45. (a) $E = \frac{hc}{\lambda} \Rightarrow \lambda = \frac{hc}{E} = \frac{6.6\times10^{-34}\times3\times10^8}{11\times1000\times1.6\times10^{-19}} = 12.4$ Å

46. (b) The wavelength of radiowaves being much larger than light, has a size comparable to those of buildings, hense diffract from them.

47. (b) Infrared radiation help to maintain the earth warmth through the greenhouse effect. Incoming visible light which passes relatively easily through the atmosphere is absorbed by the earth's surface and re-radiated as infrared radiation. The radiation is trapped by greenhouse gases such as carbon dioxide and water vapour and they heat up and heat their surrondings.

48. (c) 49. (a)

50. (c) Electromagnetic waves are the combination of mutually perpendicular electric and magnetic fields. So, option (c) is false.

Exercise 2 - Exemplar & Past Year Questions E&PYQs

Exemplar Questions

1. (c) As we know that,

$E = h\nu$

As given that $h = 6.62\times10^{-34}$ J-s

$E = 11\ eV = 11\times1.6\times10^{-19}$

$\nu = ?$

$11\ eV = h\nu$

So, $\nu = \frac{11\times1.6\times10^{-19}}{h}J = \frac{11\times1.6\times10^{-19}}{6.62\times10^{-34}}J$

$= 2.65\times10^{15}$ Hz

So, that frequency radiation belongs to ultraviolet region.

2. (b) The type of wave doesn't change when a wave is reflected from denser medium but only its phase changes by 180°. As E is along positive x-axis so reflected ray will be along negative x-axis and its component will also be opposite to earlier in (–z) direction and phase will change.

For the reflected wave $\hat{z} = -\hat{z}, \hat{i} = -\hat{i}$ and additional phase of π in the incident wave.

As given that the incident electromagnetic wave is,

$E = E_0\hat{i}\cos(kz-\omega t)$

So, the reflected electromagnetic wave is

$E_r = E_0(-\hat{i})\cos(k(-z)-\omega t+\pi)$

$= -E_0\hat{i}\cos(-(kz+\omega t)+\pi)$

$= -E_0\hat{i}\cos(\pi-(kz+\omega t))$

$= E_0\hat{i}\cos(kz+\omega t)$

3. (b)

4. (c) As we know that the electric field intensity on a surface due to incident radiation is,

$I_{av} \propto E_0^2$

$\frac{P_{av}}{A} \propto E_0^2$ (A is constant)

Here, $P_{av} \propto E_0^2$

So, $E_0 \propto \sqrt{P_{av}}$

$\therefore \frac{(E_0)_1}{(E_0)_2} = \sqrt{\frac{(P_{av})_1}{(P_{av})_2}}$

$\frac{(E_0)_1}{(E_0)_2} = \sqrt{\frac{100}{50}} = \left[\frac{\sqrt{2}}{1}\right]$

$(E_0)_2 = (E_0)_1/\sqrt{2}$

5. (d) The direction of propagation of electromagnetic wave is perpendicular to both electric field E and magnetic field B, i.e., in the direction of E × B by right thumb rule.

The diagram given below

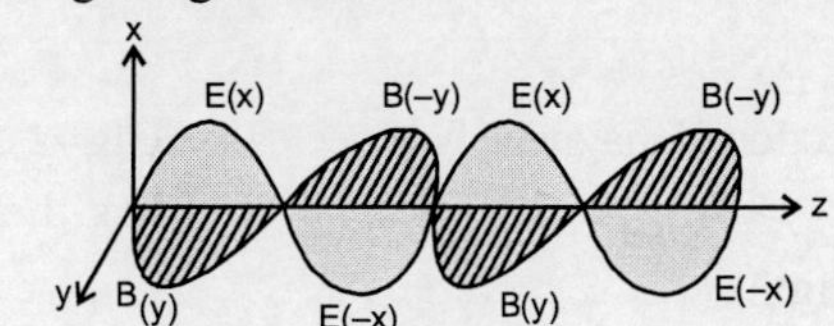

So, electromagnetic wave is along the z-direction which is give the cross product of E and B direction is perpendicular to E and B from $\vec{E}$ to $\vec{B}$. i.e., (E × B) in z-direction.

6. (c) As we know that, the electric field is inversly proportional to r, so $\left(E_0 \propto \frac{1}{r}\right)$

From a diode antenna, an electromagnetic waves are radiated outwards from dipole antenna with the amplitude of electric field vector (E_0) which transports significant energy from the source falls off intensity inversely as the distance (r) from the antenna, i.e.,

radiated energy $\left(E_0 \propto \frac{1}{r}\right)$

NEET/AIPMT (2013-2020) Questions

7. (c) Given: frequency f = 2MHz, relative permittivity $\in_r = 4$

From formula,

velocity $v = \frac{c}{\sqrt{\in_r}} = \frac{c}{2} \Rightarrow \lambda' = \frac{\lambda}{2}$

[Since frequency remains unchanged]

8. (b) Average force $F_{av} = \frac{\Delta p}{\Delta t} = \frac{2IA}{c}$ ($\because$ Power = F.V)

$= \frac{2 \times 25 \times 10^4 \times 15 \times 10^{-4}}{3 \times 10^8}$

$= 2.50 \times 10^{-6}$ N

9. (d) Energy of x-ray is (100 ev to 100 kev)

Hence energy of the order of 15 kev belongs to x-rays.

10. (a) Momentum of light falling on reflecting surface

$p = \frac{E}{C}$

As surface is perfectly reflecting so momentum reflect

$p^1 = -\frac{E}{C}$

$= P - P^1 = \frac{E}{C} - \left(-\frac{E}{C}\right) = \frac{2E}{C}$

$\frac{E}{C}$ ↓ ↑ $\frac{E}{C} = P$

So, momentum transferred

11. (d) To generate electromagnetic waves we need accelerating charge particle.

12. (a) Given, $E_{rms} = 6$ V/m

$\frac{E_{rms}}{B_{rms}} = c \Rightarrow B_{rms} = \frac{E_{rms}}{c}$ ...(i)

$B_{rms} = \frac{B_0}{\sqrt{2}} \Rightarrow B_0 = \sqrt{2}\, B_{rms}$

$B_0 = \sqrt{2} \times \frac{E_{rms}}{C}$ From equation (i)

$= \frac{\sqrt{2} \times 6}{3 \times 10^8} = 2.83 \times 10^{-8}$ T

13. (b) As we know, $\vec{E} \times \vec{B} = \vec{V}$

$(E\hat{j}) \times (\vec{B}) = V\hat{i}$ ($\because$ Electric field vector is along +y axis)

So, $\vec{B} = B\hat{k}$

i.e., direction of magnetic field vector is along +z direction.

14. (a) $\lambda_{Red} > \lambda_{Green} > \lambda_{Blue} > \lambda_{Violet.}$ Red has the longest wavelength.

15. (a) The energy in electromagnetic wave is divided equally between the electric and magnetic field.

So, in an electromagnetic wave, half of the intensity is provided by the electric field and half by the magnetic field.

Hence, required ratio should be 1 : 1.

Exercise 3 - Concept Application Problems CAP

1. (c) $\vec{E}$ and $\vec{B}$ are mutually perpendicular to each other and are in phase i.e., they become a zero and minimum at the same place and at the same time.

2. (a) Displacement current is set up in a region where the electric field is changing with time.

3. (d)

4. (b) Here, $k = \frac{2\pi}{\lambda}$, $\omega = 2\pi\upsilon$

$\therefore \frac{k}{\omega} = \frac{2\pi/\lambda}{2\pi\upsilon} = \frac{1}{\pi\upsilon} = \frac{1}{c}$ ($\because c = \upsilon\lambda$)

where c is the speed of electromagnetic wave in vacuum. It is a constant whose value is $3 \times 10^6\ ms^{-1}$

5. (b)

6. (a) Velocity of light

$C = \frac{E}{B} \Rightarrow B = \frac{E}{C} = \frac{9.3}{3 \times 10^8} = 3.1 \times 10^{-8} T$

7. (a) E.M. wave always propagates in a direction perpendicular to both electric and magnetic fields. So, electric and magnetic fields should be along + X– and + Y–directions respectively. Therefore, option (a) is the correct option.

8. (a) Here, amplitude of electric field, E_0 = 100 V/m; amplitude of magnetic field, H_0 = 0.265 A/m. We know that the maximum rate of energy flow,

$S = E_0 \times H_0 = 100 \times 0.265 = 26.5$ W/m^2.

9. (a) The speed of light $C = \frac{1}{\sqrt{\mu_0 \varepsilon_0}} = \frac{1}{\sqrt{2 \times 8}} = \frac{1}{4} = 0.25$

10. (a) Direction of energy progratiom of EM-waves is given by

$\vec{D} = K(\vec{E} \times \vec{B})$ or $-\hat{k} = K(E\,\hat{j} \times \vec{B})$

Clearly direction of magnetic field is along positive x-axis.

11. (d)

12. (d) The frequency of electromagnetic wave remains unchanged but the wavelength of electromagnetic wave changes when it passes from one medium to another.

$c = \frac{1}{\sqrt{\mu_0 \varepsilon_0}}$ $\therefore$ $c \propto \frac{1}{\sqrt{\varepsilon_0}}$ and $v \propto \frac{1}{\sqrt{\varepsilon}}$

$\therefore \frac{c}{v} = \sqrt{\frac{\varepsilon}{\varepsilon_0}} = \sqrt{\frac{4}{1}} = 2$

$\frac{c}{v} = \frac{\upsilon\lambda}{\upsilon\lambda'} = \frac{\lambda}{\lambda'} = 2$ or $\lambda' = \frac{\lambda}{2}$

13. (c) Magnetic field vector, $\vec{B} = \frac{2E_0}{c}\hat{j}\sin kz \sin \omega t$

14. (d) $B_y = 2 \times 10^{-7} \sin(0.5 \times 10^3 z + 1.5 \times 10^{11} t)$ T

The electric vector is perpendicular to B as well as direction of propagation of electromagnetic wave.

Therefore Ex has to be taken.

Further, $E_0 = B_0 \times c = 2 \times 10^{-7} \times 3 \times 10^8$ V/m

$E_0 = 2 \times 10^{-7} \times 3 \times 10^8 = 60$ V/m

$\therefore$ The corresponding value of the electric field is

$Ex = 60 \sin(0.5 \times 10^3 z + 1.5 \times 10^{11} t)$ V/m

15. (a) As $B \propto r$, since the point is on the axis where $r = 0$, So $B = 0$

16. (b) Energy density $= \frac{1}{2}\varepsilon_0 E_0^2 = 1.1 \times 10^{-8}$ J m^{-3}

Volume of cylinder = A × L = 5×10^{-4} m^3

So, required energy = $1.1 \times 10^{-8} \times 5 \times 10^{-4} = 5.5 \times 10^{-12}$ J

17. (b) As we know that,

The standard equation of magnetic field

$B = B_0 \sin(kx - \omega t)$

And, the given equation is

$B = 12 \times 10^{-8} \sin(1.20 \times 10^7 z - 3.60 \times 10^{15} t)$T.

On comparing this equation with standard equation (i), we have

$B_0 = 12 \times 10^{-8}$

So, the average intensity of the beam

$$I_{av} = \frac{1}{2}\frac{B_0^2}{\mu_0} \cdot c = \frac{1}{2} \times \frac{(12 \times 10^{-8})^2 \times 3 \times 10^8}{4\pi \times 10^{-7}} = 1.72 \text{ W/m}^2$$

18. (b)

19. (c) Average energy density corresponding to maximum electric field,

$$u_{av} = \frac{B_0^2}{2\mu_0} = \frac{(200 \times 10^{-6})^2}{2 \times 4\pi \times 10^{-7}} \cong 0.016 \text{ Jm}^{-3}$$

20. (b) 21. (d) 22. (d)

23. (c) Light waves and X-rays are electromagnetic waves.

24. (c)

25. (c) Speed of EM waves in vacuum $= \frac{1}{\sqrt{\mu_0 \epsilon_0}}$ = constant

26. (b)

27. (c) In vacuum X-rays, gamma rays and microwaves travel with same velocity, *i.e.*, with the velocity of light c ($= 3 \times 10^8$ m s^{-1}) but have different wavelengths.

28. (d) Now a days microwaves are used to locate the flying objects by Radar.

29. (a) In vacuum velocity of all EM waves are same but their wavelengths are different.

30. (a) Every body at all time, at all temperature emit radiation (except at $T = 0$), which fall in the infrared region.

31. (c) Given: Amplitude of electric field, $E_0 = 4$ v/m

Absolute permitivity, $\varepsilon_0 = 8.8 \times 10^{-12}$ c^2/N-m^2

Average energy density u_E = ?

Applying formula,

Average energy density $u_E = \frac{1}{4}\varepsilon_0 E^2$

$\Rightarrow u_E = \frac{1}{4} \times 8.8 \times 10^{-12} \times (4)^2 = 35.2 \times 10^{-12}$ J/m^3

32. (d) Intensity of EM wave is given by

$$I = \frac{P}{4\pi R^2} = v_{av} \cdot c = \frac{1}{2}\varepsilon_0 E_0^2 \times c \Rightarrow E_0 = \sqrt{\frac{P}{2\pi R^2 \varepsilon_0 c}}$$

$$= \sqrt{\frac{800}{2 \times 3.14 \times (4)^2 \times 8.85 \times 10^{-12} \times 3 \times 10^8}} = 54.77 \frac{\text{V}}{\text{m}}$$

33. (b)

34. (d) Given: $\vec{B} = 1.2 \times 10^{-8} \hat{k} T$

$\vec{E} = ?$

From formula,

$E = Bc = (1.2 \times 10^{-8}\text{T})(3 \times 10^8 \text{ ms}^{-1}) = 3.6$ Vm^{-1}

$\vec{B}$ is along Z-direction and the wave propagates along X-direction. Therefore $\vec{E}$ should be along Y-direction.

Thus, $\vec{E} = 3.6\hat{j}$ Vm^{-1}

35. (a) On comparing the given equation to

$\vec{E} = a_0 \hat{i} \cos(\omega t - kz)$, $\omega = 6 \times 10^{8z}$,

$$k = \frac{2\pi}{r} = \frac{\omega}{c}, \quad k = \frac{\omega}{c} = \frac{6 \times 10^8}{3 \times 10^8} = 2 \text{ m}^{-1}$$

36. (b)

37. (b) $\because$ The E.M. wave are transverse in nature i.e.,

$$= \frac{\vec{k} \times \vec{E}}{\mu\omega} = \vec{H} \quad \ldots\text{(i)}$$

$$\text{where } \vec{H} = \frac{\vec{B}}{\mu} \text{ and } \frac{\vec{k} \times \vec{H}}{\omega\varepsilon} = -\vec{E} \quad \ldots\text{(ii)}$$

$\vec{k}$ is $\perp$ $\vec{H}$ and $\vec{k}$ is also $\perp$ to $\vec{E}$

or In other words $\vec{X} \parallel \vec{E}$ and $\vec{k} \parallel \vec{E} \times \vec{B}$

38. (b) Displacement current, I_D = conduction current, I_C

$$\therefore \frac{dq}{dt} = \frac{d}{dt}[q_0 \cos 2\pi\upsilon t] = -q_0\, 2\pi\upsilon \sin 2\pi\upsilon t$$

39. (a)

40. (a) $E_{rms} = 720$

The average total energy density

$$= \frac{1}{2}\epsilon_0 E_0^2 = \frac{1}{2}\epsilon_0 [\sqrt{2}E_{rms}]^2 = \epsilon_0 E_{rms}^2$$

$= 8.85 \times 10^{-12} \times (720)^2 = 4.58 \times 10^{-6}$ J/m^3

41. (b)

42. (b) Comparing with the equation of wave.

$E_y = E_0 \cos(\omega t - kx)$

$\omega = 2\pi f = 2\pi \times 10^6 \quad \therefore f = 10^6$ Hz

$\frac{2\pi}{\lambda} = k = \pi \times 10^{-2}$ m^{-1}, $\lambda = 200$ m

43. (d) $I_d = 1$ mA $= 10^{-3}$ A

$C = 2\mu\text{F} = 2 \times 10^{-6}$ F

$$I_D = I_C = \frac{d}{dt}(CV) = C\frac{dV}{dt}$$

$$\text{Therefore, } \frac{dV}{dt} = \frac{I_D}{C} = \frac{10^{-3}}{2 \times 10^{-6}} = 500 \text{ Vs}^{-1}$$

Therefore, applying a varying potential difference of 500 Vs^{-1} would produce a displacement current of desired value.

44. (a) Intensity of light

$$I = \frac{B_0^2 c}{2\mu_0} = \frac{(4 \times 10^{-6})^2 \times (3 \times 10^8)}{2 \times (4\pi \times 10^{-7})} = 1900 \text{ W/m}^2.$$

45. (b) For electromagnetic waves we know that, $\frac{E}{B} = c$

$\therefore \frac{9 \times 10^{-4}}{B} = 3 \times 10^8$ ms^{-1} $\quad B = 3 \times 10^{-12}$ T.

24 Ray Optics and Optical Instruments

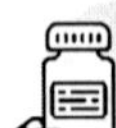

Topic 24.1 : Reflection of Light, Reflection from Plane Surface and Mirror Formula

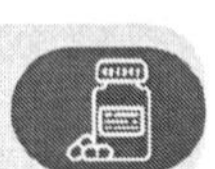

REFLECTION OF LIGHT

It is the turning back of light in the same medium.

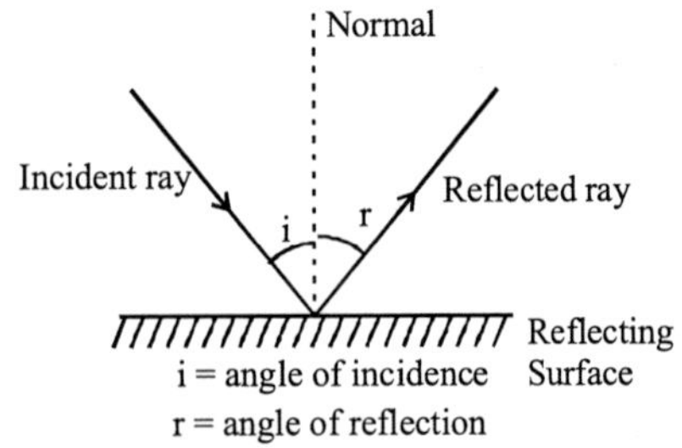

Laws of Reflection

(i) Angle of incidence (i) = angle of reflection (r)

(ii) The incident ray, reflected ray and normal are always in same plane.

REFLECTION FROM PLANE SURFACE

Plane mirror has infinitely large radius of curvature. It produces virtual image of same size but laterally inverted. Image is as much behind the mirror as much is the object in front of it.

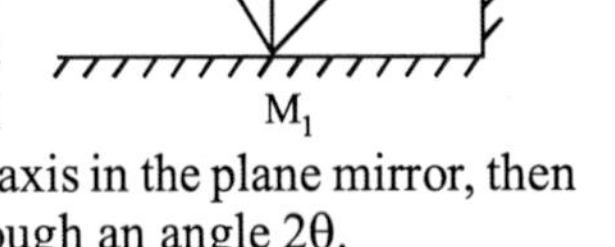

(i) If the direction of the incident ray is kept constant and the mirror is rotated through an angle θ about an axis in the plane mirror, then the reflected ray rotates through an angle 2θ.

(ii) If an object moves towards (or away from) a plane mirror at a speed v, the image will also approach (or recede) at the same speed v, i.e. the speed of image relative to object will be v – (–v) = 2v.

(iii) If two plane mirrors are inclined to each other at 90°, the emergent ray is always antiparallel to incident ray if it suffers one reflection from each whatever be the angle of incidence. The same is found to hold good for three-plane mirrors forming the corner of a cube if the incident light suffers one reflection from each of them.

(iv) If there are two plane mirrors inclined to each other at an angle θ, the no. of images of a point object formed are determined as follows :

(a) If $\frac{360°}{\theta}$ is even integer (say m), no. of images formed = (m – 1), for all positions of object.

(b) If $\left(\frac{360°}{\theta}\right)$ is odd integer (say m), no. of images formed, n = m, if the object is not on the bisector of mirrors and n = (m – 1), if the object is on the bisector of mirrors.

(c) If $\left(\frac{360°}{\theta}\right)$ is a fraction, the no. of images formed will be equal to its integral part.

Note : A plane mirror always forms a virtual image if object is real and forms a real image if the object is virtual.

MIRROR FORMULA

$$\frac{1}{v}+\frac{1}{u}=\frac{1}{f}$$

where, u = distance of the object from the pole of mirror
v = distance of the image from the pole of mirror
f = focal length of the mirror.

Note : Mirror formula is valid only when the following conditions are satisfied :

(a) Object is placed very near to the principal axis.

(b) Object is placed far from the mirror.

Magnification

$$m=\frac{v}{u}=\frac{v-f}{f}=\frac{f}{u-f} \text{ or } m=\frac{I}{O}=-\left[\frac{v}{u}\right]$$

where, I = size of the image and O = size of the object and negative sign implies that image is inverted w.r.t the object. The above formulae are applicable only for paraxial rays (the rays which makes very small angle with the principal axis).

Areal magnification : When a two dimensional object is placed with its plane perpendicular to the principal axis, its magnification called superficial magnification or aerial magnification and is given by

$$M_s=\frac{Area\ of\ image}{Area\ of\ object}=m^2=\left(\frac{v}{u}\right)^2$$

Sign Conventions for Mirror and Lenses

New cartesian sign conventions :

1. All the distances are measured from pole of spherical mirror and optical centre in case of lenses.
2. The distances measured in a direction opposite to the direction of incident light is taken as negative and vice-versa.
3. The heights measured upward and perpendicular to the principal axis of mirror are taken as positive and vice - versa.
4. Angle measured from the normal in the anticlockwise direction is positive and vice-versa.

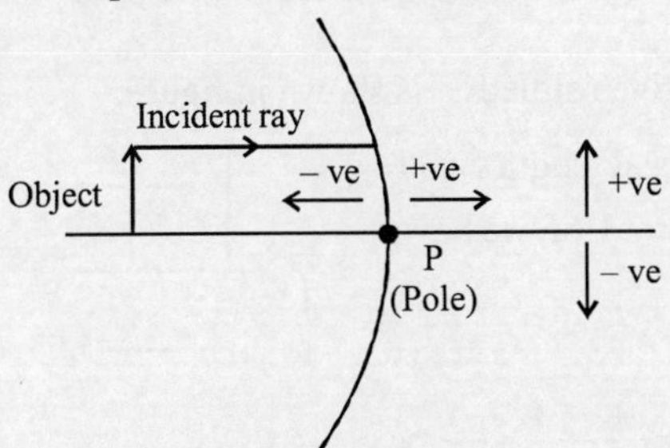

IMAGE FORMED BY CONCAVE AND CONVEX MIRROR

Image Formed by Concave Mirror

Position of object	Position of image	Magnification	Nature of image
Between P and F	Behind the mirror	+ve, m > 1	Virtual and erect
At F	At infinity	– ve, Highly magnified	Real and inverted
Between F and C	Beyond C	– ve, Magnified	Real and inverted
At C	At C	m = –1	Real and inverted
Beyond C	between F and C	Dismished	Real and inverted
At infinity	At F	Highly diminshed	Real and inverted

Image Formed by Convex Mirror

Position of object	Position of image	Magnification	Nature of image
Infront of mirror	Between P and F	m<+1	Virual and erect
At infinity	At F	m<<+1	Virtual and erect

Problem Solving Tips

1. Rays retrace their path when their direction is reversed.
2. Focal length of a mirror depends only on the curvature of the mirror $\left(f = \frac{R}{2}\right)$. It does not depend on the material of the mirror or on the wavelength of incident light.
3. Focal length of concave mirror is always negative. Focal length of convex mirror is always positive.
4. The graph of $\frac{1}{v}$ versus $\frac{1}{u}$ for a concave mirror, if real image is formed.

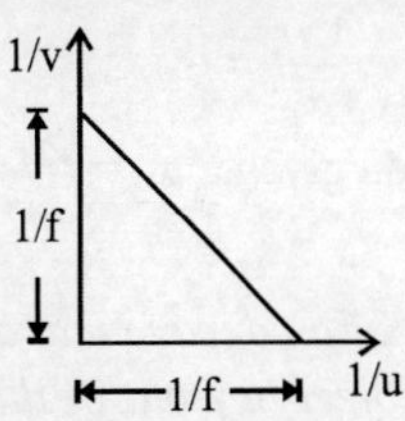

5. The graph shows variation of v with change in u for a mirror.

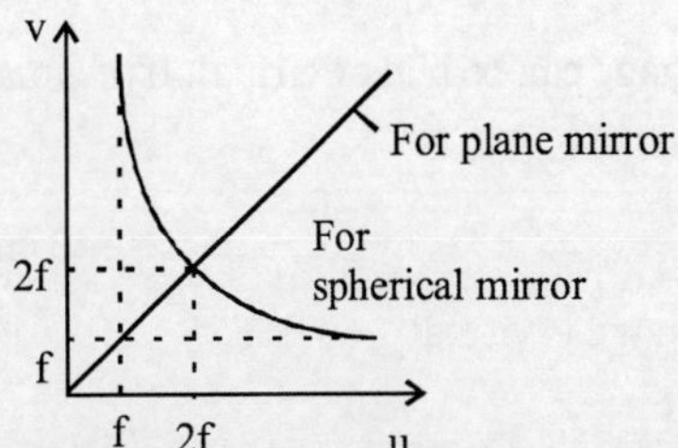

6. A person needs a plane mirror of minimum half of his height to see his full image.
7. A person standing in the middle of room can see complete wall behind him if the mirror in front of him is $\frac{1}{3}$rd of height of wall.
8. A convex mirror is used as a rear view mirror (called driver mirror).
9. If two or more optical components produce magnification, then overall magnification (m) is the product of magnification due to each component, i.e., $m = m_1 \times m_2 \times \ldots$
   - If m is negative, the image is inverted
   - If m is positive, the image is erect.
10. When an object moves with constant speed towards a concave mirror from infinity to focus, the image will move away from the mirror slower in the beginning and with the speed of the object when it is at centre of curvature C and faster later on.
11. Concave mirrors are used as reflectors, as objective in reflecting telescope and by doctors (ENT) to examine ears, nose and throat. It is also used as shaving mirrors.
12. The inability of a spherical mirror (or lens) of large aperture to focus the paraxial rays and marginal rays to the same point on the principal axis is called spherical aberration. Due to this defect the image formed is blurred. This defect can be removed by using parabolic mirror.
13. Chromatic aberration is absent in mirrors but present in lenses. This is because the focal length of mirror is independent of wavelength of light $\left(f = \frac{R}{2}\right)$ but that of lens is dependent on wavelength.
14. Different colour rays travel with different velocity in a medium but velocity of all coloured rays is same in vacuum (and air).
15. If a hole is formed in a mirror, then also we will get full image with no hole in the image. The hole will only reduce the intensity of rays forming the image.

Newton's Formula

In case of spherical mirrors if object distance (x_1) and image distance (x_2) are measured from focus instead of pole, $u = (f + x_1)$ and $v = (f + x_2)$, the mirror formula $\frac{1}{v} + \frac{1}{u} = \frac{1}{f}$

reduces to $\frac{1}{(f+x_2)}+\frac{1}{(f+x_1)}=\frac{1}{f}$

which on simplification gives $x_1 x_2=f^2$

Example 1.

The focal length of a concave mirror is 30 cm. Find the position of the object in front of the mirror, so that the image is three times the size of the object.

Solution :

Here image can be real or virtual. If the image is real

$f=-30, u=?, m=-3$

$$m=\frac{f}{f-u} \Rightarrow -3=\frac{-30}{-30-u} \Rightarrow u=-40 \text{ cm.}$$

If the image is virtual

$$m=\frac{f}{f-u} \Rightarrow 3=\frac{-30}{-30-u} \Rightarrow u=-20 \text{ cm.}$$

Example 2.

A square ABCD of side 1mm is kept at distance 15 cm infront of the concave mirror as shown in the figure. The focal length of the mirror is 10 cm.

Find the perimeter of its image.

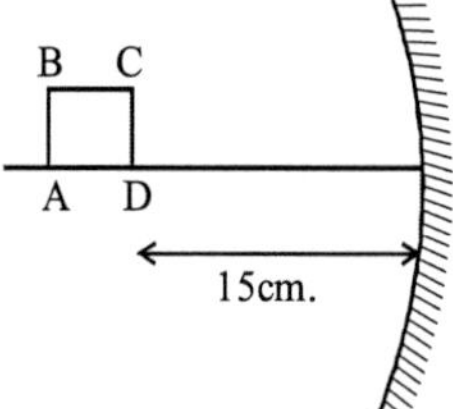

Solution :

$v=-30,\ m=-\frac{v}{u}=-2$

$\therefore A'B'=C'D'=2\times 1=2\text{mm}$

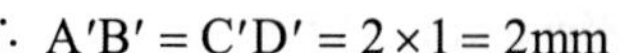

Now $\frac{B'C'}{BC}=\frac{A'D'}{AD}=\frac{v^2}{u^2}=4 \Rightarrow B'C'=A'D'=4$ mm

$\therefore$ Perimeter $=2+2+4+4=12$ mm

Example 3.

An object of length 2.5 cm is placed at a distance of 1.5 f from a concave mirror where f is the magnitude of the focal length of the mirror. The length of the object is perpendicular to the principal axis. Find the length of the image. Is the image erect or inverted?

Solution :

The given situation is shown in figure.

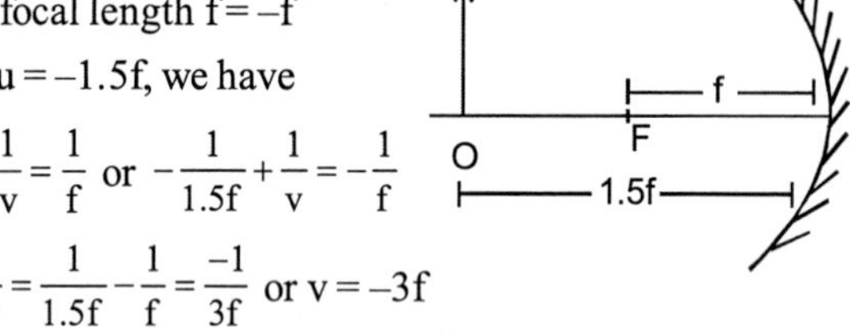

The focal length $f=-f$

and $u=-1.5f$, we have

$\frac{1}{u}+\frac{1}{v}=\frac{1}{f}$ or $-\frac{1}{1.5f}+\frac{1}{v}=-\frac{1}{f}$

or $\frac{1}{v}=\frac{1}{1.5f}-\frac{1}{f}=\frac{-1}{3f}$ or $v=-3f$

Now $m=-\frac{v}{u}=\frac{3f}{-1.5f}=-2$ or $\frac{h_2}{h_1}=-2$

or $h_2=-2h_1=-5.0$ cm

The image is 5.0 cm long. The minus sign shows that it is inverted.

24.1 Concept Practice Problems CPP

1. A convex mirror of focal length f produces an image (1/n)th of the size of the object. The distance of the object from the mirror is
(a) $(n-1)f$ (b) f/n (c) $(n+1)f$ (d) nf

2. If two mirrors are kept at 60º to each other, then the number of images formed by them is
(a) 5 (b) 6 (c) 7 (d) 8

3. A concave mirror of focal length f produces an image n times the size of object. If image is real, then distance of object from mirror, is
(a) $(n-1)f$ (b) $\{(n-1)/n\}f$
(c) $\{(n+1)/n\}f$ (d) $(n+1)f$

4. In a concave mirror, an object is placed at a distance x_1 from focus, and image is formed at a distance x_2 from focus. Then focal length of mirror is
(a) $\sqrt{x_1 x_2}$ (b) $\frac{x_1-x_2}{2}$ (c) $\frac{x_1+x_2}{2}$ (d) $\sqrt{\frac{x_1}{x_2}}$

5. A plane mirror reflects a beam of light to form a real image. The incident beam is
(a) parallel (b) convergent
(c) divergent (d) any one of the above

6. An object is placed at a distance 2f from the pole of a convex mirror of focal length f. The linear magnification is
(a) $\frac{1}{3}$ (b) $\frac{2}{3}$ (c) $\frac{3}{4}$ (d) 1

7. A concave mirror of focal length f. in vacuum is placed in a medium of refractive index 2. Its focal length in the medium is
(a) $\frac{f}{2}$ (b) f (c) 2f (d) 4f

8. An object is placed at a distance of 40 cm in front of a concave mirror of focal length 20 cm. The image produced is
(a) real, inverted and smaller in size
(b) real, inverted and of same size
(c) real and erect
(d) virtual and inverted

9. A concave mirror forms the image of an object on a screen. If the lower half of the mirror is covered with an opaque card, the effect would be to make the
(a) image less bright.
(b) lower half of the image disappear.
(c) upper half of the image disappear.
(d) image blurred.

10. A person is six feet tall. How tall must a vertical mirror be if he is able to see his entire length?
(a) 3 ft (b) 4.5 ft
(c) 7.5 ft (d) 6 ft

ANSWER KEY

1	(a)	2	(a)	3	(c)	4	(a)	5	(b)	6	(a)	7	(b)	8	(b)	9	(a)	10	(a)

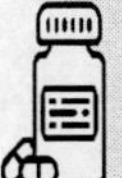

Topic 24.2 : Refraction, Total Internal Reflection, Refraction at a Spherical Surface, Refraction by a Lens, Combination of Lenses and Refraction through a Prism

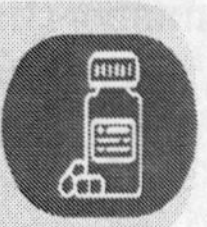

REFRACTION

Whenever a wave is bounced back into same medium at an interface reflection is said to have occurred. Transmission of a wave into the second medium at an interface is called refraction. When a ray of light is passing from denser to rarer medium, it bends away from the normal and when passing from rarer to denser medium, it bends towards the normal.

- When a ray of light passing from one medium to another medium frequency and phase do not change while wavelength and velocity changes.
- Twinkling of stars, appearance of sun before actual sunrise and after actual sunset etc. are due to atmospheric refraction.

Laws of Refraction

(i) **Snell's Law :** When a light ray is incident on a surface separating two transparent media, the ray bends at the time of changing the medium.

i.e. $\frac{\sin i}{\sin r} = \frac{v_1}{v_2} = \frac{\mu_2}{\mu_1} = {}_1\mu_2,$

where i = angle of incidence

r = angle of refraction

v_1 = vel. of light in 1st medium

v_2 = vel. of light in 2nd medium

${}_2^1\mu$ or ${}_1\mu_2$ = refractive index of 2nd medium w.r.t. the 1st medium.

μ_1 = refractive index of 1st medium w.r.t vacuum (or air)

μ_2 = refractive index of 2nd medium w.r.t vacuum (or air)

(ii) The incident ray, the normal and the refracted ray at the interface all lie in the same plane.

Refractive Index of the Medium

(a) Refractive index of second medium w.r.t. first medium

$${}_1\mu_2 = \frac{\mu_2}{\mu_1} = \frac{c/v_2}{c/v_1} = \frac{v_1}{v_2}$$

$$= \frac{\textit{Velocity of light in first medium}}{\textit{Velocity of light in second medium}}$$

(b) Absolute refractive index of medium (n or μ)

$$\frac{\textit{Velocity of light in vacuum}}{\textit{Velocity of light in medium}} = \frac{c}{v} = \frac{\sin i}{\sin r} = n = \mu$$

Refractive index is the relative property of two media. *If the first medium carrying the incident ray is a vacuum, then the ratio* $\frac{\text{Sin}\, i}{\text{Sin}\, r}$ *is called the 'absolute refractive index of the second medium'.* The relative refractive index of any two media is equal to the ratio of their absolute refractive indices. Therefore, if the absolute refractive index of medium 1 and 2 be n_1 and n_2 respectively, then the refractive index of medium 2 with respect to medium 1 is

$${}_1n_2 = n_{12} = \frac{n_2}{n_1} = \frac{\text{Sin}\, i}{\text{Sin}\, r}$$

$$n_1 \sin i = n_2 \sin r$$

According to **cauchy's formula**

$$\mu = A + \frac{B}{\lambda^2}$$

where, A and B are cauchy's constant.

$$\lambda_{red} > \lambda_{violet}$$

so, $\mu_{red} < \mu_{violet}$

(c) ${}_1n_2 = \frac{1}{{}_2n_1}$

(d) For three mediums 1, 2 and 3 due to successive refraction.

$${}_1n_2 \times {}_2n_3 \times {}_3n_1 = 1$$

$$\frac{n_2}{n_1} \times \frac{n_3}{n_2} \times \frac{n_1}{n_3} = 1$$

(e) For two mediums, n_1 and n_2 are refractive indices with respect to vacuum, the incident and emergent rays are parallel then

$$n_1 \sin\phi_1 = n_2 \sin\phi_2.$$

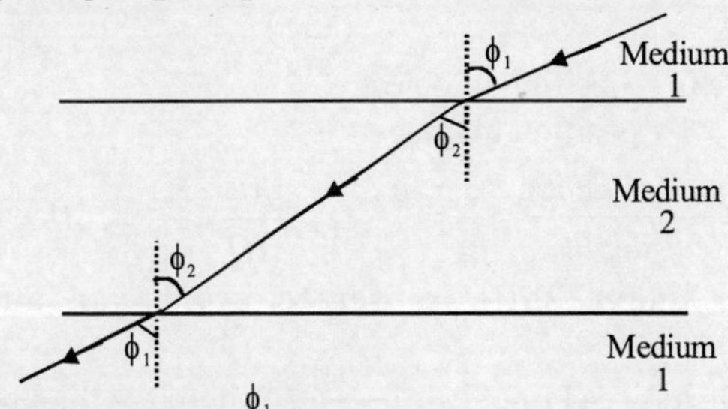

Factors affecting refractive index :

(i) Nature of the medium

(ii) Wavelength

(iii) Temperature of the medium-with increase in temperature, refractive index of medium decreases.

Transmission of Wave

(i) The equation of the wave refracted or transmitted to the next medium is given by : $y = A'' \sin(\omega t - k_0' x)$. This is independent of the nature (rarer/denser) of the medium. The wave is not inverted.

(ii) The amplitude (A″) of the transmitted wave is less than that (A) of the incident wave.

(iii) The angular frequency remains unchanged. However the wave number changes. Note that the phase of the transmitted wave is $(\omega t - k_0' x)$ and that of the incident wave is $(\omega t - kx)$.

(iv) The compression or rarefaction are transmitted as such and same is the case with the crest or trough.

The wave velocity (v_p), the angular frequency (ω) and the wave number (k) are related as $v_p = \omega/k = n\lambda$. Let the wave velocity in the medium to which the wave is transmitted be $v'_p = \omega/k' = n\lambda'$.

(i) If second medium is denser, in comparison to first medium (i.e. $\mu_2 > \mu_1$), then from Snell's law

$$\frac{\sin i}{\sin r} = \frac{\mu_2}{\mu_1} = \frac{v_2}{v_1} \quad \text{here } \mu_2 > \mu_1 \text{ so } v_1 > v_2$$

$\Rightarrow k_1 < k_2$ and $\lambda_1 > \lambda_2$.

It means that *if ray goes from rarer medium to denser medium (i.e. from first medium to second medium), then wave number increases & wavelength decreases.*

(ii) If second medium is rarer in comparison to first medium, then from Snell's law

$$\frac{\sin i}{\sin r} = \frac{\mu_2}{\mu_1} = \frac{v_1}{v_2} \quad \text{here } \mu_2 < \mu_1 \text{ so } v_1 < v_2$$

$\Rightarrow k_1 > k_2$ and $\lambda_1 < \lambda_2$.

It means that *when ray goes from denser to rarer medium, then wave number decreases & wavelength increases.*

(iii) *No change in wave number k occurs on reflection.*

Image due to refraction at a plane surface, Apparent shift

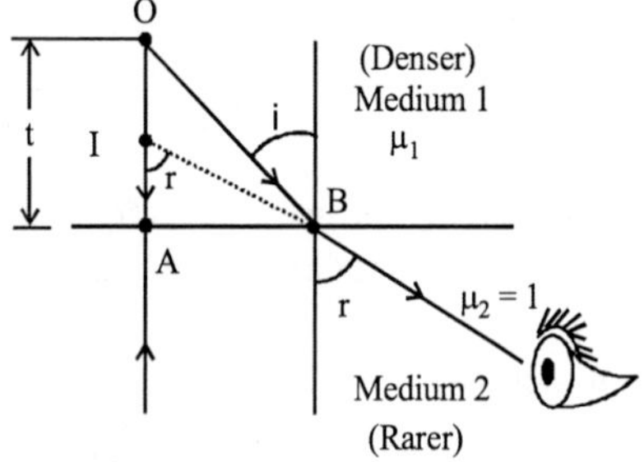

(a) Here O = position of object
I = position of image

$$\frac{\textit{Apparent depth}}{\textit{Real depth}} = \frac{1}{\mu} = \frac{\mu_2}{\mu_1} \quad \text{i.e.} \quad \frac{AI}{AO} = \frac{1}{\mu} \Rightarrow AI = \frac{t}{\mu}$$

(b) The image shifts closer to eye by an amount

$OI = AO - AI$ or $\Delta t = \left(1 - \frac{1}{\mu}\right) t$ where t = thickness of medium over the object and Δt = apparent shift in its position towards the observer.

When an object in denser medium is seen through rarer medium, then apparent depth is less than real depth. But when an aeroplane or bird flying is seen by an observers in denser medium, the apparent height is more by $(\mu - 1)t$

Lateral shift by a slab of uniform thickness t, is

$$x = \frac{t}{\cos r}\sin(i - r)$$

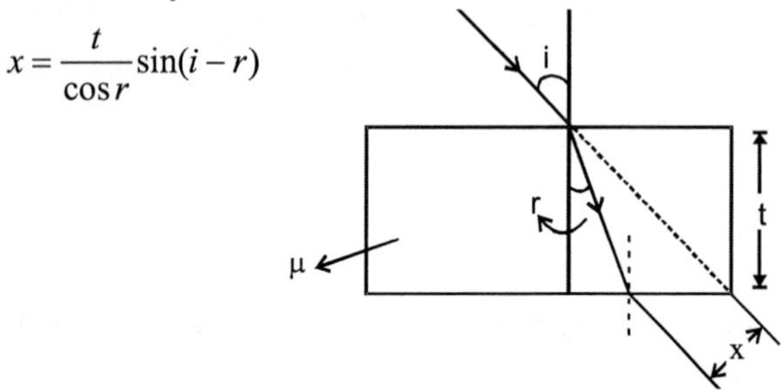

The **apparent shift** through a glass slab is in the direction of light

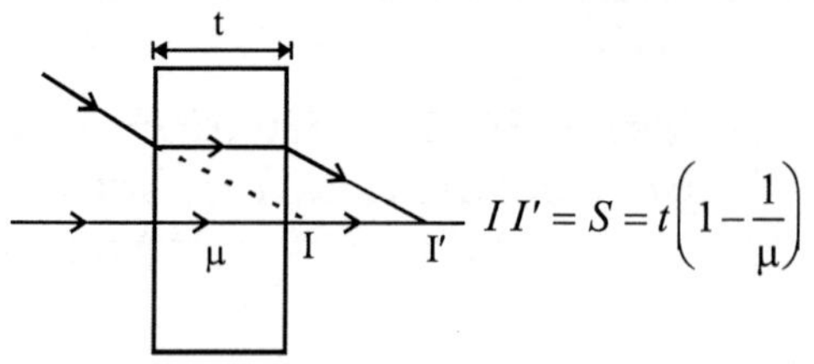

TOTAL INTERNAL REFLECTION (TIR)

When the object is placed in an optically denser medium and if the incident angle is greater than the critical angle then the ray of light gets reflected back to the originating medium. This phenomenon is called total internal reflection.

Critical angle (i_c) : When a ray passes from an optically denser medium to an optically rarer medium, the angle of refraction r is greater than the corresponding angle of incidence i. From Snell's law

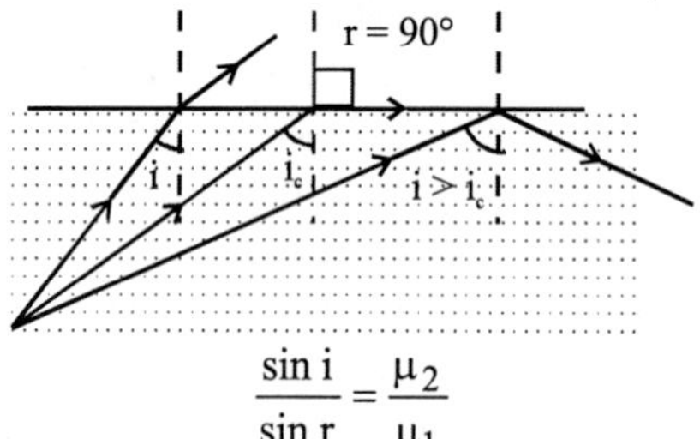

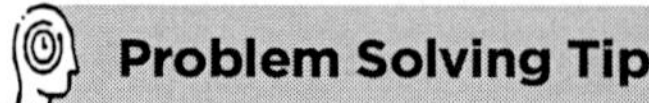

$$\frac{\sin i}{\sin r} = \frac{\mu_2}{\mu_1}$$

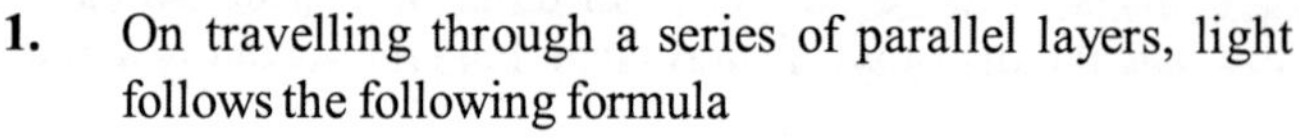

Let $\mu_1 = \mu$ and $\mu_2 = 1$ and let for $i = i_c$, $r = 90°$ then $\sin i_c = 1/\mu$

$\therefore i_c = \sin^{-1}\frac{1}{\mu}$; *$i_c$ is called the critical angle*

This phenomenon takes place in shining of air bubble, sparkling of diamond, mirage and looming, in optical communication using optical fibre.

Problem Solving Tips

1. On travelling through a series of parallel layers, light follows the following formula
$\mu \sin\theta = \text{constant} = \mu_1 \sin\theta_1 = \mu_2 \sin\theta_2 = \mu_3 \sin\theta_3$

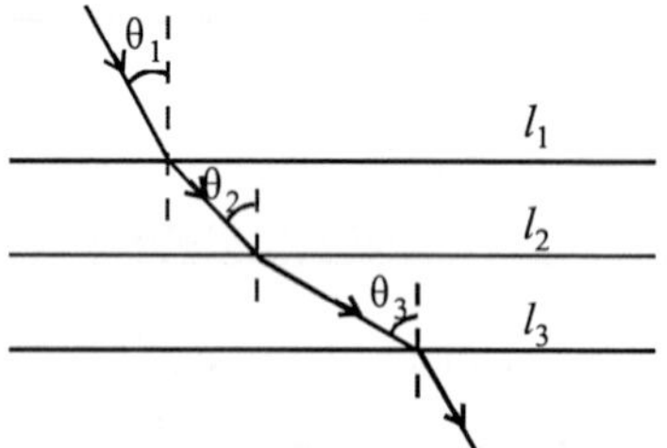

- It is important to note that the above relationship is valid only when boundaries undeviated.

2. In case of refraction, if i = 0 then r = 0. This means that the ray which strikes to a boundary at 90° passes through the boundary undeviated.
3. If an object moves towards a denser medium with a velocity v then the image moves faster with speed of μv as seen by the observer in denser medium.

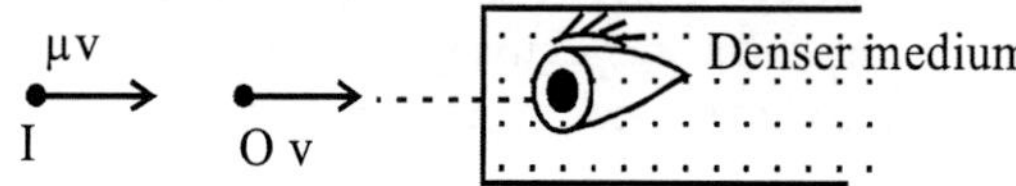

If an object moves towards a rarer medium with a velocity v then the image moves slower with a speed v/μ as seen by the observer in rarer medium.

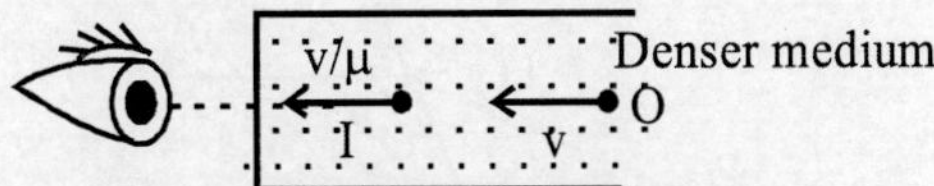

4. Denser the medium, smaller is the wavelength.
5. When light travels from one medium to another the wavelength and velocity changes proportionally but frequency of rays remains the same
6. ${}_2^1\mu = \frac{\mu_2}{\mu_1}$ and ${}_c^b\mu = \frac{{}^a\mu_c}{{}^a\mu_b}$ ('a' for air/vacuum)
7. When a parallel compound slab consists of two media of equal thickness and refractive indices μ_1 and μ_2 then the equivalent refractive index $\mu = \frac{2\mu_1\mu_2}{\mu_1 + \mu_2}$

MISCONCEPTION

✗ ***Incorrect :*** If a mirror or a lens is painted black on one half, then half of image will be formed.

✓ ***Correct :*** If half of the mirror or lens is blackened, we get full image but with half the intensity.

REFRACTION AT A SPHERICAL SURFACE

For any curved spherical surfaces. Relation between u and v in terms of refractive indices of the mediums and the radius of curvature of the curved spherical surface.

$$\frac{\mu_2}{v} - \frac{\mu_1}{u} = \frac{\mu_2 - \mu_1}{R}$$

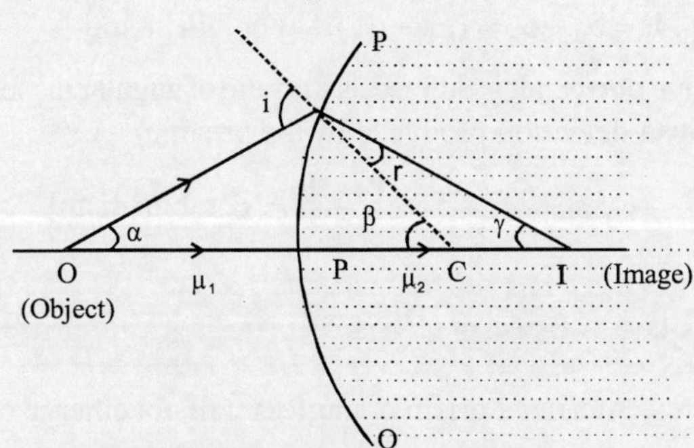

Spherical surface separating two media

(i) The **lateral magnification** in case of refraction from curved surfaces $m = \frac{\mu_1}{\mu_2}\left(\frac{v}{u}\right)$

(ii) **Longitudinal magnification** $m' = \frac{\mu_2}{\mu_1} m^2$

Note : μ_1 is refractive index of medium 1 through which light passes first before meeting the interface and μ_2 is the refractive index of medium 2 to which light encounters after it passes through the interface.

REFRACTION BY A LENS

The **focus point** of a lens is the point where image of an object placed at infinity is formed. And its distance from optical centre of the lens is called **focal length.**

Focal length of convex lens is +ve, and of concave lens is –ve.

(i) **Lens formula or thin lens formula**

$$\frac{1}{v} - \frac{1}{u} = \frac{1}{f}$$

(ii) **Lens maker's formula,**

$$\frac{1}{f} = \left(\frac{\mu_2}{\mu_1} - 1\right)\left(\frac{1}{R_1} - \frac{1}{R_2}\right) = (\mu - 1)\left[\frac{1}{R_1} - \frac{1}{R_2}\right]$$

where ${}_2^1\mu = \frac{\mu_2}{\mu_1}$

In the above formula μ_2 is refractive index of lens whereas μ_1 is the refractive index of surrounding medium.

R_1 is the radius of curvature of the lens reached first by light and R_2 is the radius of curvature of the other surface.

Magnification : m = v/u

This relation holds for both convex and concave lenses for real as well as virtual images.

Power of a lens, P = reciprocal of focal length expressed in metres. *i.e.,* $P = \frac{1}{f\,(\text{in metre})}$. Its **unit :** dioptre(D).

Note : To solve numerical problems use sign conventions while substituting values in above equations.

Equivalent focal length of two lenses separated by distance d

$$\frac{1}{F} = \frac{1}{f_1} + \frac{1}{f_2} - \frac{d}{f_1 f_2}$$

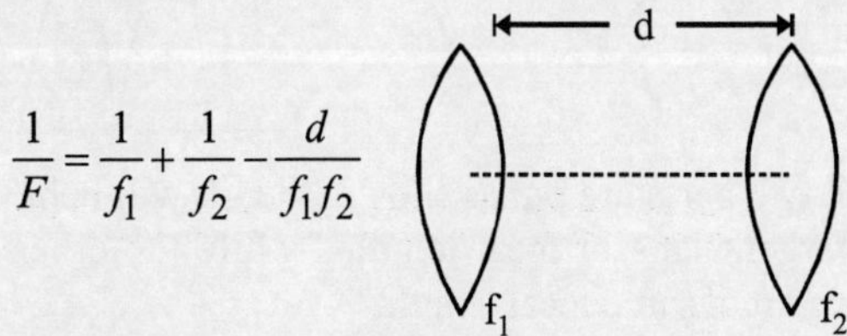

Equivalent focal length of lens - mirror combination :

In such a case, the ray of light suffers two refraction from the lens and one reflection from the mirror. The combination behaves as a mirror whose focal length is given by

$$\frac{1}{F} = \frac{2}{f_1} + \frac{1}{f_m}$$

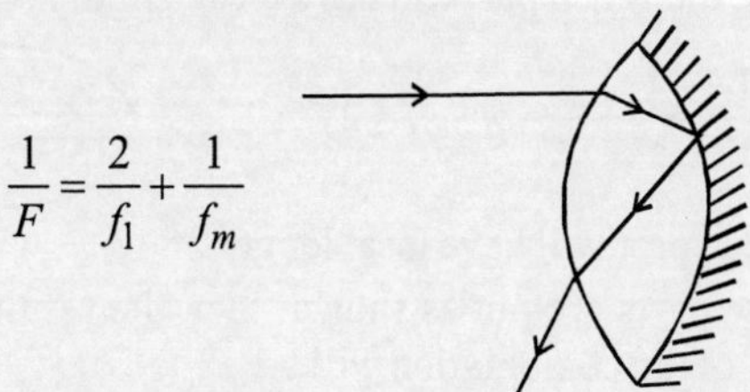

f_1 = focal length of lens, f_m = focal length of mirror

It is important that in the above formula, we cannot apply the sign conventions of cartesian system rather **following sign conventions are followed.**

Focal length of a converging lens / mirror is taken as positive and focal length of diverging lens/mirror is taken as negative.

Focal Length by Displacement Method

$$f = \frac{D^2 - d^2}{4D}$$

where D = distance between an object and screen and d = distance between two positions of lens.

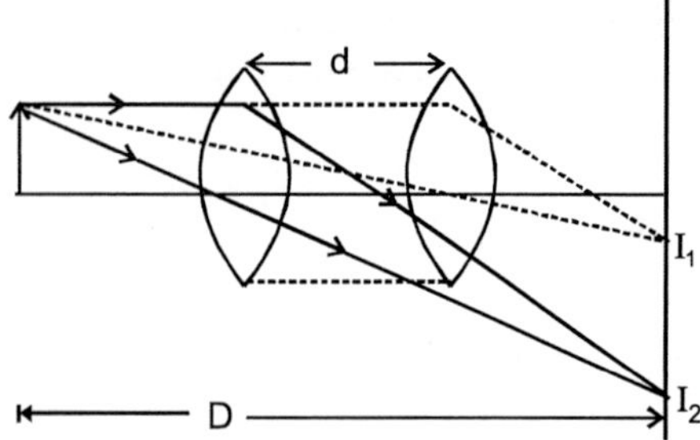

Aperture of a lens : With reference to a lens, aperture means the effective diameter of its light transmitting area. So the brightness i.e. intensity of image formed by a lens which depends on the light passing through the lens will depend on the square of aperture i.e. I ∝ (aperture)^2

COMBINATION OF LENSES

(i) If a lens of focal length f is cut in two equal parts as shown in figure, each part will have focal length = f

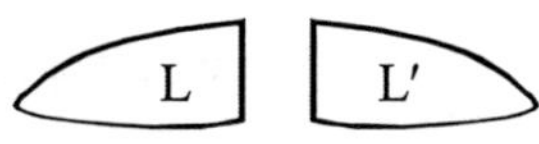

(ii) If the above parts of lens are put in contact as shown then the resultant focal length will be,

$$\frac{1}{F}=\frac{1}{f}+\frac{1}{f}=\frac{2}{f} \text{ i.e. } F=\frac{f}{2}$$

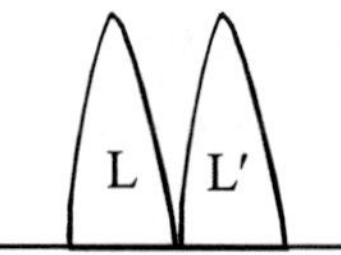

(iii) If the two parts are put as shown, then L will behave as convergent lens of focal length f while the other (L′) divergent of same focal length,

$$\therefore \frac{1}{F}=\frac{1}{+f}+\frac{1}{-f} \text{ or } F=\infty \therefore P=0$$

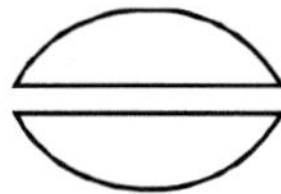

(iv) If a lens of focal length f is divided into equal parts as shown, then each part will have focal length f′,

i.e. $\frac{1}{f}=\frac{1}{f'}+\frac{1}{f'}$ or $f'=2f$

i.e., each part will have focal length 2f.

(v) If these parts are put as shown, then the resultant focal length of the combination will be

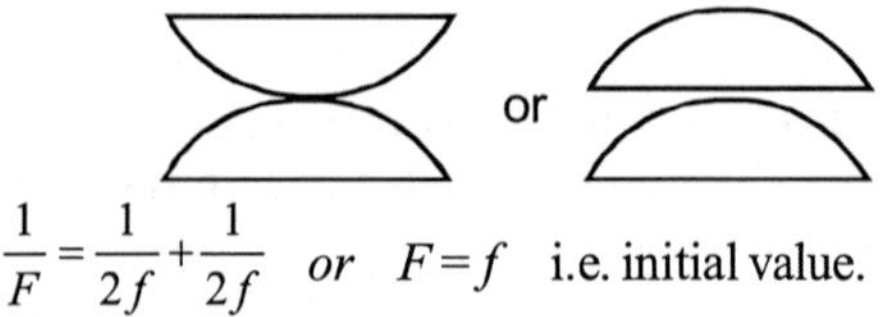

$\frac{1}{F}=\frac{1}{2f}+\frac{1}{2f}$ or $F=f$ i.e. initial value.

REFRACTION THROUGH A PRISM

Prism is a transparent medium whose refracting surfaces are inclined to each other.

(i) The angle of deviation is given by $\delta = i + i' - A$ where A= angle of prism. For δ to be minimum, $i = i'$ and $r = r'$

$\delta_m = A(\mu - 1)$

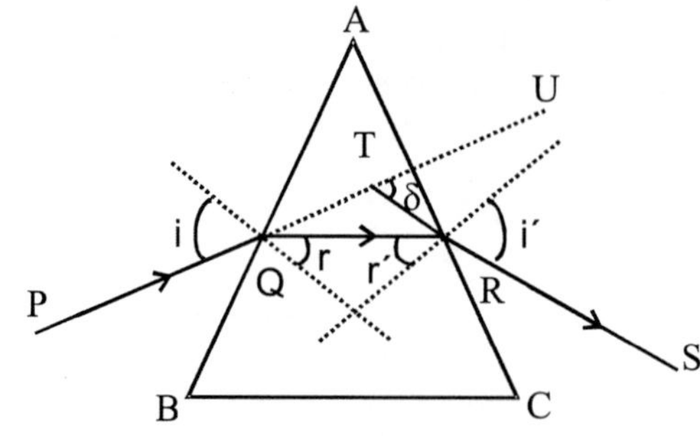

Refractive index of prism, $\mu = \dfrac{\sin\left(\dfrac{A+\delta_m}{2}\right)}{\sin\left(\dfrac{A}{2}\right)}$

where δ_m = minimum angle of deviation

If angle of prism A is small, than δ_m is also small.

$$\therefore \mu = \frac{(A+\delta_m)/2}{A/2}$$

Plot of angle of deviation (δ) versus angle of incidence (i) for a triangular prism.

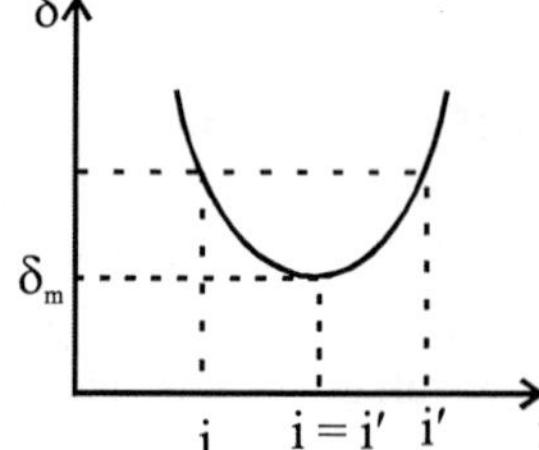

Dispersion

It is the breaking up of white ray of light into its constituents colours VIBGYOR. The band of seven constituents colours is called **spectrum.**

Angular dispersion : It is defined as the difference of deviations suffered by the extreme colours.

i.e., $\theta = \delta_v - \delta_r = (\mu_v - \mu_r)A$ [For thin prism]

Dispersive power : It is defined as the ratio of angular dispersion to the mean deviation produced by the prism.

i.e., $\omega = \dfrac{\delta_v - \delta_r}{\delta} = \dfrac{\mu_v - \mu_r}{\mu}$ [For thin prism]

Problem Solving Tips

1. A ray entering a prism of angle A will not emerge out of prism if $A > 2\theta_c$ where θ_c = critical angle
2. Maximum deviation through a prism will occur when angle of incidence is 90°.

   For this prism $\delta = (\mu - 1)A$

   This shows that for a small angled prism, deviation is independent of angle of incidence.
3. Angle of emergence of a prism is 90° (called grazing emergence) when angle of incidence

   $i = \sin^{-1}[\sqrt{(\mu^2 - 1)}\sin A - \cos A]$
4. A single prism produces deviation and dispersion simultaneously.
5. **Dispersion without deviation :** When white light is incident on a combination of two prisms of different materials and of suitable angles placed opposite to each

other, the emergent light may have only dispersion without any deviation (of mean colour yellow).

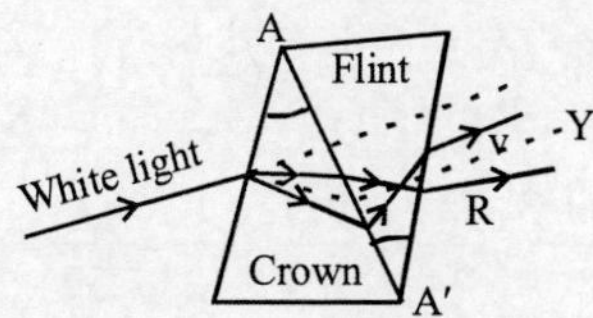

For this to happen the conditions is

$$\frac{A}{A'} = -\frac{(\mu'-1)}{(\mu-1)} \quad \text{(For thin lenses)}$$

The net angular dispersion produced

$$\theta = (\omega - \omega')\delta \quad \text{(For thin lenses)}$$

6. **Deviation without dispersion**

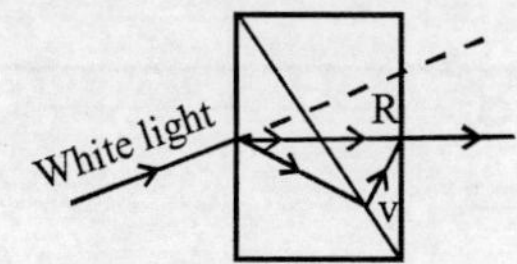

For this to happen $\frac{A'}{A} = \frac{-(\mu_v - \mu_r)}{(\mu_v' - \mu_r')}$ .... (1)

Net deviation $\delta_{net} = \delta\left(1 - \frac{\omega}{\omega'}\right)$

Equation (1) is said to be the **condition of achromatism** for combination of two prisms.

7. Variation of refractive index of a medium with wavelength causing incident light to split into constituent colours is dispersion.

Cauchy's equation : $\mu = a + \frac{b}{\lambda^2} + \frac{c}{\lambda^4}$, where *a*, *b* and *c* are constants.

8. Rayleigh scattering law explains blue colour of sky. Intensity of scattered light is proportional to $1/\lambda^4$. Hence the red light having highest value of λ_R scatters less.

9. Rainbow can be observed if light source is behind and the droplets are in front of the observer, i.e. when the back of a person is towards the sun.

   It is a consequence of dispersion of sunlight by water droplets due to a combinations of refraction and total internal reflection. If the rainbow is formed after one internal reflection in the droplets, it is called a **primary rainbow**. In this the violet ray emerges at an angle of 40.8° and red rays at an angle of 42.8°. If the rainbow is formed after two internal reflections, it is called a **secondary rainbow.** In this the violet rays emerge at 54° and red at 51°, i.e. the order of colours is reversed. The primary rainbow is brighter than the secondary.

10. When a point source of light is placed at a depth h below the surface of water of refractive index m, then radius of bright circular patch on the surface of water is given by

$$R = \frac{h}{\sqrt{\mu^2 - 1}}$$

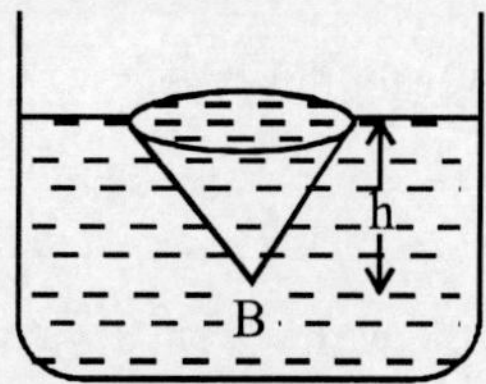

11. When a lens made up of glass is immersed in water, its focal length changes.

$$\frac{1}{f} = \left({}^a_g\mu - 1\right)\left(\frac{1}{R_1} - \frac{1}{R_2}\right) \quad \frac{1}{f'} = \left({}^w_g\mu - 1\right)\left(\frac{1}{R_1} - \frac{1}{R_2}\right)$$

$$\frac{f'}{f} = \frac{{}^a_g\mu - 1}{{}^\omega_g\mu - 1} = \frac{{}_g\mu/\mu_a - 1}{{}_g\mu/\mu_\omega - 1} = \frac{({}_g\mu - {}_a\mu)\mu_\omega}{({}_g\mu - {}_\omega\mu)\mu_a}$$

12. For achromatic combination of these lenses in contact, the necessary condition is $\frac{\omega_1}{f_1} + \frac{\omega_2}{f_2} = 0$

13. For two lenses separated by distance d, spherical aberration is minimum when $d = f_1 - f_2$.

14. A convex lens forms a real image when the object is placed beyond focus. When the object is placed between optical centre and focus, convex lens forms a virtual image.

15. A concave lens always form a virtual image for a real object.

16. A lens is called thin when the thickness of the lens is small compared to the object distance, image distance, radii of curvatures of the lens.

    In the case of thick lens, the problem has to be solved using formula for each interface one by one.

17.

Real image (inverted)	**Virtual image (erect)**
Real image is formed by intersection of rays.	Virtual image is formed by actual extending the rays in the back direction.
This image can be brought on a screen.	This image cannot be brought on screen.

MISCONCEPTIONS

✗ *Incorrect :* Using thin lens formula while the lens given in the numerical problem is thick.

✓ *Correct :* The lens formula $\left(\frac{1}{v} - \frac{1}{u} = \frac{1}{f}\right)$ and lens maker's formula $\left[\frac{1}{f} = (\mu - 1)\left(\frac{1}{R_1} - \frac{1}{R_2}\right)\right]$ are valid only for thin lenses.

Example 4.

Consider the situation shown in figure. Find maximum angle for which the light suffers total internal reflection at the vertical surface.

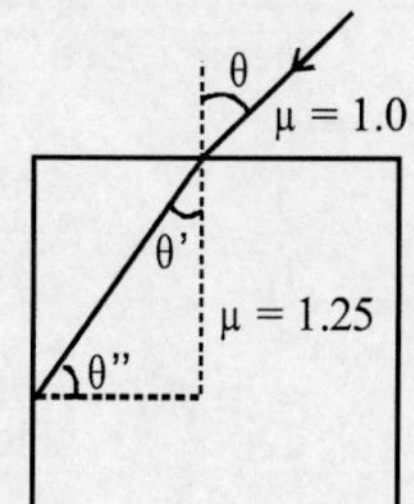

Solution :

The critical angle for this case is

$$\theta'' = \sin^{-1}\frac{1}{1.25} = \sin^{-1}\frac{4}{5} \text{ or } \sin\theta'' = \frac{4}{5}$$

Since $\theta'' = \frac{\pi}{2} - \theta'$, we have $\sin\theta' = \cos\theta'' = \frac{3}{5}$

From Snell's law,

$$\frac{\sin\theta}{\sin\theta'} = 1.25 \text{ or } \sin\theta = 1.25 \times \sin\theta' = 1.25 \times \frac{3}{5} = \frac{3}{4}$$

$$\text{or } \theta = \sin^{-1}\frac{3}{4}$$

If θ'' is greater than the critical angle, θ will be smaller than this value. Thus, the maximum value of θ' for which total internal reflection takes place at the vertical surface is $\sin^{-1}(3/4)$.

$$\frac{BO_1}{BI} = \mu \text{ or, } \frac{AB + AO_1}{BI} = \mu \text{ or } \frac{t + \mu x}{BI} = \mu$$

$$\text{or } BI = x + \frac{t}{\mu}$$

The net shift is

$$OI = OB - BI = (x + t) - \left(x + \frac{t}{\mu}\right) = t\left(1 - \frac{1}{\mu}\right)$$

which is independent of x.

Example 5.

A tank is filled with water to a height of 12.5 cm. The apparent depth of a needle lying at the bottom of full tank is measured by a microscope to be 9.4 cm. What is the refractive index of water? If water is replaced by a liquid of refractive index 1.63 upto the same height, by what distance would the microscope have to be moved to focus the needle again?

Solution :

Here real depth = 12.5 cm : apparent depth = 9.4 cm; μ = ?

$$\mu = \frac{\text{real depth}}{\text{Apparent depth}} = \frac{12.5}{9.4} = 1.33$$

Now in second case, μ = 1.63, real depth = 12.5 cm, apparent depth = ?

$$1.63 = \frac{12.5}{y} \text{ or } y = \frac{12.5}{1.63} = 7.67\text{ cm}.$$

Distance through which microscope has to be moved up = 9.4 – 7.67 = 1.73 cm.

Example 6.

A converging lens has a focal length of 20 cm in air. It is made of a material of refractive index 1.6. If the lens is immersed in a liquid of refractive index 1.3. What will be the new focal length of the lens?

Solution :

$$\frac{1}{f_1} = (\mu_1 - 1)\frac{2}{R} \qquad \mu_1 = 1.6,\ f_1 = 20$$

$$\frac{1}{f_1} = (1.6 - 1)\frac{2}{R}$$

$$\text{or } \frac{1}{20} = \frac{0.6 \times 2}{R} \therefore R = \frac{0.6 \times 2 \times 20}{10} = 24\text{cm}$$

$$\frac{1}{f_2} = (\mu_1 - 1) \times \frac{2}{R} \quad \therefore \frac{1}{f_2} = \left(\frac{1.6}{1.3} - 1\right) = \frac{2}{R}$$

$$\frac{1}{f_2} = \left(\frac{1.6 - 1.3}{1.3}\right)\frac{2}{24} = \frac{0.3}{1.3} \times \frac{1}{12} = \frac{1}{52}$$

f_2 = 52 cm.

Example 7.

Locate the image formed by refraction in the situation shown in figure. The point C is the centre of curvature.

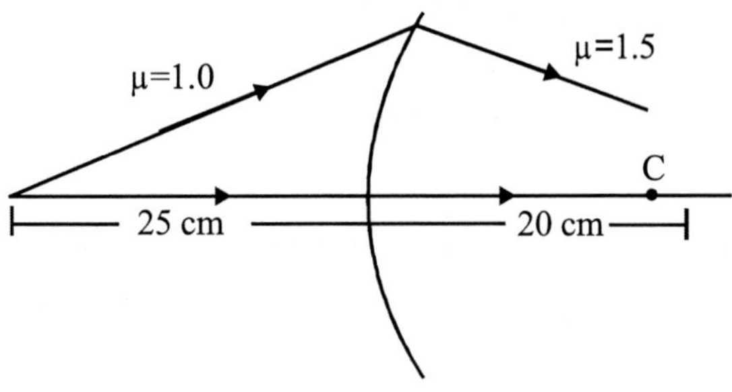

Solution :

$$\text{We have, } \frac{\mu_2}{v} - \frac{\mu_1}{u} = \frac{\mu_2 - \mu_1}{R} \quad ....(1)$$

Here u = –25 cm, R = 20 cm, μ_1 = 1.0 and μ_2 = 1.5

Putting the values in (1),

$$\frac{1.5}{v} + \frac{1.0}{25\text{ cm}} = \frac{1.5 - 1.0}{20\text{ cm}} \text{ or, } \frac{1.5}{v} = \frac{1}{40\text{ cm}} - \frac{1}{25\text{ cm}}$$

or, v = –100 cm.

As v is negative, the image is formed to the left of the separating surface at a distance of 100 cm from it.

Example 8.

One end of a horizontal cylindrical glass rod (μ = 1.5) of radius 5.0 cm is rounded in the shape of a hemisphere. An object 0.5 mm high is placed perpendicular to the axis of the rod at a distance of 20.0 cm from the rounded edge. Locate the image of the object and find its height.

Solution :

Taking the origin at the vertex, u = –20.0 cm and R = 5.0 cm.

$$\text{We have, } \frac{\mu_2}{v} - \frac{\mu_1}{u} = \frac{\mu_2 - \mu_1}{R}$$

$$\text{or } \frac{1.5}{v} = \frac{1}{-20.0\text{ cm}} + \frac{0.5}{5.0\text{ cm}} = \frac{1}{20\text{ cm}} \text{ or } v = 30\text{ cm}$$

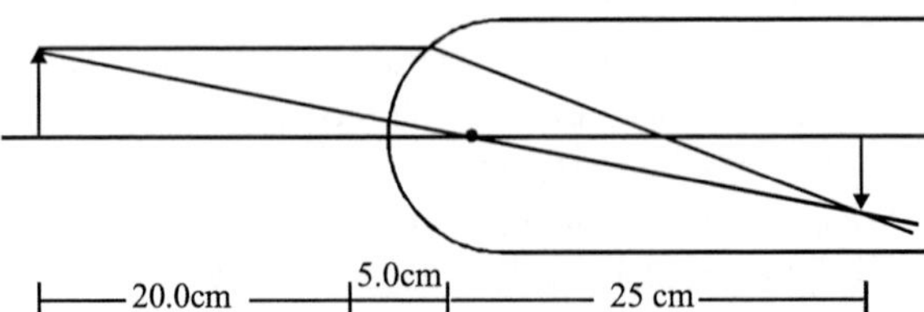

The image is formed inside the rod at a distance of 30 cm from the vertex.

The magnification is $m = \frac{\mu_1 v}{\mu_2 u} = \frac{30\text{ cm}}{-1.5 \times 20\text{ cm}} = -1$

Thus, the image will be of same height (0.5 mm) as the object but it will be inverted.

Example 9.

A convex lens focuses a distant object on a screen placed 10 cm away from it. A glass plate (μ = 1.5) of thickness 1.5 cm is inserted between the lens and the screen. Where should the object be placed so that its image is again focused on the screen.

Solution :

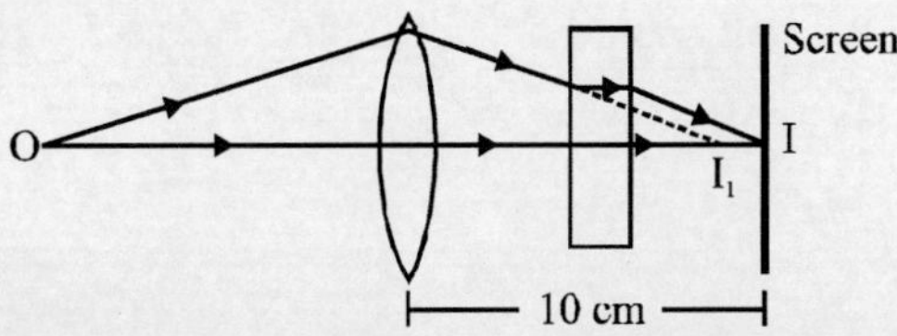

The focal length of the lens is 10 cm. The situation with the glass plate inserted is shown in figure. The object is placed at O. The lens would form the image at I_1 but the glass plate intercepts the rays and forms the image at I on the screen.

The shift

$$I_1I = t\left(1-\frac{1}{\mu}\right) = (1.5\text{ cm})\left(1-\frac{1}{1.5}\right) = 0.5\text{ cm}.$$

Thus, the lens forms the image at a distance of 9.5 cm from itself. Using

$$\frac{1}{v}-\frac{1}{u}=\frac{1}{f} \Rightarrow \frac{1}{u}=\frac{1}{v}-\frac{1}{f}=\frac{1}{9.5\text{ cm}}-\frac{1}{10\text{ cm}}$$

$\Rightarrow u = 190$ cm

Thus, the object should be placed at a distance of 190 cm from the lens.

Example 10.

A lens is cut into two equal pieces and they are placed as shown in figure. An object is placed at a distance of 12 cm left from the first half lens. The focal length of original lens was 30 cm. Find the position of final image.

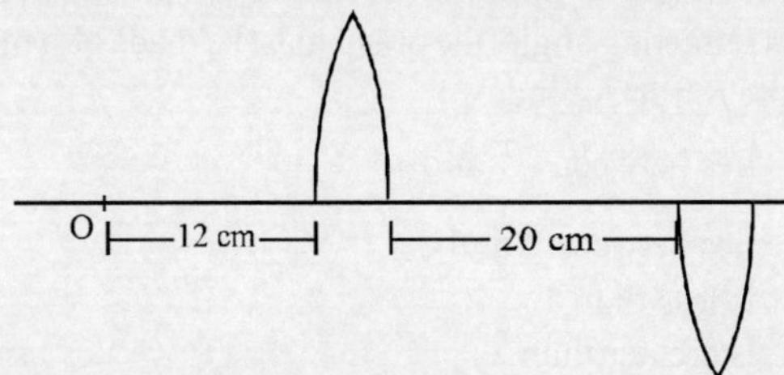

Solution :

Focal length of each lens is 30 cm

For first lens u = – 12, f = 30 cm

$$\frac{1}{v_1}-\frac{1}{u}=\frac{1}{f} \Rightarrow \frac{1}{v_1}=\frac{1}{u}+\frac{1}{f}=-\frac{1}{12}+\frac{1}{30}$$

or, $v_1 = -20$ cm.

For the second half lens image formed at v_1 acts as object.

Therefore object distance from second lens is = 20 + 20 = 40 cm or $v_1' = -40$ cm

f of this lens = 30 cm

$$\therefore \frac{1}{v}-\frac{1}{v'_1}=\frac{1}{f} \Rightarrow \frac{1}{v}=\frac{1}{v'_1}+\frac{1}{f} \Rightarrow \frac{1}{v}=-\frac{1}{40}+\frac{1}{30}=\frac{1}{120}$$

or v = 120 cm.

Final image is 120 cm right from second lens.

Example 11.

Consider the situation in figure. The bottom of the plot is a reflecting plane mirror. S is a small fish and T is a human eye, refractive index of water is μ (a) At what distance (s) from itself, will the fish see the image (s) of the eye (b) At what distance (s) from itself will the eye see the image (s) of the fish.

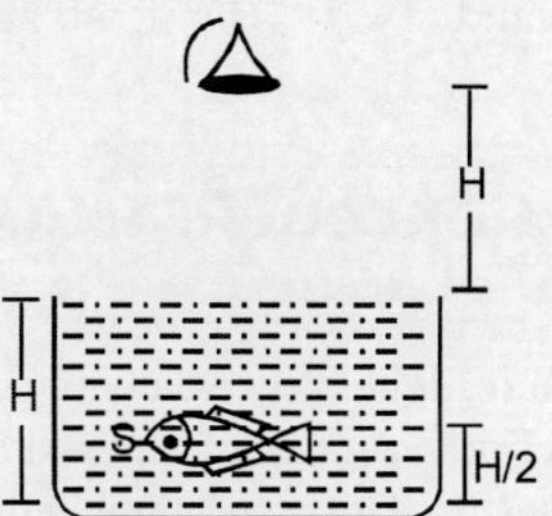

Solution :

(a) We have the formula

$$\frac{h_{app}}{h_{real}} = \frac{\mu}{1} = h_{app} = \mu H \text{ (from the surface of water)}$$

Now distance of fish from surface is H/2

∴ Image of eye as seen by fish is = H(μ + ½) above the fish.

also the apparent image of eye, again makes an image with the plane mirror, the apparent distance of eye is μH + H from the plane mirror

∴ Now image formed is μH + H below the plane mirror.

Distance of fish from the mirror is H/2

∴ Distance of image from the fish is μH + H + H/2 = H (μ + 3/2) below the fish.

(b) Here we have to find the images of fish as seen by the eye.

Let $h_{apparent}$ be the apparent distance of the fish from the surface

$$\therefore \frac{h_{app.}}{h_{real}} = \frac{1}{\mu};\ h_{app} = \frac{\mu H}{2\mu}$$

∴ Image formed is (H + H/2μ) below the, eye,

i.e, $H\left(1+\frac{1}{2\mu}\right)$ below the eye.

Also image of fish, formed by plane mirror is H/2 below the mirror.

$\therefore h_{real} = H + H/2 = 3H/2$

($\because h_{real}$ is distance of fish image formed by the mirror from the surface)

Now $\frac{h_{app}}{h_{real.}} = \frac{1}{\mu} \Rightarrow h_{app} = \frac{3H}{2\mu}$

$\therefore$ Image formed is $\left(H+\frac{3H}{2\mu}\right)$ below the eye i.e, $H\left(1+\frac{3}{2\mu}\right)$ below the eye.

Example 12.

A lens has a power of +5 diopter in air. What will be its power if completely immersed in water?

Given $\mu_g = \frac{3}{2}; \mu_w = \frac{4}{3}$

Solution :

Let f_a and f_w be the focal lengths of the lens in air water respectively, then

$$P_a = \frac{1}{f_a} \text{ and } P_w = \frac{\mu_w}{f_w}; \; f_a = 0.2 \text{ m} = 20 \text{ cm}$$

Using lens maker's formula

$$P_a = \frac{1}{f_a} = (\mu_g - 1)\left[\frac{1}{R_1} - \frac{1}{R_2}\right] \quad ...(i)$$

$$\frac{1}{f_w} = \left(\frac{\mu_g}{\mu_w} - 1\right)\left[\frac{1}{R_1} - \frac{1}{R_2}\right]$$

$$\Rightarrow P_w = \frac{\mu_w}{f_w} = (\mu_g - \mu_w)\left[\frac{1}{R_1} - \frac{1}{R_2}\right] \quad ...(ii)$$

Dividing equation (ii) by equation (i), we get,

$$\frac{P_w}{P_a} = \frac{(\mu_g - \mu_w)}{(\mu_g - 1)} = \frac{1}{3} \text{ or } P_w = \frac{P_a}{3} = \frac{+5}{3} = \frac{10}{3}\text{D}$$

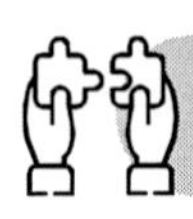

24.2 Concept Practice Problems

CPP

11. Monochromatic light of wavelength λ_1 travelling in a medium of refractive index μ_1 enters a denser medium of refractive index μ_2. The wavelength in the second medium is

(a) $\lambda_1 (\mu_1/\mu_2)$ (b) $\lambda_1 (\mu_2/\mu_1)$

(c) $\lambda_1 (\mu_2 - \mu_1)/\mu_2$ (d) $\lambda_1 (\mu_2 - \mu_1)/\mu_1$

12. A vessel of depth 2d cm is half filled with a liquid of refractive index μ_1 and the upper half with a liquid of refractive index μ_2. The apparent depth of the vessel seen perpendicularly is

(a) $\left(\frac{\mu_1 \mu_2}{\mu_1 + \mu_2}\right)d$ (b) $\left(\frac{1}{\mu_1} + \frac{1}{\mu_2}\right)d$

(c) $\left(\frac{1}{\mu_1} + \frac{1}{\mu_2}\right)2d$ (d) $\left(\frac{1}{\mu_1 \mu_2}\right)2d$

13. Which of the following is not the case with the image formed by a concave lens?

(a) It may be erect or inverted

(b) It may be magnified or diminished

(c) It may be real or virtual

(d) Real image may be between the pole and focus or beyond focus

14. Critical angle of light passing from glass to water is minimum for

(a) red colour (b) green colour

(c) yellow colour (d) violet colour

15. Light travels through a glass plate of thickness t and having refractive index μ. If c be the velocity of light in vacuum, the time taken by the light to travel this thickness of glass is

(a) $\frac{t}{\mu c}$ (b) $t\mu c$ (c) $\frac{\mu t}{c}$ (d) $\frac{tc}{\mu}$

16. The distance between an object and its real image formed by a convex lens cannot be

(a) greater than 2 f (b) less than 2 f

(c) greater than 4 f (d) less than 4 f

17. An electromagnetic radiation of frequency n, wavelength λ, travelling with velocity v in air enters in a glass slab of refractive index (μ). The frequency, wavelength and velocity of light in the glass slab will be respectively

(a) $n, \frac{\lambda}{\mu}$ and $\frac{v}{\mu}$ (b) $n, 2\lambda$ and $\frac{v}{\mu}$

(c) $\frac{n}{\mu}, \frac{\lambda}{\mu}$ and $\frac{v}{\mu}$ (d) $\frac{2\pi}{\mu}, \frac{\lambda}{\mu}$ and v

18. Two thin lenses of focal lengths f_1 and f_2 are in contact and coaxial. Its power is same as power of a single lens given by

(a) $\frac{f_1 + f_2}{f_1 f_2}$ (b) $\sqrt{\left(\frac{f_1}{f_2}\right)}$ (c) $\sqrt{\left(\frac{f_2}{f_1}\right)}$ (d) $\frac{f_1 + f_2}{2}$

19. For the angle of minimum deviation of a prism to be equal to its refracting angle, the prism must be made of a material whose refractive index

(a) lies between $\sqrt{2}$ and 1

(b) lies between 2 and $\sqrt{2}$

(c) is less than 1

(d) is greater than 2

20. Which of the following is not due to total internal reflection?

(a) Working of optical fibre

(b) Difference between apparent and real depth of pond

(c) Mirage on hot summer days

(d) Brilliance of diamond

ANSWER KEY

11	(a)	12	(b)	13	(d)	14	(d)	15	(c)	16	(d)	17	(a)	18	(a)	19	(b)	20	(b)

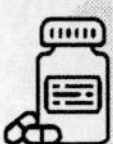

Topic 24.3 : Optical Instruments

OPTICAL INSTRUMENTS

(i) Simple Microscope

It is known as simple magnifier & consist of a convergent lens with object between its focus & optical centre & eye close to it.

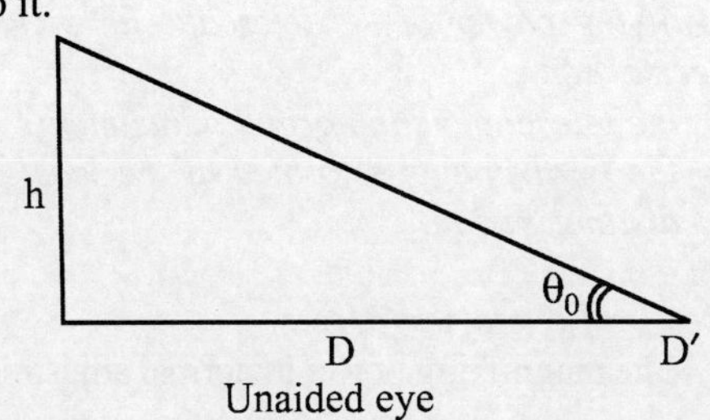

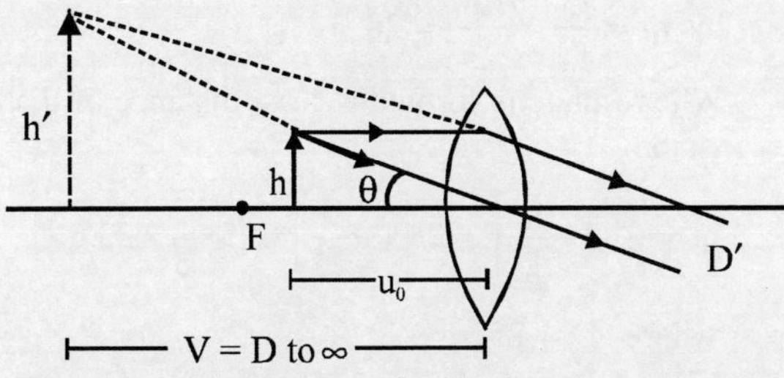

The magnifying power of a simple microscope (M.P.) is

$$M.P. = \frac{\textit{visual angle with instrument}}{\textit{max visual angle for unaided eye}} = \frac{\theta}{\theta_0}$$

Here $\theta_0 = \frac{h}{D}, \theta = \frac{h_1}{v} = \frac{h}{u}$ so $\text{M.P.} = \frac{\theta}{\theta_0} = \frac{h}{v} \times \frac{D}{h} = \frac{D}{u}$

(a) If image is at infinity [far point] then from lens formula

$$\frac{1}{v} - \frac{1}{u} = \frac{1}{f} \Rightarrow \frac{1}{\alpha} - \frac{1}{-u} = \frac{1}{f} \text{ i.e., } u = f \text{ \& } M.P. = \frac{D}{f}$$

In this case M.P. is minimum if eye is least strained.

(b) If image is at D [near point] then u = –D

and from lens formula $\frac{1}{v} - \frac{1}{u} = \frac{1}{f}$

we get $\frac{D}{u} = (1 + \frac{D}{f})$ so, $M.P = \left(1 + \frac{D}{f}\right)$

In this case M.P. is maximum and as final image is close to eye, eye is under maximum strain.

(ii) Compound Microscope

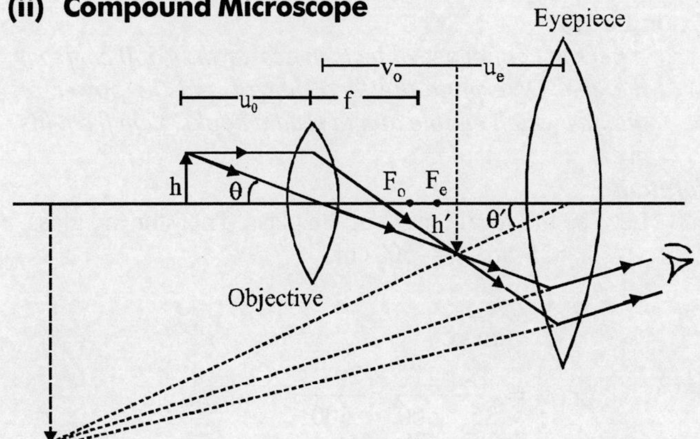

M.P. of compound microscope is defined as

$$M.P = \frac{\textit{visual angle with the instrument}}{\textit{max. visual angle for unaided eye}} = \frac{\theta}{\theta_0}$$

where $\theta_0 = \frac{h}{D}$, $\theta = \frac{h_1}{u_e}$

so $\text{M.P.} = \frac{h_1}{u_e} \times \frac{D}{h} = \left(\frac{h_1}{h}\right)\left(\frac{D}{u_e}\right)$

(since for objective $m = \frac{T}{o} = \frac{v}{u} \Rightarrow \frac{h^1}{h} = -\frac{v}{u}$, as u is –ive)

so $M.P. = \frac{-v}{u}\left(\frac{D}{u_e}\right)$

(a) **When image is formed at least distance of distinct vision,** $M = \frac{v_0}{u_0}\left(1 + \frac{D}{f_e}\right) = M_0 \times M_e$

(b) **When the final image is formed at infinity**

$$M = \frac{-v_0}{u_0}\left(\frac{D}{f_e}\right)$$

(iii) Astronomical Telescope

(a) **If the final image is formed at a distance D,**

$$M = \frac{-f_0}{f_e}\left(1 + \frac{f_e}{D}\right)$$

and **length of tube** is $L = f_0 + \frac{f_e D}{f_e + D}$

(b) **If the final image is formed at infinity** then

$M = \frac{f_0}{f_e}$ and the **length of tube** is $\ell = f_0 + f_e$

(iv) Galilean Telescope

$M = \frac{f_0}{f_e}$; **Length of tube** $L = f_o - f_e$

(v) Terrestrial Telescope

$M = \frac{f_0}{f_e}$;

Length of tube $L = f_o + f_e + 4f$, where f is the focal length of erecting lens, which is used in this telescope.

Resolving Power of Microscope and Telescope

(i) The **resolving power of microscope** is $R = \frac{2\mu \sin\theta}{\lambda}$

where μ = refractive index of medium between object and objective of microscope and θ = angle subtended by a radius of the objective on one of the objects. (When both objects are not self illuminous).

(ii) The **resolving power of a telescope** is $R = \frac{a}{1.22\lambda}$ where a = diameter of objective of telescope.

Problem Solving Tips

1.

	Refracting type telescope (use of lenses)		Reflecting type telescope (use of mirrors)
1	It suffers from spherical aberration and chromatic aberration.	1	It is almost free from spherical aberration and asbolutely free from chromatic aberration.
2	The lenses used have small aperature and therefore light gathering power is small.	2	The aperature of mirrors used is large and therefore light gathering power is large.

2.

	Simple microscope		Compound microscope
1	Use of single lens of small focal length.	1	Use of two lenses $f_0 < f_e$.
2	Magnifying power $M = \left(1 + \frac{D}{f}\right)$ When image formed at D $M = \frac{D}{f}$ When Image formed at infinite.	2	Magnifying power $M = -\frac{v_0}{u_0}\left(1 + \frac{D}{f_e}\right)$ When image formed at D $M = -\frac{v_0}{u_0}\frac{D}{f_e}$ When image formed at infinite.
3	Object is placed between optical centre and focus.	3	Object is placed just outside the principle focus.

3.

	Astronomical telescope		Galilean telescope
1	Both lenses are convex lens.	1	Objective is convex lens and eye piece is concave lens
2	Magnifying power $M = -\frac{f_0}{f_e}$ for normal adjustment.	2	Magnifying power $M = +\frac{f_0}{f_e}$ for normal adjustment.
3	Length of telescope $L = f_0 + f_e$	3	Length of telescope $L = f_0 - f_e$

4. Some common eye defects are myopia, hypermetropia, astigmatism and presbyopia.

5.

	Myopia (or short sightedness)		Hypermetropia (or long - sightedness)
1	Eye can see near objects clearly but cannot see far objects clearly because the light from the for off object arriving the eye lens may get converged in front of retina.	1	Eye can see far off objects clearly but cannot see near objects clearly because the light from the near by object arriving the eye lens may get converged at a point behind the retina.
2	It can be corrected by concave lens (power of concave lens is –ve).	2	It can be corrected by convex lens (Power of convex lens is +ve).

6. **Astigmatism :** It is due to different curvature of cornea in horizontal and vertical plane. It is corrected by using **cylindrical lens.**

7. **Presbyopia :** The eye with this defect cannot see near objects as well as far off objects clearly.

Example 13.

A small telescope has an objective of focal length 140cm and an eye piece of focal length 5.0cm. What is the magnifying power of the telescope for viewing distant objects when

(a) the telescope is in normal adjustment?

(b) the final image is formed at the least distance of distinct vision?

Solution :

Here, $f_0 = 140$ cm, $f_e = 5.0$ cm

(a) The magnifying power in normal adjustment is given by $m = \frac{f_0}{f_e} = \frac{140}{5} = 28$

(b) When image is formed at least distance of distinct vision

$$m = \frac{f_0}{f_e}\left[1 + \frac{f_e}{D}\right] = 28\left[1 + \frac{5}{25}\right] = 25 \times \frac{6}{5} = 33.6$$

where D = 25cm

Example 14.

A compound microscope has an objective of focal length 1 cm and an eyepiece of focal length 2.5 cm. An object has to be placed at a distance of 1.2 cm away from the objective, for normal adjustment. Find (a) the angular magnification and (b) the length of the microscope tube.

Solution :

(a) If the first image is formed at a distance v from the objective, then we have

$$\frac{1}{v} - \frac{1}{(-1.2\text{ cm})} = \frac{1}{1\text{ cm}} \text{ or } v = 6\text{ cm}.$$

The angular magnification in normal adjustment is,

$$m = \frac{v}{u}\frac{D}{f_e} = -\frac{6\text{ cm}}{1.2\text{ cm}} \cdot \frac{25\text{ cm}}{2.5\text{ cm}} = -50.$$

(b) For normal adjustment, the first image must be in the focal plane of the eyepiece.

The length of the tube is, therefore,

$$L = v + f_e = 6\text{ cm} + 2.5\text{ cm} = 8.5\text{ cm}$$

Example 15.

A person cannot see objects in nearer than 500 cm from the eye. Determine the focal length and the power of glasses which enable him to read a book 25 cm from his eye.

Solution :

Let f be the focal length of the glass. Then for the glass, u = 25 cm, v = –500 cm

$$\because \frac{1}{f} = \frac{1}{u} + \frac{1}{v}$$

$$\text{or, } \frac{1}{f} = \frac{1}{25} - \frac{1}{500} = \frac{20 - 1}{500}$$

or, $f = \frac{500}{19} = 26.3 \text{ cm} = 0.263 \text{ m}$

$$P(\text{power}) = \frac{1}{f} = \frac{1}{0.263} = 3.8 \text{ dioptre}$$

Example 16.

What is the power of the spectacles required (a) by a hypermetropic eye whose near point is 125 cm (b) by a myopic eye whose far point is 50 cm ?

Solution :

(a) u = 25 cm, v = –125 cm

$$\frac{1}{f} = \frac{1}{u} + \frac{1}{v}$$

or, $\frac{1}{f} = \frac{1}{25} - \frac{1}{125} = \frac{5-1}{125}$

or, $f = \frac{125}{4} = 31.25 \text{ cm} = 0.3125 \text{ m}$

$$P = \frac{1}{f} = \frac{1}{0.3125} = 3.2 \text{ dioptre}$$

(b) u = ∞, v = –50 cm

$$\because \frac{1}{f} = \frac{1}{u} + \frac{1}{v}$$

$$\frac{1}{f} = \frac{1}{\infty} + \frac{1}{v}$$

or, $\frac{1}{f} = \frac{1}{\infty} - \frac{1}{50} = -\frac{1}{50}$

$\Rightarrow f = -50 \text{ cm} = -0.5 \text{ m}$

$$P = \frac{1}{f} = -\frac{1}{0.5} = -2 \text{ dioptre}$$

Example 17.

A person with normal vision has a range of accommodation from 25 cm to infinity. Over what range would he be able to see objects distinctly when wearing the spectacles of a friend whose correction is +4 dioptres.

Solution :

P = 4 dioptres, $\therefore f = \frac{1}{4} \text{m} = 25 \text{ cm}$

For near point, v = –25 cm,

$$u = \frac{vf}{v-f} = \frac{-25 \times 25}{-25-25} = 12.5 \text{cm}$$

For far point, v = ∞

$$\because \frac{1}{u} + \frac{1}{v} = \frac{1}{f}$$

$$\frac{1}{u} + \frac{1}{\infty} = \frac{1}{25}$$

or u = 25 cm

Hence, the range of distinct vision is from 12.5 cm to 25 cm.

Example 18.

Where is the near point of an eye for which a spectacle lens of +1 dioptre is prescribed ?

Solution :

P = +1 dioptre.

$$\therefore f = \frac{1}{P} = \frac{1}{1} = 1 \text{ m} = 100 \text{ cm}$$

For the spectacle lens,

u = 25 cm, f = 100 cm, v = ?

$$\because \frac{1}{u} + \frac{1}{v} = \frac{1}{f}$$

or $\frac{1}{v} = \frac{1}{f} - \frac{1}{u} = \frac{u-f}{uf}$

or $v = \frac{uf}{u-f} = \frac{25 \times 100}{25-100} = -33.33 \text{cm}$

i.e., the near point is 33.33 cm from the eye.

Example 19.

A certain person can see clearly at distance between 20 cm and 200 cm from his eye. What sepctacles are required to enable him to see distant objects clearly and what will be his least distance of distinct vision when he is wearing them?

Solution :

For seeing distant objects

u = ∞, v = –200 cm, f = ?

$$\because \frac{1}{f} = \frac{1}{u} + \frac{1}{v}$$

or, $\frac{1}{f} = \frac{1}{\infty} - \frac{1}{200} = -\frac{1}{200}$ or f = –200cm

For finding the least distance of distinct vision

u = ?, v = –20 cm, f = –200cm.

$$u = \frac{vf}{v-f} = \frac{-20(-200)}{-20-(-200)} = \frac{(20 \times 200)}{180} = 22.2 \text{cm}$$

i.e., his least distance of distinct vision is 22.2 cm when he is wearing spectacles.

Example 20.

An elderly person cannot see clearly, without the use of spectacles, objects nearer than 200 cm. What spectacles will he need to reduce this distance to 25 cm ? If his eyes can focus rays which are converging to points not less than 150 cm behind them, calculate his range of distinct vision when using the spectacles.

Solution :

Here u = 25 cm, v = – 200 cm

$$\because \frac{1}{f} = \frac{1}{u} + \frac{1}{v}$$

or, $\frac{1}{f} = \frac{1}{25} - \frac{1}{200} = \frac{8-1}{200}$

$\Rightarrow f = \frac{200}{7} = 28.6 \text{ cm}$

i.e., he should use the converging lens of focal length 28.6 cm.

Let x be the object distance for v = 150 cm, then

$$\frac{1}{x} + \frac{1}{150} = \frac{1}{f} = \frac{7}{200}$$

$$\Rightarrow \frac{1}{x} = \frac{7}{200} - \frac{1}{150} = \frac{21-4}{600}$$

$$\Rightarrow x = \frac{600}{17} = 35.3 \text{cm}$$

∴ Range of distinct vision is 25 cm to 35.3 cm.

Example 21.

An angular magnification (magnifying power) of 30 × is desired using an objective of focal length 1.25 cm. and an eyepiece of focal length 5 cm. in a compound microscope. What is the separation between objective and the eyepiece ?

Solution :

Let final image be formed at lease distance of distinct vision

For eyepiece, $M_e = \left(1+\frac{25}{f_e}\right) = \left(1+\frac{25}{5}\right) = 6$

Now, $M = M_0 \times M_e$

For objective, $M_0 = \frac{M}{M_e} = \frac{-30}{6} = -5$,

For objective, if $u_0 = -x$ cm, $v_0 = 5x$ cm.

Again, $\frac{1}{v} - \frac{1}{u} = \frac{1}{f}$ or $\frac{1}{5x} - \frac{1}{-x} = \frac{1}{1.25}$

On simplification, $x = 1.5$

$\therefore$ $u_0 = -1.5$ cm, $v_0 = 7.5$ cm.

For eyepiece, $M_e = \frac{v_e}{u_e}$

or $u_e = \frac{v_e}{M_e} = \frac{-25}{6} = -4.17$ cm.

Distance between objective and eyepiece

$= v_{objective} + |u_{eyepiece}| = 7.5 + 4.17 = 11.67$ cm.

Example 22.

A small telescope has an objective lens of focal length 144 cm. and eye-piece of focal length 6.0 cm. What is the magnifying power of the telescope ? What is the separation between objective and eye-piece ? Assume normal adjustment.

Solution :

$M = \frac{f_0}{f_e} = \frac{144}{6} = 24$

$L = f_0 + f_e = (144 + 6)$ cm. $= 150$ cm.

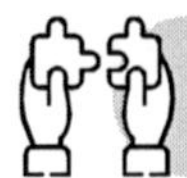

24.3 Concept Practice Problems

CPP

21. The image formed by an objective of a compound microscope is
(a) real and diminished (b) real and enlarged
(c) virtual and enlarged (d) virtual and diminished

22. To increase the angular magnification of a simple microscope, one should increase
(a) the focal length of the lens
(b) the power of the lens
(c) the aperture of the lens
(d) the object size

23. In a compound microscope, the focal length of objective lens is 1.2 cm and focal length of eye piece is 3.0 cm. When object is kept at 1.25 cm in front of objective, final image is formed at infinity. Magnifying power of the compound microscope should be:
(a) 200 (b) 100 (c) 400 (d) 150

24. An astronomical telescope has a large aperture to
(a) reduce spherical aberration
(b) have high resolution
(c) increase span of observation
(d) have low dispersion

25. A student look at distant tree of height 15m with a telescope of magnifying power 25. To the student, the tree appears.
(a) 20 times taller (b) 15 times taller
(c) 15 times nearer (d) 25 times nearer

26. A normal eye has retina 2cm behind the eye lens. What is the power of the eye-lens when the eye is fully relaxed?
(a) 50 D (b) 54 D (c) 40 D (d) 45 D

27. The magnifying power of a telescope is 9. When it is adjusted for parallel rays, the distance between the objective and the eye piece is found to be 20 cm. The focal length of lenses are
(a) 18 cm, 2 cm (b) 11 cm, 9 cm
(c) 10 cm, 10 cm (d) 15 cm, 5 cm

28. The focal length of the objective of a telescope is 60 cm. To obtain a magnification of 20, the focal length of the eye piece should be
(a) 2 cm (b) 3 cm (c) 4 cm (d) 5 cm

29. The focal lengths of objective and eye lens of an astronomical telelscope are respectively 2 meter and 5 cm. Final image is formed at (i) least distance of distinct vision (ii) infinity Magnifying power in two cases will be
(a) $-48, -40$ (b) $-40, -48$
(c) $-40, +48$ (d) $-48, +40$

30. An astronomical telescope has an angular magnification of magnitude 5 for distant objects. The separation between the objective and the eye-piece is 36 cms and the final image is formed at infinity. The focal length f_0 of the objective and f_e of the eye piece are
(a) $f_0 = 45$ cm and $f_2 = -9$ cm
(b) $f_0 = 50$ cm and $f_e = 10$ cm
(c) $f_0 = 7.2$ cm and $f_e = 5$ cm
(d) $f_0 = 30$ cm and $f_e = 6$ cm

ANSWER KEY

21	(b)	22	(b)	23	(a)	24	(b)	25	(d)	26	(a)	27	(a)	28	(b)	29	(a)	30	(d)

CONCEPT MAP

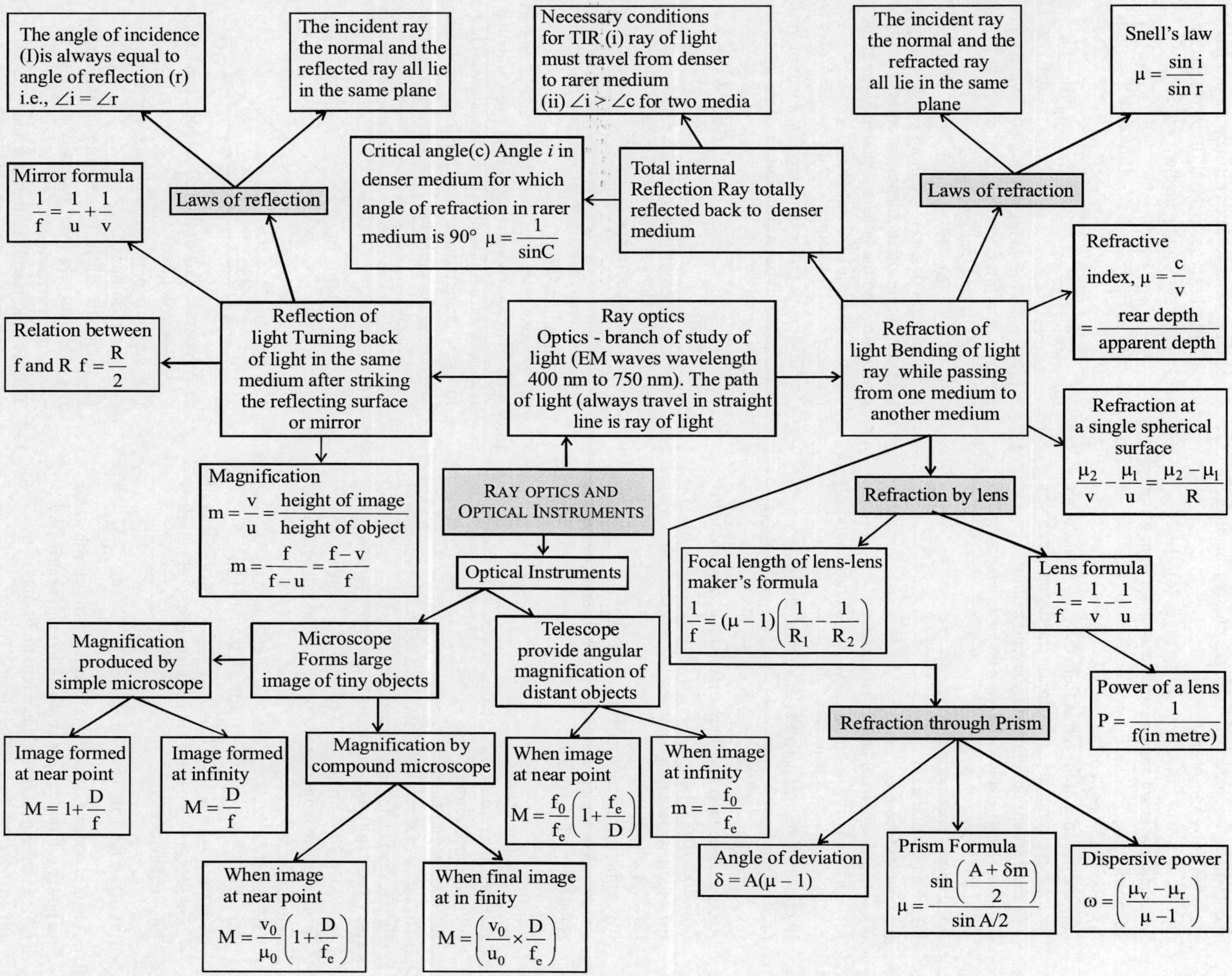

RAY OPTICS AND OPTICAL INSTRUMENTS

Ray optics
Optics - branch of study of light (EM waves wavelength 400 nm to 750 nm). The path of light (always travel in straight line is ray of light

Reflection of light Turning back of light in the same medium after striking the reflecting surface or mirror

- **Laws of reflection**
  - The angle of incidence (I)is always equal to angle of reflection (r) i.e., $\angle i = \angle r$
  - The incident ray the normal and the reflected ray all lie in the same plane
- Mirror formula $\frac{1}{f} = \frac{1}{u} + \frac{1}{v}$
- Relation between f and R $f = \frac{R}{2}$
- Magnification $m = -\frac{v}{u} = \frac{\text{height of image}}{\text{height of object}}$, $m = \frac{f}{f-u} = \frac{f-v}{f}$

Refraction of light Bending of light ray while passing from one medium to another medium

- **Laws of refraction**
  - The incident ray the normal and the refracted ray all lie in the same plane
  - Snell's law $\mu = \frac{\sin i}{\sin r}$
- Refractive index, $\mu = \frac{c}{v}$ $= \frac{\text{rear depth}}{\text{apparent depth}}$
- Refraction at a single spherical surface $\frac{\mu_2}{v} - \frac{\mu_1}{u} = \frac{\mu_2 - \mu_1}{R}$
- Total internal Reflection Ray totally reflected back to denser medium
  - Necessary conditions for TIR (i) ray of light must travel from denser to rarer medium (ii) $\angle i > \angle c$ for two media
  - Critical angle(c) Angle *i* in denser medium for which angle of refraction in rarer medium is 90° $\mu = \frac{1}{\sin C}$
- **Refraction by lens**
  - Focal length of lens-lens maker's formula $\frac{1}{f} = (\mu - 1)\left(\frac{1}{R_1} - \frac{1}{R_2}\right)$
  - Lens formula $\frac{1}{f} = \frac{1}{v} - \frac{1}{u}$
    - Power of a lens $P = \frac{1}{f(\text{in metre})}$
- **Refraction through Prism**
  - Angle of deviation $\delta = A(\mu - 1)$
  - Prism Formula $\mu = \frac{\sin\left(\frac{A + \delta m}{2}\right)}{\sin A/2}$
  - Dispersive power $\omega = \left(\frac{\mu_v - \mu_r}{\mu - 1}\right)$

Optical Instruments

- Microscope Forms large image of tiny objects
  - Magnification produced by simple microscope
    - Image formed at near point $M = 1 + \frac{D}{f}$
    - Image formed at infinity $M = \frac{D}{f}$
  - Magnification by compound microscope
    - When image at near point $M = \frac{v_0}{\mu_0}\left(1 + \frac{D}{f_e}\right)$
    - When final image at in finity $M = \left(\frac{v_0}{u_0} \times \frac{D}{f_e}\right)$
- Telescope provide angular magnification of distant objects
  - When image at near point $M = \frac{f_0}{f_e}\left(1 + \frac{f_e}{D}\right)$
  - When image at infinity $m = -\frac{f_0}{f_e}$

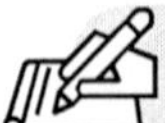

Exercise 1 - Chapter Revision Problems

CRP

1. What will be the colour of the sky as seen from the earth if there were no atmosphere?
(a) Black (b) Blue (c) Orange (d) Red

2. A normal eye is not able to see objects closer than 25 cm because
(a) the focal length of the eye is 25 cm
(b) the distance of the retina from the eye-lens is 25 cm
(c) the eye is not able to decrease the distance between the eye-lens and the retina beyond a limit
(d) the eye is not able to decrease the focal length beyond a limit

3. What causes chromatic aberration?
(a) Non - paraxial rays
(b) Paraxial rays
(c) Variation of focal length with colour
(d) Difference in radii of curvature of the bounding surfaces of the lens

4. In optical fibres, propagation of light is due to
(a) diffraction (b) total internal reflection
(c) reflection (d) refraction

5. Rectilinear motion of light in a medium is caused due to
(a) high frequency
(b) short wavelength
(c) velocity of light
(d) uniform refractive index of the medium

6. A convex lens is dipped in a liquid whose refractive index is equal to the refractive index of the lens. Then its focal length will
(a) remain unchanged
(b) become zero
(c) become infinite
(d) become small, but non-zero

7. The index of refraction of diamond is 2.0. The velocity of light in diamond is approximately
(a) 1.5×10^{10} cm/sec (b) 2×10^{10} cm/sec
(c) 3.0×10^{10} cm/sec (d) 6×10^{10} cm/sec

8. The refractive index of water is 1.33. What will be speed of light in water ?
(a) 3×10^8 m/s (b) 2.25×10^8 m/s
(c) 4×10^8 m/s (d) 1.33×10^8 m/s

9. A convex lens of focal length f_1 and a concave lens of focal length f_2 are placed in contact. The focal length of the combination is
(a) $(f_1 + f_2)$ (b) $(f_1 - f_2)$ (c) $\frac{f_1 f_2}{f_2 - f_1}$ (d) $\frac{f_1 f_2}{f_1 + f_2}$

10. A lens of power + 2 diopter is placed in contact with a lens of power – 1 diopter. The combination will behave like
(a) a convergent lens of focal length 50 cm
(b) a divergent lens of focal length 100 cm
(c) a convergent lens of focal length 100 cm
(d) a convergent lens of focal length 200 cm

11. Light takes t_1 sec to travel a distance x in vacuum and the same light takes t_2 sec to travel 10 cm in a medium. Critical angle for corresponding medium will be
(a) $\sin^{-1}\left(\frac{10 t_2}{t_1 x}\right)$ (b) $\sin^{-1}\left(\frac{t_2 x}{10 t_1}\right)$
(c) $\sin^{-1}\left(\frac{10 t_1}{t_2 x}\right)$ (d) $\sin^{-1}\left(\frac{t_1 x}{10 t_2}\right)$

12. A prism has a refracting angle of 60°. When placed in the position of minimum deviation, it produces a deviation of 30°. The angle of incidence is
(a) 30° (b) 45° (c) 15° (d) 60°

13. A ray of light passes through an equilateral prism such that the angle of incidence is equal to the angle of emergence and the latter is equal to 3/4th of the angle of prism. The angle of deviation is
(a) 45° (b) 39° (c) 20° (d) 30°

14. The dispersive power of material of a lens of focal length 20 cm is 0.08. What is the longitudinal chromatic aberration of the lens ?
(a) 0.08 cm (b) 0.08/20 cm
(c) 1.6 cm (d) 0.16 cm

15. Which of the following is false ?
(a) Convex lens always forms image with m < 1
(b) A simple mirror produces virtual, erect and same-sized image
(c) A concave mirror produces virtual, erect and magnified image
(d) A convex lens can produce real and same-sized image

16. A beam of light consisting of red, green and blue colours is incident on a right-angled prism as shown. The refractive index of the material of the prism for the above red, green and blue wavelengths are 1.39, 1.44 and 1.47 respectively. The prism will

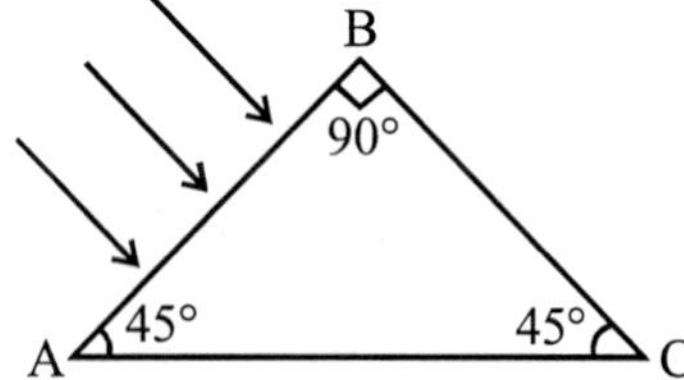

(a) separate part of the red colour from the green and blue colours.
(b) separate part of the blue colour from the red and green colours.
(c) separate all the three colours from one another.
(d) not separate even partially any colour from the other two colours.

17. The maximum and minimum distance between a convex lens and an object, for the magnification of a real image to be greater than one are
(a) 2f and f (b) f and zero
(c) ∞ and 2f (d) 4f and 2f

18. A plane convex lens of focal length 16 cm, is to be made of glass of refractive index 1.5. The radius of curvature of the curved surface should be

(a) 8 cm (b) 12 cm (c) 16 cm (d) 24 cm

19. A real image is formed by a convex lens. If we put a concave lens in contact with it, the combination again forms a real image. The new image

(a) is closer to the lens system.
(b) is farther form the lens system.
(c) is at the original position.
(d) may be anywhere depending on the focal length of the concave lens.

20. A plano-convex lens of focal length 30 cm has its plane surface silvered. An object is placed 40 cm from the lens on the convex side. The distance of the image from the lens is

(a) 18 cm (b) 24 cm (c) 30 cm (d) 40 cm

21. If D is the deviation of a normally falling light beam on a thin prism of angle A and δ is the dispersive power of the same prism then

(a) D is independent of A.
(b) D is independent of refractive Index.
(c) δ is independent of refractive index.
(d) δ is independent of A.

22. Why is refractive index in a transparent medium greater than one ?

(a) Because the speed of light in vaccum is always less than speed in a transparent medium
(b) Because the speed of light in vaccum is always greater than speed in a transparent medium
(c) Frequency of wave changes when it crosses medium
(d) None of these

23. Two convex lenses of focal lengths 0.3 m and 0.05 m are used to make a telescope. The distance kept between the two in order to obtain an image at infinity is

(a) 0.35m (b) 0.25m (c) 0.175m (d) 0.15m

24. The refractive indices of glass and water with respect to air are 3/2 and 4/3 respectively. Then the refractive index of glass with respect to water is

(a) 8/9 (b) 9/8 (c) 7/6 (d) 2

25. The frequency of a light wave in a material is 2×10^{14} Hz and wavelength is 5000 Å. The refractive index of material will be

(a) 1.50 (b) 3.00 (c) 1.33 (d) 1.40

26. A ray incident at 15° on one refracting surface of a prism of angle 60° suffers a deviation of 55°. What is the angle of emergence ?

(a) 95° (b) 45°
(c) 30° (d) None of these

27. A man's near point is 0.5 m and far point is 3 m. Power of spectacle lenses required for (i) reading purposes, (ii) seeing distant objects, respectively, are

(a) –2 D and + 3 D (b) +2 D and –3 D
(c) +2 D and –0.33 D (d) –2 D and + 0.33 D

28. Light passes through a glass plate of thickness d and refractive index μ. For small angle of incidence i, the lateral displacement is

(a) id (b) $id(\mu-1)$
(c) $\dfrac{id(\mu-1)}{\mu}$ (d) $\dfrac{id\mu}{\mu-1}$

29. A glass slab of thickness 4 cm contains the same number of waves as 5 cm of water when both are traversed by the same monochromatic light. If the refractive index of water is 4/3, what is that of glass?

(a) 5/3 (b) 5/4 (c) 16/15 (d) 1.5

30. An air bubble in glass slab ($\mu = 1.5$) from one side is 6 cm and from other side is 4 cm. The thickness of glass slab is

(a) 10 cm (b) 6.67 cm
(c) 15 cm (d) None of these

31. A man 160 cm high stands in front of a plane mirror. His eyes are at a height of 150 cm from the floor. Then the minimum length of the plane mirror for him to see his full length image is

(a) 85 cm (b) 170 cm (c) 80 cm (d) 340 cm

32. Two thin lenses are in contact and the focal length of the combination is 80 cm. If the focal length of one lens is 20 cm, then the power of the other lens will be

(a) 1.66 D (b) 4.00 D (c) – 100 D (d) – 3.75 D

33. The angle of prism is 60° and angle of deviation is 30°. In the position of minimum deviation, the values of angle of incidence and angle of emergence are:

(a) $i = 45°; e = 50°$ (b) $i = 30°; e = 45°$
(c) $i = 45°; e = 45°$ (d) $i = 30°; e = 30°$

34. Light travels in two media *A* and *B* with speeds 1.8×10^8 m s^{-1} and 2.4×10^8 m s^{-1} respectively. Then the critical angle between them is

(a) $\sin^{-1}\left(\dfrac{2}{3}\right)$ (b) $\tan^{-1}\left(\dfrac{3}{4}\right)$
(c) $\tan^{-1}\left(\dfrac{2}{3}\right)$ (d) $\sin^{-1}\left(\dfrac{3}{4}\right)$

35. A convex lens is immersed in a liquid of refractive index greater than that of glass. It will behave as a

(a) convergent lens (b) divergent lens
(c) plane glass (d) homogeneous liquid

36. A parallel beam of light is incident on the surface of a transparent hemisphere of radius *R* and refractive index 2.0 as shown in figure. The position of the image formed by refraction at the first surface is :

(a) *R*/2
(b) *R*
(c) 2*R*
(d) 3*R*

37. Yellow light is refracted through a prism producing minimum deviation. If i_1 and i_2 denote the angle of incidence and emergence for this prism, then

(a) $i_1 = i_2$ (b) $i_1 > i_2$
(c) $i_1 < i_2$ (d) $i_1 + i_2 = 90°$

38. The graph between angle of deviation (δ) and angle of incidence (i) for a triangular prism is represented by

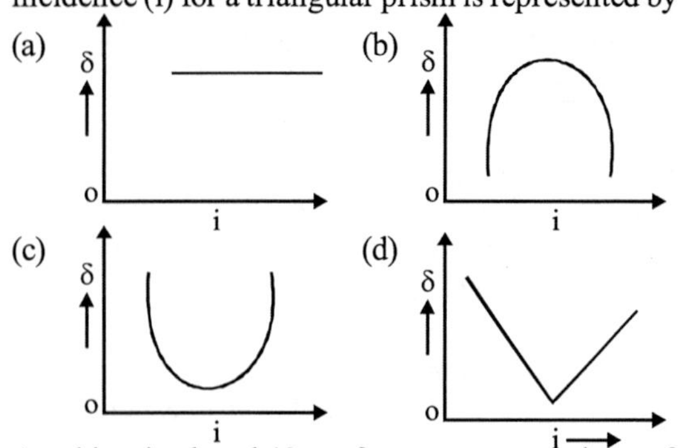

39. An object is placed 40 cm from a concave mirror of focal length 20 cm. The image formed is
(a) real, inverted and same in size
(b) real, inverted and smaller
(c) virtual, erect and larger
(d) virtual, erect and smaller

40. A thin convergent glass lens (μ_g = 1.5) has a power of + 5.0 D. When this lens is immersed in a liquid of refractive index μ, it acts as a divergent lens of focal length 100 cm. The value of μ must be
(a) 4/3 (b) 5/3 (c) 5/4 (d) 6/5

41. A ray of light passes through an equilateral prism (μ = 1.5). The angle of minimum deviation is
(a) 45° (b) 37° 12' (c) 20° (d) 30°

42. Two lenses in contact form an achromatic lens. Their focal lengths are in the ratio 2 : 3. Their dispersive powers must be in the ratio of
(a) 1 : 3 (b) 2 : 3 (c) 3 : 2 (d) 3 : 1

43. An achromatic convergent lens of focal length 20 cms is made of two lenses (in contact) of materials having dispersive powers in the ratio of 1 : 2 and having focal lengths f_1 and f_2. Which of the following is true ?
(a) $f_1 = 10$ cms, $f_2 = -20$ cms
(b) $f_1 = 20$ cms, $f_2 = 10$cms
(c) $f_1 = -10$ cms, $f_2 = -20$ cms
(d) $f_1 = 20$ cms, $f_2 = -20$ cms

44. Two lens of focal length f_1 and f_2 are kept in contact coaxially. The resultant power of combination will be
(a) $\dfrac{f_1 f_2}{f_1 - f_2}$ (b) $\dfrac{f_1 + f_2}{f_1 f_2}$ (c) $f_1 + f_2$ (d) $\dfrac{f_1}{f_2} + \dfrac{f_2}{f_1}$

45. When white light enters a prism, its gets split into its constituent colours. This is due to
(a) high density of prism material
(b) because μ is different for different wavelength
(c) diffraction of light
(d) velocity changes for different frequency

46. A pencil of light rays falls on a plane mirror and form a real image, so the incident rays are
(a) parallel (b) diverging
(c) converging (d) statement is false

47. Spherical aberration in a thin lens can be reduced by
(a) using a monochromatic light
(b) using a doublet combination
(c) using a circular annular mark over the lens
(d) increasing the size of the lens

48. A lens produces an image of an object on a screen. If a slab of refractive index *n* is placed in between lens and screen, the screen has to be moved by distance *d* behind. The thickness of slab is
(a) nd (b) $\dfrac{n-1}{nd}$ (c) $\dfrac{(n-1)d}{n}$ (d) $\dfrac{nd}{n-1}$

49. An object is moved along the principal axis of a converging lens from a position 5 focal lengths from the lens to a position that is 2 focal lengths from the lens. Which statement about the resulting image is most accurate?
(a) The image increases in size and decreases in distance from the lens
(b) The image increases in size and increases in distance from the lens
(c) The image decreases in size and decreases in distance from the lens
(d) The image decreases in size and increases in distance from the lens

50. An object is placed upright on the axis of a thin convex lens at a distance of four focal lengths (4f) from the center of the lens. An inverted image appears at a distance of 4/3 f on the other side of the lens. What is the ratio of the height of he image of the height of the object?
(a) 1/3 (b) 3/4 (c) 4/3 (d) 3/1

51. A diver inside water sees the setting sun at
(a) 41° to the horizon (b) 49° to the horizon
(c) 0° to the horizon (d) 45° to the horizon

52. The layered lens as shown is made of two types of transparent materials-one indicated by horizontal lines and the other by vertical lines. The number of images formed of an object will be
(a) 1
(b) 2
(c) 3
(d) 6

53. A ray of light traveling in water is incident on its surface open to air. The angle of incidence is θ, which is less than the critical angle. Then there will be
(a) only a reflected ray and no refracted ray
(b) only a refracted ray and no reflected ray
(c) a reflected ray and a refracted ray and the angle between them would be less than 180°–2θ
(d) a reflected ray and a refracted ray and the angle between them would be greater than 180°–2θ

54. Air has refractive index 1.0003. The thickness of air column, which will have one more wavelength of yellow light (6000 Å) than in the same thickness of vacuum is
(a) 2mm (b) 2 cm (c) 2m (d) 2km.

55. If f_V and f_R are the focal lengths of a convex lens for violet and red light respectively and F_V and F_R are the focal lengths of concave lens for violet and red light respectively, then we have

(a) $f_V < f_R$ and $F_V > F_R$ (b) $f_V < f_R$ and $F_V < F_R$
(c) $f_V > f_R$ and $F_V > F_R$ (d) $f_V > f_R$ and $F_V < F_R$

56. A ray is incident at an angle of incidence i on one surface of a prism of small angle A and emerges normally from the opposite surface. If the refractive index of the material of prism is μ, the angle of incidence i is nearly equal to
(a) $\frac{A}{\mu}$ (b) $\frac{A}{2\mu}$ (c) μA (d) $\frac{\mu A}{2}$

57. One face of a rectangular glass plate 6 cm thick is silvered. An object held 8 cm in front of the first face, forms an image 12 cm behind the silvered face. The refractive index of the glass is
(a) 0.4 (b) 0.8 (c) 1.2 (d) 1.6

58. A convex lens of focal length 80 cm and a concave lens of focal length 50 cm are combined together. What will be their resulting power?
(a) +6.5 D (b) –6.5 D (c) +7.5 D (d) –0.75 D

59. The radius of curvature of a thin plano-convex lens is 10 cm (of curved surface) and the refractive index is 1.5. If the plane surface is silvered, then it behaves like a concave mirror of focal length
(a) 10 cm (b) 15 cm (c) 20 cm (d) 5 cm

60. An air bubble in a glass slab (μ = 1.5) is 5 cm deep when viewed from one face and 2 cm deep when viewed from the opposite face. The thickness of the slab is
(a) 7.5 cm (b) 10.5 cm (c) 7 cm (d) 10 cm

61. A plano-convex lens is made of material of refractive index 1.6. The radius of curvature of the curved surface is 60 cm. The focal length of the lens is
(a) 50 cm (b) 100 cm (c) 200 cm (d) 400 cm

62. The refractive index of the material of the prism is $\sqrt{3}$; then the angle of minimum deviation of the prism is
(a) 30° (b) 45° (c) 60° (d) 75°

63. A ray of light travelling in a transparent medium of refractive index μ, falls on a surface separating the medium from air at an angle of incidence of 45°. For which of the following value of μ the ray can undergo total internal reflection?
(a) μ = 1.33 (b) μ = 1.40 (c) μ = 1.50 (d) μ = 1.25

64. A biconvex lens has a radius of curvature of magnitude 20 cm. Which one of the following options best describe the image formed of an object of height 2 cm placed 30 cm from the lens?
(a) Virtual, upright, height = 1 cm
(b) Virtual, upright, height = 0.5 cm
(c) Real, inverted, height = 4 cm
(d) Real, inverted, height = 1cm

65. A thin prism of angle 15° made of glass of refractive index μ_1 = 1.5 is combined with another prism of glass of refractive index μ_2 = 1.75. The combination of the prism produces dispersion without deviation. The angle of the second prism should be
(a) 7° (b) 10° (c) 12° (d) 5°

66.

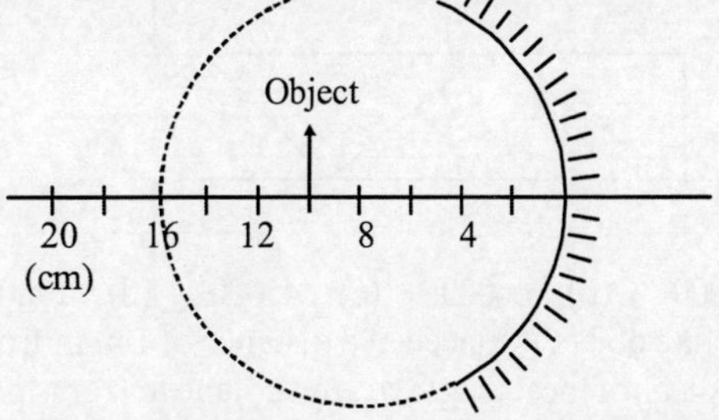

A spherical mirror is obtained as shown in the figure from a hollow glass sphere. If an object is positioned in front of the mirror, what will be the nature and magnification of the image of the object? (Figure drawn as schematic and not to scale)
(a) Inverted, real and magnified
(b) Erect, virtual and magnified
(c) Erect, virtual and unmagnified
(d) Inverted, real and unmagnified

67. A concave mirror for face viewing has focal length of 0.4 m. The distance at which you hold the mirror from your face in order to see your image upright with a magnification of 5 is:
(a) 0.24m (b) 1.60m (c) 0.32m (d) 0.16m

68. A vessel of depth 2h is half filled with a liquid of refractive index $2\sqrt{2}$ and the upper half with another liquid of refractive index $\sqrt{2}$. The liquids are immiscible. The apparent depth of the inner surface of the bottom of vessel will be:
(a) $\frac{h}{\sqrt{2}}$ (b) $\frac{h}{2(\sqrt{2}+1)}$ (c) $\frac{h}{3\sqrt{2}}$ (d) $\frac{3}{4}h\sqrt{2}$

69. The critical angle of a medium for a specific wavelength, if the medium has relative permittivity 3 and relative permeability $\frac{4}{3}$ for this wavelength, will be:
(a) 15° (b) 30° (c) 45° (d) 60°

70. A concave mirror has radius of curvature of 40 cm. It is at the bottom of a glass that has water filled up to 5 cm (see figure). If a small partricle is floating on the surface of water, its image as seen, from directly above the glass, is at a distance d from the surface of water. The value of d is close to : (Refractive index of water = 1.33)

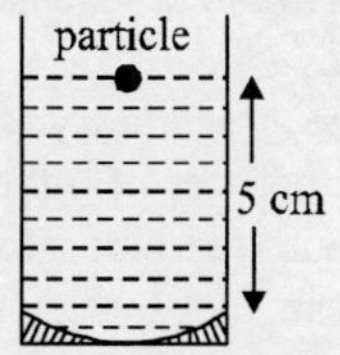

(a) 6.7 cm (b) 13.4 cm (c) 8.8 cm (d) 11.7 cm

71. In figure, the optical fiber is l = 2 m long and has a diameter of d = 20 μm. If a ray of light is incident on one end of the fiber at angle θ_1 = 40°, the number of reflections it makes before emerging from the other end is close to :
(refractive index of fiber is 1.31 and sin 40° = 0.64)

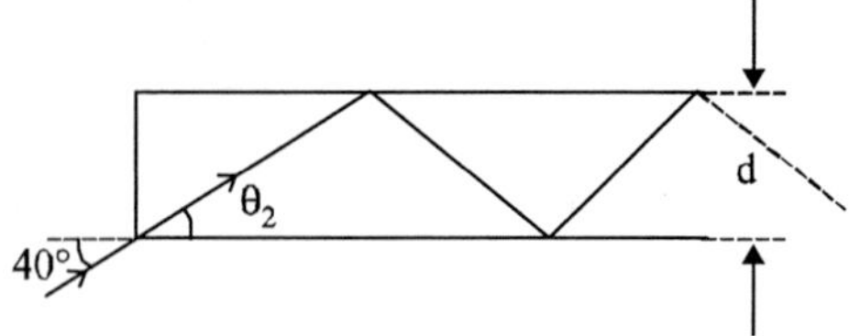

(a) 55000 (b) 66000 (c) 45000 (d) 57000

72. A point like object is placed at a distance of 1 m in front of a convex lens of focal length 0.5 m. A plane mirror is placed at a distance of 2 m behind the lens. The position and nature of the final image formed by the system is :
(a) 2.6 m from the mirror, real
(b) 1 m from the mirror, virtual
(c) 1 m from the mirror, real
(d) 2.6 m from the mirror, virtual

73. A double convex lens has power P and same radii of curvature R of both the surfaces. The radius of curvature of a surface of a plano-convex lens made of the same material with power 1.5 P is :
(a) $2R$ (b) $\frac{R}{2}$ (c) $\frac{3R}{2}$ (d) $\frac{R}{3}$

74. A thin lens made of glass (refractive index = 1.5) of focal length f = 16 cm is immersed in a liquid of refractive index 1.42. If its focal length in liquid is f_l, then the ratio f_l/f is closest to the integer:
(a) 1 (b) 9 (c) 5 (d) 17

75. The magnifying power of a telescope with tube length 60 cm is 5. What is the focal length of its eye piece?
(a) 20 cm (b) 40 cm (c) 30 cm (d) 10 cm

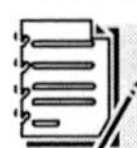

Exercise 2 - Exemplar & Past Year Questions

E&PYQs

Exemplar Questions

1. A ray of light incident at an angle θ on a refracting face of a prism emerges from the other face normally. If the angle of the prism is 5° and the prism is made of a material of refractive index 1.5, the angle of incidence is
(a) 7.5° (b) 5° (c) 15° (d) 2.5°

2. A short pulse of white light is incident from air to a glass slab at normal incidence. After travelling through the slab, the first colour to emerge is
(a) blue (b) green (c) violet (d) red

3. An object approaches a convergent lens from the left of the lens with a uniform speed 5 m/s and stops at the focus. The image
(a) moves away from the lens with an uniform speed 5 m/s
(b) moves away from the lens with an uniform acceleration
(c) moves away from the lens with a non-uniform acceleration
(d) moves towards the lens with a non-uniform acceleration

4. A passenger in an aeroplane shall
(a) never see a rainbow
(b) may see a primary and a secondary rainbow as concentric circles
(c) may see a primary and a secondary rainbow as concentric arcs
(d) shall never see a secondary rainbow

5. You are given four sources of light each one providing a light of a single colour - red, blue, green and yellow. Suppose the angle of refraction for a beam of yellow light corresponding to a particular angle of incidence at the interface of two media is 90°. Which of the following statements is correct if the source of yellow light is replaced with that of other lights without changing the angle of incidence?
(a) The beam of red light would undergo total internal reflection
(b) The beam of red light would bend towards normal while it gets refracted through the second medium
(c) The beam of blue light would undergo total internal reflection
(d) The beam of green light would bend away from the normal as it gets refracted through the second medium

6. The radius of curvature of the curved surface of a plano-convex lens is 20 cm. If the refractive index of the material of the lens be 1.5, it will
(a) act as a convex lens only for the objects that lie on its curved side
(b) act as a concave lens for the objects that lie on its curved side
(c) act as a convex lens irrespective of the side on which the object lies
(d) act as a concave lens irrespective of side on which the object lies

7. The phenomena involved in the reflection of radiowaves by ionosphere is similar to
(a) reflection of light by a plane mirror
(b) total internal reflection of light in air during a mirage
(c) dispersion of light by water molecules during the formation of a rainbow
(d) scattering of light by the particles of air

8. The direction of ray of light incident on a concave mirror is shown by PQ while directions in which the ray would travel after reflection is shown by four rays marked 1, 2, 3 and 4 (figure). Which of the four rays correctly shows the direction of reflected ray?

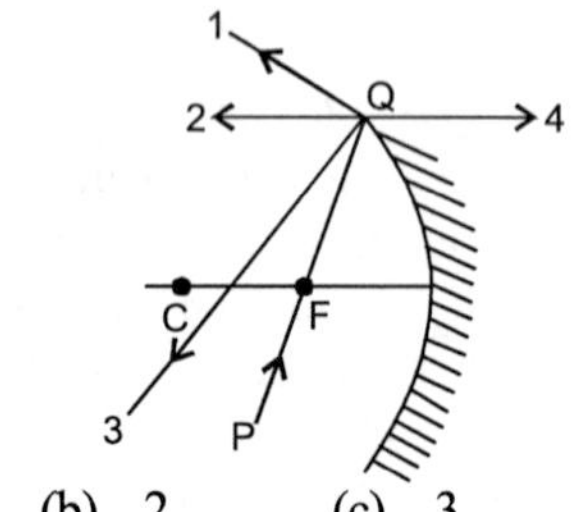

(a) 1 (b) 2 (c) 3 (d) 4

9. The optical density of turpentine is higher than tnat of water while its mass density is lower. Figure shows a layer of turpentine floating over water in a container. For which one of the four rays incident on turpentine in figure, the path shown is correct?
(a) 1
(b) 2
(c) 3
(d) 4

1 2 3 4
Air
T
W G

NEET/AIPMT (2013-2020) Questions

10. A plano convex lens fits exactly into a plano concave lens. Their plane surfaces are parallel to each other. If lenses are made of different materials of refractive indices μ_1 and μ_2 and R is the radius of curvature of the curved surface of the lenses, then the focal length of the combination is *[2013]*

(a) $\frac{R}{2(\mu_1-\mu_2)}$ (b) $\frac{R}{(\mu_1-\mu_2)}$
(c) $\frac{2R}{(\mu_2-\mu_1)}$ (d) $\frac{R}{2(\mu_1+\mu_2)}$

11. For a normal eye, the cornea of eye provides a converging power of 40D and the least converging power of the eye lens behind the cornea is 20D. Using this information, the distance between the retina and the eye lens of the eye can be estimated to be *[2013]*
(a) 2.5 cm (b) 1.67 cm (c) 1.5 cm (d) 5 cm

12. Two plane mirrors are inclined at 70°. A ray incident on one mirror at angle θ after reflection falls on second mirror and is reflected from there parallel to first mirror. The value of θ is *[NEET Kar. 2013]*
(a) 50° (b) 45° (c) 30° (d) 55°

13. The reddish appearance of the sun at sunrise and sunset is due to *[NEET Kar. 2013]*
(a) the colour of the sky (b) the scattering of light
(c) the polarisation of light (d) the colour of the sun

14. If the focal length of objective lens is increased then magnefying power of: *[2014]*
(a) microscope will increase but that of telescope decrease.
(b) microscope and telescope both will increase.
(c) microscope and telescope both will decrease
(d) microscope will decrease but that of telescope increase.

15. The angle of a prism is 'A'. One of its refracting surfaces is silvered. Light rays falling at an angle of incidence 2A on the first surface returns back through the same path after suffering reflection at the silvered surface. The refractive index μ, of the prism is: *[2014]*

(a) 2 sin A (b) 2 cos A (c) $\frac{1}{2}\cos A$ (d) tan A

16. The refracting angle of a prism is 'A', and refractive index of the material of the prism is cot(A/2). The angle of minimum deviation is: *[2015]*
(a) 180° – 2A (b) 90° – A
(c) 180° + 2A (d) 180° – 3A

17. Two identical thin plano-convex glass lenses (refractive index 1.5) each having radius of curvature of 20 cm are placed with their convex surfaces in contact at the centre. The intervening space is filled with oil of refractive index 1.7. The focal length of the combination is *[2015]*
(a) –25 cm (b) –50 cm (c) 50 cm (d) –20 cm

18. In an astronomical telescope in normal adjustment a straight black line of lenght L is drawn on inside part of objective lens. The eye-piece forms a real image of this line. The length of this image is *l*. The magnification of the telescope is : *[2015 RS]*

(a) $\frac{L}{I}-1$ (b) $\frac{L+I}{L-I}$ (c) $\frac{L}{I}$ (d) $\frac{L}{I}+1$

19. The angle of incidence for a ray of light at a refracting surface of a prism is 45°. The angle of prism is 60°. If the ray suffers minimum deviation through the prism, the angle of minimum deviation and refractive index of the material of the prism respectively, are : *[2016]*

(a) $45°, \frac{1}{\sqrt{2}}$ (b) $30°, \sqrt{2}$ (c) $45°, \sqrt{2}$ (d) $30°, \frac{1}{\sqrt{2}}$

20. A astronomical telescope has objective and eyepiece of focal lengths 40 cm and 4 cm respectively. To view an object 200 cm away from the objective, the lenses must be separated by a distance : *[2016]*
(a) 37.3 cm (b) 46.0 cm (c) 50.0 cm (d) 54.0 cm

21. A beam of light from a source L is incident normally on a plane mirror fixed at a certain distance x from the source. The beam is reflected back as a spot on a scale placed just above the source I. When the mirror is rotated through a small angle θ, the spot of the light is found to move through a distance y on the scale. The angle θ is given by *[2017]*

(a) $\frac{y}{x}$ (b) $\frac{x}{2y}$ (c) $\frac{x}{y}$ (d) $\frac{y}{2x}$

22. A thin prism having refracting angle 10° is made of glass of refractive index 1.42. This prism is combined with another thin prism of glass of refractive index 1.7. This combination produces dispersion without deviation. The refracting angle of second prism should be *[2017]*
(a) 6° (b) 8° (c) 10° (d) 4°

23. An astronomical refracting telescope will have large angular magnification and high angular resolution, when it has an objective lens of *[2018]*
(a) small focal length and large diameter
(b) large focal length and small diameter
(c) small focal length and small diameter
(d) large focal length and large diameter

24. In total internal reflection when the angle of incidence is equal to the critical angle for the pair of media in contact, what will be angle of refraction ? *[2019]*
(a) 180°
(b) 0°
(c) equal to angle of incidence
(d) 90°

25. Two similar thin equi-convex lenses, of focal length f each, are kept coaxially in contact with each other such that the focal length of the combination is F_1. When the space between the two lenses is filled with glycerin (which has the same refractive index (= 1.5) as that of glass) then the equivalent focal length is F_2. The ratio $F_1 : F_2$ will be : *[2019]*

(a) 2 : 1 (b) 1 : 2 (c) 2 : 3 (d) 3 : 4

26. An equiconvex lens has power *P*. It is cut into two symmetrical halves by a plane containing the principal axis. The power of one part will be, *[NEET Odisha 2019]*

(a) P (b) 0 (c) $\frac{P}{2}$ (d) $\frac{P}{4}$

27. A double convex lens has focal length 25 cm. The radius of curvature of one of the surfaces is double of the other. Find the radii if the refractive index of the material of the lens is 1.5. *[NEET Odisha 2019]*

(a) 50 cm, 100 cm (b) 100 cm, 50 cm
(c) 25 cm, 50 cm (d) 18.75 cm, 37.5 cm

28. Pick the wrong answer in the context with rainbow. *[2019]*

(a) When the light rays undergo two internal reflections in a water drop, a secondary rainbow is formed.
(b) The order of colours is reversed in the secondary rainbow.
(c) An observer can see a rainbow when his front is towards the sun.
(d) Rainbow is a combined effect of dispersion, refraction and reflection of sunlight.

29. A ray is incident at an angle of incidence i on one surface of a small angle prism (with angle of prism A) and emerges normally from the opposite surface. If the refractive index of the material of the prism is μ, then the angle of incidence is nearly equal to : *[2020]*

(a) $\frac{2A}{\mu}$ (b) μA (c) $\frac{\mu A}{2}$ (d) $\frac{A}{2\mu}$

Exercise 3 - Concept Application Problems CAP

1. A double convex lens of focal length 6 cm is made of glass of refractive index 1.5. The radius of curvature of one surface is double that of other surface. The value of small radius of curvature is

(a) 6 cm (b) 4.5 cm (c) 9 cm (d) 4 cm

2. The critical angle for light going from medium X into medium Y is θ. The speed of light in medium X is v, then speed of light in medium Y is

(a) $v(1 - \cos\theta)$ (b) $v/\sin\theta$
(c) $v/\cos\theta$ (d) $v\cos\theta$

3. An achromatic convergent doublet of two lenses in contact has a power of + 2D. The convex lens has power + 5D. What is the ratio of dispersive powers of convergent and divergent lenses ?

(a) 2 : 5 (b) 3 : 5 (c) 5 : 2 (d) 5 : 3

4. Two convex lenses of focal lengths f_1 and f_2 are mounted coaxially separated by a distance. If the power of the combination is zero, the distance between the lenses is

(a) $|f_1 - f_2|$ (b) $f_1 + f_2$ (c) $\frac{f_1 f_2}{|f_1 - f_2|}$ (d) $\frac{f_1 f_2}{f_1 + f_2}$

5. The wavelength of a monochromatic light in vacuum is λ. It travels from vacuum to a medium of absolute refractive index μ. The ratio of wavelength of the incident and refracted wave is

(a) $\mu^2 : 1$ (b) 1 : 1 (c) μ : 1 (d) 1 : μ

6. A rectangular block of glass is placed on a mark made on the surface of the table and it is viewed from the vertical position of eye. If refractive index of glass be μ and its thickness d, then the mark will appear to be raised up by

(a) $\frac{(\mu+1)d}{\mu}$ (b) $\frac{(\mu-1)d}{\mu}$
(c) $\frac{(\mu+1)}{\mu d}$ (d) $\frac{(\mu-1)\mu}{d}$

7. A vessel is half filled with a liquid of refractive index μ. The other half of the vessel is filled with an immiscible liquid of refrative index 1.5 μ. The apparent depth of the vessel is 50% of the actual depth. Then μ is

(a) 1.4 (b) 1.5 (c) 1.6 (d) 1.67

8. It is desired to photograph the image of an object placed at a distance of 3 m from plane mirror. The camera, which is at a distance of 4.5 m from mirror should be focussed for a distance of

(a) 3m (b) 4.5m (c) 6m (d) 7.5m

9. A combination is made of two lenses of focal length f and f' in contact, the dispersive powers of the materials of the lenses are ω and ω'. The combination is achromatic, when

(a) $\omega = \omega_0, \omega' = 2\omega_0 \quad f' = 2f$
(b) $\omega = \omega_0, \omega' = 2\omega_0 \quad f' = f/2$
(c) $\omega = \omega_0, \omega' = 2\omega_0 \quad f' = -f/2$
(d) $\omega = \omega_0, \omega' = 2\omega_0 \quad f' = -2f$

10. A simple telescope, consisting of an objective of focal length 60 cm and a single eye lens of focal length 5 cm is focussed on a distant object in such a way that parallel rays emerge from the eye lens. If the object subtends an angle of 2° at the objective, the angular width of the image is

(a) 10° (b) 24° (c) 50° (d) (1/6)°

11. In the displacement method, a concave lens is placed in between an object and a screen. If the magnification in the two positions are m_1 and m_2 ($m_1 > m_2$), and the distance between the two positions of the lens is x, the focal length of the lens is

(a) $\frac{x}{m_1 + m_2}$ (b) $\frac{x}{m_1 - m_2}$
(c) $\frac{x}{(m_1 + m_2)^2}$ (d) $\frac{x}{(m_1 - m_2)^2}$

12. A thin lens has focal length f, and its aperture has diameter D. It forms an image of intensity I. If the central part of the aperture, of diameter $\frac{D}{2}$, is blocked by an opaque paper, the focal length of the lens and the intensity of image will become

(a) $\frac{f}{2}, \frac{I}{2}$ (b) $f, \frac{I}{4}$ (c) $\frac{3f}{4}, \frac{I}{2}$ (d) $f, \frac{3I}{4}$

13. The graph shows the variation of magnification m produced by a convex lens with the image distance v. The focal length of the lens is

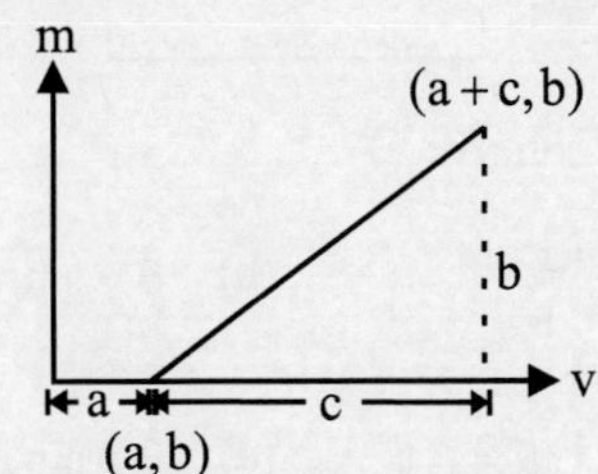

(a) $\frac{b}{c}$ (b) $\frac{c}{b}$ (c) b (d) $\frac{ab}{c}$

14. The position of final image formed by the given lens combination from the third lens will be at a distance of ($f_1 = +10$ cm, $f_2 = -10$ cm and $f_3 = +30$ cm).

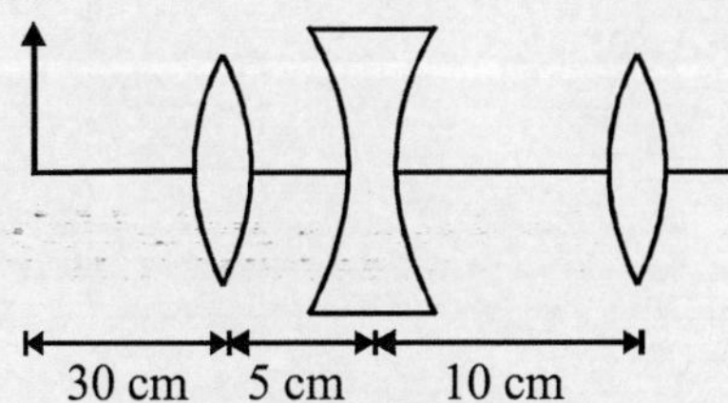

(a) 15 cm (b) infinity (c) 45 cm (d) 30 cm

15. A ray of light is travelling from glass to air. (Refractive index of glass = 1.5). The angle of incidence is 50°. The deviation of the ray is

(a) 0° (b) 80°

(c) $50° - \sin^{-1}\left[\frac{\sin 50°}{1.5}\right]$ (d) $\sin^{-1}\left[\frac{\sin 50°}{1.5}\right] - 50°$

16. A luminous object is placed at a distance of 30 cm from the convex lens of focal length 20 cm. On the other side of the lens, at what distance from the lens a convex mirror of radius of curvature 10 cm be placed in order to have an upright image of the object coincident with it?

(a) 12 cm (b) 30 cm (c) 50 cm (d) 60 cm

17. Light enters at an angle of incidence in a transparent rod of refractive index ***n***. For what value of the refractive index of the material of the rod the light once entered into it will not leave it through its lateral face whatsoever be the value of angle of incidence?

(a) $n > \sqrt{2}$ (b) $n = 1$ (c) $n = 1.1$ (d) $n = 1.3$

18. A light ray falls on a rectangular glass slab as shown. The index of refraction of the glass, if total internal reflection is to occur at the vertical face, is

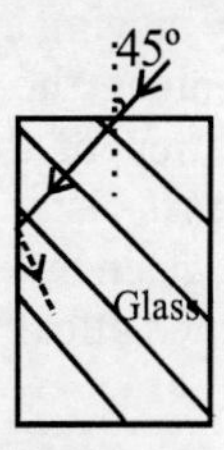

(a) $\sqrt{3/2}$ (b) $\frac{(\sqrt{3}+1)}{2}$ (c) $\frac{(\sqrt{2}+1)}{2}$ (d) $\sqrt{5}/2$

19. An equiconvex lens is cut into two halves along (i) XOX' and (ii) YOY' as shown in the figure. Let f, f', f'' be the focal lengths of the complete lens, of each half in case (i), and of each half in case (ii), respectively

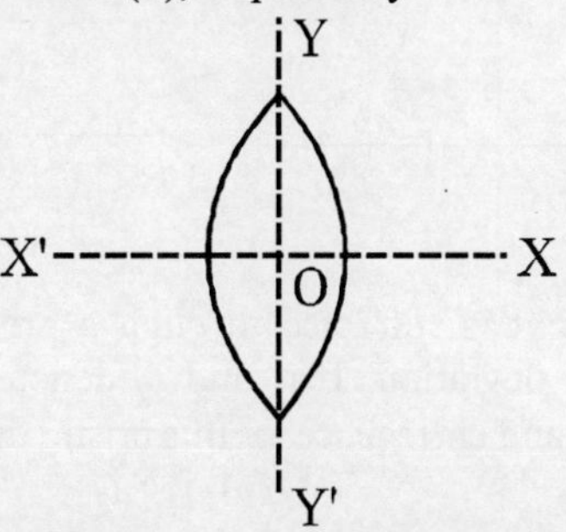

Choose the correct statement from the following

(a) f' = 2f, f'' = 2f (b) f' = f, f'' = 2f
(c) f' = 2f, f'' = f (d) f' = f, f'' = f

20. The refractive index of the material of a prism is √2 and its refracting angle is 30°. One of the refracting surfaces of the prism is made a mirror inwards. A beam of monochromatic light enters the prism from the mirrored surface if its angle of incidence of the prism is

(a) 30° (b) 45° (c) 60° (d) 0°

21. A telescope has an objective lens of 10 cm diameter and is situated at a distance of one kilometer from two objects. The minimum distance between these two objects, which can be resolved by the telescope, when the mean wavelength of light is 5000 Å, is of the order of

(a) 5 cm (b) 0.5 m (c) 5 m (d) 5 mm

22. A point source of light, S is placed at a distance L in front of the centre of plane mirror of width d which is hanging vertically on a wall. A man walks in front of the mirror along a line parallel to the mirror, at a distance 2L as shown below. The distance over which the man can see the image of the light source in the mirror is:

(a) d
(b) 2d
(c) 3d
(d) $\frac{d}{2}$

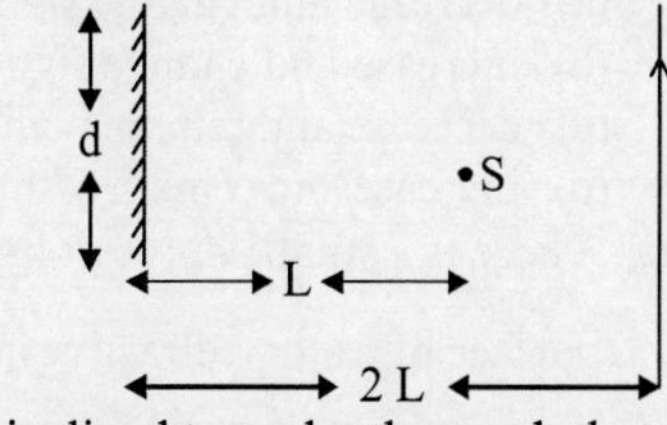

23. Two plane mirrors are inclined to each other such that a ray of light incident on the first mirror (M_1) and parallel to the second mirror (M_2) is finally reflected from the second mirror (M_2) parallel to the first mirror (M_1). The angle between the two mirrors will be:

(a) 45° (b) 60° (c) 75° (d) 90°

24. An object is gradually moving away from the focal point of a concave mirror along the axis of the mirror. The graphical representation of the magnitude of linear magnification (m) versus distance of the object from the mirror (x) is correctly given by
(Graphs are drawn schematically and are not to scale)

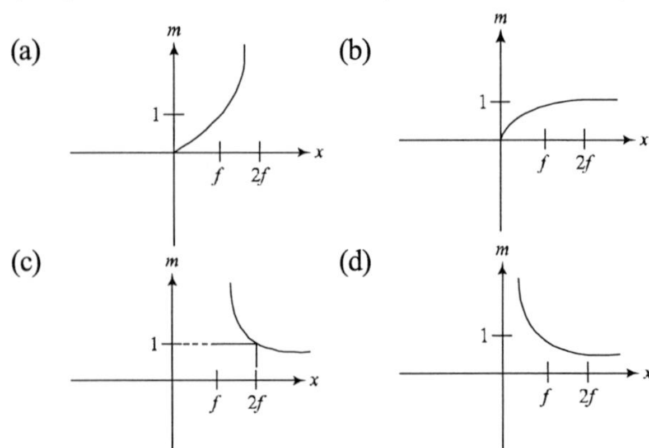

25. Yellow light is refracted through a prism producing minimum deviation. If i_1 and i_2 denote the angle of incidence and emergence for this prism, then
(a) $i_1 = i_2$ (b) $i_1 > i_2$
(c) $i_1 < i_2$ (d) $i_1 + i_2 = 90°$

26. A ray of light passes from vacuum into a medium of refractive index μ, the angle of incidence is found to be twice the angle of refraction. Then the angle of incidence is
(a) $2\cos^{-1}\left(\frac{\mu}{2}\right)$ (b) $\sin^{-1}(\mu)$
(c) $\sin^{-1}\left(\frac{\mu}{2}\right)$ (d) $\cos^{-1}\left(\frac{\mu}{2}\right)$

27. A concave mirror is used for face viewing has focal length of 0.6m. At whay distance you should hold the mirror from your face to get an upright image with a magnification of 4?
(a) 0.20m (b) 0.25m (c) 0.40m (d) 0.45m

28. If two + 5 diopter lenses are mounted at some distance apart, the equivalent power will always be negative if the distance is
(a) greater than 40 cm (b) equal to 40 cm
(c) equal to 10 cm (d) less than 10 cm

29. A bi-convex lens made of glass (refractive index 1.5) is put in a liquid of refractive index 1.7. Its focal length will
(a) decrease and change sign
(b) increase and change sign
(c) decrease and remain of the same sign
(d) increase and remain of the same sign

30. There is a small source of light at some depth below the surface of water (refractive index = $\frac{4}{3}$) in a tank of large cross sectional surface area. Neglecting any reflection from the bottom and absorption by water, percentage of light that emerges out of surface is (nearly):
[Use the fact that surface area of a spherical cap of height h and radius of curvature r is $2\pi rh$]
(a) 21% (b) 34% (c) 17% (d) 50%

31. A transparent cube of side d, made of a material of refractive index μ_2, is immersed in a liquid of refractive index $\mu_1(\mu_1 < \mu_2)$. A ray is incident on the face AB at an angle θ (shown in the figure). Total internal reflection takes place at point E on the face BC.

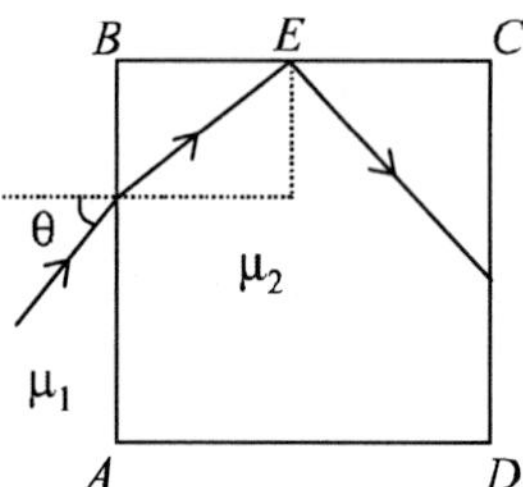

Then θ must satisfy :
(a) $\theta < \sin^{-1}\frac{\mu_1}{\mu_2}$ (b) $\theta > \sin^{-1}\sqrt{\frac{\mu_2^2}{\mu_1^2} - 1}$
(c) $\theta < \sin^{-1}\sqrt{\frac{\mu_2^2}{\mu_1^2} - 1}$ (d) $\theta > \sin^{-1}\frac{\mu_1}{\mu_2}$

32. A ray of light AO in vacuum is incident on a glass slab at angle 60° and refracted at angle 30° along OB as shown in the figure. The optical path length of light ray from A to B is :
(a) $\frac{2\sqrt{3}}{a} + 2b$
(b) $2a + \frac{2b}{3}$
(c) $2a + \frac{2b}{\sqrt{3}}$
(d) $2a + 2b$

A
60°
O
Vacuum
a
b
glass
30°
B

33. For a concave lens of focal length f, the relation between object and image distances u and v, respectively, from its pole can best be represented by ($u = v$ is the reference line) :

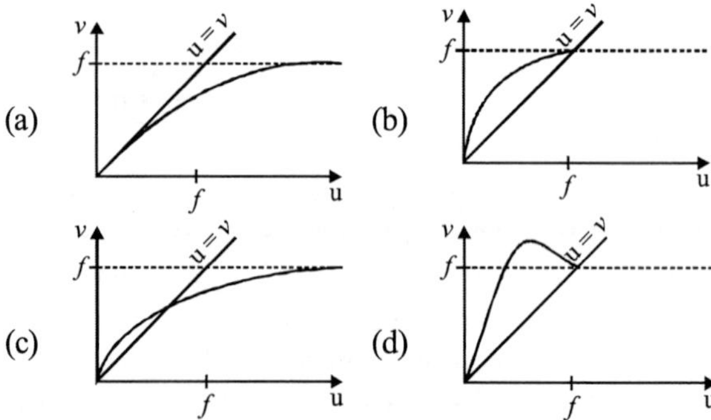

34. One plano-convex and one plano-concave lens of same radius of curvature 'R' but of different materials are joined side by side as shown in the figure. If the refractive index of the material of 1 is μ_1 and that of 2 is μ_2, then the focal length of the combination is :

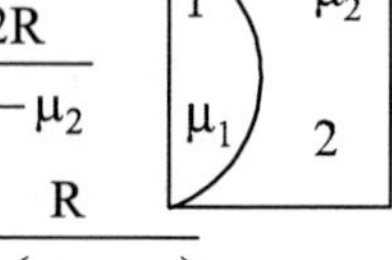

(a) $\frac{R}{\mu_1 - \mu_2}$ (b) $\frac{2R}{\mu_1 - \mu_2}$
(c) $\frac{2R}{2(\mu_1 - \mu_2)}$ (d) $\frac{R}{2-(\mu_1 - \mu_2)}$

35. The graph shows how the magnification m produced by a thin lens varies with image distance v. What is the focal length of the lens used ?

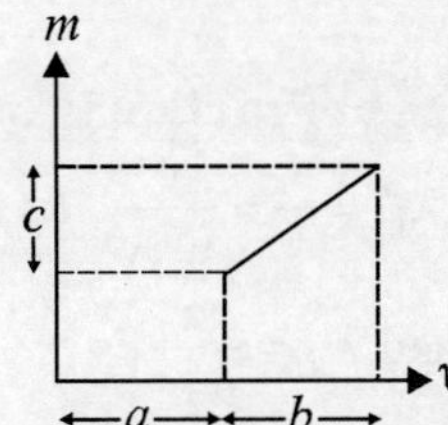

(a) $\frac{b^2}{ac}$ (b) $\frac{b^2c}{a}$ (c) $\frac{a}{c}$ (d) $\frac{b}{c}$

36. A convex lens of focal length 20 cm produces images of the same magnification 2 when an object is kept at two distances x_1 and x_2 $(x_1 > x_2)$ from the lens. The ratio of x_1 and x_2 is:

(a) 2 : 1 (b) 3 : 1 (c) 5 : 3 (d) 4 : 3

37. A thin convex lens L (refractive index = 1.5) is placed on a plane mirror M. When a pin is placed at A, such that OA = 18 cm, its real inverted image is formed at A itself, as shown in figure. When a liquid of refractive index μ_i is put between the lens and the mirror, the pin has to be moved to A', such that OA' = 27 cm, to get its inverted real image at A' itself. The value of μ_i will be:

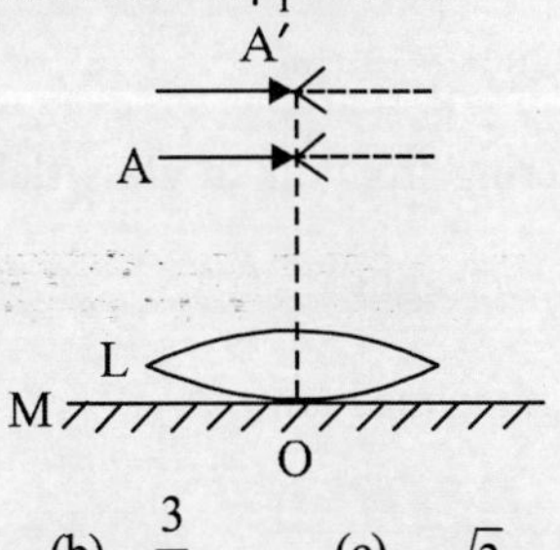

(a) $\frac{4}{3}$ (b) $\frac{3}{2}$ (c) $\sqrt{3}$ (d) $\sqrt{2}$

38. What is the position and nature of image formed by lens combination shown in figure? (f_1, f_2 are focal lengths)

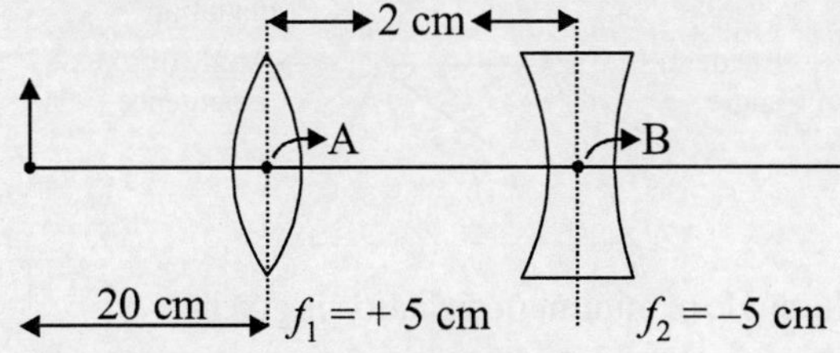

(a) 70 cm from point B at left; virtual

(b) 40 cm from point B at right; real

(c) $\frac{20}{3}$ cm from point B at right, real

(d) 70 cm from point B at right; real

39. Formation of real image using a biconvex lens is shown below :

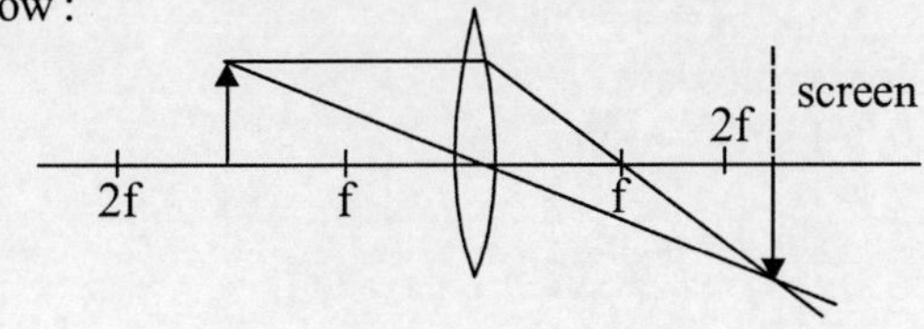

If the whole set up is immersed in water without disturbing the object and the screen positions, what will one observe on the screen ?

(a) Image disappears (b) Magnified image

(c) Erect real image (d) No change

40. An object is at a distance of 20 m from a convex lens of focal length 0.3 m. The lens forms an image of the object. If the object moves away from the lens at a speed of 5m/s, the speed and direction of the image will be :

(a) 2.26×10^{-3} m/s away from the lens

(b) 0.92×10^{-3} m/s away from the lens

(c) 3.22×10^{-3} m/s towards the lens

(d) 1.16×10^{-3} m/s towards the lens

41. A plano convex lens of refractive index μ_1 and focal length f_1 is kept in contact with another plano concave lens of refractive index μ_2 and focal length f_2 If the radius of curvature of their spherical faces is R each and $f_1 = 2f_2$, then μ_1 and μ_2 are related as:

(a) $\mu_1 + \mu_2 = 3$ (b) $2\mu_1 - \mu_2 = 1$

(c) $3\mu_2 - 2\mu_1 = 1$ (d) $2\mu_2 - \mu_1 = 1$

42. The eye can be regarded as a single refracting surface. The radius of curvature of this surface is equal to that of cornea (7.8 mm). This surface separates two media of refractive indices 1 and 1.34. Calculate the distance from the refracting surface at which a parallel beam of light will come to focus.

(a) 1 cm (b) 2 cm (c) 4.0 cm (d) 3.1 cm

43. A monochromatic light is incident at a certain angle on an equilateral triangular prism and suffers minimum deviation. If the refractive index of the material of the prism is $\sqrt{3}$, then the angle of incidence is :

(a) 90° (b) 30° (c) 60° (d) 45°

44. If we need a magnification of 375 from a compound microscope of tube length 150 mm and an objective of focal length 5 mm, the focal length of the eye-piece, should be close to:

(a) 22mm (b) 12mm (c) 2mm (d) 33mm

45. An upright object is placed at a distance of 40 cm in front of a convergent lens of focal length 20 cm. A convergent mirror of focal length 10 cm is placed at a distance of 60 cm on the other side of the lens. The position and size of the final image will be :

(a) 20 cm from the convergent mirror, same size as the object

(b) 40 cm from the convergent mirror, same size as the object

(c) 40 cm from the convergent lens, twice the size of the object

(d) 20 cm from the convergent mirror, twice the size of the object

Hints & Solutions

24.1 Concept Practice Problems

1. (a) $m = \frac{1}{n} = \frac{-v}{(-u)} \Rightarrow v = \frac{u}{n}$

As $\frac{1}{v} + \frac{1}{u} = \frac{1}{f}$ $\quad \therefore \frac{n}{u} - \frac{1}{u} = \frac{1}{f}$

$u = (n-1)f$

2. (a) Number of images $(n_1) = \frac{360^\circ}{\theta} - 1$

where θ = angle between mirrors

Here, $\theta = 60^\circ$

So, number of images $n_1 = \frac{360^\circ}{60^\circ} - 1 = 5$

3. (c) Given $v = nu$ As $\frac{1}{v} + \frac{1}{u} = \frac{1}{f}$

$\therefore \frac{1}{nu} + \frac{1}{u} = \frac{1}{f}$ or $u = \frac{(n+1)f}{n}$

4. (a) Here, $u = f + x_1$, $v = f + x_2$

use $f = \frac{uv}{u+v}$ and solve to get $f = \sqrt{x_1 x_2}$

5. (b) Virtual object forms real image on a plane mirror, so rays convergent.

6. (a) $\frac{1}{v} - \frac{1}{2f} = \frac{1}{f} \Rightarrow \frac{1}{v} = \frac{3}{2f} \Rightarrow v = \frac{2}{3}f$

$\therefore m = \frac{v}{u} = \frac{2}{3}\frac{f}{2f} = \frac{1}{3}$

7. (b) Medium doesn't effect focal length of a mirror.

8. (b) Object distance u = – 40 cm

Focal length f = – 20 cm

According to mirror formula

$\frac{1}{u} + \frac{1}{v} = \frac{1}{f}$ or $\frac{1}{v} = \frac{1}{f} - \frac{1}{u}$

or $\frac{1}{v} + \frac{1}{-20} - \frac{1}{(-40)} = \frac{1}{-20} + \frac{1}{40}$

$\frac{1}{v} = \frac{-2+1}{40} = -\frac{1}{40}$ or $v = -40$ cm.

Negative sign shows that image is infront of concave mirror. The image is real.

Magnification, $m = \frac{-v}{u} = -\frac{(-40)}{(-40)} = -1$

The image is of the same size and inverted.

9. (a) Due to covering the reflection from lower part is not there so it makes the image less bright.

10. (a) To see his full image in a plane mirror a person requires a mirror of at least half of his height.

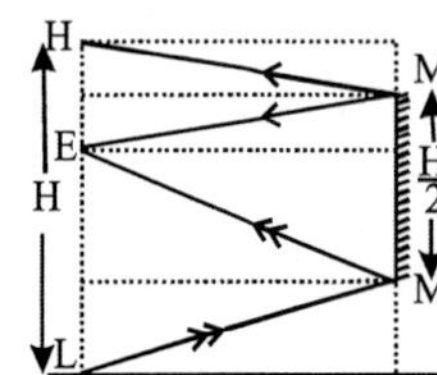

24.2 Concept Practice Problems

11. (a) $\lambda_a = \frac{c}{\nu}$ or $\lambda_m = \frac{v}{\nu} = \frac{c}{\mu_m \nu}$ $\quad (\because \mu_m = \frac{c}{v})$

$\therefore \lambda_1 = \frac{c}{\mu_1 \nu}$ and $\lambda_2 = \frac{c}{\mu_2 \nu}$

or $\lambda_1 \mu_1 = \lambda_2 \mu_2$ or $\lambda_2 = \lambda_1 (\mu_1 / \mu_2)$

12. (b) Apparent depth = $d/\mu_1 + d/\mu_2$

13. (d) 14. (d)

15. (c) $\mu = \frac{\text{velocity of light in vacuum}}{\text{velocity of light in glass plate}}$

or $\mu = \frac{c}{c'}$ or $c' = \frac{c}{\mu}$

Time taken = distance/velocity = $t/(c/\mu) = \frac{\mu t}{c}$

16. (d) Least distance is 4f when object is at radius of curvature, and greatest is infinity.

17. (a) When electromagnetic wave enters in other medium, frequency reamains unchanged while wavelength and velocity become $\frac{1}{\mu}$ times.

so, e.m. entering from air to glass slab (μ), frequency remains n, wavelength $\lambda' = \frac{\lambda}{\mu}$

velocity of light in medium $v' = \frac{v}{\mu}$

18. (a) $\frac{1}{F} = \frac{1}{f_1} + \frac{1}{f_2} = \frac{f_2 + f_1}{f_1 f_2}$; $\quad P = \frac{1}{F} = \frac{f_1 + f_2}{f_1 f_2}$

19. (b)

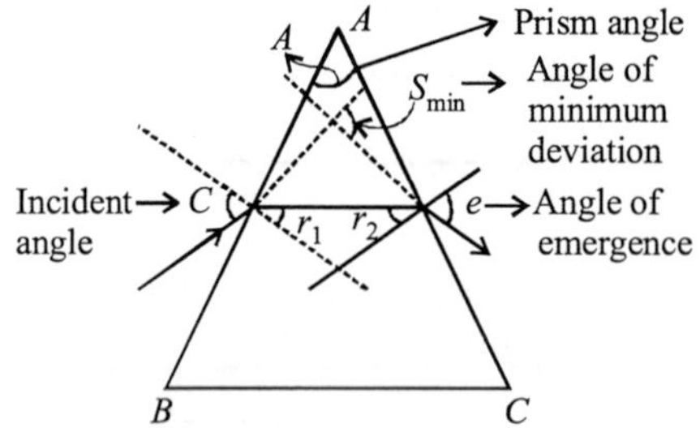

The angle of minimum deviation is given as

$\delta_{min} = i + e - A$

for minimum deviation

$\delta_{min} = A$ then

$2A = i + e$

in case of δ_{min} $i = e$

$2A = 2i \quad r_1 = r_2 = \frac{A}{2}$

$i = A = 90^\circ$

from smell's law

$1 \sin i = n \sin r_1$

$\sin A = n \sin \frac{A}{2}$

$$2\sin\frac{A}{2}\cos\frac{A}{2}=n\sin\frac{A}{2}$$

$$2\cos\frac{A}{2}=n$$

when $A=90°=i_{min}$

then $n_{min}=\sqrt{2}$

$$i=A=0\ n_{max}=2$$

20. (b) Difference between apparent and real depth of a pond is due to the refraction of light, not due to the total internal reflection. Other three phenomena are due to the total internal reflection.

24.3 Concept Practice Problems 

21. (b) The image formed by objective lens of compound microscope is real and enlarged, while final image formed by compound microscope is inverted, virtual, enlarged and at a distance D to infinite or from an eye, on same side of eye piece.

22. (b) 23. (a)

24. (b) Large aperture increases the amount of light gathered by the telescope increasing the resolution.

25. (d) 26. (a)

27. (a) $\frac{f_0}{f_e}=9, \therefore f_0=9f_e$

Also $f_0+f_e=20$ ($\because$ final image is at infinity)

$9f_e+f_e=20, f_e=2$ cm,

$\therefore$ $f_0=18$ cm

28. (b) In normal adjustment,

$$M=\frac{f_0}{f_e}=20,\ f_e=\frac{f_0}{20}=\frac{60}{20}=3\text{ cm}$$

29. (a) (i) $M=-\frac{f_0}{f_e}\left(1+\frac{f_e}{d}\right)=-\frac{200}{5}\left(1+\frac{5}{25}\right)=-48$

(since least distance d = 25cm)

(ii) $M=-\frac{f_0}{f_e}=-\frac{200}{5}=-40$

30. (d) $M=\frac{f_0}{f_e}=5, L=f_0+f_e=36$

$\therefore$ $f_e=6$ cm, $f_0=30$ cm

Exercise 1 - Chapter Revision Problems CRP

1. (a) As no scattering of light occurs, sky appears dark.

2. (d) Because, the focal length of eye lens can not decrease beyond a certain limit.

3. (c)

4. (b) Optical fibre is a device which transmits light introduced at one end to the opposite end, with little loss of the light through the sides of the fibre. It is possible with the help of total internal reflection.

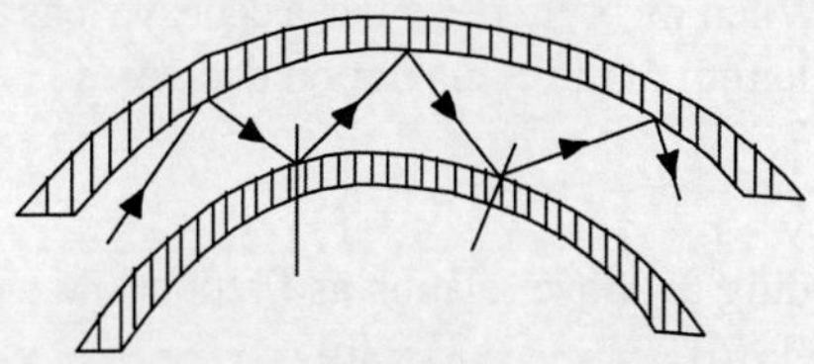

5. (d) If the medium is heterogeneous having a gradient of refractive index. Then light rays will not follow a rectilinear (straight line path).

6. (c) $\frac{1}{f}=\left({}_\ell\mu_g-1\right)\left(\frac{1}{R}-\frac{1}{R_2}\right)$ where ${}_\ell\mu_g=1$ is given, we get

$$\Rightarrow \frac{1}{f}=(1-1)\left(\frac{1}{R_1}-\frac{1}{R_2}\right)=0 \text{ or } \Rightarrow f=\infty$$

7. (a)

8. (b) $\frac{v_2}{v_1}=\frac{\mu_1}{\mu_2}=\frac{1}{1.33}$ or $v_2=\frac{v_1}{1.33}=2.25\times10^8$ m/s

9. (c) $\frac{1}{f}=\frac{1}{f_1}+\frac{1}{-f_2}=\frac{f_2-f_1}{f_1f_2}$; $f=\frac{f_1f_2}{f_2-f_1}$

10. (c) $P=P_1+P_2=+2-1=+1$ dioptre, lens behaves as convergent

$$F=\frac{1}{P}=\frac{1}{1}=1\text{ m}=100\text{ cm}$$

11. (c) $c=\frac{x}{t_1}$, $v=\frac{10}{t_2}$

$$\sin i_c=\frac{1}{\mu}=\frac{v}{c}=\frac{10}{t_2}\times\frac{t_1}{x};\ i_c=\sin^{-1}\left(\frac{10t_1}{t_2x}\right)$$

12. (b) $i=\frac{A+\delta_m}{2}=\frac{60+30}{2}=45°$

13. (d) $i_1=i_2=\frac{3}{4}A$

As $A+\delta=i_1+i_2$

$$\therefore\ \delta=i_1+i_2-A=\frac{3}{4}A+\frac{3}{4}A-A=\frac{A}{2}=\frac{60°}{2}=30°$$

14. (c) Longitudinal chromatic aberration $=\omega f$ $=0.08\times20=1.6$ cm

15. (a) Convex lens can form image with m < 1, m > 1 and m = 1 depending upon the position of the object. Convex lens forms magnified image (m > 1) when the object is pole and 2f, same size as the object (m = 1) when the object is at 2f and smaller image (m < 1), when the object is beyond 2f.

16. (a) Difference in refractive indices of blue and green colour are less so they are seen together and red is seen separate because deviation depends on refractive index.

17. (a)

18. (a) $\frac{1}{f}=(\mu-1)\left(\frac{1}{R_1}-\frac{1}{R_2}\right)$

$$\frac{1}{16} = (1.5-1)\left(\frac{1}{R} - \frac{1}{\infty}\right)$$

$$\Rightarrow \frac{1}{16} = 0.5 \times \frac{1}{R} \Rightarrow R = 8 \text{ cm}$$

19. (b) When we bring in contact a concave lens the effective focal length of the combination decreases.

$$\frac{1}{v} - \frac{1}{u} = \frac{1}{f} \Rightarrow \frac{1}{v} = \frac{1}{u} + \frac{1}{f}$$

according to above relation as f reduces, v increases.

20. (b) 21. (d) 22. (b)

23. (a) In a telescope, to obtain an image at infinity or in normal adjustment, the distance between two convex lenses one called objective (greater focal length) and the other called eye piece (shorter focal length) is L.

$L = f_0 + f_e = 0.3 + 0.05 = 0.35$ m.

24. (b) given : ${}^{a}\mu_g = \frac{3}{2}, {}^{a}\mu_w = \frac{4}{3}$

$$\because {}^{a}\mu_w \times {}^{w}\mu_g = {}^{a}\mu_g$$

$$\therefore {}^{w}\mu_g = \frac{{}^{a}\mu_g}{{}^{a}\mu_w} = \frac{3/2}{4/3} = \frac{9}{8}.$$

25. (b) $\mu = \dfrac{\text{velocity of light in vacuum (c)}}{\text{velocity of light in medium (v)}}$

But $v = \upsilon\lambda = 2 \times 10^{14} \times 5000 \times 10^{-10}$

In the medium, $v = 10^8$ m/s.

$$\therefore \mu = \frac{v_{vac}}{v_{med}} = \frac{3 \times 10^8}{10^8} = 3.$$

26. (d) Here, $i_1 = 15°, A = 60°, \delta = 55°, i_2 = e = ?$

As $i_1 + i_2 = A + \delta$

$i_2 = A + \delta - i_1 = 60° + 55° - 15° = 100°.$

27. (c) For reading purposes :

$u = -25$ cm, $v = -50$ cm, $f = ?$

$$\frac{1}{f} = \frac{1}{v} - \frac{1}{u} = -\frac{1}{50} + \frac{1}{25} = \frac{1}{50}\ ;\ P = \frac{100}{f} = +2\,\text{D}$$

For distant vision, f' = distance of far point = –3 m

$$P = \frac{1}{f'} = -\frac{1}{3}\text{D} = -0.33 \text{ D}$$

28. (c) From figure

$$\frac{x}{BC} = \sin(i-r) \approx (i-r) \quad ...(1)$$

Further, $\dfrac{d}{BC} = \cos r \approx 1$

(When i is small r is small)

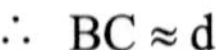

$\therefore$ BC $\approx$ d

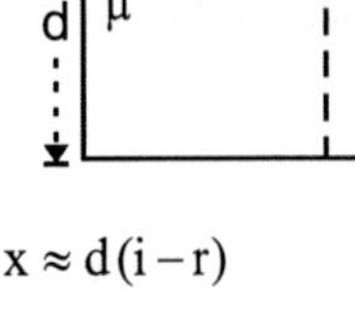

From eq. (1), $\dfrac{x}{d} \approx (i-r)$ or $x \approx d(i-r)$

or $\quad x \approx id\left(1 - \dfrac{r}{i}\right)$

Now $\dfrac{\sin i}{\sin r} = \dfrac{i}{r} = \mu \qquad \therefore x \approx id\left(1 - \dfrac{1}{\mu}\right)$

29. (a) Given that ${}_{w}\mu_g = \frac{5}{4}$ and ${}_{a}\mu_w = \frac{4}{3}$

$$\therefore \quad {}_{a}\mu_g = {}_{w}\mu_g \times {}_{a}\mu_w = \frac{5}{4} \times \frac{4}{3} = \frac{5}{3}$$

30. (c) We know that $\mu = \dfrac{\text{real depth}}{\text{apparent depth}}$

Let the thickness of the slab be t and real depth of the bubble from one side be x. Then

$$\mu = \frac{x}{6} = \frac{(t-x)}{4} \text{ or } 1.5 = \frac{x}{6} = \frac{t-x}{4}.$$

This gives x = 9 and $1.5 = \dfrac{t-9}{4}$ or t = 15 cm

31. (c) The minimum length of the mirror is half the length of the man. This can be proved from the fact that $\angle i = \angle r$.

32. (d) $P_2 = P - P_1 = \dfrac{100}{80} - \dfrac{100}{20} = -3.75$ D

33. (c) In the position of minimum deviation

$$i = e = \frac{A + \delta m}{2} = \frac{60 + 30}{2} = 45°$$

34. (d)

35. (b) $\dfrac{1}{f} = \left(\dfrac{\mu_2}{\mu_1} - 1\right)\left(\dfrac{1}{R_1} - \dfrac{1}{R_2}\right)$

As $\dfrac{\mu_2}{\mu_1} < 1$

$\therefore$ f is negative. It acts as divergent lens.

36. (c) Using, $\dfrac{\mu}{v} - \dfrac{1}{u} = \dfrac{\mu - 1}{R}$ or $\dfrac{2}{v} - \dfrac{1}{\infty} = \dfrac{2-1}{R}$

$$\therefore \quad v = 2R$$

37. (a) In the position of minimum deviation, $i_1 = i_2$.

38. (c) For the prism as the angle of incidence (i) increases, the angle of deviation (δ) first decreases goes to minimum value and then increases.

39. (a)

40. (b) $\dfrac{P_a}{P_l} = \dfrac{\left(\dfrac{\mu_g}{\mu_a} - 1\right)}{\left(\dfrac{\mu_g}{\mu_l} - 1\right)} = \dfrac{+5}{-100/100} = -5$

$$-5\left(\frac{\mu_g}{\mu_l} - 1\right) = \frac{\mu_g}{\mu_a} - 1$$

$$\frac{1.5}{\mu_l} - 1 = \frac{-1}{5}(1.5 - 1) = -0.1\ ;\ \mu_l = \frac{1.5}{0.9} = \frac{5}{3}$$

41. (b) $\mu = \dfrac{\sin(A + \delta_m)/2}{\sin A/2}$

$$\Rightarrow \frac{\sin(A + \delta_m)}{2} = \mu \sin A/2` = 1.5 \times \sin 30° = 0.75$$

$$\frac{A + \delta_m}{2} = \sin^{-1}(0.75) = 48°36' \quad \therefore \delta_m = 37°12'$$

42. (b) Condition for achromatism is $\frac{\omega_1}{f_1}+\frac{\omega_2}{f_2}=0$

$\therefore \frac{f_1}{f_2}=-\frac{\omega_1}{\omega_2}=\frac{2}{3}$ (leaving sign)

43. (a) $\frac{f_1}{f_2}=-\frac{\omega_1}{\omega_2}=-\frac{1}{2} \quad \therefore f_2=-2f_1$

As $\frac{1}{F}=\frac{1}{f_1}+\frac{1}{f_2}$

$\therefore \frac{1}{20}=\frac{1}{f_1}-\frac{1}{2f_1}=\frac{1}{2f_1} \quad \therefore f_1=10\text{ cm}$

$f_2=-20$ cm

44. (b) When two lenses are placed coaxially then their equivalent focal length F is given as

$\frac{1}{F}=\frac{1}{f_1}+\frac{1}{f_2} \Rightarrow F=\frac{f_1 f_2}{f_1+f_2}$

$f_1 \; f_2$

Now power $=\frac{1}{\text{focal length}}=\frac{f_1+f_2}{f_1 f_2}$

45. (b) Refractive index of medium is given by

$\mu=A+\frac{B}{\lambda^2}$ (where A and B are constant).

Light has seven different colour, so its each colour has different wavelength and so different refractive index. Due to difference in refractive index different refractive angle $\left(\mu=\frac{\sin i}{\sin r}\right)$.

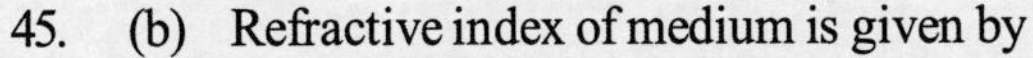

So this is due to dependence on wavelength of refractive index.

46. (c) When a object is real plane mirror form a virtual image and when object is virtual image will be real. Thus in this question object is virtual. Virtual object means object is at infinity. So rays (incident) converge on the mirror.

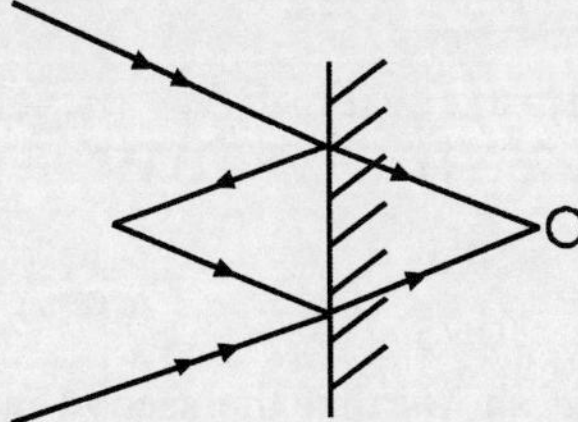

47. (c) Spherical abberation occurs due to the inability of a lens to coverage marginal rays of the same wavelength to the focus as it converges the paraxial rays, This defect can be removed by blocking marginal rays. This can be done by using a circular annular mask over the lens.

48. (d) Shift in the position of image after introducing slab,

$(d)=t\left(1-\frac{1}{n}\right)$

$nd=t(n-1) \Rightarrow t=\frac{nd}{(n-1)}$

49. (b) The easiest way to answer this question is with a fast sketch. For a given object's position, draw two rays from the top of the object. One ray is parallel to the principal axis and passes through the focal point on the opposite side of the lens. The other ray passes through the center of the lens. The top of the image appears where these two rays intersect.

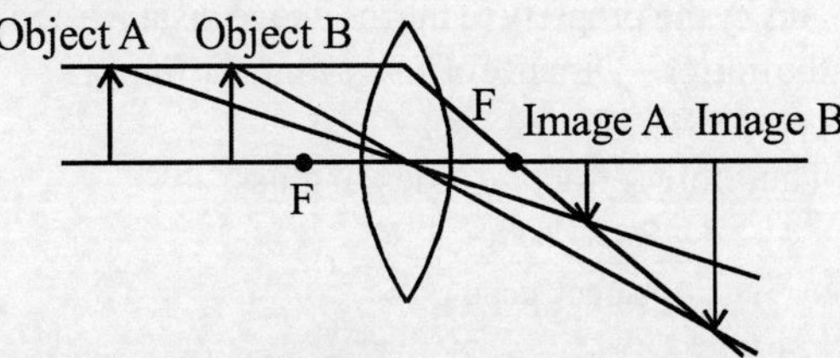

Change the object's position and repeat the process. You will observe that as the object approaches the lens while remaining beyond the focal length, the image produced on the opposite side of the lens moves away from the lens and increases in size. As an aside, the image is real and inverted.

50. (a) The ratio of object to image distance equals the ratio of object to image height. The ratio of image to object height is found by rearranging the ratios to give $4f/(4/3)f=1/3$. The image is demagnified by a factor of 3. Thus, answer choice A is the best answer.

51. (a)

52. (b) Due to difference in refractive indices images obtained will be two. Two mediums will form images at two different points due to difference in focal lengths.

53. (c) The ray is partly reflected and partly refracted.

$\angle MOB=180-2\theta$

But the angle between refracted and reflected ray is $\angle POB$. Clearly $\angle POB$ is less than $\angle MOB$.

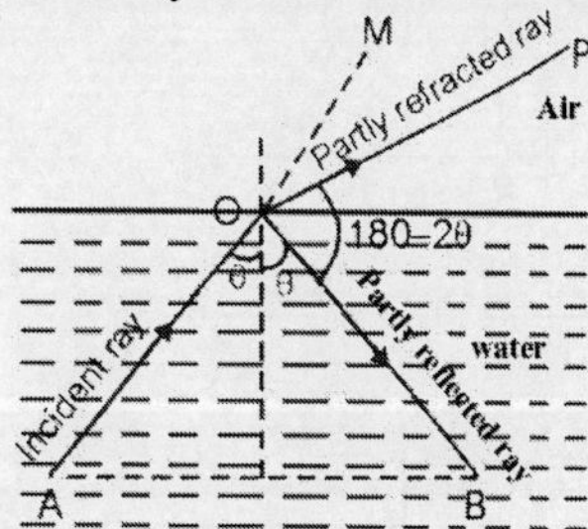

54. (a)

55. (b) $\frac{1}{f}=(\mu-1)\left(\frac{1}{R_1}-\frac{1}{R_2}\right)$

According to Cauchy relation $\mu=A+\frac{B}{\lambda^2}+\frac{C}{\lambda^4}$......

Hence $f \propto \lambda$.

Hence red light having maximum wavelength has maximum focal length.

$f_v<f_R$ and also $F_V<F_R$

56. (c) As refracted ray emerges normally from oppostite surface, $r_2=0$

As $A=r_1+r_2 \qquad \therefore r_1=A$

Now, $\mu=\frac{\sin i_1}{\sin r_1}=\frac{i_1}{r_1}=\frac{i}{A}; i=\mu A$

(where t = thickness of glass plate)

57. (c) Thickness of glass plate (t) = 6 cm;

Distance of the object (u) = 8 cm. and distance of the image (v) = 12 cm.

Let x = Apparent position of the silvered surface in cm.

Since the image is formed due to relfection at the silvered face and by the property of mirror image distance of object from the mirror = Distance of image from the mirror

or $x+8=12+6-x$ or $x=5$ cm.

Therefore refractive index of glass

$$=\frac{\text{Real depth}}{\text{Apparent depth}}=\frac{6}{5}=1.2.$$

58. (d) We know that $\frac{1}{f}=\sum_{i=1}^{n}\frac{1}{f_i}$

$$\frac{1}{f}=\frac{1}{f_1}+\frac{1}{f_2}$$

$f_1=80$ cm, $f_2=-50$ cm

$$\frac{1}{f}=\frac{1}{\frac{80}{100}}-\frac{1}{\frac{50}{100}} \Rightarrow P=\frac{1}{f}=1.25-2=-0.75D$$

59. (c) The silvered plano convex lens behaves as a concave mirror; whose focal length is given by

$$\frac{1}{F}=\frac{2}{f_1}+\frac{1}{f_m}$$

If plane surface is silvered

$$f_m=\frac{R_2}{2}=\frac{\infty}{2}=\infty$$

$$\therefore \frac{1}{f_1}=(\mu-1)\left(\frac{1}{R_1}-\frac{1}{R_2}\right)$$

$$=(\mu-1)\left(\frac{1}{R}-\frac{1}{\infty}\right)=\frac{\mu-1}{R}$$

$$\therefore \quad \frac{1}{F}=\frac{2(\mu-1)}{R}+\frac{1}{\infty}=\frac{2(\mu-1)}{R}$$

$$F=\frac{R}{2(\mu-1)}$$

Here $R=20$ cm, $\mu=1.5$

$$\therefore \quad F=\frac{20}{2(1.5-1)}=20\text{cm}$$

60. (b) $1.5=\frac{\text{Real depth }(R_1)}{\text{Apparent depth }(5\text{ cm})}$

$\therefore R_1=1.5\times 5=7.5$ cm

For opposite face,

$$1.5=\frac{R_2}{2}$$

$\Rightarrow R_2=3.0$ cm

$\therefore$ Thickness of the slab

$=R_1+R_2=7.5+3=10.5$ cm

61. (b) $R_1=60$ cm, $R_2=\infty$, $\mu=1.6$

$$\frac{1}{f}=(\mu-1)\left(\frac{1}{R_1}-\frac{1}{R_2}\right)$$

$$\frac{1}{f}=(1.6-1)\left(\frac{1}{60}\right) \Rightarrow f=100\text{ cm}.$$

62. (c) Angle of minimum deviation

$$\mu=\frac{\sin\left(\frac{A+\delta_m}{2}\right)}{\sin\left(\frac{A}{2}\right)} \Rightarrow \sqrt{3}=\frac{\sin\left(\frac{60°+\delta_m}{2}\right)}{\sin\left(\frac{60°}{2}\right)}$$

$$\Rightarrow \sin\left(30°+\frac{\delta_m}{2}\right)=\frac{\sqrt{3}}{2} \Rightarrow 30°+\frac{\delta_m}{2}=60°$$

$\Rightarrow \quad \delta_m=60°$.

63. (c) For total internal reflection,

$$\mu \geq \frac{1}{\sin C} \geq \sqrt{2} \geq 1.414$$

$\Rightarrow \quad \mu=1.50$

64. (c) $R=20$ cm, $h_0=2$, $u=-30$ cm

We have, $\frac{1}{f}=(\mu-1)\left(\frac{1}{R_1}-\frac{1}{R_2}\right)$

$$=\left(\frac{3}{2}-1\right)\left[\frac{1}{20}-\left(-\frac{1}{20}\right)\right]$$

$$\Rightarrow \frac{1}{f}=\left(\frac{3}{2}-1\right)\times\frac{2}{20}$$

$\therefore \quad f=20$ cm

$$\frac{1}{f}=\frac{1}{v}-\frac{1}{u} \Rightarrow \frac{1}{20}=\frac{1}{v}+\frac{1}{30}$$

$$\frac{1}{v}=\frac{1}{20}-\frac{1}{30}=\frac{10}{600}$$

$v=60$ cm

$$m=\frac{h_i}{h_0}=\frac{v}{u} \Rightarrow h_i=\frac{v}{u}\times h_0=\frac{60}{30}\times 2=-4\text{ cm}$$

So, image is inverted.

65. (b) Deviation = zero

So, $\delta=\delta_1+\delta_2=0 \Rightarrow (\mu_1-1)A_1+(\mu_2-1)A_2=0$

$\Rightarrow A_2(1.75-1)=-(1.5-1)\,15°$

$$\Rightarrow A_2=-\frac{0.5}{0.75}\times 15° \qquad \text{or } A_2=-10°.$$

Negative sign shows that the second prism is inverted with respect to the first.

66. (d) Object is placed beyond radius of curvature (*R*) of concave mirror hence image formed is real, inverted and diminished or unmagnified.

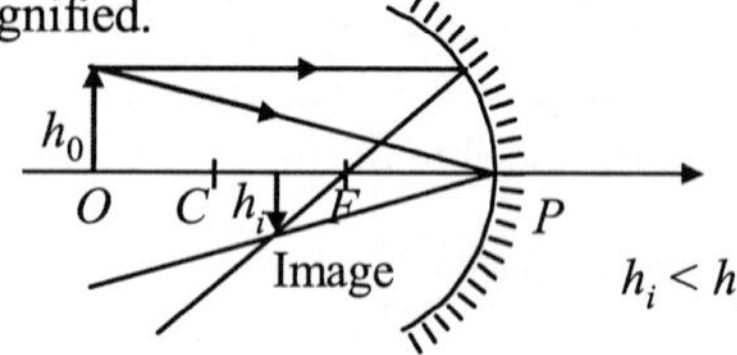

67. (c) $+5=-\frac{v}{u} \Rightarrow v=-5u$

Using $\frac{1}{v}+\frac{1}{u}=\frac{1}{f}$

or $\frac{1}{-5u}+\frac{1}{u}=\frac{1}{0.4}$

$\therefore$ u = 0.32 m

68. (d) Apparent depth,

h $\mu_1=\sqrt{2}$

$\mu_2=2\sqrt{2}$ h

$$D=\frac{t_1}{\mu_1}+\frac{t_2}{\mu_2}=\frac{h}{\sqrt{2}}+\frac{h}{2\sqrt{2}}=\frac{3h}{2\sqrt{2}}=\frac{3h\sqrt{2}}{4}$$

69. (b) Here, from question, relative permittivity

$\varepsilon_r=\frac{\varepsilon}{\varepsilon_0}=3\Rightarrow\varepsilon=3\varepsilon_0$

Relative permeability $\mu_r=\frac{\mu}{\mu_0}=\frac{4}{3}\Rightarrow\mu=\frac{4}{3}\mu_0$

$\therefore \mu\varepsilon=4\mu_0\varepsilon_0$

$\sqrt{\frac{\mu_0\varepsilon_0}{\mu\varepsilon}}=\frac{v}{c}=\frac{1}{2}\left(\because c=\frac{1}{\sqrt{\mu_0\varepsilon_0}}\right)$

$n=\sqrt{\mu_r\varepsilon_r}=\sqrt{\frac{4}{3}\times 3}=2$

And $n=\frac{1}{\sin\theta_c}$

$\Rightarrow \sin\theta_c=\frac{1}{n}=\frac{1}{2}$

$\therefore$ Critical angle, $\theta_c=30°$

70. (c) If v is the distance of image formed by mirror, then

$\frac{1}{v}+\frac{1}{u}=\frac{1}{f}$

or $\frac{1}{v}+\frac{1}{-5}=\frac{1}{-20}$

$\therefore\quad v=\frac{20}{3}$ cm

Distance of this image from water surface

$=\frac{20}{3}+5=\frac{35}{3}$ cm

Using, $\frac{RD}{AD}=\mu$

$\therefore\quad AD=d=\frac{RD}{\mu}=\frac{(35/3)}{1.33}=8.8$ cm

71. (d) Using Snell's law of refraction,

$1\times\sin 40°=1.31\sin\theta$

$\Rightarrow \sin\theta=\frac{0.64}{1.31}=0.49\approx 0.5$

$\Rightarrow \quad \theta=30°$

$x=20\ \mu\text{m}\times\cot\theta$

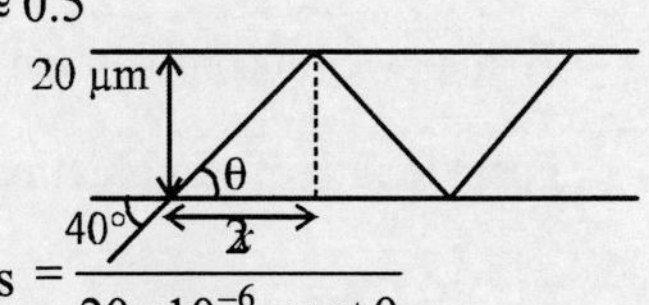

$\therefore$ Number of reflections $=\frac{2}{20\times 10^{-6}\times\cot\theta}$

$=\frac{2\times 10^6}{20\times\sqrt{3}}=57735\approx 57000$

72. (d) Focal length of the convex lens, $f=0.5$ m

Object is at $2f$ so, image (I_1) will also be at $2f$.

Image of I_1 i.e., I_2 will be 1 m behind mirror.

Now I_2 will be object for lens.

1m 1m 1m 1m
Object I_1 I_2
$f=0.5$m Mirror

$\therefore u=(-1)+(-1)+(-1)=-3$ m

Using lens formula, $\frac{1}{v}-\frac{1}{u}=\frac{1}{f}$

$\frac{1}{v}=\frac{1}{f}+\frac{1}{u}=\frac{1}{+0.5}+\frac{1}{-3}$ or $v=\frac{3}{5}=0.6$ m

Hence, distance of image from mirror

$=2+0.6=2.6$ m and real.

73. (d) Given, using lens maker's formula

$\frac{1}{f}=(k-1)\left(\frac{1}{R_1}-\frac{1}{R_2}\right)$

Here, $R_1=R_2=R$ (For double convex lens)

$\therefore\frac{1}{f}=(\mu-1)\left(\frac{1}{R}-\frac{1}{-R}\right)$

$\Rightarrow P=\frac{1}{f}=(\mu-1)\frac{2}{R}$ ...(i)

For plano convex lens,

$R_1=R',\ R_2=\infty$

Using lens maker's formula again, we have

$1.5P=(\mu-1)\left(\frac{1}{R'}-\frac{1}{\infty}\right)$ ...(ii)

$\Rightarrow\frac{3}{2}P=\frac{\mu-1}{R'}$

From (i) and (ii),

$\frac{3}{2}=\frac{R'}{2R}\Rightarrow R'=\frac{R}{3}$

74. (b) Using lens maker's formula

$\frac{1}{f}=\left(\frac{\mu_g}{\mu_a}-1\right)\left[\frac{1}{R_1}-\frac{1}{R_2}\right]$

Here, μ_g and μ_a are the refractive index of glass and air respectively

$\Rightarrow\quad\frac{1}{f}=(1.5-1)\left(\frac{1}{R_1}-\frac{1}{R_2}\right)$ ...(i)

When immersed in liquid

$\frac{1}{f_l}=\left(\frac{\mu_g}{\mu_l}-1\right)\left(\frac{1}{R_1}-\frac{1}{R_2}\right)$

[Here, μ_l = refractive index of liquid]

$\Rightarrow\frac{1}{f_l}=\left(\frac{1.5}{1.42}-1\right)\left(\frac{1}{R_1}-\frac{1}{R_2}\right)$ ...(ii)

Dividing (i) by (ii)

$$\Rightarrow \frac{f_l}{f} = \frac{(1.5-1)1.42}{0.08} = \frac{1.42}{0.16} = \frac{142}{16} \approx 9$$

75. (d) For telescope
Tube length (L) $= f_o + f_e = 60$
and magnification $(m) = \frac{f_o}{f_e} = 5 \Rightarrow f_0 = 5f_e$
$\therefore \quad f_0 = 50$ cm and $f_e = 10$ cm
Hence focal length of eye-piece, $f_e = 10$ cm

Exercise 2 - Exemplar & Past Year Questions 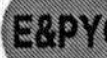

Exemplar Questions

1. (a) As we know that the deviation
$\delta = (\mu - 1)A$ ..... (i)
By geometry, the angle of refraction by first surface is 5° and given $\mu = 1.5$
So, $\delta = (1.5 - 1) \times 5° = 2.5°$
also, $\delta = \theta - r$, ... (ii)
By putting the value of δ and r in equation (ii)
$2.5° = \theta - 5°$
So, $\theta = 5 + 2.5 = 7.5°$

2. (d) As we know that when light ray goes from one medium to other medium, the frequency of light remains unchanged.
And, $c = \nu\lambda$
So, $c \propto \lambda$ the light of red colour is of highest wavelength and therefore of highest speed. Thus, after travelling through the slab, the red colour emerge first,

3. (c) According to the question, when object is at different position, and if an object approaches towards a convergent lens from the left of the lens with a uniform speed of 5 m/s, the image move away from the lens to infinity with a non-uniform acceleration.

4. (b) When a passenger in an aeroplane then he may see primary and secondary rainbow such as concentric circles.

5. (c) Among all given sources of light, the bule light have smallest wavelength.According to Cauchy relationship, smaller the wavelength higher the refractive index and consequently smaller the critical angle as $\mu = \frac{1}{\sin c}$.
Hence, corresponding to blue colour, the critical angle is least which facilitates total internal reflection for the beam of blue light and the beam of green light would also undergo total internal reflection.

6. (c) Using lens maker's formula for plano-convex lens, so focal length is
$$\frac{1}{f} = (\mu_2 - \mu_1)\left(\frac{1}{R_1} - \frac{1}{R_2}\right)$$
If object on curved suface
so, $R_2 = \infty$
then, $f = \frac{R_1}{(\mu_2 - \mu_1)}$
Lens placed in air, $\mu_1 = 1$.
(As given that, R = 20cm, $\mu_2 = 1.5$, on substituting the values in)
$$f = \frac{R_1}{\mu - 1} = \frac{20}{1.5 - 1}$$
$= 40$ cm
So, f is converging nature, as f > 0. Hence, lens will always act as a convex lens irrespective of the side on which the object lies.

7. (b) The reflection of radiowaves by ionosphere is similar to total internal reflection of light in air during a mirage because angle of incidence is greater than critical angle so that internal reflection of radio wave, take place.

8. (b) The incident PQ ray of light passes through focus F on the concave mirror, after reflection should become parallel to the principal axis, i.e., ray-2.

9. (b) As we know, when the ray goes from rarer medium air to optically denser turpentine, then it bends towards the normal i.e., i > r whereas when it goes from optically denser medium turpentine to rarer medium water, then it bends away from normal i.e., i < r.
So, the path of ray 2 is correct.

NEET/AIPMT (2013-2020) Questions

10. (d)

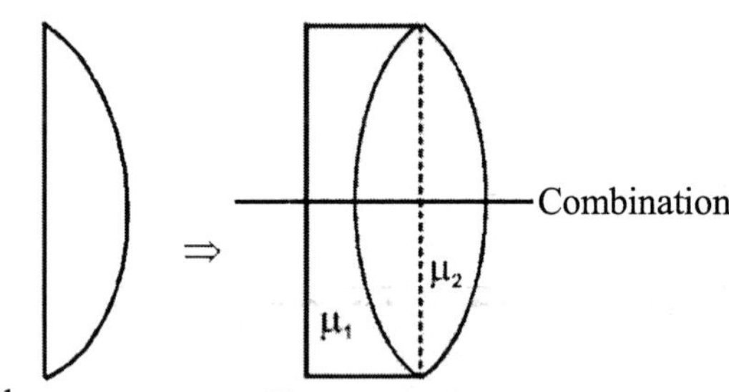

$$\frac{1}{f} = \frac{1}{f_1} + \frac{1}{f_2}$$
$$= (\mu_1 - 1)\left(\frac{1}{\infty} - \frac{1}{-R}\right) + (\mu_2 - 1)\left(\frac{1}{\infty} - \frac{1}{R}\right)$$
$$= \frac{(\mu_1 - 1)}{R} - \frac{(\mu_2 - 1)}{R} \Rightarrow \frac{1}{f} = \frac{\mu_1 - \mu_2}{R}$$
$$\Rightarrow f = \frac{R}{\mu_1 - \mu_2}$$
Hence, focal length of the combination is $\frac{R}{\mu_1 - \mu_2}$.

11. (b) $P_{cornea} = +40$ D
$P_e = +20$ D
Total power of combination = 40 + 20 = 60 D
Focal length of combination $= \frac{1}{60} \times 100$ cm
$= \frac{5}{3}$ cm
For minimum converging state of eye lens,
$u = -\infty \quad v = ? \quad f = \frac{5}{3}$

From lens formula,

$$\frac{1}{f}=\frac{1}{v}-\frac{1}{u}\Rightarrow v=\frac{5}{3}\text{ cm}$$

Distance between retina and cornea-eye lens

$$=\frac{5}{3}=1.67\text{ m}$$

12. (a)

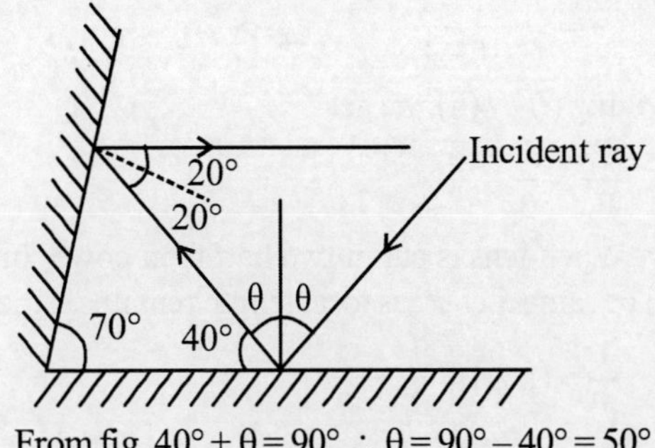

From fig. $40°+\theta=90°\ \therefore\ \theta=90°-40°=50°$

13. (b) It is due to scattering of light. Scattering $\propto\frac{1}{\lambda^4}$.
Hence the light reaches us is rich in red.

14. (d) Magnifying power of microscope

$$=\frac{LD}{f_0f_e}\propto\frac{1}{f_0}$$

Hence with increase f_0 magnifyig power of microscope decreases.

Magnifying power of telescope $=\frac{f_0}{f_e}\propto f_0$

Hence with increase f_0 magnifying power of telescope increases.

15. (b)

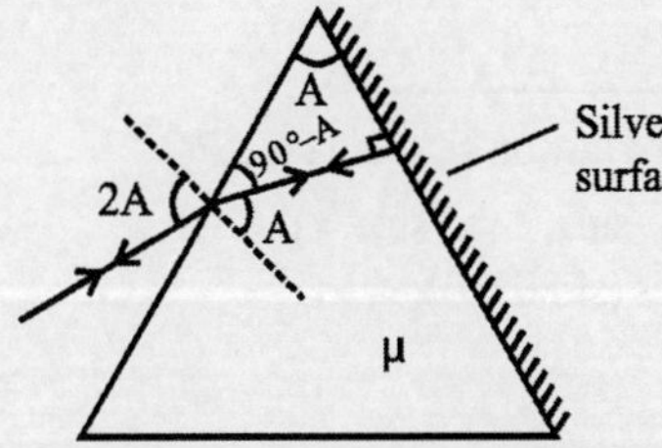

According to Snell's law $\mu=\frac{\sin i}{\sin r}$

$\Rightarrow$ (1) $\sin 2A=(\mu)\sin A\ \Rightarrow\ \mu=2\cos A$

16. (a) As we know, the refractive index of the material of the prism

$$\mu=\frac{\sin\left(\frac{\delta_m+A}{2}\right)}{\sin(A/2)}$$

$$\cot A/2=\frac{\sin\left(\frac{A+\delta_m}{2}\right)}{\sin A/2}=\frac{\cos(A/2)}{\sin(A/2)}$$

$[\because\ \mu=\cot(A/2)]$

$$\Rightarrow\ \text{Sin}\left(\frac{\delta_m+A}{2}\right)=\sin(90°+A/2)$$

$$\Rightarrow\ \delta_{min}=180°-2A$$

17. (b) Using lens maker's formula,

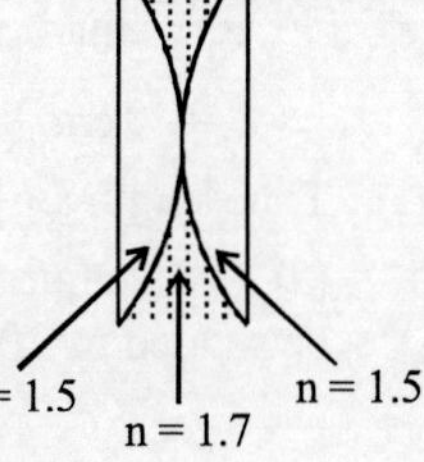

$$\frac{1}{f}=(\mu-1)\left(\frac{1}{R_1}-\frac{1}{R_2}\right)$$

$$\frac{1}{f_1}=\left(\frac{1.5}{1}-1\right)\left(\frac{1}{\infty}-\frac{1}{-20}\right)$$

$\Rightarrow\ f_1=40\text{cm}$

$$\frac{1}{f_2}=\left(\frac{1.7}{1}-1\right)\left(\frac{1}{-20}-\frac{1}{+20}\right)$$

$$\Rightarrow f_2=-\frac{100}{7}\text{ cm}$$

and $$\frac{1}{f_3}=\left(\frac{1.5}{1}-1\right)\left(\frac{1}{\infty}-\frac{1}{-20}\right)$$

$\Rightarrow f_3=40$ cm

$$\frac{1}{f_{eq}}=\frac{1}{f_1}+\frac{1}{f_2}+\frac{1}{f_3}$$

$$\Rightarrow\frac{1}{f_{eq}}=\frac{1}{40}+\frac{1}{-100/7}+\frac{1}{40}$$

$\therefore\quad f_{eq}=-50$ cm

Therefore, the focal length of the combination is – 50 cm.

18. (c)

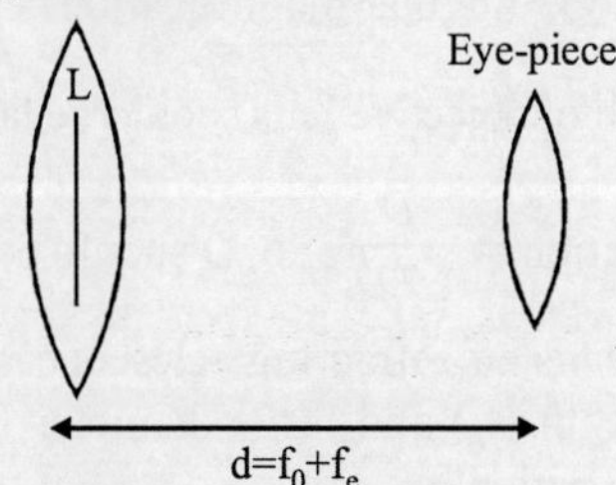

Magnification by eye piece

$$m=\frac{f}{f+u}$$

$$-\frac{I}{L}=\frac{f_e}{f_e+[-(f_0+f_e)]}=-\frac{f_e}{f_0}\quad\text{or,}\quad\frac{I}{L}=\frac{f_e}{f_0}$$

Magnification, $M=\frac{f_0}{f_e}=\frac{L}{I}$

19. (b) Given: Angle of incidence angle of prism,

$i=45°$;

$A=60°$;

Angle of minimum deviation,

$\delta_m=2i-A=30°$

Refractive index of material of prism.

$$\mu=\frac{\sin\left(\frac{A+\delta_m}{2}\right)}{\sin A/2}=\frac{\sin 45°}{\sin 30°}=\frac{1}{\sqrt{2}}\cdot\frac{2}{1}=\sqrt{2}$$

20. (d) **Given:** Focal length of objective, $f_0=40$cm
Focal length of eye – piece $f_e=4$ cm
image distance, $v_0=200$ cm
Using lens formula for objective lens

$$\frac{1}{v_0}-\frac{1}{u_0}=\frac{1}{f_0}\quad\Rightarrow\quad\frac{1}{v_0}=\frac{1}{f_0}+\frac{1}{u_0}$$

$\Rightarrow \frac{1}{v_0} = \frac{1}{40} + \frac{1}{-200} = \frac{+5-1}{200}$

$\Rightarrow v_0 = 50$ cm

Tube length $\ell = |v_0| + f_e = 50 + 4 = 54$ cm.

21. (d) When mirror is rotated by angle θ reflected ray will be rotated by 2θ.

$\frac{y}{x} = 2\theta$

$\Rightarrow \theta = \frac{y}{2x}$

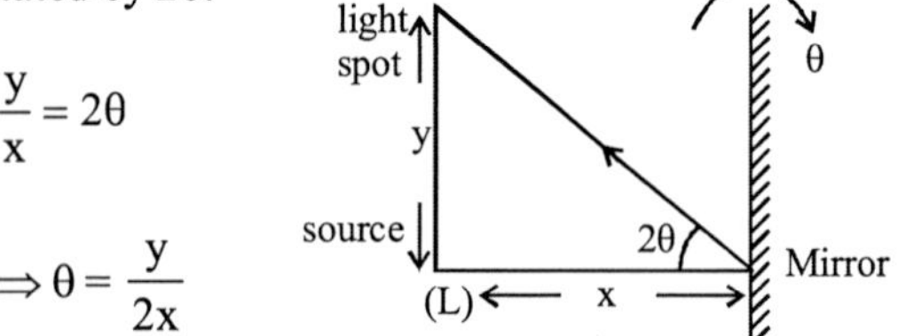

22. (a) For dispersion without deviation

$(\mu-1)A_1 + (\mu'-1)A_2 = 0$

$|(\mu-1)A_1| = |(\mu'-1)A_2|$

$(1.42-1) \times 10° = (1.7-1)A_2$

$4.2 = 0.7A_2$

$A_2 = 6°$

23. (d) For telescope, angular magnification $= \frac{f_0}{f_E}$

So, focal length of objective lens should be large.

Angular resolution $= \frac{D}{1.22\lambda}$ So, D should be large.

So, objective lens of refracting telescope should have large focal length (f_0) and large diameter D for larger angular magnification.

24. (d) For total internal reflection when $i = i_c$, then

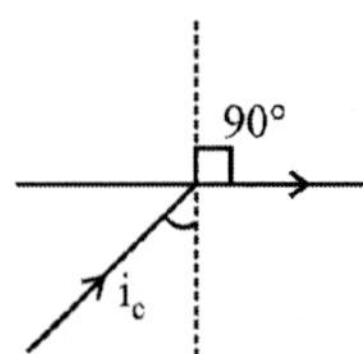

refracted ray grazes with the surface. That means the angle of refraction $r = 90°$.

25. (b)

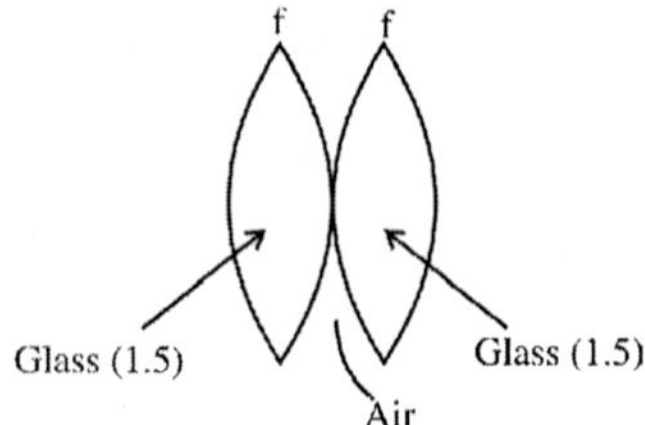

Equivalent focal length in air

$\frac{1}{F_1} = \frac{1}{f} + \frac{1}{f} = \frac{2}{f}$

$\Rightarrow F_1 = \frac{f}{2}$ ...(i)

When glycerin is filled inside, it behaves like a concave lens of focal length (–f)

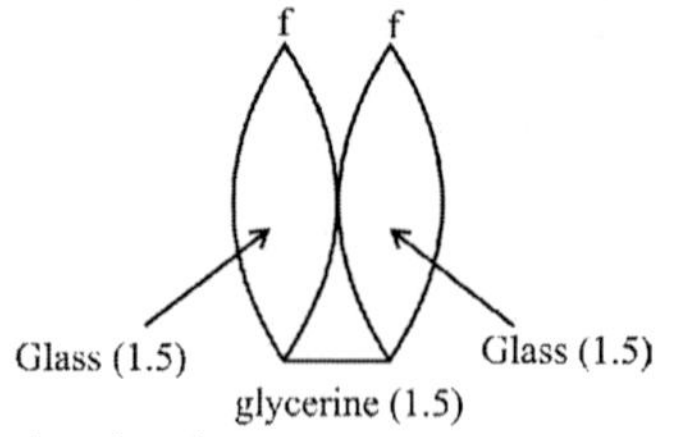

$\therefore \frac{1}{F_2} = \frac{1}{f} + \frac{1}{f} - \frac{1}{f}$ $\Rightarrow F_2 = f$ ...(ii)

Dividing (i) by (ii), we get

$\frac{F_1}{F_2} = \frac{1}{2}$

26. (a) When lens is cut in two half then power of one part will be same. i.e., *P*, as focal length remains same.

27. (d) $\frac{1}{f} = (\mu-1)\left(\frac{1}{R_1} - \frac{1}{R_2}\right)$

$\frac{1}{25} = (1.5-1)\left(\frac{1}{R} + \frac{1}{2R}\right)$ $\frac{1}{25} = 0.5\left(\frac{3}{2R}\right)$

$2R = 37.5$ cm $R = 18.75$ cm

28. (c) Rainbow will be observed only when the sun is at the back side of observer.

29. (b) Light ray emerges normally from another surface, hence, *e* (angle of emergence) = 0

$\therefore r_2 = 0$ $r_1 + r_2 = A \Rightarrow r_1 = A$

$\mu_1 \cdot \sin i = \mu_2 \cdot \sin r$

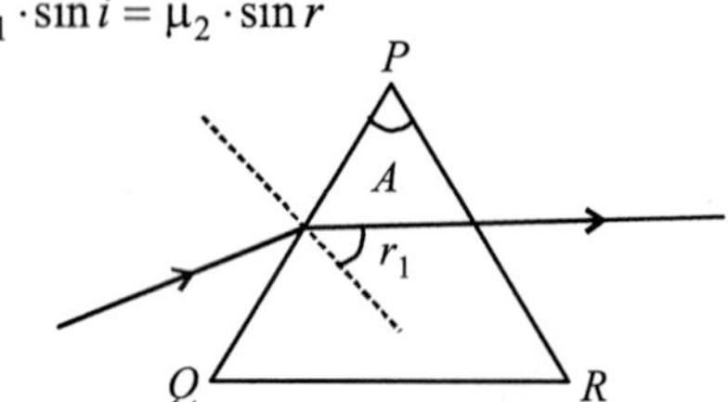

Applying Snell's law on first surface *PQ*

$\Rightarrow \mu_1 \cdot \sin i = \mu_2 \cdot \sin r_1 \Rightarrow \sin i = \mu \sin A$

For small angles ($\sin\theta \approx \theta$)

$\therefore i = \mu A$

Exercise 3 - Concept Application Problems CAP

1. (b) If $R_1 = R, R_2 = -2R$

$\frac{1}{f} = (\mu-1)\left(\frac{1}{R_1} - \frac{1}{R_2}\right)$

$\frac{1}{6} = (1.5-1)\left(\frac{1}{R} + \frac{1}{2R}\right) = \frac{0.5 \times 3}{2R}$

$R = 4.5$ cm

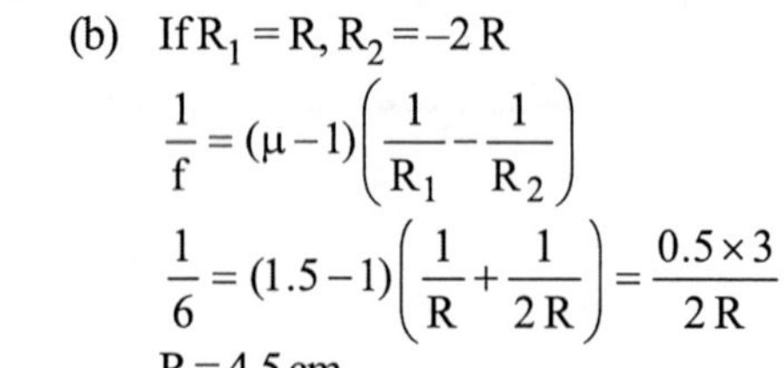

2. (b)

3. (b) Here, $P_1 = 5$ D

$P_2 = P - P_1 = 2 - 5 = -3$ D

$\frac{\omega_1}{\omega_2} = -\frac{f_1}{f_2} = \frac{-P_2}{P_1} = \frac{3}{5}$

4. (b) 5. (c)

6. (b) Since $\frac{\text{Apparent depth}}{\text{Real depth}} = \frac{1}{\mu}$

$\Rightarrow$ Apparent depth = d/μ

So mark raised up = Real depth – Apparent depth

$$= d - \frac{d}{\mu} = d\left(1 - \frac{1}{\mu}\right) = \left(\frac{\mu - 1}{\mu}\right)d$$

7. (d) Let d be the depth of two liquids.
Then apparent depth

$$\frac{(d/2)}{\mu} + \frac{(d/2)}{1.5\mu} = \frac{d}{2} \text{ or } \frac{1}{\mu} + \frac{2}{3\mu} = 1$$

Solving we get $\mu = 1.671$

8. (d) Distance of image from plane mirror = 3 m at the back. To photograph the image, camera must be focussed for a distance of 4.5 + 3 = 7.5 m.

9. (d) The necessary condition is

$$\frac{\omega}{\omega'} = -\frac{f}{f'} \text{ which is satisfied by (d)}$$

10. (b) $M = \frac{\beta}{\alpha} = \frac{f_0}{f_e}$ $\therefore$ $\beta = \frac{f_0}{f_e}\alpha = \frac{60}{5} \times 2° = 24°$

11. (b) 12. (d)

13. (b) $m = \frac{v}{u}$

$$\frac{1}{v} - \frac{1}{u} = \frac{1}{f}$$

Multiply the equation by v

$$1 - \frac{v}{u} = \frac{v}{f} \Rightarrow \frac{v}{u} = 1 - \frac{v}{f}$$

$$\therefore m = 1 - \frac{v}{f}$$

$$\text{Slope} = -\frac{1}{f} = \frac{b}{c} \Rightarrow f = \frac{c}{b}$$

14. (d) For 1st lens, $u_1 = -30$, $f_1 = +10$cm,

Formula of lens, $\frac{1}{v_1} + \frac{1}{30} = \frac{1}{10}$

or, $v_1 = 15$ cm at I_1 behind the lens.

The images I_1 serves as virtual object for concave lens. For second lens, which is concave, $u_2 = (15 - 5) = 10$ cm. I_1 acts as object. $f_2 = -10$ cm.

The rays will emerge parallel to axis as the virtual object is at focus of concave lens, as shown in the figure. Image of I_1 will be at infinity. These parallel rays are incident on the third lens viz the convex lens, $f_3 = +30$ cm. These parallel rays will be brought to convergence at the focus of the third lens.

$\therefore$ Image distance from third lens = f_3 = 30 cm

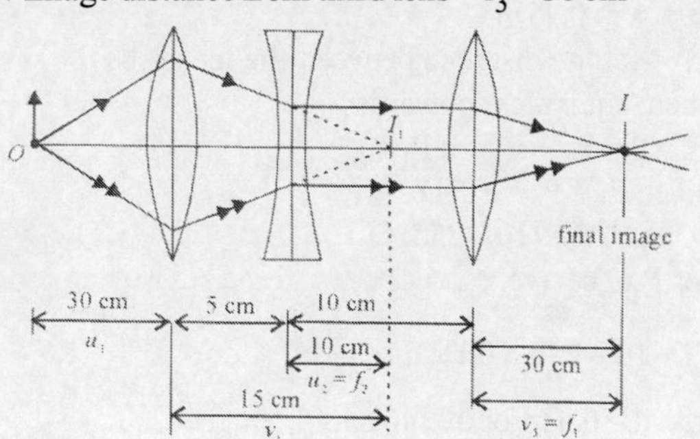

15. (b) ${}^a\mu_g = 1.5$

$\therefore$ 1.5 = cosecC or C = 42°. Critical angle for glass = 42°. Hence a ray of light incident at 50° in glass medium undergoes total internal reflection. δ denotes the deviation of the ray.

$\therefore$ δ = 180° – (50° + 50°) or δ = 80°.

16. (c)

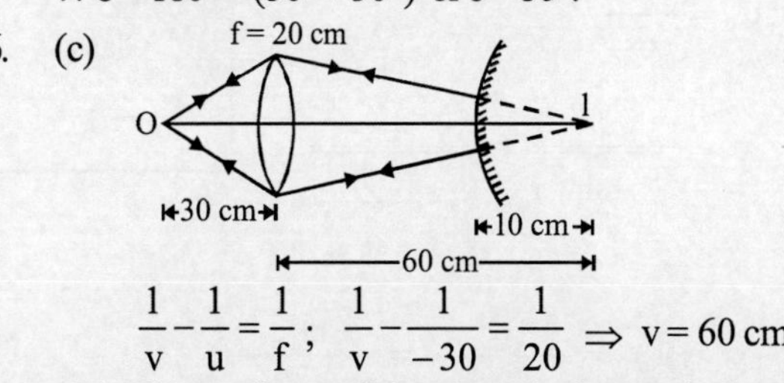

$$\frac{1}{v} - \frac{1}{u} = \frac{1}{f};\ \frac{1}{v} - \frac{1}{-30} = \frac{1}{20} \Rightarrow v = 60 \text{ cm}$$

Coincidence is possible when the image is formed at the centre of curvature of the mirror. Only then the rays refracting through the lens will fall normally on the convex mirror and retrace their path to form the image at O. So the distance between lens and mirror = 60 – 10 = 50 cm.

17. (a) Let a ray of light enter at A and refracted beam is AB. This is incident at an angle θ. For no refraction at the lateral face θ > C

sin θ > sin C But θ + r = (90°)

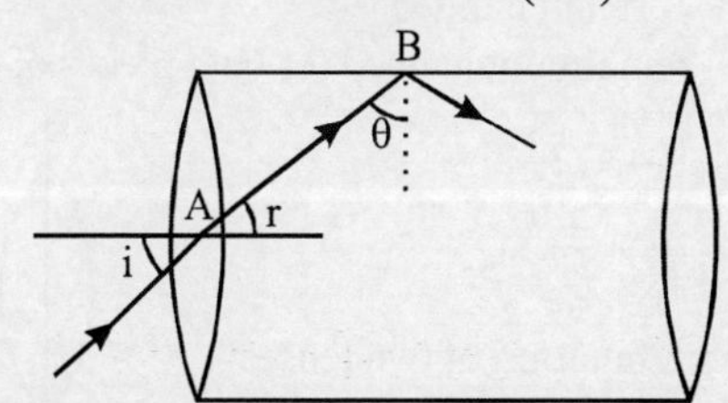

$\therefore$ sin (90° – r) > sin C or cos r > sin C ..(1)

From Snell's law $n = \frac{\sin i}{\sin r} \Rightarrow \sin r = \frac{\sin i}{n}$

$$\therefore \cos r = \sqrt{1 - \sin^2 r} = \sqrt{\left(1 - \frac{\sin^2 i}{n^2}\right)}$$

$\therefore$ equation (1) gives, $\sqrt{1 - \frac{\sin^2 i}{n^2}} > \sin C$

$$\Rightarrow 1 - \frac{\sin^2 i}{n^2} > \sin^2 C$$

Also $\sin C = \frac{1}{n}$

$$\therefore 1 - \frac{\sin^2 i}{n^2} > \frac{1}{n^2} \text{ or } 1 > \frac{\sin^2 i}{n^2} + \frac{1}{n^2}$$

$$\text{or } \frac{1}{n^2}(\sin^2 i + 1) < 1 \text{ or } n^2 > \sin^2 i + 1$$

Maximum value of sin i = 1

$$\therefore \quad n^2 > 2 \Rightarrow n > \sqrt{2}$$

18. (a) For point A, ${}_a\mu_g = \frac{\sin 45}{\sin r}$ $\Rightarrow$ $\sin r = \frac{1}{\sqrt{2}\,{}_a\mu_g}$

for point B, sin (90 – r) = ${}_g\mu_a$

$(90 - r)$ is critical angle.

$\therefore \cos r = {}_g\mu_a = \dfrac{1}{{}_a\mu_g}$

$\Rightarrow {}_a\mu_g = \dfrac{1}{\cos r}$

$= \dfrac{1}{\sqrt{1-\sin^2 r}} = \dfrac{1}{\sqrt{1-\dfrac{1}{2\,{}_a\mu_g^{\,2}}}}$

$\Rightarrow {}_a\mu_g^{\,2} = \dfrac{1}{1-\dfrac{1}{2\,{}_a\mu_g^2}} = \dfrac{2\,{}_a\mu_g^2}{2\,{}_a\mu_g^2 - 1}$

$\Rightarrow 2\,{}_a\mu_g^2 - 1 = 2 \Rightarrow {}_a\mu_g = \sqrt{\dfrac{3}{2}}$

19. (b) $\dfrac{1}{f} = (\mu-1)\left(\dfrac{1}{R_1} - \dfrac{1}{R_2}\right)$

in this case,

R_1 and R_2 are unchanged

So, f will remain unchanged for both pieces of the lens

$\therefore f = f'$

$\dfrac{1}{f} = \dfrac{1}{f_1} + \dfrac{1}{f_2}$

This is combination of two lenses of equal focal length

$\therefore \left[\dfrac{1}{f} = \dfrac{1}{f'} + \dfrac{1}{f'} = \dfrac{2}{f'}\right] \Rightarrow f'' = 2f$

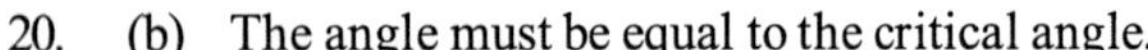

20. (b) The angle must be equal to the critical angle,

$C = \sin^{-1}\left(\dfrac{1}{\mu}\right) = \sin^{-1}\left(\dfrac{1}{\sqrt{2}}\right) = 45°$

21. (d) Here $\dfrac{x}{1000} = \dfrac{1.22\lambda}{D}$ or $x = \dfrac{1.22 \times 5 \times 10^3 \times 10^{-10} \times 10^3}{10 \times 10^{-2}}$

or $x = 1.22 \times 5 \times 10^{-3}\,m = 6.1\,m$

x is of the order of 5 mm.

22. (c)

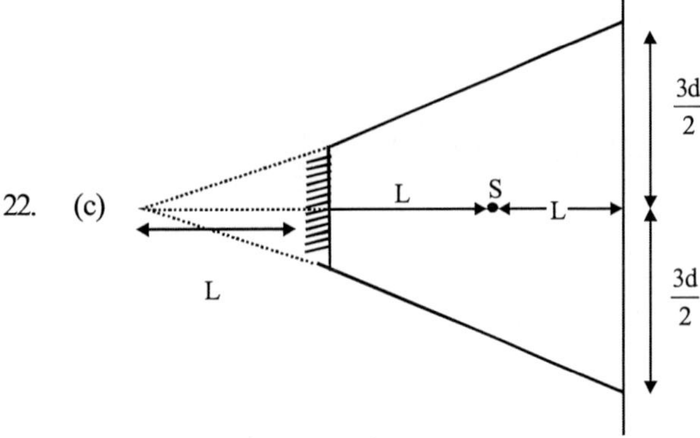

Total distance $= \dfrac{3d}{2} + \dfrac{3d}{2} = 3d$

23. (b)

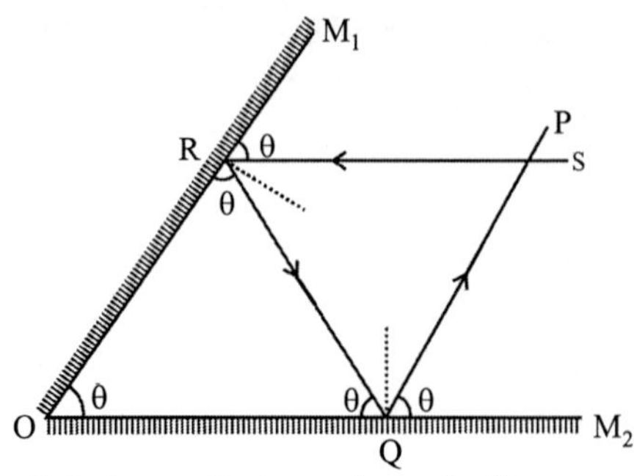

Let angle between the two mirrors be θ.

Ray PQ ∥ mirror M_1 and Rs ∥ mirror M_2

$\therefore \quad M_1Rs = \angle ORQ = \angle M_1OM_2 = \theta$

Similarly, $\angle M_2QP = \angle OQR = \angle M_2OM_1 = \theta$

$\therefore \quad$ In ΔORQ, $3\theta = 180° \Rightarrow \theta = \dfrac{180°}{3} = 60°$

24. (c) Using mirror formula, magnification is given by

$m = \dfrac{f}{u-f} = \dfrac{-1}{1-\dfrac{u}{f}}$

At focus magnification is ∞

And at $u = 2f$, magnification is 1.

Hence graph (d) correctly depicts 'm' versus distance of object 'x' graph.

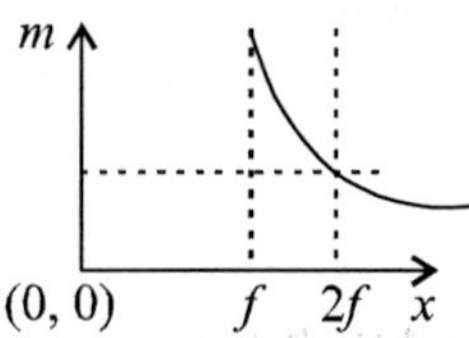

25. (a) In the position of minimum deviation, $i_1 = i_2$.

26. (a) $\mu = \dfrac{\sin i}{\sin r} \quad \because i = 2r$

$\Rightarrow \mu = \dfrac{\sin 2r}{\sin r} = \dfrac{2\sin r.\cos r}{\sin r}$

$r = \cos^{-1}\left(\dfrac{\mu}{2}\right), \quad \therefore \quad i = 2\cos^{-1}\left(\dfrac{\mu}{2}\right)$

27. (d) $M = 4 = -\dfrac{V}{4}$

$\Rightarrow V = -4u$

Using mirror formula

$\dfrac{1}{V} + \dfrac{1}{4} = \dfrac{1}{F} \Rightarrow \dfrac{1}{-4u} + \dfrac{1}{4} = \dfrac{-1}{0.6}$

$\Rightarrow \dfrac{1-40}{-44} = \dfrac{-1}{0.6}$

$\Rightarrow 4 = -0.45\,m$

28. (a) Let the distance between the lenses be d.

Then, equivalent power is

$P = P_1 + P_2 - d\,P_1 P_2$

Given $P_1 = P_2 = +5\,D$

$\therefore \quad P = (10 - 25d)\,D$

For P to be –ve,

$10 - 25d < 0 \Rightarrow d > \dfrac{2}{5}\,m$

or, $d > 0.4\,m$ or $d > 40\,cm$

29. (b)

30. (c) Given,

Refractive index, $\mu = \frac{4}{3}$

$\frac{4}{3}\sin\theta = 1\sin 90°$

$\Rightarrow \sin\theta = \frac{3}{4}$

$\cos\theta = \frac{\sqrt{7}}{4}$

Solid angle, $\Omega = 2\pi(1-\cos\theta) = 2\pi(1-\sqrt{7}/4)$

Fraction of energy transmitted

$= \frac{2\pi(1-\cos\theta)}{4\pi} = \frac{1-\sqrt{7}/4}{2} = 0.17$

Percentage of light emerges out of surface

$= 0.17 \times 100 = 17\%$

31. (c) Using, $\sin\theta_{max} = \mu_1\sqrt{\mu_2^2 - \mu_1^2} = \sqrt{\frac{\mu_2^2}{\mu_1^2} - 1}$

or $\theta_{max} = \sin^{-1}\left(\sqrt{\frac{\mu_2^2}{\mu_1^2} - 1}\right)$

For $T_1 R, \theta < \sin^{-1}\left(\sqrt{\frac{\mu_2^2}{\mu_1^2} - 1}\right)$

32. (d) From the given figure

As $\sin 60° = \mu \sin 30°$

$\Rightarrow \mu = \frac{\sin 60°}{\sin 30°} = \sqrt{3}$

$\frac{a}{AO} = \cos 60° \Rightarrow AO = 2a$

$\frac{b}{BO} = \cos 30° \Rightarrow BO = \frac{2b}{\sqrt{3}}$

Optical path length $= AO + \mu BO$

$= 2a + (\sqrt{3})\frac{2b}{\sqrt{3}} = 2a + 2b$

33. (d) From lens formula,

$\frac{1}{v} - \frac{1}{u} = \frac{1}{f} \Rightarrow v = \frac{uf}{u+f}$

Case-I : If $v = u \Rightarrow f + u = f \Rightarrow u = 0$

Case-II : If $u = \infty$ then $v = f$.

Hence, correct u versus v graph, that satisfies this condition is (a).

34. (a) Focal length of plano-convex lens-

$\frac{1}{f_1} = (\mu_1 - 1)\left(\frac{1}{\infty} - \frac{1}{-R}\right) = \frac{\mu_1 - 1}{R}$

$\Rightarrow f_1 = \frac{R}{(\mu_1 - 1)}$

Focal length of plano-concave lens -

$\frac{1}{f_2} = (\mu_2 - 1)\left(\frac{1}{-R} - \frac{1}{\infty}\right) = \frac{\mu_2 - 1}{-R}$

$\Rightarrow f_2 = \frac{-R}{(\mu_2 - 1)}$

For the combination of two lens-

$\frac{1}{f_{eq}} = \frac{1}{f_1} + \frac{1}{f_2} = \frac{\mu_1 - 1}{R} - \frac{\mu_2 - 1}{R}$

$= \frac{\mu_1 - \mu_2}{R}$

$\Rightarrow f_{eq} = \frac{R}{\mu_1 - \mu_2}$

35. (d) From the equation of line

$m = k_1 v + k_2 \quad (\because y = mx + c)$

$\Rightarrow \frac{v}{u} = k_1 v + k_2 \quad \left(\because m = \frac{v}{u}\right)$

$\Rightarrow \frac{1}{u} = k_1 + \frac{k_2}{v}$ (Dividing both sides by v)

$\Rightarrow \frac{k_2}{v} - \frac{1}{u} - k_1$

Comparing with lens formula $\frac{1}{v} - \frac{1}{u} = \frac{1}{f}$, we get

$k_1 = \frac{1}{-f}$ and $k_2 = 1$

$\therefore f = \frac{1}{\text{slope of } m - v \text{ graph}} = -\frac{b}{c}$

36. (b) Using, $M = \frac{v}{u}$

or $-2 = \frac{v_1}{x_1} \Rightarrow v_1 = -2x_1$

We have $\frac{1}{v} - \frac{1}{u} = \frac{1}{f}$

or $\frac{1}{-2x_1} - \frac{1}{x_1} = \frac{1}{20}$

$x_1 = 30$ cm

And $\frac{1}{2x_2} - \frac{1}{x_2} = \frac{1}{20}$

or $x_2 = -10$ cm

So, $\frac{x_1}{x_2} = \frac{30}{10} = 3$

37. (a) $\frac{1}{f_1} = \frac{2}{f_\ell}$

Here $2f_1 = 18$ cm or $f_1 = 9$ cm

So, $\frac{1}{9} = \frac{2}{f_\ell}$ or $f_\ell = 18$ cm

Using, $\frac{1}{f_\ell} = (\mu - 1)\left(\frac{2}{R}\right)$

or $\frac{1}{18} = (1.5 - 1)\left(\frac{2}{R}\right)$

$\therefore R = 18$ cm

when liquid is put between, then

$\frac{1}{f_2} = \frac{2}{f_\ell} + \frac{2}{f}$

or $\frac{1}{(27/2)} = \frac{2}{18} + \frac{2}{f}$

or $f = -54$ cm

Now $-\frac{1}{54} = (\mu_1 - 1) \times \frac{1}{R} = (\mu_1 - 1) \times \left(\frac{1}{-18}\right)$

$\therefore \mu_1 = \frac{1}{3} + 1 = \frac{4}{3}$

38. (d) By lens's formula, $\frac{1}{V} - \frac{1}{u} = \frac{1}{f}$

For first lens, $[u_1 = -20]$

$$\frac{1}{V_1} - \frac{1}{-20} = \frac{1}{5} \Rightarrow V_I = \frac{20}{3}$$

Image formed by first lense will behave as an object for second lens

so, $u_2 = \frac{20}{3} - 2 = \frac{14}{3}$

$$\frac{1}{V_2} - \frac{1}{\frac{14}{3}} = \frac{1}{-5} \Rightarrow V_2 = 70\,\text{cm}$$

39. (a) According to lens maker's formula,

$$\frac{1}{f} = (\mu_{rel} - 1)\left(\frac{1}{R_1} - \frac{1}{R_2}\right)$$

Focal length of lens will change due to change in refractive index μ_{rel}. So, image will be formed at new position. Hence image disappears

40. (d) By lens formula

$$\frac{1}{v} - \frac{1}{u} = \frac{1}{f}$$

$$\frac{1}{v} - \frac{1}{(-20)} = \frac{10}{3}$$

$$\frac{1}{v} = \frac{10}{3} - \frac{1}{20}$$

$$\frac{1}{v} = \frac{197}{60};\ v = \frac{60}{197}$$

Magnification of lens (m) is given by

$$m = \left(\frac{v}{u}\right) = \frac{\left(\frac{60}{197}\right)}{20}$$

velocity of image wrt. to lens is given by

$v_{I/L} = m^2 v_{O/L}$

direction of velocity of image is same as that of object

$v_{O/L} = 5$ m/s

$$v_{I/L} = \left(\frac{60 \times 1}{197 \times 20}\right)^2 (5)$$

$= 1.16 \times 10^{-3}$ m/s towards the lens

41. (b) From lens maker's formula,

$$\frac{1}{f} = (\mu - 1)\left(\frac{1}{R_1} - \frac{1}{R_2}\right)$$

$$\frac{1}{f_1} = (\mu_1 - 1)\left(\frac{1}{\infty} - \frac{1}{-R}\right) = \frac{1}{2f_2}$$

Similarly, for plano-concave lens

$$\frac{1}{f_2} = (\mu_2 - 1)\left(\frac{1}{-R} - \frac{1}{\infty}\right)$$

Dividing $\frac{1}{f_1}$ by $\frac{1}{f_2}$ we get,

$$\frac{(\mu_1 - 1)}{R} = \frac{(\mu_2 - 1)}{2R}$$

or, $2\mu_1 - \mu_2 = 1$

42. (d) using, $\frac{\mu_2}{v} - \frac{\mu_1}{u} = \frac{\mu_2 - \mu_1}{R}$

$R = 7.8$ mm

$\mu_1 = 1$ $\mu_2 = 1.34$

$$\Rightarrow \frac{1.34}{V} - \frac{1}{\infty} = \frac{1.34 - 1}{7.8} [\because u = \infty]$$

$\therefore V = 30.7$ mm $= 3.07$ cm $\simeq 3.1$ cm

43. (c) For minimum deviation:

$$r_1 = r_2 = \frac{A}{2} = 30^\circ$$

by Snell's law $\mu_1 \sin i = \mu_2 \sin r$

$$1 \times \sin i = \sqrt{3} \times \frac{1}{2} = \frac{\sqrt{3}}{2} \Rightarrow i = 60$$

44. (a) According question, $M = 375$

$L = 150$ mm, $f_0 = 5$ mm and $f_e = ?$

Using, magnification, $M \simeq \frac{L}{f_0}\left(1 + \frac{D}{f_e}\right)$

$$\Rightarrow 375 = \frac{150}{5}\left(1 + \frac{250}{f_e}\right) \quad (\because D = 25\,\text{cm} = 250\,\text{mm})$$

$$\Rightarrow 12.5 = 1 + \frac{250}{f_e}$$

$$\Rightarrow f_e = \frac{250}{11.5} = 21.7 \approx 22\,mm$$

45. (Bouns) $v_1 = \frac{40 \times 20}{(40 - 20)} = 40\,cm$

$u_2 = 60 - 40 = 20$ cm

$$\therefore v_2 = \frac{20 \times 10}{(20 - 10)} = 20\,cm$$

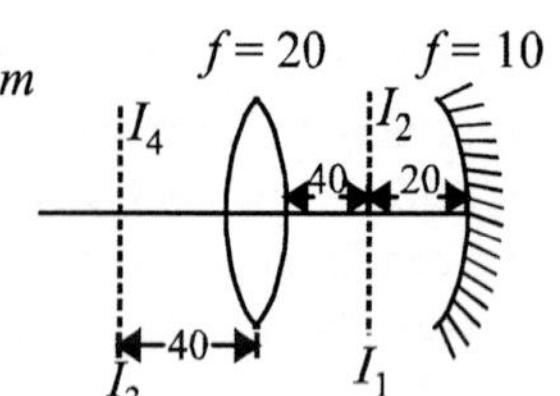

$\therefore$ Image traces back to object itself as image formed by lens is a centre of curvature of mirror.

25 Wave Optics

Topic 25.1 : Wavefront, Huygens Wave Theory, Interference of Light and Young's Double Slit Experiment

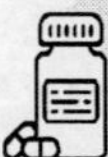

WAVEFRONT

The locus of all particles of the medium vibrating in the same phase at a given instant is called a wavefront. Depending on the shape of source of light, **wavefront can be of three types.**

(i) Spherical wavefront: A spherical wavefront is produced by a point source of light. This is because the locus of all such points which are equidistant from the point source will be a sphere. Spherical wavefronts are further divided into two headings: (i) converging spherical and (ii) diverging spherical wavefront.

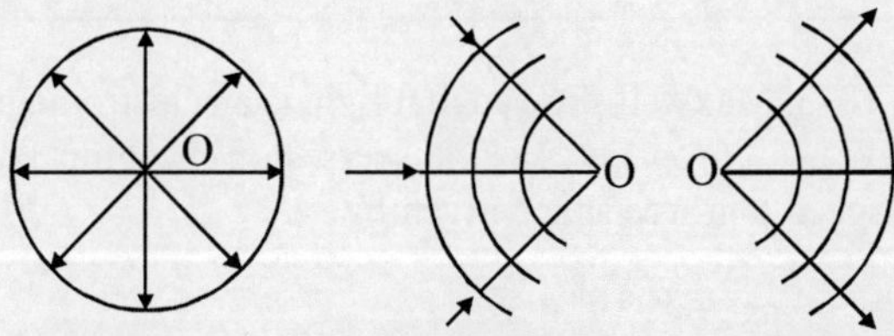

Spherical wavefront Converging spherical wavefront Diverging spherical wavefront

(ii) Cylindrical wavefront: When the source of light is linear in shape such as a slit, the cylindrical wavefront is produced. This is because all the points equidistant from a line source lie on the surface of a cylinder.

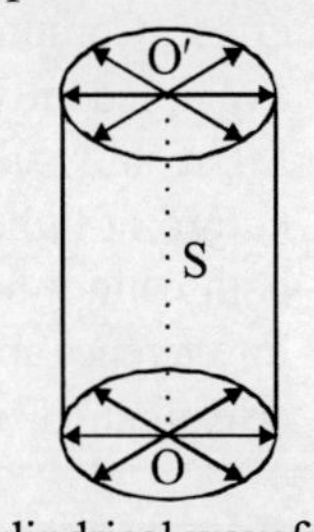

Cylindrical wavefront

(iii) Plane wavefront: A small part of a spherical or cylindrical wavefront due to a distant source will appear plane and hence it is called plane wavefront. The wavefront of parallel rays is a plane wavefront.

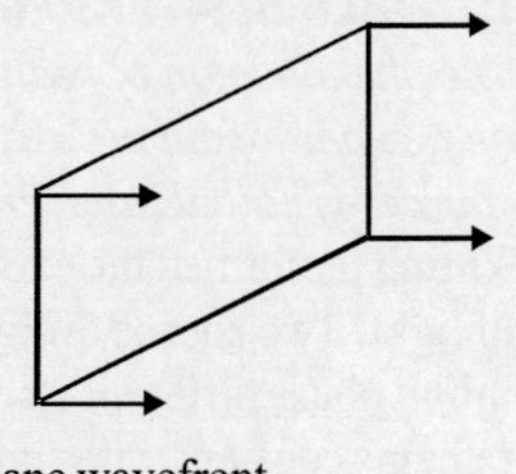

Plane wavefront

HUYGENS WAVE THEORY

(Geometrical method to find the secondary wavefront)

(i) Each point source of light is a centre of disturbance from which waves spread in all directions.

(ii) Each point on primary wavelets acts as a new source of distrubance and produces secondary wavelets which travel in space with the speed of light.

(iii) The forward envelope of the secondary wavelets at any instant gives the new wavefront.

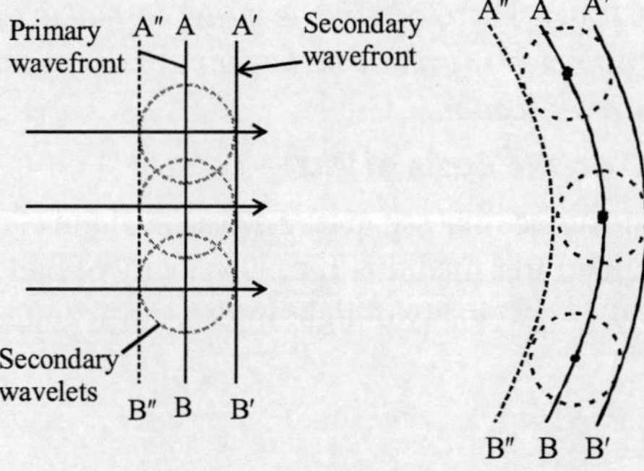

(iv) In a homogeneous medium the wavefront is always perpendicular to the direction of wave propagation.

Note : With the help of Huygen's wave theory, law of reflection and refraction, total internal reflection and dispersion can be explained easily. This theory also explain interference, diffraction and polarization successfully.

Drawbacks of Huygens Wave Theory

(a) This theory cannot explain photo-electric effect, compton, and Raman effect.

(b) Hypothetical medium in vacuum is not true imagination.

(c) The theory predicted the presence of back wave, which proved to be failure.

REFLECTION AND REFRACTION OF PLANE WAVES USING HUYGENS PRINCIPLE

Reflection on the Basis of Wave Theory

According to Huygens principle, every point on AB is a source of secondary wavelets. Let the secondary wavelets from B strike reflecting surface M_1M_2 at A′ in t seconds.

$\therefore \quad BA' = c \times t \qquad \ldots$ (i)

where c is the velocity of light in the medium.

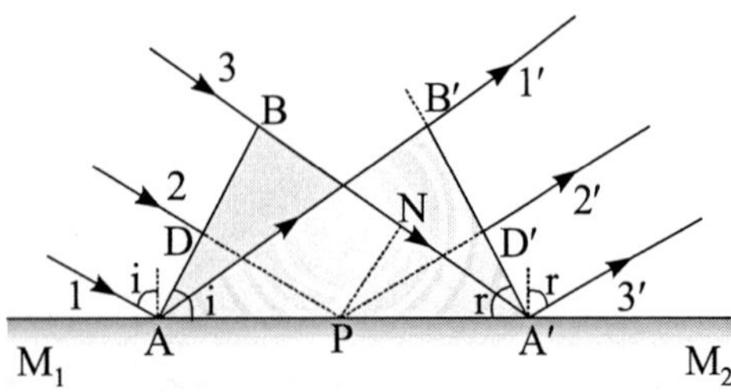

The secondary wavelets from A will travel the same distance c × t in the same time. Therefore, with A as centre and c × t as radius, draw an arc B′, so that

$AB' = c \times t \qquad \ldots$ (ii)

A′B′ is the true reflected wavefront.

angle of incidence, i = $\angle BAA'$

and angle of reflection, r = $\angle B'A'A$

In ∆s AA′B and AA′B′,

AA′ is common, $BA' = AB' = c \times t$, and $\angle B = \angle B' = 90°$

$\therefore$ ∆s are congruent $\therefore$ $\angle BAA' = \angle B'A'A$, *i.e.*, $\angle i = \angle r$ ... (iii)

Which is the *first law of reflection.*

Further, the incident wavefront AB, the reflecting surface M_1M_2 and the reflected wavefront A′B′ are all perpendicular to the plane of the paper. Therefore, *incident ray, normal to the mirror M_1M_2 and reflected ray all lie in the plane of the paper. This is second law of reflection.*

Refraction on the Basis of Wave Theory

XY is a plane surface that separates a denser medium of refractive index μ from a rarer medium. If c_1 is velocity of light in rarer medium and c_2 is velocity of light in denser medium, then by definition.

$$\mu = \frac{c_1}{c_2} \qquad \ldots \text{(iv)}$$

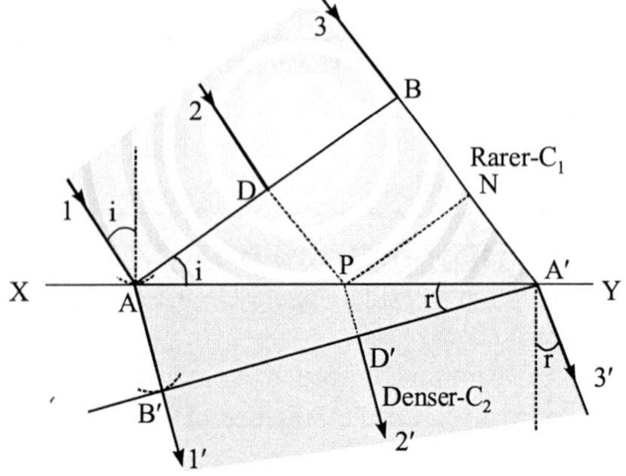

AB is a plane wave front incident on XY at $\angle BAA' = \angle i$. 1, 2, 3 are the corresponding incident rays normal to AB.

According to Huygens principle, every point on AB is a source of secondary wavelets. Let the secondary wavelets from B strike XY at A′ in t seconds.

$\therefore \quad BA' = c_1 \times t \qquad \ldots$ (v)

The secondary wavelets from A travel in the denser medium with a velocity c_2 and would cover a distance $(c_2 \times t)$ in t seconds. A′B′ is the true refracted wavefront. Let r be the angle of refraction. As angle of refraction is equal to the angle which the refracted plane wavefront A′B′ makes with the refracting surface AA′, therefore, $\angle AA'B' = r$.

Let $\angle AA'B' = r$, angle of refraction.

In ∆AA′B, $\sin i = \frac{BA'}{AA'} = \frac{c_1 \times t}{AA'}$

In ∆ AA′B′, $\sin r = \frac{AB'}{AA'} = \frac{c_2 \times t}{AA'}$

$\therefore \quad \frac{\sin i}{\sin r} = \frac{c_1}{c_2} = \mu$ [using (iv)]

Hence $\mu = \frac{\sin i}{\sin r} \qquad \ldots$ (vi)

which proves *Snell's law of refraction.*

It is clear from fig. that the incident rays, normal to the interface XY and refracted rays, all lie in the same plane (i.e., in the plane of the paper). This is the second law of refraction.

Hence laws of refraction are established on the basis of wave theory.

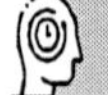

Problem Solving Tips

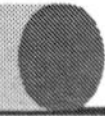

1. In 1873, Maxwell showed that light is an electromegnetic wave i.e. it propagates as transverse non-mechnical wave at speed c in free space given by

   $$c = \frac{1}{\sqrt{\mu_0 \varepsilon_0}} = 3 \times 10^8 \text{ ms}^{-1}$$

2. There are some phenomenon of light like photoelectric effect, Compton effect, Raman effect etc. which can be explained only on the basis of particle nature of light.
3. Light shows the dual nature i.e. particle as well as wave nature of light. But the wave nature and particle nature both cannot be possible simultaneously.
4. Interference and diffraction are the two phenomena that can be explained only on the basis of wave nature of light.

INTERFERENCE OF LIGHT WAVES AND YOUNG'S DOUBLE SLIT EXPERIMENT

The phenomenon of redistribution of light energy in a medium on account of superposition of light waves from two coherent sources is called ***interference of light waves.***

Young performed the experiment by taking two coherent sources of light. Two source of light waves are said to be coherent if the initial phase difference between the waves emitted by the source remains constant with time.

(i) The rays of light from two coherent sources S_1 and S_2 superpose each other on the screen forming alternately maxima and minima (constructive and destructive interference).

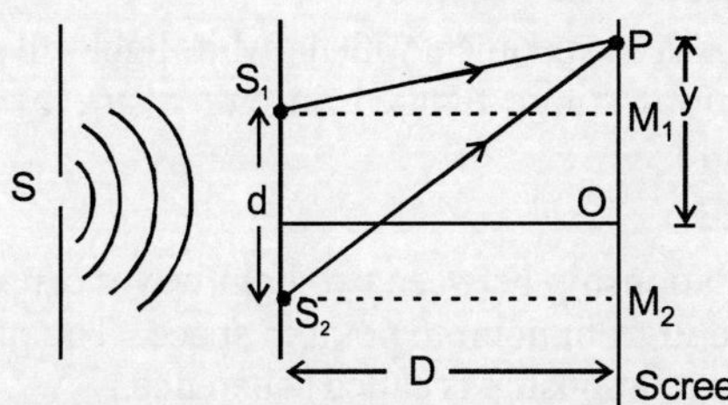

(ii) Let the equation of waves travelling from S_1 & S_2 are

$$y_1 = A_1 \text{Sin } \omega t \quad ...(1)$$

$$y_2 = A_2 \text{Sin } \omega t \quad ...(2)$$

where A_1 & A_2 are amplitudes of waves starting from S_1 & S_2 respectively. These two waves arrive at P by traversing different distances S_2P & S_1P. Hence they are superimposed with a phase difference (at point P) given by

$$\delta(\text{phase difference}) = \frac{2\pi}{\lambda} \times \Delta(\text{path difference})$$

$$= \frac{2\pi}{\lambda}(S_2P - S_1P). \quad ....(3)$$

where S_2P (from fig) $= D^2 + \left(y + \frac{d}{2}\right)^2$

$$\approx D + \frac{1}{2}\frac{(y+d/2)^2}{2D} \quad [\therefore D >> (y+d)]$$

Similarly, $S_1P \approx D + \frac{(y - d/2)^2}{4D}$

so, $S_2P - S_1P = \frac{yd}{D}$ ....(4)

(A) Conditions for maximum & minimum intensity :

(i) **Conditions for maximum intensity or constructive interference :** If phase difference $\delta = 0, 2\pi, 4\pi --- 2n\pi$

or, path difference $\Delta = S_2P - S_1P = 0, \lambda, 2\lambda --- n\lambda$ then resultant intensity at point P due two waves emanating from S_1 & S_2 is

$$I = A^2 = A_1^2 + A_2^2 + 2A_1A_2\cos\delta \quad (\therefore I \propto A^2)$$

or $I = (A_1 + A_2)^2$

or $I = I_1 + I_2 + 2\sqrt{I_1 I_2}$ ....(5)

It means that resultant intensity is greater than the sum of individual intensity (where A is the amplitude of resultant wave at point P).

(ii) **Conditions for minimum intensity or destructive interference :** If phase difference,

$$\delta = \pi, 3\pi, 5\pi ---- (2n+1)\pi$$

or, path difference

$$\Delta = S_2P - S_1P = \frac{\lambda}{2}, \frac{3\lambda}{2} --- (2n+1)\frac{\lambda}{2}$$

then resultant intensity at point P is

$$I = A^2 = A_1^2 + A_2^2 - 2A_1A_2\cos\delta$$

or $I = (A_1 - A_2)^2$

or $I = I_1 + I_2 - 2\sqrt{I_1}\sqrt{I_2}$ ...(6)

It means that resultant intensity I is less than the sum of individual intensities. Now as the position of point P on the screen changes, then the path difference at point P due to these two waves also changes & intensity alternately becomes maximum or minimum. These bright fringes (max. intensity) & dark fringes (min. intensity) make an interference pattern.

It must be clear that there is no loss of energy (at dark fringe) & no gain of energy (at bright fringe), but, only there is a redistribution of energy.

The shape of fringe obtained on the screen is approximately linear.

(B) Position of fringe:

(i) If $\Delta = S_2P - S_1P = n\lambda$, then we obtain bright fringes at point P on the screen and it corresponds to constructive interference. So from equation (4) the position of nth bright fringe

$$\Delta = S_2P - S_1P = n\lambda = \frac{yd}{D}$$

or $y = \left(\frac{nD}{d}\right)\lambda$ ...(7)

(Position of nth bright fringe)

(ii) If $\Delta = S_2P - S_1P = (2n+1)\frac{\lambda}{2}$, then we obtain dark fringe at point P on the screen and corresponds to destructive interference. So from equation(4), the position of, n^{th} dark fringe is

$$\Delta = S_2P - S_1P = (2n+1)\frac{\lambda}{2} = \frac{yd}{D}$$

or $y = \frac{(2n+1)D\lambda}{2d}$ ...(8)

(Position of nth dark fringe)

(C) Spacing or fringe width :

Let y_n and y_{n+1} are the distance of nth and $(n+1)^{th}$ bright fringe from point O then

$$y_n = \frac{Dn\lambda}{d} \ \& \ y_{n+1} = \frac{D(n+1)\lambda}{d}$$

So spacing β between n^{th} and $(n+1)^{th}$ bright fringe is

$$\beta = y_{n+1} - y_n = \frac{D\lambda}{d} \quad ...(9)$$

Since it is independent of n, so fringe width or spacing between any two consecutive bright fringes is same.

Similarly the fringe width between any two consecutive dark fringe is

$$\beta = \frac{D\lambda}{d} \quad ...(10)$$

(D) Conditions for sustained interference:

(i) The two sources should be coherent i.e they should have a constant phase difference between them.

(ii) The two sources should give light of same frequency (or wavelength).

(iii) If the interfering waves are polarized, then they must be in same state of polarization.

(E) Conditions for good observation of fringe:

(i) The distance between two sources i.e. d should be small.

(ii) The distance of screen D from the sources should be quite large.

(iii) The two interfering wavefronts must intersect at a very small angle.

(F) Conditions for good contrast of fringe :

(i) Sources must be monochromatic i.e they emit waves of single wavelength.

(ii) The amplitude of two interfering waves should be equal or nearly equal.

(iii) Both sources must be narrow.

(iv) As Intensity I is directly proportional to the square of amplitude, hence Intensity of resultant wave at P,

$I = I_1 + I_2 + 2\sqrt{I_1 I_2}\cos\phi$; if $I_1 = I_2 = I_0$., then

$I = 4I_0 \cos^2\left(\phi/2\right)$

(v) $I_{max} = \left(\sqrt{I_1}+\sqrt{I_2}\right)^2$.

If $I_1 = I_2 = I_0$, then $I_{max} = 4I_0$

$I_{min} = \left(\sqrt{I_1}-\sqrt{I_2}\right)^2$, if $I_1 = I_2 = I_0$, then $I_{min} = 0$

(vi) $\dfrac{I_{max}}{I_{min}} = \left(\dfrac{\sqrt{I_1}+\sqrt{I_2}}{\sqrt{I_1}-\sqrt{I_2}}\right)^2$.

(vii) Angular fringe-width $\theta_0 = \dfrac{\beta}{D} = \dfrac{\lambda}{d}$

(viii) The width of all interference fringes are same. Since fringe width β is proportional to λ, hence fringes with red light are wider than those for blue light.

(ix) If the interference experiment is performed in a medium of refractive index μ instead of air, the wavelength of light will change from λ to $\dfrac{\lambda}{\mu}$.

i.e. $\beta' = \dfrac{D}{d}\left(\dfrac{\lambda}{\mu}\right) = \dfrac{\beta}{\mu}$

(x) If a transparent sheet of refractive index μ and thickness t is introduced in one of the paths of interfering waves, then due to its presence optical path will become μt instead of t. Due to this a given fringe from present position shifts to a new position. So the lateral shift of the fringe,

$$y_0 = \frac{D}{d}(\mu-1)t = \frac{\beta}{\lambda}(\mu-1)t$$

(xi) In **Young's double slit experiment** (coherent sources in phase): Central fringe is a bright fringe. It is on the prerpendicular bisector of coherent sources. Central fringe position is at a place where two waves having equal phase superpose.

(xii) Young's experiment with the white light will give white central fringe flanked on either side by coloured bands.

COHERENCE

The phase relationship between two light waves can very from time to time and from point to point in space. The property of definite phase relationship is called coherence.

1. **Temporal coherence :** A light wave (photon) is produced when an excited atom goes to the ground state and emits light.

   (i) The duration of this transition is about 10^{-9} to 10^{-10} sec. Thus the emitted wave remains sinusoidal for this much time. This time is known as coherence time (τ_c).

   (ii) Definite phase relationship is maintained for a length $L = c\tau_c$ called coherence length.

   For neon $\lambda = 6238$ Å, $\tau_c \approx 10^{-10}$ sec. and L = 0.03 m.

   For cadmium $\lambda = 6238$ Å, $\tau_c = 10^{-9}$ and L = 0.3 m

   For Laser $\tau_c = 10^{-5}$ sec and L = 3 km.

   (iii) The spectral lines width $\Delta\lambda$ is related to coherence length L and coherence time τ_c.

   $$\Delta\lambda \approx \frac{\lambda^2}{c\tau_c} \quad \text{or} \quad \Delta\lambda \approx \frac{\lambda^2}{L}$$

2. **Spatial coherence :** Two points in space are said to be spatially coherence if the waves reaching there maintains a constant phase difference. Points P and Q are at the same distance from S, they will always be having the same phase. Points P and P′ will be spatially coherent if the distance between P and P′ is much less than the coherence length i.e. $PP' << c\tau_c$

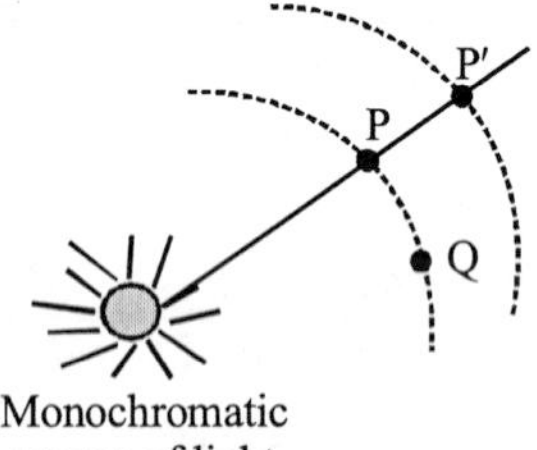

Methods of Obtaining Coherent Sources

Two coherent sources are produced from a single source of light by two methods :

(i) By division of wavefront and (ii) By division of amplitude.

(i) Division of wavefront : The wavefront emitted by a narrow source is divided in two parts by reflection, refraction or diffraction. The coherent sources so obtained are imaginary. **Example :** Fresnel's biprism, Llyod's mirror, Young's double slit, etc.

(ii) Division of amplitude : In this arrangement light wave is partly reflected (50%) and partly transmitted (50%) to produced two light rays. The amplitude of wave emitted by an extended source of light is divided in two parts by partial reflection and partial refraction. The coherent sources obtained are real and are obtained in Newton's rings, Michelson's interferometer, etc.

Incoherence of Two Conventional Light Sources

Let two conventional light sources L_1 and L_2 (like two sodium lamps or two monochromatic bulbs) illuminate two pin holes S_1 and S_2. Then we will find that no interference pattern is seen on the screen.

The reason is as follows : In conventional light source, light comes from a large number of independent atoms, each atom emitting light for about 10^{-9} seconds i.e., light emitted by an atom is essentially a pulse lasting for only 10^{-9} seconds.

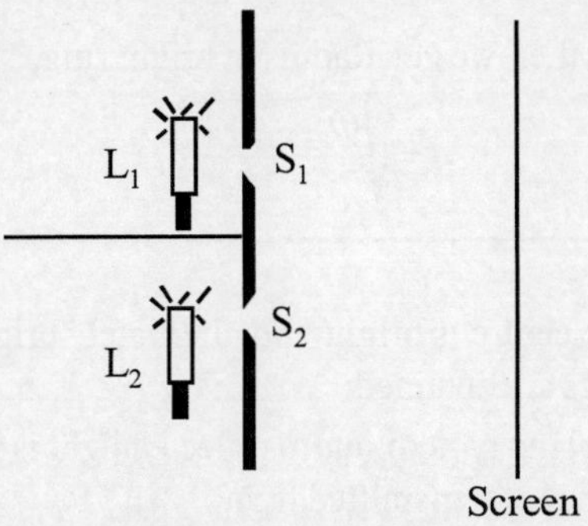

Even if all the atoms were emitting light pulses under similar conditions, waves from different atoms would differ in their initial phases. Consequently light coming out from the holes S_1 and S_2 will have a fixed phase relationship only for 10^{-9} sec. Hence any interference pattern formed on the screen would last only for 10^{-9} sec. (a billionth of a second), and then the pattern will change. The human eye can notice intensity changes which last at least for a tenth of a second and hence we will not be able to see any interference pattern. Instead due to rapid changes in the pattern, we will only observe a uniform intensity over the screen.

Lloyd's Mirror

The two sources are slit S (parallel to mirror) and its virtual image S′.

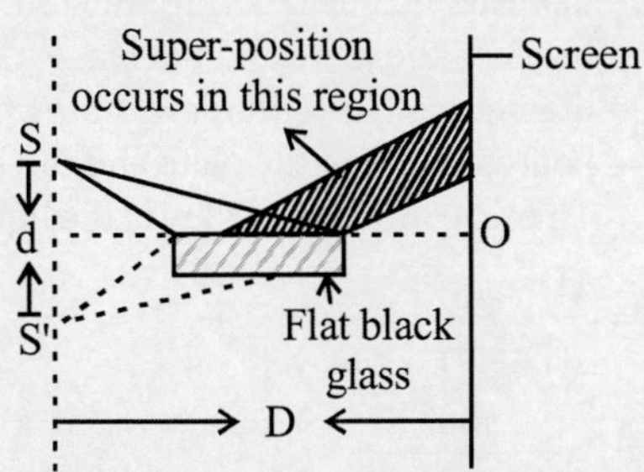

Lloyd mirror arrangement

(i) If screen is moved so that, point O touches the edge of glass plate, the geometrical path difference for two wave trains is zero. The phase change of π radian on reflection at denser medium causes a dark fringe to be formed.

- The fring width remains unchanged on introduction of transparent film.
- If the film is placed in front of upper slit S_1, the fringe pattern will shift upwards. On the other hand if the film is placed in front of lower slit S_2, the fringe pattern shifts downwards.

(ii) This interference pattern is frequently seen in a ripple tank when one uses a wave train to demonstrate the law of reflection.

(iii) In this case, fringe width $\beta = \frac{D\lambda}{d}$

Optical path : (Equivalent path in vacuum or air) In case of medium of refractive index μ and thickness t, the optical path = μt.

Interference in Thin Films

We are familiar with the colours produced by a thin film of oil on the surface of water and also by the thin film of a soap bubble. Hooke observed such colours in thin films of mica and similar thin transparent plates. Young was able to explain the phenomenon on the basis of interference between light reflected from the top and bottom surface of a thin film. It has been observed that interference in the case of thin films takes place due to (i) *reflected light and* (ii) *transmitted light.*

Interference due to reflected light

From the figure, the optical path difference between the reflected ray (AT) from the top surface and the reflected ray (CQ) from the bottom surface can be calculated. Let it be x, then

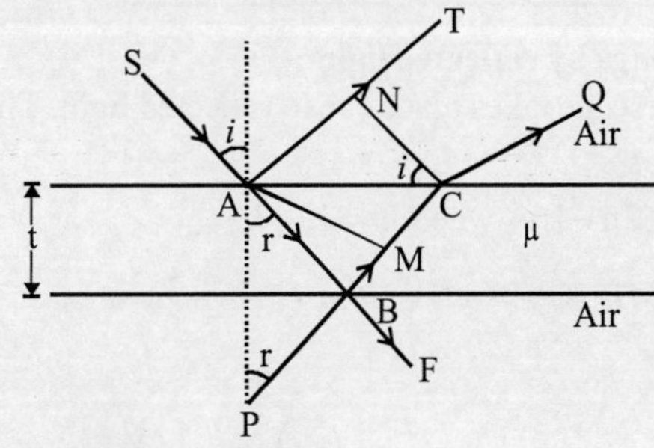

$x = \mu(AB + BC) - AN$

On simplification, we get

$x = 2\mu t \cos r$

1. If $2\mu t \cos r = (2n+1)\frac{\lambda}{2}$, where n = 0,1,2, ...then **constructive interference** takes place and the film appears bright.
2. If $2\mu t \cos r = n\lambda$, where n = 0, 1, 2, 3,............ then destructive interference takes place and the film appears dark.

Interference due to transmitted light

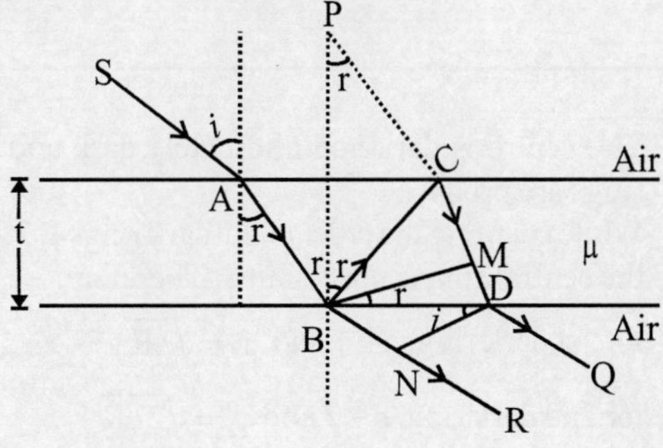

The optical path difference between the reflected ray (DQ) and the transmitted ray (NR) is given by

$$x = \mu(BC + CD) - BN$$

On simplification, we get

$$x = 2\mu t \cos r$$

1. If $2\mu t \cos r = n\lambda$, where n = 0, 1, 2, 3, ...then **constructive interference** takes place and the film appears bright.
2. If $2\mu t \cos r = (2n+1)\frac{\lambda}{2}$, $n = 0, 1, 2, ...$ then **destructive interference** takes place and the film appears dark.

Newton's Rings

Newton observed the formation of interference rings when a plano-convex lens is placed on a plane glass plate. When viewed with white light, the fringes are coloured while with monochromatic light, the fringes are bright and dark. These fringes are produced due to interference between the light reflected from the lower surface of the lens and the upper surface of the glass plate. Interference can also take place due to transmitted light.

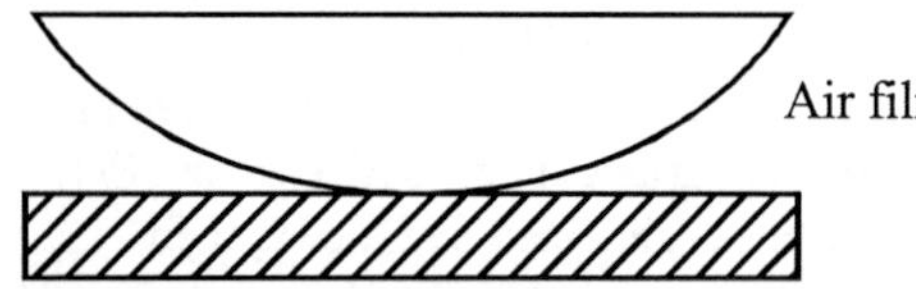

Newton's rings by reflected light :

Here, interference takes place due to reflected light. Therefore, for bright rings,

$$2\mu t \cos\theta = (2n-1)\frac{\lambda}{2} \text{ where } n = 1, 2, 3, ...$$

And for dark rings, $2\mu t \cos\theta = n\lambda, n = 1, 2, 3, ...$

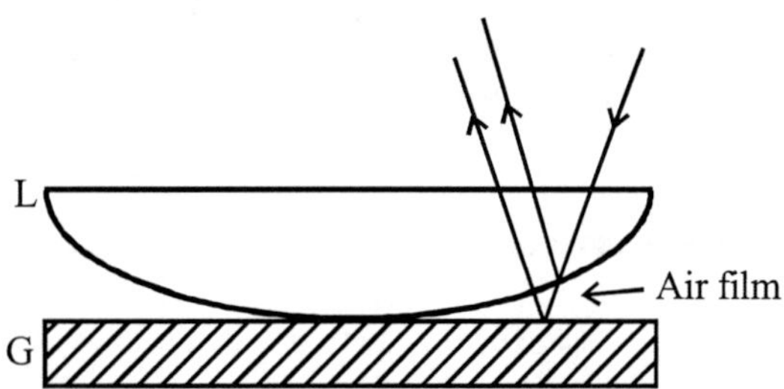

Proceeding further, we get the radius of rings as follows:

For bright rings, $r = \sqrt{\frac{(2n-1)\lambda R}{2}}$

For dark rings, $r = \sqrt{n\lambda R}$, where R = radius of curvature of lens.

Note :

(i) The centre is dark and alternately dark and bright rings are produced.

(ii) While counting the order of the dark rings 1, 2, 3, etc. the central ring is not counted. Therefore,

for 1st dark ring, n = 1 and $r_1 = \sqrt{\lambda R}$

for 2nd dark ring, n = 2 and $r_2 = \sqrt{2\lambda R}$

Newton's rings by transmitted light

Here, interference takes place due to transmitted light.

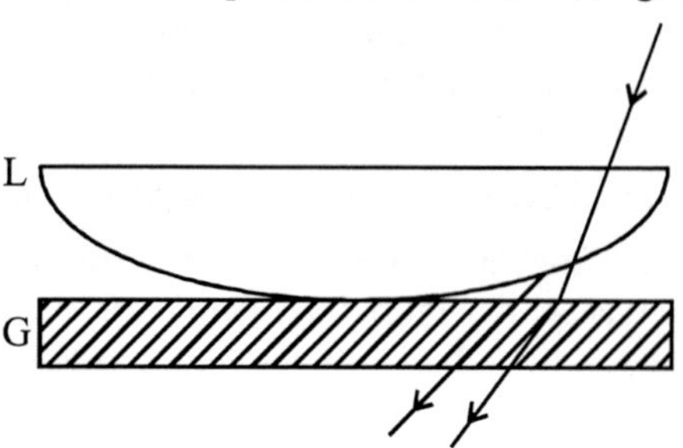

Therefore,

For bright rings, $2\mu t \cos\theta = n\lambda, n = 0, 1, 2, ...$

For dark rings, $2\mu t \cos\theta = (2n-1)\frac{\lambda}{2}$, $n = 0, 1, 2, ...$

Proceeding further, we get Radius of bright ring,

$$r = \sqrt{\frac{(2n-1)\lambda R}{2}}$$

Note :

(i) The centre is bright and alternately bright and dark rings are obtained.

(ii) The ring pattern due to reflected light is just opposite to that of transmitted light.

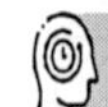 **Problem Solving Tips** 

1. If D_n and D_{n+m} be the diameters of n th and (n + m)th dark rings then the wavelength of light used is given by

$$\lambda = \frac{(D_{n+m})^2 - (D_n)^2}{4mR}$$

where, R is the radius of curvature of the lens.

2. If D_n = diameter of nth dark ring when air is present betwen the glass plate and the lens

D_{n+m} = diameter of (n+m)th dark ring when air is present between the glass plate and the lens

D'_n = diameter of n th dark ring when a liquid is poured between the plate and the lens

D'_{n+m} = diameter of (n+m)th dark ring when a liquid is poured between the plate and the lens

Then the refractive index of the liquid is given by

$$\mu = \frac{(D_{n+m})^2 - (D_n)^2}{(D'_{n+m})^2 - (D'_n)^2} \text{ or, }$$

$$\mu = \frac{4m\lambda R}{(D'_{n+m})^2 - (D'_n)^2}$$

Example 1.

In Young's expt., two coherent sources are placed 0.90 mm apart and fringes are observed one metre away. If it produces second dark fringe at a distance of 1 mm from central fringe, what would be the wavelength of monochromatic light used?

Solution :

For dark fringes, $x = (2n-1)\frac{\lambda D}{2d}$

$\therefore\ \lambda = \frac{2xd}{(2n-1)D} = \frac{2\times10^{-3}\times0.9\times10^{-3}}{(2\times2-1)\times1}$

or, $\lambda = 0.6\times10^{-6}\ m = 6\times10^{-5}$ cm.

Example 2.

Two beam of light having intensities I and 4 I interfere to produce a fringe pattern on a screen. The phase difference between the beams is π/2 at point A and π at point B. Then find the difference between the resultant intensities at A and B.

Solution :

Here, $I_1 = I;\ I_2 = 4I;\ \theta_1 = \pi/2,\ \theta_2 = \pi$

$I_A = I_1 + I_2 + 2\sqrt{I_1 I_2}\cos\theta_1$

$= I + 4I + 2\sqrt{I\times4\,I}\cos\pi/2 = 5I$

$I_B = I_1 + I_2 + 2\sqrt{I_1 I_2}\cos\theta_2$

$= I + 4I + 2\sqrt{I4I}\cos\pi = 5I - 4I = I;$

$\therefore\ I_A - I_B = 5I - I = 4I$

Example 3.

In a biprism experiment, 5th dark fringe is obtained at a point. If a thin transparent film is placed in the path of one of waves, then 7th bright fringe is obtained at the same point. Determine the thickness of the film in terms of wavelength λ and refractive index μ.

Solution :

For 5th dark fringe, $x_1 = (2n-1)\frac{\lambda}{2}\frac{D}{d} = \frac{9\lambda D}{2d}$

For 7th bright fringe, $x_2 = n\lambda\frac{D}{d} = \frac{7\lambda D}{d}$

but $x_2 - x_1 = (\mu-1)t\frac{D}{d};\ \frac{\lambda D}{d}\left[7-\frac{9}{2}\right] = (\mu-1)t\frac{D}{d}$

$\therefore$ Thickness, $t = \frac{2.5\lambda}{(\mu-1)}$

Example 4.

In a Young's double slit experiment the angular width of a fringe formed on a distant screen is 1°. The wavelength of the light used is 6280 Å. What is the distance between the two coherent sources ?

Solution :

The angular fringe width is given by $\alpha = \frac{\lambda}{d}$

where λ is wavelength and d is the distance between two coherent sources. Thus $d = \frac{\lambda}{\alpha}$

Given, $\lambda = 6280$ Å, $\alpha = 1° = \frac{\pi}{180}$ radian

Thus $d = \frac{6280\times10^{-10}}{3.14}\times180 = 3.6\times10^{-5}\ m = 0.036$ mm

25.1 Concept Practice Problems CPP

1. Light of wavelength 6.5×10^{-7} m is made incident on two slits 1 mm apart. The distance between third dark fringe and fifth bright fringe on a screen distant 1 m from the slits will be
   (a) 0.325 mm (b) 0.65 mm
   (c) 1.625 mm (d) 3.25 mm
2. If the intensities of the two interfering beams in Young's double-slit experiment are I_1 and I_2, then the contrast between the maximum and minimum intensities is good when
   (a) $|I_1$ and $I_2|$ is large (b) $|I_1$ and $I_2|$ is small
   (c) either I_1 or I_2 is zero (d) $I_1 = I_2$
3. To demonstrate the phenomenon of interference, we require two sources which emit radiation of
   (a) nearly the same frequency
   (b) the same frequency
   (c) different wavelengths
   (d) the same frequency and having a definite phase relationship
4. In Young's double slit expt. the distance between two sources is 0.1 mm. The distance of the screen from the source is 20 cm. Wavelength of light used is 5460 Å. The angular position of the first dark fringe is
   (a) 0.08° (b) 0.16° (c) 0.20° (d) 0.32°
5. The separation between successive fringes in a double slit arrangement is x. If the whole arrangement is dipped under water what will be the new fringe separation? [The wavelenght of light being used is 5000 Å]
   (a) 1.5x (b) x (c) 0.75x (d) 2x
6. Light from two coherent sources of the same amplitude A and wavelength λ illuminates the screen. The intensity of the central maximum is I_0. If the sources were incoherent, the intensity at the same point will be
   (a) $4I_0$ (b) $1I_0$ (c) I_0 (d) $I_0/2$
7. In Young's double slit experiment with sodium vapour lamp of wavelength 589 nm and the slits 0.589 mm apart, the half angular width of the central maximum is
   (a) $\sin^{-1}(0.01)$ (b) $\sin^{-1}(0.0001)$
   (c) $\sin^{-1}(0.001)$ (d) $\sin^{-1}(0.1)$
8. In young's double-slit experiment, the intensity of light at a point on the screen where the path difference is λ is I, λ being the wavelength of light used. The intensity at a point where the path difference is $\frac{\lambda}{4}$ will be
   (a) $\frac{I}{4}$ (b) $\frac{I}{2}$ (c) I (d) zero

9. In Young's double slit experiment, the fringes are displaced by a distance x when a glass plate of refractive index 1.5 is introduced in the path of one of the beams. When this plate is replaced by another plate of the same thickness, the shift of fringes is (3/2) x. The refractive index of the second plate is
(a) 1.75 (b) 1.50 (c) 1.25 (d) 1.00

10. In Young's double slit experiment, the slits are 2 mm apart and are illuminated by photons of two wavelengths $\lambda_1 = 12000Å$ and $\lambda_2 = 10000Å$. At what minimum distance from the common central bright fringe on the screen 2 m from the slit will a bright fringe from one interference pattern coincide with a bright fringe from the other ?
(a) 6mm (b) 4mm (c) 3mm (d) 8mm

ANSWER KEY

1	(c)	2	(d)	3	(d)	4	(b)	5	(c)	6	(d)	7	(c)	8	(b)	9	(a)	10	(a)

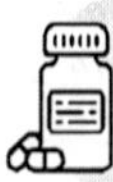

Topic 25.2 : Diffraction, Polarisation & Resolving Power of an Optical Instruments

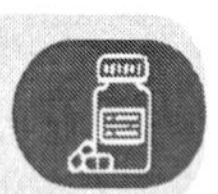

DIFFRACTION

When a wave is obstructed by an obstacle, the rays bend round the corner. This phenomenon is known as ***diffraction.***

Fraunhoffer Diffraction by Single Slit

In Fraunhoffer diffraction experiment, the source and the screen are effectively at infinite distance from the diffracting element.

In single slit diffraction, imagine aperature to be divided into two equal halves. Secondary sources in these two halves give first minima at b sin θ = λ

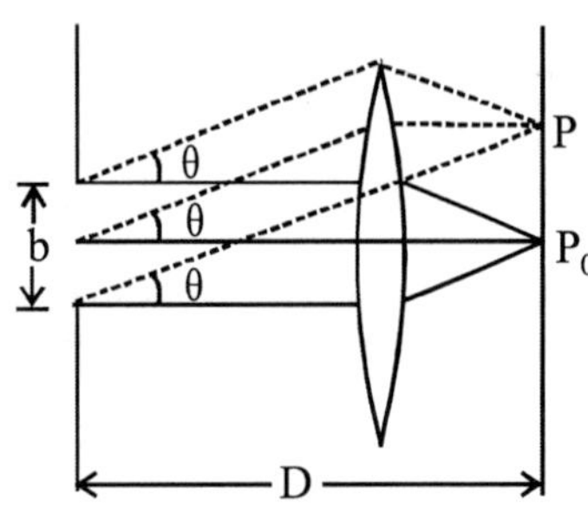

In general, $b\sin\theta = n\lambda$ *for minima and,* $b\sin\theta = (2n+1)\frac{\lambda}{2}$ *for maxima.*

(i) The points of the maximum intensity lie nearly midway between the successive minima. The amplitude E_0' of the electric field at a general point P is

$$E_0' = E_0\frac{\sin\beta}{\beta} \text{ where } \beta = \frac{\pi\, b\sin\theta}{\lambda} \text{ and}$$

E_0 = amplitude at the point P_0 i.e. at $\theta = 0$

The intensity at a general point P is given as $I = I_0\frac{\sin^2\beta}{\beta^2}$

(ii) The graph for the variation of intensity as a function of sinθ is as follows :

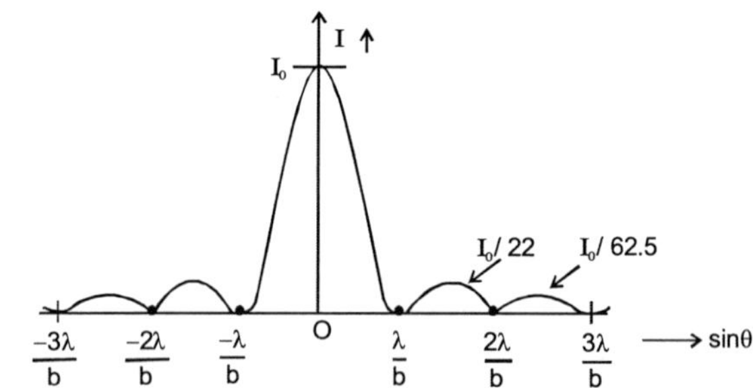

(iii) The width of the central maxima is $\left(\frac{2\lambda D}{b}\right)$ and angular width of central maxima is $\left(\frac{2\lambda}{b}\right)$.

Fraunh offer Diffraction by a Circular Aperture

(i) The 1st dark ring is formed by the light diffracted from the circular aperture at an angle θ with the axis where

$\sin\theta \approx \frac{1.22\lambda}{b}$ where λ = wavelength of light used,
b = diameter of circular aperture

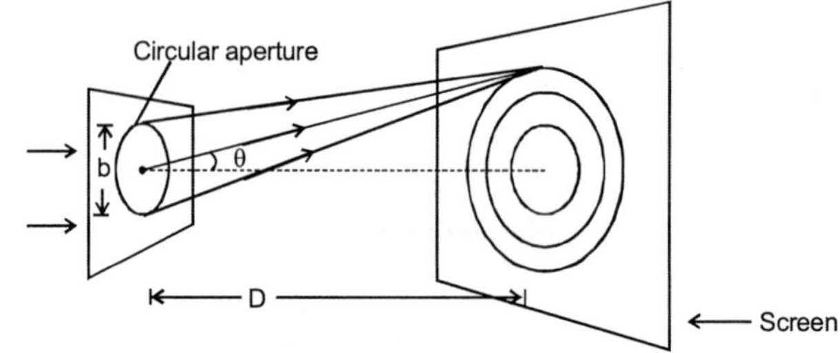

(ii) If the screen is at a distance D (D >> b) from the circular aperture, the radius of the 1st dark ring is,

$$R \approx \frac{1.22\lambda D}{b}$$

(iii) If the light transmitted by the hole is converged by a converging lens at the screen placed at the focal plane of the lens, the radius of the 1st dark ring is $R = \frac{1.22\lambda f}{b}$

This radius is also called the **radius of diffraction disc.**
For plane transmission diffraction grating
$(a+b)\sin\theta_n = n\lambda$ for maxima, where a = width of transparent portion, b = width of opaque portion.

Difference between Interference and Diffraction of light

Interference	Diffraction
1. Interference is due to the superposition of two wavefronts originating from two coherent sources.	1. Diffraction is due to the superposition of two secondary wavelets originating from the different points of the same wavefront.
2. In Interference pattern, all the maxima i.e. bright fringes are of the same intensity.	2. In diffraction pattern, the bright fringes are of varying intensity.
3. In Interference pattern, the dark fringes are usually almost perfectly dark.	3. In diffraction pattern, the dark fringes are not perfectly dark.
4. In Interference pattern, the width of fringes (bright and dark) is equal.	4. In diffraction pattern, the widths of fringes are not equal.
5. In Interference, bands are large in number.	5. In diffraction, bands are a few in number.
6. In Interference, bands are equally spaced.	6. In diffraction, bands are unequally spaced.

Example 5.

In a single slit diffraction experiment, the angular position of the first (secondary) maximum is found to be 5.2°, when the slit width is 0.01 mm. If sin 52° = 0.0906, then find the wavelength of light used.

Solution :

For single-slit diffraction, the angular position of the first maximum is determined from the relation

$$a\sin\theta_1' = \frac{3\lambda}{2}$$

It is given that a = 0.01 mm

$= 1 \times 10^{-5}$, $\theta_1' = 5.2°$, $\sin\theta_1' = 0.0906$. Therefore,

$$\lambda = \frac{2}{3}a\sin\theta_1' = \frac{2}{3}\times 10^{-5}\times 0.0906 = 6040\ \text{Å}$$

Example 6.

In Fraunhaufer diffraction from a single slit of width 0.3 mm the diffraction pattern is formed in the focal plane of a lens of focal length 1m. If the distance of third minimum from the central maximum is 5mm, then find the wavelength of light used.

Solution :

The distance of nth minimum from the central maximum is given by $X_n = \frac{n\lambda f}{a}$

where it is given that

$a = 0.3 \times 10^{-3}$ m, n = 3, f = 1m, $X_n = 5 \times 10^{-3}$ m

Therefore,

$$\lambda = \frac{aX_n}{nf} = \frac{0.3\times 10^{-3}\times 5\times 10^{-3}}{3\times 1} = 5\times 10^{-7}\ \text{m} = 500\ \text{nm}$$

POLARISATION

An ordinary source such as bulb consists of a large number of waves emitted by atoms or molecules in all directions symmetrically. Such light is called **unpolarized** light (see fig - a)

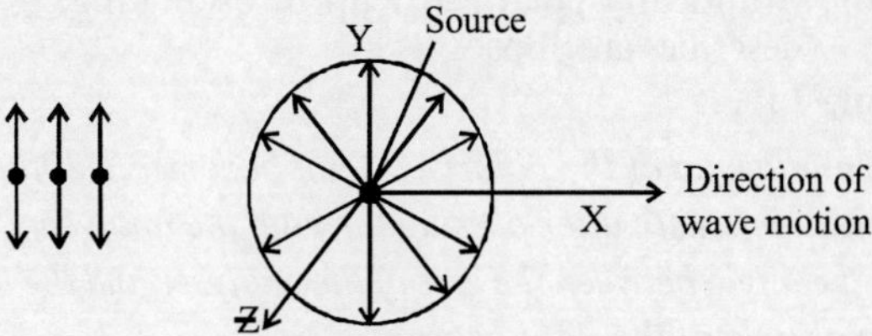

Fig (a) Unpolarised light

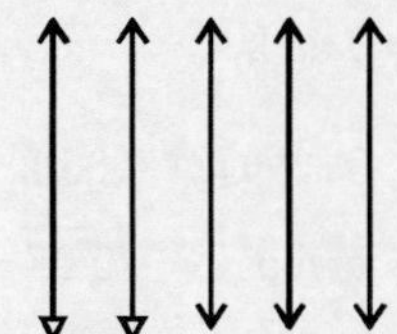

Fig (b) Polarised light

If we confine the direction of wave vibration of electric vector in one direction perpendicular to direction of wave propagation, then such type of light is called **plane polarised** or linearly polarised (with the help of polaroids or Nicol prism). *The phenomenon by which, we restrict the vibrations of wave in a particular direction (see fig-b) ⊥ to direction of wave propagation is called* ***polarization.***

The plane of vibration is that which contains the vibrations of electric vector $\vec{E}$ and plane of polarisation is perpendicular to the plane of vibration

- Tourmaline and calcite polarizes an e.m. wave passing through it.

Polarization by Reflection (Brewster's Law)

During reflection of a wave, we obtain a particular angle called angle of polarisation, for which the reflected light is completely plane polarised.

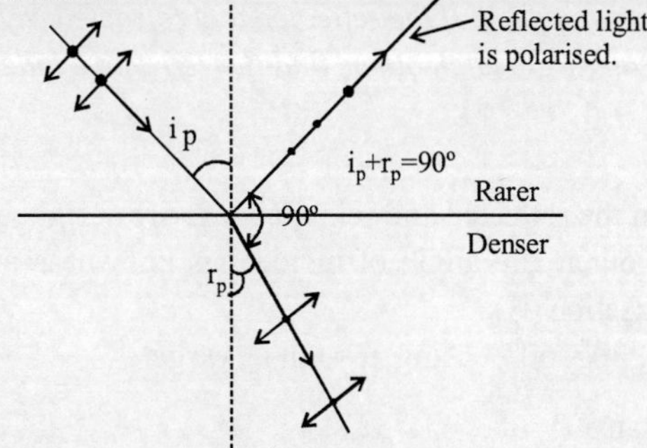

$\mu = \tan(i_p)$

where, i_p = angle of incidence, such that the reflected and refracted waves are perpendicular to each other.

Law of Malus : If the electric vector is at angle θ with the transmission axis, light is partially transmitted. The intensity of transmitted light is

$I = I_0\cos^2\theta$ where I_0 is the intensity when the incident electric vector is parallel to the transmission axis.

- Polarization can also be achieved by scattering of light
- (a) Plane polarized : oscillating $\vec{E}$ field is in a single plane.
  (b) Circularly polarized : tip of oscillating $\vec{E}$ field describes a circle.
  (c) Elliptically polarized : tip of oscillating $\vec{E}$ field describes an ellipse.

Example 7 :

The intensity of the polarised light becomes 1/20th of its initial intensity after passing through the analyser. What is the angle between the axis of the analyser and the initial amplitude of the light beam ?

Solution :

Here $I = \frac{1}{20} I_0 = 0.05\, I_0$

Using $I = I_0 \cos^2\theta$, we get $0.05\, I_0 = I_0 \cos^2\theta$

$\Rightarrow \cos^2\theta = 0.05$ or $\cos\theta = \sqrt{0.05} = 0.2236$

$\therefore\ \theta = \cos^{-1}(0.2236) = 76°9'$

Example 8 :

A beam of polarised light makes an angle of 60° with the axis of the polaroid sheet. How much is the intensity of light transmitted through the sheet ?

Solution :

Here $\theta = 60°$,
Using $I = I_0 \cos^2\theta$, we get

$$I = I_0 (\cos 60°)^2 = \frac{1}{4} I_0 \left(\because \cos 60° = \frac{1}{2}\right)$$

$\therefore$ Intensity of transmitted light $= \frac{1}{4} \times 100 = 25\%$

Thus, the intensity of the transmitted light is 25% of the intensity of incident light.

Example 9:

A ray of light strikes a glass plate at an angle of 60° with the glass surface. If the reflected and refracted rays are at right angles to each other, find the refractive index of the glass.

Solution.

When the reflected and refracted rays are at right angle to each other, the angle of incident is known as angle of polarisation (i_p).
Here, $\theta = 60°$, Using $\mu = \tan i_p$, we get

$\mu = \tan 60° = \sqrt{3} = 1.732$

RESOLVING POWER OF AN OPTICAL INSTRUMENT

The resolving power of an optical instrument, is its ability to distinguish between two closely spaced objects.

Diffraction occurs when light passes through the circular, or nearly circular, openings that admit light into cameras, telescopes, microscopes, and human eyes. The resulting diffraction pattern places a natural limit on the resolving power of these instruments.

For example, for normal vision, the limit of resolution of normal human eye is ~0.1 mm from 25 cm. (i.e., distances less than 0.1 mm cannot be resolved). For optical microscope the limit of resolution ~ 10^{-5} cm and for electron microscope ~5 Å or less.

The limit of resolution of a microscope $x = \frac{0.61\lambda}{a}$ where a is the aperture of the microscope.

DOPPLER'S EFFECT FOR LIGHT WAVES

(a) When the source moves towards the stationary observer or the observer moves towards the source, the apparent frequency.

$$\nu' = \nu\left(1 + \frac{v}{c}\right) \text{ (Blue shift)}$$

(b) When the source moves away from the stationary observer or vice-versa, $\nu' = \nu\left(1 - \frac{v}{c}\right)$ (Red shift)

where ν' = apparent frequency, ν = active frequency
v = velocity of source, c = velocity of light
But in both cases, the relative velocity v is small.

Example 10 :

The time period of rotation of the sun is 25 days and its radius is 7 × 10⁸ m. What will be the Doppler shift for the light of wavelength 6000 Å emitted from the surface of the sun?

Solution :

$$\text{Doppler's shift } d\lambda = \frac{v}{c} \times \lambda = R\,\omega\left(\frac{\lambda}{c}\right) = R\left(\frac{2\pi}{T}\right)\left(\frac{\lambda}{c}\right)$$

$$= \frac{7\times10^8 \times 2\times22}{25\times24\times60\times60\times7} \times \frac{6000}{3\times10^8}\text{Å} = 0.04\,\text{Å}$$

Example 11 :

How far in advance can one detect two headlights of a car if they are separated by a distance of 1.57 m ?

Solution :

The human eye can resolve two objects when the angle between them is 1 minute of arc. Thus, we have

$$D = \frac{x}{\theta}$$

Here $x = 1.57$ m, $\theta = 1' = \frac{1}{60} \times \frac{\pi}{180}$ rad,

$$\text{Thus } D = \frac{1.57}{\frac{1}{60} \times \frac{\pi}{180}} = \frac{10800 \times 1.57}{3.14} = 5400 \text{ m} = 5.4 \text{ km}$$

Example 12 :

The numerical aperture of a microscope is 0.12, and the wavelength of light used is 600 nm. Then find its limit of resolution.

Solution :

The limit of resolution of a microscope is given by

$$x = \frac{0.61\,\lambda}{\mu \sin\theta}$$

It is given that $\lambda = 6 \times 10^{-7}$m, and the numerical aperture $\mu \sin\theta = 0.12$.

$$\text{Therefore, } x = \frac{0.61 \times 6 \times 10^{-7}}{0.12} = 3.05 \times 10^{-6}\text{m} \approx 3\,\mu\text{m}$$

Example 13 :

A person wants to resolve two thin poles standing near each other at a distance of 1 km. What should be the minimum separation between them?

Solution :

Angular limit of resolution of eye θ = 1 minute of arc = 1/60 degree.

Therefore, the minimum separation should be such that

$$x = D\theta$$

with D = 1 km. = 10^3 m and $\theta = \frac{1}{60} \times \frac{\pi}{180}$ radian

Thus $x = \frac{10^3 \times 3.14}{60 \times 180} = \frac{31.4}{108} = 0.29$ m

or $x \approx 30$ cm.

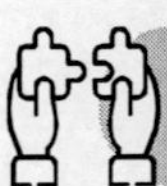

25.2 Concept Practice Problems

CPP

11. Light of wavelength 6328 Å is incident normally on a slit having a width of 0.2 mm. The angular width of the central maximum measured from minimum to minimum of diffraction pattern on a screen 9.0 metres away will be about

(a) 0.36 degree (b) 0.18 degree
(c) 0.72 degree (d) 0.09 degree

12. If a wave can be polarized, it must be

(a) a transverse wave (b) a longitudinal wave
(c) a sound wave (d) a stationary wave

13. When the light is incident at the polarizing angle on the transparent medium, then the completely polarized light is

(a) refracted light
(b) reflected light
(c) refracted and reflected light
(d) neither reflected nor refracted light

14. The Fraunhoffer 'diffraction' pattern of a single slit is formed in the focal plane of a lens of focal length 1 m. The width of slit is 0.3 mm. If third minimum is formed at a distance of 5 mm from central maximum, then wavelength of light will be

(a) 5000 Å (b) 2500 Å
(c) 7500 Å (d) 8500 Å

15. The figure shows Fraunhoffer's diffraction due to a single slit. If first minimum is obtained in the direction shown, then the path difference between rays 1 and 3 is

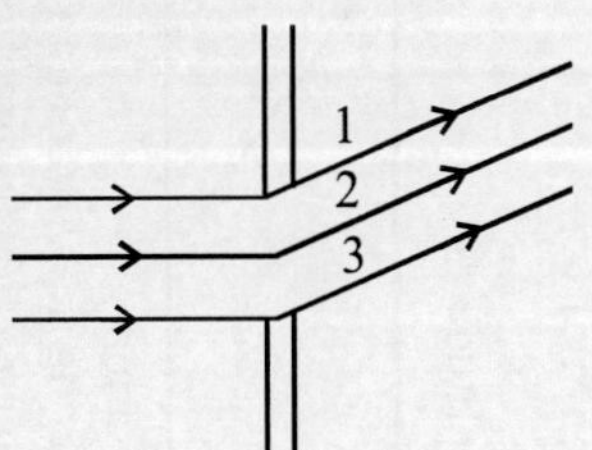

(a) 0 (b) $\lambda/4$
(c) $\lambda/2$ (d) λ

16. When unpolarised light is incident on a plane glass plate of refractive index μ, it is found that reflected and refracted rays are perpendicular to each other. Then which of the following statements is correct?

(a) Reflected and refracted rays are completely polarised with their planes of polarization parallel to each other
(b) Reflected and refracted rays are completely polarised with their planes of polarization perpendicular to each other
(c) Reflected light is plane polarised but transmitted light is partially polarised
(d) Reflected light is partially polarised but refracted light is plane polarised

17. An unpolarised beam of intensity $2a^2$ passes through a thin polaroid. Assuming zero absorption in the polaroid, the intensity of emergent plane polarised light will be

(a) $2a^2$ (b) a^2 (c) $\sqrt{2}\,a^2$ (d) $\frac{a^2}{\sqrt{2}}$

18. Which of the following diagrams represent the variation of electric field vector with time for a circularly polarised light?

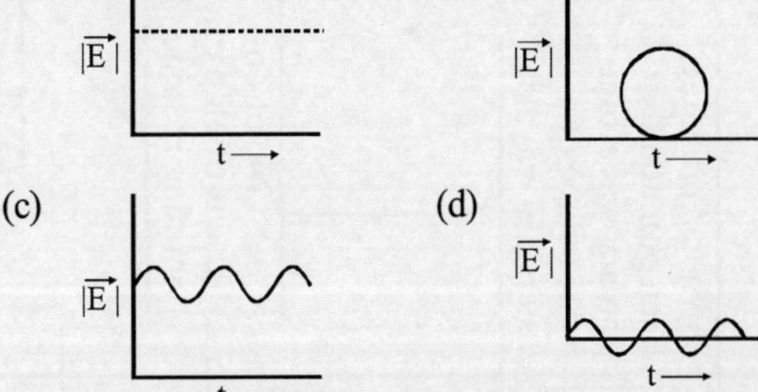

19. When the diffraction pattern from a certain slit illuminated with laser light (λ = 6330 Å) is projected on a screen 150 cm from the slit, the second minima on each side are separated by 8 cm. This tells us that :

(a) the slit is approximately 0.005 cm wide
(b) the slit is approximately 0.05 cm wide
(c) a/λ is approximately 7.5 (a is the slit width)
(d) a/λ is approximately 750

20. If the polarizing angle of a piece of glass for green light is 54.74°, then the angle of minimum deviation for an equilateral prism made of same glass is
[Given, tan 54.74° = 1.414]

(a) 45° (b) 54.74° (c) 60° (d) 30°

ANSWER KEY

11	(a)	12	(a)	13	(b)	14	(a)	15	(c)	16	(c)	17	(b)	18	(a)	19	(a)	20	(d)

CONCEPT MAP

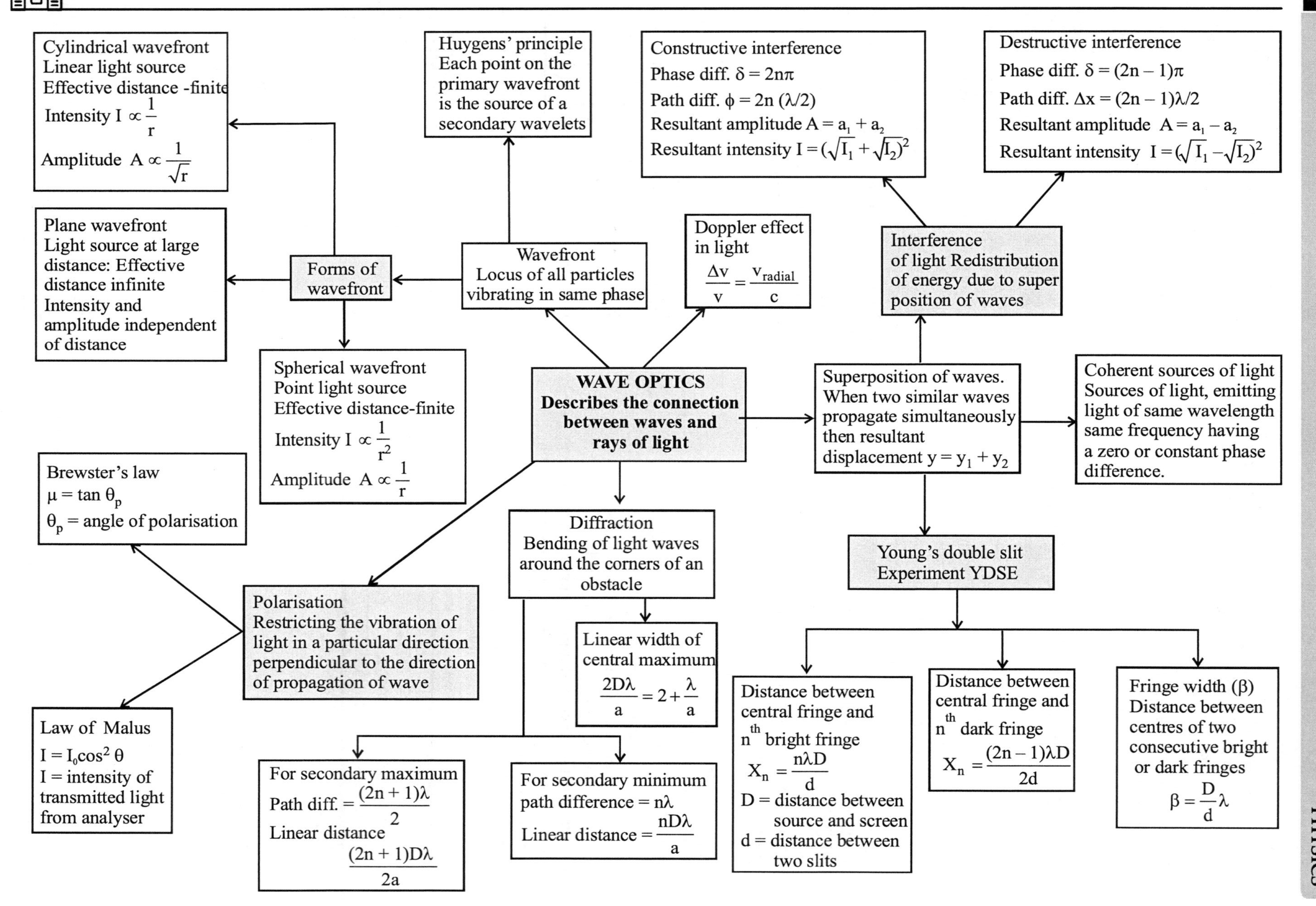
Cylindrical wavefront
Linear light source
Effective distance -finite
Intensity $I \propto \frac{1}{r}$
Amplitude $A \propto \frac{1}{\sqrt{r}}$
Huygens' principle
Each point on the primary wavefront is the source of a secondary wavelets
Constructive interference
Phase diff. $\delta = 2n\pi$
Path diff. $\phi = 2n(\lambda/2)$
Resultant amplitude $A = a_1 + a_2$
Resultant intensity $I = (\sqrt{I_1} + \sqrt{I_2})^2$
Destructive interference
Phase diff. $\delta = (2n-1)\pi$
Path diff. $\Delta x = (2n-1)\lambda/2$
Resultant amplitude $A = a_1 - a_2$
Resultant intensity $I = (\sqrt{I_1} - \sqrt{I_2})^2$
Plane wavefront
Light source at large distance: Effective distance infinite
Intensity and amplitude independent of distance
Forms of wavefront
Wavefront
Locus of all particles vibrating in same phase
Doppler effect in light
$\frac{\Delta v}{v} = \frac{v_{radial}}{c}$
Interference of light Redistribution of energy due to super position of waves
Spherical wavefront
Point light source
Effective distance-finite
Intensity $I \propto \frac{1}{r^2}$
Amplitude $A \propto \frac{1}{r}$
WAVE OPTICS
Describes the connection between waves and rays of light
Superposition of waves.
When two similar waves propagate simultaneously then resultant displacement $y = y_1 + y_2$
Coherent sources of light
Sources of light, emitting light of same wavelength same frequency having a zero or constant phase difference.
Brewster's law
$\mu = \tan\theta_p$
θ_p = angle of polarisation
Diffraction
Bending of light waves around the corners of an obstacle
Young's double slit Experiment YDSE
Polarisation
Restricting the vibration of light in a particular direction perpendicular to the direction of propagation of wave
Linear width of central maximum
$\frac{2D\lambda}{a} = 2 + \frac{\lambda}{a}$
Law of Malus
$I = I_0\cos^2\theta$
I = intensity of transmitted light from analyser
For secondary maximum
Path diff. $= \frac{(2n+1)\lambda}{2}$
Linear distance $\frac{(2n+1)D\lambda}{2a}$
For secondary minimum
path difference $= n\lambda$
Linear distance $= \frac{nD\lambda}{a}$
Distance between central fringe and n^{th} bright fringe
$X_n = \frac{n\lambda D}{d}$
D = distance between source and screen
d = distance between two slits
Distance between central fringe and n^{th} dark fringe
$X_n = \frac{(2n-1)\lambda D}{2d}$
Fringe width (β)
Distance between centres of two consecutive bright or dark fringes
$\beta = \frac{D}{d}\lambda$

Exercise 1 - Chapter Revision Problems

CRP

1. Angular width (B) of central maxima of a diffraction pattern of a single slit does not depend upon
(a) distance between slit and source
(b) wavelength of the light used
(c) width of slit
(d) frequency of light used

2. Which one of the following phenomena is not explained by Huygen's construction of wavefront?
(a) Refraction (b) Reflection
(c) Diffraction (d) Origin of spectra

3. The phenomenon by which stars recedes from each other is explained by
(a) black hole theory (b) neutron star theory
(c) white dwarf (d) red shift

4. Which of the following phenomena is not common to sound and light waves ?
(a) Interference (b) Diffraction
(c) Coherence (d) Polarisation

5. Interference is possible in
(a) light waves only
(b) sound waves only
(c) both light and sound waves
(d) neither light nor sound waves

6. A single slit diffraction pattern is obtained using a beam of red light. If the red light is replaced by the blue light, then the diffraction pattern
(a) remains unchanged (b) becomes narrower
(c) becomes broader (d) will disappear

7. The colours seen in the reflected white light from a thin oil film are due to
(a) diffraction (b) interference
(c) polarisation (d) dispersion

8. Which of the following cannot be polarised ?
(a) Radio waves (b) β rays
(c) Infrared rays (d) γ rays

9. The phenomenon of interference is shown by
(a) longitudinal mechanical waves only
(b) transverse mechanical waves only
(c) non-mechanical transverse waves only
(d) All of the above

10. The transverse nature of light is shown by
(a) interference of light (b) refraction of light
(c) polarization of light (d) dispersion of light

11. The idea of the quantum nature of light has emerged in an attempt to explain
(a) interference
(b) diffraction
(b) polarization
(d) radiation spectrum of a black body

12. Polarisation of light establishes
(a) corpuscular theory of light
(b) quantum nature of light
(c) transverse nature of light
(d) all of the three

13. When a compact disc is illuminated by small source of white light, coloured bands are observed. This is due to
(a) dispersion (b) diffraction
(c) interference (d) reflection

14. A nicol prism is based on the action of
(a) refraction (b) double refraction
(c) dichroism (d) both (b) and (c)

15. The deflection of light in a gravitational field was predicted first by
(a) Einstein (b) Newton
(c) Max Planck (d) Maxwell

16. In refraction, light waves are bent on passing from one medium to the second medium, because, in the second medium
(a) the frequency is different
(b) the coefficient of elasticity is different
(c) the speed is different
(d) the amplitude is smaller

17. The width of a slit is 0.012 mm. Monochromatic light is incident on it. The angular position of first bright line is 5.2°. The wavelength of incident light is [sin 5.2° = 0.0906].
(a) 6040 Å (b) 4026 Å (c) 5890 Å (d) 7248 Å

18. The max. intensity produced by two coherent sources of intensity I_1 and I_2 will be
(a) $I_1 + I_2$ (b) $I_1^2 + I_2^2$
(c) $I_1 + I_2 + 2\sqrt{I_1 I_2}$ (d) zero

19. The path difference between two wavefronts emitted by coherent sources of wavelength 5460Å is 2.1 micron. The phase difference between the wavefronts at that point is
(a) 7.692 (b) 7.692π (c) $\frac{7.692}{\pi}$ (d) $\frac{7.692}{3\pi}$

20. In Young's expt., the distance between two slits is $\frac{d}{3}$ and the distance between the screen and the slits is 3 D. The number of fringes in $\frac{1}{3}$m on the screen, formed by monochromatic light of wavelength 3λ, will be
(a) $\frac{d}{9D\lambda}$ (b) $\frac{d}{27D\lambda}$ (c) $\frac{d}{81 D\lambda}$ (d) $\frac{d}{D\lambda}$

21. A ray of light strikes a glass plate at an angle of 60°. If the reflected and refracted rays are perpendicular to each other, the index of refraction of glass is
(a) $\frac{1}{2}$ (b) $\sqrt{\frac{3}{2}}$ (c) $\frac{3}{2}$ (d) 1.732

22. The wavelength of H_α line in hydrogen spectrum was found to be 6563 Å in the laboratory. If the wavelength of same line in the spectrum of a milky way is observed to be 6568Å, then recession velocity of milky way will be
(a) 105 m/s (b) 1.05×10^6 m/s
(c) 10.5×10^6 m/s (d) 0.105×10^6 m/s

23. A star is receding away from earth with a velocity of 10^5 m/s. If the wavelength of its spectral line is 5700 Å, then Doppler shift will be
(a) 200 Å (b) 1.9 Å (c) 20 Å (d) 0.2 Å

24. In Fresnel's biprism expt., a mica sheet of refractive index 1.5 and thickness 6×10^{-6} m is placed in the path of one of interfering beams as a result of which the central fringe gets shifted through 5 fringe widths. The wavelength of light used is
(a) 6000 Å (b) 8000 Å (c) 4000 Å (d) 2000 Å

25. A radar sends radiowaves of frequency v towards an aeroplane moving with velocity v_a. A change Δv is observed in the frequency of reflected waves which is higher than original frequency. The velocity of aeroplane is ($v_a << c$)
(a) $\frac{c\Delta v}{v}$ (b) $\frac{2c\Delta v}{\Delta v}$ (c) $\frac{c\Delta v}{2v}$ (d) $\frac{\Delta v}{2cv}$

26. In Young's double slit experiment, we get 10 fringes in the field of view of monochromatic light of wavelength 4000Å. If we use monochromatic light of wavelength 5000Å, then the number of fringes obtained in the same field of view is
(a) 8 (b) 10 (c) 40 (d) 50

27. With a monochromatic light, the fringe-width obtained in a Young's double slit experiment is 0.133 cm. The whole set-up is immersed in water of refractive index 1.33, then the new fringe-width is
(a) 0.133 cm (b) 0.1 cm
(c) 1.33 × 1.33 cm (d) $\frac{1.33}{2}$ cm

28. A slit of width a is illuminated by white light. The first minimum for red light (λ = 6500 Å) will fall at θ = 30° when a will be
(a) 3250 Å (b) 6.5×10^{-4} cm
(c) 1.3 micron (d) 2.6×10^{-4} cm

29. Two points separated by a distance of 0.1 mm can just be inspected in a microscope, when light of wavelength 600Å is used. If the light of wavelength 4800 Å is used, the limit of resolution will become
(a) 0.80mm (b) 0.12mm (c) 0.10mm (d) 0.08mm

30. Unpolarised light of intensity 32 W m^{-2} passes through three polarizers such that the transmission axis of the last polarizer is crossed with that of the first. The intensity of final emerging light is 3 W m^{-2}. The intensity of light transmitted by first polarizer will be
(a) 32 W m^{-2} (b) 16 W m^{-2}
(c) 8 W m^{-2} (d) 4 W m^{-2}

31. Two nicols are oriented with their principal planes making an angle of 60°. Then the percentage of incident unpolarised light which passes through the system is
(a) 100 (b) 50 (c) 12.5 (d) 37.5

32. A rocket is receding away from earth with velocity 0.2 c. The rocket emits signal of frequency 4×10^7 Hz. The apparent frequency observed by the observer on earth will be
(a) 4×10^6 Hz (b) 3.2×10^7 Hz
(c) 3×10^6 Hz (d) 5×10^7 Hz

33. The heavenly body is receding from earth, such that the fractional change in λ is 1, then its velocity is
(a) c (b) $\frac{3c}{5}$ (c) $\frac{c}{5}$ (d) $\frac{2c}{5}$

34. Fluorescent tubes give more light than a filament bulb of same power because
(a) the tube contains gas at low temperature
(b) ultraviolet light is converted into visible light by fluorescence
(c) light is diffused through the walls of the tube
(d) it produces more heat than bulb

35. If the polarizing angle of a piece of glass for green light is 54.74°, then the angle of minimum deviation for an equilateral prism made of same glass is
[Given, tan 54.74° = 1.414]
(a) 45° (b) 54.74° (c) 60° (d) 30°

36. A single slit Fraunhoffer diffraction pattern is formed with white light. For what wavelength of light the third secondary maximum in the diffraction pattern coincides with the second secondary maximum in the pattern for red light of wavelength 6500 Å?
(a) 4400 Å (b) 4100 Å (c) 4642.8 Å (d) 9100 Å

37. When the angle of incidence is 60° on the surface of a glass slab, it is found that the reflected ray is completely polarised. The velocity of light in glass is
(a) $\sqrt{2} \times 10^8 \text{ms}^{-1}$ (b) $\sqrt{3} \times 10^8 \text{ms}^{-1}$
(c) $2 \times 10^8 \text{ms}^{-1}$ (d) $3 \times 10^8 \text{ms}^{-1}$

38. A lens having focal length f and aperture of diameter d forms an image of intensity I. Aperture of diameter $\frac{d}{2}$ in central region of lens is covered by a black paper. Focal length of lens and intensity of image now will be respectively
(a) f and $\frac{I}{4}$ (b) $\frac{3f}{4}$ and $\frac{I}{2}$
(c) f and $\frac{3I}{4}$ (d) $\frac{f}{2}$ and $\frac{I}{2}$

39. A parallel beam of fast moving electrons is incident normally on a narrow slit. A fluorescent screen is placed at a large distance from the slit. If the speed of the electrons is increased, which of the following statements is correct ?
(a) The angular width of the central maximum of the diffraction pattern will increase.
(b) The angular width of the central maximum will decrease.
(c) The angular width of the central maximum will be unaffected.
(d) Diffraction pattern is not observed on the screen in case of electrons.

40. In the figure below, P and Q are two equally intense coherent sources emitting radiation of wavelength 20 m. The separation between P and Q is 5 m and the phase of P is ahead of that of Q by 90°. A, B and C are three distinct points of observation, each equidistant from the midpoint of PQ. The intensities of radiation at A, B, C will be in the ratio :

(a) 0 : 1 : 4

(b) 2 : 1 : 0

(c) 0 : 1 : 2

(d) 4 : 1 : 0

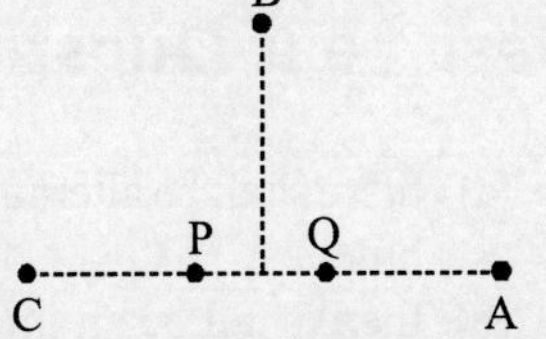

41. Two coherent sources of sound, S_1 and S_2, produce sound waves of the same wavelength, $\lambda = 1$ m, in phase. S_1 and S_2 are placed 1.5 m apart (see fig.). A listener, located at L, directly in front of S_2 finds that the intensity is at a minimum when he is 2 m away from S_2. The listener moves away from S_1, keeping his distance from S_2 fixed. The adjacent maximum of intensity is observed when the listener is at a distance d from S_1. Then, d is :

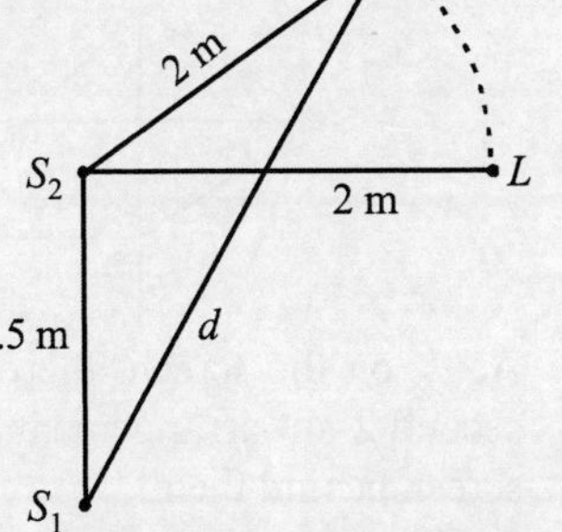

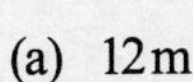

(a) 12m

(b) 5m

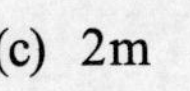

(c) 2m

(d) 3m

42. Interference pattern is observed at 'P' due to superimposition of two rays coming out from a source 'S' as shown in the figure. The value of '1' for which maxima is obtained at 'P' is:

(R is perfect reflecting surface)

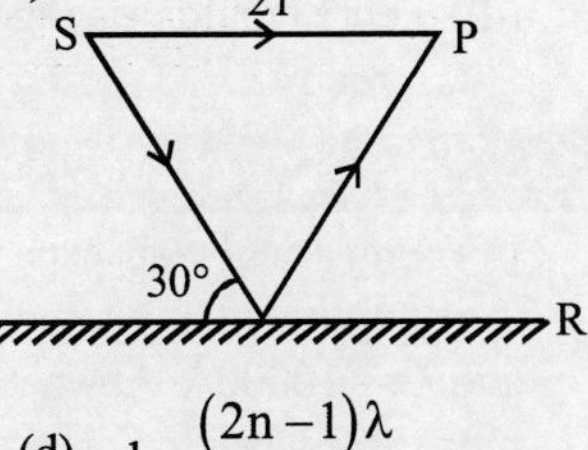

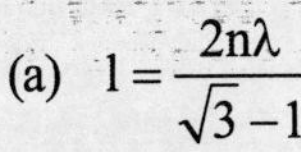

(a) $1 = \frac{2n\lambda}{\sqrt{3}-1}$

(b) $1 = \frac{(2n-1)\lambda}{2(\sqrt{3}-1)}$

(c) $1 = \frac{(2n-1)\lambda\sqrt{3}}{4(2-\sqrt{3})}$ (d) $1 = \frac{(2n-1)\lambda}{\sqrt{3}-1}$

43. Interference fringes are observed on a screen by illuminating two thin slits 1 mm apart with a light source ($\lambda = 632.8$ nm). The distance between the screen and the slits is 100 cm. If a bright fringe is observed on a screen at a distance of 1.27 mm from the central bright fringe, then the path difference between the waves, which are reaching this point from the slits is close to :

(a) 1.27 μm (b) 2.87 nm (c) 2 nm (d) 2.05 μm

44. The figure shows a Young's double slit experimental setup. It is observed that when a thin transparent sheet of thickness t and refractive index ¼ is put in front of one of the slits, the central maximum gets shifted by a distance equal to n fringe widths. If the wavelength of light used is ≈, t will be:

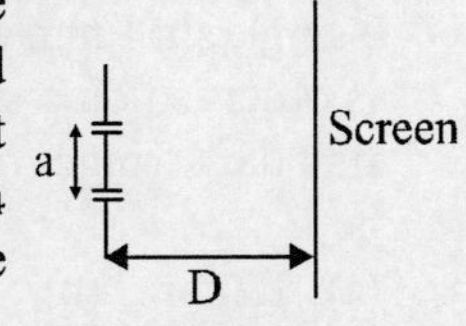

(a) $\frac{2nD\lambda}{a(\mu-1)}$ (b) $\frac{nD\lambda}{a(\mu-1)}$ (c) $\frac{D\lambda}{a(\mu-1)}$ (d) $\frac{2D\lambda}{a(\mu-1)}$

45. Consider a Young's double slit experiment as shown in figure. What should be the slit separation d in terms of wavelength λ such that the first minima occurs directly in front of the slit (S_1)?

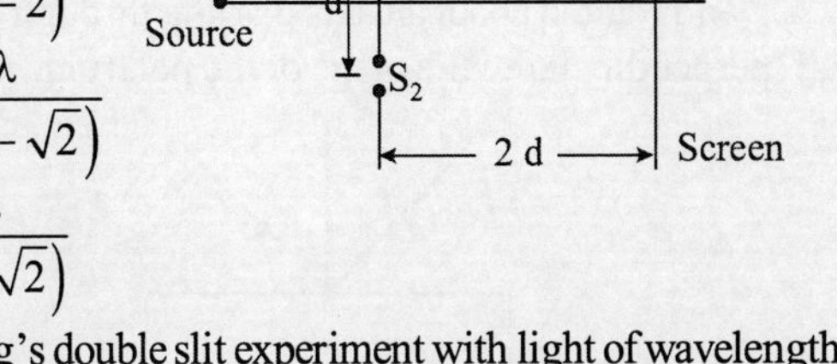

(a) $\frac{\lambda}{2(\sqrt{5}-2)}$

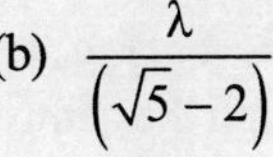

(b) $\frac{\lambda}{(\sqrt{5}-2)}$

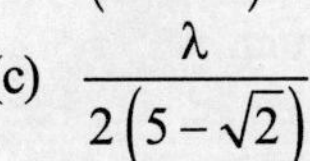

(c) $\frac{\lambda}{2(5-\sqrt{2})}$

(d) $\frac{\lambda}{(5-\sqrt{2})}$

46. In a Young's double slit experiment with light of wavelength λ, fringe pattern on the screen has fringe width β. When two thin transparent glass (refractive index μ) plates of thickness t_1 and t_2 ($t_1 > t_2$) are placed in the path of the two beams respectively, the fringe pattern will shift by a distance

(a) $\frac{\beta(\mu-1)}{\lambda}\left(\frac{t_1}{t_2}\right)$ (b) $\frac{\mu\beta}{\lambda}\frac{t_1}{t_2}$

(c) $\frac{\beta(\mu-1)}{\lambda}(t_1 - t_2)$ (d) $(\mu-1)\frac{\lambda}{\beta}(t_1 + t_2)$

47. The aperture diameter of telescope is 5m. The separation between the moon and the earth is 4×10^5 km. With light of wavelength of 5500 Å, the minimum separation between objects on the surface of moon, so that they are just resolved, is close to:

(a) 60 m (b) 20 m (c) 200 m (d) 600 m

48. Diameter of the objective lens of a telescope is 250 cm. For light of wavelength 600 nm. Coming from a distant object, the limit of resolution of the telescope is close to:

(a) 1.5×10^{-7} rad (b) 2.0×10^{-7} rad

(c) 3.0×10^{-7} rad (d) 4.5×10^{-7} rad

49. Consider a tank made of glass (refractive index 1.5) with a thick bottom. It is filled with a liquid of refractive index μ. A student finds that, irrespective of what the incident angle i (see figure) is for a beam of light entering the liquid, the light reflected from the liquid glass interface is never completely polarized. For this to happen, the minimum value of μ is:

(a) $\sqrt{\frac{5}{3}}$ (b) $\frac{3}{\sqrt{5}}$

(c) $\frac{5}{\sqrt{3}}$ (d) $\frac{4}{3}$

i

n = 1.5

50. The angular width of the central maximum in a single slit diffraction pattern is 60°. The width of the slit is 1 μm. The slit is illuminated by monochromatic plane waves. If another slit of same width is made near it, Young's fringes can be observed on a screen placed at a distance 50 cm from the slits. If the observed fringe width is 1 cm, what is slit separation distance?

(i.e. distance between the centres of each slit.)

(a) 25 μm (b) 50 μm (c) 75 μm (d) 100 μm

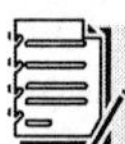

Exercise 2 - Exemplar & Past Year Questions

E&PYQs

Exemplar Questions

1. Consider a light beam incident from air to a glass slab at Brewster's angle as shown in figure.
A polaroid is placed in the path of the emergent ray at point P and rotated about an axis passing through the centre and perpendicular to the plane of the polaroid.

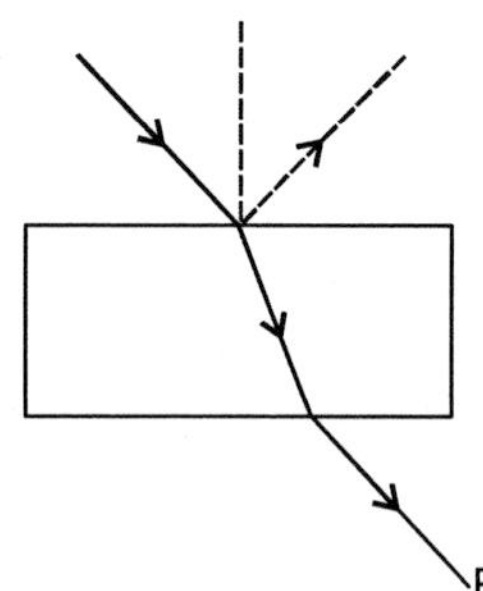

(a) For a particular orientation, there shall be darkness as observed through the polaroid
(b) The intensity of light as seen through the polaroid shall be independent of the rotation
(c) The intensity of light as seen through the polaroid shall go through a minimum but not zero for two orientations of the polaroid
(d) The intensity of light as seen through the polaroid shall go through a minimum for four orientations of the polaroid

2. Consider sunlight incident on a slit of width 10^4 Å. The image seen through the slit shall
(a) be a fine sharp slit white in colour at the centre
(b) a bright slit white at the centre diffusing to zero intensities at the edges
(c) a bright slit white at the centre diffusing to regions of different colours
(d) only be a diffused slit white in colour

3. Consider a ray of light incident from air onto a slab of glass (refractive index n) of width d, at an angle θ. The phase difference between the ray reflected bv the top surface of the glass and the bottom surface is

(a) $\frac{2\pi d}{\lambda}\left(1-\frac{1}{n^2}\sin^2\theta\right)^{1/2}+\pi$

(b) $\frac{4\pi d}{\lambda}\left(1-\frac{1}{n^2}\sin^2\theta\right)^{1/2}$

(c) $\frac{4\pi d}{\lambda}\left(1-\frac{1}{n^2}\sin^2\theta\right)^{1/2}+\frac{\pi}{2}$

(d) $\frac{4\pi d}{\lambda}\left(1-\frac{1}{n^2}\sin^2\theta\right)^{1/2}+2\pi$

4. In a Young's double-slit experiment, the source is white light. One of the holes is covered by a red filter and another by a blue filter. In this case,
(a) there shall be alternate interference patterns of red and blue
(b) there shall be an interference pattern for red distinct from that for blue
(c) there shall be no interference fringes
(d) there shall be an interference pattern for red mixing with one for blue

5. Figure shows a standard two slit arrangement witn slits S_1, S_2, P_1, P_2 are the two minima points on either side of P (figure).

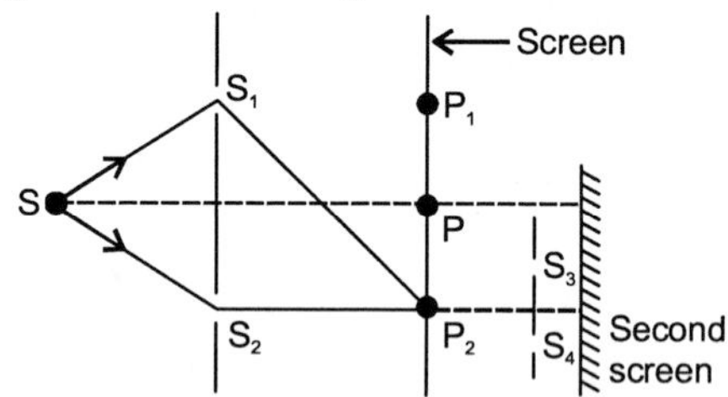

At P_2 on the screen, there is a hole and behind P_2 is a second 2-slit arrangement with slits S_3, S_4 and a second screen behind them.
(a) There would be no interference pattern on the second screen but it would be lighted
(b) The second screen would be totally dark
(c) There would be a single bright point on the second screen
(d) There would be a regular two slit pattern on the second screen

NEET/AIPMT (2013-2020) Questions

6. In Young's double slit experiment, the slits are 2 mm apart and are illuminated by photons of two wavelengths $\lambda_1 = 12000$Å and $\lambda_2 = 10000$Å. At what minimum distance from the common central bright fringe on the screen 2 m from the slit will a bright fringe from one interference pattern coincide with a bright fringe from the other ? *[2013]*
(a) 6mm (b) 4mm (c) 3mm (d) 8mm

7. In Young's double slit experiment the distance between the slits and the screen is doubled. The separation between the slits is reduced to half. As a result the fringe width *[NEET Kar. 2013]*
(a) is doubled (b) is halved
(c) becomes four times (d) remains unchanged

8. A beam of light of $\lambda = 600$ nm from a distant source falls on a single slit 1 mm wide and the resulting diffraction pattern is observed on a screen 2 m away. The distance between first dark fringes on either side of the central bright fringe is: *[2014]*
(a) 1.2 cm (b) 1.2 mm (c) 2.4 cm (d) 2.4 mm

9. In the Young's double-slit experiment, the intensity of light at a point on the screen where the path difference is λ is K, (λ being the wave length of light used). The intensity at a point where the path difference is λ/4, will be: *[2014]*
(a) K (b) K/4 (c) K/2 (d) Zero

10. In a double slit experiment, the two slits are 1 mm apart and the screen is placed 1 m away. A monochromatic light wavelength 500 nm is used. What will be the width of each slit for obtaining ten maxima of double slit within the central maxima of single slit pattern ? ***[2015]***

(a) 0.1 mm (b) 0.5 mm (c) 0.02 mm (d) 0.2 mm

11. For a parallel beam of monochromatic light of wavelength 'λ', diffraction is produced by a single slit whose width 'a' is of the wavelength of the light. If 'D' is the distance of the screen from the slit, the width of the central maxima will be: ***[2015]***

(a) $\frac{D\lambda}{a}$ (b) $\frac{Da}{\lambda}$ (c) $\frac{2Da}{\lambda}$ (d) $\frac{2D\lambda}{a}$

12. At the first minimum adjacent to the central maximum of a single-slit diffraction pattern, the phase difference between the Huygen's wavelet from the edge of the slit and the wavelet from the midpoint of the slit is : ***[2015 RS]***

(a) $\frac{\pi}{2}$ radian (b) π radian

(c) $\frac{\pi}{8}$ radian (d) $\frac{\pi}{4}$ radian

13. In a diffraction pattern due to a single slit of width 'a', the first minimum is observed at an angle 30° when light of wavelength 5000 Å is incident on the slit. The first secondary maximum is observed at an angle of : ***[2016]***

(a) $\sin^{-1}\left(\frac{1}{4}\right)$ (b) $\sin^{-1}\left(\frac{2}{3}\right)$

(c) $\sin^{-1}\left(\frac{1}{2}\right)$ (d) $\sin^{-1}\left(\frac{3}{4}\right)$

14. The intensity at the maximum in a Young's double slit experiment is I_0. Distance between two slits is $d = 5\lambda$, where λ is the wavelength of light used in the experiment. What will be the intensity in front of one of the slits on the screen placed at a distance D = 10 d ? ***[2016]***

(a) I_0 (b) $\frac{I_0}{4}$ (c) $\frac{3}{4}I_0$ (d) $\frac{I_0}{2}$

15. The ratio of resolving powers of an optical microscope for two wavelengths $\lambda_1 = 4000$ Å and $\lambda_2 = 6000$ Å is ***[2017]***

(a) 9 : 4 (b) 3 : 2 (c) 16 : 81 (d) 8 : 27

16. Young's double slit experment is first performed in air and then in a medium other than air. It is found that 8th bright fringe in the medium lies where 5th dark fringe lies in air. The refractive index of the medium is nearly ***[2017]***

(a) 1.59 (b) 1.69 (c) 1.78 (d) 1.25

17. Two Polaroids P_1 and P_2 are placed with their axis perpendicular to each other. Unpolarised light I_0 is incident on P_1. A third polaroid P_3 is kept in between P_1 and P_2 such that its axis makes an angle 45° with that of P_1. The intensity of transmitted light through P_2 is ***[2017]***

(a) $\frac{I_0}{4}$ (b) $\frac{I_0}{8}$ (c) $\frac{I_0}{16}$ (d) $\frac{I_0}{2}$

18. Unpolarised light is incident from air on a plane surface of a material of refractive index 'μ'. At a particular angle of incidence 'i', it is found that the reflected and refracted rays are perpendicular to each other. Which of the following options is correct for this situation? ***[2018]***

(a) Reflected light is polarised with its electric vector parallel to the plane of incidence

(b) Reflected light is polarised with its electric vector perpendicular to the plane of incidence

(c) $i = \tan^{-1}\left(\frac{1}{\mu}\right)$

(d) $i = \sin^{-1}\left(\frac{1}{\mu}\right)$

19. In Young's double slit experiment the separation d between the slits is 2 mm, the wavelength λ of the light used is 5896 Å and distance D between the screen and slits is100 cm. It is found that the angular width of the fringes is 0.20°. To increase the fringe angular width to 0.21° (with same λ and D) the separation between the slits needs to be changed to ***[2018]***

(a) 1.8 mm (b) 1.9 mm (c) 1.7 mm (d) 2.1 mm

20. In a double slit experiment, when light of wavelength 400 nm was used, the angular width of the first minima formed on a screen placed 1 m away, was found to be 0.2°. What will be the angular width of the first minima, if the entire experimental apparatus is immersed in water? ($\mu_{water} = 4/3$) ***[2019]***

(a) 0.266° (b) 0.15° (c) 0.05° (d) 0.1°

21. Angular width of the central maxima in the Fraunhofer diffraction for λ = 6000Å is θ_0. When the same slit is illuminated by another monochromatic light, the angular width decreases by 30%. The wavelength of this light is ***[NEET Odisha 2019]***

(a) 420 Å (b) 1800 Å (c) 4200 Å (d) 6000 Å

22. In Young's double slit experiment, if the separation between coherent sources is halved and the distance of the screen from the coherent sources is doubled, then the fringe width becomes : ***[2020]***

(a) half (b) four times

(c) one-fourth (d) double

23. The Brewsters angle i_b for an interface should be ***[2020]***

(a) $30° < i_b < 45°$ (b) $45° < i_b < 90°$

(c) $i_b = 90°$ (d) $0° < i_b < 30°$

24. Assume that light of wavelength 600 nm is coming from a star. The limit of resolution of telescope whose objective has a diameter of 2 m is : ***[2020]***

(a) 1.83×10^{-7} rad (b) 7.32×10^{-7} rad

(c) 6.00×10^{-7} rad (d) 3.66×10^{-7} rad

Exercise 3 - Concept Application Problems CAP

1. A slit of width a is illuminated by red light of wavelength 6500 Å. If the first minimum falls at $\theta = 30°$, the value of a is
(a) 6.5×10^{-4} mm (b) 1.3 micron
(c) 3250 Å (d) 2.6×10^{-4} cm

2. Which of the following does not support the wave nature of light?
(a) Interference (b) Diffraction
(c) Polarisation (d) Photoelectric effect.

3. The contrast in the fringes in an interference pattern depends on
(a) fringe width
(b) wavelength
(c) intensity ratio of the sources
(d) distance between the slits

4. Huygen's concept of wavelets is useful in
(a) explaining polarisation
(b) determining focal length of the lenses
(c) determining chromatic aberration
(d) geometrical reconstruction of a wavefront

5. When light passing through rotating nicol is observed, no change in intensity is seen. What inference can be drawn ?
(a) The incident light is unpolarized.
(b) The incident light is circularly polarized.
(c) The incident light is unpolarized or circularly polarized.
(d) The incident light is unpolarized or circularly polarized or combination of both.

6. Interference was observed in an interference chamber when air was present. Now, the chamber is evacuated and if the same light is used, a careful observation will show
(a) no interference
(b) interference with bright bands
(c) interference with dark bands
(d) interference in which breadth of the fringe will be slightly increased

7. A ray of light is incident on the surface of a glass plate at an angle of incidence equal to Brewster's angel ϕ. If μ represents the refractive index of glass with respect to air, then the angle between the reflected and the refracted rays is
(a) $90° + \phi$ (b) $\sin^{-1}(\mu \cos \phi)$
(c) $90°$ (d) $90° - \sin^{-1}\left(\frac{\sin \phi}{\mu}\right)$

8. A plane wave of wavelength 6250 Å is incident normally on a slit of width 2×10^{-2} cm. The width of the principal maximum on a screen distant 50 cm will be
(a) 312.5×10^{-3} cm (b) 312.5×10^{-3} m
(c) 312.5×10^{-3} m (d) 312m

9. In Young's double slit experiment, if the slit widths are in the ratio 1 : 2, the ratio of the intensities at minima and maxima will be
(a) 1:2 (b) 1:3 (c) 1:4 (d) 1:9

10. Two beams of light of intensity I_1 and I_2 interfere to give an interference pattern. If the ratio of maximum intensity to that of minimum intensity is 25/9, then I_1/I_2 is
(a) 5/3 (b) 4 (c) 81/625 (d) 16

11. The condition for obtaining secondary maxima in the diffraction pattern due to single slit is
(a) $a \sin \theta = n\lambda$ (b) $a \sin \theta = (2n-1)\frac{\lambda}{2}$
(c) $a \sin \theta = (2n-1)\lambda$ (d) $a \sin \theta = \frac{n\lambda}{2}$

12. In Young's double slit experiment with sodium vapour lamp of wavelength 589 nm and the slits 0.589 mm apart, the half angular width of the central maximum is
(a) $\sin^{-1} 0.01$ (b) $\sin^{-1} 0.0001$
(c) $\sin^{-1} 0.001$ (d) $\sin^{-1} 0.1$

13. In the phenomena of diffraction of light, when blue light is used in the experiment in spite of red light, then
(a) fringes will become narrower
(b) fringes will become broader
(c) no change in fringe width
(d) None of these

14. The wavefronts of a light wave travelling in vacuum are given by $x + y + z = c$. The angle made by the direction of propagation of light with the X-axis is
(a) 0° (b) 45°
(c) 90° (d) $\cos^{-1}(1/\sqrt{3})$

15. Two sources of light of wavelengths 2500 Å and 3500 Å are used in Young's double slit expt. simultaneously. Which orders of fringes of two wavelength patterns coincide?
(a) 3rd order of 1st source and 5th of the 2nd
(b) 7th order of 1st and 5th order of 2nd
(c) 5th order of 1st and 3rd order of 2nd
(d) 5th order of 1st and 7th order of 2nd

16. A parallel beam of monochromatic unpolarised light is incident on a transparent dielectric plate of refractive index $\frac{1}{\sqrt{3}}$. The reflected beam is completely polarised. Then the angle of incidence is
(a) 30° (b) 60° (c) 45° (d) 75°

17. A beam of unpolarised light passes through a tourmaline crystal A and then through another such crystal B oriented so that the principal plane is parallel to A. The intensity of emergent light is I_0. Now B is rotated by 45° about the ray. The emergent light will have intensity
(a) $I_0/2$ (b) $I_0/\sqrt{2}$ (c) $I_0\sqrt{2}$ (d) $2I_0$

18. Aperture of the human eye is 2 mm. Assuming the mean wavelength of light to be 5000 Å, the angular resolution limit of the eye is nearly
(a) 2 minute (b) 1 minute
(c) 0.5 minute (d) 1.5 minute

19. Two light waves having the same wavelength λ in vacuum are in phase initially. Then the first wave travels a path L_1 through a medium of refractive index n_1 while the second wave travels a path of length L_2 through a medium of refractive index n_2. After this the phase difference between the two waves is :

(a) $\frac{2\pi}{\lambda}\left(\frac{L_2}{n_1}-\frac{L_1}{n_2}\right)$ (b) $\frac{2\pi}{\lambda}\left(\frac{L_1}{n_1}-\frac{L_2}{n_2}\right)$

(c) $\frac{2\pi}{\lambda}(n_1L_1-n_2L_2)$ (d) $\frac{2\pi}{\lambda}(n_2L_1-n_1L_2)$

20. In an interference experiment the ratio of amplitudes of coherent waves is $\frac{a_1}{a_2}=\frac{1}{3}$. The ratio of maximum and minimum intensities of fringes will be :

(a) 2 (b) 18 (c) 4 (d) 9

21. Two coherent sources produce waves of different intensities which interfere. After interference, the ratio of the maximum intensity to the minimum intensity is 16. The intensity of the waves are in the ratio:

(a) 16 : 9 (b) 25 : 9 (c) 4 : 1 (d) 5 : 3

22. On a hot summer night, the refractive index of air is smallest near the ground and increases with height from the ground. When a light beam is directed horizontally, the Huygens' principle leads us to conclude that as it travels, the light beam :

(a) bends downwards
(b) bends upwards
(c) becomes narrower
(d) goes horizontally without any deflection

23. n identical waves each of intensity I_0 interfere with each other. The ratio of maximum intensities if the interference is (i) coherent and (ii) incoherent is :

(a) n^2 (b) $\frac{1}{n}$ (c) $\frac{1}{n^2}$ (d) n

24. A ray of light of intensity I is incident on a parallel glass slab at point A as shown in diagram. It undergoes partial reflection and refraction. At each reflection, 25% of incident energy is reflected. The rays AB and A'B' undergo interference. The ratio of I_{max} and I_{min} is :

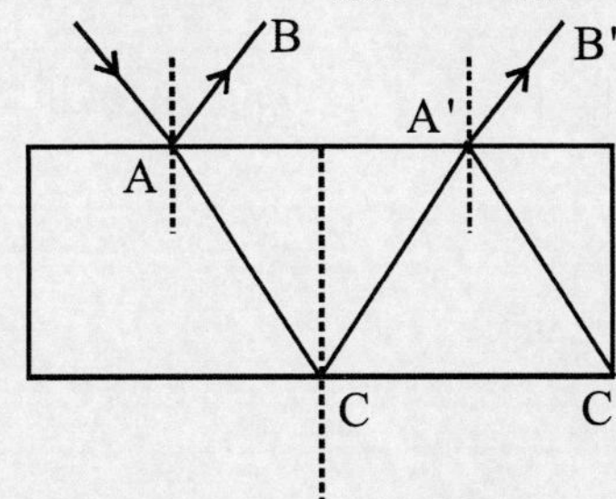

(a) 49 : 1 (b) 7 : 1 (c) 4 : 1 (d) 8 : 1

25. Two coherent plane light waves of equal amplitude makes a small angle α (<< 1) with each other. They fall almost normally on a screen. If λ is the wavelength of light waves, the fringe width Δx of interference patterns of the two sets of waves on the screen is

(a) $\frac{2\lambda}{\alpha}$ (b) $\frac{\lambda}{\alpha}$ (c) $\frac{\lambda}{(2\alpha)}$ (d) $\frac{\lambda}{\sqrt{\alpha}}$

26. In a Young's double slit experiment, light of 500 nm is used to produce an interference pattern. When the distance between the slits is 0.05 mm, the angular width (in degree) of the fringes formed on the distance screen is close to :

(a) 0.17° (b) 0.57° (c) 1.7° (d) 0.07°

27. In a Young's double slit experiment, 16 fringes are observed in a certain segment of the screen when light of wavelength 700 nm is used. If the wavelength of light is changed to 400 nm, the number of fringes observed in the same segment of the screen would be :

(a) 24 (b) 30 (c) 18 (d) 28

28. In a double-slit experiment, at a certain point on the screen the path difference between the two interfering waves is $\frac{1}{8}$ th of a wavelength. The ratio of the intensity of light at that point to that at the centre of a bright fringe is:

(a) 0.853 (b) 0.672 (c) 0.568 (d) 0.760

29. In a Young's double slit experiment, the separation between the slits is 0.15 mm. In the experiment, a source of light of wavelength 589 nm is used and the interference pattern is observed on a screen kept 1.5 m away. The separation between the successive bright fringes on the screen is:

(a) 6.9 mm (b) 3.9 mm (c) 5.9 mm (d) 4.9 mm

30. In a double slit experiment, when a thin film of thickness t having refractive index μ is introduced in front of one of the slits, the maximum at the centre of the fringe pattern shifts by one fringe width. The value of t is ($\approx$ is the wavelength of the light used) :

(a) $\frac{2\lambda}{(\mu-1)}$ (b) $\frac{\lambda}{2(\mu-1)}$ (c) $\frac{\lambda}{(\mu-1)}$ (d) $\frac{\lambda}{(2\mu-1)}$

31. In a Young's double slit experiment, the path difference, at a certain point on the screen, betwen two interfering waves is $\frac{1}{8}$th of wavelength. The ratio of the intensity at this point to that at the centre of a bright fringe is close to:

(a) 0.74 (b) 0.85 (c) 0.94 (d) 0.80

32. In a Young's double slit experiment with slit separation 0.1 mm, one observes a bright fringe at angle $\frac{1}{40}$ rad by using light of wavelength λ_1 When the light of wavelength λ_2 is used a bright fringe is seen at the same angle in the same set up. Given that λ_1 and λ_2 are in visible range (380 nm to 740 nm), their values are:

(a) 625 nm, 500 nm (b) 380 nm, 525 nm
(c) 380 nm, 500 nm (d) 400 nm, 500 nm

33. In a Young's double slit experiment, the slits are placed 0.320 mm apart. Light of wavelength λ = 500 nm is incident on the slits. The total number of bright fringes that are observed in the angular range $-30° \le \theta \le 30°$ is

(a) 640 (b) 320 (c) 321 (d) 641

34. In a Young's double slit experiment with light of wavelength λ the separation of slits is d and distance of screen is D such that D >> d >> λ. If the fringe width is β, the distance from point of maximum intensity to the point where intensity falls to half of maximum intensity on either side is:

(a) $\frac{\beta}{6}$ (b) $\frac{\beta}{3}$ (c) $\frac{\beta}{4}$ (d) $\frac{\beta}{2}$

35. The maximum number of possible interference maxima for slit separation equal to 1.8λ, where λ is the wavelength of light used, in a Young's double slit experiment is

(a) zero (b) 3 (c) infinite (d) 5

36. A beam of plane polarised light of large cross-sectional area and uniform intensity of 3.3 Wm^{-2} falls normally on a polariser (cross sectional area 3×10^{-4} m^2) which rotates about its axis with an angular speed of 31.4 rad/s. The energy of light passing through the polariser per revolution, is close to :

(a) 1.0×10^{-5} J (b) 1.0×10^{-4} J
(c) 1.5×10^{-4} J (d) 5.0×10^{-4} J

37. A polarizer - analyser set is adjusted such that the intensity of light coming out of the analyser is just 10% of the original intensity. Assuming that the polarizer - analyser set does not absorb any light, the angle by which the analyser need to be rotated further to reduce the output intensity to be zero, is:

(a) 71.6° (b) 18.4° (c) 90° (d) 45°

38. The value of numerical aperature of the objective lens of a microscope is 1.25. If light of wavelength 5000 Å is used, the minimum separation between two points, to be seen as distinct, will be :

(a) 0.24 μm (b) 0.38 μm (c) 0.12 μm (d) 0.48 μm

39. A system of three polarizers P_1, P_2, P_3 is set up such that the pass axis of P_3 is crossed with respect to that of P_1. The pass axis of P_2 is inclined at 60° to the pass axis of P_3. When a beam of unpolarized light of intensity I_0 is incident on P_1, the intensity of light transmitted by the three polarizers is I. The ratio (I_0/I) equals (nearly) :

(a) 5.33 (b) 16.00 (c) 10.67 (d) 1.80

40. Calculate the limit of resolution of a telescope objective having a diameter of 200 cm, if it has to detect light of wavelength 500 nm coming from a star.

(a) 305×10^{-9} radian (b) 610×10^{-9} radian
(c) 152.5×10^{-9} radian (d) 457.5×10^{-9} radian

41. In a double-slit experiment, green light (5303Å) falls on a double slit having a separation of 19.44 μm and a width of 4.05 μm. The number of bright fringes between the first and the second diffraction minima is :

(a) 10 (b) 05 (c) 04 (d) 09

42. Unpolarized light of intensity I passes through an ideal polarizer A. Another indentical polarizer B is placed behind A. The intensity of light beyond B is found to be $\frac{I}{2}$. Now another identical polarizer C is placed between A and B. The intensity beyond B is now found to be $\frac{I}{8}$. The angle between polarizer A and C is:

(a) 0° (b) 30° (c) 45° (d) 60°

43. Light of wavelength 550 nm falls normally on a slit of width 22.0×10^{-5}cm. The angular position of the second minima from the central maximum will be (in radians)

(a) $\frac{\pi}{8}$ (b) $\frac{\pi}{12}$ (c) $\frac{\pi}{4}$ (d) $\frac{\pi}{6}$

44. A plane polarized light is incident on a polariser with its pass axis making angle θ with x-axis, as shown in the figure. At four different values of θ, $\theta = 8°, 38°, 188°$ and 218°, the observed intensities are same. What is the angle between the direction of polarization and x-axis

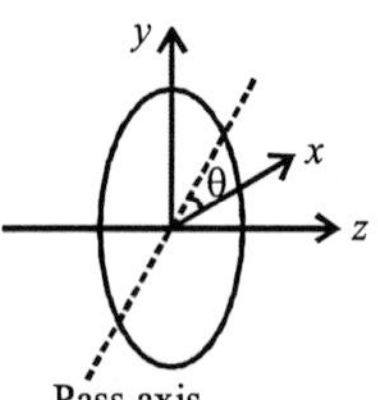

(a) 203° (b) 45° (c) 98° (d) 128°

45. Unpolarized light of intensity I is incident on a system of two polarizers, A followed by B. The intensity of emergent light is I/2. If a third polarizer C is placed between A and B, the intensity of emergent light is reduced to I/3. The angle between the polarizers A and C is θ. Then

(a) $\cos\theta = \left(\frac{2}{3}\right)^{1/4}$ (b) $\cos\theta = \left(\frac{1}{3}\right)^{1/4}$

(c) $\cos\theta = \left(\frac{1}{3}\right)^{1/2}$ (d) $\cos\theta = \left(\frac{2}{3}\right)^{1/2}$

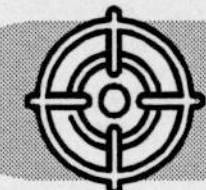

Hints & Solutions

25.1 Concept Practice Problems CPP

1. (c) $x_5 = n\lambda\frac{D}{d} = \frac{5\times 6.5\times 10^{-7}\times 1}{10^{-3}} = 32.5\times 10^{-4}\,m$

$x_3 = (2n-1)\frac{1}{2}\frac{D\lambda}{d} = \frac{5\times 6.5\times 10^{-7}\times 1}{2\times 10^{-3}} = 16.25\times 10^{-4}\,m$

$x_5 - x_3 = 16.25\times 10^{-4}\,m = 1.625\text{ mm.}$

2. (d) 3. (d)

4. (b) The position of nth dark fringe. So position of first dark fringe in $x_1 = \lambda D/2d$.

$d = 20\text{ cm}, D = 0.1\text{mm}, \lambda = 5460\text{ Å}, x_1 = 0.16$

5. (c) When the arrangement is dipped in water;

$\beta' = \beta/\mu = \frac{x}{4/3} = \frac{3}{4}x = 0.75x$

6. (d) For two coherent sources, $I_1 = I_2$

$I_{max} = (A_1 + A_2)^2 = \left(\sqrt{I_1} + \sqrt{I_2}\right)^2$

This is given as I_0 for maximum and zero for minimum. If there are two noncoherent sources, there will be no maximum and minimum intensities. Instead of all the intensity I_0 at maximum and zero for minimum, it will be just $I_0/2$.

7. (c) $\sin\theta = \frac{\lambda}{d} = \frac{589\times 10^{-9}}{0.589\times 10^{-3}} = 10^{-3} = \frac{1}{1000} = 0.0001$

8. (b) For path difference λ, phase

$\text{difference} = 2\pi\left(Q = \frac{2\pi}{\lambda}x = \frac{2\pi}{\lambda}.\lambda = 2\pi\right)$

$\Rightarrow I = I_0 + I_0 + 2I_0\cos 2\pi \Rightarrow I = 4I_0 \quad (\therefore \cos 2\pi = 1)$

For $x = \frac{\lambda}{4}$, phase difference $= \frac{\pi}{2}$

$\therefore I' = I_1 + I_2 + 2\sqrt{I_1}\sqrt{I_2}\cos\frac{\pi}{2}$

If $I_1 = I_2 = I_0$ then $I' = 2I_0 = 2.\frac{I}{4} = \frac{I}{2}$

9. (a)

10. (a) $\because y = \frac{n\lambda D}{d}$

$\therefore \quad n_1\lambda_1 = n_2\lambda_2$

$\Rightarrow \quad n_1\times 12000\times 10^{-10} = n_2\times 10000\times 10^{-10}$

or, $n(12000\times 10^{-10}) = (n+1)(10000\times 10^{-10}) \Rightarrow n = 5$

$\left(\because \lambda_1 = 12000\times 10^{-10}m;\ \lambda_2 = 10000\times 10^{-10}m\right)$

Hence, $y_{common} = \frac{n\lambda_1 D}{d}$

$= \frac{5\left(12000\times 10^{-10}\right)\times 2}{2\times 10^{-3}}$

$(\because d = 2\text{ mm and } D = 2m)$

$= 5\times 12\times 10^{-4}\,m$

$= 60\times 10^{-4}\,m$

$= 6\times 10^{-3}m = 6\,mm$

S₁ 2mm S₂ 2m y

25.2 Concept Practice Problems CPP

11. (a) The angular width of central maxi. is

$2\theta = 2\frac{\lambda}{a} = \frac{2\times 6328\times 10^{-10}}{2\times 10^{-4}}\text{radian.}$

$= 6328\times 10^{-6}\times\frac{180}{\pi}\text{degree} = 0.36°$

12. (a)

13. (b) When the light is incident at the polarising angle on the transparent medium, the reflected light is completely polarised.

14. (a) $a\sin\theta = n\lambda$

$\frac{ax}{f} = 3\lambda$

(since θ is very small so $\sin\theta \approx \tan\theta \approx \theta = x/f$)

or $\lambda = \frac{ax}{3f} = \frac{0.3\times 10^{-3}\times 5\times 10^{-3}}{3\times 1} = 5\times 10^{-7}m = 5000\text{ Å}.$

15. (c) In Fraunhoffer diffraction, for minimum intensity, $\Delta x = m\frac{\lambda}{2}$

For first minimum, m = 1 $\quad\therefore\quad \Delta x = \frac{\lambda}{2}$

16. (c) At Brewster's angle, only the reflected light is plane polarised, but transmitted light is partially polarised.

17. (b) Intensity of light transmitted by polariser is half of intensity of unpolarised light.

18. (a) For a circularly polarised light electric field remains constant with time.

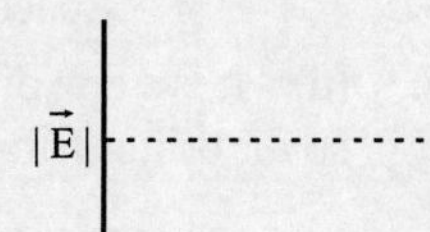

19. (a) $\sin\theta_2 = \frac{2\lambda}{d}$

or $\theta_2 = \sin^{-1}\left(\frac{2\lambda}{d}\right)$

Given $\quad y = D(2\theta_2) = 8\times 10^{-2}$

or $\quad 1.5\times 2\times\sin^{-1}\left(\frac{2\lambda}{d}\right) = 8\times 10^{-2} \Rightarrow d \simeq 0.005\text{ cm}$

20. (d) By principle of polarization, $\mu = \tan\theta_p$

or $\quad \mu = \tan 54.74°$ or $\mu = 1.414$

For an equilateral prism, $\angle A = 60°$

$\therefore\ \mu = \frac{\sin\left(\frac{A+\delta}{2}\right)}{\sin(A/2)} = \frac{\sin\left(\frac{60°+\delta}{2}\right)}{\sin(60°/2)}$

or, $\frac{1.141\times 1}{2} = \sin\left(\frac{60°+\delta}{2}\right)\left[\because 1.414 = \sqrt{2}\right]$

$\Rightarrow \frac{1}{\sqrt{2}} = \sin\left(\frac{60°+\delta}{2}\right)$ or, $\sin 45° = \sin\left(\frac{60°+\delta}{2}\right)$

$\Rightarrow \delta = 30°$

Exercise 1 - Chapter Revision Problems CRP

1. (a) For single s`lit diffraction pattern $e\sin\theta = \lambda$ Angular width, e = slit width

$$\therefore \quad \theta = \sin^{-1}\left(\frac{\lambda}{e}\right)$$

It is independent of D, distance between screen and slit.

2. (d)
3. (d) Doppler effect in light explains the phenomenon of receding of stars and approaching of star by red shift and blue shift respectively.
4. (d) 5. (c) 6. (b) 7. (b)
8. (b) Longitudinal waves cannot be polarised.
9. (d) 10. (c) 11. (d) 12. (c)
13. (b) The line rulings, each of 0.5 μm width, on a compact disc function as a diffraction grating. When a small source of light illuminates a disc, diffracted light forms coloured 'lanes' that are the composite of the diffraction patterns from the ruling.
14. (d) When a ray of light enters nicol prism, it splits into two plane polarised light in mutually perpendicular direction. One of this light undergoes total reflection and absorption whereas other comes out as a plane polarised light.
15. (b) Newton first predicted deflection of light by gravitational field.
16. (c) Speed of light is different in different media and different medium has different refractive index.

$${}^1\mu_2 = \frac{\text{Speed of light in medium 1}}{\text{Speed of light in medium 2}}$$

17. (d) It is a one of Fraunhoffer diffraction from single slit. so for bright fringe where a is the width of slit.

$$a\sin\theta = (2n+1)\frac{\lambda}{2}$$

$$\lambda = \frac{2a\sin\theta}{2n+1} = \frac{2\times1.2\times10^{-5}\times0.0906}{2\times1+1}$$

$$= 7248\times10^{-10}\ \text{m} = 7248\text{Å}.$$

18. (c) As $R^2 = a^2 + b^2 + 2ab\cos\phi$

$$\therefore \quad I_{max} = I_1 + I_2 + 2\sqrt{I_1 I_2}\cos 0^\circ = I_1 + I_2 + 2\sqrt{I_1 I_2}$$

19. (b) Phase diff. $= \frac{2\pi}{\lambda}x$

$$\text{Path difference} = \frac{2\pi\times2.1\times10^{-6}}{5460\times10^{-10}} = 7.692\,\pi\,\text{radian}.$$

20. (c) $\beta = \frac{\lambda' D'}{d'} = \frac{3\lambda 3D}{d/3} = 27\frac{\lambda D}{d}$.

No. of fringes $= \frac{1/3}{\beta} = \frac{d}{81\lambda D}$.

21. (d) As reflected and refracted rays are perpendicular to each other, therefore, $i_p = i = 60^\circ$, where i_p is called angle of polarisation.

$\mu = \tan i_p = \tan 60^\circ = \sqrt{3} = 1.732$.

22. (b) $\upsilon = \frac{\Delta\lambda}{\lambda}\times c = \frac{(6586-6263)}{6563}\times3\times10^8$

$= 1.05\times10^6$ m/s.

23. (b) $\Delta\lambda = \frac{\upsilon}{c}\times\lambda = \frac{10^5}{3\times10^8}\times5700 = 1.9\,\text{Å}$.

24. (a) Where n is equivalent number of fringe by which the centre fringe is shifted due to mica sheet

$$\lambda = \frac{(\mu-1)t}{n} = \frac{(1.5-1)6\times10^{-6}}{5} = 6\times10^{-7}\,\text{m} = 6000\ \text{Å}$$

25. (c) In Radar, the source & receiver are together, the receiver being turned for frequencies other than the source or radar frequency.

To measure the speed of helicopter

(i) The moving object of speed v_a receive a frequency

$$\nu' = \nu\left(1 + \frac{v_a}{c}\right)$$

(ii) The object which receives ν' frequency now acts as a moving source. The detector observes a frequency ν_0

$$\nu_0 = \nu'\left(\frac{1}{1-\frac{v_a}{c}}\right) = \left(\frac{1+\frac{v_a}{c}}{1-\frac{v_a}{c}}\right)$$

$$\Rightarrow (\nu_0 - \nu) = \Delta\nu = (\nu_0 + \nu)\frac{v_a}{c}$$

$$\text{or } v_a = \frac{\Delta\nu c}{2\nu} \qquad \left(\begin{array}{l}\therefore \nu_0 \approx \nu \\ \Rightarrow \nu_0 + \nu \approx 2\nu\end{array}\right)$$

26. (a) As $\beta \propto \lambda$

$\therefore$ fringe width becomes $\frac{5}{4}$ times,

No, of fringes $= \frac{4}{5}\times10 = 8$

27. (b) $\beta' = \frac{\beta}{\mu} = \frac{0.133}{1.33} = 0.1$ cm

28. (c) The position of nth dark fringe in Fraunhoffer Diffraction from a single slit is

$a\sin\theta = n\lambda$

$$a = \frac{n\lambda}{\sin\theta} = \frac{1\times6.5\times10^{-7}}{\sin 30^\circ},\ \text{(for first min. n = 1)}$$

$$= \frac{6.5\times10^{-7}}{1/2} = 13\times10^{-7}\,\text{m} = 1.3\,\mu\text{m}.$$

29. (d) Limit of resolution L.R $\propto \lambda$

$$\therefore \quad L.R' = L.R\times\frac{\lambda'}{\lambda} = 0.1\times\frac{4800}{6000} = 0.08\,\text{mm}.$$

$\therefore$ Resolution improves when light of lower wavelength is used.

30. (b) Intensity of polarised light transmitted from 1st polariser,

$I_1 = I_0\cos^2\theta$

but $(\cos^2\theta)_{av} = \frac{1}{2}$

So $I_1 = \frac{1}{2}I_0 = \frac{32}{2} = 16\,\text{Wm}^{-2}$

31. (c) Suppose intensity of unpolarised light = 100.
$\therefore$ Intensity of polarised light from first nicol prism
$= \frac{I_0}{2} = \frac{1}{2} \times 100 = 50$
According to law of Malus,
$I = I_0 \cos^2 \theta = 50\ (\cos 60°)^2 = 50 \times \left(\frac{1}{2}\right)^2 = 12.5$

32. (b) $\Delta\nu = \frac{\upsilon}{c} \times \nu = \frac{0.2\,c}{c} \times 4 \times 10^7 = 0.8 \times 10^7$ Hz
$\nu' = \nu - \Delta\nu = 4 \times 10^7 - 0.8 \times 10^7 = 3.2 \times 10^7$ Hz.

33. (a) When planet or stars are receding away from earth. If f is frequency of vibration.
Then, $f = \frac{c}{\lambda}$
If v = velocity of body moving away
λ' = apparent wavelength to an observer on the earth
$\lambda' = \frac{(c+v)}{f}$ (c and v are in opposite to each other)
$= \left(\frac{c+v}{c}\right)\lambda \qquad \lambda' = \left(1 + \frac{v}{c}\right)\lambda$
$\frac{\lambda' - \lambda}{\lambda} = \frac{v}{c}$
Fractional change in wavelength
$\therefore \quad 1 = \frac{v}{c} \Rightarrow v = c$

34. (b) The fluorescent material present in the tube converts u.v. rays into visible light.

35. (d) By principle of polarization, $\mu = \tan\theta_p$
or $\mu = \tan 54.74°$ or $\mu = 1.414$
For an equilateral prism, $\angle A = 60°$
$\therefore \mu = \frac{\sin\left(\frac{A+\delta}{2}\right)}{\sin(A/2)} = \frac{\sin\left(\frac{60°+\delta}{2}\right)}{\sin(60°/2)}$
or, $\frac{1.141 \times 1}{2} = \sin\left(\frac{60°+\delta}{2}\right) \left[\because 1.414 = \sqrt{2}\right]$
or, $\frac{\sqrt{2}}{2} = \sin\left(\frac{60°+\delta}{2}\right)$ or $\frac{1}{\sqrt{2}} = \sin\left(\frac{60°+\delta}{2}\right)$
or, $\sin 45° = \sin\left(\frac{60°+\delta}{2}\right)$ or $45° = \left(\frac{60°+\delta}{2}\right)$

36. (c) $x = \frac{(2n+1)\lambda\, D}{2a}$
For red light, $x = \frac{(4+1)D}{2a} \times 6500$Å
For other light, $x = \frac{(6+1)D}{2a} \times \lambda$Å
x is same for each.
$\therefore\ 5 \times 6500 = 7 \times \lambda \Rightarrow \lambda = \frac{5}{7} \times 6500 = 4642.8$ Å.

37. (b) ${}^a\mu_g = \tan\theta_P$ where θ_P = polarising angle.
or, ${}^a\mu_g = \tan 60°$
or, $\frac{c}{v_g} = \sqrt{3}$ or, $v_g = \frac{c}{\sqrt{3}} = \frac{3 \times 10^8}{\sqrt{3}} = \sqrt{3} \times 10^8\ \text{ms}^{-1}$

38. (c) By covering aperture, focal length does not change. But intensity is reduced by $\frac{1}{4}$ times, as aperture diameter $\frac{d}{2}$ is covered.
$\therefore \quad I' = I - \frac{I}{4} = \frac{3I}{4}$
$\therefore \quad$ New focal length = f and intensity = $\frac{3I}{4}$.

39. (b)
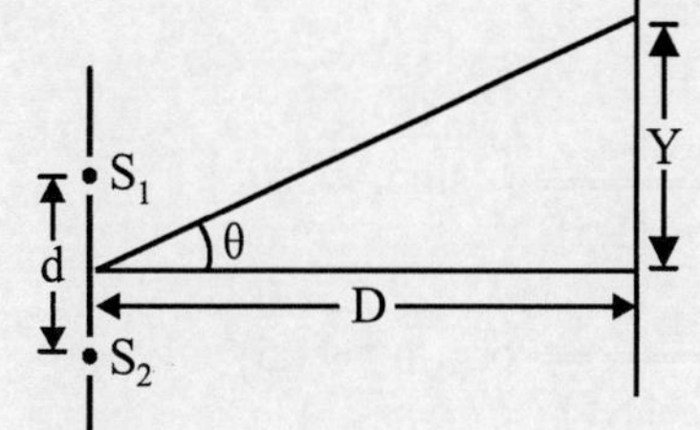

Angular width, $\theta = \frac{Y}{D} = \frac{n\lambda D}{dD} \left[\because Y = \frac{D\lambda}{d}\right]$
so, $\theta = \frac{\lambda}{d}$, $v \uparrow \lambda \downarrow \theta \downarrow$ [For central maxima n = 1]
Hence, with increase in speed of electrons angular width of central maximum decreases.

40. (b)

41. (d) Initially, $S_2L = 2$ m
$S_1L = \sqrt{2^2 + \left(\frac{3}{2}\right)^2} = \frac{5}{2} = 2.5$ m
Path difference,
$\Delta x = S_1L - S_2L = 0.5\ \text{m} = \frac{\lambda}{2}$
When the listner move from L, first maxima will appear if path difference is integral multiple of wavelength.
For example
$\Delta x = n\lambda = 1\lambda$ ($n = 1$ for first maxima)
$\therefore\ \Delta x = \lambda = S_1L' - S_2L \Rightarrow 1 = d - 2 \Rightarrow d = 3$ m

42. (c)

43. (a) Path difference, $\Delta P = d \sin\theta = d\theta$
d = distance between slits = 1 mm = 10^{-3} mm
D = distance between the slits and screen = 100 cm = 1 m
y = distance between central bright fringe and observed fringe = 1.27 mm
$\therefore \Delta P = \frac{dy}{D} = \frac{10^{-3} \times 1.270\ \text{mm}}{1\ \text{m}} = 1.27\ \mu\text{m}$

44. (Bonus) Shift = nβ (given)
$\therefore \quad D\frac{(\mu-1)t}{a} = \frac{n\lambda D}{a} \left[\because \text{Shift} = \frac{D(\mu-1)t}{a}\right]$
or $\quad t = \frac{n\lambda}{(\mu-1)}$

45. (a) Here, $x_1 = 2d$ and $x_2 = \sqrt{5}d$
For, first minima, $\Delta x = \frac{\lambda}{2}$
$\therefore \Delta x = x_2 - x_1 = \sqrt{5}d - 2d = \frac{\lambda}{2} \Rightarrow d = \frac{\lambda}{2(\sqrt{5}-2)}$

46. (c) Shift $= \frac{\beta(\mu-1)}{\lambda}t_1 - \frac{\beta(\mu-1)}{\lambda}t_2 = \frac{\beta(\mu-1)}{\lambda}(t_1 - t_2)$

47. (a)

48. (c) $\theta = \frac{1.22\lambda}{d} = \frac{1.22 \times 600 \times 10^{-9}}{250 \times 10^{-2}} = 3.0 \times 10^{-7}\text{rad}$

49. (b) According to Brewster's law, refractive index of material (μ) is equal to tangent of polarising angle

$$\because \tan i_b = \mu = \frac{1.5}{\mu}$$

$$\frac{1}{\mu} < \frac{1.5}{\sqrt{\mu^2 + (1.5)^2}} \quad (\because \sin i_c < \sin i_b)$$

$$\therefore \sin i_b = \frac{1.5}{\sqrt{\mu^2 + (1.5)^2}} \text{ or, } \sqrt{\mu^2 + (1.5)^2} < 1.5 \times \mu$$

$$\Rightarrow \mu^2 + (1.5)^2 < (\mu \times 1.5)^2$$

$$\Rightarrow \mu < \frac{3}{\sqrt{5}} \text{ i.e. minimum value of } \mu \text{ should be } \frac{3}{\sqrt{5}}$$

50. (a) Angular width of central maxima $= \frac{2\lambda}{d}$

or, $\lambda = \frac{d}{2}$; Fringe width, $\beta = \frac{\lambda \times D}{d'}$

$$10^{-2} = \frac{d}{2} \times \frac{50 \times 10^{-2}}{d'} = \frac{10^{-6} \times 50 \times 10^{-2}}{2 \times d'}$$

Therefore, slit separation distance, d' = 25μm

Exercise 2 - Exemplar & Past Year Questions 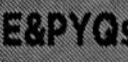

Exemplar Questions

1. (c) Let us consider the diagram shown below the light beam incident from air to the glass slab at Brewster's angle (i_p). The angle between reflected ray BE and BC is 90°. Then only reflected ray is plane polarised represented by arrows.

As the emergent and incident ray are unpolarised, so, polaroid rotated in the way of CD then the intensity cannot be zero but varies in one complete rotation.

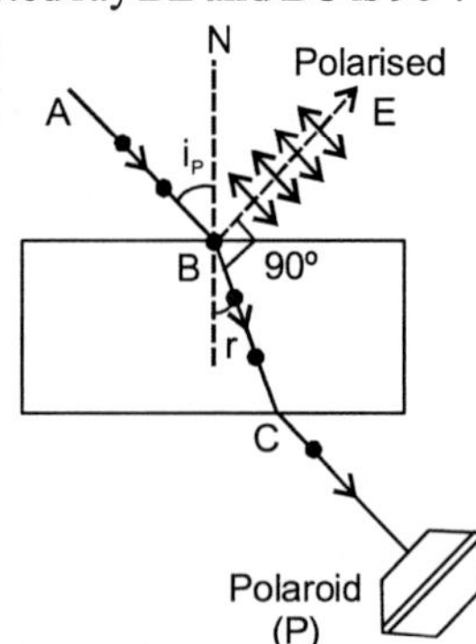

2. (a) As given that the width of the slit

$= 10^4$ Å $= 10000$ Å

$= 10^4 \times 10^{-10}\text{m} = 10^{-6}\text{m} = 1\ \mu\text{m}$

Wavelength of visible sunlight varies from 4000 Å to 8000 Å.

Thus the width of slit is 10000 Å comparable to that of wavelength visible light i.e., 8000 Å. So diffraction occurs with maxima at centre. Hence at the centre all colours appear i.e., mixing of colours form white patch at the centre.

3. (a)

4. (c) For sustained interference pattern to be formed on the screen, the sources must be coherent and emits lights of same frequency and wavelength.

In a Young's double-slit experiment, when one of the holes is covered by a red filter and another by a blue filter. In this case due to filteration only red and blue lights are present which has different frequency. In this monochromatic light is used for the formation of fringes on the screen. So, in that case there shall be no interference fringes.

5. (d) Consider the given figure there is a hole at point P_2. By Huygen's principle, wave will propagates from the sources S_1 and S_2. Each point on the screen will acts as sources of secondary wavelets.

Wavefront starting from P_2 reaches at S_3 and S_4 which will again act as two monochromatic or coherent sources. Hence, there will be always a regular two slit pattern on the second screen.

Past Years (2013-2020) NEET/AIPMT

6. (a) $\because y = \frac{n\lambda D}{d}$

$\therefore n_1 \lambda_1 = n_2 \lambda_2$

$\Rightarrow n_1 \times 12000 \times 10^{-10} = n_2 \times 10000 \times 10^{-10}$

or, $n(12000 \times 10^{-10}) = (n+1)(10000 \times 10^{-10})$

$\Rightarrow n = 5$

$(\because \lambda_1 = 12000 \times 10^{-10}\text{m};\ \lambda_2 = 10000 \times 10^{-10}\text{m})$

Hence, $y_{common} = \frac{n\lambda_1 D}{d}$

$= \frac{5(12000 \times 10^{-10}) \times 2}{2 \times 10^{-3}}$

$(\because d = 2\text{ mm and } D = 2\text{m})$

$= 5 \times 12 \times 10^{-4}\text{ m}$

$= 60 \times 10^{-4}\text{ m}$

$= 6 \times 10^{-3}\text{m} = 6\text{mm}$

S_1 2mm S_2 2m y

7. (c) Fringe width $\beta = \frac{\lambda D}{d}$;

From question $D' = 2D$ and $d' = \frac{d}{2}$

$\therefore \beta' = \frac{\lambda D^1}{d^1} = 4\beta$

8. (d) Given: $D = 2\text{m}; d = 1\text{ mm} = 1 \times 10^{-3}\text{m}$

$\lambda = 600\text{ nm} = 600 \times 10^{-6}\text{m}$

Width of central bright fringe ($= 2\beta$)

$= \frac{2\lambda D}{d} = \frac{2 \times 600 \times 10^{-6} \times 2}{1 \times 10^{-3}}\text{m} = 2.4 \times 10^{-3}\text{m} = 2.4\text{mm}$

9. (c) For path difference λ, phase difference $= 2\pi$ rad.

For path difference $\frac{\lambda}{4}$, phase difference $= \frac{\pi}{2}$ rad.

As $K = 4I_0$ so intensity at given point where path difference is $\frac{\lambda}{4}$

$$K' = 4I_0 \cos^2\left(\frac{\pi}{4}\right)\left(\cos\frac{\pi}{4} = \cos 45^\circ\right) = 2I_0 = \frac{K}{2}$$

10. (d) Here, distance between two slits,
$d = 1\text{mm} = 10^{-3}\text{m}$
distance of screen from slits, D = 1 m
wavelength of monochromatic light used,
$\lambda = 500\text{nm} = 500 \times 10^{-9}\text{m}$
width of each slit a = ?
Width of central maxima in single slit pattern $= \frac{2\lambda D}{a}$
Fringe width in double slit experiment $\beta = \frac{\lambda D}{d}$
So, required condition $\frac{10\lambda D}{d} = \frac{2\lambda D}{a}$
$\Rightarrow \quad a = \frac{d}{5D} = \frac{1}{5} \times 10^{-3}\text{m} = 0.2\,\text{mm}$

11. (d) Linear width of central maxima y
$= D(2q) = 2Dq = \frac{2D\lambda}{a} \qquad \therefore q = \frac{\lambda}{a}$

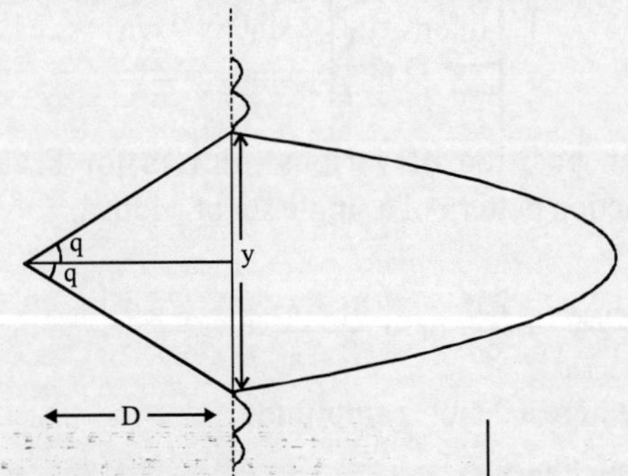

12. (b) For first minima at P
$AP - BP = \lambda$
$AP - MP = \frac{\lambda}{2}$
So phase difference,
$\phi = \frac{2\pi}{\lambda} \times \frac{\lambda}{2} = \pi\,\text{radian}$

13. (d) For the first minima,
$\theta = \frac{\eta\lambda}{a} \quad \Rightarrow \quad \sin 30^\circ = \frac{\lambda}{a} = \frac{1}{2}$
First secondary maxima will be at
$\sin\theta = \frac{3\lambda}{2a} = \frac{3}{2}\left(\frac{1}{2}\right) \quad \Rightarrow \quad \theta = \sin^{-1}\left(\frac{3}{4}\right)$

14. (d) Let P is a point infront of one slit at which intensity is to be calculated. From figure,
Path difference $= S_2P - S_1P$

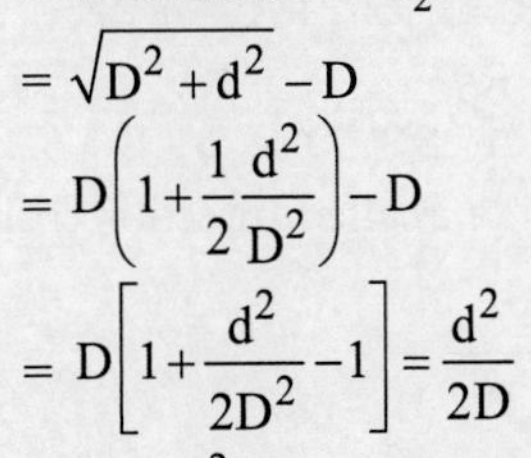

$= \sqrt{D^2 + d^2} - D$
$= D\left(1 + \frac{1}{2}\frac{d^2}{D^2}\right) - D$
$= D\left[1 + \frac{d^2}{2D^2} - 1\right] = \frac{d^2}{2D}$

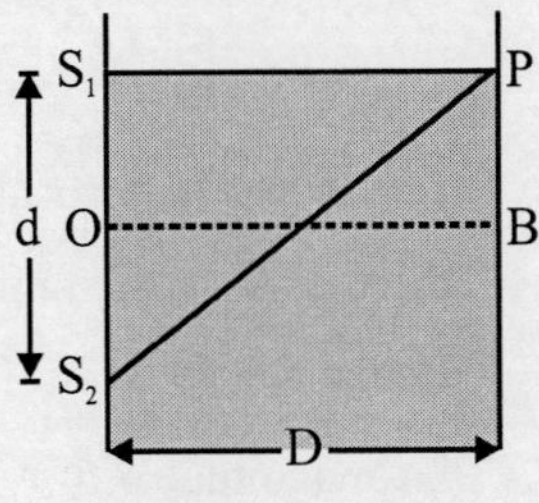

$\Delta x = \frac{d^2}{2 \times 10d} = \frac{d}{20} = \frac{5\lambda}{20} = \frac{\lambda}{4}$

Phase difference,
$\Delta\phi = \frac{2\pi}{\lambda} \times \frac{\lambda}{4} = \frac{\pi}{2}$
So, resultant intensity at the desired point 'p' is
$I = I_0 \cos^2\frac{\phi}{2} = I_0 \cos^2\frac{\pi}{4} = \frac{I_0}{2}$

15. (b) Resolving power of a microscope $= \frac{2\mu\sin\theta}{\lambda}$
i.e., $R \propto \frac{1}{\lambda}$ or, $\frac{R_1}{R_2} = \frac{\lambda_2}{\lambda_1}$
Given that the two wavelengths,
$\lambda_1 = 4000\text{Å}$
$\lambda_2 = 6000\text{Å}$
$\therefore \quad \frac{R_1}{R_2} = \frac{6000\text{Å}}{4000\text{Å}} = \frac{3}{2}$

16. (c) According to question
8th bright fringe in medium = 5th dark fring in air
$Y_{8\text{th bright}} = 8\frac{\lambda D}{\mu d}$
$Y_{5\text{th dark}} = (2 \times 5 - 1)\frac{\lambda D}{2d} = \frac{9}{2}\frac{\lambda D}{d}$
$\Rightarrow \quad \frac{9}{2}\frac{\lambda D}{d} = 8\frac{\lambda D}{\mu d}$
or, refractive index $\mu = \frac{16}{9} = 1.78$

17. (b) According to malus law, $I = I_0\cos^2\theta$
$I_1 = \frac{I_0}{2}$
$I_2 = \frac{I_0}{2}\cos^2 45^\circ$
$= \frac{I_0}{2} \times \frac{1}{2} = \frac{I_0}{4}$
$I_3 = \frac{I_0}{4}\cos^2 45^\circ$
$I_3 = \frac{I_0}{8}$

18. (b) When reflected light rays and refracted rays are perpendicular, reflected light is polarised with electric field vector perpendicular to the plane of incidence.

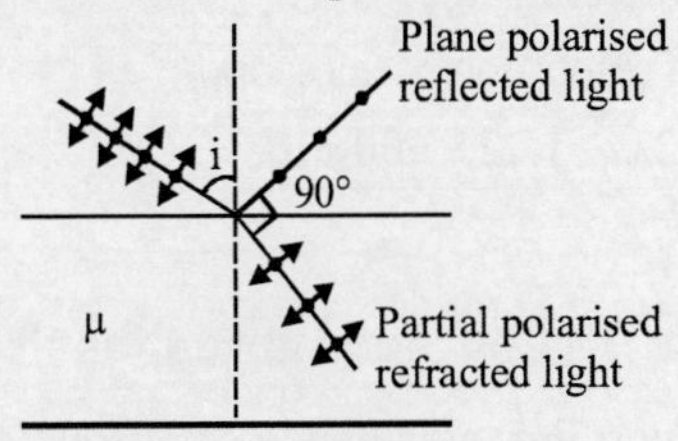

Also, tan i = μ (i = Brewester angle)

19. (b) Angular width $= \frac{\lambda}{d}$
So, $0.20^\circ = \frac{\lambda}{2\text{mm}} \Rightarrow \lambda = 0.20^\circ \times 2$
Again, $0.21^\circ = \frac{\lambda}{d}$

Now putting the value of λ

$$d = \frac{0.20° \times 2\text{mm}}{0.21°}$$

$\therefore \quad d = 1.9\,\text{mm}$

20. (b) For double slit experiment angular fringe width

$$\theta_0 = \frac{\beta}{D}$$

Angular fringe width (in water)

$$\theta_w = \frac{\beta}{\mu D} = \frac{\theta_0}{\mu} = \frac{0.2°}{\left(\frac{4}{3}\right)} = 0.15°$$

21. (c) As $\theta = \frac{2\lambda}{a}$

$$\theta_0 = \frac{2 \times 6000}{a} \quad ...(i)$$

$$\frac{\theta_1}{\theta_0} = \frac{\lambda_1}{6000} \quad ...(ii)$$

$\Rightarrow \lambda_1 = 0.7 \times 6000$ (as $\theta_1 = 0.7\,\theta_0$) $\Rightarrow 4200$ Å

22. (b) Fringe width $\beta = \frac{\lambda D}{d}$

Here, λ = wavelength of light from coherent sources,
D = distance of screen from the coherent sources,
d = separation between coherent sources

When, $d' = \frac{d}{2}$ and $D' = 2D$

New Fringe width, $\beta' = \frac{\lambda(2D)}{d/2} = \frac{4\lambda D}{d} \Rightarrow \beta' = 4\beta$

Fringe width becomes 4 times.

23. (b) According to Brewster's law, when a beam of unpolarised light is reflected from a transparent medium of refractive index (μ_2), the reflected light is completely polarised at certain angle of incidence called the angle of polarisation (i_b).

$$\tan i_b = \frac{\mu_2}{\mu_1}$$

For air, $\mu_1 = 1$

$\therefore \tan i_b = \mu_2 > 1 \Rightarrow \tan i_b > 1 \Rightarrow 90° > i_b > 45°$

24. (d) Given :

Wavelength, $\lambda = 600$ nm $= 600 \times 10^{-9}$ m

and diameter of objective, $d = 2$ m

Limit of resolution of telescope,

$$\theta = \frac{1.22\lambda}{d} = \frac{1.22 \times 600 \times 10^{-9}}{2} = 3.66 \times 10^{-7}\,\text{rad}$$

Exercise 3 - Concept Application Problems CAP

1. (b) According to principle of diffraction, a sin θ = nλ where, n = order of secondary minimum

or, $a \sin 30° = 1 \times (6500 \times 10^{-10})$

or, $a = 1.3 \times 10^{-6}$ m, or, a = 1.3 micron.

2. (d) Photoelectric effect does not support the wave nature of light.

3. (c) 4. (d) 5. (c)

6. (d) As fringe width $\beta = \frac{D}{d}\lambda$

$$\mu = A + \frac{B}{\lambda^2} + \frac{C}{\lambda^4} + ...$$

$$\mu_{Vacuum} < \mu_{Air} \text{ so } \lambda_{Vacuum} > \lambda_{Air}$$

Therefore when chamber is evacuated fringe width β slightly increases.

7. (c) $\because i_p = \phi$, therefore, angle between reflected and refracted rays is 90°.

8. (a) Width of central maximum

$$= \frac{2\lambda D}{a} = \frac{2 \times 6250 \times 10^{-10} \times 0.5}{2 \times 10^{-4}}$$

$$= 3125 \times 10^{-6}\,\text{m} = 312.5 \times 10^{-3}\,\text{cm.}$$

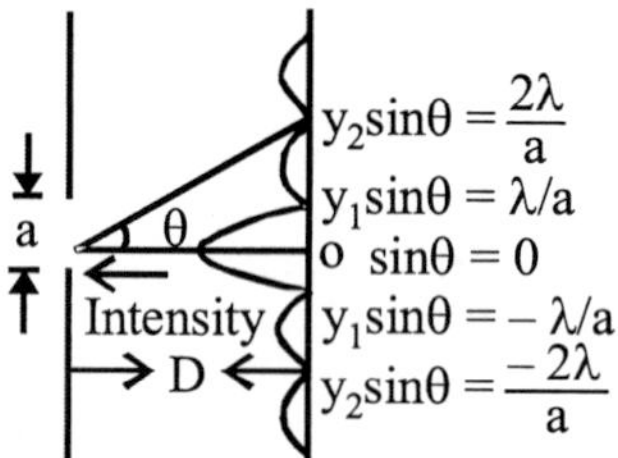

Screen position of various minima for Fraunhoffer diffraction pattern of a single slit of width a.

9. (d)

10. (d) $\frac{I_{max}}{I_{min}} = \frac{25}{9}$ or $\left(\frac{a_1 + a_2}{a_1 - a_2}\right)^2 = \frac{25}{9}$

where a denotes amplitude.

$\frac{a_1 + a_2}{a_1 - a_2} = \frac{5}{3}$ or $5a_1 - 5a_2 = 3a_1 + 3a_2$

or, $5a_1 - 5a_2 = 3a_1 + 3a_2$ or $2a_1 = 8a_2$

or, $\frac{a_1}{a_2} = 4$ or $\left(\frac{a_1}{a_2}\right)^2 = 16 = \frac{I_1}{I_2}$.

11. (b)

12. (c) In Young's double slit experiment, half angular width (θ) is given by

$$\sin\theta = \frac{\lambda}{d} = \frac{589 \times 10^{-9}}{0.589 \times 10^{-3}} = 10^{-3}$$

$\therefore \quad \theta = \sin^{-1} 0.001$

13. (a)

14. (d) Let any $\vec{R}$ its components are

$$\vec{R} = \vec{R}x + \vec{R}y + \vec{R}z$$

with $|\vec{R}| = \vec{R} = |\vec{R}| = \vec{R} = \sqrt{Rx^2 + Ry^2 + Rz}$

& $\cos\theta_x = \frac{Rx}{R}$, $\cos\theta_y \frac{Ry}{R}$, $\cos\theta_z = \frac{Rz}{R}$

there $\cos\theta_x$, $\cos\theta_y$ and $\cos\theta_z$ one called direction cosines.

Hence $x + y + z = c \quad (= \vec{R})$

So, magnitude of $c = \sqrt{I^2 + I^2 + I^2} = \sqrt{3}$

and $\cos\theta_x = \frac{1}{\sqrt{3}}$

15. (b) Let nth fringe of 2500 Å coincide with (n – 2)th fringe of 3500Å.

$\therefore$ 3500 (n – 2) = 2500 × n

1000 n = 7000, n = 7

$\therefore$ 7th order fringe of 1st source will coincide with 5th order fringe of 2nd source.

16. (a) When angle of incidence i is equal to angle of polarisation i.e, then reflected light is completely plane-polarised whose vibration is perpendicular to plane of incidence.

17. (a) According to law of Malus

$$\mathbf{I} = \mathbf{I_0}\cos^2\theta = \mathbf{I_0}(\cos 45^\circ)^2 = \mathbf{I_0}\left(\frac{1}{\sqrt{2}}\right)^2 = \frac{\mathbf{I_0}}{2}$$

18. (b) If the angular limit of resolution of human eye is R then

$$R = \frac{1.22\lambda}{a} = \frac{1.22\times5\times10^{-7}}{2\times10^{-3}}\text{ rad}$$

$$= \frac{1.22\times5\times10^{-7}}{2\times10^{-3}}\times\frac{180}{\pi}\times 60\text{ minute} = 1\text{ minute}$$

19. (c)

20. (c) Given amplitude ratio of waves is $\frac{a_1}{a_2} = \frac{3}{1}$

so, $\frac{I_{max}}{I_{min}} - \left(\frac{a_2+a_1}{a_2-a_1}\right)^2$

$$= \left(\frac{\frac{a_2}{a_1}+1}{\frac{a_2}{a_1}-1}\right)^2 = \left(\frac{3+1}{3-1}\right)^2 = \left(\frac{4}{2}\right)^2 = \frac{4}{1} = 4$$

21. (b) As we know, $\frac{I_{max}}{I_{min}} = \left(\frac{A_1+A_2}{A_1-A_2}\right)^2$

and $\sqrt{\frac{I_1}{I_2}} = \frac{A_1}{A_2}$

$$\frac{I_{max}}{I_{min}} = 16 \Rightarrow \frac{A_{max}}{A_{min}} = 4 \Rightarrow \frac{A_1+A_2}{A_1-A_2} = \frac{4}{1}$$

Using componendo and dividendo.

$$\frac{A_1}{A_2} = \frac{5}{3} \Rightarrow \frac{I_1}{I_2} = \left(\frac{5}{3}\right)^2 = \frac{25}{9}$$

22. (b)

23. (d) $\frac{\text{(Maximum intensity) coherent interference}}{\text{(Maximum intensity) in coherent interference}} = \frac{n^2 I_0}{n I_0} = n$

24. (a)

25. (c) $\Delta x = \frac{\lambda}{(2\alpha)}$

26. (b) Given : Wavelength of light, λ = 500 nm

Distance between the slits, d = 0.05 mm

Angular width of the fringe formed,

$$\theta = \frac{\lambda}{d} = \frac{500\times10^{-9}}{0.05\times10^{-3}} = 0.01\text{ rad} = 0.57^\circ.$$

27. (d) Let n_1 fringes are visible with light of wavelength λ_1 and n_2 with light of wavelength λ_2. Then

$$\beta = \frac{n_1 D\lambda_1}{d} = \frac{n_2 D\lambda_2}{d} \qquad \left(\because \beta = \frac{n\lambda D}{d}\right)$$

$$\Rightarrow \frac{n_2}{n_1} = \frac{\lambda_1}{\lambda_2} \Rightarrow n_2 = \frac{700}{400}\times 16 = 28$$

28. (a) Given, Path difference, $\Delta x = \frac{\lambda}{8}$

Phase differences, $\Delta\phi = \frac{2\pi}{\lambda}\Delta x = \frac{2\pi}{\lambda}\times\frac{\lambda}{8} = \frac{\pi}{4}$

$$I = I_0\cos^2\left(\frac{\Delta\phi}{2}\right) \Rightarrow \frac{I}{I_0} = \cos^2\left(\frac{\frac{\pi}{4}}{2}\right) = \cos^2\left(\frac{\pi}{8}\right)$$

$$\Rightarrow \frac{I}{I_0} = 0.853$$

29. (c) Given, distance between screen and slits, D = 1.5 m

Seperation between slits, d = 0.15 mm

Wavelength of source of light, λ = 589 nm

Fringe-width,

$$w = \frac{D}{d}\lambda = \frac{1.5}{0.15\times10^{-3}}\times589\times10^{-9}\,m$$

$$= 589\times10^{-2}\text{ mm} = 5.89\text{ mm} \approx 5.9\text{ mm}$$

30. (c) Given, $\Delta = \beta$

or $\frac{D(\mu-1)t}{d} = \frac{D\lambda}{d}$

$\therefore\ t = \frac{\lambda}{(\mu-1)}$

31. (b) Given, path difference, $\Delta x = \frac{\lambda}{8}$

Phase difference ($\Delta\phi$) is given by

$$\Delta\phi = \frac{2\pi}{\lambda}(\Delta x) \Rightarrow \Delta\phi = \frac{(2\pi)}{\lambda}\frac{\lambda}{8} = \frac{\pi}{4}$$

For two sources in different phases,

$$I = I_0\cos^2\left(\frac{\pi}{8}\right) \Rightarrow \frac{I}{I_0} = \cos^2\left(\frac{\pi}{8}\right)$$

$$= \frac{1+\cos\frac{\pi}{4}}{2} = \frac{1+\frac{1}{\sqrt{2}}}{2} = 0.85$$

32. (a) Path difference = d sin$\theta \approx$ dθ

$= 0.1\times\frac{1}{40}$ mm = 2500nm

For bright fringe, path difference must be integral multiple of λ.

$\therefore$ 2500 = nλ_1 = mλ_2

$\therefore$ λ_1 = 625 (for n = 4), λ_2 = 500 (for m = 5)

33. (d) For 'n' number of maximas

$d \sin\theta = n\lambda$

$0.32 \times 10^{-3} \sin 30° = n \times 500 \times 10^{-9}$

$\therefore \quad n = \dfrac{0.32 \times 10^{-3}}{500 \times 10^{-9}} \times \dfrac{1}{2} = 320$

Hence total no. of maximas observed in angular range $-30° \le \theta \le 30°$

$= 320 + 1 + 320 = 641$

34. (c) $2I_0 = 4I_0 \cos^2\left(\dfrac{\Delta\phi}{2}\right)$ here, $\Delta\phi = \dfrac{\pi}{2}$

But, $\Delta\phi = \dfrac{2\pi}{\lambda}\Delta x$ so, $\Delta x = \dfrac{\lambda}{4}$

$\dfrac{dy}{D} = \dfrac{\lambda}{4}$ ....(i)

$\dfrac{\lambda D}{d} = \beta$ ....(ii)

Multiplying equation (i) and (ii) we get,

$y = \dfrac{\beta}{4}$

35. (b) As $\sin\theta = \dfrac{n\lambda}{d}$ and $\sin\theta$ cannot be $\not> 1$

$\therefore 1 = \dfrac{n\lambda}{1.8\lambda}$ or $n = 1.8$

Hence maximum number of possible interference maximas, $0, \pm 1$ i.e. 3

36. (d) Given :

Intensity, $I_0 = 3.3$ Wm^{-2}

Area, $A = 3 \times 10^{-4}$ m^2

Angular speed, $\omega = 31.4$ rad/s

Average energy $= I_0 A < \cos^2\theta >$

$\because < \cos^2\theta > = \dfrac{1}{2}$ per revolution

$\therefore$ Average energy $= \dfrac{(3.3)(3 \times 10^{-4})}{2} \simeq 5 \times 10^{-4}$ J

37. (b) According to question, the intensity of light coming out of the analyser is just 10% of the original intensity (I_0)

Using, $I = I_0 \cos^2\theta$

$\Rightarrow \dfrac{I_0}{10} = I_0 \cos^2\theta \Rightarrow \dfrac{1}{10} = \cos^2\theta$

$\Rightarrow \cos\theta = \dfrac{1}{\sqrt{10}} = 0.316 \Rightarrow \theta \approx 71.6°$

Therefore, the angle by which the analyser need to be rotated further to reduced the output intensity to be zero

$\phi = 90° - \theta = 90° - 71.6° = 18.4°$

38. (a) $x = \dfrac{1.22\lambda}{2\mu\sin\theta} = \dfrac{1.22 \times 5000}{2 \times 1.25} = 0.24\ \mu$m

39. (c) $I = \left(\dfrac{I_0}{2}\right) \cos^2 30° \cos^2 60°$

$= \dfrac{I_0}{2} \times \dfrac{3}{4} \times \dfrac{1}{4}$

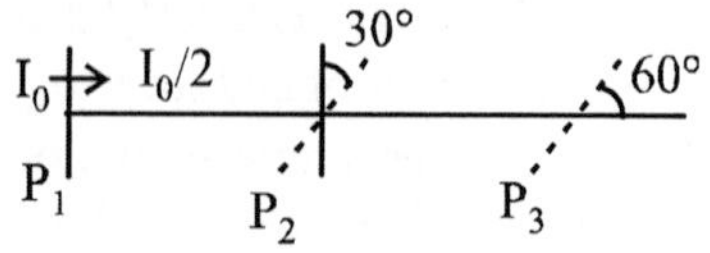

$\therefore \quad \dfrac{I_0}{I} = \dfrac{32}{3} = 10.67$

40. (a) $\theta = \dfrac{1.22\lambda}{d} = \dfrac{1.22 \times 500 \times 10^{-9}}{2} = 305 \times 10^{-9}$ rad.

41. (b)

42. (c) Axis of transmission of A & B are parallel.

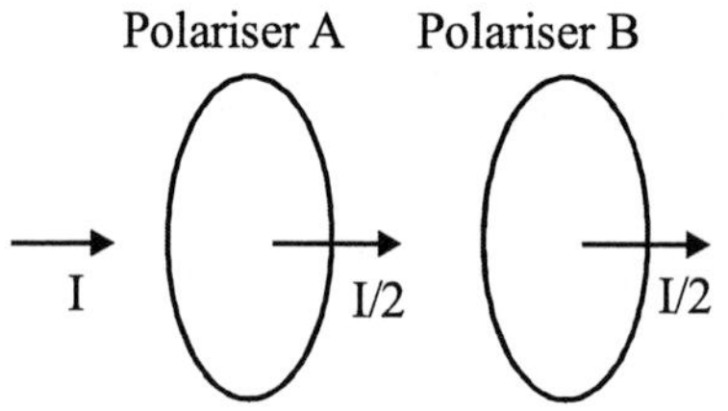

After introducing polariser C between A and B,

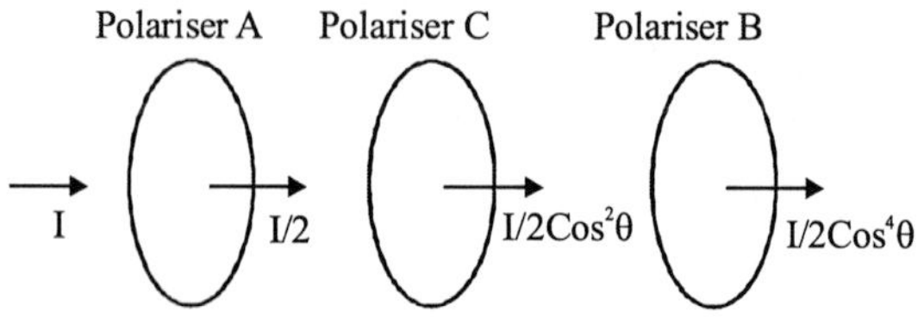

$\dfrac{I}{2}\cos^4\theta = \dfrac{I}{8} \Rightarrow \cos^4\theta = \dfrac{1}{4}$

$\Rightarrow \cos\theta = \dfrac{1}{\sqrt{2}}$ or, $\theta = 45°$

43. (a) If angular position of 2nd maxima from central maxima is θ then

$\sin\theta = \dfrac{(2n-1)\lambda}{2a} = \dfrac{3\lambda}{20} = \dfrac{3 \times 550 \times 10^{-9}}{2 \times 22 \times 10^{-7}}$

$\therefore \quad \theta \simeq \dfrac{\pi}{8}$ rad

44. (a)

45. (a) Polariser A and B have same alignment of transmission axis.

Lets assume polariser c is introduced at θ angle

$\dfrac{1}{2}\cos^2\theta \times \cos^2\theta = \dfrac{1}{3}$

or, $\cos^4\theta = \dfrac{2}{3} \Rightarrow \cos\theta = \left(\dfrac{2}{3}\right)^{1/4}$

26 Dual Nature of Radiation and Matter

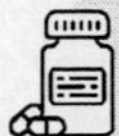

Topic 26.1 : Cathode Rays, Emission of Electron and Photoelectric Effect

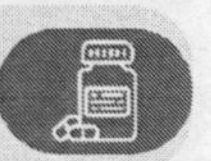

CATHODE RAYS

Discharge Tube Experiments

When a very strong potential difference is applied across the two electrodes in a discharge tube and the pressure of the air is lowered gradually, then a stage is reached at which the current begins to flow through the air with cracking noise. The potential at which this happens is called **sparking potential.**

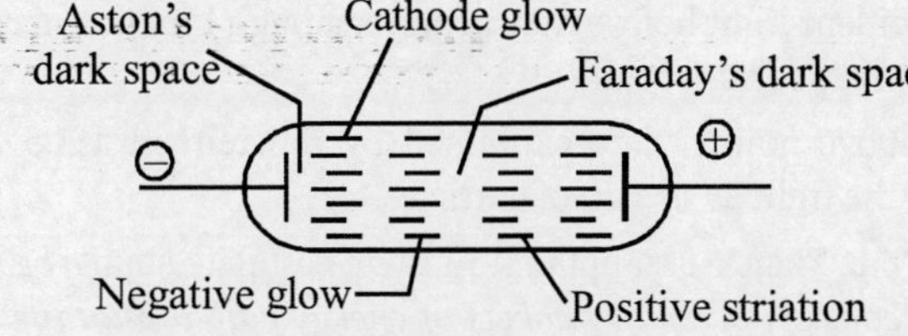

- As pressure is lowered to 0.1 m.m. Hg – cathode glow, Crooke's dark space, negative glow, Faraday's dark space and striations are observed.
- At a pressure 0.01 m.m. Hg entire tube is dark (Crooke's dark space) except the glass wall behind anode. Colour is yellowish-green for soda glass and greyish-blue for lead glass.
- The luminous streaks travelling from cathode to anode, below the pressure 0.01 m.m. Hg, are called **cathode rays.**

Properties of Cathode Ray :

(i) Emitted perpendicularly to cathode, (ii) Travel in straight lines (iii) Carry energy (iv) Possesses momentum (v) Deflected by electric and magnetic fields (vi) Excite fluroescence (vii) Ionise gas (viii) Produce highly penetrating secondary radiation when suddenly stopped (ix) Effect photographic plate etc.

J.J. Thomson's e/m value of electron :

$e/m = \dfrac{E^2}{2VB^2} = 1.76 \times 10^{11}\ C\ kg^{-1}$. This value of $\left(\dfrac{e}{m}\right)$ is for electron.

Millikan's oil drop method for e/ m :

In fig.(a) we consider a single drop of mass m carrying a negative charge –q in the absence of electric field. Then

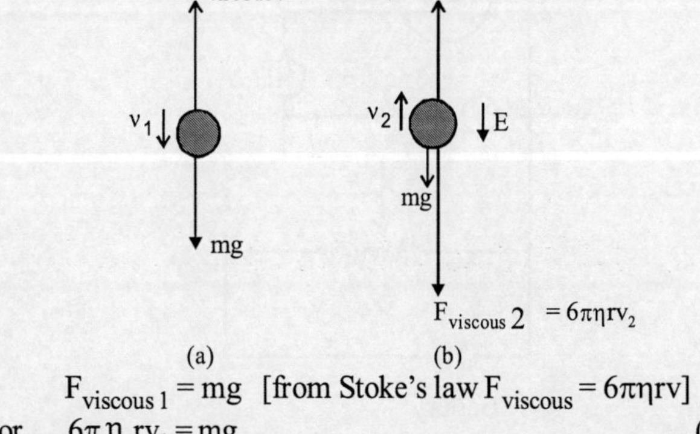

$F_{viscous\,1} = mg$ [from Stoke's law $F_{viscous} = 6\pi\eta rv$]

or $6\pi\eta\, rv_1 = mg$ ...(1)

where η is coefficient of viscocity of air, r is radius of drop and v_1 is the terminal velocity of drop.

In fig. (b) we consider a single drop of mass m, radius r carrying a negative charge –q in the presence of electric field acting downward. Then by free body diagram (fig. (b)), we get

$$(-q)E = mg + F_{viscous\,2} = mg + 6\pi\eta rv_2 \quad ...(2)$$

where v_2 is the terminal speed in this case. Then from eqn (1), we have.

$$(-q) = \frac{6\pi\eta r(v_1 + v_2)}{E} \quad ...(3)$$

and radius of drop from equation (1)

$$6\pi\eta rv_1 = mg = \frac{4}{3}\pi r^3 \rho g \text{ or } r = \sqrt{\frac{9\eta v_1}{2\rho g}} \quad ...(4)$$

where ρ is density of drop.

Millikan repeated these measurements on thousands of drops and he found that the charge q calculated for each drop was some integral multiple of an elementary charge e. ($e = 1.6 \times 10^{-19}$C).

Hence, $q = ne,\ n = 0, \pm1, \pm2$ ...(5)

This experiment gives the evidence of **quantisation of charge**.

EMISSION OF ELECTRON

Electrons from the metal surface are emitted by anyone of the following physical processes :

(i) **Thermionic emission :** The emission of electrons by suitably heating the metal surface.

(ii) **Field emission :** The emission of electrons by applying very strong field of the order of 10^8 Vm^{-1} to a metal.

(iii) **Photo-electric emission :** The emission of electrons when light of suitable frequency illuminates metal surface.

PHOTOELECTRIC EFFECT (EINSTEIN'S PHOTOELECTRIC EQUATION

In 19th century, experiments showed that *when light is incident on certain metallic surfaces, electrons are emitted from the surfaces. This phenomenon is known as the* ***photoelectric effect*** *& emitted electrons are called* ***photoelectrons.*** The first discovery of this phenomenon was made by Hertz.

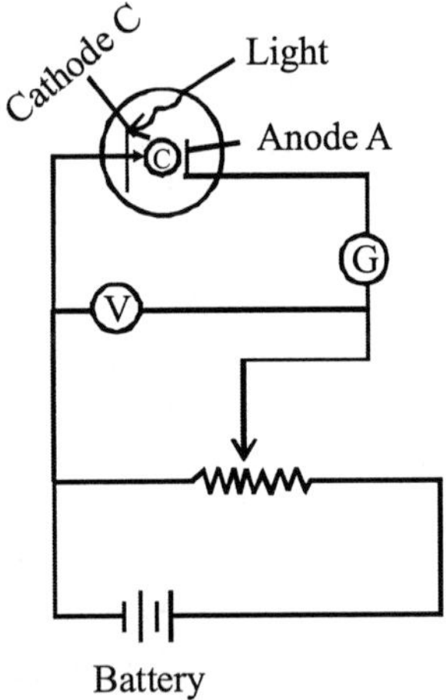

When light strikes the cathode C (metallic surface), photo electrons are ejected. Electrons are collected at anode A, constituting a current in the circuit. (Photoelectric effect)

Fig. shows, when light strikes the cathode C, electrons are emitted & they are collected on anode A due to potential difference provided by battery and constitutes the current in the circuit (observed by Galvanometer G.)

A plot of photoelecric current versus the potential difference V between cathode & anode is shown in fig below.

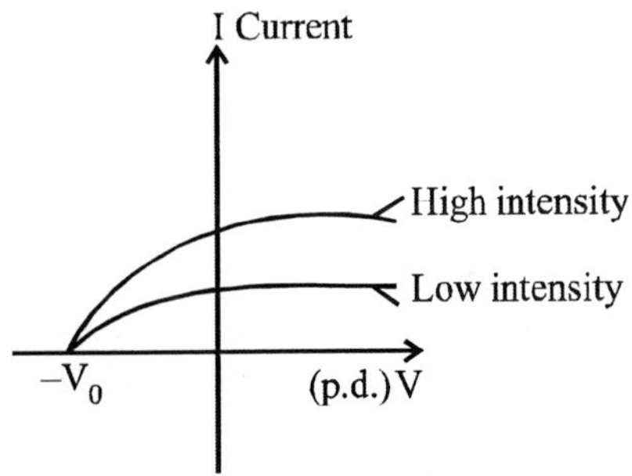

Photoelectric current versus voltage for two light intensities. At a voltage less than $-V_0$ the current is zero.

It is clear from fig. that photoelectric current increases as we increase the intensity of light & obtain saturation value at larger value of potential difference V between cathode & anode. If V is negative then, photoelectrons are repelled by negative cathode and only those electrons reaches anode, who have energy equal to or greater than eV. But if V is equal to V_0, called **stopping potential** (i.e., cut off. potential), no electrons will reach the anode

i.e., Maximum kinetic energy of electron = eV_0

or $$K_{max} = eV_0 \qquad ...(1)$$

where *e* is charge of electron ($e = 1.6 \times 10^{-19}$ coulomb).

But some features of photoelectric effect cannot be explained by classical physics & the wave theory of light.

(1) No photoelectrons are emitted, if the frequency of incident light is less than some **cut-off frequency** (i.e., **threshold frequency**) ν_0. It is inconsistent with the wave theory of light, which predicts that photoelectric effect occurs at any frequency provided intensity of incident light is sufficiently high.

(2) The maximum kinetic energy of the photoelectrons is independent of light intensiy, but increases with increasing the frequency of incident light.

(3) Electrons are emitted from surface almost instantaneously (less than 10^{-9} sec after the surface illumination), even at low intensity of incident light(classicaly we assume that the electrons would require some time to absorb the incident light before they acquire enough kinetic energy to escape from metal).

These above points were explained by Einstein in 1905 by treating the light as stream of particles.

Taking Max Planck assumptions, Einstein postulated that *a beam of light consists of small packets of energy called* ***photons or quanta.*** The energy E of a photon is equal to a constant h times its frequency ν

i.e., $$E = h\nu = \frac{hc}{\lambda} \qquad ...(2)$$

where h is a universal constant called **Planck's constant** & numerical value of $h = 6.62607 \times 10^{-34}$ J.s

When a photon arrives at surface, it is absorbed by an electron. This energy transfer is an **All-or-None process**, in contrast to continuous transfer of energy in classical theory; the electrons get all photon's energy or none at all. If this energy is greater than the **work function (ϕ)** of the metal (*ϕ is the minimum energy required to remove the electron from metal surface*), the electron may escape from the surface. Greater intensity at a particular frequency means greater number of photons per second absorbed & consequently greater number of electrons emitted per second & so greater current.

To obtain maximum kinetic energy $K_{max} = \frac{1}{2}mv_{max}^2$

for an emitted electron, applying law of conservation of energy.

According to it

$$K_{max} = \frac{1}{2}mv_{max}^2 = h\nu - \phi \quad [\phi = h\nu_0]$$

$$K_{max} = h(\nu - \nu_0) \qquad ...(3)$$

or $$eV_0 = K_{max} = h(\nu - \nu_0) \qquad ...(4)$$

or, $$\frac{1}{2}mv_{max}^2 = h(\nu - \nu_0) = hc\left(\frac{1}{\lambda} - \frac{1}{\lambda_0}\right) = ev_s$$

This is the **Einstein's photoelectric equation.**

where V_0 = cut-off potential

v_{max} = maximum velocity obtained by photoelectrons

ν = frequency of incident light i.e., photon

ν_0 = cut off frequency or threshold frequency.

ν_0 is different for different metallic surfaces. For most metals the threshold frequency is in ultarviolet region of spectrum. (Corresponding to λ between 200 & 300 nm), but for potassium & cesium oxides, it is in the visible spectrum (λ between 400 & 700 nm).

Work Function (ϕ) of Some Elements Given in Brackets :

Al	(4.3eV)	Ni	(5.1 eV)
C	(5.0 eV)	Si	(4.8 eV)
Cu	(4.7 eV)	Ag	(4.3 eV)
Au	(5.1eV)	Na	(2.7 eV)

where 1 eV = 1.602×10^{-19} joule.

Within the framework of **photon theory of light** (Quantum theory of light) we can explain above failures of classical physics.

(1) It is clear from eq. (3) that if energy of photon is less than the work function of metallic surface, the electrons will never be ejected from the surface regardless of intensity of incident light.

(2) K_{max} is independent of intensity of incident light, but it depends on the frequency of incident light i.e., $K_{max} \propto \nu$ (frequency of light).

(3) Electrons are emitted almost instantaneously consistent with particle view of light in which incident energy is concentrated in small packets (called photons) rather than over a large area (as in wave theory).

Various Graphs Related to Photoelectric Effect

1. Photocurrent versus intensity of light graph

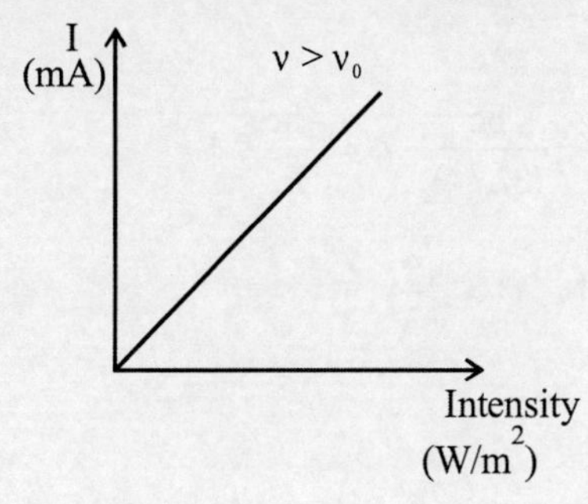

2. Photocurrent versus potential graph

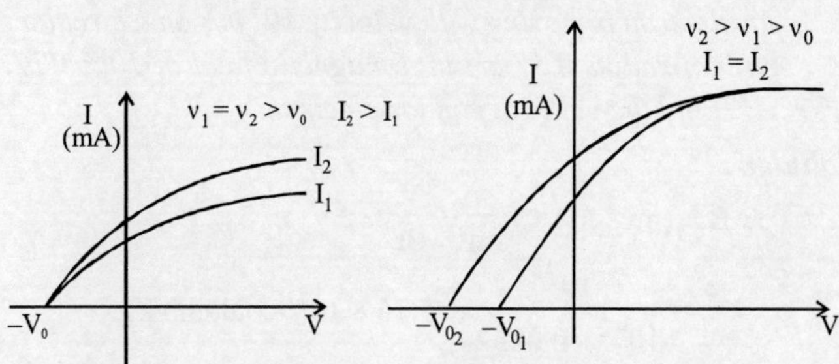

3. Maximum kinetic energy versus potential graph.

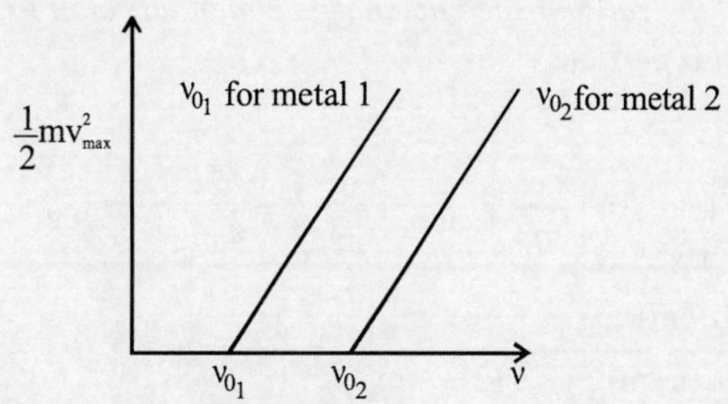

Problem Solving Tips

1. **Mass spectrograph** is an appratus used to determine the mass or the specific charge (e/m) of positive ions. Examples are (a) Thomson mass spectrograph (b) Bain bridge mass spectrograph (c) Aston mass spectrograph (d) Dempster mass spectrograph etc.

2. In photoelectric effect all photoelectrons do not have same kinetic energy. Their KE ranges from zero to E_{max} which depends on frequency of incident radiation and nature of cathode.

3. The photoelectric effect takes place only when photons strike bound electrons because for free electrons energy and momentum conservations do not hold together.

4. Cesium is the best photo sensitive material.

5. Efficiency of photoemission,

$$\eta = \frac{\textit{Number of photoelectrons emitted per unit area per unit time}}{\textit{Number of photons incident per unit area per unit time}} = \frac{n_e}{n_p}$$

$$\eta = \frac{\textit{Intensity of emitted electrons}}{\textit{Intensity of incident radiation}} = \frac{I_e}{I_p}$$

Therefore, $\eta = \frac{n_e}{n_p} = \frac{I_e}{I_p}$

6. Maximum velocity of emitted electrons

$$v_{max} = \sqrt{\frac{2h(\nu - \nu_0)}{m}} = \sqrt{\frac{2hc(\lambda_0 - \lambda)}{m\lambda\lambda_0}} = \sqrt{\frac{2ev_s}{m}}$$

7. Stopping potential

$$V_s = \frac{h(\nu - \nu_0)}{e} = \frac{hc(\lambda - \lambda_0)}{e\lambda\lambda_0}$$

Example 1.

An electron is moving with velocity 10^7 m/s on a circular path of radius 0.57 cm in a magnetic field of 10^{-2} Wb/m^2. Find the value of e/m for electron.

Solution :

$$evB = (mv^2/r) \text{ or } \frac{e}{m} = \frac{v}{Br}$$

$$\therefore \frac{e}{m} = \frac{10^7}{10^{-2} \times 0.0057} = 1.76 \times 10^{11} \text{ coulomb/kg.}$$

Example 2.

Find the ratio of specific charge e/m of a proton to that of an α particle.

Solution :

$$\left(\frac{e}{m}\right)_{proton} = \left(\frac{e}{m_p}\right) \text{ and } \left(\frac{e}{m}\right)_{\alpha} = \frac{2e}{4m_p}$$

$$\therefore \frac{(e/m)_{proton}}{(e/m)_{\alpha}} = \frac{(e/m_p)}{(2e/4m_p)} = \frac{2}{1} \text{ or } 2:1$$

Example 3.

The work function of cesium is 1.8 eV. Light of 5000 Å is incident on it. Calculate (a) threshold frequency and threshold wavelength. (b) maximum K.E. of emitted electrons. (c) maximum velocity of emitted electrons (d) if the intensity of the incident light be doubled, then what will be the maximum K.E. of the emitted electrons? (h = 6.6 × 10^{-34} joule second, mass of electron m = 9.0×10^{-31} kg and speed of light c = 3 x 10^8 m/s).

Solution :

(a) $W_0 = h\nu_0$ or $\nu_0 = h/W_0$

$$W_0 = 1.8 \times (1.6 \times 10^{-19}) = 2.9 \times 10^{-19} \text{ joule}$$

$$\therefore \nu_0 = \frac{W_0}{h} = \frac{2.9 \times 10^{-19} \text{ joule}}{6.6 \times 10^{-34} \text{ joule second}}$$

$\therefore$ Threshold frequency = 4.4 × 10^{14} sec^{-1}

Threshold wavelength

$$\lambda_0 = \frac{c}{\nu_0} = \frac{3.0 \times 10^8 \text{ m/s}}{4.4 \times 10^{14} \text{ s}^{-1}}$$

$$= 6.8 \times 10^{-7} \text{ metre} = 6800 \text{ Å}$$

(b) $E_k = h\nu - W_0 = \frac{hc}{\lambda} - W_0$

$$= \frac{(6.63 \times 10^{-34})(3 \times 10^8)}{5000 \times 10^{-10}} - (2.9 \times 10^{-19} \text{ joule})$$

$$= (4.0 - 2.9) \times 10^{-19} = 1.1 \times 10^{-19} \text{ joule.}$$

(c) $E_k = \frac{1}{2} m v_{max}^2$

$$\therefore v_{max} = \sqrt{\left(\frac{2E_k}{m}\right)} = \sqrt{\left[\frac{2 \times (1.1 \times 10^{-19})}{9.0 \times 10^{-31}}\right]}$$

$$= 5.0 \times 10^5 \text{ m/sec.}$$

(d) The K.E. of emitted electrons does not depend upon the intensity of light. Hence if the intensity of incident light be doubled, the energy will remain unchanged.

Example 4.

Calculate the energy and momentum of a photon of wavelength 6600Å.

Solution :

Energy of photon

$$E = \frac{hc}{\lambda} = \frac{6.62 \times 10^{-34} \times 3 \times 10^8}{6600 \times 10^{-10}} = 3 \times 10^{-19} \text{ J}$$

Momentum of photon

$$p = \frac{h}{\lambda} = \frac{6.6 \times 10^{-34}}{6600 \times 10^{-10}} = 10^{-27} \text{ kg m/sec}$$

Example 5.

Find the number of photons emitted per second by a 25 watt source of monochromatic light of wavelength 6000Å.

Solution :

Energy of one photon

$$E = h\nu = \frac{hc}{\lambda} = \frac{6.62 \times 10^{-34} \times 3 \times 10^8}{6000 \times 10^{-10}} = 3.315 \times 10^{-19} \text{ J}$$

No. of photons emitted per second

$$= \frac{\text{Total energy emitted per second}}{\text{Energy of the photon}} = \frac{P}{E}$$

$$= \frac{25}{3.315} \times 10^{-19} = 7.54 \times 10^{19}$$

Example 6.

In a photoelectric experiment, with light of wavelength λ, the fastest electron has speed v. If the exciting wavelength is changed to 3λ/4, then find the speed of the fastest emitted electron.

Solution :

$$\frac{1}{2} mv^2 = \frac{hc}{\lambda} - \phi$$

$$\frac{1}{2} m' = \frac{hc}{(3\lambda/4)} - \phi = \frac{4hc}{3\lambda} - \phi$$

Clearly, $v' > \sqrt{\frac{4}{3}} v$

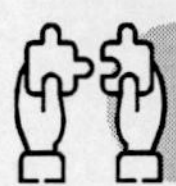

26.1 Concept Practice Problems

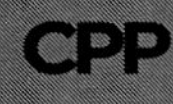

1. Einstein's work on photoelectric effect provided support for the equation
(a) E = hν (b) $E = mc^2$
(c) $E = \frac{-Rhc}{n^2}$ (d) $K.E. = \frac{1}{2}mv^2$

2. In which of the following, emission of electrons does not take place?
(a) Thermionic emission (b) X-rays emission
(c) Photoelectric emission (d) Secondary emission

3. The maximum velocity of an electron emitted by light of wavelength λ incident on the surface of a metal of work-function φ is
(a) $\sqrt{\frac{2(hc + \lambda\phi)}{m\lambda}}$ (b) $\frac{2(hc + \lambda\phi)}{m\lambda}$
(c) $\sqrt{\frac{2(hc - \lambda\phi)}{m\lambda}}$ (d) $\sqrt{\frac{2(h\lambda - \phi)}{m}}$

4. Photoelectric effect is the phenomenon in which
(a) photons come out of a metal when it is hit by a beam of electrons.
(b) photons come out of the nucleus of an atom under the action of an electric field.
(c) electrons come out of a metal with a constant velocity which depends on the frequency and intensity of incident light wave.
(d) electons come out of a metal with different velocities not greater than a certain value which depends only on the frequency of the incident light wave and not on its intensity.

5. The momentum of a photon of wavelength λ is
(a) hλ (b) h/λ (c) λ/h (d) h/cλ

6. A photo sensitive metal is not emitting photo-electrons when irradiated. It will do so when threshold is crossed. To cross the threshold we need to increase
(a) intensity (b) frequency
(c) wavelength (d) None of these

7. As intensity of incident light increases
(a) photoelectric current increase
(b) K.E. of emitted photoelectron increases
(c) photoelectric current decreases
(d) K.E. of emitted photoelectrons decreases

8. Einstein's photoelectric equation is $E_k = h\nu - \phi$. In this equation E_k refers to
(a) kinetic energy of all the emitted electrons
(b) mean kinetic energy of emitted electrons
(c) maximum kinetic energy of emitted electrons
(d) minimum kinetic energy of emitted electrons

9. Which of the following when falls on a metal will emit photoelectrons ?
(a) UV radiations (b) Infrared radiation
(c) Radio waves (d) Microwaves

10. Light of frequency ν falls on a material of threshold frequency ν_0. Maximum kinetic energy of emitted electron is proportional to
(a) $\nu - \nu_0$ (b) ν (c) $\sqrt{\nu - \nu_0}$ (d) ν_0

ANSWER KEY

1	(a)	2	(b)	3	(c)	4	(d)	5	(b)	6	(b)	7	(a)	8	(c)	9	(a)	10	(a)

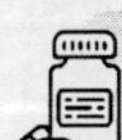

Topic 26.2 : de-Broglie Equation, Davisson-Germer Experiment and X-rays

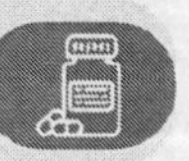

de-BROGLIE EQUATION (DUAL NATURE OF MATTER)

In 1924, Louis de Broglie, wrote a doctoral dissertation in which he proposed that since photons have wave and particle characterstics, perhaps all forms of matter have wave as well as particle properties.

This is called **dual nature of matter.** According to which A matter particle moving with a velocity v can be treated as a wave of wavelength λ. This λ is called de-Broglie wavelength & it is defined as :

$$\lambda = \frac{h}{P} = \frac{h}{mv} \quad ...(1)$$

where m is the mass of matter particle & these waves are called matter waves.

Further with the analogy of photon, the frequency of matter waves is

$$\nu = \frac{E}{h} \quad ...(2)$$

The **dual nature of matter** is quite apparent in these two equations (equations (1) & (2)). i.e., each equation contains both particle concepts (mv & E) & wave concepts (λ & ν). It is clear from next topic that Compton effect confirm the validity of p = h/λ for photons, and the photoelectric effect confirms the validity and E = hν for photons.

de-Broglie wavelength associated with electron accelerated under a potential difference V volt is given by $\lambda = \frac{12.27}{\sqrt{V}} Å$

de-Broglie wave is not an electromagnetic wave but the matter wave.

Wavelength of matter waves associated with accelerated charged particles :

If V is the accelerating voltage applied then :

(a) For the **charged particle** :

Energy $E = qV$;

Velocity $v = \sqrt{\frac{2qV}{m}} = \sqrt{\frac{2E}{m}}$

Momentum $p = \sqrt{2mE} = \sqrt{2mqV}$;

Wavelength $\lambda = \frac{h}{\sqrt{2mqV}} = \frac{h}{\sqrt{2mE}}$

(b) For **electron** $\lambda_e = \frac{12.27}{\sqrt{V}}$ Å

(c) For **proton** $\lambda_p = \frac{0.286}{\sqrt{V}}$ Å

(d) For **alpha particle** $\lambda_\alpha = \frac{0.101}{\sqrt{V}}$ Å

(e) For **deuteron** $\lambda_d = \frac{0.202}{\sqrt{V}}$ Å

For neutral particles (neutron, atom or molecule) :

(a) If E is the energy of the particle, then, $\frac{h}{p} = \frac{h}{\sqrt{2mE}}$

(b) If T is the temperature, then, $\lambda = \frac{h}{\sqrt{3mkT}}$

DAVISSON-GERMER EXPERIMENT

Idea of de-Broglie wave was tested beautifully in 1926 in an experiment performed by C. Davission (1881-1958) and L.H. Jermer (1896-1971). They directed a beam of electrons at a crystal and observed that the electrons scattered in various directions for a given crystal orientation.

In this experiment the pattern formed by the electrons reflected from the crystal lattice of aluminium is almost identical to that produced by X-rays. This strongly suggests that the electrons have a wavelength λ associated with them and that the **Bragg condition for X-ray diffraction** holds true for electron also :

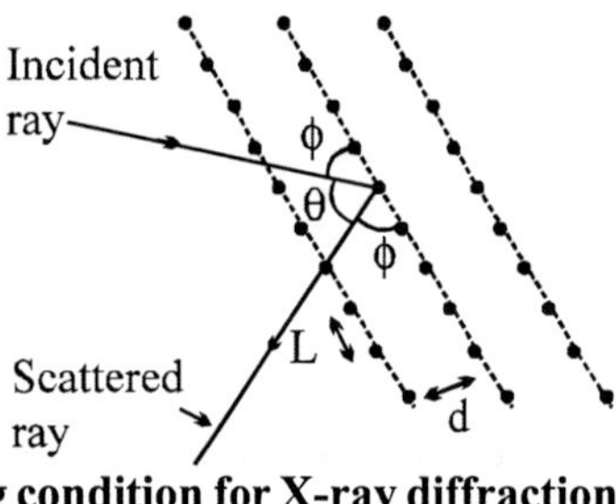

Bragg's equation

$n\lambda = D \sin\theta$ or $n\lambda = 2d \sin\phi$.

Diffraction maximum of electrons accelerated with 54 volt is obtained at $\theta = 50°$ for the Nickel crystal.

Explanation of Bohr's quantum condition :

(a) According to Bohr's quantum conditions :

Angular momentum, $mvr_n = n\frac{h}{2\pi}$

(b) Matter waves associated with the electrons moving in an orbit are stationary waves.

(c) For the production of stationary waves in the orbit the circumference of the orbit should be integral multiple of wavelength of waves associated with the electron,

i.e., $2\pi r_n = n\lambda$, where $\lambda = \frac{h}{mv}$

$\therefore\ mvr_n = \frac{nh}{2\pi}$

Compton Effect

Further experimental proof for photon concept(i.e., particle nature of light) was discovered in 1923 by American Physicist, A.H. Compton. According to which, when a monochromatic beam of X-rays (wavelength λ_0) strikes the electron in a carbon target, two types of X-rays are scattered. The first type of scattered wave has same wavelength (λ_0) as the incoming X-rays, while second type has a longer wavelength (λ) than incident rays (First type of X-rays are called unmodified x-rays, while second type of X-rays are called modified X-rays.) This change in wavelength i.e. $\Delta\lambda = \lambda - \lambda_0$ is called **Compton shift** & this effect is called **Compton effect"**.

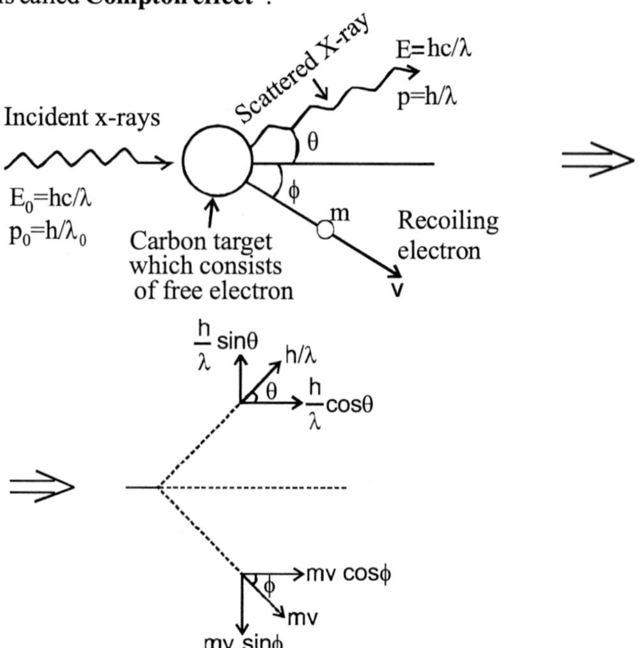

Diagram shows compton scattering of an x-rays by free electron in a carbon target. The scattered x-rays has less energy than the incident x-rays. The excess energy is taken by recoiling electrons.

This effect cannot be explained by classical theory (by wave nature of light). According to classical model, when X-rays of frequency ν_0 is incident on the material containing electrons, then electrons do oscillate & reradiate electromagnetic waves of same frequency ν_0. Hence scattered X-rays has same frequency ν_0 & same wavelength as that of incident X-rays.

Compton treated this processes as a collision between a photon & an electron. In this treatment, the photon is assumed as a particle of energy

$$E = h\nu_0 = hc/\lambda_0 \qquad ...(1)$$

Further, the rest mass of photon is zero (because photon travels with the speed of light) hence the momentum of photon can be written as

$$p = \frac{E}{c} = \frac{hc}{c\lambda} = \frac{h}{\lambda} \qquad ...(2)$$

To dervie the compton shift. $\Delta\lambda$, we apply both conservation of energy & momentum.

Conservation of energy :

$$\frac{hc}{\lambda_0} = \frac{hc}{\lambda} + K_e \quad ...(3)$$

Where hc/λ is energy of scattered X-rays, K_e is kinetic energy of recoling electron & hc/λ_0 is the energy of incoming X-rays. Since the electron may travel with the speed of light, so we must use relativistic expression of K_e in equation (3), and we obtain

$$\frac{hc}{\lambda_0} = \frac{hc}{\lambda} + \gamma\, mc^2 - mc^2 \quad ...(4)$$

where m is rest mass of electron and mc^2 is the rest mass energy of the electron

where $\gamma = \frac{1}{\sqrt{1 - v^2/c^2}}$

Conservation of momentum :

$$\frac{h}{\lambda_0} = \frac{h}{\lambda}\cos\theta + \gamma mv\cos\phi \quad \text{x - component} \quad ...(5)$$

$$0 = \frac{h}{\lambda}\sin\theta - \gamma mv\sin\phi \quad \text{y - component} \quad ...(6)$$

where $p_e = \gamma mv$ is the relativistic expression for momentum of recoiling electron.

By eliminating v & ϕ from equation (4) to (6), we obtain

$$\Delta\lambda = \lambda - \lambda_0 = \frac{h}{mc}(1 - \cos\theta) \quad ...(7)$$

$$\text{or } \Delta\lambda = 0.0243(1 - \cos\theta)\text{Å} \quad ...(8)$$

It is clear from expression (7) that compton shift $\Delta\lambda$ depends on scattering angle θ & not on the wavelength.

Problem Solving Tips

1. The wave nature of light shows up in the phenomena of interference, diffraction and polarisation whereas photoelectric effect and compton effect shows particle nature of light.
2. The maximum kinetic energy of the photoelectrons varies linearly with the frequency of incident radiation but is independent of its intensity.

X-RAYS

- The X-rays were discvoered by Prof. Roentgen, a German scientist in 1885. He was awarded Nobel Prize for this discovery in 1901. X-rays are electromagnetic waves.
- The modern apparatus for the production of X-rays was developed by Dr. Coolidge in 1913.
- X-rays are produced when fast moving electrons are suddenly stopped on a metal of high atomic number.

Properties of X-rays

(i) They are not deflected by electric or magnetic field.
(ii) They travel with the speed of light.
(iii) There is no charge on X-rays.
(iv) X-rays show both particle and wave nature.
(v) They are invisible.

Continuous and Characteristic X-rays

Experimental observation and studies of spectra of X-rays reveal that X-rays are of two types and so are their respective spectras. Characteristic X-rays and Continuous X-rays.

Characteristic X-rays: The spectra of this group consists of several radiations with specific sharp wavelengths and frequency similar to the spectrum (line) of atoms like hydrogen. The wavelengths of this group show characteristic discrete radiations emitted by the atoms of the target material. The characteristic X-rays spectra helps us to identify the element of target material. When the atoms of the target material are bombard with high energy electrons (or hard X-rays), which posses enough energy to penetrate into the atom, knock out the electron of inner shell (say K shell, n = 1). When an electron is missing in the 'K' shell, an electron from next upper shell makes a quantum jump to fill the vacancy in 'K' shell. In the transition process the electron radiates energy whose frequency lies in the X-rays region. The frequency of emitted radiation (i.e. of photon) is given by

$\nu = RZ_e^2\left(\frac{1}{n_1^2} - \frac{1}{n_2^2}\right)$; where R is constant and Z_e is effective atomic number. Generally Z_e is taken to be equal to $Z - \sigma$, where Z is proton number or atomic number of the element and σ is called the screening constant. Due to the presence of the other electrons. The charge of the nucleus as seen by the electron will be different in different shells.

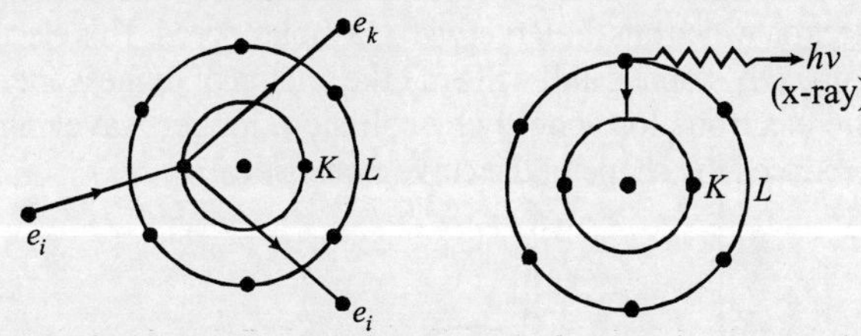

Knocking out e^- of K shell by incident electron e_i emission of X-ray photon (K_α- series)

Another vacancy is now created in the 'L' shell which is again filled up by another electron jump from one of the upper shell (M) which results in the emission of another photon, but of different X-rays frequency. This transition continues till outer shells are reached. Thus resulting in the emission of series of spectral line.

The transitions of electrons from various outer shells to the inner most 'K' shell produces a group of X-rays lines called as K-series. These radiations are most energetic and most penetrating. K-series is further divided into $K_\alpha, K_\beta, K_\gamma$ .... depending upon the outer shell from which the transition is made.

The jump of electrons from outer shells to 'L' shell results in L-Series X-rays

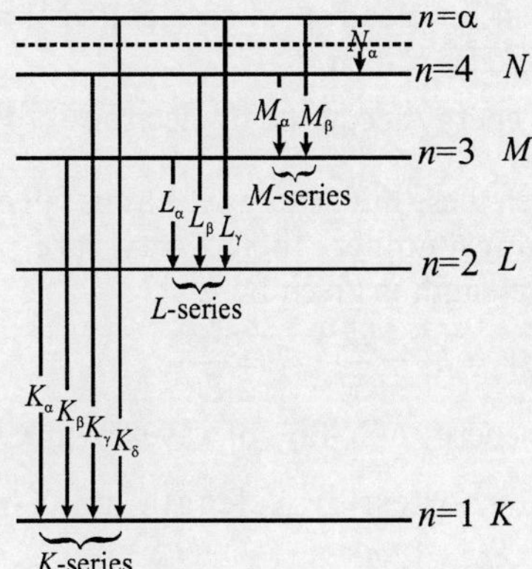

and so on.

Continuous X-rays : In addition to characteristic X-rays tubes emit a continuous spectrum also. The characteristic line spectra is superimposed on a continuous X-rays spectra of varying intensities. The wavelength of the continuous X-rays spectra are independent of material. One important feature of continuous X-rays is that they end abruptly at a certain lower wavelength for a given voltage. If an electron beam of energy eV (electron volts) is incident on the target material; the electrons are suddenly stopped. If the whole of the energy is converted to continuous radiation, then λ_{min} (corresponding to energy maximum) = hc/Ve where V is the voltage applied.

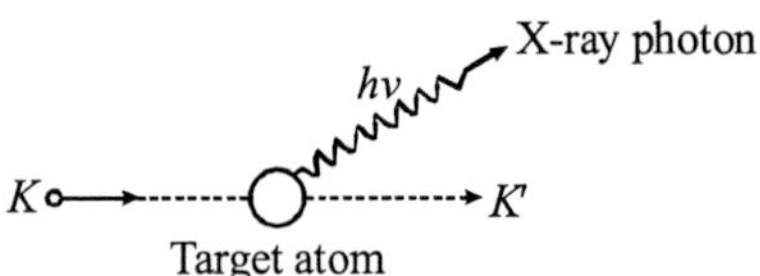

The classical theory of electromagnetism states that the suddenly accelerated or decelerated electrons emit radiations of electromagnetic nature called as bremsstrahlung **(braking radiation)** and wavelength of such radiation is continuous because the loss in energy is statistical. At the peak, the probability of maximum number of electrons producing radiation. The wavelength of X-rays emitted is minimum corresponding to the electron which hits the target with maximum speed. This electron is completely stopped and will emit the photon of highest energy. As the electrons lose energy by collision, longer wavelengths are produced the shape of the curve is statistical.

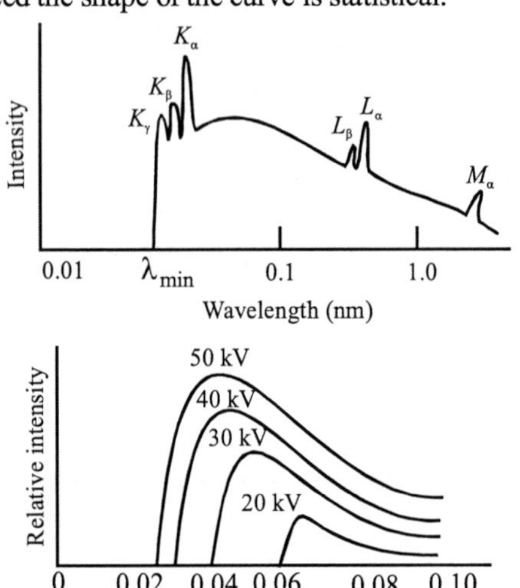

Wavelength of X-Rays (Daume Hunt Law)

(i) When an electron is accelerated through a potential difference V then
the energy accquired by electron $= eV = \frac{1}{2}mv^2$.

(ii) When these high energy electrons fall on target T of high atomic number, then X-rays are produced, whose wavelength is given by
$\therefore\ eV = h\nu = \frac{hc}{\lambda}$; $\lambda = \frac{hc}{eV}$.

(iii) The energy of X-rays of wavelength λ is $E = h\nu = \frac{hc}{\lambda}$

(iv) The shortest wavelength of X-rays emitted is $\lambda = \frac{hc}{eV} = \frac{1240}{V} nm$ i.e. $\lambda \propto \frac{1}{V}$.

It is called **Daume Hunt law.**

Types of X-Rays

1. **Hard X- rays :** *The X-rays of high frequency or low wavelength are said to be hard X-rays.* They have higher penetrating power.
2. **Soft X-rays :** *The X-rays of longer wavelength are called soft X-rays.*

Moseley's Law

Moseley used different elements as target in the X-ray tube. He found that K_α radiation of different elements were different

Mathematically, $\sqrt{\nu} = a(Z - b)$

where a and b depend on the particular line of the radiation

For Kα, $a = \sqrt{\frac{3}{4}Rc}$ and $b = 1$

where R = Rydberg constant and c = speed of light

In general the wavelength of K - lines are given as

$$\frac{1}{\lambda} = R(Z-1)^2\left[1 - \frac{1}{n^2}\right] \text{ where } n = 2, 3, ...$$

Absorption of X-rays

- X-rays are absorbed by the materials according to the relation $I = I_0\, e^{-\mu x}$, where μ is absorption coefficient and x is the thickness of the mateiral. Here I is the intensity after penetrating the material through distance x and I_0 is the initial intensity of the X-rays.
- The coefficient of absorption (μ) of the material is given by $\mu = \frac{0.6931}{x_{1/2}}$ where $x_{1/2}$ is the distance after traversing which the intensity of X-rays is reduced to half.
- Absorption coefficient depends on the nature of material and wavelength of X-rays i.e. $\mu = cZ^4\lambda^3$.
  It means that (a) $\mu \propto z^4$ (b) $\mu \propto \lambda^3$ (c) $\mu \propto \nu^{-3}$.

Fluorescence : Certain substances (like quinine sulphate, fluoricine, barium platinocyanide, uranium oxide etc.), when illuminated with light of high frequency (ultraviolet, violet, etc.) emit light of lower frequency. The phenomenon is called fluorescence.

- When quinine sulphate is illuminated with ultraviolet or violet light it gives out blue light. The fluroescence of barium sulphate as well as uranium oxide gives out green light when illuminated with ultraviolet or violet light.
- The house hold tubes are painted from inside with magnesium tungstate or zinc-beryllium silicate. They are fluorescent materials. The ultraviolet light generated inside the tube falls on the walls, where magnesium tungstate gives blue light and zinc beryllium silicate gives yellow orange light. The mixture of the two produces white light. If the inner side of the tube is painted with cadmium borate it gives fluorescence of pink light and when painted with zinc silicate, it gives fluorescence of green light.
- The fluorescence occurs as long as the material is illuminated.

Phosphorescence : Fluorescent materials emit light only so long as light is incident on them. There are certain susbstances which continue emitting light for some time after the light incident on them is stopped. This phenomenon is called phosphorescence. For example, if we make blue light incident on a zinc-sulphide (ZnS) screen, then it produces phosphorescence of green colour.

Calcium sulpide and barium sulphide, after absorbing sunlight, produce blue phosphorescence for some time. Time of phosphorescence is different for different materials.

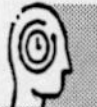

Problem Solving Tips

1. The stopping potential (and hence the maximum kinetic energy of emitted electrons) is independent of the intensity of light but that the saturation current (and hence the number of emitted photoelectrons) is proportional to the intensity.
2. Photoelctric effect doesn't take place below the threshold frequency for the photometal used.
3. In compton effect, the change in wavelength is independent of incident photon as well as of the nature of the scatterer, but depends only on the angle of scattering (θ).
4. The quantity $\frac{h}{mc}$ (= 0.02426Å) is called Compton wavelength.
5. The maximum wavelength change possible in compton effect is 0.05Å.
6. Compton effect can't be observed for visible light rays.
7. In compton effect, the direction of recoil electron is given by $\tan\phi = \frac{\lambda\sin\theta}{\lambda' - \lambda\cos\theta}$.
8. The kinetic energy of recoil electron is given by $T = h\nu\left[\frac{x(1-\cos\theta)}{1+x(1-\cos\theta)}\right]$, where $x = \frac{h\nu}{mc^2}$
9. de-Broglie wavelength of a particle of K.E., E_k is given by $\lambda = \frac{h}{\sqrt{2mE_k}}$.
10. de-Broglie wavelength for a charged particle with charge q and accelerated through a potental difference V is given by $\lambda = \frac{h}{\sqrt{2mqV}}$.
11. de-Broglie wavelength of a material particle at temperature T is given by
$\lambda = \frac{h}{\sqrt{2mkT}}$, where k is Boltzmann's constant.

Application of X-rays

Following are some important and useful applications of X-rays.

1. **Scientific applications:** The diffraction of X-rays at crystals opened new dimension to X-rays crystallography. Various diffraction patterns are used to determine internal structure of crystals. The spacing and dispositions of atoms of a crystal can be precisely determined by using Bragg's law : $n\lambda = 2d\sin\theta$.
2. **Industrial applications:** Since X-rays can penetrate through various materials, they are used in industry to detect defects in metallic structures in big machines, railway tracks and bridges. X-rays are used to analyse the composition of alloys and pearls.
3. **In radio therapy:** X-rays can cause damage to the tissues of body (cells are ionized and molecules are broken). So X-rays damages the malignant growths like cancer and tumors which are dangerous to life, when is used in proper and controlled intensities.
4. **In medicine and surgery:** X-rays are absorbed more in heavy elements than the lighter ones. Since bones (containing calcium and phosphorus) absorb more X-rays than the surrounding tissues (containing light elements like H, C, O), their shadow is casted on the photographic plate. So the cracks or fracture in bones can be easily located. Similarly intestine and digestive system abnormalities are also detected by X-rays.

Example 7.

Determine the ratio of momentum of an electron and an alpha particle which are accelerated from rest by a potential difference of 100 V.

Solution :

$$\because \frac{1}{2}mv^2 = eV \text{ or } v = (2eV/m)^{1/2}$$

$$\therefore p = mv = (2meV)^{1/2}$$

Now $p_e = (2m_e \times e \times 100)^{1/2}$ and $p_\alpha = (4m_\alpha \times e \times 100)^{1/2}$

$$\therefore p_e / p_\alpha = \sqrt{(m_e / 2m_\alpha)}$$

Example 8.

What will be the ratio of the de-Broglie wavelength of proton and α particle of same energy?

Solution :

$$\lambda = \frac{h}{mv} = \frac{h}{\sqrt{2mE}}$$

$$\therefore E = \frac{1}{2}mv^2 \text{ or } 2mE = m^2v^2 \text{ or } mv = \sqrt{2mE}$$

$$\text{so, } \frac{\lambda_p}{\lambda\alpha} = \sqrt{\left(\frac{m_\alpha}{m_p}\right)} = \sqrt{\frac{4}{1}} = 2 \text{ or } \lambda_p : \lambda_\alpha = 2:1$$

Example 9.

What is the de-Broglie wavelength associated with (a) an electron moving with a speed of 5.4×10^6 m/s, and (b) a ball of mass 150 g travelling at 30.0 m/s?

Solution :

(a) For the electron

Mass $m = 9.11 \times 10^{-31}$ kg, speed $v = 5.4 \times 10^6$ m/s.

Then, momentum $p = mv$

$= 9.11 \times 10^{-31}$ (kg) $\times 5.4 \times 10^6$ (m/s)

$p = 4.92 \times 10^{-24}$ kg m/s

de-Broglie wavelength, $\lambda = h/p = \frac{6.63' \, 10^{-34} \text{Js}}{4.92' \, 10^{-24} \text{kg m/s}}$

$= 0.135$ nm

(b) For the ball: Mass m' = 0.150 kg,

Speed v' = 30.0 m/s.

Then momentum $p' = m'v'$

$= 0.150$ (kg) $\times 30.0$ (m/s)

$p' = 4.50$ kg m/s

de Broglie wavelength $\lambda' = h/p'$

$$= \frac{6.63' \, 10^{-34} \text{Js}}{4.50 \text{ kg m/s}} = 1.47 \times 10^{-34} \text{ m}$$

The de-Broglie wavelength of electron is comparable with X-ray wavelengths. However, for the ball it is about 10^{-19} times the size of the proton, quite beyond experimental measurement.

Example 10.

What is the de Broglie wavelength associated with an electron, accelerated through a potential difference of 100 volt?

Solution :

Accelerating potential V = 100 V. The de Broglie wavelength,

$$1 = \frac{h}{p} = \frac{1.227}{\sqrt{V}} \text{nm}$$

$$1 = \frac{1.227}{\sqrt{100}} \text{nm} = 0.123\text{nm}$$

The de-Broglie wavelength associated with an electron in this case is of the order of X-ray wavelengths.

Example 11.

If the K_α radiation of Mo (Z = 42) has a wavelength of 0.71 Å, calculate wavelength of the corresponding radiation of Cu, i.e., K_α for Cu (Z = 29) assuming σ = 1.

Solution :

According to Moseley's law : $\sqrt{v} = a(Z-1)$

$\Rightarrow \ (Z-1)^2 \propto v \qquad$ or $\qquad (Z-1)^2 \propto 1/\lambda$

$$\Rightarrow \frac{(Z_{M0}-1)^2}{(Z_{Cu}-1)^2} = \frac{\lambda_{Cu}}{\lambda_{Mo}}$$

$$\Rightarrow \lambda_{Cu} = \lambda_{Mo}\frac{(Z_{M0}-1)^2}{(Z_{Cu}-1)^2} = 0.71\times\left(\frac{41}{28}\right)^2 \text{Å} = 1.52\text{Å}$$

Example 12.

The wavelength of K_α x-rays of two metals 'A' and 'B' are $\frac{4}{1875R}$ and $\frac{1}{675R}$ respectively, where 'R' is Rydberg constant. Find the number of elements lying between A and B according to their atomic numbers.

Solution :

Using $\qquad \frac{1}{\lambda} = R(Z-1)^2\left[\frac{1}{n_2^2} - \frac{1}{n_1^2}\right]$

For α particle, $n_1 = 2$, $n_2 = 1$

For metal A : $\frac{1875\ R}{4} = R\ (Z_1-1)^2\left(\frac{3}{4}\right) \Rightarrow Z_1 = 26$

For metal B : $675\ R = R\ (Z_2-1)^2\left(\frac{3}{4}\right) \Rightarrow Z_2 = 31$

Therefore, 4 elements lie between A and B.

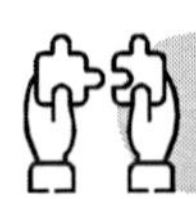

26.2 Concept Practice Problems

CPP

11. A particle with rest mass m_0 is moving with speed of light c. The de-Broglie wavelength associated with it will be

(a) $m_0 ch$ (b) zero (c) $m_0 c/h$ (d) $h\nu/m_0 c$

12. If E_1, E_2, E_3 are the respective kinetic energies of an electron, an alpha-particle and a proton, each having the same de-Broglie wavelength, then

(a) $E_1 > E_3 > E_2$ (b) $E_2 > E_3 > E_1$
(c) $E_1 > E_2 > E_3$ (d) $E_1 = E_2 = E_3$

13. In Davison-Germer experiment, an electron beam is incident on a crystal. The reflected beam consists of

(a) photons (b) protons (c) x-rays (d) electrons

14. For an electron accelerated from rest through a potential V, the de Broglie wavelength associated will be

(a) $\frac{1.772}{\sqrt{V}}$ nm (b) $\frac{1.227}{\sqrt{V}}$ μm

(c) $\frac{1.227}{\sqrt{V}}$ nm (d) $\frac{1.772}{\sqrt{V}}$ μm

15. X-rays are produced in X-ray tube operating at a given accelerating voltage. The wavelength of the continuous X-rays has values from

(a) 0 to ∞
(b) λ_{min} to ∞, where $\lambda_{min} > 0$
(c) 0 to λ_{max}, where $\lambda_{max} < \infty$
(d) λ_{min} to λ_{max}, where $0 < \lambda_{min} < \lambda_{max} < \infty$

16. The ratio of de-Broglie wavelengths of proton and α-particle having same kinetic energy is

(a) $\sqrt{2}:1$ (b) $2\sqrt{2}:1$ (c) $2:1$ (d) $4:1$

17. White X-rays are called white due to the fact that

(a) they are electromagnetic radiations having nature same as that of white light.
(b) they are produced most abundantly in X ray tubes.
(c) they have a continuous wavelength range.
(d) they can be converted to visible light using coated screens and photographic plates are affected by them just like light.

18. In case of electrons and photons having the same wavelength. What is same for them?

(a) Energy (b) Velocity
(c) Momentum (d) Angular momentum

19. In the Davisson and Germer experiment, the velocity of electrons emitted from the electron gun can be increased by

(a) increasing the potential difference between the anode and filament
(b) increasing the filament current
(c) decreasing the filament current
(d) decreasing the potential difference between the anode and filament

20. A proton and α-particle are accelerated through the same potential difference. The ratio of their de-Broglie wavelength will be

(a) $1:1$ (b) $1:2$ (c) $2:1$ (d) $2\sqrt{2}:1$

ANSWER KEY

11	(b)	12	(a)	13	(d)	14	(c)	15	(b)	16	(c)	17	(c)	18	(c)	19	(a)	20	(d)

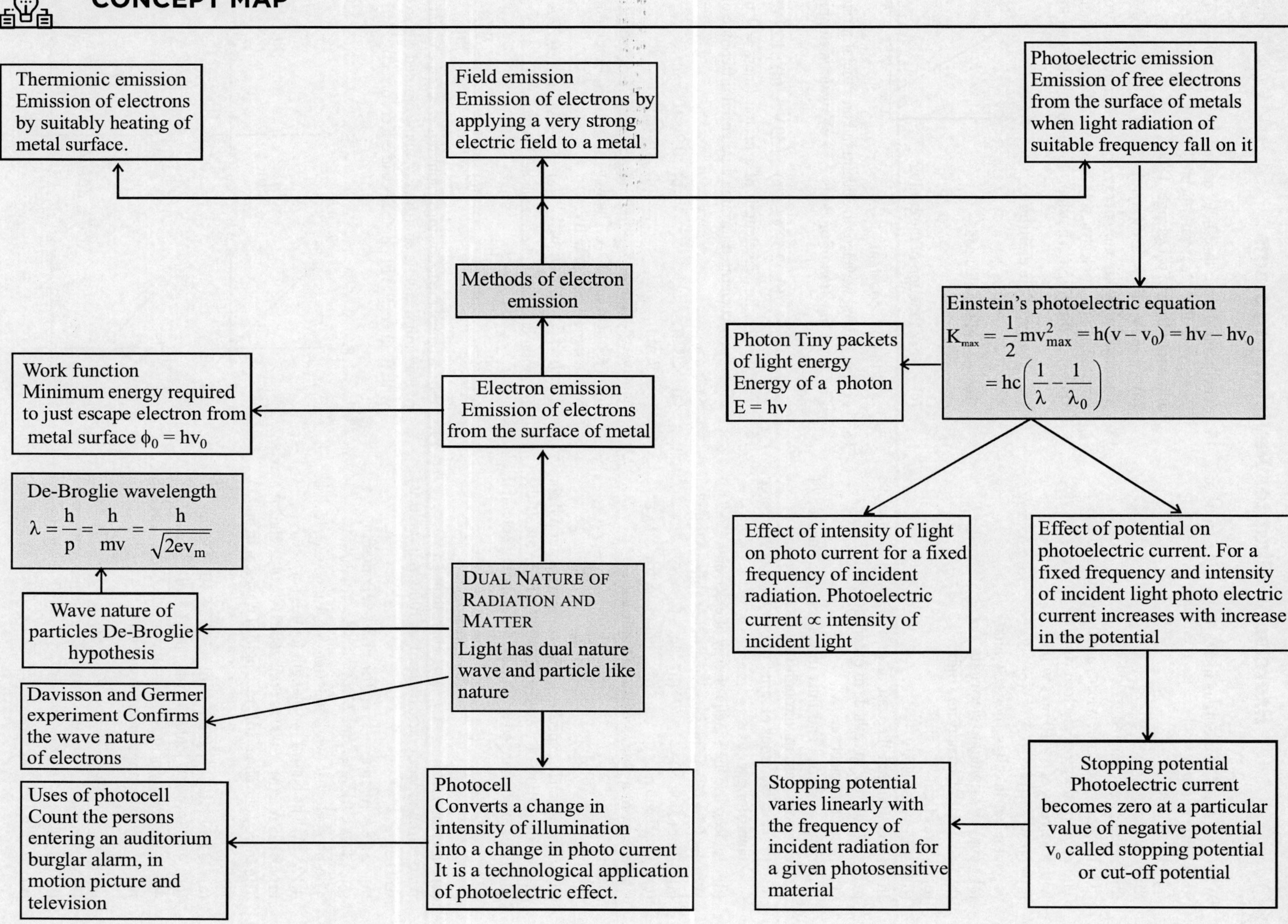
CONCEPT MAP
Thermionic emission Emission of electrons by suitably heating of metal surface.
Field emission Emission of electrons by applying a very strong electric field to a metal
Photoelectric emission Emission of free electrons from the surface of metals when light radiation of suitable frequency fall on it
Methods of electron emission
Einstein's photoelectric equation $K_{max} = \frac{1}{2}mv_{max}^2 = h(v - v_0) = hv - hv_0$ $= hc\left(\frac{1}{\lambda} - \frac{1}{\lambda_0}\right)$
Photon Tiny packets of light energy Energy of a photon E = hv
Work function Minimum energy required to just escape electron from metal surface $\phi_0 = hv_0$
Electron emission Emission of electrons from the surface of metal
De-Broglie wavelength $\lambda = \frac{h}{p} = \frac{h}{mv} = \frac{h}{\sqrt{2ev_m}}$
Effect of intensity of light on photo current for a fixed frequency of incident radiation. Photoelectric current ∝ intensity of incident light
Effect of potential on photoelectric current. For a fixed frequency and intensity of incident light photo electric current increases with increase in the potential
DUAL NATURE OF RADIATION AND MATTER Light has dual nature wave and particle like nature
Wave nature of particles De-Broglie hypothesis
Davisson and Germer experiment Confirms the wave nature of electrons
Uses of photocell Count the persons entering an auditorium burglar alarm, in motion picture and television
Photocell Converts a change in intensity of illumination into a change in photo current It is a technological application of photoelectric effect.
Stopping potential varies linearly with the frequency of incident radiation for a given photosensitive material
Stopping potential Photoelectric current becomes zero at a particular value of negative potential v_0 called stopping potential or cut-off potential

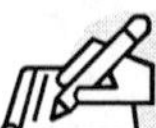

Exercise 1 - Chapter Revision Problems

CRP

1. When the speed of electrons increase, then the value of its specific charge
   (a) increases
   (b) decreases
   (c) ramains unchanged
   (d) increases upto some velocity and then begins to decrease
2. The kinetic energy of electron (in electron volt) moving with a velocity of 4×10^6 m/s will be
   (a) 60 eV (b) 50 eV (c) 30 eV (d) 45.5 eV
3. A photoelectric cell is a device which
   (a) converts light into electricity
   (b) converts electricity into light
   (c) stores light
   (d) stores electricity
4. In an electron gun the control grid is given a negative potential relative to cathode in order to
   (a) decelerate electrons
   (b) repel electrons and thus to control the number of electrons passing through it
   (c) to select electrons of same velocity and to converge them along the axis.
   (d) to decrease the kinetic energy of electrons
5. Which of the following shows par.ticle nature of light?
   (a) Refraction (b) Interference
   (c) Polarization (d) Photoelectric effect
6. The energy of a photon of wavelength λ is
   (a) $hc\lambda$ (b) $\frac{hc}{\lambda}$ (c) $\frac{\lambda}{hc}$ (d) $\frac{\lambda h}{c}$
7. In a photoelectric experiment the stopping potential for the incident light of wavelength 4000Å is 2 volt. If the wavelength be changed to 3000 Å, the stopping potential will be
   (a) 2V (b) zero
   (c) less than 2 V (d) more than 2 V
8. An electron is accelerated by a p.d. of 1000 V. Its velocity will be
   (a) 3.78×10^7 m/s (b) 1.89×10^7 m/s
   (c) 5.67×10^7 m/s (d) 0.95×10^7 m/s
9. The photoelectric work function for a metal surface is 4.125 eV. The cut-off wavelength for this surface is
   (a) 4125 Å (b) 3000 Å (c) 6000 Å (d) 2062 Å
10. The energy of a photon of green light of wavelength 5000Å is
   (a) 3.459×10^{-19} joule (b) 3.973×10^{-19} joule
   (c) 4.132×10^{-19} joule (d) 8453×10^{-19} joule
11. 4eV is the energy of incident photon and the work function is 2eV. The stopping potential will be
   (a) 2V (b) 4V (c) 6V (d) $2\sqrt{2}$V
12. If the energy of a photon is 10 eV, then its momentum is
   (a) 5.33×10^{-23} kg m/s (b) 5.33×10^{-25} kg m/s
   (c) 5.33×10^{-29} kg m/s (d) 5.33×10^{-27} kg m/s
13. The photoelectric threshold of Tungsten is 2300Å. The energy of the electrons ejected from the surface by ultraviolet light of wavelength 1800Å is
   (a) 0.15 eV (b) 1.5 eV (c) 15 eV (d) 150 eV
14. The maximum kinetic energy (E_{max}) of photoelectrons emitted in a photoelectric cell varies with frequency (ν) as shown in the graph. The slope of the graph is equal to
   (a) charge of the electron
   (b) $\frac{e}{m}$ of the electron
   (c) work function of the emitter
   (d) Plank's constant

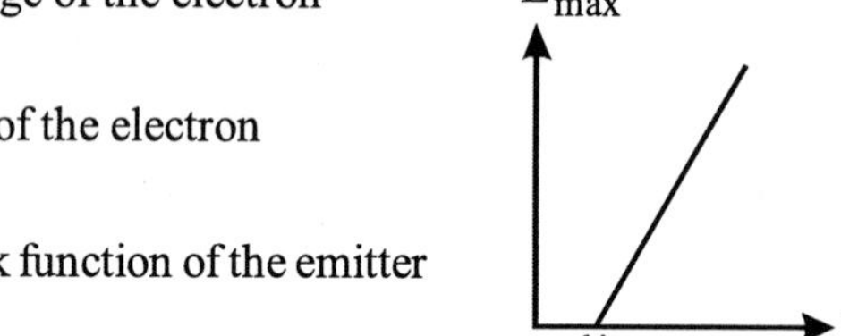

15. A light having wavelength 300 nm fall on a metal surface. The work function of metal is 2.54 eV, what is stopping potential ?
   (a) 2.3 V (b) 2.59 V (c) 1.59 V (d) 1.29 V
16. The de-Broglie wavelength of a proton (mass = 1.6×10^{-27} kg) accelerated through a potential difference of 1 kV is
   (a) 600 A (b) 0.9×10^{-12}m
   (c) 7 Å (d) 0.9 nm.
17. The wavelength of K_α-line characteristic X-rays emitted by an element is 0.32 Å. The wavelength of K_β-line emitted by the same element will be
   (a) 0.32 Å (b) 0.39 Å (c) 0.49 Å (d) 0.27 Å
18. The momentum of photon whose frequency f is
   (a) $\frac{hf}{c}$ (b) $\frac{hc}{f}$ (c) $\frac{h}{f}$ (d) $\frac{c}{hf}$
19. Which one of the following graphs represents the variation of maximum kinetic energy (E_K) of the emitted electrons with frequency υ in photoelectric effect correctly ?

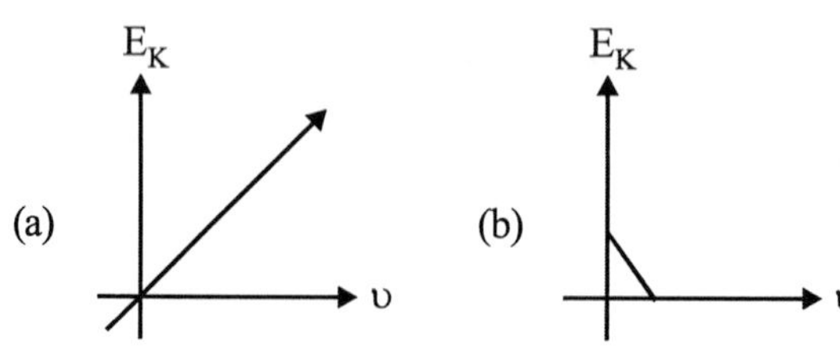

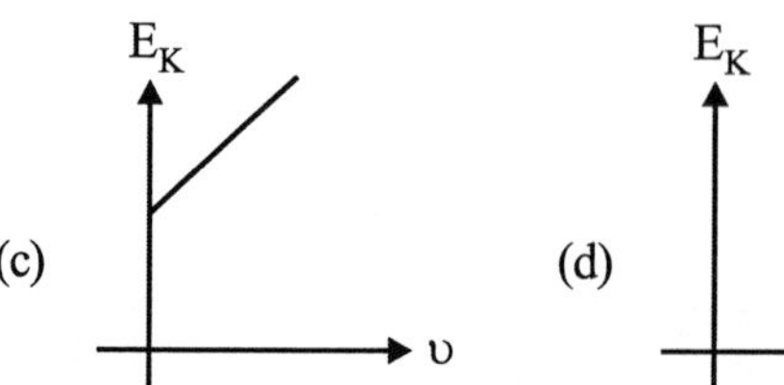

20. A steel ball of mass m is moving with a kinetic energy K. The de-Broglie wavelength associated with the ball is

(a) $\frac{h}{2mK}$ (b) $\sqrt{\frac{h}{2mK}}$

(c) $\frac{h}{\sqrt{2mK}}$ (d) meaningless

21. If the X-ray tube is working at 20 kV then the minimum wavelength of X-rays will be

(a) 0.31 Å (b) 0.62 Å (c) 0.93 Å (d) 0.47 Å

22. In an electron gun, the potential difference between the filament and plate is 3000 V. What will be the velocity of electron emitting from the gun?

(a) 3×10^8 m/s (b) 3.18×10^7 m/s

(c) 3.52×10^7 m/s (d) 3.26×10^7 m/s

23. What is the energy of k_α X-ray photon of copper (Z = 29) ?

(a) 7.99 keV (b) 8.29 keV (c) 8.25 keV (d) 7.19 keV

24. The de-Broglie wavelength of a neutron at 927°C is λ. What will be its wavelength at 27 °C ?

(a) $\frac{\lambda}{2}$ (b) λ (c) 2λ (d) 4λ

25. A monochromatic source of light operating at 200 W emits 4×10^{20} photons per second. Find the wavelength of light.

(a) 400mm (b) 200nm

(c) 4×10^{-10} Å (d) None of these

26. An X-ray tube is operated at 15 kV. Calculate the upper limit of the speed of the electrons striking the target.

(a) 7.26×10^7 m/s (b) 7.62×10^7 m/s

(c) 7.62×10^7 cm/s (d) 7.26×10^9 m/s

27. The stopping potential (V_0) versus frequency (v) plot of a substance is shown in figure, the threshold wavelength is

(a) 5×10^{14}m

(b) 6000 Å

(c) 5000 Å

(d) Cannot be estimated from given data

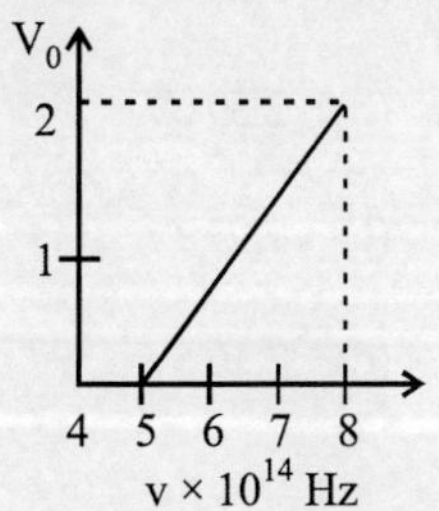

28. A photon of 1.7×10^{-13} joule is absorbed by a material under special circumstances. The correct statement is

(a) Electrons of the atom of absorbed material will go the higher energy states

(b) Electron and positron pair will be created

(c) Only positron will be produced

(d) Photoelectric effect will occur and electron will be produced

29. The glancing angle in a X-ray diffraction is 30° and the wavelength of X-rays used is 20 nm. The interplanar spacing of the crystal dffracting these X-rays will be

(a) 40nm (b) 20nm (c) 15nm (d) 10nm

30. The frequency and work function of an incident photon are v and ϕ_0. If v_0 is the threshold frequency then necessary condition for the emission of photoelectron is

(a) $v < v_0$ (b) $v = \frac{v_0}{2}$

(c) $v \geq v_0$ (d) None of these

31. The work function of aluminium is 4.2 eV. If two photons, each of energy 3.5 eV strike an electron of aluminium, then emission of electrons

(a) will be possible

(b) will not be possible

(c) Data is incomplete

(d) Depends upon the density of the surface

32. For intensity I of a light of wavelenght 5000Å the photoelectron saturation current is 0.40 μA and stopping potential is 1.36 V, the work function of metal is

(a) 2.47 eV (b) 1.36 eV (c) 1.10 eV (d) 0.43 eV

33. Photoelectric emmision occurs only when the incident light has more than a certain minimum

(a) power (b) wavelength

(c) intensity (d) frequency

34. The threshold frequency for a photosensitive metal is 3.3×10^{14} Hz. If light of frequency 8.2×10^{14} Hz is incident on this metal, the cut-off voltage for the photoelectric emission is nearly

(a) 2V (b) 3V (c) 5V (d) 1V

35. Two radiations of photons energies 1 eV and 2.5 eV, successively illuminate a photosensitive metallic surface of work function 0.5 eV. The ratio of the maximum speeds of the emitted electrons is

(a) 1 : 4 (b) 1 : 2 (c) 1 : 1 (d) 1 : 5

36. For a given photosensitive material and frequency (> threshold frequency) of incident radiation, the photoelectric current varies with the intensity of incident light as

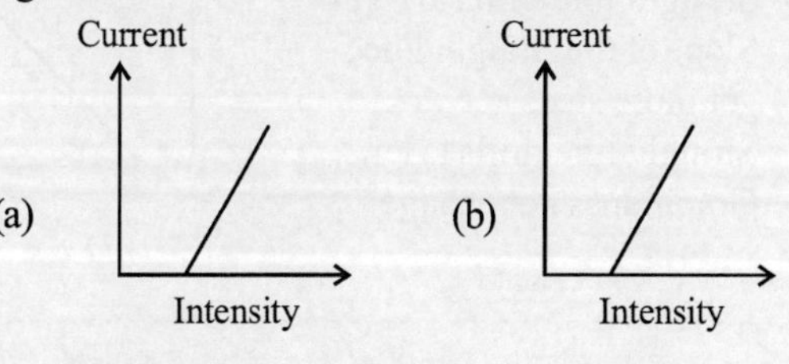

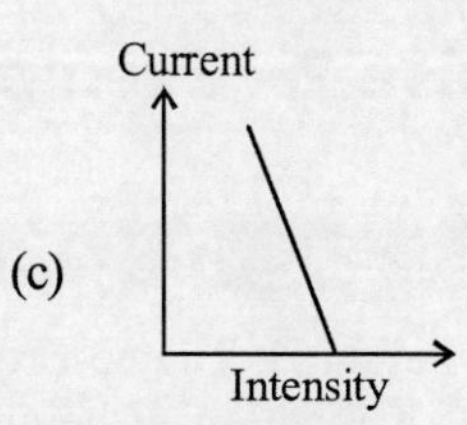

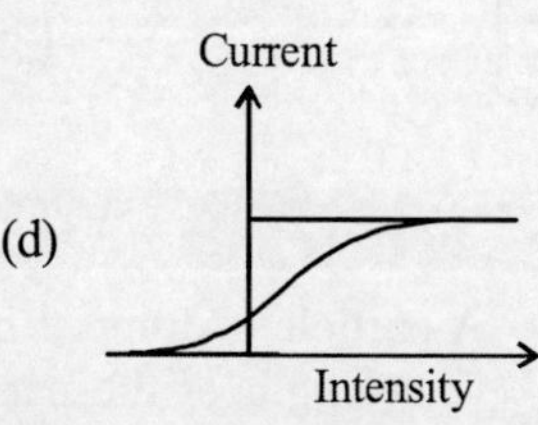

37. The wavelength of a 1 keV photon is 1.24×10^{-9} m. What is the frequency of 1 MeV photon ?

(a) 1.24×10^{15} (b) 2.4×10^{20}

(c) 1.24×10^{18} (d) $2 \times 4 \times 10^{23}$

38. Photoelectric work function of a metal is 1eV. Light of wavelength λ = 3000 Å falls on it. The photo electrons come out with velocity

(a) 10 metres/sec (b) 10^2 metres/sec

(c) 10^4 metres/sec (d) 10^6 metres/sec

39. The quantity $\frac{e^2}{2h\varepsilon_0 c}$ has a value

(a) $\frac{1}{137}\text{ ms}^{-1}$ (b) $\frac{2}{137}\text{ ms}^{-1}$

(c) $\frac{1}{137}$ (d) $\frac{2}{137}$

40. The threshold frequency for photoelectric effect on sodium corresponds to a wavelength of 5000 Å. Its work function is

(a) 4×10^{-19} J (b) 1 J

(c) 2×10^{-19} J (d) 3×10^{-19} J

41. A particle is moving 5 times as fast as an electron. The ratio of the de-Broglie wavelength of the particle to that of the electron is 1.878×10^{-4}. The mass of the particle is close to :

(a) 4.8×10^{-27} kg (b) 9.1×10^{-31} kg

(c) 1.2×10^{-28} kg (d) 9.7×10^{-28} kg

42. A particle moving with kinetic energy E has de Broglie wavelength λ. If energy ΔE is added to its energy, the wavelength become $\frac{\lambda}{2}$. Value of ΔE, is:

(a) E (b) 4E (c) 3E (d) 2E

43. An electron, a doubly ionized helium ion (He^{++}) and a proton are having the same kinetic energy. The relation between their respective de-Broglie wavelengths $\lambda_e, \lambda_{He++}$ and λ_p is :

(a) $\lambda_e > \lambda_{He++} > \lambda_p$ (b) $\lambda_e < \lambda_{He++} = \lambda_p$

(c) $\lambda_e > \lambda_p > \lambda_{He++}$ (d) $\lambda_e < \lambda_p < \lambda_{He++}$

44. In a photoelectric effect experiment, the graph of stopping potential V versus reciprocal of wavelength obtained is shown in the figure. As the intensity of incident radiation is increased :

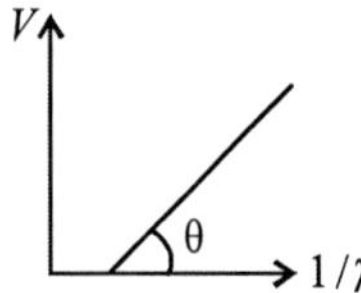

(a) Straight line shifts to right

(b) Slope of the straight line get more steep

(c) Straight line shifts to left

(d) Graph does not change

45. When the wavelength of radiation falling on a metal is changed from 500 nm to 200 nm, the maximum kinetic energy of the photoelectrons becomes three times larger. The work function of the metal is close to :

(a) 0.81 eV (b) 1.02 eV (c) 0.52 eV (d) 0.61 eV

46. In a photoelectric effect experiment the threshold wavelength of light is 380 nm. If the wavelength of incident light is 260 nm, the maximum kinetic energy of emitted electrons will be: Given E (in eV) =

(a) 1.5 eV (b) 3.0 eV (c) 4.5 eV (d) 15.1 eV

47. A 2 mW laser operates at a wavelength of 500 nm. The number of photons that will be emitted per second is : [Given Planck's constant h= 6.6×10^{-34} Js, speed of light $c = 3.0\times10^8$ m/s]

(a) 5×10^{15} (b) 1.5×10^{16}

(c) 2×10^{16} (d) 1×10^{16}

48. In a Frank-Hertz experiment, an electron of energy 5.6 eV passes through mercury vapour and emerges with an energy 0.7 eV. The minimum wavelength of photons emitted by mercury atoms is close to :

(a) 1700 nm (b) 2020 nm (c) 220 nm (d) 250 nm

49. In a photoelectric experiment, the wavelength of the light incident on a metal is changed from 300 nm to 400 nm. The decrease in the stopping potential is close to : $\left(\frac{hc}{e} = 1240\text{ nm-V}\right)$

(a) 0.5 V (b) 1.5 V (c) 1.0 V (d) 2.0 V

50. Given figure shows few data points in a photo electric effect experiment for a certain metal. The minimum energy for ejection of electron from its surface is : (Plancks constant $h = 6.62\times10^{-34}$ J.s)

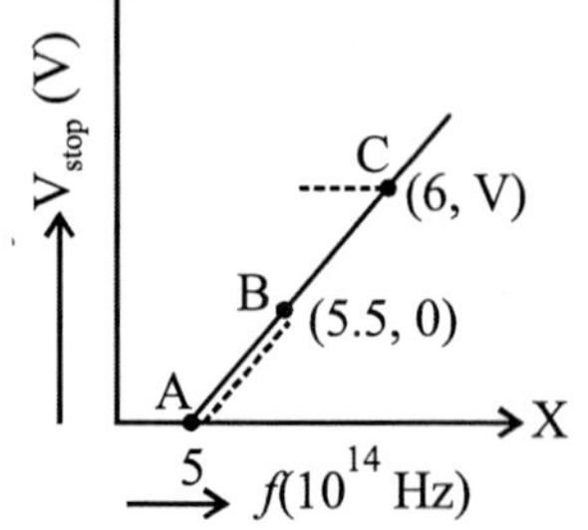

(a) 2.27 eV

(b) 2.59 eV

(c) 1.93 eV

(d) 2.10 eV

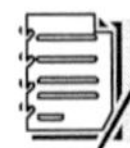

Exercise 2 - Exemplar & Past Year Questions

E&PYQs

Exemplar Questions

1. A particle is dropped from a height H. The de-Broglie wavelength of the particle as a function of height is proportional to

(a) H (b) $H^{1/2}$ (c) H^0 (d) $H^{-1/2}$

2. The wavelength of a photon needed to remove a proton from a nucleus which is bound to the nuclear with 1 MeV energy is nearly

(a) 1.2 nm (b) 1.2×10^{-3} nm

(c) 1.2×10^{-6} nm (d) 1.2×10 nm

3. Consider a beam of electrons (each electron with energy E_0) incident on a metal surface kept in an evacuated chamber. Then,

(a) no electrons will be emitted as only photons can emit electrons

(b) electrons can be emitted but all with an energy, E_0

(c) electrons can be emitted with any energy, with a maximum of $E_0 - \phi$ (ϕ is the work function)

(d) electrons can be emitted with any energy, with a maximum of E_0

4. Consider figure given below. Suppose the voltage applied to A is increased. The diffracted beam will have the maximum at value of θ that
(a) will be larger than the earlier value
(b) will be the same as the earlier value
(c) will be less than the earlier value
(d) will depend on the target

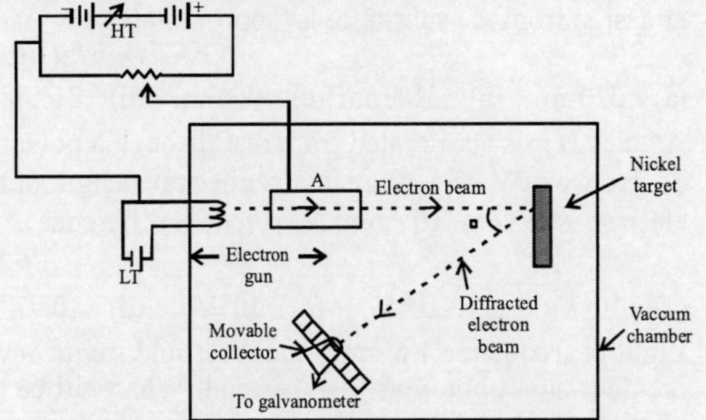

5. A proton, a neutron, an electron and an α-particle have same energy. Then, their de-Broglie wavelengths compare as
(a) $\lambda_p = \lambda_n > \lambda_e > \lambda_\alpha$ (b) $\lambda_\alpha < \lambda_p = \lambda_n > \lambda_e$
(c) $\lambda_e < \lambda_p = \lambda_n > \lambda_\alpha$ (d) $\lambda_e = \lambda_p = \lambda_n = \lambda_\alpha$

6. An electron is moving with an initial velocity $v = v_0 \vec{i}$ and is in a magnetic field $B = B_0 \vec{j}$. Then, it's de-Broglie wavelength
(a) remains constant
(b) increases with time
(c) decreases with me
(d) increases and decreases periodically

7. An electron (mass m) with an initial velocity $v = v_0 i\ (v_0 > 0)$ is in an electric field $E = -E_0\ \hat{i}\ (E_0 = \text{constant} > 0)$. It's de-Broglie wavelength at time t is given by
(a) $\dfrac{\lambda_0}{\left(1+\dfrac{eE_0}{m}\dfrac{t}{v_0}\right)}$ (b) $\left(1+\dfrac{eE_0 t}{mv_0}\right)$
(c) λ_0 (d) $\lambda_0 t$

8. An electron (mass m) with an initial velocity $v = v_0\hat{i}$ is in an electric field $E = E_0\hat{j}$. If $\lambda_0 = h/mv$, it's de-Broglie wavelnegth at time t is given by
(a) λ_0 (b) $\lambda_0\sqrt{1+\dfrac{e^2E_0^2t^2}{m^2v_0^2}}$
(c) $\dfrac{\lambda_0}{\sqrt{1+\dfrac{e^2E_0^2t^2}{m^2v_0^2}}}$ (d) $\dfrac{\lambda_0}{\left(1+\dfrac{e^2E_0^2t^2}{m^2v_0^2}\right)}$

NEET/AIPMT (2013-2020) Questions

9. For photoelectric emission from certain metal the cut-off frequency is ν. If radiation of frequency 2ν impinges on the metal plate, the maximum possible velocity of the emitted electron will be (m is the electron mass) *[2013]*
(a) $\sqrt{h\nu/m}$ (b) $\sqrt{2h\nu/m}$
(c) $2\sqrt{h\nu/m}$ (d) $\sqrt{h\nu/(2m)}$

10. The wavelength λ_e of an electron and λ_p of a photon are of same energy E are related by *[2013]*
(a) $\lambda_p \propto \lambda_e$ (b) $\lambda_p \propto \sqrt{\lambda_e}$
(c) $\lambda_p \propto \dfrac{1}{\sqrt{\lambda_e}}$ (d) $\lambda_p \propto \lambda_e^2$

11. When the energy of the incident radiation is incredased by 20%, the kinetic energy of the photoelectrons emitted from a metal surface increased from 0.5 eV to 0.8 eV. The work function of the metal is : *[2014]*
(a) 0.65 eV (b) 1.0 eV (c) 1.3 eV (d) 1.5 eV

12. If the kinetic energy of the particle is increased to 16 times its previous value, the percentage change in the de-Broglie wavelength of the particle is : *[2014]*
(a) 25 (b) 75 (c) 60 (d) 50

13. Which of the following figures represents the variation of particle momentum and the associated de-Broglie wavelength? *[2015]*

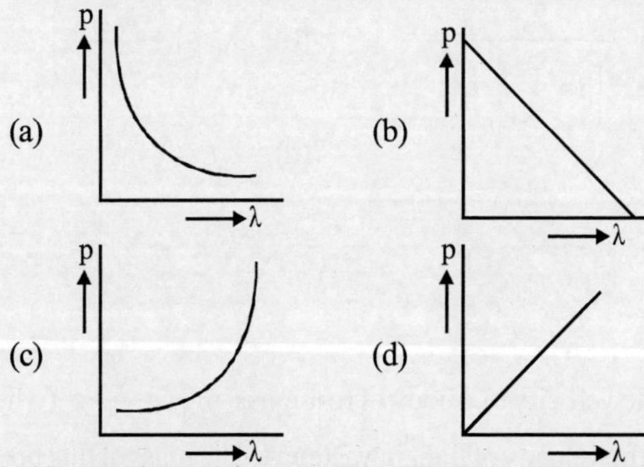

14. A certain metallic surface is illuminated with monochromatic light of wavelength λ. The stopping potential for photo-electric current for this light is $3V_0$. If the same surface is illuminated with light of wavelength 2λ, the stopping potential is V_0. The threshold wavelength for this surface for photo-electric effect is *[2015]*
(a) 4λ (b) $\dfrac{\lambda}{4}$ (c) $\dfrac{\lambda}{6}$ (d) 6λ

15. Light of wavelength 500 nm is incident on a metal with work function 2.28 eV. The de Broglie wavelength of the emitted electron is: *[2015 RS]*
(a) $< 2.8 \times 10^{-9}\ m$ (b) $\geq 2.8 \times 10^{-9}\ m$
(c) $\leq 2.8 \times 10^{-12}\ m$ (d) $< 2.8 \times 10^{-10}\ m$

16. An electron of mass m and a photon have same energy E. The ratio of de-Broglie wavelengths associated with them is : *[2016]*
(a) $\dfrac{1}{c}\left(\dfrac{E}{2m}\right)^{\frac{1}{2}}$ (b) $\left(\dfrac{E}{2m}\right)^{\frac{1}{2}}$
(c) $c(2mE)^{\frac{1}{2}}$ (d) $\dfrac{1}{xc}\left(\dfrac{2m}{E}\right)^{\frac{1}{2}}$

17. When a metallic surface is illuminated with radiation of wavelength λ, the stopping potential is V. If the same surface is illuminated with radiation of wavelength 2λ, the stopping potential is $\dfrac{V}{4}$. The threshold wavelength for the metallic surface is : *[2016]*

(a) 4λ (b) 5λ (c) $\frac{5}{2}\lambda$ (d) 3λ

18. The de-Broglie wavelength of a neutron in thermal equilibrium with heavy water at a temperature T (Kelvin) and mass m, is :- *[2017]*

(a) $\frac{h}{\sqrt{3mkT}}$ (b) $\frac{2h}{\sqrt{3mkT}}$ (c) $\frac{2h}{\sqrt{mkT}}$ (d) $\frac{h}{\sqrt{mkT}}$

19. The photoelectric threshold wavelength of silver is 3250×10^{-10}m. The velocity of the electron ejected from a silver surface by ultraviolet light of wavelength 2536×10^{-10} m is (Given $h = 4.14 \times 10^{-15}$ eVs and $c = 3 \times 10^8$ ms^{-1}) *[2017]*

(a) $\approx 0.6 \times 10^6$ ms^{-1} (b) $\approx 61 \times 10^3$ ms^{-1}
(c) $\approx 0.3 \times 10^6$ ms^{-1} (d) $\approx 6 \times 10^5$ ms^{-1}

20. An electron of mass m with an initial velocity $\vec{V} = V_0\hat{i}$ ($V_0 > 0$) enters an electric field $\vec{E} = -E_0\hat{i}$ (E_0 = constant > 0) at t = 0. If λ_0 is its de-Broglie wavelength initially, then its de-Broglie wavelength at time t is *[2018]*

(a) $\frac{\lambda_0}{\left(1+\frac{eE_0}{mV_0}t\right)}$ (b) $\lambda_0\left(1+\frac{eE_0}{mV_0}t\right)$

(c) λ_0 (d) $\lambda_0 t$

21. An electron is accelerated through a potential difference of 10,000 V. Its de Broglie wavelength is, (nearly): ($m_e = 9$ 10^{-31} kg) *[2019]*

(a) 12.2 10^{-13} m (b) 12.2 10^{-12} m
(c) 12.2 10^{-14} m (d) 12.2 nm

22. The work function of a photosensitive material is 4.0 eV. The longest wavelength of light that can cause photon emission from the substance is (approximately) *[NEET Odisha 2019]*

(a) 310 nm (b) 3100 nm (c) 966 nm (d) 31 nm

23. An electron is accelerated from rest through a potential difference of V volt. If the de Broglie wavelength of the electron is 1.227×10^{-2} nm, the potential difference is : *[2020]*

(a) 10^2 V (b) 10^3 V (c) 10^4 V (d) 10 V

24. Light of frequency 1.5 times the threshold frequency is incident on a photosensitive material. What will be the photoelectric current if the frequency is halved and intensity is doubled? *[2020]*

(a) four times (b) one-fourth
(c) zero (d) doubled

Exercise 3 - Concept Application Problems CAP

1. The velocity of a body of rest mass m_o is $\frac{\sqrt{3}}{2}$c (where c is the velocity of light in vacuum). The mass of this body is:

(a) $\left(\frac{\sqrt{3}}{2}\right)m_o$ (b) $\left(\frac{1}{2}\right)m_o$

(c) $3m_o$ (d) $2m_0$

2. Ultraviolet radiation of 6.2 eV falls on an aluminium surface (workfunction 4.2 eV). The kinetic energy in joule of the faster electron emitted is approximately

(a) 3×10^{-21} (b) 3×10^{-19}
(c) 3×10^{-17} (d) 3×10^{-15}

3. A and B are two metals with threshold frequencies 1.8×10^{14} Hz and 2.2×10^{14} Hz. Two identical photons of energy 0.825 eV each are incident on them. Then photoelectrons are emitted in (Take $h = 6.6 \times 10^{-34}$ Js)

(a) B alone (b) A alone
(c) neither A nor B (d) both A and B.

4. An ionisation chamber, with parallel conducting plates as anode and cathodes has singly charged positive ions per cm^3. The electrons are moving toward the anode with velocity 0.4 m/s. The current density from anode to cathode is X10^4 m A/m^2. The velocity of positive ions moving towards cathode is

(a) 0.1 m/s (b) 0.4 m/s (c) zero (d) 1.6 m/s

5. A parallel beam of light is incident normally on a plane surface absorbing 40% of the light and reflecting the rest. If the incident beam carries 60 watt of power, the force exerted by it on the surface is

(a) 3.2×10^{-8} N (b) 3.2×10^{-7} N
(c) 5.12×10^{-7} N (d) 5.12×10^{-8} N

6. Radiations of two photon's energy, twice and ten times the work function of metal are incident on the metal surface successsively. The ratio of maximum velocities of photoelectrons emitted in two cases is

(a) 1 : 2 (b) 1 : 3 (c) 1 : 4 (d) 1 : 1

7. A photocell is illuminated by a small bright source placed 1 m away. When the same source of light is placed 2 m away, the number of electrons emitted by photocathode are reduced by a factor of

(a) 1/8 (b) 1/16 (c) 1/2 (d) 1/4

8. In a photoelectric effect measurement, the stopping potential for a given metal is found to be V_0 volt when radiation of wavelength λ_0 is used. If radiation of wavelength 2 λ_0 is used with the same metal then the stopping potential (in volt) will be

(a) $\frac{V_0}{2}$ (b) $2V_0$

(c) $V_0 + \frac{hc}{2e\lambda_0}$ (d) $V_0 - \frac{hc}{2e\lambda_0}$

9. An electron of mass m and charge e initially at rest gets accelerated by a constant electric field E. The rate of change of de-Broglie wavelength of this electron at time t ignoring relativistic effects is

(a) $\frac{-h}{eEt^2}$ (b) $\frac{-eht}{E}$ (c) $\frac{-mh}{eEt^2}$ (d) $\frac{-h}{eE}$

10. The X-rays of wavelength 0.5 Å are scattered by a target. What will be the energy of incident X-rays, if these are scattered at an angle of 72° ?

(a) 12.41 keV (b) 6.2 keV (c) 18.6 keV (d) 24.82 keV

11. In a photo-emissive cell with exciting wavelength λ, the fastest electron has speed V. If the exciting wavelength is changed to $3\lambda/4$, the speed of the fastest emitted electron will be :

(a) $v(3/4)^{1/2}$ (b) $v(4/3)^{1/2}$

(c) less the $v(4/3)^{1/2}$ (d) greater than $v(4/3)^{1/2}$

12. A small photocell is placed at a distance of 4 m from a photosensitive surface. When light falls on the surface the current is 5 mA. If the distance of cell is decreased to 1 m, the current will become

(a) 1.25 mA (b) $\left(\frac{5}{16}\right)$ mA (c) 20 mA (d) 80 mA

13. If 5% of the energy supplied to a bulb is radiated as visible light, the number of visible quanta emitted per second by a 100 W bulb, assuming the wavelength of visible light to be 5.6×10^{-5} cm, is

(a) 1.4×10^{19} (b) 1.4×10^{20}

(c) 2×10^{19} (d) 2×10^{20}

14. A material particle with a rest mass m_0 is moving with speed of light c. The de-Broglie wavelength associated is given by

(a) $\frac{h}{m_0 c}$ (b) $\frac{m_0 c}{h}$ (c) zero (d) ∞

15. In a photoelectric effect experiment, for radiation with frequency υ_0 with $h\upsilon_0 = 8$eV, electrons are emitted with energy 2 eV. What is the energy of the electrons emitted for incoming radiation of frequency $1.25\ \upsilon_0$?

(a) 1 eV (b) 3.25 eV (c) 4 eV (d) 9.25 eV.

16. Two insulating plates are both uniformly charged in such a way that the potential difference between them is $V_2 - V_1 = 20$ V. (i.e., plate 2 is at a higher potential). The plates are separated by d = 0.1 m and can be treated as infinitely large. An electron is released from rest on the inner surface of plate 1. What is its speed when it hits plate 2? $(e = 1.6 \times 10^{-19}$ C, $m_e = 9.11 \times 10^{-31}$ kg)

(a) 2.65×10^6 m/s

(b) 7.02×10^{12} m/s

(c) 1.87×10^6 m/s

(d) 32×10^{-19} m/s

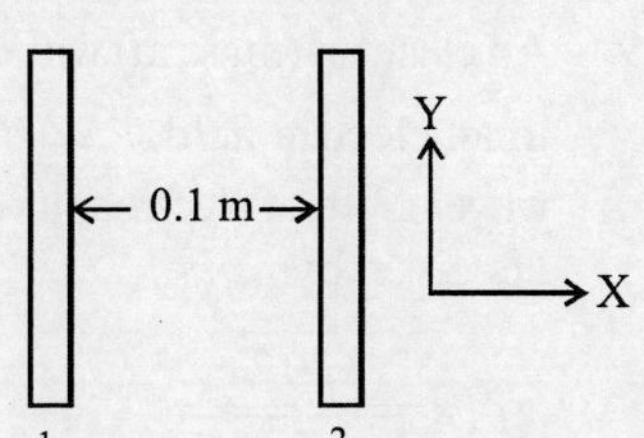

17. Which metal will be suitable for a photoelectric cell using light of wavelength 4000Å. The work functions of sodium and copper are respectively 2.0 eV and 4.0 eV.

(a) Sodium (b) Copper

(c) Both (d) None of these

18. When X-rays of wavelength 0.5 Å would be transmitted by an aluminium tube of thickness 7 mm, its intensity remains one-fourth. The attenuation coefficient of aluminium for these X-rays is

(a) 0.188 mm^{-1} (b) 0.189 mm^{-1}

(c) 0.198 mm^{-1} (d) None of these

19. An X-ray tube with Cu target is operated at 25 kV. The glancing angle for a NaCl. Crystal for the Cu k_α line is 15.8°. Find the wavelength of this line.

(d for NaCl = 2.82 Å, $h = 6.62 \times 10^{-27}$ erg-sec)

(a) 3.06 Å (b) 1.53 Å

(c) 0.75 Å (d) None of these

20. The maximum distance between interatomic lattice planes is 15 Å. The maximum wavelength of X-rays which are diffracted by this crystal will be

(a) 15 Å (b) 20 Å (c) 30 Å (d) 45 Å

21. All electrons ejected from a surface by incident light of wavelength 200nm can be stopped before travelling 1m in the direction of uniform electric field of 4N/C. The work function of the surface is

(a) 4 eV (b) 6.2 eV (c) 2 eV (d) 2.2 eV

22. Light from a hydrogen discharge tube is incident on the cathode of a photoelectric cell, the work function of the cathode surface is 4.2 eV. In order to reduce the photocurrent to zero the voltage of the anode relative to the cathode must be made

(a) −4.2 V (b) −9.4 V (c) −17.8 V (d) +9.4 V

23. A source S_1 is producing, 10^{15} photons per second of wavelength 5000 Å. Another source S_2 is producing 1.02×10^{15} photons per second of wavelength 5100Å Then, (power of S_2) to the (power of S_1) is equal to :

(a) 1.00 (b) 1.02 (c) 1.04 (d) 0.98

24. The potential difference that must be applied to stop the fastest photoelectrons emitted by a nickel surface, having work function 5.01 eV, when ultraviolet light of 200 nm falls on it, must be

(a) 2.4 V (b) −1.2 V (c) −2.4 V (d) 1.2 V

25. In photoelectric emission process from a metal of work function 1.8 eV, the kinetic energy of most energetic electrons is 0.5 eV. The corresponding stopping potential is

(a) 1.8 V (b) 1.2 V (c) 0.5 V (d) 2.3 V

26. If the momentum of electron is changed by P, then the de Broglie wavelength associated with it changes by 0.5%. The initial momentum of electron will be

(a) $200P$ (b) $400P$ (c) $\frac{P}{200}$ (d) $100P$

27. A 200 W sodium street lamp emits yellow light of wavelength 0.6 μm. Assuming it to be 25% efficient in converting electrical energy to light, the number of photons of yellow light it emits per second is

(a) 1.5×10^{20} (b) 6×10^{18} (c) 62×10^{20} (d) 3×10^{19}

28. Monochromatic radiation emitted when electron on hydrogen atom jumps from first excited to the ground state irradiates a photosensitive material. The stopping potential is measured to be 3.57 V. The threshold frequency of the materials is

(a) 4×10^{15} Hz (b) 5×10^{15} Hz
(c) 1.6×10^{15} Hz (d) 2.5×10^{15} Hz

29. The magnitude of the de-Broglie wavelength (λ) of electron (e), proton (p), neutron (n) and α-particle (α) all having the same energy of 1 MeV, in the increasing order will follow the sequence

(a) $\lambda_e, \lambda_p, \lambda_n, \lambda_\alpha$ (b) $\lambda_e, \lambda_n, \lambda_p, \lambda_\alpha$
(c) $\lambda_\alpha, \lambda_n, \lambda_p, \lambda_e$ (d) $\lambda_p, \lambda_e, \lambda_\alpha, \lambda_n$

30. The anode voltage of a photocell is kept fixed. The wavelength λ of the light falling on the cathode is gradually changed. The plate current I of the photocell varies as follows

(a) 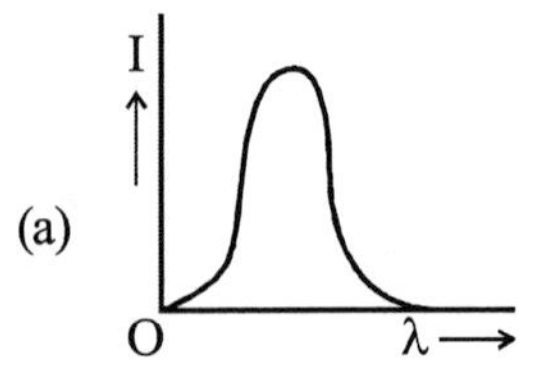

(b) 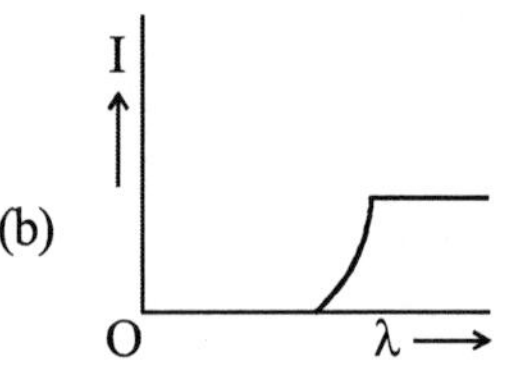

(c) 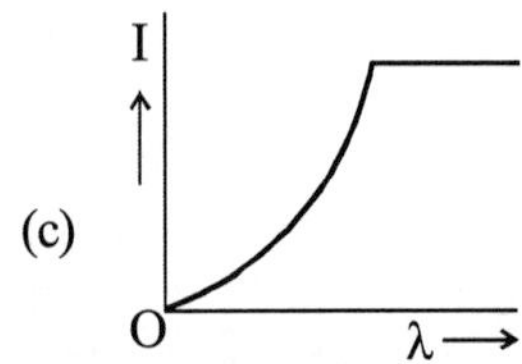

(d) 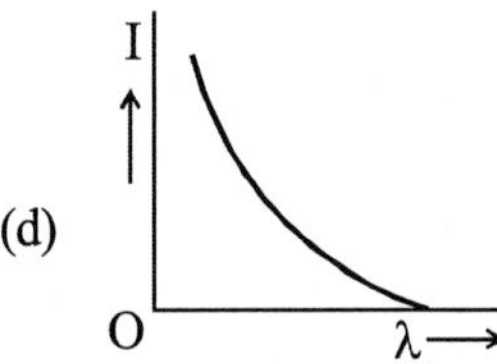

31. Radiations of intensity 0.5 W/m^2 are striking a metal plate. The pressure on the plate is

(a) 0.166×10^{-8} N/m^2 (b) 0.332×10^{-8} N/m^2
(c) 0.111×10^{-8} N/m^2 (d) 0.083×10^{-8} N/m^2

32. Hard X-rays for the study of fractures in bones should have a minimum wavelength of 10^{-11} m. The accelerating voltage for electrons in X-ray machine should be

(a) < 124 kV
(b) > 124 kV
(c) between 60 kV and 70 kV
(d) $= 100$ kV

33. Energy levels A, B, C of a certain atom correspond to increasing values of energy i.e., $E_A < E_B < E_C$. If $\lambda_1, \lambda_2, \lambda_3$ are the wavelengths of radiation corresponding to the transitions C to B, B to A and C to A respectively, which of the following relation is correct?

(a) $\lambda_3 = \lambda_1 + \lambda_2$ (b) $\lambda_3 = \dfrac{\lambda_1 \lambda_2}{\lambda_1 + \lambda_2}$
(c) $\lambda_1 + \lambda_2 + \lambda_3 = 0$ (d) $\lambda_3^2 = \lambda_1^2 + \lambda_2^2$

34. A radio transmitter operates at a freqency 880 kHz and a power of 10 kW. The number of photons emitted per second is

(a) 1.72×10^{31} (b) 1.327×10^{25}
(c) 1.327×10^{37} (d) 1.327×10^{45}

35. The momentum of a photon of an electromagnetic radiation is 3.3×10^{-29} kgms^{-1}. What is the frequency of the associated waves ?
[h = 6.6×10^{-34} Js; c = 3×10^8 ms^{-1})

(a) 1.5×10^{13} Hz (b) 7.5×10^{12} Hz
(c) 6.0×10^3 Hz (d) 3.0×10^3 Hz

36. As suming the nitrogen molecule is moving with r.m.s.velocity at 400 K, the de-Broglie wavelength of nitrongen molecule is close to :
(Given : nitrogen molecule weight : 4.64×10^{-26} kg, Boltzman constant : 1.38×10^{-23} J/K, Planck constant : 6.63×10^{-34} J.s)

(a) 0.24 Å (b) 0.20 Å (c) 0.34 Å (d) 0.44 Å

37. Particle A of mass $m_A = \dfrac{m}{2}$ moving along the x-axis with velocity v_0 collides elastically with another particle B at rest having mass $m_B = \dfrac{m}{3}$. If both particles move along the x-axis after the collision, the change $\Delta\lambda$ in de-Broglie wavelength of particle A, in terms of its de-Broglie wavelength (λ_0) before collision is :

(a) $\Delta\lambda = \dfrac{3}{2}\lambda_0$ (b) $\Delta\lambda = \dfrac{5}{2}\lambda_0$
(c) $\Delta\lambda = 2\lambda_0$ (d) $\Delta\lambda = 4\lambda_0$

38. An electron of mass m and magnitude of charge $|e|$ initially at rest gets accelerated by a constant electric field E. The rate of change of de-Broglie wavelength of this electron at time t ignoring relativistic effects is:

(a) $-\dfrac{h}{|e|E\sqrt{t}}$ (b) $\dfrac{|e|Et}{h}$
(c) $-\dfrac{h}{|e|Et}$ (d) $\dfrac{-h}{|e|Et^2}$

39. An electron (mass m) with initial velocity $\vec{v} = v_0\hat{i} + v_0\hat{j}$ is in an electric field $\vec{E} = -E_0\hat{k}$. If λ_0 is initial de-Broglie wavelength of electron, its de-Broglie wave length at time t is given by:

(a) $\dfrac{\lambda_0\sqrt{2}}{\sqrt{1+\dfrac{e^2E^2t^2}{m^2v_0^2}}}$ (b) $\dfrac{\lambda_0}{\sqrt{1+\dfrac{e^2E_0^2t^2}{m^2v_0^2}}}$
(c) $\dfrac{\lambda_0}{\sqrt{1+\dfrac{e^2E^2t^2}{2m^2v_0^2}}}$ (d) $\dfrac{\lambda_0}{\sqrt{2+\dfrac{e^2E^2t^2}{m^2v_0^2}}}$

40. A particle 'P' is formed due to a completely inelastic collision of particles 'x' and 'y' having de-Broglie wavelengths 'γ_x' and 'γ_y' respectively. If x and y were moving in opposite directions, then the de-Broglie wavelength of 'P' is:

(a) $\frac{\gamma_x \gamma_y}{\gamma_x + \gamma_y}$ (b) $\frac{\gamma_x \gamma_y}{|\gamma_x - \gamma_y|}$

(c) $\gamma_x - \gamma_y$ (d) $\gamma_x + \gamma_y$

41. A particle A of mass 'm' and charge 'q' is accelerated by a potential difference of 50v Another particle B of mass '4m' and charge'q' is accelerated by a potential differnce of 2500V. The ratio of de-Broglie wavelength $\frac{\lambda_A}{\lambda_B}$ is

(a) 10.00 (b) 0.07

(c) 14.14 (d) 4.47

42. If the deBroglie wavelength of an electron is equal to 10^{-3} times the wavelength of a photon of frequency 6×10^{14} Hz, then the speed of electron is equal to :

(Speed of light = 3×10^8 m/s)

Planck's constant = 6.63×10^{-34}J.s

Mass of electron = 9.1×10^{-31} kg)

(a) 1.1×10^6 m/s (b) 1.7×10^6 m/s

(c) 1.8×10^6 m/s (d) 1.45×10^6 m/s

43. Radiation, with wavelength 6561 Å falls on a metal surface to produce photoelectrons. The electrons are made to enter a uniform magnetic field of 3×10^{-4} T. If the radius of the largest circular path followed by the electrons is 10 mm, the work function of the metal is close to:

(a) 1.1 ev (b) 0.8 ev (c) 1.6 ev (d) 1.8 ev

44. When photon of energy 4.0 eV strikes the surface of a metal A, the ejected photoelectrons have maximum kinetic energy T_A eV and de-Broglie wavelength λ_A. The maximum kinetic energy of photoelectrons liberated from another metal B by photon of energy 4.50 eV is $T_B=(T_A-1.5)$eV. If the de-Broglie wavelength of these photoelectrons $\lambda_B = 2\lambda_A$, then the work function of metal B is:

(a) 4 eV (b) 2 eV (c) 1.5 eV (d) 3 eV

45. The stopping potential V_0 (in volt) as a function of frequency (v) for a sodium emitter, is shown in the figure. The work function of sodium, from the data plotted in the figure, will be: (Given : Planck's constant (h) = 6.63×10^{-34} Js, electron charge $e = 1.6 \times 10^{-19}$ C)

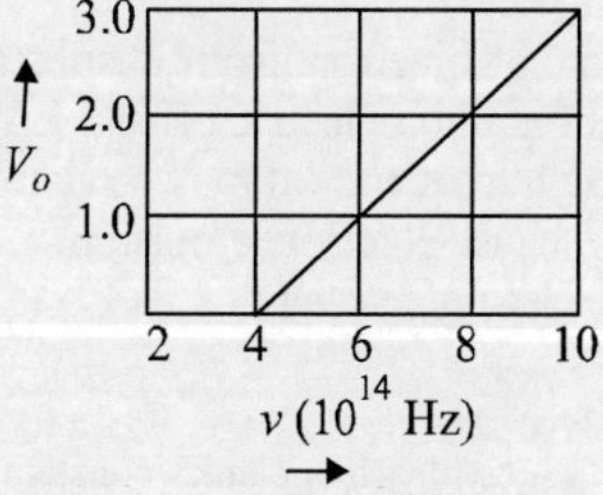

(a) 1.82 eV (b) 1.66 eV (c) 1.95 eV (d) 2.12 eV

Hints & Solutions

26.1 Concept Practice Problems CPP

1. (a) Einstein's photo electric effect & compton effect established particle nature of light. These effects can be explained only, when we assume that the light has particle nature (To explain, Interference & Diffraction the light must have wave nature. It means that light has both particle and wave nature, so it is called dual nature of light)
2. (b)
3. (c) $\frac{1}{2}mv^2 = \frac{hc}{\lambda} - \phi \Rightarrow v = \sqrt{\frac{2(hc - \lambda\phi)}{\lambda m}}$
4. (d) 5. (b) 6. (b)
7. (a) Because when intensity of incident light increases, it means that number of photons increases in incident light. If number of incident photons increases, then number of emitted photo electrons also increases, consequently the photo electric current increases.
8. (c)
9. (a) Emission of electron from a substance under the action of light is photoelectric effect. Light must be at a sufficiently high frequency. It may be visible light, U.V, X-rays. So U.V. cause electron emission.
10. (a) By photoelectric equation:
$h\nu = h\nu_0 + K.E_{electron}$
$K.E_{electron} = h\nu - h\nu_0$
$K.E_{electron} \propto (\nu - \nu_0)$ [$\because$ h is plank's constant]

26.2 Concept Practice Problems 

11. (b) $\lambda = \frac{h}{mv} = \frac{h\sqrt{1-v^2/c^2}}{m_0 v} = 0$ $(\because v = c)$
12. (a) According to relation, $E = \frac{1}{2}mv^2$
$$\sqrt{\frac{2E}{m}} = v$$
$$\lambda = \frac{h}{\sqrt{2mE}}$$
Because $m_1 < m_3 < m_2$
So for same λ, $E_1 > E_3 > E_2$.
13. (d) 14. (c) 15. (b)
16. (c) de-Broglie wavelength, $\lambda = \frac{h}{\sqrt{2mE_{K.E}}}$
$$\therefore \frac{\lambda_p}{\lambda_\alpha} = \sqrt{\frac{m_\alpha}{m_p}} = \sqrt{\frac{4m_p}{m_p}} \quad [\because E_{K.E(\alpha)} = E_{K.E(p)}]$$
$$\therefore \frac{\lambda_p}{\lambda_\alpha} = \frac{2}{1}$$
17. (c)
18. (c) Momentum $p = \frac{h}{\lambda} \Rightarrow \lambda = \frac{h}{p}$ (photon)
If $\lambda_{photon} = \lambda_{electron}$
p(momentum) will become same.
19. (a) In the Davisson and Germer experiment, the velocity of electrons emitted from the electron gun can be increased by increasing the potential difference between the anode and filament.
20. (d) $qV = \frac{1}{2}mv^2$ or $mv = \sqrt{2qVm}$;
So $\lambda = \frac{h}{mv} = \frac{h}{\sqrt{2qVm}}$ i.e. $\lambda \propto \frac{1}{\sqrt{qm}}$;
so $\frac{\lambda_p}{\lambda_\alpha} = \sqrt{\frac{q_\alpha m_\alpha}{q_p m_p}} = \sqrt{2 \times 4} = 2\sqrt{2}$

Exercise 1 - Chapter Revision Problems 

1. (b) Here the velocity of electron increases, so as per Einstein's equation mass of the electron increases, hence the specific charge $\frac{e}{m}$ decreases.
2. (d) 3. (a) 4. (b) 5. (d)
6. (b) Energy of a photon $E = h\nu = \frac{hc}{\lambda}$
7. (d) $eV_s = \frac{hc}{\lambda} - W_0$. If λ decreases, V_s increases
8. (b) $eV = \frac{1}{2}mv^2$ or $v = \sqrt{2eV/m}$
9. (b) Since work function for a metal surface is $W = \frac{hc}{\lambda_0}$
where λ_0 is threshold wavelength or cut-off wavelength for a metal surface.
here $W = 4.125\ eV = 4.125 \times 1.6 \times 10^{-19}$ Joule
so $\lambda_0 = \frac{6.6 \times 10^{-34} \times 3 \times 10^8}{4.125 \times 1.6 \times 10^{-19}} = 3000Å$
10. (b) $E = hc/\lambda = 6.6 \times 10^{-34} \times 3 \times 10^8 / 5000 \times 10^{-10}$
$= 3.973 \times 10^{-19}$ J
11. (a) Einstein equation $E = h\upsilon_o + K.E$
where E = energy of incident photon.
$h\upsilon_o$ = work function of metal
K.E = max. kinetic energy of e^-
$\therefore 4\ eV = 2\ eV + K.E$ or $K.E = 2\ eV$
Stopping potential is the potential difference which may stop this e^-.
Let it be V, then $eV = 2e \Rightarrow V = 2$ volt.
12. (d) Momentum of a photon $= \frac{E}{c} = \frac{10 \times 1.6 \times 10^{-19}}{3 \times 10^8}$
$= 5.33 \times 10^{-27}$ kg ms^{-1}
13. (a) $E_k = \frac{hc}{c}\left(\frac{1}{\lambda} - \frac{1}{\lambda_0}\right)$ (in eV)

$$= \frac{6.6\times10^{-34}\times3\times10^{8}}{1.6\times10^{-19}}\left(\frac{10^{10}}{1800}-\frac{10^{10}}{2300}\right)=0.15\text{eV}$$

14. (d) 15. (c)

16. (b) $\lambda = \frac{h}{p} = \frac{h}{\sqrt{2mE}} = \frac{h}{\sqrt{2mqV}}$

$\therefore \lambda = \frac{6.6\times10^{-34}}{\sqrt{2\times(1.6\times10^{-27})\times(1.6\times10^{-19})\times1000}}$

or $\lambda = \frac{6.6\times10^{-34}\times10^{22}}{\sqrt{1.6\sqrt{20}}} = 0.9\times10^{-12}\text{ m}$

17. (d) $\frac{1}{\lambda_\alpha} = R(Z-\alpha)^2\left[\frac{1}{1^2}-\frac{1}{2^2}\right] = \frac{3R}{4}(Z-\alpha)^2$

$\frac{1}{\lambda_\beta} = R(Z-\alpha)^2\left[\frac{1}{1^2}-\frac{1}{3^2}\right] = \frac{8}{9}R(Z-\alpha)^2$

$\therefore \frac{\lambda_\beta}{\lambda_\alpha} = \frac{27}{32}$ or $\lambda_\beta = \frac{27}{32}\lambda_\alpha = \frac{27}{32}\times0.32 = 0.27\text{ Å}$

18. (a) Moment of photon $= p = \frac{h}{\lambda}$ $\because E = mc^2$

But, $p = mc$

$\therefore E = mc.c$

So, $E = pc$ or $E = \frac{hc}{\lambda}$ $\therefore \frac{hc}{\lambda} = pc$ or $p = \frac{h}{\lambda}$ and $\lambda = \frac{c}{f}$

$\therefore p = \frac{hf}{c}$

19. (d) $h\upsilon - h\upsilon_0 = E_K$, according to photoelectric equation, when $\upsilon = \upsilon_0$, $E_K = 0$.
Graph (d) represents $E_K - \upsilon$ relationship.

20. (c) de-Broglie's relation, $\lambda = \frac{h}{p}$

momentum $p = \sqrt{2mE}$

$\Rightarrow \lambda = \frac{h}{\sqrt{2mE}} = \frac{h}{\sqrt{2mK}}$ $(\because E = K)$

21. (b) $\lambda_{min.} = \frac{hc}{eV} = \frac{12400}{V} = \frac{12400}{20\times10^3} = 0.62\text{Å}$

22. (d) V = 3000 volt.

$\frac{1}{2}mv^2 = eV \Rightarrow v = \sqrt{\frac{2eV}{m}}$

$\therefore v = \sqrt{\frac{2\times1.6\times10^{-19}\times3000}{9.1\times10^{-31}}}$

$= 32.6\times10^6 = 3.26\times10^7$ m/s.

23. (a) $E(k_\alpha) = 10.2\,(Z-1)^2$ eV
$= 10.2\times28^2$
$= 10.2\times784$
$= 7.997$ keV = 8 KeV

24. (c) de-Broglie wavelength of a material particle at temperature T is given by

$\lambda = \frac{h}{\sqrt{2mkT}}$, where k is Boltzmann's constant.

$\Rightarrow \lambda \propto \frac{1}{\sqrt{T}}$

$\therefore \frac{\lambda_2}{\lambda_1} = \sqrt{\frac{T_1}{T_2}}$

or $\frac{\lambda_2}{\lambda_1} = \sqrt{\frac{1200}{300}} = 2$

$\therefore \lambda_2 = 2\lambda_1 = 2\lambda$

25. (a) The energy of each photon $= \frac{200}{4\times10^{20}} = 5\times10^{-19}$ J

Wavelength $= \lambda = \frac{hc}{E}$

$= \frac{(6.63\times10^{-34})\times(3\times10^8)}{5\times10^{-19}}$

$\Rightarrow \lambda = 4.0\times10^{-7} = 400$ nm

26. (a) The maximum kinetic energy of an electron accelerated through a potential difference of V volt is

$\frac{1}{2}mv^2 = eV$

$\therefore$ maximum velocity $v = \sqrt{\frac{2eV}{m}}$

$v = \sqrt{\frac{2\times1.6\times10^{-19}\times15000}{9.1\times10^{-31}}} = 7.26\times10^7$ m/s

27. (b) $\lambda_0 = \frac{c}{v_0} = \frac{3\times10^8}{5\times10^{14}} = 6\times10^{-7}\text{ m} = 6000\text{Å}$

28. (b) For electron and positron pair production, minimum energy is 1.02 MeV.

Energy of photon is given $1.7\times10^{-3}\text{ J} = \frac{1.7\times10^{-13}}{1.6\times10^{-19}}$

= 1.06 MeV.

Since energy of photon is greater than 1.02 MeV. so electron positron pair will be created.

29. (b) $2d\sin\theta = n\lambda$ or $d = \frac{n\lambda}{2\sin\theta} = \frac{1\times20}{2\times\sin30^\circ} = 20$ nm

30. (c)

31. (b) For emission of electrons incident energy of each photon must be greater than work function (threshold energy).

32. (c) By using $E = W_0 + K_{max}$

$E = \frac{12375}{5000} = 2.475$ eV and $K_{max} = eV_0 = 1.36$ eV

So $2.475 = W_0 + 1.36 \Rightarrow W_0 = 1.1$ eV.

33. (d) For occurence of photoelectric effect, the incident light should have frequency more than a certain minimum which is called the threshold frequency (ν_0).

We have, $\frac{1}{2}mv^2 = h\nu - h\nu_0$

For photoelectric effect emission $\nu > \nu_0$ where ν is the frequency of the incident light.

34. (a) $K.E. = h\nu - h\nu_{th} = eV_0$ (V_0 = cut off voltage)

$$\Rightarrow V_0 = \frac{h}{e}(8.2\times10^{14} - 3.3\times10^{14})$$

$$= \frac{6.6\times10^{-34}\times4.9\times10^{14}}{1.6\times10^{-19}} \approx 2V.$$

35. (b) According to Einsten's photoelectric effect, the K.E. of the radiated electrons

$K.E_{max} = E - W$

$$\frac{1}{2}mv_1^2 = (1 - 0.5)\,eV = 0.5\,eV$$

$$\frac{1}{2}mv_2^2 = (2.5 - 0.5)\,eV = 2\,eV$$

$$\frac{v_1}{v_2} = \sqrt{\frac{0.5}{2}} = \frac{1}{\sqrt{4}} = \frac{1}{2}$$

36. (a) For a given photosensitive material and µ frequency > threshold frequency photoelectric current µ intensity.

37. (b) Here, $\frac{hc}{\lambda} = 10^3$ eV and $h\nu = 10^6$ eV

Hence, $\nu = \frac{10^3 c}{\lambda} = \frac{10^3\times3\times10^8}{1.24\times10^{-9}}$

$= 2.4\times10^{20}$ Hz

38. (d) $h\nu = W + \frac{1}{2}mv^2$ or $\frac{hc}{\lambda} = W + \frac{1}{2}mv^2$

Here $\lambda = 3000$ Å $= 3000\times10^{-10}$ m

and $W = 1$ eV $= 1.6\times10^{-19}$ joule

$$\therefore \frac{(6.6\times10^{-34})(3\times10^8)}{3000\times10^{-10}}$$

$$= (1.6\times10^{-19}) + \frac{1}{2}\times(9.1\times10^{-31})v^2$$

Solving we get, $v \cong 10^6$ m/s

39. (c) $$\frac{e^2}{2h\varepsilon_0 c} = \frac{(1.6\times10^{-19})^2}{2\times6.26\times10^{-34}\times8.857\times10^{-12}\times3\times10^8}$$

$= \frac{1}{137}$ it is unit less quantity.

40. (a) $W_0 = \frac{hc}{\lambda_0}$

$$= \frac{6.63\times10^{-34}\times3\times10^8}{5000\times10^{-10}} = 4\times10^{-19}\,J$$

41. (d) de Broglie wavelength

$$\lambda = \frac{h}{mv} \Rightarrow m = \frac{h}{\lambda v}$$

Clearly, $m \propto \frac{1}{\lambda v}$

If λ and v be the wavelength and velocity of electron and λ' and v' be the wavelength and velocity of the particle then

$$\Rightarrow \frac{m'}{m} = \frac{v\lambda}{v'\lambda'} = \frac{1}{5}\times\frac{1}{1.878}\times10^{-4}$$

$$\Rightarrow m = 9.7\times10^{-28}\text{ kg}$$

42. (c) As per question, when KE of particle E, wavelength λ and when KE becomes $E + \Delta E$ wavelength becomes $\lambda/2$

Using, $\lambda = \frac{h}{\sqrt{2mKE}}$

$$\frac{\lambda}{2} = \frac{h}{\sqrt{2m(KE + \Delta E)}}$$

$$\Rightarrow \frac{\lambda}{\lambda/2} = \sqrt{\frac{KE + \Delta E}{KE}}$$

$$\Rightarrow 4 = \frac{KE + \Delta E}{KE}$$

$\Rightarrow$ $4KE - KE = \Delta E$

$\therefore$ $\Delta E = 3\,KE = 3\,E$

43. (c) de-Broglie wavelength, $\lambda = \frac{h}{P} = \frac{h}{\sqrt{2m(KE)}}$

$$\therefore \lambda \propto \frac{1}{\sqrt{m}}$$

As $m_{He^{++}} > m_P > m_e$

$\lambda_{He^{++}} > \lambda_P > \lambda_e$ or $\lambda_e > \lambda_P > \lambda_{He^{++}}$

44. (d) According to Einstein's photoelectric equation

$K_{max} = h\nu - \phi_0$

$$\Rightarrow eV_s = \frac{hc}{\lambda} - \phi_0$$

$$\Rightarrow V_s = \frac{hc}{\lambda e} - \frac{\phi_0}{e}$$

where λ = wavelength of incident light

ϕ_0 = work function

V_s = stopping potential

Comparing the above equation with $y = mx + c$, we get

slope $= \frac{hc}{e}$

Increasing the frequency of incident radiation has no effect on work function and frequency. So, graph will not change.

45. (d) Using equation, $= \frac{hc}{\lambda} - \phi$

$$KE_{max} = \frac{hc}{\lambda} - \phi = \frac{hc}{500} - \phi \quad ...(1)$$

Again, $3KE_{max} = \frac{hc}{200} - \phi$ ...(2)

Dividing equation (2) by (1),

$$\frac{3KE_{max}}{KE_{max}} = \frac{3}{1} = \frac{\frac{hc}{200} - \phi}{\frac{hc}{500} - \phi}$$

Putting the value of $hc = 1237.5$ and solving we get, work function, $\phi = 0.61$ eV.

46. (a) $KE_{max} = E - \phi_0$

(where E = energy of incident light ϕ_0 = work function)

$= \frac{hc}{\lambda} - \frac{hc}{\lambda_0}$

$= 1237\left[\frac{1}{260} - \frac{1}{380}\right]$

$= \frac{1237 \times 120}{380 \times 260} = 1.5\text{eV}$

47. (a) Energy of photon (E) is given by

$E = \frac{hc}{\lambda}$

Number of photons of wavelength λ emitted in t second from laser of power P is given by

$n = \frac{Pt\lambda}{hc}$

$\Rightarrow n = \frac{2 \times \lambda}{hc} = \frac{2 \times 10^{-3} \times 5 \times 10^{-7}}{2 \times 10^{-25}}$ $(\because t = 1S)$

$\Rightarrow n = 5 \times 10^{15}$

48. (d) Using, wavelength, $\lambda = \frac{12375}{\Delta E}$

or, $\lambda = \frac{12375}{4.9} \simeq 250\text{nm}$

49. (c) Let ϕ = work function of the metal,

$\frac{hc}{\lambda_1} = \phi + eV_1$ ......(i)

$\frac{hc}{\lambda_2} = \phi + eV_2$ ......(ii)

Sutracting (ii) from (i) we get

$hc\left(\frac{1}{\lambda_1} - \frac{1}{\lambda_2}\right) = e(V_1 - V_2)$

$\Rightarrow V_1 - V_2 = \frac{hc}{e}\left(\frac{\lambda_2 - \lambda_1}{\lambda_1 \cdot \lambda_2}\right)$ $\left[\begin{array}{l}\lambda_1 = 300\text{nm} \\ \lambda_2 = 400\text{nm} \\ \frac{hc}{e} = 1240\text{nm} - V\end{array}\right]$

$= (1240\,\text{nm} - v)\left(\frac{100\text{nm}}{300\text{ nm} \times 400\text{nm}}\right)$

$= 1.03\text{ V} \approx 1\text{V}$

50. (a) Graph of V_s and f given at $B\,(5.5, 0)$

Minimum energy for ejection of electron = Work function (ϕ).

$\phi = hV$ joule or $\phi = \frac{hV}{e}$ eV (for $V = 0$)

$\therefore \phi = \frac{6.62 \times 10^{-34} \times 5.5 \times 10^{14}}{1.6 \times 10^{-19}}\text{eV} = 2.27\,\text{eV}$

Exercise 2 - Exemplar & Past Year Questions E&PYQs

Exemplar Questions

1. (d) Velocity of a body freely falling from a height H is

$v = \sqrt{2gH}$

So, $\lambda = \frac{h}{mv} = \frac{h}{m\sqrt{2gH}} \Rightarrow = \frac{h}{m\sqrt{2g}\sqrt{H}}$

(h, m and g are constant)

Here, $\frac{h}{m\sqrt{2g}}$ is also constant

So, $h \propto \frac{1}{\sqrt{H}}$ $\Rightarrow$ or $\boxed{\lambda \propto H^{-1/2}}$

2. (b) Energy of a photon is $E = \frac{hc}{\lambda}$

Where λ is the minimum wavelength of the photon required to eject the proton from nucleus.

Energy of photon must be equal to the binding energy of proton.

So, energy of a photon, E = 1 MeV ⇒ 10^6eV (given)

Now, $\left(E = \frac{hc}{\lambda}\right)$

So, $\lambda = \frac{hc}{E} = \left(\frac{6.63 \times 10^{-34} \times 3 \times 10^8}{10^6\text{eV}}\right)$

$\Rightarrow$ So, $\lambda = \frac{hc}{E} = \frac{6.63 \times 10^{-34} \times 3 \times 10^8}{10^6 \times 1.6 \times 10^{-19}\text{ J}}$

$= 1.24 \times 10^{-9} \times 10^{-3}$

$= 1.24 \times 10^{-3}\text{ nm}$

3. (d) When a beam of electrons of energy E_0 is incident on a metal surface kept in vacuum or evacuated chamber so electrons can be emitted with maximum energy E_0 (due to elastic collision) and with any energy less than E_0, when part of incident energy of electron is used in liberating the electrons from the surface of metal. So maximum energy of emitted electrons can be E_0.

4. (c)

5. (b) The relation between λ and K is given by

$\lambda = \frac{h}{\sqrt{2mK}}$

So, for the given value of kinetic energy K,

$\frac{h}{\sqrt{2K}}$ is a constant.

Thus, $\lambda \propto \frac{1}{\sqrt{m}}$

$\therefore \Rightarrow \lambda_p : \lambda_n : \lambda_e : \lambda_\alpha$

$\Rightarrow = \frac{1}{\sqrt{m_p}} : \frac{1}{\sqrt{m_n}} : \frac{1}{\sqrt{m_e}} : \frac{1}{\sqrt{m_\alpha}}$

if $(m_p = m_n)$, then $\lambda_p = \lambda_n$

if $(m_\alpha > m_p)$, then $\lambda_\alpha < \lambda_p$

if $(m_e < m_n)$, then $\lambda_e > \lambda_n$

Hence, $\lambda_\alpha < \lambda_p = \lambda_n < \lambda_e$.

6. (a) As given that, $v = v_0\,\vec{i}$ and $B = B_0\,\vec{j}$

Force on moving electron due to perpendicular magnetic field B is, F = –e (v × B)

$F = -e\left[v_0\hat{i} \times B_0\hat{i}\right] = -e\,v_0\,B_0\,(\hat{i} \times \hat{j})$

$\Rightarrow = -ev_0B_0\hat{k}$ $(\because \hat{k} = \hat{i} \times \hat{j})$

So, the force is perpendicular to v and B, both as the force is ⊥ to the velocity so the magnitude of v will not change, so momentum is (= mv) will remain same or constant in magnitude. Hence, de-Broglie wavelength $\lambda = \frac{h}{mv}$ remians constant.

7. (a)

8. (c) We know that,
de-Broglie wavelength of electron,

$$\lambda_0 = \frac{h}{mv_0}$$

Force on moving electron due to eletric field,

$$E = F = -eF = -eE_0\hat{j}$$

Acceleration in electron due to force

$$F = ma \text{ or } a = \frac{F}{m} = \frac{-eE_0\hat{j}}{m}$$

It is acting along negative y – axis direction and the initial velocity of electron along x – axis, $v_{x_0} = v_0\hat{i}$

Initial velocity of electron along y – axis,

$v_{y_0} = 0$.

So, velocity of electron after time t along y – axis,

$v = u + at \qquad (\because u = 0)$

$$v_y = 0 + \left(\frac{eE_0}{m}\hat{j}\right)t = -\frac{eE_0}{m}t\hat{j}$$

Magnitude of velocity of electron after time t is

$$v = \sqrt{v_x^2 + v_y^2} = \sqrt{v_0^2 + \left(\frac{-eE_0}{m}t\right)^2}$$

So, $|v| = v_0\sqrt{1 + \frac{e^2E_0^2t^2}{m^2v_0^2}}$

de-Broglie wavelength, $\lambda' = \frac{h}{mv}$

So, $= \frac{h}{mv_0\sqrt{1 + e^2E_0^2t^2/(m^2v_0^2)}} \qquad \left[\because \lambda_0 = \frac{h}{mv_0}\right]$

$$\lambda' = \frac{\lambda_0}{\sqrt{1 + e^2E_0^2t^2/m^2v_0^2}}$$

Hence, option (c) is verified.

NEET/AIPMT (2013-2020) Questions

9. (b) From photo-electric equation,

$h\nu' = h\nu + K_{max} \qquad$ ...(i)

$h.2\nu = h\nu + \frac{1}{2}mV^2_{max} \qquad [\therefore \nu' = 2\nu]$

$\Rightarrow h\nu = \frac{1}{2}mV^2_{max} \Rightarrow V_{max} = \sqrt{\frac{2h\nu}{m}}$

10. (d) As $P = \frac{E}{c}$

$\lambda_p = \frac{hc}{E} \qquad$ ...(i)

$\lambda_e = \frac{h}{\sqrt{2mE}} \Rightarrow \lambda_e^2 = \frac{h^2}{2mE} \qquad$ ...(ii)

From equations (i) and (ii)

$\lambda_p \propto \lambda_e^2$

11. (b) According to Einstein's photoelectric equation,

$h\nu = \phi_0 + K_{max}$

We have

$h\nu = \phi_0 + 0.5 \qquad$ ...(i)

and $1.2h\nu = \phi_0 + 0.8 \qquad$ ...(ii)

Therefore, from above two equations $\phi_0 = 1.0$ eV.

12. (b) As we know

$$\lambda = \frac{h}{P} = \frac{h}{\sqrt{2mK}} \qquad (\because P = \sqrt{2mKE})$$

or $\frac{\lambda_1}{\lambda_2} = \sqrt{\frac{K_2}{K_1}} = \sqrt{\frac{16K}{K}} = \frac{4}{1}$

Therefore the percentage change in de-Broglie wavelength $= \frac{1-4}{4} \times 100 = -75\%$

13. (a) According to De-broglie $p = \frac{h}{\lambda}$ or $P \propto \frac{1}{\lambda}$

where

P = particle momentum;
λ = de-Broglie wavelength
h = Plank's constant

$P \propto \frac{1}{\lambda}$ represents rectangular hyperbola.

14. (a) As we know,

$$eV_s = \frac{hc}{\lambda} - \Psi$$

$3eV_o = \frac{hc}{\lambda} - \Psi \qquad$ ...(1)

$eV_o = \frac{hc}{2\lambda} - \Psi \qquad$ ...(2)

$3eV_o = \frac{3hc}{2\lambda} - 3\Psi \qquad$ ...(3)

Multiplying eqn. (2) by (3) and subtracting it from eqn (1)

$$\Psi = \frac{hc}{4\lambda}$$

So, threshold wavelength,

$$\lambda_{th} = \frac{hc}{\Psi} = \frac{hc}{hc/4\lambda} = 4\lambda$$

15. (b) **Given :** Work function ϕ of metal = 2.28 eV
Wavelength of light $\lambda = 500 \text{ nm} = 500 \times 10^{-9}$m

$$KE_{max} = \frac{hc}{\lambda} - \phi$$

$$KE_{max} = \frac{6.6 \times 10^{-34} \times 3 \times 10^8}{5 \times 10^{-7} \times 1.6 \times 10^{-19}} - 2.28$$

$$KE_{max} = 2.48 - 2.28 = 0.2 \text{ ev}$$

$$\lambda_{min} = \frac{h}{p} = \frac{h}{\sqrt{2m(KE)_{max}}}$$

$$= \frac{\frac{20}{3} \times 10^{-34}}{\sqrt{2 \times 9 \times 10^{-31} \times 0.2 \times 1.6 \times 10^{-19}}}$$

$$\lambda_{min} = \frac{25}{9} \times 10^{-9}$$

$= 2.80 \times 10^{-9}$ nm $\therefore \lambda \geq 2.8 \times 10^{-9}$ m

16. (a) For electron De-Broglie wavelength,

$$\lambda_e = \frac{h}{\sqrt{2mE}}$$

For photon E = pc

$\Rightarrow$ De-Broglie wavelength, $\lambda_{Ph} = \frac{hc}{E}$

$$\therefore \frac{\lambda_e}{\lambda_{Ph}} = \frac{h}{\sqrt{2mE}} \times \frac{E}{hc} = \left(\frac{E}{2m}\right)^{1/2} \frac{1}{c}$$

17. (d) According to Einstein's photoelectric effect,

$$eV = \frac{hc}{\lambda} - \frac{hc}{\lambda_0} \quad \ldots(i)$$

$$eV/4 = \frac{hc}{2\lambda} - \frac{hc}{\lambda_0} \quad \ldots(ii)$$

Dividing equation (i) by (ii) by

$$\Rightarrow 4 = \frac{\frac{1}{\lambda} - \frac{1}{\lambda_0}}{\frac{1}{2\lambda} - \frac{1}{\lambda_0}}$$ on solving we get,

$$\lambda_0 = 3\lambda$$

18. (a) We know that,

de-Broglie wavelength $\lambda = \frac{\hbar}{P} = \frac{h}{\sqrt{2m(KE)}}$

K.E. of thermal neutron $= \frac{3}{2}kT$

$$= \frac{h}{\sqrt{2m\left(\frac{3}{2}kT\right)}}$$

$$\lambda = \frac{h}{\sqrt{3mkT}}$$

19. (a, d) Both answers are correct

Given,

$\lambda_0 = 3250 \times 10^{-10}$ m

$\lambda = 2536 \times 10^{-10}$ m

$$\phi = \frac{hc}{\lambda_0} = \frac{4.14 \times 10^{-15} \times 3 \times 10^8}{3250 \times 10^{-10}} = 3.82\text{eV}$$

$$hv = \frac{hc}{\lambda} = \frac{4.14 \times 10^{-15} \times 3 \times 10^8}{2536 \times 10^{-10}} = 4.89\text{eV}$$

According to Einstein's photoelectric equation,

$K_{max} = hv - \phi$

$KE_{max} = (4.89-3.82)\text{eV} = 1.077$ eV

$\frac{1}{2}mv^2 = 1.077 \times 1.6 \times 10^{-19}$

$$\Rightarrow v = \sqrt{\frac{2 \times 1.077 \times 1.6 \times 10^{-19}}{9.1 \times 10^{-31}}}$$

or, $v = 0.6 \times 10^6$ m/s or 6×10^5 m/s

20. (a)

21. (b) de-Broglie wavelength of electron

$$\lambda = \frac{12.27}{\sqrt{V}}\text{Å} = \frac{12.27 \times 10^{-10}}{\sqrt{10000}} = 12.27 \times 10^{-12}\text{ m}$$

22. (a) As $E = \frac{12400}{\lambda}$

$$\lambda = \frac{12400}{4} = 3100\text{ Å}$$

$\therefore \lambda = 310$ nm

23. (c) Using, $\lambda = \frac{12.27}{\sqrt{V}}$ Å

$$\Rightarrow \sqrt{V} = \frac{12.27 \times 10^{-10}}{1.227 \times 10^{-11}} = 10^2$$

[Given, $\lambda = 1.227 \times 10^{-11}$ m]

$\therefore V = 10^4$ volt

24. (c) For photoelectric emission, photoelectric current, incident light frequency should be greater than threshold frequency.

Light of frequency 1.5 times the threshold frequency v_0 incident.

$$v = \frac{3}{2}v_0$$

If frequency is halved,

$\therefore v' = \frac{v}{2} = \frac{3}{4}v_0 \qquad \because v' < v_0$

$\therefore$ No photoelectric emission will take place.

Exercise 3 - Concept Application Problems CAP

1. (d) $m = \frac{m_o}{\left(1 - \frac{v^2}{c^2}\right)^{1/2}} = \frac{m_o}{(1-3/4)^{1/2}} = 2m_o$

2. (b) $E_k = E - W_0 = 6.2 - 4.2 = 2.0$ eV

$= 2.0 \times 1.6 \times 10^{-19} = 3.2 \times 10^{-19}$ J

3. (b) Photoelectrons are emitted in A alone. Energy of electron needed if emitted from A $= \frac{h\upsilon}{e}$eV

$$\therefore E_A = \frac{(6.6 \times 10^{-34}) \times (1.8 \times 10^{14})}{1.6 \times 10^{-19}} = 0.74\text{eV}$$

$$E_B = \frac{(6.6 \times 10^{-34}) \times (2.2 \times 10^{14})}{1.6 \times 10^{-19}} = 0.91\text{ eV}$$

Incident energy 0.825 eV is greater than E_A (0.74 eV) but less than E_B (0.91 eV).

4. (a) Here, No. of electrons
$n_e = 5 \times 10^7/\text{cm}^3 = 5 \times 10^7 \times 10^6/\text{m}^3$
No. of positive ions,
$n_p = 5 \times 10^7 \times 10^6 = 5 \times 10^{13}/\text{m}^3$
$v = 0.4$ m/s ; $J = 4 \times 10^{-6}$ A/m^2 ; $v_p = ?$
Use the relation $J = n_e e v_e + n_p e v_p$ and solve it for v_p

5. (b) Momentum of incident light per second

$$P_1 = \frac{E}{c} = \frac{60}{3\times10^8} = 2\times10^{-7}$$

Momentum of reflected light per sec

$$P_2 = \frac{60}{100}\times\frac{E}{c} = \frac{60}{100}\times\frac{60}{3\times10^8} = 1.2\times10^{-7}$$

Force on the surface = change in momentum per sec
$= P_2 - (-P_1) = P_2 + P_1 = (2 + 1.2) \times 10^{-7} = 3.2 \times 10^{-7}$ N

6. (b) $\frac{1}{2}mv_1^2 = 2W_0 - W_0 = W_0$ and

$$\frac{1}{2}mv_2^2 = 10W_0 - W_0 = 9W_0$$

$$\therefore \quad \frac{v_1}{v_2} = \sqrt{\frac{W_0}{9W_0}} = \frac{1}{3}$$

7. (d) Intensity $\propto 1/(\text{distance})^2$; No. of photoelectrons emitted is proportional to intensity of incident light.

8. (d) $eV_0 = \frac{hc}{\lambda_0} - W_0$ and $eV' = \frac{hc}{2\lambda_0} - W_0$

Subtracting them we have

$$e(V_0 - V') = \frac{hc}{\lambda_0}\left[1 - \frac{1}{2}\right] = \frac{hc}{2\lambda_0} \text{ or } V' = V_0 - \frac{hc}{2e\lambda_0}$$

9. (a) Here, $u = 0$; $a = \frac{eE}{m}$; $v = ?$; $t = t$

$$\therefore \quad v = u + at = 0 + \frac{eE}{m}t$$

de-Broglie wavelength, $\lambda = \frac{h}{mv} = \frac{h}{m(eEt/m)} = \frac{h}{eEt}$

Rate of change of de-Broglie wavelength

$$\frac{d\lambda}{dt} = \frac{h}{eE}\left(-\frac{1}{t^2}\right) = \frac{-h}{eEt^2}$$

10. (d) Energy $= \frac{hc}{\lambda} = \frac{6.6\times10^{-34}\times3\times10^8}{0.5\times10^{-10}}$ J

$$= \frac{6.6\times10^{-34}\times3\times10^8}{5\times10^{-11}\times1.6\times10^{-19}} \text{eV} = 24.82 \text{ keV}$$

11. (d) $\frac{1}{2}mv^2 = \frac{hc}{\lambda} - \frac{hc}{\lambda_0}$ Where λ is exciting wavelength,

λ_0 is threshold wavelength & v is speed of fastest electron.

12. (d) $I \propto \frac{1}{d^2}$

13. (a) Energy associated with wave.
Let number of quanta = x

$$5\% \text{ of } 100 = \frac{nhc}{\lambda}$$

$$\Rightarrow 100 \times \frac{5}{100} = \frac{n\times6.26\times10^{-34}\times3\times10^{-8}}{5.6\times10^{-7}}$$

$$\Rightarrow n = \frac{5}{3.35\times10^{-19}} \Rightarrow n = 1.4\times10^{19}$$

14. (c) $\lambda = \frac{h}{mv}$, $v = \frac{m_0}{\sqrt{1-\left(\frac{v}{c}\right)^2}}$, $v \to c$, $m \to \infty$

hence, $\lambda \to 0$.

15. (c) $h\upsilon = W_{ex}$ + maximum kinetic energy
$h\upsilon_0 = 8 \text{ eV} = W_{ex} + 2 \text{ eV} \Rightarrow W_{ex} = 6$ eV
For incoming radiation, energy is
$h \times 1.25\,\upsilon_0 = 10$ eV, $W_{ex} = 6$ eV
$\therefore$ Kinetic energy (maximum) = 4 eV.

16. (a) $eV = \frac{1}{2}mv^2$

$$\Rightarrow v = \sqrt{\frac{2eV}{m}} = \sqrt{\frac{2\times1.6\times10^{-19}\times20}{9.1\times10^{-31}}}$$

$$= 2.65\times10^6 \text{ m/s}$$

17. (a) $\because \lambda_0 = \frac{hc}{\phi}$

$$\therefore (\lambda_0)_{sodium} = \frac{6.6\times10^{-34}\times3\times10^8}{2\times1.6\times10^{-19}} = 6188 \text{ Å}$$

$$\because \lambda_0 \propto \frac{1}{\phi} \Rightarrow \frac{(\lambda_0)_{sodium}}{(\lambda_0)_{copper}} = \frac{(\phi)_{copper}}{(\phi)_{sodium}}$$

$$\Rightarrow (\lambda_0)_{copper} = \frac{2}{4}\times6188 = 3094 \text{ Å}$$

To eject photo-electrons from sodium the longest wavelength is 6188 Å and that for copper is 3094 Å. Hence for light of wavelength 4000 Å, sodium is suitable.

18. (c) $\frac{I_0}{I} = 4$, x = 7mm (given)

$$\Rightarrow \mu = \frac{2.303 \log_{10}\frac{I_0}{I}}{x}$$

$$\mu = \frac{2.303\log_{10}4}{7} = \frac{2.303\times0.6023}{7}$$

$\mu = 0.198 \text{ mm}^{-1}$

19. (b) According to Bragg's law, $\Rightarrow 2d\sin\theta = n\lambda$,
n = 1 for first order
$\Rightarrow 2\times2.82\sin15.8 = \lambda \Rightarrow \lambda = 5.64\times0.2723 = 1.53$ Å

20. (c) $\lambda_{max.} = \frac{2d\sin\theta}{n_{min.}} = \frac{2\times15\times\sin90^\circ}{1} = 30\text{Å}$

21. (d) The electron ejected with maximum speed v_{max} are stopped by electric field E = 4N/C after travelling a distance d = 1m

$$\frac{1}{2}mv_{max}^2 = eEd = 4eV$$

The energy of incident photon $= \frac{1240}{200} = 6.2$ eV

From equation of photo electric effect

$\frac{1}{2}mv_{max}^2 = h\nu - \phi_0$

$\therefore \phi_0 = 6.2 - 4 = 2.2$ eV

22. (b) $E = W_0 + eV_0$

For hydrogen atom, $E = +13.6$ eV

$\therefore +13.6 = 4.2 + eV_0$

$\Rightarrow V_0 = \frac{(13.6-4.2)eV}{e} = 9.4V$

Potential at anode $= -9.4$ V

23. (a) Energy emitted/sec by $S_1, P_1 = n_1 \frac{hc}{\lambda_1}$

Energy emitted/sec by $S_2, P_2 = n_2 \frac{hc}{\lambda_2}$

$\therefore \frac{P_2}{P_1} = \frac{n_2}{n_1} \cdot \frac{\lambda_1}{\lambda_2}$

$= \frac{1.02 \times 10^{15}}{10^{15}} \cdot \frac{5000}{5100} = 1.0$

24. (d) $K_{max} = \frac{hc}{\lambda} - W = \frac{hc}{\lambda} - 5.01 = \frac{12375}{\lambda(\text{in Å})} - 5.01$

$= \frac{12375}{2000} - 5.01 = 6.1875 - 5.01 = 1.17775 \simeq 1.2$ V

25. (c) The stopping potential is equal to maximum kinetic energy.

26. (a) The de-Broglie's wavelength associated with the moving electron $\lambda = \frac{h}{P}$

Now, according to problem

$\frac{d\lambda}{\lambda} = -\frac{dp}{P}$

$\frac{0.5}{100} = \frac{P}{P'}$

$P' = 200P$

27. (a) Give that, only 25% of 200W converter electrical energy into light of yellow colour

$\left(\frac{hc}{\lambda}\right) \times N = 200 \times \frac{25}{100}$

Where N is the No. of photons emitted per second, h = plank's constant, c, speed of light.

$N = \frac{200 \times 25}{100} \times \frac{\lambda}{hc}$

$= \frac{200 \times 25 \times 0.6 \times 10^{-6}}{100 \times 6.2 \times 10^{-34} \times 3 \times 10^8}$

$= 1.5 \times 10^{20}$

28. (c) $n \to 2 - 1$

$E = 10.2$ eV

$kE = E - \phi$

$Q = 10.20 - 3.57$

$h\upsilon_0 = 6.63$ eV

$\upsilon_0 = \frac{6.63 \times 1.6 \times 10^{-19}}{6.67 \times 10^{-34}} = 1.6 \times 10^{15}$ Hz

29. (c) $\lambda = \frac{h}{\sqrt{2mE}}$ So $h \propto \frac{1}{\sqrt{m}}$

since $m_\alpha > m_n > m_p > m_e$

so de-Broglie wave length in increasing order will be λ_d, λ_m, λ_p, λ_e

30. (d) As λ is increased, there will be a value of λ above which photoelectrons will be cease to come out so photocurrent will become zero. Hence (d) is correct answer.

31. (a) We know that $P = Fv$ or $F = P/v$

$F = \frac{0.5}{3 \times 10^8} = 0.166 \times 10^{-8} N/m^2$

32. (a) Accelerating voltage $= \frac{hc}{\lambda} \times e$

$= \frac{6.6 \times 10^{-34} \times 3 \times 10^8 \times 1.6 \times 10^{-19}}{10^{-11}}$

$= 123.75$ KV < 124 KV

33. (b) $(E_2 - E_1) = h\nu = \frac{hc}{\lambda}$

$\therefore \frac{hc}{\lambda_1} = (E_C - E_B), \frac{hc}{\lambda_2} = (E_B - E_A)$

and $\frac{hc}{\lambda_3} = (E_C - E_A)$

Now,

$(E_C - E_A) = (E_C - E_B) + (E_B - E_A)$

or, $\frac{hc}{\lambda_3} = \frac{hc}{\lambda_1} + \frac{hc}{\lambda_2}$ or $\frac{1}{\lambda_3} = \frac{1}{\lambda_1} + \frac{1}{\lambda_2}$

$\therefore \frac{1}{\lambda_3} = \frac{\lambda_1 + \lambda_2}{\lambda_1 \lambda_2}$ or $\lambda_3 = \frac{\lambda_1 \lambda_2}{\lambda_1 + \lambda_2}$

34. (a) No. of photons emitted per sec,

$n = \frac{\text{Power}}{\text{Energy of photon}}$

$= \frac{P}{h\nu} = \frac{10000}{6.6 \times 10^{-34} \times 880 \times 10^3}$

$= 1.72 \times 10^{31}$

35. (a) As $\lambda = \frac{h}{p}$ and $\lambda = \frac{c}{\nu}$; so

$\nu = \frac{c}{\lambda} = \frac{cP}{h} = 3 \times 10^8 \times \frac{3.3 \times 10^{-29}}{6.6 \times 10^{-34}}$

$= 1.5 \times 10^{13}$ Hz

36. (a) Rms speed of gas molecule, $V_{rms} = \sqrt{\frac{3kT}{m}}$

de Broglie wavelength, $\lambda = \frac{h}{p} = \frac{h}{\sqrt{2mk}}$

$$\therefore \lambda = \frac{h}{\sqrt{2m \times \frac{1}{2} m V_{rms}^2}} = \frac{h}{\sqrt{m \times \frac{3}{2} kT}} = \frac{h}{\sqrt{3mkT}}$$

Substituting the respective values we get

$$\lambda = \frac{6.63 \times 10^{-34}}{\sqrt{3 \times 4.64 \times 10^{-26} \times 1.38 \times 10^{-13} \times 400}} = 0.24\text{Å}$$

37. (d)

38. (d) Acceleration of electron in electric field, $a = \frac{eE}{m}$

Using equation

$v = u + at$

$$\Rightarrow \quad v = 0 + \frac{eE}{m} t$$

$$\Rightarrow \quad v = \frac{eEt}{m} \qquad \text{..... (i)}$$

De-broglie wavelength λ is given by

$$\lambda = \frac{h}{mv} = \frac{h}{m\left(\frac{eEt}{m}\right)} \qquad \text{[using (i)]}$$

$$\Rightarrow \quad \lambda = \frac{h}{eEt}$$

Differentiating w.r.t. t

$$\frac{d\lambda}{dt} = \frac{d\left(\frac{h}{eEt}\right)}{dt} \Rightarrow \frac{d\lambda}{dt} = \frac{-h}{eEt^2}$$

39. (c)

40. (b) $P_1 - P_2 = (P_1 + P_2) = P$

As $P \propto \frac{1}{\lambda}$

or $\frac{1}{\lambda_x} - \frac{1}{\lambda_y} = \frac{1}{\lambda}$

or $\frac{\lambda_y - \lambda_x}{\lambda_x \lambda_y} = \frac{1}{\lambda}$

41. (c) de Broglie wavelength (λ) is given by

K = qV

$$\lambda = \frac{h}{p} = \frac{h}{\sqrt{2mK}} = \frac{h}{\sqrt{2mqV}} \left(\because p = \sqrt{2mK}\right)$$

Substituting the values we get

$$\therefore \frac{\lambda_A}{\lambda_B} = \frac{\sqrt{2m_B q_B V_B}}{\sqrt{2m_A q_A V_A}} = \sqrt{\frac{4m.q.2500}{m.q.50}}$$

$$= 2\sqrt{50} = 2 \times 7.07 = 14.14$$

42. (d) de-Broglie wavelength,

$$\lambda = \frac{h}{mv} = 10^{-3}\left(\frac{3 \times 10^8}{6 \times 10^{14}}\right) \qquad \left[\because \lambda = \frac{c}{v}\right]$$

$$v = \frac{6.63 \times 10^{-34} \times 6 \times 10^{14}}{9.1 \times 10^{-31} \times 3 \times 10^5}$$

$v = 1.45 \times 10^6$ m/s

43. (a) Using Einstein's photoelectric equation,

$E = \omega_0 + KE_{max}$

$\Rightarrow \omega_0 = KE_{max} - E$

$$p = \sqrt{2mKE} \Rightarrow KE = \frac{p^2}{2m}$$

$$r = \frac{p}{eB} \Rightarrow p = reB$$

$$K_{max} = \frac{r^2 e^2 B^2}{2m} \qquad KE_{max} = \frac{12420}{\lambda} - \omega_0$$

$$\Rightarrow \omega_0 = \frac{12420}{6561} - \frac{r^2 eB^2}{2m} (In\, \text{eV})$$

$$= 1.89(eV) - \frac{\left(10^{-4}\right)\left(1.6 \times 10^{-19}\right) 9 \times 10^5}{2 \times 9.07 \times 10^{-31}}$$

$$= 1.89(eV) - \frac{\left(10^{-4}\right)\left(1.6 \times 10^{-19}\right) 9 \times 10^5}{2 \times 9.07 \times 10^{-31}}$$

$= (1.89 - 0.79)\, eV = 1.1\, eV$

44. (a) de-Broglie wavelength (λ),

Momentum, $mv = \frac{h}{\lambda} = p = \sqrt{2m(KE)}$

$$\therefore \lambda = \frac{h}{\sqrt{2mKE}} \Rightarrow \lambda \propto \frac{1}{\sqrt{KE}}$$

$$\therefore \frac{\lambda_A}{\lambda_B} = \sqrt{\frac{K_B}{K_A}} = \sqrt{\frac{T_A - 1.5}{T_A}} \qquad \text{(as given)}$$

Also, $\frac{\lambda_A}{\lambda_B} = \frac{1}{2}$

On solving we get, $T_A = 2\, eV$

$\therefore KE_B = T_A - 1.5 = 2 - 1.5 = 0.5\, eV$

∴ Work function of metal B is

$\phi_B = E_B - KE_B = 4.5 - 0.5 = 4\, eV$

45. (b) $f_0 = 4 \times 10^{14}$ Hz

$W_0 = hf_0 = 6.63 \times 10^{-34} \times (4 \times 10^{14})$ J

$$= \frac{(6.63 \times 10^{-34}) \times (4 \times 10^{14})}{1.6 \times 10^{-19}}$$

$= 1.66$ eV

27 Atoms

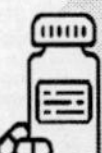

Topic 27.1 : Thomson's Atomic Model, Rutherford Alpha-Particle Scattering Experiment and Nuclear Model of Atom

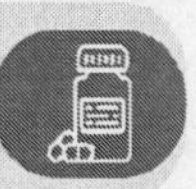

THOMSON'S ATOMIC MODEL

This model suggests an atom to be a tiny sphere of radius $\approx 10^{-10}$ m, containing the positive charge. The atom is electrically neutral. It contains an equal negative charge in the form of electrons, which are embedded randomly in this sphere, like seeds in a watermelon.

This model failed to explain (i) large scattering angle of α-particle and (ii) origin of spectral lines observed in the spectrum of hydrogen atom.

RUTHERFORD ALPHA-PARTICLE SCATTERING EXPERIMENT AND NUCLEAR MODEL OF ATOM

In Rutherford α- particle scattering experiment a very fine beam of α-particle passes through a small hole in the lead screen. This well collimated beam is then allowed to fall on a thin gold foil. While passing through the gold foil, α-particles are scattered through different angles. A zinc sulphide screen is placed out the other side of the gold foil, this screen is movable, so as to receive the α-particles, scattered from the gold foil at angles varying from 0 to 180°. When an α-particle strikes the screen, it produces a flash of light.

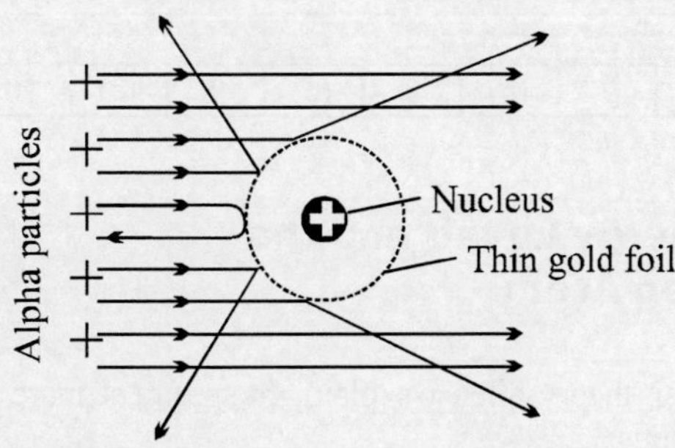

It was found that :

- Most of the α-particles went straight through the gold foil and produced flashes on the screen as if there were nothing inside gold foil. This suggests that *the most part of the atom is empty*.
- Few particles collided with the atoms of the foil which have scattered or deflected through considerable large angles. Very few particles even turned back towards source itself.

Conclusions :

- *The entire positive charge and almost whole mass of the atom is concentrated in small centre called a nucleus.*
- *The electrons revolving round the nucleus* could not deflected the path of α-particles. This suggests that electrons are very light.

In 1911 Rutherford , proposed a new type of model of the atom. According to this model, the positive charge of the atom, instead of being uniformly distributed throughout a sphere of atomic dimension is concentrated in a very small volume at its centre. This central core, called **nucleus**, is surrounded by clouds of electrons makes the entire atom electrically neutral.

According to Rutherford scattering formula, the number of α-particles scattered at angle θ by a target,

$$N \propto \text{cosec}^4 (\theta/2)$$

α

b

Nucleus

Impact parameter $b = \dfrac{2Ze^2 \cot(\theta/2)}{4\pi\varepsilon_0 m v_0^2}$

Distance of closest approach

$$r_0 = \frac{2Zeq}{4\pi\varepsilon_0 m v_0^2} = \frac{2(Ze)(2e)}{4\pi\varepsilon_0 m v_0^2}$$

Result of Rutherford scattering experiment : Nucleus- is central, massive, positively charged core, its size of the order of 10^{-15} m, number of electrons surrounding nucleus is such that atom is electrically neutral.

Unit for nuclear dimension measurement : 1 fermi = 10^{-15}m.

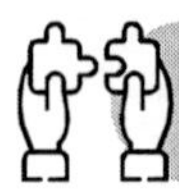

27.1 Concept Practice Problems

CPP

1. In a Rutherford experiment, the number of particles scattered at 90° angle are 28 per minute then number of scattered particles at an angle 60° and 120° will be
   (a) 117 per minute, 25 per minute
   (b) 50 per minute, 12.5 per minute
   (c) 100 per minute, 200 per minute
   (d) 112 per minute, 12.4 per minute
2. The following statements are all true. Which one did Rutherford consider to be supported by the results of experiments in which α-particles were scattered by gold foil?
   (a) The nucleus of an atom is held together by forces which are much stronger than electrical or gravitational forces.
   (b) The force of repulsion between an atomic nucleus and an α-particle varies with distance according to inverse square law.
   (c) α-particles are nuclei of Helium atoms.
   (d) Atoms can exist with a series of discrete energy levels.
3. According to the Rutherford's atomic model, the electrons inside the atom are
   (a) stationary (b) not stationary
   (c) centralized (d) None of these
4. According to classical theory, the circular path of an electron in Rutherford atom is
   (a) spiral (b) circular
   (c) parabolic (d) straight line
5. Rutherford's α-particle experiment showed that the atoms have
   (a) Proton (b) Nucleus
   (c) Neutron (d) Electrons
6. The Rutherford α-particle experiment shows that most of the α-particles pass through almost unscattered while some are scattered through large angles. What information does it give about the structure of the atom?
   (a) Atom is hollow.
   (b) The whole mass of the atom is concentrated in a small centre called nucleus
   (c) Nucleus is positively charged
   (d) All the above
7. In Rutherford scattering experiment, the number of α-particles scattered at 60° is 5×10^6. The number of α-particles scattered at 120° will be
   (a) 15×10^6 (b) $\frac{3}{5} \times 10^6$
   (c) $\frac{5}{9} \times 10^6$ (d) None of these
8. An alpha nucleus of energy $\frac{1}{2}mv^2$ bombards a heavy nuclear target of charge Ze. Then the distance of closest approach for the alpha nucleus will be proportional to
   (a) $\frac{1}{Ze}$ (b) v^2 (c) $\frac{1}{m}$ (d) $\frac{1}{v^4}$
9. In the Rutherford experiment, α-particles are scattered from a nucleus as shown. Out of the four paths, which path is not possible?

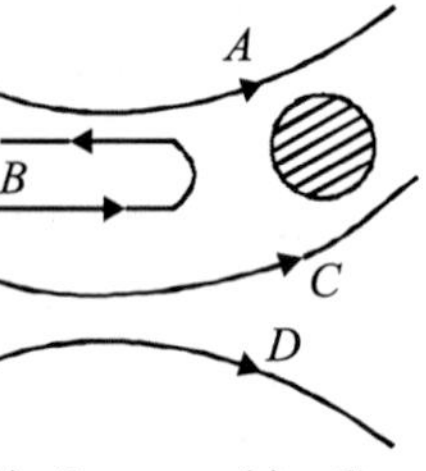

   (a) D (b) B (c) C (d) A
10. An α-particle of energy 5 MeV is scattered through 180° by a fixed uranium nucleus. The distance of closest approach is of the order of
   (a) 10^{-12} cm (b) 10^{-10} cm
   (c) 10^{-14} cm (d) 10^{-15} cm

ANSWER KEY

1	(d)	2	(b)	3	(b)	4	(a)	5	(b)	6	(d)	7	(c)	8	(c)	9	(c)	10	(a)

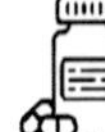

Topic 27.2 : Bohr's Atomic Model, Energy Levels and the Lines Spectra of Hydrogen Atom

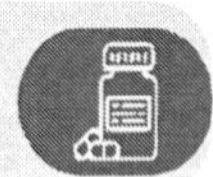

BOHR'S ATOMIC (HYDROGEN ATOM) MODEL

In 1913 Bohr gave his atomic theory primarily to explain, the spectra of hydrogen and hydrogen-like atoms. His theory, contained a combination of views from Plank's quantum theory, Einstein's photon concept and Rutherford model of atom. The Bohr theory can explain, the atomic spectra of hydrogen atom and hydrogen-like ions such as He^+, Li^{2+}, Be^{3+}.......(one electron ions). But his theory failed to explain, the spectra of more complex atom and ions.

The basic postulates of Bohr's model are :

(i) The electron moves in circular orbits around the nucleus under the influence of coulombic force of attraction between the electron and the positively charged nucleus (as shown in figure below).

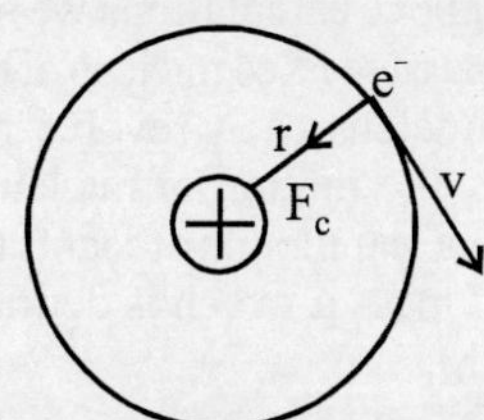

Bohr's model of hydrogen atom

(ii) The electron rotates about the nucleus in certain stationary circular orbits, for which the angular momentum of electron about the nucleus is an integral multiple of $\frac{h}{2\pi} = \hbar$, where h is plank's constant

i.e., Angular Momentum, $mvr = \frac{nh}{2\pi} = n\hbar$ ...(1)

(where n = 1, 2, 3......... principal quantum number)

(iii) When the electron is in one of its stationary orbits, it does not radiate energy, hence the atom is stable. These stationary orbits are called allowed orbits.

(iv) The atom radiates energy when the electron "jumps" from one allowed stationery state to another. The frequency of radiation follows the condition

$h\nu = E_i - E_f$ ...(2)

Where E_i and E_f are total energies of initial and final stationary states. This difference in energy (E_i - E_f) between two allowed stationory states is radiated/absorbed in the form of a packet of electromagnetic energy ($h\nu$ - one photon of frequency ν) called a photon.

Now we calculate the allowed energies of hydrogen atom, For moving an electron in a circular orbit the required centripetal force is provided by the coulomb force of attraction which acts between nucleus [Ze^+, here Z = 1 (atomic number) for hydrogen atom] & electron (e^-),

i.e., $\frac{mv^2}{r} = \frac{k\,e^2}{r^2}$ ...(3)

where $k = \frac{1}{4\pi\varepsilon_o}$ is electrostatic constant & ε_o is permittivity of free space.

Eliminating v from eqn. (1) and (3) we obtain radius of nth orbit

$$r = \frac{n^2h^2}{mke^2} = \frac{\varepsilon_o n^2 h^2}{\pi m e^2} \text{ (where n = 1, 2, 3 .....)} \quad ...(4)$$

Equation (4) gives the radii of various orbits (have discrete values).

The **smallest radius** (also called **Bohr radius**) corresponds to $n = 1$ is

$$r_0 = \frac{h^2}{mke^2} \cong 0.527 \text{Å} \quad ...(5)$$

$\Rightarrow$ r = 0.529 n^2 Å for hydrogen atom and

$r = 0.529 \times \frac{n^2}{Z}$ for hydrogen like ions.

From equation (4) & (1) we obtain,

Velocity of electron in n^{th} state

$$v^2 = \frac{n^2\hbar^2}{m^2r^2} = \frac{k^2e^4}{n^2\hbar^2} \Rightarrow v = \frac{ke^2}{n\hbar}$$

$$\text{or } v = \frac{e^2}{2\varepsilon_o nh} = \left(\frac{C}{137}\right) \times \frac{1}{n} \text{ (for hydrogen atom)} \quad ...(6)$$

$v = \left(\frac{C}{137}\right)\frac{Z}{n}$ *for hydrogen like ions*

$\frac{C}{137} = 2.19 \times 10^6 \, ms^{-1}$

The **total energy of electron** is given by

E = K.E. + P.E. = Kinetic energy + Potential energy

$= \frac{1}{2}mv^2 + \frac{ke(-e)}{r}$

$$E = \frac{-ke^2}{2r} = \frac{-me^4}{8\varepsilon_o n^2 h^2} \quad ...(7)$$

(Allowed energy state)

After substituting numerical values in eqn.(7), we obtain

$$E = \frac{-13.6}{n^2} eV \quad \textit{(for hydrogen atom)} \quad ...(8)$$

$E = \frac{-13.6Z^2}{n^2}$ eV/atom *for hydrogen like ions.*

The **lowest energy state, or ground state**, corresponds to n = 1 is

$$E_0 = \frac{-me^4}{8\varepsilon_o h^2} = -13.6 eV$$

The next state corresponds to n = 2 i.e., first excited state has an energy, E = –3.4 eV

Limitations of Bohr's Model

1. It could not explain the spectra of atoms containing more than one electron.
2. There was no theoretical basis for selecting mvr to be an integral multiple of $h/2\pi$.
3. It involved the orbit concept which could not be checked experimentally.
4. It could not explain Zeeman & Stark effect and fine lines of spectra.
5. It was against de-Broglie concept and uncertainty principle.

Problem Solving Tips

1. Total energy of electron = – Kinetic energy $= \frac{\text{Potential energy}}{2}$
2. The reference level for potential energy has been taken as infinity
3. The energy gap between two successive levels decreases as the value of n increases
4. The radius difference between the successive orbit (or shells) increases as the value of n increases

5. The velocity of electrons around the nucleus goes on decreasing as n increases
6. The time period of the electron in an orbit $T^2 \propto r^3$
7. Maximum number of spectral lines that can be emitted when an electron jumps from n^{th} orbit is $\frac{n(n-1)}{2}$

ENERGY LEVELS AND THE LINES SPECTRA OF HYDROGEN ATOM

An energy level diagram of the hydrogen atom is shown in figure. The upper most level corresponding to $n \to \infty$, represents the state for which the electron is completely removed from the atom.

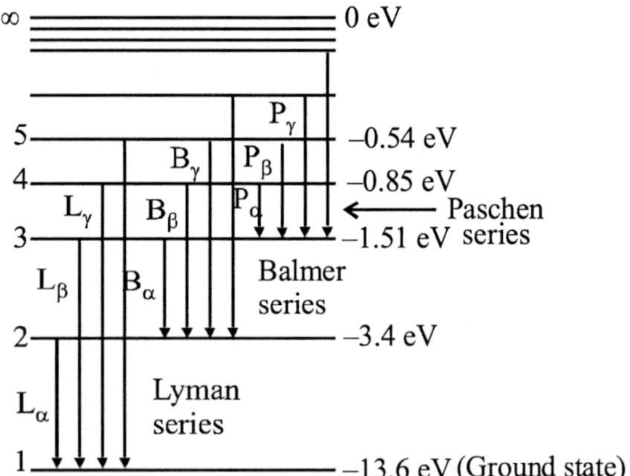

Some transitions for Lyman, Balmer & Paschen series are shown. The quantum numbers are at left & energies of levels are at right. E = 0 for r = ∞ (Since n = ∞)

If the electron jumps from allowed state n_i to allowed state n_f, then **frequency of emitted photon** is given by

$$\nu = \frac{E_f - E_i}{h} = \frac{me^4}{8\varepsilon_o h^3}\left(\frac{1}{n_i^2} - \frac{1}{n_f^2}\right) \quad ...(1)$$

and the **wavelength of emitted photon** is

$$\frac{1}{\lambda} = \frac{\nu}{c} = \frac{me^4}{8\varepsilon_o ch^3}\left(\frac{1}{n_i^2} - \frac{1}{n_f^2}\right)$$

$$\frac{1}{\lambda} = R\left(\frac{1}{n_i^2} - \frac{1}{n_f^2}\right) \text{ for hydrogen atom} \quad ...(2)$$

and $\bar{\nu} = \frac{1}{\lambda} = RZ^2\left[\frac{1}{n_1^2} - \frac{1}{n_2^2}\right]$ (*for H-like atoms*)

where $R = 1.096776 \times 10^7 m^{-1}$ is known as Rydberg constant. By using this expression we can calculate the wavelengths for various series (Lyman, Balmer...) in hydrogen spectrum, i.e.

(i) Lyman series $n_i = 1$ & $n_f = 2, 3, 4$...............
(ii) Balmer series $n_i = 2$, & $n_f = 3, 4, 5$..............
(iii) Paschen series $n_i = 3$ & $n_f = 4, 5, 6$..............
(iv) Bracett series $n_i = 4$ & $n_f = 5, 6, 7$..............
(v) P fund series $n_i = 5$ & $n_f = 6, 7, 8$...............

First three series of hydrogen atom are shown in figure.

But in practice, the value of Rydberg constant varies between $\frac{R}{2}$ and R

This is because in above calculations we assumed that electron revolves around a massive fixed nucleus of mass M. But in reality, the electron and nucleus each revolve round their common center of mass i.e., the motion of nucleus cannot be ignored. The correction for nuclear motion amounts to replacing electronic mass m by reduced mass μ which is defined as

$$\mu = \frac{mM}{m+M} \quad ...(3)$$

So total energy by taking this correction is

$$E = \frac{-\mu e^4}{8\varepsilon_o^2 h^2 n^2} \quad ...(4)$$

If we are dealing with hydrogen like ions such as – He^+, Li^{2+}, Be^{3+}, Be^{4+} (one electron ions), each can be considered as a system of two charges, the electron of mass m & charge –e & nucleus of mass M and charge +Ze, where Z is atomic number. The radii of circular orbits for these one electron ions can be written as

$$r = \frac{\varepsilon_o n^2 h^2}{\pi\mu Ze^2} = \frac{n^2\hbar^2}{\mu kZe^2} \text{ (n = 1, 2, 3............)} \quad ...(5)$$

and the allowed energies are given by

$$E \cong \frac{-\mu Z^2 e^4}{8\varepsilon_o h^2 n^2} \text{ (n = 1, 2, 3.........)} \quad ...(6)$$

Wavelength Limits in Various Spectral Series of Hydrogen Atom

(i) For **Lyman series (lies in ultraviolet region)**
$\lambda_{max} = 1216$ Å, $\lambda_{min} = 912$ Å
Here $n_i = 1$, $n_f = 2, 3$..............

(ii) For **Balmer series (lies in visible region)**
$\lambda_{max} = 6563$ Å and $\lambda_{min} = 3646$ Å
Here $n_i = 2$, $n_f = 3, 4, 5$...............

(iii) For **Paschen series (lies in infrared region)**
$\lambda_{max} = 18751$ Å and $\lambda_{min} = 8107$ Å
Here $n_i = 3$, $n_f = 4, 5, 6$...............

(iv) For **Brackett series (lies in infrared region)**
$\lambda_{max} = 40477$ Å and $\lambda_{min} = 14572$ Å
Here $n_i = 4$, $n_f = 5, 6, 7$...............

(v) For **p-fund series (lies in infrared region)**
$\lambda_{max} = 74515$ Å and $\lambda_{min} = 22768$ Å
Here $n_i = 5$, $n_f = 6, 7, 8$..............

Problem Solving Tips

1. The first line of Lyman series is when electron jumps from $2 \to 1$, It is also called α – line
   The second line of lyman series is when electron jumps from $3 \to 1$, It is also called β – line
   The limiting line of lyman series is when electron jumps from $\infty \to 1$
2. Energy of electrons in different orbits in an atom varies inversely with the square of the number of orbits. So, energy of electrons increases (decreases in negative) as the orbit becomes higher.
3. If energy of a particular orbit is E for H-atom then its value for a H-like atom with atomic number Z is given by $E' = E \times Z^2$.

4. If the radius of a particular orbit of H-atom is R then its valu for a H-like atom is given by

$$R' = \frac{R}{Z}.$$

5. If velocity of an electron in a particular orbit of H-atom be v then its value for a H-like atom is given by

$$v' = v \times Z.$$

6. If kinetic energy and potential energy of an electron in a particular orbit of H-atom be T and V respectively then their corresponding values for H-like atom are given by $T' = T \times Z^2$ and $V' = V \times Z^2$.

MISCONCEPTION

✗ *Incorrect.* Bohr's formula for spectral lines does not differentiate between isotopes. For example the first line of Lyman series in hydrogen and deuterium will have same wavelength because

$$\frac{1}{\lambda} = R(1^2)\left[\frac{1}{1^2} - \frac{1}{2^2}\right]$$

✓ *Correct.* The value of R will be different for hydrogen and deuterium and therefore λ will be different for the two cases. In fact $\lambda_D < \lambda_H$ ($\because R_D > R_H$)

Example 1.

A hydrogen atom in the ground state is excited by radiations of wavelength 975Å. Find (a) the energy state to which the atom is excited. (b) how many lines will be possible in emission spectrum ?

Solution :

(a) $\lambda = 975\text{Å} = 975 \times 10^{-10}\,\text{m}$

$$\frac{1}{\lambda} = R\left[\frac{1}{1^2} - \frac{1}{n^2}\right]$$

$$\therefore \quad \frac{1}{975 \times 10^{-10}} = 1.1 \times 10^{-7}\left[\frac{1}{1^2} - \frac{1}{n^2}\right]$$

or $n = 4$

(b) $\because$ Number of spectral lines $(N) = \dfrac{n(n-1)}{2}$

$$\therefore \quad N = \frac{4 \times (4-1)}{2} = 6$$

Possible transition

$4 \to 3, 4 \to 2, 4 \to 1, 3 \to 2, 3 \to 1, 2 \to 1.$

Example 2.

Find the longest and shortest wavelength when a hydrogen atom in the ground state is excited by radiations of wavelength 975Å.

Solution :

$$\lambda = \frac{hc}{eE} \approx \frac{12400}{E\,(eV)}\text{Å}\left[\because h = 6.6 \times 10^{-34}\,Js; C = 3 \times 10^8\,\text{m/s}\right]$$

$\therefore$ For longest wavelength

$$\lambda_{max} = \frac{12400}{E_{4\to3}} = \frac{12400}{0.66} = 18787.8\ \text{Å}$$

For smallest wavelength

$$\lambda_{min} = \frac{hc}{eE} = \frac{12400}{E_{4\to1}} = \frac{12400}{12.75} \approx 973\ \text{Å}$$

Example 3.

If the wavelength of the first line of the Lyman series for the hydrogen atom is 1210 Å, then what will be the wavelength of the first line of the Balmer series of the hydrogen spectrum?

Solution :

We know that, $\dfrac{1}{\lambda} = R\left[\dfrac{1}{n_1^2} - \dfrac{1}{n_2^2}\right]$

For first line of Lyman series, $n_1 = 1$ and $n_2 = 2$

$$\therefore \quad \frac{1}{\lambda_1} = R\left[\frac{1}{1} - \frac{1}{4}\right] = \frac{3R}{4} \text{ or } R = \frac{4}{3\lambda_1}$$

For first line of Balmer series $n_1 = 2$ and $n_2 = 3$

$$\therefore \quad \frac{1}{\lambda_2} = R\left[\frac{1}{4} - \frac{1}{9}\right] = \frac{5R}{36} = \frac{5}{36}\left[\frac{4}{3\lambda_1}\right]$$

$$\text{or, } \frac{1}{\lambda_2} = \frac{5}{36} \times \frac{4}{3} \times \frac{1}{1210}$$

$$\text{or, } \lambda_2 = \frac{36 \times 3 \times 1210}{5 \times 4} = 6434\,\text{Å}$$

Example 4.

If the electron in hydrogen atom jumps from the third orbit to second orbit, then find the wavelength of the emitted radiation.

Solution :

$$\frac{1}{\lambda} = R\left[\frac{1}{n_1^2} - \frac{1}{n_2^2}\right] \text{ or } \frac{1}{\lambda} = R\left[\frac{1}{4} - \frac{1}{9}\right] = \frac{5R}{36}$$

$$\therefore \quad \lambda = \frac{36}{5R}$$

Example 5 :

How many different wavelengths may be observed in the spectrum from a hydrogen sample if the atoms are excited to states with principal quantum number n ?

Solution :

From the nth state, the atom may go to (n – 1)th state, ..., 2nd state or 1st state. So there are (n – 1)th possible transitions starting from the *n* th sate. The atoms reaching (n – 1)th state may make (n – 2) different transitions. Similarly for other lower states, the total number of possible transitions are

$$(n-1) + (n-2) + (n-3) + ...2 + 1 = \frac{n(n-1)}{2}$$

Example 6.

In the hydrogen atom, an electron makes a transition from n = 2 to n = 1. The magnetic field produced by the circulating electron at the nucleus

(a) decreases 16 times *(b) increases 4 times*

(c) decreases 4 times *(d) increases 32 times*

Solution : (d)

$$\because \quad B = \frac{\mu_0 I}{2r} \text{ and } I = \frac{e}{T}$$

$$B = \frac{\mu_0 e}{2rT} \Rightarrow B \propto \frac{1}{n^5} \quad [\because r \propto n^2, T \propto n^5];$$

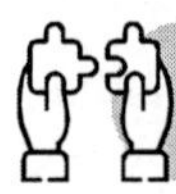

27.2 Concept Practice Problems

CPP

11. In an atom, the two electrons move round the nucleus in circular orbits of radii R and 4R. The ratio of the time taken by them to complete one revolution is

(a) 1/4 (b) 4/1 (c) 8/1 (d) 1/8

12. The angular speed of the electron in the nth orbit of Bohr hydrogen atom is

(a) directly proportional to n
(b) inversely proportional to $\sqrt{n}$
(c) inversely proportional to n^2
(d) inversely proportional to n^3

13. The ratio of the energies of the hydrogen atom in its first to second excited states is

(a) 1/4 (b) 4/9 (c) 9/4 (d) 4

14. According to Bohr's model of hydrogen atom

(a) the linear velocity of the electron is quantised.
(b) the angular velocity of the electron is quantised.
(c) the linear momentum of the electron is quantised.
(d) the angular momentum of the electron is quantised.

15. As the quantum number increases, the difference of energy between consecutive energy levels

(a) remain the same
(b) increases
(c) decreases
(d) sometimes increases and sometimes decreases.

16. According to the Bohr theory of H-atom, the speed of the electron, its energy and the radius of its orbit varies with the principal quantum number n, respectively, as

(a) $\frac{1}{n}, n^2, \frac{1}{n^2}$ (b) $n, \frac{1}{n^2}, n^2$
(c) $n, \frac{1}{n^2}, \frac{1}{n^2}$ (d) $\frac{1}{n}, \frac{1}{n^2}, n^2$

17. In a hydrogen atom following the Bohr's postulates the product of linear momentum and angular momentum is proportional to $(n)^x$ where 'n' is the orbit number. Then 'x' is

(a) 0 (b) 2 (c) –2 (d) 1

18. For the principal quantum number n = 4, the total number of different possible values of the azimuthal quantum number l, is

(a) 2 (b) 8 (c) 4 (d) 3

19. The angular momentum of the electron in hydrogen atom in the ground state is

(a) 2h (b) $\frac{h}{2}$ (c) $\frac{h}{2\pi}$ (d) $\frac{h}{4\pi}$

20. In which of the following series, does the 121.5 nm line of the spectrum of the hydrogen atom lie ?

(a) Lyman series (b) Balmer series
(c) Paschen series (d) Brackett series.

ANSWER KEY

11	(d)	12	(d)	13	(c)	14	(d)	15	(c)	16	(d)	17	(a)	18	(c)	19	(c)	20	(a)

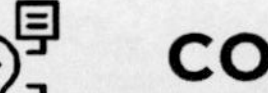

CONCEPT MAP

Model of atom

ATOMS
Consists of three elementary particles electrons, protons and neutrons

Bohr model of Hydrogen atom Electron can revolve only in those orbits in which angular momentum about the nucleus is an integral multiple of $\frac{h}{2\pi}$ i.e., $mvr = \frac{nh}{2\pi}$

J.J Thomson model of atom First model of atom plum pudding model- positive charge is uniformly distributed and negatively charged electrons are embedded in it like seeds in a watermelon

Rutherford nuclear model entire positive charge and most of the mass of the atom is concentrated in nucleus and electrons revolving around the nucleus

Drawbacks of Bohr model
- unable to explain the fine structure of spectral lines
- Valid only for single electron system

Various parameters

Radius of n-th or bit
$$r_n = \frac{n^2 h^2}{4\pi^2 KZe^2 m} = 0.53\frac{n^2}{Z}\text{Å}$$

Velocity of electron in n-th orbit
$$v_n = \frac{2\pi KZe^2}{nh} = 2.2 \times 10^6 \frac{Z}{n}\text{ m/s}$$

Potential energy (Un) in n-th orbit
$$U_n = \frac{-KZe^2}{r_n} = \frac{-27.2}{n^2}Z^2\text{ev}$$

Kinetic energy
$$E_k = \frac{KZe^2}{2r_n} = \frac{13.6Z^2}{n^2}\text{ev}$$

Rutherford α- particle scattering experiment Most of the α-particles passed through the gold foil i.e., atom has lot of empty space
- Only about 0.14% of the α-particles scatter by more than 1° and one α-particle in every 8000 α-particles deflected by > 90° positively charged particles protons confined to core called nucleus, size about 10^{-15} to 10^{-14} m

Number of a-particles scattered per unit area
$$N(\theta) \propto \frac{1}{\sin^4 \theta/2}$$

Impact parameter
$$b = \frac{1}{4\pi\epsilon_0}\frac{Ze^2 \cot\frac{\theta}{2}}{\frac{1}{2}mv^2}$$
θ = angle of scattering

Various series of line spectra of hydrogen atom

Lyman series
$$\overline{v} = \frac{1}{\lambda} = R\left[\frac{1}{1^2} - \frac{1}{n^2}\right]$$
n = 2, 3, 4.........
in uv-region

Balmer series
$$\overline{v} = \frac{1}{\lambda} = R\left[\frac{1}{2^2} - \frac{1}{n^2}\right]$$
n = 3, 4, 5
in visible region

In infra-red region

Paschem series
$$\overline{v} = \frac{1}{\lambda} = R\left[\frac{1}{3^2} - \frac{1}{n^2}\right]$$
n = 4, 5, 6, ...

Brackett series
$$\overline{v} = \frac{1}{\lambda} = R\left[\frac{1}{4^2} - \frac{1}{n^2}\right]$$
n = 5, 6, 7, ...

P-fond series
$$\overline{v} = \frac{1}{\lambda} = R\left[\frac{1}{5^2} - \frac{1}{n^2}\right]$$
n = 6, 7, 8, ...

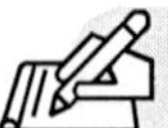

Exercise 1 - Chapter Revision Problems

CRP

1. With increasing quantum number, the energy difference between adjacent energy levels in atoms
(a) decreases
(b) increases
(c) remains constant
(d) decreases for low Z and increases for high Z

2. If e is electronic charge, the equivalent current for an electron revolving with a frequency n in the ground state of hydrogen atom is
(a) $2\pi ne$ (b) $\frac{e}{\pi n}$ (c) $\frac{e}{2\pi n}$ (d) en

3. In Millikan's oil drop experiment, an oil drop is observed to move vertically upward. The upward motion of the drop is due to
(a) gravity (b) viscosity
(c) buoyancy (d) electric field

4. The proof of quantization of energy states in an atom is obtained by the experiment performed by
(a) Thomson (b) Millikan
(c) Rutherford (d) Franck and Hertz

5. Line spectrum is obtained whenever the incandescent vapours at low pressure of the excited substance are in their
(a) atomic state (b) molecular state
(c) nuclear state (d) None of these

6. The principle of LASER action involves
(a) amplification of particular frequency emitted by the system
(b) population inversion
(c) stimulated emissin
(d) All of the above.

7. For the azimuthal quantum number $l = 3$, the total number of different possible values of the magnetic azimuthal quantum number m_l, is
(a) 3 (b) 4 (c) 5 (d) 7

8. The ratio between Bohr radii is
(a) 1 : 2 : 3 (b) 2 : 4 : 6 (c) 1 : 4 : 9 (d) 1 : 3 : 5

9. The kinetic energy of the electorn in an orbit of radius r in hydrogen atom is (e = electronic charge)
(a) $\frac{e^2}{r^2}$ (b) $\frac{e^2}{2r}$ (c) $\frac{e^2}{r}$ (d) $\frac{e^2}{2r^2}$

10. Electrons in the atom are held to the nucleus by
(a) coulomb's force (b) nuclear force
(c) vander waal's force (d) gravitational force

11. The angular momentum of electron in n^{th} orbit is given by
(a) nh (b) $\frac{h}{2\pi n}$ (c) $n\frac{h}{2\pi}$ (d) $n^2\frac{h}{2\pi}$

12. In a hypothetical Bohr hydrogen atom, the mass of the electron is doubled. The energy E_0' and radius r_0' of the first orbit will be (r_0 is the Bohr radius)
(a) –11.2 eV (b) –6.8 eV
(c) –13.6 eV (d) –27.2 eV

13. A 15.0 eV photon collides with and ionizes a hydrogen atom. If the atom was originally in the ground state (ionization potential = 13.6 eV), what is the kinetic energy of the ejected electron?
(a) 1.4 eV (b) 13.6 eV (c) 15.0 eV (d) 28.6 eV

14. The ratio of areas between the electron orbits for the first excited state to the ground state for the hydrogen atom is
(a) 2 : 1 (b) 4 : 1 (c) 8 : 1 (d) 16 : 1

15. The potential energy associated with an electron in the orbit
(a) increases with the increases in radii of the orbit
(b) decreases with the increase in the radii of the orbit
(c) remains the same with the change in the radii of the orbit
(d) None of these

16. A hydrogen atom emits a photon corresponding to an electron transition from n = 5 to n = 1. The recoil speed of hydrogen atom is almost
(a) $10^{-4}\,ms^{-1}$ (b) $2 \times 10^{-2}\,ms^{-1}$
(c) $4\,ms^{-1}$ (d) $8 \times 10^{2}\,ms^{-1}$

17. The approximate value of quantum number n for the circular orbit of hydrogen 0.0001 mm in diameter is
(a) 1000 (b) 60 (c) 10000 (d) 31

18. The ionization energy of Li^{++} is equal to
(a) 9hcR (b) 6hcR (c) 2hcR (d) hcR.

19. Which of the following series in the spectrum of hydrogen atom lies in the visible region of the electromagnetic spectrum?
(a) Paschen series (b) Balmer series
(c) Lyman series (d) Brackett series

20. The ratio of maximum to minimum wavelength in Balmer series is
(a) 3 : 4 (b) 1 : 4 (c) 5 : 36 (d) 5 : 9

21. What element has k_α line of wavelength 1.785 Å? $R = 109737\,cm^{-1}$.
(a) Platinum (b) Zinc (c) Iron (d) Cobalt

22. If the k_α radiation of Mo (Z = 42) has a wavelength of 0.71Å. Calculate the wavelength of the corresponding radiation of Cu (Z = 29).
(a) 1.52Å (b) 2.52Å (c) 0.52Å (d) 4.52Å

23. The extreme wavelengths of Paschen series are
(a) 0.365 μm and 0.565 μm (b) 0.818 μm and 1.89 μm
(c) 1.45 μm and 4.04 μm (d) 2.27 μm and 7.43 μm

24. The first line of Balmer series has wavelength 6563 Å. What will be the wavelength of the first member of Lyman series
(a) 1215.4 Å (b) 2500 Å (c) 7500 Å (d) 600 Å

25. Hydrogen atom excites energy level from fundamental state to n = 3. Number of spectral lines according to Bohr, is
(a) 4 (b) 3 (c) 1 (d) 2

26. The ratio of the longest to shortest wavelengths in Brackett series of hydrogen spectra is
(a) $\frac{25}{9}$ (b) $\frac{17}{6}$ (c) $\frac{9}{5}$ (d) $\frac{4}{3}$

27. The energy levels of the hydrogen spectrum is shown in figure. There are some transitions A, B, C, D and E. Transition A, B and C respectively represent

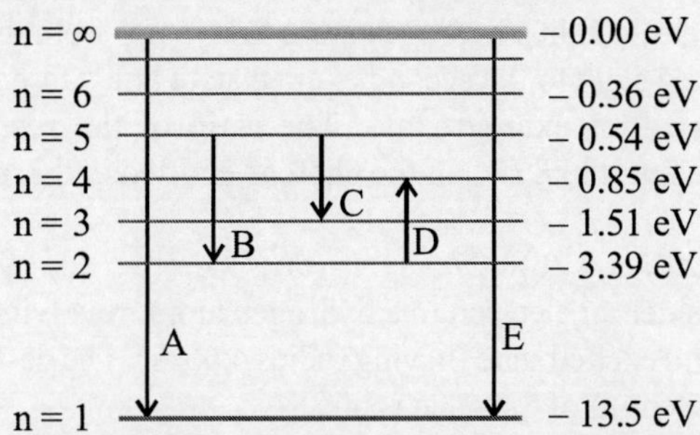

(a) first member of Lyman series, third spectral line of Balmer series and the second spectral line of Paschen series
(b) ionization potential of hydrogen, second spectral line of Balmer series, third spectral line of Paschen series
(c) series limit of Lyman series, third spectral line of Balmer series and second spectral line of Paschen series
(d) series limit of Lyman series, second spectral line of Balmer series and third spectral line of Paschen series

28. Which of the following statements are true regarding Bohr's model of hydrogen atom?
(I) Orbiting speed of electron decreases as it shifts to discrete orbits away from the nucleus
(II) Radii of allowed orbits of electron are proportional to the principal quantum number
(III) Frequency with which electrons orbit around the nucleus in discrete orbits is inversely proportional to the cube of principal quantum number
(IV) Binding force with which the electron is bound to the nucleus increases as it shifts to outer orbits
Select correct answer using the codes given below.
Codes :
(a) I and II (b) II and IV
(c) I, II and III (d) II, III and IV

29. If in hydrogen atom, radius of nth Bohr orbit is r_n, frequency of revolution of electron in n^{th} orbit is f_n, choose the correct option.

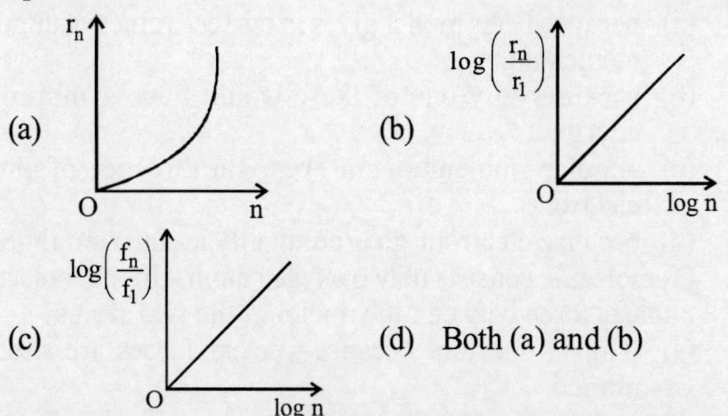

30. Excitation energy of a hydrogen like ion in its excitation state is 40.8 eV. Energy needed to remove the electron from the ion in ground state is
(a) 54.4 eV (b) 13.6 eV (c) 40.8 eV (d) 27.2 eV

31. The energy of electron in the nth orbit of hydrogen atom is expressed as $E_n = \frac{-13.6}{n^2}$ eV. The shortest and longest wavelength of Lyman series will be
(a) 910 Å, 1213 Å (b) 5463 Å, 7858 Å
(c) 1315 Å, 1530 Å (d) None of these

32. A hydrogen atom in its ground state absorbs 10.2 eV of energy. The orbital angular momentum is increased by
(a) 1.05×10^{-34} J-s (b) 3.16×10^{-34} J-s
(c) 2.11×10^{-34} J-s (d) 4.22×10^{-34} J-s

33. Taking Rydberg's constant $R_H = 1.097 \times 10^7$m, first and second wavelength of Balmer series in hydrogen spectrum is
(a) 2000 Å, 3000 Å (b) 1575 Å, 2960 Å
(c) 6529 Å, 4280 Å (d) 6552 Å, 4863 Å

34. If the atom ${}_{100}Fm^{257}$ follows the Bohr model and the radius of ${}_{100}Fm^{257}$ is *n* times the Bohr radius, then find *n*.
(a) 100 (b) 200 (c) 4 (d) 1/4

35. The energy of He^+ in the ground state is – 54.4 eV, then the energy of Li^{++} in the first excited state will be
(a) –30.6 eV (b) 27.2 eV
(c) –13.6 eV (d) –27.2 eV

36. A hydrogen atom is in ground state. Then to get six lines in emission spectrum, wavelength of incident radiation should be
(a) 800 Å (b) 825 Å (c) 975 Å (d) 1025 Å

37. In the hydrogen atom, an electron makes a transition from n = 2 to n = 1. The magnetic field produced by the circulating electron at the nucleus
(a) decreases 16 times (b) increases 4 times
(c) decreases 4 times (d) increases 32 times

38. Doubly ionised helium atom and hydrogen ions are accelerated, from rest, through the same potential difference. The ratio of final velocities of helium and hydrogen is
(a) $1:\sqrt{2}$ (b) $\sqrt{2}:1$ (c) $1:2$ (d) $2:1$

39. Which of the following transitions in hydrogen atoms emit photons of highest frequency?
(a) n = 1 to n = 2 (b) n = 2 to n = 6
(c) n = 6 to n = 2 (d) n = 2 to n = 1

40. The energy of a hydrogen atom in the ground state is – 13.6 *eV*. The energy of a He^+ ion in the first excited state will be
(a) –13.6 *eV* (b) –27.2 *eV*
(c) –54.4 *eV* (d) –6.8 *eV*

41. The graph which depicts the results of Rutherford gold foil experiment with α-particles is:
θ: Scattering angle
Y: Number of scattered α-particles detected
(Plots are schematic and not to scale)

(a)
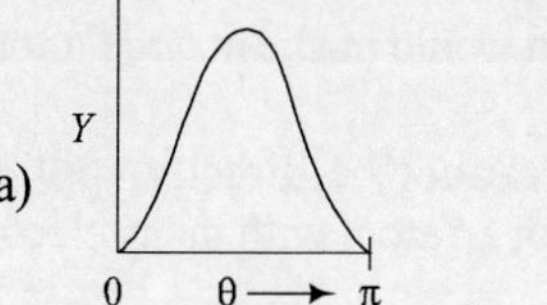

(b)
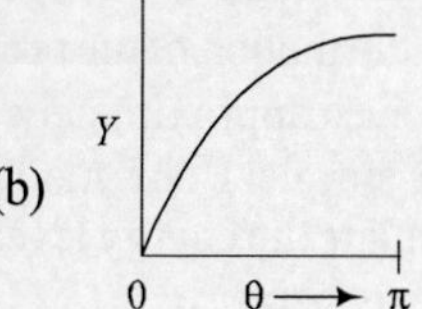

(c) 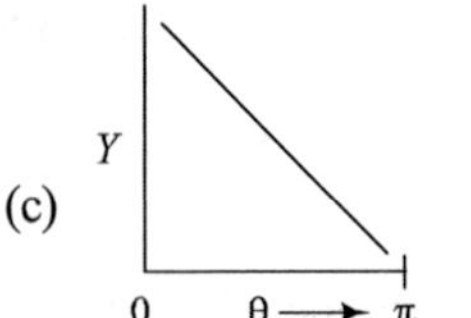

(d) 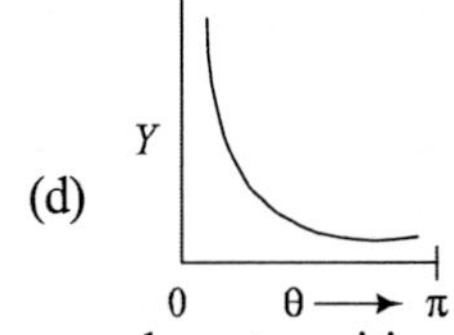

42. In a hydrogen atom the electron makes a transition from $(n+1)^{th}$ level to the nth level. If $n >> 1$, the frequency of radiation emitted is proportional to :

(a) $\frac{1}{n}$ (b) $\frac{1}{n^3}$ (c) $\frac{1}{n^2}$ (d) $\frac{1}{n^4}$

43. The energy required to ionise a hydrogen like ion in its ground state is 9 Rydbergs. What is the wavelength of the radiation emitted when the electron in this ion jumps from the second excited state to the ground state?

(a) 24.2 nm (b) 11.4 nm (c) 35.8 nm (d) 8.6 nm

44. The time period of revolution of electron in its ground state orbit in a hydrogen atom is 1.6×10^{-16} s. The frequency of revolution of the electron in its first excited state (in s^{-1}) is:

(a) 1.6×10^{14} (b) 7.8×10^{14}
(c) 6.2×10^{15} (d) 5.6×10^{12}

45. An excited He^+ ion emits two photons in succession, with wavelengths 108.5 nm and 30.4 nm, in making a transition to ground state. The quantum number *n*, corresponding to its initial excited state is (for photon of wavelength ≈, energy $E = \frac{1240eV}{\lambda(innm)}$

(a) $n=4$ (b) $n=5$ (c) $n=7$ (d) $n=6$

46. The electron in a hydrogen atom first jumps from the third excited state to the second excited state and subsequently to the first excited state. The ratio of the respective wavelengths, λ_1/λ_2, of the photons emitted in this process is :

(a) 20/7 (b) 27/5 (c) 7/5 (d) 9/7

47. Consider an electron in a hydrogen atom, revolving in its second excited state (having radius 4.65 Å). The de-Broglie wavelength of this electron is :

(a) 3.5 Å (b) 6.6 Å (c) 12.9 Å (d) 9.7 Å

48. Taking the wavelength of first Balmer line in hydrogen spectrum (n = 3 to n = 2) as 660 nm, the wavelength of the 2nd Balmer line (n = 4 to n = 2) will be;

(a) 889.2 nm (b) 488.9 nm
(c) 642.7 nm (d) 388.9 nm

49. A He^+ ion is in its first excited state. Its ionization energy is:

(a) 48.36 eV (b) 54.40 eV
(c) 13.60 eV (d) 6.04 eV

50. A hydrogen atom, initially in the ground state is excited by absorbing a photon of wavelength 980Å. The radius of the atom in the excited state, in terms of Bohr radius a_0, will be:

(a) $25a_0$ (b) $9a_0$ (c) $16a_0$ (d) $4a_0$

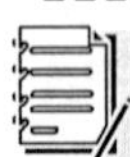

Exercise 2 - Exemplar & Past Year Questions

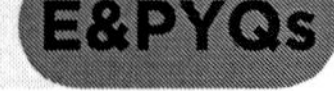

Exemplar Questions

1. Taking the Bohr radius as $a_0 = 53$ pm, the radius of Li^{++} ion in its ground state, on the basis of Bohr's model, will be about

(a) 53 pm (b) 27 pm (c) 18 pm (d) 13 pm

2. The binding energy of a H – atom, considering an electron moving around a fixed nuclei (proton), is

$$B = -\frac{me^4}{8n^2\varepsilon_0^2h^2} (m = \text{electron mass})$$

If one decides to work in a frame of reference where the electron is at rest, the proton would be moving around it. By similar arguments, the binding energy would be

$$B = -\frac{me^4}{8n^2\varepsilon_0^2h^2} (m = \text{proton mass})$$

This last expression is not correct, because

(a) n would not be integral
(b) Bohr – quantisation applies only two electron
(c) the frame in which the electron is at rest is not inertial
(d) the motion of the proton would not be in circular orbits, even approximately.

3. The simple Bohr model cannot be directly applied to calculate the energy levels of an atom with many electrons. This is because

(a) of the electrons not being subject to a central force
(b) of the electrons colliding with each other
(c) of screening effects
(d) the force between the nucleus and an electron will no longer be given by Coulomb's law

4. For the ground state, the electron in the H – atom has an angular momentum = h, according to the simple Bohr model. Angular momentum is a vector and hence there will be infinitely many orbits with the vector pointing in all possible directions. In actuality, this is not true,

(a) because Bohr model gives in correct values of angular momentum
(b) because only one of these would have a minimum energy
(c) angular momentum must be in the direction of spin of electron
(d) because electrons go around only in horizontal orbits

5. O_2 molecule consists of two oxygen atoms. In the molecule, nuclear force between the nuclei of the two atoms

(a) is not important because nuclear forces are short – ranged
(b) is as important as electrostatic force for binding the two atoms
(c) cancels the repulsive electrostatic force between the nuclei
(d) is not important because oxygen nucleus have equal number of neutrons and protons

6. Two H atoms in the ground state collide inelastically. The maximum amount by which their combined kinetic energy is reduced, is
(a) 10.20 eV (b) 20.40 eV (c) 13.6 eV (d) 27.2 eV

NEET/AIPMT (2013-2020) Questions

7. An electron in hydrogen atom makes a transition $n_1 \rightarrow n_2$ where n_1 and n_2 are principal quantum numbers of the two states. Assuming Bohr's model to be valid the time period of the electron in the initial state is eight times that in the final state. The possible values of n_1 and n_2 are *[NEET Kar. 2013]*
(a) $n_1 = 4$ and $n_2 = 2$ (b) $n_1 = 6$ and $n_2 = 2$
(c) $n_1 = 8$ and $n_2 = 1$ (d) $n_1 = 8$ and $n_2 = 2$

8. Hydrogen atom in ground state is excited by a monochromatic radiation of $\lambda = 975$ Å. Number of spectral lines in the resulting spectrum emitted will be *[2014]*
(a) 3 (b) 2 (c) 6 (d) 10

9. Consider 3rd orbit of He^+ (Helium), using non-relativistic approach, the speed of electron in this orbit will be [given K = 9 × 10^9 constant, Z = 2 and h (Plank's Constant) = 6.6×10^{-34} J s] *[2015]*
(a) 1.46×10^6 m/s (b) 0.73×10^6 m/s
(c) 3.0×10^8 m/s (d) 2.92×10^6 m/s

10. Two particles of masses m_1, m_2 move with initial velocities u_1 and u_2. On collision, one of the particles get excited to higher level, after absorbing energy ε. If final velocities of particles be v_1 and v_2 then we must have *[2015]*
(a) $\frac{1}{2}m_1u_1^2 + \frac{1}{2}m_2u_2^2 = \frac{1}{2}m_1v_1^2 + \frac{1}{2}m_2v_2^2 - \varepsilon$
(b) $\frac{1}{2}m_1u_1^2 + \frac{1}{2}m_2u_2^2 - \varepsilon = \frac{1}{2}m_1v_1^2 + \frac{1}{2}m_2V_2^2$
(c) $\frac{1}{2}m_1^2u_1^2 + \frac{1}{2}m_2^2u_2^2 + \varepsilon = \frac{1}{2}m_1^2v_1^2 + \frac{1}{2}m_2^2v_2^2$
(d) $m_1^2u_1 + m_2^2u_2 - \varepsilon = m_1^2v_1 + m_2^2v_2$

11. In the spectrum of hydrogen, the ratio of the longest wavelength in the Lyman series to the longest wavelength in the Balmer series is *[2015 RS, 2013]*
(a) $\frac{9}{4}$ (b) $\frac{27}{5}$ (c) $\frac{5}{27}$ (d) $\frac{4}{9}$

12. When an α-particle of mass 'm' moving with velocity 'v' bombards on a heavy nucleus of charge 'Ze', its distance of closest approach from the nucleus depends on m as : *[2016]*
(a) $\frac{1}{m}$ (b) $\frac{1}{\sqrt{m}}$ (c) $\frac{1}{m^2}$ (d) m

13. Given the value of Rydberg constant is $10^7 m^{-1}$, the wave number of the last line of the Balmer series in hydrogen spectrum will be : *[2016]*
(a) $0.025 \times 10^4 m^{-1}$ (b) $0.5 \times 10^7 m^{-1}$
(c) $0.25 \times 10^7 m^{-1}$ (d) $2.5 \times 10^7 m^{-1}$

14. The ratio of wavelengths of the last line of Balmer series and the last line of Lyman series is : *[2017]*
(a) 1 (b) 4 (c) 0.5 (d) 2

15. The ratio of kinetic energy to the total energy of an electron in a Bohr orbit of the hydrogen atom, is *[2018]*
(a) 1 : 1 (b) 1 : –1 (c) 1 : –2 (d) 2 : –1

16. The total energy of an electron in an atom in an orbit is – 3.4 eV. Its kinetic and potential energies are, respectively: *[2019]*
(a) –3.4 eV, –3.4 eV (b) –3.4 eV, –6.8 eV
(c) 3.4 eV, –6.8 eV (d) 3.4 eV, 3.4 eV

17. The radius of the first permitted Bohr orbit, for the electron, in a hydrogen atom equals 0.51 Å and its ground state energy equals –13.6 eV. If the electron in the hydrogen atom is replaced by muon (μ^-) [charge same as electron and mass 207 m_e], the first Bohr radius and ground state energy will be, *[NEET Odisha 2019]*
(a) 2.56×10^{-13} m, –13.6 eV (b) 0.53×10^{-13} m, –3.6 eV
(c) 25.6×10^{-13} m, –2.8 eV (d) 2.56×10^{-13} m, –2.8 eV

18. For which one of the following, Bohr model is **not** valid ? *[2020]*
(a) Singly ionised helium atom (He^+)
(b) Deuteron atom
(c) Singly ionised neon atom (Ne^+)
(d) Hydrogen atom

Exercise 3 - Concept Application Problems CAP

1. Energy levels, A, B, C of a certain atom correspond to increasing values of energy i.e. $E_A < E_B < E_C$. If $\lambda_1, \lambda_2, \lambda_3$ are the wavelengths of radiations corresponding to the transitions C to B, B to A and C to A respectively, which of the following relations is correct ?
(a) $\lambda_3 = \lambda_1 + \lambda_2$ (b) $\lambda_3 = \frac{\lambda_1\lambda_2}{\lambda_1 + \lambda_2}$
(c) $\lambda_1 + \lambda_2 + \lambda_3 = 0$ (d) $\lambda_3^3 = \lambda_1^2 + \lambda_2^2$

2. Consider the spectral line resulting from the transition n = 2 → n = 1 in the atoms and ions given below. The shortest wavelength is produced by
(a) hydrogen atom (b) deuterium atom
(c) singly ionized Helium (d) doubly ionised Lithium

3. In Bohr's model of the hydrogen atom, let R, V, T and E represent the radius of the orbit, speed of the electron, time period of revolution of electron and the total energy of the electron respectively. The quantity proportional to the quantum number n is
(a) VR (b) E (c) r (d) T

4. Let v_1 be the frequency of the series limit of the Lyman series, v_2 be the frequency of the first line of the Lyman series, and v_3 be the frequency of the series limit of the Balmer series.
(a) $v_1 - v_2 = v_3$ (b) $v_2 - v_1 = v_3$
(c) $v_3 = \frac{1}{2}(v_1 + v_2)$ (d) $v_1 + v_2 = v_3$

5. The third line of Balmer series of an ion equivalnet to hydrogen atom has wavelength of 108.5 nm. The ground state energy of an electron of this ion will be
(a) 3.4 eV (b) 13.6 eV
(c) 54.4 eV (d) 122.4 eV

6. In Hydrogen spectrum, the wavelength of H_α line is 656 nm, whereas in the spectrum of a distant galaxy, H_α line wavelength is 706 nm. Estimated speed of the galaxy with respect to earth is
(a) 2×10^8 m/s (b) 2×10^7 m/s
(c) 2×10^6 m/s (d) 2×10^5 m/s

7. The ionisation potential of H-atom is 13.6 V. When it is excited from ground state by monochromatic radiations of 970.6 Å, the number of emission lines will be (according to Bohr's theory)
(a) 10 (b) 8 (c) 6 (d) 4

8. Electrons in a certain energy level $n = n_1$, can emit 3 spectral lines. When they are in another energy level, $n = n_2$. They can emit 6 spectral lines. The orbital speed of the electrons in the two orbits are in the ratio of
(a) 4 : 3 (b) 3 : 4 (c) 2 : 1 (d) 1 : 2

9. The wavelength of radiation is λ_0 when an electron jumps from third to second orbit of hydrogen atom. For the electron to jump from the fourth to the second orbit of the hydrogen atom, the wavelength of radiation emitted will be
(a) $\frac{16}{25}\lambda_0$ (b) $\frac{20}{27}\lambda_0$ (c) $\frac{27}{20}\lambda_0$ (d) $\frac{25}{16}\lambda_0$

10. If the frequency of K_α X-rays emitted from the element with atomic number 31 is ν, then the frequency of K_α X-rays emitted from the element with atomic number 51 would be
(a) $\frac{5}{3}\nu$ (b) $\frac{51}{31}\nu$ (c) $\frac{25}{9}\nu$ (d) $\frac{9}{25}\nu$

11. One of the lines in the emission spectrum of Li^{2+} has the same wavelength as that of the 2nd line of Balmer series in hydrogen spectrum. The electronic transition corresponding to this line is $n = 12 \rightarrow n = x$. Find the value of x.
(a) 8 (b) 6 (c) 7 (c) 5

12. The wavelength K_α of X-rays for two metals 'A' and 'B' are $\frac{4}{1875R}$ and $\frac{1}{675R}$ respectively, where 'R' is Rydberg constant. Find the number of elements lying between A and B according to their atomic numbers
(a) 3 (b) 1 (c) 4 (d) 5

13. Ionization potential of hydrogen atom is 13.6 eV. Hydrogen atoms in the ground state are excited by monochromatic radiation of photon energy 12.1 eV. The spectral lines emitted by hydrogen atom according to Bohr's theory will be
(a) one (b) two (c) three (d) four

14. In Li^{++}, electron in first Bohr orbit is excited to a level by a radiation of wavelength λ. When the ion gets deexcited to the ground state in all possible ways (including intermediate emissions), a total of six spectral lines are observed. What is the value of λ ?
(Given : $h = 6.63 \times 10^{-34}$ Js; $c = 3 \times 10^8$ ms^{-1})
(a) 11.4 nm (b) 9.4 nm (c) 12.3 nm (d) 10.8 nm

15. Radiation coming from transitions $n = 2$ to $n = 1$ of hydrogen atoms fall on He^+ ions in $n = 1$ and $n = 2$ states. The possible transition of helium ions as they absorb energy from the radiation is :
(a) $n = 2 \rightarrow n = 3$ (b) $n = 1 \rightarrow n = 4$
(c) $n = 2 \rightarrow n = 5$ (d) $n = 2 \rightarrow n = 4$

16. In a hydrogen like atom, when an electron jumps from the M-shell to the L-shell, the wavelength of emitted radiation is l. If an electron jumps from N-shell to the L-shell, the wavelength of emitted radiation will be:
(a) $\frac{27}{20}\lambda$ (b) $\frac{16}{25}\lambda$ (c) $\frac{25}{16}\lambda$ (d) $\frac{20}{27}\lambda$

17. An electron from various excited states of hydrogen atom emit radiation to come to the ground state. Let λ_n, λ_g be the de Broglie wavelength of the electron in the nth state and the ground state respectively. Let Λ_n be the wavelength of the emitted photon in the transition from the nth state to the ground state. For large *n*, (A, B are constants)
(a) $\Lambda_n \approx A + \frac{B}{\lambda_n^2}$ (b) $\Lambda_n \approx A + B\lambda_n$
(c) $\Lambda_n^2 \approx A + B\lambda_n^2$ (d) $\Lambda_n^2 \approx \lambda$

18. If the series limit frequency of the Lyman series is ν_1, then the series limit frequency of the P-fund series is :
(a) 25 ν_L (b) 16 ν_L (c) $\nu_L/16$ (d) $\nu_L/25$

19. The de-Broglie wavelength (λ_B) associated with the electron orbiting in the second excited state of hydrogen atom is related to that in the ground state (λ_G) by
(a) $\lambda_B = \lambda_{G/3}$ (b) $\lambda_B = \lambda_{G/2}$
(c) $\lambda_B = 2\lambda_G$ (d) $\lambda_B = 3\lambda_G$

20. The energy required to remove the electron from a singly ionized Helium atom is 2.2 times the energy required to remove an electron from Helium atom. The total energy required to ionize the Helium atom completely is:
(a) 20 eV (b) 79 eV (c) 109 eV (d) 34 eV

21. Some energy levels of a molecule are shown in the figure. The ratio of the wavelengths $r = \lambda_1/\lambda_2$, is given by

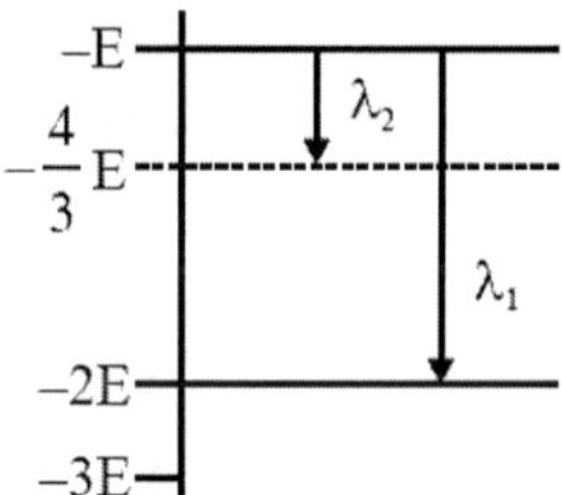

(a) $r = \frac{3}{4}$ (b) $r = \frac{1}{3}$ (c) $r = \frac{4}{3}$ (d) $r = \frac{2}{3}$

22. The acceleration of an electron in the first orbit of the hydrogen atom (z = 1) is :

(a) $\frac{h^2}{\pi^2 m^2 r^3}$ (b) $\frac{h^2}{8\pi^2 m^2 r^3}$

(c) $\frac{h^2}{4\pi^2 m^2 r^3}$ (d) $\frac{h^2}{4\pi m^2 r^3}$

23. According to Bohr's theory, the time averaged magnetic field at the centre (i.e. nucleus) of a hydrogen atom due to the motion of electrons in the nth orbit is proportional to : (n = principal quantum number)

(a) n^{-4} (b) n^{-5} (c) n^{-3} (d) n^{-2}

24. A hydrogen atom makes a transition from n = 2 to n = 1 and emits a photon. This photon strikes a doubly ionized lithium atom (z = 3) in excited state and completely removes the orbiting electron. The least quantum number for the excited state of the ion for the process is :

(a) 2 (b) 4 (c) 5 (d) 3

25. As an electron makes a transition from an excited state to the ground state of a hydrogen - like atom/ion :

(a) kinetic energy decreases, potential energy increases but total energy remains same
(b) kinetic energy and total energy decrease but potential energy increases
(c) its kinetic energy increases but potential energy and total energy decrease
(d) kinetic energy, potential energy and total energy decrease

26. The de–Broglie wavelength associated with the electron in the $n = 4$ level is :

(a) $\frac{1}{4}$ th of the de–Broglie wavelength of the electron in the ground state.
(b) four times the de–Broglie wavelength of the electron in the ground state
(c) two times the de–Broglie wavelength of the electron in the ground state
(d) half of the de–Broglie wavelength of the electron in the ground state

27. If one were to apply Bohr model to a particle of mass 'm' and charge 'q' moving in a plane under the influence of a magnetic field 'B', the energy of the charged particle in the nth level will be :

(a) $n\left(\frac{hqB}{2\pi m}\right)$ (b) $n\left(\frac{hqB}{8\pi m}\right)$

(c) $n\left(\frac{hqB}{4\pi m}\right)$ (d) $n\left(\frac{hqB}{\pi m}\right)$

28. Hydrogen $({}_1H^1)$, Deuterium $({}_1H^2)$, singly ionised Helium $({}_2He^4)^+$ and doubly ionised lithium $({}_3Li^6)^{++}$ all have one electron around the nucleus. Consider an electron transition from n = 2 to n = 1. If the wavelengths of emitted radiation are λ_1, λ_2, λ_3 and λ_4 respectively then approximately which one of the following is correct?

(a) $4\lambda_1 = 2\lambda_2 = 2\lambda_3 = \lambda_4$ (b) $\lambda_1 = 2\lambda_2 = 2\lambda_3 = \lambda_4$
(c) $\lambda_1 = \lambda_2 = 4\lambda_3 = 9\lambda_4$ (d) $\lambda_1 = 2\lambda_2 = 3\lambda_3 = 4\lambda_4$

29. A 12.5 eV electron beam is used to bombard gaseous hydrogen at room temperature. It will emit :

(a) 2 lines in the Lyman series and 1 line in the Balmar series
(b) 3 lines in the Lyman series
(c) 1 line in the Lyman series and 2 lines in the Balmar series
(d) 3 lines in the Balmer series

30. In the Bohr's model of hydrogen-like atom the force between the nucleus and the electron is modified as $F = \frac{e^2}{4\pi\varepsilon_0}\left(\frac{1}{r^2} + \frac{\beta}{r^3}\right)$, where β is a constant. For this atom, the radius of the nth orbit in terms of the Bohr radius $\left(a_0 = \frac{\varepsilon_0 h^2}{m\pi e^2}\right)$ is :

(a) $r_n = a_0 n - \beta$ (b) $r_n = a_0 n^2 + \beta$
(c) $r_n = a_0 n^2 - \beta$ (d) $r_n = a_0 n + \beta$

31. Orbits of a particle moving in a circle are such that the perimeter of the orbit equals an integer number of de-Broglie wavelengths of the particle. For a charged particle moving in a plane perpendicular to a magnetic field, the radius of the nth orbital will therefore be proportional to :

(a) n^2 (b) n (c) $n^{1/2}$ (d) $n^{1/4}$

32. In the Bohr model an electron moves in a circular orbit around the proton. Considering the orbiting electron to be a circular current loop, the magnetic moment of the hydrogen atom, when the electron is in n^{th} excited state, is :

(a) $\left(\frac{e}{2m}\frac{n^2 h}{2\pi}\right)$ (b) $\left(\frac{e}{m}\right)\frac{nh}{2\pi}$

(c) $\left(\frac{e}{2m}\right)\frac{nh}{2\pi}$ (d) $\left(\frac{e}{m}\right)\frac{n^2 h}{2\pi}$

33. A diatomic molecule is made of two masses m_1 and m_2 which are separated by a distance r. If we calculate its rotational energy by applying Bohr's rule of angular momentum quantization, its energy will be given by : (n is an integer)

(a) $\frac{(m_1+m_2)^2 n^2 h^2}{2m_1^2 m_2^2 r^2}$ (b) $\frac{n^2 h^2}{2(m_1+m_2) r^2}$

(c) $\frac{2n^2 h^2}{(m_1+m_2) r^2}$ (d) $\frac{(m_1+m_2) n^2 \hbar^2}{2m_1 m_2 r^2}$

34. Which of the plots shown in the figure represents speed (v_n) of the electron in a hydrogen atom as a function of the principal quantum number (n)?

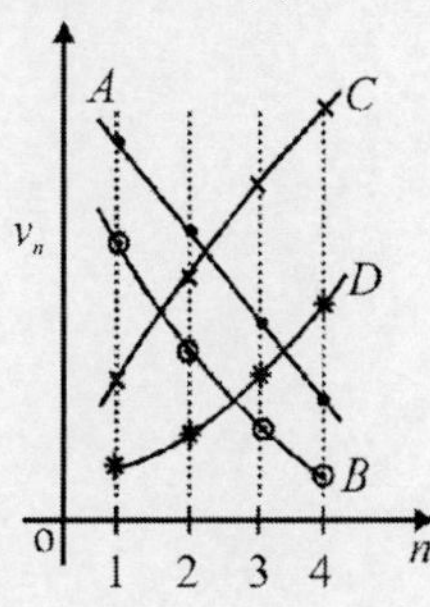

(a) B (b) D (c) C (d) A

35. A doubly ionised Li atom is excited from its ground state ($n = 1$) to $n = 3$ state. The wavelengths of the spectral lines are given by λ_{32}, λ_{31} and λ_{21}. The ratio $\lambda_{32}/\lambda_{31}$ and $\lambda_{21}/\lambda_{31}$ are, respectively

(a) 8.1, 0.67 (b) 8.1, 1.2
(c) 6.4, 1.2 (d) 6.4, 0.67

36. The electron of a hydrogen atom makes a transition from the $(n+1)^{th}$ orbit to the nth orbit. For large n the wavelength of the emitted radiation is proportional to

(a) n (b) n^3 (c) n^4 (d) n^2

37. The transition from the state $n = 4$ to $n = 3$ in a hydrogen like atom results in ultraviolet radiation. Infrared radiation will be obtained in the transition from :

(a) $3 \to 2$ (b) $4 \to 2$ (c) $5 \to 4$ (d) $2 \to 1$

38. Suppose an electron is attracted towards the origin by a force $\frac{k}{r}$ where 'k' is a constant and 'r' is the distance of the electron from the origin. By applying Bohr model to this system, the radius of the nth orbital of the electron is found to be 'r_n' and the kinetic energy of the electron to be 'T_n'. Then which of the following is true?

(a) $T_n \propto \frac{1}{n^2}, r_n \propto n^2$

(b) T_n independent of n, $r_n \propto n$

(c) $T_n \propto \frac{1}{n}, r_n \propto n$

(d) $T_n \propto \frac{1}{n^3}, r_n \propto n^2$

39. The diagram shows the energy levels for an electron in a certain atom. Which transition shown represents the emission of a photon with the most energy?

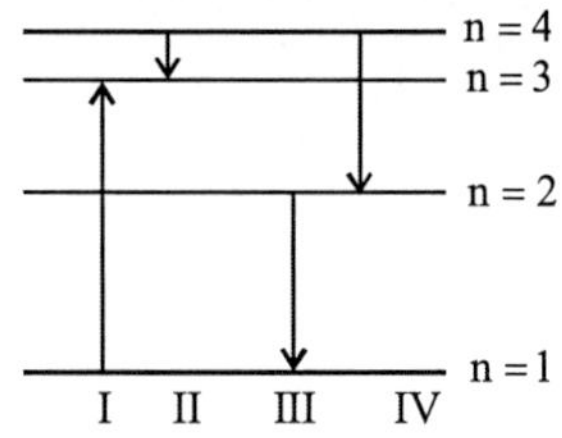

(a) IV (b) III (c) II (d) I

40. The wavelengths involved in the spectrum of deuterium $\left({}_1^2D\right)$ are slightly different from that of hydrogen spectrum, because

(a) the size of the two nuclei are different
(b) the nuclear forces are different in the two cases
(c) the masses of the two nuclei are different
(d) the attraction between the electron and the nucleus is differernt in the two cases

41. If 13.6 eV energy is required to ionize the hydrogen atom, then the energy required to remove an electron from $n = 2$ is

(a) 10.2 eV (b) 0 eV
(c) 3.4 eV (d) 6.8 eV

42. Hydrogen (${}_1H^1$), Deuterium (${}_1H^2$), singly ionised Helium $({}_2He^4)^+$ and doubly ionised lithium $({}_3Li^6)^{++}$ all have one electron around the nucleus. Consider an electron transition from n = 2 to n = 1. If the wavelengths of emitted radiation are λ_1, λ_2, λ_3 and λ_4 respectively then approximately which one of the following is correct?

(a) $4\lambda_1 = 2\lambda_2 = 2\lambda_3 = \lambda_4$ (b) $\lambda_1 = 2\lambda_2 = 2\lambda_3 = \lambda_4$
(c) $\lambda_1 = \lambda_2 = 4\lambda_3 = 9\lambda_4$ (d) $\lambda_1 = 2\lambda_2 = 3\lambda_3 = 4\lambda_4$

43. The radiation corresponding to $3 \to 2$ transition of hydrogen atom falls on a metal surface to produce photoelectrons. These electrons are made to enter a magnetic field of 3×10^{-4} T. If the radius of the largest circular path followed by these electrons is 10.0 mm, the work function of the metal is close to:

(a) 1.8 eV (b) 1.1 eV (c) 0.8 eV (d) 1.6 eV

44. The energy required to remove the electron from a singly ionized Helium atom is 2.2 times the energy required to remove an electron from Helium atom. The total energy required to ionize the Helium atom completely is:

(a) 20 eV (b) 79 eV (c) 109 eV (d) 34 eV

45. A hypothetical atom has only three energy levels. The ground level has energy, $E_1 = -8$ eV. The two excited states have energies, $E_2 = -6$ eV and $E_3 = -2$ eV. Then which of the following wavelengths will not be present in the emission spectrum of this atom?

(a) 207 nm (b) 465 nm (c) 310 nm (d) 620 nm

Hints & Solutions

27.1 Concept Practice Problems CPP

1. (d) No. of particles scattered through an angle

$$\theta = N(\theta) = \frac{kZ^2}{\sin^4\left(\frac{\theta}{2}\right)(K.E.)^2}$$

$$\therefore 28 = \frac{4kcz^2}{(K.E.)^2} \text{ for } \theta = 90^\circ \quad \therefore \frac{kz^2}{(K.E.)^2} = \frac{28}{4} = 7$$

$$\therefore N(60^\circ) = \frac{7}{\sin^4\left(\frac{60^\circ}{2}\right)} = 16 \times 7 = 112\,/\text{min.}$$

$$N(120^\circ) = \frac{7}{\sin^4\left(\frac{120^\circ}{2}\right)} = 12.4\,/\,\text{min}$$

2. (b) 3. (b) 4. (a) 5. (b)

6. (d)

7. (c) $N \propto \frac{1}{\sin^4\theta/2}$; $\frac{N_2}{N_1} = \frac{\sin^4(\theta_1/2)}{\sin^4(\theta_2/2)}$

or $\frac{N_2}{5\times10^6} = \frac{\sin^4(60^\circ/2)}{\sin^4(120^\circ/2)}$ or $\frac{N_2}{5\times10^6} = \frac{\sin^4 30^\circ}{\sin^4 60^\circ}$

or $N_2 = 5\times10^6 \times \left(\frac{1}{2}\right)^4\left(\frac{2}{\sqrt{3}}\right)^4 = \frac{5}{9}\times10^6$

8. (c) Kinetic energy of alpha nucleus is equall to electrostatic potential energy of the system of the alpha particle and the heavy nucleus. That is,

$$\frac{1}{2}mv^2 = \frac{1}{4\pi\varepsilon_0}\frac{q_\alpha Ze}{r_0}$$

where r_0 is the distance of closest approach

$$r_0 = \frac{2}{4\pi\varepsilon_0}\frac{q_\alpha Ze}{mv^2}$$

$$\Rightarrow r_0 \propto Ze \propto q_\alpha \propto \frac{1}{m} \propto \frac{1}{v^2}$$

Hence, correct option is (c).

9. (c) As α-particles are doubly ionised helium He^{++} i.e. Positively charged and nucleus is also positively charged and we know that like charges repel each other.

10. (a) Distance of closest approach

$$r_0 = \frac{Ze(2e)}{4\pi\varepsilon_0\left(\frac{1}{2}mv^2\right)}$$

Energy, $E = 5\times10^6\times1.6\times10^{-19}$ J

$$\therefore r_0 = \frac{9\times10^9\times(92\times1.6\times10^{-19})(2\times1.6\times10^{-19})}{5\times10^6\times1.6\times10^{-19}}$$

$$\Rightarrow r_h = 5.2\times10^{-14}\,m = 5.3\times10^{-12}\text{ cm}$$

27.2 Concept Practice Problems CPP

11. (d) $\frac{R_1}{R_2} = \frac{n_1^2}{n_2^2} = \frac{1}{4} \quad \therefore \frac{n_1}{n_2} = \frac{1}{2}$

$$\frac{T_1}{T_2} = \left(\frac{n_1}{n_2}\right)^3 = \left(\frac{1}{2}\right)^3 = \frac{1}{8}$$

12. (d)

13. (c) Ist excited state corresponds to n = 2
2nd excited state corresponds to n = 3

$$\therefore \frac{E_1}{E_2} = \frac{n_2^2}{n_1^2} = \frac{3^2}{2^2} = \frac{9}{4}$$

14. (d) 15. (c) 16. (d) 17. (a)

18. (c) $\ell = 0$ to $(n-1)$ i.e. 0, 1, 2, 3,. In all 4 values.

19. (c) According to Bohr's theory,

Angular momentum, $mvr = \frac{nh}{2\pi}$

So in ground state, angular momentum $= \frac{h}{2\pi}$.

20. (a) Since 121.5 nm line of spectrum of hydrogen atom lies in ultraviolet region, therefore it is Lyman series.

Exercise 1 - Chapter Revision Problems

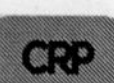

1. (a) As n increases, energy difference between adjacent energy levels decreases.

2. (d) Charge = e, frequency = n, time period = $\frac{1}{n}$

So, equivalent current $= \frac{e}{1/n} = en$

3. (d) 4. (d) 5. (a)

6. (d) Laser action involves all of the following.
(i) Amplification of particular frequency.
(ii) Population inversion.
(iii) Stimulated emission

7. (d) Different values of magnetic azimuthals quantum number are $m_l = 2\ell + 1 = 2(3) + 1 = 7$

8. (c)

9. (b) Potential energy of electron in n^{th} orbit of radius r in H-atom $U = -\frac{e^2}{r}$ (in CGS)

$\because$ K.E. $= \frac{1}{2}|$P.E.$| \Rightarrow K = \frac{e^2}{2r}$

10. (a)

11. (c) According to Bohr's second postulate.

12. (d) As $r \propto \frac{1}{m} \quad \therefore r_0' = \frac{1}{2}r_0$

As $E \propto m \quad \therefore E_0' = 2(-13.6) = -27.2$ eV

13. (a) Conservation of energy requires that the 15.0 eV photon energy first provides the ionization energy to unbind the electron, and then allows any excess energy to become the electron's kinetic energy. The kinetic energy in this case is 15.0 eV – 13.6 eV = 1.4 eV.

14. (d) $r \propto n^2 \Rightarrow \pi r^2 \propto n^4$

So area $\propto n^4 \Rightarrow$ Ratio is $2^4 : 1 \Rightarrow 16 : 1$.

15. (b) $P.E. = \frac{-Ze^2}{4\pi\varepsilon_0 r}$. Negative sign indicates that revolving electron is bound to the positive nucleus.
So, it decreases with increase in radii of orbit.

16. (c) $\Delta p \times \lambda \sim h \Rightarrow \frac{1}{\lambda} = \frac{\Delta p}{h}$

We know that $\frac{1}{\lambda} = R\left(\frac{1}{n_1^2} - \frac{1}{n_2^2}\right)$

$$\Rightarrow m_H v_H = hR_H\left(\frac{1}{n_1^2} - \frac{1}{n_2^2}\right)$$

$$v = 6.26 \times 10^{-34} \times R_H\left(\frac{24}{25}\right) = 4 \text{ ms}^{-1}$$

17. (d) $r = 0.528 n^2 \times 10^{-10}$

$$\left(\frac{1 \times 10^{-7}}{2}\right) = 0.528 n^2 \times 10^{-10}$$

$$\Rightarrow n^2 = \frac{5 \times 10^{-8}}{0.528 \times 10^{-10}} \Rightarrow n \approx 31$$

18. (a) Ionisation energy of Li^{++} = 9hcR
Ionisation energy = $RchZ^2 = Rch(3)^2$

(as Z = 3 for Li^{++})

= 9hcR.

19. (b) Transition from higher states to n = 2 lead to emission of radiation with wavelengths 656.3 nm and 365.0 nm. These wavelengths fall in the visible region and constitute the Balmer series.

20. (d) $\frac{1}{\lambda} = RZ^2\left(\frac{1}{n_1^2} - \frac{1}{n_2^2}\right)$

For Balmer series n = 2

$$\frac{1}{\lambda_{max}} = RZ^2\left(\frac{1}{2^2} - \frac{1}{\infty^2}\right) \text{ and } \frac{1}{\lambda_{min}} = RZ^2\left(\frac{1}{2^2} - \frac{1}{3^2}\right)$$

or $$\frac{1/\lambda_{min}}{1/\lambda_{max}} = \frac{(1/2^2 - 1/3^2)}{(1/2^2)} = \frac{\frac{1}{4} - \frac{1}{9}}{1/4} = 1 - \frac{4}{9} = 5/9$$

$$\Rightarrow \frac{\lambda_{max}}{\lambda_{min}} = \frac{5}{9}$$

21. (d) For k_α line $\frac{1}{\lambda_{k_\alpha}} = R(Z-1)^2\left[\frac{1}{1^2} - \frac{1}{2^2}\right]$

$$(Z-1)^2 = \frac{4}{3}\frac{1}{\lambda_{k_\alpha}}\frac{1}{R} = \frac{4}{3} \times \frac{1}{1.785 \times 10^{-8}} \times \frac{1}{109737}$$

$\Rightarrow (Z-1)^2 = 680.6 \Rightarrow Z - 1 = 26 \Rightarrow Z = 27$
Thus, the element is cobalt.

22. (a) From Mosley's law, we have,

$$(Z-1)^2 \propto \nu \therefore (Z-1)^2 = A\frac{c}{\lambda_{k_\alpha}}$$

where A is some constant,

$$\therefore \frac{(Z_{MO} - 1)^2}{(Z_{Cu} - 1)^2} = \frac{\lambda_{Cu}}{\lambda_{MO}} \text{ or } \left(\frac{41}{28}\right)^2 = \frac{\lambda_{Cu}}{0.71}$$

$$\therefore \lambda_{Cu} = 0.71 \times \left(\frac{41}{28}\right)^2 = 1.52 Å$$

23. (b) In Paschen series $\frac{1}{\lambda_{max}} = R\left[\frac{1}{(3)^2} - \frac{1}{(4)^2}\right]$

$$\Rightarrow \lambda_{max} = \frac{144}{7R} = \frac{144}{7 \times 1.1 \times 10^7} = 1.89 \times 10^{-6} \text{m} = 1.89 \ \mu\text{m}$$

Similarly $\lambda_{min} = \frac{9}{R} = \frac{9}{1.1 \times 10^7} = 0.818 \ \mu m$

24. (a) $\frac{1}{\lambda_{Balmer}} = R\left[\frac{1}{2^2} - \frac{1}{3^2}\right] = \frac{5R}{36}$,

$$\frac{1}{\lambda_{Lyman}} = R\left[\frac{1}{1^2} - \frac{1}{2^2}\right] = \frac{3R}{4}$$

$$\therefore \lambda_{Lyman} = \lambda_{Balmer} \times \frac{5}{27} = 1215.4 Å$$

25. (b) No. of lines $N_E = \frac{n(n-1)}{2} = \frac{3(3-1)}{2} = 3$

26. (a) For Bracket series $\frac{1}{\lambda_{max}} = R\left[\frac{1}{4^2} - \frac{1}{5^2}\right] = \frac{9}{25 \times 16}R$

and $\frac{1}{\lambda_{min}} = R\left[\frac{1}{4^2} - \frac{1}{\infty^2}\right] = \frac{R}{16} \Rightarrow \frac{\lambda_{max}}{\lambda_{min}} = \frac{25}{9}$

27. (c) Transition A ($n = \infty$ to 1) : Series lime of Lyman series
Transition B (n = 5 to n = 2) : Third spectral lien of Balmer series
Transition C (n = 5 to n = 3) : Second spectral line of Paschen series

28. (a) Orbital speed varies inversely as the radius of the orbit.

$$v \propto \frac{1}{n}$$

29. (d)

30. (a) Excitation energy $\Delta E = E_2 - E_1 = 13.6 Z^2\left[\frac{1}{1^2} - \frac{1}{2^2}\right]$

$$\Rightarrow 40.8 = 13.6 \times \frac{3}{4} \times Z^2 \Rightarrow Z = 2.$$

Now required energy to remove the electron from ground state $= \frac{+13.6Z^2}{(1)^2} = 13.6(Z)^2 = 54.4$ eV.

31. (a) $\frac{1}{\lambda_{max}} = R\left[\frac{1}{(1)^2} - \frac{1}{(2)^2}\right] \Rightarrow \lambda_{max} = \frac{4}{3R} \approx 1213 Å$

and $\frac{1}{\lambda_{min}} = R\left[\frac{1}{(1)^2} - \frac{1}{\infty}\right] \Rightarrow \lambda_{min} = \frac{1}{R} \approx 910Å.$

32. (a) Electron after absorbing 10.2 eV energy goes to its first excited state (n = 2) from ground state (n = 1).

$\therefore$ Increase in momentum $= \frac{h}{2\pi}$

$= \frac{6.6 \times 10^{-34}}{6.28} = 1.05 \times 10^{-34}$ J-s.

33. (d) $\frac{1}{\lambda} = R\left[\frac{1}{n_1^2} - \frac{1}{n_2^2}\right]$. For first wavelength, $n_1 = 2, n_2 = 3$ $\Rightarrow \lambda_1 = 6563$ Å. For second wavelength, $n_1 = 2, n_2 = 4 \Rightarrow \lambda_2 = 4861$ Å

34. (d) For an atom following Bohr's model, the radius is given by $r_m = \frac{r_0 m^2}{Z}$ where r_0 = Bohr's radius and m = orbit number.
For *Fm*, $m = 5$ (Fifth orbit in which the outermost electron is present)

$\therefore \quad r_m = \frac{r_0 5^2}{100} = nr_0$ (given) $\Rightarrow n = \frac{1}{4}$

35. (a) Energy of electron in n^{th} orbit is

$E_n = -(Rch)\frac{Z^2}{n^2} = -54.4$ eV

For He^+ is ground state

$E_1 = -(Rch)\frac{(2)^2}{(1)^2} = -54.4 \Rightarrow Rch = 13.6$

$\therefore$ For Li^{++} in first excited state (n = 2)

$E' = -13.6 \times \frac{(3)^2}{(2)^2} = -30.6$ eV

36. (c) Number of possible spectral lines emitted when an electron jumps back to ground state from n^{th} orbit $= \frac{n(n-1)}{2}$

Here, $\frac{n(n-1)}{2} = 6 \Rightarrow n = 4$

Wavelength λ from transition from n = 1 to n = 4 is given by,

$\frac{1}{\lambda} = R\left(\frac{1}{1} - \frac{1}{4^2}\right) \Rightarrow \lambda = \frac{16}{15R} = 975$ Å

37. (d) $\because \quad B = \frac{\mu_0 I}{2r}$ and $I = \frac{e}{T}$

$B = \frac{\mu_0 e}{2rT}$ $[r \propto n^2, T \propto n^5]$; $B \propto \frac{1}{n^5}$

38. (a) $qV = \frac{1}{2}mv^2$ or $v = \sqrt{\frac{2qV}{m}}$ i.e. $v \propto \sqrt{\frac{q}{m}}$

$\therefore \quad \frac{v_{He}}{v_H} = \sqrt{\frac{q_{He}}{q_H} \times \frac{m_H}{m_{He}}} = \sqrt{\frac{2e}{e} \times \frac{m}{4m}} = \frac{1}{\sqrt{2}}$

39. (d)

40. (a) Energy of a H-like atom in it's n^{th} state is given by

$E_n = -Z^2 \times \frac{13.6}{n^2} eV$

For, first excited state of He^+, n = 2, Z = 2

$\therefore \quad E_{He^+} = -\frac{4}{2^2} \times 13.6 = -13.6 eV$

41. (c)

42. (b) Total energy of electron in n^{th} orbit of hydrogen atom

$E_n = -\frac{Rhc}{n^2}$

Total energy of electron in $(n+1)^{th}$ level of hydrogen atom

$E_{n+1} = -\frac{Rhc}{(n+1)^2}$

When electron makes a transition from $(n+1)^{th}$ level to n^{th} level

Change in energy,

$\Delta E = E_{n+1} - E_n$

$h\nu = Rhc \cdot \left[\frac{1}{n^2} - \frac{1}{(n+1)^2}\right]$ $\quad (\because E = h\nu)$

$\nu = R \cdot c\left[\frac{(n+1)^2 - n^2}{n^2(n+1)^2}\right]$

$\nu = R \cdot c\left[\frac{1+2n}{n^2(n+1)^2}\right]$

For $n >> 1$

$\Rightarrow \nu = R \cdot c\left[\frac{2n}{n^2 \times n^2}\right] = \frac{2RC}{n^3}$

$\Rightarrow \nu \propto \frac{1}{n^3}$

43. (b) According to Bohr's Theory the wavelength of the radiation emitted from hydrogen atom is given by

$\frac{1}{\lambda} = RZ^2\left[\frac{1}{n_1^2} - \frac{1}{n_2^2}\right]$

$\because \quad Z = 3$

$\therefore \quad \frac{1}{\lambda} = 9R\left(1 - \frac{1}{9}\right)$

$\Rightarrow \lambda = \frac{1}{8R} = \frac{1}{8 \times 10973731.6}$ $\quad$ (R = 10973731.6 m–1)

$\Rightarrow \lambda = 11.39$ nm

44. (b) For first excited state n' = 3

Time period $T \propto \frac{n^3}{z^2}$

$\Rightarrow \frac{T_2}{T_1} = \frac{n'^3}{n^3}$

$\therefore$ T2 = 8T1 = 8 × 1.6 × 10–16s

$\therefore$ Frequency, $\nu = \frac{1}{T_2} = \frac{1}{8 \times 1.6 \times 10^{-16}}$

$\approx$ 7.8 × 1014 Hz

45. (b) $E = E_1 + E_2$

$13.6\frac{z^2}{n^2} = \frac{1240}{\lambda_1} + \frac{1240}{\lambda_2}$

or $\frac{13.6(2)^2}{n^2} = 1240\left(\frac{1}{108.5} + \frac{1}{30.4}\right) \times \frac{1}{10^{-9}}$

On solving, n = 5

46. (a) $\frac{1}{\lambda_1} = R\left(\frac{1}{3^2} - \frac{1}{4^2}\right) = \frac{7R}{16 \times 9}$

And $\frac{1}{\lambda_2} = R\left(\frac{1}{2^2} - \frac{1}{3^2}\right) = \frac{5R}{36}$

Now $\frac{\lambda_1}{\lambda_2} = \frac{(5R/36)}{7R/(16 \times 9)} = \frac{20}{7}$

47. (d) $v = \frac{c}{137n} = \frac{c}{137 \times 3}$

$\lambda = \frac{h}{p} = \frac{h}{mv} = \frac{h}{\left(\frac{m \times c}{3 \times 137}\right)} = \frac{h}{mc} \times (3 \times 137) = 9.7 \text{ Å}$

48. (b) $\frac{1}{\lambda_1} = -R\left(\frac{1}{2^2} - \frac{1}{3^2}\right) = \frac{5R}{36}$

$\frac{1}{\lambda_2} = R\left(\frac{1}{2^2} - \frac{1}{4^2}\right) = \frac{3R}{16}$

$\therefore \frac{\lambda_2}{\lambda_1} = \frac{80}{108}$

$\lambda_2 = \frac{80}{108}\lambda_1 = \frac{80}{108} \times 660 = 488.9 \text{ nm.}$

49. (c) $E_n = -13.6\frac{Z^2}{n^2}$

For He$^+$, $E_2 = \frac{-13.6(2)^2}{2^2} = -13.60 \text{ eV}$

Ionization energy = 0 – E2 = 13.60 eV

50. (c) Energy of photon = $\frac{hc}{\lambda} = \frac{12500}{980} = 12.75 \text{ eV}$

Energy of electron in nth orbit is given by

$E_n = \frac{-13.6}{n^2} \Rightarrow E_n - E_1 = -13.6\left[\frac{1}{n^2} \frac{-1}{1^2}\right]$

$\Rightarrow 12.75 = 13.6\left[\frac{1}{1^2} \frac{-1}{n^2}\right] \Rightarrow n = 4$

$\therefore$ Electron will excite to n = 4

We know that 'R' $\propto n^2$

$\therefore$ Radius of atom will be $16a_0$

Exercise 2 - Exemplar & Past Year Questions 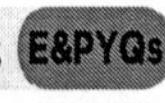

Exemplar Questions

1. (c) According to Bohr's model of atom rading of an atom in ground state is $r = \frac{r_0}{z}$ where r_0 is Bohr's radius and z is a atomic number. Given $r_0 = 53$ pm

The atomic number of lithium is 3, therefore, the radius of Li^{++} ion in its ground state, on the basis of Bohr's model, will be about $\frac{1}{3}$ times to that of Bohr radius.

So, the radius of lithium ion is $= \frac{r_0}{z} = \frac{53}{3} \approx 18$ pm.

2. (c) If one decides to work in a frame of reference where the electron is at rest, the given expression is not true as it forms the non – inertial frame of reference.

3. (a) The simple Bohr model cannot be directly applied to calculate the energy levels of an atom with many electrons. So the nuclear the electrons not being subject to a central force.

4. (a) Accroding Bohr's second postulate states that the electron evolves around the nucleus only in those orbits for which the angular momentum is some integral multiple of $\frac{h}{2\pi}$ where h is the Planck's constant (= 6.6 × 10^{-34} J-s). So, the magnitude of angular momentum is kept equal to some integral multiple of $\frac{h}{2\pi}$, where, h is Planck's constant and thus, the Bohr model does not gives correct value of angular momentum.

5. (a) As we know that, the nuclear force is too much stronger than the Coulomb force acting between charges or the gravitational forces between masses. The nuclear binding force has to dominate over the Coulomb repulsive force between protons inside the nucleus.
The nuclear force between two nucleons falls rapidly to zero as their distance is increase than a few femtometres. So in case of oxygen molecule, the distance between atoms of oxygen is larger as compared to the distance between nuclears in a necleus. So, nuclear force between the nuclei of the two oxygen atoms is not important because nuclear forces are short – ranged.

6. (a) We know that, electron on the lowest state of the atom, called the ground state have the lowest energy and the electron revolving in the orbit of smallest radius, the Bohr radius, r. The energy of this state (n = 1), E_1 is – 13.6 eV.
Total energy of two H – atoms in the ground state collide in elastically = 2 × (–13.6 eV) = –27.2 eV.
The maximum amount by which their combined kinetic energy is reduced when any one H–atom goes into first excited state after the inelastic collision. So that the total

energy of the two H – atoms after the inelastic collision

$$=\left(\frac{13.6}{2^2}\right)+(13.6)=17.0\text{eV}$$

[$\because$ for excited state (n = 2)].

So, maximum loss of their combined kinetic energy.

Due to inelastic collision

$=27.2-17.0=10.2\text{ eV}$

NEET/AIPMT (2013-2020) Questions

7. (a) $\because T\propto n^3$

$$\frac{T_1}{T_2}=\frac{8T_2}{T_2}=\left(\frac{n_1}{n_2}\right)^3$$

Hence, $n_1=2n_2$

8. (c) For the $\lambda=975$ Å

$$\frac{1}{\lambda}=R\left(\frac{1}{n_1^2}-\frac{1}{n_2^2}\right)$$

where R is the Rydberg constant

Solving we get $n_2=n=4$

($\because n_1=1$ ground state)

Therefore number of spectral lines

$$=\frac{n(n-1)}{2}=\frac{4(4-1)}{2}=6$$

9. (a) Speed of electron in nth orbit

$$V_n=\frac{2\pi KZe^2}{nh}$$

$$V=(2.19\times10^6\,\text{m/s})\,\frac{Z}{n}$$

$$V=(2.19\times10^6)\,\frac{2}{3}\ (Z=2\ \&\ n=3)$$

$V=1.46\times10^6$ m/s

10. (b) By law of conservation of energy,

$K.E_f=K.E_i-\text{excitation energy }(\varepsilon)$

or $\frac{1}{2}mv_1^2+\frac{1}{2}mv_2^2=\frac{1}{2}m_1u_1^2+\frac{1}{2}m_2u_2^2-\varepsilon$

11. (d) For Lyman series $(2\rightarrow1)$

$$\frac{1}{\lambda_L}=R\left[1-\frac{1}{2^2}\right]=\frac{3R}{4}$$

For Balmer series $(3\rightarrow2)$

$$\frac{1}{\lambda_B}=R\left[\frac{1}{4}-\frac{1}{9}\right]=\frac{5R}{36}$$

$$\Rightarrow\frac{\lambda_L}{\lambda_B}=\frac{\frac{4}{3R}}{\frac{36}{5R}}=\frac{4}{36}\left(\frac{5}{3}\right)=\frac{5}{27}$$

12. (a) At closest distance of approach, the kinetic energy of the particle will convert completely into electrostatic potential energy.

Kinetic energy $K.E.=\frac{1}{2}mv^2$

Potential energy $P.E.=\frac{KQq}{r}$

$$\frac{1}{2}mv^2=\frac{KQq}{r}\quad\Rightarrow\quad r\propto\frac{1}{m}$$

13. (c) According to Bohr's theory, the wave number of the last line of the Balmer series in hydrogen spectrum,

For hydrogen atom z = 1

$$\frac{1}{\lambda}=RZ^2\left(\frac{1}{n_2^2}-\frac{1}{n_1^2}\right)$$

$$=10^7\times1^2\left(\frac{1}{2^2}-\frac{1}{\infty^2}\right)$$

$\Rightarrow$ wave number $\frac{1}{\lambda}=0.25\times10^7\,\text{m}^{-1}$

14. (b) For last line of Balmer series : $n_1=2$ and $n_2=\infty$

$$\frac{1}{\lambda_B}=RZ^2\left[\frac{1}{n_1^2}-\frac{1}{n_2^2}\right]=R_1^2\left[\frac{1}{2^2}-\frac{1}{\infty^2}\right]$$

$$\lambda_B=\frac{4}{R}\qquad\text{...(1)}$$

For last line of Lyman series : $n_1=1$ and $n_2=\infty$

$$\frac{1}{\lambda_L}=RZ^2\left[\frac{1}{n_1^2}-\frac{1}{n_2^2}\right]=RZ^2\left[\frac{1}{1^2}-\frac{1}{\infty^2}\right]$$

$$\lambda_L=\frac{1}{R}\qquad\text{...(ii)}$$

Dividing equation (i) by (ii)

$$\frac{\lambda_B}{\lambda_L}=\frac{\frac{4}{R}}{\frac{1}{R}}$$

Ratio of wavelengths is $\frac{\lambda_B}{\lambda_L}=4$

15. (b) In a Bohr orbit of the hydrogen atom

Kinetic energy,

$$k=\frac{kze^2}{2r_n}$$

Total energy, $E=\frac{-kze^2}{2r_n}$

So, Kinetic energy : total energy = 1 : –1

16. (c) According to Bohr's model of H-atom, the relation between kinetic energy, potential energy and total energy

$$K.E.=|TE|=\frac{|P.E.|}{2}$$

so, K.E. = – (T.E.)

$\therefore$ K.E. = 3.4 eV

and P.E. = 2 (T.E)

$\Rightarrow$ P.E. = – 6.8 eV

17. (d) $r \propto \frac{1}{m}$

$R = \frac{0.51}{207}$ $\therefore$ 2.56×10^{-13} m

$E \propto m$

$\therefore$ $(E)_\mu = -13.6 \times 207 = -2.8$ keV

18. (c) Bohr model is only valid for single electron species i.e., Hydrogen or hydrogen like atom – He^+, deuteron, etc. Singly ionised neon atom has more than one electron in orbit. Hence, Bohr model is not valid.

 Exercise 3 - Concept Application Problems CAP

1. (b) As energy emitted varies inversely as wavelength, therefore

$$\frac{1}{\lambda_3} = \frac{1}{\lambda_1} + \frac{1}{\lambda_2} = \frac{\lambda_2 + \lambda_1}{\lambda_1 \lambda_2} \Rightarrow \lambda_3 = \frac{\lambda_1 \lambda_2}{\lambda_1 + \lambda_2}$$

2. (d) We know that, $\frac{1}{\lambda} = RZ^2\left[\frac{1}{n_2^2} - \frac{1}{n_1^2}\right] \Rightarrow \frac{1}{\lambda} \propto Z^2$

λ is shortest when $\frac{1}{\lambda}$ is largest i.e., when Z is big . Z is highest for lithium.

3. (a) $R \propto n^2$

$V \propto \frac{1}{n}$ so VR is $\propto n$

$T \propto n^3 \Rightarrow E \propto \frac{1}{n^2}$

4. (a) Series limit of Lyman series is $\infty \to 1$ ν_1
First line of Lyman series is $2 \to 1$ ν_2
Series limit for Balmer series $\infty \to 2$
$\therefore \nu_1 - \nu_2 = \nu_3$

5. (c) For third line of Balmer series $n_1 = 2, n_2 = 5$

$$\therefore \frac{1}{\lambda} = RZ^2\left[\frac{1}{n_1^2} - \frac{1}{n_2^2}\right] \text{gives } Z^2 = \frac{n_1^2 n_2^2}{(n_2^2 - n_1^2)\lambda R}$$

On putting values Z = 2

$$\text{From } E = -\frac{13.6Z^2}{n^2} = \frac{-13.6(2)^2}{(1)^2} = -54.4 \text{ eV}$$

6. (b) $\frac{1}{\lambda'} = \frac{1}{\lambda}\sqrt{\frac{c-v}{c+v}}$

Here, $\lambda' = 706$ nm, $\lambda = 656$ nm

$$\therefore \quad \frac{c-v}{c+v} = \left(\frac{\lambda}{\lambda'}\right)^2 = \left(\frac{656}{706}\right)^2 = 0.86$$

$$\Rightarrow \quad \frac{v}{c} = \frac{0.14}{1.86} \Rightarrow v = 0.075 \times 3 \times 10^8 = 2.25 \times 10^7 \text{m/s}$$

7. (c) $\frac{1}{\lambda} = R\left[\frac{1}{n_1^2} - \frac{1}{n_2^2}\right]$

$$\Rightarrow \frac{1}{970.6 \times 10^{-10}} = 1.097 \times 10^7 \left[\frac{1}{1^2} - \frac{1}{n_2^2}\right] \Rightarrow n_2 = 4$$

$$\therefore \text{Number of emission line } N = \frac{n(n-1)}{2} = \frac{4 \times 3}{2} = 6$$

8. (a)

9. (b) $\frac{1}{\lambda} = R\left(\frac{1}{n_1^2} - \frac{1}{n_2^2}\right)$

$$\frac{1}{\lambda_0} = R\left(\frac{1}{2^2} - \frac{1}{3^2}\right) = R\left(\frac{1}{4} - \frac{1}{9}\right) = \frac{5R}{36}$$

$$\frac{1}{\lambda} = R\left(\frac{1}{2^2} - \frac{1}{4^2}\right) = R\left(\frac{1}{4} - \frac{1}{16}\right) = \frac{3R}{16}$$

$$\frac{\lambda}{\lambda_0} = \frac{5}{36} \times \frac{16}{3} = \frac{20}{27}$$

10. (c) $\sqrt{\nu} \propto (Z-1)$ for K_α X-ray

$$\Rightarrow \frac{\nu_2}{\nu_1} = \left(\frac{Z_2 - 1}{Z_1 - 1}\right)^2 \Rightarrow \nu_2 = \left(\frac{51-1}{31-1}\right)^2 \nu = \frac{25}{9}\nu$$

11. (b) For 2nd line of Balmer series in hydrogen spectrum

$$\frac{1}{\lambda} = R\,(1)\left(\frac{1}{2^2} - \frac{1}{4^2}\right) = \frac{3}{16}R$$

$$\text{For } Li^{2+} \left[\frac{1}{\lambda} = R \times 9\left(\frac{1}{x^2} - \frac{1}{12^2}\right) = \frac{3R}{16}\right]$$

which is satisfied by n = 12 $\to$ n = 6.

12. (c) Using $\frac{1}{\lambda} = R(Z-1)^2\left[\frac{1}{n_2^2} - \frac{1}{n_1^2}\right]$

For α particle, $n_1 = 2$, $n_2 = 1$

$$\text{For metal A}: \frac{1875\,R}{4} = R\,(Z_1 - 1)^2\left(\frac{3}{4}\right) \Rightarrow Z_1 = 26$$

$$\text{For metal B}: 675\,R = R\,(Z_2 - 1)^2\left(\frac{3}{4}\right) \Rightarrow Z_2 = 31$$

Therefore, 4 elements lie between A and B.
= 220 MeV.

13. (c) Total energy of electron in excited state = –13.6 + 12.1 = –1.5 eV, which corresponds to third orbit. The possible spectral lines are when electron jumps from orbit 3rd to 2nd ; 3rd to 1st and 2nd to 1st.

14. (d) Spectral lines obtained on account of transition from nth orbit to various lower orbits is $\frac{n(n-1)}{2}$

$$\Rightarrow 6 = \frac{n(n-1)}{2}$$

$\Rightarrow n = 4$

$$\Delta E = \frac{hc}{\lambda} = \frac{-Z^2}{n^2}(13.6eV)$$

$$\Rightarrow \frac{1}{\lambda}=Z^2\left(\frac{13.6eV}{hc}\right)\left(\frac{1}{n_2^2}-\frac{1}{n_1^2}\right)$$

$$=(13.4)(3)^2\left[1-\frac{1}{16}\right]eV$$

$$\Rightarrow \lambda=\frac{1242\times16}{(13.4)\times(9)(15)}\text{nm}\simeq 10.8\text{nm}$$

15. (d) Energy released by hydrogen atom for transition n = 2 to n = 1

$$\therefore\ \Delta E_1=13.6\times\left(\frac{1}{1^2}-\frac{1}{2^2}\right)=\frac{3}{4}\times13.6\text{ eV}$$

$= 10.2$ eV

This energy is absorbed by He+ ion in transition from n = 2 to n = n1 (say)

$$\therefore\ \Delta E_2=13.6\times4\times\left(\frac{1}{4}-\frac{1}{n_1^2}\right)=10.2\text{ eV}$$

$\Rightarrow$ n1 = 4

So, possible transition is $n=2\rightarrow n=4$

16. (d) When electron jumps from $M\rightarrow L$ shell

$$\frac{1}{\lambda}=K\left(\frac{1}{2^2}-\frac{1}{3^2}\right)=\frac{K\times5}{36}\quad\text{..... (i)}$$

When eletron jumps from $N\rightarrow L$ shell

$$\frac{1}{\lambda'}=K\left(\frac{1}{2^2}-\frac{1}{4^2}\right)=\frac{K\times3}{16}\quad\text{....(ii)}$$

solving equation (i) and (ii) we get

$$\lambda'=\frac{20}{27}\lambda$$

17. (a)

18. (d) $h\nu_L=E_\infty-E_1$ ...(i)

$h\nu_f=E_\infty-E_5$ ...(ii)

$$E\propto\frac{z^2}{n^2}\Rightarrow\frac{E_5}{E_1}=\left(\frac{1}{5}\right)^2=\frac{1}{25}$$

$$\text{Eqn (i)/(ii)}\Rightarrow\frac{h\nu_L}{h\nu_f}=\frac{E_1}{E_5}$$

$$\Rightarrow\frac{\nu_L}{\nu_f}=\frac{25}{1}\Rightarrow\nu_f=\frac{\nu_L}{25}$$

19. (d) de-Broglie wavelength, $\lambda=\frac{h}{P}$

$$\frac{\lambda_B}{\lambda_G}=\frac{P_a}{P_B}=\frac{mv_G}{mv_B}$$

Speed of electron $V\propto\frac{z}{n}$

$$\text{so}\quad\frac{\lambda_B}{\lambda_G}=\frac{n_B}{n_G}=\frac{3}{1}\Rightarrow\lambda_B=3\lambda_G$$

20. (b) Energy required to remove e^- from singly ionized helium atom $=\frac{(13.6)Z^2}{1^2}=54.4$ eV $(\because Z=2)$

Energy required to remove e^- from helium atom = x eV

According to question, $54.4\text{ eV}=2.2x\Rightarrow x=24.73$ eV

Therefore, energy required to ionize helium atom $=(54.4+24.73)\text{ eV}=79.12$ eV

21. (b) From energy level diagram, using $\Delta E=\frac{hc}{\lambda}$

For wavelength $\lambda_1, \Delta E=-E-(-2E)=\frac{hc}{\lambda_1}$

$$\therefore\quad\lambda_1=\frac{hc}{E}$$

For wavelength $\lambda_2, \Delta E=-E-\left(-\frac{4E}{3}\right)=\frac{hc}{\lambda_2}$

$$\therefore\quad\lambda_2=\frac{hc}{\left(\frac{E}{3}\right)}\qquad\therefore r=\frac{\lambda_1}{\lambda_2}=\frac{1}{3}$$

22. (c)

23. (d) Magnetic field at the centre of nucleus of H-atom,

$$B=\frac{\mu_0 I}{2r}\quad\text{..... (i)}$$

According to Bohr's model, radius of orbit $r\propto n^2$

from eq. (i) we can also write as $B\propto n^{-2}$

24. (b) A hydrogen atom makes a transition from n = 2 to n = 1

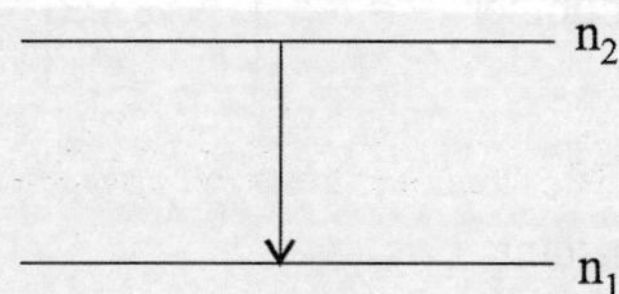

$$\text{Then wavelength}=Rcz^2\left[\frac{1}{n_1^2}-\frac{1}{n_2^2}\right]=Rc(1)^2\left[1-\frac{1}{4}\right]$$

$$\lambda=Rc\left[\frac{3}{4}\right]\quad\text{...(1)}$$

For ionized lithium

$$\lambda=Rc(3)^2\left[\frac{1}{n^2}\right]=Rc9\left[\frac{1}{n^2}\right]\quad\text{...(2)}$$

$$Rc\left[\frac{3}{4}\right]=Rc9\left[\frac{1}{n^2}\right]$$

$$\Rightarrow\frac{3}{4}=\frac{9}{n^2}\Rightarrow n=\sqrt{12}=2\sqrt{3}$$

$\therefore$ The least quantum number must be 4.

25. (c) Kinetic energy of electron is

$$\text{K.E.}\propto\left(\frac{Z}{N}\right)^2$$

When the electron makes transition from excited state to ground state, then n increases and kinetic energy increases.

Total energy = – KE

$\therefore$ Total energy also decreases.

Potential energy is lowest for ground state.

26. (b) De-Broglie wavelength of electron $\lambda = \frac{h}{mV}$

As we know, $V \propto \frac{1}{n}$

So, $\lambda \propto n$

$\lambda_4 = 4\lambda_1$

λ_1 is the de-Broglie wavelength of the electron in the ground state.

27. (c) $qVB = \frac{mv^2}{r}$ ....(i)

$\frac{nh}{2\pi} = mvr$ ....(ii)

Multiplying equation (i) and (ii),

$\frac{qBnh}{2\pi} = m^2v^2$

Now multiplying both sides by $\frac{1}{2m}$,

$n\frac{qBh}{4\pi m} = \frac{1}{2}mv^2$

i.e. KE $= n\left[\frac{qBh}{4\pi m}\right]$

28. (c) Wave number $\frac{1}{\lambda} = RZ^2\left[\frac{1}{n_1^2} - \frac{1}{n^2}\right]$

$\Rightarrow \lambda \propto \frac{1}{Z^2}$

$\therefore \lambda Z^2 =$ constant

By question $n = 1$ and $n_1 = 2$

Then, $\lambda_1 = \lambda_2 = 4\lambda_3 = 9\lambda_4$

29. (a) $E = \frac{hc}{\lambda} \Rightarrow \lambda = \frac{hc}{E} = \frac{6.62\times10^{-34}\times3\times10^8}{12.5\times1.6\times10^{-19}} = 993\,Å$

$\frac{1}{\lambda} = R\left(\frac{1}{n_1^2} - \frac{1}{n_2^2}\right)$

(where Rydberg constant, $R = 1.097 \times 10^7$)

or, $\frac{1}{993\times10^{-10}} = 1.097\times10^7\left(\frac{1}{1^2} - \frac{1}{n_2^2}\right)$

Solving we get $n_2 = 3$

Spectral lines

Total number of spectral lines = 3

Two lines in Lyman series for $n_1 = 1, n_2 = 2$ and $n_1 = 1, n_2 = 3$ and one in Balmer series for $n_1 = 2, n_2 = 3$

n = 3 — Balmer
n = 2
Lyman | Lyman
n = 1

30. (c) As $F = \frac{mv^2}{r} = \frac{e^2}{4\pi\epsilon_0}\left(\frac{1}{r^2} + \frac{\beta}{r^3}\right)$

and $mvr = \frac{nh}{2\pi} \Rightarrow v = \frac{nh}{2\pi mr}$

$\therefore m\left(\frac{nh}{2\pi mr}\right)^2 \times \frac{1}{r} = \frac{e^2}{4\pi\epsilon_0}\left(\frac{1}{r^2} + \frac{\beta}{r^3}\right)$

or, $\frac{1}{r^2} + \frac{\beta}{r^3} = \frac{mn^2h^2 4\pi\epsilon_0}{4\pi^2m^2e^2r^3}$

or, $\frac{a_0n^2}{r^3} = \frac{1}{r^2} + \frac{\beta}{r^3}$ $\left(\because a_0 = \frac{\epsilon_0 h^2}{m\pi e^2} \text{ Given}\right)$

For n^{th} atom

$\therefore r_n = a_0n^2 - \beta$

31. (c) According to the question,

$2\pi r = n\lambda = \frac{nh}{p} = \frac{nh}{mv}$

or $mvr = \frac{nh}{2\pi}$ or $mv = \frac{nh}{2\pi r}$

$F = qv_B = \frac{mv^2}{r}$ or, $q_B = \frac{mv}{r} = \frac{nh}{2\pi r.r}$

or, $r^2 = \frac{nh}{2\pi qB}$ or, $r = \sqrt{\frac{nh}{2\pi qB}}$

i.e., $r \propto n^{1/2}$

32. (c) Magnetic moment of the hydrogen atom, when the electron is in n^{th} excited state, i.e., $n' = (n+1)$

As magnetic moment $M_n = I_nA = i_n(\pi r_n^2)$

$i_n = eV_n = \frac{mz^2e^5}{4\varepsilon_0^2n^3h^3}$

$r_n = \frac{n^2h^2}{4\pi^2kzme^2}\left(k = \frac{1}{4\pi\epsilon_0}\right)$

Solving we get magnetic moment of the hydrogen atom for n^{th} excited state

$M_{n'} = \left(\frac{e}{2m}\right)\frac{nh}{2\pi}$

33. (d)

34. (a) Velocity of electron in n^{th} orbit of hydrogen atom is given by :

$V_n = \frac{2\pi KZe^2}{nh}$

Substituting the values we get,

$V_n = \frac{2.2\times10^6}{n}$ m/s or $V_n \propto \frac{1}{n}$

As principal quantum number increases, velocity decreases.

35. (c) $\frac{1}{\lambda} = R\left(\frac{1}{n_1^2} - \frac{1}{n_2^2}\right)$ where R = Rydberg constant

$\frac{1}{\lambda_{32}} = \left(\frac{1}{4} - \frac{1}{9}\right) = \frac{5}{36}$ $\Rightarrow \lambda_{32} = \frac{36}{5}$

Similarly solving for λ_{31} and λ_{21}

$\lambda_{31} = \frac{9}{8}$ and $\lambda_{21} = \frac{4}{3}$

$\therefore \quad \frac{\lambda_{32}}{\lambda_{31}} = 6.4$ and $\frac{\lambda_{21}}{\lambda_{31}} \simeq 1.2$

36. (b) If $n_1 = n$ and $n_2 = n+1$

Maximum wavelength $\lambda_{max} = \frac{n^2(n+1)^2}{(2n+1)R}$

Therefore, for large n, $\lambda_{max} \propto n^3$

37. (c) It is given that transition from the state $n = 4$ to $n = 3$ in a hydrogen like atom result in ultraviolet radiation. For infrared radiation $\left(\frac{1}{n_1^2} - \frac{1}{n_2^2}\right)$ should be less. The only option is $5 \to 4$.

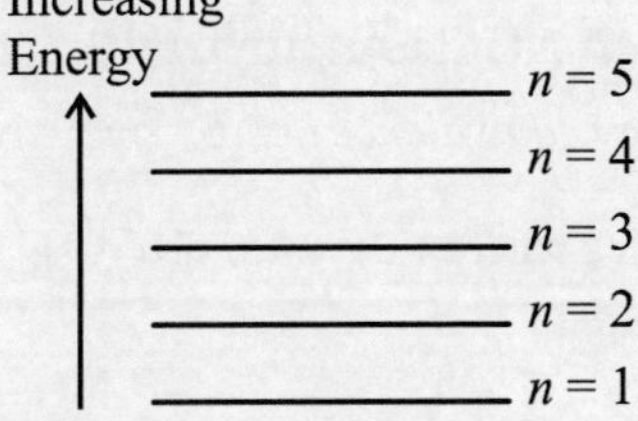

38. (b) Given,

Centripetal force $= \frac{k}{r}$

Then

$\frac{k}{r} = \frac{mv^2}{r}$

$\Rightarrow \quad k = mv^2 \quad \Rightarrow \quad Tn = \frac{1}{2}mv^2 = \frac{1}{2}k$

Tn is independent of *n*

Also,

Angular momentum, $L = \frac{nh}{2\pi}$

$\Rightarrow \quad mvr_n = \frac{nh}{2\pi} \quad (\because L = mvr)$

$\Rightarrow \quad r_n = \frac{nh}{2\pi\sqrt{km}} \quad \left(\begin{array}{l}\because m^2v^2 = km \\ \text{or } mv = \sqrt{km}\end{array}\right)$

Clearly, $r_n \propto n$

39. (b) Eenrgy of radiation that corresponds to energy difference between two energy levels n_1 and n_2 is given as

$E = Rhc\left[\frac{1}{n_1^2} - \frac{1}{n_2^2}\right] \qquad \therefore \quad E \propto \left(\frac{1}{n_1^2} - \frac{1}{n_2^2}\right)$

E will be maximum for the transition for which $\left[\frac{1}{n_1^2} - \frac{1}{n_2^2}\right]$ is maximum. Here n_2 is the higher energy level.

Clearly, $\left[\frac{1}{n_1^2} - \frac{1}{n_2^2}\right]$ is maximum for the third transition, *i.e.*, $2 \to 1$. I transition is showing the absorption of energy.

40. (c) The wavelength of spectrum is given by

$\frac{1}{\lambda} = Rz^2\left(\frac{1}{n_1^2} - \frac{1}{n_2^2}\right)$

where $R = \frac{1.097 \times 10^7}{1 + \frac{m}{M}}$

where m = mass of electron

M = mass of nucleus.

Thus, wavelength involved in the spectrum of hudrogen like atom depends upon masses of nucleus. The mass number of hydrogen and deuterium is 1 and 2 respectively, so spectrum of deuterium will be different from hydrogen.

41. (c) The energy required to remove the electron from the nth orbit of hydrogen is given by

$E_n = \frac{13.6}{n^2}$ eV /atom

For $n = 2$, $E_n = \frac{13.6}{4} = 3.4\,eV$

Therefore the energy required to remove electron from $n = 2$ is $+3.4$ eV.

42. (c) Wave number $\frac{1}{\lambda} = RZ^2\left[\frac{1}{n_1^2} - \frac{1}{n^2}\right]$

$\Rightarrow \lambda \propto \frac{1}{Z^2}$

$\therefore \lambda Z^2 = \text{constant}$

By question $n = 1$ and $n_1 = 2$

Then, $\lambda_1 = \lambda_2 = 4\lambda_3 = 9\lambda_4$

43. (b) Radius of circular path followed by electron is given by,

$r = \frac{mv}{qB} = \frac{\sqrt{2meV}}{eB} = \frac{1}{B}\sqrt{\frac{2m}{e}V}$

$\Rightarrow \quad V = \frac{B^2r^2e}{2m} = 0.8V$

For transition between 3 to 2.

$E = 13.6\left(\frac{1}{4} - \frac{1}{9}\right) = \frac{13.6 \times 5}{36} = 1.88eV$

Work function = 1.88 eV – 0.8 eV = 1.08 eV ≈ 1.1eV

44. (b) Energy required to remove e^- from singly ionized helium atom $= \frac{(13.6)Z^2}{1^2} = 54.4$ eV $(\because Z = 2)$

Energy required to remove e^- from helium atom = x eV

According to question, 54.4 eV = 2.2x ⇒ x = 24.73 eV

Therefore, energy required to ionize helium atom = (54.4 + 24.73) eV = 79.12 eV

45. (b) $E = \frac{hc}{\lambda}$

28 Nuclei

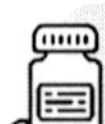

Topic 28.1 : Atomic Mass, Size & Composition of Nucleus, Mass Energy, Nuclear Binding Energy and Nuclear Force

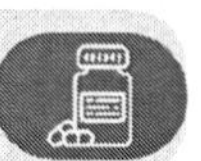

ATOMIC MASS, SIZE AND COMPOSITION OF NUCLEUS

1. Proton was discovered by **Goldstein**
2. **Atomic mass unit, 1.a.m.u** = 1/12th of mass of C-12 isotope, 1 a.m.u = 1.660565×10^{-27} kg
3. Mass of a proton, $m_p = 1.0073$ a.m.u $= 1.6726 \times 10^{-27}$ kg
4. **Chadwick's experiment :** Neutrons were detected.
   $\left[{}_2^4\text{He} + {}_4^9\text{Be} \rightarrow {}_6^{12}\text{C} + {}_0^1\text{n}\right]$
5. Mass of neutron, $m_n = 1.00866$ a.m.u $= 1.6749 \times 10^{-27}$ kg
6. Mass of electron $= 9.1 \times 10^{-31}$ kg
7. ***Mass number,*** *A = total number of nucleons (neutrons + protons present in the nucleus of an atom)*
8. ***Atomic number,*** *Z = number of protons = number of electrons*
9. **Types of nuclei :**
   (i) **Isotopes :** The atoms of the element which have the same atomic number but different atomic mass numbers. e.g., ${}_1H^1, {}_1H^2, {}_1H^3; {}_8O^{16}, {}_8O^{17}, {}_8O^{18}$
   (ii) **Isobars :** The atoms of differents element which have the same atomic mass number but different atomic numbers. e.g., ${}_6C^{14}, {}_7N^{14}, {}_{18}Ar^{40}, {}_{20}Ca^{40}$ etc.
   (iii) **Isotones :** The nuclides which contain the same number of neutrons e.g., ${}_2H_2^3, {}_2He_2^4$; ${}_2Be_5^9, {}_5Be_5^{10}$ etc.
   (iv) **Isomers :** having same mass number, same atomic number but different radioactive properties.
10. Rest mass of nucleus is less than sum of rest masses of constituent nucleons, the difference is called **mass defect**.
11. **Size of the nucleus : Radius of nucleus,** $R = R_0 A^{1/3}$ where $R_0 = 1.1 \times 10^{-15}$ m.
   Nuclear density of all elements ~ 10^{17} kg m^{-3}.

MASS ENERGY AND NUCLEAR BINDING ENERGY

Einstein's mass energy equivalence i.e., $E = mc^2$ gives :

1 a.m.u ≡ 931.5 Me.V, where 1 eV $= 1.6 \times 10^{-19}$ J.

and 1Mev = 1.6×10^{-13} J

Binding Energy

Binding energy of a nucleus is the energy with which nucleons are bound in the nucleus. It is measured by the work required to be done to separate the nucleons an infinite distance apart from the nucleus, so that they may not interact with one another.

Total $BE = \left[Zm_P + (A - Z)m_n - m_N\right]c^2$

m_p = mass of proton; m_n = mass of neutron
m_N = mass of nucleons (protons + neutrons); Z = Atomic number; A = atomic mass

Binding Energy per Nucleon

The binding energy per nucleon of a nucleus is the average energy required to extract a nucleon from the nucleus. Binding energy per nucleon

$$\bar{B} = \frac{\textit{Total binding energy}}{\textit{Total number of nucleons}} = \frac{BE}{A} = \frac{\Delta mc^2}{A}$$

$$= \frac{c^2}{A}[Zm_p + (A - Z)m_n - M({}_Z X^A)]$$

The graph of binding energy per nucleon with mass number A is as shown below.

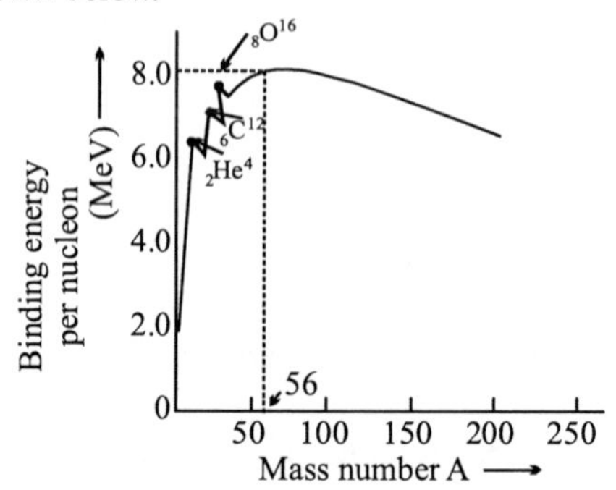

Binding energy per nucleon gives a measure of stability of nucleus. More is binding energy per nucleon more is the stability of nucleus. Binding energy per nucleon is small for lighter nuclei i.e. $_1H^1$, $_1H^2$ etc.

For A < 28 at A = 4n the curve shows some peaks at $_2He^4$, $_4Be^8$, $_6C^{16}$, $_8O^{16}$, $_{10}Ne^{20}$, $_{12}Mg^{24}$.

This represents extra stability of these elements with respect to their neighbours.

Problem Solving Tips

1. A nuclide is a specific nucleus of an atom characterised as $_ZX^A$ where A = mass number and Z = atomic number.
2. Binding energy per nucleon is nearly 8.4 MeV for nuclei in the range of mass number 40 to 120.
3. Binding energy is highest in Fe^{56}.(8.8 MeV)
4. **Binding energy curve predicts :**
   (a) **Fission :** Breaking up of a heavy nucleus (A > 200) into two nuclei of approximately equal size, and release of energy.
   (b) **Fusion :** Lighter nuclei (A < 20) combine together to form heavier nucleus and release of energy.
   (c) BE/ A varies by less than 10% above A = 10 suggests that each nucleon interacts with its neighbouring nucleon only.
   (d) For A > 56, BE/A decreases because of the destabilising effect of long-range coloumbic force.

NUCLEAR FORCE

It is the force acts in the nucleus between the nucleons and is responsible for binding the nucleon.

Characteristics of Nuclear Force :

1. It is a short range force effective only in range 10^{-15} m
2. It is charge independent. It acts between proton-proton, proton-neutron and neutron – neutron.
3. It is not a central force.
4. It is spin dependent.
5. It is 10^{38} times stronger than gravitational force and 10^2 times stronger than electric force.
6. The main cause of nuclear force is the exchange of π– mesons between nucleus

$$p \to n + \pi^+, \; p \to p + \pi^\circ, \; n \to p + \pi^-$$

Example 1.

The radius of a nucleus with nucleon number 16 is 3×10^{-15} m. What would be the radius of other nucleus with nucleon number 128?

Solution :

We know that

$$R \propto A^{1/3}$$

$$\therefore \frac{R_2}{R_1} = \left(\frac{A_2}{A_1}\right)^{1/3} \quad \text{or } R_2 = R_1\left(\frac{A_2}{A_1}\right)^{1/3}$$

so, $R_2 = 3 \times 10^{-15} \times (128/16)^{1/3}$
$= (3 \times 10^{-15}) \times 2 = 6 \times 10^{-15}$ m

Example 2.

A nucleus breaks into two parts whose velocity is in ratio of 2:1. Find the ratio of their radius.

Solution :

As per conservation of momentum $m_1v_1 + m_2v_2 = 0$

so $\frac{m_1}{m_2} = \frac{v_2}{v_1}$

Ratio of radii $\frac{R_1}{R_2} = \left(\frac{A_1}{A_2}\right)^{1/3} = \left(\frac{m_1}{m_2}\right)^{1/3} = \left(\frac{1}{2}\right)^{1/3}$

$\therefore \; R_1 : R_2 = 1 : 2^{1/3}$

Example 3.

Calculate the binding energy per nucleon for $_{17}C^{35}$. Given M (Cl^{35}) = 34.9800 amu. m_n = 1.008665 amu and m_P = 1.007825 amu.

Solution :

$BE = Zm_P + (A - Z)\,m_n - M(Cl^{35}) = 17 \times 1.007825 + 18 \times 1.008665 - 34.9800 = 0.308995$ amu

$BE = 0.308995 \times 931.5 = 287.83$ MeV

$$\bar{B} = \frac{BE}{A} = \frac{287.75}{35} = 8.22 \text{ MeV}$$

28.1 Concept Practice Problems

CPP

1. Nuclear forces are
   (a) spin dependent and have no non-central part
   (b) spin dependent and have a non-central part
   (c) spin independent and have no non-central part
   (d) spin independent and have a non-central part
2. The curve of binding energy per nucleon as a function of atomic mass number has a sharp peak for helium nucleus. This implies that helium
   (a) can easily be broken up
   (b) is very stable
   (c) can be used as fissionable meterial
   (d) is radioactive
3. The volume of a nucleus is directly proportional to
   (a) A (b) A^3 (c) $\sqrt{A}$ (d) $A^{1/3}$
4. Nucleus of an atom whose atomic mass is 24 consists of
   (a) 11 electrons, 11 protons and 13 neutrons
   (b) 11 electrons, 13 protons and 11 neutrons
   (c) 11 protons and 13 neutrons
   (d) 11 protons and 13 electrons
5. Outside a nucleus
   (a) neutron is stable
   (b) proton and neutron both are stable
   (c) neutron is unstable
   (d) neither neutron nor proton is stable

6. Atomic number of a nucleus is Z and atomic mass is M. The number of neutron is
(a) M – Z (b) M (c) Z (d) M + Z

7. If the distance between nuclei is 2×10^{-13} cm, the density of nuclear material is
(a) 3.21×10^{-12} kg/m^3 (b) 1.6×10^{-3} kg/m^3
(c) 2×10^9 kg/m^3 (d) 1×10^{17} kg/m^3

8. If the radius of a nucleus ^{256}X is 8 fermi, then the radius of ^4He nucleus will be
(a) 16 fermi (b) 2 fermi (c) 32 fermi (d) 4 fermi

9. Order of magnitude of density of uranium nucleus is ($m_p = 1.67 \times 10^{-27}$ kg)
(a) 10^{20} kg / m^3 (b) 10^{17} kg / m^3
(c) 10^{14} kg / m^3 (d) 10^{11} kg / m^3

10. The average binding energy per nucleon is maximum for the nucleus
(a) $_2He^4$ (b) $_8O^{16}$
(c) $_{26}Fe^{56}$ (d) $_{92}U^{238}$

ANSWER KEY

1	(b)	2	(b)	3	(a)	4	(c)	5	(c)	6	(a)	7	(d)	8	(b)	9	(b)	10	(c)

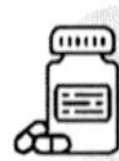

Topic 28.2 : Radioactivity, Radioactive Series and Nuclear Reaction

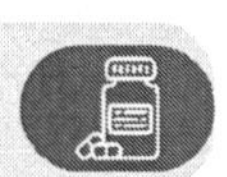

RADIOACTIVITY

It is the spontaneous disintegration of the heavy nucleus of an atom (It occurs without external provocation).

There are three main types of radioactive radiations.

(i) α-rays (i.e., Helium nuclei or α – particles)
(ii) β-rays (i.e., electron or positron or β – particles)
(iii) γ-rays (photons or gamma radiations)

It is a process by which an unstable nuclei achieves stability. This process is not affected by

(a) chemical combination
(b) changing physical environment other than nuclear bombardment.

Features of Radioactivity :

(i) It is a statistical process.

(ii) When a nucleus undergoes alpha or beta decay, its atomic number and mass number changes (in β-decay only atomic number changes) & it transforms into a new element.

(a) $_ZX^A = _{Z-2}Y^{A-4} + _2He^4$ (α-particle), it means that *by emission of alpha particle (α-particle), it loses 2 units of charge and 4 units of mass.*

(b) $_ZX^A = _{Z-1}Y^A + \beta^+$ (positron). It means that *by emission of beta particle (β⁺-particle), nucleus loses one unit of charge.* It is surprising to note that a nucleus does not contain β^+ then how is it emitted. Reason : During a β^+ particle(i.e., positron) decay, a protron converts into a neutron

$p^+ = n^0 + \beta^+ + \upsilon$ (neutrino).

A β^- particle (i.e., electron) decays, when inside the nucleus a neutron converts into a proton i.e.,

$n^0 = p^+ + \beta^- + \bar{\upsilon}$ (antineutrino)

Since β^-particle is an electron(or positron), so the loss of mass in this decay is negligible.

In β^+decay the daughter element is one place forward in the periodic table.

(iii) *When a nucleus emits a gamma ray, neither the mass nor the charge of the nucleus changes*

i.e., $\underset{\text{Excited state}}{Z^{X^A}} = \underset{\text{Ground state}}{Z^{X^A}} + \gamma$ (gamma ray or photon)

The gamma ray(γ-ray) is photon & it carries away some energy from the nucleus & nucleus returns from excited state(unstable state) to ground state (stable state)

α and β-particles are not emitted simultaneously.

γ rays are emitted after the emission of α and β-particle.

α, β and γ-rays are known as **Bequerel rays**

The energy spectrum in the case of β-particles is continous but that of α and γ-rays is a line spectrum. This means that β particles are emitted with any amount of kinetic energy.

Properties of α, β & γ-rays or α-particles

(A) Properties of α–rays or α-particles

(a) It is a positively charged particle & contains a charge of 3.2×10^{-19} coulomb(exactly double the charge of electron).

(b) The mass of α-particles is 6.645×10^{-27}kg(It is equal to mass of a helium nucleus). Actually α-particle is nucleus of helium, hence it is called doubly ionised helium.

(c) They (α-particles) get deflected in both electric & magnetic fields.

(d) The velocity of α-particle is very less than the velocity of light i.e., $V_\alpha \approx \frac{c}{10}$, where c is velocity of light.

(e) The range of α-particle in air depends on radioactive substance.

(f) The ionisation power of α-particle is higher than both β (100 times of β & 10,000 times of γ) and γ particle.

(g) The penetrating power of α particle is lowest (in comparison to β & γ particles). It is 1/100 times of β-particles & 1/10,000 times of γ-rays.

(h) The α-particles can produce fluorescence in barium platinocynide and zinc sulphide.

(i) They show little effect on photographic plate.

(j) They show heating effect on stopping.

(B) **Properties of β rays or β-particles :**

(a) The beta particles (i.e., β^- or β^+) may be positive & negative particle & contain $\pm 1.6 \times 10^{-19}$C of charge. Actually β^- is electron & β^+ is positron.

(b) They get deflected in both electric & magnetic field.

(c) The velocity of β-particle varies between 0.01c to .99c, where c is velocity of light.

(d) The mass of β particle is relativistic, because its velocity is comparable to velocity of light

(e) They have both ionisation & penetration power. Ionisation power less than α-particle and penetration power more than α-particle.

(f) They produce fluorescence on barium platinocynide & zinc sulphide.

(C) **Properties of γ-rays (or gamma radiation):**

(a) They are electromagnetic waves as x-rays.

(b) They are not deflected in electric & magnetic field, it means that they are chargeless.

(c) The velocity of γ-particle is equal to velocity of light.

(d) The ionisation power of gamma rays is less than β & α rays but penetration power more than β and α-rays.

(e) The γ-particles are emitted from the nucleus, while X-rays are obtained, when electron goes from one state to another in an atom.

(f) When γ-rays photon strikes nucleus in a substance, then it gives rise to a phenomenon of pair production i.e.,

$$\underset{(\gamma\text{-rays or photon})}{h\nu} \longrightarrow \beta^- + \beta^+ \quad \text{(Pair production)}$$

The minimum energy of γ-rays required for this phenomena is 1.02 MeV, because the rest mass energy of $\beta^{\pm}$ particle is 0 .51 MeV.

Property	α -rays	β -rays	γ -rays
Mass	$4m_p$	m_e	Zero
Charge	+2e	e	Neutral
Velocity	≈ 2×10^2 m/s	0.33 to 0.99c	c
Penetrating power	1	100	1000
Ionisation power	10,000	100	1
Spectrum	Line	Continuous	Line

Rutherford and Soddy law for radioactive decay

It states that "*at any time the rate at which particular decay occurs in a radioactive substance is proportional to number of radioactive nuclei present.*

If N is the number of nuclei at any time t & at t + dt time, it decrease to N-dN then the rate of decay of these nuclei is $\frac{-dN}{dt}$ (negative sign comes because N decreases as t increases).

So according to Rutherford & Sodi,

$$\frac{-dN}{dt} \propto N \text{ or } \frac{dN}{dt} = \lambda N \quad ...(1)$$

Where λ is decay constant (i.e., probabilily per unit time for a nucleus to decay) and it is constant for a particular nuclei, but different for different nuclei. By integration of equation (1) w.r. to time we get

$$N = N_o e^{-\lambda t} \quad ...(2)$$

where N_o is the number of nuclei at t = 0.

Activity : *The number of decays per unit time or decay rate is called activity(R)*

$$[R] = \left[\frac{dN}{dt}\right] = N_o \lambda e^{-\lambda t} = R_o e^{-\lambda t} \text{ where } R_o = N_o \lambda .$$

The **S.I. unit** of R is **bequerel,**

1 bequerel = 1 Bq = 1 decay/sec

and 1 curie = 1Ci = 3.7 × 10^{10} decay/sec

The other unit of radioactivity is rutherford.

1 rutherford = 10^6 dacay/sec

$$\Rightarrow \quad t = \frac{2.303}{\lambda} \log \frac{N_0}{N} \left[\text{and } \frac{N_0}{N} = \frac{m_0}{m}\right]$$

m_0 = mass at t =0 and m = mass at t = t

MISCONCEPTION

✗ *Incorrect.* Since β-particles (electrons) are emitted from the nucleus shows that electrons exist in nucleus

✓ *Correct.* β-particle cannot exists in nucleus. It is created and ejected at once at the time of β-decay. β-particle cannot exist in the nucleus because its wavelength is greater than the size of nucleus

Half Life of a Radioactive Substance

Half life of a substance is the time, it takes for half of a given number of radioactive nuclei to dacay

Let at = $T_{1/2}$ $N = \frac{N_o}{2}$ then by eq. (2)

$$\frac{N_o}{2} = N_o e^{-\lambda T\frac{1}{2}}$$

$$\text{or} \quad T_{1/2} = \frac{0.693}{\lambda} = \frac{\log_e 2}{\lambda}$$

Also $N = \frac{N_0}{2^n}$

for n half-lives

$\Rightarrow m = \frac{m_0}{2^n}$ where m_0 is mass of radioacive substance at t = 0 and m is mass at t = t.

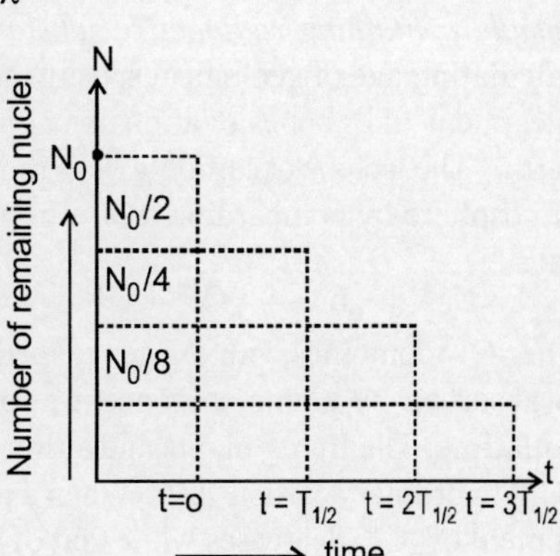

Mean Life of a Radioactive Substance:

Mean life (average life) τ is defined as the averge time the nucleus survive before it decays.

It is given as : $\tau = \frac{1}{\lambda} = \frac{T_{1/2}}{0.693}$

The equivalent λ and τ for two nuclei A and B,

$$\lambda = \lambda_A + \lambda_B \text{ and } \tau = \frac{\tau_A \tau_B}{\tau_A + \tau_B}$$

RADIOACTIVE SERIES

The heavy nuclides change their mass number by α decay and atomic number by α and β decay.

They can decay to stable end products by four paths. The four paths have mass numbers given as 4n, 4n + 1, 4n + 2, 4n + 3 where n is integer.

Last element of series is stable and has a decay constant zero.

There are **four radioactive series :**

Uranium $_{92}U^{238} \rightarrow {}_{82}Pb^{206}$

(Half life $T_{1/2} = 4.47 \times 10^9$ years)

Actinium (natural) $_{92}U^{235} \rightarrow {}_{82}Pb^{207}$

(Half life $T_{1/2} = 7.04 \times 10^8$ years)

Thorium $_{92}Th^{232} \rightarrow {}_{82}Pb^{208}$

(Half life $T_{1/2} = 1.41 \times 10^{10}$ years)

Neptunium $_{93}Nb^{237} \rightarrow {}_{83}Bi^{209}$

(Half life $T_{1/2} = 2.14 \times 10^6$ years)

But only first three series occur in nature & fourth one is artificial.

Series	Mass number	Starting isotope	Stable end product	Natural / Artificial
Thorium	4n	$_{90}Th^{232}$	$_{82}Pb^{208}$	Natural
Neptunium	4n+1	$_{93}Np^{237}$	$_{83}Bi^{209}$	Artificial
Uranium	4n+2	$_{92}U^{238}$	$_{82}Pb^{206}$	Natural
Actinium	4n+3	$_{92}U^{235}$	$_{82}Pb^{207}$	Natural

Radioactive Equilibrium

When the rate of formation of daughter nuclei becomes equal to rate of its decay then this is called as state of radioactive equilibrium

$$N_A \lambda_A = N_B \lambda_B = ... \quad \text{or} \quad \frac{N_A}{T_A} = \frac{N_B}{T_B} = ...$$

Carbon Dating

Carbon dating is the process of determination of time interval which has passed by making use of radioactive decay of a sample containing radioactive substance ($_6C^{14}$). It helps in calculating age of geological specimens like rocks, biological specimens likes bones of animals or trunk of trees and age of earth. The isotope of carbon $_6C^{14}$ is radioactive. It is formed in atmosphere by bombardment of nitrogen atoms with cosmic rays

$$_7N^{14} + {}_0n^1 \rightarrow {}_6C^{14} + {}_1H^1$$

The $_6C^{14}$ combines with oxygen to form carbondioxide which is absorbed by plants so concentration of $_6C^{14}$ is constant with time. The living plants and animals have a fixed ratio of $_6C^{14}$ to ordinary carbon $_6C^{12}$. When a plant or animal dies the content of $_6C^{14}$ decreases while that of $_6C^{12}$ remains constant.

The ratio of two indicates the time that has passed since death of plant or animal. The time interval is calculated from the laws of radioactive disintegration

$$t = \frac{1}{\lambda}\log_e \frac{N_0}{N} = \frac{2.303}{\lambda}\log_{10}\frac{N_0}{N} \quad \left(\frac{N_0}{N} = \frac{A_0}{A}\right)$$

where N_0 is number of $_6C^{14}$ nuclei at time of death, λ is decay constant of $_6C^{14}$ and N is number of $_6C^{14}$ nuclei currently present in sample.

Problem Solving Tips

1. Specific activity is the activity of 1 gram of material.
2. **Geiger Muller Counter** is used for detecting α and β particles.
3. **Cloud chamber** is used for detecting radioactive radiations and for determining their paths, range and energy.
4. **Baryon number** B = 1, for a neutron and a proton.
5. **Lepton number (L)** :L = 1 for electron, and neutrino
   L = –1 for positron and antineutrino.
6. **Radioactive isotope** — **Uses**

Radioactive isotope	Uses
Iodine-131	For detecting the activity of thyroid gland
Chromium-51	To locate the exact position of haemorrhage
Phosphorous-32	In agriculture
C – 14	Carbon dating, Photosynthesis in plants
Co^{60}	Cancer treatment
Na^{24}	For circulation of blood

NUCLEAR REACTION

Nuclear reaction obeys following conservation laws :

(1) Charge conservation
(2) Conservation of linear momentum
(3) Conservation of angular momentum
(4) Conservation of energy (Rest mass energy + K.E.)

Standard way of representing a nuclear reaction

For a nuclear reaction

$$^A_Z X + {}^4_2 He \longrightarrow {}^1_1 H + {}^{A+3}_{Z+1} Y$$

Standard way $^A_Z X(\alpha, p)\, ^{A+3}_{Z+1} Y$

Nuclear Fission (By Otto Hans and Fstrassmann)

Nuclear fission is the disintegration of a heavy nucleus upon bombardment by a projectile, such that the heavy nucleus splits up into two or more segments of comparable masses with an enormous release of energy.

$$^{235}_{92}U + {}^1_0 n \rightarrow {}^{141}_{53}Ba + {}^{92}_{36}Kr + 3\left({}^1_0 n\right) + 200 \text{ MeV}$$

The most of the energy released is by the mode of kinetic energy of fission segment.

Uncontrolled Chain Reaction : It is the principle of atom bomb (destructive use). The number of fission in this case goes on increasing at a tremendous rate leading to the creation of a huge amount of energy in a very small time.

The number of fissions in this case is maintained constant. **Nuclear reactor** has beed devised for this purpose.

The main parts of nuclear reactor are

(a) **Nuclear fuel :** $U^{233}, U^{235}, Pu^{239}$ etc.

(b) **Moderator :** Graphite, heavy water (D_2O). To slow down the neutrons (or slow down the nuclear reaction).

(c) **Control rods :** (Cadmium, boron). To absorb excess neutrons. It controls the chain reaction.

(d) **Coolant :** (water etc). To remove the heat produced in the core to heat exchanger for production of electricity.

The reaction of controlled chain reactor is also called **critical reaction**.

Critical mass : *It is the minimum amount of fissionable material required to carry out fission reaction.* It is 10 kg for ^{236}U

$$Reproduction\ factor\ K = \frac{Rate\ of\ neutron\ production}{Rate\ of\ neutron\ absorption}$$

k = 1 for controlled reaction

$k \geq 1$ for uncontrolled reaction

Breeder reactor :It converts U^{238} non-fissionable to a fissionable material ^{239}Pu or ^{235}U.

Nuclear Fusion :

Nuclear fusion is the fusion of two or more light nuclei to form a heavy nucleus with a release of huge amount of energy. For a nuclear fusion to take place, very high temperature is required to overcome the coulombic repulsive forces acting between the nuclei. It is the principle of hydrogen bomb.

The nuclear fusion reaction, which is the source of the energy of sun/ star are proton-proton cycle.

$${}_1^1H + {}_1^1H \longrightarrow {}_1^2H + {}_1^0e + \nu + 0.42MeV$$

$${}_1^2H + {}_1^1H \longrightarrow {}_2^3He + \gamma + 5.5MeV$$

$${}_2^3He + {}_2^3He \longrightarrow {}_2^4He + {}_1^1H + {}_1^1H + 12.8MeV$$

$$4{}_1^1H \longrightarrow {}_2^4He + 2{}_1^0e + 2\nu + 2\gamma + 24.6\ MeV$$

Stars with mass 0.4 to 2.5 solar mass produce energy by carbon-nitrogen cycle. Stars with lower mas produce energy by proton-proton cycle.

Nuclear holocaust : It is the name given to large scale destruction which will be created upon the use of piled up nuclear weapons. It is believed that if the existing nuclear weapons are used, then the radioactive waste will hang like a cloud in the earth's atmosphere. This clould will be capable to absorb solar radiation due to which these radiation will not reach earth. This would result to a long nuclear winter.

Radiation hazards : The γ-radiations are highly energetic and causes pathological and genetic damage.

Example 4.

The activity of a radioactive element decreased to one third of the original activity I_0 in a period of nine years. What will be its activity after a further lapse of nine years?

Solution :

$$\left(\frac{I}{I_0}\right) = \left(\frac{1}{2}\right)^{t/T} \quad \text{or} \quad \frac{1}{3} = \left(\frac{1}{2}\right)^{9/T}$$

$$\left(\frac{I'}{I_0}\right) = \left(\frac{1}{2}\right)^{18/T} = \left[\left(\frac{1}{2}\right)^{9/T}\right]^2 = \left(\frac{1}{3}\right)^2$$

$$\therefore\ I' = I_0/9$$

Example 5.

At any instant, the ratio of the amount of radioactive substances is 2 : 1. If their half lives be respectively 12 and 16 hours, then after two days, what will be the ratio of amount of the substances?

Solution :

For first substance $n = \frac{48}{12} = 4$

$$\therefore\ N_1 = N_{01}\left(\frac{1}{2}\right)^4 = N_{01}/16 \quad ...(1)$$

For second substance, $n = \frac{48}{16} = 3$

$$N_2 = N_{02}\left(\frac{1}{2}\right)^3 = N_{02}/8 \quad ...(2)$$

Now, $\frac{N_1}{N_2} = \frac{N_{01}}{N_{02}} \times \frac{1}{2} = 2 \times \frac{1}{2} = 1 \ (\because N_{01} = 2N_{02})$

$\therefore\ N_1 : N_2 = 1 : 1$

Example 6.

The half life of radium is 1620 years and its atomic weight is 226. Find the number of atoms that will decay from its 1 gm sample per second.

Solution :

According to Avogadro's hypothesis,

$$N_0 = \frac{6.02 \times 10^{23}}{226} = 2.66 \times 10^{21}$$

$$\text{Half life} = T = \frac{0.6931}{\lambda} = 1620\ \text{years}$$

$$\therefore\ \lambda = \frac{0.6931}{1620 \times 3.16 \times 10^7} = 1.35 \times 10^{-11}\ s^{-1}$$

Because half life is very much large as compared to its time interval, hence $N \approx N_0$

$$\frac{dN}{dt} = \lambda N = \lambda N_0 \quad \text{or} \quad dN = \lambda N_0 dt$$

$$\therefore\ dN = (1.35 \times 10^{-11})(2.66 \times 10^{21})(1) = 3.61 \times 10^{10}.$$

Example 7.

A star initially has 10^{40} deutrons. It produces energy by processes

$${}_1H^2 + {}_1H^2 \longrightarrow {}_1H^3 + p$$

and $${}_1H^2 + {}_1H^3 \longrightarrow {}_2He^4 + n$$

If average power radiated by star is $10^{16}W$ then find time in which deutron is exhausted.

$M({}_1H^2) = 2.01471$ amu *$M({}_2He^4) = 4.00388$ amu*

$m_p = 1.00783$ amu and *$m_n = 1.00866$ amu*

Solution :

Adding the two equation $3\,{}_1H^2 \longrightarrow {}_2He^4 + p + n$

mass defect $= 3 \times 2.01471 - 4.00388 - 1.00783 - 1.00866$

$= 0.02376\ \text{amu} = 0.02376 \times 931.5\ \text{MeV}$

$= 22.13\ \text{MeV}$

Power of star $= 10^{16}W = 10^{16}\ J/s$

Number of deutrons used per second

$$= \frac{10^{16}}{1.6 \times 10^{-19} \times 22.13 \times 10^{6}} = 2.82 \times 10^{27}$$

Time in which deutrons will be used

$$= \frac{\text{Number of deutrons}}{\text{Number of deutrons used per second}}$$

$$= \frac{10^{40}}{2.82 \times 10^{27}} = 3.5 \times 10^{12} \text{ sec}$$

Example 8.

One gram of Radium emits 3.7 × 10^{10} α particles per second. Calculate half life and mean life of Radium. Given: Atomic mass of Radium = 226.

Solution :

Rate of decay of Radium = rate of emission of α particles

or $\frac{-dN}{dt} = \lambda N = 3.7 \times 10^{10}$ per second

Number of active atoms $N = \frac{6.023 \times 10^{23} \times 1}{226}$

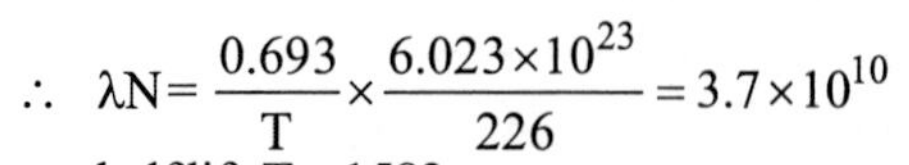

$$\therefore \lambda N = \frac{0.693}{T} \times \frac{6.023 \times 10^{23}}{226} = 3.7 \times 10^{10}$$

or half life T = 1583 years

Mean life τ = 1.44 T = 1.44 × 1580 = 2279 years

Example 9.

Determine the disintegration energy of the process $_{84}Po_0^{210} \longrightarrow {}_{82}Pb^{206} + {}_2He^4 + Q$ *if an α particle of energy 5.3 MeV is emitted in it.*

Solution :

Kinetic energy of α particle $E_\alpha = \frac{A-4}{A} Q$

so $Q = \frac{A}{A-4} E_\alpha = \frac{210}{210-4} \times 5.3 = 5.40$ MeV

Example 10.

The activity of a radioactive substance drops to 1/32 of its initial value in 7.5 h. Find the half life.

Solution :

Using $\frac{A}{A_0} = \left(\frac{1}{2}\right)^{t/T}$ or $\frac{1}{32} = \left(\frac{1}{2}\right)^{7.5/T}$

or $\left(\frac{1}{2}\right)^5 = \left(\frac{1}{2}\right)^{7.5/T}$ or $5 = \frac{7.5}{T}$ i.e. T = 1.5 hour

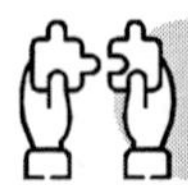

28.2 Concept Practice Problems

CPP

11. A radioactive substance has a half life of four months. Three fourth of the substance will decay in
(a) three months (b) four months
(c) eight months (d) twelve months

12. In gamma ray emission from a nucleus
(a) only the proton number changes
(b) both the neutron number and the proton number change
(c) there is no change in the proton number and the neutron number
(d) only the neutron number changes

13. In which sequence the radioactive radiations are emitted in the following nuclear reaction?

$$_ZX^A \longrightarrow {}_{Z+1}Y^A \longrightarrow$$

$$_{Z-1}K^{A-4} \longrightarrow {}_{Z-1}K^{A-4}$$

(a) γ, α, β (b) α, β, γ (c) β, γ, α (d) β, α, γ

14. Radioactive substance emits
(a) α-rays (b) β-rays
(c) γ-rays (d) All of the above

15. A nucleus ^m_nX emits one α-particle and two β-particles. The resulting nucleus is
(a) $^{m-6}_{n-4}Z$ (b) $^{m-6}_{n}Z$ (c) $^{m-4}_{n}X$ (d) $^{m-4}_{n-2}Y$

16 One curie is equal to
(a) 3.7 × 10^{10} disintegration/sec
(b) 3.2 × 10^{8} disintegration/sec
(c) 2.8 × 10^{10} disintegration/sec
(d) None of these

17. Half life of radioactive element depends upon
(a) amount of element present
(b) temperature
(c) pressure
(d) nature of element

18. A radioactive substance contains 10000 nuclei and its half-life period is 20 days. The number of nuclei present at the end of 10 days is
(a) 7070 (b) 9000 (c) 8000 (d) 7500

19. A radioactive element forms its own isotope after 3 consecutive disintegrations. The particles emitted are
(a) 3 β–particles
(b) 2 β–particles and 1 α–particle
(c) 3 β–particles and 1 α–particle
(d) 2 α–particles and 1 β–particle.

20. Consider a radioactive material of half-life 1.0 minute. If one of the nuclei decays now, the next one will decay
(a) after 1 minute
(b) after $\frac{1}{\log_e 2}$ minute
(c) after $\frac{1}{N}$ minute, where N is the number of nuclei present at that moment
(d) after any time

ANSWER KEY

11	(c)	12	(c)	13	(d)	14	(d)	15	(c)	16	(a)	17	(d)	18	(a)	19	(b)	20	(d)

CONCEPT MAP

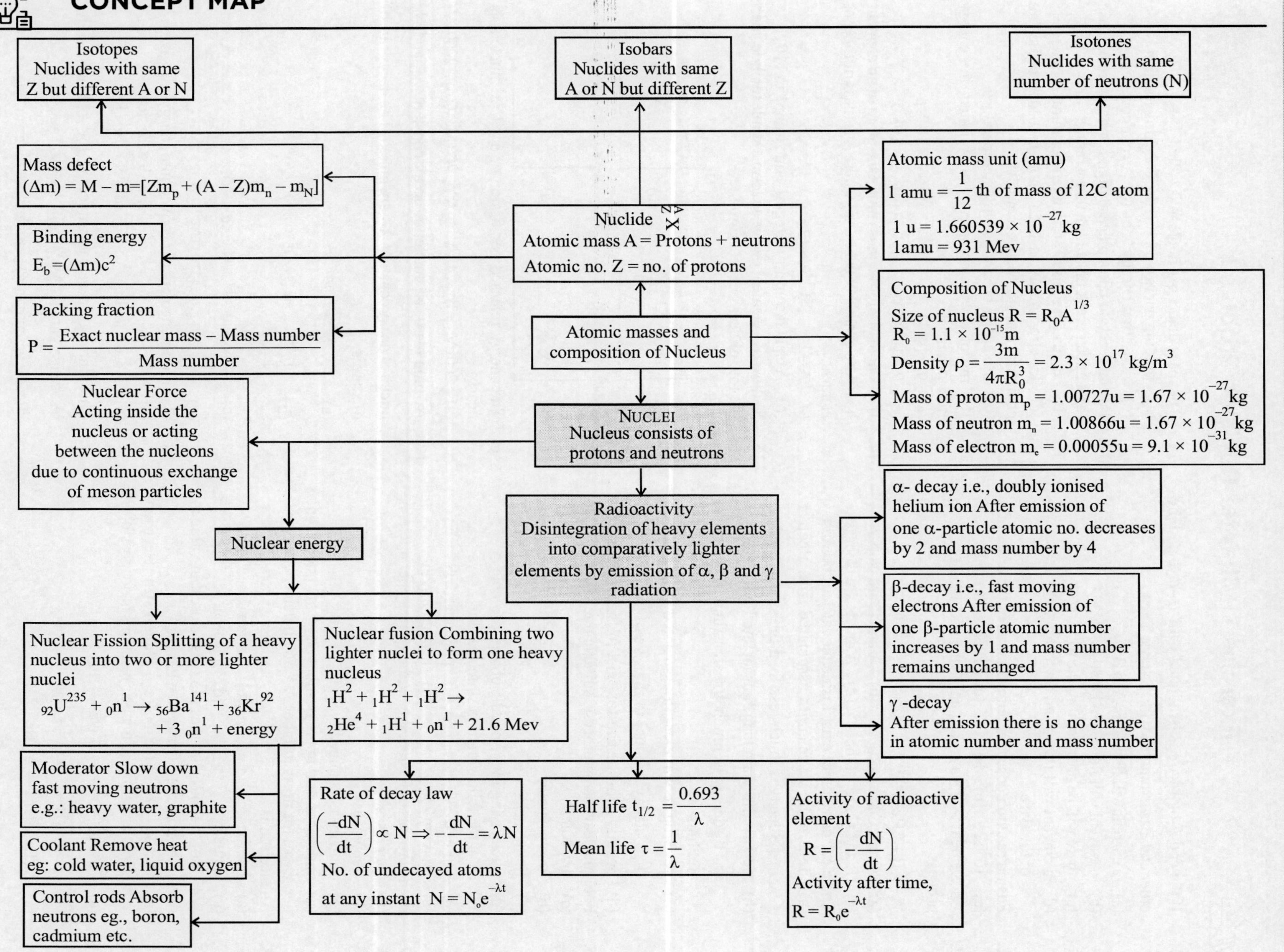
Isotopes
Nuclides with same Z but different A or N
Isobars
Nuclides with same A or N but different Z
Isotones
Nuclides with same number of neutrons (N)
Mass defect
$(\Delta m) = M - m = [Zm_p + (A - Z)m_n - m_N]$
Binding energy
$E_b = (\Delta m)c^2$
Packing fraction
$P = \frac{\text{Exact nuclear mass} - \text{Mass number}}{\text{Mass number}}$
Nuclear Force
Acting inside the nucleus or acting between the nucleons due to continuous exchange of meson particles
Nuclide $^{A}_{Z}X$
Atomic mass A = Protons + neutrons
Atomic no. Z = no. of protons
Atomic masses and composition of Nucleus
NUCLEI
Nucleus consists of protons and neutrons
Atomic mass unit (amu)
1 amu = $\frac{1}{12}$ th of mass of 12C atom
$1\ u = 1.660539 \times 10^{-27}$ kg
1amu = 931 Mev
Composition of Nucleus
Size of nucleus $R = R_0A^{1/3}$
$R_0 = 1.1 \times 10^{-15}$ m
Density $\rho = \frac{3m}{4\pi R_0^3} = 2.3 \times 10^{17}$ kg/m^3
Mass of proton $m_p = 1.00727u = 1.67 \times 10^{-27}$ kg
Mass of neutron $m_n = 1.00866u = 1.67 \times 10^{-27}$ kg
Mass of electron $m_e = 0.00055u = 9.1 \times 10^{-31}$ kg
Nuclear energy
Radioactivity
Disintegration of heavy elements into comparatively lighter elements by emission of α, β and γ radiation
α- decay i.e., doubly ionised helium ion After emission of one α-particle atomic no. decreases by 2 and mass number by 4
β-decay i.e., fast moving electrons After emission of one β-particle atomic number increases by 1 and mass number remains unchanged
γ -decay
After emission there is no change in atomic number and mass number
Nuclear Fission Splitting of a heavy nucleus into two or more lighter nuclei
$_{92}U^{235} + {_0n^1} \rightarrow {_{56}Ba^{141}} + {_{36}Kr^{92}} + 3\ {_0n^1}$ + energy
Nuclear fusion Combining two lighter nuclei to form one heavy nucleus
$_1H^2 + {_1H^2} + {_1H^2} \rightarrow {_2He^4} + {_1H^1} + {_0n^1}$ + 21.6 Mev
Moderator Slow down fast moving neutrons e.g.: heavy water, graphite
Coolant Remove heat eg: cold water, liquid oxygen
Control rods Absorb neutrons eg., boron, cadmium etc.
Rate of decay law
$\left(\frac{-dN}{dt}\right) \propto N \Rightarrow -\frac{dN}{dt} = \lambda N$
No. of undecayed atoms at any instant $N = N_0e^{-\lambda t}$
Half life $t_{1/2} = \frac{0.693}{\lambda}$
Mean life $\tau = \frac{1}{\lambda}$
Activity of radioactive element
$R = \left(-\frac{dN}{dt}\right)$
Activity after time,
$R = R_0e^{-\lambda t}$

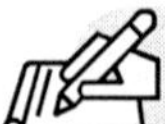

Exercise 1 - Chapter Revision Problems

CRP

1. If the end A of a wire is irradiated with α-rays and the other end B is irradiated with β-rays. Then
(a) a current will flow from A to B
(b) a current will flow from B to A
(c) there will be no current in the wire
(d) a current will flow from each end to the mid-point of the wire

2. Fusion reaction occurs at temperatures of the order of
(a) 10^3 K (b) 10^7 K (c) 10 K (d) 10^4 K

3. An element A decays into an element C by a two step process
$A \rightarrow B + 2He^4$ and $B \rightarrow C + 2e^-$. Then,
(a) A and C are isotopes (b) A and C are isobars
(c) B and C are isotopes (d) A and B are isobars

4. The electrons cannot exist inside the nucleus because
(a) de-Broglie wavelength associated with electron in β-decay is much less than the size of nucleus
(b) de-Broglie wavelength associated with electron in β-decay is much greater than the size of nucleus
(c) de-Broglie wavelength associated with electron in β-decay is equal to the size of nucleus
(d) negative charge cannot exist in the nucleus

5. For a nuclear fusion process, suitable nuclei are
(a) any Nuclei
(b) heavy Nuclei
(c) light Nuclei
(d) nuclei lying in the middle of periodic table

6. Which of the following is best nuclear fuel
(a) thorium 236 (b) plutonium 239
(c) uranium 236 (d) neptunium 239

7. In the process of fission, the binding energy per nucleon
(a) increases
(b) decreases
(c) remains unchanged
(d) increases for mass number A < 56 nuclei but decreases for mass number A > 56 nuclei

8. An electron is
(a) hadron (b) baryon
(c) a nucleon (d) a lepton.

9. Which of the following has the mass closest in value to that of the positron? (1 a.m.u. = 931 MeV)
(a) Proton (b) Electron (c) Photon (d) Neutrino

10. Which of the following nuclear reactions is not possible?
(a) ${}^{12}_{6}C + {}^{12}_{6}C \longrightarrow {}^{20}_{10}Ne + {}^{4}_{2}He$
(b) ${}^{9}_{4}Be + {}^{1}_{1}H \longrightarrow {}^{6}_{3}Li + {}^{4}_{2}He$
(c) ${}^{11}_{5}Be + {}^{1}_{1}H \longrightarrow {}^{9}_{4}Be + {}^{4}_{2}He$
(d) ${}^{7}_{3}Li + {}^{4}_{2}He \longrightarrow {}^{1}_{1}H + {}^{10}_{4}B$

11. The mass defect per nucleon is called
(a) binding energy (b) packing fraction
(c) ionisation energy (d) excitation energy

12. Fusion reaction takes place at high temperature because
(a) nuclei break up at high temperature
(b) atoms get ionised at high temperature
(c) kinetic energy is high enough to overcome the coulomb repulsion between nuclei
(d) molecules break up at high temperature

13. If 1 mg of U^{235} is completely annihilated, the energy liberated is
(a) 9×10^{10} J (b) 9×10^{19} J
(c) 9×10^{18} J (d) 9×10^{17} J

14. If u denotes 1 atomic mass unit. One atom of an element has mass exactly equal to Au, where A is mass number of element.
(a) A = 1 (b) A = 12 (c) A = 16
(d) A can take up any integral value from 1 to 110

15. Radioactive element decays to form a stable nuclide, then the rate of decay of reactant is

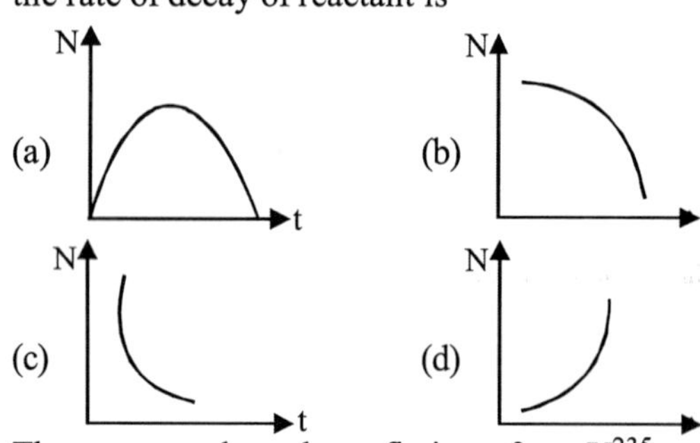

16. The energy released per fission of a ${}_{92}U^{235}$ nucleus is nearly
(a) 200 eV (b) 20 eV (c) 200 MeV (d) 2000 eV

17. At time t = 0, N_1 nuclei of decay constant λ_1 and N_2 nuclei of decay constant λ_2 are mixed. The decay rate of mixture is
(a) $-N_1N_2e^{-(\lambda_1+\lambda_2)t}$
(b) $-\left(\frac{N_1}{N_2}\right)e^{-(\lambda_1+\lambda_2)t}$
(c) $-(N_1\lambda_1e^{-\lambda_1 t} + N_1\lambda_2e^{-\lambda_2 t})$
(d) $-N_1\lambda_1N_2\lambda_2e^{(-\lambda_1+\lambda_2)t}$

18. One milligram of matter convert into energy will give
(a) 90 joule (b) 9×10^3 joule
(c) 9×10^5 joule (d) 9×10^{10} joule

19. The binding energy per nucleon for ${}^{2}_{1}H$ and ${}^{4}_{2}He$ respectively are 1.1 MeV and 7.1 MeV. The energy released in MeV when two ${}^{2}_{1}H$ nuclei fuse to form ${}^{4}_{2}He$ is
(a) 4.4 (b) 8.2 (c) 24 (d) 28.4

20. The rest energy of an electron is
(a) 510 KeV (b) 931 KeV (c) 510 MeV (d) 931 MeV

21. From the following equations, pick out the possible nuclear reactions.
(a) ${}_6C^{13} + {}_1H^1 \rightarrow {}_6C^{14} + 4.3\text{ MeV}$
(b) ${}_6C^{12} + {}_1H^1 \rightarrow {}_7N^{13} + 2\text{ MeV}$
(c) ${}_7N^{14} + {}_1H^1 \rightarrow {}_8O^{15} + 7.3\text{ MeV}$
(d) ${}_{92}U^{235} + {}_0n^1 \rightarrow {}_{54}X^{140} + {}_{38}Si^{94} + {}_{20}n^1 + \gamma + 200\text{ MeV}$

22. The fossil bone has a $^{14}C : {}^{12}C$ ratio, which is $\left[\frac{1}{16}\right]$ of that in a living animal bone. If the half-life of ^{14}C is 5730 years, then the age of the fossil bone is
(a) 11460 years (b) 17190 years
(c) 22920 years (d) 45840 years

23. The ratio of half-life times of two elements A and B is $\frac{T_A}{T_B}$.
The ratio of respective decay constant $\frac{\lambda_A}{\lambda_B}$, is
(a) T_B/T_A (b) T_A/T_B (c) $\frac{T_A + T_B}{T_A}$ (d) $\frac{T_A - T_B}{T_A}$

24. A radioactive nucleus undergoes a series of decay according to the scheme
$$A \xrightarrow{a} A_1 \xrightarrow{\beta} A_2 \xrightarrow{\alpha} A_3 \xrightarrow{\gamma} A_4$$
If the mass number and atomic number of 'A' are 180 and 72 respectively, then what are these numbers for A_4
(a) 172 and 69 (b) 174 and 70
(c) 176 and 69 (d) 176 and 70

25. The mass defect in a particular nuclear reaction is 0.3 grams. The amount of energy liberated in kilowatt hour is (Velocity of light $= 3 \times 10^8$ m/s)
(a) 1.5×10^6 (b) 2.5×10^6 (c) 3×10^6 (d) 7.5×10^6

26. The binding energies per nucleon for a deuteron and an α-particle are x_1 and x_2 respectively. What will be the energy Q released in the reaction ${}_1H^2 + {}_1H^2 \rightarrow {}_2He^4 + Q$
(a) $4(x_1 + x_2)$ (b) $4(x_2 - x_1)$
(c) $2(x_1 + x_2)$ (d) $2(x_2 - x_1)$

27. After 150 days, the activity of a radioactive sample is 5000 dps. The activity becomes 2500 dps after another 75 days. The initial activity of the sample is
(a) 20000 dps (b) 40000 dps
(c) 7500 dps (d) 10000 dps

28. If the total binding energies of ${}^2_1H$, ${}^4_2He$, ${}^{56}_{26}Fe$ & ${}^{235}_{92}U$ nuclei are 2.22, 28.3, 492 and 1786 MeV respectively, identify the most stable nucleus of the following.
(a) ${}^{56}_{26}Fe$ (b) ${}^2_1H$ (c) ${}^{235}_{92}U$ (d) ${}^4_2He$

29. M_p denotes the mass of a proton and M_n that of a neutron. A given nucleus, of binding energy B, contains Z protons and N neutrons. The mass M(N, Z) of the nucleus is given by (c is the velocity of light)
(a) $M(N, Z) = NM_n + ZM_p + B/c^2$
(b) $M(N, Z) = NM_n + ZM_p - Bc^2$
(c) $M(N, Z) = NM_n + ZM_p + Bc^2$
(d) $M(N, Z) = NM_n + ZM_p - B/c^2$

30. The mass of a ${}^7_3Li$ nucleus is 0.042 u less than the sum of the masses of all its nucleons. The binding energy per nucleon of ${}^7_3Li$ nucleus is nearly
(a) 46 MeV (b) 5.6 MeV (c) 3.9 MeV (d) 23 MeV

31. A radioactive nucleus of mass M emits a photon of frequency ν and the nucleus recoils. The recoil energy will be
(a) $Mc^2 - h\nu$ (b) $h^2\nu^2 / 2Mc^2$
(c) zero (d) $h\nu$

32. If the nuclear radius of ^{27}Al is 3.6 fermi, the approximate nuclear radius of ^{64}Cu in fermi is
(a) 2.4 (b) 1.2 (c) 4.8 (d) 3.6

33. A mixture consists of two radioactive materials A_1 and A_2 with half lives of 20 s and 10 s respectively. Initially the mixture has 40 g of A_1 and 160 g of A_2. The amount of the two in the mixture will become equal after
(a) 60 s (b) 80 s (c) 20 s (d) 40 s

34. A certain mass of Hydrogen is changed to Helium by the process of fusion. The mass defect in fusion reaction is 0.02866 a.m.u. The energy liberated per a.m.u. is (Given : 1 a.m.u = 931 MeV)
(a) 26.7 MeV (b) 6.675 MeV
(c) 13.35 MeV (d) 2.67 MeV

35. Fraction of tritium left after 150 years (half life of tritium is 12.5 years) is
(a) 1/1024 (b) 1/2048 (c) 1/4096 (d) 1/8192

36. A duetron strikes ${}_8O^{16}$ nucleus with subsequent emission of alpha particle. Identify the nucleus so produced
(a) ${}_3Li^7$ (b) ${}_5B^{10}$ (c) ${}_7N^{13}$ (d) ${}_7N^{14}$

37. The more readily fissionable isotope of uranium has an atomic mass of
(a) 234 (b) 235 (c) 236 (d) 238

38. A nuclear reaction is given by
${}_ZX^A \rightarrow {}_{Z+1}Y^A + {}_{-1}e^0 + \bar{\nu}$, represents
(a) fission (b) β-decay
(c) σ-decay (d) fusion

39. The half life of the radioactive substance is 40 days. The substance will disintegrate completely in
(a) 40 days (b) 400 days
(c) 4000 days (d) infinite time

40. They decay constant of radium is 4.28×10^{-4} per year. Its half life will be
(a) 2000 years (b) 1240 years
(c) 63 years (d) 1620 years

41. The radius *R* of a nucleus of mass number *A* can be estimated by the formula $R = (1.3 \times 10^{-15})A^{1/3}$ m. It follows that the mass density of a nucleus is of the order of :
$(M_{prot.} \cong M_{neut.} \simeq 1.67 \times 10^{-27}\text{ kg})$
(a) 10^3 kg m^{-3} (b) 10^{10} kg m^{-3}
(c) 10^{24} kg m^{-3} (d) 10^{17} kg m^{-3}

42. The ratio of the mass densities of nuclei of ^{40}Ca and ^{16}O is close to :
(a) 1 (b) 0.1 (c) 5 (d) 2

43. In a radioactive material, fraction of active material remaining after time t is 9/16. The fraction that was remaining after $t/2$ is :
(a) $\frac{4}{5}$ (b) $\frac{3}{5}$ (c) $\frac{3}{4}$ (d) $\frac{7}{8}$

44. The activity of a radioactive sample falls from 700 s^{-1} to 500 s^{-1} in 30 minutes. Its half life is close to:
(a) 72 min (b) 62 min (c) 66 min (d) 52 min

45. Two radioactive materials A and B have decay constants 10 λ and λ, respectively. If initially they have the same number of nuclei, then the ratio of the number of nuclei of A to that of B will be 1/e after a time :
(a) $\frac{1}{9\lambda}$ (b) $\frac{1}{11\lambda}$ (c) $\frac{11}{10\lambda}$ (d) $\frac{1}{10\lambda}$

46. A radioactive nucleus decays by two different processes. The half life for the first process is 10 s and that for the second is 100 s. The effective half life of the nucleus is close to :
(a) 9 sec. (b) 6 sec. (c) 55 sec. (d) 12 sec.

47. An unstable heavy nucleus at rest breaks into two nuclei which move away with velocities in the ratio of 8:27. The ratio of the radii of the nuclei (assumed to be spherical) is:
(a) 8 : 27 (b) 2 : 3 (c) 3 : 2 (d) 4 : 9

48. You are given that mass of $^7_3\text{Li} = 7.0160$ u,
Mass of $^4_2\text{He} = 4.0026$ u
and Mass of $^1_1\text{H} = 1.0079$ u.
When 20 g of ^7_3Li is converted into ^4_2He by proton capture, the energy liberated, (in kWh), is :
[Mass of nucleon = 1 GeV/c^2]
(a) 4.5×10^5 (b) 8×10^6
(c) 6.82×10^5 (d) 1.33×10^6

49. Find the Binding energy per neucleon for $^{120}_{50}$Sn. Mass of proton $m_p = 1.00783$ U, mass of neutron $m_n = 1.00867$ U and mass of tin nucleus $m_{Sn} = 119.902199$ U.
(take 1U = 931 MeV)
(a) 7.5 MeV (b) 9.0 MeV
(c) 8.0 MeV (d) 8.5 MeV

50. At some instant, a radioactive sample S_1 having an activity 5μCi has twice the number of nuclei as another sample S_2 which has an activity of 10μCi. The half lives of S_1 and S_2 are
(a) 10 years and 20 years, respectively
(b) 5 years and 20 years, respectively
(c) 20 years and 10 years, respectively
(d) 20 years and 5 years, respectively

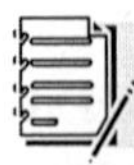

Exercise 2 - Exemplar & Past Year Questions

E&PYQs

Exemplar MCQs

1. Suppose we consider a large number of containers each containing initially 10000 atoms of a radioactive material with a half life of 1 yr. After 1 year,
(a) all the containers will have 5000 atoms of the material
(b) all the contains will conatin the same number of atoms of the material but that number will only be approximately 5000
(c) the containers will in general have different numbers of the atoms of the material but their average will be close to 5000
(d) none of the containers can have more than 5000 atoms.

2. The gravitational force between a H-atom and another particle of mass m will be given by Newton's law
$F = G\frac{M.m}{r^2}$, where r is in km and
(a) $M = m_{proton} + m_{electron}$
(b) $M = m_{proton} + m_{electron} - \frac{B}{c^2}$ (B = 13.6 eV)
(c) M is not related to the mass of the hydrogen atom
(d) $M = m_{proton} + m_{electron} - \frac{|V|}{c^2}$ (|V| = magnitude of the potential energy of electron in the H-atom.

3. When a nucleus in an atom undergoes a radioactive decay, the electronic energy levels of the atom
(a) do not change for any type of radioactivity
(b) change for α and β-radioactivity but not for γ-radioactivity
(c) change for α-radioactivity but not for others
(d) change for β-radioactivity but not for others

4. M_x and M_y denote the atomic masses of the parent and the daughter nuclei respectively in radioactive decay. The Q – value for a β^- decay is Q_1 and that for a β^+ decay is Q_2. If m_e denotes the mass of an electron, then which of the following statements is correct?
(a) $Q_1 = (M_x - M_y)c^2$ and $Q_2 = [M_x - M_y - 2m_e]c^2$
(b) $Q_1 = (M_x - M_y)c^2$ and $Q_2 = (M_x - M_y)c^2$
(c) $Q_1 = (M_x - M_y - 2m_e)c^2$ and $Q_2 = (M_x - M_y + 2c_e)c^2$
(d) $Q_1 = (M_x - M_y + 2m_e)c^2$ and $Q_2 = (M_x - M_y + 2m_e)c^2$

5. Tritium is an isotope of hydrogen whose nucleus triton contains neutrons and 1 proton. Free neutrons decay into $p + \bar{e} + \bar{n}$. If one of the neutrons is Triton decays, it would transform into He^3 nucleus. This does not happen. This is because
(a) Triton energy is less than that of a He^3 nucleus
(b) The electron created in the beta decay process cannot remain in the nucleus
(c) both the neutrons in triton have to decay simultaneously resulting in a nucleus with 3 protons, which is not a He^3 nucleus.
(d) free neutrons decay due to external perturbations which is absent in triton nucleus

6. Heavy stable nuclei have more neutrons than protons. this is because of the fact that
(a) neutrons are heavier than protons
(b) electrostatic force between protons are repulsive
(c) neutrons decay into protons through beta decay
(d) nuclear force between neutrons are weaker than that between protons

7. In a nuclear reactor, moderators slow down the neutrons which come out in a fission process. the moderator used have light nuclei. Heavy nuclei will not serve the purpose, because
(a) they will break up
(b) elastic collision of neutrons with heavy nuclei will not slow them down
(c) the net weight of the reactor would be unbearably high
(d) substances with heavy nuclei do not occur in liquid or gaseous state at room temperature

NEET/AIPMT (2013-2020) Questions

8. A certain mass of Hydrogen is changed to Helium by the process of fusion. The mass defect in fusion reaction is 0.02866 a.m.u. The energy liberated per a.m.u. is *[2013]*
(Given : 1 a.m.u = 931 MeV)
(a) 26.7 MeV (b) 6.675 MeV
(c) 13.35 MeV (d) 2.67 MeV

9. The half life of a radioactive isotope 'X' is 20 years. It decays to another element 'Y' which is stable. The two elements 'X' and 'Y' were found to be in the ratio of 1 : 7 in a sample of a the given rock. The age of the rock is estimated to be *[2013]*
(a) 60 years (b) 80 years (c) 100 years (d) 40 years

10. α-particles, β-particles and γ-rays are all having same energy. Their penetrating power in a given medium in increasing order will be *[NEET Kar. 2013]*
(a) β, γ, α (b) γ, α, β (c) α, β, γ (d) β, α, γ

11. How does the binding energy per nucleon vary with the increase in the number of nucleons? *[NEET Kar. 2013]*
(a) Increases continuously with mass number
(b) Decreases continuously with mass number
(c) First decreases and then increases with increase in mass number
(d) First increases and then decreases with increase in mass number

12. The Binding energy per nucleon of ${}^7_3Li$ and ${}^4_2He$ nuclei are 5.60 MeV and 7.06 MeV, respectively.
In the nuclear reaction ${}^7_3Li + {}^1_1H \rightarrow {}^4_2He + Q$, the value of energy Q released is : *[2014]*
(a) 19.6 MeV (b) –2.4 MeV
(c) 8.4 MeV (d) 17.3 MeV

13. A radio isotope 'X' with a half life 1.4×10^9 years decays to 'Y' which is stable. A sample of the rock from a cave was found to contain 'X' and 'Y' in the ratio 1 : 7. The age of the rock is : *[2014]*
(a) 1.96×10^9 years (b) 3.92×10^9 years
(c) 4.20×10^9 years (d) 8.40×10^9 years

14. If radius of the ${}^{27}_{12}Al$ nucleus is taken to be R_{Al}, then the radius of ${}^{125}_{53}Te$ nucleus is nearly: *[2015]*
(a) $\frac{5}{3}R_{Al}$ (b) $\frac{3}{5}R_{Al}$
(c) $\left(\frac{13}{53}\right)^{1/3} R_{Al}$ (d) $\left(\frac{53}{13}\right)^{1/3} R_{Al}$

15. A nucleus of uranium decays at rest into nuclei of thorium and helium. Then : *[2015 RS]*
(a) the helium nucleus has less momentum than the thorium nucleus.
(b) the helium nucleus has more momentum than the thorium nucleus.
(c) the helium nucleus has less kinetic energy than the thorium nucleus.
(d) the helium nucleus has more kinetic energy than the thorium nucleus.

16. Radioactive material 'A' has decay constant '8 λ' and material 'B' has decay constant 'λ'. Initially they have same number of nuclei. After what time, the ratio of number of nuclei of material 'B' to that 'A' will be $\frac{1}{e}$? *[2017]*
(a) $\frac{1}{7\lambda}$ (b) $\frac{1}{8\lambda}$ (c) $\frac{1}{9\lambda}$ (d) $\frac{1}{\lambda}$

17. For a radioactive material, half-life is 10 minutes. If initially there are 600 number of nuclei, the time taken (in minutes) for the disintegration of 450 nuclei is *[2018]*
(a) 20 (b) 10 (c) 15 (d) 30

18. α-particle consists of: *[2019]*
(a) 2 protons and 2 neutrons only
(b) 2 electrons, 2 protons and 2 neutrons
(c) 2 electrons and 4 protons only
(d) 2 protons only

19. The rate of radioactive disintegration at an instant for a radioactive sample of half life 2.2×10^9 s is 10^{10} s^{-1}. The number of radioactive atoms in that sample at that instant is, *[NEET Odisha 2019]*
(a) 3.17×10^{19} (b) 3.17×10^{20}
(c) 3.17×10^{17} (d) 3.17×10^{18}

20. When a uranium isotope ${}^{235}_{92}U$ is bombarded with a neutron, it generates ${}^{89}_{36}kr$, three neutrons and : *[2020]*
(a) ${}^{91}_{40}Zr$ (b) ${}^{101}_{36}Kr$ (c) ${}^{103}_{36}Kr$ (d) ${}^{144}_{56}Ba$

21. The energy equivalent of 0.5 g of a substance is : *[2020]*
(a) 4.5×10^{13} J (b) 1.5×10^{13} J
(c) 0.5×10^{13} J (d) 4.5×10^{16} J

Exercise 3 - Concept Application Problems CAP

1. If Avogadro number is 6×10^{23}, then number of protons, neutrons and electrons in 14 gms of $_6C^{14}$ are respecitvely
(a) $36 \times 10^{23}, 48 \times 10^{23}, 36 \times 10^{23}$
(b) $36 \times 10^{23}, 36 \times 10^{23}, 36 \times 10^{23}$
(c) $48 \times 10^{23}, 36 \times 10^{23}, 48 \times 10^{23}$
(d) $48 \times 10^{23}, 48 \times 10^{23}, 36 \times 10^{23}$

2. Actinium 231, $^{231}AC_{89}$, emit in succession two β particles, four α-particles, one β and one α plus several γ rays. What is the resultant isotope?
(a) $^{221}Au_{79}$ (b) $^{211}Au_{79}$
(c) $^{221}Pb_{82}$ (d) $^{211}Pb_{82}$

3. A gamma ray photon creates an electron-positron pair. If the rest mass energy of an electron is 0.5 MeV and the total kinetic energy of the electron-positron pair is 0.78 MeV, then the energy of the gamma ray photon must be
(a) 0.78 MeV (b) 1.78 MeV
(c) 1.28 MeV (d) 0.28 MeV

4. The half-life of radioactive Radon is 3.8 days. The time at the end of which (1/20)th of the Radon sample will remain undecayed is (given $\log_{10}e = 0.4343$)
(a) 13.8 days (b) 16.5 days
(c) 33 days (d) 76 days

5. A freshly prepared radioactive source of half life 2 hr emits radiation of intensity which is 64 times the permissible safe level. The minimum time after which it would be possible to work safely with this source is
(a) 6 hr (b) 12 hr (c) 24 hr (d) 128 hr

6. The intensity of gamma radiation from a given source is I_0. On passing through 37.5 mm of lead it is reduced to $I_0/8$. The thickness of lead which will reduce it to $I_0/2$ is
(a) $(37.5)^{1/3}$ mm (b) $(37.5)^{1/4}$ mm
(c) 37.5/3 mm (d) (37.5/4) mm

7. In the uranium radioactive series, the initial nucleus is $_{92}U^{238}$ and that the final nucleus is $_{82}Pb^{206}$. When uranium nucleus decays to lead, the number of α particles and β particles emitted are
(a) 8α, 6β (b) 6α, 7β (c) 6α, 8β (d) 4α, 3β

8. A radioactive nucleus undergoes α-emission to form a stable element. What will be the recoil velocity of the daughter nucleus if v is the velocity of α emission?
(a) $\frac{4v}{A-4}$ (b) $\frac{2v}{A-4}$ (c) $\frac{4v}{A+4}$ (d) $\frac{2v}{A+4}$

9. If an electron and positron annihilate, then the energy released is
(a) 3.2×10^{-13} J (b) 1.6×10^{-13} J
(c) 4.8×10^{-13} J (d) 6.4×10^{-13} J

10. Radium ^{226}Ra, spontaneously decays to radon with the emission of an α-particle and a γ ray. If the speed of the α particle upon emission from an initially stationary radium nucleus is 1.5×10^7 m/s, what is the recoil speed of the resultant radon nucleus? Assume the momentum of γ ray is negligible compared to that of α particle.
(a) $2..0 \times 10^5$ m/s (b) 2.7×10^5 m/s
(c) 3.5×10^5 m/s (d) 1.5×10^7 m/s

11. A radioactive nuclide is produced at the constant rate of n per second (say, by bombarding a target with neutrons). The expected number N of nuclei in existence t seconds after the number is N_0 is given by
(a) $N = N_0e^{-\lambda t}$
(b) $N = \frac{n}{\lambda} + N_0e^{-\lambda t}$
(c) $N = \frac{n}{\lambda} + \left(N_0 - \frac{n}{\lambda}\right)e^{-\lambda t}$
(d) $N = \frac{n}{\lambda} + \left(N_0 + \frac{n}{\lambda}\right)e^{-\lambda t}$
Where λ is the decay constant of the sample

12. Which one is correct about fission?
(a) Approx. 0.1% mass converts into energy
(b) Most of energy of fission is in the form of heat
(c) In a fission of U^{235} about 200 eV energy is released
(d) On an average, one neutron is released per fission of U^{235}

13. The mass and energy equivalent to 1 amu are respectively
(a) 1.67×10^{-27} gm, 9.30 MeV
(b) 1.67×10^{-27} kg, 930 MeV
(c) 1.67×10^{-27} kg, 1 MeV
(d) 1.67×10^{-34} kg, 1 MeV

14. Which of the following statements is true?
(a) $_{78}Pt^{192}$ has 78 neutrons
(b) $_{84}Po^{214} \rightarrow {}_{82}Pb^{210} + \beta^-$
(c) $_{92}U^{238} \rightarrow {}_{90}Th^{234} + {}_2He^4$
(d) $_{90}Th^{234} \rightarrow {}_{91}Pa^{234} + {}_2He^4$

15. If 200 MeV energy is released in the fission of a single U^{235} nucleus, the number of fissions required per second to produce 1 kilowatt power shall be
(Given 1 eV = 1.6×10^{-19} J)
(a) 3.125×10^{13} (b) 3.125×10^{14}
(c) 3.125×10^{15} (d) 3.125×10^{16}

16. An archaeologist analyses the wood in a prehistoric structure and finds that C^{14} (Half life = 5700 years) to C^{12} is only one-fourth of that found in the cells of buried plants. The age of the wood is about
(a) 5700 years (b) 2850 years
(c) 11,400 years (d) 22,800 years

17. 1 g of hydrogen is converted into 0.993 g of helium in a thermonuclear reaction. The energy released is
(a) 63×10^7 J (b) 63×10^{10} J
(c) 63×10^{14} J (d) 63×10^{20} J

18. Atomic weight of boron is 10.81 and it has two isotopes $_5B^{10}$ and $_5B^{11}$. Then ratio of $_5B^{10} : {}_5B^{11}$ in nature would be
(a) 19 : 81 (b) 10 : 11 (c) 15 : 16 (d) 81 : 19

19. The masses of neutron and proton are 1.0087 a.m.u. and 1.0073 a.m.u. respectively. If the neutrons and protons combine to form a helium nucleus (alpha particles) of mass 4.0015 a.m.u the binding energy fo the helium nucleus will be (1 a.m.u. = 931 MeV)
(a) 28.4 MeV (b) 20.8 MeV
(c) 27.3 MeV (d) 14.2 MeV

20. The radioactivity of a sample is R_1 at a time T_1 and R_2 at a time T_2. If the half-life of the specimen is T, the number of atoms that have disintegrated in the time $(T_1 - T_2)$ is proportional to
(a) $(R_1T_1 - R_2T_2)$ (b) $(R_1 - R_2)$
(c) $(R_1 - R_2)/T$ (d) $(R_1 - R_2)\,T$

21. A radioactive element X converts into another stable element Y. Half life of X is 2 hrs. Initially only X is present. After time t, the ratio of atoms of X and Y is found to be 1 : 4, then t in hours is
(a) 2 (b) 4
(c) between 4 and 6 (d) 6

22. A neutron travelling with a velocity v and kinetic energy E has a perfectly elastic head-on collision with a nucleus of an atom of mass number A at rest. The fraction of total energy retained by the neutron is approximately
(a) $[(A-1)/(A+1)]^2$ (b) $[(A+1)/(A-1)]^2$
(c) $[(A-1)/A]^2$ (d) $[(A+1)/A]^2$

23. At any instant, the ratio of the amount of radioactive substances is 2 : 1. If their half lives be respectively 12 and 16 hours, then after two days, what will be the ratio of the substances ?
(a) 1 : 1 (b) 2 : 1 (c) 1 : 2 (d) 1 : 4

24. Half lives for α and β emission of a radioactive material are 16 years and 48 years respectively. When material decays giving α and β emission simultaneously, time in which $3/4^{th}$ material decays is
(a) 29 years (b) 24 years
(c) 64 years (d) 12 years

25. In an α-decay the kinetic energy of α-particle is 48 MeV and Q-value of the reaction is 50 MeV. The mass number of the mother nucleus is X. Find value of X/25.
(Assume that daughter nucleus is in ground state)
(a) 2 (b) 4 (c) 6 (d) 8

26. A heavy nucleus having mass number 200 gets disintegrated into two small fragments of mass number 80 and 120. If binding energy per nucleon for parent atom is 6.5 MeV and for daughter nuclei is 7 MeV and 8 MeV respectively, then the energy released in the decay is X × 110 MeV. Find the value of X.
(a) 3 (b) 4 (c) 2 (d) 1

27. The activity of a radioactive sample is measured as 9750 counts per minute at t = 0 & 975 counts per minute at T = 5 minutes. The decay constant is approximately.
(a) 0.922 per minutes (b) 0.691 per minutes
(c) 0.461 per minutes (d) 0.230 per minutes

28. In a fission reaction

$${}^{236}_{92}\text{U} \rightarrow {}^{117}\text{X} + {}^{117}\text{Y} + \text{n} + \text{n}$$

the binding energy per nucleon of X & Y is 8.5 MeV. Whereas of ^{236}U is 7.6 MeV. The total energy liberated will be about
(a) 2000 MeV (b) 200 MeV
(c) 2 MwV (d) 200 KeV

29. Half lives of two radio active substance A & B are respectively 20 minutes & 40 minutes. Initially the samples of A & B have equal numbers of nulcei. After 80 minutes the ratio of remaining numbers of A & B nuclei is
(a) 1 : 16 (b) 4 : 1 (c) 1 : 4 (d) 1 : 1

30. The activity of a radioactive sample is measured as N_0 counts per minute at $t = 0$ and N_0/e counts per minute at $t = 5$ minutes. The time (in minutes) at which the activity reduces to half its value is
(a) $\log_e 2/5$ (b) $\dfrac{5}{\log_e 2}$
(c) $5 \log_{10} 2$ (d) $5 \log_e 2$

31. The half life of a radioactive isotope 'X' is 50 years. It decays to another element 'Y' which is stable. The two elements 'X' and 'Y' were found to be in the ratio of 1 : 15 in a sample of a given rock. The age of the rock was estimated to be
(a) 150 years (b) 200 years
(c) 250 years (d) 100 years

32. Two radioactive nuclei P and Q, in a given sample decay into a stable nucleus R. At time t = 0, number of P species are 4 N_0 and that of Q are N_0. Half-life of P (for conversion to R) is 1 minute where as that of Q is 2 minutes. Initially there are no nuclei of R present in the sample. When number of nuclei of P and Q are equal, the number of nuclei of R present in the sample would be
(a) $3N_0$ (b) $\dfrac{9N_0}{2}$ (c) $\dfrac{5N_0}{2}$ (d) $2N_0$

33. The half life of a radioactive nucleus is 50 days. The time interval $(t_2 - t_1)$ between the time t_2 when $\frac{2}{3}$ of it has decayed and the time t_1 when $\frac{1}{3}$ of it had decayed is
(a) 30 days (b) 50 days (c) 60 days (d) 15 days

34. The half life of a radioactive isotope 'X' is 20 years. It decays to another element 'Y' which is stable. The two elements 'X' and 'Y' were found to be in the ratio of 1 : 7 in a sample of a the given rock. The age of the rock is estimated to be
(a) 60 years (b) 80 years (c) 100 years (d) 40 years

35. Activity of a radioactive sample decreases to (1/3) rd of its original value in 3 days. Then, in 9 days its activity will become
(a) (1/27) of the orginal value
(b) (1/9) of the original value
(c) (1/18) of the original value
(d) (1/3) of the orignal value

36. A radioactive sample with a half life of 1 month has the label 'Activity = 2 micro curies on 1–8–1991. What would be its activity two months earlier ?
(a) 1.0 micro curie (b) 0.5 micro curie
(c) 4 micro curie (d) 8 micro curie

37. The nucleus $^{115}_{48}\text{Cd}$, after two successive β– decay will give

(a) $^{115}_{46}\text{Pa}$ (b) $^{114}_{49}\text{In}$ (c) $^{113}_{50}\text{Sn}$ (d) $^{115}_{50}\text{Sn}$

38. Given the masses of various atomic particles $m_p = 1.0072$ u, $m_n = 1.0087$ u, $m_e = 0.000548$ u, $m_{\bar{\nu}} = 0$, $m_d = 2.0141$ u, where p ≡ proton, n ≡ neutron, e ≡ electron, $\bar{\nu}$ ≡ antineutrino and d ≡ deuteron. Which of the following process is allowed by momentum and energy conservation?

(a) n + n → deuterium atom (electron bound to the nucleus)

(b) $p \to n + e^+ + \bar{\nu}$

(c) $n + p \to d + \gamma$

(d) $e^+ + e^- \to \gamma$

39. In a reactor, 2 kg of $_{92}U^{235}$ fuel is fully used up in 30 days. The energy released per fission is 200 MeV. Given that the Avogadro number, $N = 6.023 \times 10^{26}$ per kilo mole and $1 \text{ eV} = 1.6 \times 10^{-19}$ J. The power output of the reactor is close to:

(a) 35 MW (b) 60 MW (c) 125 MW (d) 54 MW

40. Consider the nuclear fission

$Ne^{20} \to 2He^4 + C^{12}$

Given that the binding energy/nucleon of Ne^{20}, He^4 and C^{12} are, respectively, 8.03 MeV, 7.07 MeV and 7.86 MeV, identify the correct statement:

(a) energy of 12.4 MeV will be supplied

(b) 8.3 MeV energy will be released

(c) energy of 3.6 MeV will be released

(d) energy of 11.9 MeV has to be supplied

41. Acitvities of three radioactive substances A, B and C are represented by the curves A, B and C, in the figure. Then their half-lives $T_{\frac{1}{2}}(A) : T_{\frac{1}{2}}(B) : T_{\frac{1}{2}}(C)$ are in the ratio :

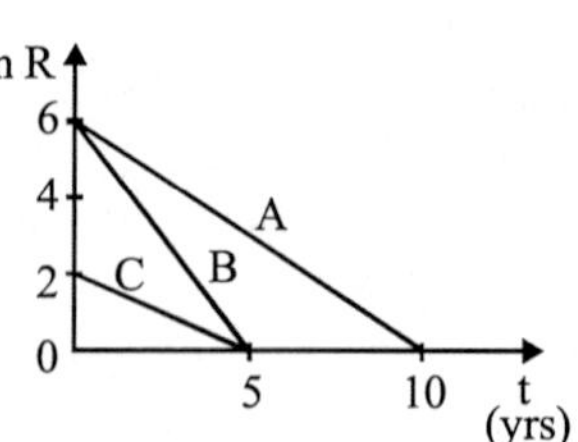

(a) 2:1:1 (b) 3:2:1 (c) 2:1:3 (d) 4:3:1

42. Two radioactive substances A and B have decay constants 5λ and λ respectively. At $t = 0$, a sample has the same number of the two nuclei. The time taken for the ratio of the number of nuclei to become $\left(\frac{1}{e}\right)^2$ will be :

(a) 1/2λ (b) 1/4λ (c) 1/λ (d) 2/λ

43. In a radioactive decay chain, the initial nucleus is $^{232}_{90}\text{Th}$. At the end there are 6 α-particles and 4 β-particles which are emitted. If the end nucleus is $^{A}_{Z}X$, A and Z are given by:

(a) A = 208 ; Z = 80 (b) A = 202 ; Z = 80

(c) A = 208 ; Z = 82 (d) A = 200; Z = 81

44. Using a nuclear counter the count rate of emitted particles from a radioactive source is measured. At t = 0 it was 1600 counts per second and t = 8 seconds it was 100 counts per second. The count rate observed, as counts per second, at t = 6 seconds is close to:

(a) 200 (b) 150 (c) 400 (d) 360

45. A sample of radioactive material A, that has an activity of 10 mCi (1 Ci = 3.7×10^{10} decays/s), has twice the number of nuclei as another sample of a different radioactive material B which has an acitvity of 20 mCi. The correct choices for half-lives of A and B would then be respectively:

(a) 5 days and 10 days (b) 10 days and 40 days

(c) 20 days and 5 days (d) 20 days and 10 days

Hints & Solutions

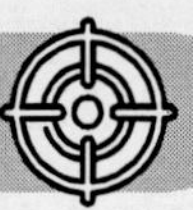

28.1 Concept Practice Problems CPP

1. (b) Nuclear force is spin dependent and non-central.
2. (b)
3. (a) Radius of nucleus $R = R_0 A^{1/3}$ where A is the mass number of nucleus.

$\therefore$ Volume of nucleus $= \frac{4}{3}\pi R^3 = \left(\frac{4}{3}\pi R_0^3\right)A$

$\therefore$ Volume is proportional to A.

4. (c) Nucleus does not contain electron.
5. (c) Out side the nucleus, neutron is unstable (life ≈ 932 s).
6. (a) $N = M - Z$ = Total no. of nucleons – no. of protons.
7. (d) Density of nuclear material = mass/volume

$$= \frac{10^{-27}}{\frac{4}{3}\pi r^3} = \frac{3\times10^{-27}}{4\pi(2\times10^{-15})^3} = 10^{17}\ \text{kg/m}^3$$

8. (b) $R = R_0(A)^{1/3}$

$$\therefore \frac{R_1}{R_2} = \left(\frac{A_1}{A_2}\right)^{1/3} = \left(\frac{256}{4}\right)^{1/3} = 4$$

$$R_2 = \frac{R_1}{4} = 2\ \text{fermi}$$

9. (b) The order of magnitude of mass and volume of uranium nucleus will be

$m \simeq A(1.67\times10^{-27}\ \text{kg})$ (A is atomic number)

$$V = \frac{4}{3}\pi r^3 \simeq \frac{4}{3}\pi[(1.25\times10^{-15}\text{m})A^{1/3}]^3$$

$$\simeq (8.2\times10^{-45}\text{m}^3)A$$

Hence, $\rho = \frac{m}{V} = \frac{A(1.67\times10^{-27}\text{kg})}{(8.2\times10^{-45}\text{m}^3)A} \simeq 2.0\times10^{17}\ \text{kg/m}^3$.

10. (c) Binding energy per nucleon increases with atomic number. The greater the binding energy per nucleon the more stable is the nucleus.

For $_{26}Fe^{56}$ number of nucleons is 56.

This is most stable nucleus, since maximum energy is needed to pull a nucleon away from it.

28.2 Concept Practice Problems CPP

11. (c) Substance left undecayed, $N_0 - \frac{3}{4}N_0 = \frac{1}{4}N_0$

$$\frac{N}{N_0} = \frac{1}{4} = \left(\frac{1}{2}\right)^n$$

$\therefore$ Number of atoms left undecayed,

$n = 2$ i.e. in two half lives

$\therefore$ $t = nT = 2\times4 = 8$ months

12. (c) 13. (d) 14. (d)
15. (c) When ^m_nX emits one α-particle then its atomic mass decreases by 4 units and atomic number by 2. Therefore, the new nucleus becomes $^{m-4}_{n-2}Y$. But as it emits two β^- particles, its atomic number increases by 2. Thus the resulting nucleus is $^{m-4}_{n}X$.
16. (a)
17. (d) Half life of a substance doesn't depends upon amount, temperature and pressure. It depends upon the nature of the substance.
18. (a) $\frac{N}{N_0} = \left(\frac{1}{2}\right)^{\frac{t}{T}}$ or $\frac{N}{10000} = \left(\frac{1}{2}\right)^{\frac{10}{20}}$

or $N = \frac{10000\times1}{\sqrt{2}} = \frac{10000}{1.414} = 7070.$

19. (b) A nucleus is denoted by $_ZX^A$

An isotope should have same Z.

α–particle $= {}_2He^4$; β–particle $= {}_{-1}\beta^0$

The emission of one α particle and the emission of two β particles maintain the Z same.

Hence, for isotope formation 2β particles and one α particle are emitted.

20. (d) Because radioactivity is a spontaneous phenomenon.

Exercise 1 - Chapter Revision Problems CRP

1. (a) Due to irradiation of α-rays on end A will make it (positive) and irradiation of β-rays on end B will make it (negative) hence current will flow from A to B (or from positive to negative).
2. (b) 3. (a) 4. (b) 5. (c)
6. (b) Plutonium 239 is processed by breeder mechanism to be used as nuclear feul.
7. (a)
8. (d) An electron is a lepton.
9. (b) Positron is the antiparticle of electron.
10. (c) In this reaction mass is not conserved.
11. (b)
12. (c) When the coulomb repulsion between the nuclei is overcome then nuclear fusion reaction takes place. This is possible when temperature is too high.
13. (a) $E = mc^2 = 10^{-6}\times(3\times10^8)^2 = 10^{-6}\times9\times10^{16} = 9\times10^{10}$ J
14. (b)
15. (c) No. of nuclide at time t is given by $N = N_oe^{-\lambda t}$

Where N_o = initial nuclide

thus this equation is equivalent to

$y = ae^{-kx}$

thus correct graph is

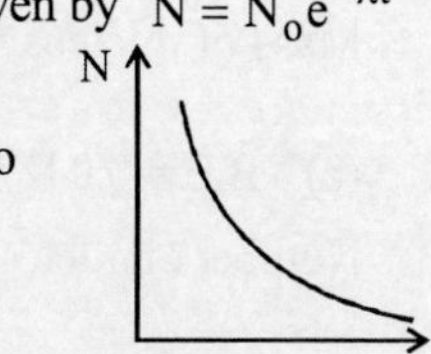

16. (c) Energy released per fission is ≈ 200 MeV
17. (d)
18. (d) $E = mc^2 = 10^{-3}\times10^{-3}(3\times10^8)^2 = 9\times10^{10}$ J
19. (c) The chemical reaction of process is $2\,^2_1H \rightarrow \,^4_2He$

Energy released $= 4\times(7.1) - 4(1.1) = 24$ eV

20. (a) Rest energy of an electron $= m_ec^2$

Here $m_e = 9.1\times10^{-31}$ kg and C = velocity of light

$\therefore$ Rest energy $= 9.1 \times 10^{-31} \times (3 \times 10^8)^2$ joule

$$= \frac{9.1 \times 10^{-31} \times (3 \times 10^8)^2}{1.6 \times 10^{-19}} \text{eV} \approx 510 \text{ KeV}$$

21. (b, c)

22. (c) $\frac{^{14}C}{^{12}C} = \frac{1}{16} = \frac{N}{N_0}$

$\because \frac{N}{N_0} = \left(\frac{1}{2}\right)^n \Rightarrow \frac{1}{16} = \left(\frac{1}{2}\right)^n \Rightarrow \left(\frac{1}{2}\right)^4 = \left(\frac{1}{2}\right)^n$

or, $n = 4$ or $\frac{t}{T} = 4$

or $t = 4 \times T = 4 \times 5730 = 22920$ years

23. (a) $T_{1/2} = \frac{\ln 2}{\lambda} \therefore \lambda = \frac{\ln 2}{T_{1/2}}$

$\Rightarrow \lambda_A = \frac{\ln 2}{T_A}, \lambda_B = \frac{\ln 2}{T_B} \Rightarrow \frac{\lambda_A}{\lambda_B} = \frac{T_B}{T_A}$.

24. (a) ${}_{72}A^{180} \xrightarrow{\alpha} {}_{70}A_1^{176} \xrightarrow{\beta} {}_{71}A_2^{176}$

$\xrightarrow{\alpha} {}_{69}A_3^{172} \xrightarrow{\gamma} {}_{69}A_4^{172}$

25. (d) $E = \Delta m.c^2 \Rightarrow E = \frac{0.3}{1000} \times (3 \times 10^8)^2 = 2.7 \times 10^{13}$ J

$= \frac{2.7 \times 10^{13}}{3.6 \times 10^6} = 7.5 \times 10^6$ kWh.

26. (b) $Q = 4(x_2 - x_1)$

27. (a) Activity of sample becomes 2500 from 5000 in 75 days therefore its half life is 75 days, so

$R = \frac{R_0}{2^{\frac{150}{75}}} = 5000 \Rightarrow R_0 = 5000 \times 4 = 20,000$

28. (a) $B.E_H = \frac{2.22}{2} = 1.11$

$B.E_{He} = \frac{28.3}{4} = 7.08$

$B.E_{Fe} = \frac{492}{56} = 8.78 =$ maximum

$B.E_U = \frac{1786}{235} = 7.6$

${}^{56}_{26}Fe$ is most stable as it has maximum binding energy per nucleon.

29. (d) Mass defect $= \frac{B.E}{c^2}$

Mass of nucleus = Mass of proton + mass of neutron – mass defect

30. (b) B.E. $= 0.042 \times 931 \simeq 42$ MeV

Number of nucleons in ${}^7_3Li$ is 7.

$\therefore$ B.E./nucleon $= \frac{42}{7} = 6$ MeV $\simeq 5.6$ MeV

31. (b) Momentum

$Mu = \frac{E}{c} = \frac{h\nu}{c}$

Recoil energy

$\frac{1}{2}Mu^2 = \frac{1}{2}\frac{M^2u^2}{M} = \frac{1}{2M}\left(\frac{h\nu}{c}\right)^2 = \frac{h^2\nu^2}{2Mc^2}$

32. (c) The radius of the nuclears is directly proportional to cube root of atomic number i.e. $R \propto A^{1/3}$

$\Rightarrow R = R_0 A^{1/3}$, where R_0 is a constant of proportionality

$\frac{R_2}{R_1} = \left(\frac{A_2}{A_1}\right)^{1/3} \left(\frac{64}{27}\right)^{1/3} = \frac{4}{3}$

where R_1 = the radius of ^{27}Al, and

A_1 = Atomic mass number of Al

R_2 = the radius of ^{64}Cu

and A_2 = Atomic mass number of C4

$R_2 = 3.6 \times \frac{4}{3} = 4.8$m

33. (d)

34. (b) Mass defect $\Delta m = 0.02866$ a.m.u.

Energy $= 0.02866 \times 931 = 26.7$ MeV

As ${}_1H^2 + {}_1H^2 \longrightarrow {}_2He^4$

Energy liberated per a.m.u = 13.35/2 MeV = 6.675 MeV

35. (c) $n = \frac{150}{12.5} = 12$

$\frac{N}{N_0} = \left(\frac{1}{2}\right)^{12}$

36. (d) ${}_8O^{16} + {}_1H^2 \rightarrow {}_7N^{14} + {}_2He^4$

37. (b)

38. (b) ${}_{-1}e^0$ is known as β^- particle & $\bar{\nu}$ is known as antineutrino. Since in this reaction $\bar{\nu}$ is emitted with ${}_{-1}e^0$ (β^- particle or electron), so it is known as β-decay.

39. (d) Time taken to disintegrate completely by a substance is infinity as $\log\frac{N_0}{N} = \lambda t \Rightarrow \log\frac{N_0}{0} = \lambda t$

$\log\infty = \lambda t$

hence when $N \to 0$, $t \to \infty$.

40. (d) $T = \frac{0.6931 \times 1}{\lambda} = \frac{0.6931}{4.28 \times 10^{-4}}$ year $= 1620$ years

41. (d) Density of nucleus, $\rho = \frac{\text{Mass}}{\text{Volume}} = \frac{mA}{\frac{4}{3}\pi R^3}$

$\Rightarrow \rho = \frac{mA}{\frac{4}{3}\pi(R_0A^{1/3})^3}$ $(\because R = R_0A^{1/3})$

Here m = mass of a nucleon

$\therefore \rho = \frac{3 \times 1.67 \times 10^{-27}}{4 \times 3.14 \times (1.3 \times 10^{-15})^3}$ (Given, $R_0 = 1.3 \times 10^{-15}$)

$\Rightarrow \rho = 2.38 \times 10^{17}$ kg/m^3

42. (a) Nuclear density is independent of atomic number.

43. (c) As we know, for first order decay, $N(t) = N_0e^{-\lambda t}$

According to question, $\frac{N(t)}{N_0} = \frac{9}{16} = e^{-\lambda t}$

After time, $t/2$;

$N(t/2) = N_0e^{-\lambda(t/2)}$

$\frac{N(t/2)}{N_0} = \sqrt{e^{-\lambda t}} = \sqrt{\frac{9}{16}}$ $\quad \therefore N(t/2) = \frac{3}{4}N_0$

44. (b) We know that

Activity, $A = A_0 e^{-\lambda t}$

$$A = A_0 e^{-tIn2/T_{1/2}} \left(\because \lambda = \frac{In_2}{T_{1/2}}\right)$$

$$\Rightarrow 500 = 700\, e^{-tIn2/T_{1/2}}$$

$$\Rightarrow In\frac{7}{5} = \frac{30 In2}{T_{1/2}} \quad (\because t = 30 \text{ minute})$$

$$\Rightarrow T_{1/2} = 30\frac{In\ 2}{In\ 1.4} = 61.8 \text{ minute}$$

$(\because \ln 2 = 0.693 \text{ and } \ln.1.4 = 0.336)$

$$\Rightarrow T_{1/2} \approx 62 \text{ minute}$$

45. (a) As, $N = N_0 e^{-\lambda t}$

so, $\frac{N_A}{N_B} = e^{(\lambda_B - \lambda_A)t} = \frac{1}{e} \Rightarrow (\lambda_B - \lambda_A)t = -1$

$\Rightarrow (\lambda_A - \lambda_B).t = 1 \Rightarrow t = \frac{1}{(\lambda_B - \lambda_A)}\ t = \frac{1}{10\lambda - \lambda} = \frac{1}{9\lambda}$

46. (a)

47. (c) Let heavy nucleus breaks into two nuclei of mass m_1 and m_2 and move away with velocities V_1 and V_2 respectively.

According to question, $\frac{V_1}{V_2} = \frac{8}{27}$

$m_1 V_1 = m_2 V_2$ (Law of momentum conservation)

$$\Rightarrow \frac{m_1}{m_2} = \frac{V_2}{V_1} = \frac{27}{8}$$

$$\frac{\rho \times \frac{4}{3}\pi R_1^3}{\rho \times \frac{4}{3}\pi R_2^3} \left(\because \text{density } \rho = \frac{\text{mass}}{\text{volume}}\right)$$

$$\Rightarrow \left(\frac{R_1}{R_2}\right) = \left(\frac{27}{8}\right)^{\frac{1}{3}} = \left(\frac{3}{2}\right)^{3 \times \frac{1}{3}} \quad \therefore \frac{R_1}{R_2} = \frac{3}{2}$$

48. (d) ${}^7_3\text{Li} + {}^1_1\text{H} \longrightarrow 2\left({}^4_2\text{He}\right)$

$\Delta m \to [m_{\text{Li}} + m_{\text{H}}] - 2[M_{\text{He}}]$

Energy released $= \Delta mc^2$

In use of 1 g Li energy released $= \frac{\Delta mc^2}{m_{\text{Li}}}$

In use of 20 g energy released $= \frac{\Delta mc^2}{m_{\text{Li}}} \times 20$ g

$$= \frac{[(7.016 + 1.0079) - 2 \times 4.0026]u \times c^2}{7.016 \times 1.6 \times 10^{-24}} \times 20 \text{ g}$$

$$= \left(\frac{0.0187 \times 1.6 \times 10^{-19} \times 10^9}{7.016 \times 1.6 \times 10^{-24}} \times 20\right) = 480 \times 10^{10}\text{ J}$$

$\because 1\text{ J} = 2.778 \times 10^{-7}$ kWh

$\therefore$ Energy released $= 480 \times 10^{10} \times 2.778 \times 10^{-7}$
$= 1.33 \times 10^6$ kWh

49. (d) Mass defect,

$\Delta m = (50m_p + 70m_n) - (m_{sn})$

$= (50 \times 1.00783 + 70 \times 1.008) - (119.902199) = 1.096$

Binding energy $= (\Delta m)C^2 = (\Delta m) \times 931 = 1020.56$

$$\frac{\text{Binding energy}}{\text{Nucleon}} = \frac{1020.5631}{120} = 8.5 \text{ MeV}$$

50. (b) Given : $N_1 = 2N_2$

Activity of radioactive substance $= \lambda N$

Half life period $t = \frac{\ln 2}{\lambda}$ or, $\lambda = \frac{\ln 2}{T}$

$$\lambda_1 N_1 = \frac{\ln 2}{t_1} \times N_1 = 5\,\mu c_i \quad \text{..... (i)}$$

$$\lambda_2 N_2 = \frac{\ln 2}{t_2} \times N_2 = 10\,\mu c_i \quad \text{..... (ii)}$$

Dividing equation (ii) by (i)

$$\frac{t_2}{t_1} \times \frac{N_1}{N_2} = \frac{1}{2}$$

$$\frac{t_2}{t_1} = \frac{1}{4} \Rightarrow t_1 = 4t_2$$

i.e., Half life of S_1 is four times of sample S_2.

Hence 5 years and 20 years.

Exercise 2 - Exemplar & Past Year Questions E&PYQs

Exemplar Questions

1. (c) Radioactivity is a process due to which a radiactive material spontaneously decays. Half-life time for a radioactive remain average half of its or of radioactive atoms will decay. So, the containers will in general have different number of atoms of the material,after one year means one half life i.e., average atom of radioactive subtance remain after 1 year, in each container is equal to

$\frac{1}{2}$ of 10000 = 5000 atoms.

2. (b) Due my formation of H-atom some mass of necleons convert into energy by $E = mc^2$, this energy is used to bind the nucleons along with nucleus, so mass of atom becomes slightly less than sum of actual masses of electron and nucleons.

Given, $F = \frac{GMm}{r^2}$

M = effective mass of hydrogen atom

Actual mass of H-atom $\left(\because \frac{B}{c^2} \text{is binding energy}\right)$

$= \underset{(\text{Me})}{\text{mass of electron}} + \underset{(\text{Mp})}{\text{mass of proton}} - \frac{B}{c^2}$

where B is BE of hydrogen atom = 13.6 eV.

3. (b) β-particle carries one unit of negative charge and α-particle carries 2 units of positive charge and γ-particle carries no charge, so electronic energy levels of the atom charges in emission of α and β particle, but not in γ-decay.

4. (a)

5. (a) Tritium $({}_1H^3)$ has proton and 2 neutrons. If a neutron decays as $n \to P + \bar{e} + \bar{v}$, then the nucleus may have 2 protons and neutron, i.e., tritium atom will convert into ${}_2He^3$ (2 protons and 1 neutron).

Binding energy of ${}_1H^3$ is less than that of ${}_2He^3$ nucleus, So, transformation is not possible energetically.

6. (b) Stable heavy nuclei have more neutrons than protons because electrostatic force between protons is repulsive, which causes unstability of nucleus.

7. (b) The moderator used have light nuclei (like proton). When protons undergo perfectly elastic collision with the neutron emitted their velocities are exchanged, i.e., neutrons come to rest and protons move with the velocity of neutrons. To slowdown the speed of neutrons substance should be made up of proton for perfectly elastic i.e., we need light nuclei not heavy nuclei because heavy nuclei will not serve the purpose because elastic collisions of neutrons with heavy nuclei will not slow them down or speed but only direction will change.

NEET/AIPMT (2013-2020) Questions

8. (b) Mass defect $\Delta m = 0.02866$ a.m.u.
Energy $= 0.02866 \times 931 = 26.7$ MeV
As ${}_1H^2 + {}_1H^2 \longrightarrow {}_2He^4$
Energy liberated per a.m.u $= 13.35/2$ MeV
$= 6.675$ MeV

9. (a) The value of x is $\frac{1}{8}$

$$= \frac{x_0}{8} = \frac{x_0}{2^3} \Rightarrow t = 3T = 3 \times 20 = 60 \text{ years}$$

Hence the estimated age of the rock is 60 years

10. (c) Increasing order of penetrating power :
$\alpha < \beta < \gamma$.
For same energy, lighter particle has higher penentrating power.

11. (d) From the graph of BE/A versus mass number A it is clear that, BE/A first increases and then decreases with increase in mass number.

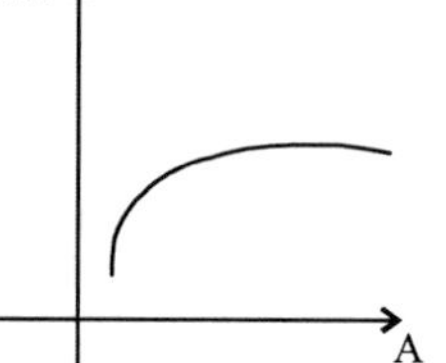

12. (d) BE of ${}_2He^4 = 4 \times 7.06 = 28.24$ MeV

BE of ${}_3^7Li = 7 \times 5.60 = 39.20$ MeV

$${}_3^7Li + {}_1^1H \rightarrow {}_2He^4 + {}_2He^4 + Q$$

39.20 $\quad$ $28.24 \times 2 (= 56.48 \text{ MeV})$

Therefore, $Q = 56.48 - 39.20 = 17.28$ MeV.

13. (c) As $\frac{N_x}{N_y} = \frac{1}{7}$ (Given) $\Rightarrow \frac{N_x}{N_x + N_y} = \frac{1}{8} = \left(\frac{1}{2}\right)^3$

Therefore, age of the rock
$t = 3T_{1/2} = 3 \times 1.4 \times 10^9$ yrs $= 4.2 \times 10^9$ yrs.

14. (a) As we know, $R = R_0 (A)^{1/3}$
where A = mass number
$R_{Al} = R_0 (27)^{1/3} = 3R_0$

$$R_{Te} = R_0 (125)^{1/3} = 5R_0 = \frac{5}{3} R_{Al}$$

15. (d) In an explosion a body breaks up into two pieces of unequal masses both part will have numerically equal momentum and lighter part will have more velocity.
$U \rightarrow Th + He$

$$KE_{Th} = \frac{p^2}{2m_{Th}}, KE_{He} = \frac{p^2}{2m_{He}}$$

since m_{He} is less so KE_{He} will be more.

16. (a) Given, $\lambda_A = 8\lambda, \lambda_B = \lambda$

$$N_B = \frac{N_A}{e} \Rightarrow N_o e^{-\lambda_B t} = N_o \frac{e^{-\lambda_A t}}{e}$$

$$e^{-\lambda t} = e^{-8\lambda t} e^{-1}$$

$$e^{-\lambda t} = e^{-8\lambda t - 1}$$

Comparing both side powers

$$-\lambda t = -8\lambda t - 1 \Rightarrow -1 = 7\lambda t \Rightarrow t = -\frac{1}{7\lambda}$$

The best possible answer is $t = \frac{1}{7\lambda}$

17. (a) Number of nuclei remaining, $N = 600 - 450 = 150$ after time 't'

$$\frac{N}{N_0} = \frac{150}{600} = \frac{1}{4}$$

$$N = N_0 e^{-\lambda t} \Rightarrow \ell n \frac{N_0}{N} = \lambda t \Rightarrow t = \frac{1}{\lambda} \ell n \frac{N_0}{N}$$

$$\Rightarrow t = \frac{2.303 \times T_{\frac{1}{2}}}{0.693} \log_{10} \frac{N_0}{N} = \frac{2.303 \times 10}{0.693} \log_{10} 4$$

18. (a) α-particle is nucleus of helium He^{++} which has two protons and two neutrons.

19. (a) $t_{1/2} = \frac{ln 2}{\lambda} = \frac{0.693}{\lambda}$ $\quad \lambda = \frac{0.693}{2.2 \times 10^9} = 3.15 \times 10^{-10}$

$R = \lambda N$

$$N = \frac{R}{\lambda} = \frac{10^{10}}{3.15 \times 10^{-10}} = 3.17 \times 10^{19}$$

20. (d) It is a nuclear fission reaction.

$${}_{92}^{235}U + {}_0^1n \longrightarrow {}_{36}^{89}Kr + {}_{56}^{144}Ba + {}_3^1n + Q$$

21. (a) From the Einstein's mass-energy equivalence, the relation between the mass of a substance m and its energy E is
$E = mc^2$
Here, c = speed of light
$\therefore E = 0.5 \times 10^{-3} \times (3 \times 10^8)^2 = 0.5 \times 10^{-3} \times 9 \times 10^{16}$
$= 4.5 \times 10^{13}$ J.

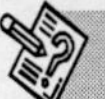

Exercise 3 - Concept Application Problems CAP

1. (a) Each atom of $_6C^{14}$ contains 6 p, 6 e and 8 n
$\therefore$ In 14 gram of $_6C^{14}$
$p = 6 \times 6 \times 10^{23} = 36 \times 10^{23}$
$n = 8 \times 6 \times 10^{23} = 48 \times 10^{23}$
$e = p = 36 \times 10^{23}$

2. (d)

3. (b) Energy of γ-ray photon = Rest mass energy + K.E.
$= 2(0.5) + 0.78 = 1.78$ MeV

4. (b) $\left(\frac{1}{2}\right)^n = \frac{N}{N_0} = \frac{1}{20}$ gives $n = 4.32$
$t = nT = 4.3 \times 3.8 = 16.5$ days

5. (b) To work safely, intensity must reduce by 1/64
$\therefore \frac{N}{N_0} = \frac{1}{64} = \left(\frac{1}{2}\right)^{t/T}$ i.e. $\left(\frac{1}{2}\right)^6 = \left(\frac{1}{2}\right)^{t/T}$
or $\frac{t}{T} = 6$ or $t = 6T = 12$ hrs

6. (c) As $\frac{I}{I_0} = e^{-\mu x}$
$\therefore \frac{1}{8} = e^{-\mu 37.5}$ ....(i) and $\frac{1}{2} = e^{-\mu x}$ ....(ii)
Put (ii) in (i), $e^{-3\mu x} = e^{-\mu(37.5)}$
$x = \frac{37.5}{3} = 12.5$ mm

7. (a) Let no. of α-particles emitted be x and no. of β particles emitted be y.
Diff. in mass no. $4x = 238 - 206 = 32 \Rightarrow x = 8$
Diff. in charge no. $2x - 1y = 92 - 82 = 10$
$16 - y = 10, y = 6$

8. (a) We assume that mass number of nucleus when it was at rest = A
$\because$ mass number of α-particle = 4
$\therefore$ mass number of remaining nucleus = A - 4
As there is no external force, so momentum of the system will remain conserved
$\Rightarrow 0 = (A-4)v' + 4v \Rightarrow v' = -\frac{4v}{(A-4)}$
negative sign represents that direction is opposite to the direction of motion of α-particle.

9. (b) Energy of electron $= m_e c^2$
Energy of positron $= m_p c^2$
$m_e = m_p$, c = speed of light.
Thus according to conservation of energy released
$= 2m_e c^2 = 2 \times 9.1 \times 10^{-31}(3 \times 10^8)^2 = 1.6 \times 10^{-13}$ Joules.

10. (b) Conservation of linear momentum requires: $m_{radon}v_{radon} = m_{helium}v_{helium}$ with helium identified as the alpha particle. The nuclear masses can be approximated by their mass numbers (222 and 4). Thus, the recoil speed of the radon is $(4/222) \times 1.5 \times 10^7$ m/s $= 2.7 \times 10^5$ m/s.

11. (c) 12. (a) 13. (b) 14. (c)

15. (a) $P = n\left(\frac{E}{t}\right) \Rightarrow 1000 = \frac{n \times 200 \times 10^6 \times 1.6 \times 10^{-19}}{t}$
$\Rightarrow \frac{n}{t} = 3.125 \times 10^{13}$.

16. (c) $\frac{C_{14}}{C_{12}} = \frac{1}{4} = \left(\frac{1}{2}\right)^{t/5700}$
$\Rightarrow \frac{t}{5700} = 2 \Rightarrow t = 11400$ years

17. (b) $\Delta m = 1 - 0.993 = 0.007$ gm
$\therefore E = (\Delta m)c^2 = (0.007 \times 10^{-3})(3 \times 10^8)^2 = 63 \times 10^{10}$ J.

18. (a) Let the percentage of B^{10} atoms be x, then average atomic weight
$= \frac{10x + 11(100 - x)}{100} = 10.81 \Rightarrow x = 19$
$\therefore \frac{N_{B^{10}}}{N_{B^{11}}} = \frac{19}{81}$

19. (a) B.E. $= \Delta mc^2 = \Delta \times 931$ MeV
$= [2(1.0087 + 1.0073) - 4.0015] \times 931 = 28.4$ MeV

20. (d) Radioactivity at T_1, $R_1 = \lambda N_1$
Radioactivity at T_2, $R_2 = \lambda N_2$
$\therefore$ Number of atoms decayed in time
$(T_1 - T_2) = (N_1 - N_2)$
$= \frac{(R_1 - R_2)}{\lambda} = \frac{(R_1 - R_2)T}{0.693} \propto (R_1 - R_2)T$

21. (c) Let N_0 be the number of atoms of X at time t = 0.
Then at t = 4 hrs (two half lives)
$N_x = \frac{N_0}{4}$ and $N_y = \frac{3N_0}{4}$
$\therefore N_x/N_y = 1/3$
and at t = 6 hrs (three half lives)
$N_x = \frac{N_0}{8}$ and $N_y = \frac{7N_0}{8}$
or $\frac{N_x}{N_y} = \frac{1}{7}$
The given ratio $\frac{1}{4}$ lies between $\frac{1}{3}$ and $\frac{1}{7}$.
Therefore, t lies between 4 hrs and 6 hrs.

22. (a) $v'_1 = \frac{(m_1 - m_2)v_1 + 2m_2v_2}{m_1 + m_2}$

As v_2 is zero, $m_2 > m_1$, v'_1 is in the opposite direction.
$m_1 = 1, m_2 = A.$

$\therefore \quad |v'_1| = \frac{(A-1)}{(A+1)} v_1$

The fraction of total energy retained is

$$\frac{1/2mv_1'^2}{1/2mv_1^2} = \frac{(A-1)^2}{(A+1)^2}$$

23. (a) For substance A :

$$2N_0 \to N_A = 2N_0\left(\frac{1}{2}\right)^{48/12} = \frac{N_0}{2^3} = \frac{N_0}{8}$$

For substance B :

$$N_0 \to N_B = N_0\left(\frac{1}{2}\right)^{48/16} = \frac{N_0}{2^3} = \frac{N_0}{8}$$

$N_A : N_B = 1 : 1$

24. (b) Effective half life is calculated as

$$\frac{1}{T} = \frac{1}{T_1} + \frac{1}{T_2}$$

$$\frac{1}{T} = \frac{1}{16} + \frac{1}{48} \Rightarrow T = 12 \text{ years}$$

Time in which $\frac{3}{4}$ will decay is 2 half lives = 24 years

25. (b) We have $K_\alpha = \frac{m_y}{m_y + m_\alpha}.Q$

$$\Rightarrow \quad K_\alpha = \frac{A-4}{A}.Q \Rightarrow 48 = \frac{A-4}{A}.50 \Rightarrow A = 100$$

26. (c) Energy released = $(80 \times 7 + 120 \times 8 - 200 \times 6.5)$

27. (c) $\frac{dN}{dt} = \lambda N = \text{activity } R$

$R_0 = \lambda N_0$ at $t = 0$, $R_1 = \lambda N_1$ at $t = 5$ minutes

where $\lambda = \frac{2.303}{t}\log\frac{N_0}{N_1}$

28. (b) Liberated energy $Q = 117 \times 8.5 + 117 \times 8.5 - 236 \times 7.6 = 200$ MeV. Thus, in fission of one Uranium nuclei nearly 200 MeV energy is liberated.

29. (c) $\frac{N_A}{N_B} = \frac{(1/2)^{n_A}}{(1/2)^{n_B}} = \frac{(1/2)^4}{(1/2)^2} = \frac{1}{4}$, where n_A & n_B are number of half lives of samples A & B respectively. N_A & N_B are the remaining numbers of A & B after 80 minutes in this case.

30. (d) $N = N_0 e^{-\lambda t}$

Here, $t = 5$ minutes

$$\frac{N_0}{e} = N_0 \cdot e^{-5\lambda} \Rightarrow 5\lambda = 1, \text{ or } \lambda = \frac{1}{5},$$

Now, $T_{1/2} = \frac{\ell n2}{\lambda} = 5\ \ell n2$

31. (b) Let number of atoms in X = N_x

Number of atoms in Y = N_y

By question

$$\frac{N_x}{N_y} = \frac{1}{15}$$

$\therefore$ Part of $N_x = \frac{1}{16}(N_x + N_y) = \frac{1}{2^4}(N_x + N_y)$

So, total 4 half lives are passed, so, age of rock is $4 \times 50 = 200$ years

32. (b) Initially $P \to 4N_0$

$Q \to N_0$

Half life $T_P = 1$ min.

$T_Q = 2$ min.

Let after time t number of nuclei of P and Q are equal, that is

$$\frac{4N_0}{2^{t/1}} = \frac{N_0}{2^{t/2}} \text{ Þ } \frac{4N}{2^{t/1}} = \frac{1}{2^{t/2}} \Rightarrow 2^{t/1} = 4.2^{t/2}$$

$$2^2.2^{t/2} = 2^{(2+t/2)}$$

$$\Rightarrow \frac{t}{1} = 2 + \frac{t}{2} \Rightarrow \frac{t}{2} = 2 \Rightarrow t = 4 \text{ min}$$

$$N_P = \frac{(4N_0)}{2^{4/1}} = \frac{N_0}{4}$$

at $t = 4$ min.

$$N_0 = \frac{N_0}{4} = \frac{N_0}{4}$$

or population of R

$$\left(4N_0 - \frac{N_0}{4}\right) + \left(N_0 - \frac{N_0}{4}\right) = \frac{9N_0}{2}$$

33. (b) $N_1 = N_0 e^{-\lambda t} \quad N_1 = \frac{1}{3}N_0$

$$\frac{N_0}{3} = N_0 e^{-\lambda t_2} \Rightarrow \frac{1}{3} = e^{-\lambda t^2} \quad ...(i)$$

$$N_2 = \frac{2}{3}N_0$$

$$\frac{2}{3}N_0 = N_0 e^{-\lambda t_1} \Rightarrow \frac{2}{3} = e^{-\lambda t_1} \quad ...(ii)$$

Dividing equation (i) by equation (ii)

$$\frac{1}{2} = e^{-\lambda(t_2 - t_1)}$$

$$\lambda(t_2 - t_1) = \ln 2$$

$$t_2 - t_1 = \frac{\ln 2}{\lambda} = T_{1/2} = 50 \text{ days}$$

34. (a) The value of x is $\frac{1}{8}$

$$= \frac{x_0}{8} = \frac{x_0}{2^3} \Rightarrow t = 3T = 3 \times 20 = 60 \text{ years}$$

Hence the estimated age of the rock is 60 years

35. (a) By Radioactive decay law, $N = N_0 e^{-\lambda t}$

Taking log on both sides, we get $\lambda t = \log_e \frac{N_0}{N}$

As $N_a = \frac{1}{3} N_0$ and, $t = 3 \times 24 \times 60 \times 60$ sec

$\therefore \lambda = \frac{0.477}{3 \times 24 \times 60 \times 60} = 1.8 \times 10^{-6}/\text{sec}$

Now in 9 days, activity becomes,

$N = N_0 e^{-(1.8 \times 10^{-6}) \times (9 \times 24 \times 60 \times 60)}$

on solving we get,

$N = \frac{N_0}{27}$

Hence, in 9 days activity will become $\frac{1}{27}$ of the original value.

36. (d) In two half lives, the activity becomes one fourth. Activity on 1–8–91 was 2 micro–curie

$\therefore$ Activity before two months,

4×2 micro-curie $= 8$ micro curie

37. (d) Two successive β decay increases the atomic number by 2. Therefore, (d) is correct.

38. (c) For the momentum and energy conservation, mass defect (Δm) should be positive. Since some energy is lost in every process.

$(m_p + m_n) > m_d$

39. (b) Power output of the reactor,

$P = \frac{\text{energy}}{\text{time}}$

$= \frac{2}{235} \times \frac{6.023 \times 10^{26} \times 200 \times 1.6 \times 10^{-19}}{30 \times 24 \times 60 \times 60} \simeq 60\,\text{MW}$

40. (d)

41. (c) Since, $R = R_0 e^{-\lambda t}$

$\ln R = \ln R_0 + (-\lambda \ln t)$

$\lambda = \frac{\ln 2}{t_{1/2}} = \text{Slope}$

$\lambda_A = \frac{6}{10} \Rightarrow T_A = \frac{10}{6} \ln 2$

$\lambda_B = \frac{6}{5} \Rightarrow T_B = \frac{5 \ln 2}{6}$

$\lambda_C = \frac{2}{5} \Rightarrow T_C = \frac{5 \ln 2}{6}$

$\therefore T_{\frac{1}{2}A} : T_{\frac{1}{2}B} : T_{\frac{1}{2}C} = \frac{10}{6} : \frac{5}{6} : \frac{15}{6} = 2:1:3$

42. (a) Let N_1 and N_2 be the number of radioactive nuclei of substance at anytime t.

$N_1 (\text{at } t) = N_0 e^{-5\lambda t}$ (i)

$N_2 (\text{at } t) = N_0 e^{-\lambda t}$ (ii)

Dividing equation (i) by (ii), we get

$\frac{N_1}{N_2} = \frac{1}{e^2} = e^{-4\lambda t} \Rightarrow 4\lambda t = 2 \Rightarrow t = \frac{2}{4\lambda} = \left(\frac{1}{2\lambda}\right)$

43. (c) When one α- particle emitted then danghter nuclei has 4 unit less mass number (A) and 2 unit less atomic (z) number (z).

${}^{232}_{90}\text{Th} \rightarrow {}^{208}_{78}\text{Y} + 6{}^{4}_{2}\text{He}$

${}^{208}_{78}\text{Y} \rightarrow {}^{208}_{82}\text{X} + 4\beta$ praticle

44. (a) According to question, at t = 0, A0 = $\frac{dN}{dt}$ =1600 C/s and at t = 8s, A = 100 C/s

$\therefore \frac{A}{A_0} = \frac{1}{16}$ in 8s

Therefore half life period, t1/2 = 2s

$\therefore$ Activity at t = 6s = $1600 \left(\frac{1}{2}\right)^3 = 200$C/s

45. (c) Activity A = 1 N

For material, A   10 = (2 N0)lA

For material, B   20 = N0lB

$\Rightarrow \lambda_B = 4\lambda_A \therefore T_{½A} = 4T_{½B} \left[\because T_{½} = \frac{0.693}{\lambda}\right]$

i.e. 20 days half-lives for A and 5 days $\left(T_{½}\right)_B$ for material B.

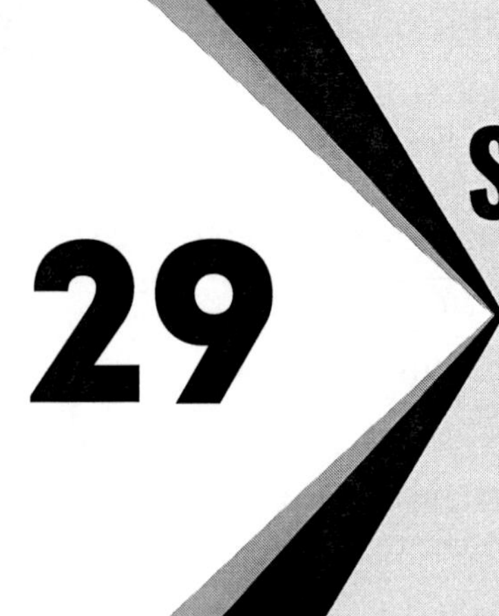

29 Semiconductor Electronics : Materials, Devices and Simple Circuits

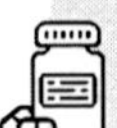

Topic 29.1 : Energy Band Theory of Solids, Conductors, Insulators & Semiconductors, p-n Junction Diode, Forward and Reverse Bias of p-n Junction Diode

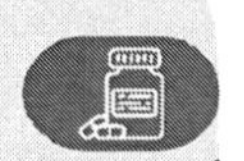

ENERGY BAND THEORY OF SOLIDS

When two identical atoms, are far apart, the electronic levels (or electronic wave functions) in one are not disturbed by the presence of other atom fig 1(a). For example, the 3s electron of each sodium atom has a single energy with respect to its nucleus. But when the two atoms come closer, these electron's wave function starts to overlap and each electron revolves round both nuclei.

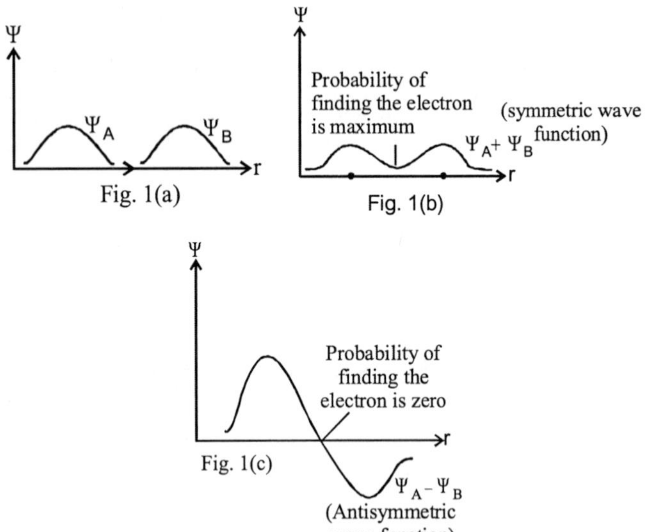

Fig. 1 : Wave functions of two sodium atoms (each in G-state) :

(a) : At wide separation

(b) : Small separation : Isolated wave function combined with same sign (i.e., lower energy)

(c) : Small separation : Isolated wave function combined with opposite sign i.e., antisymmetric state of joint wave functions Ψ_A & Ψ_B(higher energy state)

Splitting of 3s levels when two atoms are brought together.

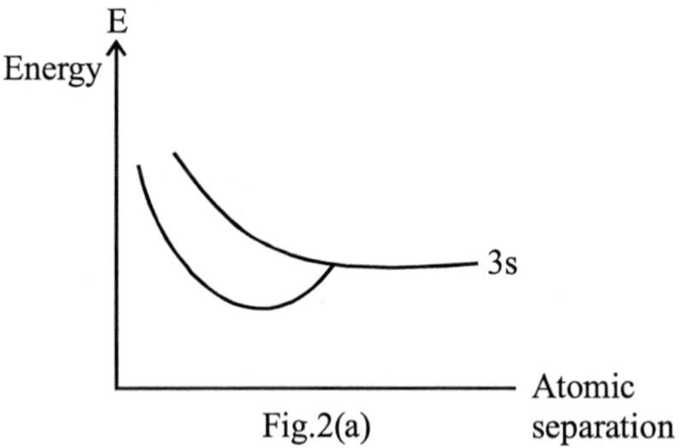

Fig.2(a)

Splitting of 3s levels when four atoms are brought together.

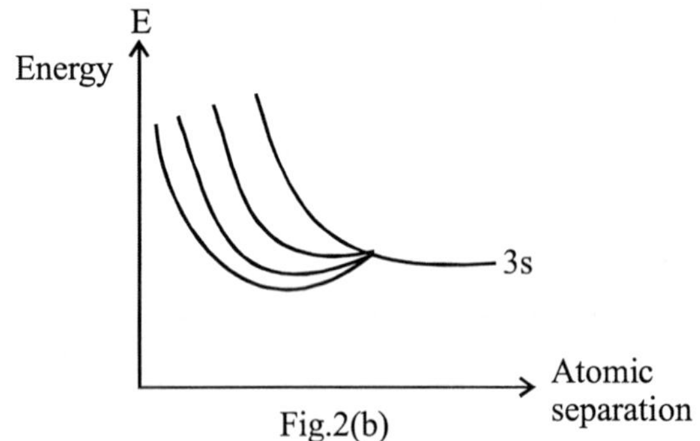

Fig.2(b)

Formation of 3s band by a larger number of atoms.(G-state)

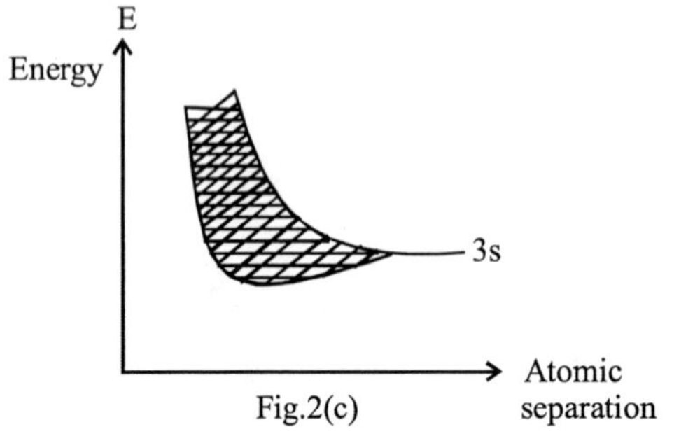

Fig.2(c)

The wave function of each electron is roughly, a combination of the wave functions of isolated atoms : Fig 1(b) & (c) show two possible wave functions. In the first, the two isolated wave functions are combined with (make symmetric state) same sign, in the second with opposite signs(antisymmetic state). The symmetric state has lower energy as compared to antisymmetric state, because the electron is more likely to be found midway between the nuclei, which leads to lower coulomb energy. This is the effect, responsible for molecular bonding. Representation of energy level (when two sodium atoms come closer) is shown in fig 2(a).

As we bring together a large number of atoms to form a solid, the same sort of effect occurs. When the sodium atoms are far apart, all 3s electrons have same energy & as we begin to move them together, the energy levels begin to "split". The situation for four sodium atoms is shown in fig 2(b). As the number of atoms is increased (may be 10^{20} atoms), the levels become so numerous & so close that we can no longer distinguish the individual levels as shown in fig 2(c). We can regard the N atoms as forming an almost continuous band of energy. Since those levels were identified with 3s atomic levels of sodium, we refer to the 3s band.

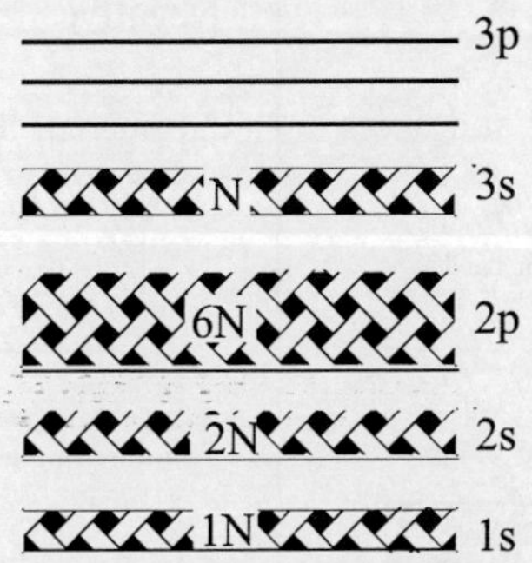

Fig. 3- Energy bands in sodium metal (G-state)

Each band has a total of N individual levels. Each level can hold $2 \times (2\ell + 1)$ electrons (ℓ is azimuthal quantum number), so the capacity of each band is $2(2\ell + 1)$N electrons.

Fig - 3 shows a complete representation of energy bands in sodium metal. The 1s, 2s & 2p bands are each full, 3s band is half & 3p band is completely empty. The 1s & 2s bands each contain 2N electrons & 2p band contain 6N electrons. The 3s band contain N electron, so it is half filled. The band, which can hold 6N electrons is completely empty.

When we add energy to a system i.e., to sodium metal, the electron can move from filled state to empty state. In this case, the electron can move from partially full states of 3s band to empty states of 3s band by absorbing small amount of energy or move to 3p band by absorbing larger amount of energy.

In a solid at zero temperature, the electron settle into the available states of lowest energy. The lower energy bands will therefore be completely filled & the upper most energy band will be either completely filled or partially filled, depending on the number of electrons & on the number of available states. The diffence between conductor & insulator arises from a partially filled or a completely filled upper most energy band.

CONDUCTORS, INSLULATORS AND SEMICONDUCTORS

Conductors

A conductor such as sodium, has a partially filled band (in sodium, the upper most band 3s is half filled). In these substance, electrons are free to move by applying an electric field, because un-occupied states are available in upper most band (in 3s band of sodium only half states are completely filled & half states are empty or un-occupied). Therefore these electrons are mobile & can contribute to electrical & thermal conductivity. For example the energy bands of sodium metal are shown in fig. 4.

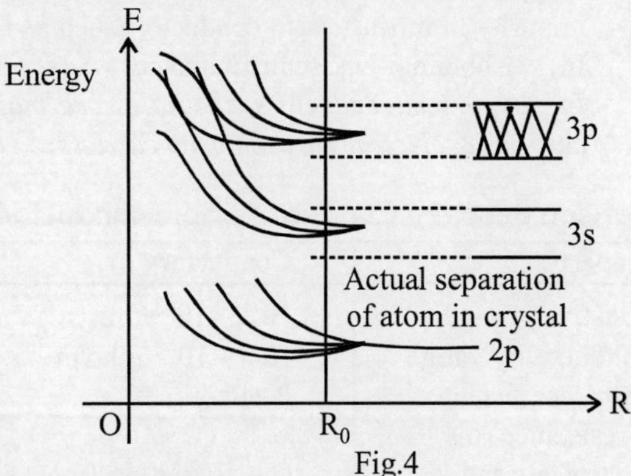

Fig.4

Origin of energy bands in sodium metals, as atoms move together the energy level spreads into bands.

In an isolated sodium atom, the six 3p lowest excited state for valence electrons are about 2.1 eV above two 3s G-states. But in solid sodium the 3s & 3p bands are spread out enough so that they actually overlap, forming a single band.

Because each sodium atom has only one valence electron but eight 3s & 3p states, that single band is only 1/8 filled & other states are unoccupied.

Insulators

In these substances (such as diamond), the upper most level is compeletely filled i.e., no unoccupied state is available for electron to move. The nearest unoccupied states are in next band(called C.B.), but this is separated from filled band (called V.B.) by an energy gap (Eg) of about 6eV. Hence electron refuses to carry an electric current.

Semiconductors

A semiconductor, has a completely filled valence band i.e., it resembles an insulator at zero temperature. However, the gap between this filled valence band & next band (C.B.) is small, about 1eV or less. Hence electrons can easily make the transitions from one band to another at room temperature & then carry an electric current (Silicon and germanium are semiconductors).

In a semiconductors, in thermal equilibrium, $n_e n_h = ni^2$

There are **two types of semiconductor**.

(i) **Intrinsic (or pure) semiconductors :** These semiconductors are pure materials in which the thermal vibrations of the lattice have liberated charge carriers (i.e., electrons & holes). In intrinsic semiconductor, the number of electrons (n_e) are equal to the number of holes (n_h).

(ii) **Extrinsic (or impure or doped) semiconductors :** They are impure semiconductors in which minutes traces of impurity introduces mobile charge carriers [which may be +ive (holes) or -ive (electrons)] in addition to those liberated by thermal vibration.

Again there are **two types of extrinsic semiconductors**.

(a) **N-type semiconductor :** When we add a pentavalent impurity in intrinsic semiconductor, then we obtain N-type semi-conductor. The pentavalent impurity substances are P, As & Sb. I*n N-type semi-conductors, the electrons are majority carriers & holes are minority carriers.*

i.e., $n_e >> n_h$

(b) **P-type semiconductor :** When we add a trivalent impurity in intrinsic semiconductor (such as B, Al, In), we obtain p-type semiconductor.

In p-type semiconductors, the holes are majority carriers & electrons are minority carriers.

i.e., $n_h >> n_e$

In acceptor impurity (trivalent element) energy level is just above the top of valence band (V.B.)

C.B.

$^*E_F$ ↑ Acceptor energy level

V.B.

($^*E_F$ is called fermi level & at T = 0 all the states below are completely filled. In N-type semiconductor it lies between conduction band & donor energy level E_d & in case of P-type, it lies between acceptor level E_a & valence band. In intrinsic semiconductor the E_F level lies in midway between C.B. & V.B.)

Comparison Between Conductors, Semiconductors and Insulators

Property	Conductors	Semiconductors	Insulators
Resistivity range	$10^{-6} - 10^{-8}\ \Omega$m	$10^{-4} - 0.5\ \Omega$m	$10^{7} - 10^{16}\ \Omega$m
Conductivity range	$10^{-6} - 10^{-8}$ mho/m	$10^{4} - 0.5$ mho/m	$10^{-7} - 10^{-16}$ mho/m
Temp. coefficient of resistance (α)	Positive	Negative	Negative
Flow of current	Due to free electrons	Due to electrons and holes	No current flow
Energy band diagram	Electron energy; Conduction band (CB); No gap; Overlapping region; Valence band (VB)	Electron energy; Conduction band (CB); Forbidden gap; $\Delta E_g \cong 1$eV; Valence band (VB)	Electron energy; Conduction band (CB); Forbidden gap; $\Delta E_g \geq 6$eV; Valence band (VB)
Forbidden energy gap	$\cong$ 0eV	$\cong$ 0.1 – 3eV	$\geq$6eV
Examples	Pt, Al, Cu, Ag etc.	Ge, Si, C, Ga, As GaF_2 etc.	Wood, plastic diamond, mica

MISCONCEPTIONS

× *Incorrect.* N–type semiconductors are negatively and P–type semiconductors are positively charged.

√ *Correct.* Both N–type and P–type semiconductors are neutral because these are made up of neutral atoms.

× *Incorrect.* Mobility of holes is greater than mobility of electrons

√ *Correct.* Mobility of holes is less than mobility of electrons because mobility of holes takes place in valance band and mobility of electrons takes place in conduction band.

Problem Solving Tips

1. Width of forbidden energy gap = Spacing between the top of valence band and the bottom of conduction band.
2. At absolute zero temperature (0 K), there are no free electrons in the conduction band of a semi-conductor.
3. A good number of semi-conductors (elemental and compound) have been discovered but the most frequently used are germanium (Ge) and silicon (Si) of group-IV of periodic table because the forbidden energy gap of them is small (of the order of 1 eV) so that at ordinary room temperature covalent bonds break easily and free electrons become available in the conduction band.
4. Important compound semi-conductors are gallium arsenide (GaAs), lead sulphide (Pbs), cadmium sulphide (Cds), indium phosphide (InP), etc.
5. Holes doesn't exist in conductors but only in semi-conductors. They are deflected by electric and magnetic fields like electrons. Their movement contributes to electric current similar to electrons.

Example 1.

Find the current produced at the room temperature in a pure germanium plate of area 2×10^{-4} m^2 and of thickness 1.2×10^{-3} m when a potential of 5 V is applied across the faces. Concentration of carriers in germanium at room temperature is 1.6×10^6 per cubic metre. The mobility of electrons and holes are $0.4\ m^2V^{-1}s^{-1}$ and $0.2\ m^2V^{-1}s^{-1}$ respectively. How much heat is generated in the plate in 100 second?

Solution :

Here, $n_i = 1.6 \times 10^6\ m^{-3}$

$\mu_e = 0.4\ m^2V^{-1}s^{-1}$

$\mu_h = 0.2\ m^2\ V^2\ s^{-1}$;

$A = 2 \times 10^{-4}\ m^2$ and $d = 1.2 \times 10^{-3} m$; $V = 5\ V$

As $\sigma = n_i e(\mu_e + \mu_h)$

$= \left(1.6 \times 10^6\right) \times (1.6 \times 10^{-19})(0.4 + 0.2)$

$= 1.53 \times 10^{-13}\ Sm^{-1}$

Current produced in germanium plate

$$I = JA = \sigma EA = \sigma\left(\frac{V}{d}\right)A$$

$$= 1.53 \times 10^{-13} \times \frac{5}{(1.2 \times 10^{-3})} \times 2 \times 10^{-4} = 1.28 \times 10^{-13}\ A$$

Heat generated in plate,

$H = VIt = 5 \times 1.28 \times 10^{-13} \times 100 = 6.4 \times 10^{-11}$ J.

p-n JUNCTION DIODE

If we join a piece of n-type to a piece of p-type semiconductor by appropriate method, then we obtain p-n junction diode. The two ends of p-n junction is provided with metallic conductors for the application of an external voltage. It is clear that p-type has more holes concentration but less concentration of electrons than n-type semicondutor.

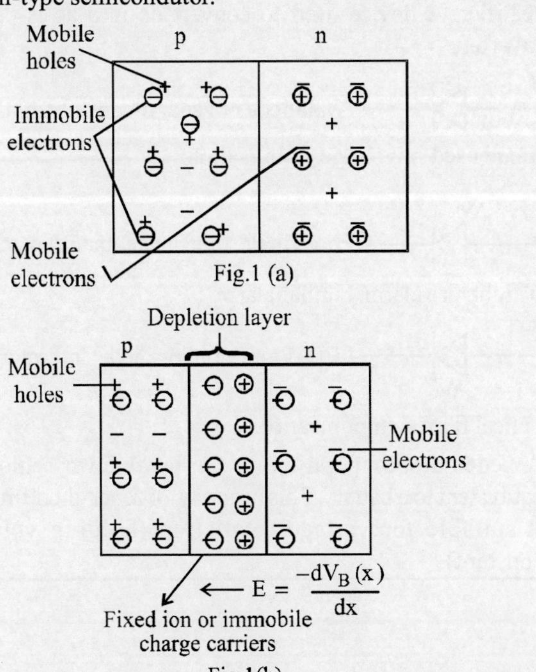

Fig.1 (a)

Fig.1(b)

Due to this difference in concentration, density gradient is established across the junction resulting in majority carriers diffusion : Holes (+ive ions) diffuses from p-type to n-type & electrons (–ive ions) from n-type to p-type (shown in fig (a)) & terminating their existence by recombination.

Diffusion and Drift Current

Diffusion current : We know that due to concentration difference, holes diffuse from p-side to n-side (in figure -1(a)) they move from left to right) & electron diffuse from n-side to p-side (in fig 1(a) they move from right to left). But electric field at junction repels the holes as they come to depletion layer & only those holes which have high kinetic energy are able to cross the potential barrier. Similarly electric field at junction repels electrons & those having high kinetic energy cross the junction.

The electric potential of n-side is more +ive (or higher) than p-side –ive (or lower). The variation of potential barrier V_B is shown in fig (c).

The potential difference created across the p-n junction due to the diffusion of electrons and holes is called **potential barrier**. So diffusion results in an electric current from p-side to n-side known as **diffusion current**.

Drift current : Due to thermal collision, some times a covalent bond is broken & electron-hole pair is created. But those electron-hole pairs are destroyed easily due to recombination. This process [generation of electron-hole (e-h) pair] occurs in the whole part of material.

But, if e-h pair is created in depletion region, the electron is quickly pushed by electric field towards n-side & holes towards p-side. As e-h pairs are continuously created in depletion region, there is a regular flow of electron towards n-side & holes towards p-side & so current flows from n-side to p-side. This current is drift current.

In steady state the magnitude of drift current is equal to diffusion current & since they are in opposite direction, hence there is no net transfer of charge at any cross section.

This recombination produces narrow region near junction called depletion layer. Since this region is depleted of free or mobile charge carrier and contains only immobile charge carriers, hence it is called **depletion region**. Due to these immobile charge carriers, a potential barrier V_B is established & further diffusion is stopped & equilibrium is reached (shown by fig. 1(b)). The sign of V_B is +ive towards the n-type & –ive towards p-type.

The schematic symbol of diode & corresponding equivalance in terms of V_B are shown below in fig. 2 (a) & (b).

Cathode (p) — Anode (n) (a) V_B (b) Depletion layer V_B o x (c)

Fig (2)

In fig-2(a) the triangle shows the direction of current. *For Si diode the value of V_B is 0.7V & for Ge diode the value of V_B is 0.3V.*

FORWARD AND REVERSE BIAS OF p-n JUNCTION DIODE

Forward Bias

When p-side of the p-n junction is connected to the +ve terminal of a battery and n to –ve terminal, conduction takes place and the diode is said to be forward biased.

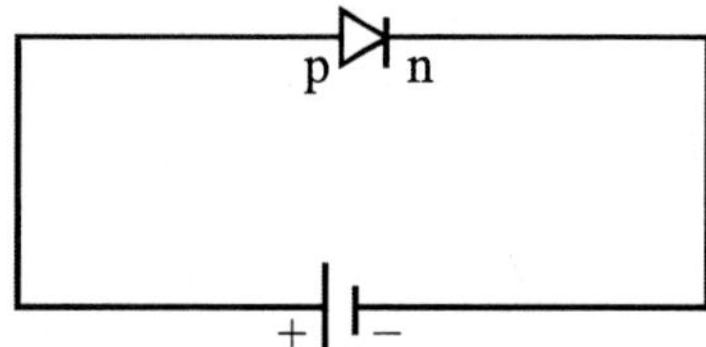

Reverse Bias

When p-side of he p-n junction is connected to the -ve terminal of a battery and n-side to the +ve terminal, there is no conduction takes place and diode is said to be reverse biased.

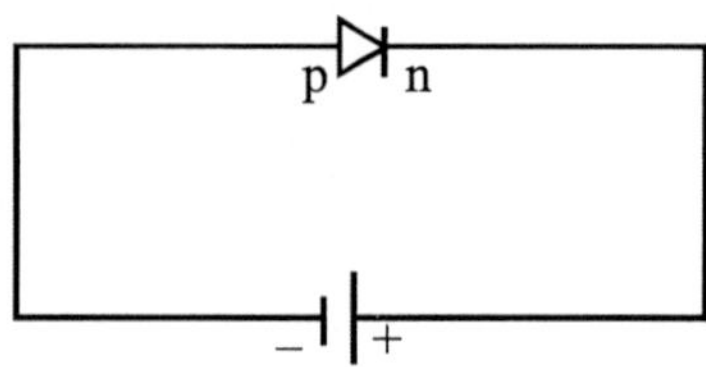

Effect of biasing : In forward bias, the thickness of depletion layer decreases and potential barrier reduces, while in reverse bias, the thickness of depletion layer increases and potential barrier also increases. In forward bias the current increases exponentially & in reverse bias, the current remains constant at very small magnitude upto breakdown voltage V_0 & after that it increases sharply without any further increase of reverse voltage shown in fig.1.

V-I characteristics of a p-n junction diode in forward and reverse bias.

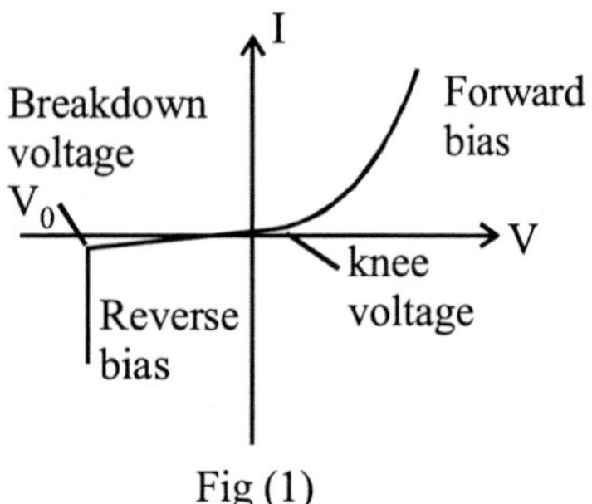

Fig (1)

The effect of forward biasing & reverse biasing on potential barrier are shown in fig.(2).

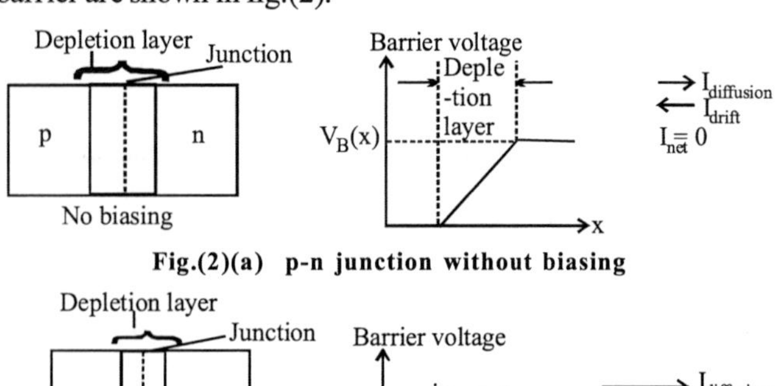

Fig.(2)(a) p-n junction without biasing

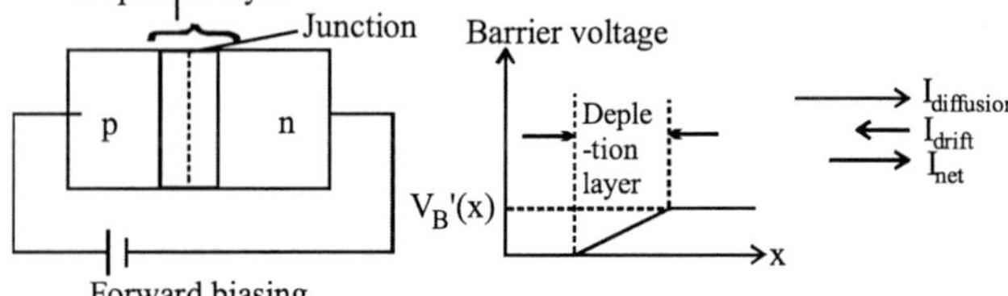

Fig.(2)(b) p-n junction with forward biasing

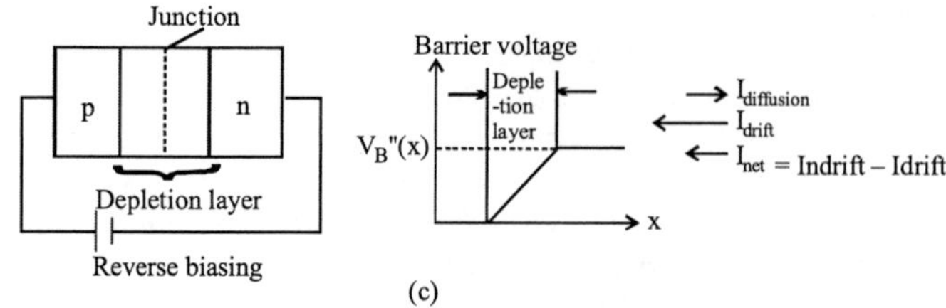

(c)

Fig.(2) (c) p-n junction with reverse biasing

In forward bias the expression of current is $I = I_0 (\exp \frac{eV}{K_B T} - 1)$

where V is applied voltage

I_0 is reverse saturation current

e is fundamental electronic charge

K_B is Boltzmann constant and

T is temperature

Problem Solving Tips

1. Width of depletion layer $\propto \frac{1}{\text{Doping}}$
2. Depletion is directly proportional to temperature.
3. Resistance is forward bias $R_{forward} \approx 10\Omega - 25\Omega$ and resistance in reverse bias $R_{reverse} \approx 10^5\Omega$.
4. Under suitable reverse bias break down occurs and voltage gets stabilized at Zener voltage.
5. Junction diode (p-n junction) can be used to convert the a.c. current to d.c. current i.e. as a **rectifier**. The process of conversion from a.c. to d.c. is called rectification.
6. p-n junction diode can be used as a half wave or full wave rectifier. A device used to convert dc into ac is called **inverter**.
7. 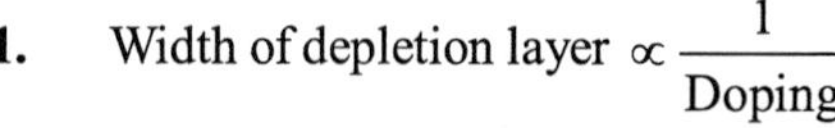 Avalanche or zener diode or breakdown diode used in voltage stabilisation.
8. 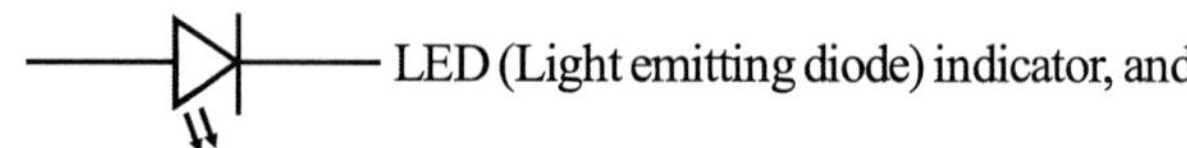 Photodiode, used in automatic switching of light, fire alarm, burglar alarm

   LED (Light emitting diode) indicator, and optical fibre communication.
9. A zener diode operating in the breakdown region is equivalent to a battery. This property of zener diode makes it suitable for voltage regulation (holding voltage constant).

Some Important Results of Half-wave and Full-wave Rectifier

	Circuit and Quantity	Half wave rectifier	Full wave rectifier
1.	Circuit	I/P, diode, R_L, V_0	I/P, D_1, D_2, R_L, V_0
2.	Input voltage (V_{in}, t)	Output voltage (V_0, t)	Output voltage (V_0, t)
3.	The value of I_{rms} of input alternating current $I = I_0 \sin \omega t$	$I_0 / 2$	$I_0 / \sqrt{2}$
4.	Peak inverse voltage (i.e. maximum voltage across diode when it is not conducting)	E_0	$2E_0$
5.	Output direct current	I_0 / π	$2I_0 / \pi$
6.	Ripple factor $\gamma = \sqrt{\left(\frac{I_{rms}}{I_{dc}}\right)^2 - 1}$	1.21	0.48
7.	Efficiency $\eta = \frac{\text{Output d.c. power}}{\text{Input a.c. power}}$	40.6%	81.2%
8.	Form factor $= \frac{I_{rms}}{I_{dc}} = \frac{E_{rms}}{E_{dc}}$	1.57	1.11
9.	The value of d.c. component in output voltage as compared to input a.c. voltage	Less	More

Example 2.

The diode used in the circuit shown has a constant voltage drop at 0.5 V at all currents and a maximum power rating of 100 milli-watt. What should be the value of the resistor R, connected in series with diode to obtain maximum current?

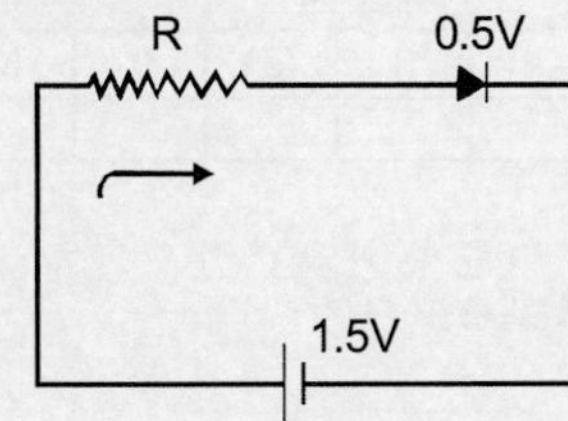

Solution :

$V_P = 0.5$ V, Maximum power rating P = 100 mW = 100×10^{-3} W and source voltage $V_s = 1.5$ V.

Now diode resistance $R_D = \frac{V_P^2}{P} = \frac{(0.5)^2}{100 \times 10^{-3}} = 2.5\Omega$

Current in diode $I_D = \frac{V_D}{R_D} = \frac{0.5}{2.5} = 0.2$A

$\therefore$ Total resistance in the circuit

$$R_T = \frac{V_s}{I_D} = \frac{1.5}{0.2} = 7.5\Omega$$

So, resistance R in circuit = $R_T - R_D = 7.5 - 2.5 = 5\Omega$

Example 3.

In p-n junction diode the reverse saturation current is 10^{-5} A at 27ºC. Find the forward current for a voltage of 0.2 V. [exp (7.62) = 2038.6, k = 1.4×10^{-23} J/K]

Solution :

$\because \; I = I_0 (e^{eV/kT} - 1)$

By solving we get,

$I = 10^{-5} [e^{7.62} - 1] = 10^{-5} [2038.6 - 1] = 20.376 \times 10^{-3}$ A

So the forward current for voltage 0.2V is 20.376×10^{-3}A

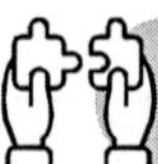

29.1 Concept Practice Problems

CPP

1. By increasing the temperature, the specific resistance of a conductor and a semiconductor
   (a) increases for both (b) decreases for both
   (c) increases, decreases (d) decreases, increases
2. Application of a forward bias to a p–n junction
   (a) widens the depletion zone.
   (b) increases the potential difference across the depletion zone
   (c) increases the number of donors on the n side.
   (d) increases the electric field in the depletion zone.
3. In a semiconductor diode, the barrier potential offers opposition to
   (a) holes in P-region only
   (b) free electrons in N-region only
   (c) majority carriers in both regions
   (d) majority as well as minority carriers in both regions
4. In a junction diode, the holes are due to
   (a) protons (b) extra electrons
   (c) neutrons (d) missing electrons
5. Choose the only false statement from the following.
   (a) In conductors, the valence and conduction bands may overlap.
   (b) Substances with energy gap of the order of 10 eV are insulators.
   (c) The resistivity of a semiconductor increases with increase in temperature.
   (d) The conductivity of a semiconductor increases with increase in temperature.
6. The energy band gap is maximum in
   (a) metals (b) superconductors
   (c) insulators (d) semiconductors.
7. Minority carriers in a p-type semiconductor are
   (a) free electrons
   (b) holes
   (c) neither holes nor free electron
   (d) both holes and free electrons.
8. In insulator
   (a) valence band is partially filled with electrons
   (b) conduction band is partially filled with electrons
   (c) conduction band is filled with electrons and valence band is empty
   (d) conduction band is empty and valence band is filled with electrons.
9. The intrinsic semi conductor becomes an insulator at
   (a) 0ºC (b) 0 K (c) 300 K (d) –100ºC
10. One serious drawback of semi-conductor devices is
    (a) they do not last for long time.
    (b) they are costly
    (c) they cannot be used with high voltage.
    (d) they pollute the environment.
11. At absolute zero, Si acts as
    (a) non-metal (b) metal
    (c) insulator (d) none of these
12. The drift current in a p-n junction is from the
    (a) n-side to the p-side
    (b) p-side to the n-side
    (c) n-side to the p-side if the junction is forward-biased and in the opposite direction if it is reverse biased
    (d) p-side to the n-side if the junction is forward-biased and in the opposite direction if it is reverse-biased
13. In forward biasing of the p–n junction
    (a) the positive terminal of the battery is connected to p–side and the depletion region becomes thick
    (b) the positive terminal of the battery is connected to n–side and the depletion region becomes thin
    (c) the positive terminal of the battery is connected to n–side and the depletion region becomes thick
    (d) the positive terminal of the battery is connected to p–side and the depletion region becomes thin
14. If a small amount of antimony is added to germanium crystal
    (a) it becomes a p–type semiconductor
    (b) the antimony becomes an acceptor atom
    (c) there will be more free electrons than holes in the semiconductor
    (d) its resistance is increased
15. A hole in a *P*-type semiconductor is
    (a) an excess electron (b) a missing electron
    (c) a missing atom (d) a donor level

ANSWER KEY

1	(c)	2	(c)	3	(c)	4	(d)	5	(c)	6	(c)	7	(a)	8	(d)	9	(b)	10	(c)
11	(c)	12	(a)	13	(d)	14	(c)	15	(b)										

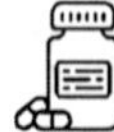

Topic 29.2 : Transistor and Logic Gates

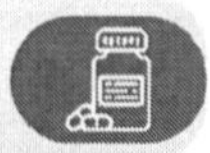

TRANSISTOR

Transistors are three terminal (solid state) devices just like triode. It can be assumed to consist of two back to back p-n junctions. In practice a junction transistor (p-n-p) consists of silicon (or germanium) bar crystal in which a layer of n-type silicon (or Ge) is sandwiched between two layers of p-type silicon & we get p-n-p transistor. Alternatively it may consist of a layer of p-type between two layers of n-type material & we get a n-p-n transister as shown by fig. (1).

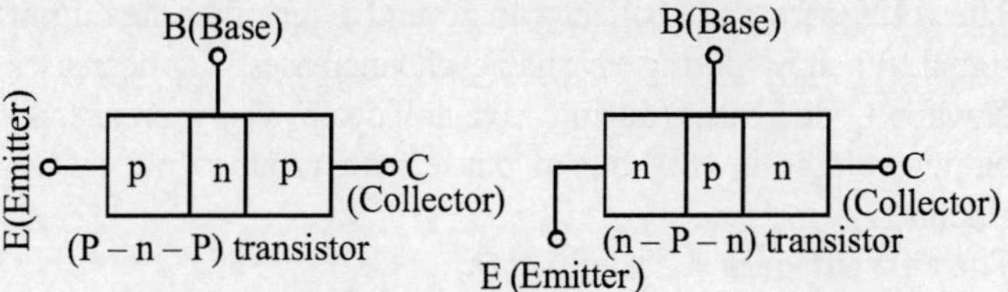

Fig. (1)

The **schematic symbols of transistor are**

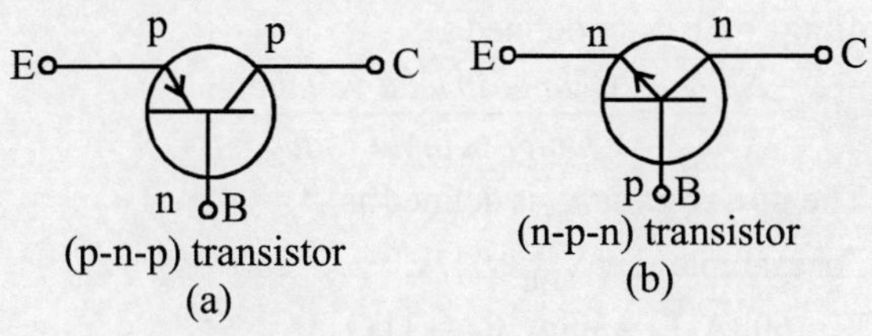

Fig. (2)

Components of Transistor :

Emitter (E) : It supplies charge carriers (electron in n-p-n transistor and holes in p-n-p transistor) & it has high density of impurity concentration i.e., highly doped. It is always forward biased.

Collector (C) : It is a region on other side of base. It has maximum area out of other sections(emitter & base) of transistor to dissipate the heat. It collects the charge carriers & it is always reverse biased.

Base (B) : It is middle region which forms the two junctions between emitter & collector. It is very lightly doped.

Biasing of Transistor

In proper biasing of transistor the input (i.e., base emitter junction) is always forward biased & output (i.e., collector base junction) is always reverse biased as shown in fig.(3)

This scheme of biasing is same for all three transistor configurations; Common base configuration (CB), common emitter configuration (CE) & common collector configuration (CC)]

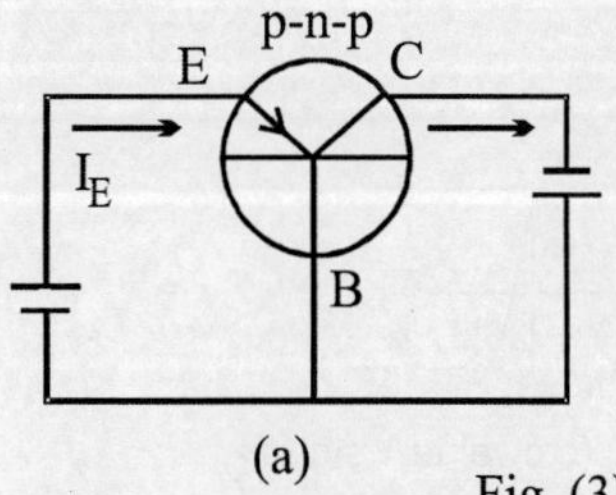

(a)

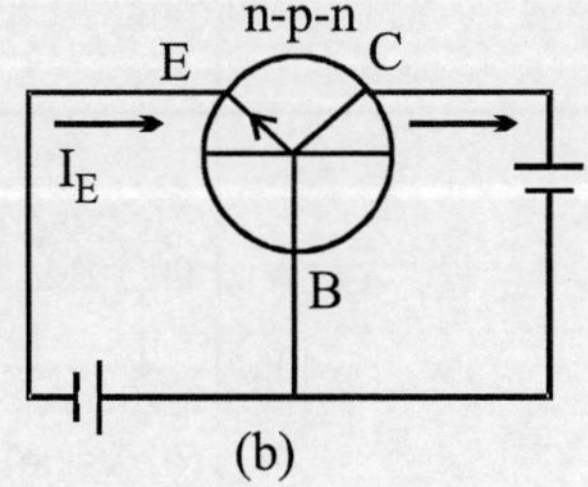

(b)

Fig. (3)

Working of Transistor

Fig. (4) shows a common base (C.B.) configuration of p-n-p transistor. The forward biasing of emitter junction lowers the emitter base potential barrier, whereas the reverse biasing of collector junction increases the collector-base potential barrier. Hence holes (majority carriers in p-type) flows through emitter to base & constitutes an emitter current I_E. Since emitter is heavily doped in comparison to base, so approximately (only 5% holes recombine with electrons in base region & constitute base current I_B) 95% holes reach to collector & constitute collector current I_C.

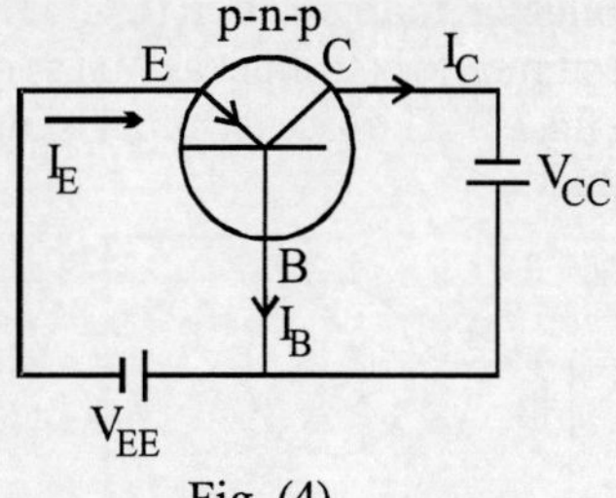

Fig. (4)

From Kirch off's current law,

$$I_E = I_C + I_B \quad ...(1)$$

Eq. (1) holds true regardless of circuit configuration or transistor type (p-n-p or n-p-n) that is used.

The **current gain (B)** *of transistor is defined as ratio of collector current I_C to base current I_B*

$$\text{i.e., } \beta = \frac{I_C}{I_B} \quad ...(2)$$

The value of β lies between 10 and 100. Since $I_E \approx I_C$

Current gain (α) *is defined as the ratio of collector current I_C to emitter current I_E.* The value of α is always less than unity.

$$\alpha = \frac{I_C}{I_E} \quad ...(3)$$

Relation between α and β

$$\alpha = \frac{\beta}{1+\beta} \quad \text{or} \quad \beta = \frac{\alpha}{1-\alpha} \quad ...(4)$$

Configurations of Transistor

There are three types of transistor configuration. We can take either terminal as input terminal and other terminal as output.

(i) **Common base configuration (CB) :** Here base terminal is common to both input & output terminals. The emitter terminal is taken as input.

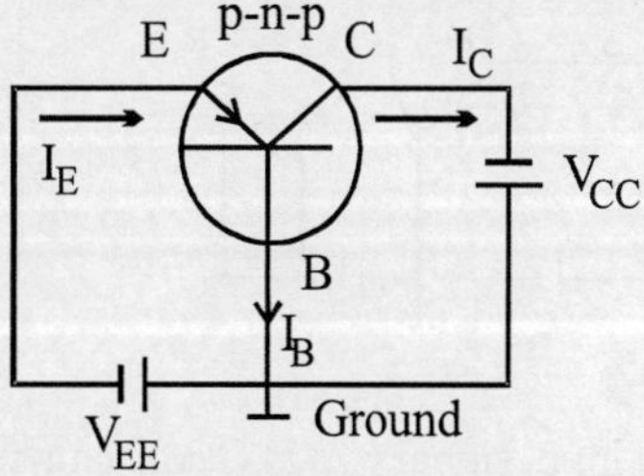

Fig. (5)

(ii) **Common emitter configuration (CE) :** Here emitter terminal is common to both input and output terminals as shown in fig. (6). The base terminal is taken as input and collector is taken as output.

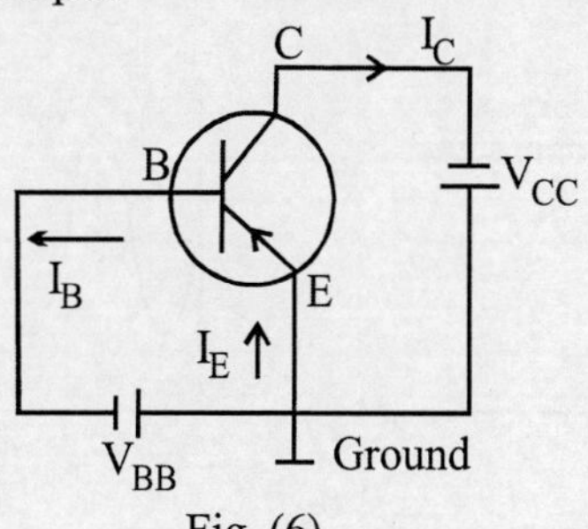

Fig. (6)

(iii) **Common collector configuration (CC) :** Here the collector terminal is common to both input as well as output terminals as shown in fig. (7). The base terminal is input & emitter is output terminal.

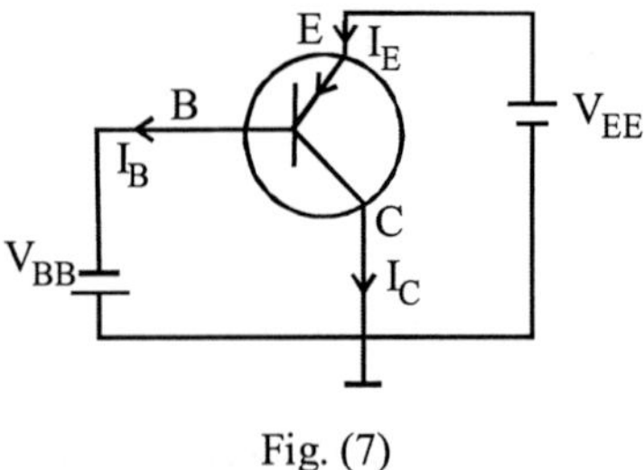

Fig. (7)

Transistor as an Amplifier

Amplification is the process of linearly increasing the amplitude of a signal. It is one of the major properties of a transistor.

This amplifing action was produced by transfering a current from a low (base emitter loop is forward biased & hence provide low resistance path and collector base junction is reverse biased & hence gives high resistance path in common emitter configuration) to a high resistance circuit.

Common-Emitter (CE) Amplifier : Fig. 8 shows a basic common-emitter amplifier circuit in which we connect a signal source V_s. The input voltage loop is V_s, then from base to emitter through transister to ground (common refrence point) & then through V_{BE} back to V_s. The output voltage loop consists ground, then from emitter to collector through R_C. The emitter is connected to ground. During a +ive half cycle of V_s, the forward bias across the emitter base junction will be increased, while during – ive half cycle of V_s (signal source), the forward bias across emitter base junction will be decreased. Hence more electrons flow during +ive half cycle and so we obtain more collector current and so large voltage drop across R_C and less value and V_{CE}. In negative half cycle collector current decreases.

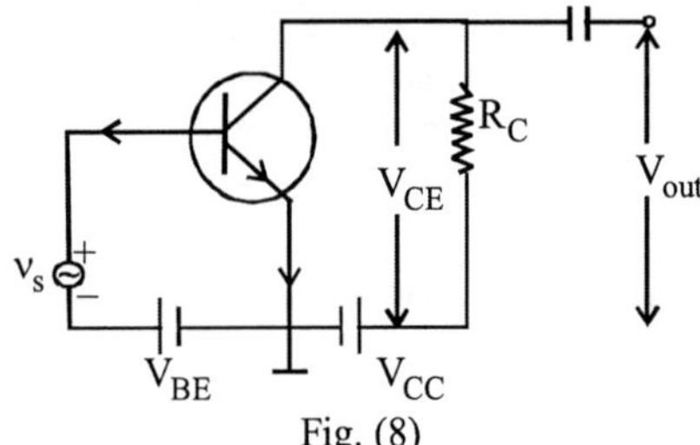

Fig. (8)

In the absence of input signal v_s, a D.C collector current I_C flows in collector circuit due to forward biased battery V_{BE}. This is called **zero signal collector current**. So total collector current is

$$I_{\text{total collector current}} = \underset{\text{d.c. collector current}}{I_C} + \underset{\text{a.c. collector current}}{I_c}$$

(a) V_s, Curve & input signal, $+V_s$, V_{BE}, $-V_s$, O, t

(b) V_{out}, $V_s = V_{ce}$, Curve of output signal, V_{CE}, t, $-V_s = -V_{ce}$

Fig. (9)

(a) Input signal superimposed on V_{BE}
(b) Output amplifying signal wave from super imposed on V_{CE}

The voltage from the collector to ground determines the output signal. When I_C (during +ive half cycle) increases, V_{CE} decreases & when I_C decreases (during – ive half cycle) V_{CE} increase. So output voltage is 180° out of phase with input signal in CE amplifier:

The **current gain A_i** is defined as,

$$A_i = \frac{\Delta I_C}{\Delta I_B} = \frac{\text{Change in load current/collector current}}{\text{Change in input current/base current}}$$

The **voltage gain A_v** is defined as,

$$A_v = \frac{\Delta V_{CE}}{\Delta V_{BE}} = \frac{\text{Change in load voltage}}{\text{Change in input voltage}}$$

The **power gain A_p** is defined as, $A_p = A_i \times A_v$

For example : Let $V_{BE} = 0.7V$, $V_{CC} = 20V$

$I_B = 60\mu A$, $I_C = 3mA$, $R_C = 3\,k\Omega$

Then $\beta_{d.c} = \frac{I_C}{I_B} = \frac{3mA}{60\mu A} = 50$

The collector current flowing through R_C results in voltage drop:

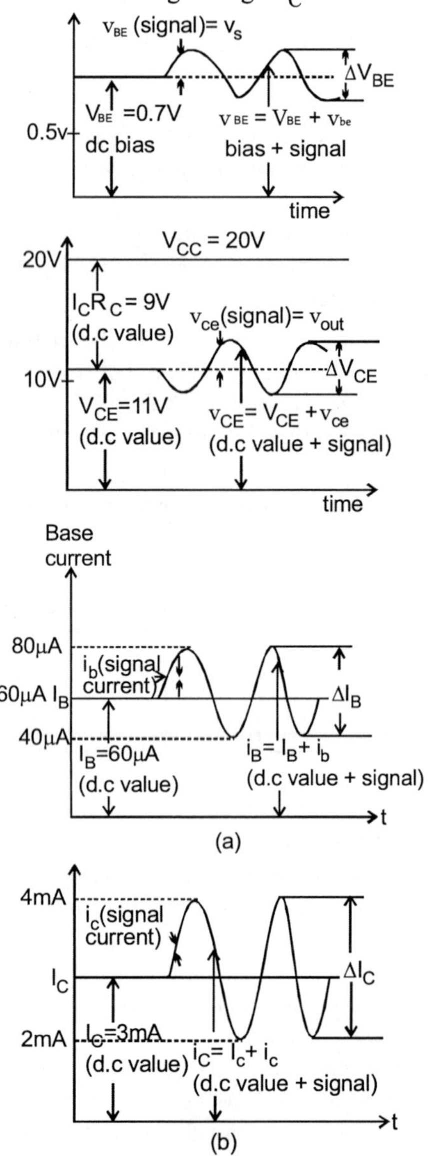

Fig. (a) Base wave forms or input wave forms
(b) Collector wave froms or output wave forms.

$I_C R_C = .003A \times 3000\Omega = 9.0V$

So by K.V.L the voltage from collector to emitter is

$V_{CE} = V_{CC} - I_C R_C = 20 - 9 = 11.0V$

Now we introduce signal voltage v_s, which has peak value 50mV. During +ive half cycle of $v_s = +50mV$, I_B rises to 80μA & during –ive half cycle of $v_s = -50mV$. I_B decreases to 40μA.

So change in base current is ΔI_B (80 – 60) μA = 20μA

and change in collector current is $\Delta I_C (\beta_{ac} \Delta I_B) = 50 \times 20 = 1mA$

It means during +ive half cycle I_C becomes 4mA hence

$V_{CE} = V_{CC} - I_C R_C = 20 - 12 = 8.V$

During the negative half cycle I_C becomes 2mA, hence

$V_{CE} = 20 - 6 = 14V.$

so $\Delta V_{CE} = 3V$

so $A_i = \dfrac{\Delta I_C}{\Delta I_B} = \dfrac{1mA}{20\mu A} = 50$

$A_v = \dfrac{\Delta V_{CE}}{\Delta V_{BE}} = \dfrac{3V}{50mV} = 60$

and $A_p = A_i \times A_v = 3000$

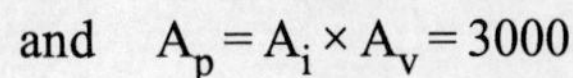

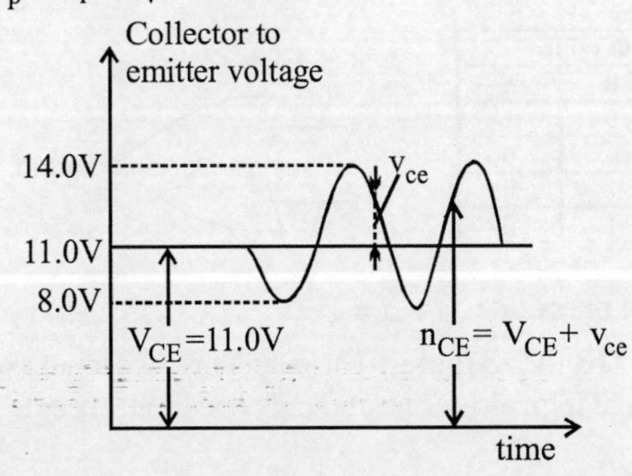

Problem Solving Tips

1. Amplifier is a device used to increase the amplitude of input signal.
2. Amplification factor of triode valve $\mu = g_m \times R_p$ where g_m = mutual or transconductance and R_p = plate resistance.
3. Transistor is also used as an oscillator.
   Frequency of transistor LC oscillator is given by,
   $f = \dfrac{1}{2\pi\sqrt{LC}}$
4. In phase shift oscillator (which consists of three RC section), the frequency is given by $f = \dfrac{1}{2\pi\sqrt{6RC}}$
5. **Oscillator** gives continuous, undamped oscillating output.
6. **Inverter :** An oscillator which converts d.c. into a.c.
7. An amplifier with feed back in proper phase and magnitude behaves as an oscillator.
8. **Berkhausen criteria :** for amplifier to act as oscillator :
   Gain with feed back, A′ = A/[1 - KA], K = feed back ratio.
   Criteria to become oscillator, (1 - KA) = 0.
   "Where A' is called closed loop gain & A is called open loop gain.
9. The basic rules for normal operation of a transistor are
   (i) the emitter-base junction is forward blased to offer a low resistance to the flow of current.
   (ii) the collector-base junction is reverse biased to offer a high resistance to the flow of current.

Comparative study of CB, CE and CC Amplifier

Use and property	Common base (CB) amplifier	Common emitter (CE) amplifier	Common collector (CC) amplifier
Used for	Voltage amplification	Power amplification	Current amplification
Impedance	Low	High	Low
Output Impedance	High	High	Low
Current gain	$A_i < 1$ (α)	$A_i < 1$ (β) (β ≈ 20 – 100)	A_i (B + 1)> 1 (20 – 200)
Voltage gain	$A_v > 1$	$A_v > 1$	$A_v < 1$
Power gain	$A_p > 1$	$A_p > 1$	$A_v > 1$
Phase shift	Nil	180°	Nil

Example 4.

The correct relationship between two current gains α and β in a transistor is

(a) $\beta = \dfrac{\alpha}{1+\alpha}$ (b) $\beta = \dfrac{1+\alpha}{\alpha}$

(c) $\alpha = \dfrac{\beta}{1+\beta}$ (d) $\alpha = \dfrac{1+\beta}{\beta}$

Solution : (c)

$\beta = \dfrac{\alpha}{1-\alpha}$ or $\beta(1-\alpha) = \alpha$ or $\beta - \beta\alpha = \alpha$

or $\beta = \alpha(1+\beta)$; $\therefore \alpha = \beta/(1+\beta)$

Example 5.

The current gain of a transistor in common base mode is 0.99. To change the emitter current by 5 mA, what will be the necessary change in collector current?

Solution :

$\dfrac{\Delta I_c}{\Delta I_e} = \alpha$ or $\Delta I_c = \alpha \Delta I_e$; $\Delta Ic = .99 \times 5 = 4.95$ mA

Example 6.

For a transistor, the current amplification factor is 0.8, the transistor is connected in common emitter configuration. Find the change in the collector current when the base current changes by 6 mA.

Solution :

$\alpha = 0.8$; $\beta = \dfrac{\alpha}{1-\alpha} = \dfrac{0.8}{1-0.8} = 4$;

$\beta = \Delta I_c / \Delta I_b$ or $\Delta I_c = \beta \Delta I_b = 4 \times 6 = 24$ mA

Example 7.

The current gain of a transistor in a common emitter configuration is 40. If the emitter current is 8.2 mA, then find the base current.

Solution :

$$\beta = \frac{I_c}{I_b} = \frac{I_e - I_b}{I_b} = \frac{I_e}{I_b} - 1 \text{ or } \frac{I_e}{I_b} = 1 + \beta$$

$$\text{or} \quad I_b = \frac{I_e}{1+\beta} = \frac{8.2}{1+40} = \frac{8.2}{41} = .20\,\text{mA}$$

Example 8.

In a common emitter transistor amplifier $\beta = 60$, $R_0 = 5000\ \Omega$ and internal resistance of a trnasistor is $500\ \Omega$. What will be the voltage amplification of amplifier?

Solution :

$$A_v = \beta \frac{R_0}{R_i} = 60 \times \frac{5000}{500} = 600$$

Example 9.

A p-n-p transistor is used in common-emitter mode in an amplifier circuit. A change of 40 μA in the base current brings a change of 2 mA in collector current and 0.04 V in base emitter voltage. Find the (i) input resistance R_i (ii) the base current amplification factor (β). (iii) If a load resistance of 6 kΩ is used, then also find the voltage gain of the amplifier.

Solution :

Here, $\Delta I_b = 40 \times 10^{-6}$ A; $\Delta I_c = 2 \times 10^{-3}$ A;
$\Delta V_i = 0.04$ V; $R_0 = 6000\Omega$

(i) Input resistance, $R_i = \frac{\Delta V_i}{\Delta I_b} = \frac{0.04}{40 \times 10^{-6}} = 10^3 \Omega$

(ii) Base current amplification factor,

$$\beta = \frac{\Delta I_c}{\Delta I_b} = \frac{2 \times 10^{-3}}{40 \times 10^{-6}} = 50$$

(iii) Voltage gain, $Av = \beta \frac{R_0}{R_i} = 50 \times \frac{6000}{10^3} = 300$.

LOGIC GATES

A logic gate is a digital circuit that follow certain logical relationship between input and output voltages. They control the flow of information.

Basic logic gates are : AND, OR and NOT gates.

AND gate : The output is high or 1 when all inputs are high.

Truth table

A	B	Y
0	0	0
0	1	0
1	0	0

Logic symbol

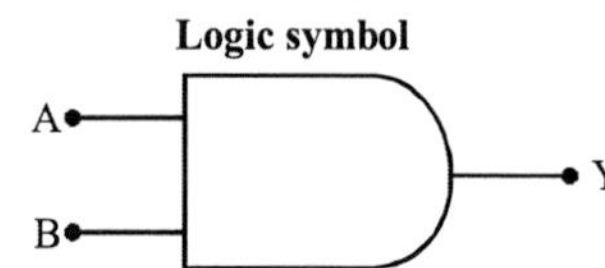

Boolean expression : $A \, . \, B = y$

OR gate : Output is high even if one of the inputs is high.

Truth table

A	B	Y
0	0	0
0	1	1
1	0	1
1	1	1

Logic symbol

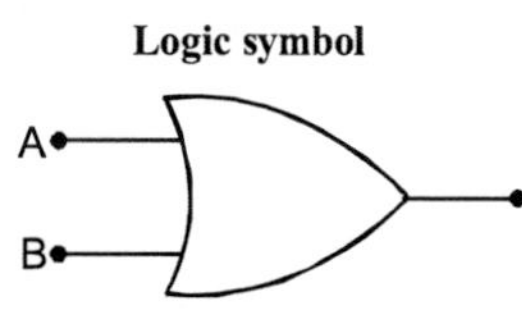

Boolean expression : $A + B = y$

NOT gate : Output is not the input.

Truth table

A	Y
0	1
1	0

Logic symbol

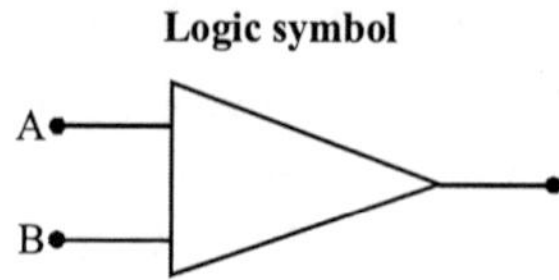

Boolean expression : $y = \overline{A}$

NAND gate : It is the combinatin of AND and NOT gate. The output is high, even if all inputs are low (i.e., 0) or one input is low.

Truth table

A	B	Y
0	0	1
1	0	1
0	1	1
1	1	0

Logic symbol

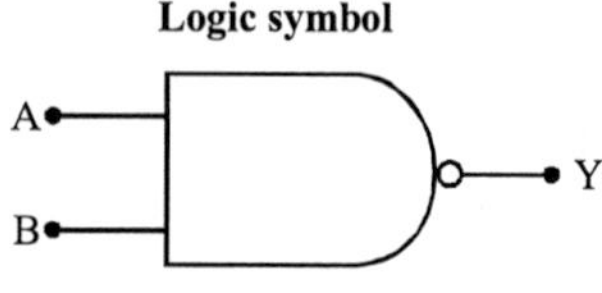

Boolean expression : $\overline{A.B} = Y$

NAND gate is called the building block of all digital circuits.

NOR gate : It is the combination of NOT and OR gate. The output is high, when all inputs are low.

Truth table

A	B	Y
0	0	1
1	0	0
0	1	0
1	1	0

Logic symbol

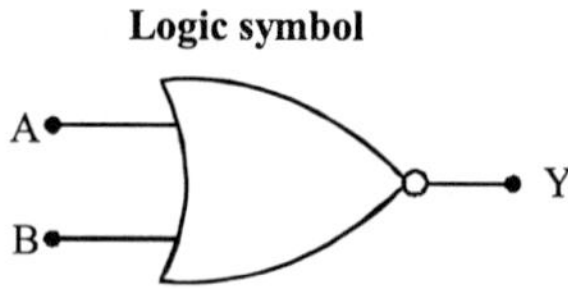

Boolean expression : $\overline{A + B} = Y$

Exclusive OR (XOR) gate : The output of a two input exclusive OR gate is at logical 1 if one and only one input accepts logical 0 (zero)

Logic symbol:

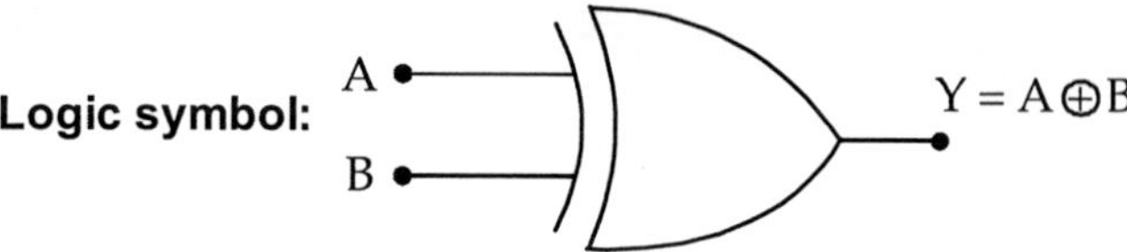

Truth table

Input		Output
A	**B**	**$Y = A \oplus B$**
0	0	0
0	1	1
1	0	1
1	1	0

Logic expression : $Y = A \oplus B = \overline{A}B + A\overline{B}$

Note : This circuit is also called inequality **comparator** or **detector** because it produces an output only when the two inputs are different.

Demorgan Theorems

(i) $\overline{A.B} = \overline{A} + \overline{B}$ (ii) $\overline{A + B} = \overline{A}.\overline{B}$

These theorems are self proved.

Some basic boolean identies :

OR operation	**AND operation**	**NOT operation**
$A+0=A$	$A.0=0$	$A+\overline{A}=1$
$A+1=1$	$A.1=A$	$A\overline{A}=0$
$A+A=A$	$A.A=A$	$\overline{\overline{A}}=A$
$A+\overline{A}=1$	$A.\overline{A}=0$	

$A+B=B+A \quad A.B=B.A$

$A(B+C)=AB+ACA+BC=(A+B)(A+C)$

$A+AB=A \qquad A(A+B)=A$

$A+\overline{A}B=A+B \qquad A(\overline{A}+B)=AB$

These above theorems, identities & relations can be easily proved.

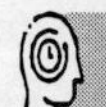

Problem Solving Tips

1. The basic concept of digital circuit has been provided by George Boole.
2. Claude shanon established an analogy between function of mechanical switches and Boolean algebra.
3. Series combination of switches is equivalent to AND logic operation.
4. Parallel combination of switches is equivalent to OR logic operation.
5. NOT logic operation is performed on a single variable. That's why it is called unary operation.
6. AND, OR and NOT logic operations follow closure property, i.e., input as well as output are in either of the binary states.
7. NAND and NOR gates are universal gates
8. If the logic gate is changed from positive to negative or vice-versa; AND changes into OR, OR changes into AND, NAND changes into NOR and NOR charges into NAND.

Example 10.

Identify the gate represented by the block diagram shown in fig. Write the Boolean expression and truth table.

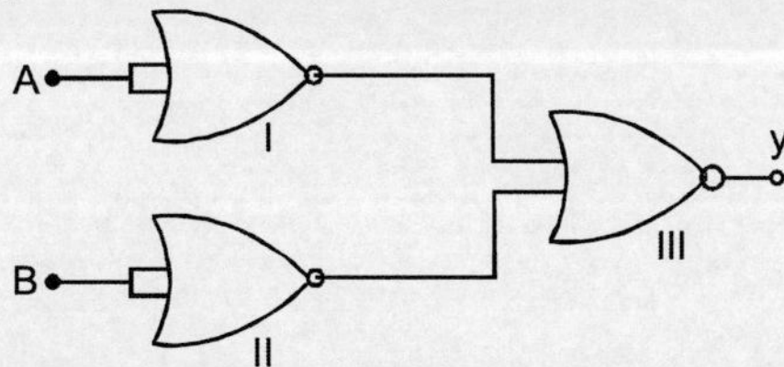

Solution :

Here for the input, the two NOR gates have been used as NOT gates (by joining the input terminals of NOR gate). Their outputs are jointly fed to the NOR gate. From the NOR gate I, for the input A, the output is $\overline{A}$. From the NOR gate II, for the input B, the output is $\overline{B}$. From NOR gate III, the output is given by $Y=\overline{\overline{A}+\overline{B}}=A.B$

Thus Boolean expression for this combination of gate is

$Y=\overline{\overline{A}+\overline{B}}=A.B$

which is for AND gate. Thus the combination will work as AND gate. The truth table of the combination of gates is

A	B	$\overline{A}$	$\overline{B}$	Y
0	0	1	1	0
1	0	0	1	0
0	1	1	0	0
1	1	0	0	1

Example 11.

The combinations of the 'NAND' gates shown here in fig. are equivalent to

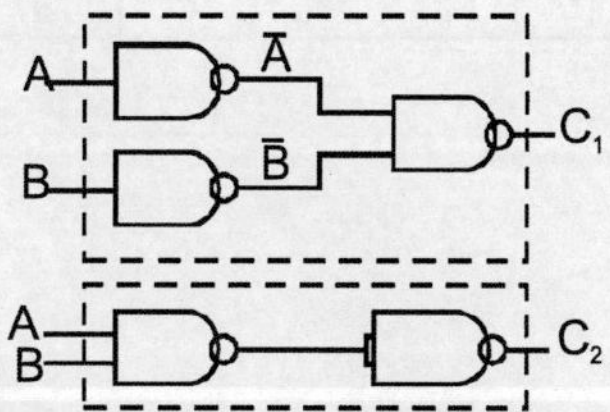

(a) an 'OR' gate and an 'AND' gate respectively
(b) an 'AND' gate and a 'NOT' gate respectively
(c) an 'AND' gate and an 'OR' gate respectively
(d) an 'OR' gate and a 'NOT' gate respectively

Solution : **(a)**

For first case, $C_1=\overline{\overline{A}.\overline{B}}=(A+B)$ (by Demorgan's theorem)

The truth table is shown below

A	B	$\overline{A}$	$\overline{B}$	$\overline{A}.\overline{B}$	$\overline{\overline{A}.\overline{B}}$
1	0	0	1	0	1
0	1	1	0	0	1
0	0	1	1	1	0
1	1	0	0	0	1

This is truth table for $C_1=A+B$ i.e. OR gate

For second case, $C_2=\overline{\overline{A.B}}=A.B$ i.e., AND gate.

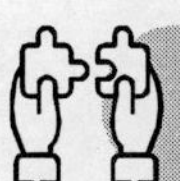

29.2 Concept Practice Problems

CPP

16. A transistor has three impurity regions. All the three regions have different doping levels. In order of increasing doping level, the regions are

(a) emitter, base and collector
(b) collector, base and emitter
(c) base, emitter and collector
(d) base, collector and emitter

17. In Boolean algebra, $Y=A+B$ implies that

(a) output Y exists when both inputs A and B exist
(b) output Y exists when either input A exists or input B exists or both inputs A and B exist
(c) output Y exists when either input A exists or input B exists but not when both inputs A and B exist
(d) output Y exists when both inputs A and B exists but not when either input A or B exist

18. Which of the following is unipolar transistor?
(a) $p-n-p$ transistor (b) $n-p-n$ transistor
(c) Field effect transistor (d) Point contact transistor

19. When n-P-n transistor is used as an amplifier, then
(a) electrons move from collector to emitter
(b) electrons move from emitter to collector
(c) electrons move from collector to base
(d) holes move from emitter to collector

20. An oscillator is nothing but an amplifier with
(a) positive feedback (b) large gain
(c) no feedback (d) negative feedback

21. NAND and NOR gates are called universal gates primarily because they
(a) are available universally
(b) can be combined to produce OR, AND and NOT gates
(c) are widely used in Integrated circuit packages
(d) are easiest to manufacture

22. Radiowaves of constant amplitude can be generated with
(a) FET (b) filter
(c) rectifier (d) oscillator

23. The transistor are usually made of
(a) metal oxides with high temperature coefficient of resistivity
(b) metals with high temperature coefficient of resistivity
(c) metals with low temperature coefficient of resistivity
(d) semiconducting materials having low temperature coefficient of resistivity

24. The device that can act as a complete electronic circuit is
(a) junction diode (b) integrated circuit
(c) junction transistor (d) zener diode

25. Current gain of a transistor in common base mode is 0.95. Its value in common emitter mode is
(a) 0.95 (b) 1.5 (c) 19 (d) $(19)^{-1}$

ANSWER KEY																			
16	(d)	**17**	(b)	**18**	(c)	**19**	(b)	**20**	(a)	**21**	(b)	**22**	(d)	**23**	(a)	**24**	(b)	**25**	(c)

CONCEPT MAP

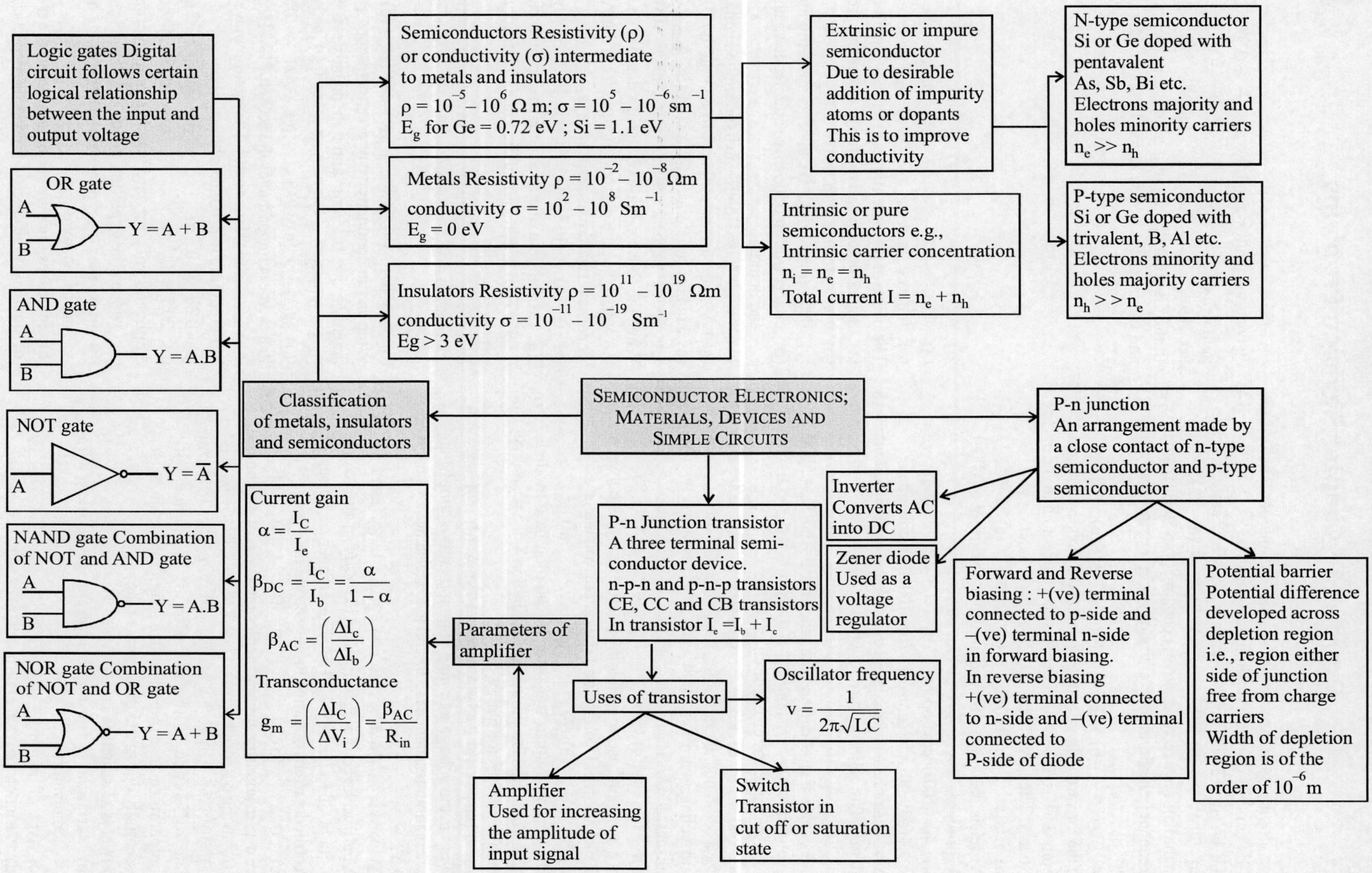

SEMICONDUCTOR ELECTRONICS; MATERIALS, DEVICES AND SIMPLE CIRCUITS

Classification of metals, insulators and semiconductors

Semiconductors Resistivity (ρ) or conductivity (σ) intermediate to metals and insulators
$\rho = 10^{-5} - 10^{6}\ \Omega$ m; $\sigma = 10^{5} - 10^{-6}$ sm^{-1}
E_g for Ge = 0.72 eV ; Si = 1.1 eV

Extrinsic or impure semiconductor
Due to desirable addition of impurity atoms or dopants
This is to improve conductivity

N-type semiconductor
Si or Ge doped with pentavalent
As, Sb, Bi etc.
Electrons majority and holes minority carriers
$n_e >> n_h$

P-type semiconductor
Si or Ge doped with trivalent, B, Al etc.
Electrons minority and holes majority carriers
$n_h >> n_e$

Intrinsic or pure semiconductors e.g.,
Intrinsic carrier concentration
$n_i = n_e = n_h$
Total current $I = n_e + n_h$

Metals Resistivity $\rho = 10^{-2} - 10^{-8}\ \Omega m$
conductivity $\sigma = 10^{2} - 10^{8}\ Sm^{-1}$
$E_g = 0$ eV

Insulators Resistivity $\rho = 10^{11} - 10^{19}\ \Omega m$
conductivity $\sigma = 10^{-11} - 10^{-19}\ Sm^{-1}$
Eg > 3 eV

Logic gates Digital circuit follows certain logical relationship between the input and output voltage

OR gate: A, B — $Y = A + B$

AND gate: A, B — $Y = A.B$

NOT gate: A — $Y = \overline{A}$

NAND gate Combination of NOT and AND gate: A, B — $Y = \overline{A.B}$

NOR gate Combination of NOT and OR gate: A, B — $Y = \overline{A + B}$

P-n junction
An arrangement made by a close contact of n-type semiconductor and p-type semiconductor

Inverter
Converts AC into DC

Zener diode
Used as a voltage regulator

Forward and Reverse biasing : +(ve) terminal connected to p-side and –(ve) terminal n-side in forward biasing.
In reverse biasing +(ve) terminal connected to n-side and –(ve) terminal connected to P-side of diode

Potential barrier
Potential difference developed across depletion region i.e., region either side of junction free from charge carriers
Width of depletion region is of the order of 10^{-6} m

P-n Junction transistor
A three terminal semi-conductor device.
n-p-n and p-n-p transistors
CE, CC and CB transistors
In transistor $I_e = I_b + I_c$

Uses of transistor

Oscillator frequency
$$v = \frac{1}{2\pi\sqrt{LC}}$$

Amplifier
Used for increasing the amplitude of input signal

Switch
Transistor in cut off or saturation state

Parameters of amplifier

Current gain
$$\alpha = \frac{I_C}{I_e}$$
$$\beta_{DC} = \frac{I_C}{I_b} = \frac{\alpha}{1-\alpha}$$
$$\beta_{AC} = \left(\frac{\Delta I_c}{\Delta I_b}\right)$$
Transconductance
$$g_m = \left(\frac{\Delta I_C}{\Delta V_i}\right) = \frac{\beta_{AC}}{R_{in}}$$

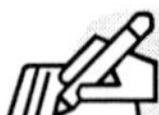

Exercise 1 - Chapter Revision Problems

CRP

1. On doping germanium with donor atoms of density 10^{17} cm^{-3} its conductivity in mho/cm will be [Given : $\mu_e = 3800$ cm^2/V–s and $n_i = 2.5 \times 10^{13}$ cm^{-13}]
   (a) 30.4 (b) 60.8 (c) 91.2 (d) 121.6
2. In the half wave rectifier circuit operating from 50 Hz mains frequency, the fundamental frequency in the ripple would be
   (a) 25 Hz (b) 50 Hz (c) 70.7 Hz (d) 100 Hz
3. If the forward voltage in a semiconductor diode is changed from 0.5V to 0.7 V, then the forward current changes by 1.0 mA. The forward resistance of diode junction will be
   (a) 100 Ω (b) 120 Ω (c) 200 Ω (d) 240 Ω
4. A transistor has $\beta = 40$. A change in base current of 100 μ A, produces change in collector current
   (a) 40×100 microampere (b) $(100 - 40)$ microampere
   (c) $(100 + 40)$ microampere (d) 100/40 microampere
5. A transistor has a base current of 1 mA and emitter current 90 mA. The collector current will be
   (a) 90 mA (b) 1 mA (c) 89 mA (d) 91 mA
6. In a common emitter transistor amplifier $\beta = 60$, $R_o = 5000$ Ω and internal resistance of a transistor is 500 Ω. The voltage amplification of amplifier will be
   (a) 500 (b) 460 (c) 600 (d) 560
7. For a common base amplifier, the values of resistance gain and voltage gain are 3000 and 2800 respectively. The current gain will be
   (a) 1.1 (b) 0.98 (c) 0.93 (d) 0.83
8. In a common base amplifier the phase difference between the input signal voltage and the output voltage is
   (a) 0 (b) π/4 (c) π/2 (d) π
9. The current gain in transistor in common base mode is 0.99. To change the emitter current by 5 mA, the necessary change in collector will be
   (a) 0.196 mA (b) 2.45 mA (c) 4.95 mA (d) 5.1 mA
10. What is the voltage gain in a common emitter amplifier, where input resistance is 3 Ω and load resistance 24 Ω, $\beta = 0.6$?
    (a) 8.4 (b) 4.8 (c) 2.4 (d) 480
11. A half-wave rectifier is being used to rectify an alternating voltage of frequency 50 Hz. The number of pulses of rectified current obtained in one second is
    (a) 50 (b) 25 (c) 100 (d) 2000
12. In a p-n junction having depletion layer of thickness 10^{-6} m the potential across it is 0.1 V. The electric field is
    (a) 10^7 V/m (b) 10^{-6} V/m (c) 10^5 V/m (d) 10^{-5} V/m
13. The difference in the variation of resistance with temperature in a metal and a semiconductor arises essentially due to the difference in the
    (a) crystal structure
    (b) variation of the number of charge carriers with temperature
    (c) type of bonding
    (d) variation of scattering mechanism with temperature
14. In common emitter amplifier the $\frac{I_c}{I_e}$ is 0.98. The current gain will be
    (a) 4.9 (b) 7.8 (c) 49 (d) 78
15. In the diagram, the input is across the terminals A and C and the output is across B and D. Then the output is

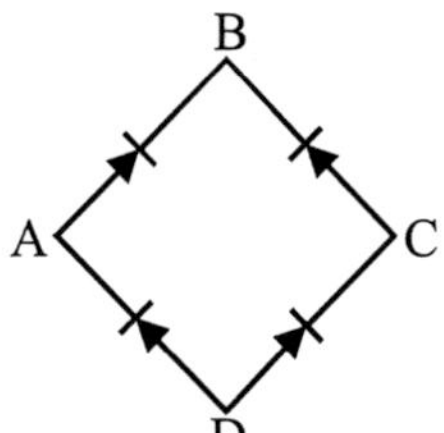

    (a) zero (b) same as the input
    (c) full wave rectifier (d) half wave rectifier
16. The cause of the potential barrier in a p-n diode is
    (a) depletion of positive charges near the junction
    (b) concentration of positive charges near the junction
    (c) depletion of negative charges near the junction
    (d) concentration of positive and negative charges near the junction
17. In a reverse biased diode when the applied voltage changes by 1 V, the current is found to change by 0.5 μA. The reverse bias resistance of the diode is
    (a) 2×10^5 Ω (b) 2×10^6 Ω (c) 200 Ω (d) 2 Ω.
18. When the forward bias voltage of a diode is changed from 0.6 V to 0.7 V, the current changes from 5 mA to 15 mA. Then its forward bias resistance is
    (a) 0.01 Ω (b) 0.1 Ω (c) 10 Ω (d) 100 Ω
19. The current gain of a transistor in common base mode is 0.995. The current gain of the same transistor in common emitter mode is
    (a) 197 (b) 201 (c) 198 (d) 199
20. The gate for which output is high if atleast one input is low?
    (a) NAND (b) NOR (c) AND (d) OR
21. What is the conductivity of a semiconductor if electron density = 5×10^{12}/cm^3 and hole density = 8×10^{13}/cm^3 ($\mu_e = 2.3$ m^2 V^{-1} s^{-1}, $\mu_h = 0.01$ m^{2}V^{-1} s^{-1})
    (a) 5.634 (b) 1.968 (c) 3.421 (d) 8.964.
22. In a p-type semiconductor the acceptor level is situated 60 meV above the valence band. The maximum wavelength of light required to produce a hole will be
    (a) 0.207×10^{-5} m (b) 2.07×10^{-5} m
    (c) 20.7×10^{-5} m (d) 2075×10^{-5} m
23. Application of a forward bias to a p–n junction
    (a) widens the depletion zone
    (b) increases the potential difference across the depletion zone
    (c) increases the number of donors on the n side
    (d) increases the electric field in the depletion zone.

24. A semi-conducting device is connected in a series circuit with a battery and a resistance. A current is found to pass through the circuit. If the polarity of the battery is reversed, the current drops to almost zero. The device may be
(a) a p-n junction
(b) an intrinsic semi-conductor
(c) a p-type semi-conductor
(d) an n-type semi-conductor

25. Which of the following gates will have an output of 1?

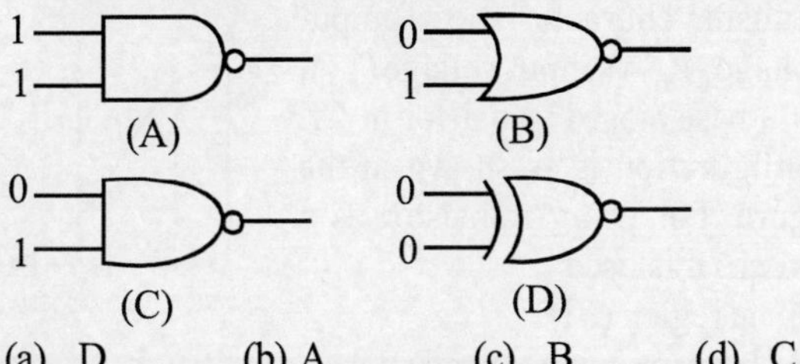

(a) D (b) A (c) B (d) C

26. The following circut represents

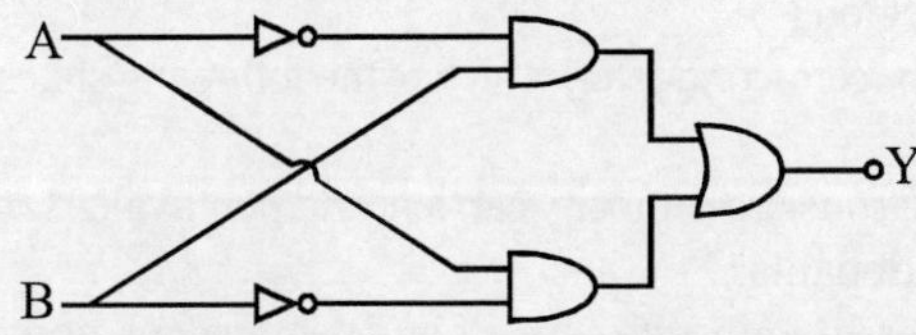

(a) OR gate (b) XOR gate
(c) AND gate (d) NAND gate

27. The diagram of a logic circuit is given below. The output F of the circuit is represented by

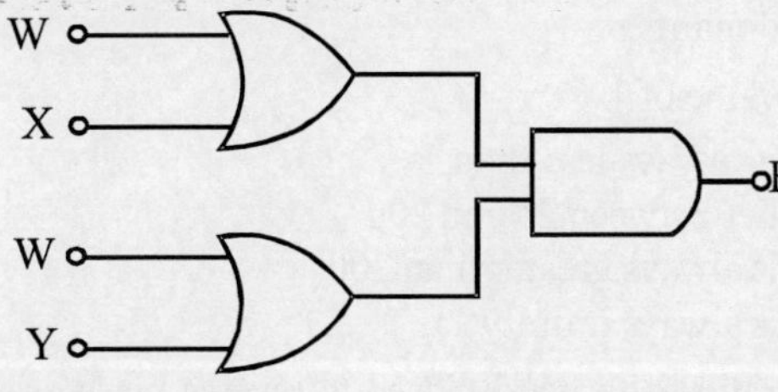

(a) W.(X+Y) (b) W.(X.Y)
(c) W+(X.Y) (d) W+(X+Y)

28. Assuming that the silicon diode having resistance of 20 Ω, the current through the diode is (knee voltage 0.7 V)

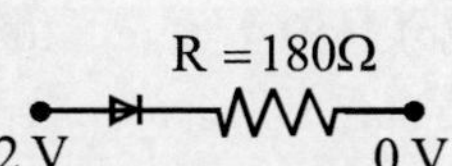

(a) 0 mA (b) 10 mA (c) 6.5 mA (d) 13.5 mA

29. The current gain β may be defined as
(a) the ratio of change in collector current to the change in emitter current for a constant collector voltage in a common base arrangement.
(b) the ratio of change in collector current to the change in the base current at constant collector voltage in a common emitter circuit
(c) the ratio of change in emitter current to the change in base current for constant emitter voltage in common emitter circuit.
(d) the ratio of change in base current to the change in collector current at constant collector voltage in common emitter circuit.

30. In common emitter amplifier, the current gain is 62. The collector resistance and input resistance are 5 kΩ an 500Ω respectively. If the input voltage is 0.01 V, the output voltage is
(a) 0.62 V (b) 6.2 V (c) 62 V (d) 620 V

31. The time variations of signals are given as in A, B and C. Point out the true statement from the following :

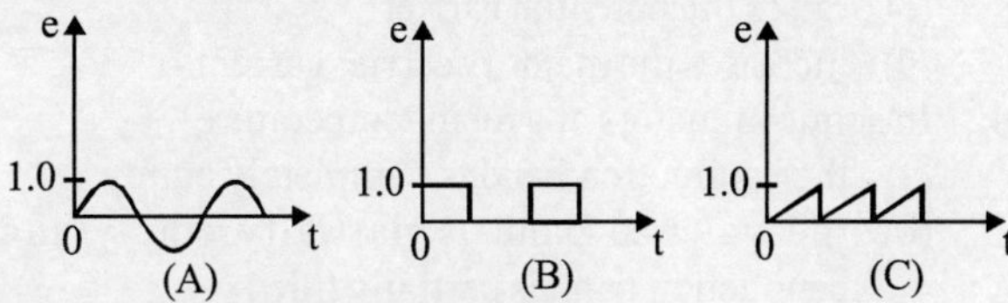

(a) A, B and C are analogue signals
(b) A and B are analogue, but C is digital signal
(c) A and C are digital, but B is analogue signal
(d) A and C are analogue, but B is digital signal

32. If the ratio of the concentration of electrons to that of holes in a semiconductor is $\frac{7}{5}$ and the ratio of currents is $\frac{7}{4}$, then what is the ratio of their drift velocities?
(a) $\frac{5}{8}$ (b) $\frac{4}{5}$ (c) $\frac{5}{4}$ (d) $\frac{4}{7}$

33. In the energy band diagram of a material shown below, the open circles and filled circles denote holes and electrons respectively. The material is
(a) an insulator
(b) a metal
(c) an *n*-type semiconductor
(d) a *p*-type semiconductor

34. In a P -N junction
(a) the potential of P & N sides becomes higher alternately
(b) the P side is at higher electrical potential than N side.
(c) the N side is at higher electric potential than P side.
(d) both P & N sides are at same potential.

35. In the case of a common emitter transistor amplifier the ratio of the collector current to the emitter current I_c/I_e is 0.96. The current gain of the amplifier is
(a) 6 (b) 48 (c) 24 (d) 12

36. Barrier potential of a P-N junction diode does not depend on
(a) doping density (b) diode design
(c) temperature (d) forward bias

37. A n-p-n transistor conducts when
(a) both collector and emitter are negative with respect to the base
(b) both collector and emitter are positive with respect to the base
(c) collector is positive and emitter is negative with respect to the base
(d) collector is positive and emitter is at same potential as the base

38. Following diagram performs the logic function of

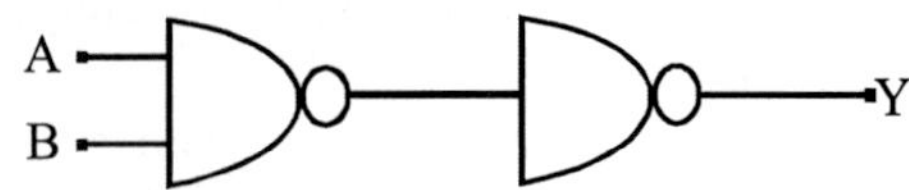

(a) XOR gate (b) AND gate
(c) NAND gate (d) OR gate

39. Reverse bias applied to a junction diode
(a) increases the minority carrier current
(b) lowers the potential barrier
(c) raises the potential barrier
(d) increases the majority carrier current

40. In semiconductors at a room temperature
(a) the conduction band is completely empty
(b) the valence band is partially empty and the conduction band is partially filled
(c) the valence band is completely filled and the conduction band is partially filled
(d) the valence band is completely filled

41. In a p-n junction photo cell, the value of the photo-electromotive force produced by monochromatic light is proportional to
(a) the voltage applied at the p-n junction
(b) the barrier voltage at the p-n junction
(c) the intensity of the light falling on the cell
(d) the frequency of the light falling on the cell

42. Of the diodes shown in the following diagrams, which one is reverse biased?

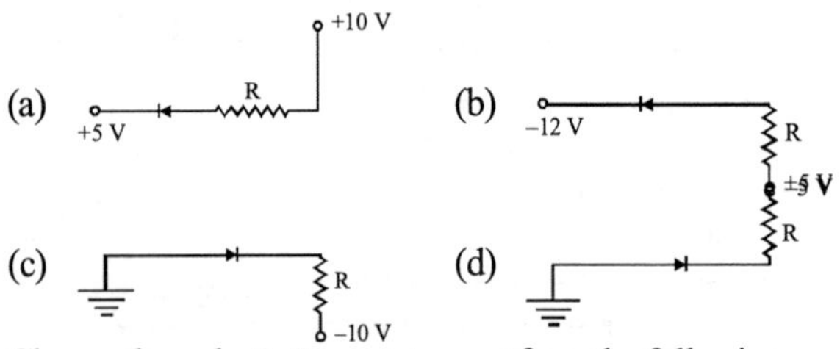

43. Choose the only **false** statement from the following.
(a) In conductors the valence and conduction bands may overlap.
(b) Substances with energy gap of the order of 10 eV are insulators.
(c) The resistivity of a semiconductor increases with increase in temperature.
(d) The conductivity of a semiconductor increases with increase in temperature.

44. Which one of the following statement is false ?
(a) Pure Si doped with trivalent impurities gives a p-type semiconductor
(b) Majority carriers in a n-type semiconductor are holes
(c) Minority carriers in a p-type semiconductor are electrons
(d) The resistance of intrinsic semiconductor decreases with increase of temperature

45. A common emitter amplifier has a voltage gain of 50, an input impedance of 100Ω and an output impedance of 200Ω. The power gain of the amplifier is
(a) 500 (b) 1000 (c) 1250 (d) 50

46. For transistor action
(1) Base, emitter and collector regions should have similar size and doping concentrations.
(2) The base region must be very thin and lightly doped.
(3) The eimtter-base junction is forward biased and base-collector junction is reverse based.
(4) Both the emitter-base junction as well as the base-collector junction are forward biased.
(a) (3) and (4) (b) (4) and (1)
(c) (1) and (2) (d) (2) and (3)

47. Transfer characteristics [output voltage (V_0) vs input voltage (V_1)] for a base biased transistor in CE configuration is as shown in the figure. For using transistor as a switch, it is used

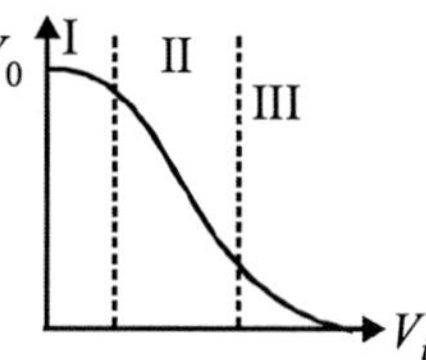

(a) in region (III)
(b) both in region (I) and (III)
(c) in region (II)
(d) in region (I)

48. In a n-type semiconductor, which of the following statement is true?
(a) Electrons are minority carriers and pentavalent atoms are dopants.
(b) Holes are minority carriers and pentavalent atoms are dopants.
(c) Holes are majority carriers and trivalent atoms are dopants.
(d) Electrons are majority carriers and trivalent atoms are dopants.

49. The value of β
(a) is always less than 1
(b) lies between 20 and 200
(c) is always greater than 200
(d) is always infinity

50. The ratio of forward biased to reverse biased resistance for pn junction diode is
(a) $10^{-1} : 1$ (b) $10^{-2} : 1$ (c) $10^{4} : 1$ (d) $10^{-4} : 1$

51. In germanium the energy gap is about 0.75 eV. The wavelength of light which germanium starts absorbing is
(a) 5000 Å (b) 1650 Å (c) 16500 Å (d) 165000 Å

52. With increasing biasing voltage of a photodiode, the photocurrent magnitude :
(a) remains constant
(b) increases initially and after attaining certain value, it decreases
(c) Increases linearly
(d) increases initially and saturates finally

53. If a semiconductor photodiode can detect a photon with a maximum wavelength of 400 nm, then its band gap energy is:
Planck's constant, $h = 6.63 \times 10^{-34}$ J.s.
Speed of light, $c = 3 \times 10^{8}$ m/s
(a) 1.1 eV (b) 2.0 eV (c) 1.5 eV (d) 3.1 eV

54. In the figure, potential difference between A and B is:

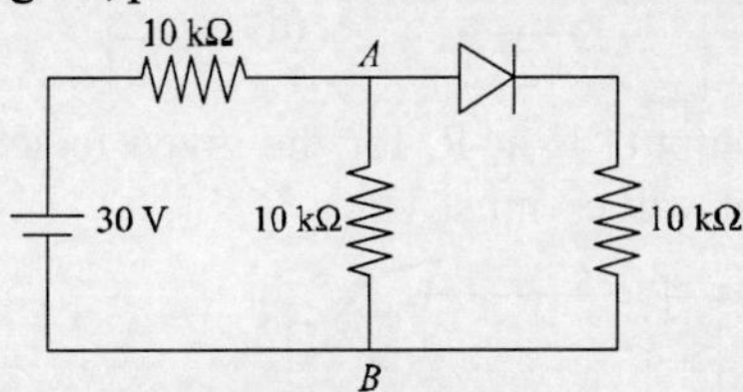

(a) 10V (b) 5V (c) 15V (d) zero

55. The reverse breakdown voltage of a Zener diode is 5.6 V in the given circuit.

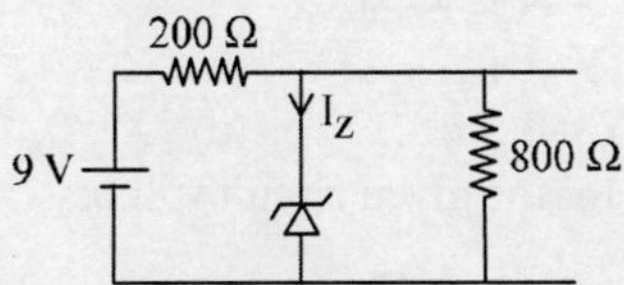

The current I_z through the Zener is :

(a) 10 mA (b) 17 mA (c) 15 mA (d) 7 mA

56. The transfer characteristic curve of a transistor, having input and output resistance 100 Ω and 100 k Ω respectively, is shown in the figure. The Voltage and Power gain, are respectively :

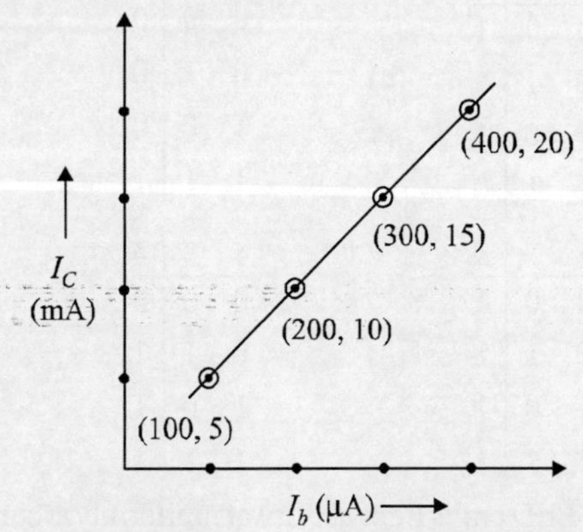

(a) $2.5\times10^4, 2.5\times10^6$ (b) $5\times10^4, 5\times10^6$
(c) $5\times10^4, 5\times10^5$ (d) $5\times10^4, 2.5\times10^6$

57. An npn transistor operates as a common emitter amplifier, with a power gain of 60 dB. The input circuit resistance is 100Ω and the output load resistance is 10 kΩ. The common emitter current gain β is :

(a) 10^2 (b) 60 (c) 6×10^2 (d) 10^4

58. In a common emitter configuration with suitable bias, it is given than R_L is the load resistance and R_{BE} is small signal dynamic resistance (input side). Then, voltage gain, current gain and power gain are given, respectively, by:
(β is current gain, I_B, I_C, I_E are respectively base, collector and emitter currents:)

(a) $\beta\frac{R_L}{R_{BE}}, \frac{\Delta I_E}{\Delta I_B}, \beta^2\frac{R_L}{R_{BE}}$

(b) $\beta^2\frac{R_L}{R_{BE}}, \frac{\Delta I_C}{\Delta I_B}, \beta\frac{R_L}{R_{BE}}$

(c) $\beta^2\frac{R_L}{R_{BE}}, \frac{\Delta I_C}{\Delta I_E}, \beta^2\frac{R_L}{R_{BE}}$

(d) $\beta\frac{R_L}{R_{BE}}, \frac{\Delta I_C}{\Delta I_B}, \beta^2\frac{R_L}{R_{BE}}$

59. Take the breakdown voltage of the zener diode used in the given circuit as 6V. For the input voltage shown in figure below, the time variation of the output voltage is : (Graphs drawn are schematic and not to scale)

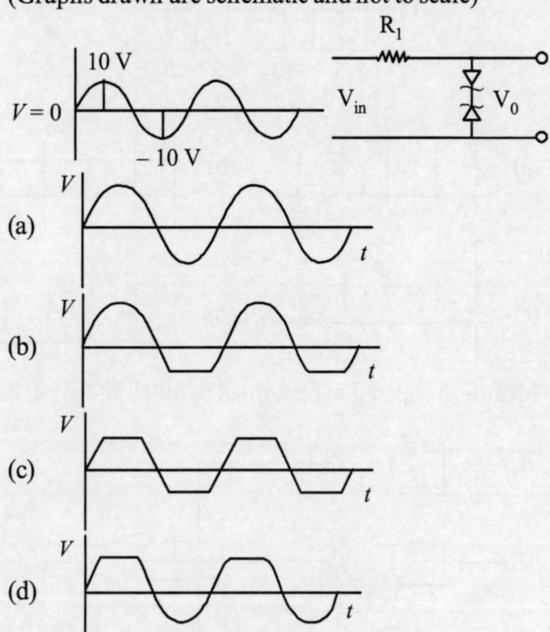

60. The current i in the network is:

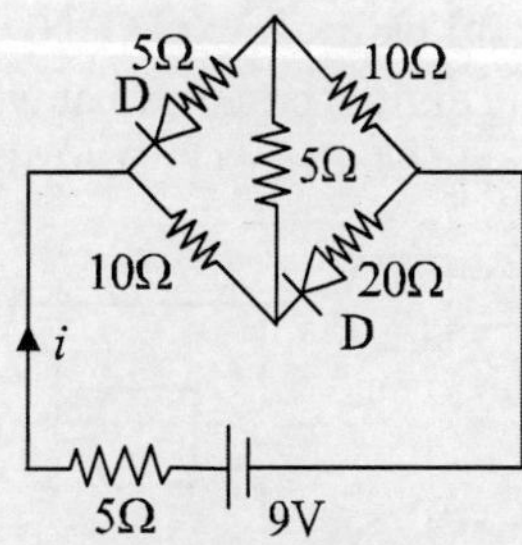

(a) 0.2 A (b) 0.6 A (c) 0.3 A (d) 0 A

61. A common emitter amplifier circuit, built using an npn transistor, is shown in the figure. Its dc current gain is 250, R_C = 1 k&! and V_{CC} = 10V. What is the minimum base current for V_{CE} to reach saturation ?

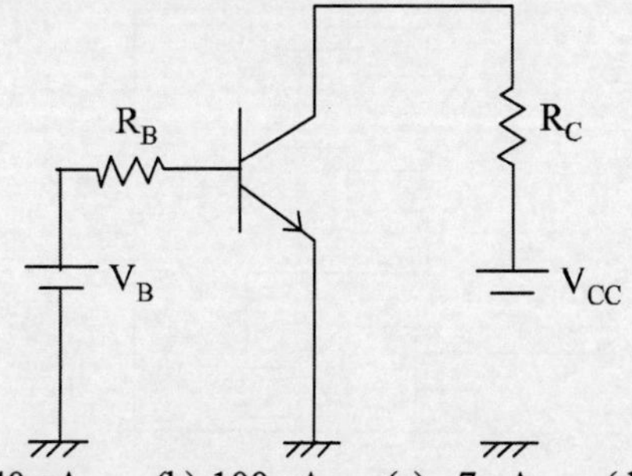

(a) 40 μA (b) 100 μA (c) 7 μA (d) 10 μA

62. Identify the correct output signal Y in the given combination of gates (as shown) for the given inputs A and B.

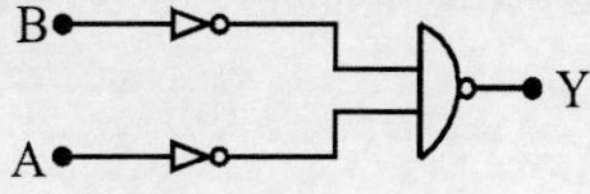

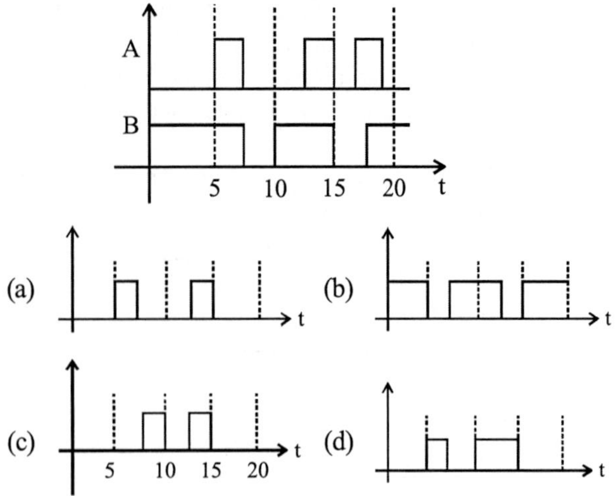

63. Identify the operation performed by the circuit given below:

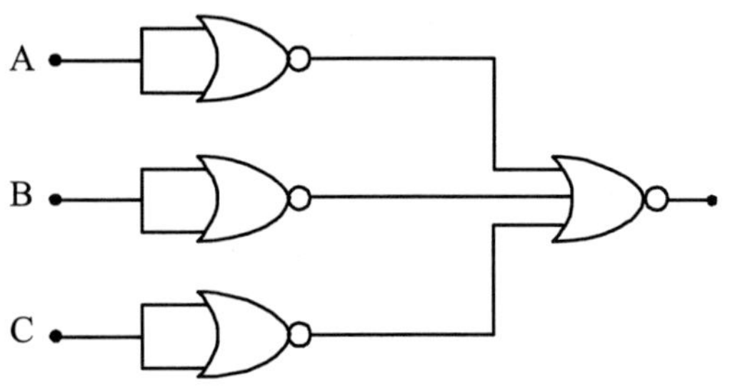

(a) NAND (b) OR (c) AND (d) NOT

64. In the following digitial circuit, what will be the output at 'Z', when the input (A, B) are (1, 0), (0, 0), (1, 1), (0, 1) :

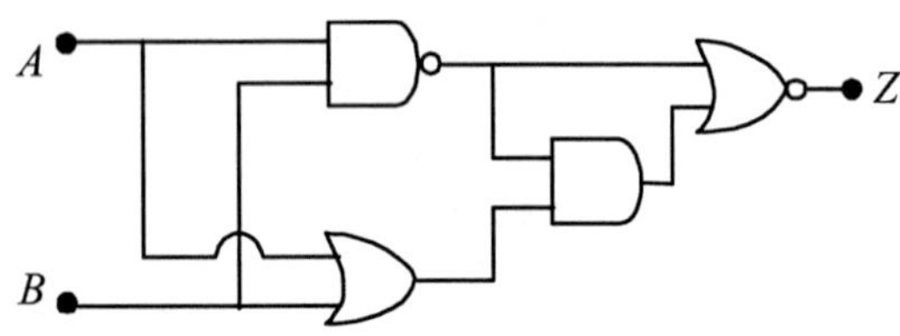

(a) 0, 0, 1, 0 (b) 1, 0, 1, 1 (c) 1, 1, 0, 1 (d) 0, 1, 0, 0

65. In the given circuit, value of Y is:

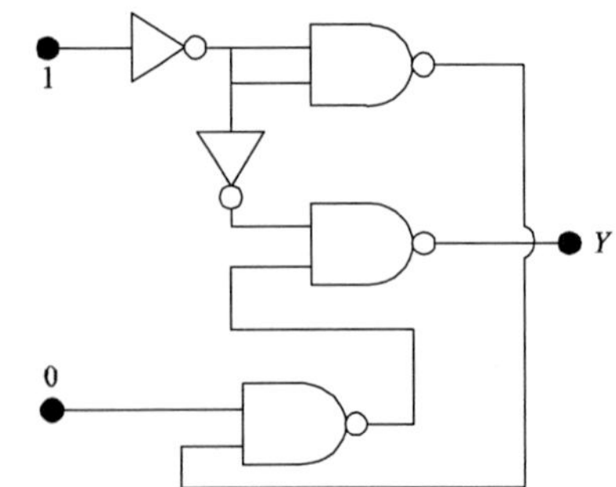

(a) 0
(b) toggles between 0 and 1
(c) will not execute
(d) 1

66. Which of the following gives a reversible operation?

(a) 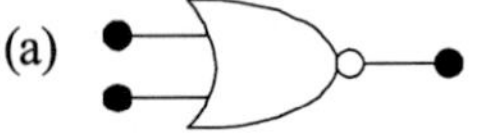 (b) 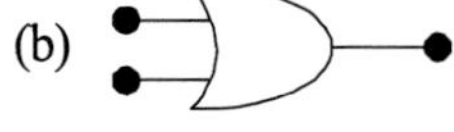

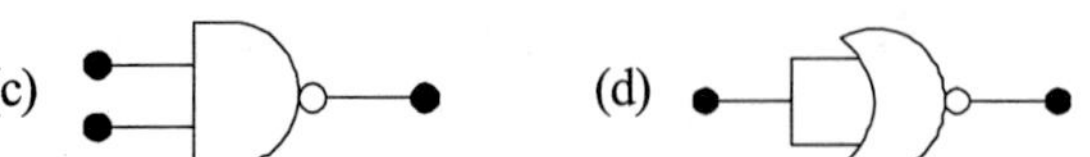

67. To get output '1' at R, for the given logic gate circuit the input values must be:

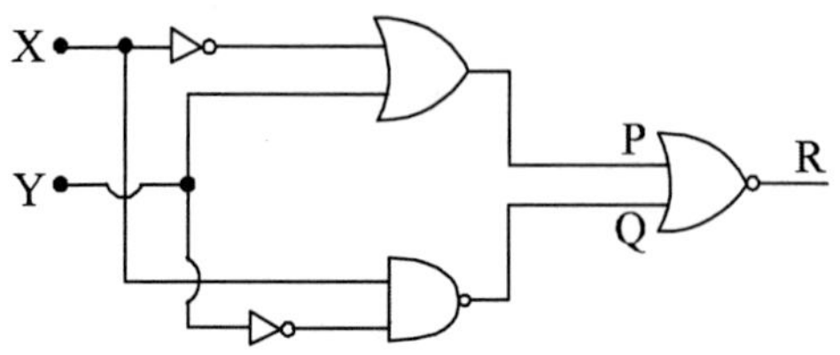

(a) X = 0, Y = 1 (b) X = 1, Y = 1
(c) X = 1, Y = 0 (d) X = 0, Y = 0

68. Truth table for the given circuit will be

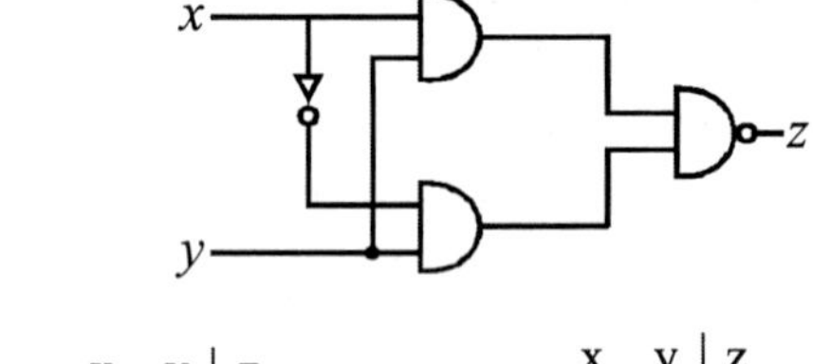

(a)

x	y	z
0	0	1
0	1	1
1	0	1
1	1	0

(b)

x	y	z
0	0	0
0	1	0
1	0	0
1	1	1

(c)

x	y	z
0	0	1
0	1	1
1	0	1
1	1	1

(d)

x	y	z
0	0	0
0	1	1
1	0	1
1	1	1

69. A red LED emits light at 0.1 watt uniformly around it. The amplitude of the electric field of the light at a distance of 1 m from the diode is :

(a) 5.48 V/m (b) 7.75 V/m (c) 1.73 V/m (d) 2.45 V/m

70. The forward biased diode connection is:

(a) +2V —▷|— −2V
(b) −3V —▷|— −3V
(c) 2V —▷|— 4V
(d) −2V —▷|— +2V

71. Identify the semiconductor devices whose characteristics are given below, in the order (i), (ii), (iii), (iv) :

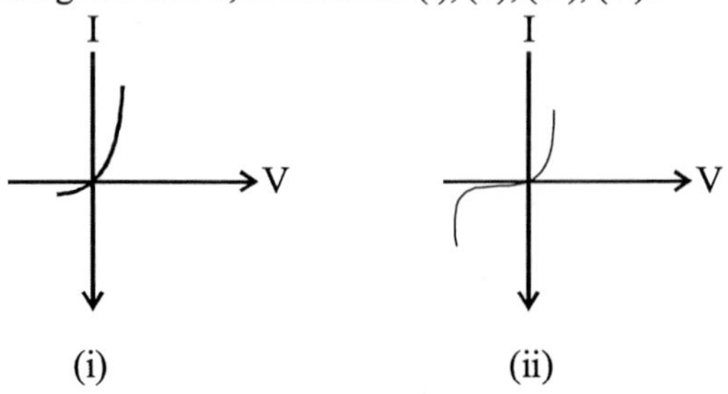

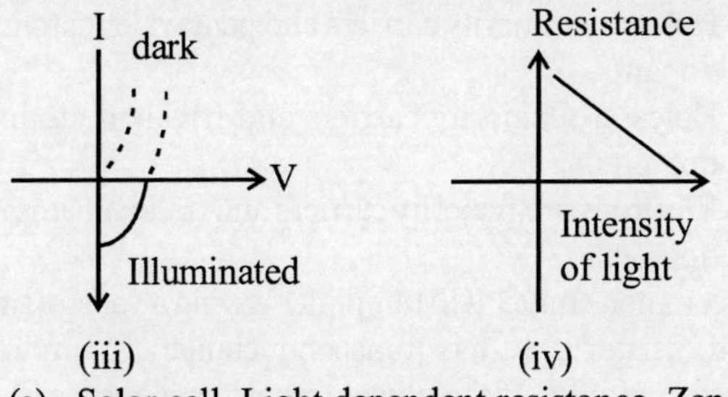

(a) Solar cell, Light dependent resistance, Zener diode, simple diode
(b) Zener diode, Solar cell, simple diode, Light dependent resistance
(c) Simple diode, Zener diode, Solar cell, Light dependent resistance
(d) Zener diode, Simple diode, Light dependent resistance, Solar cell

72. If in a *p-n* junction diode, a square input signal of 10 V is applied as shown

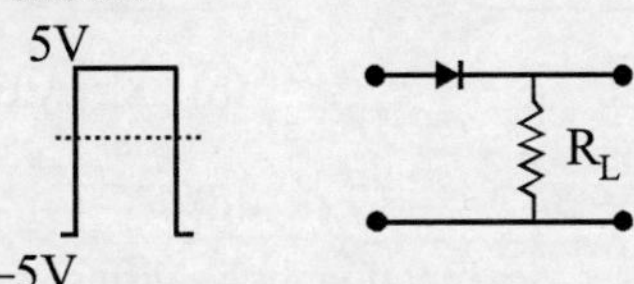

Then the output signal across R_L will be

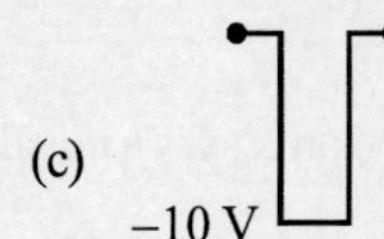

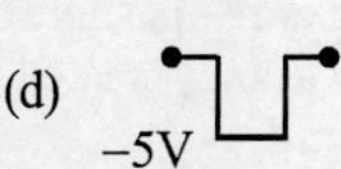

73. Carbon, silicon and germanium have four valence electrons each. At room temperature which one of the following statements is most appropriate ?
(a) The number of free electrons for conduction is significant only in Si and Ge but small in C.
(b) The number of free conduction electrons is significant in C but small in Si and Ge.
(c) The number of free conduction electrons is negligibly small in all the three.
(d) The number of free electrons for conduction is significant in all the three.

74. The electrical conductivity of a semiconductor increases when electromagnetic radiation of wavelength shorter than 2480 nm is incident on it. The band gap in (eV) for the semiconductor is
(a) 2.5 eV (b) 1.1 eV (c) 0.7 eV (d) 0.5 eV

75. The temperature dependence of resistances of Cu and undoped Si in the temperature range 300-400 K, is best described by
(a) linear increase for Cu, exponential decrease of Si
(b) linear decrease for Cu, linear decrease for Si
(c) linear increase for Cu, linear increase for Si
(d) linear increase for Cu, exponential increase for Si

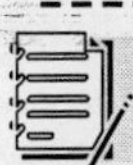

Exercise 2 - Exemplar & Past Year Questions

E&PYQs

Exemplar Questions

1. The conductivity of a semiconductor increases with increase in temperature because
(a) number density of free current carries increases
(b) relaxation time increases
(c) both number density of carries and relaxation time increase
(d) number density of carries increases, relaxation time decreases but effect of decrease in relaxation time is much less than increase in number density

2. In figure given below V_0 is the potential barrier across a p–n junction, when no battary is connected across the junction

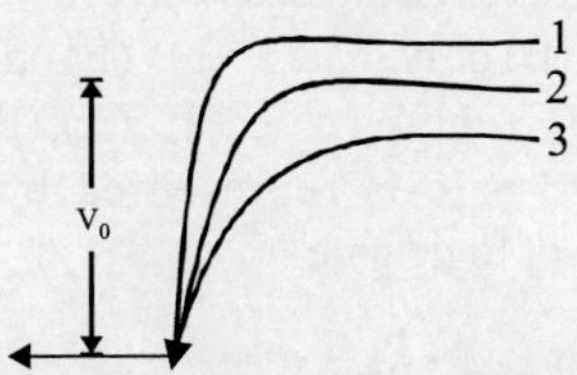

(a) 1 and 3 both correspond to forward bias of junction
(b) 3 corresponds to forward bias of junction and 1 corresponds to reverse bias of junctions
(c) 1 corresponds to forward bias and 3 corresponds to reverse bias of junction
(d) 3 and 1 both correspond to reverse bias of junction

3. In figure given below, assuming the diodes to be ideal
(a) D_1 is forward biased and D_2 is reverse biased and hence current flows from A to B
(b) D_2 is forward biased and D_1 is reverse biased and hence no current flows from B to A and vice–versa
(c) D_1 and D_2 are both forward biased and hence current flows from A to B
(d) D_1 and D_2 are both reverse biased and hence no current flows from A to B and vice – versa

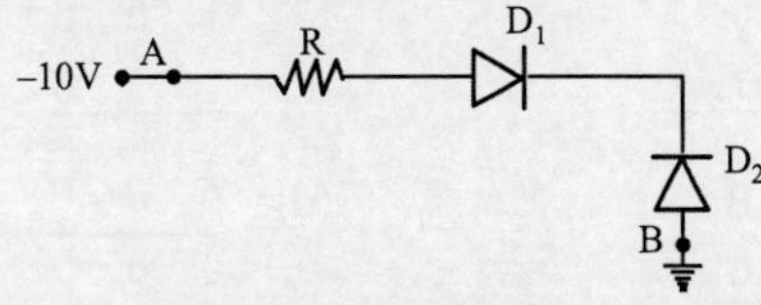

4. A 220 V AC supply is connected between points A and B (figure). What will be the potential difference V across the capacitor?

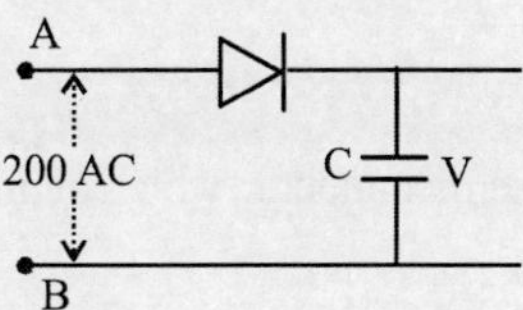

(a) 220V (b) 110V (c) 0V (d) $220\sqrt{2}$V

5. Hole in semiconductor is
(a) an anti – particle of electron
(b) a vacancy created when an electron leaves a covalent bond
(c) absence of free electrons
(d) an artificially created particle

6. The output of the given circuit in figure given below,

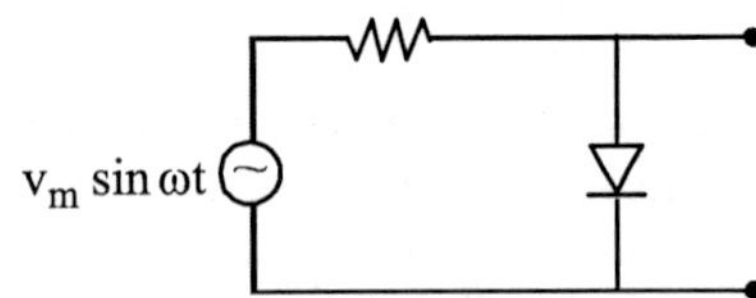

(a) would be zero at all times
(b) would be like a half wave rectifier with positive cycles in output
(c) would be like a half wave rectifier with negative cycles in output
(d) would be like that of a full wave rectifier

7. In the circuit shown in figure given below, if the diode forward voltage drop is 0.3 V, the voltage difference between A and B is

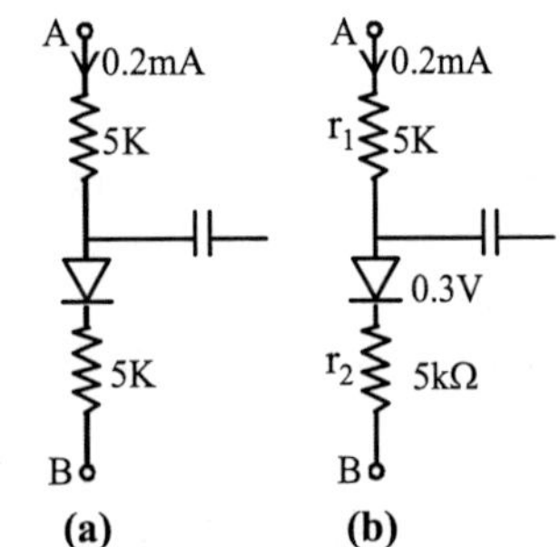

(a) 1.3 V (b) 2.3 V (c) 0 (d) 0.5 V

8. Truth table for the given circuit is

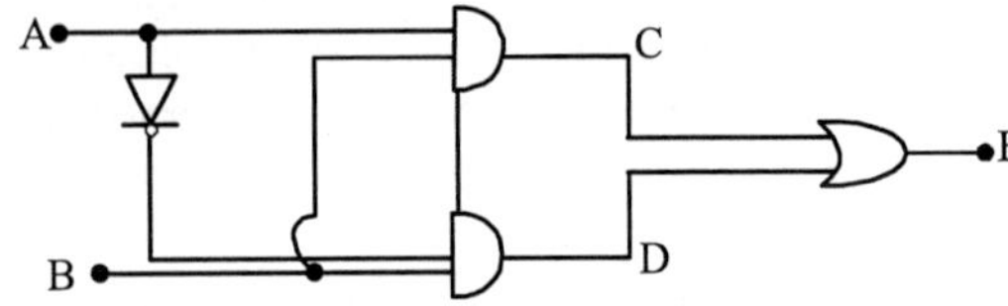

(a)

A	B	E
0	0	1
0	1	0
1	0	1
1	1	0

(b)

A	B	E
0	0	1
0	1	0
1	0	0
1	1	0

(c)

A	B	E
0	0	0
0	1	1
1	0	0
1	1	1

(d)

A	B	E
0	0	0
0	1	1
1	0	1
1	1	0

NEET/AIPMT (2013-2020) Questions

9. In a n-type semiconductor, which of the following statement is true? ***[2013]***
(a) Electrons are minority carriers and pentavalent atoms are dopants.
(b) Holes are minority carriers and pentavalent atoms are dopants.
(c) Holes are majority carriers and trivalent atoms are dopants.
(d) Electrons are majority carriers and trivalent atoms are dopants.

10. In a common emitter (CE) amplifier having a voltage gain G, the transistor used has transconductance 0.03 mho and current gain 25. If the above transistor is replaced with another one with transconductance 0.02 mho and current gain 20, the voltage gain will be ***[2013]***

(a) 1.5G (b) $\frac{1}{3}$G (c) $\frac{5}{4}$G (d) $\frac{2}{3}$G

11. The output(X) of the logic circuit shown in figure will be ***[2013]***

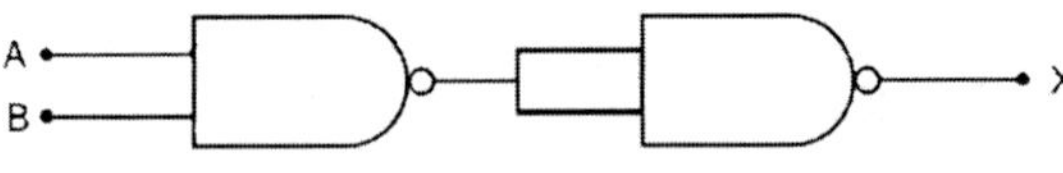

(a) X = $\overline{A.B}$ (b) X = A.B
(c) X = $\overline{A+B}$ (d) X = $\overline{\overline{A}}, \overline{\overline{B}}$

12. In an unbiased p-n junction, holes diffuse from the p-region to n-region because of ***[NEET Kar. 2013]***
(a) the potential difference across the p-n junction
(b) the attraction of free electrons of n-region
(c) the higher hole concentration in p-region than that in n-region
(d) the higher concentration of electrons in the n-region than that in the p-region

13. One way in which the operation of a n-p-n transistor differs from that of a p-n-p ***[NEET Kar. 2013]***
(a) the emitter junction is reversed biased in n-p-n
(b) the emitter junction injects minority carriers into the base region of the p-n-p
(c) the emitter injects holes into the base of the p-n-p and electrons into the base region of n-p-n
(d) the emitter injects holes into the base of n-p-n

14. The barrier potential of a p-n junction depends on: ***[2014]***
(A) type of semi conductor material
(B) amount of doping
(C) temperature
Which one of the following is correct ?
(a) (A) and (B) only (b) (B) only
(c) (B) and (C) only (d) (A), (B) and (C)

15. Which logic gate is represented by the following combination of logic gate ? ***[2015]***

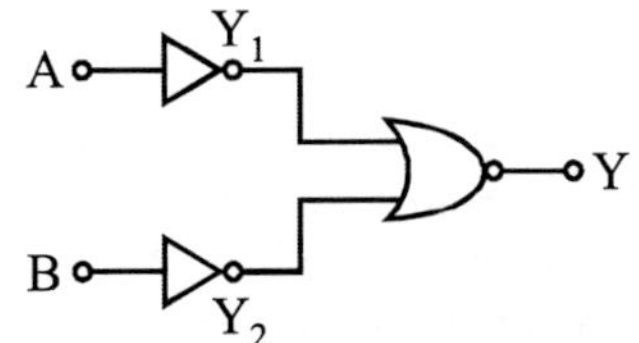

(a) NAND (b) AND (c) NOR (d) OR

16. If in a p-n junction, a square input signal of 10 V is applied as shown, then the output across R_L will be *[2015]*

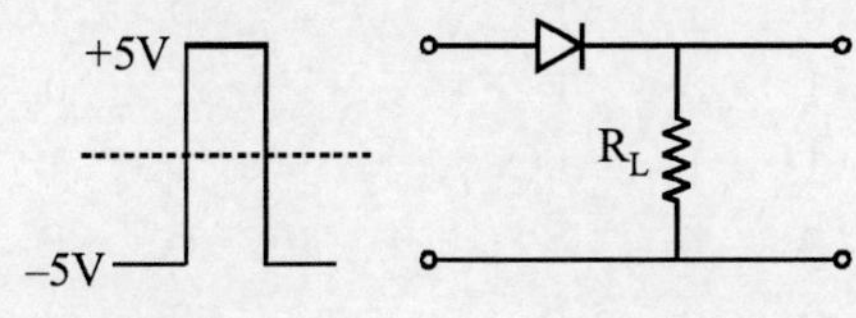

(a) 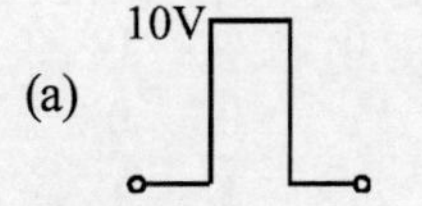

(b) 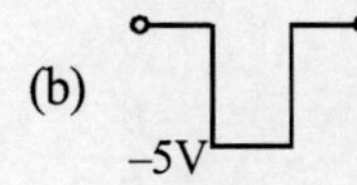

(c) 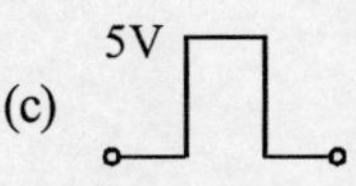

(d) 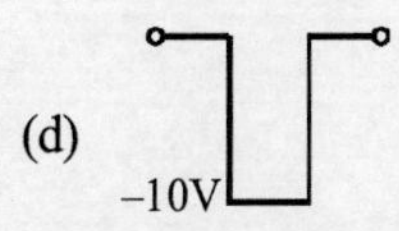

17. Consider the junction diode as ideal. The value of current flowing through AB is : *[2016]*

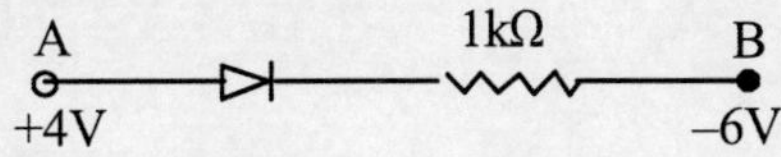

(a) 0 A (b) 10^{-2} A (c) 10^{-1} A (d) 10^{-3} A

18. A npn transistor is connected in common emitter configuration in a given amplifier. A load resistance of 800 Ω is connected in the collector circuit and the voltage drop across it is 0.8 V. If the current amplification factor is 0.96 and the input resistance of the circuit is 192Ω, the voltage gain and the power gain of the amplifier will respectively be: *[2016]*

(a) 4, 3.84 (b) 3.69, 3.84
(c) 4, 4 (d) 4, 3.69

19. To get output 1 for the following circuit, the correct choice for the input is *[2016]*

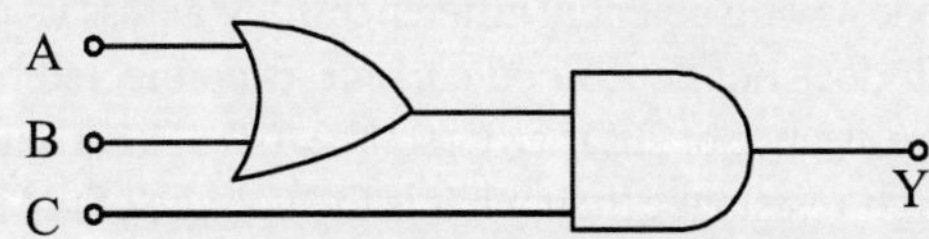

(a) A = 0, B = 1, C = 0 (b) A = 1, B = 0, C = 0
(c) A = 1, B = 1, C = 0 (d) A = 1, B = 0, C = 1

20. In a common emitter transistor amplifier the audio signal voltage across the collector is 3V. The resistance of collector is 3 kΩ. If current gain is 100 and the base resistance is 2 kΩ, the voltage and power gain of the amplifier is *[2017]*

(a) 15 and 200 (b) 150 and 15000
(c) 20 and 2000 (d) 200 and 1000

21. The given electrical network is equivalent to : *[2017]*

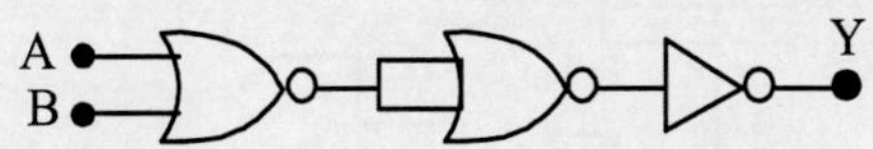

(a) OR gate (b) NOR gate
(c) NOT gate (d) AND gate

22. Which one of the following represents forward bias diode? *[2017]*

(a) –4V R –3V
(b) –2V R +2V
(c) 3V R 5V
(d) 0V R –2V

23. In a p-n junction diode, change in temperature due to heating *[2018]*

(a) Affects only reverse resistance
(b) Affects only forward resistance
(c) Affects the overall V-I characteristics of p-n junction
(d) Does not affect resistance of p-n junction

24. In the combination of the following gates the output Y can be written in terms of inputs A and B as *[2018]*

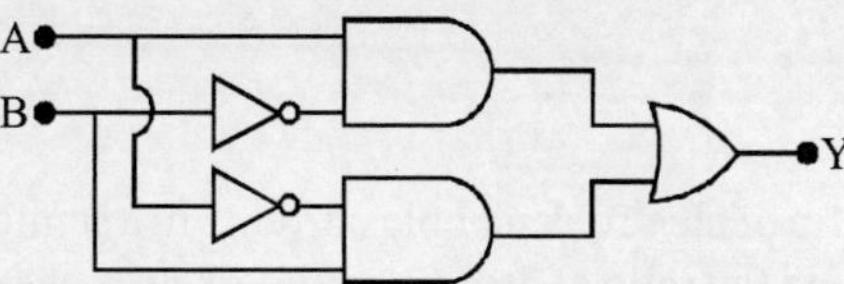

(a) $\overline{A \cdot B}$ (b) $A \cdot \overline{B} + \overline{A} \cdot B$
(c) $\overline{A + B}$ (d) $\overline{A \cdot B + A \cdot B}$

25. For a p-type semiconductor, which of the following statements is **true** ? *[2019]*

(a) Electrons are the majority carriers and trivalent atoms are the dopants.
(b) Holes are the majority carriers and trivalent atoms are the dopants.
(c) Holes are the majority carriers and pentavalent atoms are the dopants.
(d) Electrons are the majority carriers and pentavalent atoms are the dopants.

26. An LED is constructed from a p-n junction diode using GaAsP. The energy gap is 1.9 eV. The wavelength of the light emitted will be equal to *[NEET Odisha 2019]*

(a) 654×10^{-11} m (b) 10.4×10^{-26} m
(c) 654 nm (d) 654 Å

27.

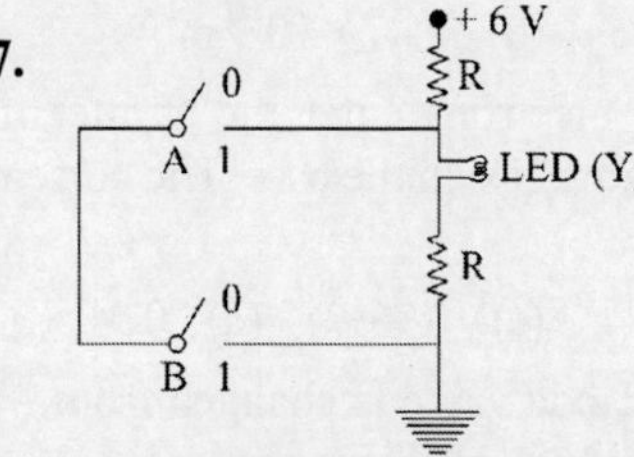

The **correct** Boolean operation represented by the circuit diagram drawn is : *[2019]*

(a) AND (b) OR (c) NAND (d) NOR

28. The increase in the width of the depletion region in a p-n junction diode is due to : *[2020]*

(a) reverse bias only
(b) both forward bias and reverse bias
(c) increase in forward current
(d) forward bias only

29. For transistor action, which of the following statements is **correct**? *[2020]*
(a) Base, emitter and collector regions should have same size.
(b) Both emitter junction as well as the collector junction are forward biased.
(c) The base region must be very thin and lightly doped.
(d) Base, emitter and collector regions should have same doping concentrations.

30. For the logic circuit shown, the truth table is: *[2020]*

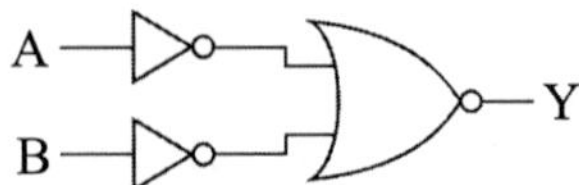

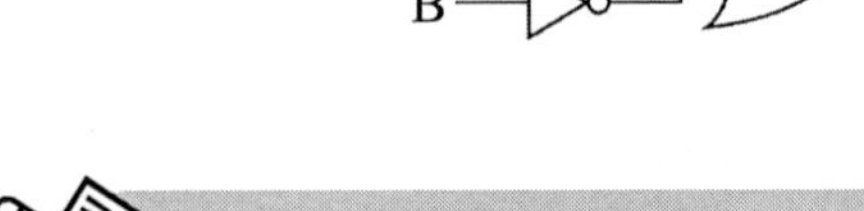

(a)

A	B	Y
0	0	0
0	1	1
1	0	1
1	1	1

(b)

A	B	Y
0	0	1
0	1	1
1	0	1
1	1	0

(c)

A	B	Y
0	0	1
0	1	0
1	0	0
1	1	0

(d)

A	B	Y
0	0	0
0	1	0
1	0	0
1	1	1

Exercise 3 - Concept Application Problems CAP

1. The ratio of electron and hole currents in a semiconductor is 7/4 and the ratio of drift velocities of electrons and holes is 5/4, then the ratio of concentrations of electrons and holes will be
(a) 5/7 (b) 7/5 (c) 25/49 (d) 49/25

2. In a full wave rectifier circuit operating from 50 Hz mains frequency, the fundamental frequency in the ripple would be
(a) 25 Hz (b) 50 Hz (c) 70.7 Hz (d) 100 Hz

3. The electrical conductivity of a semiconductor increases when electromagnetic radiation of wavelength shorter than 2480 nm is incident on it. The band gap (in eV) for the semiconductor is
(a) 0.9 (b) 0.7 (c) 0.5 (d) 1.1

4. The intrinsic conductivity of germanium at 27° is 2.13 mho m^{-1} and mobilities of electrons and holes are 0.38 and 0.18 $m^2V^{-1}s^{-1}$ respectively. The density of charge carriers is
(a) $2.37 \times 10^{19}\, m^{-3}$ (b) $3.28 \times 10^{19}\, m^{-3}$
(c) $7.83 \times 10^{19}\, m^{-3}$ (d) $8.47 \times 10^{19}\, m^{-3}$

5. In a npn transistor 10^{10} electrons enter the emitter in 10^{-6} s. 4% of the electrons are lost in the base. The current transfer ratio will be
(a) 0.98 (b) 0.97 (c) 0.96 (d) 0.94

6. The grid voltage of any triode valve is changed from –1 volt to –3 volt and the mutual conductance is 3×10^{-4} mho. The change in plate circuit current will be
(a) 0.8 mA (b) 0.6 mA (c) 0.4 mA (d) 1 mA

7. The transfer ratio β of transistor is 50. The input resistance of a transistor when used in C.E. (Common Emitter) configuration is 1kΩ. The peak value of the collector A.C current for an A.C input voltage of 0.01V peak is
(a) 100 μA (b) .01 mA (c) .25 mA (d) 500 μA

8. The frequency response curve of RC coupled amplifier is shown in figure. The band with of the amplifier will be

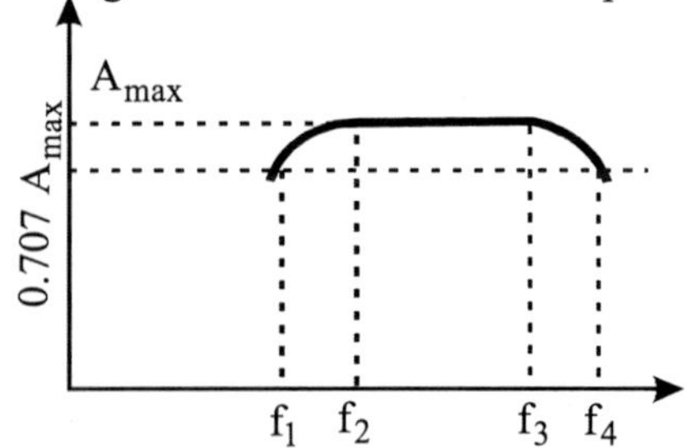

(a) $f_3 - f_2$ (b) $f_4 - f_1$ (c) $\frac{f_4 - f_2}{2}$ (d) $f_3 - f_1$

9. A diode having potential difference 0.5 V across its junction which does not depend on current, is connected in series with resistance of 20Ω across source. If 0.1 A current passes through resistance then what is the voltage of the source?
(a) 1.5 V (b) 2.0 V (c) 2.5 V (d) 5 V

10. Carbon, Silicon and Germanium atoms have four valence electrons each. Their valence and conduction bands are separated by energy band gaps represented by $(E_g)_C$, $(E_g)_{Si}$ and $(E_g)_{Ge}$ respectively. Which one of the following relationship is true in their case?
(a) $(E_g)_C > (E_g)_{Si}$ (b) $(E_g)_C < (E_g)_{Si}$
(c) $(E_g)_C = (E_g)_{Si}$ (d) $(E_g)_C < (E_g)_{Ge}$

11. The following configuration of gate is equivalent to

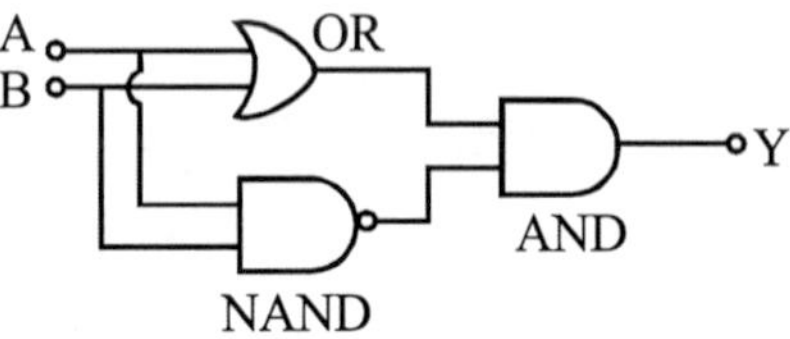

(a) NAND gate (b) XOR gate
(c) OR gate (d) NOR gate

12. Two junction diodes one of Germanium (Ge) and other of silicon (Si) are connected as shown in figure to a battery of emf 12 V and a load resistance 10 k Ω. The germanium diode conducts at 0.3 V and silicon diode at 0.7 V. When a current flows in the circuit, the potential of terminal Y will be

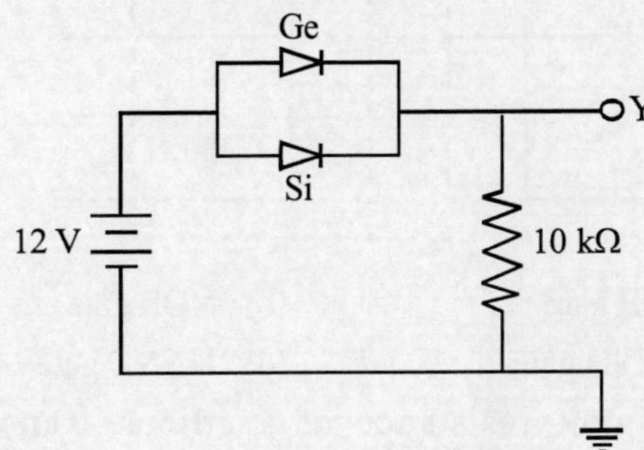

(a) 12 V (b) 11 V (c) 11.3 V (d) 11.7 V

13. In a transistor, the change in base current from 100 μA to 125 μA causes a change in collector current from 5 mA to 7.5 mA, keeping collector-to-emitter voltage constant at 10 V. What is the current gain of the transistor?

(a) 200 (b) 100 (c) 50 (d) 25

14. The truth table given below is for

(a) NOR

(b) AND

(c) XOR

(d) NAND

A	B	Y
0	0	1
0	1	1
1	0	1
1	1	0

15. In the following circuit, the output Y for all possible inputs A and B is expressed by the truth table.

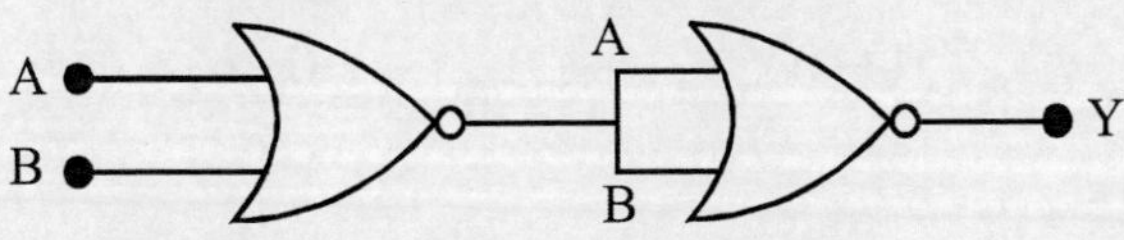

(a)

A	B	Y
0	0	1
0	1	1
1	0	1
1	1	0

(b)

A	B	Y
0	0	1
0	1	0
1	0	0
1	1	0

(c)

A	B	Y
0	0	0
0	1	1
1	0	1
1	1	1

(d)

A	B	Y
0	0	0
0	1	0
1	0	0
1	1	1

16. The real time variation of input signals A and B are as shown below. If the inputs are fed into NAND gate, then select the output signal from the following.

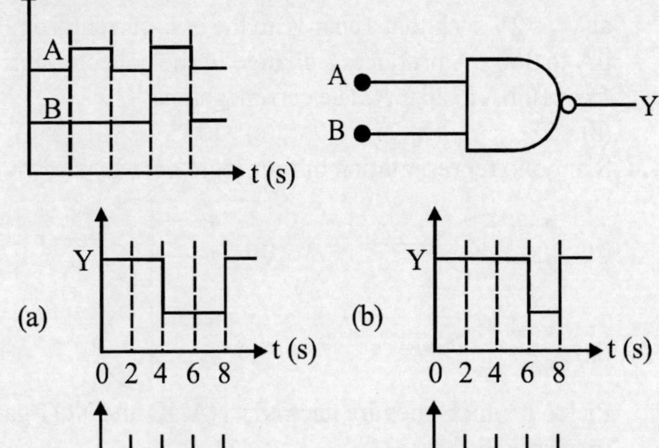

(c) (d)

17. The circuit has two oppositively connected ideal diodes in parallel. What is the current flowing in the circuit?

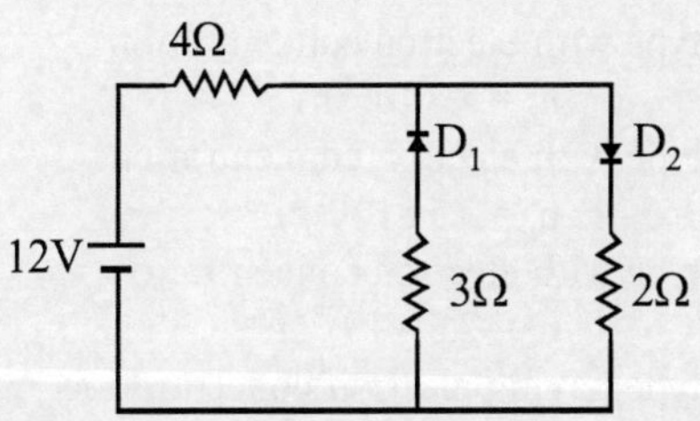

(a) 1.71 A (b) 2.00 A (c) 2.31 A (d) 1.33 A

18. The peak voltage in the output of a half-wave diode rectifier fed with a sinusoidal signal without filter is 10V. The d.c. component of the output voltage is

(a) $20/\pi$ V (b) $10/\sqrt{2}$ V (c) $10/\pi$ V (d) 10V

19. The following figure shows a logic gate circuit with two inputs *A* and *B* and the output *Y*. The voltage waveforms of A, B and Y are given

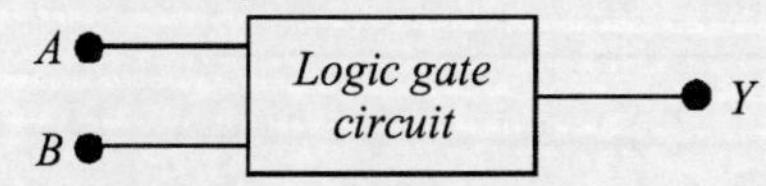

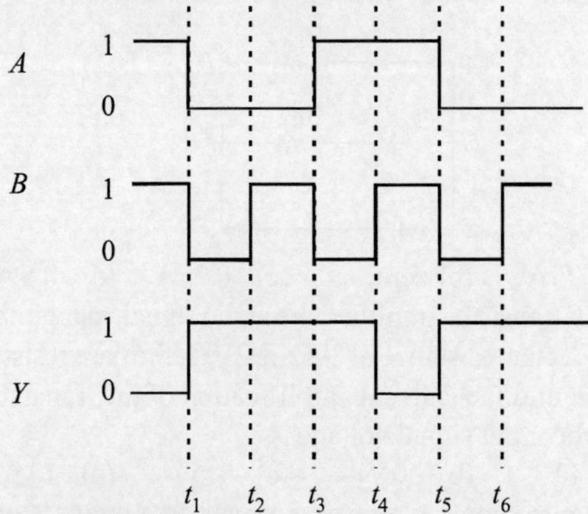

The logic gate is :

(a) NAND gate (b) NOR gate

(c) OR gate (d) AND gate

20. A transistor is operated in common emitter configuration at $V_C = 2V$ such that a change in the base current from 100 μA to 300 μA produces a change in the collector current from 10mA to 20 mA. The current gain is

(a) 50 (b) 75 (c) 100 (d) 25

21. Symbolic representation of four logic gate are shown as

(i) 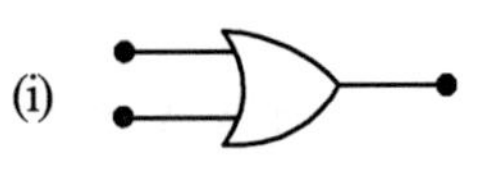 (ii) 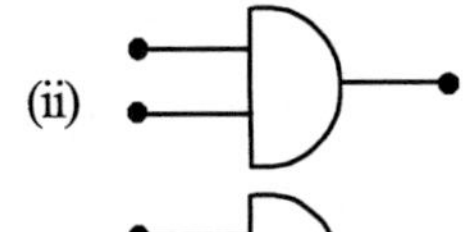

(iii) 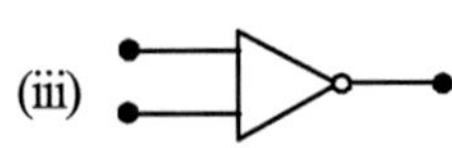 (iv) 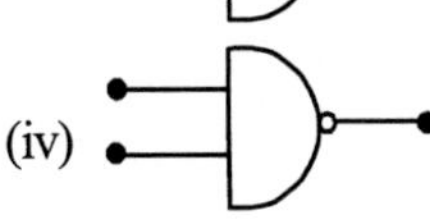

Pick out which ones are for AND, NAND and NOT gates, respectively

(a) (ii), (iii) and (iv) (b) (iii), (ii) and (i)
(c) (iii), (iii) and (iv) (d) (ii), (iv) and (iii)

22. Pure Si at 500K has equal number of electron (n_e) and hole (n_h) concentrations of 1.5×10^{16} m^{-3}. Doping by indium increases n_h to 4.5×10^{22} m^{-3}. The doped semiconductor is of

(a) n–type with electron concentration $n_e = 5 \times 10^{22}$ m^{-3}
(b) p–type with electron concentration $n_e = 2.5 \times 10^{10}$ m^{-3}
(c) n–type with electron concentration $n_e = 2.5 \times 10^{23}$ m^{-3}
(d) p–type having electron concentration $n_e = 5 \times 10^{9}$ m^{-3}

23. A zener diode, having breakdown voltage equal to 15V, is used in a voltage regulator circuit shown in figure. The current through the diode is

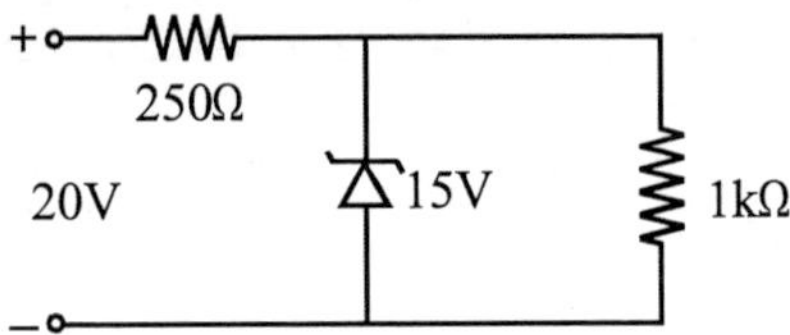

(a) 10mA (b) 15mA (c) 20mA (d) 5mA

24. Two ideal diodes are connected to a battery as shown in the circuit. The current supplied by the battery is

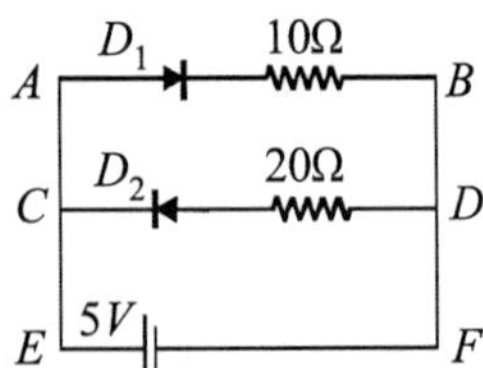

(a) 0.75 A (b) zero (c) 0.25 A (d) 0.5 A

25. In a *CE* transistor amplifier, the audio signal voltage across the collector resistance of 2kΩ is 2V. If the base resistance is 1kΩ and the current amplification of the transistor is 100, the input signal voltage is

(a) 0.1 V (b) 1.0 V (c) 1mV (d) 10 mV

26. The figure shows a logic circuit with two inputs *A* and *B* and the output *C*. The voltage wave forms across *A*, *B* and *C* are as given. The logic gate circuit is:

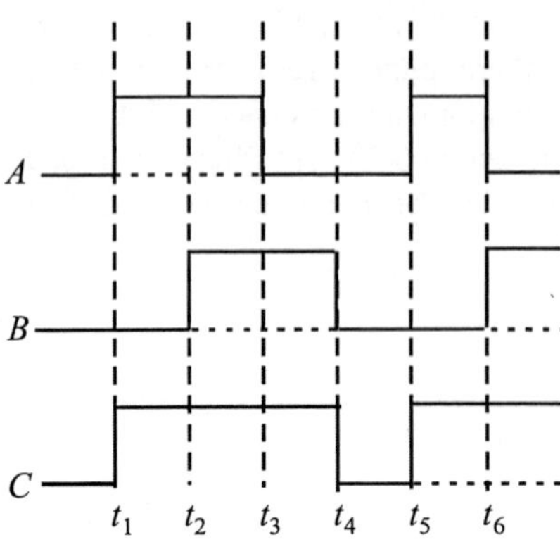

(a) OR gate (b) NOR gate
(c) AND gate (d) NAND gate

27. The input resistance of a silicon transistor is 100 W. Base current is changed by 40 μA which results in a change in collector current by 2 mA. This transistor is used as a common emitter amplifier with a load resistance of 4 KΩ. The voltage gain of the amplifier is

(a) 2000 (b) 3000 (c) 4000 (d) 1000

28. In a common emitter (CE) amplifier having a voltage gain G, the transistor used has transconductance 0.03 mho and current gain 25. If the above transistor is replaced with another one with transconductance 0.02 mho and current gain 20, the voltage gain will be

(a) 1.5G (b) $\frac{1}{3}$G (c) $\frac{5}{4}$G (d) $\frac{2}{3}$G

29. In the study of transistor as amplifier, if $\alpha = \frac{I_C}{I_E}$ and $\beta = \frac{I_C}{I_B}$, where, I_C, I_B and I_E are the collector, base and emitter currents, then

(a) $\beta = \frac{(1+\alpha)}{\alpha}$ (b) $\beta = \frac{(1-\alpha)}{\alpha}$

(c) $\beta = \frac{\alpha}{(1-\alpha)}$ (d) $\beta = \frac{\alpha}{(1+\alpha)}$

30. Two identical capacitors A and B, charged to the same potential 5V are connected in two different circuits as shown below at time $t = 0$. If the charge on capacitors A and B at time $t = CR$ is Q_A and Q_B respectively, then (Here e is the base of natural logarithm)

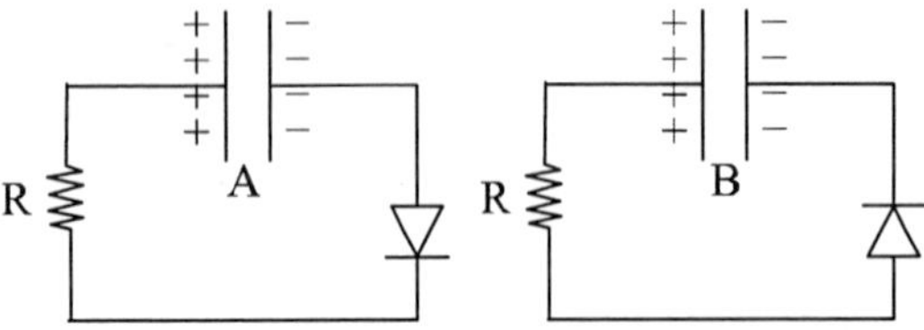

(a) $Q_A = \frac{VC}{e}, Q_B = \frac{CV}{2}$ (b) $Q_A = VC, Q_B = CV$

(c) $Q_A = VC, Q_B = \frac{VC}{e}$ (d) $Q_A = \frac{CV}{2}, Q_B = \frac{VC}{e}$

31. Figure shows a DC voltage regulator circuit, with a Zener diode of breakdown voltage = 6V. If the unregulated input voltage varies between 10 V to 16 V, then what is the maximum Zener current ?

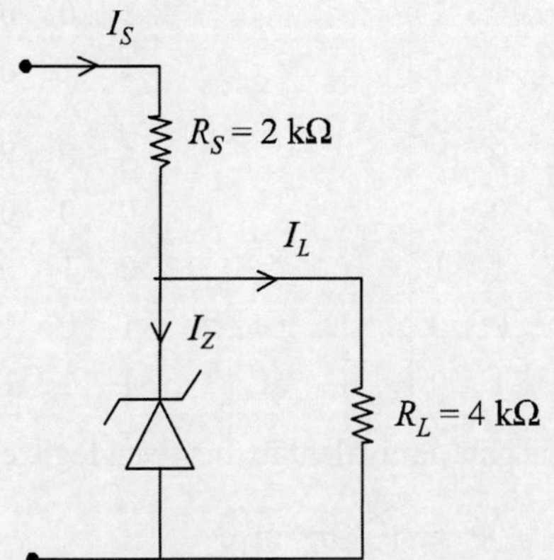

(a) 2.5 mA (b) 1.5 mA (c) 7.5 mA (d) 3.5 mA

32. The figure represents a voltage regulator circuit using a Zener diode. The breakdown voltage of the Zener diode is 6 V and the load resistance is R_L = 4 k. The series resistance of the circuit is R_i=1k. If the battery voltage V_B varies from 8 V to 16 V, what are the minimum and maximum values of the current through Zener diode ?

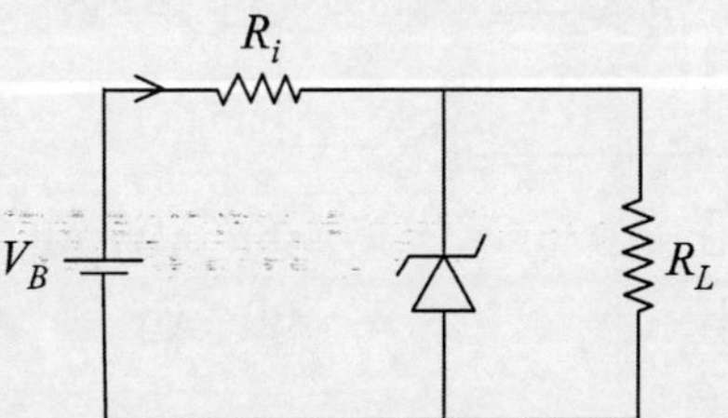

(a) 0.5 mA; 6 mA (b) 1 mA; 8.5 mA
(c) 0.5 mA; 8.5 mA (d) 1.5 mA; 8.5 mA

33. In the given circuit the current through Zener Diode is close to :

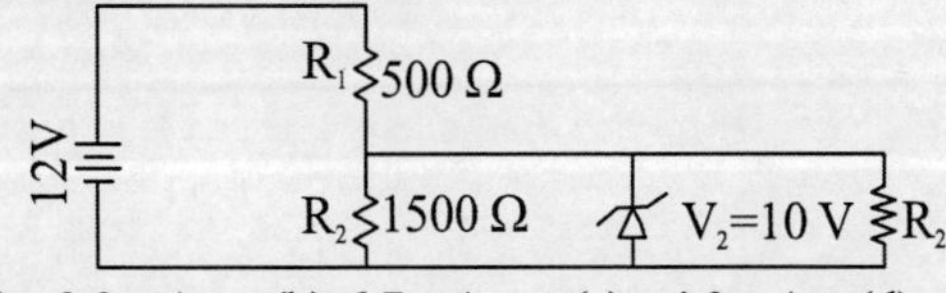

(a) 0.0 mA (b) 6.7 mA (c) 4.0 mA (d) 6.0 mA

34. The circuit shown below contains two ideal diodes, each with a forward resistance of 50 Ω. If the battery voltage is 6V, the current through the 100 Ω resistance (in Amperes) is :

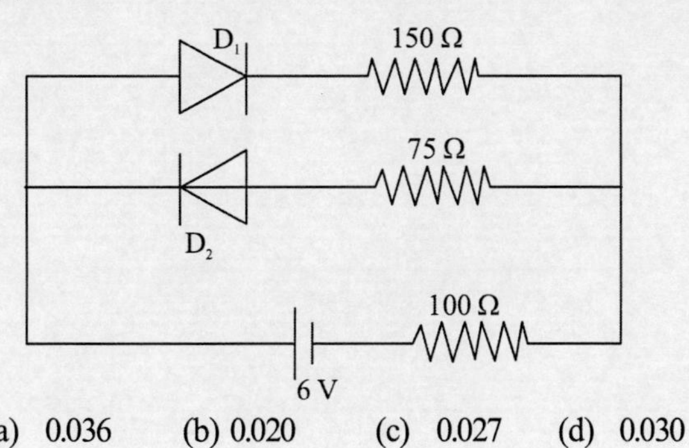

(a) 0.036 (b) 0.020 (c) 0.027 (d) 0.030

35. For the circuit shown below, the current through the Zener diode is:

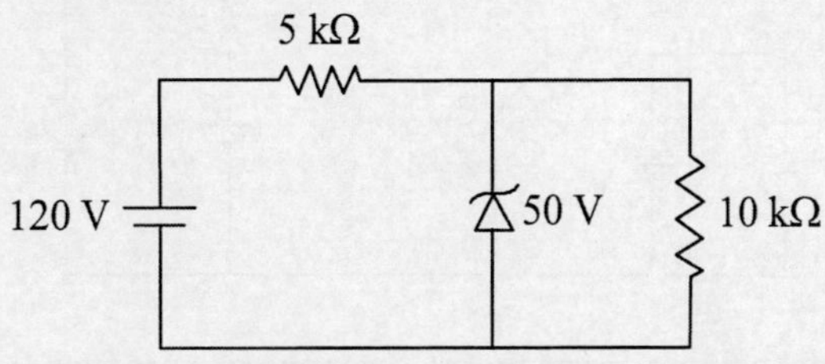

(a) 9 mA (b) 5 mA (c) Zero (d) 14 mA

36. Mobility of electrons in a semiconductor is defined as the ratio of their drift velocity to the applied electric field. If, for an n-type semiconductor, the density of electrons is 10^{19} m^{-3} and their mobility is 1.6m^2/(V.s) then the resistivity of the semiconductor (since it is an n-type semiconductor contribution of holes is ignored) is close to:

(a) 2 Ωm (b) 4 Ωm (c) 0.4 Ωm (d) 0.2 Ωm

37. Ge and Si diodes start conducting at 0.3 V and 0.7 V respectively. In the following figure if Ge diode connection are reversed, the value of V_o changes by : (assume that the Ge diode has large breakdown voltage)

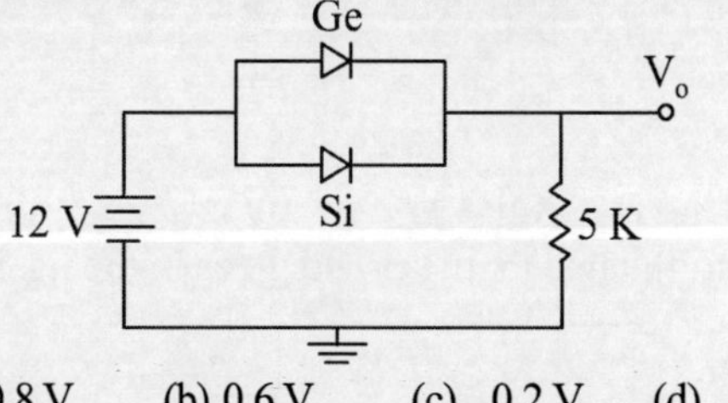

(a) 0.8 V (b) 0.6 V (c) 0.2 V (d) 0.4 V

38. The reading of the ammeter for a silicon diode in the given circuit is :

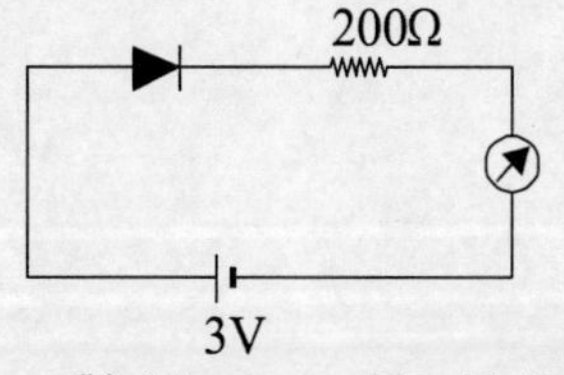

(a) 0 (b) 15 mA (c) 11.5 mA (d) 13.5 mA

39. In the given circuit, the current through zener diode is:

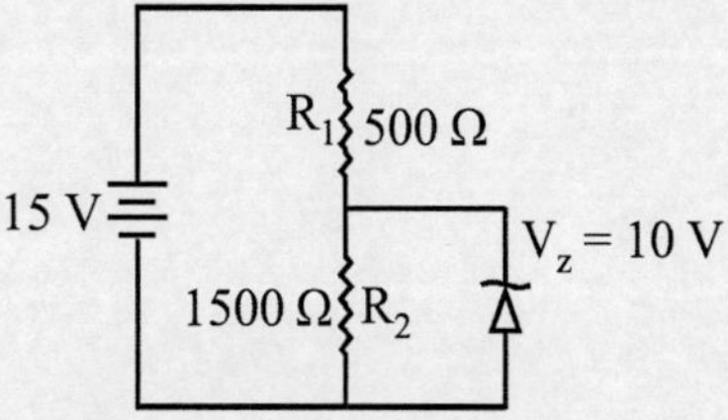

(a) 2.5mA (b) 3.3mA (c) 5.5mA (d) 6.7mA

40. An NPN transistor is used in common emitterconfiguration as an amplifier with 1 k &! load resistance. Signal voltage of 10 mV is applied across the base-emitter. This produces a 3 mA change in the collector current and 15 ¼A change in the base current of the amplifier. The input resistance and voltage gain are:

(a) 0.33 k Ω 1.5 (b) 0.67 k Ω 300
(c) 0.67 k Ω 200 (d) 0.33 k Ω 300

41. 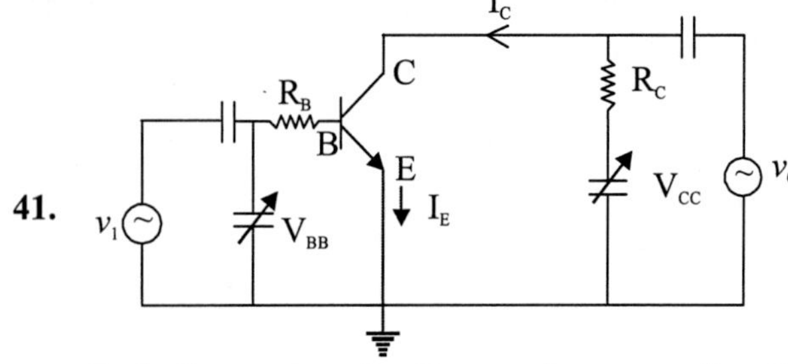

In the figure, given that V_{BB} supply can vary from 0 to 5.0 V, V_{CC} = 5 V, $\beta_{dc} = 200$, $R_B = 100\ k\Omega$, $R_C = 1\ K\Omega$ and $V_{BE} = 1.0$ V. The minimum base current and the input voltage at which the transistor will go to saturation, will be, respectively :

(a) 25 μA and 3.5 V (b) 20 μA and 3.5 V
(c) 25 μA and 2.8 V (d) 20 μA and 2.8 V

42. Boolean relation at the output stage-*Y* for the following circuit is:

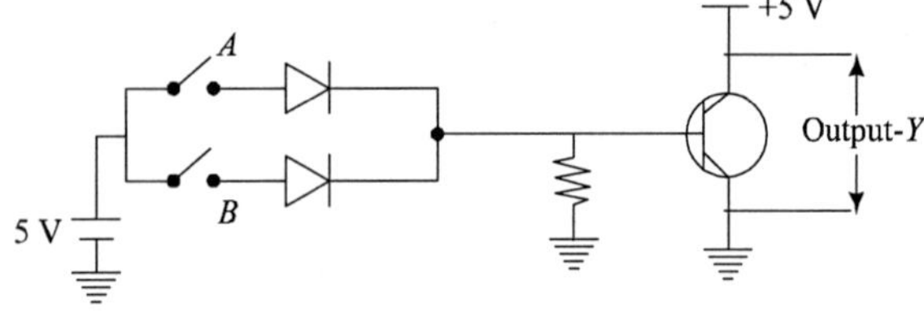

(a) $\bar{A}+\bar{B}$ (b) $A+B$ (c) $A.B$ (d) $\bar{A}.\bar{B}$

43. The truth table for the circuit given in the fig. is :

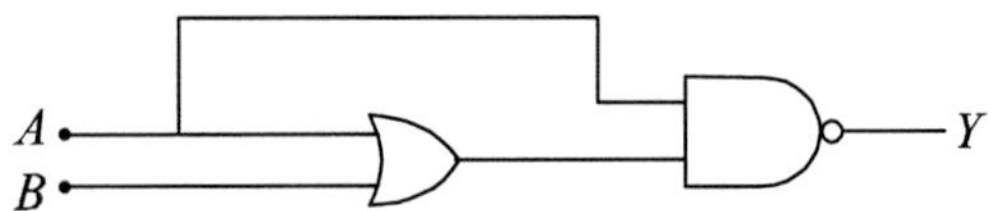

(a)

A	B	Y
0	0	1
0	1	1
1	0	1
1	1	1

(b)

A	B	Y
0	0	1
0	1	0
1	0	0
1	1	0

(c)

A	B	Y
0	0	1
0	1	1
1	0	0
1	1	0

(d)

A	B	Y
0	0	0
0	1	0
1	0	1
1	1	1

44. The logic gate equivalent to the given logic circuit is:

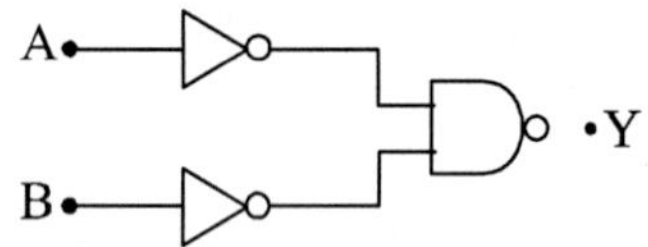

(a) NAND (b) OR (c) NOR (d) AND

45. The ouput of the given logic cirfcuit is:

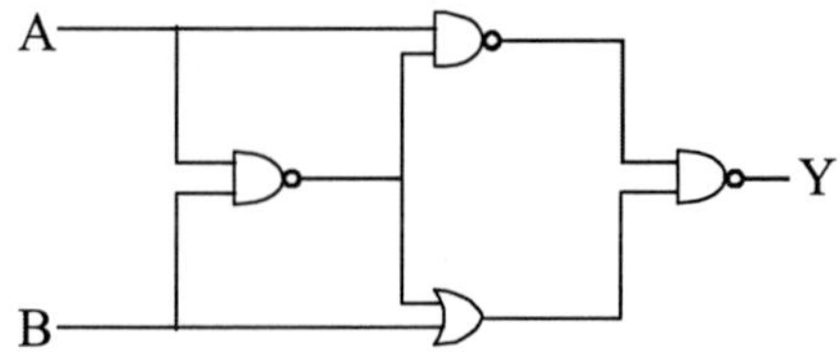

(a) $A\bar{B}+\bar{A}B$ (b) $AB+\bar{A}B$
(c) $A\bar{B}$ (d) $\overline{AB}$

Hints & Solutions

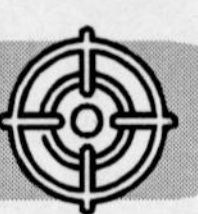

29.1 Concept Practice Problems CPP

1. (c) The resistivity of conductor increases with increase in temperature. The resistivity of semiconductor decreases as the temperature increases
2. (c) 3. (c) 4. (d) 5. (c)
6. (c) Maximum in insulators and overlaping in metals
7. (a) Minority carriers in a p-type semiconductor are free electrons.
8. (d)
9. (b) [Hint : At 0K (–273°C) motion of free electron stop i.e., there is no electron in conduction band therefore at 0K intrinsic semiconductor becomes insulator.]
10. (c)
11. (c) Semiconductors are insulators at room temperature.
12. (a)
13. (d) In forward biasing of the p-n junction, the positive terminal of the battery is connected to p-side and the negative terminal of the battery is connected to n-side. The depletion region becomes thin.
14. (c) When small amount of antimony (pentavalent) is added to germanium crystal then crystal becomes n-type semi conductor. Therefore, there will be more free electrons than holes in the semiconductor.
15. (b)

29.2 Concept Practice Problems CPP

16. (d) Doping- base > collector > emitter
17. (b)
18. (c) Field effect tansistor is unipolar in nature because in this either holes or electrons are present. But in case of BJT both holes and electrons are present due to which they are bipolar in nature.
19. (b) 20. (a)
21. (b) Combination of NAND & NOR gates can produce OR, AND & NOT gates
22. (d) Radiowaves of constant amplitude can be produced by using oscillator with proper feedback.
23. (a) Metal oxides with high temperature coefficient of resistivity.
24. (b) Integrated circuit can act as a complete electronic circuit.
25. (c) $\beta = \frac{\alpha}{1-\alpha} = \frac{0.95}{1-0.95} = \frac{0.95}{0.05} = 19$

Exercise 1 - Chapter Revision Problems CRP

1. (b) Conductivity $\sigma = n_i e\mu_e = 10^{17} \times (1.6\times10^{-19}) \times 3800$
$= 60.8$ mho/cm
2. (b) In half wave rectifier, we get the output only in one half cycle of input a.c. therefore, the frequency of the ripple of the output is same as that of input a.c. i.e. 50 Hz
3. (c) Forward resistance $= \frac{\Delta V}{\Delta I} = \frac{0.7-0.5}{1.0\times10^{-3}} = 200\,\Omega$
4. (a) $\beta = \frac{\Delta I_C}{\Delta I_B}$ or $\Delta I_C = \beta\,\Delta I_B = 40\times100\ \mu A$
5. (c) $I_C = I_E - I_B = 90-1 = 89$ mA
6. (c) Voltage amplification $A_v = \beta\frac{R_o}{R_i} = 60\times\frac{5000}{500} = 600$
7. (c) Current gain, $\alpha = \frac{A_V}{A_R} = \frac{2800}{3000} = 0.93$
8. (a) The phase difference between output voltage and input signal voltage in common base transistor circuit is zero
9. (c) $\Delta I_C = \alpha\,\Delta I_E = 0.99\times5 = 4.95$ mA
10. (b) Voltage gain, $A_v = \beta\frac{R_L}{R_i} = 0.6\times\frac{24}{3} = 4.8$
11. (b) In half wave rectifier only half of the wave is rectified
12. (c) $E = \frac{V}{d} = \frac{0.1}{10^{-6}} = 10^5$ V/m
13. (b)
14. (c) We know that for common base

$$\alpha = \frac{i_c}{i_e} = \frac{\text{collector current}}{\text{emiter current}} = 0.98$$

& for common emitter

$$\beta = \frac{i_c}{i_b} = \frac{\text{collector current}}{\text{base current}}$$

$$\beta = \frac{\alpha}{1-\alpha} = \frac{0.98}{1-0.98} = \frac{0.98}{0.02} = 49.$$

15. (c) The given circuit is a circuit of full wave rectifier.
16. (d) During the formation of a junction diode, holes from p-region diffuse into n-region and electrons from n-region diffuse into p-region. In both cases, when an electrons meets a hole, they cancel the effect at each other and as a result, a thin layer at the junction becomes free from any of charges carriers. This is called depletion layer. There is a

potential gradient in the depletion layer, negative on the p-side, and positive on the n-side. The potential difference thus developed across the junction is called potential barrier.

17. (b) Reverse resistance

$$= \frac{\Delta V}{\Delta I} = \frac{1}{0.5\times10^{-6}} = 2\times10^{6}\Omega$$

18. (c) Forward bias resistance $= \frac{\Delta V}{\Delta I}$

$$= \frac{(0.7-0.6)V}{(15-5)mA} = \frac{0.1}{10\times10^{-3}} = 10\Omega.$$

19. (d) Current gain in common emitter mode

$$= \frac{\alpha}{1-\alpha} = \frac{0.995}{1-0.995} = \frac{0.995}{0.005} = 199.$$

20. (a)

21. (b) Given : $\mu_e = 2.3\ m^2\ V^{-1}\ s^{-1}$

$\mu_h = 0.01\ m^2\ V^{-1}\ s^{-1}, n_e = 5\times10^{12}/cm^3$

$= 5\times10^{18}/m^3\ n_h = 8\times10^{13}/cm^3 = 8\times10^{19}/m^3.$

Conductivity $\sigma = e[n_e\mu_e + n_h\mu_h]$

$= 1.6\times10^{-19}[5\times10^{18}\times2.3 + 8\times10^{19}\times0.01]$

$= 1.6\times10^{-1}[11.5+0.8]$

$= 1.6\times10^{-1}\times12.3 = 1.968\ \Omega^{-1}\ m^{-1}.$

22. (b) $\lambda = \frac{hc}{E} = \frac{6.62\times10^{-34}\times3\times10^{8}}{(60\times10^{-3}\times1.6\times10^{-19})} = 2.07\times10^{-5}\ m$

23. (c)

P N

Before diffusion

● Solid dot = electron

o Hollow circle = hole

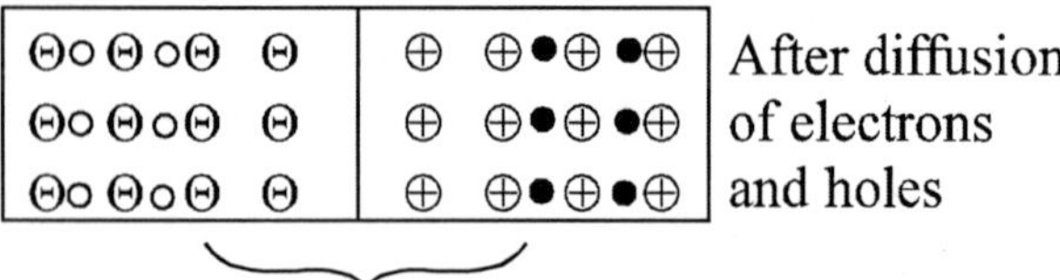

Depletion region

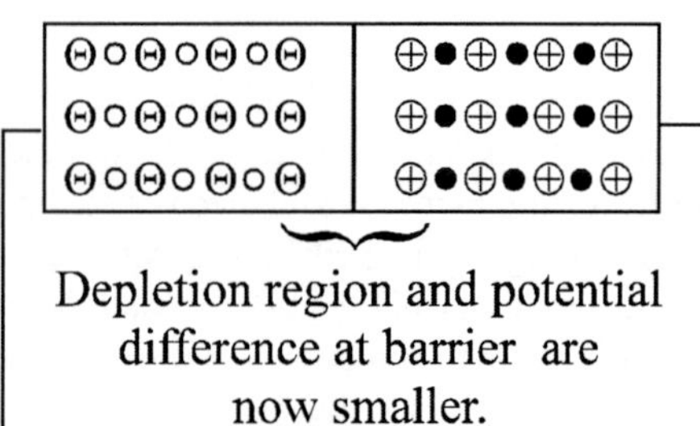

Number of donors is more because electrons from –ve terminal of the cell pushes (enters) the n side and decreases the number of uncompensated pentavalent ion due to which potential barrier is reduced. The neutralised pentavalent atom are again in position to donate electrons.

24. (a) In reverse bias the current through the p-n junction is almost zero.

25. (d) (A) is a NAND gate so output is $\overline{1\times1} = \overline{1} = 0$

(B) is a NOR gate so output is $\overline{0+1} = \overline{1} = 0$

(C) is a NAND gate so output is $\overline{0\times1} = \overline{0} = 1$

(D) is a XOR gate so output is $0\oplus0 = 0$

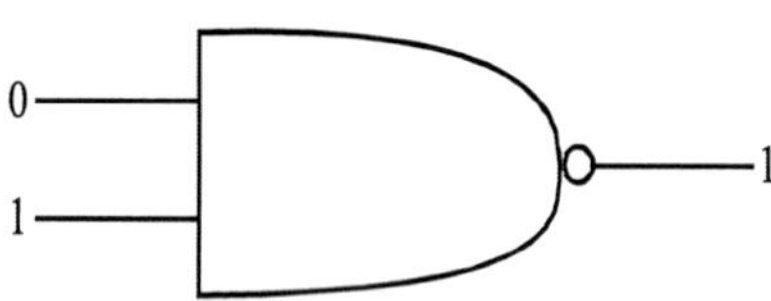

Following is NAND Gate $Y = \overline{AB}$

26. (b) Output of upper AND gate $= \overline{A}B$

Output of lower AND gate $= A\overline{B}$

$\therefore$ Output of OR gate, $Y = A\overline{B} + B\overline{A}$

This is boolean expression for XOR gate.

27. (c) $(W+X).(W+Y) = W+(X.Y)$

28. (c) Here diode is forward biased with voltage $= 2-0 = 2$ V.

$V_B = V_{knee} + IR$

$2 = 0.7 + I\times200$

($\because$ Total resistance $= 180+20 = 200\Omega$)

$\therefore\ I = \frac{1.3}{200} = 6.5mA$

29. (b)

30. (b) $\frac{V_o}{V_{in}} = \frac{R_o}{R_{in}}\times\beta = \frac{5\times10^{3}\times62}{500} = 10\times62 = 620$

$V_o = 620\times V_{in} = 620\times0.01 = 6.2\,V$

$\therefore V_o = 6.2$ volt.

31. (d) A and C are analogue but B is digital signal.

32. (c) $\frac{I_e}{I_h} = \frac{n_e e A v_e}{n_h e A v_h} \Rightarrow \frac{7}{4} = \frac{7}{5}\times\frac{v_e}{v_h}$

$\Rightarrow \frac{v_e}{v_h} = \frac{5}{4}$

33. (d) For a *p*-type semiconductor, the acceptor energy level, as shown in the diagram, is slightly above the top E_v of the valence band. With very small supply of energy an electron from the valence band can jump to the level E_A and ionise acceptor negatively.

34. (b) [Hint : For easy flow of current the P side must be connected to +ive terminal of battery i.e., it is connected to higher potential in comparison to N. This connection is called forward biased. In this case the input resistance is very low.
In reverse-biased, the P-side is connected to –ive terminal & N side to (+ive) terminal to battery. In this case input resistance is very high.

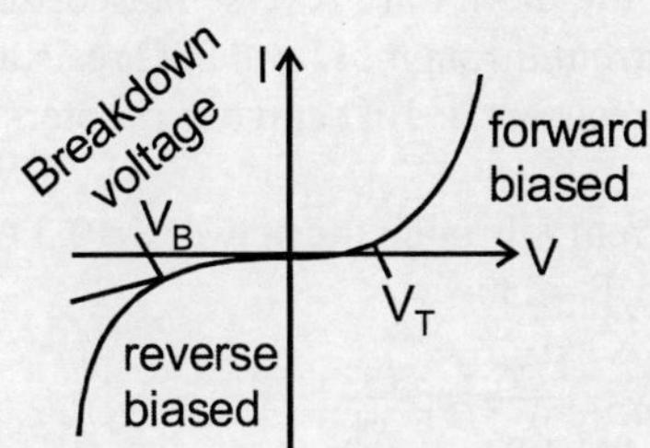

35. (c) $\frac{I_c}{I_e} = 0.96 \Rightarrow I_c = 0.96 I_e$
But $I_e = I_c + I_b = 0.96 I_e + I_b \Rightarrow I_b = 0.04 I_e$
$\therefore$ Current gain $\beta = \frac{I_c}{I_b} = \frac{0.96 I_e}{0.04 I_e} = 24$

36. (b) [Hint : Barrier potential depends on, doping density, temperature, forward/reverse bias but does not depend on diode design.]

37. (c) When the collector is positive and emitter is negative w.r.t. base it causes the forward biasing for each junction, which causes conduction of current.

38. (b)

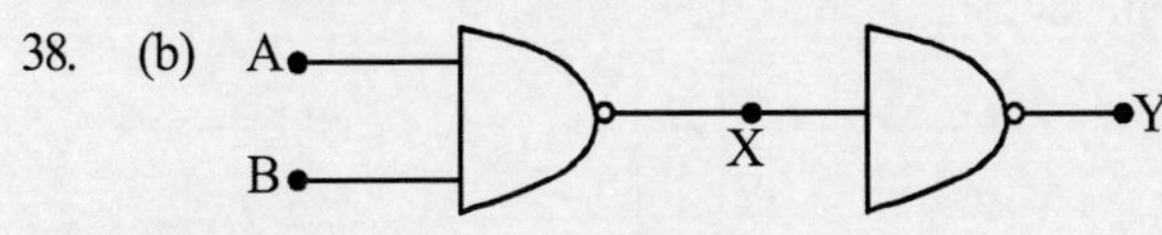

$X = \overline{AB}$
$\therefore Y = \overline{X} = \overline{\overline{AB}}$
Y = AB by Demorgan theorem
$\therefore$ This diagram performs the function of AND gate.

39. (c) In reverse biasing, the conduction across the p-n junction does not take place due to majority carriers, but takes place due to minority carriers if the voltage of external battery is large. The size of the depletion region increases thereby increasing the potential barrier.

40. (c) In semiconductors, the conduction band is empty and the valence band is completely filled at 0 K. No electron from valence band can cross over to conduction band at 0 K. But at room temperature some electrons in the valence band jump over to the conduction band due to the small forbidden gap, i.e., 1 eV.

41. (c) Electromotive force depends upon intensity of light falling, it does not depend on frequency of barrier voltage.

42. (d) Positive terminal is at lower potential (0V) and negative terminal is at higher potential 5V.

43. (c) Semiconductors have –ve temperature coefficient of resistivity.

44. (b) Majority carriers in an n-type semiconductor are electrons.

45. (c) Power gain = voltage gain × current gain
$= V_G \cdot I_G = \frac{V_0}{V_i} \cdot \frac{I_0}{I_i}$
$= \frac{V_0^2}{V_i^2} \cdot \frac{R_i}{R_0} = 50 \times 50 \times \frac{100}{200}$
$= \frac{2500}{2} = 1250$

46. (d) For transistor action, the base region must be very thin and lightly doped. Also, the emitter-base junction is forward biased and base-collector junction is reverse biased.

47. (b) I → ON
II → OFF
In IInd state it is used as a amplifier it is active region.

48. (b) In a n-type semiconductor holes are minority carriers and pentavalent atoms are dopants.

49. (b) 50. (d)

51. (c) $E = \frac{hc}{\lambda}$
$\Rightarrow \lambda = \frac{hc}{E} = \frac{6.63 \times 10^{-34} \times 3 \times 10^8}{0.75 \times 1.6 \times 10^{-19}} = 16500 Å$

52. (d) I-V characteristic of a photodiode is as follows :

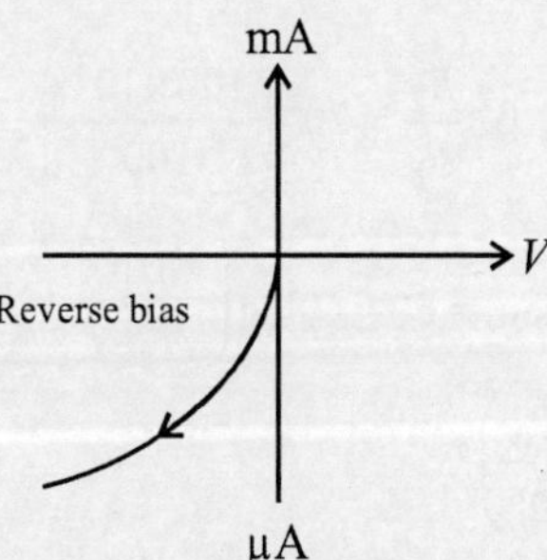

On increasing the biasing voltage of a photodiode, the magnitude of photocurrent first increases and then attains a saturation.

53. (d) Given,
Wavelength of photon, $\lambda = 400$ nm
A photodiode can detect a wavelength corresponding to the energy of band gap. If the signal is having wavelength greater than this value, photodiode cannot detect it.
$\therefore$ Band gap $E_g = \frac{hc}{\lambda} = \frac{1237.5}{400} = 3.09$ eV

54. (a) The given circuit has two $10k\Omega$ resistances in parallel, so we can reduce this parallel combination to a single equivalent resistance of $5k\Omega$.

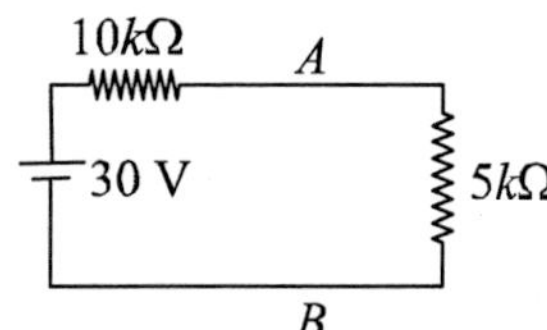

Diode is in forward bias. So it will behave like a conducting wire.

$$V_A - V_B = \frac{30}{5+10} \times 5 = 10\,V$$

55. (a)

P.D. across 800Ω resistors = 5.6 V

so, $I_{800\Omega} = \frac{5.6}{800} A = 7\text{ mA}$

Now, P.D. across 200Ω resistors = 9 – 5.6 V = 3.4 V

so, $I_{200\Omega} = \frac{9-5.6}{200} = 17\text{ mA}$

so, current through zener diode = I_2 = 17 – 7 = 10 mA

56. (Bonus) $\beta = \frac{\Delta i_c}{\Delta i_b} = \frac{200-100}{10-5} = 20$

Voltage gain = $\beta \frac{R_2}{R_1} = \frac{20 \times 100 \times 10^3}{100} = 20 \times 10^3$

Power gain = $\beta^2 \frac{R_2}{R_1} = 20^2 \left(\frac{100 \times 10^3}{100}\right) = 4 \times 10^5$

57. (a) Power gain = $60 = 10\log\left(\frac{P_0}{P_i}\right)$

$\Rightarrow 6 = \log\left(\frac{P_0}{P_i}\right)$

$\Rightarrow \frac{P_0}{P_i} = 10^6$

$= \beta^2\left(\frac{R_{out}}{R_{in}}\right)$

$\Rightarrow 10^6 = \beta^2\left(\frac{10000}{100}\right)$ [as $R_{out} = 10,000\Omega$ $R_{in} = 100\Omega$]

$\Rightarrow \beta = 100$

58. (d) Curent gain $\beta = \frac{\Delta I_C}{I_B}$

Voltage gain A_v = Current gain × Resistance gain = $\beta \frac{R_L}{R_{BE}}$

Power gain A_p = (Current gain)^2 × Resistance gain

$= \beta^2 \frac{R_L}{R_{BE}}$

59. (c) Here two zener diodes are in reverse polarity so if one is in forward bias the other will be in reverse bias and above 6V the reverse bias will too be in conduction mode. Hence when V > 6V the output will be constant. And when V < 6V it will follow the inut voltage.

60. (c) Both the diodes are reverse biased, so, there is no flow of current through 5Ω and 20Ω resistances. Now, two resistors of 10Ω and two resistors of 5Ω are in series.
Hence current I through the network = 0.3 A

61. (a) Given, β = 250

Voltage gain, $\frac{V_{CC}}{V_B} = \beta \frac{R_C}{R_B}$

$\frac{10}{V_B} = 250 \times \frac{10^3}{R_B}$

$\therefore \frac{V_B}{R_B} = \frac{1}{25 \times 10^3} = 40\mu A$

62. (a) Boolean expression,

$y = \overline{\overline{A} \cdot \overline{B}} = \overline{\overline{A}} + \overline{\overline{B}} = A + B$

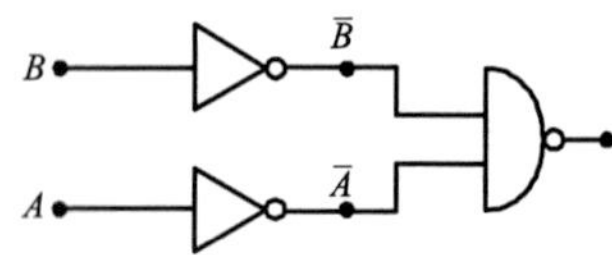

Truth table :

A	B	Y
0	1	1
1	0	1
0	0	0
1	1	1

$y = A + B$

63. (c) When two inputs of NAND gate is shorted, it behaves like a NOT gate so boolen equation will be

$y = \overline{\overline{A} + \overline{B} + \overline{C}}$

$y = A \cdot B \cdot C$

A	B	C	
0	0	0	0
1	0	0	0
0	1	0	0
0	0	1	0
1	1	0	0
1	0	1	0
0	1	1	0
1	1	1	1

Thus, whole arrangement behaves like a AND gate.

64. (a)

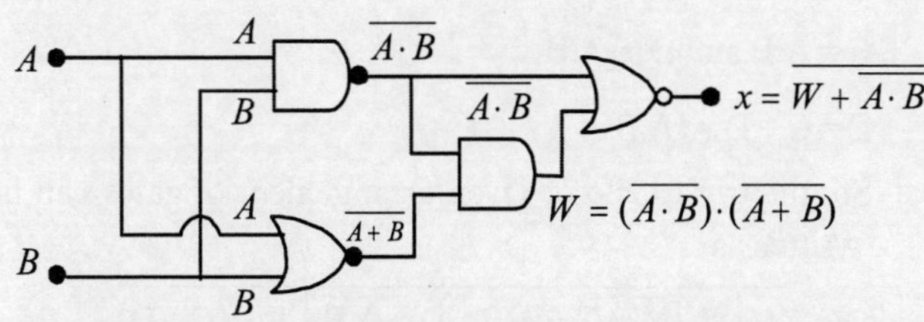

A	B	$\overline{A\cdot B}$	$\overline{A+B}$	$W=(\overline{A\cdot B})\cdot(\overline{A+B})$	$Q=\overline{W+\overline{A\cdot B}}$	$\overline{Q}=x$
1	0	1	0	0	1	0
0	1	1	0	0	1	0
1	1	0	0	0	0	1
0	0	1	1	1	0	0

65. (a)

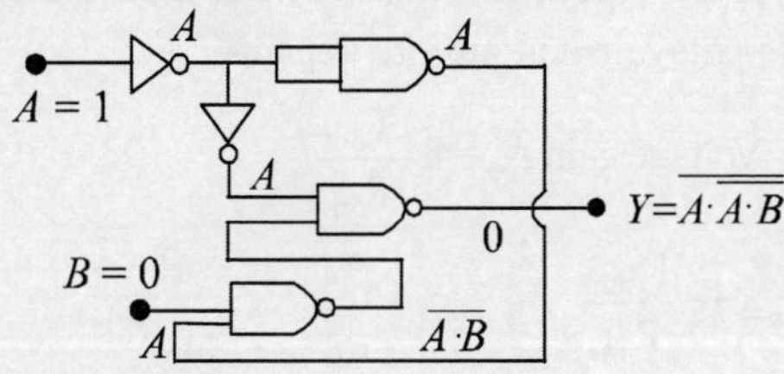

$Y=\overline{\overline{AB}.A}=\overline{\overline{AB}}+\overline{A}=AB+\overline{A}$

For $A=1, B=0$

$Y=(1)\times 0+0$

$\Rightarrow Y=0+0=0$

66. (d) A logic gate is reversible if we can recover input data from the output. Hence NOT gate.

67. (c) From the given logic circuit,

$p=\overline{x}+y$

$Q=\overline{\overline{y}.x}=y+\overline{x}$

Output, $R=\overline{P+Q}$

To make output 1

P + Q must be '0'

So, x = 1, y = 0

68. (c) Truth table of the circuit is as follows

x	y	$\overline{x}$	$a=x.y$	$b=\overline{x}.y$	$z=\overline{a.b}$
0	0	1	0	0	1
0	1	1	0	1	1
1	0	0	0	0	1
1	1	0	1	0	1

69. (d) Using $U_{av}=\frac{1}{2}\varepsilon_0 E_0^2$

But $U_{av}=\frac{P}{4\pi r^2\times c}$

$\therefore \quad \frac{P}{4\pi r^2}=\frac{1}{2}\varepsilon_0 E_0^2\times c$

$E_0^2=\frac{2P}{4pr^2 e_0 c}=\frac{2\times 0.1\times 9\times 10^9}{1\times 3\times 10^8}$

$\therefore \quad E_0=\sqrt{6}=2.45\text{V/m}$

70. (a) P ⊳| n

For forward bias, p-side must be at higher potential than n-side. $\Delta V=(+)Ve$

71. (c) Graph (p) is for a simple diode.

Graph (q) is showing the V Break down used for zener diode.

Graph (r) is for solar cell which shows cut-off voltage and open circuit current.

Graph (s) shows the variation of resistance h and hence current with intensity of light.

72. (a) The current will flow through R_L when the diode is forward biased.

73. (a) Si and Ge are semiconductors but C is an insulator. In Si and Ge at room temperature, the energy band gap is low due to which electrons in the covalent bonds gains kinetic energy and break the bond and move to conduction band. As a result, hole is created in valence band. So, the number of free electrons is significant in Si and Ge.

74. (d) Band gap = energy of photon of wavelength 2480 nm. So,

Band gap, $E_g=\frac{hc}{\lambda}$

$=\left(\frac{6.63\times 10^{-34}\times 3\times 10^8}{2480\times 10^{-9}}\right)\times\frac{1}{1.6\times 10^{-19}}eV$

$=0.5\text{ eV}$

75. (a)

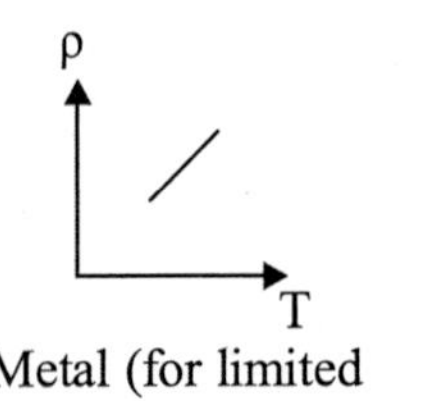

Metal (for limited range of temperature) | Semiconductor $\rho = \rho_o e^{\frac{-Eg}{K_BT}}$

Exercise 2 - Exemplar & Past Year Questions E&PYQs

Exemplar Questions

1. (d) In semiconsuctor the density of change carriers (electron hole) are very small, so its resistance is high when the conductivity of a semiconductor increases with increase in temperature, because the number density of current carries increases then the speed of free electron increase and relaxation time decreases but effect of decrease in relaxation is much less than increase in number density.
2. (b) When p–n junction is forward biased then the depleton layer is compresses or decrease so it opposes the potential junction resulting decrease in potential barrier junction when p–n junction is reverese biased, it supports the potential barrier junction, resulting increase in potential across the junction.
3. (b) As the given circuit, p–side of p–n function D_1 is connected to lower voltage and n –side of D_1 of higher voltage.
So, D_1 is reverse biased.
In circuit A is at –10V and B is at 0 (zero) V. So B is positive then A or
The p–side of p–n junction D_2 is at higher potential and n–side of D_2 is at lower potential.
So, D_2 is forward biased.
Hence, No current flows through the junction B to A and vice–versa.
4. (d) As the given figure p–n junction conducts during positive half cycyle only, then diode connected here will work is positive half cycle. Potential difference across C will be peak voltage when diode is in forword bias then the peak voltage of the given AC voltage
$$= V_0 = V_{rms}\sqrt{2} = 220\sqrt{2}V$$
5. (b) Atom of semiconductor are bounded by covalent bonds between the atoms of same or different type. The concept of hole describes the lack of an electron at a position where one could exist in an atom or atomic lattice. If an electron is excited into a higher state, it leaves a hole in its old state. So, hole can be defined as a vacancy created when an electron leaves a covalent bond.
6. (c) When the diode will be in forward biased during positive half cycle of input AC voltage, the resistance of p–n junction is low. The current in the circuit is maximum. So, a maximum potential difference will appear across resistance connected in series of circuit. So, potential across PN junction will be zero. When the diode will be in reverse biase during negative half cycle of AC voltage, the resistance of p–n juntion becomes high which will be more than resistance in series. So, there will be voltage across p–n junction with negative cycle in output.
7. (b) Let the potential difference between A and B is V, Given here $r_1 = 5\ k\Omega$ and $r_2 = 5\ k\Omega$ are resistance in series connection.
So,
$V_{AB} - 0.3 = [(r_1 + r_2)\ 10^3] \times (0.2 \times 10^{-3})]$ $[\because V = ir]$
$(V_{AB} - 0.3) = 10 \times 10^3 \times 0.2 \times 10^{-3} = 2$
So, $V_{AB} = 2 + 0.3 = 2.3$ V
8. (c) As the given figure the output of C,D and E are :
$C = A.B$ and $D = \overline{A}.B$
$E = C + D = (A.B) + (\overline{A}.B)$
So, the truth table of given arrangement of gates can be written as :

A	B	$\overline{A}$	C = A.B	D = $\overline{A}$.B	E = (C+D)
0	0	1	0	0	0
0	1	1	0	1	1
1	0	0	0	0	0
1	1	0	1	0	1

NEET/AIPMT (2013-2020) Questions

9. (b) In a n-type semiconductor holes are minority carriers and pentavalent atoms are dopants.
10. (d) Voltage gain $A_V = \beta \dfrac{R_{out}}{R_{in}}$
$$\Rightarrow G = 25\frac{R_{out}}{R_{in}} \quad ...(i)$$
Transconductance $g_m = \dfrac{\beta}{R_{in}}$
$$\Rightarrow R_{in} = \frac{\beta}{g_m} = \frac{25}{0.03}$$
Putting this value of R_{in} in eqn. (i)
$$G = 25\frac{R_{out}}{25} \times 0.03 \quad ...(ii)$$
$$\therefore \quad G' = 20\frac{R_{out}}{20} \times 0.02 \quad ...(iii)$$
From eqs. (ii) and (iii)
Voltage gain of new transistor $G' = \dfrac{2}{3}G$
11. (b)

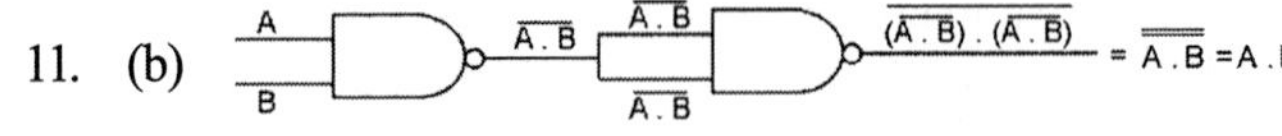

i.e., output X = A.B

12. (c) In p-region of p-n junction holes concentration > electrons concentration and in n-region electrons concentration > holes concentration.

13. (c) In p-n-p transistor holes are injected into the base while electrons are injected into the base of n-p-n transistor. Emitter-base junction is forward biased.

14. (d) The barrier potential of a p-n junction depends on amount of doping, type of semiconductor material and temperature.

15. (b) First two gates are NOT gates and the last gate is NOR gate.

Thus, $y_1 = \overline{A}$, $y_2 = \overline{B}$ and $y = \overline{y_1 + y_2}$

The truth table corresponding to this is as follows:

A	B	$y_1 = \overline{A}$	$y_2 = \overline{B}$	$y_1 + y_2$	$y = \overline{y_1 + y_2}$	A . B
0	0	1	1	1	0	0
0	1	1	0	1	0	0
1	0	0	1	1	0	0
1	1	0	0	0	1	1

Thus the combination of gate represents AND gate.

16. (c) Here P-N junction diode rectifies half of the ac wave i.e., acts as half wave rectifier. During + ve half cycle Diode → forward biased output across will be

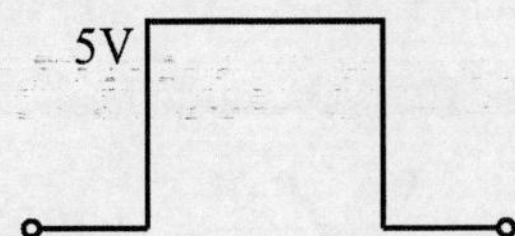

During –ve half cycle Diode → reverse biased output will not obtained.

17. (b) Since diode is in forward bias, so the value of current flowing through AB

$$i = \frac{\Delta V}{R} = \frac{4-(-6)}{1\times10^3} = \frac{10}{10^3} = 10^{-2}A$$

18. (a) Given: amplification factor $\alpha = 0.96$

load resistance, $R_L = 800\ \Omega$

input resistance, $R_i = 192\Omega$

So, $\beta = \frac{\alpha}{1-\alpha} = \frac{0.96}{0.04} \Rightarrow \beta = 24$

Voltage gain for common emitter configuration

$$A_v = \beta.\frac{R_L}{R_i} = 24 \times \frac{800}{192} = 100$$

Power gain for common emitter configuration

$P_v = \beta A_v = 24 \times 100 = 2400$

Voltage gain for common base configuration

$$A_v = \alpha, \frac{R_L}{R_P} = 0.96 \times \frac{800}{192} = 4$$

Power gain for common base configuration

$P_v = A_v\alpha = 4 \times 0.96 = 3.84$

19. (d) The Boolen expression for the given combination is output $Y = (A + B) \cdot C$

Truth table

A	B	C	$Y = (A+B) \cdot C$
0	0	0	0
1	0	0	0
0	1	0	0
0	0	1	0
1	1	0	0
0	1	1	1
1	0	1	1
1	1	1	1

Hence, A = 1, B = 0, C = 1

20. (b) Given, current gain $\beta = 100$, $R_c = 3k\Omega$, $R_b = 2k\Omega$

$$\text{Voltage gain } (A_v) = \beta\frac{R_c}{R_b} = 100\left(\frac{3}{2}\right) = 150$$

Power gain $= A_v\beta = 150\,(100) = 15000$

21. (b) A B Y_1 Y_2 Y

$y_1 = \overline{A+B}$

$y_2 = \overline{y_1 + y_1} = \overline{y_1} = A+B$

$y = \overline{y_2} = \overline{A+B}$ i.e. NOR gate

22. (d) V_1 V_2

In forward bias, $V_1 > V_2$ i.e., in figure (iv) p-type semiconductor is at higher potential w.r.t. n-type semiconductor.

23. (c) On heating, number of electron-hole pairs increases, so overall resistance of diode will change. Hence forward biasing and reversed biasing both are changed.

24. (b)

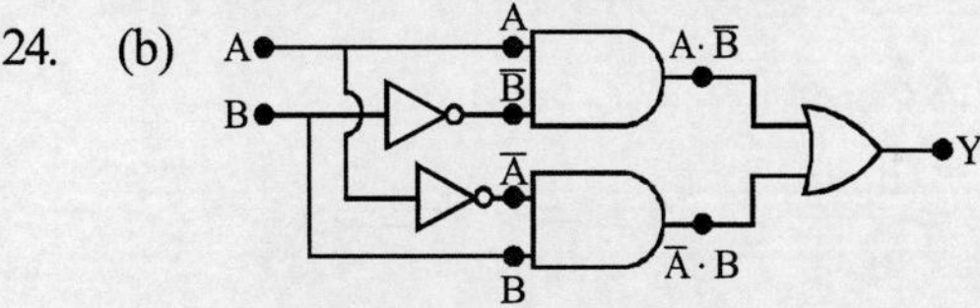

$Y = (A \cdot \overline{B} + \overline{A} \cdot B)$

25. (b) In p-type semiconductor, trivalent impurities are added to intrinsic semiconductor, which creates holes which are majority charge carriers.

26. (c) $\lambda = \frac{12400}{E_g}Å = \frac{12400}{1.9} = 6526Å \simeq 654\text{ nm}$

27. (c) From the given logic circuit, LED will glow, when voltage across LED is high.

Truth Table

A	B	Y
0	0	1
0	1	1
1	0	1
1	1	0

Boolean expression $Y = \overline{A.B}$

i.e.,circuit represents NAND gate.

28. (a) Due to reverse biasing, the width of the depletion region increases in a *p-n* junction diode.

29. (c) In a transistor, emitter is heavily doped, the base region is lightly doped and thin. The size of collector region is larger than other two regions.

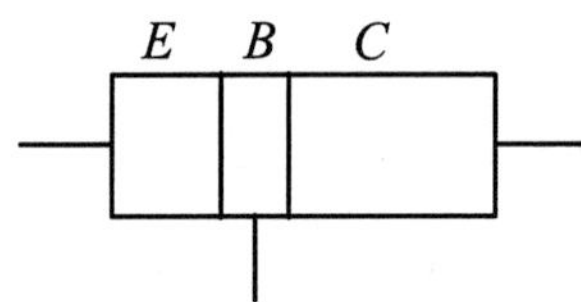

Length profile in transistor is $L_C > L_E > L_B$ and doping profile in transistor is $E > C > B$.

For transistor action Base-emitter junction is forward biased and Base-collector junction is reversed biased.

30. (d)

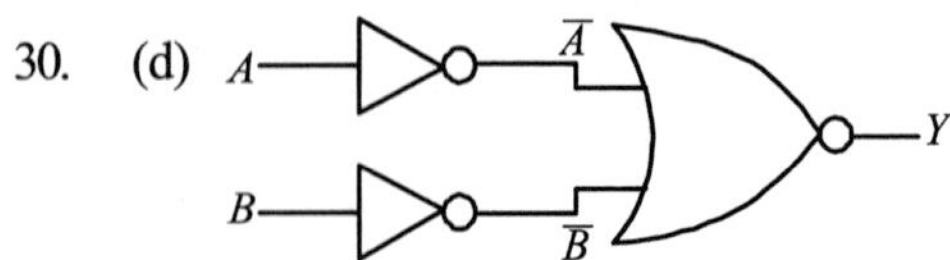

$Y = \overline{\overline{A}+\overline{B}} = \overline{\overline{A \cdot B}} = A \cdot B \Rightarrow$ AND Gate

Truth Table is :

A	B	Y
0	0	0
0	1	0
1	0	0
1	1	1

Exercise 3 - Concept Application Problems CAP

1. (b) $I = nA\,ev_d$ or $I \propto nv_d$

$$\therefore \frac{I_e}{I_h} = \frac{n_e v_e}{n_h v_h} \text{ or } \frac{n_e}{n_h} = \frac{I_e}{I_h} \times \frac{v_h}{v_e} = \frac{7}{4} \times \frac{4}{5} = \frac{7}{5}$$

2. (d) In full wave rectifier, we get the output for the positive and negative cycle of input a.c. Hence the frequency of the ripple of the output is twice than that of input a.c. i.e. 100 Hz

3. (c) Band gap,

$$E_g = \frac{hc}{\lambda} = \frac{(6.6\times10^{-34})(3\times10^8)}{2480\times10^{-9}\times1.6\times10^{-19}} eV = 0.49\,eV$$

4. (a) Conductivity, $\sigma = \frac{1}{\rho} = e(n_e\mu_e + n_h\mu_h)$

ie, $2.13 = 1.6 \times 10^{-19}(0.38 + 0.18)\,n_i$

(Since in intrinsic semi-conductor, $n_e = n_h = n_i$)

$\therefore$ density of charge carriers, n_i

$$= \frac{2.13}{1.6\times10^{-19}\times0.56} = 2.37\times10^{19}\,m^{-3}.$$

5. (c) No. of electrons reaching the collector,

$$n_C = \frac{96}{100}\times10^{10} = 0.96\times10^{10}$$

Emitter current, $I_E = \frac{n_E \times e}{t}$

Collector current, $I_C = \frac{n_C \times e}{t}$

$\therefore$ Current transfer ratio,

$$\alpha = \frac{I_C}{I_E} = \frac{n_C}{n_E} = \frac{0.96\times10^{10}}{10^{10}} = 0.96$$

6. (b) $g_m = \frac{\Delta I_p}{\Delta V_g}$

or $\Delta I_p = g_m \times \Delta V_g = 3\times10^{-4}\times[-3-(-1)]$

$= -0.6 \times 10^{-3}$ A = shortage of 0.6×10^{-3} A

7. (d) [Hint $\Rightarrow i_B = \frac{V_s}{R_{in}} = \frac{0.01}{10^3} = 1\times10^{-5}$ A

Now β of transistor is defined as $\beta_{ac} = \frac{i_c}{i_b}$

or $i_c = 50\times10^{-5} = 500\mu A$]

8. (b)

9. (c) $V' = V + IR = 0.5 + 0.1 \times 20 = 2.5$ V

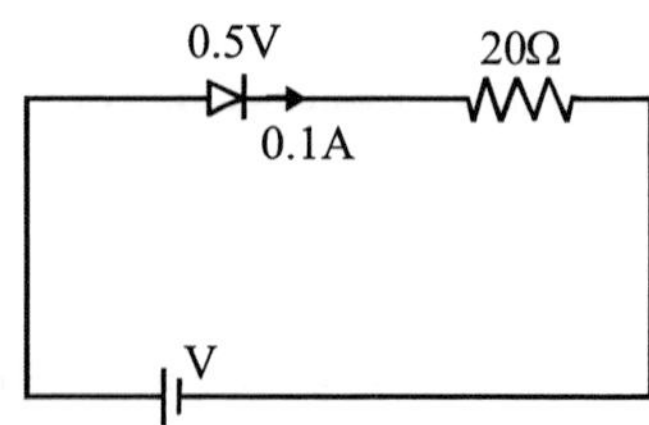

10. (a) Due to strong electronegativity of carbon.

11. (b)

$Y_1 = A + B,\ Y_2 = \overline{A.B}$

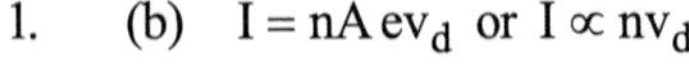

$Y = (A+B)\cdot\overline{AB} = A\cdot\overline{A} + A\cdot\overline{B} + B\cdot\overline{A} + B\cdot\overline{B}$

$= 0 + A\cdot\overline{B} + B\cdot\overline{A} + 0 = A\cdot\overline{B} + B\cdot\overline{A}$

This expression is for XOR

12. (d)

13. (b) Current gain $= \frac{\Delta I_C}{\Delta I_B}$ when V_{CE} is constant.

$= \frac{2.5\times10^{-3}}{25\times10^{-6}} = 0.1\times10^3 = 100$

$[\Delta I_B = 125\ \mu A - 100\ \mu A = 25\ \mu A$

$\Delta I_C = 7.5\ mA - 5\ mA = 2.5\ mA]$

14. (d) The given truth table is for NAND gate.

15. (c)

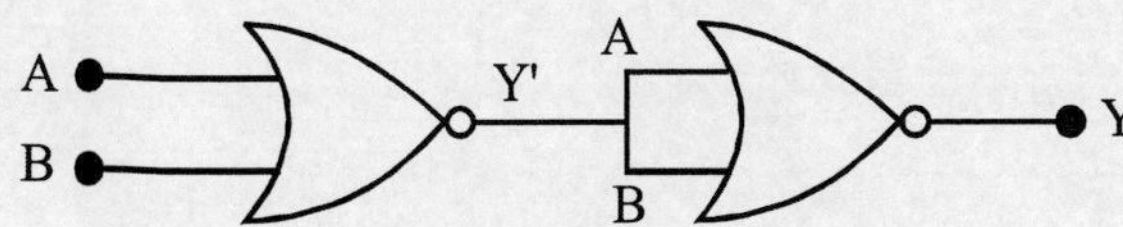

$Y' = \overline{A+B}.\quad Y = \overline{\overline{A+B}} = A+B.$

Truth table of the given circuit is given by

A	B	Y'	Y
0	0	1	0
0	1	0	1
1	0	0	1
1	1	0	1

16. (b) From input signals, we have,

A	B	Output NAND gate
0	0	1
1	0	1
0	0	1
1	1	0
0	0	1

The output signal is shown at B.

17. (b) D_2 is forward biased whereas D_1 is reversed biased. So effective resistance of the circuit $R = 4 + 2 = 6\Omega$

$\therefore i = \frac{12}{6} = 2\ A$

18. (c) $V = \frac{V_o}{\pi} = \frac{10}{\pi}V$

19. (a) From the given waveforms, the truth table is as follows.

A	*B*	*Y*
1	1	0
0	0	1
0	1	1
1	0	1

The above truth table is for NAND gate. Therefore, the logic gate is NAND gate.

20. (a) The current gain

$$\beta = \frac{\Delta I_C}{\Delta I_B} = \frac{10mA}{200\mu A} = \frac{10\times10^3}{200} = 50$$

21. (d)

22. (d) $n_i^2 = n_e n_h$

$(1.5\times10^{16})^2 = n_e(4.5\times10^{22})$

$\Rightarrow \quad n_e = 0.5\times10^{10}$

or $\quad n_e = 5\times10^9$

Given $\quad n_h = 4.5\times10^{22}$

$\Rightarrow n_h >> n_e$

$\therefore$ Semiconductor is p-type and

$n_e = 5\times10^9\ m^{-3}$.

23. (d) Voltage across zener diode is constant.

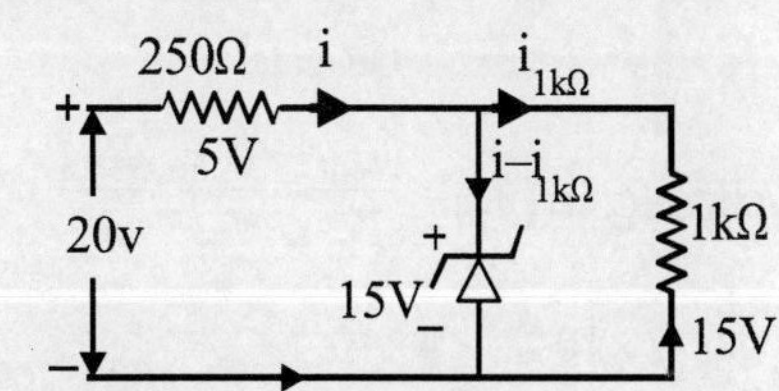

Current in 1kΩ resistor,

$(i)_{1k\Omega} = \frac{15 volt}{1k\Omega} = 15\ mA$

Current in 250Ω resistor,

$(i)_{250\Omega} = \frac{(20-15)V}{250W} = \frac{5V}{250W}$

$= \frac{20}{1000}A = 20\ mA$

$\therefore (i)_{zener\ diode} = (20-15) = 5mA.$

24. (d) Here D_1 is in forward bias and D_2 is in reverse bias so, D_1 will conduct and D_2 will not conduct. Thus, no current will flow through *DC*.

$$I = \frac{V}{R} = \frac{5}{10} = \frac{1}{2}\text{Amp.}$$

25. (d)

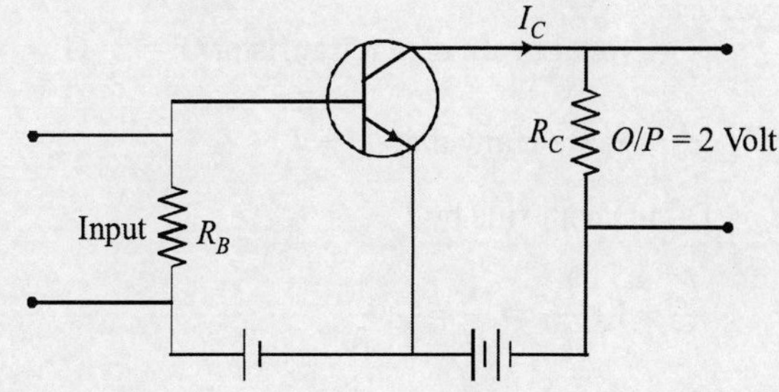

The output voltage, across the load R_C

$V_0 = I_C R_C = 2$

The collector current (I_C)

$$I_C = \frac{2}{2\times10^3} = 10^{-3}\text{ Amp}$$

Current gain (β)

$$(\beta)\text{ current gain} = \frac{I_C}{I_B} = 100$$

$$I_B = \frac{I_C}{100} = \frac{10^{-3}}{100} = 10^{-5}\text{ Amp}$$

Input voltage (V_i)

$V_i = R_B I_B = 1\times10^3\times10^{-5} = 10^{-2}$ Volt

$V_i = 10$ mV

26. (a)

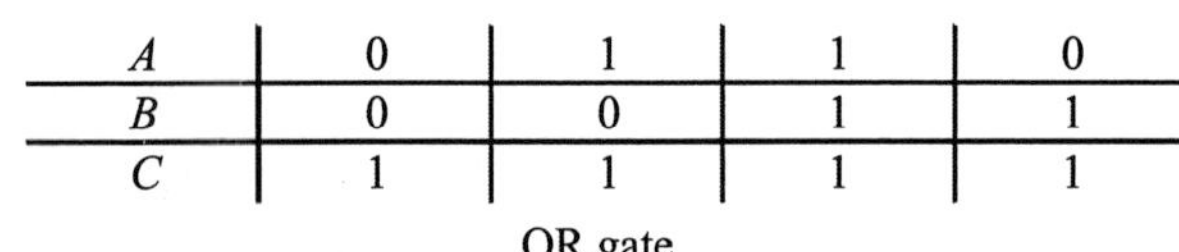

A	0	1	1	0
B	0	0	1	1
C	1	1	1	1

OR gate

27. (a) Voltage gain $(A_V) = \frac{V_{out}}{V_{in}} = \frac{I_{out}}{I_{in}} \times \frac{R_{out}}{R_{in}}$

$$A_V = \frac{2\times10^{-3}}{40\times10^{-6}} \times \frac{4\times10^3}{100} = 2\times100 = 2000$$

28. (d) Voltage gain $\Delta_V = \beta\,\frac{R_{out}}{R_{in}}$

$$\Rightarrow G = 25\,\frac{R_{out}}{R_{in}} \qquad \text{...(i)}$$

Transconductance $g_m = \frac{\beta}{R_{in}}$

$$\Rightarrow R_{in} = \frac{\beta}{g_m} = \frac{25}{0.03}$$

Putting this value of R_{in} in eqn. (i)

$$G = 25\,\frac{R_{out}}{25}\times0.03 \qquad \text{...(ii)}$$

$$\therefore\ G' = 20\,\frac{R_{out}}{20}\times0.02 \qquad \text{...(iii)}$$

From eqs. (ii) and (iii)

Voltage gain of new transistor $G' = \frac{2}{3}G$

29. (c) As we know that $I_e = I_c + I_b$

Divide both side by I_e

$$\frac{I_e}{I_c} = 1 + \frac{I_b}{I_c} \Rightarrow \frac{1}{\alpha} = 1 + \frac{1}{\beta}$$

$$\beta = \frac{\alpha}{1-\alpha}$$

30. (c) In case I diode is reverse biased, so no current flows

$\therefore\ Q_A = CV$

In case II, current will flow as diode is forward biased. So, it offers negligible resistance to the flow of current and thus be replaced by short circuit. Now, the charge of capacitor will leak through the resistance and decay exponentially with time.

During discharging of capacitor

Potential difference across the capacitor at any instant

$$V' = Ve^{-\frac{t}{CR}}$$

But $t = CR$

$$V' = Ve^{-1} = \frac{V}{e}$$

$\therefore$ Charge $Q_B = CV' = \frac{CV}{e}$

31. (d) Current in load resistance,

$$i_1 = \frac{6}{4\times10^3} = 1.5\times10^{-3}\text{ A} = 1.5\text{ mA}$$

For $V = 16$ volt,

$$i_s = \frac{(16-6)}{2\times10^3} = 5\text{ mA}$$

$\therefore\ i_2 = i_s - i_1 = 5 - 1.5 = 3.5$ mA

32. (c)

$\left(I_1 + \frac{3}{2}\right)$ 1 kΩ

$\frac{6}{4}$ mA

I_1

V

4 kΩ

For voltage, V = 8V

Current, $I_1 = \left(8 - 6 - \frac{3}{2}\right) = \frac{1}{2} = 0.5\text{mA}$

For voltage, V = 16V

Current, $I_2 = \left(16 - 6 - \frac{3}{2}\right) = 8.5\text{mA}$

33. (a) Since voltage across zener diode does not reach to breakdown voltage therefore its resistance will be infinite & current through it is 0.

34. (b) As D_2 is reversed biased, so no current through 75Ω resistor.

now $R_{eq} = 150 + 50 + 100$

$= 300\ \Omega$

So, required current $I = \dfrac{\text{Battery Voltage}}{300}$

$I = \dfrac{6}{300} = 0.02$

35. (a) The voltage across zener diode is constant

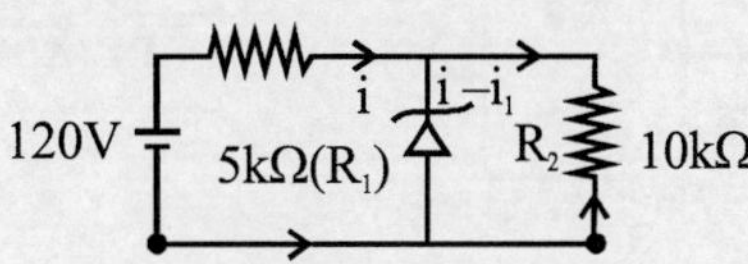

$i_{(R_2)} = \dfrac{V}{R} = \dfrac{50}{10\times10^3} = 5\times10^{-3}\,A$

$i_{(R_1)} = \dfrac{V}{R} = \dfrac{120-50}{5\times10^3} = \dfrac{70}{5\times10^3} 14\times10^{-3}\,A$

$\therefore i_{zenerdiode} = 14\times10^{-3} - 5\times10^{-3} = 9\times10^{-3}\,A = 9\,mA$

36. (c) As we know, current density,

$j = \sigma E = nev_d$

$\sigma = ne\dfrac{v_d}{E} = ne\mu$

$\dfrac{1}{\sigma} = \rho = \dfrac{1}{n_e e\mu_e}$ = Resistivity

$= \dfrac{1}{10^{19}\times1.6\times10^{19} - 19\times1.6}$

or $P = 0.4\ \Omega m$

37. (d) Initially Ge and Si are both forward biased so current will effectivily pass through Ge diode $\therefore V_o = 12 - 0.3 = 11.7\,V$

And if "Ge" is revesed then current will flow through "Si" diode

$\therefore V_o = 12 - 0.7 = 11.3\,V$

Clearly, V_o changes by $11.7 - 11.3 = 0.4\,V$

38. (c) Clearly from fig. given in question, Silicon diode is in forward bias.

$\therefore$ Potential barrier across diode

$\Delta V = 0.7$ volts

Current, $I = \dfrac{V-\Delta V}{R} = \dfrac{3-0.7}{200} = \dfrac{2.3}{200} = 11.5\text{mA}$

39. (b)

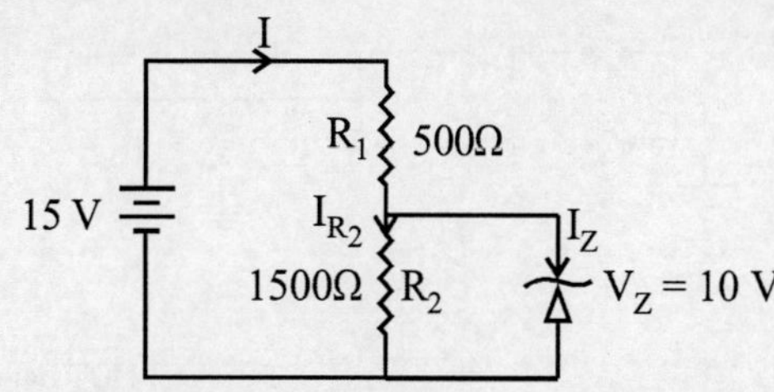

The voltage drop across R_2 is $V_{R_2} = V_Z = 10V$

The current through R_2 is

$I_{R_2} = \dfrac{V_{R_2}}{R_2} = \dfrac{10\,V}{1500\Omega} = 0.667\times10^{-2}\,A$

$= 6.67\times10^{-3}\,A = 6.67\,mA$

The voltage drop across R_1 is

$V_{R_1} = 15V - V_{R_2} = 15V - 10V = 5V$

The current through R_1 is

$I_{R_1} = \dfrac{V_{R_1}}{R_1} = \dfrac{5\,V}{500\Omega} = 10^{-2}\,A = 10\times10^{-3}\,A = 10\,mA$

The current through the zener diode is

$I_Z = I_{R_1} - I_{R_2} = (10 - 6.67)mA = 3.3mA$

40. (b) $\beta = \dfrac{\Delta lc}{\Delta lb} = \dfrac{3\times10^{-3}}{15\times10^{-6}} = 200$

We have $\dfrac{V_0}{V_i} = \beta\dfrac{R^2}{R_1}$

or $\dfrac{V_0}{V_i} = 200\left(\dfrac{1000}{R_1}\right)$

If $R_1 = 0.67k\Omega \Rightarrow \dfrac{V_0}{V_i} = 300$

41. (a) At saturation, $V_{CE} = 0$

$V_{CE} = V_{CC} - I_C R_C$

$\Rightarrow I_C = \dfrac{V_{CC}}{R_c} = 5\times10^{-3}\,A$

Current gain,

$\beta_{dc} = \dfrac{I_C}{I_B}$

$I_B = \dfrac{5\times10^{-3}}{200} = 25\ \mu A$

At input side

$V_{BB} = I_B R_B + V_{BE}$

$= (25\ mA)(100\ k\Omega) + 1V$

$V_{BB} = 3.5\ V$

42. (d)

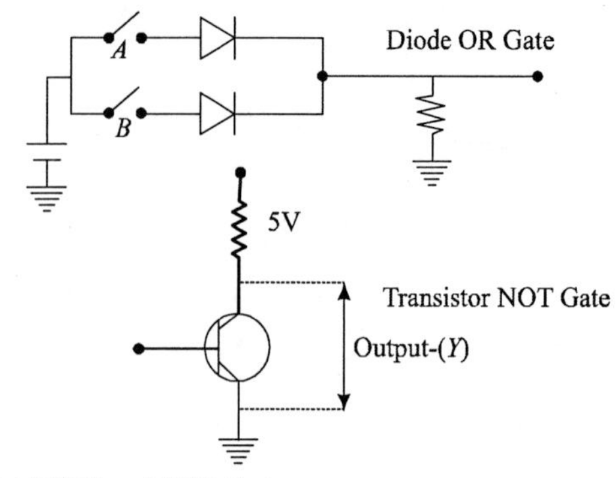

OR + NOT $\rightarrow$ NOR Gate

Hence Boolean relation at the output stage – Y for the circuit,

$$Y = \overline{A+B} = \bar{A}.\bar{B}$$

43. (c)

A	B	(A + B)	(A + B). A	$\overline{(A+B).A}$
0	0	0	0	1
0	1	1	0	1
1	0	1	1	0
1	1	1	1	0

44. (b) Truth table $\rightarrow$

The output is of OR-gate

A	B	$\bar{A}$	$\bar{B}$	$\overline{\bar{A}.\bar{B}}$
0	0	1	1	0
0	1	1	0	1
1	0	0	1	1
1	1	0	0	1

45. (c)

A, B, $\overline{A.B}$, $A.\overline{AB}$, $\overline{A.B}$, $\overline{AB}$, $(\overline{AB}+B)$

$Y = \overline{(A.\overline{AB}).(\overline{AB}+B)}$

$$Y = \left(\overline{\overline{A\cdot\overline{AB}}}\right) + \left(\overline{\overline{AB}+B}\right)$$

$$= A\cdot\overline{AB} + AB\cdot\bar{B}$$

$$= A\cdot\left(\bar{A}+\bar{B}\right) + AB\cdot\bar{B}$$

$$= A\bar{B}$$